Volume 2

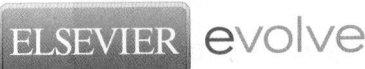
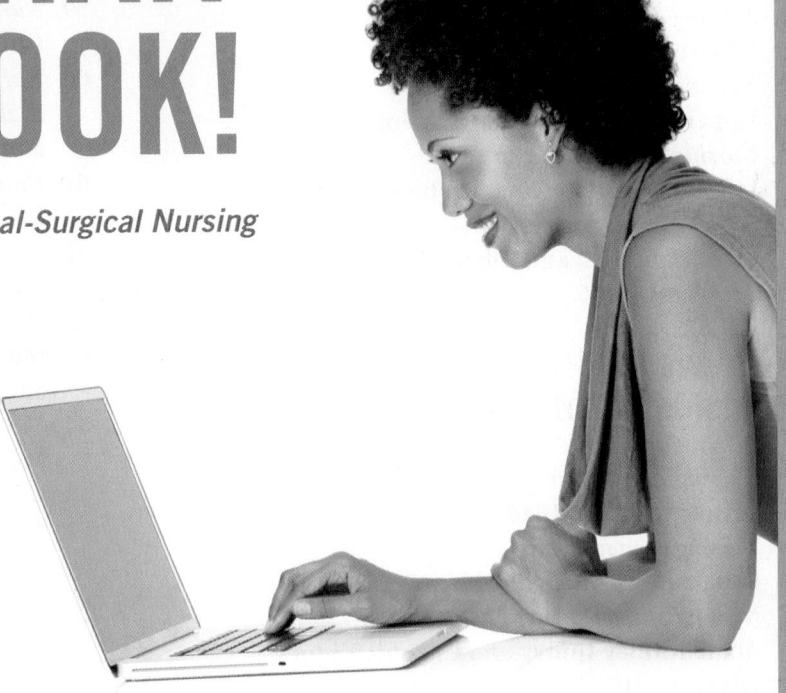
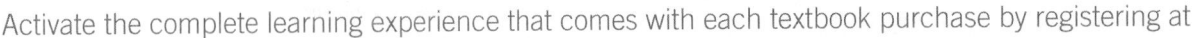

NINTH EDITION

MEDICAL-SURGICAL NURSING

Assessment and Management of Clinical Problems

Volume 2

Sharon L. Lewis, RN, PhD, FAAN
Professor Emerita
University of New Mexico
Albuquerque, New Mexico;
Former Castella Distinguished Professor
School of Nursing
University of Texas Health Science Center at San Antonio
San Antonio, Texas;
Developer and Consultant
Stress-Busting Program for Family Caregivers

Shannon Ruff Dirksen, RN, PhD, FAAN
Associate Professor
College of Nursing and Health Innovation
Arizona State University
Phoenix, Arizona

Margaret McLean Heitkemper, RN, PhD, FAAN
Professor and Chairperson, Biobehavioral Nursing and Health Systems
Elizabeth Sterling Soule Endowed Chair in Nursing
School of Nursing;
Adjunct Professor, Division of Gastroenterology
School of Medicine
University of Washington
Seattle, Washington

Linda Bucher, RN, PhD, CEN, CNE
Emerita Professor
School of Nursing
University of Delaware
Newark, Delaware;
Consultant/Mentor
W. Cary Edwards School of Nursing
Thomas Edison State College
Trenton, New Jersey;
Per Diem Staff Nurse
Emergency Department
Virtua Memorial Hospital
Mt. Holly, New Jersey

Special Editor
Mariann M. Harding, RN, PhD, CNE
Associate Professor of Nursing
Kent State University at Tuscarawas
New Philadelphia, Ohio

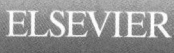

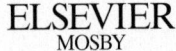

ELSEVIER
MOSBY

3251 Riverport Lane
St. Louis, Missouri 63043

MEDICAL-SURGICAL NURSING: ASSESSMENT AND MANAGEMENT OF CLINICAL PROBLEMS

ISBN: 978-0-323-10089-2

Notices

Library of Congress Cataloging-in-Publication Data

Lewis, Sharon Mantik, author.
Medical-surgical nursing : assessment and management of clinical problems / Sharon L. Lewis, Shannon Ruff Dirksen, Margaret McLean Heitkemper, Linda Bucher ; special editor, Mariann M. Harding. – Ninth edition.
    p. ; cm.
  Preceded by: Medical-surgical nursing : assessment and management of clinical problems / Sharon L. Lewis … [et al.]. 8th ed. c2011.
  Includes bibliographical references and index.
  ISBN 978-0-323-10089-2 (two volume set, pbk. : alk. paper)
  I. Dirksen, Shannon Ruff, author. II. Heitkemper, Margaret M. (Margaret McLean), author. III. Bucher, Linda, author. IV. Harding, Mariann, editor. V. Title.
  [DNLM: 1. Nursing Care. 2. Nursing Assessment. 3. Perioperative Nursing. WY 100]
  RT41
  617.0231–dc23

2013036087

Executive Content Strategist: Kristin Geen
Content Manager: Jamie Randall
Associate Content Development Specialist: Melissa Rawe
Content Coordinator: Hannah Corrier
Publishing Services Manager: Jeff Patterson
Senior Project Manager: Mary G. Stueck
Designer: Maggie Reid

Printed in Canada

Last digit is the print number: 9 8 7 6 5 4 3 2

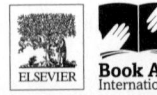
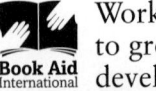

Working together
to grow libraries in
developing countries

www.elsevier.com • www.bookaid.org

SHARON L. LEWIS, RN, PhD, FAAN

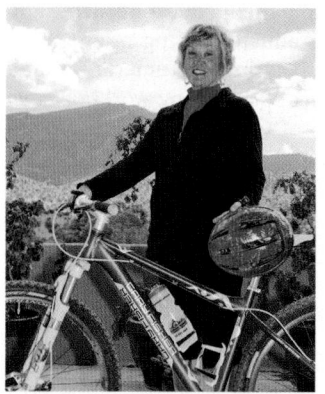

Sharon Lewis received her Bachelor of Science in nursing from the University of Wisconsin–Madison, Master of Science in nursing with a minor in biological sciences from the University of Colorado–Denver, and PhD in immunology from the Department of Pathology at the University of New Mexico School of Medicine. She had a 2-year postdoctoral fellowship from the National Kidney Foundation. Her more than 40 years of teaching experience include inservice education and teaching in associate degree, baccalaureate, master's degree, and doctoral programs in Maryland, Illinois, Wisconsin, New Mexico, and Texas. Favorite teaching areas are pathophysiology, immunology, and family caregiving. She has been actively involved in clinical research for the past 30 years, investigating altered immune responses in various disorders and developing a stress management program for family caregivers. Her primary professional responsibility is disseminating the Stress-Busting for Family Caregivers Program that she developed. Her free time is spent biking, landscaping, gardening, and being a grandmother.

SHANNON RUFF DIRKSEN, RN, PhD, FAAN

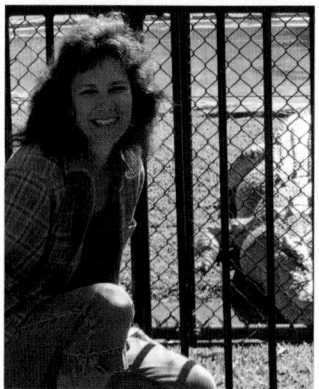

Shannon Dirksen is Associate Professor at the College of Nursing and Health Innovation, Arizona State University. She received her Bachelor of Science in nursing from Arizona State University, Master of Science in nursing from the University of Arizona, and doctorate in clinical nursing research with a minor in psychology from the University of Arizona. She has over 25 years of undergraduate and graduate teaching experience at the University of Arizona, Edith Cowan University (Western Australia), Intercollegiate College of Nursing–Washington State University, and University of New Mexico. She has been on the faculty at Arizona State University since 1996. She currently teaches nursing theory and research, including evidence-based practice. Her research for the past 25 years has focused on quality of life among individuals diagnosed with cancer. Her free time is spent traveling, gardening, bicycling, and reading.

MARGARET McLEAN HEITKEMPER, RN, PhD, FAAN

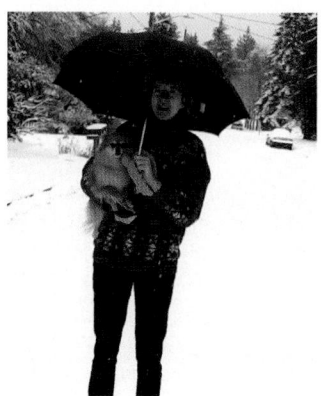

Margaret Heitkemper is Professor and Chairperson, Department of Biobehavioral Nursing and Health Systems at the School of Nursing, and Adjunct Professor, Division of Gastroenterology at the School of Medicine at the University of Washington. She is also Director of the National Institutes of Health-National Institute for Nursing Research–funded Center for Research on Management of Sleep Disturbances at the University of Washington. In the fall of 2006, Dr. Heitkemper was appointed the Elizabeth Sterling Soule Endowed Chair in Nursing. Dr. Heitkemper received her Bachelor of Science in nursing from Seattle University, a Master of Nursing in gerontologic nursing from the University of Washington, and a doctorate in Physiology and Biophysics from the University of Illinois–Chicago. She has been on faculty at the University of Washington since 1981 and has been the recipient of three School of Nursing Excellence in Teaching awards and the University of Washington Distinguished Teaching Award. In addition, in 2002 she received the Distinguished Nutrition Support Nurse Award from the American Society for Parenteral and Enteral Nutrition (ASPEN), in 2003 the American Gastroenterological Association and Janssen Award for Clinical Research in Gastroenterology, and in 2005 she was the first recipient of the Pfizer and Friends of the National Institutes for Nursing Research Award for Research in Women's Health.

LINDA BUCHER, RN, PhD, CEN, CNE

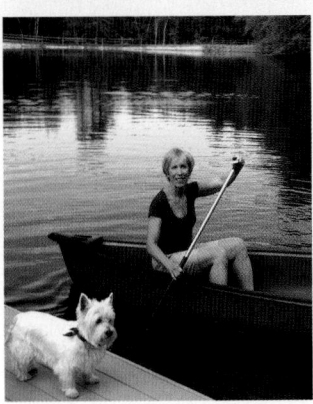

Linda Bucher is an Emerita Professor in the School of Nursing at the University of Delaware in Newark, Delaware. She also is a consultant/mentor in the W. Cary Edwards School of Nursing at Thomas Edison State College. She received her Bachelor of Science in nursing from Thomas Jefferson University in Philadelphia, her Master of Science in adult health and illness from the University of Pennsylvania in Philadelphia, and her doctorate in nursing from Widener University in Chester, Pennsylvania. Her 37 years of nursing experience has spanned staff and patient education, acute and critical care nursing, and teaching in associate, baccalaureate, and graduate nursing programs in New Jersey, Pennsylvania, and Delaware. Her preferred teaching areas include emergency and cardiac nursing and evidence-based practice. She maintains her clinical practice by working as an emergency nurse, is an active member of the American Association of Critical Care Nurses, and enjoys working as a volunteer nurse for Operation Smile. In her free time she enjoys traveling and skiing with her family.

CONTRIBUTORS

Richard Arbour, RN, MSN, CCRN, CNRN, CCNS, FAAN
Critical Care Clinical Nurse Specialist
Albert Einstein Healthcare Network
Philadelphia, Pennsylvania

Margaret Baker, RN, PhD, CNL
Associate Professor
University of Washington School of Nursing
Seattle, Washington

Elisabeth G. Bradley, RN, MS, ACNS-BC
Clinical Leader Cardiovascular Prevention
Program
Christiana Care Health System
Newark, Delaware

Lucy Bradley-Springer, RN, PhD, ACRN, FAAN
Associate Professor
University of Colorado–Denver, Anschutz
Medical Campus
Denver, Colorado

Jormain Cady, DNP, ARNP, AOCN
Nurse Practitioner
Virginia Mason Medical Center
Department of Radiation Oncology
Seattle, Washington

Paula Cox-North, RN, PhD, NP-C
Harborview Medical Center
Seattle, Washington

Anne Croghan, MN, ARNP
Nurse Practitioner
Seattle Gastroenterology Associates
Seattle, Washington

Betty Jean Reid Czarapata, MSN, ANP-BC, CUNP
Nurse Practitioner
Urology Wellness Center
Gaithersburg, Maryland

Judi Daniels, PhD, FNP, PNP
Advanced Practice Registered Nurse
Kentucky Polk-Dalton Clinic
Lexington, Kentucky;
Course Coordinator
Frontier Nursing University
Richmond, Kentucky

Rose DiMaria-Ghalili, RN, PhD, CNSC
Associate Professor of Nursing
College of Nursing and Health Professions
Drexel University
Philadelphia, Pennsylvania

Angela DiSabatino, RN, MS
Manager, Cardiovascular Clinical Trials
Christiana Care Health System
Newark, Delaware

Laura Dulski, MSN, RNC-HROB, CNE
Assistant Professor
Resurrection University
Chicago, Illinois

Susan J. Eisel, RN, MSEd
Associate Professor of Nursing
Mercy College of Ohio
Toledo, Ohio

Deborah Hamolsky, RN, MS, AOCNS
Clinical Nurse IV
Carol Franc Buck Breast Care Center
UCSF Helen Diller Family Comprehensive
Cancer Center
San Francisco, California

Mariann M. Harding, RN, PhD, CNE
Associate Professor of Nursing
Kent State University at Tuscarawas
New Philadelphia, Ohio

Jerry Harvey, RN, MS, BC
Assistant Professor of Nursing
Liberty University
Lynchburg, Virginia

Carol Headley, RN, DNSc, ACNP-BC, CNN
Nephrology Nurse Practitioner
Veterans Affairs Medical Center
Memphis, Tennessee

Teresa E. Hills, RN, MSN, ACNP-BC, CNRN
Neurosurgery Critical Care Nurse
Practitioner
Christiana Care Health System
Newark, Delaware

Christine Hoch, RN, MSN
Nursing Instructor
Delaware Technical Community College
Newark, Delaware

David M. Horner, CRNA, MS, APN
Nurse Anesthetist
Virtua Hospital
Marlton, New Jersey

Joyce Jackowski, MS, FNP-BC, AOCNP
Nurse Practitioner
Virginia Cancer Specialists
Arlington, Virginia

Kay Jarrell, RN, MS, CNE
Clinical Associate Professor
College of Nursing and Health Innovation
Arizona State University
Phoenix, Arizona

Sharmila Johnson, MSN, ACNS-BC, CCRN
Cardiovascular Clinical Nurse Specialist
Christiana Care Health System
Newark, Delaware

Jane Steinman Kaufman, RN, MS, ANP-BC, CRNP
Advanced Senior Lecturer
University of Pennsylvania School of
Nursing
Philadelphia, Pennsylvania

Katherine A. Kelly, RN, DNP, FNP-C, CEN
Assistant Professor
School of Nursing
California State University
Sacramento, California

Lindsay L. Kindler, RN, PhD, CNS
Research Associate
Kaiser Permanente Center for Health
Research
Portland, Oregon

Judy Knighton, RN, MScN
Clinical Nurse Specialist–Burns
Ross Tilley Burn Centre
Sunnybrook Health Sciences Centre
Toronto, Ontario, Canada

Mary Ann Kolis, RN, MSN, ANP-BC, APNP
Instructor
Gateway Technical College
Kenosha, Wisconsin

Catherine N. Kotecki, RN, PhD, APN
Associate Dean
W. Cary Edwards School of Nursing
Thomas Edison State College
Trenton, New Jersey

Nancy Kupper, RN, MSN
Associate Professor
Tarrant County College
Fort Worth, Texas

Jeffrey Kwong, DNP, MPH, ANP-BC
Assistant Professor of Nursing at CUMC
Program Director, Adult-Gerontology Nurse
Practitioner Program
Columbia University
New York, New York

Carol A. Landis, RN, DNSc
Professor
Biobehavioral Nursing and Health Systems
University of Washington
School of Nursing
Seattle, Washington

Susan C. Landis, RN, MSN
Lecturer
Biobehavioral Nursing and Health Systems
University of Washington School of Nursing
Seattle, Washington

Janice Lazear, DNP, CRNP, CDE
Assistant Professor
School of Nursing
University of Maryland
Baltimore, Maryland

Catherine (Kate) Lein, MS, FNP-BC
Assistant Professor
Michigan State University College of
Nursing
East Lansing, Michigan

Janet Lenart, RN, MN, MPH
Senior Lecturer
University of Washington School of Nursing
Seattle, Washington

Nancy MacMullen, PhD, APN/CNS, RNC, HR-OB, CNE
Associate Professor
Governors State University
Oak Forest, Illinois

Dorothy (Dottie) M. Mathers, RN, DNP, CNE
Professor
School of Health Sciences
Pennsylvania College of Technology
Williamsport, Pennsylvania

De Ann F. Mitchell, RN, PhD
Professor of Nursing
Tarrant County College
Trinity River East Campus
Fort Worth, Texas

Carolyn Moffa, MSN, FNP-C, CHFN
Clinical Leader
Heart Failure Program
Christiana Care Health System
Newark, Delaware

Janice Neil, RN, PhD
Associate Professor and Chair, Undergraduate
Nursing Science Junior Division
College of Nursing
East Carolina University
Greenville, North Carolina

DaiWai Olson, RN, PhD, CCRN
Associate Professor of Neurology and
Neurotherapeutics
University of Texas Southwestern
Dallas, Texas

Rosemary C. Polomano, RN, PhD, FAAN
Associate Professor of Pain Practice
Department of Biobehavioral Health
Sciences
University of Pennsylvania School of
Nursing;
Associate Professor of Anesthesiology and
Critical Care
University of Pennsylvania Perelman School
of Medicine
Philadelphia, Pennsylvania

Kathleen A. Rich, RN, PhD, CCNS, CCRN-CSC, CNN
Cardiovascular Clinical Specialist
Indiana University Health La Porte Hospital
La Porte, Indiana

Dottie Roberts, RN, MSN, MACI, CMSRN, OCNS-C, CNE
Instructor
University of South Carolina College of
Nursing
Columbia, South Carolina

Sandra Irene Rome, RN, MN, AOCN, CNS
Clinical Nurse Specialist
Hematology/Oncology/BMT
Cedars-Sinai Medical Center
Los Angeles, California

Jennifer Saylor, RN, PhD, ACNS-BC
Clinical Instructor
University of Delaware
Wilmington, Delaware

Marilee Schmelzer, RN, PhD
Associate Professor
University of Texas at Arlington College of
Nursing
Arlington, Texas

Maureen A. Seckel, RN, APN, MSN, ACNS-BC, CCNS, CCRN
Clinical Nurse Specialist Medical Pulmonary
Critical Care
Christiana Care Health System
Newark, Delaware

Virginia (Jennie) Shaw, RN, MSN
Associate Professor
University of Texas Health Science Center
School of Nursing
San Antonio, Texas

Anita Jo Shoup, RN, MSN, CNOR
Perioperative Clinical Nurse Specialist
Swedish Edmonds
Edmonds, Washington

Dierdre D. Wipke-Tevis, RN, PhD
Associate Professor
PhD Program Director, Coordinator of
Clinical Nurse Specialist Area of Study
Sinclair School of Nursing
University of Missouri
Columbia, Missouri

Mary Wollan, RN, BAN, ONC
Orthopaedic Nurse Educator
Twin Cities Orthopaedic Education
Association
Spring Park, Minnesota

Meg Zomorodi, RN, PhD, CNL
Clinical Associate Professor
University of North Carolina at Chapel Hill
School of Nursing
Chapel Hill, North Carolina

Damien Zsiros, RN, MSN, CNE, CRNP
Nursing Instructor
The Pennsylvania State University School of
Nursing
Fayette/The Eberly Campus
Uniontown, Pennsylvania

Lakshi M. Aldredge, RN, MSN, ANP-BC
Portland, Oregon

Katrina Allen, RN, MSN, CCRN
Fairhope and Bay Minette, Alabama

Carol C. Annesser, RN, MSN, BC, CNE
Toledo, Ohio

Debra Backus, RN, PhD, CNE, NEA-BC
Canton, New York

Jo Ann Baker, RN, MSN, FNP-C
Dover, Delaware

Kathleen M. Barta, RN, EdD
Fayetteville, Arkansas

Cecilia M. Bidigare, RN, MSN
Beavercreek, Ohio

Beth Perry Black, RN, PhD
Chapel Hill, North Carolina

Kathleen Blais, RN, EdD
Wilton Manors, Florida

Mary Blessing, RN, MSN
Albuquerque, New Mexico

Danese M. Boob, MSN/ED, RN-BC
Hershey, Pennsylvania

Barbara S. Broome, RN, PhD, FAAN
Mobile, Alabama

Anna M. Bruch, RN, MSN
Oglesby, Illinois

Carmen Bruni, RN, MSN
Laredo, Texas

Jean Burt, RN, MSN
Chicago, Illinois

Michelle M. Byrne, RN, PhD, CNE, CNOR
Dahlonega, Georgia

Carol Capitano, RN, PhD
Albuquerque, New Mexico

Ronald R. Castaldo, CRNA, MBA, MS, CCRN
New Castle, Delaware

Phyllis Christianson, MN, APRN-BC, GNP
Seattle, Washington

Katie Clark, RD, MPH, CDE
San Diego, California

Bernice Coleman, PhD, ACNP-BC, FAHA
Los Angeles, California

Deborah Marks Conley, RN, MSN, APRN-CNS, GCNS-BC, FNGNA
Omaha, Nebraska

Mary A. Cox, RN, MS
Dayton, Ohio

Paula Cox-North, RN, PhD, NP-C
Seattle, Washington

Betty Jean Reid Czarapata, MSN, ANP-BC, CUNP
Washington, D. C.

Julie Darby, RN, MSN
Memphis, Tennessee

Evelyn Dean, RN, MSN, ACNS-BC, CCRN
Kansas City, Missouri

Fernande E. Deno, RN, MSN, CNE
Coon Rapids, Minnesota

David J. Derrico, RN, MSN
Gainesville, Florida

Julie Dittmer, RN, MSN
Bettendorf, Iowa

Marci Ebberts, RN, BSN, CCRN
Kansas City, Missouri

Susan J. Eisel, RN, MSEd
Toledo, Ohio

Dana R. Epstein, RN, PhD
Phoenix, Arizona

Marianne Ferrin, MSN, ACNP-BC
Philadelphia, Pennsylvania

Shelley Fess, RN, MS, AOCN, CRNI
Rochester, New York

Eleanor Fitzpatrick, RN, MSN, CCRN
Philadelphia, Pennsylvania

Amanda J. Flagg, PhD, ACNS-BC, CNE
San Antonio, Texas

Jan Foecke, RN, MS, ONC
Kansas City, Missouri

Margie Francisco, RN, MSN, EdD
Oglesby, Illinois

Lori Godaire, RN-BC, MS, CCRN, CNL
Norwich, Connecticut

Debra B. Gordon, RN-BC, DNP, ACNS-BC, FAAN
Seattle, Washington

Claudia C. Grobbel, RN, DNP
Rochester, Michigan

Dianne Travers Gustafson, RN, PhD
Omaha, Nebraska

Elizabeth E. Hand, RN, MS
Tulsa, Oklahoma

Carla V. Hannon, MS, APRN, CCRN
New Haven, Connecticut

Mariann M. Harding, RN, PhD, CNE
New Philadelphia, Ohio

Shannon T. Harrington, RN, PhD
Norfolk, Virginia

Jerry Harvey, RN, MS, BC
Lynchburg, Virginia

Mimi Haskins, RN, MS, CMSRN
Buffalo, New York

Kay Helzer, RN, MSN
Phoenix, Arizona

Saundra J. Hendricks, RN, MS, FNP, BC-ADM
Houston, Texas

Margie Hesson, RN, MSN
Rapid City, South Dakota

Kathleen M. Hill, RN, MSN, CCNS
Cleveland, Ohio

Misty Hobart, RN, MSN, ARNP
Spokane, Washington

Patricia Hong, RN, MA
Seattle, Washington

Teressa Sanders Hunter, RN, PhD
Langston, Oklahoma

Janet E. Jackson, RN, MS
Peoria, Illinois

Suzanne L. Jed, MSN, FNP-BC
Los Angeles, California

**Jane Faith Kapustin, PhD, CRNP,
BC-ADM, FAANP**
Baltimore, Maryland

Nancy Karnes, RN, MSN, CCRN, CDE
Bellevue, Washington

Christina D. Keller, RN, MSN
Radford, Virginia

Katherine A. Kelly, RN, DNP, FNP-C, CEN
Sacramento, California

Lisa Kiper, RN, MSN
Morehead, Kentucky

Teri Lynn Kiss, RN, MS, MSSW, CCRN
Fairbanks, Alaska

Tracy H. Knoll, RN, MSN
St. Louis, Missouri

**Mary Ann Kolis, RN, MSN, ANP-BC,
APNP**
Kenosha, Wisconsin

Krista Krause, MSN, FNP-C
Syracuse, New York

Regina Kukulski, RN, MSN, ACNS, BC
Trenton, New Jersey

Vera Kunte, RN-BC, MSN
Trenton, New Jersey

Marci Lagenkamp, RN, MS
Piqua, Ohio

Catherine (Kate) Lein, MS, FNP-BC
East Lansing, Michigan

**Linda R. Littlejohns, RN, MSN, CNRN,
FAAN**
San Juan Capistrano, California

Sarah Livesay, RN, DNP, ACNP, CNS-A
Houston, Texas

Erin M. Loughery, MSN, APRN
Norwich, Connecticut

Beth Lucasey, RN, MA
Kansas City, Missouri

Barbara Lukert, MD
Kansas City, Kansas

Jane A. Madden, RN, MSN
Colorado Springs, Colorado

Laura Mallett, RN, MSN
Laramie, Wyoming

Angela M. Martinelli, RN, PhD, CNOR
Fort Detrick, Maryland

Carole Martz, RN, MS, AOCN, CBCN
Highland Park, Illinois

**Dorothy (Dottie) M. Mathers, RN, DNP,
CNE**
Williamsport, Pennsylvania

**Phyllis A. Matthews, RN, MS, ANCP-BC,
CUNP**
Denver, Colorado

Molly L. McClelland, RN, PhD
Detroit, Michigan

**Tara McMillan-Queen, RN, MSN, ANP,
GNP**
Charlotte, North Carolina

Molly M. McNett, RN, PhD
Cleveland, Ohio

Doreen Mingo, RN, MSN
Waterloo, Illinois

Heidi E. Monroe, RN, MSN, CPAN, CAPA
Green Bay, Wisconsin

Anna Moore, RN, MS
Richmond, Virginia

Amanda Jones Moose, RN, BSN
Taylorsville, North Carolina

Arlene H. Morris, RN, EdD, CNE
Montgomery, Alabama

Brenda C. Morris, RN, EdD, CNE
Phoenix, Arizona

Jason Mott, RN, MSN
Green Bay, Wisconsin

C. Denise Neill, RN, PhD, CNE
Victoria, Texas

Geri B. Neuberger, EdD, APRN-CNS
Kansas City, Kansas

**Lorraine Nowakowski-Grier, MSN, APRN,
BC, CDE**
Newark, Delaware

**Patricia O'Brien, RN, ACNS-BC, MA,
MSN**
Albuquerque, New Mexico

**Margaret Ochab-Ohryn, RN, MS, MBA,
CRNA**
Farmington Hills, Michigan

Devorah Overbay, RN, MSN, CNS
Newberg, Oregon

Judith A. Paice, RN, PhD
Chicago, Illinois

Steven J. Palazzo, RN, PhD
Seattle, Washington

Trevah A. Panek, RN, MSN, CCRN
Loretto, Pennsylvania

Brenda Pavill, RN, PhD, FNP
Dallas, Pennsylvania

Rosalynde D. Peterson, RN, DNP
Tuscaloosa, Alabama

Barbara Pope, RN, MSN, PPCN, CCRN
Philadelphia, Pennsylvania

Tammy Ann Ramon, RN, MSN
University Center, Michigan

Patricia S. Regojo, RN, MSN
Philadelphia, Pennsylvania

Lynn F. Reinke, PhD, ARNP
Seattle, Washington

Tammy C. Roman, RN, EdD, CNE
Rochester, New York

Susan A. Sandstrom, RN, MSN, BC, CNE
Omaha, Nebraska

Marian Sawyier, RN, MSN
Albuquerque, New Mexico

Jennifer Saylor, RN, PhD, ACNS-BC
Wilmington, Delaware

Sally P. Scavone, RN, MS
Buffalo, New York

Mary Scheid, RN, MSN, OCN, CBCN
Greeley, Colorado

Cynthia Schoonover, RN, MS, CCRN
Kettering, Ohio

Teresa J. Seright, RN, PhD, CCRN
Bozeman, Montana

Shellie Simons, RN, PhD
Lowell, Massachusetts

Sarah Smith, RN, MA, CRNO, COT
Oxford, Iowa

Clemma K. Snider, RN, MSN
Richmond, Kentucky

Helen Stegall, RN, BSN, CORLN
Iowa City, Iowa

Elaine K. Strouss, RN, MSN
Monaca, Pennsylvania

Mindy B. Tinkle, RN, PhD, WHNP-BC
Albuquerque, New Mexico

Susan Turner, RN, MSN, FNP
Gilroy, California

Mark R. Van Horn, BS
High Point, North Carolina

Cheryl A. Waklatsi, RN, MSN
Cincinnati, Ohio

Danette Y. Wall, ACRN, MSN, MBA/HCM
Tampa, Florida

Daryle Wane, PhD, ARNP, FNP-BC
New Port Richey, Florida

Lisa A. Webb, RN, MSN, CEN
Charleston, South Carolina

Judith A. Widdoss, RN, MSN, CNE
Bethlehem, Pennsylvania

Sharon A. Willadsen, RN, PhD
Cleveland, Wisconsin

Julie Willenbrink, RN, MSN
Piqua, Ohio

Linda Wilson, RN, PhD, CPAN, CAPA, BC, CNE
Philadelphia, Pennsylvania

Mary Wollan, RN, BAN, ONC
Spring Park, Minnesota

Karen M. Wood, RN, DNSc, CCRN, CNL
Evergreen Park, Illinois

Patricia Worthington, RN, MSN, CNSC
Philadelphia, Pennsylvania

Susan Yeager, RN, MS, CCRN, ACNP
Columbus, Ohio

Amber Young, RN, MSN
Green Bay, Wisconsin

Damien Zsiros, RN, MSN, CNE, CRNP
Uniontown, Pennsylvania

The ninth edition of *Medical-Surgical Nursing: Assessment and Management of Clinical Problems* has been thoroughly revised to incorporate the most current medical-surgical nursing information in an easy-to-use format. More than just a textbook, this is a comprehensive resource containing essential information that students need to prepare for lectures, classroom activities, examinations, clinical assignments, and the safe, comprehensive care of patients. In addition to the readable writing style and full-color illustrations, the text and accompanying resources include many special features to help students learn key medical-surgical nursing content, including patient and caregiver teaching, gerontology, collaborative care, cultural and ethnic considerations, patient safety, genetics, nutrition and drug therapy, evidence-based practice, and much more.

The comprehensive and timely content, special features, attractive layout, and student-friendly writing style combine to make this the number one medical-surgical nursing textbook used in more nursing schools than any other medical-surgical nursing textbook.

The strengths of the first eight editions have been retained, including the use of the nursing process as an organizational theme for nursing management. Numerous new features have been added to address some of the rapid changes in practice. Contributors have been selected for their expertise in specific content areas; one or more specialists in the subject area have thoroughly reviewed each chapter to increase accuracy. The editors have undertaken final rewriting and editing to achieve internal consistency. All efforts have been directed toward building on the strengths of the previous edition while preparing an even more effective new edition.

ORGANIZATION

Content is organized into two major divisions. The first division, Section 1 (Chapters 1 through 11), discusses general concepts related to adult patients. The second division, Sections 2 through 12 (Chapters 12 through 69), presents nursing assessment and nursing management of medical-surgical problems.

The various body systems are grouped to reflect their interrelated functions. Each section is organized around two central themes: assessment and management. Chapters dealing with assessment of a body system include a discussion of the following:

1. A brief review of anatomy and physiology, focusing on information that will promote understanding of nursing care
2. Health history and noninvasive physical assessment skills to expand the knowledge base on which treatment decisions are made
3. Common diagnostic studies, expected results, and related nursing responsibilities to provide easily accessible information

Management chapters focus on the pathophysiology, clinical manifestations, diagnostic studies, collaborative care, and nursing management of various diseases and disorders. The nursing management sections are organized into assessment,

nursing diagnoses, planning, implementation, and evaluation. To emphasize the importance of patient care in various clinical settings, nursing implementation of all major health problems is organized by the following levels of care:

1. Health Promotion
2. Acute Intervention
3. Ambulatory and Home Care

CLASSIC FEATURES

- **Nursing management** is presented in a consistent and comprehensive format, with headings for Health Promotion, Acute Intervention, and Ambulatory and Home Care. Over 60 nursing care plans on the Evolve website and in the text incorporate Nursing Interventions Classification (NIC) and Nursing Outcomes Classification (NOC) in a way that clearly shows the linkages among NIC, NOC, and nursing diagnoses, and applies them to nursing practice.
- **Cultural and ethnic health disparities** content and boxes in the text highlight risk factors and important issues related to the nursing care of various ethnic groups. A special Culturally Competent Care heading denotes cultural and ethnic content related to diseases and disorders. Chapter 2: *Health Disparities and Culturally Competent Care* discusses health status differences among groups of people related to access to care, economic aspects of health care, gender and cultural issues, and disease risk.
- **Collaborative care** is highlighted in special Collaborative Care sections in all management chapters and Collaborative Care tables throughout the text.
- **Coverage on delegation and prioritization** includes the following:
  - Delegation Decisions boxes throughout the text highlight specific topics and skills related to delegation
  - Delegation and priority questions in case studies and Bridge to NCLEX® Examination Questions
  - Nursing interventions throughout the text are listed in order of priority
  - Nursing diagnoses in the nursing care plans are listed in order of priority
- **Focused Assessment boxes** in all assessment chapters provide brief checklists that help students do a more practical "assessment on the run" or bedside approach to assessment. They can be used to evaluate the status of previously identified health problems and monitor for signs of new problems.
- **Safety Alert boxes** highlight important patient safety issues and focus on the National Patient Safety Goals.
- **Pathophysiology Maps** outline complex concepts related to diseases in flowchart format, making them easier to understand.
- **Chapter 8: *Sleep and Sleep Disorders*** expands on this key topic that impacts multiple disorders and body systems as well as nearly every aspect of daily functioning.
- **Patient and caregiver teaching** is an ongoing theme throughout the text. Chapter 4: *Patient and Caregiver Teaching* emphasizes the increasing importance and prevalence of

patient management of chronic illnesses and conditions and the role of the caregiver in patient care.

- **Gerontology and chronic illness** are discussed in Chapter 5: *Chronic Illness and Older Adults,* and included throughout the text under Gerontologic Considerations headings and in Gerontologic Assessment Differences tables.
- **Nutrition** is highlighted throughout the book. Nutritional Therapy tables summarize nutritional interventions and promote healthy lifestyles in patients with various health problems.
- *Healthy People* boxes present health care goals as they relate to specific disorders such as diabetes and cancer.
- **Extensive drug therapy content** includes Drug Therapy tables and concise Drug Alerts highlighting important safety considerations for key drugs.
- **Genetics in Clinical Practice boxes** summarize the genetic basis, genetic testing, and clinical implications for genetic disorders that affect adults.
- **Gender Differences boxes** discuss how women and men are affected differently by conditions such as pain and hypertension.
- A separate chapter on **complementary and alternative therapies** (CAT) addresses current issues in today's health care settings related to these therapies. Complementary & Alternative Therapies boxes expand on this information and summarize what nurses need to know about therapies such as herbal remedies, acupuncture, and biofeedback.
- **Ethical/Legal Dilemmas boxes** promote critical thinking for timely and sensitive issues that nursing students may deal with in clinical practice—topics such as informed consent, advance directives, and confidentiality.
- **Home care/community-based care** is found in special Ambulatory and Home Care sections in the nursing management chapters.
- **Emergency Management tables** outline the emergency treatment of health problems most likely to require emergency intervention.
- **Assessment Abnormalities tables** in assessment chapters alert the nurse to frequently encountered abnormalities and their possible etiologies.
- **Nursing Assessment tables** summarize the key subjective and objective data related to common diseases. Subjective data are organized by functional health patterns.
- **Health History tables** in assessment chapters present key questions to ask patients related to a specific disease or disorder.
- Student-friendly pedagogy includes the following:
  - **Learning Outcomes** and **Key Terms** at the beginning of each chapter help students identify the key content for that chapter.
  - **Evolve website boxes** in chapter openers alert students to supplemental online content and exercises, making it easy for students to facilitate online learning.
  - **Bridge to NCLEX® Examination Questions** at the end of each chapter are matched to the learning outcomes and help students learn the important points in the chapter. Answers are provided just below the questions for immediate feedback, and rationales are provided on the Evolve website.
  - **Case Studies with photos** at the end of chapters bring patients to life. Multiple disorders are incorporated so

students learn how to prioritize care and manage patients in the clinical setting. Discussion questions with a focus on prioritization, delegation, and evidence-based practice are included. Answer guidelines are provided on the Evolve website.
- **Resources** at the end of most chapters include websites for nursing and health care organizations that provide patient teaching and disease and disorder information.
- A **glossary** of key terms and definitions is provided at the back of the text. An expanded version of the glossary with audio pronunciations is included on the Evolve website.

NEW FEATURES

- Once again, each chapter has been carefully revised to ensure a **lower reading level** and more reader-friendly and understandable content than ever. Essential content has been streamlined to help students more effectively learn critical content.
- **Unfolding case studies** in every assessment chapter are an engaging tool that help students apply nursing concepts to real-life patient care.
- **Managing Multiple Patients Case Studies** at the end of each section help students learn to prioritize, delegate, and manage patient care.
- **Informatics boxes** discuss how technology is used by nurses and patients in health care settings.
- **Expanded evidence-based practice content** includes new Applying the Evidence boxes, updated Translating Research Into Practice boxes, and evidence-based practice-focused questions in the case studies.
- **Safety Alerts** have been expanded throughout the book to cover surveillance for high-risk situations.
- New content in Chapter 1 covers **teamwork and interdisciplinary teams,** as this is a key component of QSEN.
- An **increased focus on genetics** includes:
  - A new **genetics chapter** that focuses on practical application of nursing care as it relates to this important topic
  - **Genetic Risk Alerts** in the assessment chapters call attention to important genetic risks
  - **Genetic Link headings** in the management chapters highlight the specific genetic bases of many disorders
- **Expanded coverage of delegation** includes additional Delegation Decision boxes covering issues such as hypertension and postoperative patient care.
- Coverage of **legal considerations has been expanded** in the revised Ethical/Legal Dilemmas boxes.
- **New art** enhances the book's visual appeal and lends a more contemporary look throughout.

LEARNING SUPPLEMENTS FOR STUDENTS

- The handy *Clinical Companion* presents approximately 200 common medical-surgical conditions and procedures in a concise, alphabetical format for quick clinical reference. Designed for portability, this popular reference includes the essential, need-to-know information for treatments and procedures in which nurses play a major role. An attractive and functional two-color design highlights key information for quick, easy reference.

- An exceptionally thorough *Study Guide* contains over 500 pages of review material that reflect the content found in the book. It features a wide variety of clinically relevant exercises and activities, including NCLEX-format multiple choice and alternate format questions, case studies, anatomy review, critical thinking activities, and much more. It features an attractive two-color design and many alternate-item format questions to better prepare students for the NCLEX examination. An answer key is included to provide students with immediate feedback as they study.
- The **Evolve Student Resources** are available online at *http://evolve.elsevier.com/Lewis/medsurg* and include the following valuable learning aids organized by chapter:
  - Printable Key Points summaries for each chapter
  - 1000 NCLEX Examination Review Questions
  - Pre-Tests for every chapter
  - Answer Guidelines to the case studies in the textbook
  - Rationales for the Bridge to NCLEX® Examination Questions in the textbook
  - 55 Interactive Case Studies with state-of-the-art animations and a variety of learning activities, which provide students with immediate feedback. Ten of the case studies are enhanced with photos and narration of the clinical scenarios.
  - Customizable Nursing Care Plans
  - Concept Map Creator and concept maps for selected case studies in the textbook
  - Audio glossary of key terms, available as comprehensive alphabetical glossary and organized by chapter
  - Stress-Busting Kit
  - Animations, video clips, and audio clips
  - Fluids and Electrolytes Tutorial
  - Content Updates
  - Additional resources, including tables, figures, and clinical references
- **Virtual Clinical Excursions** (VCE) is an exciting learning tool that brings learning to life in a "virtual" hospital setting. VCE simulates a realistic, yet safe, nursing environment where the routine and rigors of the average clinical rotation abound. Students can conduct a complete assessment of a patient and set priorities for care, collect data, analyze and interpret data, prepare and administer medications, and reach conclusions about complex problems. Each lesson has a textbook reading assignment and online activities based on "visiting" patients in the hospital. Instructors receive an implementation manual with directions for using VCE as a teaching tool.
- More than just words on a screen, **Pageburst eBooks** come with a wealth of built-in study tools and interactive functionality to help students better connect with the course material and their instructors. Plus, with the ability to fit an entire library of books on one portable device, Pageburst gives students the ability to study when, where, and how they want.

TEACHING SUPPLEMENTS FOR INSTRUCTORS

- The **Evolve Instructor Resources** (available online at *http://evolve.elsevier.com/Lewis/medsurg*) remain the most comprehensive set of instructor's materials available, containing the following:

- **TEACH for Nurses Lesson Plans** with electronic resources organized by chapter to help instructors develop and manage the course curriculum. This exciting resource includes:
  - Objectives
  - Teaching focus
  - Key terms
  - Nursing curriculum standards
  - Student and instructor chapter resource listings
  - Detailed chapter outlines
  - Teaching strategies with learning activities and links to resources in the image collection, PowerPoint presentations, animations, etc.
  - Case studies with answer guidelines
- The **Test Bank** features over 2000 NCLEX Examination test questions with text page references and answers coded for NCLEX Client Needs category, nursing process, and cognitive level. The ninth edition test bank has been completely updated and reviewed, and it now includes hundreds of prioritization, delegation, and multiple patient questions. All alternate item format questions are included. The ExamView software allows instructors to create new tests; edit, add, and delete test questions; sort questions by NCLEX category, cognitive level, nursing process step, and question type; and administer and grade online tests.
- The **Image Collection** contains more than 800 full-color images from the text for use in lectures.
- An extensive collection of **PowerPoint Presentations** includes over 125 different presentations focused on the most common diseases and disorders. The presentations have been thoroughly revised to include helpful instructor notes/teaching tips, unfolding case studies, new illustrations and photos not found in the book, new animations, and updated audience response questions for use with iClicker and other audience response systems.
- Course management system.
- Access to all student resources listed above.
- The **Simulation Learning System (SLS)** is an online toolkit that helps instructors and facilitators effectively incorporate medium- to high-fidelity simulation into their nursing curriculum. Detailed patient scenarios promote and enhance the clinical decision-making skills of students at all levels. The SLS provides detailed instructions for preparation and implementation of the simulation experience, debriefing questions that encourage critical thinking, and learning resources to reinforce student comprehension. Each scenario in the SLS complements the textbook content and helps bridge the gap between lecture and clinical. The SLS provides the perfect environment for students to practice what they are learning in the text for a true-to-life, hands-on learning experience.

ACKNOWLEDGMENTS

The editors are especially grateful to many people at Elsevier who assisted with this major revision effort. In particular, we wish to thank the team of Kristin Geen, Jamie Randall, Mary Stueck, Jeff Patterson, and Maggie Reid. In addition, we want to thank the marketing team of Pat Crowe, Katie Schlesinger, and Becky McBride.

Special thanks and appreciation go to Peter Bonner who assisted with many details of manuscript preparation and review and photography for the book and interactive case studies.

We are particularly indebted to the faculty, nurses, and student nurses who have put their faith in our book to assist them on their path to excellence. The increasing use of this book throughout the United States, Canada, Australia, and other parts of the world has been gratifying. We appreciate the many users who have shared their comments and suggestions on the previous editions. All feedback is welcome.

We also wish to thank our contributors and reviewers for their assistance with the revision process. We sincerely hope that this book will assist both students and clinicians in practicing truly professional nursing.

Sharon L. Lewis
Shannon Ruff Dirksen
Margaret McLean Heitkemper
Linda Bucher

TEST BANK

Barbara Bartz, MN, ARNP, CCRN
Nursing Instructor
Yakima Valley Community College
Yakima, Washington

Linda Bucher, RN, PhD, CEN, CNE
Emerita Professor
School of Nursing, University of Delaware
Newark, Delaware;
Consultant/Mentor
W. Cary Edwards School of Nursing
Thomas Edison State College
Trenton, New Jersey;
Per Diem Staff Nurse
Emergency Department,
Virtua Memorial Hospital
Mt. Holly, New Jersey

Debra Hagler, RN, PhD, ACNS-BC, CNE, CHSE, ANEF, FAAN
Clinical Professor
College of Nursing and Healthcare Innovation
Arizona State University
Phoenix, Arizona

Christina D. Keller, RN, MSN
Instructor
Radford University School of Nursing
Clinical Simulation Center
Radford, Virginia

Jo A. Voss, RN, PhD, CNS
Associate Professor
South Dakota State University
Rapid City, South Dakota

PRE-TESTS

Debra Hagler, RN, PhD, ACNS-BC, CNE, CHSE, ANEF, FAAN
Clinical Professor
College of Nursing and Healthcare Innovation
Arizona State University
Phoenix, Arizona

CASE STUDIES

Interactive, Managing Multiple Patients, and Assessment Case Studies
Dorothy (Dottie) M. Mathers, RN, DNP, CNE
Professor
School of Health Sciences
Pennsylvania College of Technology
Williamsport, Pennsylvania

TEACH for Nurses Case Studies
Elizabeth Day, RN, MSN, CHPN
Nursing Faculty
Fresno City College and Madera Center
Fresno, California

Heidi E. Monroe, RN-BC, MSN, CPAN, CAPA
Assistant Professor of Nursing
Bellin College
Green Bay, Wisconsin

POWERPOINT PRESENTATIONS

Dorothy (Dottie) M. Mathers, RN, DNP, CNE
Professor
School of Health Sciences
Pennsylvania College of Technology
Williamsport, Pennsylvania

Jane E. Oehme, RN, MS
Associate Professor of Nursing
Pennsylvania College of Technology
Williamsport, Pennsylvania

Michelle A. Latshaw, RN, MSN
Associate Professor of Nursing
Williamsport, Pennsylvania

PowerPoint Presentations and Glossaries
Cory Shaw Retherford, MOM, LAc.
Former Research Assistant
University of Texas Health Science Center at San Antonio
San Antonio, Texas

TEACH FOR NURSES

Mariann M. Harding, RN, PhD, CNE
Associate Professor of Nursing
Kent State University at Tuscarawas
New Philadelphia, Ohio

AUDIENCE RESPONSE QUESTIONS

Jo A. Voss, RN, PhD, CNS
Associate Professor
South Dakota State University
Rapid City, South Dakota

NCLEX® EXAMINATION REVIEW QUESTIONS

Susan A. Sandstrom, RN, MSN, BC, CNE
Associate Professor in Nursing, Retired
College of Saint Mary
Omaha, Nebraska

STUDY GUIDE

Susan A. Sandstrom, RN, MSN, BC, CNE
Associate Professor in Nursing, Retired
College of Saint Mary
Omaha, Nebraska

CLINICAL COMPANION

Shannon Ruff Dirksen, RN, PhD, FAAN
Associate Professor
College of Nursing and Health Innovation
Arizona State University
Phoenix, Arizona

Sharon L. Lewis, RN, PhD, FAAN
Professor Emerita
University of New Mexico
Albuquerque, New Mexico;
Former Castella Distinguished Professor
School of Nursing
University of Texas Health Science Center at San Antonio
San Antonio, Texas;
Developer and Consultant
Stress-Busting Program for Family Caregivers

ETHICAL/LEGAL DILEMMAS BOXES

Kathy Lucke, RN, PhD
Clinical Professor
University at Buffalo
School of Nursing
Buffalo, New York

Rosemary J. Mann, RN, CNM, MS, JD, PhD
Clinical Professor
School of Nursing
University at Buffalo
Buffalo, New York

DELEGATION DECISIONS BOXES

Barbara Bartz, MN, ARNP, CCRN
Nursing Instructor
Yakima Valley Community College
Yakima, Washington

EVIDENCE-BASED PRACTICE BOXES

Applying the Evidence Boxes

Linda Bucher, RN, PhD, CEN, CNE
Emerita Professor
School of Nursing
University of Delaware
Newark, Delaware;
Consultant/Mentor
W. Cary Edwards School of Nursing
Thomas Edison State College
Trenton, New Jersey;
Per Diem Staff Nurse
Emergency Department
Virtua Memorial Hospital
Mt. Holly, New Jersey

Translating Research Into Practice Boxes

Shannon Ruff Dirksen, RN, PhD, FAAN
Associate Professor
College of Nursing and Health Innovation
Arizona State University
Phoenix, Arizona

INFORMATICS BOXES

Mariann M. Harding, RN, PhD, CNE
Associate Professor of Nursing
Kent State University at Tuscarawas
New Philadelphia, Ohio

NURSING CARE PLANS

Patricia O'Brien, RN, ACNS-BC, MA, MSN
Albuquerque, New Mexico

SPECIAL PROJECTS

Peter Bonner, MS
DSI
Placitas, New Mexico

CONTENTS

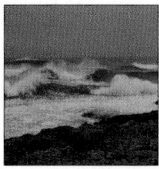
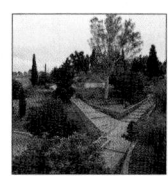
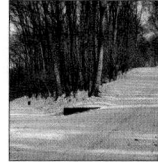
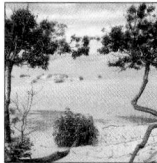
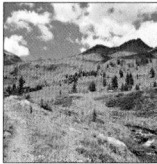
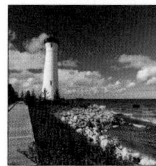

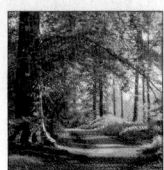

SECTION 7
Problems of Oxygenation: Perfusion

VOLUME 2

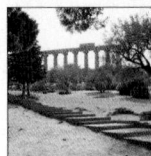

SECTION 8
Problems of Ingestion, Digestion, Absorption, and Elimination

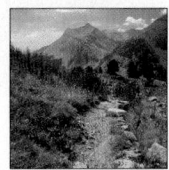

SECTION 9
Problems of Urinary Function

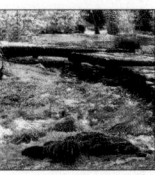

SECTION 10
Problems Related to Regulatory and Reproductive Mechanisms

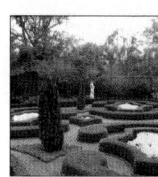

SECTION 11
Problems Related to Movement and Coordination

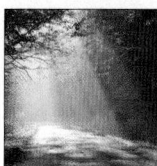

SECTION 12
Nursing Care in Critical Care Settings

APPENDIXES

COMPLEMENTARY & ALTERNATIVE THERAPIES BOXES

CULTURAL & ETHNIC HEALTH DISPARITIES BOXES

DELEGATION DECISIONS BOXES

DIAGNOSTIC STUDIES TABLES

DRUG THERAPY TABLES

EMERGENCY MANAGEMENT TABLES

ETHICAL/LEGAL DILEMMAS BOXES

EVIDENCE-BASED PRACTICE

Applying the Evidence Boxes

EVIDENCE-BASED PRACTICE

Translating Research Into Practice Boxes

NURSING CARE PLANS

NUTRITIONAL THERAPY TABLES

PATIENT & CAREGIVER TEACHING GUIDE TABLES

Problems of Ingestion, Digestion, Absorption, and Elimination

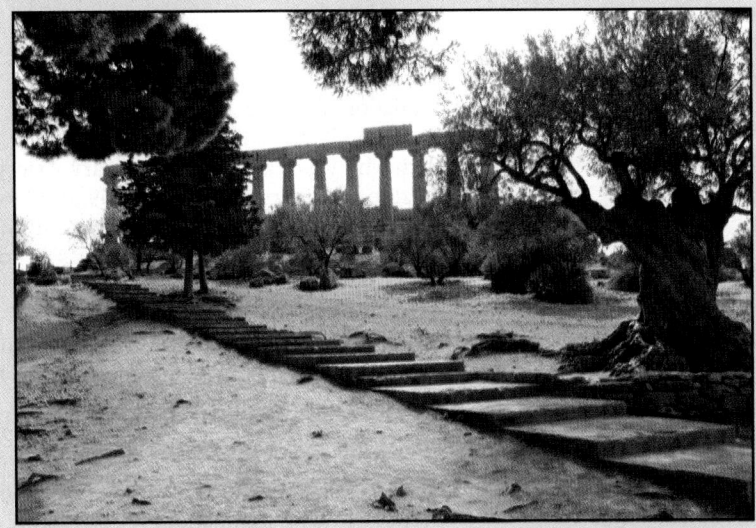

Peter Bonner

I see my path, but I don't know where it leads. Not knowing where I'm going is what inspires me to travel it.
Rosalia de Castro

It's all right to have butterflies in your stomach. Just get them to fly in formation.
Rob Gilbert

Nursing Assessment
Gastrointestinal System

Paula Cox-North

℮volve WEBSITE

http://evolve.elsevier.com/Lewis/medsurg

- NCLEX Review Questions
- Key Points
- Pre-Test
- Answer Guidelines for Case Study in this chapter
- Rationales for Bridge to NCLEX Examination Questions
- Concept Map Creator
- Glossary
- Content Updates
- Animation
  - Rectal Examination

- Videos
  - Auscultation: Abdomen, Bowel Sounds
  - Palpation: Abdomen, Superficial and Deep
  - Percussion: Abdomen
  - Percussion: Liver
  - Percussion: Spleen
  - Physical Examination: Abdomen: Inspection, Auscultation, and Percussion
  - Physical Examination: Abdomen: Palpation

eFigures
- eFig. 39-1: Omentum
- eFig. 39-2: Microscopic structure of liver lobule

LEARNING OUTCOMES

1. Describe the structures and functions of the organs of the gastrointestinal tract.
2. Describe the structures and functions of the liver, gallbladder, biliary tract, and pancreas.
3. Differentiate the processes of ingestion, digestion, absorption, and elimination.
4. Explain the processes of biliary metabolism, bile production, and bile excretion.
5. Link the age-related changes of the gastrointestinal system to the differences in assessment findings.

6. Select significant subjective and objective assessment data related to the gastrointestinal system that should be obtained from a patient.
7. Identify the appropriate techniques used in the physical assessment of the gastrointestinal system.
8. Differentiate normal from abnormal findings of a physical assessment of the gastrointestinal system.
9. Describe the purpose, significance of results, and nursing responsibilities related to diagnostic studies of the gastrointestinal system.

KEY TERMS

bilirubin, p. 870
borborygmi, Table 39-11, p. 878
cheilosis, Table 39-11, p. 878
deglutition, p. 867
endoscopy, p. 882

hematemesis, Table 39-11, p. 878
hepatocytes, p. 869
Kupffer cells, p. 870
melena, Table 39-11, p. 878
pyorrhea, Table 39-11, p. 878

pyrosis, Table 39-11, p. 878
steatorrhea, Table 39-11, p. 878
tenesmus, Table 39-11, p. 878
Valsalva maneuver, p. 869

Reviewed by Phyllis Christianson, MN, APRN-BC, GNP, Senior Lecturer, University of Washington, School of Nursing, Seattle, Washington; and Marian Sawyier, RN, MSN, Staff Nurse, University of New Mexico Hospital, Albuquerque, New Mexico.

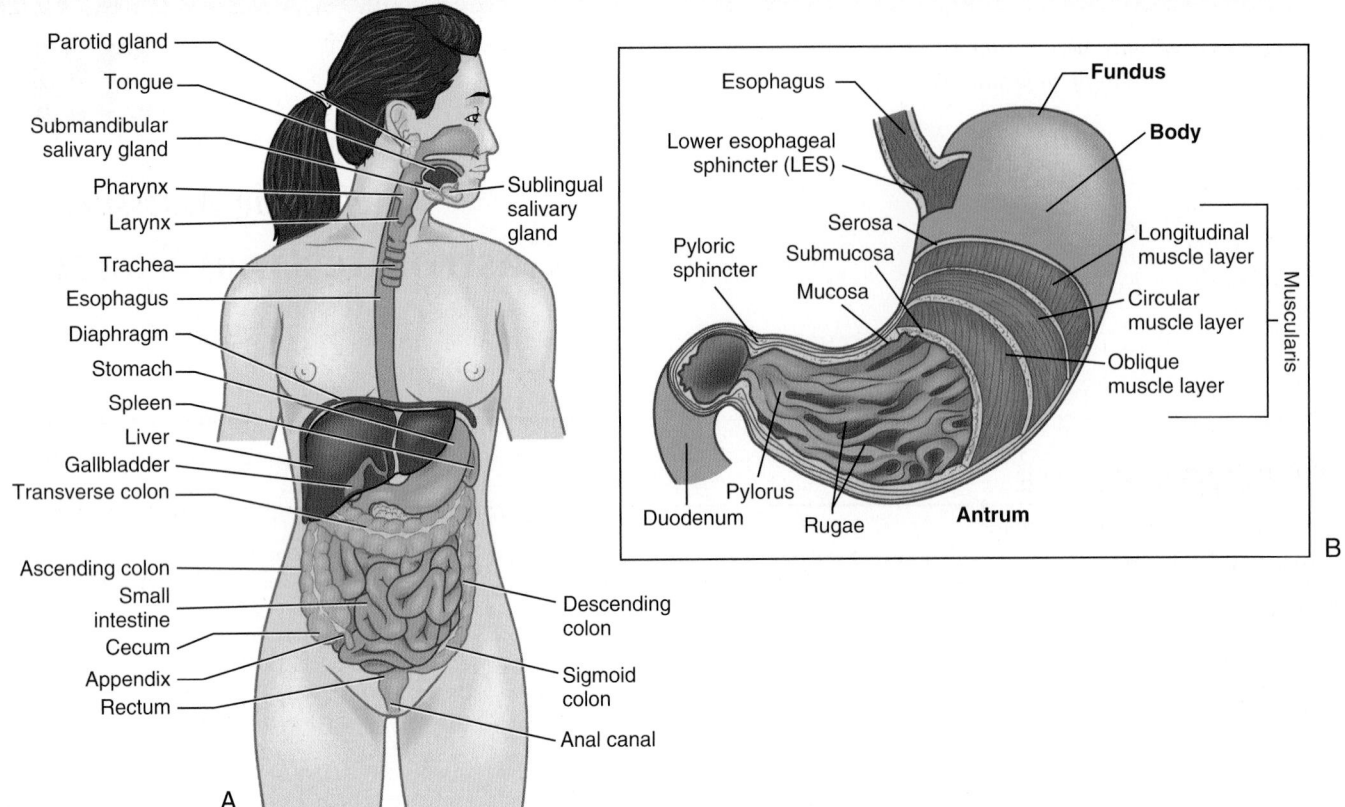

FIG. 39-1 A, Location of organs of the gastrointestinal system. **B,** Parts of the stomach.

The gastrointestinal (GI) system (also called the digestive system) consists of the GI tract and its associated organs and glands. Included in the GI tract are the mouth, esophagus, stomach, small intestine, large intestine, rectum, and anus. The associated organs are the liver, pancreas, and gallbladder (Fig. 39-1).

STRUCTURES AND FUNCTIONS OF GASTROINTESTINAL SYSTEM

The GI tract extends approximately 30 ft (9 m) from the mouth to the anus. It is composed of four common layers. From the inside to the outside, these layers are (1) mucosa, (2) submucosa, (3) muscle, and (4) serosa (see Fig. 39-1). The muscular coat consists of two layers: the circular (inner) layer and the longitudinal (outer) layer.

The GI tract is innervated by the parasympathetic and sympathetic branches of the autonomic nervous system. The parasympathetic (cholinergic) system is mainly excitatory, and the sympathetic (adrenergic) system is mainly inhibitory. For example, peristalsis is increased by parasympathetic stimulation and decreased by sympathetic stimulation. Sensory information is relayed via both sympathetic and parasympathetic afferent fibers.

The GI tract has its own nervous system: the enteric (or intrinsic) nervous system. The enteric nervous system is composed of two nerve layers that lie between the mucosa and the muscle layers. These neurons have receptors for pressure and movement.

The GI tract and accessory organs receive approximately 25% to 30% of the cardiac output at rest and 35% or more after eating. Circulation in the GI system is unique in that venous

blood draining the GI tract organs empties into the portal vein, which then perfuses the liver. The vascular supply to the GI tract includes the celiac artery, superior mesenteric artery (SMA), and the inferior mesenteric artery (IMA). The stomach and duodenum receive their blood supply from the celiac axis. The distal small intestine to mid larger intestine receives its blood supply from branches of the hepatic and SMAs. The distal large intestine through the anus receives its blood supply from the IMA. Because such a large percentage of the cardiac output perfuses these organs, the GI tract is a major source from which blood flow can be diverted during exercise, stress, or injury.

The abdominal organs are almost completely covered by the peritoneum. The two layers of the peritoneum are the *parietal layer,* which lines the abdominal cavity wall, and the *visceral layer,* which covers the abdominal organs. The peritoneal cavity is the potential space between the parietal and visceral layers. The two folds of the peritoneum are the mesentery and the omentum. The mesentery attaches the small intestine and part of the large intestine to the posterior abdominal wall and contains blood and lymph vessels. The omentum hangs like an apron from the stomach to the intestines and contains fat and lymph nodes (see eFig. 39-1 on the website for this chapter).

The main function of the GI system is to supply nutrients to body cells. This is accomplished through the processes of (1) *ingestion* (taking in food), (2) *digestion* (breaking down food), and (3) *absorption* (transferring food products into circulation). *Elimination* is the process of excreting the waste products of digestion.

Ingestion

Ingestion is the intake of food. A person's appetite or desire to ingest food influences how much food is eaten. An appetite center is located in the hypothalamus. It is directly or indirectly stimulated by hypoglycemia, an empty stomach, decrease in body temperature, and input from higher brain centers. The hormone *ghrelin* released from the stomach mucosa plays a role in appetite stimulation. Another hormone, *leptin,* is involved in appetite suppression. (Ghrelin and leptin are discussed in Chapter 41.) The sight, smell, and taste of food frequently stimulate appetite. Appetite may be inhibited by stomach distention, illness (especially accompanied by fever), hyperglycemia, nausea and vomiting, and certain drugs (e.g., amphetamines).

Deglutition (swallowing) is the mechanical component of ingestion. The organs involved in the deglutition of food are the mouth, pharynx, and esophagus.

Mouth. The mouth consists of the lips and the oral (buccal) cavity. The lips surround the orifice of the mouth and function in speech. The roof of the oral cavity is formed by the hard and soft palates. The oral cavity contains the teeth, used in mastication (chewing), and the tongue. The tongue is a solid muscle mass and assists in chewing and moving food to the back of the throat for swallowing. Taste receptors (taste buds) are found on the sides and tip of the tongue. The tongue is also important in speech.

Within the oral cavity are three pairs of salivary glands: the parotid, submaxillary, and sublingual glands. These glands produce saliva, which consists of water, protein, mucin, inorganic salts, and salivary amylase.

Pharynx. The pharynx is a musculomembranous tube that is divided into the nasopharynx, the oropharynx, and the laryngeal pharynx. The mucous membrane of the pharynx is continuous with the nasal cavity, mouth, auditory tubes, and larynx. The epiglottis is a lid of fibrocartilage that closes over the larynx during swallowing. During ingestion, the oropharynx provides a route for food from the mouth to the esophagus. When receptors in the oropharynx are stimulated by food or liquid, the swallowing reflex is initiated. The tonsils and the adenoids, composed of lymphoid tissue, assist the body in preventing infection.

Esophagus. The esophagus is a hollow, muscular tube that receives food from the pharynx and moves it to the stomach. It is 7 to 10 in (18 to 25 cm) long and 0.8 in (2 cm) in diameter. The esophagus is located in the thoracic cavity. The upper third of the esophagus is composed of striated skeletal muscle, and the distal two thirds are composed of smooth muscle.

With swallowing, the upper esophageal sphincter (cricopharyngeal muscle) relaxes and a peristaltic wave moves the bolus into the esophagus. Between swallows, the esophagus is collapsed. It is structurally composed of four layers: inner mucosa, submucosa, muscularis propria, and outermost adventitia.

The muscular layers contract *(peristalsis)* and propel the food to the stomach. There are two sphincters: the *upper esophageal sphincter* (UES) at the proximal end of the esophagus and the *lower esophageal sphincter* (LES) at the distal end. The LES remains contracted except during swallowing, belching, or vomiting. The LES is an important barrier that normally prevents reflux of acidic gastric contents into the esophagus.

Digestion and Absorption

Stomach. The stomach's functions are to store food, mix food with gastric secretions, and empty contents in small boluses into the small intestine. The stomach absorbs only small amounts of water, alcohol, electrolytes, and certain drugs.

The stomach is usually J shaped and lies obliquely in the epigastric, umbilical, and left hypochondriac regions of the abdomen (see Fig. 39-5 later in the chapter). It always contains gastric fluid and mucus. The three main parts of the stomach are the fundus (cardia), body, and antrum (see Fig. 39-1). The pylorus is a small portion of the antrum proximal to the pyloric sphincter. Sphincter muscles (the LES and the pyloric sphincter) guard the entrance to and exit from the stomach.

The serous (outer) layer of the stomach is formed by the peritoneum. The muscular layer consists of the longitudinal (outer) layer, circular (middle) layer, and oblique (inner) layer. The mucosal layer forms folds called *rugae* that contain many small glands. In the fundus the glands contain chief cells, which secrete pepsinogen, and parietal cells, which secrete hydrochloric (HCl) acid, water, and intrinsic factor. The secretion of HCl acid makes gastric juice acidic. This acidic pH aids in the protection against ingested organisms. Intrinsic factor promotes cobalamin (vitamin B_{12}) absorption in the small intestine.

Small Intestine. The two primary functions of the small intestine are digestion and *absorption* (uptake of nutrients from the gut lumen to the bloodstream). The small intestine is a coiled tube approximately 23 ft (7 m) in length and 1 to 1.1 in (2.5 to 2.8 cm) in diameter. It extends from the pylorus to the ileocecal valve. The small intestine is composed of the duodenum, jejunum, and ileum. The ileocecal valve prevents reflux of large intestine contents into the small intestine.

The mucosa of the small intestine is thick, vascular, and glandular. The functional units of the small intestine are *villi,* minute, fingerlike projections in the mucous membrane. They contain epithelial cells that produce the intestinal digestive enzymes. The epithelial cells on the villi also have *microvilli.* The circular folds in the mucous and submucous layers, along with the villi and microvilli, increase the surface area for digestion and absorption.

The digestive enzymes on the brush border of the microvilli chemically break down nutrients for absorption. The villi are surrounded by the crypts of Lieberkühn, which contain the multipotent stem cells for the other epithelial cell types. (Stem cells are discussed in Chapter 13.) Brunner's glands in the submucosa of the duodenum secrete an alkaline fluid containing bicarbonate. Intestinal goblet cells secrete mucus that protects the mucosa.

Physiology of Digestion. *Digestion* is the physical and chemical breakdown of food into absorbable substances. Digestion in the GI tract is facilitated by the timely movement of food through the GI tract and the secretion of specific enzymes. These enzymes break down foodstuffs to particles of appropriate size for absorption (Table 39-1).

The process of digestion begins in the mouth, where the food is chewed, mechanically broken down, and mixed with saliva. Approximately 1 L of saliva is produced each day. Saliva facilitates swallowing by lubricating food. Saliva contains amylase (ptyalin), which breaks down starches to maltose. Salivary gland secretion is stimulated by chewing movements and the sight, smell, thought, and taste of food. After swallowing, food is moved through the esophagus to the stomach. No digestion or absorption occurs in the esophagus.

In the stomach the digestion of proteins begins with the release of pepsinogen from chief cells. The stomach's acidic environment results in the conversion of pepsinogen to its active form, pepsin. Pepsin begins the breakdown of proteins. There is minimal digestion of starches and fats. The food is mixed with gastric secretions, which are under neural and hormonal control (Tables 39-2 and 39-3). The stomach also serves as a reservoir for food, which is slowly released into the small intestine. The length of time that food remains in the stomach depends on the composition of the food, but average meals remain from 3 to 4 hours.

In the small intestine, carbohydrates are broken down to monosaccharides, fats to glycerol and fatty acids, and proteins to amino acids. The physical presence and chemical nature of *chyme* (food mixed with gastric secretions) stimulate motility and secretion. Secretions involved in digestion include enzymes from the pancreas, bile from the liver (see Table 39-1), and enzymes from the small intestine. Enzymes on the brush border of the microvilli complete the digestion process. These enzymes break down disaccharides to monosaccharides and peptides to amino acids for absorption.

Both secretion and motility are under neural and hormonal control. When food enters the stomach and small intestine, hormones are released into the bloodstream (see Table 39-3). These hormones play important roles in the control of HCl acid secretion, production and release of digestive enzymes, and motility.

Absorption is the transfer of the end products of digestion across the intestinal wall to the circulation. Most absorption occurs in the small intestine. The movement of the villi enables the end products of digestion to come in contact with the absorbing membrane. Monosaccharides (from carbohydrates), fatty acids (from fats), amino acids (from proteins), water, electrolytes, vitamins, and minerals are absorbed.

Elimination

Large Intestine. The large intestine is a hollow, muscular tube approximately 5 to 6 ft (1.5 to 1.8 m) long and 2 in (5 cm) in diameter. The four parts of the large intestine are shown in Fig. 39-2.

The most important function of the large intestine is the absorption of water and electrolytes. The large intestine also forms feces and serves as a reservoir for the fecal mass until defecation occurs. Feces are composed of water (75%), bacteria, unabsorbed minerals, undigested foodstuffs, bile pigments, and

TABLE 39-1	GASTROINTESTINAL SECRETIONS	
Daily Amount (mL)	**Secretions, Enzymes**	**Action**
Salivary Glands		
1000-1500	Salivary amylase (ptyalin)	Initiation of starch digestion
Stomach		
2500	Pepsinogen	Protein digestion
	HCl acid	Activation of pepsinogen to pepsin
	Lipase	Fat digestion
	Intrinsic factor	Essential for cobalamin absorption in ileum
Small Intestine		
3000	Enterokinase	Activation of trypsinogen to trypsin
	Amylase	Carbohydrate digestion
	Peptidases	Protein digestion
	Aminopeptidases	Protein digestion
	Maltase	Maltose to two glucose molecules
	Sucrase	Sucrose to glucose and fructose
	Lactase	Lactose to glucose and galactose
	Lipase	Fat digestion
Pancreas		
700	Trypsinogen	Protein digestion
	Chymotrypsin	Protein digestion
	Amylase	Starch to disaccharides
	Lipase	Fat digestion
Liver and Gallbladder		
1000	Bile	Emulsification of fats and aid in absorption of fatty acids and fat-soluble vitamins (A, D, E, K)

TABLE 39-2	PHASES OF GASTRIC SECRETION
Stimulus to Secretion	**Secretion**
Cephalic (nervous) Sight, smell, taste of food (before food enters stomach). Initiated in the CNS and mediated by the vagus nerve.	HCl acid, pepsinogen, mucus
Gastric (hormonal and nervous) Food in antrum of stomach, vagal stimulation.	Release of gastrin from antrum into circulation to stimulate gastric secretions and motility
Intestinal (hormonal) Presence of chyme in small intestine.	*Acidic chyme* (pH <2): Release of secretin, gastric inhibitory polypeptide, cholecystokinin into circulation to decrease HCl acid secretion *Chyme* (pH >3): Release of gastrin from duodenum to increase acid secretion

TABLE 39-3	HORMONES CONTROLLING GI SECRETION AND MOTILITY		
Hormone	**Source**	**Activating Stimuli**	**Function**
Gastrin	Gastric and duodenal mucosa	Stomach distention, partially digested proteins in pylorus	Stimulates gastric acid secretion and motility. Maintains lower esophageal sphincter tone.
Secretin	Duodenal mucosa	Acid entering small intestine	Inhibits gastric motility and acid secretion. Stimulates pancreatic bicarbonate secretion.
Cholecystokinin	Duodenal mucosa	Fatty acids and amino acids in small intestine	Contracts gallbladder and relaxes sphincter of Oddi. Allows increased flow of bile into duodenum; release of pancreatic digestive enzymes.
Gastric inhibitory peptide	Duodenal mucosa	Fatty acids and lipids in small intestine	Inhibits gastric acid secretion and motility.

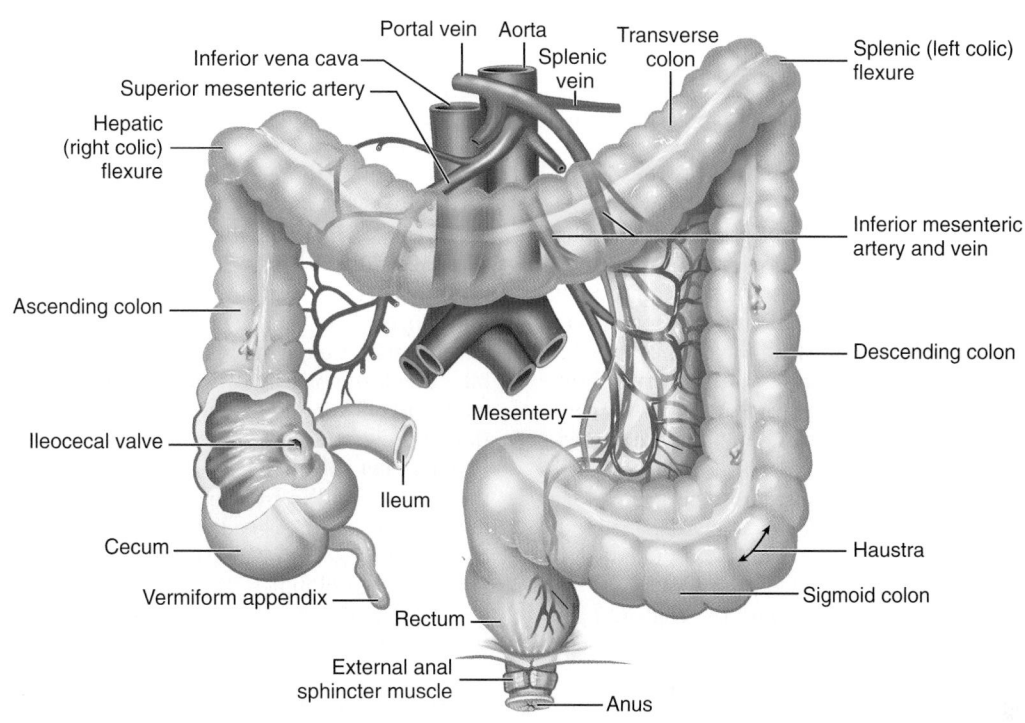

FIG. 39-2 Anatomic locations of the large intestine.

desquamated (shed) epithelial cells. The large intestine secretes mucus, which acts as a lubricant and protects the mucosa.

Microorganisms in the colon are responsible for the breakdown of proteins not digested or absorbed in the small intestine. These amino acids are deaminated by the bacteria, leaving ammonia, which is carried to the liver and converted to urea, which is excreted by the kidneys. Bacteria in the colon also synthesize vitamin K and some of the B vitamins. Bacteria also play a part in the production of flatus.

The movements of the large intestine are usually slow. However, propulsive (mass movements) peristalsis also occurs. When food enters the stomach and duodenum, gastrocolic and duodenocolic reflexes are initiated, resulting in peristalsis in the colon. These reflexes are more active after the first daily meal and frequently result in bowel evacuation.

Defecation is a reflex action involving voluntary and involuntary control. Feces in the rectum stimulate sensory nerve endings that produce the desire to defecate. The reflex center for defecation is in the sacral portion of the spinal cord (parasympathetic nerve fibers). These fibers produce contraction of the rectum and relaxation of the internal anal sphincter. Defecation is controlled voluntarily by relaxing the external anal sphincter when the desire to defecate is felt. An acceptable environment for defecation is usually necessary, or the urge to defecate will be ignored. If defecation is suppressed over long periods, problems can occur, such as constipation or fecal impaction.

Defecation can be facilitated by the Valsalva maneuver. This maneuver involves contraction of the chest muscles on a closed glottis with simultaneous contraction of the abdominal muscles. These actions result in increased intraabdominal pressure. The Valsalva maneuver may be contraindicated in the patient with a head injury, eye surgery, cardiac problems, hemorrhoids, abdominal surgery, or liver cirrhosis with portal hypertension.

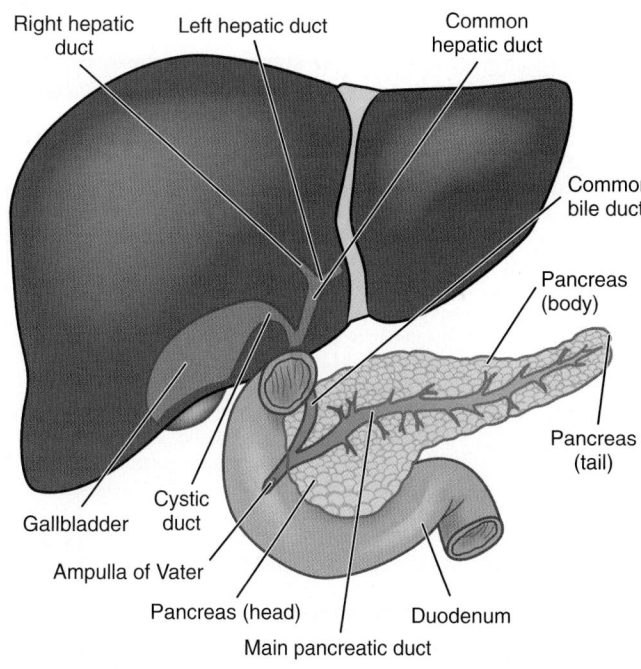

FIG. 39-3 Gross structure of the liver, gallbladder, pancreas, and duct system.

Liver, Biliary Tract, and Pancreas

Liver. The liver is the largest internal organ in the body, weighing approximately 3 lb (1.36 kg). It lies in the right epigastric region (see Fig. 39-5 later in the chapter). Most of the liver is enclosed in peritoneum. It has a fibrous capsule that divides it into right and left lobes (Fig. 39-3).

The functional units of the liver are lobules (see eFig. 39-2 on the website for this chapter). The lobule consists of rows of hepatic cells (hepatocytes) arranged around a central vein. The capillaries (sinusoids) are located between the rows of hepatocytes and are lined with Kupffer cells, which carry out phagocytic activity (removal of bacteria and toxins from the blood). Interlobular bile ducts form from bile capillaries (canaliculi). The hepatic cells secrete bile into the canaliculi.

About one fourth of the blood supply comes from the hepatic artery (branch of the celiac artery), and three fourths comes from the portal vein. The portal circulatory system (enterohepatic) brings blood to the liver from the stomach, intestines, spleen, and pancreas. The portal vein carries absorbed products of digestion directly to the liver. In the liver the portal vein branches and comes in contact with each lobule.

The liver is essential for life. It functions in the manufacture, storage, transformation, and excretion of a number of substances involved in metabolism. The liver's functions are numerous and can be classified into four main areas (Table 39-4).

Biliary Tract. The biliary tract consists of the gallbladder and the duct system. The gallbladder is a pear-shaped sac located below the liver. The gallbladder's function is to concentrate and store bile. It holds approximately 45 mL of bile.

Bile is produced by the hepatic cells and secreted into the biliary canaliculi of the lobules. Bile then drains into the interlobular bile ducts, which unite into the two main left and right hepatic ducts. The hepatic ducts merge with the cystic duct from the gallbladder to form the common bile duct (see Fig. 39-3). Most of the bile is stored and concentrated in the gallbladder. It is then released into the cystic duct and moves down the common bile duct to enter the duodenum at the ampulla of Vater. In the intestines, bilirubin is reduced to stercobilinogen and urobilinogen by bacterial action. Stercobilinogen accounts for the brown color of stool. A small amount of conjugated bilirubin is reabsorbed into the blood. Some urobilinogen is reabsorbed into the blood, returned to the liver through the portal circulation (enterohepatic), and excreted in the bile.

Bilirubin Metabolism. Bilirubin, a pigment derived from the breakdown of hemoglobin, is constantly produced (Fig. 39-4). Because it is insoluble in water, it is bound to albumin for transport to the liver. This form of bilirubin is referred to as *unconjugated*. In the liver bilirubin is conjugated with glucuronic acid. *Conjugated* bilirubin is soluble and is excreted in bile. Bile also consists of water, cholesterol, bile salts, electrolytes, and phospholipids. Bile salts are needed for fat emulsification and digestion.

Pancreas. The pancreas is a long, slender gland lying behind the stomach and in front of the first and second lumbar vertebrae. It consists of a head, body, and tail. The anterior surface of the pancreas is covered by peritoneum. The pancreas contains lobes and lobules. The pancreatic duct extends along the gland and enters the duodenum through the common bile duct (see Fig. 39-3).

The pancreas has both exocrine and endocrine functions. The exocrine function contributes to digestion through the production and release of enzymes (see Table 39-1). The endocrine function occurs in the islets of Langerhans, whose β cells secrete insulin and amylin; α cells secrete glucagon; δ cells secrete somatostatin; and F cells secrete pancreatic polypeptide.

TABLE 39-4	FUNCTIONS OF THE LIVER
Function	**Description**
Metabolic Functions	
Carbohydrate metabolism	Glycogenesis (conversion of glucose to glycogen), glycogenolysis (process of breaking down glycogen to glucose), gluconeogenesis (formation of glucose from amino acids and fatty acids).
Protein metabolism	Synthesis of nonessential amino acids, synthesis of plasma proteins (except gamma globulin), synthesis of clotting factors, urea formation from ammonia (NH_3) (NH_3 formed from deamination of amino acids by action of bacteria in colon).
Fat metabolism	Synthesis of lipoproteins, breakdown of triglycerides into fatty acids and glycerol, formation of ketone bodies, synthesis of fatty acids from amino acids and glucose, synthesis and breakdown of cholesterol.
Detoxification	Inactivation of drugs and harmful substances and excretion of their breakdown products.
Steroid metabolism	Conjugation and excretion of gonadal and adrenal corticosteroid hormones.
Bile Synthesis	
Bile production	Formation of bile, containing bile salts, bile pigments (mainly bilirubin), and cholesterol.
Bile excretion	Bile excretion by liver about 1 L/day.
Storage	Glucose in form of glycogen. Vitamins, including fat soluble (A, D, E, K) and water soluble (B_1, B_2, cobalamin, folic acid). Fatty acids. Minerals (iron, copper). Amino acids in form of albumin and beta-globulins.
Mononuclear Phagocyte System	
Kupffer cells	Breakdown of old RBCs, WBCs, bacteria, and other particles. Breakdown of hemoglobin from old RBCs to bilirubin and biliverdin.

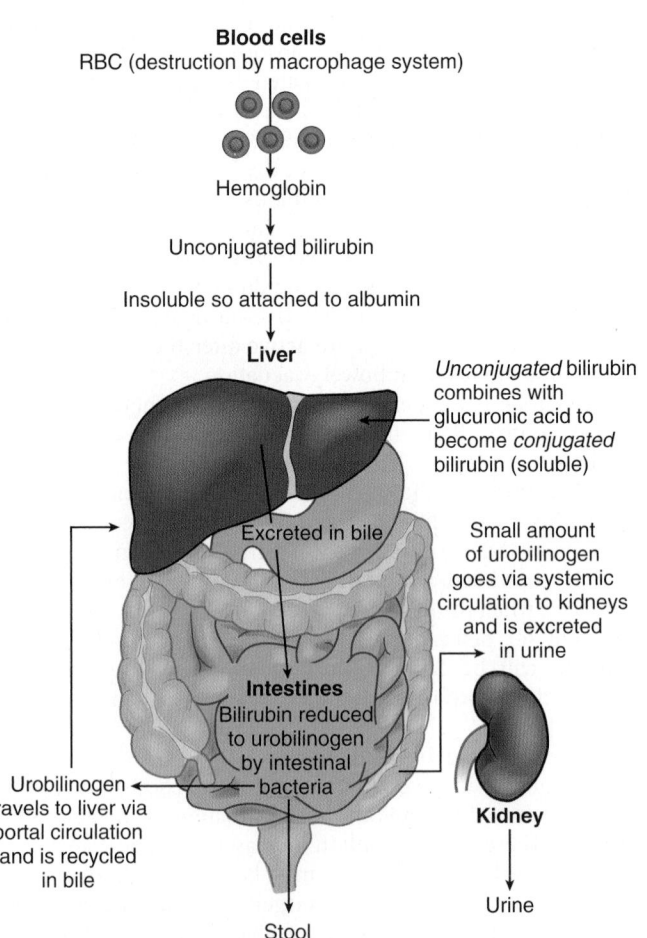

FIG. 39-4 Bilirubin metabolism and conjugation.

GERONTOLOGIC CONSIDERATIONS

EFFECTS OF AGING ON GASTROINTESTINAL SYSTEM

The process of aging changes the functional ability of the GI system (Table 39-5). Diet, alcohol intake, and obesity affect organs of the GI system, making it a challenge to separate the sole effects of aging from lifestyle. *Xerostomia* (decreased saliva production), or dry mouth, affects many older adults and may be associated with difficulty swallowing (dysphagia).[1] Many factors can lead to a decrease in appetite and make eating less

pleasurable. These include a decrease in taste buds and salivary gland secretion, diminished sense of smell, and caries and periodontal disease leading to loss of teeth.

Age-related changes in the esophagus include delayed emptying resulting from smooth muscle weakness and an incompetent LES.[2] Although motility of the GI system decreases with age, secretion and absorption are affected to a lesser extent. The older patient often has a decrease in HCl acid secretion (hypochlorhydria) and a subsequent reduction in the amount of intrinsic factor secreted.

Although constipation is a common complaint of older adults, age-related changes in colonic secretion or motility have not been consistently shown.[3] Factors that may increase the risk for constipation include slower peristalsis, inactivity, decreased dietary fiber, decreased fluid intake, constipating medications, and laxative abuse; neurologic, cognitive, and metabolic disorders may also play a role.[4,5] (Constipation is discussed in Chapter 43.)

The liver size decreases after 50 years of age, but results of liver function tests remain within normal ranges. Age-related enzyme changes in the liver decrease the liver's ability to metabolize drugs and hormones.

The size of the pancreas is unaffected by aging, but it does undergo structural changes such as fibrosis, fatty acid deposits, and atrophy. Both obstructive and nonobstructive gallbladder diseases increase with age.[6]

Older adults, especially those over 85, are at risk for decreased food intake.[7] The economic inability to purchase food supplies affects nutritional intake, especially in the older adult. Economic constraints may also reduce the number of fresh fruits and vegetables consumed and thus the amount of fiber. Immobility limits the ability to obtain and prepare meals. In the United States, approximately one third of people over 60 are obese.[7,8] Age-related changes in the GI system and differences in assessment findings are presented in Table 39-5.

TABLE 39-5   GERONTOLOGIC ASSESSMENT DIFFERENCES

Gastrointestinal System

Expected Aging Changes	Differences in Assessment Findings
Mouth	
Gingival retraction	Loss of teeth, dental implants, dentures, difficulty chewing
Decreased taste buds, decreased sense of smell	Diminished sense of taste (especially salty and sweet)
Decreased volume of saliva	Dry oral mucosa
Atrophy of gingival tissue	Poor-fitting dentures
Esophagus	
Lower esophageal sphincter pressure decreased, motility decreased	Epigastric distress, dysphagia, potential for hiatal hernia and aspiration
Abdominal Wall	
Thinner and less taut	More visible peristalsis, easier palpation of organs
Decreased number and sensitivity of sensory receptors	Less sensitivity to surface pain
Stomach	
Atrophy of gastric mucosa, decreased blood flow	Food intolerances, signs of anemia as result of cobalamin malabsorption, slower gastric emptying
Small Intestines	
Slightly decreased motility and secretion of most digestive enzymes	Complaints of indigestion, slowed intestinal transit, delayed absorption of fat-soluble vitamins
Liver	
Decreased size and lowered position	Easier palpation because of lower border extending past costal margin
Decreased protein synthesis, ability to regenerate decreased	Decreased drug and hormone metabolism
Large Intestine, Anus, Rectum	
Decreased anal sphincter tone and nerve supply to rectal area	Fecal incontinence
Decreased muscular tone, decreased motility	Flatulence, abdominal distention, relaxed perineal musculature
Increased transit time, decreased sensation to defecation	Constipation, fecal impaction
Pancreas	
Pancreatic ducts distended, lipase production decreased, pancreatic reserve impaired	Impaired fat absorption, decreased glucose tolerance

ASSESSMENT OF GASTROINTESTINAL SYSTEM

Subjective Data

Important Health Information

Past Health History. Gather information from the patient about the history or existence of the following problems related to GI functioning: abdominal pain, nausea and vomiting, diarrhea, constipation, abdominal distention, jaundice, anemia, heartburn, dyspepsia, changes in appetite, hematemesis, food intolerance or allergies, indigestion, excessive gas, bloating, lactose intolerance, melena, trouble swallowing, hemorrhoids, or rectal bleeding. In addition, ask the patient about a history or existence of diseases such as reflux, gastritis, hepatitis, colitis, gallstones, peptic ulcer, cancer, diverticuli, or hernias.

Question the patient about weight history. Explore in detail any unexplained or unplanned weight loss or gain within the past 6 to 12 months. Document a history of chronic dieting and repeated weight loss and gain.

Medications. The health history should include an assessment of the patient's past and current use of medications. The names of all drugs, their frequency of use, and their duration of use are important. This is a critical aspect of history taking because many medications may not only have an effect on the GI system but also may be affected by abnormalities of the GI system. The medication assessment should include information about over-the-counter (OTC) medications, prescription

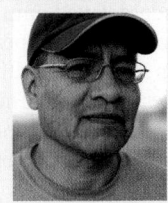
TABLE 39-6   HEPATOTOXIC CHEMICALS AND DRUGS

- acetaminophen (Tylenol)
- amiodarone (Cordarone)
- arsenic
- azathioprine (Imuran)
- carbamazepine (Tegretol)
- chloroform
- fluconazole (Diflucan)
- gold compounds
- halothane
- isoniazid (INH)
- ketoconazole (Nizoral)

- 6-mercaptopurine (6-MP)
- mercury
- methotrexate
- nevirapine (Viramune)
- niacin
- statins (e.g., simvastatin [Zocor])
- sulfonamides
- thiazide diuretics (e.g., hydrochlorothiazide)
- thiazolidinediones (e.g., pioglitazone [Actos])

TABLE 39-7   SURGERIES OF THE GASTROINTESTINAL SYSTEM

Procedure	Description
Appendectomy	Removal of appendix
Cholecystectomy	Removal of gallbladder
Choledochojejunostomy	Opening between common bile duct and jejunum
Choledocholithotomy	Opening into common bile duct for removal of stones
Colectomy	Removal of colon
Colostomy	Opening into colon
Esophagoenterostomy	Removal of portion of esophagus with segment of colon attached to remaining portion
Esophagogastrostomy	Removal of esophagus and anastomosis of remaining portion to stomach
Gastrectomy	Removal of stomach
Gastrostomy	Opening into stomach
Glossectomy	Removal of tongue
Hemiglossectomy	Removal of half of tongue
Herniorrhaphy	Removal of a hernia
Ileostomy	Opening into ileum
Mandibulectomy	Removal of mandible
Pyloroplasty	Enlargement and repair of pyloric sphincter area
Vagotomy	Resection of branch of vagus nerve

drugs, herbal products, vitamins, and nutritional supplements (see the Complementary & Alternative Therapies box in Chapter 3 on p. 39). Note the use of prescription or OTC appetite suppressants.

Many chemicals and drugs are potentially hepatotoxic (Table 39-6) and result in significant patient harm unless monitored closely. For example, chronic high doses of acetaminophen and nonsteroidal antiinflammatory drugs (NSAIDs) may be hepatotoxic. NSAIDs (including aspirin) may also predispose a patient to upper GI bleeding, with an increasing risk as the person ages. Other medications such as antibiotics may change the normal bacterial composition in the GI tract, resulting in diarrhea. Antacids and laxatives may affect the absorption of certain medications. Ask the patient if laxatives or antacids are taken, including the kind and frequency.

Surgery or Other Treatments. Obtain information about hospitalizations for any problems related to the GI system. Also obtain data related to any abdominal or rectal surgery, including the year, reason for surgery, postoperative course, and possible blood transfusions. Terms related to surgery of the GI system are presented in Table 39-7.

Functional Health Patterns. Key questions to ask a patient with a GI problem are presented in Table 39-8.

Health Perception–Health Management Pattern. Ask about the patient's health practices related to the GI system, such as maintenance of normal body weight, proper dental care, adequate nutrition, and effective elimination habits.

Query the patient about recent foreign travel with possible exposure to hepatitis or parasitic infestation. Ask about potential risk behaviors for hepatitis C exposure. Document whether the patient has received hepatitis A and B vaccination.

Assess the patient for habits that directly affect GI functioning. The intake of alcohol in large quantities or for long periods has detrimental effects on the stomach mucosa. Chronic alcohol exposure causes fatty infiltration of the liver and can cause damage, leading to cirrhosis and hepatocellular carcinoma. Obtain a history of cigarette smoking. Nicotine is irritating to the GI tract mucosa. Cigarette smoking is related to GI cancers (especially mouth and esophageal cancers), esophagitis, and ulcers. Smoking delays the healing of ulcers.

🧬 **GENETIC RISK ALERT: Colorectal Cancer**
- Colorectal cancer may run in families if first-degree relatives (parents, siblings) or many other family members (grandparents, aunts, uncles) have had colorectal cancer. This is especially true when family members are diagnosed with colorectal cancer before age 50.
- Some genetic conditions associated with an increased risk of colorectal cancer include:
  - Hereditary nonpolyposis colorectal cancer (HNPCC), which is caused by mutations in several different genes.
  - Familial adenomatous polyposis (FAP), which is characterized by multiple polyps that are noncancerous at first, but eventually develop into cancer if not treated. Most cases of FAP are due to mutations of the adenomatous polyposis coli *(APC)* gene.

🧬 **GENETIC RISK ALERT: Inflammatory Bowel Disease (IBD)**
- People with IBD have a genetic predisposition or susceptibility to the disease.
- First-degree relatives have a 5- to 20-fold increased risk of developing IBD.

Family history is an important component of this health pattern. Because of the relationship between colorectal and breast cancer, inquire about a history of either type of cancer in the family. Women with HNPCC also have an increased risk of endometrial and ovarian cancer.

TABLE 39-8   HEALTH HISTORY

Gastrointestinal System

Health Perception–Health Management
- Describe any measures used to treat GI symptoms such as diarrhea or vomiting.
- Do you smoke?* Do you drink alcohol?*
- Are you exposed to any chemicals on a regular basis?* Have you been exposed in the past?*
- Have you recently traveled outside the United States?*

Nutritional-Metabolic
- Describe your usual daily food and fluid intake.
- Do you take any supplemental vitamins or minerals?*
- Have you experienced any changes in appetite or food tolerance?*
- Has there been a weight change in the past 6-12 mo?*
- Are you allergic to any foods?*

Elimination
- Describe the frequency and time of day you have bowel movements. What is the consistency of the bowel movement?
- Do you use laxatives or enemas?* If so, how often?
- Have there been any recent changes in your bowel pattern?*
- Describe any skin problems caused by GI problems.
- Do you need any assistive equipment, such as ostomy equipment, raised toilet seat, commode?

Activity-Exercise
- Do you have limitations in mobility that make it difficult for you to procure and prepare food?*

Sleep-Rest
- Do you experience any difficulty sleeping because of a GI problem?*
- Are you awakened by symptoms such as gas, abdominal pain, diarrhea, or heartburn?*

Cognitive-Perceptual
- Have you experienced any change in taste or smell that has affected your appetite?*
- Do you have any heat or cold sensitivity that affects eating?*
- Does pain interfere with food preparation, appetite, or chewing?*
- Do pain medications cause constipation, diarrhea, or appetite suppression?*

Self-Perception–Self-Concept
- Describe any changes in your weight that have affected how you feel about yourself.
- Have you had any changes in normal elimination that have affected how you feel about yourself?*
- Have any symptoms of GI disease caused physical changes that are a problem for you?*

Role-Relationship
- Describe the impact of any GI problem on your usual roles and relationships.
- Have any changes in elimination affected your relationships?*
- Do you live alone? Describe how your family or others assist you with your GI problems.

Sexuality-Reproductive
- Describe the effect of your GI problem on your sexual activity.

Coping–Stress Tolerance
- Do you experience GI symptoms in response to stressful or emotional situations?
- Describe how you deal with any GI symptoms that result.

Value-Belief
- Describe any culturally specific health beliefs regarding food and food preparation that may influence the treatment of your GI problem.

*If yes, describe.

Nutritional-Metabolic Pattern. A thorough nutritional assessment is essential. Take a diet history and inquire about both content and amount (portion size). Food preferences and preparation may vary by culture. Open-ended questions allow the patient to express beliefs and feelings about the diet. For example, you can say, "Please tell me about your food and beverage intake over the past 24 hours." A 24-hour dietary recall can be used to analyze the adequacy of the diet. Assist the patient in recalling the preceding day's food intake, including early morning and nighttime intake, snacks, liquids, and vitamin supplements. You can then evaluate the diet in relation to recommended servings. The U.S. Department of Agriculture released MyPlate (www.choosemyplate.gov) recommendations for dietary intake. A 1-week recall may provide additional information on usual dietary patterns. Compare weekday and weekend dietary intake patterns in relation to both the quality and quantity of food.

Ask the patient about the use of sugar and salt substitutes, use of caffeine, and amount of fluid and fiber intake. Note any changes in appetite, food tolerance, and weight. Anorexia and weight loss may indicate cancer or inflammation. Decreased food intake can also be the consequence of economic problems and depression.

Ask about food allergies and what GI symptoms occur with the allergic response. Inquire about dietary intolerances, including lactose and gluten.

Elimination Pattern. Elicit a detailed account of the patient's bowel elimination pattern. Note the frequency, time of day, and usual consistency of stool. Document the use of laxatives and enemas, including type, frequency, and results. Investigate any recent change in bowel patterns.

Document the amount and type of fluid and fiber intake because these influence the frequency and consistency of stools. Inadequate intake of fiber can be associated with constipation. Investigate the possible association between a skin problem and a GI problem. Food allergies can cause skin lesions, pruritus, and edema. Diarrhea can result in redness, irritation, and pain in the perianal area. External drainage systems, such as an ileostomy or ileal conduit, may cause local skin irritation.

Activity-Exercise Pattern. Activity and exercise affect GI motility. Immobility is a risk factor for constipation.

Assess ambulatory status to determine if the patient is capable of securing and preparing food. If the patient is unable to do these tasks, determine if a family member or an outside agency is meeting this need.

Note any limitation in patients' ability to feed themselves. Assess for access to a toilet. Identify the use of and access to supplies such as a commode or ostomy supplies.

Sleep-Rest Pattern. GI symptoms can interfere with the quality of sleep. Nausea, vomiting, diarrhea, indigestion, and bloating can produce sleep problems and should be investigated. Ask the patient if GI symptoms affect sleep or rest. For example, a patient with gastroesophageal reflux disease (GERD) may be awakened because of burning, epigastric pain.

A patient may have a bedtime ritual that involves a particular food or beverage. Herbal teas may be sleep inducing. Document individual routines and comply with these whenever possible to avoid sleeplessness. Hunger can prevent sleep and should be relieved by a light, easily digested snack (unless contraindicated).

Cognitive-Perceptual Pattern. Sensory alterations can result in problems related to the acquisition, preparation, and ingestion of food. Changes in taste or smell can affect appetite and eating pleasure. Vertigo can make shopping and standing at a stove difficult and dangerous. Heat or cold sensitivity can make certain foods painful to eat. Problems in expressive communication limit the patient's ability to state personal dietary preferences. If a patient is diagnosed as having a GI disorder, ask questions to determine his or her understanding of the illness and its treatment.

Both acute and chronic pain influence dietary intake. Behaviors associated with pain include avoidance of activity, fatigue, and disruption of eating patterns. Assess patients receiving opioid medications for constipation, nausea, sedation, and appetite suppression.

Self-Perception–Self-Concept Pattern. Many GI and nutritional problems affect the patient's self-perception. Overweight and underweight persons may have problems related to self-esteem and body image. Repeated attempts to achieve a personally acceptable weight can be discouraging and depressing for some people. The way a person recounts a weight history can alert you to potential problems in this area.

The need for external devices to manage elimination, such as a colostomy or an ileostomy, may be challenging for some patients. The patient's willingness to engage in self-care and to discuss this situation provides you with valuable information related to body image and self-esteem.

The altered physical changes often associated with advanced liver disease can be disturbing for the patient. Jaundice and ascites cause significant changes in external appearance. Assess the patient's attitude toward these changes.

Role-Relationship Pattern. Problems related to the GI system such as cirrhosis, hepatitis, ostomies, obesity, and carcinoma may alter the patient's ability to maintain usual roles and relationships. A chronic illness may necessitate leaving a job or reducing work hours. Changes in body image and self-esteem can affect relationships.

Sexuality-Reproductive Pattern. Changes related to sexuality and reproductive status can result from problems of the GI system. For example, obesity, jaundice, anorexia, and ascites could decrease the acceptance of a potential sexual partner. An ostomy could affect the patient's confidence related to sexual activity. Your sensitive questioning can identify potential problems.

Anorexia can affect the reproductive status of a female patient. Obesity leads to reduced fertility and increased miscarriage rates in women.[9]

Coping–Stress Tolerance Pattern. Determine what is stressful for the patient and what coping mechanisms the patient uses. Factors outside the GI tract can influence its functioning. Both psychologic and emotional factors, such as stress and anxiety, influence GI functioning in many people. Stress may be manifested as anorexia, nausea, epigastric and abdominal pain, or diarrhea. Some diseases of the GI system, such as peptic ulcer disease, IBS, and IBD, may be aggravated by stress. However,

Subjective Data

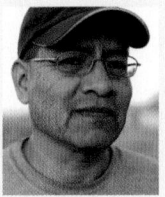
iStockphoto/Thinkstock

A focused subjective assessment of L.C. revealed the following information:
- ***PMH:*** Negative history for medical or surgical problems.
- ***Medications:*** None.
- ***Health Perception–Health Management:*** L.C. states he has not been feeling well for the past several weeks. He feels weak and is easily fatigued. Denies exposure to chemicals. No recent travel outside of the United States. Smokes approximately 1 pack of cigarettes/day for 20 yr. Drinks beer on a daily basis, typically three or four bottles per day.
- ***Nutritional-Metabolic:*** L.C. is 5 ft, 9 in tall and weighs 140 lb (BMI: 20.7 kg/m^2). States has been losing weight over the past several months and does not have an appetite. No food allergies.
- ***Elimination:*** States has had alternating episodes of constipation and diarrhea. He noticed some bright red blood in stools. Has not had a bowel movement for 4 days.
- ***Cognitive-Perceptual:*** Rates pain as a 9 on a scale of 0-10. States pain comes and goes in waves. Prefers to lie still with knees flexed and drawn into his abdomen.

GI symptoms should never be attributed solely to psychologic factors.

Value-Belief Pattern. Assess the patient's spiritual and cultural beliefs regarding food and food preparation. Whenever possible, respect these preferences. Determine if any value or belief could interfere with planned interventions. For example, if the patient with anemia is a vegetarian, the prescription of a high-meat diet would be resisted. Thoughtful assessment and consideration of the patient's beliefs and values usually increase adherence and satisfaction.

Objective Data
Physical Examination
Mouth

Inspection. Inspect the mouth for symmetry, color, and size. Observe for abnormalities such as pallor or cyanosis, cracking, ulcers, or fissures. The dorsum (top) of the tongue should have a thin white coating; the undersurface should be smooth. Observe for any lesions. Using a tongue blade, inspect the buccal mucosa and note the color, any areas of pigmentation, and any lesions. Dark-skinned individuals normally have patchy areas of pigmentation. In assessing the teeth and gums, look for caries; loose teeth; abnormal shape and position of teeth; and swelling, bleeding, discoloration, or inflammation of the gingivae. Note any distinctive breath odor.

Inspect the pharynx by tilting the patient's head back and depressing the tongue with a tongue blade. Observe the tonsils, uvula, soft palate, and anterior and posterior pillars. Instruct the patient to say "ah." The uvula and soft palate should rise and remain in the midline.

Palpation. Palpate any suspicious areas in the mouth. Note ulcers, nodules, indurations, and areas of tenderness. The mouth of the older adult requires careful assessment. Give particular attention to dentures (e.g., fit, condition), ability to swallow, the tongue, and lesions. Ask the patient with dentures to remove them during an oral examination to allow for good visualization and palpation of the area.

Abdomen. Two systems are used to anatomically describe the surface of the abdomen. One system divides the abdomen

TABLE 39-9 STRUCTURES LOCATED IN ABDOMINAL REGIONS

Right Upper Quadrant	Left Upper Quadrant	Right Lower Quadrant	Left Lower Quadrant
• Liver and gallbladder	• Left lobe of liver	• Lower pole of right kidney	• Lower pole of left kidney
• Pylorus	• Spleen	• Cecum and appendix	• Sigmoid flexure
• Duodenum	• Stomach	• Portion of ascending colon	• Portion of descending colon
• Head of pancreas	• Body of pancreas	• Bladder (if distended)	• Bladder (if distended)
• Right adrenal gland	• Left adrenal gland	• Right ovary and salpinx	• Left ovary and salpinx
• Portion of right kidney	• Portion of left kidney	• Uterus (if enlarged)	• Uterus (if enlarged)
• Hepatic flexure of colon	• Splenic flexure of colon	• Right spermatic cord	• Left spermatic cord
• Portion of ascending and transverse colon	• Portion of transverse and descending colon	• Right ureter	• Left ureter

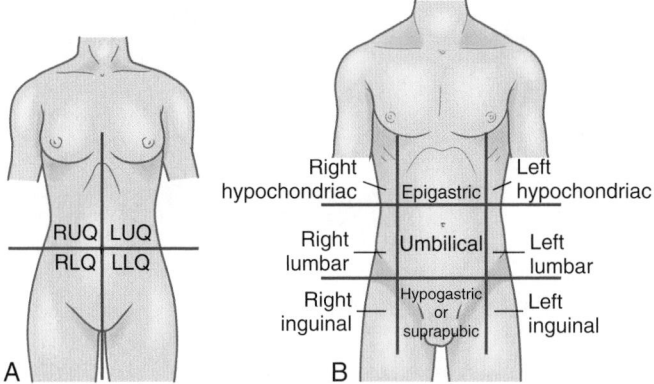

FIG. 39-5 **A,** Abdominal quadrants. **B,** Abdominal regions. *LLQ,* Left lower quadrant; *LUQ,* left upper quadrant; *RLQ,* right lower quadrant; *RUQ,* right upper quadrant.

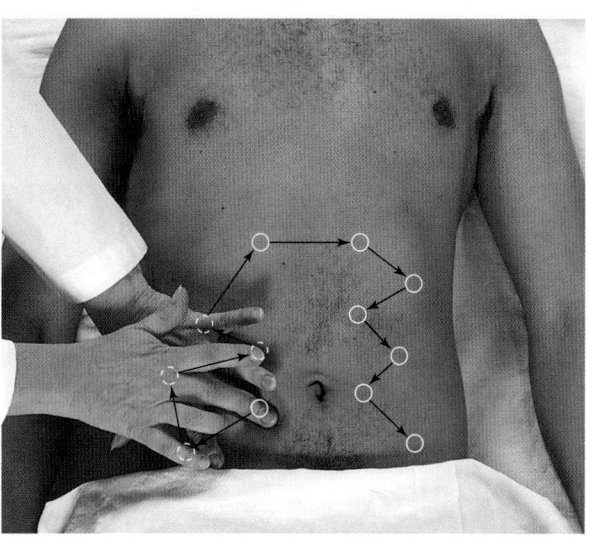

FIG. 39-6 Technique for percussion of the abdomen. Moving clockwise, percuss lightly in all four quadrants. From Jarvis C: *Physical examination and health assessment,* ed 6, St Louis, 2012, Saunders.

into four quadrants by a perpendicular line from the sternum to the pubic bone and a horizontal line across the abdomen at the umbilicus (Fig. 39-5, *A,* and Table 39-9). The other system divides the abdomen into nine regions (Fig. 39-5, *B*), but only the epigastric, umbilical, and suprapubic or hypogastric regions are commonly assessed.

For the abdominal examination, good lighting should shine across the abdomen. The patient should be in the supine position and as relaxed as possible. To help relax the abdominal muscles, have the patient slightly flex the knees and raise the head of the bed slightly. The patient should have an empty bladder. Use warm hands when doing the abdominal examination to avoid eliciting muscle guarding. Ask the patient to breathe slowly through the mouth.

Inspection. Assess the abdomen for skin changes (color, texture, scars, striae, dilated veins, rashes, lesions), umbilicus (location and contour), symmetry, contour (flat, rounded [convex], concave, protuberant, distention), observable masses (hernias or other masses), and movement (pulsations and peristalsis). A normal aortic pulsation may be seen in the epigastric area. Look across the abdomen tangentially (across the abdomen in a line) for peristalsis. Peristalsis is not normally visible in an adult but may be visible in a thin person.

Auscultation. During examination of the abdomen, auscultate before percussion and palpation because these latter procedures may alter the bowel sounds. Use the diaphragm of the stethoscope to auscultate bowel sounds because they are relatively high pitched. Use the bell of the stethoscope to detect lower-pitched sounds. Warm the stethoscope in your hands before auscultating to help prevent abdominal muscle contraction. Listen in the epigastrium and in all four quadrants (start in the lower right quadrant). Listen for bowel sounds for at least

2 minutes. A perfectly "silent abdomen" is uncommon.[10] If you are patient and listen for several minutes, you will frequently find that the sounds are not absent but are hypoactive. If you do not hear bowel sounds, note the amount of time you listened in each quadrant without hearing bowel sounds.

The frequency and intensity of bowel sounds vary depending on the phase of digestion. Normal sounds are relatively high pitched and gurgling. Loud gurgles indicate hyperperistalsis and are termed *borborygmi* (stomach growling). The bowel sounds are more high pitched (rushes and tinkling) when the intestines are under tension, as in intestinal obstruction. Listen for decreased or absent bowel sounds. Terms used to describe bowel sounds include *present, absent, increased, decreased, high pitched, tinkling, gurgling,* and *rushing.*

Also listen for vascular sounds. Normally no aortic bruits should be heard. A *bruit,* best heard with the bell of the stethoscope, is a swishing or buzzing sound and indicates turbulent blood flow.

Percussion. The purpose of percussion of the abdomen is to estimate the size of the liver and determine the presence of fluid, distention, and masses. Sound waves vary according to the density of underlying tissues. Air produces a higher-pitched, hollow sound termed *tympany.* Fluid or masses produce a short, high-pitched sound with little resonance termed *dullness.* Lightly percuss all four quadrants of the abdomen and assess the distribution of tympany and dullness (Fig. 39-6). Tympany is the predominant percussion sound of the abdomen.

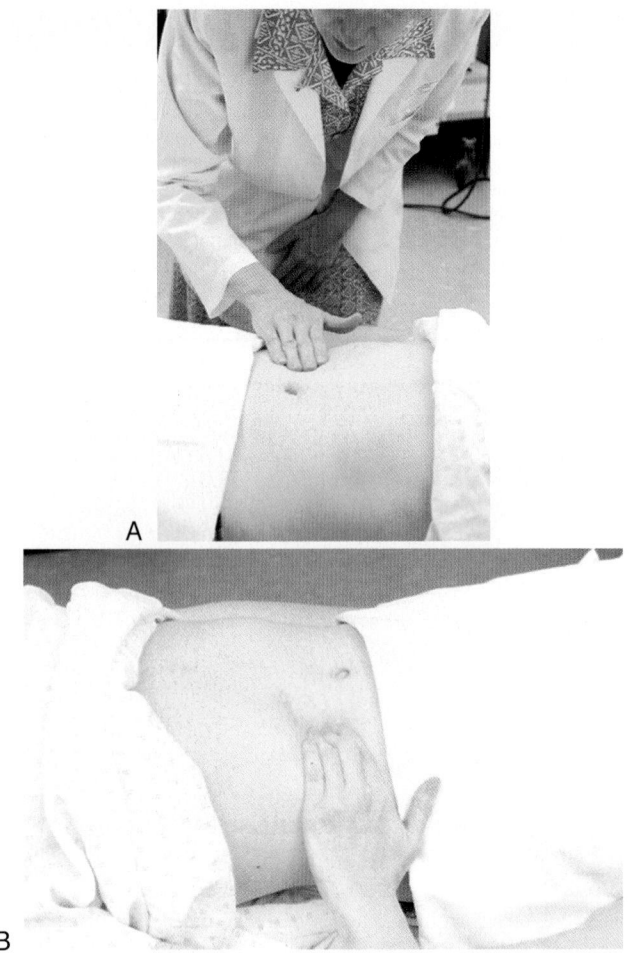

FIG. 39-7 A, Technique for light palpation of the abdomen. **B,** Technique for deep palpation.

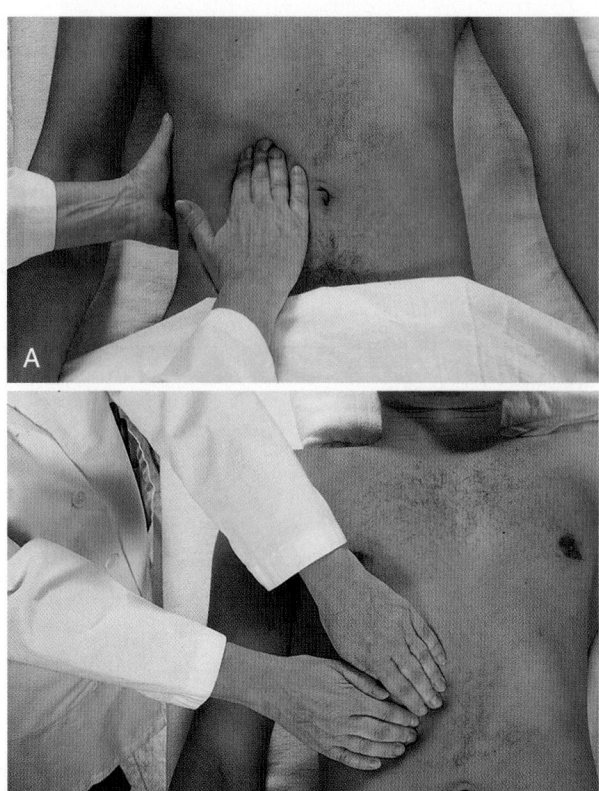

FIG. 39-8 A, Technique for liver palpation. **B,** Alternative technique to palpate liver with fingers hooked over the costal region. From Jarvis C: *Physical examination and health assessment,* ed 6, St Louis, 2012, Saunders.

To percuss the liver, start below the umbilicus in the right midclavicular line and percuss lightly upward until dullness is heard, thus determining the lower border of the liver. Next, start at the nipple line in the right midclavicular line and percuss downward between ribs to the area of dullness indicating the upper border of the liver. Measure the height or vertical space between the two borders to determine the size of the liver. The normal range of liver height in the right midclavicular line is 2.4 to 5 in (6 to 12.7 cm).

Palpation. *Light palpation* is used to detect tenderness or cutaneous hypersensitivity, muscular resistance, masses, and swelling. Help the patient relax for deeper palpation. Keep your fingers together and press gently with the pads of the fingertips, depressing the abdominal wall about 0.4 in (1 cm). Use smooth movements and palpate all quadrants (Fig. 39-7, *A*).

Deep palpation is used to delineate abdominal organs and masses (Fig. 39-7, *B*). Use the palmar surfaces of your fingers to press more deeply. Again, palpate all quadrants and note the location, size, and shape of masses, as well as the presence of tenderness. During these maneuvers, observe the patient's facial expression because it will provide nonverbal cues of discomfort or pain.

An alternative method for deep abdominal palpation is the two-hand method. Place one hand on top of the other and apply pressure to the bottom hand with the fingers of the top hand. With the fingers of the bottom hand, feel for organs and masses.

Practice both methods of palpation to determine which one is most effective.

Check a problem area on the abdomen for rebound tenderness by pressing in slowly and firmly over the painful site. Withdraw the palpating fingers quickly. Pain on withdrawal of the fingers indicates peritoneal inflammation. Because assessing for rebound tenderness may produce pain and severe muscle spasm, it should be done at the end of the examination and only by an experienced practitioner.

To palpate the liver, place your left hand behind the patient to support the right eleventh and twelfth ribs (Fig. 39-8). The patient may relax on your hand. Press the left hand forward and place the right hand on the patient's right abdomen lateral to the rectus muscle. The fingertips should be below the lower border of liver dullness and pointed toward the right costal margin. Gently press in and up. The patient should take a deep breath with the abdomen so that the liver drops and is in a better position to be palpated. Try to feel the liver edge as it comes down to the fingertips. During inspiration the liver edge should feel firm, sharp, and smooth. Describe the surface and contour and any tenderness.

To palpate the spleen, move to the patient's left side. Place your right hand under the patient, and support and press the patient's left lower rib cage forward. Place your left hand below the left costal margin, and press it in toward the spleen. Ask the patient to breathe deeply. The tip or edge of an enlarged spleen will be felt by the fingertips. The spleen is normally not palpable. If it is palpable, do not continue because manual compression of an enlarged spleen may cause it to rupture.

TABLE 39-10 NORMAL PHYSICAL ASSESSMENT OF GASTROINTESTINAL SYSTEM

Mouth
- Moist and pink lips
- Pink and moist buccal mucosa and gingivae without plaques or lesions
- Teeth in good repair
- Protrusion of tongue in midline without deviation or fasciculations
- Pink uvula (in midline), soft palate, tonsils, and posterior pharynx
- Swallows smoothly without coughing or gagging

Abdomen
- Flat without masses or scars; no bruises
- Bowel sounds in all quadrants
- No abdominal tenderness; nonpalpable liver and spleen
- Liver 10 cm in right midclavicular line
- Generalized tympany

Anus
- Absence of lesions, fissures, and hemorrhoids
- Good sphincter tone
- Rectal walls smooth and soft
- No masses
- Stool soft, brown, and heme negative

CASE STUDY—cont'd

Objective Data: Physical Examination

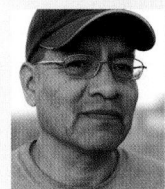

iStockphoto/Thinkstock

A focused assessment of L.C. reveals the following: BP 120/74, heart rate 110, respiratory rate 24, temp 100.4°F (38°C). Abdomen firm and slightly distended. High-pitched bowel sounds in upper quadrants. No bowel sounds auscultated in left lower quadrant. Mild abdominal palpation elicits pain.

As you continue to read this chapter, consider diagnostic studies you would anticipate being performed for L.C.

The standard approach for examining the abdomen can be used on the older adult. Palpation is important because it may reveal a tumor. The abdomen may be thinner and more lax unless the patient is obese. If the patient has chronic obstructive pulmonary disease, large lungs, or a low diaphragm, the liver may be palpated 0.4 to 0.8 in (1 to 2 cm) below the right costal margin.

Rectum and Anus. Inspect perianal and anal areas for color, texture, masses, rashes, scars, erythema, fissures, and external hemorrhoids. Palpate any masses or unusual areas with a gloved hand.

For the digital examination of the rectum, place a gloved, lubricated index finger against the anus while the patient gently bears down (Valsalva maneuver). Then, as the sphincter relaxes, insert the finger. Point the finger toward the umbilicus. Try to get the patient to relax. Insert the finger into the rectum as far as possible, and palpate all surfaces. Assess any nodules, tenderness, or irregularities. A sample of stool can be removed with the gloved finger and checked for occult blood. However, a single guaiac-based fecal occult blood test has limited sensitivity in detecting colorectal cancer.

Findings of a normal physical assessment of the GI system are given in Table 39-10. Gerontologic differences in the GI

FOCUSED ASSESSMENT
Gastrointestinal System

Use this checklist to make sure the key assessment steps have been done.

Subjective
Ask the patient about any of the following and note responses.

Loss of appetite	Y	N
Abdominal pain	Y	N
Changes in stools (e.g., color, blood, consistency, frequency)	Y	N
Nausea, vomiting	Y	N
Painful swallowing	Y	N

Objective: Diagnostic
Check the following laboratory results for critical values.

Endoscopy: colonoscopy, sigmoidoscopy, esophagogastroduodenoscopy	✓
CT scan	✓
Radiologic series: upper GI, lower GI	✓
Stool for occult blood or ova and parasites	✓
Liver function tests	✓

Objective: Physical Examination
Inspect

Skin for color, lesions, scars, petechiae, etc.	✓
Abdominal contour for symmetry and distention	✓
Perianal area for intact skin, hemorrhoids	✓

Auscultate*

Bowel sounds	✓

Palpate

Abdominal quadrants using light touch	✓
Abdominal quadrants using a deep technique	✓

*NOTE: Do auscultation before palpation.

system and differences in assessment findings are described in Table 39-5. Assessment abnormalities are presented in Table 39-11. A *focused assessment* is used to evaluate the status of previously identified GI problems and to monitor for signs of new problems (see Table 3-6). A focused assessment of the GI system is presented above.

DIAGNOSTIC STUDIES OF GASTROINTESTINAL SYSTEM

Table 39-12 presents common diagnostic studies of the GI system. Selected diagnostic studies are described in more detail below.

For most diagnostic studies, make sure a signed consent form for the procedure has been completed and is in the medical record. The health care provider doing the procedure is responsible for explaining the procedure and obtaining written consent. However, you play an important role in teaching patients about the procedures. When preparing the patient, it is important to ask about any known allergies to drugs, iodine, shellfish, or contrast media.

Many GI system diagnostic procedures require measures to cleanse the GI tract and the ingestion or injection of a contrast medium or a radiopaque tracer. Often the patient has a series of GI diagnostic tests done. Monitor the patient closely to ensure adequate hydration and nutrition during the testing period.

TABLE 39-11 **ASSESSMENT ABNORMALITIES**

Gastrointestinal System

Finding	Description	Possible Etiology and Significance
Mouth		
Ulcer, plaque on lips or in mouth	Sore or lesion	Carcinoma, viral infections
Cheilosis	Softening, fissuring, and cracking of lips at angles of mouth	Riboflavin deficiency
Cheilitis	Inflammation of lips (usually lower) with fissuring, scaling, crusting	Often unknown
Geographic tongue	Scattered red, smooth (loss of papillae) areas on dorsum of tongue	Unknown
Smooth tongue	Red, slick appearance	Cobalamin deficiency
Leukoplakia	Thickened white patches	Premalignant lesion
Pyorrhea	Recessed gingivae, purulent pockets	Periodontitis
Herpes simplex	Benign vesicular lesion	Herpesvirus
Candidiasis	White, curdlike lesions surrounded by erythematous mucosa	*Candida albicans*
Glossitis	Reddened, ulcerated, swollen tongue	Exposure to streptococci, irritation, injury, vitamin B deficiencies, anemia
Acute marginal gingivitis	Friable, edematous, painful, bleeding gingivae	Irritation from ill-fitting dentures or orthodontic appliances, calcium deposits on teeth, food impaction
Esophagus and Stomach		
Dysphagia	Difficulty swallowing, sensation of food sticking in esophagus	Esophageal problems, cancer of esophagus
Hematemesis	Vomiting of blood	Esophageal varices, bleeding peptic ulcer
Pyrosis	Heartburn, burning in epigastric or substernal area	Hiatal hernia, esophagitis, incompetent lower esophageal sphincter
Dyspepsia	Burning or indigestion	Peptic ulcer disease, gallbladder disease
Odynophagia	Painful swallowing	Cancer of esophagus, esophagitis
Eructation	Belching	Gallbladder disease
Nausea and vomiting	Feeling of impending vomiting, expulsion of gastric contents through mouth	GI infections, common manifestation of many GI diseases; stress, fear, and pathologic conditions
Abdomen		
Distention	Excessive gas accumulation, enlarged abdomen, generalized tympany	Obstruction, paralytic ileus
Ascites	Accumulated fluid within abdominal cavity, eversion of umbilicus (usually)	Peritoneal inflammation, heart failure, metastatic carcinoma, cirrhosis
Bruit	Humming or swishing sound heard through stethoscope over vessel	Partial arterial obstruction (narrowing of vessel), turbulent flow (aneurysm)
Hyperresonance	Loud, tinkling rushes	Intestinal obstruction
Borborygmi	Waves of loud, gurgling sounds	Hyperactive bowel as result of eating
Absent bowel sounds	No bowel sounds on auscultation	Peritonitis, paralytic ileus, obstruction
Absence of liver dullness	Tympany on percussion	Air from viscus (e.g., perforated ulcer)
Masses	Lump on palpation	Tumors, cysts
Rebound tenderness	Sudden pain when fingers withdrawn quickly	Peritoneal inflammation, appendicitis
Nodular liver	Enlarged, hard liver with irregular edge or surface	Cirrhosis, carcinoma
Hepatomegaly	Enlargement of liver, liver edge >1-2 cm below costal margin	Metastatic carcinoma, hepatitis, venous congestion
Splenomegaly	Enlarged spleen	Chronic leukemia, hemolytic states, portal hypertension, some infections
Hernia	Bulge or nodule in abdomen, usually appearing on straining	Inguinal (in inguinal canal), femoral (in femoral canal), umbilical (herniation of umbilicus), or incisional (defect in muscles after surgery)
Rectum and Anus		
Hemorrhoids	Thrombosed veins in rectum and anus (internal or external)	Portal hypertension, chronic constipation, prolonged sitting or standing, pregnancy
Mass	Firm, nodular edge	Tumor, carcinoma
Pilonidal cyst	Opening of sinus tract, cyst in midline just above coccyx	Probably congenital
Fissure	Ulceration in anal canal	Straining, irritation
Melena	Abnormal, black, tarry stool containing digested blood	Cancer, bleeding in upper GI tract from ulcers, varices
Tenesmus	Painful and ineffective straining at stool. Sense of incomplete evacuation	Inflammatory bowel disease, irritable bowel syndrome, diarrhea secondary to GI infection (e.g., food poisoning)
Steatorrhea	Fatty, frothy, foul-smelling stool	Chronic pancreatitis, biliary obstruction, malabsorption problems

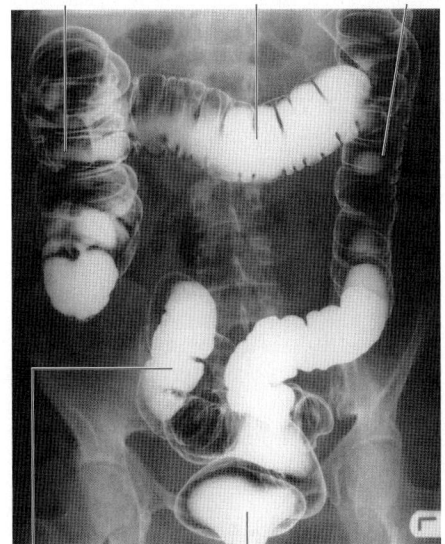

Ascending colon   Transverse colon   Descending colon

Sigmoid colon   Rectum

FIG. 39-9 Barium enema x-ray showing the large intestine.

Some diagnostic studies are especially difficult and uncomfortable for the older adult. Adjustments may be needed during the preparation to avoid dehydration or worsening renal function, and during testing for positioning. Close monitoring is needed to avoid problems such as dehydration from prolonged fluid restriction and diarrhea from bowel-cleansing procedures.

Radiologic Studies

Upper Gastrointestinal Series. An upper GI series with small bowel follow-through provides visualization of the oropharyngeal area, the esophagus, the stomach, and the small intestine via fluoroscopy and x-ray examination. The procedure consists of the patient swallowing contrast medium (a thick barium solution or gastrograffin) and then assuming different positions on the x-ray table. The movement of the contrast medium is observed with fluoroscopy, and several x-rays are taken (see Table 39-12). An upper GI series is used to identify disorders such as esophageal strictures, polyps, tumors, hiatal hernias, foreign bodies, and peptic ulcers.

Lower Gastrointestinal Series. The purpose of a lower GI series (barium enema) examination is to observe by means of fluoroscopy the colon filling with contrast medium and to

TABLE 39-12   DIAGNOSTIC STUDIES

Gastrointestinal System

Study	Description and Purpose	Nursing Responsibility
Radiology		
Upper gastrointestinal (GI) or barium swallow	Fluoroscopic x-ray study using contrast medium. Used to diagnose structural abnormalities of esophagus, stomach, and duodenum.	Explain procedure to patient, including the need to drink contrast medium and assume various positions on x-ray table. Keep patient NPO for 8-12 hr before procedure. Tell patient to avoid smoking after midnight before study. After x-ray, take measures to prevent contrast medium impaction (fluids, laxatives). Tell patient that stool may be white up to 72 hr after test.
Small bowel series	Contrast medium is ingested and films taken every 30 min until medium reaches terminal ileum.	Same as for upper GI.
Lower GI or barium enema	Fluoroscopic x-ray examination of colon using contrast medium, which is administered rectally (enema) (see Fig. 39-9). Double-contrast or air-contrast barium enema is test of choice. Air is infused after thick barium flows through transverse colon. Because of the use of endoscopy, not done as frequently.	*Before procedure:* Administer laxatives and enemas until colon is clear of stool evening before procedure. Administer clear liquid diet evening before procedure. Keep patient NPO for 8 hr before test. Instruct patient about being given barium by enema. Explain that cramping and urge to defecate may occur during procedure and that patient may be placed in various positions on tilt table. *After procedure:* Give fluids, laxatives, or suppositories to assist in expelling barium. Observe stool for passage of contrast medium.
Cholangiography		
• Percutaneous transhepatic (PTC)	After local anesthesia and monitored anesthesia care (formerly called conscious sedation), liver is entered with long needle (under fluoroscopy), bile duct is entered, bile withdrawn, and radiopaque contrast medium injected. Fluoroscopy is used to determine filling of hepatic and biliary ducts. IV antibiotics are given prophylactically.	Observe patient for signs of hemorrhage, bile leakage, and infection. Assess patient's medications for possible contraindications, precautions, or complications with use of contrast medium.
• Surgical cholangiogram	Performed during surgery on biliary structures, such as gallbladder. Contrast medium is injected into common bile duct.	Explain to patient that anesthetic will be used. Assess patient's medications for possible contraindications, precautions, or complications with use of contrast medium.
• Magnetic resonance cholangiopancreatography (MRCP)	Uses MRI technology to obtain images of biliary and pancreatic ducts.	Explain procedure to patient. Contraindicated in patient with metal implants (e.g., pacemaker) or one who is pregnant.

Continued

TABLE 39-12 DIAGNOSTIC STUDIES—cont'd

Gastrointestinal System

Study	Description and Purpose	Nursing Responsibility
Radiology—cont'd		
Ultrasound	Used to show the size and configuration of organ. Noninvasive procedure uses high-frequency sound waves (ultrasound waves), which are passed into body structures and recorded as they are reflected (bounded).	
• Abdominal ultrasound	Detects abdominal masses (tumors, cysts), biliary and liver disease, gallstones. A conductive gel (lubricant jelly) is applied to the skin and a transducer is placed on the area.	Instruct patient to be NPO 8-12 hr before ultrasound. Air or gas can reduce quality of images. Food intake can cause gallbladder contraction, resulting in suboptimal study.
• Endoscopic ultrasound (EUS)	Small ultrasound transducer is installed on tip of endoscope. Because EUS transducer gets close to the organ(s) being examined, images obtained are often more accurate and detailed than images provided by traditional ultrasound. Detects and stages esophageal, gastric, rectal, biliary, and pancreatic tumors and abnormalities. Fine-needle aspiration can be used to diagnose dysplasia or cancer.	Same as esophagogastroduodenoscopy (EGD).
• FibroScan or FibroTest	FibroScan (transient elastography) uses an ultrasound transducer to determine liver stiffness (fibrosis). It is noninvasive and is used in patients with chronic hepatitis C and cirrhosis.	Patient lies in dorsal decubitus position with the right arm in extreme abduction. A probe is positioned in an intercostal space between the ribs.
Nuclear imaging scans (scintigraphy)	Shows size, shape, and position of organ. Functional disorders and structural defects may be identified. Radionuclide (radioactive isotope) is injected IV, and a counter (scanning) device picks up radioactive emission, which is recorded on paper. Only tracer doses of radioactive isotopes are used.	Tell patient that substance to be ingested contains only traces of radioactivity and poses little to no danger. Schedule no more than one radionuclide test on the same day. Explain to patient need to lie flat during scanning.
• Gastric emptying studies	Radionuclide study (scintigraphy) is used to assess ability of stomach to empty solids. Cooked egg containing Tc-99m and toast are eaten with water. Images are obtained at 0, 1, 2, and 4 hr later. Study is used in patients with gastric emptying disorders caused by peptic ulcer, ulcer surgery, diabetes, gastric malignancies, or functional disorders.	Same as above.
• Hepatobiliary scintigraphy (HIDA)	Patient is given IV injection of Tc-99m and positioned under camera to record distribution of tracer in liver, biliary tree, gallbladder, and proximal small intestine. Used to identify obstructions of bile ducts (e.g., gallstones, tumors), diseases of gallbladder, and bile leaks.	Same as above.
• Scintigraphy of GI bleeding	Tc-99m–labeled sulfur colloid or Tc-99m labeling of the patient's own red blood cells (RBCs) to determine the site of active GI blood loss. Sulfur colloid or the patient's RBCs are injected, and images of the abdomen are obtained at intermittent intervals.	Same as above.
Computed tomography (CT)	Noninvasive radiologic examination allows for exposures at different depths. Detects biliary tract, liver, and pancreatic disorders. Use of oral and IV contrast medium accentuates density differences.	Explain procedure to patient. Determine sensitivity to iodine or shellfish if contrast material used.
Magnetic resonance imaging (MRI)	Noninvasive procedure using radiofrequency waves and a magnetic field. Used to detect hepatobiliary disease, hepatic lesions, and sources of GI bleeding and to stage colorectal cancer. IV contrast medium (gadolinium) may be used.	Explain procedure to patient. Contraindicated in patient with metal implants (e.g., pacemaker) or one who is pregnant.
Virtual colonoscopy	Combines CT scanning or MRI with computer virtual reality software to detect intestine and colon diseases, including polyps, colorectal cancer, diverticulosis, and lower GI bleeding. Air is introduced via a tube placed in rectum to enlarge colon to enhance visualization. Images obtained while patient is on back and abdomen. Computer combines images to form 2- and 3-D pictures that are viewed on monitor.	Bowel preparation similar to colonoscopy (see Colonoscopy, below). Unlike conventional colonoscopy, no sedatives are needed and no scope is used. Procedure takes about 15-20 min.

TABLE 39-12   DIAGNOSTIC STUDIES—cont'd

Gastrointestinal System

Study	Description and Purpose	Nursing Responsibility
Endoscopy		
Esophagogastroduodenoscopy (EGD)	Directly visualizes mucosal lining of esophagus, stomach, and duodenum with flexible endoscope. Test may use video imaging to visualize stomach motility. Inflammations, ulcerations, tumors, varices, or Mallory-Weiss tears may be detected. Biopsies may be taken and varices can be treated with band ligation or sclerotherapy.	*Before procedure:* Keep patient NPO for 8 hr. Make sure signed consent is on chart. Give preoperative medication if ordered. Explain to patient that local anesthesia may be sprayed on throat before insertion of scope and that patient will be sedated during the procedure. *After procedure:* Keep patient NPO until gag reflex returns. Gently tickle back of throat to determine reflex. Use warm saline gargles for relief of sore throat. Check temperature q15-30min for 1-2 hr (sudden temperature spike is sign of perforation).
Colonoscopy	Directly visualizes entire colon up to ileocecal valve with flexible fiberoptic scope. Patient's position is changed frequently during procedure to assist with advancement of scope to cecum. Used to diagnose or detect inflammatory bowel disease, polyps, tumors, and diverticulosis and dilate strictures. Procedure allows for biopsy and removal of polyps without laparotomy.	*Before procedure:* Bowel preparation is done. This varies depending on physician. For example, patients may be kept on clear liquids 1-2 days before procedure. Cathartic and/or enema given the night before. An alternative is to give 1 gal of polyethylene glycol (GoLYTELY, Colyte) evening before (8-oz glass q10min) or Prepopik, one packet the night before colonoscopy and a second packet morning of colonoscopy. Explain to patient that flexible scope will be inserted while patient in side-lying position. Explain to patient that sedation will be given. *After procedure:* Patient may experience abdominal cramps caused by stimulation of peristalsis because the bowel is constantly inflated with air during procedure. Observe for rectal bleeding and manifestations of perforation (e.g., malaise, abdominal distention, tenesmus). Check vital signs.
Video capsule endoscopy (VCE)	Patient swallows a capsule with camera (approximately the size of a large vitamin), which provides endoscopic visualization of GI tract (see Fig. 39-11). Most commonly used to visualize small intestine and diagnose diseases such as Crohn's disease, small bowel tumors, small bowel injury due to NSAIDs, celiac disease, and malabsorption syndrome and to identify sources of possible GI bleeding in areas not accessible by upper endoscopy or colonoscopy. Camera takes >50,000 images during 8-hr examination. Capsule relays images to monitoring device that patient wears on belt. After examination, images are downloaded to a workstation. Not used in patients with suspected intestinal strictures.	Instruct patient to fast overnight. Patient may have bowel preparation similar to colonoscopy. The video capsule is swallowed, and clear liquids resumed after 2 hr and food and medications after 4 hr. Procedure is comfortable for most patients. Eight hours after swallowing the capsule, the patient returns to have the monitoring device removed. A patency capsule may be used first in patients determined to be high risk for capsule retention due to strictures. Peristalsis causes passage of the disposable capsule with a bowel movement.
Sigmoidoscopy	Directly visualizes rectum and sigmoid colon with lighted flexible endoscope. Sometimes special table is used to tilt patient into knee-chest position. Used to detect tumors, polyps, inflammatory and infectious diseases, fissures, hemorrhoids.	Administer enemas evening before and morning of procedure. Patient may have clear liquids day before, or no dietary restrictions may be necessary. Explain to patient knee-chest position (unless patient is older or very ill), need to take deep breaths during insertion of scope, and possible urge to defecate as scope is passed. Encourage patient to relax and let abdomen go limp. Observe for rectal bleeding after polypectomy or biopsy.
Endoscopic retrograde cholangiopancreatography (ERCP)	Fiberoptic endoscope (using fluoroscopy) is orally inserted into descending duodenum, then common bile and pancreatic ducts are cannulated. Contrast medium is injected into ducts and allows for direct visualization of structures. Technique can also be used to retrieve a gallstone from distal common bile duct, dilate strictures, biopsy, diagnose pseudocysts.	*Before procedure:* Explain procedure to patient, including patient role. Keep patient NPO 8 hr before procedure. Ensure consent form signed. Administer sedation immediately before and during procedure. Administer antibiotics if ordered. *After procedure:* Check vital signs. Check for signs of perforation or infection. Be aware that pancreatitis is most common complication. Check for return of gag reflex.
Endoscopic ultrasound	Combined use of endoscopy and ultrasound using an ultrasound transducer attached to an endoscope. Enables visualization of esophagus, stomach, intestine, liver, pancreas, and gallstones.	Similar to EGD.

Continued

TABLE 39-12   DIAGNOSTIC STUDIES—cont'd

Gastrointestinal System

Study	Description and Purpose	Nursing Responsibility
Endoscopy—cont'd		
Laparoscopy (peritoneoscopy)	Peritoneal cavity and contents are visualized with laparoscope. Biopsy specimen may also be taken. Done with patient in operating room. Double-puncture peritoneoscopy permits better visualization of abdominal cavity, especially liver. Can eliminate need for exploratory laparotomy in many patients.	Make sure signed consent is on chart. Keep patient NPO 8 hr before study. Administer preoperative sedative medication. Ensure that bladder and bowels are emptied. Observe for possible complications of bleeding and bowel perforation after the procedure.
Blood Studies		
Amylase	Measures secretion of amylase by pancreas. Is important in diagnosing acute pancreatitis. Level of amylase peaks in 24 hr and then drops to normal in 48-72 hr. Depending on method, *reference interval* is 30-122 U/L (0.51-2.07 µkat/L).	Obtain blood sample in acute attack of pancreatitis. Explain procedure to patient.
Lipase	Measures secretion of lipase by pancreas. Level stays elevated longer than serum amylase in acute pancreatitis. *Reference interval:* 31-186 U/L (0.5-3.2 µkat/L).	Explain procedure to patient.
Gastrin	Gastrin is a hormone secreted by cells of the antrum of the stomach, the duodenum, and the pancreatic islets of Langerhans. *Reference interval:* 25-100 pg/mL when fasting.	Explain procedure to patient.
Liver Biopsy	Percutaneous procedure uses needle inserted between 6th and 7th or 8th and 9th intercostal spaces on the right side to obtain specimen of hepatic tissue. Often done using ultrasound or CT guidance.	*Before procedure:* Check patient's coagulation status (prothrombin time, clotting or bleeding time). Ensure that patient's blood is typed and crossmatched. Take vital signs as baseline data. Explain holding of breath after expiration when needle is inserted. Ensure that informed consent has been signed. *After procedure:* Check vital signs to detect internal bleeding q15min × 2, q30min × 4, q1hr × 4. Keep patient lying on right side for minimum of 2 hr to splint puncture site. Keep patient in bed in flat position for 12-14 hr. Assess patient for complications such as bile peritonitis, shock, pneumothorax.
Fecal Tests		
Fecal analysis	Form, consistency, and color are noted. Specimen examined for mucus, blood, pus, parasites, and fat content. Tests for occult blood (guaiac test, Hemoccult, Hemoccult II, Hemoccult-SENSA, Hematest) are done. Single DNA test (PreGen-Plus) is a panel of DNA markers used to detect and monitor colorectal cancer.	Observe patient's stools. Collect stool specimens. Check stools for blood. Keep diet free of red meat for 24-48 hr before occult blood test.
Stool culture	Tests for the presence of bacteria, including *Clostridium difficile.*	Collect stool specimen.

observe by x-ray the filled colon. This procedure identifies polyps, tumors, and other lesions in the colon. It consists of administering an enema of contrast medium to the patient. The air-contrast barium enema provides better visualization (Fig. 39-9). Because it requires the patient to retain the barium, it is not tolerated as well in an older or immobile patient.

Virtual Colonoscopy. *Virtual colonoscopy* combines computed tomography (CT) scanning or magnetic resonance imaging (MRI) with computer software to produce images of the colon and the rectum. The test is less invasive than a conventional colonoscopy but does require radiation and prior cleansing of the colon (the technique is described in Table 39-12).

Virtual colonoscopy enables one to better see inside a colon that is narrowed due to inflammation or a growth.[11] However,

if a polyp is discovered using virtual colonoscopy, a conventional colonoscopy will then be needed to obtain a biopsy or remove it. A disadvantage of virtual colonoscopy is that it may be less sensitive in obtaining information on the details and color of the mucosa. In addition, it is less sensitive in detecting small (less than 10 mm) or flat polyps.

Endoscopy

Endoscopy refers to the direct visualization of a body structure through a lighted fiberoptic instrument. The GI structures that can be examined by endoscopy include the esophagus, the stomach, the duodenum, and the colon. The pancreatic, hepatic, and common bile ducts can be visualized with an endoscope. This procedure is called *endoscopic retrograde cholangiopancreatography* (ERCP).

Ascending colon

Ileum

Ileocecal fold flaps

Cecum Appendix

A

Ileocecal fold

B

FIG. 39-10 A, Illustration showing the ileocecal junction and the ileocecal fold. **B,** Endoscopic image of the ileocecal fold.

CASE STUDY—cont'd

Objective Data: Diagnostic Studies

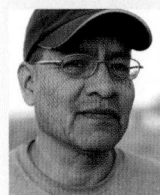

iStockphoto/Thinkstock

The ED physician performs a rectal examination and finds a palpable mass. The following diagnostic tests are ordered:

- CBC
- Electrolytes
- Liver function tests
- Urinalysis
- CT scan of the abdomen
- Colonoscopy

The CBC reveals an Hgb of 6.8 g/dL and an Hct of 20%. The white blood cell count is normal. The electrolytes, liver function tests, and urinalysis are within normal limits. The CT scan reveals pockets of gas and fluid in the ascending colon and two medium-sized tumors in the transverse colon.

This case study is continued in Chapter 43 on p. 1003.

The endoscope is an instrument through which biopsy forceps and cytology brushes may be passed. Cameras are attached, and video and still pictures can be taken (Fig. 39-10). Endoscopy is often done in combination with biopsy and cytologic studies.

The major complication of GI endoscopy is perforation through the structure being scoped. All endoscopic procedures require informed, written consent. Specific endoscopy procedures are discussed in Table 39-12. In addition to diagnostic procedures, many invasive and therapeutic procedures may be done with endoscopes. Examples include polypectomy, sclerosis or banding of varices, laser treatment, cauterization of bleeding sites, papillotomy, common bile duct stone removal, and balloon dilation. Many endoscopic procedures require IV short-acting sedation.

Capsule endoscopy is a noninvasive approach to visualize the GI tract (Fig. 39-11). (See Table 39-12 for further discussion of this diagnostic technique.) Its sensitivity in detecting the source of GI bleeding, small lesions, esophageal varices, colonic polyps, and colorectal cancer is under investigation.[12]

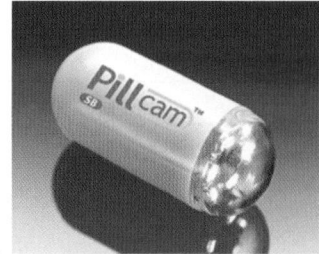

A

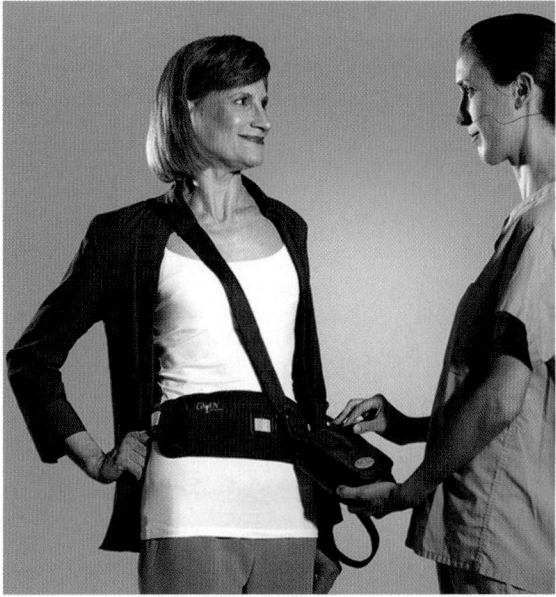

B

FIG. 39-11 Capsule endoscopy. **A,** The video capsule has its own camera and light source. After it is swallowed, it travels through the GI tract and allows visualization of the small intestine. It sends messages to a monitoring device that is worn on a waist belt **(B).** During the 8-hour examination, the patient is free to move about. After the test, the images are viewed on a video monitor.

Liver Biopsy

The purpose of a liver biopsy is to obtain hepatic tissue that can be used in establishing a diagnosis or assessing fibrosis. It may also be useful for following the progress of liver disease, such as chronic hepatitis.

The two types of liver biopsy are open and closed. The *open method* involves making an incision and removing a wedge of tissue. It is done in the operating room with the patient under general anesthesia, often concurrently with another surgical procedure. The *closed,* or *needle, biopsy* is a percutaneous procedure in which the site is infiltrated with a local anesthetic and a needle is inserted between the sixth and seventh or eighth and ninth intercostal spaces on the right side. The patient lies supine with the right arm over the head. Instruct the patient to expire fully and to not breathe while the needle is inserted (see Table 39-12).

Liver Function Studies

Liver function tests (LFTs) are laboratory (blood) studies that reflect hepatic disease. Table 39-13 describes some common LFTs.

TABLE 39-13   DIAGNOSTIC STUDIES

Liver Function Tests

Test	Description and Purpose
Bile Formation and Excretion	
Serum bilirubin	Measurement of liver's ability to conjugate and excrete bilirubin, allowing differentiation between unconjugated (indirect) and conjugated (direct) bilirubin in plasma.
• Total	Measurement of direct and indirect total bilirubin. *Reference interval:* 0.2-1.2 mg/dL (3-21 µmol/L)
• Direct	Measurement of conjugated bilirubin. Elevated in obstructive jaundice. *Reference interval:* 0.1-0.3 mg/dL (1.7-5.1 µmol/L)
• Indirect	Measurement of unconjugated bilirubin. Elevated in hepatocellular and hemolytic conditions. *Reference interval:* 0.1-1.0 mg/dL (1.7-17 µmol/L)
Urinary bilirubin	Measurement of urinary excretion of conjugated bilirubin. *Reference interval:* 0 or negative
Protein Metabolism	
Protein (serum)	Measurement of serum proteins manufactured by the liver. • Albumin, *reference interval:* 3.5-5.0 g/dL (35-50 g/L) • Globulin, *reference interval:* 2.0-3.5 g/dL (20-35 g/L) • Total protein, *reference interval:* 6.4-8.3 g/dL (64-83 g/L) • A/G ratio, *reference interval:* 1.5:1-2.5:1
α-Fetoprotein	Indication of hepatocellular cancer. *Reference interval:* <10 ng/mL (<10 mcg/L)
Ammonia	Conversion of ammonia to urea normally occurs in the liver. Increase can result in hepatic encephalopathy secondary to liver cirrhosis. *Reference interval:* 15-45 mcg N/dL (11-32 µmol N/L)

Test	Description and Purpose
Hemostatic Function	
Prothrombin time (PT)	Determination of prothrombin activity. *Reference interval:* 11-16 sec
International normalized ratio (INR)	Standardized system of reporting PT based on a reference calibration model and calculated by comparing the patient's PT with a control value. *Reference interval:* In general, 2-3 is the desired therapeutic level with warfarin (Coumadin), depending on laboratory
Vitamin K	Essential cofactor for many clotting factors. *Reference interval:* 0.1-2.2 ng/mL (0.22-4.88 nmol/L)
Serum Enzymes	
Alkaline phosphatase (ALP)	Originates from bone and liver. Serum levels rise when excretion is impaired as a result of obstruction in the biliary tract. *Reference interval:* 38-126 U/L (0.65-2.14 µkat/L), depending on method and age
Aspartate aminotransferase (AST)	Elevated in liver damage and inflammation. *Reference interval:* 10-30 U/L (0.17-0.51 µkat/L)
Alanine aminotransferase (ALT)	Elevated in liver damage and inflammation. *Reference interval:* 10-40 U/L (0.17-0.68 µkat/L)
γ-Glutamyl transpeptidase (GGT)	Present in biliary tract (not in skeletal or cardiac muscle). Increase in hepatitis and alcoholic liver disease. More sensitive for liver dysfunction than ALP. *Reference interval:* 0-30 U/L (0-0.5 µkat/L)
Lipid Metabolism	
Cholesterol (serum)	Synthesis and excretion by liver. Increase in biliary obstruction. Decrease in cirrhosis and malnutrition. *Reference interval:* <200 mg/dL (<5.2 mmol/L), varying with age

A/G, Albumin/globulin.

BRIDGE TO NCLEX EXAMINATION

The number of the question corresponds to the same-numbered outcome at the beginning of the chapter.

1. A patient is admitted to the hospital with a diagnosis of diarrhea with dehydration. The nurse recognizes that increased peristalsis resulting in diarrhea can be related to
   a. sympathetic inhibition.
   b. mixing and propulsion.
   c. sympathetic stimulation.
   d. parasympathetic stimulation.
2. A patient has an elevated blood level of indirect (unconjugated) bilirubin. One cause of this finding is that
   a. the gallbladder is unable to contract to release stored bile.
   b. bilirubin is not being conjugated and excreted into the bile by the liver.
   c. the Kupffer cells in the liver are unable to remove bilirubin from the blood.
   d. there is an obstruction in the biliary tract preventing flow of bile into the small intestine.

3. As gastric contents move into the small intestine, the bowel is normally protected from the acidity of gastric contents by the
   a. inhibition of secretin release.
   b. release of bicarbonate by the pancreas.
   c. release of pancreatic digestive enzymes.
   d. release of gastrin by the duodenal mucosa.
4. A patient is jaundiced and her stools are clay colored (gray). This is most likely related to
   a. decreased bile flow into the intestine.
   b. increased production of urobilinogen.
   c. increased production of cholecystokinin.
   d. increased bile and bilirubin in the blood.
5. An 80-year-old man states that, although he adds a lot of salt to his food, it still does not have much taste. The nurse's response is based on the knowledge that the older adult
   a. should not experience changes in taste.
   b. has a loss of taste buds, especially for sweet and salt.
   c. has some loss of taste but no difficulty chewing food.
   d. loses the sense of taste because the ability to smell is decreased.

6. When the nurse is assessing the health perception–health mainte-nance pattern as related to GI function, an appropriate question to ask is
   a. "What is your usual bowel elimination pattern?"
   b. "What percentage of your income is spent on food?"
   c. "Have you traveled to a foreign country in the last year?"
   d. "Do you have diarrhea when you are under a lot of stress?"

7. During an examination of the abdomen the nurse should
   a. position the patient in the supine position with the bed flat and knees straight.
   b. listen in the epigastrium and all four quadrants for 2 minutes for bowel sounds.
   c. use the following order of techniques: inspection, palpation, percussion, auscultation.
   d. describe bowel sounds as absent if no sound is heard in the lower right quadrant after 2 minutes.

8. A normal physical assessment finding of the GI system is/are (select all that apply)
   a. nonpalpable liver and spleen.
   b. borborygmi in upper right quadrant.
   c. tympany on percussion of the abdomen.
   d. liver edge 2 to 4 cm below the costal margin.
   e. finding of a firm, nodular edge on the rectal examination.

9. In preparing a patient for a colonoscopy, the nurse explains that
   a. a signed permit is not necessary.
   b. sedation may be used during the procedure.
   c. only one cleansing enema is necessary for preparation.
   d. a light meal should be eaten the day before the procedure.

1. d, 2. b, 3. b, 4. a, 5. b, 6. c, 7. b, 8. a, c, 9. b

ⓔvolve

For rationales to these answers and even more NCLEX review questions, visit *http://evolve.elsevier.com/Lewis/medsurg*.

REFERENCES

1. de Mata C, McKenna G, Burke FM: Caries and the older patients, *Dent Update* 38:376, 2011.
2. Gutschow CA, Leers JM, Schroder W, et al: Effect of aging on esophageal motility in patients with and without GERD, *Ger Med Sci* 9:Doc22. doi:10.3205/000145.
3. Rao SS, Go JT: Update on the management of constipation in the elderly: new treatment options, *Clin Interv Aging* 9:163, 2010.
4. Franklin LE, Spain MP, Edlund BJ: Pharmacological management of chronic constipation in older adults, *J Gerontol Nurs* 14:1, 2012.
5. Gallegos-Orozco JR, Foxx-Orenstein AE, Sterler SM, et al: Chronic constipation in the elderly, *Am J Gastroenterol* 107:18, 2012.
6. Holm AN, Gerke H: What should be done with a dilated bile duct? *Curr Gastroenterol Rep* 12:150, 2010.
7. Villareal DT, Chode S, Parimi N, et al: Weight loss, exercise or both and physical function in obese older adults, *N Engl J Med* 364:1218, 2011.
8. Zuchelli T, Myers SE: Gastrointestinal issues in the older female patient, *Gastroenterol Clin North Am* 40:449, 2011.
9. Boots C, Stephenson MD: Does obesity increase the risk of miscarriage in spontaneous conception: a systematic review, *Semin Reprod Med* 29:507, 2011.
10. Jarvis C: *Physical examination and health assessment*, ed 6, St Louis, 2012, Saunders.
11. National Digestive Diseases Information Clearinghouse: Virtual colonoscopy. Retrieved from *http://digestive.niddk.nih.gov/ddiseases/pubs/virtualcolonoscopy/index.aspx#what*.
12. Sieg A: Capsule endoscopy compared with conventional colonoscopy for detection of colorectal neoplasms, *World J Gastrointest Endosc* 3:81, 2011.

RESOURCES

Resources for this chapter are listed in Chapter 40 on p. 905, Chapter 42 on p. 960, Chapter 43 on p. 1004, and Chapter 44 on p. 1043.

40

To eat is a necessity,
but to eat intelligently is an art.
La Rochefoucauld

Nursing Management
Nutritional Problems

Rose DiMaria-Ghalili

LEARNING OUTCOMES

1. Relate the essential components of a well-balanced diet to their impact on health outcomes.
2. Describe the common etiologic factors, clinical manifestations, and management of malnutrition.
3. Describe the components of a nutritional assessment.
4. Explain the indications, complications, and nursing management principles related to the use of enteral nutrition.
5. Explain the indications, complications, and nursing management related to the use of parenteral nutrition.
6. Compare the etiologic factors, clinical manifestations, and nursing management of eating disorders.

KEY TERMS

anorexia nervosa, p. 903
bulimia nervosa, p. 903
enteral nutrition (EN), p. 897

malabsorption syndrome, p. 891
malnutrition, p. 890

parenteral nutrition (PN), p. 901
tube feeding, p. 897

This chapter focuses on problems related to nutrition. A review of normal nutrition provides a basis for evaluating nutritional status. Malnutrition and types of supplemental nutrition, including enteral and parenteral nutrition, are discussed. Obesity is discussed in Chapter 41.

NUTRITIONAL PROBLEMS

Nutrition is the sum of processes by which one takes in and utilizes nutrients.[1] Nutritional status can be viewed as a continuum from undernutrition to normal nutrition to overnutri-

tion. An alteration in the process of nutrient intake or utilization can potentially cause nutritional problems. Nutritional problems occur in all age-groups, cultures, ethnic groups, and socioeconomic classes and across all educational levels.

The nutritional status of a person or a family is influenced by many factors. Attitudes toward the importance of food and eating habits are established early. Cultural or religious preferences and requirements are frequently reflected in dietary intake. The financial status of a family or an individual may influence the type and amount of nutritionally sound food that can be purchased.[2]

Reviewed by Katie Clark, RD, MPH CDE, Assistant Clinical Professor, Nutrition, University of California San Francisco, School of Nursing, San Diego, California; Shellie Simons, RN, PhD, Assistant Professor, University of Massachusetts Lowell, Lowell, Massachusetts; and Patricia Worthington, RN, MSN, CNSC, Nutritional Support Clinical Specialist, Thomas Jefferson University Hospital, Philadelphia, Pennsylvania.

NORMAL NUTRITION

Nutrition is important for energy, growth, and maintenance and repair of body tissues. Optimal nutrition (in the absence of any underlying disease process) results from the ingestion of a balanced diet. The major components of the basic food groups are carbohydrates, fats, proteins, vitamins, minerals, and water. Optimal nutrition and daily physical activity are essential for a healthy lifestyle.

The MyPlate approach to nutritional education *(www.choosemyplate.gov)* provides a visual guideline for sensible meal planning to help Americans eat healthfully and make good food choices. MyPlate focuses on the proportions of five food groups (grains, protein, fruits, vegetables, and dairy) that you should eat at each meal (Fig. 40-1, Table 40-1). eTables 40-1 and 40-2 (available on the website for this chapter) show the recommended daily amount of food from each food group and sample meal plans.

MyPlate materials have been developed for older adults and are available at *www.nutrition.tufts.edu/research/myplate-older-adults.* Tips on how to be physically active are available at *www.choosemyplate.gov/physical-activity.html.*

A growing number of electronic and print sources are available for determining nutritional information in commonly consumed foods. Nutrition Facts labels are listed on food products (Fig. 40-2). Calories, nutrients, and ingredients of food consumed can be easily tracked for healthy weight management. Consumer and health professional educational materials on the Nutrition Facts labels are available on the U.S. Food and Drug Administration (FDA) website.[3]

A person's daily caloric requirements are influenced by body type, age, gender, medications, physical activity, and the presence or absence of disease. Adjustments in caloric intake are necessary depending on changes in health status and daily activity level. The Mifflin–St. Jeor equation is recommended to estimate daily adult energy (calorie) requirements based on resting metabolic rate for individuals[4,5] (Table 40-2).

A more convenient way to estimate daily calories is based on kilocalories per kilogram (kcal/kg). (Kilocalorie [kcal] is the correct unit to designate caloric intake and expenditure. However, calorie is more commonly used.) An average adult requires an estimated 20 to 35 cal/kg of body weight per day, using an appropriate reference weight.[6] During illness, energy

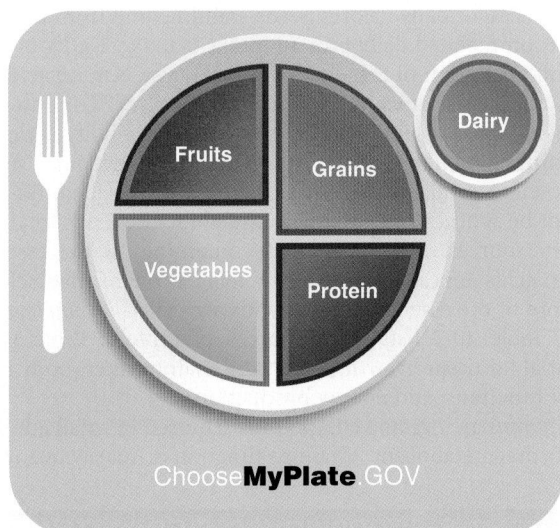

FIG. 40-1 MyPlate is the primary food group symbol that serves as a reminder to make healthy food choices and to build a healthy plate at mealtimes. It is a visual cue that identifies the five basic food groups from which to select healthy foods. The plate is divided into four slightly different-sized quadrants, with fruits and vegetables taking up half the space and grains and protein making up the other half. The vegetables and grains portions are the largest of the four. Next to the plate is a blue circle for dairy, which could be a glass of milk or a food such as cheese or yogurt. For more information, see *www.choosemyplate.gov.*

TABLE 40-1	**NUTRITIONAL THERAPY**

MyPlate Tips for a Healthy Lifestyle

Making food choices for a healthy lifestyle can be as simple as using these 10 tips. Use the ideas in this list to (1) balance your calories, (2) choose foods to eat more often, and (3) cut back on foods to eat less often.

1.	Balance calories	Find out how many calories you need for a day as a first step in managing your weight. Go to *www.choosemyplate.gov* to find your calorie level. Being physically active also helps you balance calories.
2.	Enjoy your food, but eat less	Take the time to fully enjoy your food as you eat it. Eating too fast or when your attention is elsewhere may lead to eating too many calories. Pay attention to hunger and fullness cues before, during, and after meals. Use them to recognize when to eat and when you have had enough.
3.	Avoid oversized portions	Use a smaller plate, bowl, and glass. Portion out foods before you eat. When eating out, choose a smaller size option, share a dish, or take home part of your meal.
4.	Foods to eat more often	Eat more vegetables, fruits, whole grains, and fat-free or 1% milk and dairy products. These foods have the nutrients you need for health, including potassium, calcium, vitamin D, and fiber. Make them the basis for meals and snacks.
5.	Make half your plate fruits and vegetables	Choose red, orange, and dark-green vegetables like tomatoes, sweet potatoes, and broccoli, along with other vegetables, for your meals. Add fruit to meals as part of main or side dishes or as dessert.
6.	Switch to fat-free or low-fat (1%) milk	They have the same amount of calcium and other essential nutrients as whole milk, but fewer calories and less saturated fat.
7.	Make half your grains whole grains	To eat more whole grains, substitute a whole-grain product for a refined product. For example, eat whole-wheat bread instead of white bread, or brown rice instead of white rice.
8.	Foods to eat less often	Cut back on foods high in solid fats, added sugars, and salt. They include cakes, cookies, ice cream, candies, sweetened drinks, pizza, and fatty meats like ribs, sausages, bacon, and hot dogs. Use these foods as occasional treats, not everyday foods.
9.	Compare sodium in foods	Use the Nutrition Facts label (see Fig. 40-2) to choose lower sodium versions of foods like soup, bread, and frozen meals. Select foods labeled "low sodium," "reduced sodium," or "no salt added."
10.	Drink water instead of sugary drinks	Cut calories by drinking water or unsweetened beverages. Soda, energy drinks, and sports drinks are a major source of added sugar and calories in American diets.

Source: US Department of Agriculture Center for Nutrition Policy and Promotion: Nutrition education series, DG Tips Sheet No 1, June 2011. Retrieved from *www.choosemyplate.gov* and *www.health.gov/dietaryguidelines.*

needs may be greater. Rule-of-thumb estimations are that an individual should consume 20 to 25 cal/kg body weight to lose weight, 25 to 30 cal/kg to maintain body weight, and 30 to 35 cal/kg to gain weight.

Carbohydrates, the body's primary source of energy, yield approximately 4 cal/g. Carbohydrates can be classified as either simple or complex. Simple carbohydrates come in two forms: monosaccharides (e.g., glucose, fructose), which are found in fruits and honey; and disaccharides (e.g., sucrose, maltose, lactose), which are found in foods such as table sugar, malted cereal, and milk, respectively. Complex carbohydrates or polysaccharides include starches, such as cereal grains, potatoes, and legumes.

Carbohydrates are the chief protein-sparing ingredient in a nutritionally sound diet. The Dietary Reference Intake (DRI) recommendations are that 45% to 65% of total calories should come from carbohydrates.[6] Furthermore, individuals should take approximately 14 g of dietary fiber per 1000 calories eaten per day from fruits, vegetables, and whole grains, equating to roughly 28 or 30 g for a typical 2000-calorie diet. Individuals should choose food and beverages with little added sugar or caloric sweeteners.

Fats are a major source of energy for the body. One gram of fat yields 9 calories. Fats are stored in adipose tissue and in the abdominal cavity. Fats also act as carriers of essential fatty acids and fat-soluble vitamins. Fats provide a feeling of satiety after eating. Individuals should limit their fat intake to 20% to 35% of total calories.[7]

Fats in the diet can be divided into (1) potentially harmful (saturated fat and *trans* fat) and (2) healthier dietary fat (monounsaturated and polyunsaturated fat) (see Fig. 34-3). One type of polyunsaturated fat, omega-3 fatty acids, may be especially beneficial to your heart. Omega-3 fatty acids, found in some types of fatty fish, appear to decrease the risk of coronary artery disease.[8]

Diets high in excess calories, usually in the form of fats, contribute to the development of obesity. Individuals should consume less than 10% of calories from saturated fatty acids (approximately 20 g of saturated fat per day in a 2000-calorie diet), limit intake of fat and oils high in *trans*-fatty acids, and limit intake of dietary cholesterol to 300 mg/day.

Proteins, another essential component of a well-balanced diet, are obtained from both animal and plant sources. Ideally, 10% to 35% of daily caloric needs should come from protein.[7] The recommended daily protein intake is 0.8 to 1 g/kg of body weight. One gram of protein yields 4 calories. Amino acids are the fundamental units of protein structure. The 22 amino acids are classified as essential and nonessential. The body is capable of synthesizing nonessential amino acids if an adequate supply of protein is available. However, the nine essential amino acids cannot be synthesized, and their availability depends totally on dietary sources. Protein sources containing all the essential amino acids are called *complete proteins*. Proteins that lack one or more of the essential amino acids are called *incomplete proteins*. Table 40-3 lists good sources of protein. Proteins are essential for tissue growth, repair, and maintenance; body regulatory functions; and energy production.

Vitamins are organic compounds required in small amounts for normal metabolism. Vitamins function primarily in enzyme

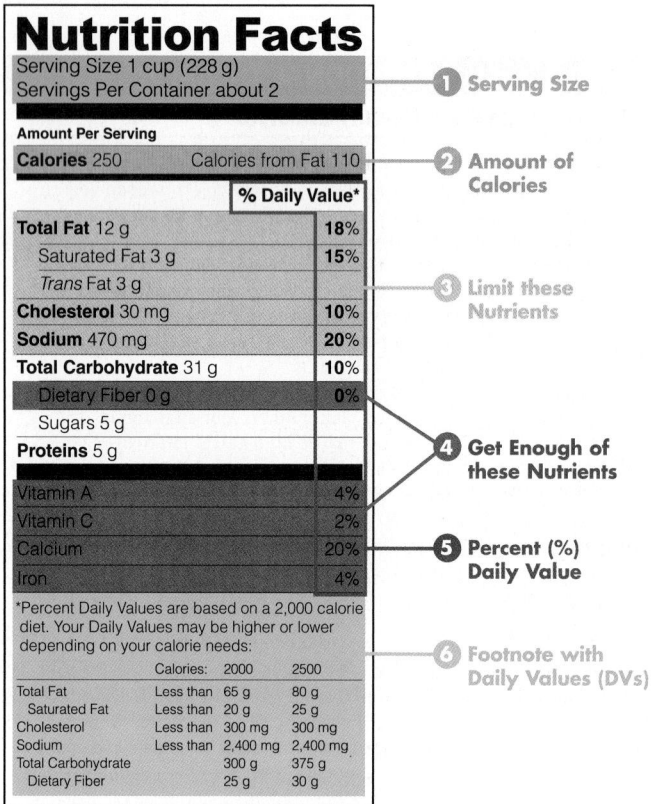

FIG. 40-2 Sample of a Nutrition Facts label.

TABLE 40-2   ESTIMATING DAILY ENERGY (CALORIE) REQUIREMENTS

Mifflin–St. Jeor Equation
Men: Energy expenditure = 5 + 10 (wt in kg) + 6.25 (ht in cm) − 5 (age)
Women: Energy expenditure = −161 + 10 (wt in kg) + 6.25 (ht in cm) − 5 (age)
To determine total daily calorie needs, the energy expenditure has to be multiplied by the appropriate activity factor, as follows:

  1.200 = sedentary (little or no exercise)
  1.375 = lightly active (light exercise/sports 1-3 days/wk)
  1.550 = moderately active (moderate exercise/sports 3-5 days/wk)
  1.725 = very active (hard exercise/sports 6-7 days a wk)
  1.900 = extra active (very hard exercise/sports and physical job)

Example
Man: Weight 180 lb, height 5 ft, 10 in, age 50, very active
Energy expenditure = 5 + 10 (82) + 6.25 (178) − 5 (50) × 1.725 = 2911
Woman: Weight 150 lb, height 5 ft,' 6 in", age 60, lightly active
Energy expenditure = −161 + 10 (68) + 6.25 (168) − 5 (60) × 1.375 = 1745

Ht, Height; *wt,* weight.

TABLE 40-3   GOOD SOURCES OF PROTEIN

Complete Proteins	Incomplete Proteins
• Milk and milk products (e.g., cheese)	• Grains (e.g., corn)
• Eggs	• Legumes (e.g., navy beans, soybeans, peas)
• Fish	• Nuts (e.g., peanuts)
• Meats	• Seeds (e.g., sesame seeds, sunflower seeds)
• Poultry	

TABLE 40-4 MAJOR MINERALS AND TRACE ELEMENTS

Major Minerals	Trace Elements
• Calcium	• Chromium
• Chloride	• Copper
• Magnesium	• Fluoride
• Phosphorus	• Iodine
• Potassium	• Iron
• Sodium	• Manganese
• Sulfur	• Molybdenum
	• Selenium
	• Zinc

TABLE 40-5 NUTRITIONAL THERAPY
Foods High in Iron*

Food	Selected Serving Size
Breads, Cereals, and Grain Products	
Farina, regular or quick cooked (enriched)	⅔ cup
Oatmeal, instant, fortified, prepared (enriched)	⅔ cup
Ready-to-eat cereals, fortified (enriched)	1 oz
Meat, Poultry, Fish, and Alternatives	
Beef liver, braised	3 oz
Pork liver, braised	3 oz
Chicken or turkey liver, braised	½ cup diced
Clams: steamed, boiled, or canned (drained)	3 oz
Oysters: baked, broiled, steamed, or canned (undrained)	3 oz
Soybeans, cooked	½ cup

*These foods provide 25%-39% of the Dietary Reference Intake (DRI) of iron.

reactions that facilitate the metabolism of amino acids, fats, and carbohydrates. Vitamins are divided into two categories: *water-soluble* vitamins (vitamin C and the B-complex vitamins) and *fat-soluble* vitamins (vitamins A, D, E, and K). Because the body stores excess fat-soluble vitamins, there is the potential for toxicity when too much is consumed. Upper limits have been established for vitamins A, D, and E.

Mineral salts (e.g., magnesium, iron, calcium) make up approximately 4% of the total body weight. Minerals present in minute amounts are referred to as *trace elements*. Minerals required in amounts greater than 100 mg/day are called *major minerals*. Table 40-4 lists the major minerals and trace elements. Minerals are necessary for the body to build and repair tissues, regulate body fluids, and assist in various functions. Some minerals are stored and can be toxic if taken in excess amounts. The amount of minerals needed in the daily diet varies greatly, from a few micrograms of trace minerals to 1 g or more of the major minerals, such as calcium, phosphorus, and sodium. A well-balanced diet can usually meet the daily requirements of minerals. However, deficiency and excess states can occur.

SPECIAL DIET: VEGETARIAN DIET

The common element among all vegetarians is the exclusion of red meat from the diet. There are many types of vegetarians and no strict definition of the word "vegetarian." Many vegetarians are *vegans,* who are pure or total vegetarians and eat only plants, and *lacto-ovo-vegetarians,* who eat plants and sometimes dairy products and eggs.

Vegetarians can have vitamin or protein deficiencies unless their diets are well planned. Plant protein, although of a lesser quality than that of animal origin, fulfills most of the protein requirements. Combinations of vegetable protein foods (e.g., cornmeal, kidney beans) can increase the nutritional value. Milk made from soybeans or almonds is also an excellent protein source and should be calcium fortified. Other deficiencies that may be present in a vegan diet include calcium, zinc, and vitamins A and D.

The primary deficiency for a strict vegan is lack of cobalamin. This vitamin can be obtained only from animal protein, special supplements, or foods that have been fortified with the vitamin. Vegans not using cobalamin supplements are susceptible to the development of megaloblastic anemia and the neurologic signs of cobalamin deficiency.

Strict vegetarians and lacto-ovo-vegetarians are also at risk for iron deficiency. Table 40-5 lists examples of foods high in iron.

CULTURALLY COMPETENT CARE

NUTRITION

People have unique cultural heritages that may affect eating customs and nutritional status. Each culture has its own beliefs and behaviors related to food and the role that food plays in the etiology and treatment of disease. In addition, culture and religion can influence what food is considered edible, how it is prepared, when it is eaten, and how and who prepares it. For example, some religions, such as Judaism and Islam, have specific laws regarding food. (The websites for Kosher Quest [www.kosherquest.org] and the Islamic Food and Nutrition Council of America [www.ifanca.org] provide detailed information.) Assess the extent to which Jewish or Muslim patients adhere to Kosher or Halal dietary practices to ensure that appropriate meals are served.

Assess the patient's diet history and implement necessary dietary changes. Avoid *cultural stereotyping* by making assumptions or generalizations about diet based on an individual's cultural background. Dietary habits differ considerably within and among ethnic groups. Acculturation, the extent to which immigrants adopt attributes of a new culture, can also affect dietary practices.[9]

It is important to know whether the patient eats "traditional foods" associated with the culture. If traditional foods are eaten, assess their impact on health. For example, "soul foods," which include traditional foods eaten by some African Americans, tend to be high in fat, cholesterol, and sodium.[10] Traditional foods eaten by some Asian Americans may be high in fiber and low in fat and cholesterol, but the diet may also be low in calcium because of limited dairy product intake.[11]

Consideration of cultural beliefs is important when planning and monitoring acceptance of dietary changes. Perception of body weight and size may also be influenced by culture. Ask the patient or family about how culture affects dietary choices and weight maintenance. For example, in some cultures overweight and obesity do not carry the stigma that they do in Western cultures.[12] This may make teaching regarding the necessity of weight reduction more challenging. A Jewish patient who eats only Kosher food may be comforted in knowing that most enteral formulas are manufactured Kosher and are labeled as such. Another example of culturally sensitive planning is adjusting meal service plans for the Muslim patient observing Ramadan (the Islamic month of *fasting*, in which Muslims refrain from eating and drinking during daylight hours).

Teaching related to dietary restrictions and recommended dietary changes should involve the patient's family. Often it is a family member who does the grocery shopping and cooking.

MALNUTRITION

Malnutrition is a deficit, excess, or imbalance of essential nutrients. It may occur with or without inflammation. Malnutrition affects body composition and functional status.[13] Imbalances in macronutrients (carbohydrates, proteins, fat) or micronutrients (electrolytes, minerals, vitamins) occur with malnutrition. Terms such as *undernutrition* and *overnutrition* are also used to describe malnutrition.

Undernutrition describes a state of poor nourishment as a result of inadequate diet or diseases that interfere with normal appetite and assimilation of ingested food. *Overnutrition* refers to the ingestion of more food than is required for body needs, as in obesity.

Malnutrition is a problem in both developing and developed countries across the care continuum (community, hospital, long-term care).[13] Twenty percent to 70% of hospitalized adults are considered malnourished or at nutritional risk.[14] The prevalence of malnutrition in older adults based on the Mini Nutritional Assessment (MNA) ranges from approximately 6% (community-dwelling older adults) to 50% (rehabilitation settings).[15]

Etiology of Malnutrition

Many terms are used to describe the types and etiologies of adult malnutrition.[16,17] Older terms that are still used in some settings include *primary* or *secondary protein-calorie malnutrition* (PCM), *marasmus*, and *kwashiorkor*. Marasmus and kwashiorkor describe forms of malnutrition seen in children in developing countries;[17] these terms should not be used to describe malnutrition in adults.

The following etiology-based terminology is the preferred terminology to use in clinical practice settings, since it indicates the interaction and importance of inflammation on nutritional status.[16,18]

- *Starvation-related malnutrition,* or primary PCM, occurs when nutritional needs are not met (Fig. 40-3). It is a clinical state in which there is chronic starvation without inflammation (e.g., anorexia nervosa).

- *Chronic disease–related malnutrition,* or secondary PCM, is associated with conditions that impose sustained inflammation of a mild to moderate degree.[16] This occurs when tissue needs are not met even though the dietary intake would be satisfactory under normal conditions. Examples of conditions associated with this type of malnutrition include organ failure, cancer, rheumatoid arthritis, obesity, and metabolic syndrome.

- *Acute disease– or injury-related malnutrition* is associated with acute disease or injury states with marked inflammatory response (e.g., major infection, burns, trauma, closed head injury).

Contributing Factors to Malnutrition

Many factors contribute to the development of malnutrition, including socioeconomic factors, physical illnesses, incomplete diets, and food-drug interactions. Table 40-6 lists conditions that increase the risk for malnutrition.

Socioeconomic Factors. *Food security* refers to access by all people, at all times, to sufficient food for an active and healthy lifestyle.[2] Individuals or families with limited financial resources may have *food insecurity* (inadequate access). Food insecurity is problematic because it affects the overall quality of food that is available in both quantity and nutritional value. Families with food insecurity usually choose less expensive "filling" foods, which are more energy dense (high fat) and lack nutritional value. This type of diet increases the risk of nutrient deficiencies.

To help them obtain food, individuals and families may use "safety net programs," including food assistance programs; housing and energy subsidies; and in-kind contributions from relatives, friends, food pantries, or charitable organizations.

Consult with social workers to help patients gain access to government and local programs such as Meals on Wheels that deliver nutritious meals to home-bound individuals. The "heat or eat" phenomenon is problematic, as families with limited economic resources struggle to pay household utility bills or put food on the table. Older adults on a fixed income have an added burden of deciding on whether to pay for medications or food. You and the registered dietitian can assist patients in making food choices that meet nutritional requirements while staying within their limited resources.

Physical Illnesses. Malnutrition is a common consequence of illness, surgery, injury, or hospitalization. The hospitalized patient, especially the older adult, is at risk of becoming malnourished. Prolonged illness, major surgery, sepsis, draining wounds, burns, hemorrhage, fractures, and immobilization can

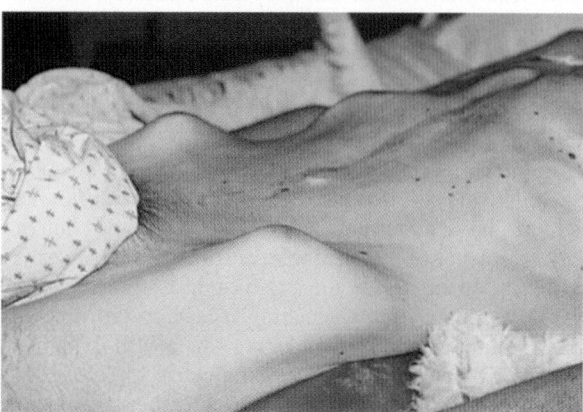

FIG. 40-3 Patient with malnutrition.

TABLE 40-6	CONDITIONS THAT INCREASE THE RISK FOR MALNUTRITION

- Dementia
- Depression
- Chronic alcoholism
- Excessive dieting to lose weight
- Swallowing disorders (e.g., head and neck cancer)
- Decreased mobility that limits access to food or its preparation
- Nutrient losses from malabsorption, dialysis, fistulas, or wounds
- Drugs with antinutrient or catabolic properties such as corticosteroids and oral antibiotics
- Extreme need for nutrients because of hypermetabolism or stresses such as infection, burns, trauma, or fever
- No oral intake and/or receiving standard IV solutions (5% dextrose) for 10 days (adults) or for 5 days (older adults)

all contribute to malnutrition. Pathologic conditions are frequently aggravated by undernutrition, and an existing deficiency state is likely to become more severe during illness.

Anorexia, nausea, vomiting, diarrhea, abdominal distention, and abdominal cramping may accompany diseases of the GI system. Any combination of these symptoms interferes with normal food consumption and metabolism. In addition, a patient may restrict dietary intake to a few foods or fluids that may not be nutritionally sound out of fear of aggravating an existing GI problem.

Malabsorption syndrome is the impaired absorption of nutrients from the GI tract. Decreases in digestive enzymes or in bowel surface area can quickly lead to a deficiency state. Many drugs have undesirable GI side effects and alter normal digestive and absorptive processes. For example, antibiotics change the normal flora of the intestines, decreasing the body's ability to synthesize biotin.

Fever accompanies many illnesses, injuries, and infections, with a concomitant increase in the body's basal metabolic rate (BMR). Each degree of temperature increase on the Fahrenheit scale raises the BMR by about 7%.[19] Without an increase in caloric intake, body protein stores will be used to supply calories, and protein depletion develops.

Assume responsibility, along with the health care provider and the registered dietitian, for meeting the patient's nutritional needs. Also consider the nutritional requirements of a patient who is not overtly ill but who is undergoing diagnostic studies. This patient may be nutritionally fit on entering the hospital but can develop nutritional problems because of the dietary restrictions imposed by multiple diagnostic studies.

Incomplete Diets. Vitamin deficiencies are rare in most developed countries, except for individuals with eating disorders and chronic abusers of alcohol. Vitamin deficiencies usually involve several vitamins, rather than a single one. The recommended dietary allowances, or DRIs, for essential vitamins and minerals (Table 40-7) can be obtained by eating a diet consisting of foods from the five basic food groups (see Fig. 40-1). DRIs from the Food and Nutrition Board have a safety margin because the levels exceed minimum daily requirements for most people.[20]

When vitamin imbalances do occur, they are usually found among persons with a pattern of alcohol and drug abuse, persons who are chronically ill, and individuals who follow poor dietary practices. Persons who have had surgery on the GI tract may be at risk for vitamin deficiencies. For example, resection of the terminal ileum poses a risk for deficiencies of fat-soluble vitamins. After a gastrectomy, patients require cobalamin supplementation because intrinsic factor (normally made in the stomach) is not available to bind with cobalamin so that this vitamin can be absorbed in the ileum. Followers of fad diets or poorly planned vegetarian diets are also at risk.

Clinical manifestations of vitamin imbalances are most commonly neurologic signs. The recommended DRIs and manifestations of imbalances are presented in eTable 40-3 (available on the website for this chapter).

Food-Drug Interactions. When the patient's health conditions require drug therapy, drug and food interactions may occur. Potential adverse interactions include incompatibilities, altered drug effectiveness, and impaired nutritional status. Food-drug interactions can also occur with the use of over-the-counter drugs and herbs and dietary supplements. Monitor and prevent these potential interactions for patients in the hospital and at home. Examples of common food-drug interactions are presented in eTable 40-4 (available on the website for this chapter). Additional information is available at *www. foodmedinteractions.com*.

Pathophysiology of Starvation

Knowing the pathophysiology of the starvation process helps to understand the physiologic changes that occur in malnutrition. Initially, the body selectively uses carbohydrates (glycogen) rather than fat and protein to meet metabolic needs. These carbohydrate stores, found in the liver and the muscles, are minimal and may be totally depleted within 18 hours. During this early phase of starvation, protein is used only in its normal participation in cellular metabolism. However, once carbohydrate stores are depleted, skeletal protein is converted to glucose for energy. Alanine and glutamine are the first amino acids to be used by the liver for the formation of glucose in a process termed *gluconeogenesis*. The resulting available plasma glucose allows the metabolic processes to continue. With these amino acids being used as energy sources, the person may be in negative nitrogen balance (nitrogen excretion exceeds nitrogen intake). Within 5 to 9 days, body fat is fully mobilized to supply much of the needed energy.

In prolonged starvation, up to 97% of calories are provided by fat, and protein is conserved. Depletion of fat stores depends on the amount available, but fat stores are generally used up in

TABLE 40-7	RECOMMENDED DAILY VITAMIN AND CALCIUM INTAKE*
Vitamin or Mineral	**Dietary Reference Intake**
Fat-Soluble Vitamins	
A	*Men:* 900 mcg/retinol equivalents *Women:* 700 mcg/retinol equivalents
D	*Adults ages 19-70:* 600 IU *Adults age >70:* 800 IU
E	*Adults:* 15 mg
K	*Men:* 120 mcg *Women:* 90 mcg
Water-Soluble Vitamins	
B_1	*Men:* 1.2 mg *Women:* 1.1 mg
B_6	*Men ages 19-50:* 1.3 mg *Men age >51:* 1.7 mg *Women ages 19-50:* 1.3 mg *Women age >51:* 1.5 mg
Cobalamin (B_{12})	*Adults:* 2-4 mcg
C	*Men:* 90 mg *Women:* 75 mg
Folate (folic acid)	*Adults:* 400 mcg
Minerals	
Calcium	*Men ages 19-70:* 1000 mg *Men age >70:* 1200 mg *Women ages 19-50:* 1000 mg *Women age >51:* 1500 mg

Source: Food and Nutrition Board, Institute of Medicine: *Dietary Reference Intakes (DRIs): recommended dietary allowance and adequate intakes, vitamins,* Washington, DC, 2006, Food and Nutrition Board, National Academies; and Institute of Medicine: *Dietary Reference Intakes for calcium and vitamin D,* Washington, DC, 2010, National Academies Press.
*See eTable 40-3 (on the website for this chapter) for Recommended Dietary Reference Intakes and Manifestations of Imbalance.

4 to 6 weeks. Once fat stores are used, body or visceral proteins, including those in internal organs and plasma, can no longer be spared and rapidly decrease because they are the only remaining body source of energy available.

If a malnourished patient has surgery, experiences physical trauma, or has an infection, the stress response is superimposed on the starvation response. Protein stores are used for body energy to meet the increased metabolic energy expenditure.

As the protein depletion continues, liver function becomes impaired, and synthesis of proteins decreases. The plasma oncotic pressure is lower because of decreased protein synthesis. A major function of plasma proteins, primarily albumin, is the maintenance of the osmotic pressure of the blood. Because of decreased oncotic pressure, body fluids shift from the vascular space into the interstitial compartment. Eventually albumin leaks into the interstitial space along with the fluid. Edema becomes clinically observable. Often the edema in the patient's face and legs masks the underlying muscle wasting.

As the total blood volume is reduced, the skin appears dry and wrinkled. As fluids shift to the interstitial space, ions also move. Sodium (a predominant extracellular ion) is found in increased amounts within the cell, and potassium (a predominant intracellular ion) and magnesium are shifted to the extracellular space. The sodium-potassium exchange pump has high energy needs, using 20% to 50% of all calories ingested. When the diet is extremely deficient in calories and essential proteins, the pump will fail, leaving sodium inside the cell (along with water), and the cell will expand.

The liver is the body organ that loses the most mass during protein deprivation. It gradually becomes infiltrated with fat secondary to decreased synthesis of lipoproteins. If dietary protein and other necessary constituents are not given, death will rapidly ensue.

Impact of Inflammation. Inflammation affects nutrient metabolism and is an important component of the nutritional status. During the starvation process, there is a decreased BMR, sparing of skeletal muscle, and decreased protein breakdown. However, in inflammatory states, there are alterations in the expression of proinflammatory (e.g., interleukin-6) and antiinflammatory cytokines (e.g., interleukin-10). These cytokine changes result in increased protein and skeletal muscle breakdown, increased BMR, increased glucose turnover, decreased negative acute phase protein (albumin, prealbumin) production, and increased positive acute phase protein (e.g., C-reactive protein [CRP]) production.[16]

Clinical Manifestations

The clinical manifestations of malnutrition range from mild to emaciation (Fig. 40-4) and death. The most obvious clinical signs on physical examination are apparent in the skin (dry and scaly skin, brittle nails, rashes, hair loss), mouth (crusting and ulceration, changes in tongue), muscles (decreased mass and weakness), and CNS (mental changes such as confusion, irritability). The speed at which the malnutrition develops depends on the quantity and quality of the protein intake, caloric value, illness, and the person's age.

Clinical manifestations of malnutrition are the result of numerous interactions at the cellular level. As protein intake is severely reduced, the muscles, which are the largest store of protein in the body, become wasted and flabby, leading to weakness and fatigability. Decreased protein is available for repair, and as a result, wound healing may be delayed. The person is

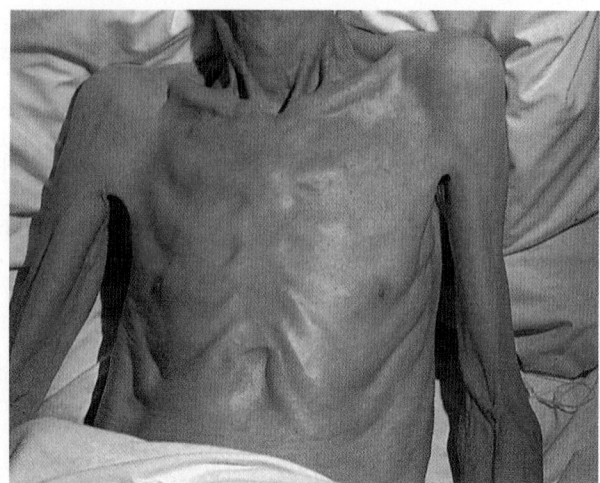
FIG. 40-4 Severe malnutrition that results in wasting and extensive loss of adipose tissue.

more susceptible to infections. Both humoral and cell-mediated immunity are deficient in malnutrition. There is a decrease in leukocytes in the peripheral blood. Phagocytosis is altered because of the lack of energy necessary to drive the process. Many malnourished individuals are anemic, generally as a result of nutritional deficiencies in iron and folic acid, the necessary building blocks for red blood cells (RBCs). A detailed listing of the clinical manifestations of malnutrition is available in eTable 40-5 (available on the website for this chapter).

Diagnostic Studies

History and Physical Examination. A diet history of foods eaten over the past week reveals a great deal about the patient's dietary habits and knowledge of good nutrition. In addition to the height, weight, and vital signs, assess and document the patient's physical state and each body system. Table 40-8 summarizes the assessment and findings of the patient with malnutrition.

Laboratory Studies. The diagnosis of malnutrition is best determined by body composition, including a thorough history of weight loss, nutrient intake, and measures of functional status and inflammation. Serum albumin has a half-life of approximately 20 to 22 days. In the absence of marked fluid loss, such as from hemorrhage or burns, the serum albumin value lags behind actual protein changes by more than 2 weeks. Therefore albumin is not a good indicator of acute changes in nutritional status.

Prealbumin, a protein synthesized by the liver, has a half-life of 2 days and is a better indicator of recent or current nutritional status. Serum transferrin level is another indicator of protein status. Transferrin, a protein synthesized by the liver and used to transport iron, decreases when protein is deficient.

However, the extent to which visceral proteins, including albumin, prealbumin, and transferrin, are true markers of malnutrition is questionable. Albumin, prealbumin, and transferrin are *negative acute phase proteins,* which mean that during an inflammatory response, the synthesis of these proteins in the liver is decreased. Therefore low or below normal levels of these negative acute phase proteins correspond to an inflammatory state rather than accurately indicating nutritional status.[16,20]

CRP, which is a *positive acute phase protein,* is typically elevated during inflammation and predicts morbidity and mortal-

TABLE 40-8 NURSING ASSESSMENT

Malnutrition

Subjective Data

Important Health Information

Past health history: Severe burns, major trauma, hemorrhage, draining wounds, bone fractures with prolonged immobility, chronic renal or liver disease, cancer, malabsorption syndromes, GI obstruction, infectious diseases (TB, AIDS), acute (e.g., trauma, sepsis) or chronic inflammatory condition (e.g., rheumatoid arthritis)

Medications: Corticosteroids, chemotherapeutic agents, diet pills

Surgery or other treatments: Recent surgery, radiation

Functional Health Patterns

Health perception–health management: Alcohol or drug abuse; malaise, apathy

Nutritional-metabolic: Increase or decrease in weight, weight problems; increase or decrease in appetite, typical dietary intake; food preferences and aversions; food allergies or intolerance; ill-fitting or absent dentures; dry mouth, difficulty in chewing or swallowing; bloating or gas; ↑ sensitivity to cold; delayed wound healing

Elimination: Constipation, diarrhea, nocturia, decreased urine output

Activity-exercise: Increase or decrease in activity patterns; weakness, fatigue, decreased endurance

Cognitive-perceptual: Pain in mouth; paresthesias; loss of position and vibratory sense

Role-relationship: Change in family (e.g., loss of a spouse); financial resources

Sexual-reproductive: Amenorrhea, impotence, decreased libido

Objective Data

General

Listless, cachectic; underweight for height

Integumentary

Dry, brittle, sparse hair with color changes and lack of luster, alopecia; dry, scaly lips, fever blisters, angular crusts and lesions at corners of mouth (cheilosis); brittle, ridged nails; decreased tone and elasticity of skin; cool, rough, dry, scaly skin with brown-gray pigment changes; reddened, scaly dermatitis, scrotal dermatitis; slight cyanosis; peripheral edema

Eyes

Pale or red conjunctivae, gray keratinized epithelium on conjunctiva (Bitot's spots); dryness and dull appearance of conjunctivae and cornea, soft cornea; blood vessel growth in cornea; redness and fissuring of eyelid corners

Respiratory

Decreased respiratory rate, ↓ vital capacity, crackles, weak cough

Cardiovascular

Increased or decreased heart rate, ↓ BP, dysrhythmias

Gastrointestinal

Swollen, smooth, raw, beefy red tongue (glossitis), hypertrophic or atrophic papillae; dental cavities, absent or loose teeth, discolored tooth enamel; spongy, pale, receded gums with a tendency to bleed easily, periodontal disease; ulcerations, white patches or plaques, redness, swelling of oral mucosa; distended, tympanic abdomen; ascites, hepatomegaly, decreased bowel sounds; steatorrhea

Neurologic

Decreased or loss of reflexes, tremor; inattention, irritability, confusion, syncope

Musculoskeletal

Decreased muscle mass with poor tone, "wasted" appearance; bowlegs, knock-knees, beaded ribs, chest deformity, prominent bony structures

Possible Diagnostic Findings

↓ Hemoglobin and hematocrit; ↓ MCV, MCH, or MCHC (iron deficiency); ↓ MCV or MCH (folic acid or cobalamin deficiency); altered serum electrolyte levels, especially hyperkalemia; ↓ BUN and creatinine; ↓ serum albumin, transferrin, and prealbumin; ↓ lymphocytes; ↑ liver enzymes; ↓ serum vitamin levels

MCH, Mean corpuscular hemoglobin; *MCHC,* mean corpuscular hemoglobin concentration; *MCV,* mean corpuscular volume; *TB,* tuberculosis.

ity.[21,22] Serum electrolyte levels reflect changes taking place between the intracellular and extracellular spaces. The serum potassium level is often elevated. The RBC count and the hemoglobin level indicate the presence and degree of anemia. The total lymphocyte count decreases with malnutrition. It is calculated by multiplying the percent of lymphocytes times the total white blood cell (WBC) count. Liver enzyme levels, a reflection of liver function, may be elevated during malnutrition. Serum levels of both fat-soluble and water-soluble vitamins are usually decreased. The lowered serum levels of the fat-soluble vitamins correlate with the clinical signs of *steatorrhea* (fatty stools).

Anthropometric Measurements. Anthropometric measurements are gross measures of fat and muscle contents. These measurements tend to be most beneficial when done serially, and by well-trained anthropometrists, to evaluate the long-term effects of malnutrition or responses to nutritional interventions. They consist of measures of skinfold thickness at various sites, which are indicators of subcutaneous fat stores, and midarm muscle circumference, an indicator of protein stores. These measurements are then compared with standards for healthy persons of the same age and gender.

The sites most reflective of body fat are those over the biceps and the triceps, below the scapula, above the iliac crest, and

over the upper thigh. Both skinfold thickness and midarm circumference measurements are decreased in malnutrition. These measurements may also be influenced by shifts in hydration status. The exact relationship of the midarm circumference measure to morbidity and mortality remains to be established.

Waist circumference and hip-to-waist ratio are used more commonly in acute care to reflect nutritional status. These measures are discussed in Chapter 41.

Functional Measurements. Measures of muscle strength are used to assess functional status, an important outcome of nutrition states. Handgrip strength is measured with a hand dynamometer. Functional performance tests such as the Short Physical Performance Battery may be ordered.[23]

NURSING AND COLLABORATIVE MANAGEMENT MALNUTRITION

NURSING ASSESSMENT

As a nurse, you are responsible for nutritional screening across care settings. Nutritional screening identifies individuals who are malnourished or at risk for malnutrition. Nutritional screening is also used to determine if a more detailed nutritional assessment is necessary. The Joint Commission requires nutritional screening for all patients within 24 hours of admission. Many nutritional screening and assessment tools are available.[24,25] Hospital-specific screening tools based on common admission assessment criteria include history of weight loss, prior intake before admission, use of nutritional support, chewing or swallowing issues, and skin breakdown. A standardized approach to nutritional screening is needed to ensure valid and reliable tools are used in the clinical setting.

In older adults the Mini Nutritional Assessment (MNA) is often used[25] (available at *www.mna-elderly.com/forms/mini/mna_mini_english.pdf*). In long-term care the Minimum Data Set (MDS) form is used to obtain information about a person's nutritional status.[26] In home care settings the Outcome and Assessment Information Set (OASIS) prompts you to collect information on diet, oral intake, dental health, swallowing difficulties, and any need for meal assistance.[27]

If the nutritional screening identifies an individual at nutritional risk, a full nutritional assessment is most often needed. A nutritional assessment is a comprehensive approach that includes medical, nutritional, and medication histories; physical examination; anthropometric measurements; and laboratory data (Table 40-9). Nutritional assessment provides the basis for nutritional intervention.

Across all care settings, be aware of the patient's nutritional status. Obtaining an accurate measure of body weight and height and recording this information are critical components of this assessment. When assessing weight, obtain a detailed weight history, noting weight loss. Ask whether the weight loss was intentional or unintentional and the period over which it took place. A loss of more than 5% of usual body weight over 6 months, whether intentional or unintentional, is a critical indicator for further assessment, especially in the older adult.[28] If an involuntary weight loss exceeds 10% of the usual weight, determine the reason. Unintentional weight loss is also important to consider in the obese individual, since latent malnutrition may be present despite excess body weight. Determine the patient's current weight in relation to ideal body weight.

When possible, measure the patient's actual height rather than using the patient's self-report. Alternatives to standing height (stature) measurements include arm demi-span and knee-height measurements. The *arm demi-span* is the distance from a point on the midline at the suprasternal notch to the web between the middle and ring fingers with the arm horizontally outstretched (*www.mna-elderly.com/forms/mna_guide_english.pdf*). For persons who are confined to bed, the use of a Luft ruler is an alternative to standing height.[29]

Body mass index (BMI) is a measure of weight for height (see Fig. 41-2). A BMI of less than 18.5 kg/m^2 is considered underweight, normal weight is a BMI between 18.5 and 24.9 kg/m^2, and overweight is a BMI between 25 and 29.9 kg/m^2. A BMI of 30 kg/m^2 or greater is obese. BMIs outside the normal weight range are associated with increased morbidity and mortality.[30]

In addition, obtain a complete diet history from the patient or caregiver. The patient's nutritional state may not be the reason medical care was sought. However, it may be a contributing factor to the disease and have an impact on management and recovery.

NURSING DIAGNOSES

Nursing diagnoses for the patient with malnutrition include, but are not limited to, the following:

- Imbalanced nutrition: less than body requirements *related to* decreased access, ingestion, digestion, or absorption of food or *related to* anorexia, dysphagia, or increased metabolic needs
- Feeding self-care deficit *related to* decreased strength and endurance, fatigue, and apathy
- Deficient fluid volume *related to* factors affecting access to or absorption of fluids
- Risk for impaired skin integrity *related to* poor nutritional state
- Noncompliance *related to* alteration in perception, lack of motivation, or incompatibility of regimen with lifestyle or resources

PLANNING

The overall goals are that the patient with malnutrition will (1) gain weight, particularly muscle mass; (2) consume a specified number of calories per day (with a diet individualized for the patient); and (3) have no adverse consequences related to malnutrition or nutritional therapies.

NURSING IMPLEMENTATION

HEALTH PROMOTION. You are in a good position to teach and reinforce healthy eating habits with individuals and groups of persons throughout their life span. Use MyPlate, Dietary Guidelines for Americans 2010, and Nutrition Facts food labels to promote healthy nutrition. Free interactive web-based programs are available to track physical activity, calories, and foods eaten (see *www.choosemyplate.gov*).

TABLE 40-9	COMPONENTS OF NUTRITIONAL ASSESSMENT
Anthropometric Measurements • Height and weight • Body mass index (BMI) • Rate of weight change • Amount of weight loss	**Diet History** • Chewing and swallowing ability • Changes in appetite or taste • Food and nutrient intake • Availability of food
Physical Examination • Physical appearance • Muscle mass and strength • Dental and oral health	**Laboratory Data** • Glucose • Electrolytes • Lipid profile • Blood urea nitrogen (BUN)
Health History • Personal and family history • Acute or chronic illnesses • Current medications, herbs, supplements • Cognitive status, depression	**Functional Status** • Ability to perform basic and instrumental activities of daily living • Handgrip strength • Performance tests (e.g., timed walk tests)

HEALTHY PEOPLE

Health Impact of a Well-Balanced Diet

- Reduces incidence of anemia
- Maintains normal body weight and prevents obesity
- Maintains good bone health and reduces risk of osteoporosis
- Lowers the risk of developing elevated cholesterol and type 2 diabetes mellitus
- Decreases the risk of heart disease, hypertension, and certain types of cancers

EVIDENCE-BASED PRACTICE
Translating Research Into Practice

Does Nutritional Education Improve Functional Outcomes in Older Adults?

Clinical Question
In older adults (P) what is the effect of nutritional education (I) on diet, physical and emotional functioning, and quality of life (O)?

Best Available Evidence
- Systematic review of randomized controlled trials (RCTs)

Critical Appraisal and Synthesis of Evidence
- Twenty-three RCTs (n = 12,610) of community-dwelling older adults (65 yr and older) with various diseases. Five trials with nutritional education only; remaining trials with nutritional and lifestyle advice, exercise advice, or screening. Education varied in format and intensity.
- Outcomes included diet, functional outcomes (e.g., strength, balance), hospital readmissions, depression, anxiety, and quality of life.
- Results showed improved body mass index, weight loss, and physical health with decreased depression.
- Brief interventions were as effective as more lengthy ones.

Conclusion
- Nutritional education alone or in combination with other interventions positively influences physical and emotional health.

Implications for Nursing Practice
- Locate nutritional educational resources for older patients residing at home.
- Help patients identify community programs to make positive changes in lifestyle and exercise.

Reference for Evidence
Young K, Bunn F, Trivedi D, et al: Nutritional education for community dwelling older people: a systematic review of randomised controlled trials, *Int J Nurs Stud* 48:751, 2011.

P, Patient population of interest; *I*, intervention or area of interest; *O*, outcomes of interest (see p. 12).

ACUTE INTERVENTION. Assess the patient's nutritional state during your assessment of the patient's other physical problems. Identify nutritional risk factors and why they might exist. In states of increased stress, such as surgery, severe trauma, and sepsis, more calories and protein are needed. Wound healing requires increased protein synthesis. For patients undergoing major surgery or those with or at risk for malnutrition, several weeks of increased protein and calorie intake are needed preoperatively to promote healing postoperatively.

When fever is present, the metabolic rate is increased and nitrogen loss is accelerated. Despite the return of body temperature to normal, the rate of protein breakdown and resynthesis may be increased for several weeks. Teach the patient and caregiver the importance of good nutrition and the rationale for recording the daily weight, intake, and output. Daily weights can give an ongoing record of body weight gain or loss. However, rapid gains and losses are usually the result of shifts in fluid balance. The body weight, in conjunction with accurate recording of food and fluid intake, provides a clearer picture of the patient's fluid and nutritional state. To obtain an accurate weight, weigh the patient at the same time each day, on the same scale, with the same type or amount of clothing, and preferably with the bladder recently emptied.

TABLE 40-10 NUTRITIONAL THERAPY*
High-Calorie, High-Protein Diet

Suggestions for high-calorie, high-protein foods include the following.

Breads and Cereals
- Hot cereals (oatmeal, cream of wheat) prepared with milk, added fat (butter or margarine), and sugar
- Potatoes prepared with added fat (butter and whole milk)
- Granola and other cereals with dried fruit
- Croissants, buttermilk biscuits, muffins, banana bread, zucchini bread

Vegetables
- Vegetables prepared with added fat (margarine, butter)
- Fried vegetables

Fruits
- Canned fruit in heavy syrup
- Dried fruit

Meat
- Fried meats
- Meats covered in cream sauces or gravy
- Casseroles

Milk and Milk Products
- Milkshakes
- Whole milk and milk products (yogurt, ice cream, cheese)
- Whipping cream or heavy cream
- Whole milk with added nutritional supplements

*Suggested meal plans for high-calorie, high-protein diet are presented in eTable 40-6 (available on the website for this chapter).

The protein and calorie intake required in the malnourished patient depends on the cause of the malnutrition, the treatment being used, and other stressors affecting the patient. If the patient is able to take food by mouth, obtain a daily calorie count and diet diary to give an accurate record of food intake. You and the registered dietitian can assist the patient and family in selecting high-calorie and high-protein foods (unless medically contraindicated). Preparation of foods preferred by the patient enhances the daily intake. Encourage the family to bring the patient's favorite foods from home while the patient is hospitalized. Table 40-10 gives examples of high-calorie, high-protein foods.

The undernourished patient usually needs to have between-meal supplements. These may consist of items prepared in the dietary department or commercially prepared products. Eating these items between meals provides extra calories, proteins, fluids, and nutrients. If the patient is unable to consume enough nutrition with a high-calorie, high-protein diet, oral liquid nutritional supplements can be added.

Some patients may benefit from appetite stimulants such as megestrol acetate (Megace) or dronabinol (Marinol) to improve nutritional intake. If the patient is still unable to take in enough calories, enteral feedings may be considered. Parenteral nutrition (PN) might need to be initiated if enteral feedings are not feasible.[31] Contraindications for enteral nutrition include GI obstruction, prolonged ileus, severe diarrhea or vomiting, and enterocutaneous fistula.

AMBULATORY AND HOME CARE. With shortened hospital stays, many patients are discharged on a therapeutic diet. Discharge preparation for both the patient and the caregiver is essential. Teach them about the cause of the undernourished state and ways to avoid the problem in the future. Individuals need to be aware that undernourishment, whatever the cause, can recur and that adhering to a diet high in protein and calories for a few weeks cannot fully restore a normal nutritional state. Many months may be needed to reach this goal. Assess the patient's understanding and reinforce the information whenever possible. Assess the patient's and caregiver's ability to comply with the dietary instructions in light of past eating habits, religious and ethnic preferences, age, income, other resources, and state of health. Emphasize the need for continual follow-up care if rehabilitation is to be accomplished and maintained. In the discharge planning, ensure proper follow-up such as visits by the home health nurse and outpatient registered dietitian referrals.

Determine the need for nutritious meals and snacks after discharge from the hospital. The ability of the patient or caregiver to access a registered dietitian may be limited. As a nurse, you may be the primary source of nutritional information. In your assessment, consider the availability and acceptability of community resources that provide meals such as Meals on Wheels, senior congregate feeding sites, and the Supplemental Nutrition Assistance Program (SNAP, formerly known as Food Stamps). Help the patient identify reliable Internet sources that provide evidence-based food and nutrition recommendations.

Keeping a diet diary for 3 days at a time is one way to analyze and reinforce healthful eating patterns. These records are also helpful to the health care team in the follow-up care. Encourage self-assessment of progress by having the patient weigh himself or herself once or twice a week and keep a weight record.

▌EVALUATION

The expected outcomes are that the patient who is malnourished will

- Achieve and maintain optimal body weight
- Consume a well-balanced diet
- Experience no adverse outcomes related to malnutrition
- Maintain optimal physical functioning

▌GERONTOLOGIC CONSIDERATIONS

MALNUTRITION

Older adults are particularly vulnerable to malnutrition across care settings.[32] Nutrition affects quality of life, functional status, and health in older adults. Older hospitalized adults with malnutrition are more likely to have poor wound healing, pressure ulcers, infections, decreased muscle strength, postoperative complications, and increased morbidity and mortality risks.[28] You play an important role in assessing the physiologic, functional, environmental, dietary, psychologic, and social factors related to nutritional risk in older adults. Older adults are also less able to regain body weight after periods of undernutrition due to illness or surgery.

Older adults may report little or no appetite, problems with eating or swallowing, inadequate servings of nutrients, and fewer than two meals per day. Limited incomes may cause them to restrict the number of meals or the dietary quality of meals eaten. Social isolation is a problem in older adults. Older adults who live alone may lose their desire to cook and report decreased appetite. Functional limitations may also affect the ability to feed one's self or to purchase food, cook, or prepare meals. Furthermore, older adults may lack transportation to buy food.

Chronic illnesses associated with aging can also affect nutritional status. For example, depression and dysphagia (secondary to stroke) can affect intake. Poor oral health from cavities, gum disease (gingivitis), and missing teeth, as well as *xerostomia* (dry mouth), can impair the older adult's ability to lubricate, masticate, and swallow food. Medications can cause dry mouth, alter the taste of food, or decrease appetite.

Physiologic changes associated with aging include a decrease in lean body mass and redistribution of fat around internal organs, which can lead to a decreased caloric requirement. Furthermore, changes in odor and taste perception (from medications, nutrient deficiencies, or taste-bud atrophy) can alter nutritional status. Sarcopenia is a loss of lean body mass with aging and affects muscle strength and function. Older adults on bed rest or prolonged inactivity lose more lean body mass than younger adults.[30]

Measure weight and height on admission, and routinely assess and document the person's weight. Determine if there is a history of voluntary or involuntary weight loss. Collaborate with the primary care provider and registered dietitian to identify the cause for weight loss and implement appropriate interventions.

Daily requirements for healthy older adults for weight maintenance include 30 cal/kg of body weight, and 0.8 to 1 g/kg of protein per day, with no more than 30% of calories from fat.[28,30] Nutritional requirements may differ depending on the degree of malnutrition and physiologic stress. To prevent loss of muscle mass and maintain function, some experts recommend older adults consume a moderate amount of high-quality protein at each meal.[33] Daily calcium and vitamin D requirements are higher for older adults (see Table 40-7).

Focus your initial care strategies on improving oral intake and providing a stimulating environment for meals. Special strategies, such as adaptive devices (e.g., large-handled eating utensils), often are helpful in increasing dietary intake.

Oral liquid supplements may have a role in improving the nutritional status of older adults.[34] Do not use supplements as meal substitutes, but use them between meals as snacks. In long-term care these beverages may be used instead of water with oral medication administration to increase caloric intake. Some older persons may require nutritional support therapies until their strength and general health improve. Before starting any nutritional support therapy (e.g., enteral or parenteral nutrition) for an older patient unable to give consent, review his or her advance directives regarding the use of artificial nutrition and hydration.

Malnourished or nutritionally at-risk older adults are vulnerable when discharged from the hospital to the home. Older adults may not be able to shop for or prepare foods during the initial recovery period.[35] Consult with the social worker and registered dietitian to ensure that older adults have access to food on discharge. Home-delivered meals or senior congregate feeding programs are an appropriate referral. Many community nutritional programs are available to the older person to make mealtime a pleasant, social event. Improving the social setting of a meal frequently improves dietary intake. The use of SNAP is another alternative that allows low-income households, regardless of age, to buy more food of a greater variety.

Older adults with dementia or a stroke present unique nursing challenges with regard to eating and feeding. (Dementia is discussed in Chapter 60, and strokes are discussed in Chapter 58.)

TYPES OF SPECIALIZED NUTRITIONAL SUPPORT

Oral Feeding

Oral supplements may be used in the patient whose nutritional intake is deficient. This may include milkshakes, puddings, or

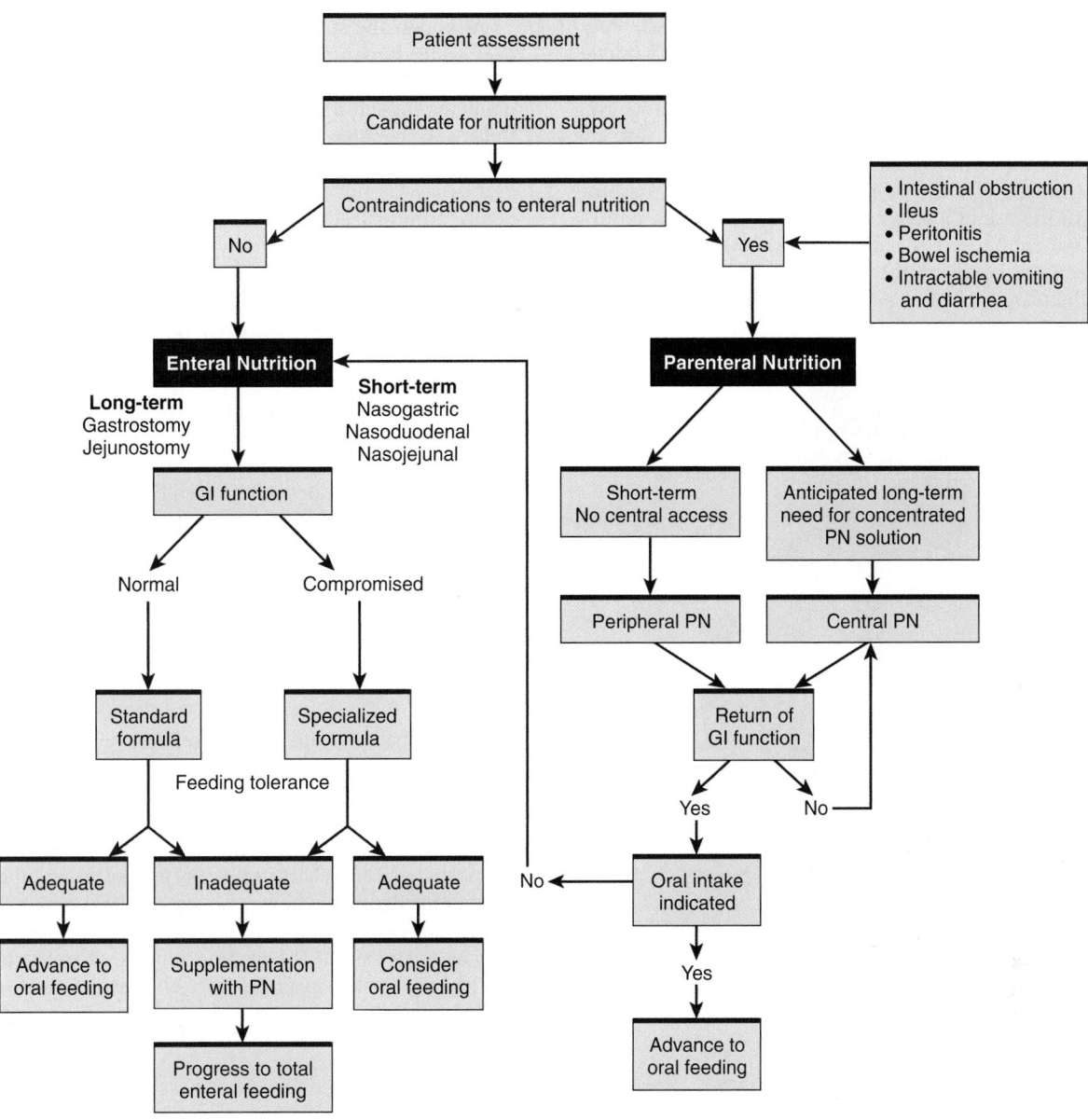

FIG. 40-5 Nutritional support algorithm.

commercially available products (e.g., Carnation Instant Breakfast, Ensure, Boost). If patients are unable to maintain or achieve adequate nutritional status, nutritional support may be necessary. For a decision-making plan related to nutritional support, see Fig. 40-5.

Enteral Nutrition

Enteral nutrition (EN), also known as tube feeding, is defined as nutrition (e.g., a nutritionally balanced liquefied food or formula) provided through the GI tract via a tube, catheter, or stoma that delivers nutrients distal to the oral cavity. EN may be ordered for the patient who has a functioning GI tract but is unable to take any or enough oral nourishment, or when it is unsafe to do so.

Indications for EN may include persons with anorexia, orofacial fractures, head and neck cancer, neurologic or psychiatric conditions that prevent oral intake, extensive burns, or critical illness (especially if mechanical ventilation is required), and those who are receiving chemotherapy or radiation therapy. EN

is considered to be easily administered, safer, more physiologically efficient, and typically less expensive than parenteral nutrition (PN).

Common delivery options are continuous infusion by pump, intermittent infusion by gravity, intermittent bolus by syringe, and cyclic feedings by infusion pump. Continuous infusion is most often used with critically ill patients. Intermittent feeding may be preferred as the patient improves or is receiving EN at home.[36]

Nasally and orally placed tubes (orogastric, nasogastric [NG], nasoduodenal, or nasojejunal) are most commonly used for short-term feeding (less than 4 weeks). Nasoduodenal and nasojejunal tubes are transpyloric tubes. These tubes are used when pathophysiologic conditions such as risk of aspiration warrant feeding the patient below the pyloric sphincter. If the feedings are necessary for an extended time, other tubes are placed in the stomach or small bowel by surgical, endoscopic, or fluoroscopic procedures. (Fig. 40-6 shows the locations of commonly used enteral feeding tubes.)

Orogastric, Nasogastric, and Nasointestinal Tubes. Polyurethane or silicone feeding tubes are long, small in diameter, soft, and flexible, thereby decreasing the risk of mucosal damage from prolonged placement. These tubes are radiopaque, making their position readily identified by x-ray. Placement into the small intestine theoretically decreases the likelihood of regurgitation of contents into the esophagus and subsequent aspiration.[37] With the use of a stylet, these tubes can be placed in a comatose patient because the ability to swallow is not essential during insertion. However, the use of a stylet has been associated with increased risk for perforation.

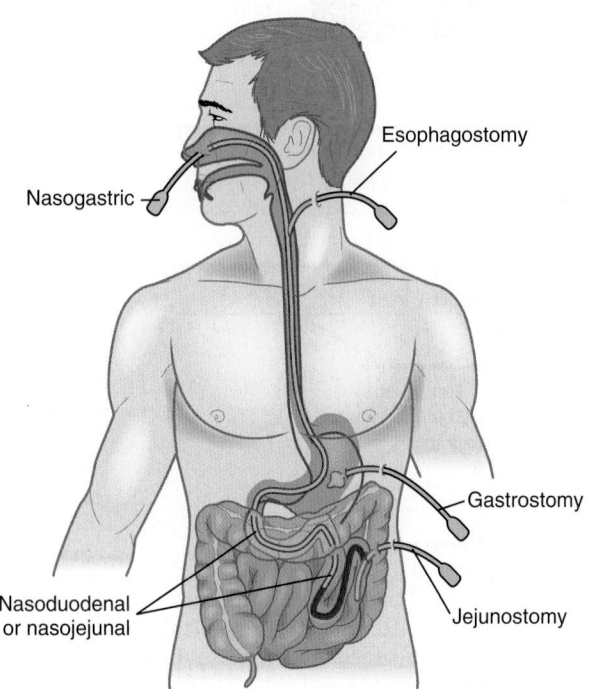

FIG. 40-6 Common enteral feeding tube placement locations.

Although the smaller feeding tubes have many advantages over wider-lumen tubes, such as the standard decompression NG tube, there are some disadvantages. Because of the small diameter, these tubes are more easily clogged when feedings are thick, and the tubes are more difficult to use for checking residual volumes. They are particularly prone to obstruction when oral drugs are not thoroughly crushed and dissolved in water before administration. Failure to flush the tubing before and after both drug administration and residual volume determinations can result in tube clogging. When the tube becomes clogged, it may necessitate removal and insertion of a new tube, adding to cost and patient discomfort. The tubes can become dislodged by vomiting or coughing and can also become knotted or kinked.

Gastrostomy and Jejunostomy Tubes. A gastrostomy tube may be used for a patient who requires EN over an extended time (see Fig. 40-6). Gastrostomy tubes can be placed surgically, radiologically, or endoscopically. The placement of a percutaneous endoscopic gastrostomy (PEG) tube is shown in Fig. 40-7. The patient must have an intact, unobstructed GI tract, and the esophageal lumen must be wide enough to pass the endoscope for PEG tube placement. PEG tube and radiologically placed gastrostomy tube procedures have fewer risks than surgical placement. The procedure requires IV sedation and local anesthesia. IV antibiotics are given before the procedure.

For the patient with chronic reflux, a jejunostomy (J-tube) with continuous feedings may be necessary to reduce the risk of aspiration.[38] Jejunostomy tubes are placed either endoscopically or with open or laparoscopic surgery.

Enteral feedings can be started within 24 to 48 hours after a surgically placed gastrostomy or jejunostomy tube without waiting for flatus or a bowel movement. PEG tube feeding may be started within 2 hours of insertion, although institutionally policies may vary.[39] The feeding tube is either premarked or marked at the skin insertion site. The tube is most often connected to a pump for continuous feeding.

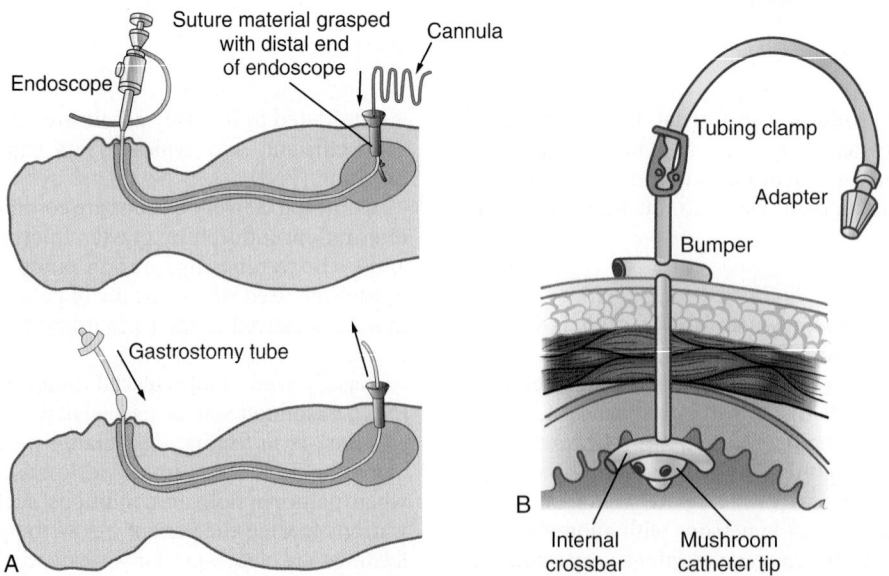

FIG. 40-7 Percutaneous endoscopic gastrostomy. **A,** Gastrostomy tube placement via percutaneous endoscopy. With use of endoscopy, a gastrostomy tube is inserted through the esophagus into the stomach and then pulled through a stab wound made in the abdominal wall. **B,** A retention disk and bumper secure the tube.

TABLE 40-11 PROBLEMS RELATED TO TUBE FEEDINGS

PROBLEMS AND CAUSES	CORRECTIVE MEASURES
Vomiting or Aspiration	
Improper placement of tube	• Replace tube in proper position. • Check tube position before beginning feeding and every 8 hr if continuous feedings.
Delayed gastric emptying, increased residual volume	• If gastric residual volume is ≥250 mL after second gastric residual check, consider a promotility agent. • If gastric residual volume is >500 mL, hold enteral nutrition and reassess patient tolerance.
Potential for aspiration	• Keep head of bed elevated to 30- to 45-degree angle. • Have patient sit up on side of bed or in chair. • Encourage ambulation unless contraindicated.
Dehydration	
Excessive diarrhea, vomiting	• Decrease rate or change formula. • Check drugs that patient is receiving, especially antibiotics. • Take care to prevent bacterial contamination of formula and equipment.
Poor fluid intake	• Increase intake and check amount and number of feedings. • Increase amount of fluid intake if appropriate.
High-protein formula	• Change formula.
Hyperosmotic diuresis	• Check blood glucose levels frequently. • Change formula.

PROBLEMS AND CAUSES	CORRECTIVE MEASURES
Diarrhea	
Feeding too fast	• Decrease rate of feeding. • Change to continuous drip feedings.
Medications	• Check for drugs that may cause diarrhea (e.g., sorbitol in liquid medications, antibiotics).
Low-fiber formula	• Change to formula with more fiber.
Tube moving distally	• Properly secure tube before beginning feeding. • Check before each feeding or at least every 24 hr if continuous feedings.

Contamination of formula	• Refrigerate unused formula and record date opened.
	• Discard outdated formula every 24 hr.
	• Discard formula left standing for longer than manufacturer's guidelines.
	  • 8 hr for ready-to-feed formulas (cans)
	  • 4 hr for reconstituted formula
	  • 24-48 hr for closed-system enteral formulas
	• Use closed system to prevent contamination.
	• Use sterile water for flushes.

Constipation	
Formula components	• Consult health care provider for change in formula to one with more fiber content. • Obtain laxative order.
Poor fluid intake	• Increase fluid intake if not contraindicated. • Give free water as well as formula. • Give total fluid intake of 30 mL/kg body weight.
Drugs	• Check for drugs that may be constipating.
Impaction	• Perform rectal examinations to check and manually remove feces if present.

Tube Feedings and Safety. You have a critical role to ensure that tube feedings are administered safely. Nursing management of tube feedings is briefly addressed in eTable 40-7 (available on the website for this chapter). Aspiration and dislodged tubes are two important safety concerns.

Patient Position. Proper patient positioning decreases the risk of aspiration. Elevate the head of bed to a minimum of 30 degrees, but preferably 45 degrees, to prevent aspiration. A reverse Trendelenburg position can be used to elevate the head of the bed, unless contraindicated, when a back rest elevation is not tolerated. If it is necessary to lower the head of the bed for a procedure, return the patient to an elevated position as soon as possible. Check institution policy for suspending feeding while the patient is supine. If intermittent delivery is used, the head should remain elevated for 30 to 60 minutes after feeding.[32]

Aspiration Risk. Evaluate all enterally fed patients for risk of aspiration. Before starting tube feedings, ensure that the tube is in the proper position. Maintain head-of-bed elevation as described above. Checking gastric residual volumes is important when feedings are administered into the stomach. For example, when the infusion rate is 100 mL/hr, the total infused volume of 400 mL may accumulate when gastric emptying is delayed. In addition, gastric secretions can increase the volume beyond 400 mL. With increased residual volume there is increased risk for aspiration of formula into the lungs.[36,37]

Residual Volumes. Check gastric residual volumes every 4 hours during the first 48 hours for gastrically fed patients. After the enteral feeding goal rate is achieved, gastric residual monitoring may be decreased to every 6 to 8 hours in non–critically ill patients or continued every 4 hours in critically ill patients. (Corrective measures for residual volume are described in Table 40-11.) Feeding tubes may need to be placed below the ligament of Treitz (jejunostomy) when gastric residual volumes consistently measure more than 500 mL. Do not obtain residual volumes for EN delivered through a jejunostomy tube.

Tube Position. Confirm tube position of newly inserted nasal or orogastric tubes before feeding or administering medications. Obtain x-ray confirmation to determine if a blindly placed NG or orogastric tube (small bore or large bore) is properly positioned in the GI tract before administering feedings or medications.

Smaller feeding tubes may be passed directly into the bronchus on insertion without any obvious respiratory manifestations. Do not rely on the auscultation method to differentiate between gastric and respiratory placement, or to differentiate between gastric and small bowel placement. Capnography, a direct monitor of breath-to-breath carbon dioxide level, may be used to detect inadvertent entry of tube into the trachea during insertion. X-ray confirmation is still needed to verify location before feeding. When in doubt, request an x-ray to determine tube location.[37,38]

Maintain proper placement of the tube after feedings are started. A small bowel tube may dislocate upward into the stomach, or the tube's tip can dislocate upward into the esophagus. To determine if a feeding tube has maintained the proper position, mark the exit site of the feeding tube at the time of the initial x-ray and observe for a change in the external tube length during feedings. Recheck the tube insertion length at regular intervals.

Observe for negative pressure when attempting to withdraw fluid from the feeding tube.[39] Negative pressure is more likely felt during attempts to aspirate fluid from a small bowel than from a gastric tube. Observe for unexpected changes in residual volume. An increase in gastric residual volume may indicate displacement of the small intestine tube into the stomach.[39] If a significant increase in the external length is observed, use other bedside tests to help determine whether the tube has become dislocated. These measures include assessment of aspirate color and pH. Because each of these measures has limitations, confirmation is done with more than one single bedside test. Use of technology such as electromagnetic tracking devices along with "tube teams" is associated with reduced tube misplacement.[40]

Complications Related to Tubes and Feedings. The types of problems in patients receiving tube feedings and corrective measures are presented in Table 40-11. When commercial products are used, the concentration, flavor, osmolarity, and amounts of protein, sodium, and fat vary according to the manufacturer. Most commercial formulas are lactose free. The concentrations range from 1 to 2 cal/mL, with most standard formulas providing between 1 and 1.5 cal/mL. Refeeding syndrome, which occasionally occurs with EN, is described below.

Osmolality of the solution is determined by the number and size of particles in solution. In feeding formulas the more hydrolyzed or broken down the nutrients, the greater the osmolality. The more calorically dense the formula, the less water it contains. Protein content greater than 16% can lead to dehydration unless the patient is given supplemental fluids or is sufficiently alert to request additional fluids.

Be aware of this potential problem and provide extra fluids through the feeding tube or, if permitted, by mouth. Tube feedings with high sodium content are contraindicated in the patient with cardiovascular problems, such as heart failure. High fat content is not advocated for a patient with short bowel syndrome or ileocecal resection because of impaired fat absorption.

The registered dietitian is an important health care team member in providing EN. Some institutions have nutritional support teams composed of a physician, nurse, dietitian, and pharmacist. The team's function is to oversee the nutritional support of select inpatients and outpatients. The nutritional support nurse on that team is a key resource for issues regarding patients' nutrition.

In patients receiving gastrostomy or jejunostomy feeding, be alert to two possible problems: (1) skin irritation and (2) dislodgment of the tube. Skin care around the tube site is important because the action of the digestive juices irritates the skin. Assess the skin around the feeding tube daily for signs of redness and maceration. To keep the skin clean and dry, initially rinse it with sterile water and then dry it. Once the site has healed, wash with mild soap and water. A protective ointment (zinc oxide, petroleum gauze) or a skin barrier (karaya, Stomahesive) may be used on the skin around the tube. Other types of drain or tube pouches may be used if the skin is irritated. An enterostomal therapist can provide assistance if these issues arise.

Teach the patient and caregiver how to care for the feeding tube. Accidental tube removal can result in delayed feedings and potential discomfort with tube replacement. Patient teaching includes skin care, care of the tube, and complete information about feeding administration and potential complications.

DELEGATION DECISIONS

Nasogastric and Gastric Tubes and Enteral Feedings

Role of Registered Nurse (RN)
- Insert nasogastric (NG) tube for unstable patient.
- Irrigate NG or gastrostomy tube for unstable patient.
- Insert nasointestinal tube.
- After tube placement is verified, administer bolus or continuous enteral feeding for unstable patient.
- Administer medications through the NG or gastrostomy tube to unstable patient.
- Evaluate nutritional status of patient receiving enteral feedings.
- Monitor for complications related to tubes and enteral feedings.
- Develop plan for gastrostomy or jejunostomy tube care.
- Teach patient and caregiver about home enteral feeding and gastrostomy or jejunostomy tube care.
- Evaluate for therapeutic effect of NG tube connected to suction (e.g., decreased nausea or distention).

Role of Licensed Practical/Vocational Nurse (LPN/LVN)
- Insert NG tube for stable patient.
- Irrigate NG and gastrostomy tubes.
- Administer bolus or continuous enteral feeding for stable patient.
- Remove NG tube.
- Administer medications through NG or gastrostomy tube to stable patient.
- Provide skin care around gastrostomy or jejunostomy tubes.

Role of Unlicensed Assistive Personnel (UAP)
- Provide oral care to patient with NG, gastrostomy, or jejunostomy tube.
- Weigh patient who is receiving enteral feeding.
- Position and maintain patient receiving enteral feeding with the head of bed elevated.
- Notify RN or LPN about patient symptoms (e.g., nausea, diarrhea) that may indicate problems with enteral feedings.
- Alert RN or LPN about enteral feeding infusion pump alarms.
- Empty drainage devices and measure output.

An *enteral feeding misconnection* is an inadvertent connection between an enteral feeding system and a nonenteral system such as an IV line, a peritoneal dialysis catheter, or a tracheostomy tube cuff.[1] With an enteral feeding misconnection, nutritional formula intended for administration into the GI tract is administered via the wrong route, resulting in serious and potentially life-threatening patient complications. Nursing interventions aimed at decreasing the risk of enteral feeding misconnections are found in Table 40-12. eNursing Care Plan 40-1 for patients receiving EN is on the website for this chapter.

GERONTOLOGIC CONSIDERATIONS

ENTERAL NUTRITION

EN strategies, including orogastric, NG, nasointestinal, and gastrostomy feedings, are used in the older patient to improve nutritional status. Because of physiologic changes associated with aging, the older adult is more vulnerable to complications associated with nutritional interventions, especially fluid and electrolyte imbalances. Complications such as diarrhea can leave the patient dehydrated. Decreased thirst perception or impaired cognitive function decreases the patient's ability to seek additional fluids.

With aging, there is an increased risk of glucose intolerance. As a result, the older patient may be more susceptible to hyperglycemia in response to the high carbohydrate load of some

TABLE 40-12	DECREASING RISK OF ENTERAL FEEDING MISCONNECTIONS

1. Teach visitors, LPN/LVNs, and UAP to notify nurse if an enteral feeding line becomes disconnected.
2. Teach visitors, LPN/LVNs, and UAP not to reconnect enteral feeding lines.
3. Do not modify or adapt IV or feeding devices because you may compromise the safety features incorporated into their design.
4. Don't force connections if device parts do not seem to fit properly. Ill-fitting pieces indicate a problem.
5. When making a reconnection, routinely trace lines back to their origins and then ensure that they are secure.
6. When patient arrives on a new unit or setting or during shift handoff, recheck connections and trace all tubes.
7. Route tubes and catheters that have different purposes in unique and standardized directions (e.g., route IV lines toward the patient's head, and route enteral lines toward the feet).
8. Package together all parts needed for enteral feeding and reduce the availability of additional adapters and connectors. This will minimize the availability of dissimilar tubes or catheters that could be improperly connected.
9. Label or color-code feeding tubes and connectors, and teach staff about the labeling or color-coding process in the institution's enteral feeding system.
10. Be sure to identify and confirm the solution's label, since a three-in-one parenteral nutrition solution can appear similar to an enteral nutrition formulation bag. Label the bags with large, bold statements such as "WARNING! For Enteral Use Only—NOT for IV Use."
11. Ensure that all connections are made under proper lighting conditions.
12. Follow your facility's protocol for reporting adverse events and near misses.

Adapted from Millin CJ, Brooks M: Reduce and report enteral feeding tube misconnections, *Nursing* 40:60, 2010; and Guenter P, Hicks RW, Simmons D, et al: Enteral feeding misconnections: a consortium position statement, *Jt Comm J Qual Patient Saf* 34:285, 2008.

TABLE 40-13	INDICATIONS FOR PARENTERAL NUTRITION*

- Chronic severe diarrhea and vomiting
- Complicated surgery or trauma
- GI obstruction
- Intractable diarrhea
- Severe anorexia nervosa
- Severe malabsorption
- Short bowel syndrome
- GI tract anomalies and fistulae

*This list is not all-inclusive.

enteral feeding formulas. If the older adult has compromised cardiovascular function (e.g., heart failure), he or she will have a decreased ability to handle large volumes of formula. In this situation the use of more concentrated formulas (2.0 cal/mL) may be warranted. The older adult also is at increased risk for aspiration caused by gastroesophageal reflux disease (GERD), delayed gastric emptying, hiatal hernia, or diminished gag reflex. Physical mobility, fine motor movement, and visual system changes associated with aging may contribute to difficulties in managing EN in the home setting.

Parenteral Nutrition

Parenteral nutrition (PN) refers to the administration of nutrients by a route other than the GI tract (e.g., the bloodstream). It is used when the GI tract cannot be used for the ingestion, digestion, and absorption of essential nutrients. PN is a relatively safe and practical method of delivering complete nutritional support.

Regular IV solutions of 5% dextrose (5 g dextrose/dL) in water (D_5W) or 5% dextrose in lactated Ringer's solution (D_5LR) contain no protein and have approximately 170 cal/L. The average adult requires a minimum of 1200 to 1500 cal/day to carry out normal physiologic functions. Patients who sustain severe injury, surgery, or burns and those who are malnourished as a result of medical treatment or disease processes have greatly increased nutritional needs. The volume of regular dextrose

solutions needed to meet the caloric requirements exceeds the capacity of the cardiovascular system. Table 40-13 lists common indications for the use of PN.

Composition. Commercially prepared PN base solutions are available. These base solutions contain dextrose and protein in the form of amino acids. The pharmacy adds the prescribed electrolytes (e.g., sodium, potassium, chloride, calcium, magnesium, and phosphate), vitamins, and trace elements (e.g., zinc, copper, chromium, and manganese) to customize and meet the patient's needs. A three-in-one or total nutrient admixture containing an IV fat emulsion, dextrose, and amino acids is widely used.

Calories. Calories in PN are supplied primarily by carbohydrates in the form of dextrose and by fat in the form of fat emulsion. The administration of 100 to 150 g of dextrose daily (1 g provides approximately 3.4 calories, as opposed to oral carbohydrates, which provide 4 calories) has a protein-sparing effect. Adequate nonprotein calories in the form of glucose and fat must be provided to allow use of amino acids for wound healing and not for energy. However, overfeeding can lead to metabolic complications. To minimize these problems, an energy intake of 25 to 35 cal/kg/day in a nonobese patient is often recommended.

The U.S. FDA has approved the use of 10%, 20%, and 30% fat-emulsion solutions. Fat emulsions provide approximately 1 cal/mL (10% solution) or 2 cal/mL (20% solution). The contents of fat emulsion are primarily soybean or safflower triglycerides with egg phospholipids added as an emulsifier.

IV fat emulsions should provide up to 30% of total calories. Most stable patients receive 1 g/kg/day, and the maximum daily lipid dose is 2.5 g/kg/day. Critically ill patients may not tolerate this dose and may receive less than 1 g/kg/day.[31,41] Serum triglyceride levels are determined at the beginning of PN and then monitored closely after that. IV fat emulsions administered separately should be administered over a course of 8 to 10 hours, and the infusion rate should not exceed 0.11 g/kg/hr.[41,42]

It is becoming more common to administer lipid-free PN for the first 3 to 5 days of a critical illness because of the potential for omega-6 fatty acids to produce proinflammatory mediators.[31,41]

Nausea, vomiting, and elevated temperature have been reported, especially when lipids are infused quickly. The administration of fat emulsion is contraindicated in the patient with a disturbance in fat metabolism such as hyperlipidemia. Fat emulsions are used cautiously in the patient at risk for fat embolism (e.g., fractured femur) and the patient with an allergy to eggs or soybeans. Lipid emulsions are also used cautiously in patients with pancreatitis, bleeding disorders, liver failure, and respiratory disease.

Protein. The normal healthy person of average body size needs approximately 45 to 65 g of protein daily. Protein should be provided at the rate of 1 to 1.5 g/kg/day depending on the patient's needs. In a nutritionally depleted patient who is also under the stress of illness or surgery, protein requirements can exceed 150 g/day (1.5 to 2 g/kg/day) to ensure a positive nitrogen balance. Burn patients, who are often on PN, EN, and oral food, may need upward of 2 g/kg protein. Protein needs may be lower than 1 g/kg and restricted in individuals with end-stage renal disease who are not on dialysis.

Electrolytes. Individual requirements should be assessed daily at the beginning of therapy and then several times a week as the treatment progresses. The following are ranges for average daily electrolyte requirements for adult patients without renal or hepatic impairment:[37]

- Sodium: 1 to 2 mEq/kg
- Potassium: 1 to 2 mEq/kg
- Chloride: as needed to maintain acid-base balance
- Magnesium: 8 to 20 mEq
- Calcium: 10 to 15 mEq
- Phosphate: 20 to 40 mmol

The exact amount of electrolytes needed depends on the patient's health problem and on electrolyte levels as determined by blood testing.

Trace Elements and Vitamins. Zinc, copper, chromium, manganese, selenium, molybdenum, and iodine supplements may be added according to the patient's condition and needs. Levels of these elements are monitored in the patient receiving PN, and the health care provider may order additional amounts added to the solutions.

The daily addition of a multivitamin preparation to the PN generally meets the vitamin requirements.

Methods of Administration. PN may be administered as central PN or peripheral parenteral nutrition (PPN). Both central PN and PPN are used in a patient who is not a candidate for EN. The patient receiving PN must be able to tolerate a large volume of fluid.

Central Parenteral Nutrition. *Central PN* is indicated when long-term support is necessary or when the patient has high protein and caloric requirements. Central PN may be given through a central venous catheter that originates at the subclavian or jugular vein and whose tip lies in the superior vena cava (see Fig. 17-18). Central PN can also be given using peripherally inserted central catheters (PICCs) that are placed into the basilic or cephalic vein and then advanced into the distal end of the superior vena cava (see Fig. 17-19).

Peripheral Parenteral Nutrition. *PPN* is administered through a peripherally inserted catheter or vascular access device, which uses a large vein. PPN is used when (1) nutritional support is needed for only a short time, (2) protein and caloric requirements are not high, (3) the risk of a central catheter is too great, or (4) PN is used to supplement inadequate oral intake.

Comparison of Central and Peripheral Parenteral Nutrition. Central PN and PPN differ in tonicity, which is measured in milliosmoles (mOsm; the concentration of particles in a fluid). Blood is isotonic and measures approximately 280 mOsm/L. The standard IV solutions of D_5W and normal saline are essentially isotonic. Central PN solutions are hypertonic, measuring at least 1600 mOsm/L. The high glucose content ranges from 20% to 50%. Central PN must be infused in a large central vein so that rapid dilution can occur. The use of a peripheral vein for hypertonic, central PN solutions would cause irritation and thrombophlebitis. Nutrients can be infused using smaller volumes than PPN. PPN solutions are also hypertonic (as much as 20% glucose), but less so than with central PN, and can be safely administered through a large peripheral vein, although

TABLE 40-14	**COMPLICATIONS OF PARENTERAL NUTRITION**
Infection	**Catheter-Related Problems**
• Fungus	• Air embolus
• Gram-positive bacteria	• Pneumothorax, hemothorax, and hydrothorax
• Gram-negative bacteria	• Hemorrhage
Metabolic Problems	• Dislodgment
• Hyperglycemia, hypoglycemia	• Thrombosis of vein
• Altered renal function	• Phlebitis
• Essential fatty acid deficiency	
• Electrolyte and vitamin excesses and deficiencies	
• Trace mineral deficiencies	
• Hyperlipidemia	

phlebitis can occur. Another potential complication of PPN is fluid overload.

NURSING MANAGEMENT PARENTERAL NUTRITION

Nursing management of patients receiving PN is presented in eTable 40-8 and eNursing Care Plan 40-2 (available on the website for this chapter).

COMPLICATIONS

Refeeding syndrome is characterized by fluid retention and electrolyte imbalances (hypophosphatemia, hypokalemia, hypomagnesemia) (Table 40-14). Conditions that predispose patients to refeeding syndrome include long-standing malnutrition states such as chronic alcoholism, vomiting and diarrhea, chemotherapy, and major surgery. Refeeding syndrome can occur any time a malnourished patient is started on aggressive nutritional support. Hypophosphatemia is the hallmark of refeeding syndrome and is associated with serious outcomes, including cardiac dysrhythmias, respiratory arrest, and neurologic disturbances (e.g., paresthesias).

HOME NUTRITIONAL SUPPORT

Home PN or EN is an accepted mode of nutritional therapy for the person who does not require hospitalization but who requires continued nutritional support. Some patients have been successfully treated at home for many months and even years. It is important for you to teach the patient and caregiver about catheter or tube care, proper technique in mixing and handling of the solutions and tubing, and side effects and complications.

Home nutritional therapies are expensive. For patients to be reimbursed for expenses, specific criteria must be met. The discharge planning team needs to be involved early in the admission to help plan for such issues. Home nutritional support may also be a burden on the patient and the caregivers and may affect quality of life. Tell the family about support groups such as the Oley Foundation *(www.oley.org)* that provide peer support and advocacy.

EATING DISORDERS

Eating disorders are primarily psychiatric disorders and occur more often in women. Men are also at risk, but are less likely to seek treatment because eating disorders are perceived to be a women's disease.[43] The notion that eating disorders occur more frequently in whites is being challenged. African Americans, Asian Americans, and Mexican Americans are also at risk for eating disorders.[44,45] Patients with eating disorders may be hospitalized for fluid and electrolyte alterations; cardiac dysrhythmias; nutritional, endocrine, and metabolic disorders; and menstrual problems.[46] A number of nutritional problems associated with these disorders require you to implement a nutritional plan of care.

The three most common types of eating disorders are anorexia nervosa, bulimia nervosa, and binge-eating disorder.

Anorexia Nervosa

Anorexia nervosa is characterized by a self-imposed weight loss, endocrine dysfunction, and a distorted psychopathologic attitude toward weight and eating.[47] Anorexia nervosa is a serious mental illness affecting 1.2% to 2.2% of people during their lifetime, and it occurs more frequently in women.[44] Anorexia nervosa clinically manifests as abnormal weight loss, deliberate self-starvation, intense fear of gaining weight, *lanugo* (soft, downy hair covering the body except the palms and soles), refusal to eat, continuous dieting, hair loss, sensitivity to cold, compulsive exercise, absent or irregular menstruation, dry and yellowish skin, and constipation. Signs of malnutrition are noted during the physical examination.

Diagnostic studies often show iron-deficiency anemia and an elevated blood urea nitrogen level that reflects marked intravascular volume depletion and abnormal renal function. Lack of potassium in the diet and loss of potassium in the urine lead to potassium deficiency. Manifestations of potassium deficiency include muscle weakness, cardiac dysrhythmias, and renal failure. Leukopenia, hypoglycemia, hyponatremia, hypomagnesemia, and hypophosphatemia may also be present.

Multidisciplinary treatment must involve a combination of nutritional support and psychiatric care.[48] Nutritional rehabilitation focuses on reaching and maintaining a healthy weight, normal eating patterns, and perception of hunger and satiety. Hospitalization may be necessary if the patient has medical complications that cannot be managed in an outpatient therapy program. Nutritional repletion must be closely supervised to ensure consistent and ongoing weight gains. Refeeding syndrome is a rare but serious complication of refeeding programs. The use of EN or PN may be necessary.

Improved nutrition, however, is not a cure for anorexia nervosa. The underlying psychiatric problem must be addressed by identification of the disturbed patterns of individual and family interactions, followed by individual and family counseling.

Bulimia Nervosa

Bulimia nervosa is a disorder characterized by frequent binge eating and self-induced vomiting associated with loss of control related to eating and a persistent concern with body image.[47] Individuals with bulimia nervosa may have normal weight for height, or their weight may fluctuate with bingeing and purging. They may also abuse laxatives, diuretics, exercise, or diet drugs. They may have signs of frequent vomiting, such as macerated knuckles, swollen salivary glands, broken blood vessels in the eyes, and dental problems. The individual with bulimia nervosa goes to great lengths to conceal abnormal eating habits. Abnormal laboratory parameters, including hypokalemia, metabolic alkalosis, and elevated serum amylase, may occur with frequent vomiting.[47]

The cause of bulimia remains unclear but is thought to be similar to that of anorexia nervosa. Substance abuse, anxiety, affective disorders, and personality disturbances have been reported among persons with bulimia. Over time, problems associated with bulimia become increasingly hard to deal with effectively. A treatment combination of psychologic counseling and diet therapy is essential.[48]

Antidepressants are helpful for some but not all patients with bulimia. Education and emotional support for the patient and family are vital. Support groups such as the National Association of Anorexia Nervosa and Associated Disorders (ANAD) *(www.anad.org)* are helpful to those affected by these disorders.

Binge-eating disorder is less severe than bulimia nervosa and anorexia nervosa. Individuals with binge-eating disorder do not have a distorted body image and are often overweight or obese.[49]

CASE STUDY

Undernutrition

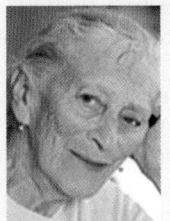

iStockphoto/Thinkstock

Patient Profile
M.S. is a 70-yr-old white woman who is 5 ft, 4 in tall and weighs 100 lb. She was recently admitted to the inpatient medical unit.

Subjective Data
- Reports 30-lb weight loss in past 2 mo
- Recently had a thrombotic stroke with hemiparesis and dysphagia
- Has a history of rheumatoid arthritis
- Has had nothing by mouth for the past 24 hr and just started enteral nutrition via PEG tube
- Lives with her daughter, who is at her bedside

Objective Data
Physical Examination
- Has left-sided weakness
- BP is 150/90 mm Hg
- A PEG tube was recently placed

Laboratory Results
- Serum albumin 2.9 g/dL
- Prealbumin 11.0 mg/dL

Discussion Questions
1. What are M.S.'s risk factors for malnutrition?
2. What is her BMI?
3. What are contributing factors to her developing dysphagia and malnutrition?
4. What should you include in a successful weight gain program for M.S.?
5. Which possible complications of enteral nutrition could M.S. be at risk for developing?
6. *Priority Decision:* What is the priority of the nursing care for M.S.?
7. *Priority Decision:* Based on the assessment data presented, write one or more appropriate nursing diagnoses. Are there any collaborative problems?
8. *Delegation Decision:* How would you use unlicensed assistive personnel (UAP) to care for M.S.?
9. *Evidence-Based Practice:* M.S.'s daughter tells you that her mother's abdomen appears bloated and she wonders if she should massage it.

▌ BRIDGE TO NCLEX EXAMINATION

The number of the question corresponds to the same-numbered outcome at the beginning of the chapter.

1. The percentage of daily calories for a healthy individual consists of
   a. 50% carbohydrates, 25% protein, 25% fat, and <10% of fat from saturated fatty acids.
   b. 65% carbohydrates, 25% protein, 25% fat, and >10% of fat from saturated fatty acids.
   c. 50% carbohydrates, 40% protein, 10% fat, and <10% of fat from saturated fatty acids.
   d. 40% carbohydrates, 30% protein, 30% fat, and >10% of fat from saturated fatty acids.

2. During starvation, the order in which the body obtains substrate for energy is
   a. visceral protein, skeletal protein, fat, glycogen.
   b. glycogen, skeletal protein, fat stores, visceral protein.
   c. visceral protein, fat stores, glycogen, skeletal protein.
   d. fat stores, skeletal protein, visceral protein, glycogen.

3. A complete nutritional assessment including anthropometric measurements is important for the patient who
   a. has a BMI of 25.5 kg/m^2.
   b. complains of frequent nocturia.
   c. reports a 5-year history of constipation.
   d. reports an unintentional weight loss of 10 lb in 2 months.

4. The nurse confirms initial placement of a blindly inserted small-bore NG feeding tube by
   a. x-ray.
   b. air insufflation.
   c. observing patient for coughing.
   d. pH measurement of gastric aspirate.

5. A patient is receiving peripheral parenteral nutrition. The parenteral nutrition solution is completed before the new solution arrives on the unit. The nurse administers
   a. 20% intralipids.
   b. 5% dextrose solution.
   c. 0.45% normal saline solution.
   d. 5% lactated Ringer's solution.

6. A patient with anorexia nervosa shows signs of malnutrition. During initial refeeding, the nurse carefully assesses the patient for
   a. hyperkalemia.
   b. hypoglycemia.
   c. hypercalcemia.
   d. hypophosphatemia.

1. a, 2. b, 3. d, 4. a, 5. b, 6. d

ⓔvolve

For rationales to these answers and even more NCLEX review questions, visit *http://evolve.elsevier.com/Lewis/medsurg.*

REFERENCES

1. ASPEN Board of Directors: Definition of terms, style, and conventions used in ASPEN. Retrieved from *www.nutritioncare. org/Professional_Resources/Guidelines_and_Standards/ Guidelines/2010_Definitions_of_Terms,_Style,_and_ Conventions_Used_in_A_S_P_E_N__Board_of_Directors.*
2. Holben D: Position of the American Dietetic Association: food insecurity in the United States, *J Am Diet Assoc* 110:1368, 2010.
3. US Food and Drug Administration: Nutrition facts label programs. Retrieved from *www.fda.gov/Food/ResourcesForYou/ Consumers/NFLPM/default.htm.*
*4. Academy of Nutrition and Dietetics: Adult weight management evidence-based nutrition practice guideline: executive summary. Retrieved from *www.adaevidencelibrary.com/ topic.cfm?cat=3014.*
5. Mifflin MD, St. Jeor ST, Hill LA, et al: A new predictive equation for resting energy expenditure in healthy individuals, *Am J Clin Nutr* 51:242, 1990. (Classic)
6. Wooley JA, Frankenfield D: Energy. In Gotschlich MM, DeLegge MH, Mattox T, et al, editors: *The A.S.P.E.N. nutrition support core curriculum: a case-based approach—the adult patient,* Silver Spring, Md, 2007, ASPEN. (Classic)
7. US Department of Agriculture and US Department of Health and Human Services: *Dietary guidelines for Americans, 2010,* ed 7, Washington, DC, 2010, US Government Printing Office.
8. Mozaffaarian D, Wu JH: Fatty acids and cardiovascular health: are effects of EPA and DHA shared or complementary? *J Nutr* 142:614S, 2012.

9. Satia J: Dietary acculturation and the nutrition transition: an overview, *Appl Physiol Nutr Metab* 35:219, 2010.
10. Spencer A, Jablonski R, Susan SJ: Hypertensive African American women and the DASH diet, *Nurse Pract* 37:41, 2012.
11. Lv N, Brown JL: Impact of a nutrition education program to increase intake of calcium-rich foods by Chinese American women, *J Am Diet Assoc* 111:143, 2011.
*12. Barroso C, Peters RJ, Kelder SH, et al: Beliefs and perceived norms concerning body image among African-American and Latino teenagers, *J Health Psych* 15:858, 2010.
13. Soeters P, Schols A: Advances in understanding and assessing malnutrition, *Curr Opin Clin Nutr Metab Care* 12:487, 2009. (Classic)
14. Heersink J, Brown C, DiMaria-Ghalili R, et al: Undernutrition in hospitalized older adults: patterns and correlates, outcomes, and opportunities for intervention with a focus on processes of care, *J Nutr Elderly* 29:4, 2010.
*15. Kaiser MJ, Bauer JM, Ramsch C, et al: Frequency of malnutrition in older adults: a multinational perspective using the Mini Nutritional Assessment, *J Am Geriatr Soc* 58:1734, 2010.
*16. Jensen GL, Mirtallo J, Compher C, et al: Adult starvation and disease-related malnutrition: a proposal for etiology-based diagnosis in the clinical practice setting from the International Consensus Guideline Committee, *JPEN J Parenter Enteral Nutr* 34:156, 2010.
17. Osorio SN: Reconsidering kwashiorkor, *Top Clin Nutr* 26:10, 2011.
18. Mueller C: Inflammation and malnutrition, *Top Clin Nutr* 26:3, 2011.
19. Wilmore DW: *The metabolic management of the critically ill,* New York, 1977, Plenum. (Classic)

*Evidence-based information for clinical practice.

20. Otten JJ, Hellwig JP, Meyers LD: *Dietary reference intakes: the essential guide to nutrient requirements*, Washington, DC, 2006, National Academies Press. (Classic)

*21. Mueller C, Compher C, Druyan ME, et al: A.S.P.E.N. clinical guidelines: nutrition screening, assessment, and intervention in adults, *JPEN J Parenter Enteral Nutr* 35:16, 2011.

22. Jensen GL: Nutrition assessment and requirements. In Marian M, Russell MK, Shikora SA, editors: *Clinical nutrition for surgical patients*, Boston, 2008, Jones & Bartlett. (Classic)

*23. Skipper A, Ferguson M, Thompson K, et al: Nutrition screening tools: an analysis of the evidence, *JPEN J Parenter Enteral Nutr* 36:292, 2012.

24. DiMaria-Ghalili RA, Guenter PA: The mini-nutritional assessment, *Am J Nurs* 108:50, 2008. (Classic)

25. Dorner B, Posthauer ME, Friedrich EK, et al: Enteral nutrition for older adults in nursing facilities, *Nutr Clin Pract* 26:261, 2011.

26. Guralnik JM, Simonsick EM, Ferrucci L, et al: Short physical performance battery. Retrieved from *www.pt.ntu.edu.tw/mhh/course/neuro/BS/mmh_geriatric/ShortPhysicalPerformance Battery%5B2%5D.pdf.*

27. Vogelzang JL: Making nutrition sense from OASIS, *Home Healthc Nurse* 21:592, 2003. (Classic)

28. DiMaria-Ghalili RA: Nutrition. In Boltz M, Capezuti E, Fulmer T, et al, editors: *Evidence-based geriatric nursing protocols for best practice*, ed 4, New York, 2012, Springer.

*29. Luft VC, Beghetto M, Castro SMJ, et al: Validation of a new method developed to measure the height of adult patients in bed, *Nutr Clin Pract* 23:424, 2008. (Classic)

*30. Gupta R, Knobel D, Gunabushanam V, et al: The effect of low body mass index on outcome in critically ill surgical patients, *Nutr Clin Pract* 26:593, 2011.

31. Worthington PH, Gilber KA: Parenteral nutrition: risks, complications, and management, *J Infus Nurs* 35:52, 2012.

32. Institute of Medicine: *Retooling for an aging America: building the health care workforce*, Washington, DC, 2008, National Academies Press. (Classic)

33. Locher JL, Wellman NS: "Never the twain shall meet": dual systems exacerbate malnutrition in older adults recently discharged from hospitals, *J Nutr Gerontol Geriatr* 30:24, 2011.

34. English K, Paddon-Jones D: Protecting muscle mass and function in older adults during bed rest, *Curr Opin Clin Nutr Metab Care* 13:34, 2010.

*35. Milne AC, Potter J, Vivanti A, et al: Protein and energy supplementation in elderly people at risk from malnutrition, *Cochrane Database Syst Rev* 2:CD003288, 2009. (Classic)

*36. Enteral Nutrition Practice Recommendations Task Force: Enteral nutrition practice recommendations, *JPEN J Parenter Enteral Nutr* 33:122, 2009. (Classic)

*37. Metheny NA, Stewart BJ, McClave SA: Relationship between feeding tube site and respiratory outcomes, *JPEN J Parenter Enteral Nutr* 35:346, 2011.

38. Bankhead RR, Fang JC: Enteral access devices. In Gotschlich MM, DeLegge MH, Mattox T, et al, editors: *The A.S.P.E.N. nutrition support core curriculum: a case-based approach—the adult patient*, Silver Spring, Md, 2007, ASPEN.

39. Boullata J, Carney LN, Guenter P: *A.S.P.E.N. enteral nutrition handbook*, Silver Springs Md, 2010, ASPEN.

40. Koopmann MC, Kudsk KA, Szotkowski MJ, et al: A team-based protocol and electromagnetic technology eliminate feeding tube placement complications, *Ann Surg* 253:287, 2011.

41. Canada T, Crill C, Guenter P: *A.S.P.E.N. parenteral nutrition handbook*, Silver Springs, Md, 2009, ASPEN. (Classic)

*42. ASPEN Board of Directors: Guidelines for the use of parenteral and enteral nutrition in adult and pediatric patients, *JPEN J Parenter Enteral Nutr* 26(Suppl 1):1SA, 2002. (Classic)

43. National Association of Anorexia Nervosa and Associated Disorders: Eating disorders statistics. Retrieved from *www.anad.org/get-information/about-eating-disorders/eating-disorders-statistics.*

44. Talleyrand RM: Eating disorders in African American girls: implications for counselors, *J Counsel Develop* 88:319, 2010.

45. National Eating Disorders Association: Research results on eating disorders in diverse populations. Retrieved from *www.nationaleatingdisorders.org.*

*46. Zhao Y, Encinosa W: *An update on hospitalizations for eating disorders, 1999 to 2009*, HCUP Statistical Brief No 120, Rockville, Md, 2011, Agency for Healthcare Research and Quality.

47. Miller CA, Golder NH: An introduction to eating disorders: clinical presentation, epidemiology, and prognosis, *Nutr Clin Pract* 25:110, 2010.

48. Reiter CS, Graves L: Nutrition therapy for eating disorders, *Nutr Clin Pract* 25:122, 2010.

49. National Institute of Mental Health: Eating disorders. Retrieved from *www.nimh.nih.gov/health/publications/eating-disorders/index.shtml.*

RESOURCES

Academy for Eating Disorders
www.aedweb.org
Academy of Nutrition and Dietetics (formerly American Dietetic Association)
www.eatright.org
American Society for Parenteral and Enteral Nutrition (ASPEN)
www.nutritioncare.org
FDA Food Safety
www.fda.gov/Food/FoodSafety/
Institute of Medicine, Food and Nutrition Board
www.iom.edu/About-IOM/Leadership-Staff/Boards/Food-and-Nutrition-Board.aspx
National Eating Disorder Information Centre
www.nedic.ca
National Eating Disorders Association
www.nationaleatingdisorders.org
U.S. Department of Agriculture, MyPlate
www.choosemyplate.gov

41

If you have a dream, don't just sit there.
Gather courage to believe that you can
succeed and leave no stone unturned
to make it a reality.
Rooplean

Nursing Management

Obesity

Judi Daniels

---

evolve WEBSITE

http://evolve.elsevier.com/Lewis/medsurg
- NCLEX Review Questions
- Key Points
- Pre-Test
- Answer Guidelines for Case Study on p. 922
- Rationales for Bridge to NCLEX Examination Questions

- Case Study
  - Patient With Obesity and Osteoarthritis
- Concept Map Creator
- Glossary
- Content Updates

eFigure
- eFig. 41-1: Obese women

eTables
- eTable 41-1: Comparison of Fad Diets
- eTable 41-2: Nutritional Therapy: Meal Plans for 1200-Calorie–Restricted Weight-Reduction Diet

LEARNING OUTCOMES

1. Discuss the epidemiology and etiology of obesity.
2. Compare the classification systems for determining a person's body size.
3. Explain the health risks associated with obesity.
4. Discuss nutritional therapy and exercise plans for the obese patient.
5. Describe the different bariatric surgical procedures used to treat obesity.
6. Describe the nursing management related to conservative and surgical therapies for obesity.
7. Describe the etiology, clinical manifestations, and nursing and collaborative management of metabolic syndrome.

KEY TERMS

bariatric surgery, p. 916
body mass index (BMI), p. 906
lipectomy, p. 917

metabolic syndrome, p. 921
obese, p. 906
overweight, p. 906

severely obese, p. 906
waist-to-hip ratio (WHR), p. 907

OBESITY

Obesity is an excessively high amount of body fat or adipose tissue (Fig. 41-1). Obesity is a major health problem because it increases the risk of numerous other diseases such as diabetes and cancer.[1]

Classifications of Body Weight and Obesity

An important part of your patient assessment is to determine and classify a patient's body weight. A number of assessment methods are available, including body mass index (BMI), waist circumference, waist-to-hip ratio (WHR), and body shape. The most widely used and endorsed measures are BMI and waist circumference.[2] These measures are cost-effective with acceptable reliability and are easily used in all practice settings.

Body Mass Index. The most common measure of obesity is the body mass index (BMI). BMI is calculated by dividing a person's weight (in kilograms) by the square of the height in meters (Fig. 41-2). Individuals with a BMI less than 18.5 kg/m^2 are considered underweight, whereas those with a BMI between 18.5 and 24.9 kg/m^2 reflect a normal body weight. A BMI of 25 to 29.9 kg/m^2 is classified as being overweight, and those with values at 30 kg/m^2 or above are considered obese. The term severely (*morbidly, extremely*) obese is used for those with a BMI greater than 40 kg/m^2 (eFig. 41-1 on the website shows individuals who are severely obese).

Table 41-1 shows the classification of overweight and obesity by BMI. The BMI, which provides an overall assessment of fat mass, must be considered in relation to the patient's age, gender, and body build. For example, a body builder may have a BMI associated with obesity but because of a high

---

Reviewed by Amanda J. Flagg, PhD, ACNS-BC, CNE, Assistant Clinical Professor, University of Texas Health Science Center at San Antonio School of Nursing, San Antonio, Texas; and Daryle Wane, PhD, ARNP, FNP-BC, Professor of Nursing, Generic Program Track Coordinator, Pasco-Hernando Community College, New Port Richey, Florida.

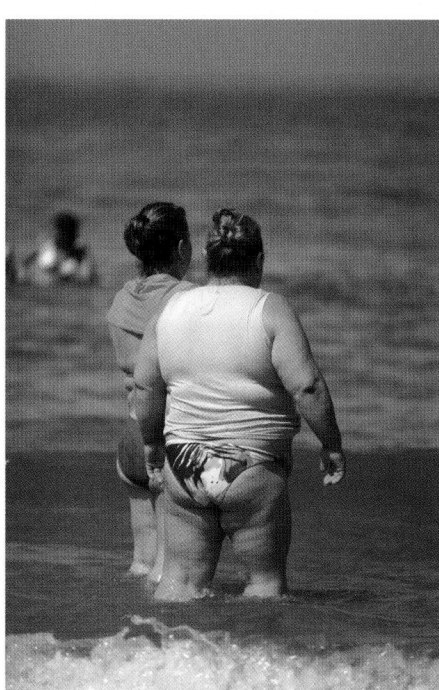

FIG. 41-1 Obesity is an epidemic in the United States. (iStockphoto/Thinkstock)

$$BMI\ (kg/m^2) = \frac{Weight\ (pounds) \times 703}{Height\ (inches)^2}$$

Weight in Pounds

Height	120	130	140	150	160	170	180	190	200	210	220	230	240	250
4'6	29	31	34	36	39	41	43	46	48	51	53	56	58	60
4'8	27	29	31	34	36	38	40	43	45	47	49	52	54	56
4'10	25	27	29	31	34	36	38	40	42	44	46	48	50	52
5'0	23	25	27	29	31	33	35	37	39	41	43	45	47	49
5'2	22	24	26	27	29	31	33	35	37	38	40	42	44	46
5'4	21	22	24	26	28	29	31	33	34	36	38	40	41	43
5'6	19	21	23	24	26	27	29	31	32	34	36	37	39	40
5'8	18	20	21	23	24	26	27	29	30	32	34	35	37	38
5'10	17	19	20	22	23	24	26	27	29	30	32	33	35	36
6'0	16	18	19	20	22	23	24	26	27	28	30	31	33	34
6'2	15	17	18	19	21	22	23	24	26	27	28	30	31	32
6'4	15	16	17	18	20	21	22	23	24	26	27	28	29	30
6'6	14	15	16	17	19	20	21	22	23	24	25	27	28	29
6'8	13	14	15	17	18	19	20	21	22	23	24	25	26	28

Height in Feet and Inches

☐ Underweight ☐ Normal weight ☐ Overweight ☐ Obese ☐ Severely obese

FIG. 41-2 Body mass index (BMI) chart. Healthy weight: BMI 18 to 24.9 kg/m²; overweight: BMI 25 to 29.9 kg/m²; obesity: BMI 30 kg/m². BMI = weight (kg)/height (m²).

muscle mass, the BMI would not be an accurate assessment. In contrast, in individuals who have lost body mass (e.g., older adults), the BMI would underestimate the degree of obesity. For this reason, other measures must be combined with the BMI for an accurate evaluation of a person's weight.

Waist Circumference. *Waist circumference* is another way to assess and classify a person's weight (see Table 41-1). People who have visceral fat with truncal obesity are at an increased risk for cardiovascular disease and metabolic syndrome (discussed later in this chapter). Health risks increase if the waist circumference is greater than 40 inches in men and greater than 35 inches in women.[1]

Waist-to-Hip Ratio. The waist-to-hip ratio (WHR) is another tool used to assess obesity. This ratio is a method of describing the distribution of both subcutaneous and visceral adipose tissue. The ratio is calculated by using the waist measurement divided by the hip measurement. A WHR less than 0.8 is optimal, and a WHR greater than 0.8 indicates more truncal fat, which puts the individual at a greater risk for health complications.

Body Shape. *Body shape* is another method of identifying those who are at a higher risk for health problems (Table 41-2). Individuals with fat located primarily in the abdominal area, an *apple-shaped body*, have *android obesity*. Those with fat distribution in the upper legs, a *pear-shaped body*, have *gynoid obesity*. Genetics has an important role in determining a person's body shape. Weight and shape are influenced by genetics.[3]

Epidemiology of Obesity

Currently, more than 35% of adults in the United States are obese. Unless Americans change their ways, 50% of the U.S. population will be obese by 2030.[4] Women having a slightly higher incidence of obesity than men. When those who are

TABLE 41-1 CLASSIFICATION OF OVERWEIGHT AND OBESITY

	BMI (kg/m²)	Obesity Class	Disease Risk Based on Waist Circumference* Men ≤40 in (102 cm) Women ≤35 in (89 cm)	Men >40 in (102 cm) Women >35 in (89 cm)
Underweight	<18.5	—	—	—
Normal†	18.5-24.9	—	—	—
Overweight	25.0-29.9	—	Increased	High
Obese	30.0-34.9	Class I	High	Very high
	35.0-39.9	Class II	Very high	Very high
Severely obese	≥40.0	Class III	Extremely high	Extremely high

Source: National Heart, Lung, and Blood Institute: Classification of overweight and obesity by BMI, waist circumference, and associated disease risks. Retrieved from *www.nhlbi.nih.gov/health/public/heart/obesity/lose_wt/bmi_dis.htm.*
*Disease risk for type 2 diabetes, hypertension, and cardiovascular disease relative to person of normal weight.
†Increased waist circumference can also be a marker for increased risk in persons of normal weight.
BMI, Body mass index.

TABLE 41-2 RELATIONSHIP BETWEEN BODY SHAPE AND HEALTH RISKS

Body Shape	Characteristics	Health Risks
Gynoid (pear) 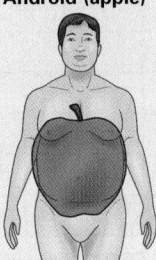	• Fat mainly located in the upper legs • Has a better prognosis but difficult to treat	• Osteoporosis • Varicose veins • Cellulite • Subcutaneous fat traps and stores dietary fat • Trapped fatty acids stored as triglycerides

Android (apple)	• Fat primarily located in abdominal area
	• Fat also distributed over upper body (neck, arms, shoulders)
	• Greater risk for obesity-related complications
		• Heart disease
		• Diabetes mellitus
		• Breast cancer
		• Endometrial cancer
		• Visceral fat more active, causing
		  • ↓ Insulin sensitivity
		  • ↑ Triglycerides
		  • ↓ HDL cholesterol
		  • ↑ BP
		  • ↑ Free fatty acid release into blood

HDL, High-density lipoprotein.

CULTURAL & ETHNIC HEALTH DISPARITIES

Obesity

- African Americans and Hispanics have a higher prevalence of obesity than whites.
- Among women, African Americans have the highest prevalence of being overweight or obese, and 15% are severely obese.
- Among men, Mexican Americans have the highest prevalence of being overweight or obese.
- African American and Hispanic women with low incomes appear to have the greatest likelihood of being overweight when compared with other socioeconomic groups.
- Native Americans have a higher prevalence of being overweight than the general population.
- Among Native Americans ages 45 to 74, more than 30% of women are overweight and more than 40% are obese.
- Asian Americans have the lowest prevalence of being overweight and obese compared with the general population.

overweight are included, the incidence of the adult population with a BMI greater than 25 kg/m² increases to more than 68%.[5]

The highest prevalence of obesity occurs between ages 40 and 59 for women and after 60 years of age for men.[5] African Americans have the highest incidence of obesity followed by Hispanics (see Cultural & Ethnic Health Disparities box above).

Obesity in adulthood is often a problem that begins in childhood or adolescence. Nearly one third of children and teens are currently obese or overweight. It is estimated that almost half of overweight adults were overweight in childhood, and two thirds of obese children remained obese into adulthood.[6] Reversing the childhood obesity crisis is key to addressing the overall obesity epidemic.

HEALTHY PEOPLE

Health Impact of Maintaining a Healthy Weight

- Reduces the risk of developing type 2 diabetes mellitus
- Increases chance of longevity and better quality of life
- Lowers the risk of hypertension and elevated cholesterol
- Reduces the risk of heart disease, stroke, and gallbladder disease
- Reduces the likelihood of breathing problems, including sleep apnea and asthma
- Decreases the risk of developing osteoarthritis, low back pain, and certain types of cancers

Etiology and Pathophysiology

Obesity is an increase in body weight beyond the body's physical requirements. This results in an abnormal increase and accumulation of fat cells. However, the processes leading to and sustaining the obese state are complex and still undergoing investigation.

In obesity, there is an increase in the number of adipocytes *(hyperplasia)* and an increase in their size *(hypertrophy).* Adipocyte *hypertrophy* is a process by which adipocytes can increase their volume several thousand–fold to accommodate large increases in lipid storage. In addition, preadipocytes are triggered to become adipocytes once storage of existing fat cells is exceeded.[2] This process primarily occurs in the visceral (intraabdominal) and subcutaneous tissues. The process of *hyperplasia* (increase in numbers) of adipocytes is greatest from infancy through adolescence.

The majority of obese persons have *primary obesity,* which is excess calorie intake over energy expenditure for the body's metabolic demands. Others have *secondary obesity,* which can result from various congenital anomalies, chromosomal anomalies, metabolic problems, or central nervous system lesions and disorders.

The cause of obesity involves significant genetic and biologic factors that are highly influenced by environmental and psychosocial factors. Each of these factors can and should be considered individually, but in reality they are interrelated.

Genetic Link

Studies of twins, adoptees, and families all suggest the existence of genetic factors in obesity.[7,8] The heritability of obesity estimated from twin studies is high, with only slightly lower values in twins raised apart than in those raised together. Similarly, in adoptees the children's BMI correlated with that of their biologic parents rather than their adoptive parents.[9] Estimates of obesity as an inherited problem are more than 50%.[8]

A number of genes have been identified as being linked to obesity. Genes actually may influence how calories are stored and energy released. "Energy-thrifty" genes, once protective against long periods where food was not available, are now maladaptive in societies where food availability is no longer a primary issue.[7] Genes may be responsible for why two individuals living in the same environment can vary considerably in body size.

A strong link exists between a gene known as *FTO* (fat mass and obesity-associated gene) and BMI. Variants of this gene may explain why some people become overweight whereas others do not. People with two copies of a certain allele at the *FTO* gene weigh 7 to 8 lb more and have a greater risk of obesity than those who do not have the risk allele.[10] More research is needed to better understand the role of genes in obesity.

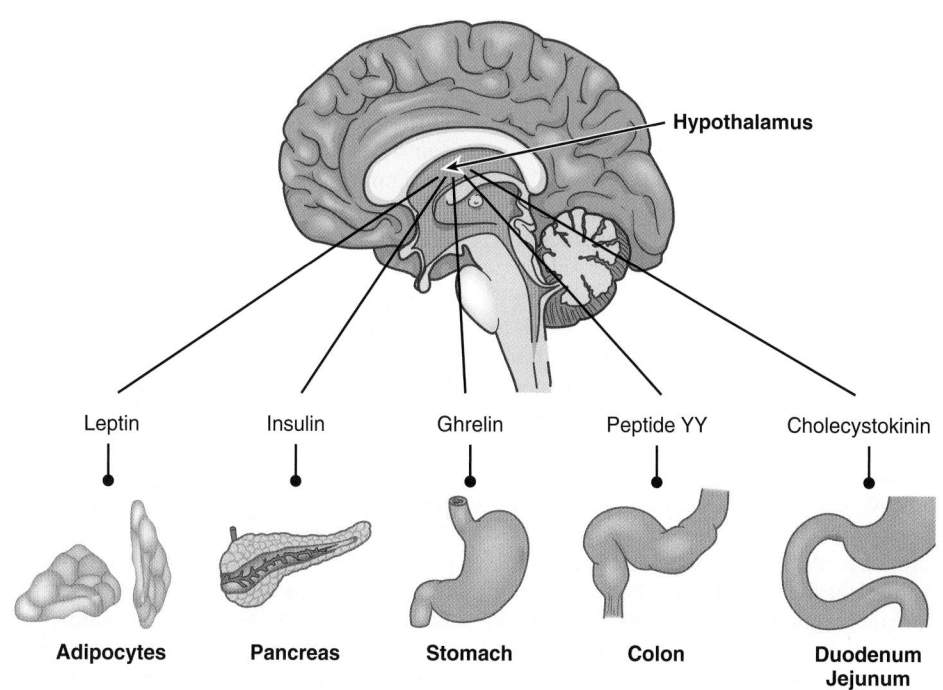

FIG. 41-3 Some of the common hormones and peptides that interact with the hypothalamus to control and influence eating patterns, metabolic activities, and digestion. Obesity disrupts this balance (see Table 41-3).

TABLE 41-3 HORMONES AND PEPTIDES IN OBESITY

Where Produced	Normal Function	Alteration in Obesity	Where Produced	Normal Function	Alteration in Obesity
Neuropeptide Y			**Insulin**		
Hypothalamus	Stimulates appetite	Imbalance causes increased appetite.	Pancreas	Decreases appetite	Increased insulin secretion which stimulates ↑ liver synthesis of triglycerides and ↓ HDL production.
Ghrelin					
Stomach (primarily)	Stimulates appetite ↑ After food deprivation ↓ In response to food in the stomach	Normal postprandial decline does not occur, which can lead to increased appetite and overeating.	**Peptide YY**		
			Colon	Inhibits appetite by slowing GI motility and gastric emptying	Circulating levels are decreased. ↓ Release after eating.
Leptin			**Cholecystokinin**		
Adipocytes	Suppresses appetite and hunger Regulates eating behavior	Obesity is associated with high levels. Leptin resistance develops; thus obese people may lose the effect of appetite suppression.	Duodenum Jejunum	Inhibits gastric emptying and sends satiety signals to hypothalamus	Unknown role

HDL, High-density lipoprotein.

Physiologic Regulatory Mechanisms in Obesity. Research has focused on the physiologic regulatory processes that control eating behavior, energy metabolism, and body fat metabolism. Knowing how appetite is triggered and energy is expended provides important information for understanding obesity and specific targets for the development of drugs.

The hypothalamus, gut, and adipose tissue synthesize hormones and peptides that inhibit or stimulate the appetite (Fig. 41-3). The hypothalamus is a major site for regulating appetite. Neuropeptide Y, produced in the hypothalamus, is a powerful appetite stimulant. When it is imbalanced, it leads to overeating and obesity. Hormones and peptides produced in the gut and adipocyte cells affect the hypothalamus and have a critical role in appetite and energy balance (Table 41-3).

Leptin, secreted from adipocytes when they fill with fat, acts in the hypothalamus to suppress appetite, increase physical activity, and increase fat metabolism. A genetic deficiency of leptin causes extreme obesity. In obesity the level of leptin is actually increased, which has raised the question of whether obese people are insensitive to leptin.[2] Possible causes include failure to produce enough leptin receptors or production of receptors that are faulty.

Ghrelin, a gut hormone, regulates appetite through inhibition of leptin. In a fasting state, ghrelin is increased. Ghrelin acts in the hypothalamus by working on the reward system that triggers overeating. Ghrelin is thought to play a part in compulsive eating. In gastric bypass surgery, ghrelin is decreased significantly, which helps suppress appetite.

The two major consequences of obesity are due to the sheer increase in fat mass and the production of adipokines produced by fat cells. Adipocytes produce at least 100 different proteins. These proteins, secreted as enzymes, adipokines, growth factors, and hormones, contribute to the development of insulin resistance and atherosclerosis.

An increased release of cytokines from fat cells may disrupt immune factors, thus predisposing the person to certain cancers. Because visceral fat accumulation is associated with more alterations of these adipokines, people with abdominal obesity have more complications of obesity.[11]

Environmental Factors. Environmental factors play an important role in obesity. In today's culture, people have greater access to food, particularly prepackaged and fast foods, and soft drinks, which have poor nutritional quality. Portion size of meals has increased dramatically (Table 41-4). The Centers for Disease Control and Prevention has developed visual programs that demonstrate how portions have increased over time.[12] Underestimating portion sizes and therefore caloric intake is common. In addition, eating outside of the home interferes with the ability to control the quality and quantity of food.

Lack of physical exercise is another factor that contributes to weight gain and obesity. With increases in use of technology, labor-saving devices, and cars, Americans are expending less energy in their everyday lives. Elimination of physical education programs in schools, along with increased time spent playing video games and watching TV, has contributed to the increase in sedentary habits.

Socioeconomic status is a known risk factor for obesity in a variety of ways.[13] People with low incomes may attempt to stretch their food dollars by purchasing less expensive foods that often have poor nutritional quality with a greater caloric content. For example, people with low incomes are more likely to purchase pasta, bread, and canned fruit packed with sugar rather than chicken and fresh fruits and vegetables. Low-income residents may also live in environments that do not accommodate outdoor activities (e.g., safe playgrounds, walking tracks, tennis, swimming pools).

TABLE 41-4	**PORTION SIZES: YESTERDAY VS TODAY**	
	25 Yr Ago	**Today**
Turkey sandwich	320 cal	820 cal
Bagel	3-in diameter, 140 cal	6-in diameter, 350 cal
Cheeseburger	333 cal	590 cal
Soda	6½ oz, 85 cal	20 oz, 250 cal

Psychosocial Factors. People use food for many reasons besides their nutritional value. Associations with food begin in childhood, such as the use of food for comfort or rewards. Furthermore, when overeating develops at an early age and continues into adulthood, one's ability to sense fullness *(satiety)* is compromised. Whether triggered by specific foods or by the wide variety of choices, some people consume more food than their bodies need. The lack of hunger that drives eating has been termed "mindless eating" and leads to consumption of unnecessary calories and increase in body weight.[13,14]

Finally, the social component of eating begins early in life when food is associated with pleasure and fun at such events as birthday parties, Thanksgiving, and religious holidays. All of these factors must be included when considering the etiology and treatment of obesity.

HEALTH RISKS ASSOCIATED WITH OBESITY

Hippocrates wrote that "corpulence is not only a disease itself, but the harbinger of others," thus recognizing that obesity has major adverse effects on health. Many problems occur in obese people at higher rates than people of normal weight (Fig. 41-4).

The medical cost of adult obesity in the United States is difficult to calculate, but estimates range from $147 billion to nearly $210 billion per year. The bulk of the spending is from treating obesity-related diseases such as diabetes. Obese people spend 42% more on health care costs than healthy-weight people.[4]

Mortality rates rise as obesity increases, especially when obesity is associated with visceral fat. For obese persons, mortality rates from all causes, especially from cardiovascular disease, are increased by 50% to 100% above those of persons with a normal BMI. Being overweight in midlife, once thought to have fewer health consequences than being obese, confers a 20% to 40% increase in mortality rate for both men and women.[11] In addition to these problems, obese patients have a reduced quality of life. Fortunately, most of these conditions can improve if an individual loses weight.

Cardiovascular Problems

Obesity is a significant risk factor for cardiovascular disease in both men and women.[11] Android obesity is the best predictor of these risks and is linked with increased low-density lipoproteins (LDLs), high triglycerides, and decreased high-density lipoproteins (HDLs). Obesity is also associated with hypertension, which can occur because of increased circulating blood volume, abnormal vasoconstriction, increased inflammation (damaging blood vessels), and increased risk of sleep apnea (raises blood pressure [BP]). Altered lipid metabolism and hypertension can increase the long-term risk of heart disease and stroke. Excess body fat can also lead to chronic inflammation throughout the body, especially in blood vessels, thus increasing the risk of heart disease.

Diabetes Mellitus

More than 80% of people with type 2 diabetes are obese or overweight.[4] Hyperinsulinemia and insulin resistance, common features of type 2 diabetes, are also found in obesity, especially when visceral fat is increased. Excess weight decreases the effectiveness of insulin. When insulin does not work effectively, too much glucose stays in the bloodstream. Thus more insulin is made to compensate. Pancreatic β cells (cells that make insulin)

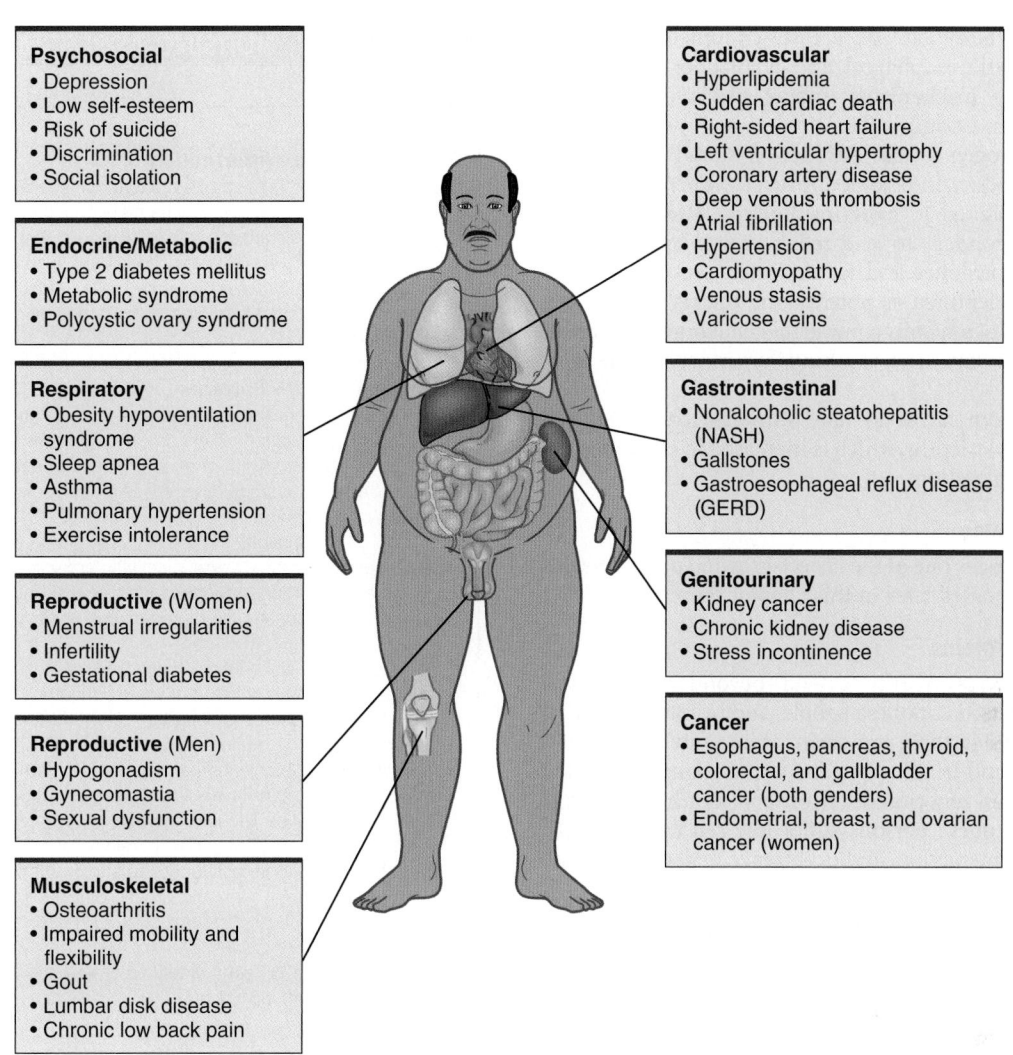

Psychosocial
- Depression
- Low self-esteem
- Risk of suicide
- Discrimination
- Social isolation

Endocrine/Metabolic
- Type 2 diabetes mellitus
- Metabolic syndrome
- Polycystic ovary syndrome

Respiratory
- Obesity hypoventilation syndrome
- Sleep apnea
- Asthma
- Pulmonary hypertension
- Exercise intolerance

Reproductive (Women)
- Menstrual irregularities
- Infertility
- Gestational diabetes

Reproductive (Men)
- Hypogonadism
- Gynecomastia
- Sexual dysfunction

Musculoskeletal
- Osteoarthritis
- Impaired mobility and flexibility
- Gout
- Lumbar disk disease
- Chronic low back pain

Cardiovascular
- Hyperlipidemia
- Sudden cardiac death
- Right-sided heart failure
- Left ventricular hypertrophy
- Coronary artery disease
- Deep venous thrombosis
- Atrial fibrillation
- Hypertension
- Cardiomyopathy
- Venous stasis
- Varicose veins

Gastrointestinal
- Nonalcoholic steatohepatitis (NASH)
- Gallstones
- Gastroesophageal reflux disease (GERD)

Genitourinary
- Kidney cancer
- Chronic kidney disease
- Stress incontinence

Cancer
- Esophagus, pancreas, thyroid, colorectal, and gallbladder cancer (both genders)
- Endometrial, breast, and ovarian cancer (women)

FIG. 41-4 Health risks associated with obesity.

may get overworked and become worn out. Over time, the pancreas is no longer able to keep blood glucose in normal range. It appears that adiponectin, a peptide that increases insulin sensitivity, is decreased in obese people.

Obesity is a major risk factor for development of type 2 diabetes. Furthermore, obesity complicates the management of type 2 diabetes by increasing insulin resistance and glucose intolerance, which makes drug treatment for diabetes less effective. A weight reduction of 7% can decrease the risk of diabetes by 58%.[15]

Gastrointestinal and Liver Problems

Gastroesophageal reflux disease (GERD) and gallstones are more prevalent in obese people. Gallstones occur due to supersaturation of the bile with cholesterol. Nonalcoholic steatohepatitis (NASH) is a condition in which lipids are deposited in the liver, resulting in a fatty liver. NASH is associated with elevated hepatic glucose production. NASH can eventually progress to cirrhosis and can be fatal. Weight loss can improve NASH.

Respiratory and Sleep Problems

The increased fat mass associated with obesity may lead to sleep apnea and obesity hypoventilation syndrome. The increased distribution of fat around the diaphragm causes a reduced chest

wall compliance, increased work of breathing, and decreased total lung capacity and functional residual capacity. Sleep apnea results from increased fat around the neck, leading to snoring and hypoventilation while sleeping. Weight loss can bring substantial improvement in lung function.

Poor sleep and sleep deprivation may increase appetite. Sleep deprivation has been associated with obesity. Building up a sleep debt over a matter of days can impair metabolism and disrupt hormone levels. The level of leptin falls in people who are sleep deprived, thus promoting appetite.

Musculoskeletal Problems

Obesity is associated with an increased incidence of osteoarthritis because of the stress put on weight-bearing joints, especially the knees and hips. Increased body fat also triggers inflammatory mediators and contributes to deterioration of cartilage. Hyperuricemia and gout are often found in people who are obese and in those who have metabolic syndrome (discussed later in this chapter).

Cancer

Obesity is one of the most important known preventable causes of cancer. About 20% of cancers in women and 15% in men are attributable to obesity.[16] The types of cancer most strongly linked to excess body fat are breast, endometrial, kidney, colorectal, pancreatic, esophageal, and gallbladder cancer.

The underlying mechanisms linking obesity and cancer remain unclear. Breast and endometrial cancer may be due to the increased estrogen levels (estrogen is stored in fat cells) associated with obesity in postmenopausal women. Colorectal cancer has been linked to hyperinsulinemia, and esophageal cancer may be secondary to acid reflux caused by abdominal obesity. Several hormones and factors often present in obese states have been identified as potentiating the risk for cancer. For example insulin, which is a powerful cellular growth factor, is increased in obesity. The resulting hyperinsulinemia may affect cancer cells.

Adipokines (from fat cells) may stimulate or inhibit cell growth. For example, leptin, which is increased in obese people, promotes cell proliferation.

Metabolic Syndrome

Metabolic syndrome is one of the fastest-growing obesity health concerns. It is discussed later in this chapter on p. 921.

Psychosocial Problems

The consequences of obesity extend beyond the physical changes. Stigmatization of obese people, and in some cases discrimination, occurs in three important areas of living: employment, education, and health care. The social stigma associated with obesity has an emotional toll on a person's psychologic well-being. Many obese persons suffer low self-esteem, withdraw from social interaction, and experience major depression.

NURSING AND COLLABORATIVE MANAGEMENT OBESITY

NURSING ASSESSMENT

The first step in the treatment of obesity is to determine whether any physical conditions are present that may be causing or contributing to obesity. This requires a thorough history and physical examination.

Table 41-5 lists information that can assist you in understanding an obese patient and provides a basis for intervention. When assessing an individual who is overweight or obese, be sensitive and nonjudgmental in asking specific and leading questions about weight, diet, and exercise (Table 41-6). In doing so, you can often obtain information that the patient might have withheld out of embarrassment or shyness. Patients need to understand the rationale for questions asked about weight or dietary habits, and you must be ready to respond to their concerns.

When obtaining the history, explore genetic and endocrine factors such as hypothyroidism, hypothalamic tumors, Cushing syndrome, hypogonadism in men, and polycystic ovary syndrome in women. Laboratory tests of liver function and thyroid function, a fasting glucose level, and a lipid panel (triglyceride level, LDL and HDL cholesterol levels) assist in evaluating the cause and effects of obesity. When no organic cause (e.g., hypothyroidism) is associated with obesity, the disorder should be considered a chronic, complex illness.

As part of the initial nursing history and physical examination, examine each body system with particular attention to the organ system in which the patient has expressed a problem or concern. Measurements used with the obese person may include skinfold thickness, waist circumference, height (without shoes), weight (obtain in a private location and in a gown if possible), and BMI. Provide specific documentation on these areas. Also assess for any co-morbid diseases associated with obesity (e.g., hypertension, sleep apnea), since these conditions require special treatment.

PLANNING

The overall goals are that the obese patient will (1) modify eating patterns, (2) participate in a regular physical activity program, (3) achieve and maintain weight loss to a specified level, and (4) minimize or prevent health problems related to obesity.

TABLE 41-5   NURSING ASSESSMENT

Obese Patient

Subjective Data
Important Health Information
Past health history: Time of obesity onset; diseases related to metabolism and obesity, such as hypertension, cardiovascular problems, stroke, cancer, chronic joint pain, respiratory problems, diabetes mellitus, cholelithiasis, metabolic syndrome
Medications: Thyroid preparations, diet pills, herbal products
Surgery or other treatments: Prior weight-reduction procedures (bariatric surgery)

Functional Health Patterns
Health perception–health management: Family history of obesity; perception of problem; methods of weight loss attempted
Nutritional-metabolic: Amount and frequency of eating; overeating in response to boredom, stress, specific times, or activities; history of weight gain and loss
Elimination: Constipation
Activity-exercise: Typical physical activity; drowsiness, somnolence; dyspnea on exertion, orthopnea, paroxysmal nocturnal dyspnea
Sleep-rest: Sleep apnea, use of continuous positive airway pressure (CPAP)
Cognitive-perceptual: Feelings of rejection, depression, isolation, guilt, or shame; meaning or value of food; adherence to prescribed reducing diets, degree of long-term commitment to a weight loss program
Role-relationship: Change in financial status or family relationships; personal, social, and financial resources to support a reducing diet
Sexuality-reproductive: Menstrual irregularity, heavy menstrual flow in women, birth control practices, infertility; effect of obesity on sexual activity and attractiveness to significant other

Objective Data
General
Body mass index $\geq$30 kg/m^2; waist circumference: woman >35 in (89 cm), man >40 in (102 cm)

Respiratory
Increased work of breathing; wheezing; rapid, shallow breathing

Cardiovascular
Hypertension, tachycardia, dysrhythmias

Musculoskeletal
Decreased joint mobility and flexibility; knee, hip, and low back pain

Reproductive
Gynecomastia and hypogonadism in men

Possible Findings
Elevated serum glucose, cholesterol, triglycerides; chest x-ray demonstrating enlarged heart; electrocardiogram showing dysrhythmia; abnormal liver function tests

TABLE 41-6 ASSESSING PATIENTS WITH OBESITY

When assessing patients with obesity and before selecting a weight loss strategy, ask the following questions.

- What is your history with weight gain and weight loss?
- What is your motivation for losing weight?
- Would you like to manage your weight differently? If so, how?
- What do you think contributes to your weight?
- What sort of barriers do you think impede your weight loss efforts?
- Are there any major stresses that will make it difficult to focus on weight control?
- What does food mean to you? How do you use food (e.g., to relieve stress, provide comfort)?
- Are other family members overweight?
- How much time can you devote to exercise on a daily or weekly basis?
- How has your health been affected by your body weight?
- What type of support do you have from family and/or friends for losing weight?

TABLE 41-7 COLLABORATIVE CARE

Obesity

Diagnostic
- History and physical examination
- BMI
- Waist-to-hip ratio

Collaborative Therapy
- Nutritional therapy
- Exercise
- Behavior modification
- Support groups
- Drug therapy
  - Appetite-suppressing drugs
  - Nutrient absorption–blocking drugs (orlistat [Xenical])
  - Serotonin agonists (lorcaserin [Belviq])
  - phentermine and topiramate (Qsymia)
- Surgical therapy (see Table 41-9)

BMI, Body mass index.

NURSING IMPLEMENTATION

Obesity is one of the most challenging health crises in the United States. It is a chronic disease, much like hypertension and diabetes. Although obese people can lose weight, they often tend to regain weight. For most patients, lifelong management is indicated.

Together with other members of the health care team, you have a major role in planning for and managing the care of an obese patient. First, examine your own personal beliefs and any potential biases related to obesity. If you associate obesity with a lack of willpower and with overindulgence, the patient can experience shame in a setting that claims to be a caring one. You are in a pivotal position to help overweight and obese individuals. Interventions include helping obese patients explore and deal with their negative experiences and educating other health professionals about stigma and biases experienced by obese patients.

Although health care for obese people has inherently greater demands, health care providers often fail to address these needs, and obese people underutilize health care opportunities available to them. Health care providers are often reluctant to counsel patients about obesity for a variety of reasons, including (1) time constraints during appointments make it difficult, (2) weight management may be viewed as professionally unrewarding, (3) reimbursement for weight management services is difficult to obtain, and (4) many providers do not feel knowledgeable about giving weight loss advice.

Despite the known benefits of weight loss, it is a difficult process for most individuals. Obesity treatment begins with patients understanding their weight history and deciding on a plan that is best for them. In general, the average weight loss program (except for bariatric surgery) results in a 10% reduction of body weight. This average reduction should not be considered a failure, since it is associated with significant health benefits.

Exploring an individual's motivation for weight loss is essential for overall success. Using principles from motivational interviewing (discussed in Chapter 11 on p. 157), you can help patients understand their desire to lose weight and gain confidence in achieving weight loss.[17]

Focusing on the reasons for wanting to lose weight may help patients develop strategies for a weight loss program. Any

supervised plan of care must be directed at two different processes: (1) successful weight loss, which requires a short-term energy deficit; and (2) successful weight control, which requires long-term behavior changes.[18]

A multifaceted approach needs to be used, including nutritional therapy, exercise, behavior modification, and for some, medication or surgical intervention (Table 41-7). Focusing on more than one aspect provides for more effective weight loss and weight control efforts. While doing patient teaching, stress healthy eating habits and adequate physical activity as lifestyle patterns to develop and maintain.

A number of smart phone applications are now available to help patients track eating patterns, calories, and exercise. These tracking systems may provide a patient with immediate access to nutritional information for better dietary decision making.

Even with a comprehensive action plan, there is a high rate of weight regain. This is discouraging when one considers the amount of time, effort, and money expended in attempts to lose weight. For successful management of obesity, it is beneficial to view obesity as a chronic life-long condition that necessitates day-to-day attention.

NUTRITIONAL THERAPY. Restricting dietary intake so that it is below energy requirements is a cornerstone for any weight loss or maintenance program. A good weight loss plan should contain foods from the basic food groups (MyPlate is presented in Fig. 40-1 and Table 40-1). A dietary reduction of at least 500 to 1000 cal/day is recommended for an expected weight loss of 1 to 2 lb/wk.[18] (Table 41-8 presents an example of a 1200-calorie diet.)

A supervised diet plan may be prescribed limiting calories to a total of 800 or less calories per day, but this is not sustainable on a long-term basis. Persons on low-calorie and very-low-calorie diets need frequent professional monitoring because the severe energy restriction places them at risk for multiple nutrient deficiencies.

In general, it is best to recommend a diet that includes adequate amounts of fruits and vegetables, provides enough bulk to prevent constipation, and meets daily vitamin A and vitamin C requirements. Lean meat, fish, and eggs provide sufficient protein and the B-complex vitamins.

It is rare to find an overweight person who has not at some time attempted to lose weight. Some people met with limited

TABLE 41-8 NUTRITIONAL THERAPY

1200-Calorie–Restricted Weight-Reduction Diet*

General Principles
1. Eat regularly. Do not skip meals.
2. Measure foods to determine the correct portion size.
3. Avoid concentrated sweets, such as sugar, candy, honey, pies, cakes, cookies, and regular sodas.
4. Reduce fat intake by baking, broiling, or steaming foods.
5. Maintain a regular exercise program for successful weight loss.

Meal	Exchanges	Menu Plan†
Breakfast	1 meat	1 hard-boiled egg
	2 bread	1 slice toast
		¾ cup dry cereal (unsweetened)
	1 fruit	½ small banana
	1 fat	1 tsp margarine
	1 dairy‡	1 cup low-fat milk
	Beverage	Coffee
Lunch	2 meat	Cheese enchiladas (made with 2 oz
	2 bread	cheese, two corn tortillas, lettuce,
	Vegetable	chili sauce)
	1 fruit	Fresh grapes (12)
	Beverage	Diet soda
Dinner	2 meat	2 oz baked chicken
	1 bread	Corn on the cob with 1 tsp margarine
	Vegetable	Tossed salad and 1 tbs salad dressing
	1 fruit	¾ cup strawberries
	1 milk	1 cup low-fat milk

*For 1000 cal, omit 1 fruit exchange and change low-fat milk to skim milk. For 1500 cal, add 1 meat exchange, 1 fruit exchange, and 2 fat exchanges; change low-fat milk to whole milk. For 1800 cal, add 2 bread exchanges, 3 meat exchanges, 3 fat exchanges, and 1 fruit exchange; change low-fat milk to whole milk.
†Additional sample meal plans are presented in eTable 41-2 available on the website for this chapter.
‡One extra fat exchange allowed for each cup of 2% low-fat milk; 2 extra fat exchanges allowed for each cup of skim milk.

and temporary success, and others have met only with failure. Many individuals attempt weight loss by trying one of the many fad diets that offer the enticement of quick weight loss with little effort (see eTable 41-1 on the website). Often these quick weight-reduction diets (found in the popular media) advocate the elimination of one category of foods (e.g., carbohydrates). Therefore these should be discouraged. Low-carbohydrate diets do produce a rapid weight loss, but reduce the opportunity to get adequate amounts of fiber, vitamins, and minerals. These restrictive diets are difficult to maintain in the long term. It is best to recommend a dietary approach in which calorie restriction includes all food groups. Patients will find it easier to incorporate such a change into their lifestyle and not become as bored with their food options.

The weight loss associated with fad diets is generally short lived. The MyPlate guidelines have longer-lasting results. However, the degree of weight loss strongly depends on the patient's ability to adhere to the diet. The more restrictive the regimen, the greater the demand for intense discipline in the face of an intense desire to eat foods not allowed on the diet.[19]

The degree of success of any reducing diet depends in part on the amount of weight to be lost. A moderately obese person will obviously attain his or her goal more easily than a severely obese person. Because men have a higher percentage of lean body mass, they are often able to lose weight more quickly than women. Women have a higher percentage of body fat, which is metabolically less active than muscle tissue. Postmenopausal women are particularly prone to weight gain, including increased abdominal fat.

Motivation is an essential ingredient for successful weight loss. The obese patient must recognize the advantages of weight loss and weight control. You can assist by helping the patient track eating patterns with a diet diary. Through a frank discussion of eating patterns, the patient often realizes that eating is "mindless" and the result of bad habits picked up over time. These eating behaviors must be changed, or any weight loss will only be temporary.

Setting a realistic and healthy goal, such as losing 1 to 2 lb/wk, should be mutually agreed on at the beginning of counseling. Trying to lose too much too fast usually results in a sense of frustration and failure for the patient. You can help patients understand that losing large amounts of weight in a short period causes skin and underlying tissue to lose elasticity and tone. Slower weight loss offers better cosmetic results.

Inevitably, the patient reaches plateau periods during which no weight is lost. These plateaus may last from several days to several weeks. Remind the patient that plateaus are normal occurrences during weight reduction. A weekly check of body weight is a good method of monitoring progress. Daily weighing is not recommended because of the frequent fluctuations resulting from retained water (including urine) and elimination of feces. Instruct the patient to record the weight at the same time of the day, wearing the same type of clothing.

Experts disagree on the number of meals to be eaten when a person is on a diet. Some nutritionists advocate several small meals per day because the body's metabolic rate is temporarily increased immediately after eating. However, when eating several small meals a day, patients may consume more calories unless they carefully adhere to portion sizes and total daily calorie allotment.

When a person first starts a weight-reduction program, food portion sizes need to be carefully determined to stay within the dietary guidelines. Portion sizes over the past 20 years have increased considerably[12] (see Table 41-4). Food portions can be weighed using a scale, or everyday objects can be used as a visual cue to determine portion sizes. The size of a woman's fist or a baseball is equivalent to a serving of vegetables or fruit. A serving of meat is about the size of a person's palm or a deck of cards. A serving of cheese is about the size of a thumb or six dice. A test on portion sizes is available at *http://hin.nhlbi.nih.gov/portion/index.htm*.

Another aspect of the American diet that needs to be considered is which foods contribute the most calories—animal sources, fruits, grains, or vegetables. Two thirds or more of an individual's diet should be plant-source foods, and the other one third or less should be from animal protein. Being aware of personal consumption habits and striving for the two-thirds to one-third ratio is a simple goal that can be achieved without weighing and measuring foods at every meal. Once this ratio has been adopted into the patient's meal planning, portions can gradually be reduced as activity levels are gradually increased to achieve healthy weight loss. The recommended portion size of animal protein is 3 oz. The standard size for chopped vegetables is ½ cup, according to MyPlate guidelines (see Table 40-1).

A list of healthy or low-calorie foods serves as a good reference and permits an occasional meal to be eaten at a restaurant. Furthermore, the patient who carefully follows the prescribed diet may not need to take vitamin supplements. Encourage the appropriate fluid intake in the form of water. Alcoholic and sugary beverages should be limited or avoided, since they increase caloric intake and are low in nutritional value.

EXERCISE. Exercise is an essential part of a weight control program. Patients should exercise daily, preferably 30 minutes to an hour. There is no evidence that increased activity promotes an increase in appetite or leads to dietary excess. In fact, exercise frequently has the opposite effect. The addition of exercise produces more weight loss than does dieting alone and has a favorable effect on body fat distribution. With regular exercise, WHR is reduced. Finally, exercise is especially important in maintaining weight loss.

When large muscles are involved in the exercise program, a primary benefit is cardiovascular conditioning. Overweight men and women who are active and fit have lower rates of morbidity and mortality than overweight persons who are sedentary and unfit. Therefore exercise is of benefit to overweight persons even if it does not make them lean. Many psychologic benefits can be derived from an increased physical activity program. Exercise decreases tension and stress, promotes better-quality sleep and rest, increases stamina and energy, improves self-concept and self-confidence, improves attitudes, and increases optimism about the future.[18]

Explore with the patient possible ways to incorporate exercise in daily routines. It may be as simple as parking farther from their place of employment or taking the stairs versus an elevator. Encourage individuals to wear a pedometer to track their activity with a goal of 10,000 steps a day. However, success may be walking one third of the recommended steps with incremental increases over time. Although joining a health club can be one way of getting exercise, it is not necessary. Patients can walk, swim, and cycle, all of which have long-term benefits. Stress to patients that engaging in weekend exercise only or in spurts of strenuous activity is not advantageous and can actually be dangerous.

BEHAVIOR MODIFICATION. The assumption behind behavior modification is twofold: (1) obesity is a learned disorder caused by overeating and (2) often the critical difference between an obese person and a person of normal weight is the cues that regulate eating behavior. Therefore most behavior-modification programs deemphasize the diet and focus on how and when to eat.

Teach people to restrict their eating to designated meals and to increase the amount of physical activity in their lives. Persons who participate in a behavioral therapy program are more successful in maintaining their losses over an extended time than those who do not participate in such training.

Various behavioral techniques for patients engaged in a weight loss program include (1) self-monitoring, (2) stimulus control, and (3) rewards. *Self-monitoring* may involve keeping a record of the type and time food was consumed and how the person was feeling when eating. *Stimulus control* is aimed at separating events that trigger eating from the act of eating. *Rewards* may be used as incentives for weight loss. Short- and long-term goals are useful benchmarks for earning rewards. It is important that the reward for a specified weight loss not be associated with food, such as dinner out or a favorite treat. Reward items do not have to have a monetary component. For example, time for a hot bath or an hour of pleasure reading would be an enjoyable reward for many people.

SUPPORT GROUPS. People who are on a weight management plan are often encouraged to join a group where others are also trying to modify their eating habits. Many self-help groups

are available that offer support and information on dieting tips. For example, Take Off Pounds Sensibly (TOPS) *(www.tops. org)* is the oldest nonprofit organization of this type. Behavior modification is an integral part of the program, along with nutrition education. Weight Watchers International, Inc. *(www.weightwatchers.com)* is probably the most successful commercial weight-reduction enterprise. Weight Watchers offers a food plan that is nutritionally balanced and practical to follow. Group leaders, all of whom have successfully lost weight with Weight Watchers, teach members various behavior-modification techniques.

Commercial weight-reduction centers have proliferated across the nation. Many of these programs are staffed by nurses and dietitians. An initial physical examination by a health care provider is required before a candidate is accepted for weight reduction. These weight-reduction centers are cost prohibitive for those with limited financial resources. Many of these programs also offer special prepackaged foods and supplements that must be purchased as part of the weight-reduction plan. Only these prescribed foods and drinks are to be consumed until an agreed-on amount of weight is lost. The patient is encouraged to buy the same type of foods for the maintenance phase of the program, lasting from 6 months to 1 year. Behavior-modification training is incorporated in these programs as well. Individuals must learn how to adjust their diet once they are no longer using the commercial products. This can be challenging for many, and the weight lost may be regained once the restricted food program is completed.

In recent years a number of employers have begun weight loss programs at the workplace. The rationale for such programs is that better health repays the cost of the programs through improved work performance, decreased absenteeism, less hospitalization, and lower insurance costs. Such programs have been well accepted by both employees and employers.

DRUG THERAPY

Drugs should never be used alone. Rather, they should be part of a comprehensive weight-reduction program that includes reduced-calorie diet, exercise, and behavior modification. Drugs should be reserved for adults with a BMI of 30 kg/m^2 or greater (obese), or adults with a BMI of 27 kg/m^2 or greater (overweight) who have at least one weight-related condition such as hypertension, type 2 diabetes, or dyslipidemia.

Appetite-Suppressing Drugs
The sympathomimetic amines suppress appetite by increasing the availability of norepinephrine in the brain, thus stimulating the central nervous system. The sympathomimetics fall into two groups: amphetamines and nonamphetamines. The amphetamines have a much higher abuse potential than the nonamphetamines. Amphetamines are not recommended nor are they approved by the U.S. Food and Drug Administration (FDA) for either short- or long-term weight loss.

Nonamphetamines are not usually recommended for weight loss because of the potential for abuse. If used, these drugs should only be used short term (for 3 months or less). Nonamphetamines include phentermine (Adipex-P, Fastin, Ionamin), diethylpropion (Tenuate), phendimetrazine (Bontril), and benzphetamine (Didrex). Adverse effects of these drugs include palpitations, tachycardia, overstimulation, restlessness, dizziness, insomnia, weakness, and fatigue.

Nutrient Absorption–Blocking Drugs

Orlistat (Xenical) works by blocking fat breakdown and absorption in the intestine. It inhibits the action of intestinal lipases, resulting in undigested fat excreted in the feces. Some fat-soluble vitamin levels may also decrease and may need to be supplemented. Allī, a low-dose form of orlistat, is available for over-the-counter use.

Orlistat is associated with leakage of stool, flatulence, diarrhea, and abdominal bloating, which is accentuated if a high-fat diet is consumed. These side effects limit its acceptance as a weight loss tool. Severe liver injury has been reported in patients using orlistat.[20]

Serotonin Agonist

Lorcaserin (Belviq) is a selective serotonin (5-HT) agonist that suppresses appetite and creates a sense of satiety. Lorcaserin works by activating the serotonin receptor in the brain. Activation of this receptor may help a person eat less and feel full after eating smaller amounts of food. The most common side effects are headache, dizziness, fatigue, nausea, dry mouth, and constipation.

Phentermine and Topiramate (Qsymia)

Qsymia is a combination of two drugs, phentermine and topiramate. Phentermine is a sympathomimetic agent already approved for short-term management of obesity. Topiramate is currently approved for seizure disorders and prophylaxis of migraine. In overweight patients, phentermine suppresses appetite, and topiramate induces a sense of satiety. Qsymia must not be used in patients with glaucoma or hyperthyroidism. Qsymia can increase heart rate, and its effect on the heart rate in patients at high risk for heart attack or stroke is not known.

Nursing Interventions Related to Drug Therapy

Drugs will not cure obesity, and individuals must understand that without substantial changes in food intake and increased physical activity, they will gain weight when drug therapy is stopped. As with any drug treatment, there are side effects. Careful evaluation for other medical conditions can help determine which drugs, if any, would be advisable for a given patient.

Your role related to drug therapy is to teach the patient about proper administration, side effects, and how the drugs fit into the overall weight loss plan. The modification of dosage without consultation with the health care provider can have detrimental effects. Emphasize that diet and exercise regimens are the cornerstones of permanent weight loss. Finally, discourage the purchase of over-the-counter diet aids except for Allī.

SURGICAL THERAPY

Bariatric surgery has become a viable and popular option for treating obesity.[21] Surgery is currently the only treatment that has been found to have a successful and lasting impact for sustained weight loss for severely obese individuals.[22]

The majority of people who undergo bariatric surgery successfully improve their overall quality of life. In addition to losing weight, patients often experience resolution of comorbidities such as diabetes. Although overall mortality is very low, a number of complications can arise from surgery, and the option to have surgery must be carefully considered.

Criteria guidelines for bariatric surgery include having a BMI of 40 kg/m² or a BMI of 35 kg/m² with one or more severe obesity-related medical complications (e.g., hypertension, type 2 diabetes mellitus, heart failure, sleep apnea). Many insurance carriers do not cover the cost of bariatric surgery. If they do consider reimbursing for the surgery, most of them require documentation of a medically supervised weight loss program for approximately 6 months.[23]

Before being considered candidates for surgery, patients must be screened for psychologic, physical, and behavioral conditions that have been associated with poor surgical outcomes. These include untreated depression, binge eating disorders, and drug and alcohol abuse that may interfere with a commitment to lifelong behavioral changes. Other contraindications to surgery include illnesses that are known to reduce life expectancy and are not likely to be improved with weight reduction. These conditions include advanced cancer; end-stage kidney, liver, and cardiopulmonary disease; severe coagulopathy; or inability to comply with nutritional recommendations.[24]

Bariatric surgeries fall into one of three broad categories: restrictive, malabsorptive, or a combination of malabsorptive and restrictive (Table 41-9 and Fig. 41-5). In *restrictive procedures* the stomach is reduced in size (less food eaten), and in *malabsorptive procedures* the length of the small intestine is decreased (less food absorbed).[21] The majority of procedures are performed laparoscopically, thus decreasing postoperative recuperation as compared to an open procedure. With laparoscopy, patients have fewer wound infections, shorter hospital stays, and a faster recovery period.[23]

Restrictive Surgeries

Restrictive bariatric surgery reduces either the size of the stomach, which causes the patient to feel full more quickly, or the amount allowed to enter the stomach. In these surgeries, digestion is not altered so the risk of anemia or cobalamin deficiency is low. The most common restrictive surgeries include adjustable gastric banding and vertical sleeve gastrectomy.[24]

Adjustable Gastric Banding. Laparoscopic *adjustable gastric banding* (AGB), the most common restrictive procedure done, involves limiting the stomach size with an inflatable band placed around the fundus of the stomach (Fig. 41-5, *A*). This restrictive procedure can be done using a Lap-Band or Realize Band system. The band is connected to a subcutaneous port and can be inflated or deflated (by fluid injection in the health care provider's office) to change the stoma size to meet the patient's needs as weight is lost. The restrictive effect of the band creates a sense of fullness as the upper portion of the stomach now accommodates less than the average stomach. The band then causes a delay in stomach emptying, providing patients with further satiety.

The procedure can be either modified or reversed at a later date if necessary. AGB is the preferred option for patients who are surgical risks because it is a less invasive approach.

Vertical Sleeve Gastrectomy. In the vertical sleeve gastrectomy, about 85% of the stomach is removed, leaving a sleeve-shaped stomach (Fig. 41-5, *B*). Although the stomach is drastically reduced in size, its function is preserved. The procedure is not reversible. The removal of the majority of the stomach also results in the elimination of hormones produced in the stomach that stimulate hunger, such as ghrelin.

Combination of Restrictive and Malabsorptive Surgery

Roux-en-Y Gastric Bypass. The Roux-en-Y gastric bypass (RYGB) procedure is a combination of restrictive and malab-

TABLE 41-9 SURGICAL INTERVENTIONS FOR OBESITY*

Procedure	Anatomic Changes	Advantages	Complications
Restrictive Surgery			
Adjustable gastric banding (AGB) (Lap-Band, Realize Band)	Band encircles the stomach, creating a stoma and a gastric pouch with about 30 mL capacity	• Food digestion occurs through normal process • Band can be adjusted to ↑ or ↓ restriction • Surgery can be reversed • Absence of dumping syndrome • Lack of malabsorption	• Low complication rate • Some nausea and vomiting initially • Problems with adjustment device • Band may slip or erode into stomach wall • Gastric perforation
Vertical sleeve gastrectomy	About 85% of stomach removed, leaving a sleeve-shaped stomach with 60-150 mL capacity	• Function of stomach preserved • No bypass of intestine • Avoids complications of obstruction, anemia, vitamin deficiencies	• Weight loss may be limited • Leakage related to stapling
Vertical banded gastroplasty (VBG)	Band placed around stomach, and staples used above band to create a small gastric pouch	• No surgical anastomosis • More normal anatomy and physiology maintained • Lower risk of infection	• High complication rate • Slow weight loss • Rupture of staple line • Dilated pouch • Dumping syndrome (nausea, vomiting, and/or diarrhea related to ingestion of sweets, high-calorie liquids, or dairy products)
Malabsorptive Surgery			
Biliopancreatic diversion (BPD) with or without duodenal switch	70% of the stomach removed horizontally Anastomosis between the stomach and the intestine Decreases the amount of small intestine available for nutrient absorption Duodenal switch cuts the stomach vertically and is shaped like a tube	• Increased amount of food intake • Less food intolerance • Greater long-term weight loss • Rapid weight loss	• Abdominal bloating, diarrhea, and foul-smelling gas (steatorrhea) • Three or four loose bowel movements a day • Malabsorption of fat-soluble vitamins • Iron deficiency • Protein-calorie malnutrition • Dumping syndrome (with duodenal switch, last two problems are less common)
Combination of Restrictive and Malabsorptive Surgery			
Roux-en-Y gastric bypass (RYGB)	Restrictive surgery on stomach creating pouch Small gastric pouch connected to jejunum Remaining stomach and first segment of small intestine are bypassed	• Better weight loss results than with gastric restrictive procedures • Lower incidence of malnutrition and diarrhea • Rapid improvement of weight-related co-morbidities	• Leak at site of anastomosis • Anemia: iron deficiency, cobalamin deficiency, folic acid deficiency • Calcium deficiency • Dumping syndrome

*See Fig. 41-5.

sorptive surgery. This surgical procedure is the most common bariatric procedure performed in the United States and is considered the gold standard among bariatric procedures.

This procedure, which is irreversible, involves creating a small gastric pouch and attaching it directly to the small intestine using a Y-shaped limb of the small bowel. After the procedure, food bypasses 90% of the stomach, the duodenum, and a small segment of jejunum.

Overall, it has low complication rates, has excellent patient tolerance, and sustains long-term weight loss. Outcomes include improved glucose control with improvement or reversal of diabetes, normalization of BP, decreased total cholesterol and triglycerides, decreased GERD, and decreased sleep apnea.[25]

A complication of the RYGB is *dumping syndrome,* in which gastric contents empty too rapidly into the small intestine, overwhelming its ability to digest nutrients. Symptoms can include vomiting, nausea, weakness, sweating, faintness, and, on occasion, diarrhea. Patients are discouraged from eating sugary foods after surgery to avoid dumping syndrome.[25] Because sections of the small intestine are bypassed, poor absorption of iron can cause iron-deficiency anemia. Patients need to take a multivitamin with iron and calcium supplements. Chronic anemia caused by cobalamin deficiency may also occur. This

problem can usually be managed with parenteral or intranasal cobalamin.

Cosmetic Surgeries to Reduce Fatty Tissue and Skinfolds

Lipectomy. Lipectomy (adipectomy) is performed to remove unsightly flabby folds of adipose tissue (Fig. 41-6). In some patients, up to 15% of the total fat cells can be removed from the breasts, abdomen, and lumbar and femoral areas. There is no evidence that a regeneration of adipose tissue occurs at the surgical sites. However, emphasize to the patient that surgical removal does not prevent obesity from recurring, especially if lifetime eating habits remain the same. Although body image and self-esteem may be enhanced by such procedures, these operations are not without complications. The dangerous effects of anesthesia and the potential for poor wound healing in the obese patient cannot be overemphasized.

Liposuction. Another cosmetic surgical procedure is liposuction, or suction-assisted lipectomy. It is used for cosmetic purposes and not for weight reduction. This surgical intervention helps improve facial appearance or body contours. A good candidate for this type of surgery is a person who has achieved weight reduction but who has excess fat under the chin, along the jaw line, in the nasolabial folds, over the abdomen, or

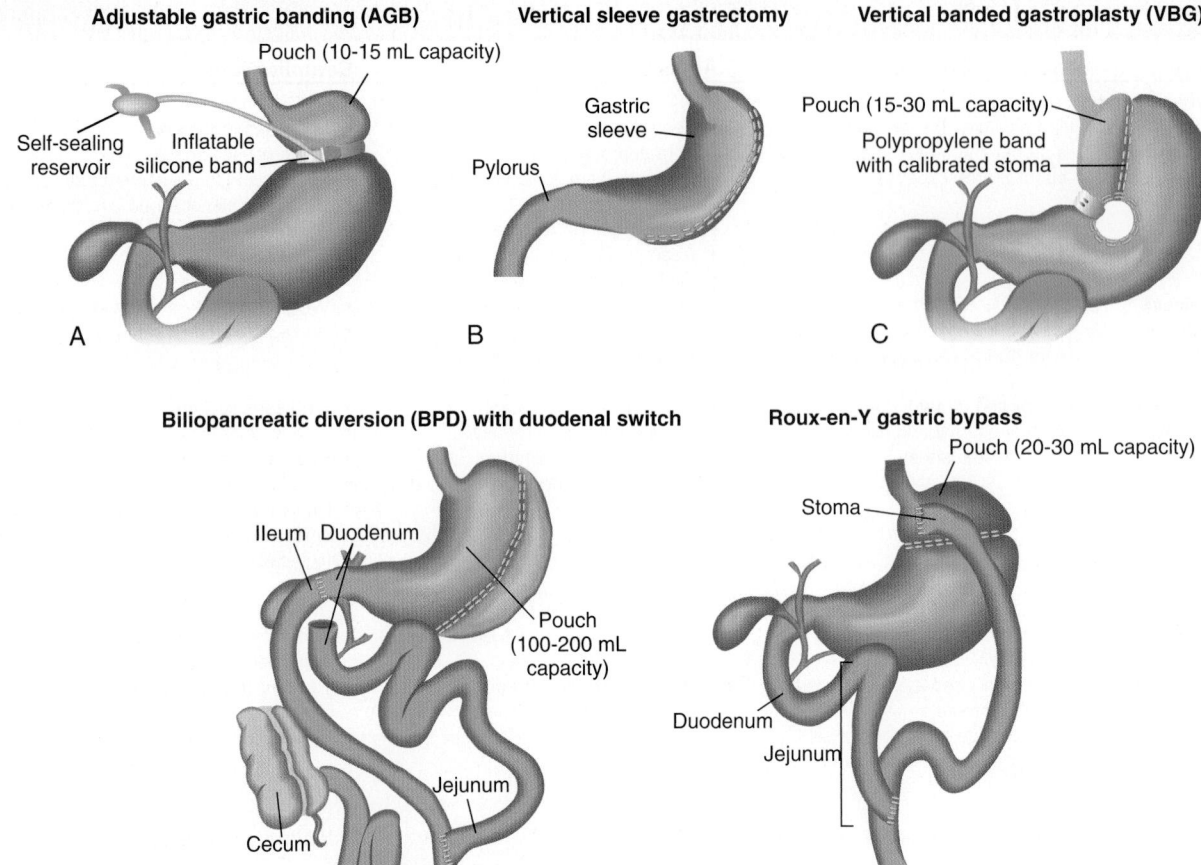

FIG. 41-5 Bariatric surgical procedures. **A,** Adjustable gastric banding (AGB) uses a band to create a gastric pouch. **B,** Vertical sleeve gastrectomy involves creating a sleeve-shaped stomach by removing about 80% of the stomach. **C,** Vertical banded gastroplasty (VBG) involves creating a small gastric pouch. **D,** Biliopancreatic diversion (BPD) with duodenal switch procedure creates an anastomosis between the stomach and the intestine. **E,** Roux-en-Y gastric bypass procedure involves constructing a gastric pouch whose outlet is a Y-shaped limb of small intestine.

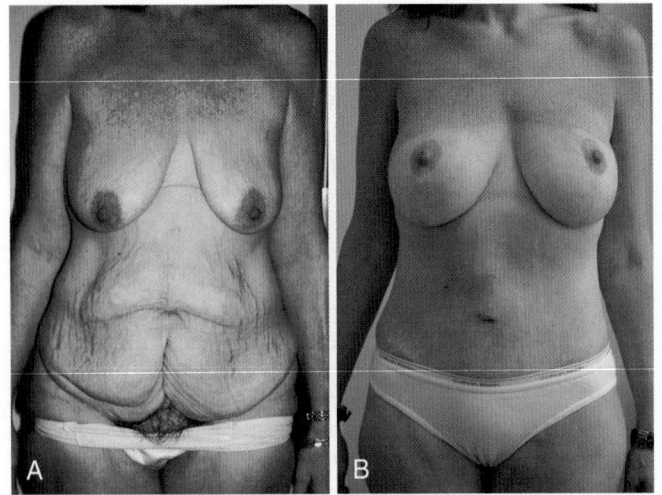

FIG. 41-6 A, Preoperative view of a 37-year-old woman with massive weight loss who had gastric bypass surgery. **B,** Postoperative view 2½ years after abdominoplasty. She also underwent breast surgery, thighlift, backlift with excision of excess skin of the lower back and upper buttocks, and upper arm surgery.

around the waist and upper thighs. A long, hollow, stainless steel cannula is inserted through a small incision over the fatty tissue to be suctioned. This surgical procedure is not usually recommended for the older person because the skin is less elastic and will not accommodate the new underlying shape.

NURSING MANAGEMENT
PERIOPERATIVE CARE OF THE OBESE PATIENT

NURSING IMPLEMENTATION

This section discusses general nursing considerations for the care of the obese patient who is having surgery. Special nursing considerations are described for the patient who is having bariatric surgery. (Care of the surgical patient is discussed in Chapters 18 to 20.)

PREOPERATIVE CARE. Special considerations are necessary for the obese patient, especially the severely obese individual, who is admitted to the hospital for surgery.[26] Before surgery, interview the patient to identify past and current health information and any assistive devices currently in use (e.g., continuous positive airway pressure [CPAP] for sleep apnea). Co-morbidities secondary to obesity increase the risk for complications in the perioperative period. It may be necessary to coordinate care with the patient's cardiologist, pulmonologist, gynecologist, gastroenterologist, or other specialists.

Have a plan in place before the patients arrive so they receive optimal care and do not feel like they are a burden to the nursing staff. Nursing units must have available appropriate size hospital gowns, beds that accommodate an increased body size, and necessary patient transfer equipment. To correctly measure BP in obese people, a larger cuff size is needed to avoid artifactual errors. Ensure that oversized BP cuffs are available and placed in the patient's room.

Consider how the patient will be weighed and transported throughout the hospital. A wheelchair with removable arms that is large enough to safely accommodate the patient and pass easily through doorways should be available.

Preoperative and postoperative assessment of heart, lung, and bowel sounds may require the use of alternative assessment techniques. For example, because of the large chest wall, breath and heart sounds are often distant. Electronic stethoscopes can be used to amplify lung, heart, and bowel sounds. Pulse oximetry may also be used to assess oxygenation status.

Instruct the patient in the proper coughing and deep breathing techniques and methods of turning and positioning to prevent pulmonary complications after surgery. If possible, demonstrate the use of a spirometer before surgery. Use of the spirometer helps prevent and treat postoperative lung congestion. Practicing these strategies preoperatively can help the patient perform them correctly postoperatively. Furthermore, if the patient uses CPAP at home for sleep apnea, make arrangements for the use of a machine while the patient is hospitalized.

Obtaining venous access may be complicated by excess adipose tissue. A longer IV catheter is helpful (longer than 1 in) to go through the overlying tissue to the vein. It is important that the cannula is far enough into the vein to ensure that it is not dislodged or infiltrated.

Special Considerations for Bariatric Surgery. Ensure that the patient scheduled for bariatric surgery understands the surgical procedure. Your teaching depends on the type of procedure and surgical approach.

Prepare the patient before surgery for the possibility of returning with one or more of the following: urinary catheter, IV catheter, compression stockings, and nasogastric tube. Emphasize that vital signs and a general assessment will be conducted frequently to monitor for complications. Further, the patient must understand that he or she will be assisted with ambulation soon after surgery and encouraged to cough and deep breathe to prevent pulmonary complications. Liquids will be started early but only after the patient is fully awake and there is no evidence of any anastomosis leaks.

POSTOPERATIVE CARE. The initial postoperative care focuses on careful assessment and immediate intervention for cardiopulmonary complications, thrombus formation, anastomosis leaks, and electrolyte imbalances. The transfer from surgery may require many trained staff members. During the transfer, the patient's airway should remain stabilized and attention given to managing the patient's pain. Maintain the patient's head at a 35- to 40-degree angle to reduce abdominal pressure and increase lung expansion.

The body stores anesthetics in adipose tissue, thus placing patients with excess adipose tissue at risk for re-sedation. As adipose cells release anesthetics back into the bloodstream, the patient may become sedated after surgery. If this happens, be prepared to perform a head-tilt or jaw-thrust maneuver and keep the patient's oral and nasal airways open.[27]

Diligence in turning and ambulation postoperatively will prevent complications from surgery. Tell the patient that typically he or she will be assisted in walking the evening after surgery and then at least three or four times each day. The patient may be reluctant to move or may not have the stamina to walk even a short distance. In either situation, you will need additional help in facilitating movement in an obese patient.

Obesity can cause a patient's breathing to become shallow and rapid. The extra adipose tissue in the chest and abdomen compresses the diaphragmatic, thoracic, and abdominal structures. This compression restricts the chest's ability to expand, preventing the lungs from working as efficiently as they would otherwise. The patient retains more carbon dioxide with less oxygen delivered to the lungs. This results in hypoxemia, pulmonary hypertension, and polycythemia.

Postoperatively the risk for deep venous thrombosis (DVT) is increased. Venous stasis is common due to the pressure on the veins. Antiembolic stockings or sequential compression stockings may be ordered along with low-dose heparin to minimize the risk of a DVT. Active and passive range-of-motion exercises are a frequent part of daily care.

Wound infection, dehiscence, and delayed healing are potential problems for all obese patients. Assess the patient's skin for any complications related to wound healing. Keep skinfolds clean and dry to prevent dermatitis and secondary bacterial or fungal infections.

Special Considerations for Bariatric Surgery. Patients experience considerable abdominal pain after bariatric surgery. Give pain medications as necessary during the immediate postoperative period (first 24 hours). Be aware that pain could be from an anastomosis leak rather than typical surgical pain.

Abdominal wounds require frequent observation for the amount and type of drainage, condition of the incision, and signs of infection. Protect the incision against undue straining that accompanies turning and coughing. Monitor vital signs to assist in identifying problems such as infection.

If a nasogastric tube is inserted, monitor it for patency and keep it in the correct position. If the patient vomits with a nasogastric tube in place, it may require repositioning; notify the surgeon immediately. The upper gastric pouch is small, and irrigating the tube with too much solution or manipulating the tube position can lead to disruption of the anastomosis or staple line.

During the immediate postoperative period water and sugar-free clear liquids are given (30 mL every 2 hours while awake). Before discharge, instruct patients on a measured amount of a high-protein liquid diet. The patient is taught to eat slowly, stop eating when feeling full, and not consume liquids with solid food. Vomiting is a common complication during this time. A dietitian is usually part of the bariatric team and assists the patient with the transition to the new diet.

AMBULATORY AND HOME CARE

Special Considerations for Bariatric Surgery. The patient who has undergone major surgical treatment for obesity has not been successful in the past in following or maintaining a prescribed diet. Now the patient is forced to reduce oral intake because of the anatomic changes from the surgical procedure. The patient's adherence to a reduced intake is necessary because of the concern for abdominal distention, cramping abdominal pain, and perhaps diarrhea.

Weight loss is considerable during the first 6 to 12 months. During this time the patient must learn to adjust intake sufficiently to maintain a stable weight. Although behavior modification is not necessarily an intended outcome with these surgical procedures, it becomes an unexpected secondary gain. For example, a person who has had bariatric surgery cannot overeat or binge eat without consequences.

The diet generally prescribed should be high in protein and low in carbohydrates, fat, and roughage and consist of six small feedings daily. Fluids should not be ingested with the meal, and in some cases, fluids should be restricted to less than 1000 mL/day. Fluids and foods high in carbohydrate tend to promote diarrhea and symptoms of the dumping syndrome. Generally, calorically dense foods (foods high in fat) should be avoided to permit more nutritionally sound food to be consumed.

The patient must clearly understand the proper diet. Late complications can be anticipated after bariatric surgery, including anemia, vitamin deficiencies, diarrhea, and psychologic problems. Failure to lose weight or loss of too much weight may be caused by the surgical formation of too large a stomach pouch or of an outlet that is much too small, respectively. Peptic ulcer formation, dumping syndrome, and small bowel obstruction may be seen late in the recovery and rehabilitation stage.

Emphasize the importance of long-term follow-up care, in part because of potential complications late in the recovery period. Encourage patients to adhere strictly to the prescribed diet and to inform the health care provider of any changes in their physical or emotional condition. Some patients have been known to overeat when they return home and gain rather than lose weight.

Several potential psychologic problems may arise after surgery. Some patients express guilt feelings that weight loss was achieved by surgical interventions rather than by the "sheer willpower" of reduced dietary intake and exercise. Be ready to provide support and assist the patient in moving away from such negative feelings.

By 6 to 8 months after surgery, considerable weight loss has occurred, and patients are able to see how much their appearance has changed. Discussion of this possible outcome with the patient before surgery and again during the rehabilitation phase facilitates the patient's adjustment to a new body image. Do not hesitate to encourage counseling for unresolved psychologic issues.

Massive weight loss often leaves the patient with large quantities of flabby skin that can result in problems related to altered body image. Reconstructive surgery may alleviate this situation. Reductions of the breasts, upper arms, thighs, and excess abdominal skinfolds are possible solutions.

Often one result of bariatric surgery is the return of fertility in women. Pregnancy complications can result from anemia and nutritional deficiencies. Furthermore, depending on the type of surgery, intestinal obstructions and hernias are commonly experienced in pregnancy.[28] Gallbladder problems may also arise, leading to pancreatitis. Women must carefully consider the risk of pregnancy after bariatric surgery. In general, encourage women to postpone pregnancy for 12 to 18 months after bariatric surgery.[28]

▌EVALUATION

The expected outcomes are that the obese patient will

- Experience long-term weight loss
- Have improvement in obesity-related co-morbidities

- Integrate healthy practices into daily routines
- Monitor for adverse side effects of surgical therapy
- Have an improved self-image

▌GERONTOLOGIC CONSIDERATIONS

OBESITY IN OLDER ADULTS

The prevalence of obesity is increasing in all age-groups, including older people. The number of obese older persons has markedly risen because of increases in both the total number of older persons and the percentage of the older adults who are obese. Obesity is more common in older women than in older men. A decrease in energy expenditure is an important contributor to a gradual increase in body fat with age.

Obesity in older adults can exacerbate age-related declines in physical function and lead to frailty and disability. Obesity is associated with decreased survival. Individuals who are obese live 6 to 7 years less than people of normal weight do.

Many of the changes associated with aging are exacerbated by obesity. Excess body weight places more demands on arthritic joints. The mechanical strain on weight-bearing joints can lead to premature immobility. Excess weight also affects other body systems. Older adults may find that excess intraabdominal weight causes problems with urinary incontinence. In addition, excess weight may contribute to hypoventilation and sleep apnea.

TABLE 41-10	CRITERIA FOR METABOLIC SYNDROME*
Measure	**Criteria**
Waist circumference	≥40 in (102 cm) in men
	≥35 in (89 cm) in women
Triglycerides	>150 mg/dL (1.7 mmol/L)
	OR
	Drug treatment for elevated triglycerides
High-density lipoprotein (HDL) cholesterol	<40 mg/dL (0.9 mmol/L) in men
	<50 mg/dL (1.1 mmol/L) in women
	OR
	Drug treatment for reduced HDL cholesterol
BP	≥130 mm Hg systolic BP
	OR
	≥85 mm Hg diastolic BP
	OR
	Drug treatment for hypertension
Fasting blood glucose	≥110 mg/dL
	OR
	Drug treatment for elevated glucose

Source: National Heart, Lung, and Blood Institute: How is metabolic syndrome diagnosed? Retrieved from *www.nhlbi.nih.gov/health/dci/Diseases/ms/ms_diagnosis.html*.
*Any three of the five measures are needed for a diagnosis of metabolic syndrome.

PATHOPHYSIOLOGY MAP

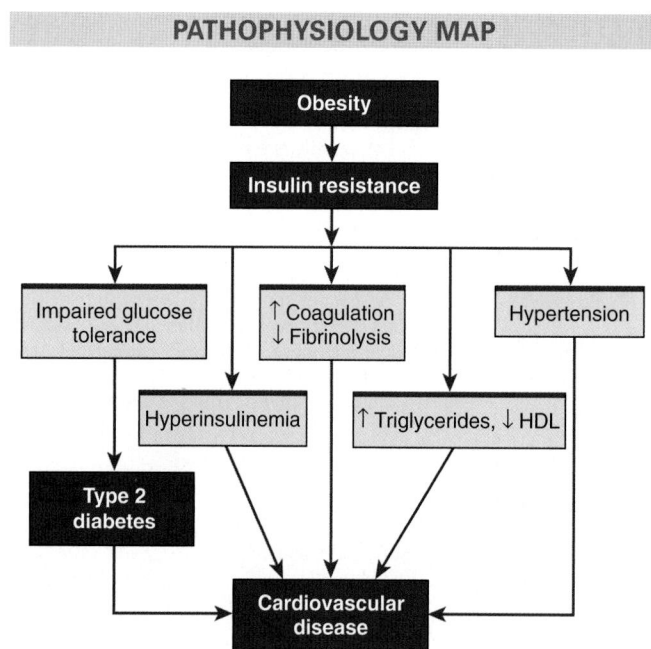

FIG. 41-7 Relationship among insulin resistance, obesity, diabetes mellitus, and cardiovascular disease. *HDL,* High-density lipoprotein.

Obesity affects the quality of life for older adults. Weight loss can improve physical functioning and obesity-related health complications. The same therapeutic approaches for obesity as were discussed earlier also apply to the older adult.

METABOLIC SYNDROME

Metabolic syndrome, also known as *syndrome X, insulin resistance syndrome,* and *dysmetabolic syndrome,* is a collection of risk factors that increase an individual's chance of developing cardiovascular disease, stroke, and diabetes mellitus. It is estimated that around 70 million to 80 million, or about 25%, of Americans have metabolic syndrome.[29] The syndrome is more prevalent in those 60 years of age and older.[30]

Metabolic syndrome is characterized by a cluster of health problems, including obesity, hypertension, abnormal lipid levels, and high blood glucose. Metabolic syndrome is diagnosed if an individual has three or more of the conditions listed in Table 41-10.

Currently health professionals are debating the usefulness of focusing attention on the syndrome itself. The interventions are focused on each risk factor, since there is not one standard treatment for the syndrome itself.[30]

Etiology and Pathophysiology

The main underlying risk factor for metabolic syndrome is insulin resistance related to excessive visceral fat (Fig. 41-7). Insulin resistance is the body's cells diminished ability to respond to the action of insulin. The pancreas compensates by secreting more insulin, resulting in hyperinsulinemia.

Other characteristics of metabolic syndrome include hypertension, increased risk for clotting, and abnormalities in cholesterol levels. The net effect of these conditions is an increased prevalence of coronary artery disease.

Genetics and environment have important roles in the development of metabolic syndrome. African Americans, Hispanics, Native Americans, and Asians are at an increased risk for metabolic syndrome. Environmental factors that influence the chances of having the syndrome are the same involved in the development of obesity. Metabolic syndrome is also associated with aging.

Clinical Manifestations and Diagnostic Studies

The signs of metabolic syndrome are impaired fasting blood glucose, hypertension, abnormal cholesterol levels, and obesity. Medical problems develop over time if the condition remains unaddressed. Patients with this syndrome are at a higher risk of heart disease, stroke, diabetes, renal disease, and polycystic ovary syndrome. Patients who have metabolic syndrome and smoke are at an even higher risk.

NURSING AND COLLABORATIVE MANAGEMENT METABOLIC SYNDROME

Lifestyle modifications are the first-line interventions to reduce the risk factors for metabolic syndrome. Management or reversal of metabolic syndrome can be achieved by reducing the major risk factors of cardiovascular disease: reducing LDL cholesterol, stopping smoking, lowering BP, and reducing glucose levels. For long-term risk reduction, weight should be decreased, physical activity increased, and healthy dietary habits established.

There is no specific management of metabolic syndrome. You can assist patients by providing information on healthy diets, exercise, and positive lifestyle changes. The diet, which should be low in saturated fats, should promote weight loss. Weight reduction and maintenance of a lower weight should be the first priority in those with abdominal obesity and metabolic syndrome.

Because sedentary lifestyles contribute to metabolic syndrome, increasing regular physical activity will lower a patient's risk factors. In addition to assisting in weight reduction, regular

CASE STUDY

Obesity

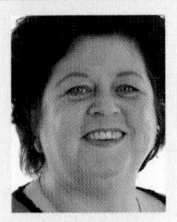

Hemera/Thinkstock

Patient Profile

S.R. is a 48-yr-old white woman.

Subjective Data

- Reports gradual weight gain of 40 lb during past 40 yr
- Lives in a rural community with no sidewalks
- Spends most of her free time watching television
- Reports health problems related to type 2 diabetes mellitus, shortness of breath, hypertension, and osteoarthritis
- Had knee replacement surgery at age 46 for osteoarthritis

Objective Data

Physical Examination

- 5 ft, 4 in tall; weighs 210 lb; waist circumference of 39 in
- Has obese, nontender, soft round, abdomen
- BP 160/100 mm Hg

Laboratory Results

- Fasting blood glucose 250 mg/dL (13.9 mmol/L)
- Total cholesterol 205 mg/dL (5.3 mmol/L)
- Triglyceride 298 mg/dL (3.36 mmol/L)
- HDL cholesterol 31 mg/dL (0.8 mmol/L)
- LDL cholesterol 114 mg/dL

Discussion Questions

1. What are S.R.'s risk factors for obesity?
2. What is her estimated BMI?
3. Of the possible complications of obesity, which ones does S.R. have? Why did she develop them?
4. ***Priority Decision:*** How would you assist S.R. in designing a successful weight loss and weight management program?
5. What are S.R.'s risk factors for metabolic syndrome?
6. Is S.R. a candidate for surgical intervention for obesity? Why or why not?
7. ***Evidence-Based Practice:*** S.R. tells you that she is motivated to lose weight and thinks that she can "do it on her own." Based on your understanding of the evidence, is this the best approach for her to be successful in losing weight?

Ⓔvolve Answers available at *http://evolve.elsevier.com/Lewis/medsurg.*

---

exercise has been found to decrease the triglyceride level and increase the HDL cholesterol level in patients with metabolic syndrome.

Patients unable to lower risk factors with lifestyle therapies alone or those at high risk for a coronary event or diabetes may be considered for drug therapy. Although there is no specific medication for metabolic syndrome, cholesterol-lowering and antihypertensive drugs can be used. Metformin (Glucophage) has also been used to prevent diabetes by lowering glucose levels and enhancing the cells' sensitivity to insulin.

▌ BRIDGE TO NCLEX EXAMINATION

The number of the question corresponds to the same-numbered outcome at the beginning of the chapter.

1. Which statement best describes the etiology of obesity?
   a. Obesity primarily results from a genetic predisposition.
   b. Psychosocial factors can override the effects of genetics in the etiology of obesity.
   c. Obesity is the result of complex interactions between genetic and environmental factors.
   d. Genetic factors are more important than environmental factors in the etiology of obesity.

2. The obesity classification that is most often associated with cardiovascular health problems is
   a. primary obesity.
   b. secondary obesity.
   c. gynoid fat distribution.
   d. android fat distribution.

3. Health risks associated with obesity include *(select all that apply)*
   a. colorectal cancer.
   b. rheumatoid arthritis.
   c. polycystic ovary syndrome.
   d. nonalcoholic steatohepatitis.
   e. systemic lupus erythematosus.

4. The best nutritional therapy plan for a person who is obese is
   a. the Zone diet.
   b. the Atkins diet.
   c. Sugar Busters.
   d. foods from the basic food groups.

5. This bariatric surgical procedure involves creating a stoma and gastric pouch that is reversible, and no malabsorption occurs. What surgical procedure is this?
   a. Vertical gastric banding
   b. Biliopancreatic diversion
   c. Roux-en-Y gastric bypass
   d. Adjustable gastric banding

6. A severely obese patient has undergone Roux-en-Y gastric bypass surgery. In planning postoperative care, the nurse anticipates that the patient
   a. may have severe diarrhea early in the postoperative period.
   b. will not be allowed to ambulate for 1 to 2 days postoperatively.
   c. will require nasogastric suction until the incision heals.
   d. may have only liquids orally, and in very limited amounts, during the early postoperative period.

7. Which of the following criteria must be met for a diagnosis of metabolic syndrome *(select all that apply)*?
   a. Hypertension
   b. Elevated triglycerides
   c. Elevated plasma glucose
   d. Increased waist circumference
   e. Decreased low-density lipoproteins

1. c, 2. d, 3. a, c, d, 4. d, 5. d, 6. d, 7. a, b, c, d

Ⓔvolve

For rationales to these answers and even more NCLEX review questions, visit *http://evolve.elsever.com/Lewis/medsurg.*

REFERENCES

1. Achike F, To P, Wang H, et al: Obesity, metabolic syndrome, adipocytes, and vascular function: a holistic viewpoint, *Clin Exper Pharmacol Physiol* 38:1, 2011.
*2. Cornier MA, Depres JP, Davis N, et al: Assessing adiposity: a scientific statement from the American Heart Association, *Circulation* 124(18):1996, 2011.
3. Spanos A: Do weight and shape concerns exhibit genetic effects? Investigating discrepant findings, *Int J Eat Disord* 43(1):29, 2010.
*4. Robert Wood Johnson Foundation: F as in fat: how obesity threatens America's future, Trust for America's Health, 2011. Retrieved from *www.healthyamericans.org/assets/files/TFAH2011FasInFat10.pdf.*
5. Flegal KM, Carroll MD, Ogden C, et al: Prevalence and trends in obesity among US adults, 1999-2008, *JAMA* 303(3):235, 2010.
6. Biro FM, Wien M: Childhood obesity and adult morbidities, *Am J Clin Nutr* 91(5):1499S, 2010.
7. Centers for Disease Control and Prevention: Genomics and health. Retrieved from *www.cdc.gov/genomics/resources/diseases/obesity/obesedit.htm.*
8. Malis C, Rasmussen EL, Foulsen P, et al: Total and regional fat distribution is strongly influenced by genetic factors in young and elderly twins, *Obesity Res* 13:2139, 2005. (Classic)
9. Stunkard A, Sorensen TI, Hanis C, et al: An adoption study of human obesity, *N Engl J Med* 314(4):1483, 1986. (Classic)
10. University of Oxford: Overactive FTO gene does cause overeating and obesity, *Science Daily*, 2010. Retrieved from *www.sciencedaily.com/releases/2010/11/101116220332.htm.*
11. Bray G: Obesity. In Feldman M, Friedman LS, Brandt LJ, editors: *Sleisenger and Fordtran's gastrointestinal and liver disease,* ed 9, Philadelphia, 2010, Saunders.
12. Centers for Disease Control and Prevention: Healthy weight: it's not a diet, it's a lifestyle. Retrieved from *www.cdc.gov/hgov/healthyweight/healthy_eating/portion_size.html.*
13. Davis N, Forges B, Wylie-Rosett J: Role of obesity and lifestyle interventions in the prevention and management of type 2 diabetes, *Minerva Med* 100(3):221, 2009.
14. Popkin BM, Duffey KL: Does hunger and satiety drive eating anymore? Increasing eating occasions and decreasing time between eating occasions in the United States, *Am J Clin Nutr* 91:1342, 2010.
15. Franklin J, Thanavaro J, Ellis P: Body mass index as a guide for diagnosing prediabetes and diabetes, *J Nurse Pract* 7(8):634, 2011.
16. American Institute for Cancer Research: Excess body fat alone causes over 100,000 cancers in US each year. Retrieved from *www.aicr.org/assets/docs/pdf/research/2010pdfs/HarrisonGail_Intro.pdf.*

*17. Appel LJ, Clark JM, Yeh H, et al: Comparative effectiveness of weight-loss interventions in clinical practice, *N Engl J Med* 365(21):1959, 2011.
18. National Heart, Lung, and Blood Institute, North American Association for the Study of Obesity: *The practical guide: identification, evaluation, and treatment of overweight and obesity in adults,* Pub No 00-4084, Washington, DC, 2000, US Department of Health and Human Services.
*19. Sacks F, Bray G, Carey V, et al: Comparison of weight-loss diets with different compositions of fat, protein, and carbohydrates, *N Engl J Med* 360(9):859, 2009.
20. US Food and Drug Administration: Early communication about an ongoing safety review: orlistat (marketed as Alli and Xenical). Retrieved from *www.fda.gov/Drugs/DrugSafety/PostmarketDrugSafetyInformationforPatientsandProviders/DrugSafetyInformationforHealthcareProfessionals/ucm179166.htm.*
21. National Institutes of Health: Bariatric surgery for severe obesity. Retrieved from *http://win.niddk.nih.gov/publications/PDFs/Bariatric_Surgery_508.pdf.*
22. DeMaria EJ: Baseline data from American Society for Metabolic and Bariatric Surgery–designated Bariatric Surgery Centers of Excellence using the Bariatric Outcomes Longitudinal Database, *Surg Obesity Rel Dis* 6(4):347, 2010.
23. Schroeder R, Garrison JM, Johnson MS: Treatment of adult obesity with bariatric surgery, *Am Fam Physician* 84(7):805, 2011.
24. Saver A: Bariatric surgery. Retrieved from *http://emedicine.medscape.com/article/197081-overview#aw2aab6b2b1aa.*
25. Gagnon L, Karwacki Sheff EJ: Outcomes and complications after bariatric surgery, *Am J Nurs* 112:26, 2012.
26. Al-Benna S: Perioperative management of morbid obesity, *J Periop Pract* 21(7):225, 2011.
27. Rowen L, Hunt D, Johnson KL: Managing obese patients in the OR, *OR Nurse* 6:26, 2012.
28. Conrad K, Russell A, Keister K: Bariatric surgery and its impact on childbearing, *Nurs Women's Health* 15(3):228, 2011.
29. Lau DC: Metabolic syndrome: perception or reality? *Curr Atheroscl Rep* 11:264, 2009.
30. Sinclair A, Viljoen A: The metabolic syndrome in older persons, *Clin Geriatr Med* 26(2):261, 2010.

RESOURCES

American Society for Metabolic and Bariatric Surgery
http://asmbs.org
Obesity Society
www.obesity.org
Overeaters Anonymous Headquarters
www.oa.org
Weight Control Information Network
www.win.niddk.nih.gov

*Evidence-based information for clinical practice.

42

When I repress my emotions, my stomach keeps score.
John Powell

Nursing Management
Upper Gastrointestinal Problems

Paula Cox-North

⊖volve WEBSITE

http://evolve.elsevier.com/Lewis/medsurg

- NCLEX Review Questions
- Key Points
- Pre-Test
- Answer Guidelines for Case Study on p. 957
- Rationales for Bridge to NCLEX Examination Questions

- Case Studies
  - Patient With Oral Cancer
  - Patient With Peptic Ulcer Disease
- Nursing Care Plans (Customizable)
  - eNCP 42-1: Patient With Nausea and Vomiting
  - eNCP 42-2: Patient With Peptic Ulcer Disease

- Concept Map Creator
- Glossary
- Content Updates

eFigures
- eFig. 42-1: Billroth I and II
- eFig. 42-2: Stress ulcers

LEARNING OUTCOMES

1. Describe the etiology, complications, collaborative care, and nursing management of nausea and vomiting.
2. Describe the etiology, clinical manifestations, and treatment of common oral inflammations and infections.
3. Describe the etiology, clinical manifestations, complications, collaborative care, and nursing management of oral cancer.
4. Explain the types, pathophysiology, clinical manifestations, complications, and collaborative care (including surgical therapy and nursing management) of gastroesophageal reflux disease (GERD) and hiatal hernia.
5. Describe the pathophysiology, clinical manifestations, complications, and collaborative care of esophageal cancer, diverticula, achalasia, and esophageal strictures.
6. Differentiate between acute and chronic gastritis, including the etiology, pathophysiology, collaborative care, and nursing management.
7. Compare and contrast gastric and duodenal ulcers, including the etiology, pathophysiology, clinical manifestations, complications, collaborative care, and nursing management.
8. Describe the clinical manifestations, collaborative care, and nursing management of stomach cancer.
9. Explain the common etiologies, clinical manifestations, collaborative care, and nursing management of upper gastrointestinal bleeding.
10. Identify common types of foodborne illnesses and nursing responsibilities related to food poisoning.

KEY TERMS

NAUSEA AND VOMITING

Nausea and vomiting are the most common manifestations of gastrointestinal (GI) diseases. Although nausea and vomiting can occur independently, they are usually closely related and treated as one problem. Nausea is a feeling of discomfort in the epigastrium with a conscious desire to vomit. Vomiting is the forceful ejection of partially digested food and secretions *(emesis)* from the upper GI tract.

Vomiting is a complex act that requires the coordinated activities of several structures: closure of the glottis, deep inspiration with contraction of the diaphragm in the inspiratory position, closure of the pylorus, relaxation of the stomach and lower esophageal sphincter (LES), and contraction of the abdominal muscles with increasing intraabdominal pressure. These simultaneous activities force the stomach contents up through the esophagus, into the pharynx, and out the mouth.

Etiology and Pathophysiology

Nausea and vomiting occur in a wide variety of GI disorders and in conditions that are unrelated to GI disease. These include pregnancy; infection; central nervous system (CNS)

Reviewed by Marian Sawyier, RN, MSN, Staff Nurse, University of New Mexico Hospital, Albuquerque, New Mexico.

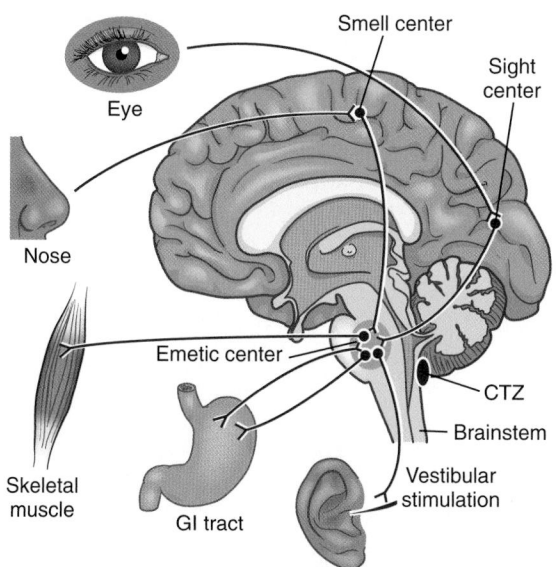

FIG. 42-1 Stimuli involved in the act of vomiting. *CTZ,* Chemoreceptor trigger zone.

disorders (e.g., meningitis, tumor); cardiovascular problems (e.g., myocardial infarction, heart failure); metabolic disorders (e.g., diabetes mellitus, Addison's disease, renal failure); postoperatively after general anesthesia; side effects of drugs (e.g., chemotherapy, opioids, digitalis); psychologic factors (e.g., stress, fear); and conditions in which the GI tract becomes overly irritated, excited, or distended.

A vomiting center in the brainstem coordinates the multiple components involved in vomiting. This center receives input from various stimuli. Neural impulses reach the vomiting center via afferent pathways through branches of the autonomic nervous system. Receptors for these afferent fibers are located in the GI tract, kidneys, heart, and uterus. When stimulated, these receptors relay information to the vomiting center, which then initiates the vomiting reflex (Fig. 42-1).

The chemoreceptor trigger zone (CTZ) located in the brainstem responds to chemical stimuli of drugs, toxins, and labyrinthine stimulation (e.g., motion sickness). Once stimulated, the CTZ transmits impulses directly to the vomiting center. This action activates the autonomic nervous system, resulting in both parasympathetic and sympathetic stimulation. Sympathetic activation produces tachycardia, tachypnea, and diaphoresis. Parasympathetic stimulation causes relaxation of the LES, an increase in gastric motility, and a pronounced increase in salivation.

Clinical Manifestations

Nausea is a subjective complaint. *Anorexia* (lack of appetite) usually accompanies nausea. When nausea and vomiting occur over a long period, dehydration can develop rapidly. Water and essential electrolytes (e.g., potassium, sodium, chloride, hydrogen) are lost. As vomiting persists, the patient may have severe electrolyte imbalances, loss of extracellular fluid volume, decreased plasma volume, and eventually circulatory failure.

Metabolic alkalosis can result from loss of gastric hydrochloric (HCl) acid. When contents of the small intestine are vomited, metabolic acidosis can occur. However, metabolic acidosis is less common than metabolic alkalosis. Weight loss resulting from fluid loss is evident in a short time when vomiting is severe.

The threat of pulmonary aspiration is a concern when vomiting occurs in older or unconscious patients or in patients with other conditions that impair the gag reflex. To prevent aspiration, put the patient who cannot adequately manage self-care in a semi-Fowler's or side-lying position.

Collaborative Care

The goals of collaborative care are to determine and treat the underlying cause of the nausea and vomiting and to provide symptomatic relief. Assess the patient for precipitating factors, and describe the contents of the emesis. Women are more likely to suffer from nausea and vomiting associated with surgical procedures and motion sickness.[1]

It is important to differentiate among vomiting, regurgitation, and projectile vomiting. *Regurgitation* is an effortless process in which partially digested food slowly comes up from the stomach. Retching or vomiting rarely occurs before it. *Projectile vomiting* is a forceful expulsion of stomach contents without nausea and is characteristic of CNS (brain and spinal cord) tumors.

Emesis containing partially digested food several hours after a meal is indicative of gastric outlet obstruction or delayed gastric emptying. The presence of fecal odor and bile after prolonged vomiting suggests intestinal obstruction below the level of the pylorus. Bile in the emesis may suggest obstruction below the ampulla of Vater. The color of the emesis aids in identifying the presence and source of bleeding. Vomitus with a "coffee ground" appearance is related to gastric bleeding, where blood changes to dark brown as a result of its interaction with HCl acid. Bright red blood indicates active bleeding. This could be due to a Mallory-Weiss tear (disruption of the mucosal lining near the esophagogastric junction), esophageal varices, gastric or duodenal ulcer, or neoplasm. A Mallory-Weiss tear is most often related to severe retching and vomiting.

The time of day at which the vomiting occurs is often helpful in determining the cause. Early morning vomiting is common in pregnancy. Emotional stressors with no evident pathologic disorder may elicit vomiting during or immediately after eating.

Drug Therapy. The use of drugs (Table 42-1) in the treatment of nausea and vomiting depends on the cause of the problem. Because the cause cannot always be readily determined, use drugs with caution. Using antiemetics before determining the cause can mask the underlying disease process and delay diagnosis and treatment. Many antiemetic drugs act in the CNS via the CTZ to block the neurochemicals that trigger nausea and vomiting.

> **DRUG ALERT: Promethazine Injection**
> - Promethazine should not be administered into an artery or under the skin because of the risk of severe tissue injury, including gangrene.
> - When promethazine is administered IV, it can leach out from the vein and cause serious damage to surrounding tissue.
> - Deep muscle injection is the preferred route of injection administration.

> **DRUG ALERT: Metoclopramide (Reglan)**
> - Chronic use or high doses of metoclopramide carry the risk of tardive dyskinesia.
> - Tardive dyskinesia is a neurologic condition characterized by involuntary and repetitive movements of the body (e.g., extremity movements, lip smacking).
> - With discontinuation of the drug, the tardive dyskinesia persists.

The serotonin (5-HT₃) receptor antagonists are effective in reducing cancer chemotherapy–induced vomiting caused by delayed gastric emptying and also the nausea and vomiting

TABLE 42-1   DRUG THERAPY

Nausea and Vomiting

Drug	Mechanism of Action	Side Effects
Phenothiazines chlorpromazine (Thorazine) perphenazine (Trilafon) prochlorperazine (Compazine) trifluoperazine (Stelazine) promethazine (Phenergan)	Act in the CNS level of the CTZ Block dopamine receptors that trigger nausea and vomiting	Dry mouth, hypotension, sedative effects, rashes, constipation
Antihistamines meclizine (Bonine, Antivert) dimenhydrinate (Dramamine) hydroxyzine (Vistaril) diphenhydramine (Benadryl)	Block the histamine receptors that trigger nausea and vomiting	Dry mouth, hypotension, sedative effects, rashes, constipation
Prokinetic Agents domperidone (Motilium) metoclopramide (Reglan)	Inhibit action of dopamine ↑ Gastric motility and emptying	CNS side effects ranging from anxiety to hallucinations Extrapyramidal side effects, including tremor and dyskinesias (similar to Parkinson's disease)
Serotonin (5-HT$_3$) Antagonists dolasetron (Anzemet) granisetron (Kytril) ondansetron (Zofran) palonosetron (Aloxi)	Block the action of serotonin (substance that causes nausea and vomiting)	Constipation, diarrhea, headache, fatigue, malaise, elevated liver function tests
Anticholinergic (Antimuscarinic) scopolamine transdermal	Blocks the cholinergic pathways to the vomiting center	Xerostomia, somnolence
Butyrophenone droperidol (Inapsine)	Blocks the neurochemicals that trigger nausea and vomiting	Dry mouth, hypotension, sedative effects, rashes, constipation
Others aprepitant (Emend) dexamethasone (Decadron) dronabinol (Marinol) nabilone (Cesamet) thiethylperazine (Torecan) trimethobenzamide (Tigan)		

CTZ, Chemoreceptor trigger zone.

related to migraine headache and anxiety.[2] 5-HT$_3$ antagonists are also used in prevention and treatment of postoperative nausea and vomiting. Dexamethasone (Decadron) is used in the management of both acute and delayed cancer chemotherapy–induced emesis, usually in combination with other antiemetics such as ondansetron (Zofran). Aprepitant (Emend), a substance P/neurokinin-1 receptor antagonist, is used for the prevention of chemotherapy-induced and postoperative nausea and vomiting.

Dronabinol (Marinol) is an orally active cannabinoid that is used alone or in combination with other antiemetics for the prevention of chemotherapy-induced emesis. Because of the potential for abuse, as well as drowsiness and sedation, this drug is used only when other therapies are ineffective.

Nutritional Therapy. The patient with severe vomiting requires IV fluid therapy with electrolyte and glucose replacement until able to tolerate oral intake. In some cases a nasogastric (NG) tube and suction are used to decompress the stomach. Start oral nutrition beginning with clear liquids once symptoms have subsided. Extremely hot or cold liquids are often difficult to tolerate. Carbonated beverages at room temperature and with

the carbonation gone and warm tea are easier to tolerate. The addition of dry toast or crackers may be helpful. Water is the initial fluid of choice for rehydration by mouth. Sipping small amounts of fluid (5 to 15 mL) every 15 to 20 minutes is usually better tolerated than drinking large amounts less frequently. Broth and Gatorade are high in sodium, so administer them with caution.

As the patient's condition improves, provide a diet high in carbohydrates and low in fat. Items such as a baked potato, plain gelatin, cereal, and hard candy are ideal. Coffee, spicy foods, highly acidic foods, and those with strong odors are often poorly tolerated. Tell the patient to eat food slowly and in small amounts to prevent overdistention of the stomach. Liquids taken between meals rather than with meals also reduce overdistention. Consult a dietitian regarding appropriate foods that have nutritional value and are well tolerated by the patient.

Nondrug Therapy. For some patients, acupressure or acupuncture at specific points is effective in reducing postoperative nausea and vomiting.[3] Some patients use herbs such as ginger and peppermint oil. Relaxation breathing exercises, changes in body position, or exercise may be helpful for some patients.

COMPLEMENTARY & ALTERNATIVE THERAPIES

Ginger

Scientific Evidence
- Some evidence that ginger may be effective for nausea and vomiting of pregnancy when used at recommended doses for short periods
- Unclear scientific evidence for the use of ginger for nausea and vomiting related to other conditions

Nursing Implications
- Few adverse effects have been reported with short-term use.
- Ginger may inhibit platelet aggregation and increase risk of bleeding.
- It may lower blood glucose levels.

Source: Based on a systematic review of scientific literature. Retrieved from *www.naturalstandard.com.*

NURSING MANAGEMENT
NAUSEA AND VOMITING

NURSING ASSESSMENT

Each patient with a history of prolonged and persistent nausea or vomiting requires a thorough nursing assessment before you develop a specific plan of care. Although numerous conditions are associated with nausea and vomiting, you should have a basic understanding of the more common conditions and be able to identify the patient who is at high risk. Knowledge of the physiologic mechanisms involved in nausea and vomiting is important in the assessment process. Table 42-2 presents subjective and objective data to be obtained from a patient with nausea and vomiting.

NURSING DIAGNOSES

Nursing diagnoses for the patient with nausea and vomiting may include, but are not limited to, the following:
- Nausea *related to* multiple etiologies
- Deficient fluid volume *related to* prolonged vomiting
- Imbalanced nutrition: less than body requirements *related to* nausea and vomiting

Additional information on nursing diagnoses is presented in eNursing Care Plan 42-1 on the website for this chapter.

PLANNING

The overall goals are that the patient with nausea and vomiting will (1) experience minimal or no nausea and vomiting, (2) have normal electrolyte levels and hydration status, and (3) return to a normal pattern of fluid balance and nutrient intake.

NURSING IMPLEMENTATION

ACUTE INTERVENTION. Most people with nausea and vomiting can be managed at home. When nausea and vomiting persist, hospitalization may be necessary for diagnosis of the underlying problem. Until a diagnosis is confirmed, the patient is on nothing-by-mouth (NPO) status and given IV fluids. An NG tube connected to suction may be needed for the patient with persistent vomiting or when a bowel obstruction or paralytic ileus is suspected. Secure the NG tube to prevent its movement in the nose and back of the throat because this can stimulate nausea and vomiting.

With prolonged vomiting, there is a probability of dehydration and acid-base and electrolyte imbalances. Provide explanations regarding diagnostic tests or procedures performed. Record intake and output, position the patient to prevent

---

TABLE 42-2 NURSING ASSESSMENT

Nausea and Vomiting

Subjective Data
Important Health Information
Past health history: GI disorders, chronic indigestion, food allergies, pregnancy, infection, CNS disorders, recent travel, bulimia, metabolic disorders, cancer, cardiovascular disease, renal disease
Medications: Antiemetics, digitalis, opioids, ferrous sulfate, aspirin, aminophylline, alcohol, antibiotics; general anesthesia; chemotherapy
Surgery or other treatments: Recent surgery

Functional Health Patterns
Nutritional-metabolic: Amount, frequency, character, and color of vomitus; dry heaves; anorexia; weight loss
Activity-exercise: Weakness, fatigue
Cognitive-perceptual: Abdominal tenderness or pain
Coping–stress tolerance: Stress, fear

Objective Data
General
Lethargy, sunken eyeballs

Integumentary
Pallor, dry mucous membranes, poor skin turgor

Gastrointestinal
Amount, frequency, character (e.g., projectile), content (undigested food, blood, bile, feces), and color of vomitus (red, "coffee ground," green-yellow)

Urinary
Decreased output, concentrated urine

Possible Diagnostic Findings
Altered serum electrolytes (especially hypokalemia), metabolic alkalosis, abnormal upper GI findings on endoscopy or abdominal x-rays

---

aspiration, and monitor vital signs. Assess for signs of dehydration, and observe for changes in the patient's physical comfort and mentation. Provide physical and emotional support, and maintain a quiet, odor-free environment.

AMBULATORY AND HOME CARE. Teach the patient and the caregiver (1) how to manage the unpleasant sensation of nausea, (2) methods to prevent nausea and vomiting, and (3) strategies to maintain fluid and nutritional intake. You can minimize the occurrence of nausea or vomiting by keeping the immediate environment quiet, free of noxious odors, and well ventilated. Avoiding sudden changes of position and unnecessary activity is also helpful. Use of relaxation techniques, frequent rest periods, effective pain management strategies, and diversional tactics can prevent or reduce nausea and vomiting. Cleansing the face and hands with a cool washcloth and providing mouth care between episodes increase the person's comfort level. When symptoms occur, stop all foods and drugs until the acute phase is over.

If you suspect a medication is the cause, notify the health care provider immediately so that either the dosage can be altered or a new drug prescribed. Advise the patient that stopping the drug without consulting the health care provider may have detrimental effects on the person's health.

When food is the precipitating cause of nausea and vomiting, help the patient identify the specific food. In addition, determine when it was eaten, prior history with that food, and whether anyone else in the family is sick.

A patient may be reluctant to resume fluid intake because of fear of nausea recurring. Suggest that he or she begin with clear liquids or cola beverages, Gatorade, tea or broth, dry crackers or toast, and then plain gelatin. Bland foods, such as pasta, rice, and cooked chicken, are generally well tolerated in small amounts. An antiemetic drug is taken only if prescribed by the health care provider. Taking over-the-counter (OTC) drugs for relief of symptoms may make the problem worse.

EVALUATION

The expected outcomes are that the patient with nausea and vomiting will

- Be comfortable with minimal or no nausea and vomiting
- Have electrolyte levels within normal range
- Be able to maintain adequate intake of fluids and nutrients

GERONTOLOGIC CONSIDERATIONS

NAUSEA AND VOMITING

The older adult experiencing nausea and vomiting requires careful assessment and monitoring, particularly during periods of fluid loss and subsequent rehydration therapy. Older patients are more likely to have cardiac or renal insufficiency that places them at greater risk for life-threatening fluid and electrolyte imbalances. Excessive replacement of fluid and electrolytes may result in adverse consequences for the person who has heart failure or renal disease. The older adult with a decreased level of consciousness may be at high risk for aspiration of vomitus. Close monitoring of the patient's physical status and level of consciousness during episodes of vomiting is important.

Older adults are particularly susceptible to the CNS side effects of antiemetic drugs, since these drugs may produce confusion and increase their risk for falls. Dosages should be reduced and efficacy closely evaluated. Institute safety precautions for these patients (e.g., removing rugs that may cause slipping).

ORAL INFLAMMATION AND INFECTIONS

Oral inflammation and infections may be due to specific mouth diseases or secondary to systemic disorders such as leukemia or vitamin deficiency. Oral inflammation and infections can severely impair oral ingestion. Common inflammations and infections of the oral cavity are presented in Table 42-3. The patient who is immunosuppressed (e.g., receiving chemotherapy for cancer) or using corticosteroid inhalant treatment for asthma is at risk for oral infections (e.g., candidiasis).

TABLE 42-3   INFECTIONS AND INFLAMMATION OF THE MOUTH

Infection or Inflammation	Etiology	Clinical Manifestations	Treatment
Gingivitis	Neglected oral hygiene, malocclusion, missing or irregular teeth, faulty dentistry, eating of soft rather than fibrous foods.	Inflamed gingivae and interdental papillae, bleeding during tooth brushing, development of pus, formation of abscess with loosening of teeth (periodontitis).	Prevention through health teaching, dental care, gingival massage, professional cleaning of teeth, fibrous foods, conscientious brushing habits with flossing.
Vincent's infection (acute necrotizing ulcerative gingivitis, trench mouth)	Fusiform bacteria, Vincent spirochetes; predisposing factors of stress, excessive fatigue, poor oral hygiene, nutritional deficiencies (B and C vitamins).	Painful, bleeding gingivae. Eroding necrotic lesions of interdental papillae, ulcerations that bleed, increased saliva with metallic taste, fetid mouth odor, anorexia, fever, general malaise.	Rest (physical and mental); avoidance of smoking and alcoholic beverages. Soft, nutritious diet. Correct oral hygiene habits. Topical applications of antibiotics. Mouth irrigations with chlorhexidine (Hibiclens) and saline solutions.
Oral candidiasis (moniliasis or thrush)	*Candida albicans* (a yeastlike fungus), debilitation, prolonged high-dose antibiotic or corticosteroid therapy.	Pearly, bluish white "milk-curd" membranous lesions on mucosa of mouth and larynx. Sore mouth, yeasty halitosis.	Miconazole buccal tablets (Oravig), nystatin or amphotericin B as oral suspension or buccal tablets. Good oral hygiene.
Herpes simplex (cold sore, fever blister)*	Herpes simplex virus (type 1 or 2), predisposing factors of upper respiratory tract infections, excessive exposure to sunlight, food allergies, emotional tension, onset of menstruation.	Lip lesions, mouth lesions, vesicle formation (single or clustered). Shallow, painful ulcers.	Spirits of camphor, corticosteroid cream, mild antiseptic mouthwash, viscous lidocaine; removal or control of predisposing factors, antiviral agents (e.g., acyclovir [Zovirax], famciclovir [Famvir], penciclovir [Denavir], valacyclovir [Valtrex]).
Aphthous stomatitis (canker sore)	Recurrent and chronic form of infection secondary to systemic disease, trauma, stress, or unknown causes.	Ulcers of mouth and lips, causing extreme pain. Ulcers surrounded by erythematous base.	Corticosteroids (topical or systemic), tetracycline oral suspension.
Parotitis (inflammation of parotid gland, surgical mumps)	Usually *Staphylococcus* species, *Streptococcus* species occasionally, debilitation and dehydration with poor oral hygiene, NPO status for an extended time.	Pain in area of gland and ear, absence of salivation, purulent exudate from gland, erythema, ulcers.	Antibiotics, mouthwashes, warm compresses; preventive measures such as chewing gum, sucking on hard candy (lemon drops), adequate fluid intake.
Stomatitis (inflammation of mouth)	Trauma, pathogens, irritants (tobacco, alcohol). Renal, liver, and hematologic diseases. Side effect of many cancer chemotherapy drugs and radiation.	Excessive salivation, halitosis, sore mouth.	Removal or treatment of cause, oral hygiene with soothing solutions, topical medications. Soft, bland diet.

*See Table 24-5.

Oral infections may predispose the patient to infections in other body organs. For example, the oral cavity is a potential reservoir for respiratory pathogens. In addition, oral pathogens have been associated with diabetes and heart disease.[4]

Regular and good oral and dental hygiene reduces oral infections and inflammation. Management of these conditions focuses on identification of the cause, elimination of infection, provision of comfort measures, and maintenance of nutritional intake.

ORAL CANCER

There are two types of oral cancer: *oral cavity cancer*, which starts in the mouth, and *oropharyngeal cancer*, which develops in the part of the throat just behind the mouth (called the oropharynx). *Head and neck squamous cell carcinoma* (HNSCC) is a term used for cancers of the oral cavity, pharynx, and larynx, which account for 90% of malignant oral tumors. Annually, oral cancer is diagnosed in 40,250 Americans, and it is estimated that 7850 people die from the disease.[5]

Oral cancer is more prevalent in African American men, and their survival rate is lower than that of white men. Oral cancer is more common after age 35, with 65 years being the average age of diagnosis. It is two times more common in men than in women. The 5-year survival rate is 83% for localized cancer and 61% for all stages of cancer of the oral cavity and pharynx combined.[5]

Most oral malignant lesions occur on the lower lip. Other common sites are the lateral border and undersurface of the tongue, the labial commissure, and the buccal mucosa. Carcinoma of the lip has the most favorable prognosis of any of the oral tumors because lip lesions are usually diagnosed earlier.

Etiology and Pathophysiology

Although the definitive cause of oral cancer is unknown, it has a number of predisposing factors (Table 42-4). The risk of developing oral cancer is related to the duration of tobacco use. A history of frequent alcohol consumption is reported by 75% to 80% of patients who develop oral cancer. More than 30% of patients with cancer of the lip have outdoor occupations, indicating that prolonged exposure to sunlight is a risk factor. Irritation from the pipe stem resting on the lip is a factor in pipe smokers. Human papillomavirus (HPV) contributes to 25% of oral cancer cases.[5] HPV-associated oropharyngeal cancer is associated with multiple sexual partners, especially multiple oral sex partners.[6]

Clinical Manifestations

The common manifestations of oral cancer are shown in Table 42-4. Patients may also report nonspecific symptoms such as chronic sore throat, sore mouth, and voice changes. *Leukoplakia*, called "smoker's patch," is a white patch on the mouth mucosa or tongue. It is often considered a precancerous lesion, although less than 15% of these lesions actually transform into malignant cells. The patch becomes *keratinized* (hard and leathery) and is sometimes described as hyperkeratosis. Leukoplakia is the result of chronic irritation, especially from smoking. *Erythroplasia* (erythroplakia), which is a red velvety patch on the mouth or tongue, is also a precancerous lesion. More than 50% of cases of erythroplakia progress to squamous cell carcinoma.

Cancer of the lip usually appears as an indurated, painless ulcer on the lip. The first sign of carcinoma of the tongue is an ulcer or area of thickening. Soreness or pain of the tongue may occur, especially when eating hot or highly seasoned foods. Cancerous lesions are most likely to develop in the proximal half of the tongue. Some patients experience limitation of movement of the tongue. Later symptoms of cancer of the tongue include increased salivation, slurred speech, dysphagia (difficulty swallowing), toothache, and earache. Approximately 30% of patients with oral cancer have an asymptomatic neck mass.

CULTURAL & ETHNIC HEALTH DISPARITIES
Oral, Pharyngeal, and Esophageal Problems

Nausea and Vomiting
- Asian Americans, Middle Easterners, and African Americans are more likely to experience nausea and vomiting than whites.

Cancers of Oral Cavity and Pharynx
- The incidence and mortality rates are higher in African American men than in whites.
- Death rates as a result of oral cancer are decreasing in whites but increasing in nonwhites.

Esophageal Cancer
- Highest incidence is in non-Hispanic white men.
- Higher incidence occurs in Alaska Natives than in whites.

Stomach Cancer
- Asian Americans and Pacific Islanders, Hispanics, and African Americans have higher rates of stomach cancer than non-Hispanic whites.
- Asian Americans show significantly higher survival rates than other ethnic groups.

TABLE 42-4   TYPES AND CHARACTERISTICS OF ORAL CANCER

Location	Predisposing Factors	Clinical Manifestations	Treatment
Lip	Constant overexposure to sun, ruddy and fair complexion, recurrent herpetic lesions, irritation from pipe stem, syphilis, immunosuppression	Indurated, painless ulcer	Surgical excision, radiation
Tongue	Tobacco, alcohol, chronic irritation, syphilis	Ulcer or area of thickening, soreness or pain. Increased salivation, slurred speech, dysphagia, toothache, earache (later signs)	Surgery (hemiglossectomy or glossectomy), radiation
Oral cavity	Poor oral hygiene, tobacco usage (pipe and cigar smoking, snuff, chewing tobacco), chronic alcohol intake, chronic irritation (jagged tooth, ill-fitting prosthesis, chemical or mechanical irritants), human papillomavirus (HPV)	Leukoplakia, erythroplakia, ulcerations, sore spot, rough area, pain, dysphagia, a lump or thickening in the cheek. A sore throat or a feeling that something is stuck. Difficulty chewing and speaking (later signs)	Surgery (mandibulectomy, radical neck dissection, resection of buccal mucosa), internal and external radiation

---

TABLE 42-5   COLLABORATIVE CARE

Oral Cancer

Diagnostic	Collaborative Therapy*

• History and physical examination
• Biopsy
• Oral exfoliative cytology
• Toluidine blue test
• CT, MRI, PET
	• Surgery
	  • Surgical excision of the tumor
	  • Radical neck dissection
	• Radiation (internal or external)
	• Combined surgical resection with radiation
	• Chemotherapy

*Any of these approaches may be used, depending on the primary lesion and the extent of metastasis.

Diagnostic Studies

Diagnostic tests are performed to identify oral dysplasias, which are precursors to oral cancer. Oral exfoliative cytologic study involves scraping the suspicious lesion and spreading this scraping on a slide for microscopic examination. The toluidine blue test is also used as a screening test for oral cancer. Toluidine blue is applied topically to stain an area, and cancer cells preferentially take up the dye. A negative cytologic smear or negative toluidine blue test does not necessarily rule out a malignant condition. Once cancer is diagnosed, computed tomography (CT), magnetic resonance imaging (MRI), and positron emission tomography (PET) are used in staging the oral cancer.[7]

Collaborative Care

Collaborative care of the patient with oral carcinoma usually consists of surgery, radiation, chemotherapy, or a combination of these (Table 42-5).

Surgical Therapy. Surgery remains the most effective treatment, especially for early-stage disease. Various surgical procedures may be performed, depending on the location and extent of the tumor. Many of the operations are radical procedures involving extensive resections. Some examples are partial *mandibulectomy* (removal of the mandible), *hemiglossectomy* (removal of half of the tongue), *glossectomy* (removal of the tongue), resections of the buccal mucosa and floor of the mouth, and radical neck dissection.

Radical neck dissection includes wide excision of the primary lesion with removal of the regional lymph nodes, the deep cervical lymph nodes, and their lymphatic channels. The following structures may also be removed or transected (depending on the extent of the primary lesion): sternocleidomastoid muscle and other closely associated muscles, internal jugular vein, mandible, submaxillary gland, part of the thyroid and parathyroid glands, and spinal accessory nerve. A tracheostomy is commonly performed along with the radical neck dissection. Drainage tubes are inserted into the surgical area and connected to suction to remove fluid and blood.

Nonsurgical Therapy. Chemotherapy and radiation therapy are used together when there are positive margins, bone erosion, or positive lymph nodes. Chemotherapeutic agents used include 5-fluorouracil (5-FU), methotrexate, cisplatin (Platinol), carboplatin (Paraplatin), paclitaxel (Taxol), docetaxel (Taxotere), cetuximab (Erbitux), and bleomycin (Blenoxane). Combination drug therapies are also used.[8] (Chemotherapy is discussed in Chapter 16.) Brachytherapy with implantations of radioactive seeds may be used to treat early-stage oral cancer.

Palliative treatment is often the best management when the prognosis is poor, the cancer is inoperable, or the patient decides against surgery. Palliation aims to treat the symptoms and make the patient more comfortable. If it becomes difficult for the patient to swallow, a gastrostomy tube may be inserted to allow for adequate nutritional intake. (Enteral nutrition is discussed in Chapter 40.) Analgesic medication should be given freely. Frequent suctioning of the oral cavity is necessary when swallowing becomes difficult. (Other palliative and end-of-life nursing measures are discussed in Chapter 10.)

Nutritional Therapy. Because of depression, alcoholism, or presurgery radiation treatment, patients may be malnourished before surgery. A percutaneous endoscopic gastrostomy (PEG) placement may be considered before radiation treatment or surgery. After radical neck surgery, the patient may be unable to orally ingest nutrients because of mucositis, swelling, location of sutures, or difficulty swallowing. Parenteral fluids are given for the first 24 to 48 hours. After this time, enteral nutrition is given via an NG, gastrostomy, or nasointestinal tube. (PEG and parenteral and enteral feedings are discussed in Chapter 40.) Cervical esophagostomy and pharyngostomy have also been used.

Observe for feeding tolerance and adjust the amount, time, and formula if nausea, vomiting, diarrhea, or distention occurs. Give small amounts of water when the patient can swallow. Observe for choking. Suctioning may be necessary to prevent aspiration.

NURSING MANAGEMENT
ORAL CANCER

NURSING ASSESSMENT

Subjective and objective data to obtain from a patient with oral cancer are presented in Table 42-6.

TABLE 42-6   NURSING ASSESSMENT

Oral Cancer

Subjective Data
Important Health Information
Past health history: Recurrent oral herpetic lesions, human papillomavirus (HPV) infection or vaccination, syphilis, exposure to sunlight
Medications: Immunosuppressants
Surgery or other treatments: Removal of prior tumors or lesions

Functional Health Patterns
Health perception–health management: Use of alcohol and tobacco, pipe smoking; poor oral hygiene
Nutritional-metabolic: Reductions in oral intake, weight loss; difficulty chewing food; increased salivation; intolerance to certain foods or temperatures of food
Cognitive-perceptual: Mouth or tongue soreness or pain, toothache, earache, neck stiffness, dysphagia, difficulty speaking

Objective Data
Integumentary
Indurated, painless ulcer on lip; painless neck mass

Gastrointestinal
Areas of thickening or roughness, ulcers, leukoplakia, or erythroplakia on the tongue or oral mucosa; limited movement of the tongue; increased salivation, drooling; slurred speech; foul breath odor

Possible Diagnostic Findings
Positive exfoliative smear cytology (microscopic examination of cells removed by scraping); positive biopsy

NURSING DIAGNOSES

Nursing diagnoses for the patient with oral cancer may include, but are not limited to, the following:

- Imbalanced nutrition: less than body requirements *related to* oral pain, difficulty chewing and swallowing, surgical resection, and radiation treatment
- Chronic pain *related to* the tumor, surgery, or radiation
- Anxiety *related to* diagnosis of cancer, uncertain future, potential for disfiguring surgery, potential for recurrence, and prognosis
- Ineffective health maintenance *related to* lack of knowledge of disease process and therapeutic regimen and unavailability of a support system

PLANNING

The overall goals are that the patient with carcinoma of the oral cavity will (1) have a patent airway, (2) be able to communicate, (3) have adequate nutritional intake to promote wound healing, and (4) have relief of pain and discomfort.

NURSING IMPLEMENTATION

You have a significant role in early detection and treatment of oral cancer. Identify patients at risk (see Table 42-4) and provide information regarding predisposing factors. Inform the patient who smokes about smoking cessation programs available in the community. Warn adolescents and teenagers about the danger of using snuff or chewing tobacco. (Smoking cessation is discussed in Chapter 11 and Tables 11-4 to 11-6.)

Because early detection of oral cancer is important, teach the patient to report unexplained pain or soreness of the mouth, unusual bleeding, dysphagia, sore throat, voice changes, or swelling or lump in the neck. Refer any individual with an ulcerative lesion that does not heal within 2 to 3 weeks to a health care provider.

Preoperative care for the patient who will have a radical neck dissection involves consideration of the patient's physical and psychosocial needs. Physical preparation is the same as that for any major surgery, with special emphasis on oral hygiene. Explanations and emotional support should include information on postoperative communication and feeding. Explain the surgical procedure, and ensure that the patient understands the information. Radical neck dissection and related nursing management are discussed in Chapter 27 and eNursing Care Plan 27-2.

EVALUATION

The expected outcomes are that the patient with oral cancer will

- Have no respiratory complications
- Be able to communicate
- Maintain an adequate nutritional intake to promote wound healing
- Experience minimal pain and discomfort with eating, drinking, and talking

ESOFHAGEAL DISORDERS

GASTROESOPHAGEAL REFLUX DISEASE

Gastroesophageal reflux disease (GERD) is a chronic symptom of mucosal damage caused by reflux of stomach acid into the lower esophagus. GERD is not a disease but a syndrome. GERD is the most common upper GI problem. Approximately 10% to

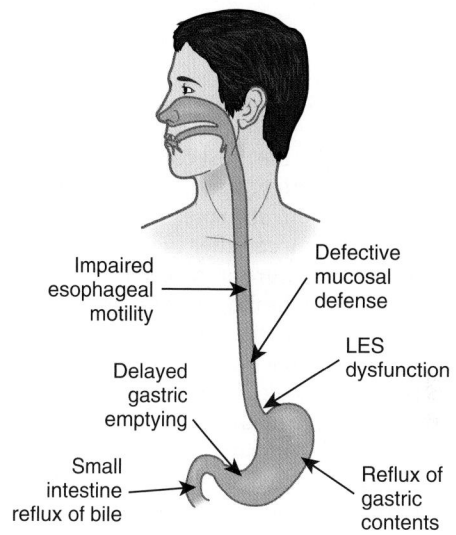

FIG. 42-2 Factors involved in the pathogenesis of gastroesophageal reflux disease (GERD). *LES,* Lower esophageal sphincter.

20% of the U.S. population experience GERD symptoms (heartburn or regurgitation) at least once a week.[9]

Etiology and Pathophysiology

GERD has no one single cause (Fig. 42-2). GERD results when the defenses of the esophagus are overwhelmed by the reflux of acidic gastric contents into the esophagus. Gastric HCl acid and pepsin secretions that reflux cause esophageal irritation and inflammation *(esophagitis)*. If the refluxate contains intestinal proteolytic enzymes (e.g., trypsin) and bile, this further irritates the esophageal mucosa. The degree of inflammation depends on the amount and composition of the gastric reflux and on the esophagus's mucosal defense mechanisms.

One of the primary etiologic factors in GERD is an incompetent LES. Under normal conditions, the LES acts as an antireflux barrier. An incompetent LES lets gastric contents move from the stomach to the esophagus when the patient is supine or has an increase in intraabdominal pressure.

Decreased LES pressure can be due to certain foods (e.g., caffeine, chocolate, peppermint) and drugs (e.g., anticholinergics). Obesity is a risk factor for GERD, although the specific mechanism remains to be determined.[10] In an obese person the intraabdominal pressure is increased, which can exacerbate GERD. Cigarette and cigar smoking can also contribute to GERD. A common cause of GERD is a hiatal hernia, which is discussed in the next section.

Clinical Manifestations

The symptoms of GERD vary from person to person. The persistence of mild symptoms (i.e., more than twice a week) or moderate to severe symptoms once a week is considered GERD.

TABLE 42-7	FACTORS AFFECTING LOWER ESOPHAGEAL SPHINCTER PRESSURE

Increase Pressure
- bethanechol (Urecholine)
- metoclopramide (Reglan)

Decrease Pressure
- Alcohol
- Anticholinergics
- Chocolate (theobromine)
- Fatty foods
- Nicotine
- Peppermint, spearmint

- Tea, coffee (caffeine)
- Drugs
  - β-Adrenergic blockers
  - Calcium channel blockers
  - diazepam (Valium)
  - morphine sulfate
  - Nitrates
  - progesterone
  - theophylline

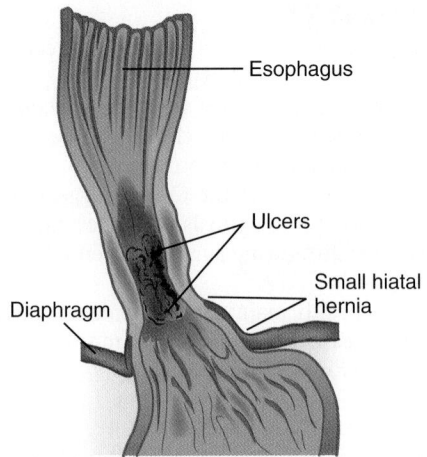

FIG. 42-3 Esophagitis with esophageal ulcerations.

Heartburn *(pyrosis)* is the most common clinical manifestation. Heartburn is a burning, tight sensation felt intermittently beneath the lower sternum and spreading upward to the throat or jaw. Heartburn may occur after ingestion of food or drugs that decrease the LES pressure or directly irritate the esophageal mucosa (Table 42-7). A health care provider should evaluate heartburn that occurs more than twice a week, is rated as severe, occurs at night and wakes a person from sleep, or is associated with dysphagia. Older adults who complain of recent onset of heartburn should receive medical evaluation.

Patients may also complain of dyspepsia. *Dyspepsia* is pain or discomfort centered in the upper abdomen (mainly in or around the midline as opposed to the right or left hypochondrium).

Regurgitation is a fairly common manifestation of GERD. It is often described as hot, bitter, or sour liquid coming into the throat or mouth. Hypersalivation (water brash) may also be reported.

An individual with GERD may also report respiratory symptoms, including wheezing, coughing, and dyspnea. Nocturnal discomfort and coughing can awaken the patient, resulting in disturbed sleep patterns. Otolaryngologic symptoms include hoarseness, sore throat, a *globus sensation* (sense of a lump in the throat), and choking.

GERD-related chest pain can mimic angina and is described as burning; squeezing; or radiating to the back, neck, jaw, or arms. Complaints of chest pain are more common in older adults with GERD. Unlike angina, GERD-related chest pain is relieved with antacids.

Complications

Complications of GERD are due to the direct local effects of gastric acid on the esophageal mucosa. Esophagitis (inflammation of the esophagus) is a common complication of GERD. Esophagitis with esophageal ulcerations is shown in Fig. 42-3. Repeated esophagitis may lead to scar tissue formation, stricture, and ultimately dysphagia.

Another complication of chronic GERD is Barrett's esophagus (esophageal metaplasia). (*Metaplasia* is the reversible change from one type of cell to another type and is generally caused by some sort of abnormal stimulus.) In Barrett's esophagus the flat epithelial cells in the distal esophagus change to columnar epithelial cells. These cell changes are thought to be due primarily to GERD. However, people with no history of reflux symptoms can develop Barrett's esophagus.

Barrett's esophagus is considered a precancerous lesion that increases the patient's risk for esophageal adenocarcinoma.

Approximately 5% to 15% of patients with chronic reflux have Barrett's esophagus.[11] Compared with whites, African Americans and Asians are at lower risk for Barrett's esophagus. Because patients with evidence of metaplasia on an initial endoscopic examination are at risk for esophageal cancer, a surveillance endoscopy every 2 to 3 years is often recommended.[12]

Respiratory complications of GERD include cough, bronchospasm, laryngospasm, and cricopharyngeal spasm. These complications are due to irritation of the upper airway by gastric secretions. Asthma, chronic bronchitis, and pneumonia may develop as a result of aspiration into the respiratory system. Dental erosion, especially in the posterior teeth, may result from acid reflux into the mouth.[12]

Diagnostic Studies

GERD is usually diagnosed on the basis of symptoms and the patient's response to behavioral and drug therapies. Diagnostic tests are done when these therapies are refractory or when complications are suspected. Diagnostic studies performed to determine the cause of the GERD are shown in Table 42-8.

Endoscopy is useful in assessing the LES competence and the degree of inflammation (if present), potential scarring, and strictures. Biopsy and cytologic specimens can differentiate stomach or esophageal carcinoma from Barrett's esophagus. In addition, the degree of dysplasia (low grade versus high grade) is determined. Manometric studies measure pressure in the esophagus and LES and esophageal motility function. Ambulatory esophageal pH monitoring may be done for patients with refractory symptoms and no evidence of mucosal inflammation. Radionuclide tests can also detect reflux of gastric contents and the rate of esophageal clearance.

Collaborative Care

Most patients with GERD can successfully manage this condition through lifestyle modifications and drug therapy. These long-term approaches require patient teaching and adherence to therapies. When these therapies are ineffective, surgery is an option (see Table 42-8).

Lifestyle Modifications. Teach the patient with GERD to avoid factors that trigger symptoms (see Table 42-7). Give particular attention to diet and drugs that may affect the LES, acid secretion, or gastric emptying. Recommend weight reduction if the patient is overweight. A patient and caregiver teaching guide is provided in Table 42-9.

Encourage patients who smoke to stop. If needed, refer the patient to community resources for assistance in stopping smoking. (See Chapter 11 for additional information related to smoking cessation.) If stress seems to cause symptoms, discuss measures to cope with stress. (See Chapter 7 for stress management techniques.)

Nutritional Therapy. Diet does not cause GERD, but food can aggravate symptoms. No specific diet is necessary. Teach patients to avoid foods that decrease LES pressure, such as chocolate, peppermint, tomatoes, fatty foods, coffee, and tea (see Table 42-7), which predispose them to reflux. Also teach patients with GERD to avoid milk, especially at bedtime, since it increases gastric acid secretion. Small, frequent meals help prevent overdistention of the stomach. Saliva production can be increased by chewing gum and oral lozenges, which may help patients with mild symptoms of GERD.

Tell the patient to avoid late evening meals and nocturnal snacking, and to take fluids between rather than with meals to reduce gastric distention. Certain foods (e.g., tomato-based products, orange juice, cola, red wine) may irritate the esophagus.

Drug Therapy. Drug therapy for GERD focuses on decreasing volume and acidity of reflux, improving LES function, increasing esophageal clearance, and protecting the esophageal mucosa[13] (Table 42-10). Proton pump inhibitors (PPIs) and histamine (H_2)-receptor blockers are common and effective treatments for symptomatic GERD. The goal of HCl acid suppression treatment is to reduce the acidity of the gastric refluxate. Patients who are symptomatic with GERD but do not have evidence of esophagitis *(nonerosive GERD)* achieve symptom relief with PPIs and H_2-receptor blockers. The PPIs are more effective in healing esophagitis than H_2-receptor blockers. PPIs are also beneficial in decreasing the incidence of esophageal strictures, a complication of chronic GERD. Omeprazole is available as a prescription as well as an OTC preparation (Prilosec OTC) and in an immediate-release form (Zegerid).

TABLE 42-8 COLLABORATIVE CARE

Gastroesophageal Reflux Disease (GERD) and Hiatal Hernia

Diagnostic
- History and physical examination
- Upper GI endoscopy with biopsy and cytologic analysis
- Esophagram (barium swallow)
- Motility (manometry) studies
- pH monitoring (laboratory or 24 hr ambulatory)
- Radionuclide studies

Collaborative Therapy
Conservative
- Elevation of head of bed on 4- to 6-in blocks
- Avoid reflux-inducing foods (fatty foods, chocolate, peppermint)
- Avoid alcohol
- Reduce or avoid acidic pH beverages (colas, red wine, orange juice)
- Antacids
- Drug therapy (see Table 42-10)
  - Proton pump inhibitors
  - H_2-receptor blockers
  - Prokinetic drug therapy
  - Cholinergic drugs

Surgical
- Nissen fundoplication
- Toupet fundoplication

Endoscopic
- Intraluminal valvuloplasty
- Radiofrequency therapy

LES, Lower esophageal sphincter.

TABLE 42-9 PATIENT & CAREGIVER TEACHING GUIDE

Gastroesophageal Reflux Disease (GERD)

Include the following instructions when teaching the patient and caregiver about management of GERD.
1. Explain the rationale for a low-fat diet.
2. Encourage the patient to eat small, frequent meals to prevent gastric distention.
3. Explain the rationale for avoiding alcohol, smoking (causes an almost immediate, marked decrease in LES pressure), and beverages that contain caffeine.
4. Advise the patient to not lie down for 2-3 hr after eating, wear tight clothing around the waist, or bend over (especially after eating).
5. Have the patient avoid eating within 3 hr of bedtime.
6. Encourage the patient to sleep with head of bed elevated on 4- to 8-inch blocks (gravity fosters esophageal emptying).
7. Provide information regarding drugs, including rationale for their use and common side effects.
8. Discuss strategies for weight reduction if appropriate.
9. Encourage patient and caregiver to share concerns about lifestyle changes and living with a chronic problem.

LES, Lower esophageal sphincter.

EVIDENCE-BASED PRACTICE

Translating Research Into Practice

Are Proton Pump Inhibitors Associated With Increased Risk of Diarrhea?

Clinical Question
Among hospitalized patients (P), does the use of proton pump inhibitor drugs (I) increase the risk of *Clostridium difficile*–associated diarrhea (O)?

Best Available Evidence
Meta-analysis of case-control and cohort studies

Critical Appraisal and Synthesis of Evidence
- Twenty-three studies examined hospitalized patient medical records (n = 300,000) for proton pump inhibitor (PPI) exposure and confirmation of acute diarrhea due to *C. difficile.*
- Patients taking PPIs have a greater risk (65%) of *C. difficile*–associated diarrhea (CDAD).

Conclusion
- There is a significant positive association between PPIs and the incidence of CDAD.

Implications for Nursing Practice
- Advise patients taking PPIs of the risk for diarrhea and to contact their health care provider if it does not improve.
- Inform patients that CDAD symptoms include watery stool, abdominal pain, and fever.
- Institute infection control procedures in hospitalized patients suspected of having *C. difficile* infection.

Reference for Evidence
Janarthanan S, Ditah I, Adler D, et al: *Clostridium difficile*–associated diarrhea and proton pump inhibitor therapy: a meta-analysis, *Am J Gastroenterol* 107:1001, 2012.

P, Patient population of interest; *I,* intervention or area of interest; *O,* outcomes of interest (see p.12).

TABLE 42-10   **DRUG THERAPY**

Gastroesophageal Reflux Disease (GERD) and Peptic Ulcer Disease (PUD)

Drug	Mechanism of Action	Side Effects
Proton Pump Inhibitors (PPIs) dexlansoprazole (Dexilant) esomeprazole (Nexium) lansoprazole (Prevacid) omeprazole (Prilosec) pantoprazole (Protonix) rabeprazole (AcipHex)	↓ HCl acid secretion by inhibiting the proton pump (H⁺-K⁺-ATPase) responsible for the secretion of H⁺ ↓ Irritation of the esophageal and gastric mucosa	Headache, abdominal pain, nausea, diarrhea, vomiting, flatulence
Histamine (H₂)-Receptor Blockers cimetidine (Tagamet) famotidine (Pepcid) nizatidine (Axid) ranitidine (Zantac)	Blocks the action of histamine on the H₂ receptors to ↓ HCl acid secretion ↓ Conversion of pepsinogen to pepsin ↓ Irritation of the esophageal and gastric mucosa	Headache, abdominal pain, constipation, diarrhea
Prokinetic Agents metoclopramide (Reglan)	Blocks effect of dopamine ↑ Gastric motility and emptying Reduces reflux	CNS side effects ranging from anxiety to hallucinations Extrapyramidal side effects (tremor and dyskinesias similar to Parkinson's disease)
Antiulcer, Protectants sucralfate (Carafate)	Acts to form a protective layer and serves as a barrier against acid, bile salts, and enzymes in the stomach	Constipation
Cholinergic bethanechol (Urecholine)	↑ LES pressure, improves esophageal emptying, increases gastric emptying	Lightheadedness, syncope, flushing diarrhea, stomach cramps, dizziness
Antacids, Acid Neutralizers *Single Substance* aluminum carbonate (Basaljel) aluminum hydroxide (Amphojel) calcium carbonate (Tums, Titralac) magnesium oxide (MagOx) sodium bicarbonate (Alka-Seltzer) sodium citrate (Bicitra) *Aluminum and Magnesium* Gelusil, Maalox, Mylanta, Aludrox aluminum/magnesium trisilicate (Gaviscon)	Neutralizes HCl acid Taken 1-3 hr after meals and at bedtime	*Aluminum hydroxide:* Constipation, phosphorus depletion with chronic use *Calcium carbonate:* Constipation or diarrhea, hypercalcemia, milk-alkali syndrome, renal calculi *Magnesium preparations:* Diarrhea, hypermagnesemia *Sodium preparations:* Milk-alkali syndrome if used with large amounts of calcium; use with caution in patients on sodium restrictions
Prostaglandin (Synthetic) misoprostol (Cytotec)	Protects lining of stomach *Cytoprotective:* Increases production of gastric mucus and mucosal secretion of bicarbonate *Antisecretory:* ↓ HCl acid secretion	Abdominal pain, diarrhea, GI bleeding, uterine rupture if pregnant

LES, Lower esophageal sphincter.

Long-term use of PPIs has been associated with decreased bone density,[14] chronic hypochlorhydria, and increased risk of *Clostridium difficile* in hospitalized patients.[15] Long-term PPI use has also been associated with pneumonia.

DRUG ALERT: Proton Pump Inhibitors (PPIs)
- Long-term use or high doses of PPIs may increase the risk of fractures of hip, wrist, and spine.
- Lower doses or shorter duration of therapy should be considered.
- PPIs are associated with increased risk of *C. difficile* infection in hospitalized patients.

H₂-receptor blockers reduce symptoms and promote esophageal healing in 50% of patients. These drugs are available in OTC and prescription formulations. OTC preparations have lower drug dosages compared with prescription drugs. Some formulations include an H₂-receptor blocker plus antacid combination. For example, Pepcid Complete includes famotidine, calcium carbonate, and magnesium hydroxide. (Antihistamine drugs used to treat allergies are H₁-receptor blockers and have no effect on HCl acid secretion.)

Sucralfate (Carafate), an antiulcer drug, is used in some patients with GERD for its cytoprotective properties. Cholinergic drugs (e.g., bethanechol [Urecholine]) increase LES pressure, improve esophageal emptying in the supine position, and increase gastric emptying. However, cholinergic drugs also increase HCl acid secretion. Prokinetic (motility-enhancing) drugs (metoclopramide [Reglan]) promote gastric emptying and reduce the risk of gastric acid reflux (see Table 42-10) but are not used as primary therapies for GERD.

Antacids produce quick but short-lived relief of heartburn. They should be taken 1 to 3 hours after meals and at bedtime.

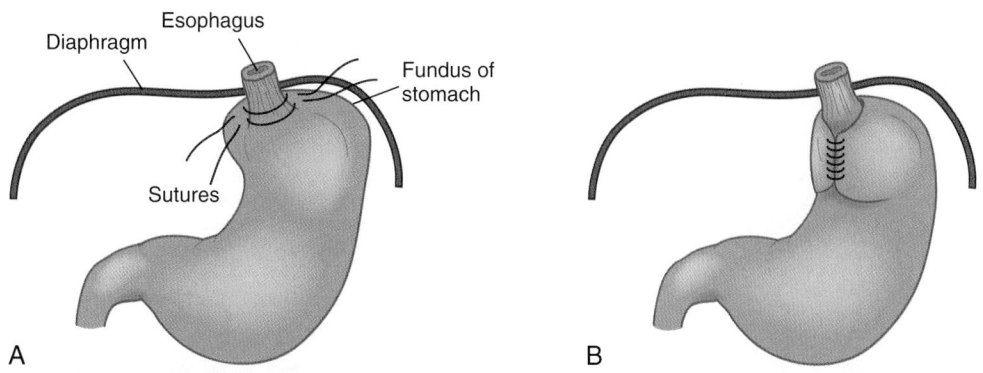

FIG. 42-4 Nissen fundoplication for repair of hiatal hernia. **A,** Fundus of stomach is wrapped around distal esophagus. **B,** The fundus is then sutured to itself.

Antacids with or without alginic acid (e.g., Gaviscon) may be useful in patients with mild, intermittent heartburn. However, in patients with moderate to severe or frequent symptoms or patients with documented esophagitis, antacids are not effective in relieving symptoms or healing lesions.

Surgical Therapy. Surgical therapy (*antireflux* surgery) is reserved for patients with complications of reflux, including esophagitis, intolerance of medications, stricture, Barrett's metaplasia, and persistence of severe symptoms. Most surgical procedures are performed laparoscopically. The goal of surgical interventions is to reduce reflux by enhancing the integrity of the LES. In these procedures the fundus of the stomach is wrapped around the lower portion of the esophagus to reinforce and repair the defective barrier. Laparoscopically performed Nissen and Toupet fundoplications are common antireflux surgeries (Fig. 42-4).

The LINX Reflux Management System is used for patients who continue to have symptoms despite maximum medical management. In this system, titanium beads with a magnetic core are strung together and implanted laparoscopically into the LES. Once implanted, the ring provides strength (augmentation) to a weakened LES. Under resting, nonswallowing conditions the ring tightens due to the magnetic attraction of the beads. When the individual swallows, the force of pressure associated with the movement of the fluids or foods overwhelms the magnetic forces such that the fluid or food passes to the stomach. Adverse events experienced with the system include difficulty swallowing, vomiting, nausea, chest pain, and pain when swallowing food.

Endoscopic Therapy. Alternatives to surgical therapy include endoscopic mucosal resection (EMR), photodynamic therapy, cryotherapy, and radiofrequency ablation (image-guided technique that kills cells through heating). For patients with high-grade dysplasia, EMR can also be used as a diagnostic test to obtain biopsy samples. The results of the biopsy can determine whether adenocarcinoma is present.

NURSING MANAGEMENT
GASTROESOPHAGEAL REFLUX DISEASE

Nursing care for the patient with acute symptoms of GERD consists of encouraging the patient to follow the necessary regimen. The head of the bed is elevated to approximately 30 degrees. This can be done using pillows or with 4- to 8-in blocks under the bed. For 2 to 3 hours after a meal the patient should not be supine. Teach the patient to avoid food and activities that cause reflux (e.g., late-night eating). Instruct patients to contact their health care provider if symptoms persist.

The patient on a PPI needs to take medication before the first meal of the day. Instruct the patient about possible medication side effects (see Table 42-10). Tell the patient on a prescription H$_2$-receptor agent to take the medication as prescribed and not to stop without checking with his or her health care provider.

Postoperative care focuses on prevention of respiratory complications, maintenance of fluid and electrolyte balance, and prevention of infection. If an open high abdominal incision is used, respiratory complications can occur. Respiratory assessment includes respiratory rate and rhythm, pulse rate and rhythm, and signs of pneumothorax (e.g., dyspnea, chest pain, cyanosis). Deep breathing is essential to fully expand the lungs. Because most procedures are performed laparoscopically, the risk of respiratory complications is reduced. The laparoscopic fundoplication is often performed as an outpatient procedure. However, patients at risk for complications, including those with prior upper abdominal surgeries or co-morbidities (e.g., cardiac disease, obesity), may be hospitalized after the procedure. During the postoperative phase, patients require medications to prevent nausea and vomiting and to control pain. A small percentage of patients experience complications, including gastric or esophageal injury, splenic injury, pneumothorax, perforation, bleeding, infection, and pneumonia.

When peristalsis returns, only fluids are given initially. Measure and record the intake and output. Solids are added gradually with the goal of resuming a normal diet. Teach the patient to avoid foods that are gas forming to prevent gastric distention and to chew food thoroughly.

After surgery, reflux symptoms should decrease. However, the recurrence rate may range from 10% to 30% over a 20-year period. In the first month after surgery the patient may report mild dysphagia caused by edema, but it should resolve. Instruct the patient to report persistent symptoms such as heartburn and regurgitation.

HIATAL HERNIA

Hiatal hernia is herniation of a portion of the stomach into the esophagus through an opening, or hiatus, in the diaphragm. It is also referred to as diaphragmatic hernia and esophageal hernia. It is the most common abnormality found on x-ray examination of the upper GI tract. Hiatal hernias are common in older adults and occur more often in women than in men.

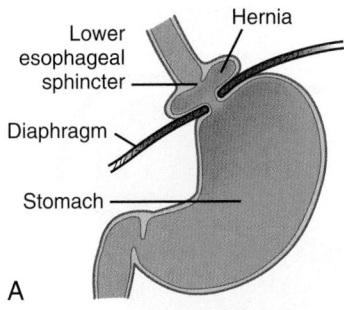

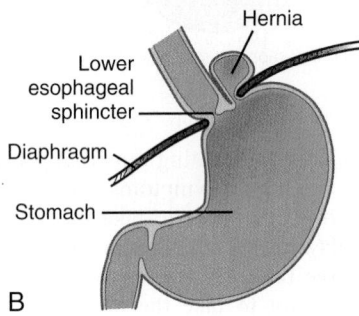

FIG. 42-5 **A,** Sliding hiatal hernia. **B,** Rolling or paraesophageal hernia.

Hiatal hernias are classified into the following two types (Fig. 42-5):

1. *Sliding:* The junction of the stomach and the esophagus is above the diaphragm, and a part of the stomach slides through the hiatal opening in the diaphragm. This occurs when the patient is supine, and the hernia usually goes back into the abdominal cavity when the patient is standing upright. This is the most common type of hiatal hernia.

2. *Paraesophageal,* or *rolling:* The esophagogastric junction remains in the normal position, but the fundus and the greater curvature of the stomach roll up through the diaphragm, forming a pocket alongside the esophagus. Acute paraesophageal hernia is a medical emergency.

Etiology and Pathophysiology

Many factors contribute to the development of hiatal hernia. Structural changes, such as weakening of the muscles in the diaphragm around the esophagogastric opening, occur with aging. Factors that increase intraabdominal pressure, including obesity, pregnancy, ascites, tumors, intense physical exertion, and heavy lifting on a continual basis, may also predispose patients to development of a hiatal hernia.

Clinical Manifestations and Complications

Some individuals with hiatal hernia are asymptomatic. When present, signs and symptoms of hiatal hernia are similar to those described for GERD on pp. 931-932.

Complications that may occur with hiatal hernia include GERD, esophagitis, hemorrhage from erosion, stenosis (narrowing of the esophagus), ulcerations of the herniated portion of the stomach, strangulation of the hernia, and regurgitation with tracheal aspiration.

Diagnostic Studies

An esophagram (barium swallow) may show the protrusion of gastric mucosa through the esophageal hiatus. Endoscopic visualization of the lower esophagus provides information on the

degree of mucosal inflammation or other abnormalities. Other tests are listed in Table 42-8.

NURSING AND COLLABORATIVE MANAGEMENT HIATAL HERNIA

Conservative therapy of hiatal hernia is similar to that described for GERD (pp. 932-935). Teach the patient to reduce intraabdominal pressure by eliminating constricting garments and avoiding lifting and straining.

Surgical approaches to hiatal hernias can include reduction of the herniated stomach into the abdomen, *herniotomy* (excision of the hernia sac), *herniorrhaphy* (closure of the hiatal defect), an antireflux procedure, and *gastropexy* (attachment of the stomach subdiaphragmatically to prevent reherniation). The goals are to reduce the hernia, provide an acceptable LES pressure, and prevent movement of the gastroesophageal junction. Antireflux surgeries for hiatal hernia are laparoscopically performed Nissen and Toupet techniques (see Fig. 42-4). A thoracic or an open abdominal approach may be done, depending on the patient.

GERONTOLOGIC CONSIDERATIONS

GASTROESOPHAGEAL REFLUX DISEASE AND HIATAL HERNIA

The incidence of hiatal hernia and GERD increases with age. Hiatal hernia is associated with weakening of the diaphragm, obesity, kyphosis, or other factors (e.g., wearing girdles) that increase intraabdominal pressure. Medications commonly taken by older patients decrease LES pressure (e.g., nitrates, calcium channel blockers, antidepressants). Other agents such as nonsteroidal antiinflammatory drugs (NSAIDs) and potassium can irritate the esophageal mucosa (medication-induced esophagitis).

Some older adults with hiatal hernia and GERD are asymptomatic or have less severe symptoms. The first indications may include esophageal bleeding secondary to esophagitis or respiratory complications (e.g., aspiration pneumonia) related to aspiration of gastric contents.

The clinical course and management of GERD and hiatal hernia in the older adult are similar to those for the younger adult. Changes in lifestyle, including eliminating dietary factors (such as caffeine-containing beverages and chocolate) and elevating the head of the bed on blocks, may be challenging for the older adult.

Laparoscopic procedures reduce the risk of surgical repair. An older patient with cardiovascular and pulmonary problems may not be a good candidate for surgical intervention.

ESOPHAGEAL CANCER

Esophageal cancer (malignant neoplasm of the esophagus) is not common. However, the rates are increasing. Annually in the United States approximately 17,460 new cases of esophageal cancer are diagnosed and 15,070 deaths occur from esophageal cancer.[5] The 5-year survival rate is 37% for localized cancer and 18% for regional cancer.

The majority of esophageal cancers are adenocarcinomas, with the remainder being squamous cell tumors. Adenocarcinomas arise from the glands lining the esophagus and resemble cancers of the stomach and small intestine. The incidence of esophageal cancer increases with age, with those between 70 and 84 at greatest risk. There is a higher incidence of esophageal cancer in non-Hispanic white men and Alaska Natives compared with other ethnic groups. The incidence of esophageal cancer is higher in men than in women.

Etiology and Pathophysiology

The cause of esophageal cancer is unknown. Several important risk factors include Barrett's metaplasia, smoking, excessive alcohol intake, and obesity. For example, current smoking or a history of smoking are associated with a 2-fold higher risk of esophageal cancer. Patients with injury to the esophageal mucosa (e.g., from occupational exposure) are at greater risk. Achalasia, a condition in which there is delayed emptying of the lower esophagus, is associated with squamous cell cancer.

Most esophageal tumors are located in the middle and lower portions of the esophagus. The malignant tumor usually appears as an ulcerated lesion and has often advanced by the time the patient experiences symptoms. The tumor may penetrate the muscular layer and even extend outside the wall of the esophagus. Obstruction of the esophagus occurs in the later stages.

Clinical Manifestations and Complications

The onset of symptoms is usually late relative to tumor growth. The majority of patients have advanced disease at diagnosis. Progressive dysphagia is the most common symptom and may be described as a substernal feeling as if food is not passing. Initially the dysphagia occurs only with meat, then with soft foods, and eventually with liquids.

Pain develops late. It is described as occurring in the substernal, epigastric, or back areas and usually increases with swallowing. The pain may radiate to the neck, jaw, ears, and shoulders. If the tumor is in the upper third of the esophagus, symptoms such as sore throat, choking, and hoarseness may occur. Weight loss is fairly common. When esophageal stenosis (narrowing) is severe, regurgitation of blood-flecked esophageal contents is common.

Hemorrhage occurs if the cancer erodes through the esophagus and into the aorta. Esophageal perforation with fistula formation into the lung or trachea sometimes develops. The tumor may enlarge enough to cause esophageal obstruction. The cancer spreads via the lymph system, with the liver and the lung being common sites of metastasis.

Diagnostic Studies

Endoscopic biopsy is necessary to make a definitive diagnosis of carcinoma by identification of malignant cells. Endoscopic ultrasonography (EUS) is an important tool used to stage esophageal cancer. Esophagram (barium swallow) may show narrowing of the esophagus at the tumor site (Table 42-11).

Collaborative Care

The treatment of esophageal cancer depends on the location of the tumor and whether invasion or metastasis has occurred. Esophageal cancer has a poor prognosis, mainly because it is often not diagnosed until the disease is advanced. The best

---

TABLE 42-11 COLLABORATIVE CARE

Esophageal Cancer

Diagnostic
- History and physical examination
- Endoscopy of esophagus with biopsy
- Endoscopic ultrasonography
- Esophagram (barium swallow)
- Bronchoscopy
- CT, MRI

Collaborative Therapy
- Surgery
  - Esophagectomy
  - Esophagogastrostomy
  - Esophagoenterostomy
- Endoscopic procedures
  - Photodynamic therapy
  - Endoscopic mucosal resection
- Radiation therapy
- Chemotherapy
- Palliative treatment
  - Dilation
  - Stent or prosthesis
  - Laser therapy
  - Gastrostomy

results are obtained with a multimodal approach, including surgery, endoscopic ablation, chemotherapy, and radiation therapy. Depending on the location and cancer spread, only chemotherapy and radiation may be used.

Surgery. The types of surgical procedures done are (1) removal of part or all of the esophagus *(esophagectomy)* with use of a Dacron graft to replace the resected part, (2) resection of a portion of the esophagus and anastomosis of the remaining portion to the stomach *(esophagogastrostomy),* and (3) resection of a portion of the esophagus and anastomosis of a segment of colon to the remaining portion *(esophagoenterostomy).* The surgical approaches may be open (thoracic, abdominal incision) or laparoscopic.

Minimally invasive esophagectomy (e.g., laparoscopic vagal nerve–sparing surgery) is being performed more frequently. It has the advantage of using smaller incisions, decreasing intensive care unit (ICU) and hospital stays, and producing fewer pulmonary complications.

Endoscopic Procedures. Endoscopic approaches using photodynamic and/or laser therapy can be performed. In photodynamic therapy, porfimer sodium (Photofrin), which is a photosensitizer, is injected IV. The porfimer is absorbed by most tissues but selectively retained to a greater degree by neoplastic tissue. The light (activator) is transmitted via a fiber passed through the endoscope. Warn patients to avoid direct sunlight for up to 4 weeks after the procedure. Other endoscopic procedures include EMR.

Radiation and Chemotherapy. Most patients with newly diagnosed esophageal cancer have local and advanced disease. Treatment includes chemotherapy with or without radiation therapy. Concurrent radiation and chemotherapy are administered for palliation of symptoms, especially dysphagia, and to increase survival. In some patients, treatment is started before surgery is performed.

Currently, no standard single-agent or combination drug therapy is recommended for esophageal cancer. Single-agent chemotherapeutic agents include bleomycin, mitomycin (Mutamycin), methotrexate, paclitaxel, docetaxel, and irinotecan (Camptosar). Combination regimens include ECF (epirubicin [Ellence], cisplatin, 5-fluorouracil [5-FU]), and taxane- and irinotecan-based combinations. Cisplatin in combination with newer fluoropyrimidine such as tegafur-uracil (Uftoral) (tegafur is a 5-FU prodrug) is also used.

Palliative therapy consists of restoration of the swallowing function and maintenance of nutrition and hydration. Dilation, stent placement, or both can relieve obstruction. Self-expandable metal stents are available with features to prevent stent migration and tumor ingrowth. Dilation is done with various types of dilators. Dilation often relieves dysphagia and allows for improved nutrition. Endoscopic placement of stents or expandable stents may help when dilation is no longer effective.[16] This allows food and liquid to pass through the stenotic segment of the esophagus. Stents may be placed before surgery to improve the patient's nutritional status.

Endoscopic laser therapy of the tumor may be used in combination with dilation. Obstruction recurs as the tumor grows, but laser therapy can be repeated. Sometimes these procedures are combined with radiation therapy. Other measures for palliation include gastrostomy or esophagostomy tube placement for nutritional support and pain management.

Nutritional Therapy. After esophageal surgery, parenteral fluids are given. A jejunostomy feeding tube may be used depending on the type of surgery (e.g., esophagogastrectomy)

performed. A swallowing study is often given before the patient is allowed to have oral fluids. When fluids are permitted, water (30 to 60 mL) is given hourly, with gradual progression to small, frequent, bland meals. The patient should be in an upright position to prevent regurgitation of the fluid. With tube feeding, observe the patient for signs of intolerance to the feeding or leakage of the feeding into the mediastinum. Symptoms that indicate leakage are pain, increased temperature, and dyspnea. A gastrostomy tube may be placed to feed the patient. (Enteral nutrition is discussed in Chapter 40.)

NURSING MANAGEMENT
ESOPHAGEAL CANCER

NURSING ASSESSMENT

Ask the patient about a history of GERD, hiatal hernia, achalasia, Barrett's esophagus, and tobacco and alcohol use. Assess the patient for progressive dysphagia and *odynophagia* (burning, squeezing pain while swallowing). Ask about the type of substances (e.g., meats, soft foods, liquids) that cause dysphagia. Also assess the patient for pain (substernal, epigastric, or back areas), choking, heartburn, hoarseness, cough, anorexia, weight loss, and regurgitation.

NURSING DIAGNOSES

Nursing diagnoses for the patient with esophageal cancer include, but are not limited to, the following:

- Chronic pain *related to* the compression of tumor on surrounding tissues, esophageal stenosis
- Imbalanced nutrition: less than body requirements *related to* dysphagia, odynophagia, weakness, chemotherapy, and radiation therapy
- Ineffective health maintenance *related to* lack of knowledge of disease process and treatment, lack of a support system, and chronic debilitating disease
- Anxiety and grieving *related to* diagnosis of cancer, uncertain future, and poor prognosis

PLANNING

The overall goals are that the patient with esophageal cancer will (1) have relief of symptoms, including pain and dysphagia; (2) achieve optimal nutritional intake; (3) understand the prognosis of the disease; and (4) experience a quality of life appropriate to disease progression.

NURSING IMPLEMENTATION

HEALTH PROMOTION. Counsel the patient with GERD, Barrett's esophagus, or hiatal hernia about the importance of regular follow-up evaluation. Health counseling should focus on elimination of smoking and excessive alcohol intake, as well as other risk factors for GERD (see Table 42-7). Maintenance of good oral hygiene and dietary habits (e.g., intake of fresh fruits and vegetables) is important. Encourage patients to seek medical attention for any esophageal problems, especially dysphagia.

ACUTE INTERVENTION

Preoperative Care. In addition to general preoperative teaching and preparation, pay particular attention to the patient's nutritional needs. Many patients are poorly nourished because of the inability to ingest adequate amounts of food and fluids before surgery. A high-calorie, high-protein diet is recommended. Some patients require a liquid form of this diet. Some patients may need IV fluid replacement or parenteral nutrition. Instruct the patient and caregiver on how to keep an intake and output record and assess for signs of fluid and electrolyte imbalance. Some treatment protocols necessitate preoperative radiation and chemotherapy.

Meticulous oral care is essential. Cleanse the mouth thoroughly, including the tongue, gingivae, and teeth or dentures. It may be necessary to use swabs or a gauze pad and to scrub the mouth, including the tongue. Milk of magnesia with mineral oil helps remove crust formation.

Teaching should include information about chest tubes (if an open thoracic approach is used), IV lines, NG tubes, pain management, gastrostomy or jejunostomy feeding, turning, coughing, and deep breathing. (General preoperative care is discussed in Chapter 18.)

Postoperative Care. The patient usually has an NG tube in place and may have bloody drainage for 8 to 12 hours. The drainage gradually changes to greenish yellow. Assessment of the drainage, maintenance of the tube, and oral and nasal care are nursing responsibilities. Do not reposition the NG tube or reinsert it without consulting the surgeon.

Because of the location of the surgery and the patient's general condition, emphasize prevention of respiratory complications. Turning and deep breathing should be done every 2 hours. Use of an incentive spirometer helps to prevent respiratory complications.

Cardiac dysrhythmias may result from the proximity of the pericardium to the surgical site. Additional complications that can occur after esophagectomy include esophageal anastomotic leaks, fistula formation, interstitial pulmonary edema, and acute respiratory distress related to the disruption of the mediastinal lymph nodes.

Position the patient in a semi-Fowler's or Fowler's position to prevent reflux and aspiration of gastric secretions. When the patient can drink fluids or eat, maintain the upright position for at least 2 hours after eating to assist with gastric emptying.

AMBULATORY AND HOME CARE. Many patients require long-term follow-up care after surgery for esophageal cancer. The patient may undergo chemotherapy and radiation treatment after surgery. Encourage and assist the patient in maintaining adequate nutrition. A permanent feeding gastrostomy may be required. The patient usually has fears and anxieties about a diagnosis of cancer. Know what the health care provider has told the patient regarding the prognosis and then provide appropriate counseling.

Referral to a palliative care or home health nurse may be needed. (See Chapter 16 for the care of the cancer patient and Chapter 10 for a discussion of palliative and end-of-life care.)

EVALUATION

The expected outcomes are that the patient with esophageal cancer will

- Maintain a patent airway
- Have relief of pain
- Be able to swallow comfortably and consume adequate nutritional intake
- Understand the prognosis of the disease
- Experience a quality of life appropriate to disease progression

OTHER ESOPHAGEAL DISORDERS

Eosinophilic Esophagitis

Eosinophilic esophagitis (EE) is characterized by swelling of the esophagus caused by an infiltration of *eosinophils*. People with

EE frequently have a personal or family history of other allergic diseases. The most common food triggers are milk, egg, wheat, rye, and beef. Environmental allergens, such as pollens, molds, cat, dog, and dust mite allergens, may be involved in the development of EE.

Clinical manifestations include severe heartburn, difficulty swallowing, food impaction in the esophagus, nausea, vomiting, and weight loss. The diagnosis is based on the symptoms and biopsy findings of eosinophils infiltrating the esophageal tissue obtained from endoscopy.

Allergy skin testing helps to determine the person's allergens. A trial of avoidance of the foods to which the person has positive allergy tests is the initial form of treatment for EE. A variety of treatment approaches, including acid suppression (see Table 42-10), corticosteroids, and endoscopic dilation, can be used alone or in combination.

Corticosteroids are frequently used to treat EE when avoidance of allergic triggers does not relieve symptoms. Corticosteroids may be used orally (prednisone) or as a topical therapy, such as inhaled corticosteroids (e.g., fluticasone [Flovent]). In asthma, where fluticasone is typically used, it is inhaled. In EE it is swallowed, and this results in the delivery of the drug directly to the esophagus.

Esophageal Diverticula

Esophageal diverticula are saclike outpouchings of one or more layers of the esophagus. They occur in three main areas: (1) above the upper esophageal sphincter *(Zenker's diverticulum)*, which is the most common location; (2) near the esophageal midpoint (traction diverticulum); and (3) above the LES (epiphrenic diverticulum) (Fig. 42-6). Pharyngeal pouches (Zenker's diverticula) occur most commonly in individuals over 60 years.

Typical symptoms include dysphagia, regurgitation, chronic cough, aspiration, and weight loss. The patient frequently complains of tasting sour food and smelling a foul odor caused by the stagnant food. Complications include malnutrition, aspiration, and perforation. Endoscopy or barium studies can easily establish a diagnosis.

There is no specific treatment for esophageal diverticula. Some patients find that they can empty the pocket of food that collects by applying pressure at a point on the neck. The diet may need to be limited to foods that pass more readily (e.g., blenderized foods). Treatment via an endoscopic or open approach may be necessary if nutrition is disrupted. Treatment

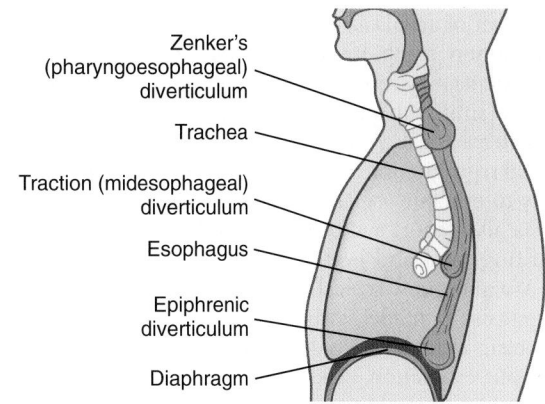

Zenker's (pharyngoesophageal) diverticulum

Trachea

Traction (midesophageal) diverticulum

Esophagus

Epiphrenic diverticulum

Diaphragm

FIG. 42-6 Possible sites for esophageal diverticula. These hollow outpouchings may occur just above the upper esophageal sphincter (Zenker's, the most common type of pulsion diverticulum), near the midpoint of the esophagus (traction), and just above the lower esophageal sphincter (epiphrenic).

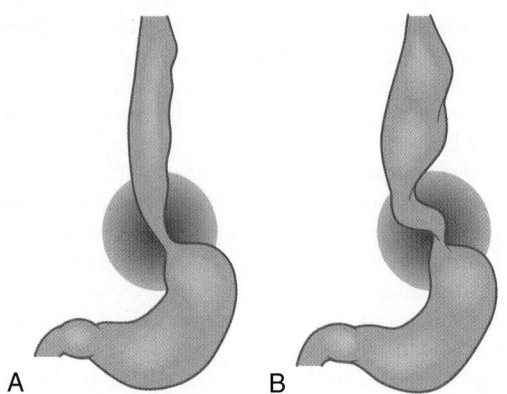

FIG. 42-7 Esophageal achalasia. **A,** Early stage, showing tapering of lower esophagus. **B,** Advanced stage, showing dilated, tortuous esophagus.

by endoscopic stapling diverticulotomy or diverticulostomy is associated with decreased complications compared with the open approaches. The most serious complication of this treatment is perforation of the esophagus.

Esophageal Strictures

The most common cause of *esophageal strictures* (or narrowing) is chronic GERD. The ingestion of strong acids or alkalis, external beam radiation, and surgical anastomosis can also create strictures. Trauma such as throat lacerations and gunshot wounds may also lead to strictures as a result of scar formation. The strictures can result in dysphagia, regurgitation, and ultimately weight loss.

Strictures can be dilated endoscopically using mechanical *bougies* (dilating instruments) or balloons. The dilation may be performed with or without endoscopy, or with fluoroscopy. Surgical excision with anastomosis is sometimes necessary. The patient may have a temporary or permanent gastrostomy.

Achalasia

In achalasia, peristalsis of the lower two thirds (smooth muscle) of the esophagus is absent. Achalasia is a rare, chronic disorder. With achalasia the pressure in the LES increases along with incomplete relaxation. Obstruction of the esophagus at or near the diaphragm occurs. Food and fluid accumulate in the lower esophagus. The result of this condition is dilation of the lower esophagus proximal to (above) the tapering affected segment of the lower esophagus (Fig. 42-7). There is a selective loss of inhibitory neurons, resulting in unopposed contraction of the LES.

The onset of achalasia is usually insidious. Dysphagia is the most common symptom and occurs with both liquids and solids. Patients may report a globus sensation and/or substernal chest pain (similar to angina pain) that occurs during or immediately after a meal. About a third of the patients experience nocturnal regurgitation. *Halitosis* (foul-smelling breath) and the inability to eructate (belch) are other symptoms. Patients with achalasia also report symptoms of GERD and regurgitation of sour-tasting food and liquids, especially when they are lying down. Weight loss is typical.

Diagnosis is made with esophagram (barium swallow), manometric evaluation (high-resolution manometry), and/or endoscopic evaluation. The exact cause of achalasia is not known, so treatment focuses on symptom management. The goals of treatment are to relieve dysphagia and regurgitation, improve esophageal emptying by disrupting the LES, and

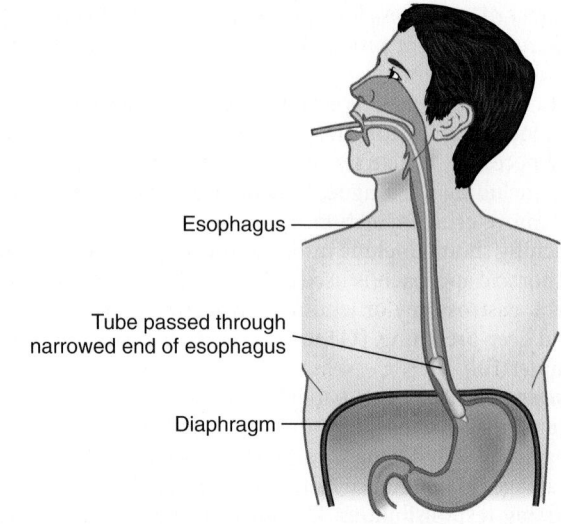

FIG. 42-8 Pneumatic dilation attempts to treat achalasia by maintaining an adequate lumen and decreasing lower esophageal sphincter (LES) tone.

prevent development of megaesophagus (enlargement of the lower esophagus).

Endoscopic pneumatic dilation is done as an outpatient procedure. The LES muscle is disrupted from within using balloons of progressively larger diameter (3.0, 3.5, and 4.0 cm) (Fig. 42-8). If this is ineffective, then a surgical procedure, Heller myotomy, is done laparoscopically. In this procedure the LES is surgically disrupted (myotomy). Because GERD with esophagitis and stricture is a common complication, the patient often has antireflux surgery performed at the same time. The patient can usually return to work 1 to 2 weeks after this procedure.

Medical therapy is less effective than invasive procedures. Smooth muscle relaxants such as nitrates (isosorbide dinitrate [Isordil]) and calcium channel blockers (e.g., nifedipine [Procardia]) taken sublingually 30 to 45 minutes before meals to improve dysphagia may be prescribed. However, side effects (e.g., headache), drug tolerance, and short duration of action limit their use.

The injection of botulinum toxin endoscopically into the LES gives short-term relief of symptoms and improves esophageal emptying. It works by promoting relaxation of the smooth muscle. This treatment is used for older patients for whom surgery and pneumatic dilation may not be appropriate due to other chronic illnesses. Symptomatic treatment consists of eating a semisoft diet, eating slowly and drinking fluid with meals, and sleeping with the head elevated.

Esophageal Varices

Esophageal varices are dilated, tortuous veins occurring in the lower portion of the esophagus as a result of portal hypertension. Esophageal varices are a common complication of liver cirrhosis and are discussed in Chapter 44.

DISORDERS OF THE STOMACH AND UPPER SMALL INTESTINE

GASTRITIS

Gastritis, an inflammation of the gastric mucosa, is one of the most common problems affecting the stomach. Gastritis may be acute or chronic and diffuse or localized.

TABLE 42-12	CAUSES OF GASTRITIS

Drugs
- Aspirin
- Corticosteroids
- Nonsteroidal antiinflammatory drugs (NSAIDs)

Diet
- Alcohol
- Spicy, irritating food

Microorganisms
- *Helicobacter pylori*
- *Salmonella* organisms
- *Staphylococcus* organisms

Environmental Factors
- Radiation
- Smoking

Pathophysiologic Conditions
- Burns
- Large hiatal hernia
- Physiologic stress
- Reflux of bile and pancreatic secretions
- Renal failure (uremia)
- Sepsis
- Shock

Other Factors
- Endoscopic procedures
- Nasogastric tube
- Psychologic stress

Etiology and Pathophysiology

Gastritis occurs as the result of a breakdown in the normal gastric mucosal barrier. This mucosal barrier normally protects the stomach tissue from the corrosive action of HCl acid and pepsin. When the barrier is broken, HCl acid and pepsin can diffuse back into the mucosa. This back diffusion results in tissue edema, disruption of capillary walls with loss of plasma into the gastric lumen, and possible hemorrhage.

Risk Factors. Risk factors and causes of gastritis are listed in Table 42-12. Some of the risk factors are discussed in this section.

Drug-Related Gastritis. Drugs contribute to the development of acute and chronic gastritis. NSAIDs, including aspirin, and corticosteroids inhibit the synthesis of prostaglandins that are protective to the gastric mucosa. Thus the mucosa is more susceptible to injury. NSAID-related gastritis is associated with many drugs, including piroxicam (Feldene), naproxen (Naprosyn), sulindac (Clinoril), indomethacin (Indocin), diclofenac (Voltaren), and ibuprofen (Motrin, Advil).[17]

Risk factors for NSAID-induced gastritis include being female; being over age 60; having a history of ulcer disease; taking anticoagulants, other NSAIDs (including low-dose aspirin), or other ulcerogenic drugs (including corticosteroids); and having a chronic debilitating disorder such as cardiovascular disease. Some drugs such as digitalis (digoxin) and alendronate (Fosamax) have direct irritating effects on the gastric mucosa.

Diet. Dietary indiscretions can also result in acute gastritis. After an alcoholic drinking binge, acute damage to the gastric mucosa can range from localized injury of superficial epithelial cells to destruction of the mucosa with mucosal congestion, edema, and hemorrhage. Prolonged damage induced by repeated alcohol abuse results in chronic gastritis. Eating large quantities of spicy, irritating foods and metabolic conditions such as renal failure can also cause acute gastritis.

Helicobacter pylori. An important cause of chronic gastritis is *Helicobacter pylori* infection. *H. pylori* infection is highest in underdeveloped countries and in people of low socioeconomic status. Infection likely occurs during childhood with transmission from family members to the child, possibly through a fecal-oral or oral-oral route.

In the United States, people born before 1940 are more likely to carry *H. pylori* than people in younger age-groups. *H. pylori* has also been linked to stomach cancer and non-Hodgkin's lymphoma. The role of *H. pylori* in ulcer development is discussed in greater detail in this chapter on p. 943.

Other Risk Factors. Although not as common, other risk factors of chronic gastritis have been identified. Bacterial, viral, and fungal infections, including *Mycobacterium* species, cytomegalovirus (CMV), and syphilis, are associated with chronic gastritis. Gastritis can occur from reflux of bile salts from the duodenum into the stomach as a result of anatomic changes following surgical procedures (e.g., gastroduodenostomy, gastrojejunostomy). Prolonged vomiting may also cause reflux of bile salts. Intense emotional responses and CNS lesions may also produce inflammation of the mucosal lining as a result of hypersecretion of HCl acid.

Autoimmune Gastritis. Autoimmune metaplastic atrophic gastritis (also called autoimmune atrophic gastritis) is an inherited condition in which there is an immune response directed against parietal cells. It most commonly affects women of northern European descent. Patients with autoimmune atrophic gastritis often have other autoimmune disorders. The loss of parietal cells leads to low chloride levels, inadequate production of intrinsic factor, cobalamin (vitamin B_{12}) malabsorption, and pernicious anemia. Atrophic gastritis is associated with an increased risk of stomach cancer.

Clinical Manifestations

In *acute gastritis* the symptoms include anorexia, nausea and vomiting, epigastric tenderness, and a feeling of fullness. Hemorrhage is commonly associated with alcohol abuse and at times is the only symptom. Acute gastritis is self-limiting, lasting from a few hours to a few days, with complete healing of the mucosa expected.

In *chronic gastritis* the manifestations are similar to those described for acute gastritis. Some patients are asymptomatic. However, when the parietal cells are lost as a result of atrophy, the source of intrinsic factor is also lost. The loss of *intrinsic factor,* a substance essential for the absorption of cobalamin in the terminal ileum, ultimately results in cobalamin deficiency. With time, the body's storage of cobalamin in the liver becomes depleted, and a state of deficiency exists. Because it is essential for the growth and maturation of red blood cells (RBCs), the lack of cobalamin results in pernicious anemia and neurologic complications. (Cobalamin deficiency anemia is discussed in Chapter 31.)

Diagnostic Studies

Diagnosis of acute gastritis is most often based on the patient's history of drug and alcohol use. Endoscopic examination with biopsy may be warranted to obtain a definitive diagnosis. Breath, urine, serum, stool, and gastric tissue biopsy tests are available for the determination of *H. pylori* infection. (These diagnostic tests are described in the section on peptic ulcer disease later in this chapter on p. 945.)

Radiologic studies are not helpful because the superficial mucosa is generally involved, and changes will not show clearly on x-ray examination. A complete blood count (CBC) may demonstrate anemia from blood loss or lack of intrinsic factor. Stools are tested for occult blood. Serum tests for antibodies to parietal cells and intrinsic factor may be performed. Tissue biopsy is necessary to rule out gastric carcinoma.

TABLE 42-13	**DRUG THERAPY**	
Helicobacter pylori Infection		
Treatment	**Duration**	**Eradication Rate**
Triple-Drug Therapy	7-14 days	70%-85%
proton pump inhibitor (PPI)*		
amoxicillin		
clarithromycin (Biaxin)		
Quadruple Therapy	10-14 days	85%
PPI*		
bismuth†		
tetracycline		
metronidazole (Flagyl)		

*See Table 42-10.
†Bismuth is part of a combination capsule (Pylera) containing bismuth, tetracycline, and metronidazole that is used in combination with a PPI (e.g., omeprazole [Prilosec]).

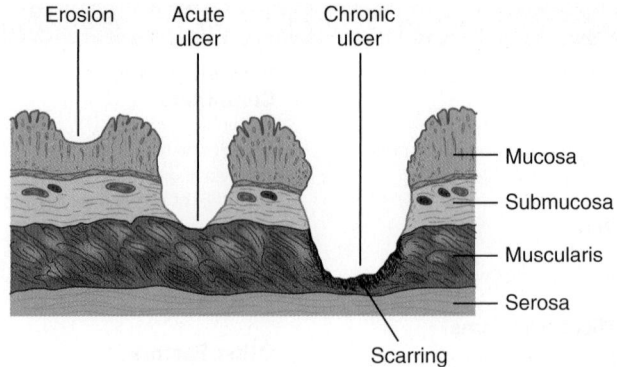

FIG. 42-9 Peptic ulcers, including an erosion, an acute ulcer, and a chronic ulcer. Both the acute ulcer and the chronic ulcer may penetrate the entire wall of the stomach.

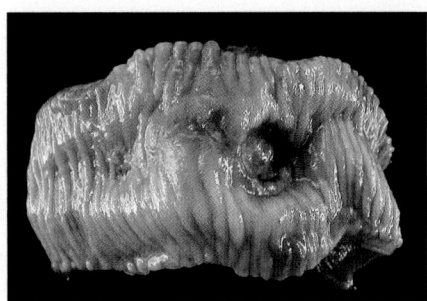

FIG. 42-10 Peptic ulcer of the duodenum.

NURSING AND COLLABORATIVE MANAGEMENT GASTRITIS

ACUTE GASTRITIS

Eliminating the cause and preventing or avoiding it in the future are generally all that is needed to treat acute gastritis. The plan of care is supportive and similar to that described for nausea and vomiting. If vomiting accompanies acute gastritis, rest, NPO status, and IV fluids may be prescribed. Dehydration can occur rapidly in acute gastritis with vomiting. Antiemetics are given for nausea and vomiting (see Table 42-1).

In severe cases of acute gastritis, an NG tube may be used (1) to monitor for bleeding, (2) to lavage the precipitating agent from the stomach, or (3) to keep the stomach empty and free of noxious stimuli. Clear liquids are resumed when symptoms have subsided, with gradual reintroduction of solids.

If hemorrhage is considered likely, frequently check vital signs and test the vomitus for blood. All of the management strategies discussed in the section on upper GI bleeding apply to the patient with severe gastritis (see p. 955).

Drug therapy focuses on reducing irritation of the gastric mucosa and providing symptomatic relief. H_2-receptor blockers (e.g., ranitidine, cimetidine) or PPIs (e.g., omeprazole, lansoprazole) reduce gastric HCl acid secretion (see Table 42-10). Teach the patient about the therapeutic effects of PPIs and H_2-receptor blockers.

CHRONIC GASTRITIS

The treatment of chronic gastritis focuses on evaluating and eliminating the specific cause (e.g., cessation of alcohol intake, abstinence from drugs, H. pylori eradication). Currently, antibiotic combinations are used to eradicate H. pylori (Table 42-13). For the patient with pernicious anemia, cobalamin (administered orally, nasally, or by injections) is needed (see Chapter 31). Discuss the need for lifelong cobalamin therapy with the patient.

The patient undergoing treatment for chronic gastritis may have to adapt to lifestyle changes and strictly adhere to a drug regimen. Some patients find a nonirritating diet consisting of six small feedings a day helpful. Smoking is contraindicated in all forms of gastritis. An interprofessional team approach in which the physician, nurse, dietitian, and pharmacist provide consistent information and support may increase the patient's success in making these alterations.

PEPTIC ULCER DISEASE

Peptic ulcer disease (PUD) is a condition characterized by erosion of the GI mucosa resulting from the digestive action of HCl acid and pepsin. Any portion of the GI tract that comes into contact with gastric secretions is susceptible to ulcer development, including the lower esophagus, stomach, duodenum, and margin of a gastrojejunal anastomosis after surgical procedures. Approximately 350,000 new cases of ulcers are diagnosed each year.

Types

Peptic ulcers can be classified as acute or chronic, depending on the degree and duration of mucosal involvement, and gastric or duodenal, according to the location. The *acute ulcer* (Fig. 42-9) is associated with superficial erosion and minimal inflammation. It is of short duration and resolves quickly when the cause is identified and removed. A chronic ulcer (Fig. 42-10) is one of long duration, eroding through the muscular wall with the formation of fibrous tissue. It is present continuously for many months or intermittently throughout the person's lifetime. Chronic ulcers are more common than acute erosions.

Gastric and duodenal ulcers, although defined as PUD, are different in their etiology and incidence (Table 42-14). Generally, the treatment of all types of ulcers is similar.

Etiology and Pathophysiology

Peptic ulcers develop only in an acid environment. However, an excess of HCl acid may not be necessary for ulcer development. Pepsinogen, the precursor of pepsin, is activated to pepsin in the presence of HCl acid and a pH of 2 to 3. When the stomach acid level is neutralized by food or antacids or acid secretion is

TABLE 42-14   COMPARISON OF GASTRIC AND DUODENAL ULCERS

Gastric Ulcers	Duodenal Ulcers
Lesion	
Superficial, smooth margins Round, oval, or cone shaped	Penetrating (associated with deformity of duodenal bulb from healing of recurrent ulcers)
Location of Lesion	
Predominantly antrum, also in body and fundus of stomach	First 1-2 cm of duodenum
Gastric Secretion	
Normal to decreased	Increased
Incidence	
Greater in women	Greater in men, but increasing in women (especially postmenopausal)
Peak age 50-60 yr	Peak age 35-45 yr
More common in people of lower socioeconomic status	Associated with psychologic stress
↑ With smoking, drug use (aspirin, NSAID), and alcohol use	↑ With smoking, drug use, and alcohol use
↑ With incompetent pyloric sphincter and bile reflux	Associated with other diseases (e.g., chronic obstructive pulmonary disease, pancreatic disease, hyperparathyroidism, Zollinger-Ellison syndrome, chronic renal failure)
Clinical Manifestations	
Burning or gaseous pressure in high left epigastrium and back and upper abdomen	Burning, cramping, pressure-like pain across midepigastrium and upper abdomen. Back pain with posterior ulcers
Pain 1-2 hr after meals. If penetrating ulcer, aggravation of discomfort with food	Pain 2-4 hr after meals and midmorning, midafternoon, middle of night. Periodic and episodic. Pain relief with antacids and food
Occasional nausea and vomiting, weight loss	Occasional nausea and vomiting
Recurrence Rate	
High	High
Complications	
Hemorrhage, perforation, gastric outlet obstruction, intractability	Hemorrhage, perforation, obstruction

PATHOPHYSIOLOGY MAP

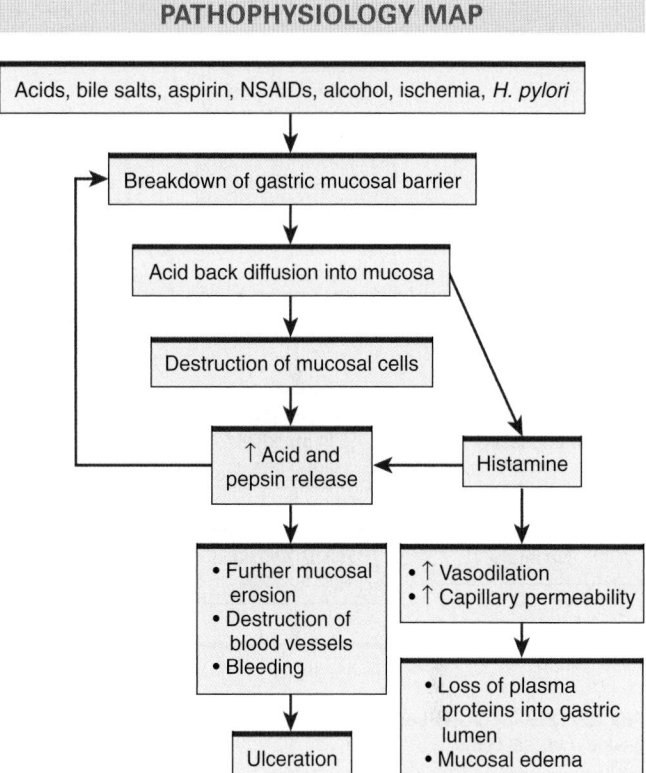

FIG. 42-11 Disruption of gastric mucosa and pathophysiologic consequences of back diffusion of acids.

blocked by drugs, the pH is increased to 3.5 or more. At a pH of 3.5 or more, pepsin has little or no proteolytic activity.

The pathophysiology of ulcer development is outlined in Fig. 42-11. The back diffusion of HCl acid into the gastric mucosa results in cellular destruction and inflammation. Histamine is released from the damaged mucosa, resulting in vasodilation and increased capillary permeability and further secretion of acid and pepsin. Fig. 42-12 depicts the interrelationship between the mucosal blood flow and disruption of the gastric mucosal barrier. As described in the section on gastritis, a variety of agents are known to damage the mucosal barrier.

Helicobacter pylori. In addition to chronic gastritis, *H. pylori* is associated with peptic ulcer development. Approximately two thirds of the world's population is infected with *H. pylori*.[18]

In the stomach the bacteria can survive a long time by colonizing the gastric epithelial cells within the mucosal layer. The bacteria also produce urease, which metabolizes urea-producing ammonium chloride and other damaging chemicals. Urease also activates the immune response with both antibody production and the release of inflammatory cytokines.

The response to *H. pylori* is variable. Not all individuals infected with *H. pylori* go on to develop ulcers. In one scenario, *H. pylori* leads to intestinal metaplasia in the stomach resulting in chronic atrophic gastritis and in some cases stomach cancer. In another scenario, *H. pylori* alters gastric secretion and produces tissue damage, leading to PUD. The response to *H. pylori* is influenced by a variety of factors, including genetics, environment, and diet.

Medication-Induced Injury. Ulcerogenic drugs, such as aspirin and NSAIDs, inhibit synthesis of prostaglandins, increase gastric acid secretion, and reduce the integrity of the mucosal barrier. The use of NSAIDs is responsible for the majority of non–*H. pylori* peptic ulcers. NSAIDs in the presence of *H. pylori* increase the risk of PUD.[17] Patients on corticosteroids, anticoagulants, and selective serotonin reuptake inhibitors (e.g., fluoxetine [Prozac]) are also at increased risk of ulcer development.[19] Corticosteroids affect mucosal cell renewal and decrease its protective effects.

Lifestyle Factors. High alcohol intake is associated with acute mucosal lesions. In addition, alcohol stimulates acid secretion. Coffee (caffeinated and decaffeinated) is a strong stimulant of gastric acid secretion. Psychologic distress, including stress and depression, can negatively influence the healing of ulcers once they have developed. Smoking also delays ulcer healing.

PATHOPHYSIOLOGY MAP

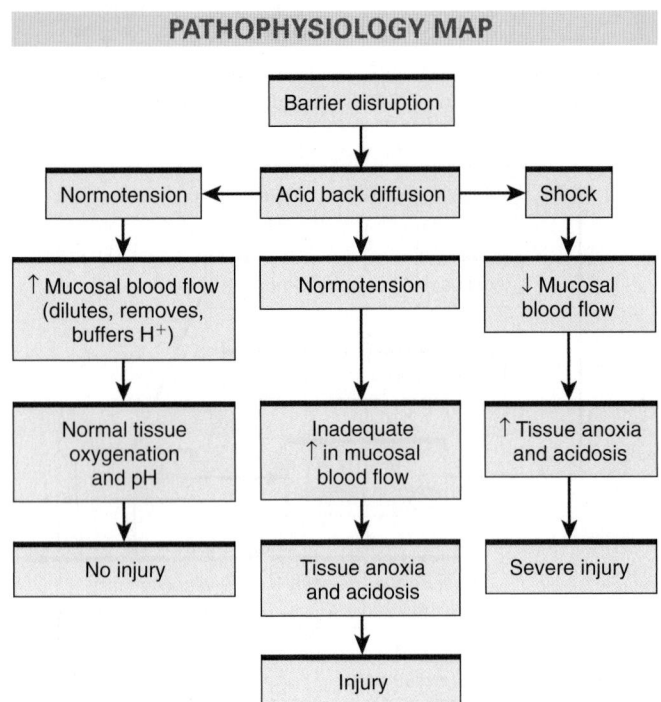

FIG. 42-12 Relationship between mucosal blood flow and disruption of the gastric mucosal barrier.

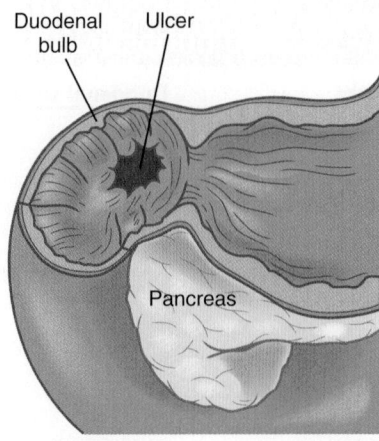

FIG. 42-13 Duodenal ulcer of the posterior wall penetrating into the head of the pancreas, resulting in walled-off perforation.

Gastric Ulcers. Although gastric ulcers can occur in any portion of the stomach, they are most commonly found in the antrum. Gastric ulcers are less common than duodenal ulcers. Gastric ulcers are more prevalent in women and in older adults. Because the peak incidence of gastric ulcers is in people over 50 years of age, the mortality rate from gastric ulcers is greater than that from duodenal ulcers. Gastric ulcers are more likely than duodenal ulcers to result in obstruction. *H. pylori*, medications, smoking, and bile reflux are risk factors for gastric ulcers.

Duodenal Ulcers. Duodenal ulcers account for about 80% of all peptic ulcers. Duodenal ulcers may occur at any age, but the incidence is especially high between 35 and 45 years of age. Duodenal ulcers can develop in anyone, regardless of occupation or socioeconomic group.

Although many factors are associated with the development of duodenal ulcers, *H. pylori* is most common. *H. pylori* infection is found in approximately 90% to 95% of patients with duodenal ulcers.

The development of duodenal ulcers is often associated with a high HCl acid secretion. Alcohol ingestion and smoking are associated with duodenal ulcer formation because both are known stimulants of acid secretion. Several patient groups are at high risk of duodenal ulcer development, including those with chronic obstructive pulmonary disease, cirrhosis of the liver, chronic pancreatitis, hyperparathyroidism, chronic kidney disease, and *Zollinger-Ellison syndrome* (a rare condition characterized by severe peptic ulceration and HCl acid hypersecretion).

Stress-Related Mucosal Disease (SRMD). SRMD is described later in this chapter in the section on acute upper GI bleeding on p. 954.

Clinical Manifestations

The discomfort generally associated with gastric ulcers is located high in the epigastrium and occurs about 1 to 2 hours after meals. The pain is described as "burning" or "gaseous." If the ulcer has eroded through the gastric mucosa, food tends to aggravate rather than alleviate the pain. For some patients, the earliest symptoms are due to a serious complication such as perforation.

The symptoms of duodenal ulcers occur when gastric acid comes in contact with the ulcers. With meal ingestion, food is present to help buffer the acid. Symptoms of duodenal ulcers occur generally 2 to 5 hours after a meal. The pain is described as "burning" or "cramplike." It is most often located in the midepigastric region beneath the xiphoid process. Duodenal ulcers can also produce back pain.

Antacids alone or in combination with an H_2-receptor blocker, as well as food, neutralize the acid to provide relief. A characteristic of duodenal ulcer is its tendency to occur continuously for a few weeks or months and then disappear for a time, only to recur some months later.

Not all patients with gastric or duodenal ulcers experience pain or discomfort. *Silent* peptic ulcers are more likely to occur in older adults and those taking NSAIDs. The presence or absence of symptoms is not directly related to the size of the ulcer or the degree of healing.

Complications

The three major complications of chronic PUD are hemorrhage, perforation, and gastric outlet obstruction. All are considered emergency situations and may require surgical intervention.

Hemorrhage. Hemorrhage is the most common complication of PUD. Duodenal ulcers account for a greater percentage of upper GI bleeding episodes than gastric ulcers.

Perforation. Perforation is considered the most lethal complication of PUD. Perforation is commonly seen in large penetrating duodenal ulcers (Fig. 42-13). Even though duodenal ulcers are more prevalent and perforate more often, mortality rates associated with perforation of gastric ulcers are higher. The patient with gastric ulcers is older and often has concurrent medical problems, which accounts for the higher mortality rate.

With perforation, the ulcer penetrates the serosal surface with spillage of either gastric or duodenal contents into the peritoneal cavity. Small perforations seal themselves, resulting in a cessation of symptoms. Larger perforations require immediate surgical closure. Spontaneous sealing occurs as a result of fibrin production in response to the perforation. This can lead to fibrinous fusion of the duodenum or gastric curvature to adjacent tissue (mainly the liver) and strictures that can obstruct the flow of intestinal contents and the passage of stool.

The clinical manifestations of perforation are sudden and dramatic in onset. During the initial phase (0 to 2 hours after perforation) the patient experiences sudden, severe upper abdominal pain that quickly spreads throughout the abdomen. The pain radiates to the back and is not relieved by food or antacids. The abdomen appears rigid and boardlike as the abdominal muscles attempt to protect from further injury. The patient's respirations become shallow and rapid. The heart rate is elevated (tachycardia), and the pulse is weak. Bowel sounds are usually absent. Nausea and vomiting may occur. Many patients report a history of ulcer disease or recent symptoms of indigestion.

The contents entering the peritoneal cavity from the stomach or duodenum may contain air, saliva, food particles, HCl acid, pepsin, bacteria, bile, and pancreatic fluid and enzymes. If the condition is untreated, bacterial peritonitis may occur within 6 to 12 hours. The intensity of the peritonitis is proportional to the amount and duration of the spillage through the perforation. It is difficult to determine from the symptoms alone whether a gastric or duodenal ulcer has perforated because the clinical characteristics of intestinal perforation are the same (see Chapter 43).

Gastric Outlet Obstruction. Both acute and chronic PUD can result in gastric outlet obstruction. Obstruction in the distal stomach and duodenum is the result of edema, inflammation, or pylorospasm and fibrous scar tissue formation. With obstruction the patient reports discomfort or pain that is worse toward the end of the day as the stomach fills and dilates. Relief may be obtained by belching or by self-induced vomiting. Vomiting is common and often projectile. The vomitus contains food particles that were ingested hours or days before the vomiting episode. Constipation occurs because of dehydration and decreased diet intake secondary to anorexia. Over time dilation of the stomach and visible swelling in the upper abdomen may occur.

Diagnostic Studies

The diagnostic tests used to determine the presence and location of an ulcer are similar to those used for acute upper GI bleeding. Endoscopy is the most accurate diagnostic procedure. Endoscopy allows for direct viewing of the gastric and duodenal mucosa (Fig. 42-14). It can be used to determine the degree of ulcer healing after treatment and to confirm the absence of malignancy. During endoscopy, tissue specimens are obtained for identification of *H. pylori* and to rule out stomach cancer.

Several diagnostic tests are available to confirm *H. pylori* infection. These are classified as noninvasive and invasive. Biopsy of the antral mucosa and testing for urease (rapid urease testing) is considered the gold standard for diagnosis of *H. pylori* infection. Noninvasive tests include stool testing or breath testing. Serum or whole blood antibody tests, particularly immunoglobulin G (IgG), do not distinguish between past and current infection. The urea breath test can identify active infection. Urea is a by-product of the metabolism of *H. pylori* bacteria. Although not as accurate as the urea breath test, stool antigen tests can also be performed.

A barium contrast study may be used in the diagnosis of gastric outlet obstruction or for ulcer detection in those patients who cannot undergo endoscopy. The presence of a possible gastrinoma (Zollinger-Ellison syndrome) can be diagnosed by measuring fasting serum gastrin levels. With a gastrinoma, the gastrin levels are elevated. A secretin stimulation test can dif-

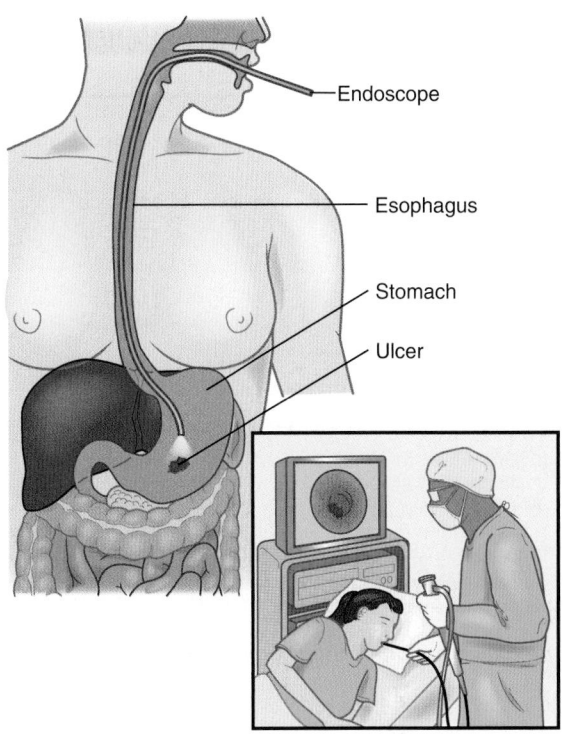

FIG. 42-14 Esophagogastroduodenoscopy (EGD) directly visualizes the mucosal lining of the stomach with a flexible endoscope. Ulcers or tumors can be directly visualized and biopsies taken.

ferentiate patients with gastrinomas from those with other causes of hypergastrinemia.

Laboratory tests, including a CBC, liver enzyme studies, serum amylase determination, and stool examination, should be performed. A CBC may indicate anemia secondary to ulcer bleeding. Liver enzyme studies help detect any liver problems (e.g., cirrhosis) that may complicate ulcer treatment. Stools are routinely tested for blood. A serum amylase determination is done to determine pancreatic function when posterior duodenal ulcer penetration of the pancreas is suspected.

Collaborative Care
Conservative Therapy

When the patient's clinical manifestations and health history suggest the diagnosis of PUD and diagnostic studies confirm it, a treatment regimen is instituted (Table 42-15). The regimen consists of adequate rest, drug therapy, elimination of smoking, dietary modifications (if needed), and long-term follow-up care. The aim of treatment is to decrease gastric acidity and enhance mucosal defense mechanisms.

Patients are generally treated in ambulatory care clinics. Pain disappears after 3 to 6 days, but ulcer healing is much slower. Complete healing may take 3 to 9 weeks, depending on ulcer size, treatment regimen, and patient adherence. Endoscopic examination is the most accurate method to monitor for ulcer healing. The usual follow-up endoscopic evaluation is performed 3 to 6 months after diagnosis and treatment.

Aspirin and nonselective NSAIDs are discontinued for 4 to 6 weeks. When aspirin must be continued, co-administration with a PPI, H_2-receptor blocker, or misoprostol (Cytotec) may be prescribed. Patients with *H. pylori* infection are treated with antibiotics and a PPI. Patients receiving low-dose aspirin for cardiovascular and stroke risk who have a history of ulcer disease or complications may need to receive long-term treatment with a PPI.[20] Enteric-coated aspirin decreases localized

TABLE 42-15 COLLABORATIVE CARE

Peptic Ulcer Disease

Diagnostic
- History and physical examination
- Upper GI endoscopy with biopsy
- *Helicobacter pylori* testing of breath, urine, blood, tissue
- Complete blood cell count
- Liver enzymes
- Serum electrolytes

Collaborative Therapy
Conservative Therapy
- Adequate rest
- Cessation of smoking
- Drug therapy (see Tables 42-9 and 42-13)
  - Proton pump inhibitors
  - H$_2$-receptor blockers
  - Antibiotics for *H. pylori*
  - Cytoprotective drugs
  - Antacids
  - Anticholinergics (used rarely)
- Stress management (see Chapter 7)

Acute Exacerbation Without Complications
- NPO
- NG suction
- Adequate rest
- IV fluid replacement
- Drug therapy
  - Proton pump inhibitors
  - H$_2$-receptor blockers
  - Antacids
  - Anticholinergics
  - Sedatives

Acute Exacerbation With Complications (Hemorrhage, Perforation, Obstruction)
- NPO
- NG suction
- IV proton pump inhibitor
- Bed rest
- IV fluid replacement (lactated Ringer's solution)
- Blood transfusions
- Stomach lavage (possible)

Surgical Therapy
- *Perforation:* Simple closure with omentum graft
- *Gastric outlet obstruction:* Pyloroplasty and vagotomy
- *Ulcer removal or reduction*
  - Billroth I and II
  - Vagotomy and pyloroplasty

irritation but has not been proved to reduce the overall risk for GI bleeding.

Smoking has an irritating effect on the mucosa and delays mucosal healing. Smoking should be eliminated completely or severely reduced. (Strategies to enhance patient smoking cessation are discussed in Chapter 11.) Adequate rest, both physical and emotional, is important for ulcer healing and may require some modifications in the patient's daily routine. Avoidance or restriction of alcohol intake will also enhance healing.

Drug Therapy. Drugs are a vital part of therapy (see Table 42-10). Strict adherence to the prescribed regimen of drugs is important. Teach the patient about each drug prescribed, why it is ordered, and the expected benefits.

Because ulcers frequently recur, interruption or discontinuation of therapy can have harmful results. Encourage the patient to adhere to therapy and continue with follow-up care as prescribed. H$_2$-receptor blockers and PPIs may be stopped after the ulcer has healed or may be prescribed as low-dose maintenance therapy. Teach the patient and the family what to do if pain and discomfort recur or blood is noted in the vomitus or stools.

Histamine (H$_2$)-Receptor Blockers. H$_2$-receptor blockers promote ulcer healing. Famotidine, ranitidine, and cimetidine can be given orally or IV, but nizatidine is only available orally. Depending on the specific drug, therapeutic effects last up to 12 hours. The onset of action of H$_2$-receptor blockers is 1 hour, which is longer than antacids.

Proton Pump Inhibitors. PPIs are more effective than H$_2$-receptor blockers in reducing gastric acid secretion and promoting ulcer healing. PPIs are also used in combination with antibiotics to treat ulcers caused by *H. pylori*. Omeprazole is available in an OTC formulation at a lower dose and in an immediate-release form.

Antibiotic Therapy. The treatment of *H. pylori* is the most important element of treating PUD in patients positive for *H. pylori*. Antibiotic therapy for *H. pylori* is shown in Table 42-13. Antibiotics are prescribed concurrently with a PPI for 7 to 14 days. Because of the development of antibiotic-resistant organisms, a growing percentage of patients do not have the *H. pylori* eradicated with a single round of therapy.

Antacids. Antacids are used as adjunct therapy for PUD. They increase gastric pH by neutralizing the HCl acid. As a result, the acid content of chyme reaching the duodenum is reduced. In addition, some antacids, such as aluminum hydroxide, can bind to bile salts, thus decreasing the damaging effects of bile on the gastric mucosa. Patients who are at risk for SRMD may be treated prophylactically with antacids along with an antisecretory agent.

The common commercial nonsystemic (poorly absorbed) antacids consist of magnesium hydroxide or aluminum hydroxide as single preparations or in various combinations (see Table 42-10). The neutralizing effects of antacids taken on an empty stomach last only 20 to 30 minutes because they are quickly evacuated. When antacids are taken after meals, the effects may last as long as 3 to 4 hours. Therapy recommending frequent dosing (e.g., hourly) often results in poor adherence.

After the acute phase of bleeding, antacids are generally administered hourly, either orally or through the NG tube. If the tube is in place, the stomach contents should be aspirated and tested periodically for pH level. If pH is less than 5, intermittent suction may be used, or the frequency or dosage of the antacid or antisecretory agent may be increased.

The type and dosage of antacid prescribed depend on side effects and potential drug interactions. Antacids high in sodium (e.g., sodium citrate [Bicitra]) need to be used with caution in older adults and patients with liver cirrhosis, hypertension, heart failure, and renal disease. Magnesium preparations should not be prescribed for patients with renal failure because of the risk of magnesium toxicity. An antacid combination of aluminum and magnesium seems to decrease the side effects of both.

Antacids can interact unfavorably with some drugs. They can enhance the absorption of drugs such as dicumarol and amphetamines. Digitalis preparations can be potentiated when taken in combination with calcium or magnesium antacids. In some instances, antacids decrease the absorption rates of prescribed drugs, such as tetracycline. Before antacid therapy begins, inform the health care provider of any drugs that a patient is taking.

Cytoprotective Drug Therapy. Sucralfate is used for the short-term treatment of ulcers. It provides cytoprotection for the esophagus, stomach, and duodenum. Sucralfate does not have acid-neutralizing capabilities. Its action is most effective at a low pH, and it should be given at least 30 minutes before or after an antacid. Adverse side effects are minimal. However, it does bind with cimetidine, digoxin, warfarin (Coumadin), phenytoin (Dilantin), and tetracycline, causing reduced bioavailability of these drugs.

Misoprostol is a synthetic prostaglandin analog prescribed for the prevention of gastric ulcers caused by NSAIDs and aspirin. It has protective and some antisecretory effects on gastric mucosa. Misoprostol does not interfere with the therapeutic effects of aspirin and NSAIDs. People who require chronic NSAID therapy, such as those with osteoarthritis, may benefit from the use of misoprostol.

Other Drugs. Tricyclic antidepressants (e.g., imipramine [Tofranil], doxepin [Sinequan]) may be prescribed for patients with PUD. Antidepressants may contribute to overall pain relief through their effects on afferent pain fiber transmission. In addition, tricyclic antidepressants have (to varying degrees) some anticholinergic properties, which result in reduced acid secretion. Selective serotonin reuptake inhibitors are associated with a modest risk for upper GI bleeding.[19]

Anticholinergic drugs are used only occasionally for PUD treatment. Anticholinergics are associated with a number of side effects, such as dry mouth, warm skin, flushing, thirst, tachycardia, dilated pupils, blurred vision, and urine retention.

Nutritional Therapy. There is no specific recommended dietary modification for PUD. Patients are taught to eat and drink foods and fluids that do not cause any distressing symptoms. Caffeine-containing beverages and foods can increase symptom distress in some patients. Teach the patient to eliminate alcohol because it can delay healing. Foods that commonly cause gastric irritation include hot, spicy foods; pepper; carbonated beverages; and broth (meat extract).

Therapy Related to Complications of Peptic Ulcer Disease

Acute Exacerbation. An acute exacerbation is frequently accompanied by bleeding, increased pain and discomfort, and nausea and vomiting. Management is similar to that described for upper GI bleeding later in this chapter (see pp. 955-957).

Perforation. The immediate focus of management of a patient with a perforation is to stop the spillage of gastric or duodenal contents into the peritoneal cavity and restore blood volume. An NG tube is inserted into the stomach to provide continuous aspiration and gastric decompression to stop spillage through the perforation. For duodenal aspiration, the tube is placed as near to the perforation site as possible to facilitate decompression.

Circulating blood volume is replaced with lactated Ringer's and albumin solutions. These solutions substitute for the fluids lost from the vascular and interstitial space as the peritonitis develops. Blood replacement in the form of packed RBCs may be necessary. A central venous pressure line and an indwelling urinary catheter may be inserted and monitored hourly. The patient with a history of cardiac disease requires electrocardiographic (ECG) monitoring or placement of a pulmonary artery catheter for accurate assessment of left ventricular function. Broad-spectrum antibiotic therapy is started immediately to treat bacterial peritonitis. Administration of pain medications provides comfort.

Either open or laparoscopic procedures are used for perforation repair depending on the location of the ulcer and the surgeon's preference. The procedure involving the least risk to the patient is simple oversewing of the perforation and reinforcement of the area with a graft of omentum. The excess gastric contents are suctioned from the peritoneal cavity during the surgical procedure.

Gastric Outlet Obstruction. The aim of therapy for obstruction is to decompress the stomach, correct any existing fluid and electrolyte imbalances, and improve the patient's general state of health. An NG tube is used as described previously. With continuous decompression for several days, the ulcer can begin healing, and the inflammation and edema will subside.

After several days of suction, clamp the NG tube and measure gastric residual volume periodically. The frequency and amount of time the tube remains clamped are related to the amount of aspirate obtained and the patient's comfort level. A method commonly followed is to clamp the tube overnight for approximately 8 to 12 hours and then measure the gastric residue in the morning. When the aspirate falls below 200 mL, this is within a normal range and the patient can begin oral intake of clear liquids. Oral fluids begin at 30 mL/hr and then gradually increase in amount. Assess the patient for signs and symptoms of distress or vomiting. As the amount of gastric residue decreases, solid foods are added and the tube removed.

IV fluids and electrolytes are administered according to the degree of dehydration, vomiting, and electrolyte imbalance indicated by laboratory studies. Pain relief results from the decompression. A PPI or H_2-receptor blocker is used if the obstruction is due to an active ulcer as determined by endoscopy. Pyloric obstruction may be treated endoscopically by balloon dilations. Surgical intervention may be necessary to remove scar tissue.

NURSING MANAGEMENT PEPTIC ULCER DISEASE

NURSING ASSESSMENT
Subjective and objective data to obtain from a patient with PUD are presented in Table 42-16.

NURSING DIAGNOSES
Nursing diagnoses related to PUD may include, but are not limited to, the following:
- Acute pain *related to* increased gastric secretions
- Ineffective self–health management *related to* lack of knowledge of long-term management of PUD
- Nausea *related to* acute exacerbation of disease process

Additional information on nursing diagnoses for the patient with PUD is presented in eNursing Care Plan 42-2 on the website for this chapter.

PLANNING
The overall goals are that the patient with PUD will (1) adhere to the prescribed therapeutic regimen, (2) experience a reduction in or absence of discomfort, (3) exhibit no signs of GI complications, (4) have complete healing of the peptic ulcer, and (5) make appropriate lifestyle changes to prevent recurrence.

NURSING IMPLEMENTATION
HEALTH PROMOTION. You have an important role in identifying patients at risk for PUD. Early detection and effective treat-

TABLE 42-16 NURSING ASSESSMENT

Peptic Ulcer Disease

Subjective Data

Important Health Information

Past health history: Chronic kidney disease, pancreatic disease, chronic obstructive pulmonary disease, serious illness or trauma, hyperparathyroidism, cirrhosis of the liver, Zollinger-Ellison syndrome

Medications: Aspirin, corticosteroids, nonsteroidal antiinflammatory drugs

Surgery or other treatments: Complicated or prolonged surgery

Functional Health Patterns

Health perception–health management: Chronic alcohol abuse, smoking, caffeine use; family history of peptic ulcer disease

Nutritional-metabolic: Weight loss, anorexia, nausea and vomiting, hematemesis, dyspepsia, heartburn, belching

Elimination: Black, tarry stools

Cognitive-perceptual

　Duodenal ulcers: Burning, midepigastric or back pain occurring 2-4 hr after meals and relieved by food; nocturnal pain common

　Gastric ulcers: High epigastric pain occurring 1-2 hr after meals; pain may be precipitated or aggravated by food

Coping-stress tolerance: Acute or chronic stress

Objective Data

General

Anxiety, irritability

Gastrointestinal

Epigastric tenderness

Possible Diagnostic Findings

Anemia; guaiac-positive stools; positive blood, urine, breath, or stool tests for *Helicobacter pylori;* abnormal upper gastrointestinal endoscopic and barium studies

---

ment of ulcers are important aspects of reducing morbidity risks associated with PUD. Patients who are taking ulcerogenic drugs (e.g., aspirin, NSAIDs) are at risk for PUD. Encourage patients to take these drugs with food. Teach patients to report symptoms related to gastric irritation, including epigastric pain, to their health care provider.

ACUTE INTERVENTION. During the acute exacerbation of an ulcer, the patient often complains of increased pain and nausea and vomiting, and some may have evidence of bleeding. Initially many patients attempt to cope with the symptoms at home before seeking medical assistance.

During this acute phase the patient may be NPO for a few days, have an NG tube inserted and connected to intermittent suction, and have IV fluid replacement. Explain to the patient and the caregiver the reasons for these therapies so they understand that the advantages far outweigh any temporary discomfort. Regular mouth care alleviates the dry mouth. Cleansing and lubrication of the nares facilitate breathing and decrease soreness. Analysis of gastric contents may include pH testing and analysis for blood, bile, or other substances. When the stomach is empty of gastric secretions, the ulcer pain diminishes and ulcer healing begins.

The volume of fluid lost, the patient's signs and symptoms, and laboratory test results (hemoglobin, hematocrit, and electrolytes) determine the type and amount of IV fluids administered. Be aware that other health problem (e.g., heart failure) may be adversely affected by the type or amount of fluid used. Take vital signs initially and at least hourly to detect and treat shock.

Physical and emotional rest is conducive to ulcer healing. The patient's immediate environment should be quiet and restful. The use of a mild sedative or tranquilizer has beneficial effects when the patient is anxious and apprehensive. Use good judgment before sedating a person who is becoming increasingly restless because the drug could mask the signs of shock secondary to upper GI bleeding.

If the patient's condition improves without worsening of symptoms (e.g., increased pain, vomiting, hemorrhage), the regimen outlined for conservative therapy is followed. However, complications such as hemorrhage, perforation, and obstruction can occur.

Hemorrhage. Changes in the vital signs and an increase in the amount and redness of the aspirate often signal massive upper GI bleeding. With bleeding, the patient's pain often decreases because the blood helps neutralize the acidic gastric contents. It is important to maintain the patency of the NG tube so that blood clots do not obstruct the tube. If the tube becomes blocked, the patient can develop abdominal distention. Use interventions similar to those described for upper GI bleeding on pp. 955-957.

Perforation. With perforation, the patient complains of sudden, severe abdominal pain. Perforation is manifested by a rigid, boardlike abdomen; severe generalized abdominal and shoulder pain; drawing up of the knees; and shallow, grunting respirations. The bowel sounds that may have been previously normal or hyperactive may diminish and become absent. When the patient with an ulcer demonstrates these changes, suspect perforation and notify the health care provider immediately.

Take vital signs promptly and record them every 15 to 30 minutes. Temporarily stop all oral or NG drugs and feedings until you can notify the health care provider and a definitive diagnosis is made. If perforation does exist, anything taken orally can add to the spillage into the peritoneal cavity and increase discomfort. If you are administering IV fluids at the time of the perforation, maintain the rate or increase it to replace the depleted plasma volume.

When perforation is confirmed, antibiotic therapy begins. When the perforation fails to seal spontaneously, surgical or laparoscopic closure is necessary and is performed as soon as possible. There may not be adequate time to thoroughly prepare the patient and family for the surgical intervention.

Gastric Outlet Obstruction. Gastric outlet obstruction can happen at any time. It is most likely to occur in the patient whose ulcer is located close to the pylorus. The onset of symptoms is usually gradual. Constant NG aspiration of stomach contents can help relieve symptoms. This allows edema and inflammation to subside and permits normal flow of gastric contents through the pylorus.

Regular irrigation of the tube with a normal saline solution per institutional policy may facilitate proper functioning. It may also be helpful to reposition the patient from side to side so that the tube tip is not constantly lying against the mucosal surface.

When the patient has resumed oral feedings and you notice symptoms of obstruction, promptly inform the health care provider. Generally, all that is necessary to treat the problem is to resume gastric aspiration so that the edema and inflammation resulting from the acute episode resolve. IV fluids with electrolyte replacement keep the patient hydrated during this period. To check for ongoing obstruction, clamp the NG tube intermittently and measure the gastric aspirate. It is important to maintain accurate intake and output records, especially of the gastric

TABLE 42-17 PATIENT & CAREGIVER TEACHING GUIDE

Peptic Ulcer Disease (PUD)

Include the following instructions when teaching the patient and caregiver about management of PUD.

1. Follow dietary modifications, including avoidance of foods that may cause epigastric distress. This may include black pepper, spicy foods, and acidic foods.
2. Avoid cigarettes. In addition to promoting ulcer development, smoking delays ulcer healing.
3. Reduce or eliminate alcohol intake.
4. Avoid OTC drugs unless approved by the health care provider. Many preparations contain ingredients, such as aspirin, that should not be taken unless approved by the health care provider. Check with the health care provider regarding the use of nonsteroidal antiinflammatory drugs.
5. Do not interchange brands of antacids, H_2-receptor blockers, and proton pump inhibitors that can be purchased OTC without checking with the health care provider. This can lead to harmful side effects.
6. Take all medications as prescribed. This includes both antisecretory and antibiotic drugs. Failure to take medications as prescribed can result in relapse.
7. It is important to report any of the following:
   - Increased nausea or vomiting
   - Increased epigastric pain
   - Bloody emesis or tarry stools
8. Stress can be related to signs and symptoms of PUD. Learn and use stress management strategies (see Chapter 7).
9. Share concerns about lifestyle changes and living with a chronic illness.

aspirate. When conservative treatment is not successful, surgery is performed after the acute phase has passed.

AMBULATORY AND HOME CARE. Patients with PUD have specific needs to prevent recurrence or complications. General instructions should cover aspects of the disease process itself, drugs, possible changes in lifestyle (alcohol intake, smoking), and regular follow-up care. Table 42-17 provides a patient and caregiver teaching guide for PUD.

Knowing the etiology and pathophysiology of PUD may motivate the patient to become involved in care and improve adherence to therapy. Work collaboratively with the dietitian to elicit a dietary history and plan ways to incorporate dietary modifications (if needed) into the patient's home and work setting.

The patient may not be honest about habitual use of alcohol or cigarettes. Provide information about the negative effects of alcohol and cigarettes on PUD and ulcer healing. Teach the patient about prescribed drugs, including their actions, side effects, and dangers if omitted for any reason. Make sure the patient knows why OTC drugs (e.g., aspirin, NSAIDs) should not be taken unless approved by the health care provider.[20] Because you can buy some H_2-receptor blockers and PPIs without a prescription, inform the patient that substituting prescription with OTC preparations without checking with the health care provider can lead to harmful side effects.

Try to obtain information about the patient's psychosocial status. Knowledge of lifestyle, occupation, and coping behaviors can be helpful in planning care. The patient may be reluctant to talk about personal subjects, the stress experienced at home or on the job, the usual methods of coping, or dependence on drugs or alcohol.

PUD is often a chronic, recurring disorder. Emphasize the need for long-term follow-up care, and encourage the

patient to seek immediate intervention if symptoms return. The patient may be frustrated, especially if the prescribed mode of therapy has been faithfully followed, yet has failed to prevent the recurrence.

Some patients do not adhere to the plan of care, and they experience repeated exacerbations. Patients quickly learn that they often experience no discomfort when they omit prescribed drugs, smoke, or drink alcohol. Consequently, they make no or little alteration in lifestyle. After an acute exacerbation, the patient is likely to be more amenable to following the plan of care and open to suggestions for changes in lifestyle.

Changes, such as smoking cessation and alcohol abstinence, are difficult for many people. The patient may do better in reducing use of these substances rather than totally eliminating them. However, the goal should always be total cessation. Inform the patient with chronic PUD about potential complications, the clinical manifestations indicating their presence, and what to do until the health care provider can be seen.

▌EVALUATION

Expected outcomes are that the patient with PUD will
- Have pain controlled without the use of analgesics
- Verbalize an understanding of the treatment regimen
- Commit to self-care and management of the disease
- Have no complications (hemorrhage, perforation)

Additional information on expected outcomes for the patient with PUD is presented in eNursing Care Plan 42-2 on the website for this chapter.

Collaborative Care
Surgical Therapy for Peptic Ulcer Disease

With the use of antisecretory and antibiotic agents, surgery for PUD is uncommon. Surgery is performed on patients with complications that are unresponsive to medical management or concerns about stomach cancer.

Surgical procedures include partial gastrectomy, vagotomy, and pyloroplasty. Partial gastrectomy with removal of the distal two thirds of the stomach and anastomosis of the gastric stump to the duodenum is called a *gastroduodenostomy* or *Billroth I* operation (see eFig. 42-1 on the website for this chapter). Partial gastrectomy with removal of the distal two thirds of the stomach and anastomosis of the gastric stump to the jejunum is called a *gastrojejunostomy* or *Billroth II* operation (see eFig. 42-1).

Vagotomy is the severing of the vagus nerve, either totally *(truncal)* or selectively *(highly selective vagotomy)*. These procedures are done to decrease gastric acid secretion. *Pyloroplasty* consists of surgical enlargement of the pyloric sphincter to facilitate the easy passage of contents from the stomach. It is commonly done after vagotomy or to enlarge an opening that has been constricted from scar tissue.

Postoperative Complications. As with all surgeries, acute postoperative bleeding at the surgical site can occur. Monitoring of patients is similar to that described under acute upper GI bleeding. The most common long-term postoperative complications from PUD surgery are (1) dumping syndrome, (2) postprandial hypoglycemia, and (3) bile reflux gastritis.

Dumping Syndrome. *Dumping syndrome* is the direct result of surgical removal of a large portion of the stomach and the pyloric sphincter. Approximately 20% of patients experience dumping syndrome after PUD surgery.

Normally, gastric chyme enters the small intestine in small amounts. However, after surgery the stomach no longer has control over the amount of gastric chyme entering the small intestine. Consequently, a large bolus of hypertonic fluid enters the intestine and results in fluid being drawn into the bowel lumen. This creates a decrease in plasma volume along with distention of the bowel lumen and rapid intestinal transit.

The onset of symptoms occurs within 15 to 30 minutes after eating. The patient usually describes feelings of generalized weakness, sweating, palpitations, and dizziness. These symptoms are due to the sudden decrease in plasma volume. The patient complains of abdominal cramps, *borborygmi* (audible abdominal sounds produced by hyperactive intestinal peristalsis), and the urge to defecate. These manifestations usually last less than 1 hour after eating.

Postprandial Hypoglycemia. Postprandial hypoglycemia is considered a variant of dumping syndrome because it is the result of uncontrolled gastric emptying of a bolus of fluid high in carbohydrate into the small intestine. The bolus of concentrated carbohydrate results in hyperglycemia and the release of excessive amounts of insulin into the circulation. This results in reflex hypoglycemia. Symptoms are similar to those of any hypoglycemic reaction and include sweating, weakness, mental confusion, palpitations, tachycardia, and anxiety. Symptoms generally occur 2 hours after eating.

Bile Reflux Gastritis. Gastric surgery that involves the pylorus, with either reconstruction or removal, can result in reflux of bile into the stomach. Prolonged contact with bile causes damage to the gastric mucosa, chronic gastritis, and recurrence of PUD.

The symptoms associated with reflux alkaline gastritis are continuous epigastric distress that increases after meals. Vomiting relieves the distress, but only temporarily. The administration of cholestyramine (Questran), either before or with meals, has been used successfully to treat this problem. Cholestyramine binds with the bile salts that are the source of gastric irritation.

Nutritional Therapy. Start discharge planning and teaching as soon as the immediate postoperative period is successfully passed. The dietitian usually gives dietary instructions, and you need to reinforce them. Because the stomach's reservoir is diminished after gastric resection, patients must reduce their meal size accordingly. Advise the patient to reduce fluids drunk with meals. Dry foods with a low carbohydrate content and moderate protein and fat content are better tolerated initially. Dietary changes, along with a short rest period after each meal, reduce the likelihood of dumping syndrome. Reassure the patient that the unpleasant symptoms are usually of short duration. Following these dietary measures will decrease symptoms within a few months and is essential to long-term adherence.

The immediate ingestion of sugared fluids or candy relieves the hypoglycemic symptoms. To avoid hypoglycemic episodes, instruct the patient to limit the amount of sugar consumed with each meal and to eat small, frequent meals with moderate amounts of protein and fat (Table 42-18). Although only a small percentage of patients experience bile reflux gastritis, caution the patient to notify the health care provider of any continuous epigastric distress after meals.

NURSING MANAGEMENT
SURGICAL THERAPY FOR PEPTIC ULCER DISEASE

PREOPERATIVE CARE
Given the greater use of endoscopic procedures for the treatment of PUD, surgical procedures are used less frequently.

TABLE 42-18 NUTRITIONAL THERAPY

Postgastrectomy Dumping Syndrome

Purposes
- To slow the rapid passage of food into the intestine
- To control symptoms of dumping syndrome (dizziness, sense of fullness, diarrhea, tachycardia), which sometimes occurs after a partial or total gastrectomy

Diet Principles
- Divide meals into six small feedings to avoid overloading the stomach and intestine at mealtimes.
- Do not take fluids with meals but at least 30-45 min before or after meals. This helps prevent distention or a feeling of fullness.
- Avoid concentrated sweets (e.g., honey, sugar, jelly, jam, candies, sweet pastries, sweetened fruit) because they sometimes cause dizziness, diarrhea, and a sense of fullness.
- Increase protein and fats to promote rebuilding of body tissues and to meet energy needs. Meat, cheese, and eggs are specific foods to increase in the diet.
- Amount of time these restrictions should be followed varies. The health care provider decides the proper amount of time to remain on this prescribed diet according to the patient's clinical condition and progress.

Surgery can involve either laparoscopic or open surgery techniques. When surgery is planned, the surgeon provides the necessary information about the procedure and the expected outcome so that the patient can make an informed decision. Help the patient and caregiver by clarifying and interpreting their questions. Instruct them on what to expect after surgery, including comfort measures, pain relief, coughing and breathing exercises, use of an NG tube, and IV fluid administration (see Chapter 18).

POSTOPERATIVE CARE
Care of the patient after major abdominal surgery is similar to the postoperative care after abdominal laparotomy (see Chapter 43). An NG tube is used to decompress the remaining portion of the stomach to decrease pressure on the suture line and to allow for resolution of edema and inflammation resulting from surgical trauma.

Observe the gastric aspirate for color, amount, and odor during the immediate postoperative period. The aspirate is usually bright red at first, with a gradual darkening within the first 24 hours after surgery. Normally the color changes to yellow-green within 36 to 48 hours. If the tube becomes clogged during this period, the health care provider may order periodic gentle irrigations with normal saline solution. It is essential that the NG suction is working and that the tube remains patent so that accumulated gastric secretions do not put a strain on the anastomosis. This can lead to distention of the remaining portion of the stomach and result in (1) rupture of the sutures, (2) leakage of gastric contents into the peritoneal cavity, (3) hemorrhage, and (4) possible abscess formation. If the tube must be replaced or repositioned, call the health care provider to perform this task because of the danger of perforating the gastric mucosa or disrupting the suture line.

Observe the patient for signs of decreased peristalsis, including abdominal distention and lower abdominal discomfort, which may indicate intestinal obstruction. Monitor and record accurate intake and output every 4 hours.

Keep the patient comfortable and free of pain by administering prescribed drugs and frequently changing position. In an open surgical approach, the incision is relatively high in the epigastrium and may interfere with deep breathing and coughing. Splinting the area with a pillow while gently and persistently encouraging the patient to deep breathe helps prevent pulmonary complications. Splinting also protects the abdominal suture line from rupturing during coughing. Observe the dressing for signs of bleeding or odor and drainage indicative of an infection. Encourage early ambulation.

While the NG tube is connected to suction, maintain IV therapy. Add potassium and vitamin supplements (as ordered) to the infusion until oral feedings are resumed. Before the NG tube is removed, the patient begins oral feedings of clear liquids to determine the tolerance level. The stomach may be aspirated within 1 or 2 hours to assess the amount remaining and its color and consistency. When fluids are well tolerated, the NG tube is removed and fluids are increased in frequency, with a slow progression to regular foods. The patient begins the regimen of six small meals a day.

Pernicious anemia is a long-term complication of total gastrectomy and may occur after partial gastrectomy. Pernicious anemia is due to the loss of intrinsic factor, which is produced by the parietal cells. The patient may require cobalamin replacement therapy (see Chapter 31). PUD is a chronic problem, and ulcers can recur, especially at the site of the anastomosis.

GERONTOLOGIC CONSIDERATIONS

PEPTIC ULCER DISEASE

The morbidity and mortality rates associated with PUD in the older patient are higher than those for younger adults because of concomitant health problems and a decreased ability to withstand hypovolemia. Monitor older adults who use NSAIDs for osteoarthritis for signs and symptoms of PUD. In older patients, pain may not be the first symptom associated with an ulcer. For some patients the first manifestation is frank gastric bleeding or a decrease in hematocrit.

The treatment and management of PUD in older adults are similar to those in younger adults. An emphasis is placed on prevention of both gastritis and PUD. This includes teaching the patient to take NSAIDs and other gastric-irritating drugs with food, milk, or antacids. Instruct the patient to avoid irritating substances, adhere to the PPI or H_2-receptor blocker therapy as prescribed, and report abdominal pain or discomfort to the health care provider.

STOMACH CANCER

Stomach (gastric) cancer is an adenocarcinoma of the stomach wall (Fig. 42-15). The rate of stomach (particularly distal) cancer has been steadily declining in the United States. However, cancer of the cardia and the gastroesophageal junction is increasing. Gastric cancer still accounts for more than 10,540 deaths and 21,320 new cancer cases annually.[5]

Asian Americans and Pacific Islanders, Hispanics, and African Americans have higher rates of stomach cancer than non-Hispanic whites. Stomach cancer is more prevalent in men of the lower socioeconomic class, primarily those living in urban areas. The incidence of stomach cancer increases with age, with the majority being diagnosed between 65 and 80. At the time of diagnosis, only 10% to 20% of patients have disease confined to the stomach, and more than 50% have advanced

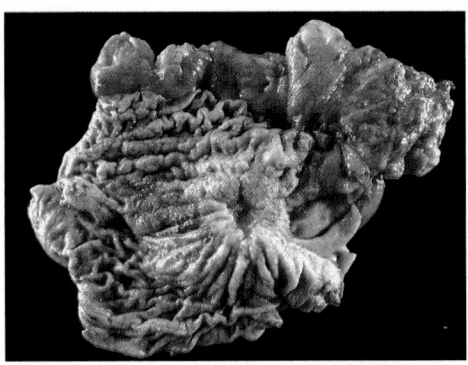

FIG. 42-15 Stomach carcinoma. Gross photograph showing an ill-defined, excavated central ulcer surrounded by irregular, heaped-up borders.

metastatic disease. The 5-year survival rate is 80% in patients with early stages (confined to the stomach) and less than 30% in those with advanced disease.[5]

Etiology and Pathophysiology

Many factors have been implicated in the development of stomach cancer, yet no single causative agent has been identified.[21] Stomach cancer probably begins with a nonspecific mucosal injury as a result of infection (*H. pylori*), autoimmune-related inflammation, repeated exposure to irritants such as bile, antiinflammatory agents, and tobacco use.

Stomach cancer has been associated with diets containing smoked foods, salted fish and meat, and pickled vegetables. Whole grains and fresh fruits and vegetables are associated with reduced rates of stomach cancer. Infection with *H. pylori*, especially at an early age, is a risk factor for stomach cancer. It is possible that *H. pylori* and resulting cell changes can induce a sequence of transitions from dysplasia to cancer. Individuals with lymphoma of the stomach (mucosa-associated lymphoid tissue [MALT]) are at higher risk of stomach cancer.

Other predisposing factors include atrophic gastritis, pernicious anemia, adenomatous polyps, hyperplastic polyps, and achlorhydria. Smoking and obesity both increase the risk of stomach cancer. Although first-degree relatives of patients with stomach cancer are at increased risk, only 8% to 10% of stomach cancers have an inherited familial component.[21]

Stomach cancer spreads by direct extension and typically infiltrates rapidly to the surrounding tissue and liver. Seeding of tumor cells into the peritoneal cavity occurs late in the course of the disease.

Clinical Manifestations

Stomach cancers often spread to adjacent organs before any distressing symptoms occur. The clinical manifestations can include unexplained weight loss, early satiety, indigestion, abdominal discomfort or pain, and signs and symptoms of anemia. The patient may report *early satiety*, or a sense of being full sooner than usual. Anemia, which is common, is caused by chronic blood loss as the lesion erodes through the mucosa or as a result of pernicious anemia (caused by loss of intrinsic factor). The person appears pale and weak and complains of fatigue, weakness, dizziness, and, in extreme cases, shortness of breath. The stool may be positive for occult blood. Supraclavicular lymph nodes that are hard and enlarged suggest metastasis via the thoracic duct. The presence of ascites is a poor prognostic sign.

TABLE 42-19   COLLABORATIVE CARE

Stomach Cancer

Diagnostic	Collaborative Therapy

• History and physical examination
• Endoscopy and biopsy
• CT
• Upper GI barium study (less frequent)
• Exfoliative cytologic study
• Endoscopic ultrasonography
• Complete blood count
• Urinalysis
• Stool examination
• Liver enzymes
• Serum amylase
• Tumor markers
  • Carcinoembryonic antigen (CEA)
  • Carbohydrate antigen (CA)–19-9, CA-125, CA 72-4
  • α-Fetoprotein
	• Surgery
	  • Subtotal gastrectomy—Billroth I or II procedure (see eFig. 42-1)
	  • Total gastrectomy with esophagojejunostomy
	• Adjuvant therapy
	  • Radiation therapy
	  • Chemotherapy
	  • Combination radiation therapy and chemotherapy

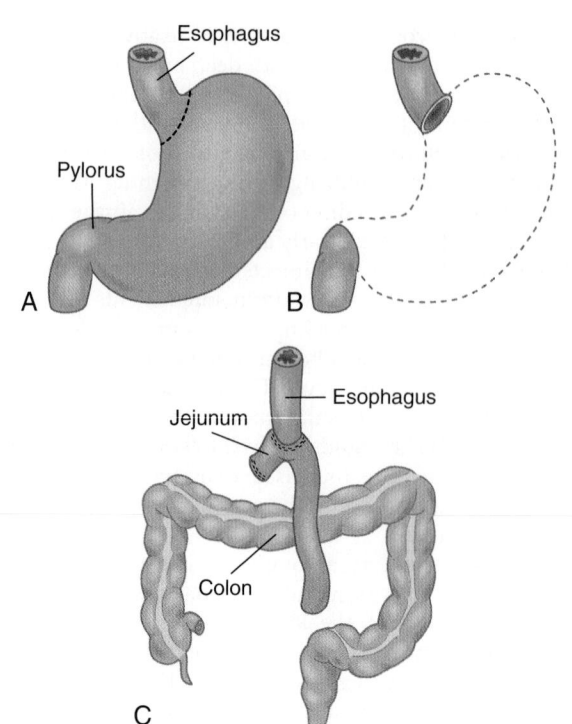

FIG. 42-16 Total gastrectomy for stomach cancer. **A,** Normal anatomic structure of the stomach. **B,** Removal of the stomach (total gastrectomy). **C,** Anastomosis of the esophagus with the jejunum (esophagojejunostomy).

Diagnostic Studies

The diagnostic studies for stomach cancer are presented in Table 42-19. Upper GI endoscopy is the best diagnostic tool. The stomach can be distended with air during the procedure so that the mucosal folds can be stretched. Biopsy of the tissue and subsequent histologic examination are important for the diagnosis of stomach cancer.

Endoscopic ultrasound, CT, and PET scanning can be used to stage the disease. Barium studies do not always detect small lesions of the cardia and the fundus. Laparoscopy is done to determine peritoneal spread.

Blood chemistry studies detect anemia and determine its severity. Elevations in liver enzymes and serum amylase levels may indicate liver and pancreatic involvement. Stool examination provides evidence of occult or gross bleeding.

Collaborative Care

The treatment of choice for stomach cancer is surgical removal of the tumor. Preoperative management of the patient focuses on the correction of nutritional deficits and treatment of anemia. Transfusions of packed RBCs correct the anemia. If a gastric outlet obstruction occurs, gastric decompression may be necessary before surgery. When the tumor has extended into the transverse colon, partial colon resection is required. Preoperative preparation for bowel surgery includes a low-residue diet, enemas to cleanse the bowel, and antibiotics to reduce the intestinal bacteria. Correction of malnutrition is important if surgery is planned.

Surgical Therapy. The surgical intervention used in the treatment of stomach cancer may be the same surgical procedures used for PUD. The location and extent of the lesion, the patient's physical condition, and the surgeon's preference determine the specific surgery used (e.g., open versus laparoscopic). For patients with localized stomach cancer, surgical treatment alone results in a greater than 50% 5-year survival rate. For patients with lymph node–positive cancer, the 5-year survival rate after surgery is 10% to 50% depending on the degree of spread. Survival rates are less when organs adjacent to the stomach show evidence of invasion at the time of surgery.

The surgical aim is to remove as much of the stomach as necessary to remove the tumor and a margin of normal tissue. When the lesion is located in the fundus, a total gastrectomy

with esophagojejunostomy is performed (Fig. 42-16). Lesions located in the antrum or the pyloric region are generally treated by either a Billroth I or II procedure. When metastasis has occurred to adjacent organs, such as the spleen, ovaries, or bowel, the surgical procedure is modified and extended as necessary.

Adjuvant Therapy. The current therapy for localized stomach cancer includes surgical resection and chemotherapy. Agents used in combination include continuous-infusion fluorouracil, epirubicin, cisplatin, etoposide, irinotecan, capecitabine (Xeloda), docetaxel, and oxaliplatin (Eloxatin).

Radiation therapy may be used together with chemotherapy to reduce recurrence and as a palliative measure to decrease tumor mass and provide temporary relief of obstruction. Additional therapies, including intraperitoneal administration of chemotherapeutic agents and immunotherapy, are undergoing evaluation. (These therapies are discussed in Chapter 16.)

NURSING MANAGEMENT STOMACH CANCER

NURSING ASSESSMENT

The assessment of a person with possible stomach cancer is similar to that for PUD (see Table 42-16). Important data to obtain from the patient and the family include a nutritional assessment, a psychosocial history, the patient's perceptions of the health problem and need for care, and a physical examination of the patient.

The nutritional assessment obtains information regarding appetite and changes in eating patterns over the previous 6 months. Determine the patient's normal weight and any recent changes in it. Unexplained weight loss is common. The patient may report a history of vague abdominal symptoms, including dyspepsia and intestinal gas discomfort or pain. If the patient reports pain, explore where and when it occurs and how it is relieved.

Determine the patient's personal perception of the health problem and method of coping with hospitalization, diagnostic tests, and procedures. The possibility of a diagnosis of cancer and a treatment regimen that may include surgery, chemotherapy, or radiation treatment is stressful.[22] It is important to support the patient and the family. If surgery is probable, assess the patient's expectations regarding surgery (cure or palliation) and how the patient has responded to previous surgical procedures.

Focus your assessment on the patient's current functional abilities, other health problems, and response to therapy. Evaluate the patient's nutritional status. Cachexia may be evident if the nutritional intake has been reduced for an extended period. A malnourished patient does not respond well to chemotherapy or radiation therapy and is a poor surgical risk.

NURSING DIAGNOSES

Nursing diagnoses for the patient with stomach cancer include, but are not limited to, the following:

- Imbalanced nutrition: less than body requirements *related to* inability to ingest, digest, or absorb nutrients
- Anxiety *related to* lack of knowledge of diagnostic tests, unknown diagnostic outcome, disease process, and therapeutic regimen
- Acute pain *related to* underlying disease process and side effects of surgery, chemotherapy, or radiation therapy
- Grieving *related to* perceived unfavorable diagnosis and impending death

PLANNING

The overall goals are that the patient with stomach cancer will (1) experience minimal discomfort, (2) achieve optimal nutritional status, and (3) maintain a degree of spiritual and psychologic well-being appropriate to the disease stage.

NURSING IMPLEMENTATION

HEALTH PROMOTION. Your role in the early detection of stomach cancer is focused on identification of the patient at risk because of specific disorders such as *H. pylori* infection, pernicious anemia, and achlorhydria. Be aware of symptoms associated with stomach cancer, method of spread, and the significant findings on physical examination. Symptoms often occur late and mimic other conditions, such as PUD. Poor appetite, weight loss, fatigue, and persistent stomach distress are symptoms of stomach cancer. Encourage patients who have a positive family history of stomach cancer to undergo diagnostic evaluation if manifestations of anemia, PUD, or vague epigastric distress are present. It is important that you recognize the possible existence of stomach cancer in a patient who is treated for PUD and who fails to have relief after 3 weeks of prescribed therapy.

ACUTE INTERVENTION

Preoperative Care. When the diagnostic tests confirm a malignancy, the patient and the caregiver generally react with shock, disbelief, and depression. Provide emotional and physical support, provide information, clarify test results, and maintain a positive attitude with respect to the patient's immediate recovery and long-term survival.

Because of changes in appetite and early satiety, the patient's current nutritional status may be poor. Surgery may be delayed while the patient becomes more physically able to withstand it.

A positive nutritional state enhances wound healing and the ability to deal with infection and other possible postoperative complications. The patient may be better able to tolerate several small meals a day than three regular meals. The diet may be supplemented by a variety of commercial liquid supplements (see Chapter 40) and vitamins. It may be challenging to persuade the patient to eat when he or she has no appetite and is depressed. Getting the patient's caregiver to assist with meals and encourage intake may be beneficial. If the patient is unable to ingest oral feedings, the health care provider may prescribe enteral (tube feeding) or parenteral nutrition.

If needed, packed RBCs and fluid volume restoration may be given during the preoperative period. Closely observe for reactions to the transfusions. Monitor hemoglobin and hematocrit levels.

The preoperative teaching plan before stomach cancer surgery is similar to that for PUD (see the section on surgical therapy for PUD on pp. 949-951).

Postoperative Care. Postoperative care of the patient with stomach cancer is similar to that following a Billroth I or II procedure (see the section on surgical therapy for PUD earlier in this chapter). When the surgical intervention involves a total gastrectomy, the plan of care is somewhat different. A total gastrectomy requires resection of the lower esophagus, removal of the entire stomach, and anastomosis of the esophagus to the jejunum. If the chest cavity is entered, postoperative drainage is accomplished by the insertion of chest tubes. (Chest surgery and drainage tubes are discussed in Chapter 28.)

After total gastrectomy, the NG tube does not drain a large quantity of secretions because removal of the stomach has eliminated the reservoir capacity. The NG tube is removed when intestinal peristalsis has resumed. Small amounts of clear fluid may then be started. Closely observe the patient for signs of leakage of the fluids at the anastomosis site as evidenced by an elevation in the temperature and increasing dyspnea. When the patient tolerates fluids without distress, fluid intake is increased along with the addition of some solid foods.

As a consequence of a total gastrectomy, a patient experiences the symptoms of dumping syndrome. Weight loss often occurs. Postoperative wound healing may be impaired because of poor nutritional intake. This necessitates IV or oral replacement of vitamins C, D, and K; the B-complex vitamins; and cobalamin. Because these vitamins (with the exception of cobalamin) are normally absorbed in the duodenum, they need to be replaced. For the patient who has had a Billroth I or II procedure (see eFig. 42-1 on the website for this chapter), the postoperative care is similar to that of the patient having this procedure for PUD.

Radiation therapy or chemotherapy is used as an adjuvant to surgery or for palliation. Your role is to provide detailed instructions, reassure the patient, and ensure completion of the designated number of treatments. Start by assessing the patient's knowledge of these therapies. Teach the patient about skin care, the need for nutrition and fluid intake during therapy, and the appropriate use of antiemetic drugs. (Specific care of the patient receiving chemotherapy and radiation therapy is discussed in Chapter 16.)

AMBULATORY AND HOME CARE. Most dietary measures useful after PUD surgery are applicable after surgery for stomach cancer. Make plans for the relief of pain, including comfort measures and the judicious use of analgesics. Teach wound care, if needed, to the primary caregiver in the home setting. Dressings, special equipment, or special services may be required for

TABLE 42-20	TYPES OF UPPER GASTROINTESTINAL BLEEDING
Type	**Manifestations**
Obvious bleeding	
Hematemesis	Bloody vomitus appearing as fresh, bright red blood or "coffee-ground" appearance (dark, grainy digested blood).
Melena	Black, tarry stools (often foul smelling) caused by digestion of blood in the GI tract. Black appearance is from the presence of iron.
Occult bleeding	Small amounts of blood in gastric secretions, vomitus, or stools not apparent by appearance. Detectable by guaiac test.

TABLE 42-21 COMMON CAUSES OF UPPER GASTROINTESTINAL BLEEDING

Drug Induced
- Corticosteroids
- Nonsteroidal antiinflammatory drugs (NSAIDs)
- Salicylates

Esophagus
- Esophageal varices
- Esophagitis
- Mallory-Weiss tear

Stomach and Duodenum
- Stomach cancer
- Hemorrhagic gastritis
- Peptic ulcer disease
- Polyps
- Stress-related mucosal disease

Systemic Diseases
- Blood dyscrasias (e.g., leukemia, aplastic anemia)
- Renal failure

the patient's care at home. Provide the patient with a list of community agencies (e.g., American Cancer Society) that are available for assistance before the patient goes home.

When chemotherapy or radiation treatment is to be continued after discharge, a referral to the home health nurse may be beneficial. The home health nurse can assist with recovery, determine the degree of patient adherence, and provide consultation to the patient and the caregivers. Encourage the patient to adhere to the prescribed therapies, to keep appointments for chemotherapy administration or radiation treatments, and to keep the health care provider informed of changes in physical condition. (Long-term management of the cancer patient is discussed in Chapter 16.)

EVALUATION

Expected outcomes are that the patient with stomach cancer will
- Experience no or minimal discomfort, pain, or nausea
- Achieve optimal nutritional status
- Maintain a degree of psychologic well-being appropriate to the disease stage

UPPER GASTROINTESTINAL BLEEDING

In the United States approximately 300,000 hospital admissions occur each year for upper GI bleeding.[23] Approximately 60% of these are adults over age 65. Despite advances in drug management of predisposing conditions and identification of risk factors, the mortality rate for upper GI bleeding has remained at approximately 6% to 13% for the past 45 years.[23]

Etiology and Pathophysiology

Although the most serious loss of blood from the upper GI tract is characterized by a sudden onset, insidious occult bleeding can also be a major problem. The severity of bleeding depends on whether the origin is venous, capillary, or arterial. (Types of upper GI bleeding are presented in Table 42-20.) Bleeding from an arterial source is profuse, and the blood is bright red, indicating it has not been in contact with gastric HCl acid secretion. In contrast, "coffee-ground" vomitus indicates that the blood has been in the stomach for some time. A massive upper GI hemorrhage is a loss of more than 1500 mL of blood or 25% of intravascular blood volume. *Melena* (black, tarry stools) indicates slow bleeding from an upper GI source. The longer the passage of blood through the intestines, the darker the stool color because of the breakdown of hemoglobin and the release of iron.

Discovering the cause of the bleeding is not always easy. A variety of areas in the GI tract may be involved. Table 42-21 lists the common causes of upper GI bleeding.

Esophageal Origin. Bleeding from the esophagus is most likely due to chronic esophagitis, Mallory-Weiss tear, or esophageal varices. Chronic esophagitis can be caused by GERD, the ingestion of drugs irritating to the mucosa, alcohol, and cigarette smoking. Esophageal varices most often occur secondary to cirrhosis of the liver. (Esophageal varices are discussed in Chapter 44.)

Stomach and Duodenal Origin. Bleeding peptic ulcers account for 40% of the cases of upper GI bleeding. Drugs (either prescription or OTC) are a major cause of upper GI bleeding. Approximately 25% of people on chronic NSAIDs (e.g., ibuprofen) develop endoscopically determined ulcer disease; of these, 2% to 4% will bleed. Aspirin, NSAIDs, and corticosteroids can cause irritation and disruption of the gastroduodenal mucosa. Even low-dose aspirin is associated with risk for GI bleeding. Many OTC preparations contain aspirin. A careful history of all commonly used drugs is necessary whenever upper GI bleeding is suspected.

Stress-related mucosal disease (SRMD), also called *physiologic stress ulcers,* occurs in patients who have had severe burns or trauma or major surgery. In SRMD, there is either diffuse superficial mucosal injury or discrete deeper ulcers in the fundus and body portions of the stomach (see eFig. 42-2 on the website for this chapter). Patients with coagulopathy and those who experience respiratory failure resulting in mechanical ventilation for more than 48 hours are at highest risk.[24]

Diagnostic Studies

Endoscopy is the primary tool for diagnosing the source (e.g., esophageal or gastric varices, gastritis) of upper GI bleeding (see below). Angiography is used in diagnosing upper GI bleeding when endoscopy cannot be done or when bleeding persists after endoscopic therapy. Angiography is an invasive procedure requiring preparation and setup time and may not be appropriate for a high-risk, unstable patient. In this procedure, a catheter is placed into the left gastric or superior mesenteric artery and advanced until the site of bleeding is discovered.

Laboratory studies include CBC, blood urea nitrogen (BUN), serum electrolytes, prothrombin time, partial thromboplastin time, liver enzymes, arterial blood gases (ABGs), and a type and crossmatch for possible blood transfusions. All vomitus and stools should be tested for gross and occult blood.

Monitor the patient's laboratory studies to estimate the effectiveness of therapy. The hemoglobin and hematocrit values are not of immediate help in estimating the degree of blood loss, but they provide a baseline for guiding further treatment. The initial hematocrit may be normal and may not reflect the loss until 4 to 6 hours after fluid replacement, since initially the loss of plasma and RBCs is equal.

Assess the patient's BUN level. During a significant hemorrhage, blood proteins are broken down by GI tract bacteria, resulting in elevated BUN levels. However, the elevated BUN level may also indicate renal hypoperfusion or renal disease.

Collaborative Care

Although approximately 80% to 85% of patients who have massive hemorrhage spontaneously stop bleeding, the cause must be identified and treatment initiated immediately.

Emergency Assessment and Management. A complete history of events leading to the bleeding episode is deferred until emergency care has been initiated. To facilitate early intervention, the physical examination should focus on early identification of signs and symptoms of shock such as tachycardia, weak pulse, hypotension, cool extremities, prolonged capillary refill, and apprehension. (Shock is discussed in Chapter 67). Monitor vital signs every 15 to 30 minutes.

The patient is at risk for gut perforation and peritonitis, which may be indicated by a tense, rigid, boardlike abdomen. Do a thorough abdominal examination, and note the presence or absence of bowel sounds.

IV lines, preferably two, with a 16- or 18-gauge needle are placed for fluid and blood replacement. The type and amount of fluids infused are dictated by physical and laboratory findings. Generally, an isotonic crystalloid solution (e.g., lactated Ringer's solution) is started. Whole blood, packed RBCs, and fresh frozen plasma may be used for replacement of volume in massive hemorrhage. (The use of blood transfusions and volume expanders is discussed in Chapter 31.)

When upper GI bleeding is less profuse, infusion of isotonic saline solution followed by packed RBCs permits restoration of the hematocrit more quickly and does not create complications related to fluid volume overload. The use of supplemental oxygen delivered by face mask or nasal cannula may help increase blood oxygen saturation.

Urine output is one of the best measures of vital organ perfusion. Therefore an indwelling urinary catheter is inserted so that output can be accurately assessed hourly. A central venous pressure line may be inserted for fluid volume status assessment. If the patient has a history of valvular heart disease, coronary artery disease, or heart failure, a pulmonary artery catheter may be necessary to monitor the patient.

Endoscopic Therapy. The first-line management of upper GI bleeding is endoscopy and endotherapy. Endoscopy performed within the first 24 hours of bleeding is important for diagnosis and the determination of the need for surgical or radiologic intervention.

The goal of endoscopic hemostasis is to coagulate or thrombose the bleeding vessel. Several techniques are used, including (1) thermal (heat) probe, (2) multipolar and bipolar electrocoagulation probe, (3) argon plasma coagulation (APC), and (4) neodymium:yttrium-aluminum-garnet (Nd:YAG) laser. Multipolar electrocoagulation and thermal probe are the two most commonly used procedures. The heat probe coagulates tissue by directly applying a heating element to the bleeding site. The APC is a noncontact coagulation that delivers mono-

TABLE 42-22 DRUG THERAPY

Acute Gastrointestinal Bleeding*

Drug	Source of GI Bleeding	Mechanism of Action
vasopressin (Pitressin)	Esophageal varices	Causes vasoconstriction. ↓ Pressure in the portal circulation and stops bleeding
octreotide (Sandostatin)	Upper GI bleeding, esophageal varices	Somatostatin analog that ↓ blood flow to GI tract ↓ HCl acid secretion by ↓ release of gastrin
epinephrine	Bleeding from ulceration	Injection during endoscopy produces hemostasis. Causes tissue edema and pressure on the source of bleeding. Injection therapy often combined with other therapies (e.g., laser)

*Other drugs used to treat GI bleeding are antacids, H_2-receptor blockers, and protein pump inhibitors (see Table 42-9).

polar current to tissue. For variceal bleeding, other strategies include variceal ligation, injection sclerotherapy, and balloon tamponade (see Chapter 44).

Surgical Therapy. Surgical intervention is indicated when bleeding continues regardless of the therapy provided and when the site of the bleeding has been identified. Surgical therapy may be necessary when the patient continues to bleed after rapid transfusion of up to 2000 mL of whole blood or remains in shock after 24 hours. The site of the hemorrhage determines the choice of operation. The mortality rates increase considerably in those over 60 years of age.

Drug Therapy. During the acute phase of upper GI bleeding, empiric PPI therapy with high-dose IV bolus and subsequent infusion is often started before endoscopy. This may decrease the amount of bleeding and the need for endoscopic therapy.

During the acute phase, drugs are used to decrease bleeding, decrease HCl acid secretion, and neutralize the HCl acid that is present. Injection therapy with epinephrine (1:10,000 dilution) during endoscopy is effective for acute hemostasis. Epinephrine produces tissue edema and, ultimately, pressure on the source of bleeding (Table 42-22).

Efforts are made to reduce acid secretion because the acidic environment can alter platelet function and interfere with clot stabilization. PPIs or H_2-receptor blockers are administered IV to decrease acid secretion (see Table 42-10). In patients with upper GI bleeding, somatostatin or its long-acting analog octreotide (Sandostatin) may be administered when endoscopy is not available. Both agents reduce blood flow to the GI organs and acid secretion. After an initial bolus, somatostatin is used for 3 to 7 days, whereas octreotide is given for 3 days after the start of bleeding.

NURSING MANAGEMENT
UPPER GASTROINTESTINAL BLEEDING

NURSING ASSESSMENT

A thorough and accurate nursing assessment is an essential first step as you begin care of the patient admitted with upper GI bleeding. The patient may not be able to provide specific information about the cause of the bleeding until immediate physical needs are met. Perform an immediate nursing assessment while you are getting the patient ready for initial treatment. The assessment includes the patient's level of consciousness, vital signs, skin color, and capillary refill. Check the abdomen for distention, guarding, and peristalsis. Immediate determination of vital signs indicates whether the patient is in shock from blood loss and also provides a baseline blood pressure (BP) and pulse for monitoring the progress of treatment. Signs and symptoms of shock include low BP; rapid, weak pulse; increased thirst; cold, clammy skin; and restlessness. Monitor the patient's vital signs every 15 to 30 minutes, and inform the health care provider of any significant changes.

Once the immediate interventions have begun, the patient or caregiver should answer the following questions: Is there a history of previous bleeding episodes? Has the patient received blood transfusions in the past, and were there any transfusion reactions? Are there any other illnesses (e.g., liver disease, cirrhosis) or medications that may contribute to bleeding or interfere with treatment? Does the patient have a religious preference that prohibits the use of blood or blood products?

Subjective and objective data that should be obtained from the patient or caregiver are presented in Table 42-23.

NURSING DIAGNOSES

Nursing diagnoses for the patient with upper GI bleeding include, but are not limited to, the following:

- Decreased cardiac output *related to* loss of blood
- Deficient fluid volume *related to* acute loss of blood and gastric secretions
- Ineffective peripheral tissue perfusion *related to* loss of circulatory volume
- Anxiety *related to* upper GI bleeding, hospitalization, uncertain outcome, source of bleeding

PLANNING

The overall goals are that the patient with upper GI bleeding will (1) have no further GI bleeding, (2) have the cause of the bleeding identified and treated, (3) experience a return to a normal hemodynamic state, and (4) experience minimal or no symptoms of pain or anxiety.

NURSING IMPLEMENTATION

HEALTH PROMOTION. Although not all cases of upper GI bleeding can be anticipated and prevented, you have an important role in identifying patients at high risk. Always consider the patient with a history of chronic gastritis or PUD at high risk. The patient who has had one major bleeding episode is more likely to have another bleed. Patients with cirrhosis and those with previous upper GI bleeding from varices are also at high risk. Instruct the at-risk patient to avoid gastric irritants such as alcohol and smoking, and to take only prescribed medications. OTC drugs can be harmful because they may contain ingredients (e.g., aspirin) that increase the risk of bleeding. Instruct the patient in the methods of testing vomitus or stools for occult blood. Promptly report positive results to the health care provider.

The patient who requires regular doses of drugs that produce gastroduodenal toxicity (peptic ulcer formation, bleeding), such as aspirin, corticosteroids, or NSAIDs, needs to be taught about the potential for GI bleeding. Patients on daily low-dose aspirin to reduce cardiovascular disease risk are at risk for upper GI bleeding, especially patients over 60 with a history of PUD.

TABLE 42-23 NURSING ASSESSMENT
Upper Gastrointestinal Bleeding

Subjective Data
Important Health Information
Past health history: Precipitating events before bleeding episode, previous bleeding episodes and treatment, peptic ulcer disease, esophageal varices, esophagitis, acute and chronic gastritis, stress-related mucosal disease
Medications: Aspirin, nonsteroidal antiinflammatory drugs, corticosteroids, anticoagulants

Functional Health Patterns
Health perception–health management: Family history of bleeding, smoking, alcohol use
Nutritional-metabolic: Nausea, vomiting, weight loss, thirst
Elimination: Diarrhea; black, tarry stools; decreased urine output; sweating
Activity-exercise: Weakness, dizziness, fainting
Cognitive-perceptual: Epigastric pain, abdominal cramps
Coping–stress tolerance: Acute or chronic stress

Objective Data
General
Fever

Integumentary
Clammy, cool, pale skin; pale mucous membranes, nail beds, and conjunctivae; spider angiomas; jaundice; peripheral edema

Respiratory
Rapid, shallow respirations

Cardiovascular
Tachycardia, weak pulse, orthostatic hypotension, slow capillary refill

Gastrointestinal
Red or "coffee-ground" vomitus; tense, rigid abdomen, ascites; hypoactive or hyperactive bowel sounds; black, tarry stools

Urinary
Decreased urine output, concentrated urine

Neurologic
Agitation, restlessness; decreasing level of consciousness

Possible Diagnostic Findings
↓ Hematocrit and hemoglobin; hematuria; guaiac-positive stools, emesis, or gastric aspirate; ↓ levels of clotting factors; ↑ liver enzymes; abnormal endoscopy results

Even the lowest dose of aspirin can cause GI bleeding. Taking these drugs with meals or snacks lessens their direct irritation. The co-administration of an NSAID with a PPI or high doses of H_2-receptor blocker can reduce bleeding risk. For the patient at risk for gastric ulcers because of NSAID use, misoprostol may also be prescribed. This prostaglandin analog inhibits acid secretion and reduces upper GI bleeding episodes associated with NSAID use. However, the drug has important side effects, including uterine cramping in women, abdominal cramping, and diarrhea.

When you are working with the patient who has a history of liver cirrhosis with esophageal or gastric varices, provide specific instructions on the importance of avoiding known irritants, such as alcohol and smoking. Emphasize the importance of treating an upper respiratory tract infection promptly. Severe coughing or sneezing can increase pressure on the already fragile varices and may result in massive hemorrhage (see Chapter 44).

Patients with blood dyscrasias (e.g., aplastic anemia) or liver dysfunction or those who are taking cancer chemotherapy drugs are at risk due to a decrease in clotting factors and platelets. Instruct these patients regarding their disease process, drugs, and increased risk of GI bleeding.

ACUTE INTERVENTION. Approach the patient in a calm manner to help decrease the level of anxiety. Use caution when administering sedatives for restlessness because it is one of the warning signs of shock and may be masked by the drugs.

Once an infusion has been started, maintain the IV line for fluid or blood replacement. An accurate intake and output record is essential so that the patient's hydration status can be assessed. Measure the urine output hourly. If the patient has a central venous pressure line or pulmonary artery catheter in place, record these readings every 1 to 2 hours. Hemodynamic monitoring provides an accurate and quick assessment of blood flow and pressure within the cardiovascular system (see Chapter 66).

Observe the older adult or the patient with a history of cardiovascular problems closely for signs of fluid overload. However, volume overload and pulmonary edema are concerns in all patients who are receiving large amounts of IV fluids within a short time. Auscultate breath sounds and closely observe the respiratory effort. Keep the head of the bed elevated to provide comfort and prevent aspiration.

ECG monitoring is also used to evaluate cardiac function. Close monitoring of vital signs, especially in the patient with cardiovascular disease, is important because dysrhythmias may occur.

When an NG tube is inserted, pay special attention to keeping it in proper position and observe the aspirate for blood. Although room-temperature, cool, or iced gastric lavage is used in some institutions, its effectiveness as a treatment for upper GI bleeding is questionable. When lavage is used, approximately 50 to 100 mL of fluid is instilled at a time into the stomach. The lavage fluid may be aspirated from the stomach or drained by gravity. When aspiration is the method used, it is important not to aspirate if resistance is felt. The tip of the NG tube may be up against the gastric mucosal lining. When resistance is a factor, use the gravity method.

Assess the stools for blood (hematochezia, black-tarry, bright red). Black, tarry stools are not usually associated with a brisk hemorrhage but are indicative of prolonged bleeding. Menses and bleeding hemorrhoids should be ruled out as possible sources of blood in the stools. When vomitus contains blood but the stool contains no gross or occult blood, the hemorrhage is considered to have been of short duration.

When oral nourishment is begun, observe the patient for symptoms of nausea and vomiting and a recurrence of bleeding. Feedings initially consist of clear fluids and are given hourly until tolerance is determined. Gradual introduction of foods follows if the patient exhibits no signs of discomfort.

When the hemorrhage is the result of chronic alcohol abuse, closely observe the patient for delirium tremens as withdrawal from alcohol takes place. Symptoms indicating the beginning of delirium tremens are agitation, uncontrolled shaking, sweating, and vivid hallucinations. (Alcohol withdrawal is discussed in Chapter 11.)

AMBULATORY AND HOME CARE. Teach the patient and the caregiver how to avoid future bleeding episodes. Ulcer disease, drug or alcohol abuse, and liver and respiratory diseases can all result in upper GI bleeding. Help the patient and the caregiver be aware of the consequences of not adhering to drug therapy. Emphasize that no drugs (especially aspirin, NSAIDs) other than those prescribed by the health care provider should be taken. Smoking and alcohol should be eliminated because they are sources of irritation and interfere with tissue repair. Long-term follow-up care may be necessary because of possible recurrence. Instruct the patient and family on what to do if an acute hemorrhage occurs in the future.

EVALUATION

The expected outcomes are that the patient with upper GI bleeding will

- Have no upper GI bleeding
- Maintain normal fluid volume
- Experience a return to a normal hemodynamic state
- Understand potential etiologic factors and make appropriate lifestyle modifications

FOODBORNE ILLNESS

Foodborne illness (food poisoning) is a nonspecific term that describes acute GI symptoms such as nausea, vomiting, diarrhea, and cramping abdominal pain caused by the intake of contaminated food or liquids.[25] There are 31 known foodborne pathogens. Each year one out of six Americans, approximately 48 million, experiences a foodborne illness. Of these, 128,000 are hospitalized and approximately 3000 die.[26]

Bacteria account for most of the foodborne illnesses. Raw foods that have become contaminated during growing, harvesting, processing, storing, shipping, or final preparation are the most common source. When food is uncooked and left out for more than 2 hours at room temperature, bacteria can multiply quickly. One example is prepackaged cookie dough. The most common bacterial food poisonings are presented in Table 42-24.

Focus interventions on prevention of infection. Teaching includes correct food preparation and cleanliness, adequate cooking, and refrigeration (Table 42-25). For the hospitalized patient, emphasize correction of fluid and electrolyte imbalance from diarrhea and vomiting. With botulism, additional assessment and care relative to neurologic symptoms are indicated (see Chapter 61).

Escherichia coli O157:H7 Poisoning

Escherichia coli O157:H7 causes hemorrhagic colitis and kidney failure. In the very young and older adults, *E. coli* O157:H7 can be life threatening. *E. coli* O157:H7 is found primarily in undercooked meats, particularly poultry and hamburger.[26] *E. coli* outbreaks have also been observed with contaminated leafy vegetables, fruits, and nuts. Person-to-person contact in families, nursing homes, and child care centers is also an important mode of transmission. Infection can also occur after drinking raw milk, unpasteurized juice, or contaminated fruit juices and after swimming in or drinking sewage-contaminated water.

Most strains of *E. coli* are harmless and live in the intestines of healthy humans and animals. *E. coli* O157:H7 produces a

TABLE 42-24   BACTERIAL FOOD POISONING

Type and Cause	Sources	Clinical Manifestations	Treatment and Prevention
Staphylococcal Toxin from *Staphylococcus aureus*	Meat, bakery products, cream fillings, salad dressings, milk. Skin and respiratory tract of food handlers	*Onset:* 30 min–7 hr Vomiting, nausea, abdominal cramping, diarrhea	*Treat:* Symptomatic, fluid and electrolyte replacement, antiemetics *Prevent:* Immediate refrigeration of foods, monitoring of food handlers
Clostridial *Clostridium perfringens*	Meat or poultry dishes cooked at lower temperature (stew, pot pie), rewarmed meat dishes, gravies, improperly canned vegetables	*Onset:* 8-24 hr Diarrhea, nausea, abdominal cramps, vomiting (rare), midepigastric pain	*Treat:* Symptomatic, fluid replacement *Prevent:* Correct preparation of meat dishes. Serving food immediately after cooking or rapid cooling of food
Salmonella *Salmonella typhimurium* (grows in gut)	Improperly cooked poultry, pork, beef, lamb, and eggs	*Onset:* 8 hr–several days Nausea and vomiting, diarrhea, abdominal cramps, fever and chills	*Treat:* Symptomatic, fluid and electrolyte replacement *Prevent:* Correct preparation of food
Botulism Toxin from *Clostridium botulinum;* ingested toxin absorbed from gut and blocks acetylcholine at neuromuscular junction	Improperly canned or preserved food, home-preserved vegetables (most common), preserved fruits and fish, canned commercial products	*Onset:* 12-36 hr *GI:* Nausea, vomiting, abdominal pain, constipation, distention *Central nervous system:* Headache, dizziness, muscular incoordination, weakness, inability to talk or swallow, diplopia, breathing difficulties, paralysis, delirium, coma	*Treat:* Maintenance of ventilation, polyvalent antitoxin, guanidine hydrochloric acid (enhances acetylcholine release) *Prevent:* Correct processing of canned foods, boiling of suspected canned foods for 15 min before serving
Escherichia coli *E. coli* O157:H7	Contaminated beef, pork, milk, cheese, fish, cookie dough	*Onset:* 8 hr–1 wk (varies by strain) Bloody stools, hemolytic uremic syndrome, abdominal cramping, profuse diarrhea	*Treat:* Symptomatic, fluid and electrolyte replacement *Prevent:* Correct preparation of food

TABLE 42-25   PATIENT & CAREGIVER TEACHING GUIDE

Prevention of Food Poisoning

Include the following instructions when teaching the patient and caregiver how to prevent food poisoning.

1. Cook all ground beef and hamburger thoroughly.
   - Use a digital instant-read meat thermometer to ensure thorough cooking (ground beef can turn brown before disease-causing bacteria are killed).
   - Cook ground beef until a thermometer inserted into several parts of the patty, including the thickest part, reads at least 160° F.
   - People who cook ground beef without using a thermometer can decrease their risk of illness by not eating ground beef patties that are still pink in the middle.
2. If you are served an undercooked hamburger or other ground beef product in a restaurant, send it back for further cooking. Also ask for a new bun and a clean plate.
3. Avoid spreading harmful bacteria. Keep raw meat separate from ready-to-eat foods. Wash hands, counters, and utensils with hot soapy water after they touch raw meat. Never place cooked hamburgers or ground beef on the unwashed plate that held raw patties. Wash meat thermometers in between tests of patties that require further cooking.
4. Drink only pasteurized milk, juice, or cider. Commercial juice with an extended shelf-life that is sold at room temperature (e.g., juice in cardboard boxes, vacuum-sealed juice in glass containers) has been pasteurized. Juice concentrates are also heated sufficiently to kill pathogens.
5. Wash fruits and vegetables thoroughly, especially those that will not be cooked.
6. Do not eat raw food products that are supposed to be cooked. Follow package directions for cooking at proper temperatures.
7. People who are immunocompromised or older adults should avoid eating alfalfa sprouts until the safety of the sprouts can be ensured.

powerful toxin and can cause severe illness. The clinical manifestations of *E. coli* O157:H7 include diarrhea (often bloody) and abdominal cramping pain for 2 to 8 days (average 3 to 4 days) after swallowing the organism. The diarrhea is variable, ranging from mild to bloody. The diarrhea may start out as watery but may progress to bloody. Systemic complications, including hemolytic uremia and thrombocytopenic purpura, and even death can occur.

Infection with *E. coli* O157:H7 is diagnosed by detecting the bacteria in the stool. All people who suddenly have diarrhea with blood should get their stool (stool culture) tested for *E. coli* O157:H7.

Treatment involves supportive care to maintain blood volume. The use of antibiotics remains controversial. Most people recover without antibiotics or other specific treatment. There is no evidence that antibiotics improve the course of disease, and it is thought that treatment with some antibiotics may precipitate kidney complications. Patients should avoid antidiarrheal agents, such as loperamide (Imodium). Other therapies may include dialysis and plasmapheresis.

In approximately 2% to 7% of infections, particularly in young children and older adults, hemolytic uremic syndrome (HUS) occurs, in which the RBCs are destroyed and the kidneys fail. HUS is a life-threatening condition usually treated in an ICU. Blood transfusions and kidney dialysis are often required. Approximately 3% to 5% of patients with HUS die. About one third of people with HUS have abnormal kidney function many years later, and a few require long-term dialysis. Additional long-term complications of HUS include hypertension, seizures, blindness, and paralysis.

CASE STUDY

Peptic Ulcer Disease

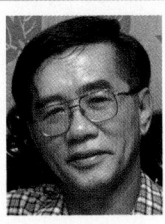

iStockphoto/Thinkstock

Patient Profile

F.H., a 40-yr-old male immigrant from Vietnam, has a 1-yr history of epigastric distress. Increasingly, it is not relieved by over-the-counter antacids and cimetidine (Tagamet). He is scheduled for an upper endoscopy this morning.

Subjective Data

• Reports increasing substernal pain, especially 2 to 3 hr after eating
• Currently avoids alcohol and is taking antacids and over-the-counter H₂-receptor blocker
• Smoking history of 1 pack of cigarettes per day for 20 yr
• Complains of increasing fatigue with exercise
• Reports occasional black bowel movement
• Takes Chinese medicine for frequent back pain

Objective Data

Physical Examination
• Height 5 ft, 5 in tall and weight 140 lb

Diagnostic Studies
• Endoscopy reveals a duodenal ulcer
• Hgb 10.2 g/dL; Hct 30%
• Histology of biopsied tissue reveals *Helicobacter pylori* infection

Collaborative Care

• omeprazole 20 mg bid × 10 days
• clarithromycin 500 mg bid × 10 days
• amoxicillin 1 g bid × 10 days

Discussion Questions

1. Explain the pathophysiology of peptic ulcer disease.
2. What are the risk factors for duodenal ulcers? Which of these did F.H. have?
3. What is the pathophysiology of *H. pylori?*
4. What lifestyle changes would you recommend for F.H.?
5. *Priority Decision:* What are the priority nursing interventions for F.H.?
6. *Delegation Decision:* For the interventions that you identified in question 5, which of the following personnel could be responsible for implementing them: registered nurse (RN), licensed practical nurse (LPN), unlicensed assistive personnel (UAP)?
7. *Priority Decision:* Based on the assessment data provided, what are the priority nursing diagnoses? Are there any collaborative problems?
8. *Evidence-Based Decision:* F.H. asks you if the treatment will work and this will be the end of his problems. How will you respond?

ⓔvolve Answers available at *http://evolve.elsevier.com/Lewis/medsurg.*

BRIDGE TO NCLEX EXAMINATION

The number of the question corresponds to the same-numbered outcome at the beginning of the chapter.

1. M.J. calls to tell the nurse that her 85-year-old mother has been nauseated all day and has vomited twice. Before the nurse hangs up and calls the health care provider, she should instruct M.J. to
   a. administer antispasmodic drugs and observe skin turgor.
   b. give her mother sips of water and elevate the head of her bed to prevent aspiration.
   c. offer her mother a high-protein liquid supplement to drink to maintain her nutritional needs.
   d. offer her mother large quantities of Gatorade to drink because older adults are at risk for sodium depletion.

2. The nurse explains to the patient with Vincent's infection that treatment will include
   a. smallpox vaccinations.
   b. viscous lidocaine rinses.
   c. amphotericin B suspension.
   d. topical application of antibiotics.

3. The nurse teaching young adults about behaviors that put them at risk for oral cancer includes
   a. discouraging use of chewing gum.
   b. avoiding use of perfumed lip gloss.
   c. avoiding use of smokeless tobacco.
   d. discouraging drinking of carbonated beverages.

4. The nurse explains to the patient with gastroesophageal reflux disease (GERD) that this disorder
   a. results in acid erosion of the esophagus from frequent vomiting.
   b. will require surgical wrapping or repair of the pyloric sphincter to control the symptoms.
   c. is the protrusion of a portion of the stomach into the esophagus through an opening in the diaphragm.
   d. often involves relaxation of the lower esophageal sphincter, allowing stomach contents to back up into the esophagus.

5. A patient who has undergone an esophagectomy for esophageal cancer develops increasing pain, fever, and dyspnea when a full liquid diet is started postoperatively. The nurse recognizes that these symptoms are most indicative of
   a. an intolerance to the feedings.
   b. extension of the tumor into the aorta.
   c. leakage of fluid or foods into the mediastinum.
   d. esophageal perforation with fistula formation into the lung.

6. The pernicious anemia that may accompany gastritis is due to
   a. chronic autoimmune destruction of cobalamin stores in the body.
   b. progressive gastric atrophy from chronic breakage in the mucosal barrier and blood loss.
   c. a lack of intrinsic factor normally produced by acid-secreting cells of the gastric mucosa.
   d. hyperchlorhydria resulting from an increase in acid-secreting parietal cells and degradation of RBCs.

7. The nurse is teaching the patient and family that peptic ulcers are
   a. caused by a stressful lifestyle and other acid-producing factors such as *H. pylori.*
   b. inherited within families and reinforced by bacterial spread of *Staphylococcus aureus* in childhood.
   c. promoted by factors that tend to cause oversecretion of acid, such as excess dietary fats, smoking, and *H. pylori.*
   d. promoted by a combination of factors that may result in erosion of the gastric mucosa, including certain drugs and alcohol.

8. An optimal teaching plan for an outpatient with stomach cancer receiving radiation therapy should include information about
   a. cancer support groups, alopecia, and stomatitis.
   b. avitaminosis, ostomy care, and community resources.
   c. prosthetic devices, skin conductance, and grief counseling.
   d. wound and skin care, nutrition, drugs, and community resources.

9. The teaching plan for the patient being discharged after an acute episode of upper GI bleeding includes information concerning the importance of *(select all that apply)*
   a. only taking aspirin with milk or bread products.
   b. avoiding taking aspirin and drugs containing aspirin.
   c. only taking drugs prescribed by the health care provider.
   d. taking all drugs 1 hour before mealtime to prevent further bleeding.
   e. reading all OTC drug labels to avoid those containing stearic acid and calcium.

10. Several patients are seen at an urgent care center with symptoms of nausea, vomiting, and diarrhea that began 2 hours ago while attending a large family reunion potluck dinner. You question the patients specifically about foods they ingested containing
    a. beef.
    b. meat and milk.
    c. poultry and eggs.
    d. home-preserved vegetables.

1. b, 2. d, 3. c, 4. d, 5. c, 6. c, 7. d, 8. d, 9. b, b, c, 10. b

ℯvolve

For rationales to these answers and even more NCLEX review questions, visit *http://evolve.elsevier.com/Lewis/medsurg.*

REFERENCES

1. Buchanan FF, Myles PS, Cicuttini F: Effect of patient sex on general anaesthesia and recovery, *Br J Anaesth* 106:832, 2011.
2. Basch E, Prestrud AA, Hesketh PJ, et al: Antiemetics: American Society of Clinical Oncology clinical practice guideline update, *J Clin Oncol* 29:4189, 2011.
3. Robinson N, Lorenc A, Liao X: The evidence for Shiatsu: a systematic review of Shiatsu and acupressure, *BMC Complement Altern Med* 11:88, 2011.
4. Bensley L, Van Eenwyk J, Ossiander EM: Associations of self-reported periodontal disease with metabolic syndrome and number of self-reported chronic conditions, *Prev Chronic Dis* 8:A50, 2011.
5. American Cancer Society: Cancer facts and figures 2012. Retrieved from *www.cancer.org.*
6. Sanders AE, Slade GD, Patton LL: National prevalence of oral HPV infection and related risk factors in the U.S. adult population, *Oral Dis* 18:430, 2012.
7. Fedele S: Diagnostic aids in the screening of oral cancer, *Head Neck Oncol* 1:5, 2009. (Classic)
8. Bhide SA, Nutting CM: Advances in chemotherapy for head and neck cancer, *Oral Oncol* 46:436, 2010.
9. Sonnenberg A: Effects of environment and lifestyle on gastroesophageal reflux disease, *Dig Dis* 29:229, 2011.
10. Anand G, Katz PO: Gastroesophageal reflux disease and obesity, *Gastroenterol Clin North Am* 39:39, 2010.
11. Robertson L: A new horizon: recommendations and treatment guidelines for Barrett's esophagus, *Gastroenterol Nurs* 32:211, 2009.
12. Ranjitkar S, Kaidonis JA, Smales RJ: Gastroesophageal reflux disease and tooth erosion, *Internat J Dentist* 1:10, 2011.
13. Kahrilas PJ, Shaheen NJ, Vaezi M: American Gastroenterological Association Institute technical review on the management of gastroesophageal reflux disease, *Gastroenterology* 135:1392, 2008. (Classic)
*14. Ngamruengphong S, Leontiadis GI, Radhi S, et al: Proton pump inhibitors and risk of fracture: a systematic review and meta-analysis of observational studies, *Am J Gastroenterol* 106:1209, 2011.
*15. Kwok CS, Arthur AK, Anibueze CI, et al: Risk of *Clostridium difficile* infection with acid suppressing drugs and antibiotics: meta-analysis, *Am J Gastroenterol* 107:1011, 2012.
16. Bower M, Jones W, Vessels B, et al: Role of esophageal stents in the nutrition support of patients with esophageal malignancy, *Nutr Clin Pract* 25:244, 2010.
*17. Lee I, Cryer B: Epidemiology and role of nonsteroidal antiinflammatory drugs in causing gastrointestinal bleeding, *Gastrointest Endosc Clin N Am* 21:597, 2011.
18. Centers for Disease Control and Prevention: *Helicobacter pylori* and peptic ulcer disease: the key to cure. Retrieved from *www.cdc.gov/ulcer/keytocure.htm.*
19. Targownik LE, Bolton JM, Metge CJ, et al: Selective serotonin reuptake inhibitors are associated with a modest increase in the risk of upper gastrointestinal bleeding, *Am J Gastroenterol* 104:1475, 2009.
*20. Thiagarajan P, Jankowski JA: Aspirin and NSAIDs: benefits and harms for the gut, *Best Pract Res Clin Gastroenterol* 26:197, 2012.
21. Blair VR: Familial gastric cancer: genetics, diagnosis, and management, *Surg Oncol Clin N Am* 21:35, 2012.
22. Qian H, Yuan C: Factors associated with self-care self-efficacy among gastric and colorectal cancer patients, *Cancer Nurs* 35:E22, 2012.
23. Holster IL, Kuipers EJ: Management of acute nonvariceal upper gastrointestinal bleeding: current policies and future perspectives, *World J Gastroenterol* 18:1202, 2012.
24. Pilkington KB, Wagstaff MJ, Greenwood JE: Prevention of gastrointestinal bleeding due to stress ulceration: a review of current literature, *Anaesth Intensive Care* 40:253, 2012.
25. National Digestive Diseases Information Clearinghouse: Bacteria and foodborne illness. Retrieved from *http:// digestive.niddk.nih.gov/ddiseases/pubs/bacteria.*
26. Centers for Disease Control and Prevention: *Escherichia coli* O157:H7. Retrieved from *www.cdc.gov/ncidod/dbmd/ diseaseinfo/escherichiacoli_g.htm.*

RESOURCES

American College of Gastroenterology
  www.acg.gi.org
American Gastroenterological Association
  www.gastro.org
Digestive Disease National Coalition
  www.ddnc.org
National Digestive Diseases Information Clearinghouse
  http://digestive.niddk.nih.gov
Society of Gastroenterology Nurses and Associates (SGNA)
  www.sgna.org

*Evidence-based information for clinical practice.

*Clouds come floating into my life, no longer
to carry rain or usher storm, but to add color
to my sunset.*
Rabindranath Tagore

Nursing Management
Lower Gastrointestinal Problems

Marilee Schmelzer

LEARNING OUTCOMES

1. Explain the common etiologies, collaborative care, and nursing management of diarrhea, fecal incontinence, and constipation.
2. Describe common causes of acute abdominal pain and nursing management of the patient after an exploratory laparotomy.
3. Describe the collaborative care and nursing management of acute appendicitis, peritonitis, and gastroenteritis.
4. Compare and contrast the inflammatory bowel diseases of ulcerative colitis and Crohn's disease, including pathophysiology, clinical manifestations, complications, collaborative care, and nursing management.
5. Differentiate among mechanical and nonmechanical bowel obstructions, including causes, collaborative care, and nursing management.
6. Describe the clinical manifestations and collaborative management of colorectal cancer.
7. Explain the anatomic and physiologic changes and nursing management of the patient with an ileostomy and a colostomy.
8. Differentiate between diverticulosis and diverticulitis, including clinical manifestations, collaborative care, and nursing management.
9. Compare and contrast the types of hernias, including etiology and surgical and nursing management.
10. Describe the types of malabsorption syndromes and collaborative care of celiac disease, lactase deficiency, and short bowel syndrome.
11. Describe the types, clinical manifestations, collaborative care, and nursing management of anorectal conditions.

KEY TERMS

anal fistula, p. 1002
appendicitis, p. 973
celiac disease, p. 997
constipation, p. 966
Crohn's disease, p. 975
diarrhea, p. 962
diverticula, p. 994
fecal incontinence, p. 964

gastroenteritis, p. 975
hemorrhoids, p. 1000
hernia, p. 996
inflammatory bowel disease (IBD), p. 975
intestinal obstruction, p. 982
irritable bowel syndrome (IBS), p. 972
lactase deficiency, p. 999

ostomy, p. 990
paralytic (adynamic) ileus, p. 982
peritonitis, p. 974
short bowel syndrome (SBS), p. 999
steatorrhea, p. 997
stoma, p. 990
ulcerative colitis, p. 975

Reviewed by Carmen Bruni, RN, MSN, Nurse Executive, Assistant Professor of Nursing, Texas A & M International University, Laredo, Texas.

The wide variety of intestinal problems presented in this chapter include the disorders of diarrhea, fecal incontinence, and constipation; inflammatory and infectious bowel disorders; bowel trauma; bowel obstructions; colorectal cancer; abdominal and bowel surgery (including ostomy formation); and malabsorption disorders.

DIARRHEA

Diarrhea is the passage of at least three loose or liquid stools per day. It may be acute, or it is considered chronic if it lasts longer than 4 weeks.[1]

Etiology and Pathophysiology

Ingestion of infectious organisms is the primary cause of acute diarrhea (Table 43-1). Viruses cause most cases of infectious diarrhea in the United States. Although viral infections can be deadly, they are usually short lived (48 hours) and mild. Therefore most patients rarely seek treatment.

Bacterial infections are also common.[2] *Escherichia coli* O157:H7, a type of enterohemorrhagic *E. coli,* is the most common cause of bloody diarrhea in the United States. It is transmitted by inadequately cooked beef or chicken contaminated with the bacteria or in fruits and vegetables exposed to contaminated manure. Other pathologic *E. coli* strains are endemic in developing countries and are common causes of traveler's diarrhea. *Giardia lamblia* is the most common intestinal parasite that causes diarrhea in the United States.

Infectious organisms attack the intestines in different ways.[3] Some organisms (e.g., *Rotavirus A, Norovirus, G. lamblia*) alter secretion and/or absorption of the enterocytes of the small intestine without causing inflammation. Other organisms (e.g., *Clostridium difficile*) impair absorption by destroying cells, cause inflammation in the colon, and produce toxins that also cause damage.

Organisms enter the body in contaminated food (e.g., *Salmonella* organisms in undercooked eggs and chicken) or contaminated drinking water (*G. lamblia* in contaminated lakes or pools). Travelers often get diarrhea, especially if they travel to countries with poorer sanitation than their own. An infection can also be transmitted from one individual to another via the fecal-oral route. For example, adult day care workers can transmit infection from one resident to another if they do not wash their hands thoroughly after changing soiled linen.

An individual's susceptibility to pathogenic organisms is influenced by age, gastric acidity, intestinal microflora, and immunocompetence. Older adults are most likely to suffer life-threatening diarrhea. Since stomach acid kills ingested pathogens, medications designed to decrease stomach acid (e.g., proton pump inhibitors and histamine [H_2]-receptor blockers) increase the likelihood that pathogens will survive.[4]

The healthy human colon contains short-chain fatty acids and bacteria such as *E. coli*. These organisms aid in fermentation and provide a microbial barrier against pathogenic bacteria. Antibiotics kill off the normal flora, making the individual more susceptible to pathogenic organisms. For example, patients receiving broad-spectrum antibiotics (e.g., clindamycin [Cleocin], cephalosporins, fluoroquinolones) are susceptible to pathogenic strains of *C. difficile*. *C. difficile* is the most serious antibiotic-associated diarrhea and is becoming more prevalent. Probiotics, in particular *Saccharomyces boulardii* and *Lactobacillus,* may be helpful in preventing antibiotic-induced diarrhea in some patients.

People who are immunocompromised because of disease (e.g., human immunodeficiency virus [HIV]) or immunosuppressive medications are susceptible to gastrointestinal (GI) tract infection. Patients who are immunocompromised and receiving jejunal enteral nutrition are especially prone to *C. difficile* and other foodborne infections. Jejunostomy and nasointestinal feedings, which bypass the stomach's acid environment, do not contain the poorly digestible fiber that is necessary for the survival of normal colonic bacteria.[5]

Not all diarrhea is due to infection. For example, drugs and specific food intolerances can cause diarrhea. Also, large amounts of undigested carbohydrate in the bowel produce an osmotic diarrhea that promotes rapid transit and prevents absorption of fluid and electrolytes. Lactose intolerance and certain laxatives (e.g., lactulose, sodium phosphate, magnesium

TABLE 43-1	CAUSES OF ACUTE INFECTIOUS DIARRHEA*
Type of Organism	**Symptoms**
Viral	
Rotavirus (e.g., Rotavirus A)	Fever, vomiting, profuse watery diarrhea. Lasts 3-8 days.
Norovirus (also called Norwalk-like virus)	Nausea, vomiting, diarrhea, stomach cramping. Rapid onset. Lasts 1-2 days.
Bacterial	
Enterotoxigenic Escherichia coli	Watery or bloody diarrhea. Abdominal cramps. Nausea, vomiting, and fever may be present. Mean duration >60 hr.
Enterohemorrhagic E. coli (e.g., E. coli O157:H7)	Severe abdominal cramping, bloody diarrhea, vomiting. Low-grade fever. Usually lasts 5-7 days.
Shigella	Diarrhea (sometimes bloody), fever, stomach cramps. Usually lasts 5-7 days. Postinfection arthritis may occur.
Salmonella	Diarrhea, fever, abdominal cramps. Lasts 4-7 days.
Staphylococcus	Nausea, vomiting, abdominal cramps, diarrhea. Usually mild. May cause illness in as little as 30 min. Lasts 1-3 days.
Campylobacter jejuni	Diarrhea, abdominal cramps, fever. Sometimes nausea and vomiting. Lasts about 7 days.
Clostridium perfringens	Diarrhea, abdominal cramps, nausea, vomiting. Occurs 8-24 hr after eating contaminated food and lasts approximately 24 hr.
Clostridium difficile	Watery diarrhea, fever, anorexia, nausea, abdominal pain.
Parasitic	
Giardia lamblia	Abdominal cramps, nausea, diarrhea. May interfere with nutrient absorption.
Entamoeba histolytica	Diarrhea, abdominal cramping. Only 10%-20% are ill, and symptoms are usually mild.
Cryptosporidium	Watery diarrhea. Lasts about 2 wk. May also have abdominal cramps, nausea, vomiting, fever, dehydration, and weight loss. Sometimes no symptoms. Long lasting and may be fatal in those who are immunocompromised (e.g., AIDS).

*An expanded version of this table (eTable 43-1) with source of infection and drug treatment is available on the website for this chapter.

citrate) produce an osmotic diarrhea. Bile salts and undigested fats also lead to excessive fluid secretion in the GI tract. The diarrhea from celiac disease and short bowel syndrome results from malabsorption in the small intestine.

Clinical Manifestations

Infections that attack the upper GI tract (e.g., *Norovirus*, *G. lamblia*) usually produce large-volume, watery stools; cramping; and periumbilical pain. Patients have either a low-grade or no fever and often experience nausea and vomiting before the diarrhea begins. Infections of the colon and distal small bowel (e.g., *Shigella, Salmonella, C. difficile*) produce fever and frequent bloody diarrhea with a small volume.

Leukocytes, blood, and mucus may be present in the stool, depending on the causative agent (see Table 43-1). Severe diarrhea produces life-threatening dehydration, electrolyte disturbances (e.g., hypokalemia), and acid-base imbalances (metabolic acidosis). *C. difficile* infection can progress to fulminant colitis and intestinal perforation.

Diagnostic Studies

Since most cases of diarrhea resolve quickly, stool cultures are indicated only for patients who are very ill, have a significant fever, or have had diarrhea longer than 3 to 5 days. Stools are examined for blood, mucus, white blood cells (WBCs), and parasites, and cultures are performed to identify infectious organisms. A multiple-pathogen test can simultaneously detect 11 common viral, bacterial, and parasitic causes of infectious gastroenteritis from a single patient sample. Toxins produced by *C. difficile* can usually be detected in a sample of a patient's stool.

Testing for ova and parasites is reserved for people who have had diarrhea more than 2 weeks. The WBC count may be elevated. People with long-standing diarrhea can develop anemia from iron and folate deficiencies. Increased hematocrit, blood urea nitrogen (BUN), and creatinine levels are signs of fluid deficit.

In patients with chronic diarrhea, measurements of stool electrolytes, pH, and osmolality help determine whether the diarrhea is related to decreased fluid absorption or increased fluid secretion. Measurement of stool fat and undigested muscle fibers may indicate fat and protein malabsorption conditions, including pancreatic insufficiency. Some patients with secretory diarrhea have elevated serum levels of GI hormones such as vasoactive intestinal polypeptide and gastrin.

Collaborative Care

Treatment depends on the cause. Foods and drugs that cause diarrhea should be avoided. Acute infectious diarrhea is usually self-limiting. The major concerns are preventing transmission, replacing fluid and electrolytes, and protecting the skin. Patients usually tolerate oral fluids. Solutions containing glucose and electrolytes (e.g., Pedialyte) may be sufficient to replace losses from mild diarrhea. Parenteral administration of fluids, electrolytes, vitamins, and nutrition is necessary if losses are severe.

Antidiarrheal agents are sometimes given to coat and protect mucous membranes, absorb irritating substances, inhibit intestinal transit, decrease intestinal secretions, or decrease central nervous system stimulation of the GI tract (Table 43-2). Antidiarrheal agents are contraindicated in the treatment of some infectious diarrheas because they potentially prolong exposure to the organism. They are used cautiously in inflammatory bowel disease (IBD) because of the danger of *toxic megacolon*

TABLE 43-2 DRUG THERAPY
Antidiarrheal Drugs

Drug	Mechanism of Action
bismuth subsalicylate (Pepto-Bismol)	Decreases secretions and has weak antibacterial activity. Used to prevent traveler's diarrhea.
calcium polycarbophil (Mitrolan)	Bulk-forming agent that absorbs excessive fluid from diarrhea to form a gel. Used when intestinal mucosa cannot absorb fluid.
loperamide (Imodium, Pepto Diarrhea Control)	Inhibits peristalsis, delays transit, increases absorption of fluid from stools.
diphenoxylate with atropine (Lomotil)	Opioid and anticholinergic. Decreases peristalsis and intestinal motility.
paregoric (camphorated tincture of opium)	Opioid. Decreases peristalsis and intestinal motility.
Donnagel-PG (combination of kaolin, pectin, and paregoric)	Decreases peristalsis and intestinal motility.
octreotide acetate (Sandostatin)	Suppresses serotonin secretion, stimulates fluid absorption from GI tract, decreases intestinal motility.

(colonic dilation greater than 5 cm). Regardless of the cause of diarrhea, antidiarrheal drugs should be given only for a short time.

Antibiotics are rarely used to treat acute diarrhea. However, they may be used for certain infections or when the infected individual is severely ill or immunosuppressed. For example, a nonabsorbable antibiotic, rifaximin (Xifaxan), is used to treat traveler's diarrhea that is caused by *E. coli.*

***Clostridium difficile* Infection.** *C. difficile* infection is a particularly hazardous health care–associated infection. Its spores can survive for up to 70 days on objects, including commodes, telephones, thermometers, bedside tables, and floors. *C. difficile* can be transmitted from patient to patient by health care workers who do not adhere to infection control precautions.

The infection is usually treated by stopping antibiotics and starting the patient on either metronidazole (Flagyl) or vancomycin (Vancocin). Metronidazole is the first line of treatment in mild disease because of concerns about vancomycin-resistant enterococcus (VRE). Since recovery rates are substantially better with vancomycin, it is preferred for serious infections. Both drugs are given orally, but metronidazole may also be given IV. Fidaxomicin (Dificid) is generally reserved for patients who are at risk for relapse or have recurrent infections.

Recurrent *C. difficile* infection occurs in about 20% of patients, and the probability of a recurrence rises with each subsequent infection. Feces transplantation is under investigation as a potential therapeutic option for patients with recurrent and resistant *C. difficile* infections.[6] In this procedure healthy person's feces are inserted into the GI tract using an enema or nasogastric tube, or during colonoscopy.

NURSING MANAGEMENT ACUTE INFECTIOUS DIARRHEA

NURSING ASSESSMENT

Begin the nursing assessment with a thorough history and physical examination (Table 43-3). Ask the patient to describe his or her stool pattern and associated symptoms. Focus on the

TABLE 43-3 NURSING ASSESSMENT

Diarrhea

Subjective Data
Important Health Information
Past health history: Recent travel, infections, stress; diverticulitis or malabsorption; metabolic disorders; inflammatory bowel disease; irritable bowel syndrome
Medications: Laxatives or enemas, magnesium-containing antacids, sorbitol-containing suspensions or elixirs, antibiotics, methyldopa, digitalis, colchicine; OTC antidiarrheal medications
Surgery or other treatments: Stomach or bowel surgery, radiation

Functional Health Patterns
Health perception–health management: Chronic laxative abuse, malaise
Nutritional-metabolic: Ingestion of fatty and spicy foods, food intolerances; anorexia, nausea, vomiting; weight loss; thirst
Elimination: Increased stool frequency, volume, and looseness; change in color and character of stools; steatorrhea, abdominal bloating; decreased urine output
Cognitive-perceptual: Abdominal tenderness, abdominal pain and cramping; tenesmus

Objective Data
General
Lethargy, sunken eyeballs, fever, malnutrition

Integumentary
Pallor, dry mucous membranes, poor skin turgor, perianal irritation

Gastrointestinal
Frequent soft to liquid stools that may alternate with constipation; altered stool color; abdominal distention, hyperactive bowel sounds; pus, blood, mucus, or fat in stools; fecal impaction

Urinary
Decreased output, concentrated urine

Possible Diagnostic Findings
Abnormal serum electrolyte levels; anemia; leukocytosis; eosinophilia; hypoalbuminemia; positive stool cultures; ova, parasites, leukocytes, blood, or fat in stool; abnormal sigmoidoscopy or colonoscopy findings; abnormal lower GI series

duration, frequency, character, and consistency of stool, and the relationship to other symptoms such as pain and vomiting. Inquire about medical conditions that might cause diarrhea and whether the person is taking medications such as antibiotics and laxatives that are known to cause diarrhea, decrease stomach acidity, or cause immunosuppression. Determine whether the patient has traveled to a foreign country or been at a day care facility recently and if family members are also ill. Ask about food preparation practices, food intolerances (e.g., milk), and changes in diet and appetite.

Assess for fever and signs of dehydration (dry skin, low-grade fever, orthostatic changes to pulse and blood pressure, decreased and concentrated urine). Assess the abdomen for distention, pain, and guarding. Inspect the perineal skin for signs of redness and breakdown from the diarrhea.

NURSING DIAGNOSES

Nursing diagnoses for the patient with acute infectious diarrhea may include, but are not limited to, the following:

- Diarrhea *related to* acute infectious process
- Deficient fluid volume *related to* excessive fluid loss and decreased fluid intake

Additional information on nursing diagnoses is presented in eNursing Care Plan 43-1 on the website for this chapter.

PLANNING

The overall goals are that the patient with diarrhea will have (1) no transmission of the microorganism causing the infectious diarrhea; (2) cessation of diarrhea and resumption of normal bowel patterns; (3) normal fluid, electrolyte, and acid-base balance; (4) normal nutritional status; and (5) no perianal skin breakdown.

NURSING IMPLEMENTATION

Consider all cases of acute diarrhea as infectious until the cause is known. Strict infection control precautions are necessary to prevent the illness from spreading to others (see eTable 15-1 on the website for Chapter 15 for CDC Isolation Precautions). Wash your hands before and after contact with each patient and when handling body fluids of any kind. Flush vomitus and stool in the toilet. Teach the patient and caregiver to wash contaminated clothing immediately with soap and water. Also teach them the principles of hygiene, infection control precautions, and the potential dangers of an illness that is infectious to themselves and others. Discuss proper food handling, cooking, and storage with the patient and the caregiver (see Chapter 42, Table 42-24).

Viruses and *C. difficile* spores are extremely difficult to kill. Alcohol-based hand cleaners and ammonia-based disinfectants are ineffective, and even vigorous cleaning with soap and water does not kill everything. Provide private rooms for patients with *C. difficile* infection, and ensure that visitors and health care providers wear gloves and gowns. Infected patients must be given their own disposable stethoscopes and thermometers. Consider all objects in the room contaminated, and ensure they are disinfected with a 10% solution of household bleach.

FECAL INCONTINENCE

Etiology and Pathophysiology

Fecal incontinence is the involuntary passage of stool. It occurs when the normal structures that maintain continence are disrupted. Defecation is a voluntary action when the neuromuscular system is intact (see Chapter 39). Problems with motor function (contraction of sphincters and rectal floor muscles) and/or sensory function (ability to perceive the presence of stool or to experience the urge to defecate) can result in fecal incontinence. Contributing factors to incontinence include weakness or disruption of the internal or external anal sphincter, damage to the pudendal nerve or other nerves that innervate the anorectum, damage to the anal tissue, and trauma to the puborectalis muscle.[7]

For women, obstetric trauma is the most common cause of sphincter disruption. Childbirth, aging, and menopause contribute to the development of fecal incontinence. Other risk factors are listed in Table 43-4. With diarrhea, the likelihood is increased that stool will be accidentally discharged. Chronic constipation can lead to *fecal impaction* (the accumulation of hardened feces in the rectum or sigmoid colon that cannot be expelled). Incontinence occurs as liquid stool seeps around the hardened feces. Fecal impaction is a common problem in older adults with limited mobility. Constipated individuals tend to strain during defecation. Straining contributes to incontinence because it weakens the pelvic floor muscles.

TABLE 43-4	CAUSES OF FECAL INCONTINENCE

Traumatic
- Anorectal surgery for hemorrhoids, fistula, and fissures
- Childbirth injury (episiotomy is a risk factor)
- Perineal trauma or pelvic fracture

Neurologic
- Brain tumor
- Cauda equina nerve injury
- Congenital abnormalities (e.g., spina bifida, myelomeningocele)
- Dementia
- Diabetes mellitus (secondary to neuropathy)
- Multiple sclerosis
- Rectal surgery
- Spinal cord injuries
- Stroke

Inflammatory
- Infection
- Inflammatory bowel disease
- Radiation

Pelvic Floor Dysfunction
- Medications
- Rectal prolapse

Functional
- Physical or mobility impairments affecting toileting ability (e.g., frail older person who cannot get to the bathroom in time)

Other
- Chronic constipation
- Denervation of pelvic muscles from chronic excessive straining
- Fecal impaction
- Loss of rectal elasticity
- Rapid transit of large diarrheal stools

Anorectal surgery such as hemorrhoidectomy and colectomy can damage the sphincters and pudendal nerves. Radiation for prostate cancer decreases rectal compliance. Neurologic conditions, including stroke, spinal cord injury, multiple sclerosis, Parkinson's disease, and diabetic neuropathy, also interfere with defecation. Even people with normally functioning defecation experience incontinence if immobility prevents timely access to a toilet.

Diagnostic Studies and Collaborative Care

The diagnosis and effective management of fecal incontinence require a thorough health history and physical examination. Ask the patient about the number of incontinent episodes per week, stool consistency and volume, and the degree that incontinence interferes with work and social activities. A rectal examination can reveal reduced anal canal muscle tone and contraction strength of the external sphincter, as well as detect internal prolapse, rectocele, hemorrhoids, fecal impaction, and masses. If the impaction is higher in the colon, an abdominal x-ray or a computed tomography (CT) scan may be helpful. Other tests include anorectal manometry, anorectal ultrasonography, and defecography. Sigmoidoscopy or colonoscopy is used to identify inflammation, tumors, fissures, and other pathologic conditions.

Treatment of incontinence depends on the underlying cause. Fecal incontinence from fecal impaction usually resolves after manual disimpaction of the hard feces and cleansing enemas. To prevent recurrence, normal stool consistency is maintained with a bowel management program that includes regular defecation practices, a high-fiber diet, and increased fluid intake. Damage to the anal sphincters may require surgical repair.

Dietary fiber supplements or bulk-forming laxatives such as psyllium in Metamucil increase stool bulk, firm stool consistency, and promote the sensation of rectal filling. Intake of foods that cause diarrhea and rectal irritation may need to be reduced or eliminated. For some patients this may include coffee, dried fruit, onions, mushrooms, green vegetables, fruit with peels, spicy foods, and foods with monosodium glutamate. An antidiarrheal agent (loperamide [Imodium]) is sometimes used to slow intestinal transit.

Kegel exercises (see Table 46-19) are used to strengthen and coordinate the pelvic floor muscles to improve continence. Biofeedback therapy may be recommended to improve awareness of rectal sensation, coordinate internal and external anal sphincters, and increase the strength of external sphincter contraction. Biofeedback training requires intact sensory and motor nerves and motivation to learn. It is a safe, painless, and relatively inexpensive treatment for fecal incontinence.[8]

An injectable treatment, dextranomer/hyaluronic acid gel (Solesta), is reserved for patients who have failed conservative fecal incontinence management. In this treatment, 4 mL of the gel is injected into the deep submucosa of the patient's anal canal. It acts through narrowing of the anal canal. No anesthesia is required. Postinjection pain and bleeding may occur.

Surgery (e.g., sphincter repair procedures) is considered only when nonsurgical conservative treatment fails, the patient has a full-thickness prolapse, and the sphincter needs repair. A colostomy is sometimes necessary.

NURSING MANAGEMENT FECAL INCONTINENCE

NURSING ASSESSMENT

Fecal incontinence is embarrassing, uncomfortable, and irritating to the skin.[9] Its unpredictable nature makes it difficult to maintain school and work activities and hampers social or intimate contact. Be sensitive to the patient's feelings when discussing incontinence. When the underlying cause cannot be corrected, help the patient reestablish a predictable pattern of defecation. Ask about bowel patterns before the incontinence developed; current bowel habits; stool consistency and frequency; and symptoms, including pain during defecation and a feeling of incomplete evacuation (tenesmus). Assess whether the patient has defecation urgency and sensation of passing flatus and leaking stool. Check the perineal area for irritation or breakdown. Ask about daily activities (mealtimes and work), diet, and family and social activities. The Bristol Stool Scale is helpful for assessing stool consistency (www.poopreport.com/Poll/bristol_scale.html).

Patients who are critically ill and have fecal incontinence are at risk for *incontinence-associated dermatitis* (IAD).[9] IAD is characterized by erythema and skin denudement (erosion) of the perianal or genital areas, buttocks, or upper thighs. It is caused by chemical irritants in feces. Dark-skinned patients may have areas of hypopigmentation. These skin changes place the patient at risk for fungal infection.

NURSING DIAGNOSES

Nursing diagnoses for the patient with fecal incontinence include, but are not limited to, the following:
- Bowel incontinence *related to* inability to control bowel function
- Self-care deficit (toileting) *related to* inability to manage bowel evacuation voluntarily
- Risk for situational low self-esteem *related to* inability to control bowel movements
- Risk for impaired skin integrity *related to* incontinence of stool

PLANNING

The overall goals are that the patient with fecal incontinence will (1) have predictable bowel elimination, (2) maintain perianal skin integrity, (3) participate in work and social activities, and (4) avoid self-esteem problems related to bowel control.

NURSING IMPLEMENTATION

Regardless of the cause of fecal incontinence, bowel training is an effective strategy for many patients. Bowel elimination occurs at regular intervals in most people. Knowing the patient's usual bowel pattern can assist you in planning a bowel program that will achieve optimal stool consistency and predictable bowel elimination patterns. For the hospitalized patient, placement on a bedpan, assistance to a bedside commode, or walks to the bathroom at a regular time daily help to establish regular defecation.[10] For many persons, a good time to schedule elimination is within 30 minutes after breakfast.

If these techniques are ineffective in reestablishing bowel regularity, a bisacodyl (Dulcolax) glycerin suppository or a small phosphate enema may be administered 15 to 30 minutes before the usual evacuation time. These preparations stimulate the anorectal reflex. Since stimulation will not occur unless the suppository or enema touches the rectal wall, first check for stool in the rectum and digitally remove it before inserting the laxative. Once a regular pattern is established, these drugs are discontinued. Digital stimulation is another method for stimulating the anorectal reflex and is commonly included in bowel programs for people with neurogenic bowels (e.g., from spinal cord injury). Irrigation of the rectum and colon (usually with tap water) at regular intervals is another method to achieve continence in patients with neurogenic bowel.[11]

Maintenance of perianal skin integrity is of utmost importance, especially in the bedridden and older adult patient. Incontinence can contaminate wounds, damage the skin, cause bladder infections, and spread infection such as *C. difficile*. Containment of the feces is essential, but it is difficult to maintain a seal with pouching systems and incontinence pads. Avoid the use of rectal tubes and urinary catheters because they can decrease responsiveness of the rectal sphincter and cause ulceration of the rectal mucosa. Fecal management systems such as the Zassi Bowel Management System, Flexi-Seal, and ActiFlo indwelling bowel catheter are designed to contain loose and liquid stools of bedridden patients without damaging the rectum or anal sphincters.[12]

Incontinence briefs may help maintain skin integrity if changed frequently. Implementation of a defined skin care program can reduce IAD. This includes prompt cleansing, moisturizing, and skin protection. The skin is cleaned with a mild soap and rinsed to remove feces, the area is dried, and a protective skin barrier cream is applied. For patients unable to care for themselves at home, teach the caregiver practices to maintain skin integrity.

Teach patients with fecal incontinence to avoid foods such as caffeine that worsen symptoms. In addition, exercising after meals can aggravate symptoms of incontinence.

CONSTIPATION

Normal bowel movements are formed and easy to pass. Frequency varies from three bowel movements daily to one bowel movement every 3 days. Constipation is characterized by absent or infrequent stools and hard, dry stools that are difficult

to defecate. Because individuals vary, it is important to compare the current symptoms with the patient's normal pattern of elimination.

Etiology and Pathophysiology

Common causes of constipation include taking in insufficient dietary fiber or fluids, decreasing physical activity, and ignoring the defecation urge. Many drugs, especially opioids, cause constipation.[13] Constipation occurs with diseases that slow GI transit and hamper neurologic function such as diabetes mellitus, Parkinson's disease, and multiple sclerosis. Emotions, including anxiety, depression, and stress, affect the GI tract and can contribute to constipation.[14] Causes of constipation are summarized in eTable 43-2 (available on the website for this chapter).

Some people believe that they are constipated if they do not have a daily bowel movement. This can result in chronic laxative use and subsequent *cathartic colon syndrome,* a condition in which the colon becomes dilated and atonic (lacking muscle tone). Ultimately, the person cannot defecate without a laxative.

Ignoring the urge to defecate for a prolonged period can cause the muscles and mucosa of the rectum to become insensitive to the presence of feces. In addition, the prolonged retention of feces results in drying of stool due to water absorption. The harder and drier the feces, the more difficult it is to expel.

Clinical Manifestations

The clinical presentation of constipation may vary from a chronic discomfort to an acute event mimicking an "acute abdomen." Stools are absent or hard, dry, and difficult to pass. Abdominal distention, bloating, increased flatulence, and increased rectal pressure may also be present.

Hemorrhoids are the most common complication of chronic constipation. They result from venous engorgement caused by repeated *Valsalva maneuvers* (straining) and venous compression from hard impacted stool. Valsalva maneuver may have serious outcomes for patients with heart failure, cerebral edema, hypertension, and coronary artery disease. During straining, the patient inspires deeply and holds the breath while contracting abdominal muscles and bearing down. This increases both intraabdominal and intrathoracic pressures and reduces venous return to the heart. The heart rate decreases (bradycardia) temporarily, the cardiac output decreases, and a transient drop in arterial pressure occurs. When the patient relaxes, thoracic pressure falls, resulting in a sudden flow of blood into the heart, increased heart rate (tachycardia), and an immediate rise in arterial pressure. These changes may be fatal for the patient who cannot compensate for the sudden increased blood flow returning to the heart.

In the presence of *obstipation* (severe constipation when no gas or stool is expelled) or fecal impaction secondary to constipation, colonic perforation may occur. Perforation, which is life threatening, causes abdominal pain, nausea, vomiting, fever, and an elevated WBC count. Rectal mucosal ulcers and fissures may also occur as a result of stool stasis or straining. Diverticulosis is another potential complication of chronic constipation and is described later in this chapter. These complications are most common in older patients.

Diagnostic Studies and Collaborative Care

Perform a thorough history and physical examination so that the underlying cause of constipation can be identified and

TABLE 43-5 DRUG THERAPY

Constipation

Mechanism of Action	Example	Comments
Bulk Forming Absorbs water; increases bulk, thereby stimulating peristalsis *Action:* Usually within 24 hr	methylcellulose (Citrucel) psyllium (Metamucil, Perdiem, Konsyl, Hydrocil, Fiberall)	Contraindicated in patients with abdominal pain, nausea, and vomiting and in patients suspected of having appendicitis, biliary tract obstruction, or acute hepatitis. Must be taken with fluids (≥8 oz); best choice for initial treatment of constipation.
Stool Softeners and Lubricants Lubricate intestinal tract and soften feces, making hard stools easier to pass; do not affect peristalsis *Action:* Softeners in 72 hr, lubricants in 8 hr	*Softeners:* docusate (Colace, Surfak, Peri-Colace) *Lubricants:* mineral oil (Fleet's Oil Retention Enema, Kondremul Plain)	Can block absorption of fat-soluble vitamins such as vitamin K, which may increase risk of bleeding in patients on anticoagulants.
Saline and Osmotic Solutions Cause retention of fluid in intestinal lumen caused by osmotic effect *Action:* Within 15 min–3 hr	Magnesium salts (magnesium citrate, Milk of Magnesia) Sodium phosphates (Fleet Enema, Phospho-soda) lactulose (Constulose) polyethylene glycol (MiraLAX, GoLYTELY, CoLyte)	Magnesium-containing products may cause hypermagnesemia in patients with renal insufficiency.
Stimulants Increase peristalsis by irritating colon wall and stimulating enteric nerves *Action:* Usually within 12 hr	cascara sagrada, senna (Senokot) phenolphthalein: sennosides (Ex-Lax), bisacodyl (Correctol, Feen-a-Mint, Dulcolax), docusate/phenolphthalein (Doxidan)	Cause melanosis coli (brown or black pigmentation of colon). Are most widely abused laxatives. Should not be used in patients with impaction or obstipation.
Selective Chloride Channel Activator Increases intestinal fluid secretion and motility *Action:* Usually within 24 hr	lubiprostone (Amitiza)	Used in the treatment of idiopathic constipation and irritable bowel syndrome with constipation (women only). Contraindicated in patients with history of mechanical GI obstruction.
Intestinal Secretagogue Increases fluid secretion and accelerates intestinal transit. *Action:* Usually within 24 hr	linaclotide (Linzess)	Used in the treatment of idiopathic constipation and irritable bowel syndrome with constipation (men and women).

treatment started. Ask the patient about usual defecation patterns and habits, diet, exercise, use of laxatives, and conditions such as obstetric injuries that could contribute to difficulties with defecation. Abdominal x-rays, barium enema, colonoscopy, sigmoidoscopy, and anorectal manometry may be performed. Many cases of constipation can be prevented by increasing dietary fiber, fluid intake, and exercise. Laxatives (Table 43-5) and enemas may be used to treat acute constipation, but are used cautiously because overuse leads to chronic constipation.[15]

The choice of laxative or enema depends on the severity of the constipation and the patient's health. Daily bulk-forming preparations are used to prevent constipation because they work like dietary fiber and do not cause dependence. Stool softeners are also used to prevent constipation. Bisacodyl tablets and suppositories, milk of magnesia, and lactulose act more rapidly. They are also more likely to cause dependence. Methylnaltrexone (Relistor) is a peripheral μ-opiate receptor antagonist that decreases constipation caused by opioid use. The drug is administered subcutaneously. This agent does not block the analgesic effects.[16]

Enemas are fast acting and beneficial for immediate treatment of constipation, but must be used cautiously. Soapsuds enemas produce inflammation of colon mucosa, tap water enemas can potentially lead to water intoxication, and sodium phosphate (e.g., Fleet) enemas may cause electrolyte imbalances in patients with cardiac and renal problems.

Biofeedback therapy may benefit patients who are constipated as a result of *anismus* (uncoordinated contraction of the anal sphincter during straining). For the patient whose perceived constipation is related to rigid beliefs regarding bowel function, initiate a discussion about these concerns. Give appropriate information on normal bowel function and discuss the adverse consequences of excessive use of laxatives and enemas.

A patient with severe constipation related to bowel motility or mechanical disorders may require more intensive treatment. Diagnostic studies include anorectal manometry, GI tract transit studies, and sigmoidoscopic rectal biopsies. In a patient with unrelenting constipation, a subtotal colectomy with ileorectal anastomosis may be performed.

Nutritional Therapy. Diet is an important factor in the prevention of constipation. Many patients experience improved symptoms when they increase their intake of dietary fiber and fluids. Dietary fiber is found in fruits, vegetables, and grains (Table 43-6). Wheat bran and prunes are especially effective for preventing and treating constipation. Insoluble fiber is found in higher concentrations in whole wheat and bran.[17]

TABLE 43-6	NUTRITIONAL THERAPY

High-Fiber Foods

High-fiber foods are especially recommended for patients with diverticulosis, irritable bowel syndrome, constipation, hemorrhoids, atherosclerosis, hyperlipidemia, and diabetes mellitus.

	Fiber/ Serving (g)	Serving Size	Calories/ Serving
Vegetables			
Asparagus	3.5	½ cup	18
Beans			
• Navy	8.4	½ cup	80
• Kidney	9.7	½ cup	94
• Lima	8.3	½ cup	63
• Pinto	8.9	½ cup	78
• String	2.1	½ cup	18
Broccoli	3.5	½ cup	18
Carrots, raw	1.8	½ cup	15
Corn	2.6	½ medium ear	72
Peas, canned	6.7	½ cup	63
Potatoes			
• Baked	1.9	½ medium	72
• Sweet	2.1	½ medium	79
Squash, acorn	7.0	1 cup	82
Tomato, raw	1.5	1 small	18
Fruits			
Apple	2.0	½ large	42
Blackberries	6.7	¾ cup	40
Orange	1.6	1 small	35
Peach	2.3	1 medium	38
Pear	2.0	½ medium	44
Raspberries	9.2	1 cup	42
Strawberries	3.1	1 cup	45
Grain Products			
Bread, whole wheat	1.3	1 slice	59
Cereal			
• All Bran (100%)	8.4	⅓ cup	70
• Corn Flakes	2.6	¾ cup	70
• Shredded Wheat	2.8	1 biscuit	70
Popcorn	3.0	3 cups	62

Dietary fiber adds to the stool bulk directly and by attracting water. Therefore adequate fluid intake (2 L/day) is essential. Large, bulky stools move through the colon much more quickly than small stools. However, the recommended fluid intake may be contraindicated in the patient with cardiac disease or renal insufficiency or failure. Inform the patient that increasing fiber intake may initially increase gas production because of fermentation in the colon, but this effect decreases with use.

NURSING MANAGEMENT CONSTIPATION

NURSING ASSESSMENT

Subjective and objective data that should be obtained from a patient with constipation are presented in Table 43-7.

NURSING DIAGNOSIS

Nursing diagnoses for the patient with constipation include, but are not limited to, the following:

• Constipation *related to* inadequate intake of dietary fiber and fluid and decreased physical activity

TABLE 43-7	NURSING ASSESSMENT

Constipation

Subjective Data
Important Health Information
Past health history: Colorectal disease, neurologic dysfunction, bowel obstruction, environmental changes, cancer, irritable bowel syndrome, diabetes mellitus
Medications: Aluminum and calcium antacids, anticholinergics, antidepressants, antihistamines, antipsychotics, diuretics, opioids, iron, laxatives, enemas

Functional Health Patterns
Health perception–health management: Chronic laxative or enema abuse; rigid beliefs regarding bowel function; malaise
Nutritional-metabolic: Changes in diet or mealtime; inadequate fiber and fluid intake; anorexia, nausea
Elimination: Change in usual elimination patterns; hard, difficult-to-pass stool, decrease in frequency and amount of stools; flatus, abdominal distention; tenesmus, rectal pressure; fecal incontinence (if impacted)
Activity-exercise: Change in daily activity routines; immobility; sedentary lifestyle
Cognitive-perceptual: Dizziness, headache, anorectal pain; abdominal pain on defecation
Coping–stress tolerance: Acute or chronic stress

Objective Data
General
Lethargy

Integumentary
Anorectal fissures, hemorrhoids, abscesses

Gastrointestinal
Abdominal distention; hypoactive or absent bowel sounds; palpable abdominal mass; fecal impaction; small, hard, dry stool; stool with blood

Possible Diagnostic Findings
Guaiac-positive stools; abdominal x-ray demonstrating stool in lower colon

PLANNING

The overall goals are that the patient with constipation will (1) increase dietary intake of fiber and fluids; (2) increase physical activity; (3) pass soft, formed stools; and (4) not have any complications, such as bleeding hemorrhoids.

NURSING IMPLEMENTATION

Nursing management should be based on the patient's symptoms and assessment (see Table 43-7). Teach the patient about the importance of diet in the prevention of constipation. A patient and caregiver teaching guide for constipation is presented in Table 43-8. Emphasize using a high-fiber diet, increasing fluid intake, and exercising regularly. Teach the patient to establish a regular time to defecate and not to suppress the urge to defecate. Discourage the use of laxatives and enemas to achieve fecal elimination.

Defecation is easiest when the person is sitting on a commode with the knees higher than the hips. The sitting position allows gravity to aid defecation, and flexing the hips straightens the angle between the anal canal and the rectum so that stool flows out more easily. Place a footstool in front of the toilet to promote flexion of the thighs. It is challenging to defecate while sitting on a bedpan. For a patient in bed, elevate the head of the bed as high as the patient can tolerate.

TABLE 43-8 **PATIENT & CAREGIVER TEACHING GUIDE**

Constipation

Include the following instructions when teaching the patient and caregiver about management of constipation.

1. Eat Dietary Fiber

Eat 20-30 g of fiber per day. Gradually increase the amount of fiber eaten over 1-2 wk. Fiber softens hard stool and adds bulk to stool, promoting evacuation.
 • Foods high in fiber: raw vegetables and fruits, beans, breakfast cereals (All Bran, oatmeal)
 • Fiber supplements: Metamucil, Citrucel, FiberCon
Eat prunes or drink prune juice daily. Prunes stimulate defecation.

2. Drink Fluids

Drink 3 quarts per day. Drink water or fruit juices. Avoid caffeinated coffee, tea, and cola. Fluid softens hard stools. Caffeine stimulates fluid loss through urination.

3. Exercise Regularly

Walk, swim, or bike at least three times per wk. Contract and relax abdominal muscles when standing or by doing sit-ups to strengthen muscles and prevent straining. Exercise stimulates bowel motility and moves stool through the colon.

4. Establish a Regular Time to Defecate

First thing in the morning or after the first meal of the day is a good time because people often have the urge to defecate at this time.

5. Do Not Delay Defecation

Respond to the urge to have a bowel movement as soon as possible. Delaying defecation results in hard stools and a decreased "urge" to defecate. Water is absorbed from stool by the intestine over time. The colon becomes less sensitive to the presence of stool in the rectum.

6. Record Your Bowel Elimination Pattern

Develop a habit of recording when you have a bowel movement on your calendar. Regular monitoring of bowel movement will assist in early identification of a problem.

7. Avoid Laxatives and Enemas

Do not overuse laxatives and enemas because they cause dependence. People who overuse them are unable to have a bowel movement without them.

TABLE 43-9 **CAUSES OF ACUTE ABDOMINAL PAIN**

• Abdominal compartment syndrome
• Acute pancreatitis
• Appendicitis
• Bowel obstruction
• Cholecystitis
• Diverticulitis
• Gastroenteritis
• Pelvic inflammatory disease
• Perforated gastric or duodenal ulcer
• Peritonitis
• Ruptured abdominal aneurysm
• Ruptured ectopic pregnancy

peritonitis cause large amounts of fluid to move from the vascular space into the abdomen (third spacing).

Clinical Manifestations

Pain is the most common symptom of an acute abdominal problem. The patient may also complain of nausea, vomiting, diarrhea, constipation, flatulence, fatigue, fever, and bloating.

Diagnostic Studies and Collaborative Care

Diagnosis begins with a complete history and physical examination. Description of the pain (frequency, timing, duration, location), accompanying symptoms, and sequence of symptoms (e.g., pain before or after vomiting) provide vital clues about the origin of the problem. Note the patient's position. The fetal posture is common with peritoneal irritation (e.g., appendicitis), a supine posture with outstretched legs is seen with visceral pain, and restlessness and a seated posture commonly occur with bowel obstructions and obstructions from kidney stones and gallstones.

Physical examination includes examination of the abdomen, rectum, and pelvis. A complete blood count (CBC), urinalysis, abdominal x-ray, and electrocardiogram are done, along with an ultrasound or CT scan. A pregnancy test is performed in women of childbearing age with acute abdominal pain to rule out ectopic pregnancy (see Table 43-9).

Emergency management of the patient with acute abdominal pain is presented in Table 43-10. The goal of management is to identify and treat the cause, and monitor and treat complications, especially shock. Careful use of pain medications (e.g., morphine) provides pain relief without interfering with diagnostic accuracy when patients have nontraumatic acute abdominal pain.

An immediate surgical consult is needed. The surgeon may perform a diagnostic laparoscopy to inspect the surface of abdominal organs, obtain biopsy specimens, perform laparoscopic ultrasounds, and remove organs. A laparotomy is used when laparoscopic techniques are inadequate. If the cause of the acute abdomen can be surgically removed (e.g., inflamed appendix) or surgically repaired (e.g., ruptured abdominal aneurysm), surgery is considered definitive therapy.

❚ NURSING MANAGEMENT ACUTE ABDOMINAL PAIN

❚ NURSING ASSESSMENT

For the patient complaining of acute abdominal pain, take vital signs immediately and again at frequent intervals. Increased pulse and decreasing blood pressure indicate impending shock. An elevated temperature suggests an inflammatory or infectious process. Intake and output measurement provides essential information about the adequacy of vascular volume. Altered

Most people are embarrassed by the sights and sounds of defecation, so provide as much privacy as possible. Encourage patients to exercise abdominal muscles and to contract abdominal muscles several times a day. Sit-ups and straight-leg raises can also help improve abdominal muscle tone.

Teach patients taking bulking products to follow product recommendations in terms of fluid intake. Patients may initially experience an increase in flatus that will decrease with use.

ACUTE ABDOMINAL PAIN

Etiology and Pathophysiology

Acute abdominal pain is pain of recent onset. It may signal a life-threatening problem and therefore requires immediate attention.[18] Causes include damage to organs in the abdomen and pelvis, which leads to inflammation, infection, obstruction, bleeding, and perforation (Fig. 43-1). The most common causes of acute abdominal pain are listed in Table 43-9. Perforation of the GI tract also results in irritation of the *peritoneum* (serous membrane lining the abdominal cavity) and peritonitis. Hypovolemic shock occurs from bleeding or when obstruction and

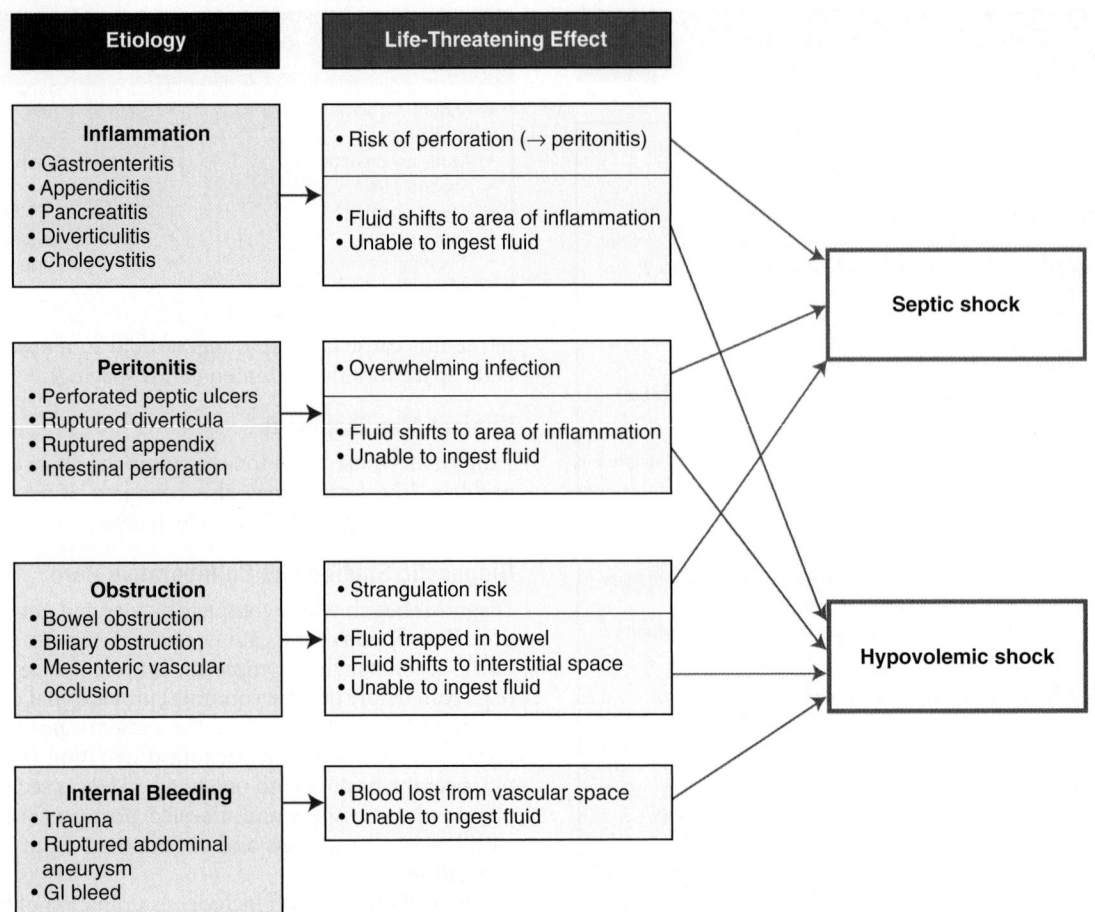

FIG. 43-1 Etiology of acute abdominal pain and pathophysiologic sequelae.

mental status indicates poor cerebral perfusion. Skin color and temperature and peripheral pulse strength provide information about skin perfusion. Inspect the abdomen for distention, masses, abnormal pulsation, symmetry, hernias, rashes, scars, and pigmentation changes. Auscultate bowel sounds. Bowel sounds that are diminished or absent in a quadrant may indicate a bowel obstruction, acute peritonitis, or paralytic ileus. Palpation should be gentle. Determine pain from peritoneal irritation by asking the person to cough, palpating the abdomen gently, or gently shaking the bed.

Ask the patient about the onset, location, intensity, duration, frequency, and character of pain. Note whether the pain has spread or moved to new sites (quadrants) and what makes the pain worse or better. Is the pain associated with other symptoms, such as nausea, vomiting, changes in bowel and bladder habits, or vaginal discharge in women? Assessment of vomiting includes the amount, color, consistency, and odor of the emesis. Also ask about usual and changes in bowel patterns and habits.

NURSING DIAGNOSES
Nursing diagnoses for the patient with acute abdominal pain include, but are not limited to, the following:
- Acute pain *related to* inflammation of the peritoneum and abdominal distention
- Risk for deficient fluid volume *related to* collection of fluid in peritoneal cavity secondary to inflammation or infection
- Anxiety *related to* pain and uncertainty of cause or outcome of condition

PLANNING
The overall goals are that the patient with acute abdominal pain will have (1) relief of abdominal pain, (2) resolution of inflammation, (3) freedom from complications (especially hypovolemic shock), and (4) normal nutritional status.

NURSING IMPLEMENTATION
General care for the patient with acute abdominal pain involves management of fluid and electrolyte imbalances, pain, and anxiety. Assess the quality and intensity of pain at regular intervals, and provide medication and other comfort measures. Maintain a calm environment and provide information to help allay anxiety. A nasogastric (NG) tube may be used to decrease vomiting and relieve discomfort from gastric distention. Conduct ongoing assessments of vital signs, intake and output, and level of consciousness, which are key indicators of hypovolemic shock.

ACUTE INTERVENTION
Preoperative Care. Preoperative care includes the emergency care of the patient described in Table 43-10 and general care of the preoperative patient (see Chapter 18).

Postoperative Care. Postoperative care depends on the type of surgical procedure performed. In some cases a laparotomy is necessary. When appropriate, a laparoscopic approach is used. Laparoscopic procedures result in lower rates of postoperative complications (poor wound healing and paralytic ileus), earlier diet advancement, and shorter hospital stays compared with open surgical procedures. eNursing Care Plan 20-1, a general plan for the postoperative patient, is presented on the website for Chapter 20.

✚ TABLE 43-10 EMERGENCY MANAGEMENT

Acute Abdominal Pain

Etiology	Assessment Findings	Interventions
Inflammation	**Abdominal and Gastrointestinal Findings**	**Initial**
• Appendicitis	• Diffuse, localized, dull, burning, or sharp abdominal pain or tenderness	• Ensure patent airway.
• Cholecystitis	• Rebound tenderness	• Administer O_2 via nasal cannula or non-rebreather mask.
• Crohn's disease	• Abdominal distention	• Establish IV access with large-bore catheter and infuse warm normal saline or lactated Ringer's solution. Insert additional large-bore catheter if shock present.
• Gastritis	• Abdominal rigidity	
• Pancreatitis	• Nausea and vomiting	
• Pyelonephritis	• Diarrhea	• Obtain blood for CBC and electrolyte levels.
• Ulcerative colitis	• Hematemesis	• Anticipate order for amylase level, pregnancy tests, clotting studies, and type and crossmatch as appropriate.
	• Melena	
Vascular Problems		• Insert indwelling urinary catheter.
• Ruptured aortic aneurysm	**Hypovolemic Shock**	• Obtain urinalysis.
• Mesenteric vascular occlusion	• ↓ Blood pressure	• Insert NG tube as needed.
	• ↓ Pulse pressure	
Gynecologic Problems	• Tachycardia	**Ongoing Monitoring**
• Pelvic inflammatory disease	• Cool, clammy skin	• Monitor vital signs, level of consciousness, O_2 saturation, and intake/output.
• Ruptured ectopic pregnancy	• ↓ Level of consciousness	• Assess quality and amount of pain.
• Ruptured ovarian cyst	• ↓ Urine output (<0.5 mL/kg/hr)	• Assess amount and character of emesis.
		• Anticipate surgical intervention.
Infectious Disease		• Keep patient NPO.
• *Escherichia coli* O157:H7		
• *Giardia*		
• *Salmonella*		
Other		
• Obstruction or perforation of abdominal organ		
• Gastrointestinal bleeding or ischemia		
• Trauma		

Postoperatively an NG tube with low suction may be used in selected patients to empty the stomach and prevent gastric dilation. If the upper GI tract has been entered, drainage from the NG tube may be dark brown to dark red for the first 12 hours. Later it should be light yellowish brown, or it may have a greenish tinge because of bile. If a dark red color continues or if bright red blood is observed, notify the surgeon because of the possibility of hemorrhage. "Coffee-ground" granules in the drainage indicate blood that has been modified by acidic gastric secretions.

Nausea and vomiting are common after a laparotomy and may be caused by the surgery, decreased peristalsis, or pain medications. Antiemetics such as ondansetron (Zofran), trimethobenzamide (Tigan), and prochlorperazine (Compazine) may be ordered. Management of nausea and vomiting is discussed in Chapter 42. Monitor fluid and electrolyte status along with blood pressure, heart rate, and respirations.

Swallowed air and reduced peristalsis from decreased mobility, manipulation of the abdominal organs during surgery, and anesthesia can result in abdominal distention and gas pains. Early ambulation helps restore peristalsis and eliminate flatus and gas pain. Gradually, as intestinal activity increases, distention and gas pain disappear.

AMBULATORY AND HOME CARE. Preparation for discharge begins soon after surgery. Teach the patient and caregiver about any modifications in activity, care of the incision, diet, and drug therapy. Clear liquids are given initially after surgery and, if tolerated, the patient progresses to a regular diet.

Early ambulation speeds recovery, but normal activities are resumed gradually, with planned rest periods. After surgery the patient is generally instructed not to lift anything heavier than a few pounds. The patient and caregiver should be aware of possible complications after surgery. Teach them to notify the surgeon immediately if fever, vomiting, pain, weight loss, incisional drainage, or changes in bowel function occur.

▌EVALUATION

The expected outcomes are that the patient with acute abdominal pain will have
- Resolution of the cause of the acute abdominal pain
- Relief of abdominal pain and discomfort
- Freedom from complications (especially hypovolemic shock and septicemia)
- Normal fluid, electrolyte, and nutritional status

▌CHRONIC ABDOMINAL PAIN

Chronic abdominal pain may originate from abdominal structures or may be referred from a site with the same or a similar nerve supply. The pain is often described as dull, aching, or diffuse. Common causes of chronic abdominal pain include irritable bowel syndrome (IBS), peptic ulcer disease, chronic pancreatitis, hepatitis, pelvic inflammatory disease, and vascular insufficiency. (Some of these disorders are discussed in this chapter).

Diagnosis of the cause of chronic abdominal pain begins with a thorough history and description of specific pain characteristics, including severity, location, frequency, duration, and onset. The assessment also includes factors that increase or decrease the pain, such as meals, defecation, and activities.

Endoscopy, CT scan, magnetic resonance imaging (MRI), laparoscopy, and barium studies may be done. Treatment for chronic abdominal pain depends on the underlying cause.

IRRITABLE BOWEL SYNDROME

Irritable bowel syndrome (IBS) is a common, chronic functional disorder, meaning that no organic cause is currently known.[19] Symptoms of IBS, including abdominal pain or discomfort and alterations in bowel patterns, are intermittent and may occur for years. Patients often report a history of GI infections and food intolerances. However, the role of food allergies in IBS is unclear. Other dietary factors that may contribute to symptoms include fermentable oligo-, di-, and monosaccharides and polyols (FODMAPs).[20] Examples include fructans (found in wheat), galactans, lactose, fructose, sorbitol, and xylitol.

Psychologic stressors (e.g., depression, anxiety, sexual abuse, posttraumatic stress disorder) are associated with development and exacerbation of IBS.[19] IBS is more frequently diagnosed in women than in men. In addition to abdominal pain and diarrhea or constipation, patients commonly experience abdominal distention, excessive flatulence, bloating, urgency, and sensation of incomplete evacuation. Non-GI symptoms may include fatigue and sleep disturbances.

There are no specific physical findings with IBS. The key to accurate diagnosis is a thorough history and physical examination. Ask patients to describe symptoms, past health history (including psychosocial factors such as stress and anxiety), family history, and drug and diet history. Determine if and how IBS symptoms interfere with school, work, or recreational activities. Diagnostic tests are selectively used to rule out other disorders such as colorectal cancer, IBD, endometriosis, and malabsorption disorders (lactose intolerance, celiac disease). Symptom-based criteria for IBS have been standardized and are referred to as the Rome criteria III (see eTable 43-3 on the website for this chapter).

Treatment is directed at psychologic and dietary factors and drugs to regulate stool output. Patients are more likely to improve with treatment if they have a trusting relationship with their health care provider. Encourage the patient to verbalize concerns. Since treatment is often focused on symptoms, patients may benefit from keeping a diary of symptoms, diet, and episodes of stress to help identify factors that seem to trigger the IBS symptoms. If tolerated, encourage the patient to have a dietary fiber intake of at least 20 g/day (see Table 43-6) or to use a stool bulking agent. Increases in dietary fiber should be started gradually to avoid bloating and abdominal discomfort from gas.

Advise the patient whose primary symptoms are abdominal distention and flatulence to avoid common gas-producing foods such as broccoli and cabbage. Yogurt may be better tolerated than milk products. Probiotics may be used because alterations in intestinal bacteria are believed to exacerbate the condition.[19]

Loperamide, a synthetic opioid that slows intestinal transit, may be used to treat diarrhea when it occurs. Alosetron (Lotronex), a serotonergic antagonist, is used for IBS patients with severe symptoms of pain and diarrhea. Because of serious side effects (e.g., severe constipation, ischemic colitis), alosetron is available only in a restricted access program for women who have not responded to other IBS therapies. Lubiprostone (Amitiza) is approved for the treatment of IBS with constipation in women. Linaclotide (Linzess) is approved for the treatment of IBS with constipation in men and women.

> **DRUG ALERT: Alosetron (Lotronex)**
> - Patients may experience severe constipation and ischemic colitis (reduced blood flow to intestines).
> - If constipation occurs, drug should be discontinued.
> - Symptoms of ischemic colitis include abdominal pain and blood in stool.

Psychologic therapies include cognitive-behavioral therapy, stress management techniques, acupuncture, and hypnosis. Low doses of tricyclic antidepressants seem beneficial, possibly because they decrease peripheral nerve sensitivity. No single therapy has been found to be effective for all patients with IBS.

ABDOMINAL TRAUMA

Etiology and Pathophysiology

Injuries to the abdominal area usually are a result of blunt trauma or penetrating injuries. Common injuries of the abdomen include lacerated liver, ruptured spleen, mesenteric artery tears, diaphragm rupture, urinary bladder rupture, great vessel tears, renal or pancreas injury, and stomach or intestine rupture. *Blunt trauma* commonly occurs with motor vehicle accidents, beatings, and falls and may not be obvious because it does not leave an open wound. Both compression injuries (e.g., direct blow to the abdomen) and shearing injuries (e.g., rapid deceleration in a motor vehicle crash allowing some tissue to move forward while other tissues are held stationary) occur with blunt trauma. *Penetrating injuries* occur when a gunshot or stabbing produces an obvious, open wound into the abdomen.[21]

When solid organs (liver, spleen) are injured, bleeding can be profuse, resulting in hypovolemic shock. When contents from hollow organs (e.g., bladder, stomach, intestines) spill into the peritoneal cavity, the patient is at risk for peritonitis. In addition, abdominal compartment syndrome can develop.

Abdominal compartment syndrome is excessively high pressure in the abdomen (abdominal hypertension). Anything that increases the volume in the abdominal cavity—including edematous organs, bleeding, and third spacing caused by obstruction and inflammation—increases abdominal pressure.[22] High abdominal pressure restricts ventilation, potentially leading to respiratory failure. The high pressure also decreases cardiac output, venous return, and arterial perfusion of organs. Decreased perfusion to the kidneys can lead to renal failure.

Clinical Manifestations

Careful assessment provides important clues to the type and severity of injury. Intraabdominal injuries are often associated with low rib fractures, fractured femur, fractured pelvis, and

✚ TABLE 43-11 EMERGENCY MANAGEMENT

Abdominal Trauma

Etiology	Assessment Findings	Interventions
Blunt • Falls • Motor vehicle collisions • Pedestrian event • Assault with blunt object • Crush injuries • Explosions **Penetrating** • Knife • Gunshot wounds • Other missiles	**Hypovolemic Shock** • ↓ Level of consciousness • Tachypnea • Tachycardia • ↓ Blood pressure • ↓ Pulse pressure **Surface Findings** • Abrasions or ecchymoses on abdominal wall, flank, or peritoneum • Open wounds: lacerations, eviscerations, puncture wounds, gunshot wounds • Impaled object • Healed incisions or old scars **Abdominal and Gastrointestinal Findings** • Nausea and vomiting • Hematemesis • Absent or decreased bowel sounds • Bloody urine (hematuria) • Abdominal distention • Abdominal rigidity • Abdominal pain with palpation • Rebound tenderness • Pain radiation to shoulder and back	**Initial** • Ensure patent airway. • Administer O_2 via non-rebreather mask. • Control external bleeding with direct pressure or sterile pressure dressing. • Establish IV access with two large-bore catheters and infuse warm normal saline or lactated Ringer's solution. • Obtain blood for type and crossmatch and CBC. • Remove clothing. • Stabilize impaled objects with bulky dressing—*do not remove.* • Cover protruding organs or tissue with sterile saline dressing. • Insert indwelling urinary catheter if there is no blood at the meatus, pelvic fracture, or boggy prostate. • Obtain urine for urinalysis. • Insert NG tube if no evidence of facial trauma. • Anticipate diagnostic peritoneal lavage. **Ongoing Monitoring** • Monitor vital signs, level of consciousness, O_2 saturation, and urine output. • Maintain patient warmth using blankets, warm IV fluids, or warm humidified O_2.

thoracic injury. If the patient was in an automobile accident, a contusion or abrasion across the lower abdomen may indicate internal organ trauma due to seat belt use. Seat belts can produce blunt trauma to abdominal organs by pressing the intestine and pancreas into the spinal column.

Clinical manifestations of abdominal trauma are (1) guarding and splinting of the abdominal wall (indicating peritonitis); (2) a hard, distended abdomen (indicating intraabdominal bleeding); (3) decreased or absent bowel sounds; (4) contusions, abrasions, or bruising over the abdomen; (5) abdominal pain; (6) pain over the scapula caused by irritation of the phrenic nerve by free blood in the abdomen; (7) hematemesis or hematuria; and (8) signs of hypovolemic shock (Table 43-11). Ecchymosis around the umbilicus (Cullen's sign) or flanks (Grey Turner's sign) may indicate retroperitoneal hemorrhage. Loss of bowel sounds occurs with peritonitis. If present, bowel sounds are heard in the chest when the diaphragm ruptures. Auscultation of bruits is indicative of arterial damage.

Diagnostic Studies

Laboratory tests include a baseline CBC and urinalysis. Even when bleeding, the patient will have normal hemoglobin and hematocrit because fluids are lost at the same rate as the red blood cells. Deficiencies are evident after fluid resuscitation begins. Blood in the urine may be a sign of damage to the kidney or bladder. Additional laboratory work includes arterial blood gases, prothrombin time, electrolytes, BUN and creatinine, and type and crossmatch (in anticipation of possible blood transfusions). An abdominal CT scan and focused abdominal sonography are the most common diagnostic methods, but the patient must be stable before going for CT. Diagnostic peritoneal lavage can be used to detect blood, bile, intestinal contents, and urine in the peritoneal cavity, but is generally used only for unstable patients to identify blood in the peritoneum.[22]

NURSING AND COLLABORATIVE MANAGEMENT ABDOMINAL TRAUMA

Emergency management of abdominal trauma focuses on establishing a patent airway and adequate breathing, fluid replacement, and prevention of hypovolemic shock (see Table 43-11). IV lines are inserted, and volume expanders or blood is given if the patient is hypotensive. An NG tube is inserted to decompress the stomach and prevent aspiration. Frequent ongoing assessment is necessary to monitor fluid status, detect deterioration in condition, and determine the necessity for surgery. An impaled object should never be removed until skilled care is available. Removal may cause further injury and bleeding. The decision about whether to do surgery depends on clinical findings, diagnostic test results, and the patient's response to conservative management.

INFLAMMATORY DISORDERS

APPENDICITIS

Appendicitis is inflammation of the appendix, a narrow blind tube that extends from the inferior part of the cecum (Fig. 43-2).

Etiology and Pathophysiology

In the United States, about 1 in 15 people will get appendicitis. It is most common in individuals 10 to 30 years of age. It is the most common cause of acute abdominal pain.[23] A common cause of appendicitis is obstruction of the lumen by a fecalith (accumulated feces) (see Fig. 43-2). Obstruction results in distention; venous engorgement; and the accumulation of mucus and bacteria, which can lead to gangrene, perforation, and peritonitis.

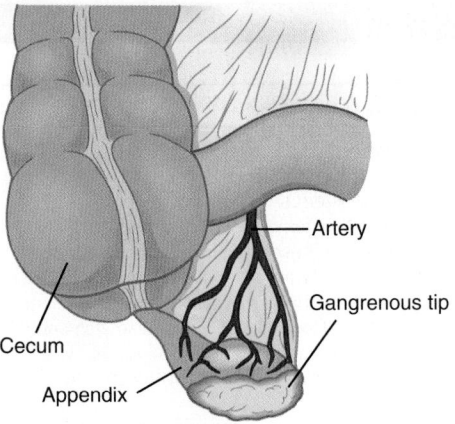

FIG. 43-2 In appendicitis the blood supply of the appendix is impaired by inflammation and bacterial infection in the wall of the appendix, which may result in gangrene.

Clinical Manifestations

Diagnosis can be difficult because many patients do not have classic symptoms. Typically appendicitis begins with periumbilical pain, followed by anorexia, nausea, and vomiting. The pain is persistent and continuous, eventually shifting to the right lower quadrant and localizing at McBurney's point (halfway between the umbilicus and the right iliac crest). Further assessment reveals localized tenderness, rebound tenderness, and muscle guarding. Coughing, sneezing, and deep inhalation magnify the pain. The patient usually prefers to lie still, often with the right leg flexed. Low-grade fever may or may not be present.[23] The older adult may report less severe pain, slight fever, and discomfort in the right iliac fossa.

Diagnostic Studies and Collaborative Care

Examination of the patient includes a complete history, physical examination, and a differential WBC count. The WBC count is mildly to moderately elevated in most cases. A urinalysis is done to rule out genitourinary conditions that mimic the manifestations of appendicitis. CT scan is the preferred diagnostic procedure, but ultrasound is also used.

If diagnosis and treatment are delayed, the appendix can rupture, and the resulting peritonitis can be fatal. The treatment of appendicitis is immediate surgical removal *(appendectomy)* if the inflammation is localized. Surgery, generally performed laparoscopically, is done as soon as the diagnosis is made. Antibiotics and fluid resuscitation are administered before surgery.

If the appendix has ruptured and there is evidence of peritonitis or an abscess, parenteral fluids and antibiotic therapy are given for 6 to 8 hours before the appendectomy to prevent dehydration and sepsis.

▍NURSING MANAGEMENT
▍APPENDICITIS

Encourage the patient with abdominal pain to see a health care provider and to avoid self-treatment. Laxatives and enemas are especially dangerous because the resulting increased peristalsis may cause perforation of the appendix. To ensure that the stomach is empty in case surgery is needed, keep patients on nothing-by-mouth (NPO) status until they can be seen by a health care provider.

TABLE 43-12	CAUSES OF PERITONITIS
Primary	**Secondary**
• Blood-borne organisms	• Appendicitis with rupture
• Genital tract organisms	• Blunt or penetrating trauma to
• Cirrhosis with ascites	abdominal organs
	• Diverticulitis with rupture
	• Ischemic bowel disorders
	• Pancreatitis
	• Perforated intestine
	• Perforated peptic ulcer
	• Peritoneal dialysis
	• Postoperative (breakage of
	anastomosis)

Postoperative nursing management for the patient who has an appendectomy is similar to postoperative care of the patient after laparotomy. Ambulation begins the day of surgery or the first postoperative day. The diet is advanced as tolerated. The patient is usually discharged on the first or second postoperative day and resumes normal activities 2 to 3 weeks after surgery.

PERITONITIS

Etiology and Pathophysiology

Peritonitis results from a localized or generalized inflammatory process of the peritoneum. Causes of peritonitis are listed in Table 43-12. Primary peritonitis occurs when blood-borne organisms enter the peritoneal cavity. For example, the ascites that occurs with cirrhosis of the liver provides an excellent liquid environment for bacteria to flourish. Organisms can also enter the peritoneum during peritoneal dialysis. (Peritoneal dialysis is described in Chapter 47.)

Secondary peritonitis is much more common. It occurs when abdominal organs perforate or rupture and release their contents (bile, enzymes, and bacteria) into the peritoneal cavity. Common causes include a ruptured appendix, perforated gastric or duodenal ulcer, severely inflamed gallbladder, and trauma from gunshot or knife wounds.

Intestinal contents and bacteria irritate the normally sterile peritoneum and produce an initial chemical peritonitis, which is followed a few hours later by a bacterial peritonitis. The resulting inflammatory response leads to massive fluid shifts (peritoneal edema) and adhesions as the body attempts to wall off the infection.

Clinical Manifestations

Abdominal pain is the most common symptom of peritonitis. A universal sign of peritonitis is tenderness over the involved area. Rebound tenderness, muscular rigidity, and spasm are other signs of irritation of the peritoneum. Patients may lie still and take only shallow breaths because movement causes pain. Abdominal distention, fever, tachycardia, tachypnea, nausea, vomiting, and altered bowel habits may also be present. These manifestations vary depending on the severity and acuteness of the underlying condition. Complications of peritonitis include hypovolemic shock, sepsis, intraabdominal abscess formation, paralytic ileus, and acute respiratory distress syndrome. If treatment is delayed, peritonitis can be fatal.

Diagnostic Studies and Collaborative Care

A CBC is done to determine elevations in WBC count and hemoconcentration from fluid shifts (Table 43-13). Peritoneal

TABLE 43-13 COLLABORATIVE CARE
Peritonitis
Diagnostic   • History and physical examination   • CBC, including WBC differential   • Serum electrolytes   • Abdominal x-ray   • Abdominal paracentesis and culture of fluid   • CT scan or ultrasound   • Peritoneoscopy   **Collaborative Therapy**   ***Preoperative or Nonoperative***   • NPO status   • IV fluid replacement   • Antibiotic therapy   • NG suction   • Analgesics (e.g., morphine)   • Oxygen PRN   • Preparation for surgery to include the above and parenteral nutrition   ***Postoperative***   • NPO status   • NG tube to low-intermittent suction   • Semi-Fowler's position   • IV fluids with electrolyte replacement   • Parenteral nutrition as needed   • Antibiotic therapy   • Blood transfusions as needed   • Sedatives and opioids

aspiration may be performed and the fluid analyzed for blood, bile, pus, bacteria, fungus, and amylase content. An x-ray of the abdomen may show dilated loops of bowel consistent with paralytic ileus, free air if perforation has occurred, or air and fluid levels if an obstruction is present. Ultrasound and CT scans may be useful in identifying ascites and abscesses. Peritoneoscopy may be helpful in the patient without ascites. Direct examination of the peritoneum can be obtained along with biopsy specimens for diagnosis.

Patients with milder cases of peritonitis or those who are poor surgical risks may be managed medically. Treatment consists of antibiotics, NG suction, analgesics, and IV fluid administration. Surgery is indicated to locate the cause of the inflammation, drain purulent fluid, and repair any damage (e.g., perforated organs).

NURSING MANAGEMENT
PERITONITIS

NURSING ASSESSMENT

Assessment of the patient's pain, including the location, is important and may help in determining the cause of peritonitis. Assess the patient for the presence and quality of bowel sounds, increasing abdominal distention, abdominal guarding, nausea, fever, and manifestations of hypovolemic shock.

NURSING DIAGNOSES

Nursing diagnoses for the patient with peritonitis include, but are not limited to, the following:

- Acute pain *related to* inflammation of the peritoneum and abdominal distention

- Risk for deficient fluid volume *related to* fluid shifts into the peritoneal cavity secondary to trauma, infection, or ischemia
- Anxiety *related to* uncertainty of cause or outcome of the condition and pain

PLANNING

The overall goals are that the patient with peritonitis will have (1) resolution of inflammation, (2) relief of abdominal pain, (3) freedom from complications (especially sepsis and hypovolemic shock), and (4) normal nutritional status.

NURSING IMPLEMENTATION

The patient with peritonitis is extremely ill and needs skilled supportive care. An IV line is inserted to replace vascular fluids lost to the peritoneal cavity and as an access for antibiotic therapy. Monitor the patient for pain and response to analgesics. The patient may be positioned with knees flexed to increase comfort. Sedatives may be given to allay anxiety.

Accurate monitoring of fluid intake and output and electrolyte status is necessary to determine replacement therapy. Monitor vital signs frequently. Antiemetics may be administered to decrease nausea and vomiting and prevent further fluid and electrolyte losses. The patient is placed on NPO status and may need an NG tube to decrease gastric distention and further leakage of bowel contents into the peritoneum. Low-flow oxygen therapy may be needed.

If the patient has an open surgical procedure, drains are inserted to remove purulent drainage and excess fluid. Postoperative care is similar to that for the patient with an exploratory laparotomy.

GASTROENTERITIS

Gastroenteritis is an inflammation of the mucosa of the stomach and small intestine. Acute gastroenteritis is defined as sudden diarrhea accompanied by nausea, vomiting, and abdominal cramping. Viruses are the most common cause of gastroenteritis. Other causes are presented in Table 43-1.

Norovirus is a leading cause of gastroenteritis from foodborne disease outbreaks in the United States. The Ridascreen Norovirus 3rd Generation EIA is used when a number of people have simultaneously contracted gastroenteritis and there is a clear avenue for virus transmission, such as a shared location or food.

Most cases of gastroenteritis are self-limiting. However, older adults and chronically ill patients may be unable to consume sufficient fluids orally to compensate for fluid loss. If dehydration occurs, IV fluid replacement may be necessary. As soon as tolerated, oral fluids containing glucose and electrolytes (e.g., Pedialyte) should be given. Nursing management of the patient with gastroenteritis is the same as for the patient with acute diarrhea (see pp. 963-964).

INFLAMMATORY BOWEL DISEASE

Inflammatory bowel disease (IBD) is a chronic inflammation of the GI tract. It is characterized by periods of remission interspersed with periods of exacerbation. The exact cause is unknown, and there is no cure. IBD is classified as either **Crohn's disease** or **ulcerative colitis** based on clinical manifestations (Table 43-14). As the name suggests, ulcerative colitis is

TABLE 43-14   COMPARISON OF ULCERATIVE COLITIS AND CROHN'S DISEASE

Characteristic	Ulcerative Colitis	Crohn's Disease
Clinical		
Usual age at onset	Teens to mid-30s*	Teens to mid-30s*
Diarrhea	Common	Common
Abdominal cramping pain	Common	Common
Fever (intermittent)	During acute attacks	Common
Weight loss	Rare	Common, may be severe
Rectal bleeding	Common	Infrequent
Tenesmus	Common	Rare
Malabsorption and nutritional deficiencies	Minimal incidence	Common
Pathologic		
Location	Usually starts in rectum and spreads in a continuous pattern up the colon	Occurs anywhere along GI tract in characteristic skip lesions. Most frequent site is terminal ileum
Distribution	Continuous areas of inflammation	Healthy tissue interspersed with areas of inflammation (skip lesions)
Depth of involvement	Mucosa and submucosa	Entire thickness of bowel wall (transmural)
Granulomas (noted on biopsy)	Occasional	Common
Cobblestoning of mucosa	Rare	Common
Pseudopolyps	Common	Rare
Small bowel involvement	Minimal	Common
Complications		
Fistulas	Rare	Common
Strictures	Occasional	Common
Anal abscesses	Rare	Common
Perforation	Common (because of toxic megacolon)	Common (because inflammation involves entire bowel wall)
Toxic megacolon	Relatively more common	Rare
Carcinoma	Increased incidence of colorectal cancer after 10 yr of disease	Increased incidence of small intestinal cancer
		Increased incidence of colorectal cancer but not as much as with ulcerative colitis
Recurrence after surgery	Cure with colectomy	Common at site of anastomosis

*Second peak in incidence after age 60.

usually limited to the colon. Crohn's disease can involve any segment of the GI tract from the mouth to the anus.

Both ulcerative colitis and Crohn's disease commonly occur during the teenage years and early adulthood, and both have a second peak in the sixth decade. IBD is more prevalent in industrialized countries and in Ashkenazi Jews. Many people with IBD have a family member with the disorder.

Etiology and Pathophysiology

IBD is an autoimmune disease involving an immune reaction to a person's own intestinal tract. Some agent or a combination of agents triggers an overactive, inappropriate, sustained immune response. The resulting inflammation causes widespread tissue destruction.

Evidence suggests that IBD is caused by a combination of factors, including environmental factors, genetic predisposition, and alterations in the function of the immune system.[24] Environmental factors such as diet, hygiene, stress, smoking, and nonsteroidal antiinflammatory drugs (NSAIDs) increase susceptibility by influencing the environment of the microbial flora and the immune system. IBD is more prevalent in industrialized regions of the world. Whether diet or other factors unique to Western countries contribute to the development of IBD is not known.[25,26] Specific dietary components have not been identified. However, high dietary intake of total fats, polyunsaturated fatty acid (PUFA), omega-6 fatty acids, and meat is associated with an increased risk of IBD.[26] High fiber and fruit intake is associated with decreased risk of Crohn's disease, whereas vegetable intake is associated with decreased risk of ulcerative colitis.[27]

CULTURAL & ETHNIC HEALTH DISPARITIES
Inflammatory Bowel Disease

- Incidence is about four times higher among whites than in other ethnic groups.
- It has the highest incidence among the Ashkenazi Jewish people and those of middle European origin.

Genetic Link

IBD occurs more frequently in whites (particularly those of Jewish descent) and in family members of persons with IBD (especially monozygotic twins). Genetic predisposition has been confirmed by numerous genome-wide association studies.[24] Certain genetic mutations are associated with Crohn's disease, others are associated with ulcerative colitis, and many are associated with both.

Recently, the first gene associated with Crohn's disease, the *NOD2* gene, was identified. Research is ongoing to understand how defects in the *NOD2* gene lead to Crohn's disease and into finding the other genes that cause IBD.

The discovery of numerous gene variations suggests that IBD is a group of diseases that produce similar types of destruction of the mucosa. A genetically susceptible person who is never exposed to the triggering agent will not become ill, and a person

Inflammatory Bowel Disease (IBD)

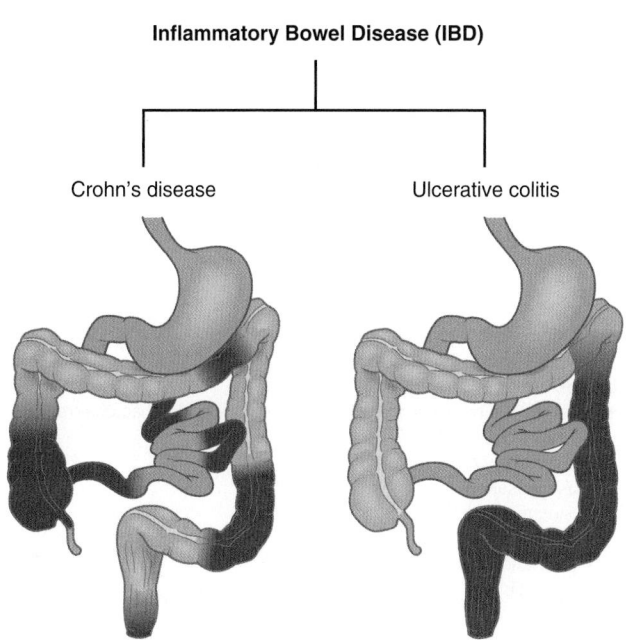

Crohn's disease   Ulcerative colitis

FIG. 43-3 Comparison of distribution patterns of Crohn's disease and ulcerative colitis.

TABLE 43-15	**EXTRAINTESTINAL COMPLICATIONS OF IBD**

- Joints
  - Peripheral arthritis (colitic)
  - Ankylosing spondylitis
  - Sacroiliitis
  - Finger clubbing
- Skin
  - Erythema nodosum
  - Pyoderma gangrenosum
- Mouth
  - Aphthous ulcers
- Eye
  - Conjunctivitis
  - Uveitis
  - Episcleritis
- Gallstones
- Kidney stones
- Liver disease: primary sclerosing cholangitis
- Osteoporosis
- Thromboembolism

who is not genetically susceptible will not develop IBD even if exposed to the triggering agent. The pathway from genetic mutation to abnormal immune responses varies depending on which gene or genes are affected. This genetic variation may explain differences in patient responses to various pharmacologic therapies for IBD.

Pattern of Inflammation in Ulcerative Colitis Versus Crohn's Disease. The pattern of inflammation differs between Crohn's disease and ulcerative colitis (Fig. 43-3). In Crohn's disease the inflammation involves all layers of the bowel wall. Crohn's disease can occur anywhere in the GI tract from the mouth to the anus, but occurs most commonly in the terminal ileum and colon. Furthermore, segments of normal bowel can occur between diseased portions, the so-called skip lesions (see Table 43-14). Typically, ulcerations are deep and longitudinal and penetrate between islands of inflamed edematous mucosa, causing the classic cobblestone appearance. Strictures at the areas of inflammation may cause bowel obstruction. Since the inflammation goes through the entire wall, microscopic leaks can allow bowel contents to enter the peritoneal cavity and form abscesses or produce peritonitis.

In Crohn's disease, fistulas can develop between adjacent areas of bowel, between the bowel and the bladder, and between the bowel and the vagina. Fistulas can also form a tract through the skin to the outside of the body. Urinary tract infections are usually the first sign of a bowel or bladder fistula, and feces is sometimes seen in the urine. Fistulas between the bowel and the vagina allow feces to leak out through the vagina, and feces leaks onto the skin if there is a skin fistula.

Ulcerative colitis usually starts in the rectum and moves in a continual fashion toward the cecum. Although sometimes mild inflammation occurs in the terminal ileum, ulcerative colitis is a disease of the colon and rectum (see Fig. 43-3). The inflammation and ulcerations occur in the mucosal layer, the innermost layer of the bowel wall. Since it does not extend through all bowel wall layers, fistulas and abscesses are rare. Water and electrolytes cannot be absorbed through inflamed

mucosa. Diarrhea with large fluid and electrolyte losses is a characteristic feature of damage to the colonic mucosa epithelium. Breakdown of cells results in protein loss through the stool. Areas of inflamed mucosa form *pseudopolyps,* tongue-like projections into the bowel lumen.

Clinical Manifestations

In ulcerative colitis and Crohn's disease, manifestations are often the same (diarrhea, bloody stools, weight loss, abdominal pain, fever, and fatigue). Bloody stools are more common with ulcerative colitis, and weight loss is more common in Crohn's disease because inflammation of the small intestine impairs nutrient absorption. Both forms of IBD are chronic disorders with mild to severe acute exacerbations that occur at unpredictable intervals over many years.

In Crohn's disease, diarrhea and crampy abdominal pain are common symptoms. If the small intestine is involved, weight loss occurs from malabsorption. Rectal bleeding sometimes occurs with Crohn's disease, although not as often as with ulcerative colitis.

In ulcerative colitis, the primary manifestations are bloody diarrhea and abdominal pain. Pain may vary from the mild lower abdominal cramping associated with diarrhea to severe, constant pain associated with acute perforations. With *mild disease,* diarrhea may consist of no more than four semiformed stools daily that contain small amounts of blood. The patient may have no other manifestations. In *moderate disease* the patient has increased stool output (up to 10 stools/day), increased bleeding, and systemic symptoms (fever, malaise, mild anemia, anorexia). In *severe disease,* diarrhea is bloody, contains mucus, and occurs 10 to 20 times a day. In addition, fever, rapid weight loss greater than 10% of total body weight, anemia, tachycardia, and dehydration are present.

Complications

Patients with IBD experience both local (confined to the GI tract) and systemic (extraintestinal) complications (Table 43-15). GI tract complications include hemorrhage, strictures, perforation (with possible peritonitis), fistulas, and colonic dilation (toxic megacolon). Patients with toxic megacolon are at risk of perforation and may need an emergency colectomy. Toxic megacolon is more common with ulcerative colitis. Hemorrhage may lead to anemia and is corrected with blood transfusions and iron supplements. Perineal abscess and fistulas occur in up to a third of patients with Crohn's disease. Some patients develop skin tags around the anus. The incidence and severity of *C. difficile* infection in patients with IBD are increasing.[27]

Nutritional problems are especially common in Crohn's disease when the terminal ileum is involved. Bile salts and cobalamin are exclusively absorbed in the terminal ileum. Thus disease in the terminal ileum can result in fat malabsorption and anemia.

Patients with a history of IBD are considered at increased or high risk for colorectal cancer. In addition, those with Crohn's disease are at increased risk for small intestinal cancer. Screening for cancer at regular intervals is important in persons with IBD.[28]

Some people with IBD suffer from systemic complications, including joint, eye, mouth, kidney, bone, vascular, and skin problems (see Table 43-15). Circulating factors such as cytokines trigger inflammation in these areas. Routine liver function tests are important because primary sclerosing cholangitis, a complication of IBD, can lead to liver failure.

Diagnostic Studies

The diagnosis of IBD includes ruling out other diseases with similar symptoms and then determining whether the patient has Crohn's disease or ulcerative colitis. In early Crohn's disease the symptoms can be similar to those of IBS. Diagnostic studies also provide information about disease severity and complications. A CBC typically shows iron-deficiency anemia from blood loss. An elevated WBC count may be an indication of toxic megacolon or perforation. Decreased serum sodium, potassium, chloride, bicarbonate, and magnesium levels are due to fluid and electrolyte losses from diarrhea and vomiting. Hypoalbuminemia is present with severe disease as a result of poor nutrition or protein loss. Elevated erythrocyte sedimentation rate, C-reactive protein, and WBCs reflect inflammation. Stool cultures are obtained to determine if infection is present. The stool is examined for blood, pus, and mucus.

Imaging studies such as double-contrast barium enema, small bowel series (small bowel follow through), transabdominal ultrasound, CT, and MRI are useful for the diagnosis of IBD. Colonoscopy allows for examination of the entire large intestine lumen and sometimes the most distal ileum. The extent of inflammation, ulcerations, pseudopolyps, and strictures is determined, and biopsy specimens are taken for a definitive diagnosis. Since a colonoscope can enter only the distal ileum, capsule endoscopy (see Chapter 39) may be used in the diagnosis of Crohn's disease in the small intestine.[29] However, biopsies cannot be obtained with either capsule endoscopy or barium enema.

Collaborative Care

The goals of treatment are to (1) rest the bowel, (2) control the inflammation, (3) combat infection, (4) correct malnutrition, (5) alleviate any stress, (6) provide symptomatic relief, and (7) improve quality of life. Since the cause is unknown, treatment relies on drugs to treat the inflammation and maintain a remission. A variety of drugs are available to treat IBD (Tables 43-16 and 43-17). Hospitalization is indicated if the patient fails to respond to drug therapy, if the disease is severe, and if complications are suspected. Since recurrence rate is high after surgical treatment of Crohn's disease, drugs are the preferred treatment.

Drug Therapy. The goals of drug treatment for IBD are to induce and then maintain a remission. Five major classes of medications used to treat IBD are aminosalicylates, antimicrobials, corticosteroids, immunosuppressants, and biologic and targeted therapy (see Table 43-17). Drugs are chosen based on

TABLE 43-16   **COLLABORATIVE CARE**
Inflammatory Bowel Disease

Diagnostic
- History and physical examination
- CBC, erythrocyte sedimentation rate
- Serum chemistries
- Testing of stool for occult blood
- Testing of stool for infection
- Capsule endoscopy
- Radiologic studies with barium contrast
- Sigmoidoscopy and colonoscopy with biopsy

Collaborative Therapy
- High-calorie, high-vitamin, high-protein, low-residue, lactose-free (if lactase deficiency) diet
- Drug therapy (see Table 43-17)
  - Aminosalicylates
  - Antimicrobials
  - Corticosteroids
  - Immunosuppressants
  - Biologic and targeted therapy (immunomodulator)
- Elemental diet or parenteral nutrition
- Physical and emotional rest
- Referral for counseling or support group
- Surgery (see Table 43-18)

the location and severity of inflammation. Depending on the severity of the disease, patients are treated with either a "step-down" or "step-up" approach. The step-up approach uses less toxic therapies (e.g., aminosalicylates and antimicrobials) first, and more toxic medications (e.g., biologic and targeted therapy) are started when initial therapies do not work. The step-down approach uses biologic and targeted therapy first.

Sulfasalazine (Azulfidine) contains sulfapyridine and 5-aminosalicylic acid (5-ASA). The 5-ASA accounts for its therapeutic benefits for IBD. Its exact mechanism of action is unknown, but topical application to the intestinal mucosa suppresses proinflammatory cytokines and other inflammatory mediators. When given orally, 5-ASA alone is absorbed before it reaches the lower GI tract where it is needed. When combined with sulfapyridine, 5-ASA reaches the colon. Because many people cannot tolerate sulfapyridine, preparations such as olsalazine (Dipentum), mesalamine (Pentasa), and balsalazide (Colazal) deliver 5-ASA to the terminal ileum and the colon. These drugs are as effective as sulfasalazine and better tolerated when administered orally.

DRUG ALERT: Sulfasalazine (Azulfidine)
- May cause yellowish orange discoloration of skin and urine.
- Avoid exposure to sunlight and ultraviolet light until photosensitivity is determined.

Preparations with 5-ASA can be administered rectally as suppositories, enemas, and foams. Topical treatment offers the advantage of delivering the 5-ASA directly to the tissue where it is needed and minimizes systemic effects. Aminosalicylates are also first-line therapies for mild to moderate Crohn's disease, especially when the colon is involved, but are more effective for ulcerative colitis. These drugs are recommended for both achieving and maintaining a remission.

Although no specific infectious agent has been identified, antimicrobials (e.g., metronidazole, ciprofloxacin [Cipro]) are used to treat IBD. Corticosteroids such as prednisolone and budesonide (Entocort) are used to achieve remission in IBD.

TABLE 43-17 DRUG THERAPY

Inflammatory Bowel Disease

Class	Action	Examples
5-Aminosalicylates (5-ASA)	Decrease GI inflammation through direct contact with bowel mucosa	*Systemic:* sulfasalazine (Azulfidine), mesalamine (Asacol, Pentasa), olsalazine (Dipentum), balsalazide (Colazal) *Topical:* 5-ASA enema (Rowasa), mesalamine suppositories (Canasa)
Antimicrobials	Prevent or treat secondary infection	metronidazole (Flagyl), ciprofloxacin (Cipro), clarithromycin (Biaxin)
Corticosteroids	Decrease inflammation	*Systemic:* corticosteroids (prednisone, budesonide [Entocort]) (oral); hydrocortisone or methylprednisolone (IV for severe IBD) *Topical:* hydrocortisone suppository or foam (Cortifoam) or enema (Cortenema)
Immunosuppressants	Suppress immune response	azathioprine (Imuran), 6-mercaptopurine (6-MP), methotrexate, cyclosporine
Biologic and targeted therapy (immunomodulators)	Inhibit the cytokine tumor necrosis factor (TNF)	infliximab (Remicade), adalimumab (Humira), certolizumab pegol (Cimzia), golimumab (Simponi)
	Prevent migration of leukocytes from bloodstream to inflamed tissue	natalizumab (Tysabri)
Antidiarrheals	Decrease GI motility*	diphenoxylate with atropine (Lomotil), loperamide (Imodium)
Hematinics and vitamins	Correct iron-deficiency anemia and promote healing	oral ferrous sulfate or gluconate, iron dextran injection (Imferon), cobalamin, zinc, folate

*Used with caution during severe disease because of potential to produce toxic megacolon.

TABLE 43-18 INDICATIONS FOR SURGICAL THERAPY FOR IBD

- Drainage of abdominal abscess
- Failure to respond to conservative therapy
- Fistulas
- Inability to decrease corticosteroids
- Intestinal obstruction
- Massive hemorrhage
- Perforation
- Severe anorectal disease
- Suspicion of carcinoma

Corticosteroids are given for the shortest possible time because of side effects associated with long-term use. Patients with disease in the left colon, sigmoid, and rectum can be given suppositories, enemas, and foams that deliver the corticosteroid directly to the inflamed tissue with minimal systemic effects. Oral prednisone is given to patients with mild to moderate disease who do not respond to either 5-ASA or topical corticosteroids. IV corticosteroids are reserved for those with severe inflammation. Corticosteroids must be tapered to very low levels when surgery is planned to prevent postoperative complications (e.g., infection, delayed wound healing).

Immunosuppressants (6-mercaptopurine, azathioprine [Imuran]) are given to maintain remission after corticosteroid induction therapy. These drugs require regular CBC monitoring because they can suppress the bone marrow and lead to inflammation of the pancreas or gallbladder. They have a delayed onset of action and are therefore useful for maintenance of remission but not for acute flare-ups.

Methotrexate has also been found to be effective for treatment of Crohn's disease, but patients may suffer flu-like symptoms, bone marrow depression, and liver dysfunction. CBCs and liver enzymes are monitored. Methotrexate should not be used in women who are pregnant because it causes birth defects and fetal death.

Currently there are five major biologic and targeted medications.[30] Four are antitumor necrosis factor (TNF) agents: infliximab (Remicade), adalimumab (Humira), certolizumab pegol (Cimzia) and golimumab (Simponi). The fifth, natalizumab (Tysabri), inhibits leukocyte adhesion by blocking α_4-integrin,

an adhesion molecule. TNF is a proinflammatory cytokine that is released during inflammation. Infliximab is a monoclonal antibody to TNF. It is given IV to induce and maintain remission in patients with Crohn's disease and in patients with draining fistulas who do not respond to conventional drug therapy. Adalimumab and certolizumab pegol have effects similar to those of infliximab. Adalimumab is self-administered subcutaneously every 1 to 2 weeks, and certolizumab pegol must be administered subcutaneously by a health care provider every 4 weeks. Golimumab is administered subcutaneously twice the first month and then every 4 weeks. Natalizumab is administered by IV infusion every 28 days.

The biologic and targeted agents do not work for everyone. They are costly and may produce allergic reactions.[30] The anti-TNF agents are immunogenic, meaning that patients receiving them frequently produce antibodies against them. Immunogenicity leads to an acute infusion reaction and delayed hypersensitivity-type reactions. The drugs are most effective when given at regular intervals and must not be discontinued unless the patient cannot tolerate them. If the drug is stopped and then restarted, infusion reactions are likely. Natalizumab is associated with increased risk of infection, hepatotoxicity, and hypersensitivity reactions. Its use requires a special safety monitoring program.

The anti-TNF agents have similar side effects. The most common adverse effects are upper respiratory and urinary tract infections, headaches, nausea, joint pain, and abdominal pain. More serious effects include reactivation of hepatitis and tuberculosis (TB); opportunistic infections; and malignancies, especially lymphoma. Patients must be tested for TB and hepatitis before treatment begins and cannot receive live virus immunizations. Patients must be informed of these risks before beginning therapy and taught methods to prevent infection and recognize early signs and symptoms (e.g., fever, cough, malaise, dyspnea).

Surgical Therapy

Ulcerative Colitis. Indications for surgery for ulcerative colitis are presented in Table 43-18. Since ulcerative colitis affects only the colon, a total proctocolectomy is curative. Surgical procedures used to treat ulcerative colitis include

(1) total proctocolectomy with ileal pouch/anal anastomosis and (2) total proctocolectomy with permanent ileostomy. Surgical procedures for ulcerative colitis can be performed laparoscopically.

Total Proctocolectomy With Ileal Pouch/Anal Anastomosis (IPAA). The most commonly used surgical procedure for ulcerative colitis is a total proctocolectomy with ileal pouch/anal anastomosis (IPAA). In this procedure a diverting ileostomy is performed, and an ileal pouch is created and anastomosed directly to the anus (Fig. 43-4). The two surgical procedures are performed approximately 8 to 12 weeks apart. The initial procedure includes colectomy, rectal mucosectomy, ileal pouch (reservoir) construction, ileoanal anastomosis, and temporary ileostomy. The second surgery involves closure of the ileostomy to direct stool toward the new pouch. Adaptation of the pouch occurs over the next 3 to 6 months, which usually results in a decreased number of bowel movements. The patient is able to control defecation at the anal sphincter. The major complication of this procedure is acute or chronic pouchitis.

Total Proctocolectomy With Permanent Ileostomy. A proctocolectomy with a permanent ileostomy is a one-stage operation involving the removal of the colon, rectum, and anus with closure of the anal opening. The end of the terminal ileum is brought out through the abdominal wall and forms a stoma, or ostomy. The stoma is usually placed in the right lower quadrant below the belt line. With a permanent ileostomy, continence is not possible.

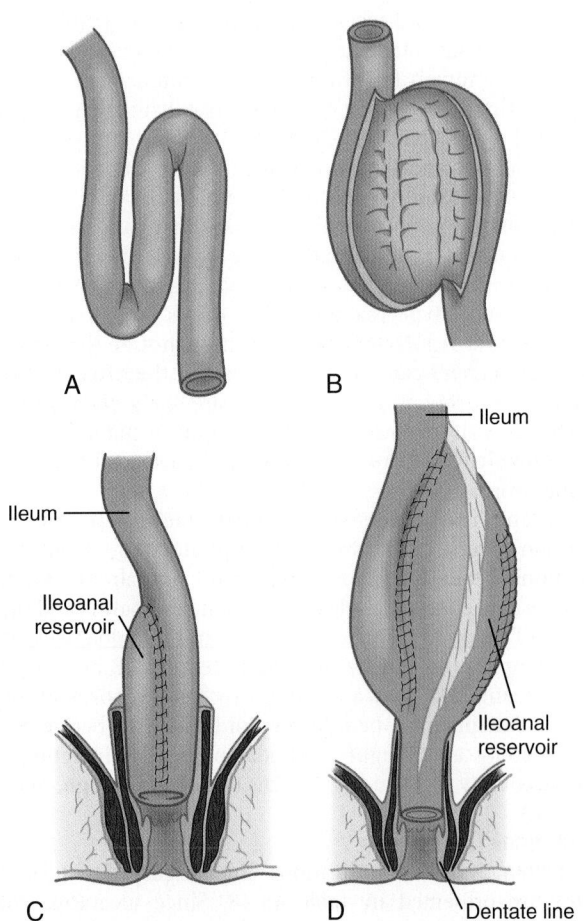

FIG. 43-4 Ileoanal pouch (reservoir). **A,** Formation of a pouch. **B,** Posterior suture lines completed. **C,** J-shaped configuration for ileoanal pouch (J-pouch). **D,** S-shaped configuration for ileoanal pouch (S-pouch).

Crohn's Disease. Surgery for Crohn's disease is usually performed for complications such as strictures, obstructions, bleeding, and fistula (see Table 43-16). Most patients with Crohn's disease eventually require surgery. When segments of the intestine are removed, the remaining intestine is reanastomosed. Unfortunately, the disease often recurs at the anastomosis site.

Repeated removal of sections of small intestine can lead to short bowel syndrome. *Short bowel syndrome* occurs when either surgery or disease leaves too little small intestine surface area to maintain life. Lifetime parenteral nutrition is necessary for survival. (Short bowel syndrome is discussed in this chapter on p. 999.

Conservative surgery is advocated instead of resective surgery in patients with Crohn's disease. Strictures obstructing the bowel can be widened with strictureplasty. If perforation allows bowel contents to drain into the abdominal cavity, the surgeon drains the purulent material, irrigates the abdomen, and makes a temporary ostomy. Abscesses are surgically drained.

Postoperative Care. Postoperative care after surgical procedures for IBD is similar to that described in the general nursing care plan for the postoperative patient (see eNursing Care Plan 20-1 on the website for Chapter 20). If an ileostomy is formed, stoma viability, the mucocutaneous juncture (the area where the mucous membrane of the bowel interfaces with the skin), and peristomal skin integrity must be monitored. (Stoma care is presented later in this chapter on pp. 991-992.)

After surgery, ileostomy output initially may be as high as 1500 to 2000 mL/24 hr. Observe the patient for signs of hemorrhage, abdominal abscess, small bowel obstruction, dehydration, and other related complications. If an NG tube is used, remove it when bowel function returns. Patients, especially those with Crohn's disease, are at risk of early (within 30 days) postoperative bowel obstruction.[31]

Transient incontinence of mucus is a result of intraoperative manipulation of the anal canal. Initial drainage through the ileoanal anastomosis will be liquid. Kegel exercises may help strengthen the pelvic floor and sphincter muscles (see Table 46-19). However, they are not recommended in the immediate postoperative period. Perianal skin care is important to protect the epidermis from mucous drainage and maceration. Instruct the patient to gently clean the skin with a mild cleanser, rinse well, and dry thoroughly. A moisture barrier ointment and a perineal pad may be used.

Nutritional Therapy. Diet is an important component in the treatment of IBD. Consult a dietitian regarding dietary recommendations. The goals of diet management are to (1) provide adequate nutrition without exacerbating symptoms, (2) correct and prevent malnutrition, (3) replace fluid and electrolyte losses, and (4) prevent weight loss.

Nutritional deficiencies are due to decreased oral intake, blood loss, and, depending on the location of the inflammation, malabsorption of nutrients. Patients may reduce food intake in an effort to reduce diarrhea. Inflammatory mediators reduce appetite. Bloody diarrhea leads to iron-deficiency anemia, which is treated with supplemental iron (ferrous sulfate or ferrous gluconate). Parenteral iron may be needed for patients who cannot tolerate oral iron. Iron dextran (Imferon) given intramuscularly by Z-track or IV injection may be necessary if anemia is severe.

Disease of the terminal ileum reduces absorption of cobalamin and bile acids. Reduced cobalamin contributes to anemia, and bile salts are important for fat absorption and contribute to osmotic diarrhea. Cobalamin is available in injection form, given monthly, or as a daily oral or nasal spray. Cholestyramine, an ion-exchange resin that binds unabsorbed bile salts, helps control the diarrhea. Zinc deficiency can result from severe or chronic diarrhea, and supplementation may be necessary.

Medications can contribute to nutritional problems. Patients receiving sulfasalazine should receive folate (folic acid) daily. Those receiving corticosteroids are prone to osteoporosis and need calcium supplements. Potassium supplements may also be necessary with corticosteroids. Corticosteroids lead to sodium retention, loss of potassium (hypokalemia), and potential toxic megacolon. Vitamin D deficiency is more common in persons with IBD. This may be due to malabsorption due to inflammation, surgical resection of intestine, reduced sunlight exposure, and decreased dietary intake.[32]

Overall, it is essential that people with IBD eat a balanced, healthy diet with sufficient calories, protein, and nutrients. Patients can use MyPlate guidelines to ensure that they get adequate portions from all of the food groups (see Fig. 40-1 and Table 40-1). The diet for each patient must be individualized.

During an acute exacerbation, patients with IBD may not be able to tolerate a regular diet. Liquid enteral feedings are preferred over parenteral nutrition because atrophy of the gut and bacterial overgrowth occur when the GI tract is not used. (Enteral and parenteral nutrition are discussed in Chapter 40.) Enteral nutrition is high in calories and nutrients, lactose free, and easily absorbed. Enteral feedings help achieve remission and improve nutritional status. When regular foods are restarted, they are added gradually to help identify food intolerances or sensitivities.

There are no universal food triggers for IBD, but individuals may find that certain foods cause diarrhea. A food diary helps to identify problem foods to avoid. Because many patients with IBD are lactose intolerant, symptoms improve when milk and milk products are avoided. Lactose-intolerant patients can use yogurt as a substitute. High-fat foods also tend to trigger diarrhea. Cold foods and high-fiber foods (cereal with bran, nuts, raw fruits with peels) may promote diarrhea. Smoking stimulates the GI tract (increases motility and secretion) and should be avoided.

NURSING MANAGEMENT
INFLAMMATORY BOWEL DISEASE

NURSING ASSESSMENT
Subjective and objective data that should be obtained from a patient with IBD are presented in Table 43-19.

NURSING DIAGNOSES
Nursing diagnoses for the patient with IBD include, but are not limited to, the following:
- Diarrhea *related to* bowel inflammation and intestinal hyperactivity
- Imbalanced nutrition: less than body requirements *related to* decreased absorption and increased nutrient loss through diarrhea
- Ineffective coping *related to* chronic disease, lifestyle changes, inadequate confidence in ability to cope

Additional information on nursing diagnoses is presented in eNursing Care Plan 43-2 on the website for this chapter.

PLANNING
The overall goals are that the patient with IBD will (1) have fewer and less severe acute exacerbations, (2) maintain normal

---

TABLE 43-19 NURSING ASSESSMENT
Inflammatory Bowel Disease

Subjective Data
Important Health Information
Past health history: Infection, autoimmune disorders
Medications: Antidiarrheal medications

Functional Health Patterns
Health perception–health management: Family history of ulcerative colitis or Crohn's disease; fatigue, malaise
Nutritional-metabolic: Nausea, vomiting; anorexia; weight loss
Elimination: Diarrhea; blood, mucus, or pus in stools
Cognitive-perceptual: Lower abdominal pain (worse before defecation), cramping, tenesmus

Objective Data
General
Intermittent fever, emaciated appearance, fatigue

Integumentary
Pale skin with poor turgor, dry mucous membranes; skin lesions; anorectal irritation, skin tags, cutaneous fistulas

Gastrointestinal
Abdominal distention, hyperactive bowel sounds, abdominal cramps

Cardiovascular
Tachycardia, hypotension

Possible Diagnostic Findings
Anemia; leukocytosis; electrolyte imbalance; hypoalbuminemia; vitamin and trace metal deficiencies; guaiac-positive stool; abnormal sigmoidoscopic, colonoscopic, and/or barium enema findings

---

fluid and electrolyte balance, (3) be free from pain or discomfort, (4) adhere to medical regimens, (5) maintain nutritional balance, and (6) have an improved quality of life.

NURSING IMPLEMENTATION
During the acute phase, focus your attention on hemodynamic stability, pain control, fluid and electrolyte balance, and nutritional support. Maintain accurate intake and output records, and monitor the number and appearance of stools. It is important to establish rapport and encourage the patient to talk about self-care strategies. An explanation of all procedures and treatment helps to build trust and decrease apprehension.

Because of the relationship between emotions and the GI tract, teach the patient strategies for managing stress (see Chapter 7). Remember that patients experiencing a relapse have been managing their disease and need to feel in control. Ask them what you can do to facilitate their self-care. Once you have established a therapeutic relationship, talk with smokers about quitting, since smoking exacerbates the disease.

IBD is a chronic illness. Given the chronicity and uncertainty related to frequency and severity of flares, the patient may experience frustration, depression, and anxiety. Psychotherapy and behavioral therapies may help the patient experiencing psychologic distress in managing his or her symptoms. Assist the patient in accepting the chronicity of IBD and learning strategies to cope with its recurrent, unpredictable nature. Inadequate coping mechanisms are sometimes result of the childhood onset of the disease before the person has the emotional and developmental maturity needed to cope. Patients may suffer severe fatigue, which limits energy for physical activity. Rest is important. Patients may lose sleep because of frequent episodes of diarrhea and abdominal pain. Nutritional deficiencies and anemia leave the patient feeling weak and listless. Schedule activities around rest periods.

Until diarrhea is controlled, help the patient stay clean, dry, and free of odor. Place a deodorizer in the room. Meticulous perianal skin care using plain water (no harsh soap) together with a skin barrier cream prevents skin breakdown. Dibucaine (Nupercainal), witch hazel, or other soothing compresses or prescribed ointment and sitz baths may reduce irritation and discomfort of the anus.

In the majority of patients with IBD the disease is characterized by intermittent exacerbation and remission of symptoms. The patient and caregiver may need help setting realistic short- and long-term goals. Teaching includes (1) the importance of rest and diet management, (2) perianal care, (3) drug action and side effects, (4) symptoms of recurrence of disease, (5) when to seek medical care, and (6) use of diversional activities to reduce stress. Excellent teaching resources written in easily comprehensible language are available from the Crohn's and Colitis Foundation of America *(www.ccfa.org)*.

▌EVALUATION

The expected outcomes are that the patient with IBD will
- Experience a decrease in the number of diarrhea stools
- Maintain body weight within a normal range
- Be free from pain and discomfort
- Demonstrate the use of effective coping strategies

Additional information on expected outcomes is presented in eNursing Care Plan 43-2 on the website for this chapter.

▌GERONTOLOGIC CONSIDERATIONS

INFLAMMATORY BOWEL DISEASE

Although IBD is considered a disease of teenagers and young adults, a second peak in occurrence is in the sixth decade. The etiology, natural history, and clinical course of IBD are similar to those observed in younger patients. However, in the older patient with ulcerative colitis, the distal colon (proctitis) is usually involved. Diagnosis is sometimes difficult in older adults, since IBD can be confused with *C. difficile* infection and the colitis associated with diverticulosis or NSAID ingestion. Older adults receive the same medical treatment as younger patients and have similar results after ileoanal reservoir surgery.[33] However, they are more prone to complications from corticosteroids than younger adults.

Collaborative care of the older patient with IBD is similar to care of the younger patient. However, because of increased risk of cardiovascular and pulmonary complications, older adults tend to have increased morbidity associated with surgical procedures.

In addition to Crohn's disease and ulcerative colitis, older adults are also vulnerable to inflammation of the colon (colitis) from drug use and systemic vascular disease. Drugs such as NSAIDs, digitalis, sumatriptan (Imitrex), vasopressin, estrogen, and allopurinol (Zyloprim) have been associated with the development of colitis in the older patient. Colitis may also be secondary to ischemic bowel disease related to atherosclerosis and heart failure.

Older adults, particularly those with diminished renal and cardiovascular function, are more vulnerable to the volume depletion consequences of diarrhea. In older adults with IBD,

focus on careful assessment of fluid and electrolyte status and evaluation of the replacement therapies.

INTESTINAL OBSTRUCTION

Intestinal obstruction occurs when intestinal contents cannot pass through the GI tract. The obstruction may occur in the small intestine or colon and can be partial or complete, simple or strangulated.[34] A partial obstruction usually resolves with conservative treatment, whereas a complete obstruction usually requires surgery. A simple obstruction has an intact blood supply, and a strangulated one does not.

TYPES OF INTESTINAL OBSTRUCTION

The causes of intestinal obstruction can be classified as mechanical or nonmechanical.

Mechanical

Mechanical obstruction is a detectable occlusion of the intestinal lumen. Most intestinal obstructions occur in the small intestine.[34] Surgical adhesion is the most common cause of small bowel obstructions and can occur within days of surgery or several years later (Fig. 43-5). Other causes of intestinal obstruction are hernia, strictures from Crohn's disease, and intussusception following bariatric abdominal surgery. The most common cause of colon obstruction is cancer, followed by diverticular disease.

Nonmechanical

Nonmechanical obstruction may result from a neuromuscular or vascular disorder. Paralytic (adynamic) ileus (lack of intestinal peristalsis and bowel sounds) is the most common form of nonmechanical obstruction. It occurs to some degree after any abdominal surgery. It can be difficult to know whether postoperative obstruction is due to paralytic ileus or adhesions. One clue is that bowel sounds usually return before postoperative adhesions develop. Other causes of paralytic ileus include peritonitis, inflammatory responses (e.g., acute pancreatitis, acute appendicitis), electrolyte abnormalities (especially hypokalemia), and thoracic or lumbar spinal fractures.

Pseudo-obstruction is a mechanical obstruction of the intestine without demonstration of obstruction by radiologic methods. Collagen vascular diseases and neurologic and endocrine disorders may cause pseudo-obstruction, but many times the cause is unknown.

Vascular obstructions are rare and are the result of an interference with the blood supply to a portion of the intestines. The most common causes are emboli and atherosclerosis of the mesenteric arteries. Emboli may originate from thrombi in patients who have chronic atrial fibrillation, diseased heart valves, and prosthetic valves. Venous thrombosis may be seen in conditions of low blood flow, such as heart failure and shock.

Etiology and Pathophysiology

About 6 to 8 L of fluid enter the small intestine daily. Most of the fluid is absorbed before it reaches the colon. Approximately 75% of intestinal gas is swallowed air. When an obstruction occurs, fluid, gas, and intestinal contents accumulate proximal to the obstruction, and the distal bowel collapses. The distention reduces the absorption of fluids and stimulates intestinal secretions. The proximal bowel becomes increasingly distended, and

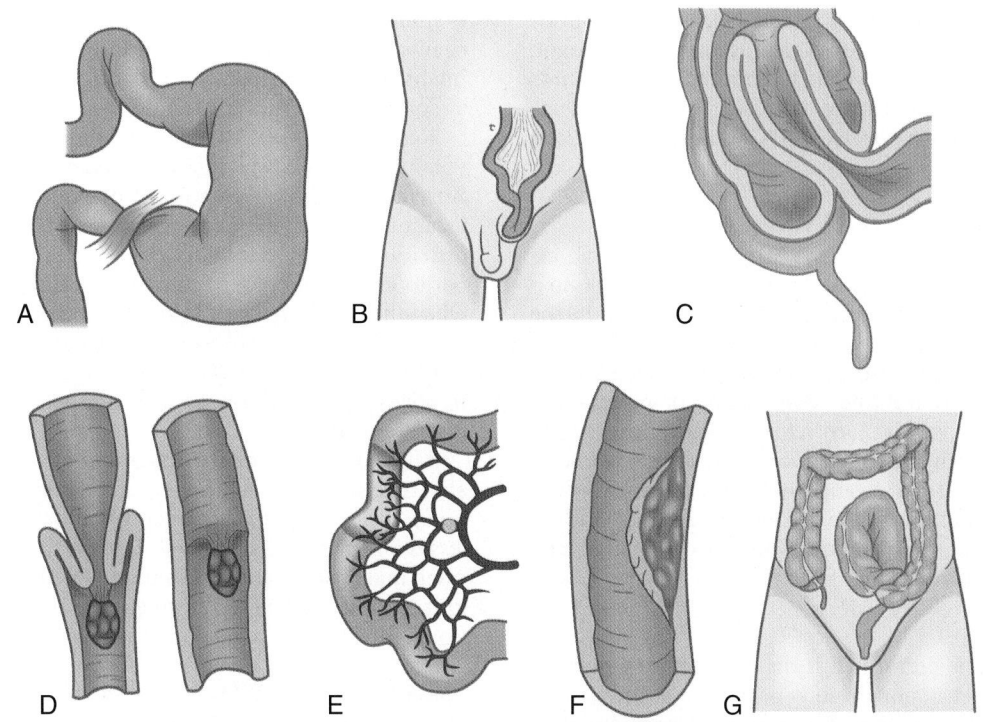

FIG. 43-5 Bowel obstructions. **A,** Adhesions. **B,** Strangulated inguinal hernia. **C,** Ileocecal intussusception. **D,** Intussusception from polyps. **E,** Mesenteric occlusion. **F,** Neoplasm. **G,** Volvulus of the sigmoid colon.

intraluminal bowel pressure rises. The increased pressure leads to an increase in capillary permeability and extravasation of fluids and electrolytes into the peritoneal cavity. Retention of fluids in the intestine and peritoneal cavity (third spacing) leads to a severe reduction in circulating blood volume and results in hypotension and hypovolemic shock.

If blood flow is inadequate, bowel tissue becomes ischemic, then necrotic, and the bowel may perforate. In the most dangerous situation the bowel becomes so distended that the blood flow stops, causing edema, cyanosis, and gangrene of a bowel segment. This is called *intestinal strangulation* or *intestinal infarction*. If it is not corrected quickly, the bowel will become necrotic and rupture, leading to infection, septic shock, and death.

The location of the obstruction determines the extent of fluid, electrolyte, and acid-base imbalances. If the obstruction is high (e.g., upper duodenum), metabolic alkalosis may result from the loss of gastric hydrochloric (HCl) acid through vomiting or NG intubation and suction. When the obstruction is located in the small intestine, dehydration occurs rapidly. Dehydration and electrolyte imbalances do not occur early in large bowel obstruction. If the obstruction is below the proximal colon, solid fecal material accumulates until symptoms of discomfort appear.

Some small intestine obstructions, especially those due to surgical adhesions, may resolve without surgery.[34] Other small intestine obstructions, such as strangulated obstructions, require emergency surgery for survival. *Volvulus* is an intestinal obstruction that occurs by the bowel twisting on itself (see Fig. 43-5). Malignant bowel obstructions are associated with colorectal and ovarian cancer.

Clinical Manifestations

The clinical manifestations of intestinal obstruction vary, depending on its location (Table 43-20). The most important early manifestations of a small bowel obstruction are colicky

TABLE 43-20	MANIFESTATIONS OF SMALL AND LARGE INTESTINAL OBSTRUCTIONS	
Manifestation	**Small Intestine**	**Large Intestine**
Onset	Rapid	Gradual
Vomiting	Frequent and copious	Rare
Pain	Colicky, cramplike, intermittent pain	Low-grade, cramping abdominal pain
Bowel movement	Feces for a short time	Absolute constipation
Abdominal distention	Absent or minimal (upper or proximal) Increased (lower or distal)	Increased

abdominal pain, nausea, vomiting, and abdominal distention. Constipation and decreased flatus occur later. Patients with obstructions in the proximal small intestine rapidly develop nausea and vomiting, which is sometimes projectile and contains bile. Vomiting from more distal obstructions of the small intestine is more gradual in onset. Foul-smelling vomitus that looks like stool indicates a long-standing obstruction requiring immediate surgery. Signs of colonic obstruction include abdominal distention, constipation (new onset), and lack of flatus.

Vomiting usually relieves abdominal pain in higher intestinal obstructions. Persistent, colicky abdominal pain is seen in patients with lower intestinal obstruction. With mechanical obstruction, pain generally comes and goes in waves. In contrast, paralytic ileus produces a more constant, generalized abdominal discomfort. Strangulation causes severe, constant pain that is rapid in onset. Abdominal distention is usually absent or minimally noticeable in proximal small intestine obstructions and markedly increased in lower intestinal obstructions. Abdominal tenderness and rigidity are usually absent unless strangulation or peritonitis has occurred.

Auscultation of bowel sounds reveals high-pitched sounds above the area of obstruction. Bowel sounds may also be absent. The patient often notes *borborygmi* (audible abdominal sounds produced by hyperactive intestinal motility). The patient's temperature rarely rises above 100° F (37.8° C) unless strangulation or peritonitis occurs.

Diagnostic Studies

Perform a thorough history and physical examination. CT scans and abdominal x-rays are ordered. Sigmoidoscopy or colonoscopy may provide direct visualization of an obstruction in the colon.

A CBC and blood chemistries may be performed. An elevated WBC count may indicate strangulation or perforation. Elevated hematocrit values may reflect hemoconcentration. Decreased hemoglobin and hematocrit values may indicate bleeding from a neoplasm or strangulation with necrosis. Serum electrolytes, BUN, and creatinine are monitored frequently to assess the degree of dehydration. Metabolic alkalosis can develop as a result of vomiting.

Collaborative Care

Emergency surgery is performed if the bowel is strangulated, but many bowel obstructions resolve with conservative treatment. Initial medical treatment of bowel obstruction caused by adhesions includes placing the patient on NPO status, inserting an NG tube for decompression, providing IV fluid therapy with either normal saline or lactated Ringer's solution (since fluid losses from the GI tract are isotonic), adding potassium to IV fluids after verifying renal function, and administering analgesics for pain control.

The treatment goal for the patient with a malignant bowel obstruction is to regain patency and resolve the obstruction. Stents can be placed via endoscopic or fluoroscopic procedures. They can be used for palliative purposes or until surgery can be performed. Corticosteroids that have antiemetic properties and decrease edema and inflammation may be used in combination with stent placement. A venting gastrostomy tube may be placed endoscopically or percutaneously.[35]

If the obstruction does not improve within 24 hours or if the patient's condition deteriorates, surgery is performed to relieve the obstruction. In some cases, parenteral nutrition may be used to improve the patient's nutritional status before surgery and promote postoperative healing. Surgery may involve simply resecting the obstructed segment of bowel and anastomosing the remaining healthy bowel back together. Partial or total colectomy, colostomy, or ileostomy may be required when extensive obstruction or necrosis is present.

Occasionally obstructions can be removed nonsurgically. A colonoscope can be used to remove polyps, dilate strictures, and remove and destroy tumors with a laser.

NURSING MANAGEMENT
INTESTINAL OBSTRUCTION

NURSING ASSESSMENT

Intestinal obstruction is a potentially life-threatening condition. Major concerns are prevention of fluid and electrolyte deficiencies and early recognition of deterioration in the patient's condition (e.g., hypovolemic shock, bowel strangulation). Nursing assessment begins with a detailed patient history and physical examination. The type and location of obstruction usually cause characteristic symptoms. Determine the location, duration, intensity, and frequency of abdominal pain and whether abdominal tenderness or rigidity is present.

Record the onset, frequency, color, odor, and amount of vomitus. Assess bowel function, including the passage of flatus. Auscultate for bowel sounds and document their character and location. Inspect the abdomen for scars, visible masses, and distention. Measure the abdominal girth, and check for signs of peritoneal irritation (e.g., muscle guarding, rebound pain, pain when the bed is shaken). If the surgeon decides to wait and see if the obstruction resolves on its own, assess the patient regularly and notify the surgeon of changes in vital signs, changes in bowel sounds, decreased urine output, increased abdominal distention, and pain.

Maintain a strict intake and output record, including emesis and tube drainage. A urinary catheter is ordered to monitor hourly urine outputs. Immediately report if the urine output is less than 0.5 mL/kg of body weight per hour because this indicates inadequate vascular volume and the potential for acute kidney injury. Rising serum creatinine and BUN levels are additional indicators of acute kidney injury.

NURSING DIAGNOSES

Nursing diagnoses for the patient with intestinal obstructions include, but are not limited to, the following:

- Acute pain *related to* abdominal distention and increased peristalsis
- Deficient fluid volume *related to* a decrease in intestinal fluid absorption, third space fluid shifts into the bowel lumen and peritoneal cavity, NG suction, and vomiting

PLANNING

The overall goals are that the patient with an intestinal obstruction will have (1) relief of the obstruction and return to normal bowel function, (2) minimal to no discomfort, and (3) normal fluid and electrolyte and acid-base status.

NURSING IMPLEMENTATION

Monitor the patient closely for signs of dehydration and electrolyte imbalances. Administer IV fluids as ordered. Watch for signs and symptoms of fluid overload, since some patients, especially older adults, may not tolerate rapid fluid replacement. Monitor serum electrolyte levels closely. A patient with a high intestinal obstruction is more likely to have metabolic alkalosis. A patient with a low obstruction is at greater risk for metabolic acidosis. The patient is often restless and constantly changes position to relieve the pain. Provide comfort measures and promote a restful environment. Nursing care of the patient after surgery for an intestinal obstruction is similar to care of the patient after a laparotomy (see pp. 970-971).

With an NG tube in place, oral care is extremely important. Vomiting leaves an unpleasant taste in the patient's mouth, and fecal odor may be present. The patient breathes through the mouth, drying the mouth and lips. Encourage and help the patient to brush the teeth frequently. Mouthwash and water for rinsing the mouth and water-soluble lubricant for the lips should be readily available to the patient. Check the nose for signs of irritation from the NG tube. Clean and dry this area daily, apply water-soluble lubricant, and retape the tube. Check the NG tube every 4 hours for patency.

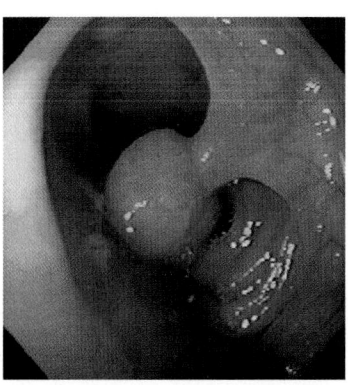

FIG. 43-6 Endoscopic image of pedunculated polyp in descending colon.

POLYPS OF LARGE INTESTINE

Colonic polyps arise from the mucosal surface of the colon and project into the lumen. They may be *sessile* (flat, broad based, and attached directly to the intestinal wall) or *pedunculated* (attached to the intestinal wall by a thin stalk). Polyps tend to be sessile when small and become pedunculated as they enlarge (Fig. 43-6). They may be found anywhere in the large intestine but are most commonly found in the rectosigmoid area. Rectal bleeding and occult blood in the stool are the most common signs. Most patients with polyps are asymptomatic.

Types of Polyps

The most common types of polyps are hyperplastic and adenomatous. *Hyperplastic polyps* are nonneoplastic growths. They rarely grow larger than 5 mm and never cause clinical symptoms. Other benign (nonneoplastic) polyps include inflammatory polyps, lipomas, and juvenile polyps.

Adenomatous polyps are neoplastic. They are closely linked to colorectal adenocarcinoma. The risk of cancer increases with polyp size. Removing adenomatous polyps decreases the occurrence of colorectal cancer.

Genetic Link

Familial adenomatous polyposis (FAP) is the most common polyposis syndrome (see the Genetics in Clinical Practice box). FAP is a genetic disorder characterized by hundreds or sometimes thousands of polyps in the colon that eventually become cancerous, usually by age 40. Since it is autosomal dominant, 50% of the offspring of a patient with FAP carry the FAP gene. Anyone with a family history of FAP should undergo genetic testing during childhood. If the FAP gene is present, colorectal screening begins at puberty, and annual colonoscopy begins at age 16. Since cancer is inevitable, the colon and rectum are removed, usually by age 25, and proctocolectomy with an IPAA or an ileostomy is performed (see p. 980). Patients with FAP are also at risk for cancers of the thyroid, small bowel, liver, and brain, so lifetime cancer surveillance is essential.[36]

Diagnostic Studies and Collaborative Care

Colonoscopy, sigmoidoscopy, barium enema, and virtual colonoscopy (CT or MRI colonography) are used to discover polyps. All polyps are considered abnormal and should be removed. Colonoscopy is preferred because it allows evaluation of the total colon, and polyps can be removed immediately *(polypectomy)*. Polyps can be detected but not removed during barium

GENETICS IN CLINICAL PRACTICE

Familial Adenomatous Polyposis (FAP)

Genetic Basis
- Classic form of disease
  - Autosomal dominant disorder.
  - Mutations in adenomatous polyposis coli *(APC)* gene.
  - Normally this is a tumor suppressor gene involved in DNA repair.
  - Normally this gene produces a special substance (a protein) that keeps polyps from developing in the colon.
- Autosomal recessive FAP
  - Autosomal recessive disorder.
  - Mutations in the *mutY* homolog *(MUTYH)* gene.
  - Normally this gene is involved in DNA repair.

Incidence
- Affects 1 in 6800 to 30,000 people.
- Men and women are affected equally.

Genetic Testing
- DNA testing is available.

Clinical Implications
- Accounts for at least 1% of all colorectal cancers.
- Classic FAP is characterized by colorectal polyps (usually hundreds to thousands).
- Polyps are not present at birth but appear during adolescence and early adulthood.
- Autosomal recessive FAP is characterized by fewer polyps, typically <100.
- If untreated, classic FAP almost always results in the development of colorectal cancer before age 40.
- With classic FAP, other benign and malignant tumors are sometimes found, especially in the duodenum, stomach, bones, skin, and other tissues.
- Many deaths related to FAP could be prevented with early and aggressive monitoring and treatment, including frequent colonoscopies and total colectomy.
- Individuals with a family history of FAP could benefit from genetic counseling.

enema and virtual colonoscopy. If the polyp is not removable during the colonoscopy, a biopsy specimen is taken to stage the cancer in preparation for surgery. After polypectomy, observe the patient for rectal bleeding, fever, severe abdominal pain, and abdominal distention, which may indicate hemorrhage or perforation.

COLORECTAL CANCER

Colorectal cancer (CRC) is the third most common form of cancer and responsible for 9% of cancer deaths. It is estimated that annually about 103,170 Americans are diagnosed with CRC.[28] The incidence of CRC is presented in eFig. 43-1 on the website for this chapter.

CRC is more common in men than in women. Mortality rates are highest among African American men and women. The risk of CRC increases with age, with about 90% of new CRC cases detected in people older than 50. However, the incidence of CRC in individuals over 50 is decreasing due to increased screening to detect precancerous lesions.

Etiology and Pathophysiology

Risk factors for CRC include a diet high in red or processed meat, obesity, physical inactivity, alcohol, long-term smoking,

🌐 CULTURAL & ETHNIC HEALTH DISPARITIES

Colorectal Cancer

- African Americans are at the highest risk compared with other ethnic groups.
- Incidence is declining in the United States except among African American men.
- Among Asian Americans, this is the second most commonly diagnosed cancer, and it is the third most frequent cause of cancer-related death.

and low intake of fruits and vegetables.[28] Genetic conditions such as FAP and a personal history of IBD place an individual at risk for CRC. About one third of cases of CRC occur in patients with a family history of CRC.

Hereditary diseases (e.g., FAP) account for about 5% to 10% of CRC cases. Hereditary nonpolyposis colorectal cancer (HNPCC) syndrome (also called Lynch syndrome) is the most common form of hereditary CRC (see the Genetics in Clinical Practice box).

Physical exercise and a diet with large amounts of fruits, vegetables, and grains may decrease the risk of CRC. Long-term use of NSAIDs (e.g., aspirin) is associated with reduced CRC risk. (See Table 43-21 for a list of risk factors.)

Adenocarcinoma is the most common type of CRC. Typically it begins as adenomatous polyps. Approximately 85% of CRCs arise from adenomatous polyps (see Fig. 43-6).

As the tumor grows, the cancer invades and penetrates the muscularis mucosae (see eFig. 43-2 on the website for this chapter). Eventually tumor cells gain access to the regional lymph nodes and vascular system and spread to distant sites. (The stages of tumor growth are shown in Fig. 43-7.) Since

🧬 GENETICS IN CLINICAL PRACTICE

Hereditary Nonpolyposis Colorectal Cancer (HNPCC) or Lynch Syndrome

Genetic Basis
- Autosomal dominant disorder.
- Mutations in *MSH2, MLH1, MSH6, PMS2* genes.
- These genes are involved in repair of mistakes when DNA is replicated.

Incidence
- Affects 1 in 500 to 2000 people.

Genetic Testing
- DNA testing is available.

Clinical Implications
- Accounts for 5% of all colorectal cancers.
- Individual with genetic mutation has 80% to 90% lifetime risk of developing colorectal cancer.
- People with HNPCC have an increased risk of cancers of stomach, small intestine, liver, gallbladder, upper urinary tract, brain, skin, and prostate. Occasionally, people with HNPCC also have colon polyps, which occur at an earlier age than do colon polyps in the general population and are more prone to become malignant.
- Individuals with known genetic mutations need to be monitored with colonoscopy every year.
- Women with HNPCC also have a greatly increased risk of endometrial and ovarian cancer.
- Examination by pelvic ultrasound and endometrial biopsy should also be considered to screen for endometrial cancer.

TABLE 43-21	RISK FACTORS FOR COLORECTAL CANCER

- Family history of colorectal cancer (first-degree relative)
- Personal history of inflammatory bowel disease
- Personal history of colorectal cancer
- Family or personal history of familial adenomatous polyposis (FAP)
- Family or personal history of hereditary nonpolyposis colorectal cancer (HNPCC) syndrome
- Obesity (body mass index ≥30 kg/m^2)
- Red meat (≥7 servings/wk)
- Cigarette smoking
- Alcohol (≥4 drinks/wk)

venous blood leaving the colon and rectum flows through the portal vein and the inferior rectal vein, the liver is a common site of metastasis. The cancer spreads from the liver to other sites, including the lungs, bones, and brain. CRC can also spread directly into adjacent structures.

Clinical Manifestations

CRC has an insidious onset, and symptoms do not appear until the disease is advanced. Common clinical manifestations include iron-deficiency anemia, rectal bleeding, abdominal pain, change in bowel habits, and intestinal obstruction or perforation.

Physical findings may include the following:
- *Early disease:* Nonspecific findings (fatigue, weight loss) or none at all
- *More advanced disease:* Abdominal tenderness, palpable abdominal mass, hepatomegaly, ascites

Right-sided lesions are more likely to bleed and cause diarrhea, while left-sided tumors are usually detected later and could present with bowel obstruction (Fig. 43-8).

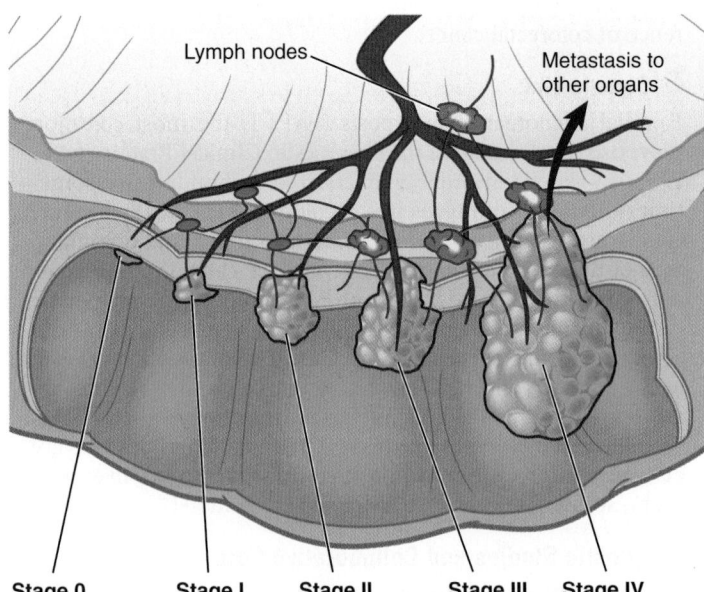

FIG. 43-7 The five stages of colorectal cancer. Stage 0 cancer has not grown beyond the mucosal layer. Stage I cancer has grown beyond the mucosa into the submucosa, but no lymph nodes are involved. Stage II cancer has grown beyond the submucosa into the muscle but there is no lymph node involvement or metastasis. Stage III cancer is any tumor with lymph node involvement but no metastasis. Stage IV cancer is any tumor with lymph node involvement and metastasis.

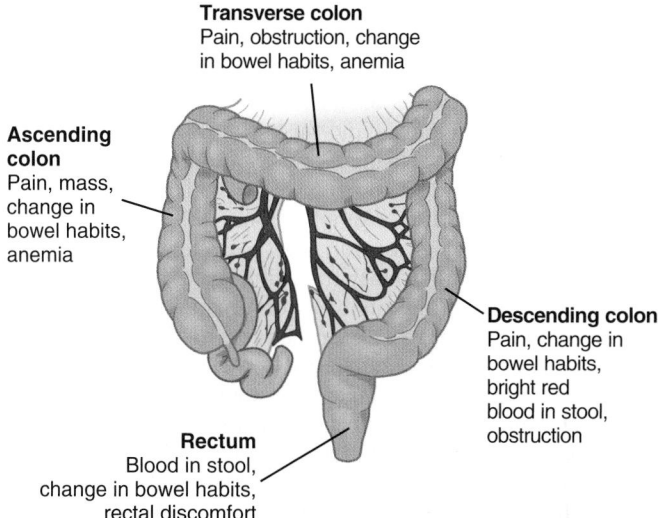

Transverse colon
Pain, obstruction, change in bowel habits, anemia

Ascending colon
Pain, mass, change in bowel habits, anemia

Descending colon
Pain, change in bowel habits, bright red blood in stool, obstruction

Rectum
Blood in stool, change in bowel habits, rectal discomfort

FIG. 43-8 Signs and symptoms of colorectal cancer by location of primary cancer.

Due to increased emphasis on screening practices, colon cancer is now often detected during screening procedures. Complications of CRC include obstruction, bleeding, perforation, peritonitis, and fistula formation.

Diagnostic Studies

Obtain a thorough history with close attention to family history (Table 43-22). Since symptoms of CRC do not become evident until the disease is advanced, regular screening is advocated to detect and remove polyps before they become cancerous. Beginning at age 50, both men and women at average risk for developing CRC should have screening tests to detect both polyps and cancer based on one of these testing schedules.[28]

Tests that find polyps and cancer include the following:
- Flexible sigmoidoscopy (done every 5 years)
- Colonoscopy (done every 10 years)
- Double-contrast barium enema (done every 5 years)
- CT colonography (virtual colonoscopy) (done every 5 years)

Tests that primarily find cancer include the following:
- Fecal occult blood test (FOBT) (done every year)
- Fecal immunochemical test (FIT) (done every year)

Colonoscopy is the gold standard for CRC screening because the entire colon is examined (only 50% of CRCs are detected by

sigmoidoscopy), biopsies can be obtained, and polyps can be immediately removed and sent to the laboratory for examination. People at average risk of CRC should have a colonoscopy every 10 years beginning at age 50, except for African Americans, who should have the first colonoscopy at age 45.[37]

Less favorable, but acceptable, screening methods include testing the stool for fecal blood. The FOBT and FIT look for blood in the stool. Stool tests must be done frequently, since tumor bleeding occurs at intervals and may easily be missed if a single test is done.

Persons at risk (see Table 43-21) should begin screening earlier and have screening done more often. Those who have a first-degree relative who developed CRC before age 60 or have two first-degree relatives with CRC should have a colonoscopy every 5 years beginning at age 40 or 10 years earlier than the youngest relative developed cancer. However, those who have one first-degree relative who had CRC after age 60 should have the same screening as the average at-risk person.

Once colonoscopy and tissue biopsies confirm the diagnosis of CRC, additional laboratory studies are done, including a CBC to check for anemia, coagulation studies, and liver function tests. A CT scan or MRI of the abdomen may be helpful in detecting liver metastases, retroperitoneal and pelvic disease, and depth of penetration of tumor into the bowel wall. However, liver function tests may be normal even when metastasis has occurred.

Carcinoembryonic antigen (CEA) is a complex glycoprotein sometimes produced by CRC cells. It may be used to monitor for disease recurrence after surgery or chemotherapy, but is not a good screening tool because of the large number of false positives.

Collaborative Care

The prognosis and treatment of CRC correlate with pathologic staging of the disease. The most commonly used staging system is the tumor, node, metastasis (TNM) staging (Table 43-23). As with other cancers, prognosis worsens with greater size and

---

TABLE 43-22 COLLABORATIVE CARE

Colorectal Cancer

Diagnostic	Collaborative Therapy
• History and physical examination	• Surgery
• Digital rectal examination	• Right hemicolectomy
• Testing of stool for occult blood	• Left hemicolectomy
• Barium enema	• Abdominal-perineal resection
• Sigmoidoscopy	• Laparoscopic colectomy
• Colonoscopy	• Chemotherapy
• CBC	• Targeted therapy
• Liver function tests	• Radiation therapy
• CT scan of abdomen	
• MRI	
• Ultrasound	
• Carcinoembryonic antigen (CEA) test	

TABLE 43-23 TNM CLASSIFICATION OF COLORECTAL CANCER

T	Primary Tumor
T_x	Primary tumor cannot be assessed because of incomplete information.
T_{is}	Carcinoma in situ. Cancer is in earliest stage and has not grown beyond mucosa layer.
T_1	Tumor has grown beyond mucosa into the submucosa.
T_2	Tumor has grown through submucosa into muscularis propria.
T_3	Tumor has grown through the muscularis propria into the subserosa but not to neighboring organs or tissues.
T_4	Tumor has spread completely through the colon or rectal wall and into nearby tissues or organs.

N	Lymph Node Involvement
N_x	Lymph nodes cannot be assessed.
N_0	No regional lymph node involvement is found.
N_1	Cancer is found in one to three nearby lymph nodes.
N_2	Cancer is found in four or more nearby lymph nodes.

M	Metastasis
M_x	Presence of distant metastasis cannot be assessed.
M_0	No distant metastasis is seen.
M_1	Distant metastasis is present.

TABLE 43-24	CLASSIFICATION SYSTEM USED TO STAGE COLORECTAL CANCER		
Stage*	TNM†	Duke's	Prognosis‡
0	$T_{is} N_0 M_0$		>96%
I	$T_1 N_0 M_0$	A	>90%
	$T_2 N_0 M_0$	B_1	85%
II	$T_3 N_0 M_0$	B_2	70%-80%
III	Any T, $N_1 M_0$	C	64%
IV	Any T, any N, M_1	D	8%

*Staging system is shown in Fig. 43-7. Staging is based on TNM classification.
†See Table 43-23.
‡Estimated 5-yr survival rates.

depth of tumor, lymph node involvement, and metastasis (Table 43-24).

Surgical Therapy. Goals of surgical therapy include (1) complete resection of the tumor together with adequate margins of healthy tissue, (2) a thorough exploration of the abdomen to determine if the cancer has spread, (3) removal of all lymph nodes that drain the area where the cancer is located, (4) restoration of bowel continuity so that normal bowel function will return, and (5) prevention of surgical complications.

Some polyps can be removed during colonoscopy, whereas others require surgery. Polypectomy during colonoscopy can be used to resect CRC in situ and is considered successful when the resected margin of the polyp is free of cancer, the cancer is well differentiated, and there is no apparent lymphatic or blood vessel involvement.

Reduction of colonic bacteria is recommended before surgery to prevent anastomotic leakage of bacteria and to decrease postoperative infection and abscess formation. The bowel is typically cleansed with a polyethylene glycol lavage solution (e.g., MiraLAX, GoLYTELY), and oral antibiotics are given to further decrease the amount of colonic and rectal bacteria.

The site of the CRC dictates the site of the resection (e.g., right hemicolectomy, left hemicolectomy). Surgical removal of stage I cancer includes removal of the tumor and at least 5 cm of intestine on either side of the tumor, plus removal of nearby lymph nodes. The remaining cancer-free ends are sewn back together. Laparoscopic surgery is sometimes used for stage I tumors, especially those in the left colon. Low-risk stage II tumors are treated with wide resection and reanastomosis, but chemotherapy is used in addition to surgery for high-risk stage II tumors.[38] Stage III tumors are treated with surgery and chemotherapy.

Once the cancer has spread to distant sites (stage IV), surgery is palliative and chemotherapy is directed at controlling the spread. Radiation may be used to provide pain relief.

If a patient has a perforation or peritonitis or is hemodynamically unstable, a temporary colostomy may be done. Then later the ends of the colon can be surgically reconnected.

In rectal cancer the surgeon has three major options: (1) local excision, (2) abdominal-perineal resection (APR) with a permanent colostomy, and (3) low anterior resection (LAR) to preserve sphincter function. The surgical decision is based on the location and staging of the cancer and ability to restore normal bowel function and continence. Most patients with rectal cancer require an APR or LAR. The LAR is used more frequently because of the potential for more normal control over defecation. When the tumor is not resectable or metastasis is present, palliative surgery is done to control hemorrhage or relieve a malignant bowel obstruction.

In APR, both the tumor and the entire rectum are removed and the person has a permanent colostomy. The perineal wound may be closed around a drain or left open with packing to allow healing by granulation. Complications that can occur are delayed wound healing, hemorrhage, persistent perineal sinus tracts, infections, and urinary tract and sexual dysfunctions.

An LAR may be indicated for tumors of the rectosigmoid and the mid to upper rectum. If the tumor is far enough from the anal sphincters, the sphincters may be left intact. The use of end-to-end anastomosis staplers has allowed lower (less than 5 cm from anus) and more secure anastomoses.

If the rectum is removed and the anal sphincters remain, an alternative reservoir with either a colonic J-pouch or coloplasty can be made. The colonic J-pouch is created by folding the distal colon back on itself and suturing it to form a pouch, which replaces the rectum as a reservoir for stool. The patient has a temporary colostomy to allow the J-pouch sutures time to heal before stool enters it. *Coloplasty* is an alternative to the pouch. It is created by slitting the side of a section of colon a short distance proximal to the anus, stretching the colon transversely to make it wider, and then suturing it closed in the new widened position. Patients with sphincter-sparing procedures may experience diarrhea, constipation, and incontinence even years after the procedure. The colonic J-pouch has decreased diarrhea and incontinence problems, but patients may have difficulty evacuating stool.

Chemotherapy and Targeted Therapy. Chemotherapy can be used to shrink the tumor before surgery, as an adjuvant therapy after colon resection, and as palliative treatment for nonresectable cancer. Adjuvant chemotherapy is recommended for patients with stage III tumors and high-risk stage II tumors. Current chemotherapy protocols include 5-fluorouracil (5-FU) and folinic acid (leucovorin) alone or in combination with oxaliplatin (Eloxatin). The preferred protocol includes oxaliplatin, but it may be omitted for patients who have too many side effects. Oral fluoropyrimidines (e.g., capecitabine [Xeloda]) have been found as effective as 5-FU/folinic acid monotherapy and can also be given in combination with oxaliplatin.[38]

DRUG ALERT: Capecitabine (Xeloda)
- Instruct patient not to get immunizations without physician's approval.
- Report temperature >100.4° F (38° C) immediately.

A variety of targeted therapies are used to treat metastatic CRC. Angiogenesis inhibitors, which inhibit the blood supply to tumors, include bevacizumab (Avastin) and ziv-aflibercept (Zaltrap). Regorafenib (Stivarga) is a multi-kinase inhibitor that blocks several enzymes that promote cancer growth. Cetuximab (Erbitux) and panitumumab (Vectibix) block the epidermal growth factor receptor.

Bevacizumab can also be used in combination with chemotherapy (e.g., fluoropyrimidine-oxaliplatin or fluoropyrimidine-irinotecan) to treat metastatic CRC. (Chemotherapy and targeted therapy are discussed in more detail in Chapter 16.)

Radiation Therapy. Radiation therapy may be used postoperatively as an adjuvant to surgery and chemotherapy or as a palliative measure for patients with metastatic cancer. As a palliative measure, its primary objective is to reduce tumor size and provide symptomatic relief. (Radiation therapy is described in Chapter 16.)

TABLE 43-25 NURSING ASSESSMENT

Colorectal Cancer

Subjective Data
Important Health Information
Past health history: Previous breast or ovarian cancer, familial polyposis, villous adenoma, adenomatous polyps, inflammatory bowel disease
Medications: Use of any medications affecting bowel function (e.g., laxatives, antidiarrheal drugs)

Functional Health Patterns
Health perception–health management: Family history of colorectal, breast, or ovarian cancer; weakness, fatigue
Nutritional-metabolic: High-calorie, high-fat, low-fiber diet; anorexia, weight loss; nausea and vomiting
Elimination: Change in bowel habits; alternating diarrhea and constipation, defecation urgency; rectal bleeding; mucoid stools; black, tarry stools; increased flatus, decrease in stool caliber; feelings of incomplete evacuation
Cognitive-perceptual: Abdominal and low back pain, tenesmus

Objective Data
General
Pallor, cachexia, lymphadenopathy (later signs)

Gastrointestinal
Palpable abdominal mass, distention, ascites, and hepatomegaly (liver metastasis)

Possible Diagnostic Findings
Anemia; guaiac-positive stools, palpable mass on digital rectal examination; positive sigmoidoscopy, colonoscopy, barium enema, or CT scan; positive biopsy

NURSING MANAGEMENT COLORECTAL CANCER

NURSING ASSESSMENT
Subjective and objective data that should be obtained from a patient with CRC are presented in Table 43-25.

NURSING DIAGNOSES
Nursing diagnoses for the patient with CRC include, but are not limited to, the following:
- Diarrhea or constipation *related to* altered bowel elimination patterns
- Fear and anxiety *related to* diagnosis of CRC, surgical or therapeutic interventions, and possible terminal illness
- Ineffective coping *related to* diagnosis of cancer and side effects of treatment

PLANNING
The overall goals are that the patient with CRC will have (1) normal bowel elimination patterns, (2) quality of life appropriate to disease progression, (3) relief of pain, and (4) feelings of comfort and well-being.

NURSING IMPLEMENTATION
HEALTH PROMOTION. Encourage all persons over 50 to have regular CRC screening. Help identify those at high risk who need screening at an earlier age. Participate in early cancer screening to help decrease mortality rates. Realize that barriers exist, including lack of information and fear of diagnosis.

Endoscopic and radiographic procedures can only reveal polyps when the bowel has been adequately prepared to eliminate stool. Provide teaching about bowel cleansing for outpatient diagnostic procedures, and administer cleansing preparations to inpatients. Generally, the patient is placed on a clear liquid diet for 24 to 48 hours before the procedure and is given 4 L of oral polyethylene glycol (PEG) lavage solution the evening before the procedure. Drinking 2 L the evening before and 2 L the morning of the procedure provides better cleansing, especially for endoscopy scheduled for the afternoon. Because many people find the PEG lavage solution difficult to drink and experience nausea and bloating, manufacturers have modified the PEG solutions to improve taste and palatability. Magnesium citrate solution or bisacodyl tablets are sometimes given before the PEG lavage to remove the bulk of stool so only 2 L of PEG are needed. Encourage the patient to drink all of the solution. Stools will be clear or clear yellow liquid when the colon is clean.

ACUTE INTERVENTION. Acute nursing care for the patient with a colon resection is similar to care of the patient having a laparotomy (see pp. 970-971). If the cancer was resected and the ends reanastomosed, bowel function is maintained and routine postoperative care is appropriate. Inform patients about prognosis and future screening. Provide support for dealing with the diagnosis of cancer. Patients who have an APR will have a permanent ostomy and need emotional support to cope with their prognosis and the radical change in body appearance and function.

Patients with more extensive surgery (e.g., APR) may have an open wound and drains (e.g., Jackson-Pratt, Hemovac) and a permanent stoma. Postoperative care includes sterile dressing changes, care of drains, and patient and caregiver teaching about the stoma. Consult with a wound, ostomy, and continence (WOC) nurse before surgery to select the ostomy site on the abdomen, and then provide follow-up care and teaching.

A patient who has open and packed wounds requires meticulous postoperative care. Reinforce dressings and change them frequently during the first several hours postoperatively when drainage is likely to be profuse. Carefully assess all drainage for amount, color, and consistency. The drainage is usually serosanguineous. Examine the wound regularly and record bleeding, excessive drainage, and unusual odor. Use aseptic technique with dressing changes.

If the patient's wound is closed or partially closed, assess the incision for suture integrity and signs and symptoms of wound inflammation and infection. Examine the drainage for amount, color, and characteristics. Observe the skin around the drain for signs of inflammation, and keep the area around the drain clean and dry. Monitor for edema, erythema, and drainage around the suture line, as well as fever and an elevated WBC count.

The patient may experience phantom rectal sensation because the sympathetic nerves responsible for rectal control are not severed during the surgery. Be astute in distinguishing phantom sensations from perineal abscess pain.

Sexual dysfunction is a possible complication of an APR. Although the likelihood of sexual dysfunction depends on the surgical technique used, the surgeon should discuss the possibility with the patient. Members of the health care team should be available to address the patient's questions and concerns. Erection, ejaculation, and orgasm involve different nerve pathways, and a dysfunction of one does not mean complete sexual dysfunction. The WOC nurse is an important source of information concerning sexual dysfunction resulting from an APR.

AMBULATORY AND HOME CARE. Psychologic support for the patient and caregiver is important. The cancer could return. Patients need much emotional support because recurrent cancer is painful, debilitating, and demoralizing. (The special needs of the cancer patient are discussed in Chapter 16.) Issues surrounding palliative care, end-of-life preparation, and hospice need to be addressed (see Chapter 10).

Patients with colostomies need to know how to care for them. Even when patients do not have stomas, they may experience diarrhea, constipation, incontinence, or difficulty passing stool depending on the section of the colon removed and the surgical procedure performed. Patients need to know about diet; incontinence products; and strategies for managing bloating, diarrhea, and bowel evacuation. Often a combination of dietary changes and drugs is used to control diarrhea and constipation.

Patients with sphincter-sparing surgery frequently experience diarrhea and incontinence of feces and gas. They often need antidiarrheal drugs or bulking agents to control the diarrhea, but may overuse them and become constipated. Consultation with a dietitian would help patients and caregivers understand how to choose foods that are less likely to cause diarrhea and odor and could help them discover which foods are problematic for them.

EVALUATION

The expected outcomes for the patient with CRC are that the patient will have

- Minimal alterations in bowel elimination patterns
- Balanced nutritional intake
- Quality of life appropriate to disease progression
- Feelings of comfort and well-being

OSTOMY SURGERY

Types

An **ostomy** is a surgical procedure that allows intestinal contents to pass from the bowel through an opening in the skin on the abdomen. The opening is called a **stoma.** The stoma is created when the intestine is brought through the abdominal wall and sutured to the skin. The intestinal contents then empty through the hole on the surface of the abdomen rather than being eliminated through the anus.

An ostomy is used when the normal elimination route is no longer possible. For example, if the person has CRC, the diseased portion is removed together with a certain margin of healthy tissue. Most stage I to III tumors of the colon can be resected, leaving enough healthy tissue to immediately *anastomose* the two remaining ends of healthy bowel, and no ostomy is necessary. If the tumor involves the rectum and is large enough to necessitate the removal of the anal sphincters, the

TABLE 43-26	**COMPARISON OF ILEOSTOMY AND COLOSTOMY**			
		Colostomy		
Characteristic	**Ileostomy**	**Ascending**	**Transverse**	**Sigmoid**
Stool consistency	Liquid to semiliquid	Semiliquid	Semiliquid to semiformed	Formed
Fluid requirement	Increased	Increased	Possibly increased	No change
Bowel regulation	No	No	No	Yes (if there is a history of a regular bowel pattern)
Pouch and skin barriers	Yes	Yes	Yes	Dependent on regulation
Irrigation	No	No	No	Possibly every 24-48 hr (if patient meets criteria)
Indications for surgery	Ulcerative colitis, Crohn's disease, diseased or injured colon, familial polyposis, trauma, cancer	Perforating diverticulum in lower colon, trauma, rectovaginal fistula, inoperable tumors of colon, rectum, or pelvis	Same as for ascending	Cancer of the rectum or rectosigmoidal area, perforating diverticulum, trauma

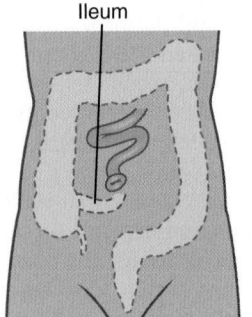

Ileostomy

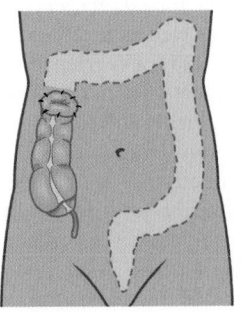

Ascending colostomy

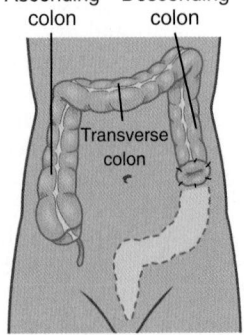

Descending colostomy

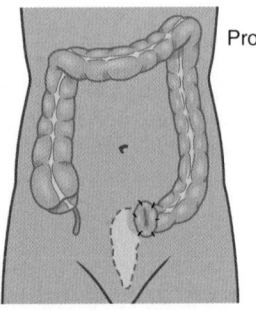

Sigmoid colostomy
single-barreled

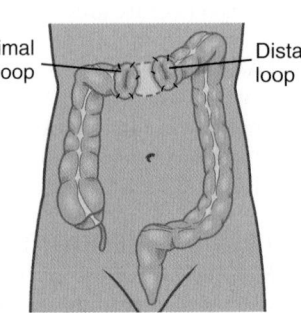

Transverse colostomy
double-barreled

FIG. 43-9 Types of ostomies.

anus is sutured shut and a permanent ostomy is created. Patients at high risk for CRC, such as those with FAP, and patients with ulcerative colitis may have a total colectomy.

Ostomies are described according to location and type (Fig. 43-9). An ostomy in the ileum is called an *ileostomy*. An ostomy in the colon is called a *colostomy*. The ostomy is further characterized by its anatomic site (e.g., sigmoid or transverse colostomy). The more distal the ostomy, the more the intestinal contents resemble feces that are eliminated from an intact colon and rectum. Output from an ileostomy has not entered the colon and thus is liquid. The ileostomy drains continuously, and the patient must constantly wear a bag to collect the drainage. In contrast, output from a sigmoid colostomy resembles normal formed stool, and some patients are able to regulate emptying time so they do not need to wear a collection bag. (See Colostomy Irrigations later in this chapter.) A comparison of colostomies and ileostomies is shown in Table 43-26.

Ostomies may be temporary or permanent. For example, the person with a draining fistula may need a temporary ostomy to prevent stool from reaching the diseased area. Patients who have trauma to the intestines (e.g., gunshot wound, stabbing) may need a temporary ostomy. Cancer involving the rectum requires a permanent ostomy because all bowel distal to the ostomy is removed.

The major types of ostomies are end stoma, double-barreled, and loop ostomy.

End Stoma. An end stoma is surgically constructed by dividing the bowel and bringing out the proximal end as a single stoma. The distal portion of the GI tract is surgically removed, or the distal segment is oversewn and left in the abdominal cavity with its mesentery intact. An end colostomy or ileostomy is then constructed. When the distal bowel is oversewn rather than removed, the procedure is known as a Hartmann's pouch (Fig. 43-10). In this procedure the potential exists for the bowel to be reanastomosed and the stoma to be closed (referred to as a *takedown*). If the distal bowel is removed, the stoma is permanent.

Loop Stoma. A loop stoma is constructed by bringing a loop of bowel to the abdominal surface and then opening the anterior wall of the bowel to provide fecal diversion. This results in one stoma with a proximal opening for feces and a distal opening for mucus drainage (from the distal colon). An intact posterior wall separates the two openings. The loop of bowel is

frequently held in place with a plastic rod for 7 to 10 days after surgery to prevent it from slipping back into the abdominal cavity (Fig. 43-11). A loop stoma is usually temporary.

Double-Barreled Stoma. When the bowel is divided, both the proximal and distal ends are brought through the abdominal wall as two separate stomas (see Fig. 43-9). The proximal one is the functioning stoma. The distal, nonfunctioning stoma is referred to as the mucus fistula. The double-barreled stoma is usually temporary.

NURSING MANAGEMENT
OSTOMY SURGERY

Two major aspects of nursing care are (1) emotional support as the patient copes with a radical change in body image and (2) patient and caregiver teaching about stoma care and the ostomy.[39] People with ostomies lose control over flatus and feces and worry about odor and leakage of feces from around the bag.[40] With time people learn to manage the stoma and make adjustments in work, social interactions, and sexual activities. People with new ostomies may be reluctant to return to work and avoid being around other people. Initially, patients may feel unattractive to their partners and unwilling to engage in sexual activities. However, with emotional support and teaching, patients can learn to manage the ostomy and return to their previous lifestyle.

PREOPERATIVE CARE

Major aspects of preoperative care that are unique to ostomy surgery include (1) psychologic preparation for the ostomy, (2) selection of a flat site on the abdomen that allows secure attachment of the collection bag, and (3) selection of a stoma site that will be clearly visible to the patient who will be taking care of it and is appropriate for clothing habits and activities.[41] Psychologic preparation and emotional support are particularly important as the person copes with the change in body image, the loss of control over elimination, and the odors. Provide the patient opportunities for verbalization of concerns and questions. This will enhance the patient's feelings of control and thus ability to cope.

A WOC nurse should select the site where the ostomy will be positioned and mark the abdomen preoperatively.[41-43] The site should be within the rectus muscle on a flat surface that the patient is able to see. Stomas placed outside the rectus muscle increase the chance of developing a hernia. A flat site makes it much easier to create a good seal and avoid leakage from

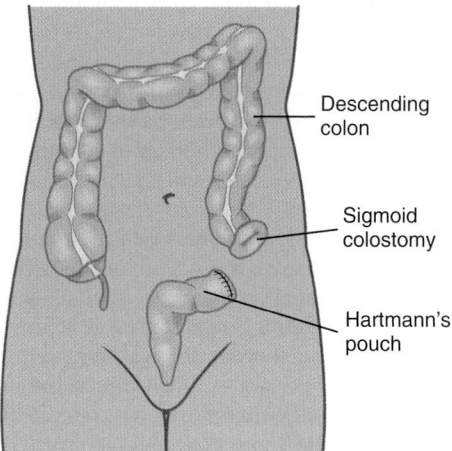

FIG. 43-10 Sigmoid colostomy. Distal bowel is oversewn and left in place to create Hartmann's pouch.

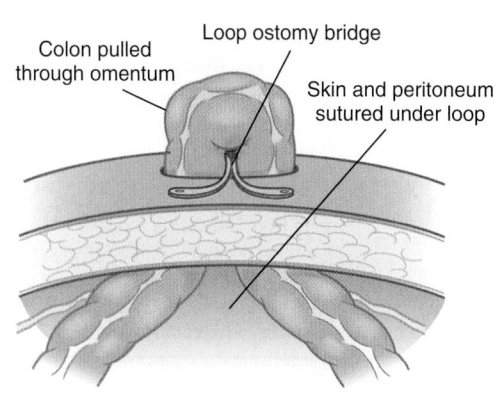

FIG. 43-11 Loop colostomy.

the bag. Patients who cannot see the stoma are unable to care for it.

The patient and caregiver usually have many questions concerning the procedures. If available, a WOC nurse should visit with the patient and the caregiver to determine the patient's ability to perform self-care, identify support systems, and determine any modifications that could facilitate learning during rehabilitation. The patient and the caregiver should understand the extent of surgery, the type of stoma, and related care.

Ask the patient if he or she would like to meet with a person who has adjusted to an ostomy. This gives the patient and caregiver an opportunity to question a person who has adjusted well to an ostomy and who has experienced some of the same feelings and concerns that they have.

POSTOPERATIVE CARE

Postoperative nursing care includes assessment of the stoma and provision of an appropriate pouching system that protects the skin and contains drainage and odor. The stoma should be dark pink to red. A dusky blue stoma indicates ischemia, and a brown-black stoma indicates necrosis. Assess and document stoma color every 4 hours and ensure that there is no excessive bleeding. Teach the patient that the stoma is mildly to moderately swollen the first 2 to 3 weeks after surgery (Table 43-27). A smaller pouch opening will be needed as the swelling goes down to accommodate the stoma's changing size. Determine the size of the stoma with a stoma-measuring card.

The colostomy starts functioning when peristalsis returns. When a temporary colostomy is performed on a colon that was not cleaned out before surgery, stool will drain when peristalsis returns. However, if the bowel was cleansed preoperatively, it will not begin producing stool until days after the surgery when the patient is eating again.

An appropriate pouching system is vital to protect the skin and provide dependable drainage collection. The various pouching systems all have an adhesive skin barrier and a bag or pouch to collect the feces. Flatus is expelled from the bag through a charcoal filter that helps control odor. The skin barrier is a piece of pectin-based or karaya wafer that has a measurable thickness and hydrocolloid adhesive properties. The adhesion occurs in two phases. First, the wafer's backing has adhesive material that forms an immediate bond with the skin. Second, the hydrocolloids interface with the moisture on the skin to form a tighter seal. If the abdominal stoma site has bends or creases, it is difficult to get a good seal and the skin barrier will pull away faster. Also, the weight of drainage from the stoma pulls the wafer away from the skin. For this reason, ostomy bags should be emptied when one-third full.

In the postoperative period an open-ended, transparent, plastic, odor-proof pouch is used to observe the stoma and collect the drainage. Record the volume, color, and consistency of the drainage. Each time the pouch is changed, observe the condition of the skin for irritation. Never place a pouch directly on irritated skin without the use of a skin barrier.

Teach the patient to perform a pouch change, provide appropriate skin care, control odor, care for the stoma, and identify signs and symptoms of complications. Instruct the patient about the importance of fluids and a healthy diet. Provide the names and addresses of United Ostomy Associations of America, and instruct the patient on when to seek health care. Home care and outpatient follow-up by a WOC nurse are highly recommended. Patients should be discharged with written information about their particular ostomy, instructions for pouch changes, a list of supplies and where to purchase them (including names and phone numbers of retailers), outpatient follow-up appointments with the surgeon and WOC nurse, and phone numbers of the surgeon and nurse. Patient and caregiver teaching guidelines are presented in Table 43-28.

Teaching is often complicated by the emotional responses to the stoma. Emotional support, interventions from skillful WOC nurses, and visits from people who have successfully learned to manage their ostomies will help patients learn to cope with and manage the new stoma.

COLOSTOMY CARE

Nursing care for the patient with a colostomy is presented in eNursing Care Plan 43-3 on the website. A colostomy in the ascending and transverse colon has semiliquid stools. Instruct the patient to use a drainable pouch. A colostomy in the sigmoid or descending colon has semiformed or formed stools and can sometimes be regulated by the irrigation method. For these patients, a drainage pouch may or may not be needed. Gas filters are available for both drainable and nondrainable pouches.

A well-balanced diet and adequate fluid intake are important, and most patients with colostomies can eat anything they choose. However, dietary modifications are helpful for decreasing gas production and odor. eTable 43-4 (on the website for this chapter) lists foods and their effects on stoma output.

Colostomy Irrigations. Colostomy irrigations may be used to stimulate emptying of the colon. When the colon is irrigated and emptied on a regular basis, no stool is eliminated between irrigation sessions. Irrigation requires manual dexterity and adequate vision. However, if bowel control is achieved, little or no spillage should occur between irrigations, and the patient may need to wear only a pad or small pouch over the stoma. Regularity is possible only when the stoma is in the distal colon. Irrigation is not used for more proximal ostomies. People who irrigate regularly should still have ostomy bags readily available in case they develop diarrhea from foods or illness. The proce-

TABLE 43-27	CHARACTERISTICS OF STOMA
Characteristic	**Description or Cause**
Color*	
Rose to brick-red	Viable stoma mucosa.
Pale	May indicate anemia.
Blanching, dark red to purple	Indicates inadequate blood supply to the stoma or bowel.
Edema†	
Mild to moderate edema	Normal in the initial postoperative period. Trauma to the stoma.
Moderate to severe edema	Obstruction of the stoma, allergic reaction to food, gastroenteritis.
Bleeding	
Small amount	Oozing from the stoma mucosa when touched is normal because of its high vascularity.
Moderate to large amount	Could indicate lower gastrointestinal bleeding, coagulation factor deficiency, stomal varices secondary to portal hypertension.

*Report sustained color changes to surgeon.
†Closely observe and report to the surgeon and adjust the stoma opening size in the pouch.

TABLE 43-28 **PATIENT & CAREGIVER TEACHING GUIDE**

Ostomy Self-Care

Include the following instructions when teaching the patient and/or caregiver about self-care of an ostomy.
1. Explain what an ostomy is and how it functions.
2. Describe the underlying condition that resulted in the need for an ostomy.
3. Demonstrate and allow the patient and caregiver to practice the following activities:
   • Remove the old skin barrier, cleanse the skin, and correctly apply new skin barriers.
   • Apply, empty, clean, and remove the pouch.
   • Empty the pouch before it is one-third full to prevent leakage.
   • Irrigate the colostomy to regulate bowel elimination (optional).
4. Explain how to contact the wound, ostomy, and continence (WOC) nurse with questions.
5. Describe how to obtain additional ostomy supplies.
6. Explain dietary and fluid management.
   • Identify a well-balanced diet and dietary supplements to prevent nutritional deficiencies.
   • Identify foods to avoid to reduce diarrhea, gas, or obstruction (with ileostomy).
   • Promote fluid intake of least 3000 mL/day to prevent dehydration (unless contraindicated).
   • Increase fluid intake during hot weather, excessive perspiration, and diarrhea to replace losses and prevent dehydration.
   • Describe symptoms of fluid and electrolyte imbalance.
   • Explain how to contact the registered dietitian with questions.
   • Explain how to recognize problems (fluid and electrolyte deficits, fever, diarrhea, skin irritation, stomal problems) and how to contact the appropriate health care provider.
7. Describe community resources to assist with emotional and psychologic adjustment to the ostomy.
8. Explain the importance of follow-up care.
9. Describe the ostomy's potential effects on sexual activity, social life, work, and recreation and strategies to manage these changes.

TABLE 43-29 **PATIENT & CAREGIVER TEACHING GUIDE**

Colostomy Irrigation

Include the following instructions when teaching the patient and caregiver to perform a colostomy irrigation.

Equipment*
Lubricant
Irrigation set (1000- to 2000-mL container, tubing with irrigating stoma cone, clamp)
Irrigating sleeve with adhesive or belt
Toilet tissue to clean around the stoma
Disposal sack for soiled dressing

Procedure
1. Place 500-1000 mL of lukewarm water (not to exceed 105° F [40.5° C]) in container. Titrate the volume for the individual; use enough irrigant to distend the bowel but not enough to cause cramping pain. Most adults use 500-1000 mL of water.
2. Ensure a comfortable position. Patient may sit in chair in front of toilet or on the toilet if the perineal wound is healed.
3. Clear tubing of all air by flushing it with fluid.
4. Hang container on hook or IV pole (18-24 in) above stoma (about shoulder height).
5. Apply irrigating sleeve and place bottom end in toilet bowl.
6. Lubricate stoma cone, insert cone tip gently into the stoma, and hold tip securely in place. The cone is designed to prevent perforation, control the depth of insertion, and prevent water from coming out of the stoma.
7. Allow irrigation solution to flow in steadily for 5-10 min.
8. If cramping occurs, stop the flow of solution for a few seconds, leaving the cone in place.
9. Clamp the tubing and remove irrigating cone when the desired amount of irrigant has been delivered or when the patient senses colonic distention.
10. Allow 30-45 min for the solution and feces to be expelled. Initial evacuation is usually complete in 10-15 min. Close off the irrigating sleeve at the bottom to allow ambulation.
11. Clean, rinse, and dry peristomal skin well.
12. Replace the colostomy drainage pouch or desired stoma covering.
13. Wash and rinse all equipment and hang to dry.

*Commercial sets usually have all the equipment that you will need.

dure for colostomy irrigation is similar to an enema and is presented in Table 43-29.

ILEOSTOMY CARE

An ileostomy stoma protrusion of at least 1 to 1.5 cm makes care easier. When the stoma is flat, seepage occurs, resulting in altered skin integrity. Drainage is frequent and extremely irritating to the skin. Since regularity cannot be established with an ileostomy, a pouch must be worn at all times. An open-ended, drainable pouch is preferable so drainage can be easily emptied. The drainable pouch is usually worn for 4 to 7 days before being changed, unless leakage occurs. In that case, the pouch should be promptly removed, the skin cleansed, and a new pouch applied. A solid skin barrier should always be used.

A transparent pouch should be used in the initial postoperative period to facilitate assessment of stoma viability and pouch application by the patient. Later on patients may prefer opaque pouches. (eNursing Care Plan 43-3 [on the website for this chapter] presents care of the patient with an ileostomy.)

Observe the patient with an ileostomy for signs and symptoms of fluid and electrolyte imbalance, particularly potassium, sodium, and fluid deficits. In the first 24 to 48 hours after surgery the amount of drainage from the stoma may be negligible. Patients with new ileostomies lose the absorptive functions provided by the colon and the delay provided by the ileocecal valve. As a result, they may experience a period of high-volume output of 1000 to 1800 mL/day when peristalsis returns. Later, as the proximal small bowel adapts, the average amount can be 500 mL/day. If the small bowel has been shortened by surgery, drainage from the ileostomy may be greater. Patients need to increase fluid intake to at least 2 to 3 L/day, or more when there are excessive fluid losses from heat and sweating. They may also need to ingest additional sodium. Patients must learn signs and symptoms of fluid and electrolyte imbalance so that they can take appropriate action.

A low-fiber diet is ordered initially, and fiber-containing foods are reintroduced gradually. The ileostomy patient is susceptible to obstruction because the lumen is less than 1 in in diameter and may narrow further at the point where the bowel passes through the fascia/muscle layer of the abdomen. Foods such as popcorn, coconut, mushrooms, olives, stringy vegetables, foods with skins, dried fruits, and meats with casings must be chewed extremely well before swallowing. The goal is for the patient to return to a normal, presurgical diet. If the terminal ileum has been removed, the patient may need cobalamin treatment.

DELEGATION DECISIONS

Ostomy Care

Although licensed practical/vocational nurses (LPN/LVNs) and unlicensed assistive personnel (UAP) provide much of the ostomy care for patients with established ostomies, patients with new ostomies have complex needs and require frequent assessment, planning, intervention, and evaluation by a registered nurse (RN).

Role of Registered Nurse (RN)
- Assess and document stoma appearance.
- For patient with a new ostomy, assess patient's psychologic preparation for ostomy care.
- Choose appropriate ostomy pouching system (skin barrier and bag or pouch) for patient.
- Place ostomy pouching system for a new ostomy.
- Develop plan of care for skin care around the ostomy.
- Teach ostomy care and skin care to patient and caregiver.
- Irrigate new colostomy.
- Teach colostomy irrigation to patient and caregiver.
- Teach patient and caregivers about appropriate dietary choices.
- Consult with wound, ostomy, and continence (WOC) nurse.

Role of Licensed Practical/Vocational Nurse (LPN/LVN)
- Monitor the volume, color, and odor of the ostomy drainage.
- Monitor the skin around the ostomy for breakdown.
- Provide skin care around the ostomy.
- Irrigate colostomy in stable patient.

Role of Unlicensed Assistive Personnel (UAP)
- Empty ostomy bag and measure liquid contents.
- Place the ostomy pouching system for an established ostomy.
- Assist stable patient with colostomy irrigation.

The stoma bleeds easily when it is touched because it has a high vascular supply. Tell the patient that minimal oozing of blood is normal.

ADAPTATION TO AN OSTOMY

Patients experience a grief reaction from the loss of a body part and an alteration in body image. They may feel like they are no longer normal and may experience shame and social isolation. People commonly feel anxiety and fear about stool leaking and the smells and sounds of flatus and stool entering the pouch. They are concerned about how the stoma will affect their lifestyle, including work, eating, sports, sex, and sleeping. They may be angry, depressed, or resentful.

Discuss the psychologic impact of the stoma and how it affects the patient's body image and self-esteem. Assist the patient in identifying ways of coping with depression and anxiety resulting from illness, surgery, or postoperative problems.[44]

Support from the caregiver, family, and friends is vitally important and reassures the patient that he or she is cherished and valued despite having the ostomy. Encourage patients to share their concerns and ask questions, provide information in a manner that is easily understood, recommend support services, and help patients develop confidence and competence in managing the stoma.

The patient can resume activities of daily living within 6 to 8 weeks but should avoid heavy lifting. The patient's physical condition determines when sports may be resumed. Some health care providers recommend avoiding participation in sports where direct trauma to the stoma is likely. Bathing and swimming may be done with or without the pouching system in place because water does not harm the stoma.

Patients want to know how to manage gas and body odors and how to choose clothing that will hide the stoma. Refer patients to the United Ostomy Associations of America (www.ostomy.org) for (1) practical information about living with an ostomy (e.g., ostomy products, irrigation, travel, sex), (2) contact information for local support groups, and (3) opportunities for online communication with other people with ostomies.

SEXUAL FUNCTION AFTER OSTOMY SURGERY

The patient with a stoma may fear rejection by a partner or that others will not find him or her desirable. Incorporate a discussion of sexuality and sexual function in the plan of care. Help the patient understand that sexual function or sexual activity may be affected, but sexuality does not have to be altered. Help the patient realize that it takes time to adjust to the pouch and to body changes before feeling secure in his or her sexual functioning. Also, a woman with an ostomy can still become pregnant.

Pelvic surgery can disrupt nerve and vascular supplies to the genitalia. Radiation therapy, chemotherapy, and medications can also alter sexual function. The patient's overall physical health influences sexual desire. Generalized fatigue caused by illness can also influence desire. Understanding this information can help patients better plan the timing of their sexual activity.

Erection of the penis depends on intact parasympathetic nerves and adequate blood supply to the pelvis and to pudendal nerves that transmit sensory responses from the genital area. Nerve-sparing surgical techniques are used when possible to preserve sexual function. Unfortunately, any pelvic surgery that removes the rectum has the potential of damaging the parasympathetic nerve plexus. Pelvic radiation can reduce blood flow to the pelvis by causing scarring in the small blood vessels. Muscle contraction and genital pleasure that occur during orgasm are not disrupted by pelvic surgery. If the sympathetic nerves in the male's presacral area are damaged, ejaculation may be disrupted. This can occur with the APR procedure.

DIVERTICULOSIS AND DIVERTICULITIS

Diverticula are saccular dilations or outpouchings of the mucosa that develop in the colon (Fig. 43-12). Multiple noninflamed diverticula are present in diverticulosis (see eFig. 43-3 on the website for this chapter). Diverticulitis is inflammation of the diverticula, resulting in perforation into the peritoneum. Clinically, diverticular disease covers a spectrum from asymptomatic, uncomplicated diverticulosis to diverticulitis with complications such as perforation, abscess, fistula, and bleeding.

Etiology and Pathophysiology

Diverticula are common, especially in older adults, but most people never develop diverticulitis.[45] Diverticula may occur anywhere in the GI tract but are most commonly found in the left (descending, sigmoid) colon. The etiology of diverticulosis of the sigmoid colon is thought to be associated with high luminal pressures from a deficiency in dietary fiber intake. The disease is more prevalent in Western, industrialized populations that consume diets low in fiber and high in refined carbohydrates. Diverticula are uncommon in vegetarians. Inadequate dietary fiber slows transit time, and more water is absorbed

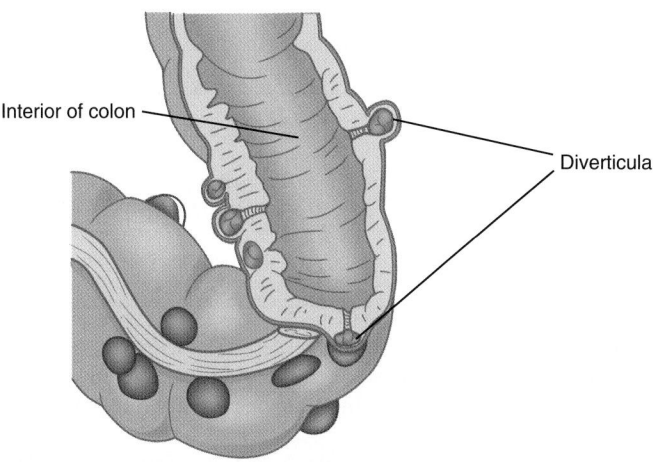

FIG. 43-12 Diverticula are outpouchings of the colon. When they become inflamed, the condition is diverticulitis. The inflammatory process can spread to the surrounding area in the intestine.

from the stool, making it more difficult to pass through the lumen. Decreased stool size raises intraluminal pressure, thus promoting diverticula formation.

Clinical Manifestations and Complications

The majority of patients with diverticulosis have no symptoms. Those with symptoms typically have abdominal pain, bloating, flatulence, or changes in bowel habits. In more serious situations, the diverticula bleed or diverticulitis develops. Diverticulitis is characterized by inflamed diverticula and increased luminal pressures that cause erosion of the bowel wall, and thus perforation into the peritoneum (Fig. 43-13). The most common symptoms of diverticulitis are acute pain in the left lower quadrant (location of sigmoid colon), a palpable abdominal mass, and systemic symptoms of infection (fever, increased C-reactive protein, and leukocytosis with a shift to the left).[45] Older adults with diverticulitis may be afebrile, with a normal WBC count and little, if any, abdominal tenderness. A localized abscess develops when the body is able to wall off the area of perfora-

TABLE 43-30 COLLABORATIVE CARE
Diverticulosis and Diverticulitis

Diagnostic
- History and physical examination
- Testing of stool for occult blood
- Barium enema
- Sigmoidoscopy
- Colonoscopy
- CBC
- Urinalysis
- Blood culture
- CT scan with oral contrast
- Abdominal x-ray
- Chest x-ray

Collaborative Therapy
Conservative Therapy
- High-fiber diet
- Dietary fiber supplements
- Stool softeners
- Anticholinergics
- Bed rest
- Clear liquid diet
- Oral antibiotics
- Mineral oil
- Bulk laxatives
- Weight reduction (if overweight)

Acute Care: Diverticulitis
- Antibiotic therapy
- NPO status
- IV fluids
- Bed rest
- NG suction
- Surgery
  - Possible resection of involved colon for obstruction or hemorrhage
  - Possible temporary colostomy

tion. Peritonitis develops if it cannot be contained. Bleeding can be extensive, but usually stops spontaneously.

Diagnostic Studies

Diverticular disease can be asymptomatic and is typically discovered during routine sigmoidoscopy or colonoscopy. Diagnosis of diverticulitis is based on the history and physical examination (Table 43-30). Abdominal and chest x-ray rule out other causes of acute abdominal pain, but the preferred diagnostic test is a CT scan with oral contrast.

NURSING AND COLLABORATIVE MANAGEMENT DIVERTICULOSIS AND DIVERTICULITIS

A high-fiber diet, mainly from fruits and vegetables, and decreased intake of fat and red meat are recommended for preventing diverticular disease. High levels of physical activity also seem to decrease the risk. A high-fiber diet (see Table 43-6) is also recommended once diverticular disease is present. Currently there is no evidence to support the theory that diverticulitis can be prevented by avoiding nuts and seeds.

Weight reduction is important for the obese person. A patient with diverticular disease should avoid increased intraabdominal pressure because it may precipitate an attack. Factors that increase intraabdominal pressure are straining at stool, vomiting, bending, lifting, and wearing tight restrictive clothing.

PATHOPHYSIOLOGY MAP

Diverticulitis

Acute → Chronic

Acute → Hemorrhage, Perforation, Pericolic abscess

Chronic → Pericolic abscess, Stricture

Perforation → General peritonitis

Pericolic abscess → Fistula

General peritonitis, Perforation, Pericolic abscess → Local suppuration

Stricture, Fistula → Intestinal obstruction

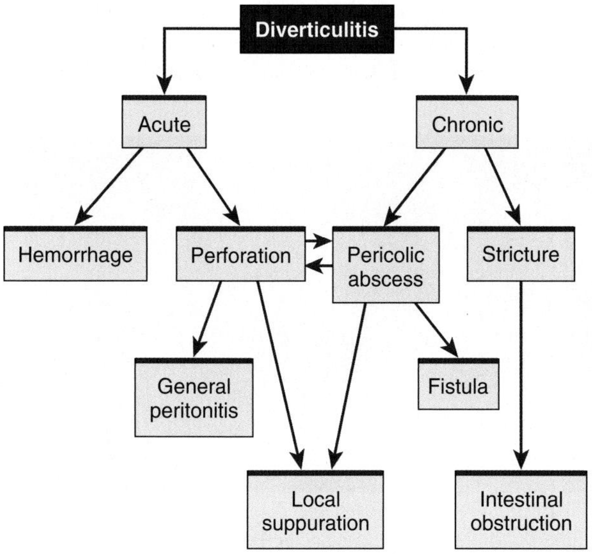

FIG. 43-13 Complications of diverticulitis.

In acute diverticulitis the goal of treatment is to let the colon rest and the inflammation subside. Some patients can be managed at home with oral antibiotics and a clear liquid diet. Hospitalization is necessary if symptoms are severe, the patient is unable to tolerate oral fluids, or the patient has co-morbid diseases.

Patients who are older, are immunosuppressed, or have systemic manifestations of infection (fever, significant leukocytosis) are hospitalized. If hospitalized, the patient is kept on NPO status and bed rest, and fluids and IV antibiotics are given. Observe for signs of abscess, bleeding, and peritonitis, and monitor the WBC count. When the acute attack subsides, give oral fluids first and then progress the diet to semisolids. Ambulation is allowed.

Surgery is reserved for patients with complications such as an abscess or obstruction that cannot be managed medically. The usual surgical procedures involve resection of the involved colon with either a primary anastomosis if adequate bowel cleansing is feasible or a temporary diverting colostomy. The colostomy is reanastomosed after the colon heals.

Provide the patient with diverticular disease with a full explanation of the condition. Patients who understand the disease process well and adhere to the prescribed regimen are less likely to experience an exacerbation of the disease and its complications.

HERNIAS

A hernia is a protrusion of the viscus (internal organ such as the intestine) through an abnormal opening or a weakened area in the wall of the cavity in which it is normally contained. A hernia may occur in any part of the body, but it usually occurs within the abdominal cavity (Fig. 43-14). Hernias that easily return to the abdominal cavity are called *reducible*. The hernia can be reduced manually or may reduce spontaneously when the person lies down. If the hernia cannot be placed back into the abdominal cavity, it is known as *irreducible* or *incarcerated*. In this situation the intestinal flow may be obstructed. When the hernia is irreducible and the intestinal flow and blood supply are obstructed, the hernia is strangulated. The result is an acute intestinal obstruction.

Types

The *inguinal hernia* is the most common type of hernia and occurs at the point of weakness in the abdominal wall where

the spermatic cord (in men) or the round ligament (in women) emerges (see Fig. 43-14, *C*). Inguinal hernias are more common in men.

A *femoral hernia* occurs when there is a protrusion through the femoral ring into the femoral canal. It appears as a bulge below the inguinal ligament. It easily becomes strangulated. It occurs more often in women (see Fig. 43-14, *B*). The *umbilical hernia* occurs when the rectus muscle is weak (as with obesity) or the umbilical opening fails to close after birth (see Fig. 43-14, *A*).

Ventral or *incisional hernias* are due to weakness of the abdominal wall at the site of a previous incision. They occur most commonly in patients who are obese, have had multiple surgical procedures in the same area, or have had inadequate wound healing because of poor nutrition or infection.

Clinical Manifestations

A hernia may be readily visible, especially when the person tenses the abdominal muscles. There may be some discomfort as a result of tension. If the hernia becomes strangulated, the patient will have severe pain and symptoms of a bowel obstruction such as vomiting, cramping abdominal pain, and distention. Strangulated hernias or painful, inflamed hernias that cannot be reduced require emergency surgery.[46]

NURSING AND COLLABORATIVE MANAGEMENT HERNIAS

Diagnosis is based on history and physical examination findings. Laparoscopic surgery is the treatment of choice for hernias. The surgical repair of a hernia, known as a *herniorrhaphy*, is usually an outpatient procedure. Reinforcement of the weakened area with wire, fascia, or mesh is known as a *hernioplasty*.

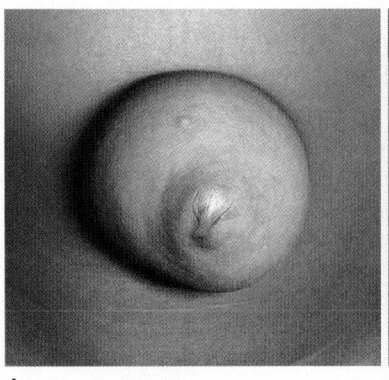
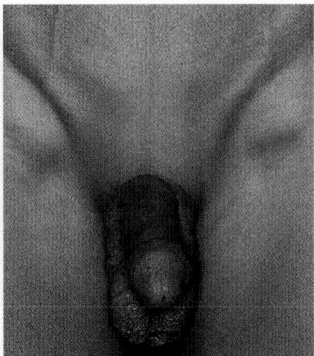
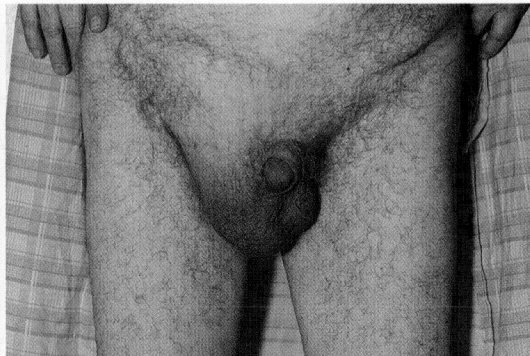

FIG. 43-14 A, Umbilical hernia. **B,** Femoral hernias (note swelling below the inguinal ligaments). **C,** Right inguinal hernia.

Strangulated hernias are treated immediately with resection of the involved area or a temporary colostomy so that necrosis and gangrene do not occur.

After a hernia repair, the patient may have difficulty voiding. Measure intake and output and observe for a distended bladder. Scrotal edema is a painful complication after an inguinal hernia repair. A scrotal support with application of an ice bag may help relieve pain and edema. Encourage deep breathing, but not coughing. Teach patients to splint the incision and keep their mouths open when coughing or sneezing are unavoidable. The patient may be restricted from heavy lifting for 6 to 8 weeks.

MALABSORPTION SYNDROME

Malabsorption results from impaired absorption of fats, carbohydrates, proteins, minerals, and vitamins. The stomach, small intestine, liver, and pancreas regulate normal digestion and absorption. Digestive enzymes ordinarily break down nutrients so that absorption can take place. If this process is interrupted at any point, malabsorption may occur. Several problems can cause malabsorption (Table 43-31). Lactose intolerance is the most common malabsorption disorder, followed by IBD, celiac disease, tropical sprue, and cystic fibrosis.

The most common signs of malabsorption are weight loss, diarrhea, and steatorrhea (bulky, foul-smelling, yellow-gray, greasy stools with putty-like consistency) (Table 43-32). Steatorrhea does not occur with lactose intolerance.

Tests used to determine the cause of malabsorption include qualitative examination of stool for fat (e.g., Sudan III stain), a 72-hour stool collection for quantitative measurement of fecal fat, serologic testing for celiac disease, and fecal elastase testing to determine if there is pancreatic insufficiency. Near-infrared reflectance analysis (NIRA) for fecal fat is available at some centers in the United States.

Other diagnostic studies include a CT scan and endoscopy to obtain a small bowel biopsy specimen. A small bowel barium enema may be performed to identify abnormal mucosal patterns. Capsule endoscopy can be used to assess the small intestine for alterations in mucosal integrity and inflammation. Tests for carbohydrate malabsorption include the D-xylose test and the lactose tolerance test. Laboratory studies that are frequently ordered include a CBC, measurement of prothrombin time (to see if vitamin K absorption is adequate), serum vitamin A and carotene levels, serum electrolytes, cholesterol, and calcium.

CELIAC DISEASE

Celiac disease is an autoimmune disease characterized by damage to the small intestinal mucosa from the ingestion of wheat, barley, and rye in genetically susceptible individuals.[47] It is a relatively common disease that occurs at all ages and has a wide variety of symptoms. *Celiac sprue* and *gluten-sensitive enteropathy* are other names for celiac disease.

Celiac disease is not the same disease as *tropical sprue*, a chronic disorder acquired in tropical areas that is characterized

TABLE 43-31	**CAUSES OF MALABSORPTION**
Biochemical or Enzyme Deficiencies	**Bacterial Proliferation**
• Lactase deficiency	• Tropical sprue
• Biliary tract obstruction	• Parasitic infection
• Pancreatic insufficiency	
• Cystic fibrosis	**Small Intestinal Mucosal Disruption**
• Chronic pancreatitis	• Celiac disease
• Zollinger-Ellison syndrome	• Whipple's disease
	• Crohn's disease
Disturbed Lymphatic and Vascular Circulation	
• Lymphoma	**Surface Area Loss**
• Ischemia	• Billroth II gastrectomy
• Lymphangiectasia	• Short bowel syndrome
• Heart failure	• Distal ileal resection, disease, or bypass

TABLE 43-32	**MANIFESTATIONS OF MALABSORPTION**
Manifestations	**Pathophysiology**
Gastrointestinal	
Weight loss	Malabsorption of fat, carbohydrates, and protein leading to loss of calories. Marked reduction in caloric intake or increased use of calories.
Diarrhea	Impaired absorption of water, sodium, fatty acids, bile salts, and carbohydrates.
Flatulence	Bacterial fermentation of unabsorbed carbohydrates.
Steatorrhea	Undigested and unabsorbed fat.
Glossitis, cheilosis, stomatitis	Deficiency of iron, riboflavin, cobalamin, folic acid, and other vitamins.
Hematologic	
Anemia	Impaired absorption of iron, cobalamin, and folic acid.
Hemorrhagic tendency	Vitamin C deficiency. Vitamin K deficiency inhibiting production of clotting factors II, VII, IX, and X.
Musculoskeletal	
Bone pain	Osteoporosis from impaired calcium absorption. Osteomalacia secondary to hypocalcemia, hypophosphatemia, inadequate vitamin D.
Tetany	Hypocalcemia, hypomagnesemia.
Weakness, muscle cramps	Anemia, electrolyte depletion (especially potassium).
Muscle wasting	Protein malabsorption.
Neurologic	
Altered mental status	Dehydration.
Paresthesias	Cobalamin deficiency.
Peripheral neuropathy	Cobalamin deficiency.
Night blindness	Thiamine deficiency, vitamin A deficiency.
Integumentary	
Bruising	Vitamin K deficiency.
Dermatitis	Fatty acid deficiency, zinc deficiency, niacin and other vitamin deficiencies.
Brittle nails	Iron deficiency.
Hair thinning and loss	Protein deficiency.
Cardiovascular	
Hypotension	Dehydration.
Tachycardia	Hypovolemia, anemia.
Peripheral edema	Protein malabsorption, protein loss in diarrhea.

by progressive disruption of jejunal and ileal tissue, resulting in nutritional difficulties. Tropical sprue is treated with folic acid and tetracycline.

Celiac disease is most common in people of European ancestry and affects about 1% of the population of the United States. High-risk groups include first- or second-degree relatives of someone with celiac disease and people with disorders associated with the disease such as migraine and myocarditis. It is slightly more common in women, and symptoms often begin in childhood.

Etiology and Pathophysiology

Three factors necessary for developing celiac disease are genetic predisposition, gluten ingestion, and an immune-mediated response.

Genetic Link

About 90% to 95% of patients with celiac disease have human leukocyte antigen (HLA) alleles HLA-DQ2, and the other 5% to 10% have HLA-DQ8. However, not everyone with these genetic markers develops celiac disease, and some people with celiac disease do not have these HLA alleles. (HLAs are discussed in Chapter 14.)

As with other autoimmune diseases, the tissue destruction that occurs with celiac disease is the result of chronic inflammation. Inflammation is activated by the ingestion of gluten found in wheat, rye, and barley. Gluten contains specific peptides called prolamines. In genetically susceptible individuals, partial digestion of gluten releases prolamine peptides, which are absorbed into the intestinal submucosa. The peptides then bind to HLA-DQ2 and/or HLA-DQ8 and activate an inflammatory response. Inflammation damages the microvilli and brush border of the small intestine, ultimately decreasing the amount of surface area available for nutrient absorption. Damage is most severe in the duodenum, probably because it has more exposure to gluten. The inflammation lasts as long as gluten ingestion continues.

Clinical Manifestations

Classic manifestations of celiac disease include foul-smelling diarrhea, steatorrhea, flatulence, abdominal distention, and malnutrition.[48] Some people have no obvious GI symptoms and may instead have atypical signs and symptoms such as decreased bone density and osteoporosis, dental enamel hypoplasia, iron and folate deficiencies, peripheral neuropathy, and reproductive problems. A pruritic, vesicular skin lesion, called *dermatitis herpetiformis,* is sometimes present and occurs as a rash on the buttocks, scalp, face, elbows, and knees.[48] Celiac disease is also associated with other autoimmune diseases, particularly rheumatoid arthritis, type 1 diabetes mellitus, and thyroid disease. The link between celiac disease and reproductive problems is less clear.

Protein, fat, and carbohydrate absorption is affected. Weight loss, muscle wasting, and other signs of malnutrition may be present. Abnormal serum folate, iron, and cobalamin levels can occur. Iron-deficiency anemia is one of the most common manifestations of celiac disease. Patients may exhibit lactose intolerance and need to refrain from lactose-containing products until the disease is under control. Inadequate calcium intake and vitamin D absorption can lead to decreased bone density and osteoporosis.

Diagnostic Studies and Collaborative Care

Early diagnosis and treatment can prevent complications. Screening is recommended for close relatives of patients known to have the disease, young patients with decreased bone density, those with anemia once other causes are ruled out, and certain autoimmune diseases.

Celiac disease is confirmed by (1) histologic evidence of the disease when a biopsy is taken from the small intestine and (2) the symptoms and histologic evidence disappearing when the person eats a gluten-free diet. Diagnostic testing must be done before the person is placed on a gluten-free diet, since the diet will alter the results. Serologic testing for immunoglobulin A (IgA) antitissue transglutaminase and IgA endomysial antibody provides good sensitivity and specificity. Histologic evidence remains the gold standard for confirming the diagnosis. Biopsies show flattened mucosa and noticeable losses of villi. Genotyping involves testing for HLA-DQ2 and/or HLA-DQ8 antigens. Many people spend years seeking treatment for nonspecific complaints before celiac disease is eventually diagnosed.

Treatment with a gluten-free diet (Table 43-33) halts the process. Most patients recover completely within 3 to 6 months of treatment, but they need to maintain a gluten-free diet for the rest of their lives. If the disease is untreated, chronic inflammation and hyperplasia continue. Individuals with celiac disease have an increased risk of non-Hodgkin's lymphoma and GI cancers.

Teach the patient to avoid wheat, barley, oats, and rye products. Although pure oats do not contain gluten, oat products can become contaminated with wheat, rye, and barley during the milling process. Gluten is also found in some medications and in many food additives, preservatives, and stabilizers. A combination of corticosteroids and a gluten-free diet is used to treat individuals with refractory celiac disease who do not respond to a gluten-free diet alone.

Maintenance of a gluten-free diet is difficult, particularly when traveling or eating in restaurants.[49-51] Therefore dietary consultation is imperative. The patient needs to know where to purchase gluten-free products. Gluten-free products are sold in health food stores, in many grocery stores, and through Internet

---

TABLE 43-33 NUTRITIONAL THERAPY

Celiac Disease

Foods to Eat*	Foods to Avoid
• Eggs	• Wheat
• Potatoes	• Barley
• Butter	• Oats
• Cheese, cottage cheese	• Rye
• Meat, fish, poultry (not marinated or breaded)	• Flour (unless it says gluten-free flour, or is made purely from a nongluten source, such as rice flour)
• Yogurt	
• Fresh fruits	
• Tapioca	• Baked goods, including muffins, cookies, cakes, pies
• Corn tortillas	
• Flax, corn, and rice	• Bread, including wheat bread, white bread, "potato" bread
• Soy products	
• Gluten-free breads, crackers, pasta, and cereals	• Pasta, pizza, bagels
• Unflavored milk	
• Peanut butter	
• Coffee, tea, and cocoa	

*Read food labels to look for gluten stabilizers or ingredients that contain gluten.

sites. Check the Internet to get a list of grocery stores that sell gluten-free products. Patients may need referral for financial assistance, since gluten-free products are more expensive than regular foods. The Celiac Sprue Association website *(www. csaceliacs.info)* and the Celiac Disease Foundation *(www. celiac.org)* provide suggestions for maintaining a gluten-free diet and living with celiac disease.

Continually encourage and motivate patients to continue the gluten-free diet. Reinforce that nonadherence to the diet will result in chronic inflammation, which can lead to complications such as anemia and osteoporosis.

LACTASE DEFICIENCY

Lactase deficiency is a condition in which the lactase enzyme is deficient or absent. Lactase is the enzyme that breaks down lactose into two simple sugars: glucose and galactose. Primary lactase insufficiency is most commonly a result of genetic factors. Certain ethnic or racial groups, especially those with Asian or African ancestry, develop low lactase levels in childhood. Less common causes include low lactase levels resulting from premature birth and congenital lactase deficiency, a rare genetic disorder. Lactose malabsorption can also occur when conditions leading to bacterial overgrowth promote lactose fermentation in the small bowel, and when intestinal mucosal damage interferes with absorption. The latter occurs with IBD and celiac disease.

The symptoms of lactose intolerance include bloating, flatulence, cramping abdominal pain, and diarrhea. Symptoms generally occur within 30 minutes to several hours after drinking a glass of milk or ingesting a milk product. The diarrhea of lactose intolerance results from fluid secretion into the small intestine, responding to the osmotic action of undigested lactose.

Many lactose-intolerant persons are aware of their milk intolerance and avoid milk and milk products. Lactose intolerance is diagnosed with a lactose tolerance test, a lactose hydrogen breath test, or genetic testing.

Treatment consists of eliminating lactose from the diet by avoiding milk and milk products and/or replacing lactase with commercially available preparations. Milk and ice cream contain more lactose than cheese. Live culture yogurt is an alternative source of calcium, but the patient needs to be sure that milk products have not been added to the yogurt.

A lactose-free diet is given initially and may be gradually advanced to a low-lactose diet as tolerated by the patient. Teach the patient that adherence to the diet is important. Many lactose-intolerant persons may not exhibit symptoms if lactose is taken in small amounts. In some persons, lactose may be tolerated better if taken with meals. Since avoidance of milk and milk products can lead to calcium deficiency, supplements may be necessary to prevent osteoporosis. Lactase enzyme (Lactaid) is available commercially as an over-the-counter (OTC) product. It is mixed with milk and breaks down the lactose before the milk is ingested.

SHORT BOWEL SYNDROME

Short bowel syndrome (SBS) is a condition in which the small intestine does not have adequate surface area to absorb enough nutrients. Thus the person is unable to meet energy, fluid, elec-trolyte, and nutritional needs on a standard diet. Causes of SBS include diseases that damage the intestinal mucosa, surgical removal of too much small intestine (primarily in patients with Crohn's disease), and congenital defects. Without adequate surface area, lifetime parenteral nutrition is necessary for survival.

Resections of up to 50% of the small intestine cause little disturbance of bowel function, especially if the terminal ileum and ileocecal valve remain intact. The remaining intestine undergoes adaptive changes that are more pronounced in the ileum. The villi and crypts increase in size, and the absorptive capacity of the remaining intestine increases.

Clinical Manifestations

The predominant manifestations of SBS are diarrhea and steatorrhea (unabsorbed fat in the stool). Signs of malnutrition as well as vitamin and mineral deficiencies include weight loss, cobalamin and zinc deficiency, and hypocalcemia. The patient may develop lactase deficiency and bacterial overgrowth. Oxalate kidney stones may form because of increased colonic absorption of oxalate.

Collaborative Care

The overall goals of treatment are that the patient with SBS will have fluid and electrolyte balance, normal nutritional status, and control of diarrhea. In the period immediately following massive bowel resection, patients receive parenteral nutrition to replace fluid, electrolyte, and nutrient losses and to rest the bowel. An antisecretory agent (histamine [H_2]-blocker or proton pump inhibitor) may be given to decrease gastric acid secretion.

A diet high in carbohydrate and low in fat supplemented with soluble fiber, pectin, and the amino acid glutamine is often recommended. The patient with SBS is encouraged to eat at least six meals per day to increase the time of contact between food and the intestine. Oral intake can be supplemented with elemental nutrient formulas and tube feeding during the night. For patients with severe malabsorption, parenteral nutrition (see Chapter 40) may be used.[52] Oral supplements of calcium, zinc, and multivitamins are typically recommended.

Teduglutide (Gattex) is used in SBS in patients who need additional nutrition from parenteral nutrition. It is a subcutaneous injection given once daily that helps to improve intestinal absorption of fluids and nutrients, reducing the frequency and volume of parenteral nutrition.

Opioid antidiarrheal drugs are the most effective in decreasing intestinal motility (see Table 43-2). For patients who have limited ileal resections (less than 39 in [99 cm]), cholestyramine (Questran) reduces diarrhea resulting from unabsorbed bile acids by increasing their excretion in feces. Bile acids stimulate intestinal fluid secretion and reduce colonic fluid absorption.

Intestinal transplantation is a procedure performed at a few specialized transplant centers in the United States. Candidates for this procedure are patients with SBS, dependence on parenteral nutrition, and chronic liver disease. It is often considered a last-resort treatment option for patients with intestinal failure who develop life-threatening complications from parenteral nutrition. Transplantation may include the intestine alone, liver and intestine, or multivisceral combinations (stomach, duodenum, jejunum, ileum, colon, and pancreas).

GASTROINTESTINAL STROMAL TUMORS

Gastrointestinal stromal tumors (GISTs) are a rare form of cancer that originates in cells found in the wall of the GI tract.[53] These cells, known as interstitial cells of Cajal, help control the movement of food and liquid through the stomach and intestines. About 55% of GISTs are found in the stomach; 35% are found in the small intestine; 5% are found in the rectum; and the rest are found in the esophagus, colon, or peritoneum.[53] GISTs are most frequently diagnosed in people between the ages of 50 and 70. Most GISTs are caused by genetic mutations.

The manifestations of GISTs depend on the part of the GI tract affected. Early manifestations are often subtle, including early satiety, bloating, nausea, and vomiting. Because these manifestations are similar to those of many other GI problems, the cancer is difficult to detect early. Later manifestations may include GI bleeding and obstruction caused by growth of the tumor. Often the GIST is found during evaluation (e.g., endoscopy, x-ray) for other problems such as CRC or stomach cancer. The diagnosis of GIST is based on histologic examination of biopsied tissue. Endoscopic ultrasound can be used to determine the extent of the tumor.

Patients initially undergo surgery to remove the tumor, but the GIST has often metastasized by the time of diagnosis or commonly recurs. GISTs are unresponsive to conventional chemotherapy. However, discovery of genetic mutations led to the development of tyrosine kinase inhibitor drugs (e.g., imatinib mesylate [Gleevec]) that are highly effective against GISTs.[43] (Targeted drug therapies are discussed in Chapter 16.)

ANORECTAL PROBLEMS

HEMORRHOIDS

Hemorrhoids are dilated hemorrhoidal veins. They may be internal (occurring above the internal sphincter) or external (occurring outside the external sphincter) (Figs. 43-15 and 43-16). Symptoms include rectal bleeding, pruritus, prolapse, and pain. In affected persons, hemorrhoids appear periodically, depending on the amount of anorectal pressure.

Etiology and Pathophysiology

Hemorrhoids develop as a result of increased anal pressure and weakened connective tissue that normally supports the hemorrhoidal veins. When supporting tissues in the anal canal weaken, usually as a result of straining at defecation, venules become dilated. In addition, blood flow through the veins of the hemorrhoidal plexus is impaired. An intravascular clot in the venule results in a thrombosed external hemorrhoid.

Hemorrhoids are the most common reason for bleeding with defecation. The amount of blood lost at one time may be small, but over time it may lead to iron-deficiency anemia. Hemorrhoids may be precipitated by many factors, including pregnancy, prolonged constipation, straining in an effort to defecate, heavy lifting, prolonged standing and sitting, and portal hypertension (as found in cirrhosis).

Clinical Manifestations

The classic manifestations of hemorrhoidal disease include bleeding, anal pruritus, prolapse, and pain. The patient with internal hemorrhoids may be asymptomatic. However, when internal hemorrhoids become constricted, the patient will

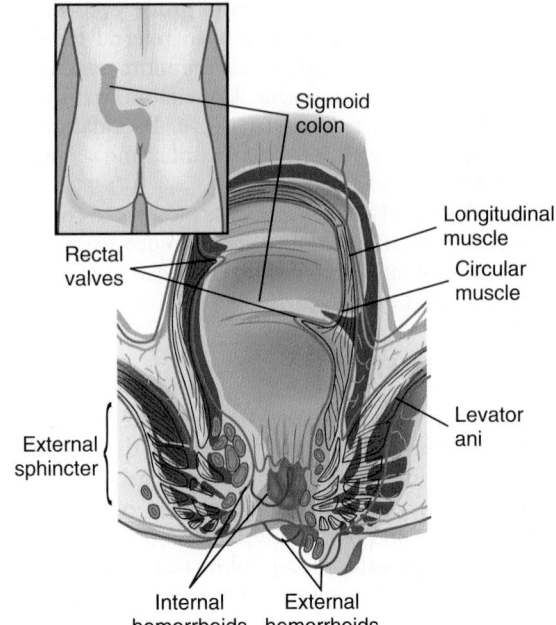

FIG. 43-15 Anatomic structures of the rectum and anus with external and internal hemorrhoids.

report pain. Internal hemorrhoids can bleed, resulting in blood on toilet paper after defecation or blood on the outside of stool. The patient may report a chronic, dull, aching discomfort, particularly when the hemorrhoids have prolapsed.

External hemorrhoids are reddish blue and seldom bleed. Blood clots in external hemorrhoids cause pain and inflammation, and the hemorrhoids are described as thrombosed. External hemorrhoids cause intermittent pain, pain on palpation, itching, and burning. Patients also report bleeding associated with defecation. Constipation or diarrhea can aggravate these symptoms.

Diagnostic Studies and Collaborative Care

Internal hemorrhoids are diagnosed by digital examination, anoscopy, and sigmoidoscopy. External hemorrhoids can be diagnosed by visual inspection and digital examination.

Therapy is directed toward the causes and the patient's symptoms. A high-fiber diet and increased fluid intake prevent constipation and reduce straining, which allows engorgement of the veins to subside. The resulting stool bulk may also decrease stool leakage and therefore itching. Ointments such as dibucaine; creams, suppositories, and impregnated pads that contain

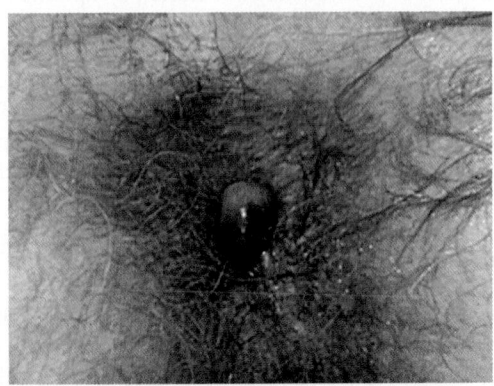

FIG. 43-16 Thrombosed external hemorrhoids.

antiinflammatory agents (e.g., hydrocortisone); or astringents and anesthetics (e.g., witch hazel, benzocaine) may be used to shrink the mucous membranes and relieve discomfort. The use of topical corticosteroids such as hydrocortisone agents should be limited to 1 week or less to prevent side effects such as contact dermatitis and mucosal atrophy. Stool softeners may be ordered to keep the stools soft, and sitz baths help relieve pain.

External hemorrhoids are usually managed by conservative therapy unless they become thrombosed. For internal hemorrhoids, nonsurgical approaches (rubber band ligation, infrared coagulation, cryotherapy, laser treatment) can be used. Rubber band ligation is the most widely used technique. An anoscope is inserted so the hemorrhoid can be identified and then ligated with a rubber band. The rubber band around the hemorrhoid constricts circulation, and the tissue becomes necrotic, separates, and sloughs off. There is some local discomfort with this procedure, but no anesthetic is required. Aspirin or acetaminophen is usually given for discomfort. Infrared coagulation can be used to treat bleeding internal hemorrhoids. In this procedure, either infrared or electric current produces local inflammation. Cryotherapy involves rapid freezing of the hemorrhoid.

A *hemorrhoidectomy* is the surgical excision of hemorrhoids. Surgery is indicated when there is prolapse, excessive pain or bleeding, or large hemorrhoids. In general, hemorrhoidectomy is reserved for patients with severe symptoms related to multiple thrombosed hemorrhoids or marked protrusion. Surgical removal may be done by cautery, clamp, or excision. One surgical approach is to leave the area open so that healing takes place by secondary intention. In another approach, the hemorrhoids are removed, the tissue is sutured, and wound healing takes place by primary intention.

NURSING MANAGEMENT
HEMORRHOIDS

Conservative nursing management for the patient with hemorrhoids includes teaching measures to prevent constipation, avoid prolonged standing or sitting, and properly use OTC drugs for hemorrhoidal symptoms. Teach the patient to seek medical care for severe symptoms of hemorrhoids (e.g., excessive pain and bleeding, prolapsed hemorrhoids). Sitz baths (15 to 20 minutes) two or three times each day for 7 to 10 days may help reduce discomfort and swelling associated with hemorrhoids.

Pain caused by sphincter spasm is a common problem after a hemorrhoidectomy. Be aware that although the procedure is minor, the pain is severe. Opioids are usually given initially. Postoperatively, topical nitroglycerin preparations may be used to decrease pain and subsequent opioid use.

Sitz baths are started 1 or 2 days after surgery. A warm sitz bath provides comfort and keeps the anal area clean. A sponge ring in the sitz bath helps relieve pressure on the area. Initially, the patient should not be left alone because of the possibility of weakness or fainting.

Packing may be inserted into the rectum to absorb drainage, with a T-binder used to hold the dressing in place. If packing is inserted, it usually is removed on the first or second postoperative day. Assess for rectal bleeding. The patient may be embarrassed when the dressing is changed, and privacy should be provided. The patient usually dreads the first bowel movement and often resists the urge to defecate. Pain medication may be given before the bowel movement to reduce discomfort.

A stool softener such as docusate (Colace) is usually ordered for the first few postoperative days. If the patient does not have a bowel movement within 2 or 3 days, an oil-retention enema is given. Teach the patient the importance of diet, care of the anal area, symptoms of complications (especially bleeding), and avoidance of constipation and straining. Sitz baths are recommended for 1 to 2 weeks. The health care provider may order a stool softener to be taken for a time. Hemorrhoids may recur. Occasionally, anal strictures develop and dilation is necessary. Regular checkups are important to prevent any further problems.

ANAL FISSURE

An *anal fissure* is a skin ulcer or a crack in the lining of the anal wall that is caused by trauma, local infection, or inflammation (Fig. 43-17). Fissures are considered either primary or secondary based on their etiology. *Primary fissures* usually occur as a result of local trauma, such as vaginal delivery. High pressure in the internal anal sphincter can result in ischemia, which can lead to fissuring. *Secondary fissures* are due to a variety of conditions, including IBD, prior anal surgery, and infection (syphilis; tuberculosis; gonorrhea; or infection with *Chlamydia*, herpes simplex virus, or HIV).

Anal tissue ulcerates because of ischemia caused by a combination of high resting anal sphincter tone and poor blood supply to the area. The ischemic tissue may ulcerate spontaneously or when traumatized by factors such as hard stools that would not normally cause tissue breakdown. If ischemia is not corrected, the anal fissures will not be able to heal.

The major symptoms are anal pain and bleeding. Pain is especially severe during and after defecation and has been described as "passing broken glass."[54] Bleeding is bright red and usually slight. Constipation results because of fear of pain associated with bowel movements.

Anal fissures are diagnosed through physical examination. Conservative care with fiber supplements, adequate fluid intake, sitz baths, and topical analgesics is successful in some cases, especially if the situation is acute. Topical preparations, including nitrates and calcium channel blockers, are used to decrease rectal anal pressure to allow the fissure to heal without sphincter damage. Local injections of botulinum toxin are also used to decrease rectal anal pressure, and are most effective when

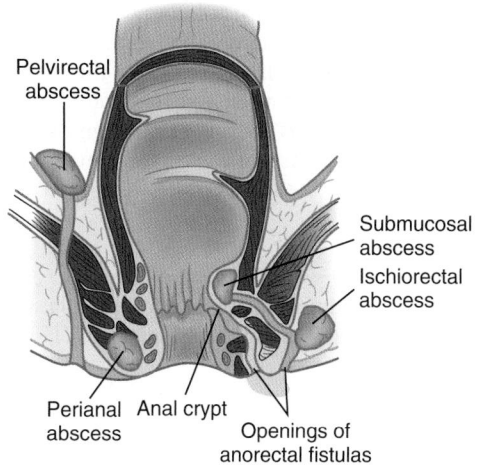

Pelvirectal abscess

Submucosal abscess

Ischiorectal abscess

Perianal abscess   Anal crypt   Openings of anorectal fistulas

FIG. 43-17 Common sites of anorectal abscesses and fistula formation.

combined with nitrates. Pain may be decreased by softening stools with mineral oil or stool softeners. Warm sitz baths (15 to 20 minutes, three times per day) and anal anesthetic suppositories with hydrocortisone (Anusol-HC) are also ordered.

If topical medications are ineffective, a lateral internal sphincterotomy is the recommended surgical procedure, but it carries the risk of postoperative incontinence. Postoperative nursing care is the same as the care for the patient who has had a hemorrhoidectomy.

ANORECTAL ABSCESS

An *anorectal abscess* is a collection of perianal pus (see Fig. 43-17). The abscess is the result of obstruction of the anal glands, leading to infection and subsequent abscess formation. Abscess formation can occur secondary to anal fissures, trauma, or IBD. The most common causative organisms are *Escherichia coli*, staphylococci, and streptococci. Clinical manifestations include local severe pain and swelling, foul-smelling drainage, tenderness, and elevated temperature. Sepsis can occur as a complication. Anorectal abscesses are diagnosed by rectal examination.

Surgical therapy consists of drainage of abscesses. If packing is used, it should be impregnated with petroleum jelly, and the area should be allowed to heal by granulation. The packing is changed every day, and moist, hot compresses are applied to the area. Care must be taken to avoid soiling the dressing during urination or defecation. A low-fiber diet is given. The patient may leave the hospital with the wound still open. Teach the patient about wound care and the importance of sitz baths, thorough cleaning after bowel movements, and follow-up visits to a health care provider.

ANAL FISTULA

An anal fistula is an abnormal tunnel leading from the anus or rectum. It may extend to the outside of the skin, vagina, or buttocks and often precedes an abscess. Anal fistulas are a complication of Crohn's disease and may resolve when drug treatment (i.e., with infliximab) achieves remission of the disease. About 50% of anal fistulas are due to anorectal abscess.

Feces may enter the fistula and cause an infection. There may be persistent, blood-stained, purulent discharge or stool leakage from the fistula. The patient may need to wear a pad to avoid staining clothes.

Surgical therapy involves a fistulotomy or a fistulectomy. In a fistulotomy the fistula is opened, and healthy tissue is allowed to granulate. A fistulectomy is an excision of the entire fistulous tract. Gauze packing is inserted, and the wound is allowed to heal by granulation. Care is the same as that given after a hemorrhoidectomy. In patients with complex fistulas, fibrin glue may be injected to seal the fistula.

ANAL CANCER

Anal cancer is uncommon in the general population, but the incidence is increasing. Human papillomavirus (HPV) is asso-ciated with about 80% of the cases of anal cancer. The American Cancer Society estimates that about 7100 people are diagnosed with anal cancer each year in the United States, with more women diagnosed than men.[55] Risk factors include having many sexual partners, genital warts (which are caused by HPV), smoking, receptive anal sex, and HIV infection. The average age at diagnosis is 60. Anal cancer is more common in African Americans than in whites.

Most frequently the initial symptom is rectal bleeding. Other symptoms include rectal pain and sensation of a rectal mass. Some patients have no symptoms, which leads to delayed diagnosis and treatment.

It is especially important to screen high-risk individuals. A swab of the anal mucosa can be obtained during a digital rectal examination. Identification of cell changes (e.g., dysplasia, neoplasia) can be determined. High-resolution anoscopy allows for visualization of the mucosa and biopsy. An endo-anal (*endorectal*) *ultrasound* may also be done.

The use of condoms to reduce the transmission of HPV is recommended. The HPV vaccine Gardasil is used for the prevention of anal cancer and associated precancerous lesions caused by HPV types 6, 11, 16, and 18. Gardasil is also approved for the prevention of cervical, vulvar, and vaginal cancer and the associated precancerous lesions caused by HPV in women. (It is also approved for the prevention of genital warts in men and women.) Another HPV vaccine, Cervarix, may also be useful in the prevention of HPV-associated anal cancer. After vaccination with HPV vaccine, patients at risk need to continue their recommended screening program.

Treatment of anal cancer depends on the size and depth of the lesions. Topical therapy with bichloroacetic or trichloroacetic acid may be used to kill the HPV virus. Imiquimod (Aldara), an immunomodulator, is also used as a topical agent. Therapy also includes surgery, radiation, and chemotherapy. Chemotherapy may include mitomycin, cisplatin (Platinol), and 5-FU.

PILONIDAL SINUS

A *pilonidal sinus* is a small tract under the skin between the buttocks in the sacrococcygeal area. It is thought to be of congenital origin. It may have several openings and is lined with epithelium and hair, hence the name *pilonidal* ("a nest of hair"). The skin is moist, and movement of the buttocks causes the short, wiry hair to penetrate the skin. The irritated skin becomes infected and forms a pilonidal cyst or abscess. There are no symptoms unless there is an infection. If it becomes infected, the patient complains of pain and swelling at the base of the spine.

The formed abscess requires incision and drainage. The wound may be closed or left open to heal by secondary intention. The wound is packed, and sitz baths are ordered. Nursing care includes warm, moist heat applications when an abscess is present. The patient is usually more comfortable lying on the abdomen or side. Teach the patient to avoid contaminating the dressing when urinating or defecating and to avoid straining whenever possible.

CASE STUDY

Colorectal Cancer

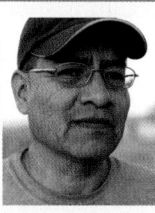

iStockphoto/Thinkstock

Patient Profile

L.C., a 58-year-old Native American man, is from a Pueblo tribe in northern New Mexico. L.C.'s wife and family drove 50 miles to take him to the Indian Health Service hospital because of his deteriorating health (see the case study in Chapter 39).

Subjective Data

See the case study in Chapter 39 on p. 874.

Objective Data

Physical Examination

See the case study in Chapter 39 on p. 877.

Laboratory Tests

- CT scan and colonoscopy show two medium-sized tumors in the transverse colon

Collaborative Care

Surgical Procedure

- Tranverse hemicolectomy performed and lymph node biopsies taken
- Pathology results indicate that the adenocarcinoma tumor has invaded the muscle wall of colon and 2 out of 5 lymph nodes are positive for cancer

Postoperative

- Feels like his life has ended and does not want to leave hospital.
- States that there is no one to take care of him at his home and he is far away from the hospital.

Follow-Up Treatment

- Scheduled for outpatient chemotherapy

Discussion Questions

1. What are the signs and symptoms of colorectal cancer that L.C. manifested (see the case study in Chapter 39 on p. 874)?
2. What types of diagnostic information are available from a colonoscopy versus a sigmoidoscopy?
3. What stage of CRC does L.C. probably have? What treatment is recommended for this stage of CRC?
4. How could you provide emotional support to L.C. and his family?
5. What is a culturally sensitive way for you to support L.C. and his family in making decisions about his continued health care?
6. **Priority Decision:** Based on the assessment data, what are the priority nursing diagnoses? Are there any collaborative problems?
7. **Priority Decision:** What are the priority nursing interventions for L.C. at this stage of his illness?
8. **Evidence-Based Practice:** L.C. had not had a previous colonoscopy. He is worried that other members of his family may have colon cancer. What can you tell him about the recommendations for colorectal cancer screening?

 Answers available at *http://evolve.elsevier.com/Lewis/medsurg.*

BRIDGE TO NCLEX EXAMINATION

The number of the question corresponds to the same-numbered outcome at the beginning of the chapter.

1. The appropriate collaborative therapy for the patient with acute diarrhea caused by a viral infection is to
   a. increase fluid intake.
   b. administer an antibiotic.
   c. administer antimotility drugs.
   d. quarantine the patient to prevent spread of the virus.

2. When a 35-year-old female patient is admitted to the emergency department with acute abdominal pain, which possible diagnosis should you consider that may be the cause of her pain *(select all that apply)?*
   a. Gastroenteritis
   b. Ectopic pregnancy
   c. Gastrointestinal bleeding
   d. Irritable bowel syndrome
   e. Inflammatory bowel disease

3. Assessment findings suggestive of peritonitis include
   a. rebound abdominal pain.
   b. a soft, distended abdomen.
   c. dull, continuous abdominal pain.
   d. observing that the patient is restless.

4. In planning care for the patient with Crohn's disease, the nurse recognizes that a major difference between ulcerative colitis and Crohn's disease is that Crohn's disease
   a. frequently results in toxic megacolon.
   b. causes fewer nutritional deficiencies than ulcerative colitis.
   c. often recurs after surgery, whereas ulcerative colitis is curable with a colectomy.
   d. is manifested by rectal bleeding and anemia more frequently than is ulcerative colitis.

5. The nurse performs a detailed assessment of the abdomen of a patient with a possible bowel obstruction, knowing that manifestations of an obstruction in the large intestine are *(select all that apply)*
   a. persistent abdominal pain.
   b. marked abdominal distention.
   c. diarrhea that is loose or liquid.
   d. colicky, severe, intermittent pain.
   e. profuse vomiting that relieves abdominal pain.

6. A patient with stage I colorectal cancer is scheduled for surgery. Patient teaching for this patient would include an explanation that
   a. chemotherapy will begin after the patient recovers from the surgery.
   b. both chemotherapy and radiation can be used as palliative treatments.
   c. follow-up colonoscopies will be needed to ensure that the cancer does not recur.
   d. a wound, ostomy, and continence nurse will visit the patient to identify an abdominal site for the ostomy.

7. The nurse explains to the patient undergoing ostomy surgery that the procedure that maintains the most normal functioning of the bowel is
   a. a sigmoid colostomy.
   b. a transverse colostomy.
   c. a descending colostomy.
   d. an ascending colostomy.

8. In contrast to diverticulitis, the patient with diverticulosis
   a. has rectal bleeding.
   b. often has no symptoms.
   c. has localized cramping pain.
   d. frequently develops peritonitis.

9. A nursing intervention that is most appropriate to decrease postoperative edema and pain after an inguinal herniorrhaphy is
   a. applying a truss to the hernia site.
   b. allowing the patient to stand to void.
   c. supporting the incision during coughing.
   d. applying a scrotal support with ice bag.

10. The nurse determines that the goals of dietary teaching have been met when the patient with celiac disease selects from the menu
    a. scrambled eggs and sausage.
    b. buckwheat pancakes with syrup.
    c. oatmeal, skim milk, and orange juice.
    d. yogurt, strawberries, and rye toast with butter.

11. What should a patient be taught after a hemorrhoidectomy?
    a. Take mineral oil before bedtime.
    b. Eat a low-fiber diet to rest the colon.
    c. Administer oil-retention enema to empty the colon.
    d. Use prescribed pain medication before a bowel movement.

1. a, 2. a, b, c, d, e, 3. a, 4. c, 5. a, b, 6. c, 7. a, 8. b, 9. d, 10. a, 11. d

evolve

For rationales to these answers and even more NCLEX review questions, visit *http://evolve.elsevier.com/Lewis/medsurg.*

REFERENCES

1. Navaneethan U, Giannella RA: Definition, epidemiology, pathophysiology, clinical classification, and differential diagnosis of diarrhea. In Guandalini S, Vaziri H, editors: *Diarrhea diagnostic and therapeutic advances*, New York, 2011, Humana.

2. McClarren RL, Lynch B, Nyayapati N: Acute infectious diarrhea, *Prim Care Clin Office Pract* 38:539, 2011.

3. Newton JM, Surawicz CM: Infectious gastroenteritis and colitis. In Guandalini S, Vaziri H, editors: *Diarrhea diagnostic and therapeutic advances*, New York, 2011, Humana.

4. Guandalini S: Probiotics for diarrheal disease. In Guandalini S, Vaziri H, editors: *Diarrhea diagnostic and therapeutic advances*, New York, 2011, Humana.

5. O'Keefe SJD: Tube feeding, the microbiota, and *Clostridium difficile* infection, *World J Gatroenterol* 16:139, 2010.

6. Weissman JS, Coyle W: Stool transplants: ready for prime time? *Curr Gastroenterol Rep* 14:313, 2012.

7. Hurnauth C: Management of faecal incontinence in acutely ill patients, *Nurs Stand* 25:48, 2011.

8. Fargo MV, Latimer KM: Evaluation and management of common anorectal conditions, *Am Fam Physician* 15:624, 2012.

*9. Bliss DZ, Savik K, Thorson MAL, et al: Incontinence-associated dermatitis in critically ill adults: time to development, severity, and risk factors, *J Wound Ostomy Continence Nurs* 38:433, 2011.

10. Chipps T: Using behavioural methods to manage faecal incontinence, *Br J Nurs* 20:1172, 2011.

11. Emmanuel A: Review of the efficacy and safety of transanal irrigation for neurogenic bowel dysfunction, *Spinal Cord* 48:664, 2010.

12. Marchetti F, Corallo JP, Ritter J, et al: Retention cuff pressure study of three indwelling stool management systems: randomized study of 10 healthy subjects, *J Wound Ostomy Continence Nurs* 38:569, 2011.

13. Apau D: Assessing the cause of constipation and appropriate interventions, *Gastrointestinal Nurs* 8:24, 2010.

*14. Zhou L, Lin Z, Lin L, et al: Functional constipation: implications for nursing interventions, *J Clin Nurs* 19:1838, 2010.

15. Roerig JL, Steffen KJ, Mitchell JE, et al: Laxative abuse: epidemiology, diagnosis, and management, *Drugs* 70:503, 2010.

*16. Michna E, Blonsky ER, Schulman S, et al: Subcutaneous methylnaltrexone for treatment of opioid-induced constipation in patients with chronic, nonmalignant pain: a randomized controlled study, *J Pain* 12:554, 2011.

17. Suares NC, Ford AC: Systematic review: the effects of fibre in the management of chronic idiopathic constipation, *Aliment Pharmacol Ther* 33:895, 2011.

18. Schein M: The acute abdomen. In Schein M, Rogers P, Assalia A, editors: *Schein's common sense emergency abdominal surgery*, Berlin, 2010, Springer Verlag.

19. Harris LA, Heitkemper MM: Practical considerations for recognizing and managing severe irritable bowel syndrome, *Gastroenterol Nurs* 35:12, 2012.

20. Gibson PR, Shepherd SJ: Evidence-based dietary management of functional gastrointestinal symptoms: the FODMAP approach, *J Gastroenterol Hepatol* 25:252, 2010.

21. Saadia R: Penetrating abdominal trauma. In Schein M, Rogers P, Assalia A, editors: *Schein's common sense emergency abdominal surgery*, Berlin, 2010, Springer Verlag.

22. Schein M: Abdominal compartment syndrome. In Schein M, Rogers P, Assalia A, editors: *Schein's common sense emergency abdominal surgery*, Berlin, 2010, Springer Verlag.

23. National Digestive Diseases Information Clearinghouse: Appendicitis. Retrieved from *http://digestive.niddk.nih.gov/ddiseases/pubs/appendicitis/appendicitis_508.pdf.*

24. Kaser A, Zeissig S, Blumberg RS: Inflammatory bowel disease, *Ann Rev Immunol* 28:573, 2010.

25. Lomer MCE: Symposium 7: nutrition in inflammatory bowel disease: dietary and nutritional considerations for inflammatory bowel disease, *Proc Nutr Soc* 70:329, 2011.

26. Hou JK, Abraham B, El-Serag H: Dietary intake and risk of developing inflammatory bowel disease: a systematic review of the literature, *Am J Gastroenterol* 106:563, 2011.

27. Berg AM, Kelly CP, Farraye FA: *Clostridium difficile* infection in the inflammatory bowel disease patients, *Inflamm Bowel Dis,* 19:194, 2013.

28. American Cancer Society: Colorectal cancer. Retrieved from *www.cancer.org/Cancer/ColonandRectumCancer/DetailedGuide/colorectal-cancer-detection.*

29. Fisher LR, Hasler WL: New vision in video capsule endoscopy: current status and future directions, *Nat Rev Gastroenterol Hepatol* 9:392, 2012.

30. Yanai H, Hanauer SB: Assessing response and loss of response to biological therapies in IBD, *Am J Gastroenterol* 106:685, 2011.

31. Masoomi H, Kang CY, Chaudhry O, et al: Predictive factors of early bowel obstruction in colon and rectal surgery: data from the Nationwide Inpatient Sample, 2006-2008, *J Am Coll Surg* 214:831, 2012.

32. Garq M, Lubel JS, Sparrow MP, et al: Review article: vitamin D and inflammatory bowel disease—established concepts and future directions, *Aliment Pharmacol Ther* 36:324, 2012.

*Evidence-based information for clinical practice.

33. del Val JH: Old-age inflammatory bowel disease onset: a different problem? *World J Gastroenterol* 17:2734, 2011.

34. Schein M: Small bowel obstruction. In Schein M, Rogers P, Assalia A, editors: *Schein's common sense emergency abdominal surgery*, Berlin, 2010, Springer Verlag.

35. Dolan EA: Malignant bowel obstruction: a review of current treatment strategies, *Am J Hospice Palliat Med* 28:576, 2011.

36. Framp A: Working toward understanding the impact of hereditary cancers, *Gastroenterol Nurs* 33:400, 2010.

37. American College of Gastroenterology: Colorectal cancer screening for African Americans. Retrieved from *http:// s3.gi.org/patients/ccrk/ColonCancerFinal.pdf*.

38. Labianca R, Nordlinger B, Beretta GD, et al: Primary colon cancer: ESMO clinical practice guidelines for diagnosis, adjuvant treatment and follow-up, *Ann Oncol* 21(Suppl 5):v70, 2010.

39. Landers M, Savage E, McCarthy G, et al: Self-care strategies for the management of bowel symptoms following sphincter-saving surgery for rectal cancer, *Clin J Oncol Nurs* 15:E105, 2011.

*40. Pittman J: Characteristics of the patient with an ostomy, *J Wound Ostomy Continence Nurs* 38:271, 2011.

41. Deitz D, Gates J: Basic ostomy management, part 1, *Nursing* 40:61, 2010.

42. Ostomy Guidelines Task Force: Management of the patient with a fecal ostomy: best practice guidelines for clinicians, *J Wound Ostomy Continence Nurs* 37:596, 2010.

43. United Ostomy Associations of America: Intimacy after ostomy surgery. Retrieved from *www.ostomy.org/ostomy_info/pubs/ uoaa_sexuality_en.pdf*.

44. Burch J: Resuming a normal life: holistic care of the person with an ostomy, *Br J Community Nurs* 16:366, 2011.

45. Weizman AV, Nguyen GC: Diverticular disease: epidemiology and management, *Can J Gastroenterol* 35:385, 2011.

*46. Mason RJ, Moazzez A, Sohn HJ, et al: Laparoscopic versus open anterior abdominal wall hernia repair: 30-day morbidity and mortality using the ACS-NSQIP data base, *Ann Surg* 254:641, 2011.

47. Ryan M, Grossman S: Celiac disease: implications for patient management, *Gastroenterol Nurs* 34:225, 2011.

48. Gainer CL: Celiac disease: helping patient live gluten-free, *Nurse Pract* 36:14, 2011.

*49. Smith MM, Goodfellow L: The relationship between quality of life and coping strategies of adults with celiac disease adhering to a gluten-free diet, *Gastroenterol Nurs* 34:460, 2011.

50. Armstrong MJ, Hegade V: Advances in coeliac disease, *Curr Opin Gastroenterol* 28:104, 2012.

51. Lee AR, Ng DL, Diamond B, et al: Living with celiac disease: survey from the USA, *J Hum Nutr Diet* 25:233, 2012.

52. Burns DL, Gill BM: Reversal of parenteral nutrition–associated liver disease with a fish oil–based lipid emulsion (Omegaven) in an adult dependent on home parenteral nutrition, *J Parenter Enteral Nutr* 37:274, 2013.

53. Joensuu H, DeMatteo RP: The management of gastrointestinal stromal tumors: a model for targeted and multidisciplinary therapy of malignancy, *Ann Rev Med* 63:247, 2012.

54. Fargo MW, Latimer KM: Evaluation and management of common anorectal conditions, *Am Fam Physician* 15:624, 2012.

55. American Cancer Society: Anal cancer. Retrieved from www.cancer.org/cancer/analcancer/detailedguide/anal-cancer -what-is-key-statistics.

RESOURCES

American Gastroenterological Association
www.gastro.org
American Society for Gastrointestinal Endoscopy (ASGE)
www.asge.org
Celiac Sprue Association
www.csaceliacs.info
Crohn's and Colitis Foundation of America (CCFA)
www.ccfa.org
International Ostomy Association
www.ostomyinternational.org
Society of Gastroenterology Nurses and Associates
www.sgna.org
Wound, Ostomy, and Continence Nurses Society
www.wocn.org

44

Life loves the liver of it.
Anne Elizabeth Alice Louise

Nursing Management
Liver, Pancreas, and Biliary Tract Problems

Anne Croghan

evolve WEBSITE

LEARNING OUTCOMES

1. Differentiate among the types of viral hepatitis, including etiology, pathophysiology, clinical manifestations, complications, and collaborative care.
2. Describe the nursing management of the patient with viral hepatitis.
3. Describe the pathophysiology, clinical manifestations, complications, and collaborative care of the patient with nonalcoholic fatty liver disease.
4. Explain the etiology, pathophysiology, clinical manifestations, complications, collaborative care, and nursing management of the patient with cirrhosis of the liver.
5. Describe the clinical manifestations and management of liver cancer.
6. Differentiate between acute and chronic pancreatitis related to pathophysiology, clinical manifestations, complications, collaborative care, and nursing management.
7. Explain the clinical manifestations, collaborative care, and nursing management of the patient with pancreatic cancer.
8. Describe the pathophysiology, clinical manifestations, complications, and collaborative care of gallbladder disorders.
9. Describe the nursing management of the patient undergoing surgical treatment of cholecystitis and cholelithiasis.

KEY TERMS

acute liver failure, p. 1027
acute pancreatitis, p. 1030
ascites, p. 1019
asterixis, p. 1021
biliary sludge, p. 1030
cholecystitis, p. 1036
cholelithiasis, p. 1036
chronic pancreatitis, p. 1034

cirrhosis, p. 1017
esophageal varices, p. 1019
gastric varices, p. 1019
hepatic encephalopathy, p. 1021
hepatitis, p. 1007
hepatorenal syndrome, p. 1021
jaundice, p. 1009

nonalcoholic fatty liver disease (NAFLD), p. 1016
nonalcoholic steatohepatitis (NASH), p. 1016
paracentesis, p. 1022
portal hypertension, p. 1019
spider angiomas, p. 1018

Reviewed by Paula Cox-North, RN, PhD, NP-C, Harborview Medical Center, Seattle, Washington; Trevah A. Panek, RN, MSN, CCRN, Assistant Professor of Nursing, Saint Francis University, Loretto, Pennsylvania; and Sally P. Scavone, RN, MS, Professor of Nursing, Erie Community College, Buffalo, New York.

Nursing management of patients with liver, pancreatic, and gallbladder problems is the focus of this chapter. Viral hepatitis, cirrhosis, acute pancreatitis, cholecystitis, and cholelithiasis are described in detail.

DISORDERS OF THE LIVER

HEPATITIS

Hepatitis is a broad term that means inflammation of the liver. Hepatitis is most commonly caused by viruses but can also be caused by drugs (alcohol), chemicals (see Table 39-6), autoimmune diseases, and metabolic abnormalities.

Viral Hepatitis

The types of viral hepatitis are A, B, C, D, and E. They differ in their modes of transmission and clinical manifestations (Table 44-1). The different hepatitis viruses can be responsible for both acute and chronic liver disease.

Other less common viruses can also cause liver disease. These include cytomegalovirus (CMV), Epstein-Barr virus (EBV), herpesvirus, coxsackievirus, and rubella virus.

Hepatitis A Virus. Hepatitis A viral infection can cause a mild flu-like illness or acute hepatitis with jaundice. It can also cause acute liver failure. It does not result in a chronic (long-term) infection. In the United States the incidence of hepatitis A viral infection has declined since vaccination was recommended for at-risk persons and children (at the age of 1 year).[1]

Hepatitis A virus (HAV) is a ribonucleic acid (RNA) virus that is transmitted primarily through the fecal-oral route. It frequently occurs in small outbreaks caused by fecal contamination of food or drinking water. Poor hygiene, improper handling of food, crowded situations, and poor sanitary conditions are contributing factors. Transmission occurs between family members, institutionalized individuals, and children in day care centers. Foodborne hepatitis A outbreaks are usually due to food contaminated by an infected food handler.

The virus is present in feces during the incubation period, so it can be carried and transmitted by persons who have undetectable, subclinical infections. The greatest risk of transmission occurs before clinical symptoms are apparent. HAV is found in feces 2 or more weeks before the onset of symptoms and up to 1 week after the onset of jaundice (Fig. 44-1). It is present only briefly in blood. Anti-HAV (antibody to HAV) immunoglobulin (Ig) M appears in the serum as the stool becomes negative for the virus. Detection of hepatitis A IgM indicates acute hepatitis. Although not commonly tested clinically, hepatitis A IgG indicates past infection. IgG antibody

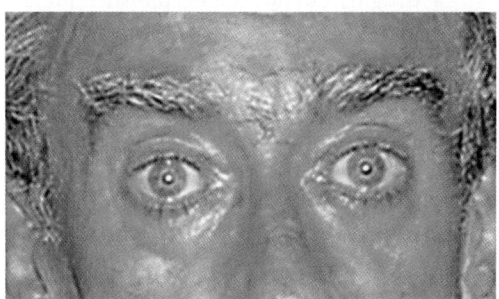

FIG. 44-1 Jaundiced patient.

TABLE 44-1 CHARACTERISTICS OF HEPATITIS VIRUSES

Incubation Period and Mode of Transmission	Sources of Infection	Infectivity
Hepatitis A Virus (HAV) 15-50 days (average 28) Fecal-oral (primarily fecal contamination and oral ingestion)	Crowded conditions (e.g., day care, nursing home). Poor personal hygiene. Poor sanitation. Contaminated food, milk, water, shellfish. Persons with subclinical infections, infected food handlers; sexual contact, IV drug users.	Most infectious during 2 wk before onset of symptoms. Infectious until 1-2 wk after the start of symptoms.
Hepatitis B Virus (HBV) 45-180 days (average 56-96) Percutaneous (parenteral) or permucosal exposure to blood or blood products Sexual contact Perinatal transmission	Contaminated needles, syringes, and blood products. Sexual activity with infected partners. Asymptomatic carriers. Tattoos or body piercing with contaminated needles.	Before and after symptoms appear. Infectious for 4-6 mo. Carriers continue to be infectious for life.
Hepatitis C Virus (HCV) 14-180 days (average 56) Percutaneous (parenteral) or mucosal exposure to blood or blood products High-risk sexual contact Perinatal contact	Blood and blood products. Needles and syringes. Sexual activity with infected partners.	1-2 wk before symptoms appear. Continues during clinical course. 75%-85% go on to develop chronic hepatitis C and remain infectious.
Hepatitis D Virus (HDV) 2-26 wk HBV must precede HDV Chronic carriers of HBV always at risk	Same as HBV. Can cause infection only when HBV is present. Routes of transmission same as for HBV.	Blood infectious at all stages of HDV infection.
Hepatitis E Virus (HEV) 15-64 days (average 26-42 days) Fecal-oral route Outbreaks associated with contaminated water supply in developing countries	Contaminated water, poor sanitation. Found in Asia, Africa, and Mexico. Not common in United States.	Not known. May be similar to HAV.

provides lifelong immunity (Fig. 44-2). Hepatitis A vaccination and thorough hand washing are the best measures to prevent outbreaks.

Hepatitis B Virus. Hepatitis B virus (HBV) can cause either acute or chronic disease. Transmission occurs when the virus (from infected blood or body fluids) enters the body of an uninfected person who has not received the HBV vaccine. Since the 1990s, the incidence of HBV infection has decreased because of the widespread use of the HBV vaccine.[1]

About 12 million Americans have been infected with HBV. In the majority of adults with acute hepatitis B, the infection completely resolves. Of the more than 1 million Americans who develop chronic infections, liver impairment may range from a normal liver to severe liver disease. Approximately 15% to 25% of chronically infected persons die from chronic liver disease.

HBV is a deoxyribonucleic acid (DNA) virus. It can be transmitted perinatally by mothers infected with HBV; percutaneously (e.g., IV drug use, accidental needle-stick punctures); or

by mucosal exposure to infectious blood, blood products, or other body fluids (e.g., semen, vaginal secretions, saliva). In people with HBV, hepatitis B surface antigen (HBsAg) has been detected in almost every body fluid. Infected semen and saliva contain much lower concentrations of HBV than blood, but the virus can be transmitted via these secretions. If gastrointestinal (GI) bleeding occurs, feces can be contaminated with the virus from the blood. There is no evidence that urine, feces (without GI bleeding), breast milk, tears, and sweat are infective. Organ and tissue transplantation is another potential source of infection. In some patients with acute hepatitis B, there is no readily identifiable risk factor.[1]

Sexual transmission is a common mode of HBV transmission. Men who have sex with men (especially those practicing unprotected anal intercourse) are at risk for HBV infection. Although the risk of transmission is much lower, kissing and sharing food items may spread the virus via saliva. Other at-risk individuals include those who live with chronically infected persons, hemodialysis patients, and health care and public safety workers. HBV can live on a dry surface for at least 7 days; it is much more infectious than human immunodeficiency virus (HIV).

HBV is a complex structure with three distinct antigens: the surface antigen (HBsAg), the core antigen (HBcAg), and the e antigen (HBeAg). HBsAg in the serum for 6 months or longer after infection indicates chronic HBV infection. Each antigen has a corresponding antibody that may develop in response to HBV infection. The presence of hepatitis B surface antibody (anti-HBs) in the blood indicates immunity from the HBV vaccine or from past HBV infection (Fig. 44-3).

Hepatitis C Virus. Infection with the hepatitis C virus (HCV) can result in both acute and chronic illness. Acute hepatitis C, which is usually asymptomatic, can be difficult to detect unless diagnosed with laboratory testing. The most common causes of acute hepatitis C are injection drug use and outbreaks among HIV-positive men who have sex with men.

The majority of patients who acquire hepatitis C usually develop chronic infection.[2] Most are unaware of their infection. Chronic HCV results in a potentially progressive liver disease, with 20% to 30% of these patients developing cirrhosis. Hepa-

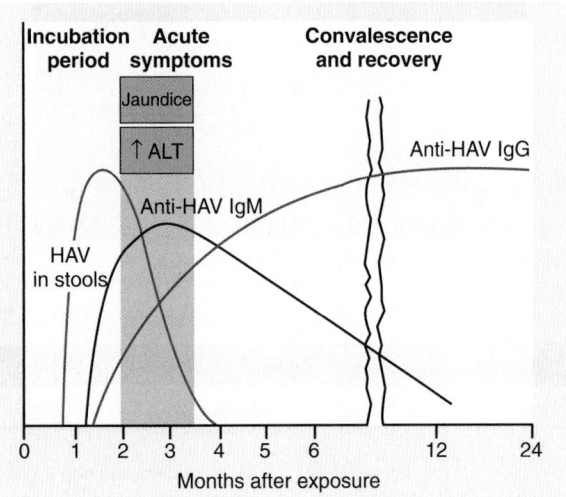

FIG. 44-2 Course of infection with hepatitis A virus *(HAV)*. *ALT,* Alanine aminotransferase.

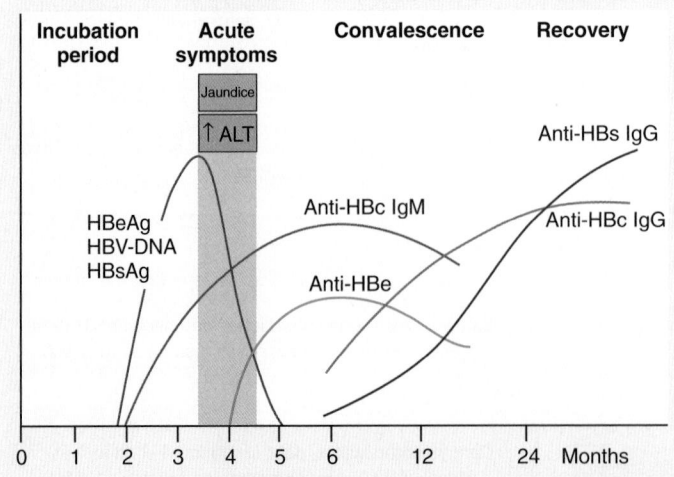

FIG. 44-3 Course of infection with hepatitis B virus *(HBV)*. *ALT,* Alanine aminotransferase; *anti-HBc,* antibody to hepatitis B core antigen; *anti-HBe,* antibody to HBeAg; *anti-HBs,* antibody to HBsAg; *HBeAg,* hepatitis B e antigen; *HBsAg,* hepatitis B surface antigen.

titis C is the most common cause of chronic liver disease and the most common indication for liver transplantation in the United States.[3]

HCV is an RNA virus that is primarily transmitted percutaneously. The most common mode of HCV transmission is the sharing of contaminated needles and equipment among IV drug users.

The proportion of cases attributed to high-risk sexual behavior (e.g., unprotected sex, multiple partners) has increased in recent years. In the United States, 10% of all cases of HCV infection are due to occupational exposure, hemodialysis, and perinatal transmission.[2] Some patients with HCV cannot identify a source. The risk of perinatal HCV transmission is higher in women who are co-infected with both HIV and HCV.

Patients given blood or blood products before 1992 (when blood product testing for HCV began) may be at risk for chronic HCV infection and should be tested. Because of the 15- to 20-year delay between infection and the clinical appearance of liver damage, long-term effects of HCV infection pose important future health care challenges. Chronic HBV and HCV account for 80% of the cases of hepatocellular cancer.

Persons at risk for HCV infection are also at risk for HBV and HIV infections. About 30% to 40% of HIV-infected patients also have HCV. This high rate of co-infection is primarily related to IV drug use. Co-infection with HIV and HCV places the patient at greater risk for progression to cirrhosis.

Hepatitis D Virus. Hepatitis D virus (HDV), also called *delta virus,* is a defective single-stranded RNA virus that cannot survive on its own. It requires hepatitis B to replicate. It can be acquired at the same time as HBV, or a person with HBV can be infected with HDV at a later time. HDV is transmitted percutaneously, similar to HBV. It can cause a spectrum of illness ranging from an asymptomatic chronic carrier state to acute liver failure. There is no vaccine for HDV. However, vaccination against HBV reduces the risk of HDV co-infection.

Hepatitis E Virus. Hepatitis E virus (HEV) is an RNA virus transmitted by the fecal-oral route. The usual mode of transmission is drinking contaminated water. Hepatitis E infection occurs primarily in developing countries, with epidemics reported in India, Asia, Mexico, and Africa. Only a few cases of HEV have been reported in the United States, primarily in persons who recently traveled to an HEV-endemic area.

Pathophysiology

Liver. During an acute viral hepatitis infection, liver damage is mediated by cytotoxic cytokines and natural killer cells that cause lysis of infected hepatocytes. Inflammation can interrupt bile flow (cholestasis). After resolution of an acute infection, liver cells can regenerate and, if no complications occur, resume their normal appearance and function.

A chronic viral hepatitis infection causes chronic inflammation and can cause fibrosis that (over decades) can progress to cirrhosis. (Cirrhosis is discussed later in this chapter.)

Systemic Effects. The antigen-antibody complexes between the virus and its corresponding antibody may form circulating immune complexes in the early phases of hepatitis. The circulating immune complexes activate the complement system (see Chapter 12). The clinical manifestations of this activation are rash, angioedema, arthritis, fever, and malaise. *Cryoglobulinemia* (abnormal proteins found in the blood), glomerulonephritis, and vasculitis have also been found secondary to immune complex activation.

TABLE 44-2	**MANIFESTATIONS OF HEPATITIS**
Acute Hepatitis	**Chronic Hepatitis**
• Anorexia	• Malaise
• Nausea, vomiting	• Easy fatigability
• Right upper quadrant discomfort	• Hepatomegaly
• Constipation or diarrhea	• Myalgias and/or arthralgias
• Decreased sense of taste and smell	• Elevated liver enzymes (aspartate aminotransferase [AST] and alanine aminotransferase [ALT])
• Malaise	
• Headache	
• Fever	
• Arthralgias	
• Urticaria	
• Hepatomegaly	
• Splenomegaly	
• Weight loss	
• Jaundice	
• Pruritus	
• Dark urine	
• Bilirubinuria	
• Light stools	
• Fatigue	
• Continued hepatomegaly with tenderness	
• Weight loss	

Clinical Manifestations

The clinical manifestations of viral hepatitis can be classified into acute and chronic phases (Table 44-2). A large number of patients with acute hepatitis have no symptoms. As a result, infection during the acute phase may not be detected in all patients. However, others may have intermittent or ongoing malaise, fatigue, myalgias, arthralgias, and hepatomegaly.

The acute phase usually lasts from 1 to 4 months. During the incubation period, symptoms may include malaise, anorexia and weight loss, fatigue, nausea, occasional vomiting, and abdominal (right upper quadrant) discomfort. The patient may find food repugnant, and smokers may have distaste for cigarettes. There is also a decreased sense of smell. Other symptoms may include headache, low-grade fever, arthralgias, and skin rashes. Physical examination may reveal hepatomegaly, lymphadenopathy, and sometimes splenomegaly. The acute phase is the period of maximal infectivity.

The acute phase may be *icteric* (jaundice) or anicteric. (Types of jaundice are presented in Table 44-3.) Jaundice, a yellowish discoloration of body tissues, results from an alteration in normal bilirubin metabolism or flow of bile into the hepatic or biliary duct systems. (Normal bilirubin metabolism is presented in Fig. 39-4.) The urine may darken because of excess bilirubin being excreted by the kidneys. If conjugated bilirubin cannot flow out of the liver because of obstruction or inflammation of the bile ducts, the stools will be light or clay colored. *Pruritus* (intense chronic itching) sometimes accompanies jaundice. The pruritus occurs as a result of the accumulation of bile salts beneath the skin.

The convalescent phase following the acute phase begins as jaundice fades and lasts for weeks to months, with an average of 2 to 4 months. During this period, the patient's major complaint is malaise and easy fatigability. Hepatomegaly remains for several weeks, but splenomegaly subsides during this period.

Prior infection with HAV or HBV can provide immunity to that virus *(homologous immunity).* However, the patient can still

TABLE 44-3	CLASSIFICATION OF JAUNDICE		
	Hemolytic Jaundice	**Hepatocellular Jaundice**	**Obstructive Jaundice**
Causes	• Blood transfusion reactions, sickle cell crisis, hemolytic anemia.	• Hepatitis, cirrhosis, hepatocellular carcinoma.	• Hepatitis, cirrhosis, hepatocellular carcinoma. Common bile duct obstruction from stone(s), biliary strictures, sclerosing cholangitis, and pancreatic cancer.
Description	• Caused by increased breakdown of RBCs, which produces an increased amount of unconjugated bilirubin in blood. • Liver is unable to handle increased load.	• Results from liver's altered ability to take up bilirubin from the blood or to conjugate or excrete it. • In hepatocellular disease, damaged hepatocytes leak bilirubin.	• Results from decreased or obstructed flow of bile through liver or biliary duct system. • Obstruction may occur in intrahepatic or extrahepatic bile ducts. Intrahepatic obstructions are due to swelling or fibrosis of the liver's canaliculi and bile ducts.
Diagnostic Findings ***Serum Bilirubin*** Unconjugated (indirect) Conjugated (direct)	 ↑ Normal	 ↑ ↑ or ↓ (severe disease)	 Somewhat ↑ Moderately ↑
Urine Bilirubin	Negative	↑	↑
Urobilinogen Stool Urine	 ↑ ↑	 Normal, ↓ Normal, ↑	 ↓ ↓

be infected with another type of viral hepatitis. An individual with hepatitis C can be reinfected with another strain of HCV.

Complications

Most patients with acute viral hepatitis recover completely. The overall mortality rate for acute hepatitis is less than 1%. The mortality rate is higher in older adults and those with underlying debilitating illnesses (including chronic liver disease). Complications that can occur include acute liver failure, chronic hepatitis, cirrhosis of the liver, and hepatocellular carcinoma.

Almost all cases of acute hepatitis A resolve, although a small number may have a viral relapse in the first 2 to 3 months after the infection. The disappearance of jaundice does not mean the patient has totally recovered. Some HBV infections and the majority of HCV infections result in chronic (lifelong) viral infection.

Chronic HBV is more likely to develop in infants born to infected mothers and in those who acquire the infection before age 5 than in those who acquire the virus after age 5.[1] Alterations in the patient's cellular immune response may be important in the development of the chronic HBsAg carrier state and the progression of acute HBV to chronic HBV. These immune system alterations may explain why the patient with chronic kidney disease who is undergoing dialysis when hepatitis B is acquired is more at risk for developing chronic infection.[4] Persons with chronic kidney disease have a depressed cellular immune response.

HCV infection is more likely than HBV to become chronic.[5] As previously mentioned, many patients with chronic HCV infection develop chronic liver disease, cirrhosis, and hepatocellular cancer.[6] Risk factors for progression to cirrhosis include male gender, alcohol consumption, and excess iron deposition in the liver. Elevated cholesterol or triglycerides, obesity, and diabetes mellitus are also risk factors for the progression of HCV to cirrhosis.

Diagnostic Studies

The only definitive way to distinguish among the various forms of viral hepatitis is by testing the patient's blood for the specific antigen or antibody. In some types of viral hepatitis, the blood can be tested for the viral level (also known as the *viral load*). Tests for the different types of viral hepatitis are presented in Table 44-4. In viral hepatitis, many of the liver function tests show significant abnormalities. The common abnormalities are shown in Table 44-5.

Several tests are available to determine the presence of HCV. Initial testing for HCV infection includes HCV antibody testing. If the antibody test is positive, HCV RNA testing should be obtained to assess for chronic infection; a positive result confirms chronic infection. A small number of patients may have a false-positive HCV antibody test with a negative HCV RNA test. If recent HCV infection is suspected, HCV RNA testing is usually obtained because it may take several weeks or longer for HCV antibodies to develop. This testing may also be helpful in the immunocompromised patient (e.g., patient with HIV). Because of altered or delayed antibody response to HCV, these patients may not have detectable antibody levels even though they are infected with HCV.

Viral genotype testing is done in patients undergoing drug therapy for HBV or HCV infection. HBV has at least eight different genotypes (A to H). In some centers, HBV genotyping is performed before starting treatment. HBV genotype may be useful in predicting disease and treatment outcomes.[6]

HCV has six genotypes and more than 50 subtypes. In the United States, 75% of HCV infections are caused by HCV genotype 1. Genotype is one of the strongest predictors of response to drug therapy.[7] For patients who test positive for HCV, genotyping is obtained before drug therapy is started.

Physical assessment may reveal hepatic tenderness, hepatomegaly, and splenomegaly. The liver is palpable. A liver biopsy is not indicated in acute hepatitis unless the diagnosis is in doubt. In chronic hepatitis a liver biopsy may be done. Biopsy of liver tissue allows for histologic examination of liver cells and characterization of the degree of inflammation, fibrosis, or cirrhosis that may be present. A patient who has a bleeding disorder may not be an appropriate candidate for biopsy because of the risk of bleeding. In these patients a transjugular biopsy may be an option.

TABLE 44-4   TESTS FOR VIRAL HEPATITIS

Virus	Tests	Significance
A	Anti-HAV immunoglobulin M (IgM)	Acute infection.
	Anti-HAV immunoglobulin G (IgG)	Previous infection or immunization. Not routinely done in clinical practice.
B	HBsAg (hepatitis B surface antigen)	Marker of infectivity.
		Present in acute or chronic infection.
		Positive in chronic carriers.
	Anti-HBs (hepatitis B surface antibody)	Indicates previous infection with HBV or immunization.
	HBeAg (hepatitis B e antigen)	Indicates high infectivity.
		Used to determine the clinical management of patients with chronic hepatitis B.
	Anti-HBe (hepatitis B e antibody)	Indicates previous infection.
		In chronic hepatitis B, indicates a low viral load and low degree of infectivity.
	Anti-HBc (antibody to hepatitis B core antigen) IgM	Indicates acute infection.
		Does not appear after vaccination.
	Anti-HBc IgG	Indicates previous infection or ongoing infection with hepatitis B.
		Does not appear after vaccination.
	HBV DNA quantitation	Indicates active ongoing viral replication.
		Best indicator of viral replication and effectiveness of therapy in patient with chronic hepatitis B.
	HBV genotyping	Indicates the genotype of HBV.
C	Anti-HCV (antibody to HCV)	Marker for acute or chronic infection with HCV.
	HCV RNA quantitation	Indicates active ongoing viral replication.
	HCV genotyping	Indicates the genotype of HCV.
D	Anti-HDV	Present in past or current infection with HDV.
	HDV Ag (hepatitis D antigen)	Present within a few days after infection.
E*	Anti-HEV IgM and IgG	Present 1 wk–2 mo after illness onset.
	HEV RNA quantitation	Indicates active ongoing viral replication.

*Currently, no serologic tests to diagnose HEV infection are commercially available in the United States. However, diagnostic tests are available in research laboratories to detect IgM and IgG anti-HEV and HEV RNA levels.
A, Hepatitis A virus (HAV); *B,* hepatitis B virus (HBV); *C,* hepatitis C virus (HCV); *D,* hepatitis D virus (HDV); *E,* hepatitis E virus (HEV).

TABLE 44-5   DIAGNOSTIC FINDINGS IN ACUTE HEPATITIS

Test	Abnormal Finding	Etiology
Transaminases (aminotransferases)		
• Aspartate aminotransferase (AST)	Increased in acute phase	Liver cell injury
	Decreases as jaundice disappears	
• Alanine aminotransferase (ALT)	Increased in acute phase	Liver cell injury
	Decreases as jaundice disappears	
γ-Glutamyl transpeptidase (GGT)	Increased	Liver cell injury
Alkaline phosphatase	Moderately increased	Impaired excretory function of the liver
Serum proteins		
• γ-Globulin	Normal or increased	Impaired clearance from liver
• Albumin	Normal or decreased	Liver cell damage
Serum bilirubin (total)	Increased to about 8-15 mg/dL (137-257 μmol/L)	Liver cell damage
Urinary bilirubin	Increased	Conjugated hyperbilirubinemia
Urinary urobilinogen	Increased 2-5 days before jaundice	Diminished reabsorption of urobilinogen
Prothrombin time	Prolonged	Decreased prothrombin production by liver

Techniques for noninvasive assessment of liver fibrosis may eventually replace the need for liver biopsy. Options include the FibroScan, which uses an ultrasound transducer to determine liver fibrosis. FibroSure (FibroTest) is a biomarker that uses the results of serum tests (e.g., liver enzyme levels) to assess the degree of hepatic fibrosis.[8]

Collaborative Care

There is no specific treatment or therapy for acute viral hepatitis. Most patients can be managed at home. Emphasis is on measures to rest the body and assist the liver in regenerating (Table 44-6). Adequate nutrition and rest seem to be most beneficial for healing and liver cell regeneration. Rest reduces the metabolic demands on the liver and promotes cell regeneration. The degree of rest ordered depends on the severity of symptoms, but usually alternating periods of activity and rest are adequate. Counseling should include the importance of avoiding alcohol and notification of possible contacts for testing and prophylaxis, if indicated.

Drug Therapy. There are no drug therapies for the treatment of acute hepatitis A infection. Treatment of acute hepatitis B is indicated only in patients with severe hepatitis and liver failure. In persons with acute hepatitis C, treatment with pegylated interferon within the first 12 to 24 weeks of infection decreases the development of chronic hepatitis C.[2] Supportive drug therapy may include antiemetics for nausea, such as prochlorperazine (Compazine), promethazine (Phenergan), or ondansetron (Zofran).

Chronic Hepatitis B. Drug therapy for chronic HBV is focused on decreasing the viral load and liver enzymes and slowing the rate of disease progression. Long-term goals are prevention of cirrhosis, liver failure, and hepatocellular cancer.

TABLE 44-6 COLLABORATIVE CARE

Viral Hepatitis

Diagnostic
- History and physical examination
- Liver function studies
- Alanine aminotransferase (ALT)
- Aspartate aminotransferase (AST)
- Serum bilirubin
- Prothrombin time (PT) and INR
- Alkaline phosphatase
- γ-Glutamyl transpeptidase
- Hepatitis testing:
  - *Hepatitis A:* Anti-HAV IgM
  - *Hepatitis B:* HBsAg, anti-HBs, HBeAg, anti-HBe, anti-HBc IgM and IgG, HBV DNA quantitation, HBV genotyping
  - *Hepatitis C:* Anti-HCV, HCV RNA quantitation, HCV genotyping
  - *Hepatitis D:* Anti-HDV, HDV Ag
- FibroScan
- FibroSure (FibroTest)

Collaborative Therapy
Acute and Chronic
- Well-balanced diet
- Vitamin supplements
- Rest (degree of strictness varies)
- Avoidance of alcohol intake and drugs detoxified by the liver

Chronic HBV
- Standard interferon (Intron A)
- Pegylated interferon (PegIntron, Pegasys)
- Nucleoside and nucleotide analogs
  - lamivudine (Epivir)
  - adefovir (Hepsera)
  - entecavir (Baraclude)
  - telbivudine (Tyzeka)
  - tenofovir (Viread)

Chronic HCV
- Pegylated interferon
- ribavirin (Rebetol, Copegus)
- Protease inhibitors
  - telaprevir (Incivek)
  - boceprevir (Victrelis)

HAV, hepatitis A virus; *HB,* hepatitis B; *HBeAg,* hepatitis B e antigen; *HBsAg,* hepatitis B surface antigen; *HBV,* hepatitis B virus; *HCV,* hepatitis C virus; *HDV Ag,* hepatitis D antigen; *HDV,* hepatitis D virus; *INR,* international normalized ratio.

COMPLEMENTARY & ALTERNATIVE THERAPIES

Milk Thistle (Silymarin)

Scientific Evidence
- Previous studies suggested that milk thistle may benefit the liver by protecting and promoting the growth of liver cells and inhibiting inflammation. These studies were small and not well designed.
- Two rigorously designed studies found no real benefit from using milk thistle:
  - Silymarin was no better than placebo for chronic hepatitis C in people who had not responded to standard antiviral treatment.*
  - Hepatitis C patients who used silymarin had fewer and milder symptoms of liver disease and somewhat better quality of life but no change in virus activity or liver inflammation.†

Nursing Implications
- Appears to be well tolerated in recommended doses for up to 6 yr.
- May lower blood glucose.
- May interfere with the liver's cytochrome P450 enzyme system.

*Fried MW, Navarro VJ, Afdhal N, et al: Effect of silymarin (milk thistle) on liver disease in patients with chronic hepatitis C who failed interferon therapy: a randomized, placebo-controlled trial, *JAMA* 308(3):274, 2012.
†Seeff LB, Curto TM, Szabo G, et al: Herbal product use by persons enrolled in the hepatitis C Antiviral Long-Term Treatment Against Cirrhosis (HALT-C) Trial, *Hepatology* 47(2):605, 2008.

Current drug therapies for chronic HBV do not eradicate the virus, but work well to suppress viral replication and prevent complications of hepatitis B.[9] First-line therapies include pegylated interferon and nucleoside and nucleotide analogs (see Table 44-6).

Interferon. Interferon has multiple effects on the viral replication cycle. After binding to receptors on host cell membranes, the drug blocks viral entry into cells, synthesis of viral proteins, and viral assembly and release (see Fig. 14-4). There are two forms of interferon: standard (Intron A) and pegylated. Standard (conventional) interferon has a short half-life, necessitating frequent subcutaneous administrations (three times per week). In contrast, the long-acting preparations (pegylated interferons) are administered subcutaneously less frequently (just once per week), making them more convenient. In addition, with the long-acting preparations, blood levels remain high between doses, and therefore clinical responses are better.

The long-acting preparations are made by conjugating a standard interferon with polyethylene glycol (PEG), in a process known as *pegylation.* Therapeutic effects of the pegylated products (Pegasys and PegIntron) are due solely to its interferon component. The PEG component serves only to delay elimination of the drug. Because of their convenience and superior efficacy, these products are preferred to standard interferon and are used in both hepatitis B and hepatitis C treatment.

In patients with HBV receiving interferon, one third will have a significant reduction of serum HBV DNA levels, normalization of alanine aminotransferase (ALT) levels, and loss of HBeAg. The response to treatment may vary based on viral genotype. Interferon treatment is associated with a number of side effects (see eTable 44-1 on the website for this chapter). These side effects are dose related and tend to decrease in severity with continued treatment. Patients receiving interferon should have blood counts and liver function tests performed every 4 to 6 weeks.

Nucleoside and Nucleotide Analogs. HBV reproduces by making copies of its viral DNA nucleosides and nucleotides. The nucleoside and nucleotide analog drugs fool the virus into thinking they are normal building blocks for DNA. Thus the virus is unable to reproduce.

Nucleoside and nucleotide analogs do not prevent all viral reproduction, but they can substantially lower the amount of virus in the body. These medications include lamivudine (Epivir), adefovir (Hepsera), entecavir (Baraclude), telbivudine (Tyzeka), and tenofovir (Viread). These oral medications are used in the treatment of chronic HBV when there is evidence of active viral replication.

Nucleoside and nucleotide analogs have beneficial effects in terms of reducing viral load, decreasing liver damage, and decreasing liver enzymes. Most patients with HBV require long-term treatment with these medications.[10] When these drugs are stopped, the majority of patients (except those who have seroconverted) have HBV DNA and liver enzyme levels that return to pretreatment levels.

Severe exacerbations of hepatitis B have developed after discontinuation of treatment. If these drugs are discontinued, monitor liver function closely for several months.

Chronic Hepatitis C. Drug therapy is directed at eradicating the virus and preventing HCV-related complications.[11] Treatment for HCV includes pegylated interferon given with ribavirin (Rebetol, Copegus). Patients who have HCV genotype 1 also receive either telaprevir (Incivek) or boceprevir (Victrelis), which are HCV protease inhibitors.[11] Protease is an enzyme that is essential in viral replication.

Treatment of chronic hepatitis C is individualized and based on the genotype, the severity of liver disease, potential side effects, presence of co-morbid conditions, patient's readiness for treatment, and presence of other health problems (e.g., HIV). Pegylated interferon is injected once a week, and ribavirin is taken orally twice daily. Both boceprevir and telaprevir are taken orally every 8 hours. Ribavirin, given in combination with pegylated interferon, has a synergistic effect and reduces the rate of relapse following hepatitis C treatment. Ribavirin has a number of side effects (see eTable 44-1 on the website for this chapter).

DRUG ALERT: Ribavirin (Rebetol, Copegus)

- During treatment, pregnancy must be avoided both by women taking the drug and by women whose male partners are taking the drug.

Many patients with HIV also have HCV. Patients who have stable HIV and relatively intact immune systems (CD4[+] counts greater than 200/μL) are treated for HCV with the goal of eradicating HCV and reducing the risk of progression to cirrhosis. HCV treatment may reduce CD4[+] counts, and increase the patient's risk for anemia and leukopenia.

Patients who have advanced fibrosis or cirrhosis can be treated with drug therapy as long as liver decompensation (e.g., ascites, esophageal hemorrhage, jaundice, wasting, encephalopathy) is not present.

Depression or mood changes are common in patients receiving treatment for HCV. Patients need to be screened for depression and other mood disorders before starting interferon-based treatment and monitored frequently while on therapy.[12]

Nutritional Therapy. No special diet is required in the treatment of viral hepatitis. Emphasis is placed on a well-balanced diet that the patient can tolerate. During acute viral hepatitis, adequate calories are important because the patient usually loses weight. If fat content is poorly tolerated because of decreased bile production, it should be reduced. Vitamin supplements, particularly B-complex vitamins and vitamin K, are frequently used. If anorexia, nausea, and vomiting are severe, IV solutions of glucose or supplemental enteral nutrition therapy may be used. Fluid and electrolyte balance must be maintained.

NURSING MANAGEMENT
VIRAL HEPATITIS

NURSING ASSESSMENT

Subjective and objective data that should be obtained from a person with hepatitis are presented in Table 44-7.

NURSING DIAGNOSES

Nursing diagnoses for the patient with viral hepatitis may include, but are not limited to, the following:

- Imbalanced nutrition: less than body requirements *related to* anorexia and nausea
- Activity intolerance *related to* fatigue and weakness
- Risk for impaired liver function *related to* viral infection

TABLE 44-7 **NURSING ASSESSMENT**
Hepatitis*

Subjective Data
Important Health Information
Past health history: Hemophilia; exposure to infected persons; ingestion of contaminated food or water; exposure to benzene, carbon tetrachloride, or other hepatotoxic agents; crowded, unsanitary living conditions; exposure to contaminated needles; recent travel; organ transplant recipient; exposure to new drug regimens, hemodialysis, transfusion of blood or blood products before 1992; HIV status (if known)
Medications: Use and misuse of acetaminophen, new prescription, over-the-counter, or herbal medications or supplements

Functional Health Patterns
Health perception–health management: IV drug and alcohol abuse; malaise, distaste for cigarettes (in smokers), high-risk sexual behaviors
Nutritional-metabolic: Weight loss, anorexia, nausea, vomiting; feeling of fullness in right upper quadrant
Elimination: Dark urine; light-colored stools, constipation or diarrhea; skin rashes, hives
Activity-exercise: Fatigue, arthralgias, myalgias
Cognitive-perceptual: Right upper quadrant pain and liver tenderness, headache; pruritus
Role-relationship: Exposure as health care worker, long-term care institution resident, incarceration, homeless

Objective Data
General
Low-grade fever, lethargy, lymphadenopathy

Integumentary
Rash or other skin changes, jaundice, icteric sclera, injection sites

Gastrointestinal
Hepatomegaly, splenomegaly

Possible Diagnostic Findings
Elevated liver enzyme levels; ↑ serum total bilirubin, hypoalbuminemia, anemia, bilirubin in urine and increased urobilinogen, prolonged prothrombin time, positive tests for hepatitis, including anti-HAV IgM, HBsAg, anti-HBs, HBeAg, anti-HBe, anti-HBc IgM and IgG, HBV DNA quantitation, anti-HCV, HCV RNA quantitation, anti-HDV; HDV Ag; abnormal liver scan; abnormal results on liver biopsy

*Hepatitis includes both viral and nonviral causes.
HAV, Hepatitis A virus; *HBcAg,* hepatitis B core antigen; *HBeAg,* hepatitis B e antigen; *HBsAg,* hepatitis B surface antigen; *HBV,* hepatitis B virus; *HCV,* hepatitis C virus; *HDV Ag,* hepatitis D antigen; *HDV,* hepatitis D virus.

Additional information is presented on nursing diagnoses for the patient with viral hepatitis in eNursing Care Plan 44-1 (on the website for this chapter).

PLANNING

The overall goals are that the patient with viral hepatitis will (1) have relief of discomfort, (2) be able to resume normal activities, and (3) return to normal liver function without complications.

NURSING IMPLEMENTATION

HEALTH PROMOTION. Viral hepatitis is a public health problem. Your role is important in the prevention and control of this disease. It is helpful to understand the epidemiology of the different types of viral hepatitis before considering appropriate control measures. Preventive and control measures for hepatitis A, B, and C are summarized in Table 44-8.

TABLE 44-8	PREVENTIVE MEASURES FOR VIRAL HEPATITIS*
Hepatitis A	**Hepatitis B and C**
General Measures	**Percutaneous Transmission**

• Hand washing
• Proper personal hygiene
• Environmental sanitation
• Control and screening (signs, symptoms) of food handlers
• Serologic screening for those carrying virus
• Active immunization: HAV vaccine
	Screening of donated blood
	  • *HBV:* HBsAg
	  • *HCV:* Anti-HCV
	Use of disposable needles and syringes
	
	Sexual Transmission

Use of Immune Globulin	• Acute exposure: HBIG administration to sexual partner of HBsAg-positive person • HBV vaccine series administered to uninfected sexual partners • Condoms used for sexual intercourse
• Early administration (1-2 wk after exposure) to those exposed • Prophylaxis for travelers to areas where hepatitis A is common if not vaccinated with HAV vaccine	
	General Measures
	• Hand washing • Avoid sharing toothbrushes and razors • HBIG administration for one-time exposure (needle stick, contact of mucous membranes with infectious material) • Active immunization: HBV vaccine
Special Considerations for Health Care Personnel	
• Wash hands after contact with a patient or removal of gloves • Use infection control precautions†	**Special Considerations for Health Care Personnel**
	• Use infection control precautions† • Reduce contact with blood or blood-containing secretions • Handle the blood of patients as potentially infective • Dispose of needles properly • Use needleless IV access devices when available

*A suggested guideline for general practice to prevent you from contracting viral hepatitis from diagnosed and undiagnosed patients and carriers is for you to wear disposable gloves, goggles, and gowns (sometimes) when fecal or blood contamination is likely in handling (1) soiled bedpans, urinals, and catheters; and (2) when the patient's bed linens are soiled by body excreta or secretions.
†See eTable 15-1 available on the website.
HAV, Hepatitis A virus; *HBIG,* hepatitis B immune globulin; *HBsAg,* hepatitis B surface antigen; *HBV,* hepatitis B virus; *HCV,* hepatitis C virus.

Hepatitis A. Outbreaks of viral hepatitis are usually due to HAV. Preventive measures include personal and environmental hygiene and health education to promote good sanitation. Hand washing is probably the most important precaution. Teach about careful hand washing after bowel movements and before eating.

Vaccination is the best protection against HAV. All children at 1 year of age should receive the vaccine. Adults at risk should also receive the vaccine. These include people who travel to areas with increased rates of hepatitis A, men who have sex with men, injecting and noninjecting drug users, persons with clotting factor disorders (e.g., hemophilia), and persons with chronic liver disease.[1]

There are currently several forms of the HAV vaccine, including Havrix, Vaqta, and Avaxim. HAV vaccine is inactivated HAV. Primary immunization consists of a single dose administered intramuscularly (IM) in the deltoid muscle. A booster is recommended 6 to 12 months after the primary dose to ensure

adequate antibody titers and long-term protection. The primary immunization provides immunity within 30 days after a single dose in more than 95% of those vaccinated.

Twinrix, a combined HAV and HBV vaccine, is available for people over 18 years of age. Immunization consists of three doses, given on a 0-, 1-, and 6-month schedule, the same schedule as that used for the single HBV vaccine. Twinrix may be given to high-risk individuals, including patients with chronic liver disease, users of illicit IV drugs, patients on hemodialysis, men who have sex with men, and people with clotting factor disorders who receive therapeutic blood products. The side effects of the vaccine are mild and usually limited to soreness and redness at the injection site.

Isolation is not required for HAV infection. For a patient with HAV infection, use infection control precautions (see eTable 15-1 available on the website for that chapter). A private room is indicated if the patient is incontinent of stool or has poor personal hygiene.

Both hepatitis A vaccine and immune globulin (IG) are used for prevention of HAV infection after exposure to an infected person *(postexposure prophylaxis).* The vaccine is used for pre-exposure prophylaxis, and IG can be used either before or after exposure. IG provides temporary (1 to 2 months) passive immunity and is effective for preventing hepatitis A if given within 2 weeks after exposure. IG is recommended for persons who do not have anti-HAV antibodies and are exposed as a result of close (household, day care center) contact with persons who have HAV or foodborne exposure. Because patients with HAV are most infectious just before the onset of symptoms (the preicteric phase), those exposed through household contact or foodborne outbreaks should receive IG. Although IG may not prevent infection in all persons, it may modify the illness to a subclinical infection. When hepatitis A occurs in a food handler, IG should be administered to all other food handlers at the establishment. Patrons may also need to be given IG.

Persons who have received a dose of HAV vaccine more than 1 month previously or who have a history of laboratory-confirmed HAV infection do not require IG.

Hepatitis B. The best way to reduce HBV infection is to identify those at risk, screen them for HBV, and vaccinate those who are not infected. Teach individuals at high risk of contracting HBV to reduce risks. Good hygienic practices, including hand washing and using gloves when expecting contact with blood, are important. Patients should not share razors, toothbrushes, and other personal items. Teach patients to use a condom for sexual intercourse, and the partner should be vaccinated.

The HBV vaccine is the best means of prevention. The HBV vaccines (Recombivax HB, Engerix-B) contain HBsAg, which promotes the synthesis of specific antibodies directed against HBV. The vaccine is given in a series of three IM injections in the deltoid muscle. The second dose is administered within 1 month of the first one, and the third one within 6 months of the first. The vaccine is more than 95% effective. Only minor adverse reactions have been reported with vaccination, including transient fever and soreness at the injection site. The vaccine is not contraindicated in pregnancy.

The first dose of hepatitis B vaccine should be given at birth, with the vaccine series completed by age 6 to 18 months. Older children and adolescents who did not previously receive the hepatitis B vaccine should also be vaccinated.[13] It is also important to vaccinate adults in the at-risk groups discussed above. Household members of the patient with HBV should be tested and vaccinated if they are HBsAg and antibody negative. Hepatitis vaccination is recommended for patients with chronic kidney disease before they start dialysis. Dialysis patients should routinely have their antibody titer levels checked to determine the need for revaccination.[13]

For postexposure prophylaxis, the HBV vaccine and hepatitis B immune globulin (HBIG) are used. HBIG contains antibodies to HBV and confers temporary passive immunity. HBIG is prepared from plasma of donors with a high titer of anti-HBs. HBIG is recommended for postexposure prophylaxis in cases of needle stick, mucous membrane contact, or sexual exposure and for infants born to mothers who are positive for HBsAg. Ideally HBIG should be given within 24 hours of exposure. The vaccine series should also be started.

According to Centers for Disease Control and Prevention (CDC) guidelines, follow infection control precautions for the patient with HBV. This includes using disposable needles and syringes and disposing of them in puncture-resistant units without recapping, bending, or breaking. (See eTable 15-1 on the website for that chapter for various types of infection control precautions.)

Hepatitis C. No vaccine is currently available for hepatitis C. The primary measures to prevent HCV transmission include screening of blood, organ, and tissue donors; use of infection control precautions; and modification of high-risk behavior. Identify individuals at high risk for contracting HCV and teach methods to reduce risks. Because of the number of people with hepatitis C who have not been diagnosed, the CDC recommends that all persons born between 1945 and 1965 undergo HCV testing regardless of risk factor status.[14] The CDC does not recommend IG or antiviral agents such as interferon for postexposure prophylaxis (e.g., needle-stick exposure from an infected patient) for HCV infection. After an acute exposure (e.g., needle stick), the person should have anti-HCV testing done. For the person exposed to HCV, baseline anti-HCV and ALT levels should be measured, with follow-up testing at 4 to 6 months. Testing for HCV RNA may be performed at 4 to 6 weeks.[15,16]

ACUTE INTERVENTION. In patients with hepatitis, assess for the presence and degree of jaundice. In light-skinned persons, jaundice is usually observed first in the sclera of the eyes and later in the skin. In dark-skinned persons, jaundice is observed in the hard palate of the mouth and inner canthus of the eyes. The urine may have a dark brown or brownish red color because of bilirubin. Comfort measures to relieve pruritus (if present), headache, and arthralgias are helpful (see eNursing Care Plan 44-1 on the website for this chapter).

Ensuring that the patient receives adequate nutrition is not always easy. The anorexia and distaste for food cause nutritional problems. Assess the patient's tolerance of specific foods and eating pattern. Small, frequent meals may be preferable to three large ones and may also help prevent nausea. Often a patient with hepatitis finds that anorexia is not as severe in the morning, so it is easier to eat a good breakfast than a large dinner. Measures to stimulate the appetite, such as mouth care, antiemetics, and attractively served meals in pleasant surroundings, should be included in your nursing care plan. Drinking carbonated beverages and avoiding very hot or very cold foods may help alleviate anorexia. Adequate fluid intake (2500 to 3000 mL/day) is important.

Rest is an important factor in promoting hepatocyte regeneration. Assess the patient's response to the rest and activity plan, and modify it accordingly. Liver function tests and symptoms are used as a guide to activity.

Psychologic and emotional rest is as essential as physical rest. Limited activity may produce anxiety and extreme restlessness in some patients. Diversional activities, such as reading and hobbies, may help.

AMBULATORY AND HOME CARE. Most patients with viral hepatitis are cared for at home, so you need to assess the patient's knowledge of nutrition and provide the necessary dietary teaching. Caution the patient about overexertion and the need to follow the health care provider's advice about when to return to work. Teach the patient and the caregiver how to prevent transmission to other family members. Also teach what symptoms should be reported to the health care provider.

Assess the patient for manifestations of complications. Bleeding tendencies with increasing prothrombin time values, symptoms of encephalopathy, or elevated liver function tests indicate problems.

Instruct the patient to have regular follow-up for at least 1 year after the diagnosis of hepatitis. Because relapses occur with hepatitis B and C, teach the patient the symptoms of recurrence and the need for follow-up evaluations. All patients with chronic HBV or HCV should avoid alcohol, since it can accelerate disease progression.

The patient who is receiving interferon for the treatment of HBV or HCV requires education regarding this drug. Because interferon is administered subcutaneously, the patient or the caregiver needs to be taught how to administer the drug. The numerous side effects with the therapy, including flu-like symptoms (e.g., fever, malaise, fatigue), make adherence to therapy challenging for some patients. Patients who are positive for HBsAg (chronic carrier status) or HCV antibody should not be blood donors.

EVALUATION

Expected outcomes are that the patient with hepatitis will
- Maintain food and fluid intake adequate to meet nutritional needs
- Demonstrate gradual increase in activity tolerance
- Perform daily activities with scheduled rest periods

Additional information on expected outcomes for the patient with hepatitis is provided in eNursing Care Plan 44-1 on the website for this chapter.

DRUG- AND CHEMICAL-INDUCED LIVER DISEASES

Alcohol consumption is a frequent cause of both acute and chronic liver disease. It can cause a spectrum of symptoms, ranging from mild elevation in liver enzymes (aspartate aminotransferase [AST] and ALT); to acute alcoholic hepatitis; to advanced fibrosis and cirrhosis, which usually occurs after decades of excessive alcohol intake. Patients may have serious liver disease caused by another chronic disease (e.g., chronic HCV infection) in combination with alcoholic liver disease.

Acute alcoholic hepatitis is a syndrome of enlarged liver (hepatomegaly), jaundice, elevation in liver enzyme tests (AST, ALT, alkaline phosphate), low-grade fever, and possibly ascites and prolonged prothrombin time. These symptoms may improve with cessation of alcohol intake.

Patients may have undetected liver disease and be seen with complications of cirrhosis. Even at this stage, abstinence can result in significant reversal in some patients. If liver function does not recover after abstaining from alcohol for several months or longer, liver transplantation may be considered.

Chemical hepatotoxicity is due to systemic poisons (e.g., carbon tetrachloride, gold compounds). However, because of their declining use, the incidence of these reactions has declined since the 1980s.

Drug-induced liver injury (DILI) is one of the more common causes of jaundice.[17] Many medications (prescription, over-the-counter [OTC], and herbal supplements) can cause an increase in liver enzymes and, in severe cases, jaundice and acute liver failure. The pattern of injury depends on the drug causing the reaction. The most common cause of DILI is acetaminophen.

DRUG ALERT: Acetaminophen (Tylenol)

- Drug is safe if taken at recommended levels. However, its prevalence in a variety of pain relievers, fever reducers, and cough medicines may mean that patients do not realize they are taking several drugs that all contain acetaminophen.
- Many Americans each year experience acute liver failure as a result of taking acetaminophen. About 100 people die annually from overdosing, either intentionally or unintentionally.
- Combining the drug with alcoholic beverages increases the risk of liver damage.

AUTOIMMUNE, GENETIC, AND METABOLIC DISEASES

Autoimmune Hepatitis

Autoimmune hepatitis is a chronic inflammatory disorder of the liver of unknown cause. It is characterized by the presence of autoantibodies, high levels of serum immunoglobulins, and frequent association with other autoimmune diseases. The majority of patients with autoimmune hepatitis are women. Laboratory tests are used to distinguish it from other forms of hepatitis. Serologic markers are often useful in the diagnosis. These include antinuclear antibodies (ANAs) and anti-DNA antibodies.

The disease process involves an autoimmune reaction against normal hepatocytes. Although it can cause acute liver failure, the course of the disease is variable, with most patients developing chronic hepatitis. Untreated autoimmune hepatitis can progress to cirrhosis. Prednisone with or without azathioprine (Imuran) is the recommended treatment for active autoimmune hepatitis. Cyclosporine (Gengraf), tacrolimus (Prograf, FK506), budesonide (Entocort), methotrexate, and mycophenolate mofetil (CellCept) have also been used in patients who do not respond to prednisone and azathioprine.

Wilson's Disease

Wilson's disease is an autosomal recessive defect in cellular copper transport. A defect in biliary excretion leads to accumulation of copper in the liver, causing progressive liver injury and cirrhosis. Approximately one in 40,000 people have Wilson's disease. It affects both men and women equally. Symptoms appear between ages 5 and 35.[18]

Once cirrhosis occurs, copper leaks into the plasma; accumulates in and damages other tissues; and can cause neurologic, hematologic, and renal disease. The hallmark of Wilson's disease is corneal Kayser-Fleischer rings. These are brownish red rings that can be seen in the cornea near the limbus on eye examination. Low serum ceruloplasmin levels and measurable copper concentrations from liver biopsy samples are also present. Diag-

nosis is based on clinical findings, including the corneal rings and neurologic symptoms. First-degree relatives of patients with Wilson's disease should be screened for the disease.

The recommended initial treatment of symptomatic patients or those with active disease is with chelating agents such as D-penicillamine (Cuprimine) or trientine (Syprine), which promote the excretion of urinary copper. Zinc acetate (Galzin), which has also been used as therapy, interferes with the absorption of copper. Liver transplantation may be required in patients who develop cirrhosis.

Hemochromatosis

Hemochromatosis is an iron overload disorder. Although it is primarily caused by a genetic defect *(hereditary hemochromatosis)*, it may also be caused by liver disease and chronic blood transfusions that are used to treat thalassemia and sickle cell disease. (Hemochromatosis is discussed in Chapter 31.)

Primary Biliary Cirrhosis

Primary biliary cirrhosis (PBC) is a chronic disease of the small bile ducts of the liver. In PBC, there is a T-cell–mediated attack of the small bile duct cells resulting in loss of bile ducts and ultimately *cholestasis* (blockage of bile flow). Over time, this leads to liver fibrosis and cirrhosis.

Most patients diagnosed with PBC are women between ages 30 and 65. The disease is associated with other autoimmune disorders such as rheumatoid arthritis, Sjögren's syndrome, and scleroderma. Elevated serum alkaline phosphatase levels, antimitochondrial antibodies (AMAs), ANAs, and serum lipid levels are seen in patients with PBC.

The goals of treatment are the suppression of ongoing liver damage, prevention of complications, and symptom management. The only approved drug for PBC is ursodeoxycholic acid (ursodiol [Actigall]). Management focuses on malabsorption, skin disorders such as pruritus and xanthomas (cholesterol deposits in the skin), hyperlipidemia, vitamin deficiencies, anemia, and fatigue. Cholestyramine (Questran) is used to treat pruritus. Patients are monitored for progression to cirrhosis. Liver transplantation is a treatment option for end-stage liver disease in patients with PBC.

Primary Sclerosing Cholangitis

Primary sclerosing cholangitis (PSC) is a disease of unknown etiology characterized by chronic inflammation, fibrosis, and strictures (narrowing) of the medium and large bile ducts. The majority of patients with PSC also have ulcerative colitis. Complications of PSC can include cholangitis, cholestasis with jaundice, cholangiocarcinoma (bile duct cancer), and cirrhosis.

Drug therapy has not been beneficial. Treatment is directed at reducing the incidence of biliary complications and screening for bile duct and colorectal cancer, which is related to the high incidence of ulcerative colitis. Patients with advanced liver disease may require liver transplantation.

Nonalcoholic Fatty Liver Disease and Nonalcoholic Steatohepatitis

Nonalcoholic fatty liver disease (NAFLD) refers to a wide spectrum of *liver diseases* ranging from a fatty liver (steatosis) to nonalcoholic steatohepatitis (NASH) to *cirrhosis*. In the spectrum of NAFLD, the common characteristic is the accumulation of fatty infiltration in the hepatocytes. In NASH the fat accumulation is associated with varying degrees of inflammation and fibrosis of the liver. NASH is a serious liver disease that can cause cirrhosis, hepatocellular cancer, and liver failure.

The term *nonalcoholic* is used because NAFLD and NASH occur in individuals who do not consume excessive amounts of alcohol. However, a pathologic analysis of liver cells in NAFLD is similar to that in alcoholic liver disease.

Currently, NAFLD affects about 10% to 20% of the U.S. population. This percentage is increasing because of the growing number of people who are obese. NAFLD should be considered in patients with risk factors such as obesity, diabetes, hyperlipidemia, and hypertension. NASH affects 2% to 5% of the U.S. population.[19] Elevations in liver function tests (ALT, AST) are often the first signs of NAFLD. Definitive diagnosis is by liver biopsy. Ultrasound and computed tomography (CT) scans are also used to diagnose NAFLD.

There is no definitive treatment, and therapy is directed at reduction of risk factors. This includes treatment of diabetes, reduction in body weight, and management of hyperlipidemia.

CIRRHOSIS

Cirrhosis is a chronic progressive disease of the liver characterized by extensive degeneration and destruction of the liver cells (Fig. 44-4). The development of cirrhosis is an insidious, prolonged course, usually after decades of chronic liver disease. Cirrhosis (combined with chronic liver diseases) ranks as the eighth leading cause of death in the United States. Cirrhosis is twice as common in men as in women.

Etiology and Pathophysiology

Any chronic liver disease, including disease from excessive alcohol intake and NAFLD, can cause cirrhosis. The specific cause of cirrhosis may not be determined in all patients. The most common causes of cirrhosis in the United States are chronic hepatitis C infection and alcohol-induced liver disease. In patients with alcohol-induced liver disease, some controversy exists as to whether the cause is the alcohol or the malnutrition that often coexists with alcoholism. A common problem in people who abuse alcohol is protein malnutrition. Some cases of nutrition-related cirrhosis have resulted from extreme dieting, malabsorption, and obesity. Environmental factors and genetic predisposition may also lead to the development of cirrhosis, regardless of dietary or alcohol intake.

Approximately 20% of patients with chronic hepatitis C and 10% to 20% of those with chronic hepatitis B develop cirrhosis.

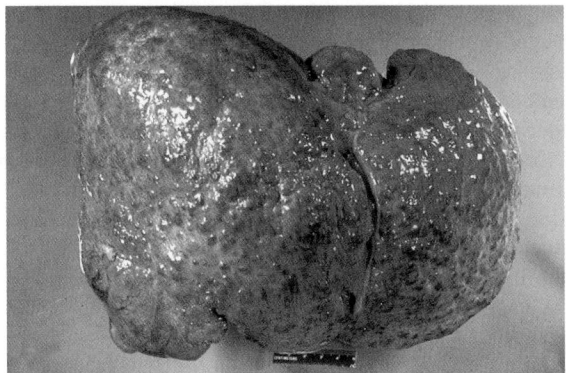

FIG. 44-4 Cirrhosis that developed secondary to alcoholism. The characteristic diffuse nodularity of the surface is due to the combination of regeneration and scarring of the liver.

Chronic inflammation and cell necrosis result in fibrosis and, ultimately, cirrhosis. Chronic hepatitis combined with alcohol ingestion is synergistic in accelerating liver damage.

Biliary causes of cirrhosis include primary biliary cirrhosis (PBC) and primary sclerosing cholangitis (PSC). Both are described earlier in this chapter on the facing page.

Cardiac cirrhosis includes a spectrum of hepatic derangements that result from long-standing, severe, right-sided heart failure. The treatment is aimed at managing the patient's underlying heart failure.

In cirrhosis the liver cells attempt to regenerate, but the regenerative process is disorganized, resulting in abnormal blood vessel and bile duct architecture. The overgrowth of new and fibrous connective tissue distorts the liver's normal lobular structure, resulting in lobules of irregular size and shape with impeded blood flow. Eventually, irregular and disorganized liver regeneration, poor cellular nutrition, and hypoxia (from inadequate blood flow and scar tissue) result in decreased functioning of the liver.

Clinical Manifestations

Early Manifestations. The onset of cirrhosis is usually insidious. Early symptoms include fatigue. Many patients with normal liver function (compensated cirrhosis) may not be aware of their liver condition. The diagnosis may not be discovered until later, when they manifest symptoms of more advanced liver disease.

Later Manifestations. Later symptoms may be severe and result from liver failure and portal hypertension (Fig. 44-5). Jaundice, peripheral edema, and ascites develop gradually. Other late symptoms include skin lesions, hematologic disorders, endocrine disturbances, and peripheral neuropathies (Fig. 44-6). In the advanced stages, the liver becomes small and nodular.

Jaundice. Jaundice results from the functional derangement of liver cells and compression of bile ducts by connective tissue overgrowth. Jaundice occurs as a result of the decreased ability to conjugate and excrete bilirubin (see Table 44-3). (Normal bilirubin metabolism is presented in Fig. 39-4.) The jaundice

PATHOPHYSIOLOGY MAP

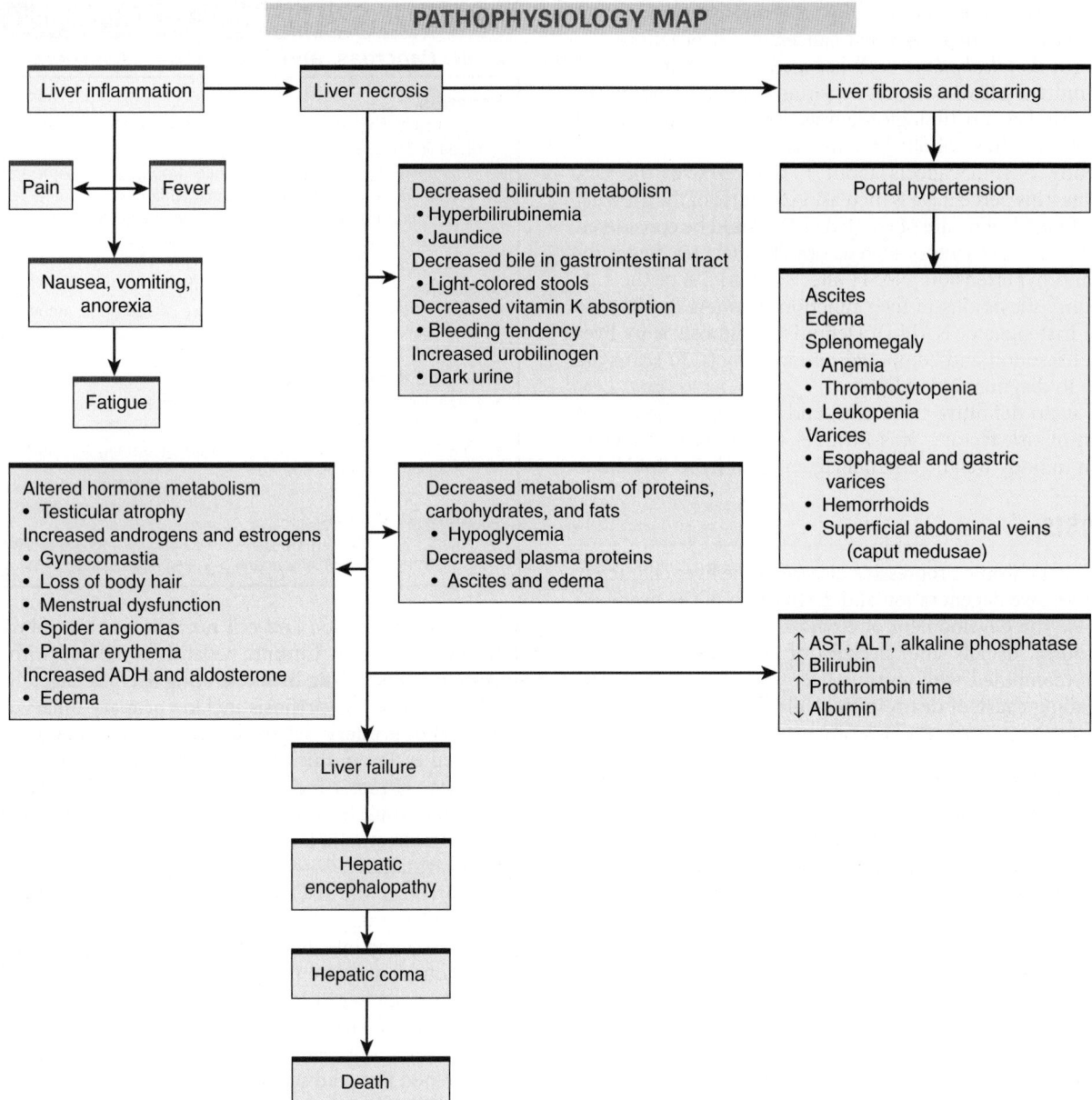

FIG. 44-5 Continuum of liver dysfunction in cirrhosis and resulting manifestations. *ADH,* Antidiuretic hormone; *ALT,* alanine aminotransferase; *AST,* aspartate aminotransferase.

may be minimal or severe, depending on the degree of liver damage.

Skin Lesions. Various skin manifestations are commonly seen in cirrhosis. Spider angiomas (*telangiectasia* or *spider nevi*) are small, dilated blood vessels with a bright red center point and spiderlike branches. They occur on the nose, cheeks, upper trunk, neck, and shoulders. *Palmar erythema* (a red area that blanches with pressure) is located on the palms of the hands. Both of these lesions are attributed to an increase in circulating estrogen as a result of the damaged liver's inability to metabolize steroid hormones.

Hematologic Problems. Hematologic problems include thrombocytopenia, leukopenia, anemia, and coagulation disorders. Thrombocytopenia, leukopenia, and anemia are probably caused by the splenomegaly that results from backup of blood from the portal vein into the spleen (portal hypertension). Overactivity of the enlarged spleen results in increased

removal of blood cells from circulation. Anemia is also due to inadequate red blood cell (RBC) production and survival, poor diet, poor absorption of folic acid, and bleeding from varices.

The coagulation problems result from the liver's inability to produce prothrombin and other factors essential for blood clotting. Coagulation problems are manifested by hemorrhage or bleeding tendencies, such as epistaxis, purpura, petechiae, easy bruising, gingival bleeding, and heavy menstrual bleeding.

Endocrine Problems. Normally the liver is important in the metabolism of adrenocortical hormones, estrogen, and testosterone. In men with cirrhosis, gynecomastia (benign growth of the glandular tissue of the male breast), loss of axillary and pubic hair, testicular atrophy, and impotence with loss of libido may occur because of increased estrogen levels. Younger women with cirrhosis may develop amenorrhea, and older women may have vaginal bleeding. The liver fails to metabolize aldosterone

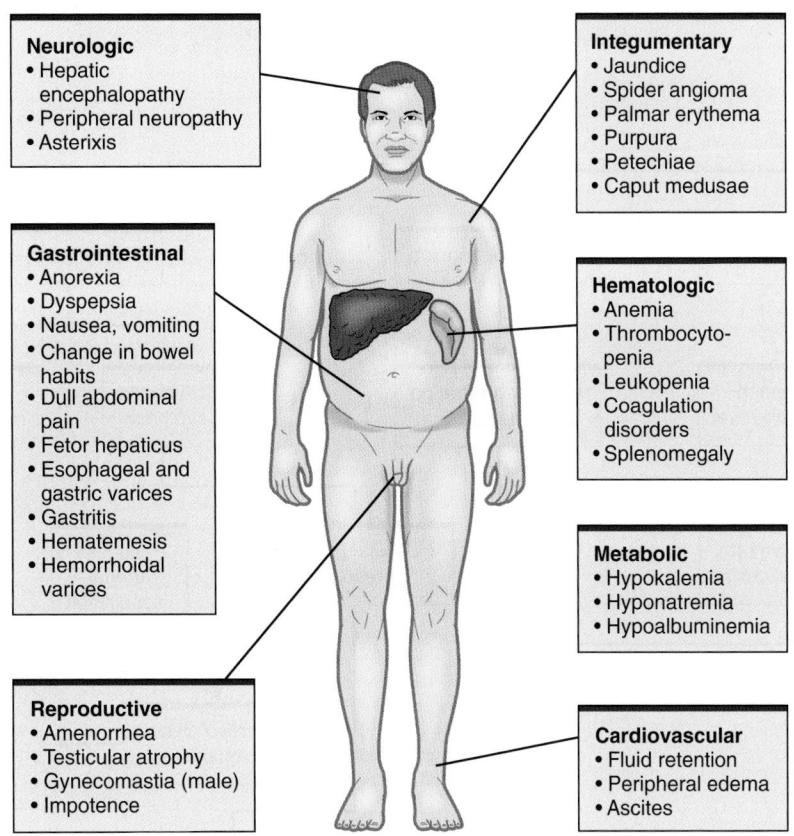

Neurologic
• Hepatic encephalopathy
• Peripheral neuropathy
• Asterixis

Integumentary
• Jaundice
• Spider angioma
• Palmar erythema
• Purpura
• Petechiae
• Caput medusae

Gastrointestinal
• Anorexia
• Dyspepsia
• Nausea, vomiting
• Change in bowel habits
• Dull abdominal pain
• Fetor hepaticus
• Esophageal and gastric varices
• Gastritis
• Hematemesis
• Hemorrhoidal varices

Hematologic
• Anemia
• Thrombocyto-penia
• Leukopenia
• Coagulation disorders
• Splenomegaly

Metabolic
• Hypokalemia
• Hyponatremia
• Hypoalbuminemia

Reproductive
• Amenorrhea
• Testicular atrophy
• Gynecomastia (male)
• Impotence

Cardiovascular
• Fluid retention
• Peripheral edema
• Ascites

FIG. 44-6 Systemic clinical manifestations of liver cirrhosis.

adequately, resulting in hyperaldosteronism with subsequent sodium and water retention and potassium loss.

Peripheral Neuropathy. Peripheral neuropathy is a common finding in alcoholic cirrhosis and is probably due to a dietary deficiency of thiamine, folic acid, and cobalamin. The neuropathy usually results in mixed nervous system symptoms, but sensory symptoms may predominate.

Complications

Major complications of cirrhosis are portal hypertension with resultant esophageal and gastric varices, peripheral edema and ascites, hepatic encephalopathy (mental status changes, including coma), and hepatorenal syndrome. Patients without complications of cirrhosis have *compensated cirrhosis.* Those who have one or more complications of their liver disease have *decompensated cirrhosis.*

Portal Hypertension and Esophageal and Gastric Varices. Structural changes in the liver result in compression and destruction of the portal and hepatic veins and sinusoids. These changes cause obstruction to the normal flow of blood through the portal system, resulting in portal hypertension. Portal hypertension is characterized by increased venous pressure in the portal circulation, splenomegaly, large collateral veins, ascites, and gastric and esophageal varices. Collateral circulation develops in an attempt to reduce high portal pressure and the increased plasma volume and lymphatic flow. The collateral channels commonly form in the lower esophagus (the anastomosis of the left gastric vein and the azygos veins), anterior abdominal wall, parietal peritoneum, and rectum. Varicosities may develop in areas where the collateral and systemic circulations communicate, resulting in esophageal and gastric varices,

caput medusae (ring of varices around the umbilicus), and hemorrhoids.

Esophageal varices are a complex of tortuous veins at the lower end of the esophagus, which are enlarged and swollen as a result of portal hypertension. Gastric varices are located in the upper portion (cardia, fundus) of the stomach. These varices contain little elastic tissue and are fragile. They tolerate high pressure poorly and, as a result, bleed easily. Large varices are more likely to bleed. Esophageal varices are responsible for approximately 80% of variceal hemorrhages. The remaining 20% of variceal hemorrhages are due to gastric varices.

Bleeding esophageal varices are the most life-threatening complication of cirrhosis. The patient may have melena or hematemesis. There may be slow oozing or massive hemorrhage. Massive hemorrhage is a medical emergency.

Peripheral Edema and Ascites. Peripheral edema sometimes precedes ascites, but in some patients its development coincides with or occurs after ascites. Edema results from decreased colloidal oncotic pressure from impaired liver synthesis of albumin and increased portacaval pressure from portal hypertension. Peripheral edema occurs as ankle and presacral edema.

Ascites is the accumulation of serous fluid in the peritoneal or abdominal cavity. It is a common manifestation of cirrhosis. With portal hypertension, proteins shift from the blood vessels via the larger pores of the sinusoids (capillaries) into the lymph space (Fig. 44-7). When the lymphatic system is unable to carry off the excess proteins and water, they leak through the liver capsule into the peritoneal cavity. The osmotic pressure of the proteins pulls additional fluid into the peritoneal cavity (Table 44-9).

PATHOPHYSIOLOGY MAP

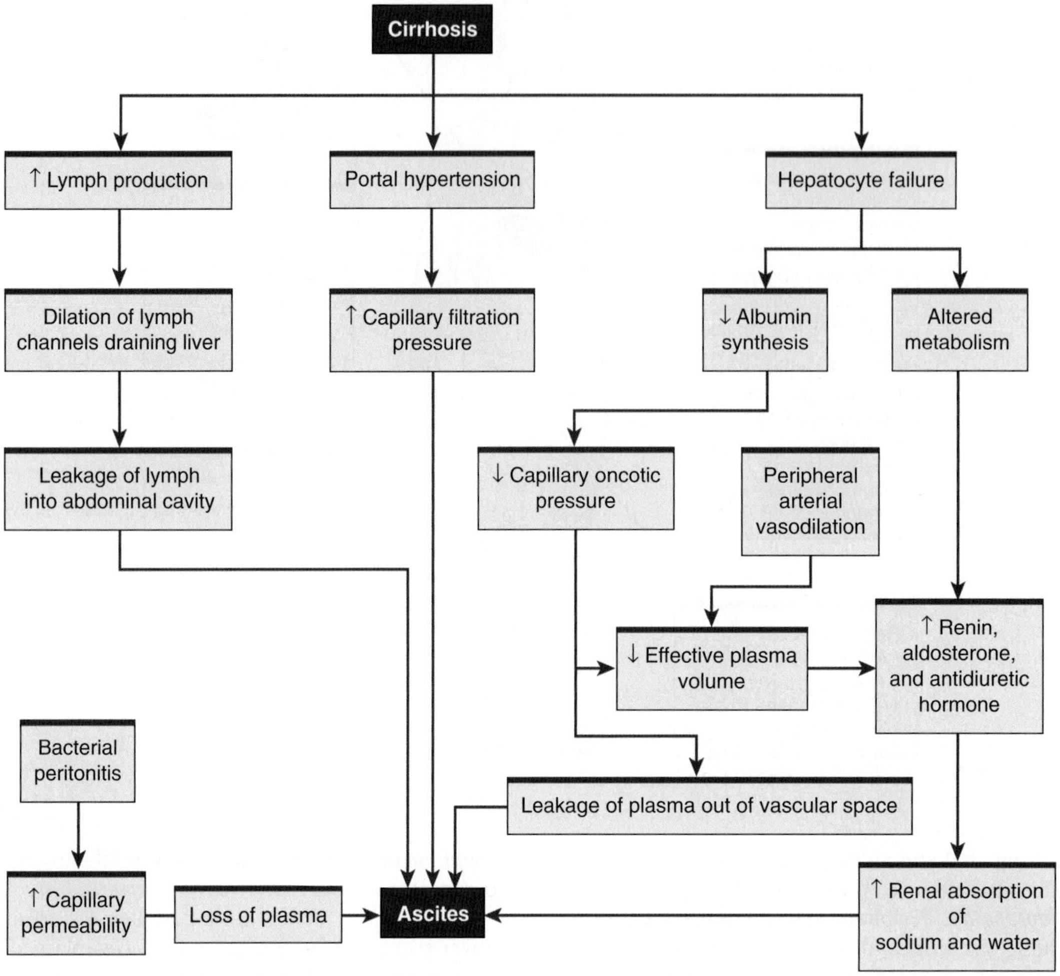

```
                              ┌──────────────┐
                              │  Cirrhosis   │
                              └──────────────┘
          ┌──────────────────────┬───────────────────────────┐
          ▼                      ▼                            ▼
  ┌─────────────────┐   ┌──────────────────┐       ┌──────────────────┐
  │ ↑ Lymph         │   │ Portal           │       │ Hepatocyte       │
  │ production      │   │ hypertension     │       │ failure          │
  └─────────────────┘   └──────────────────┘       └──────────────────┘
          │                      │                  ┌──────────┴──────────┐
          ▼                      ▼                  ▼                     ▼
  ┌─────────────────┐   ┌──────────────────┐  ┌─────────────┐   ┌─────────────┐
  │ Dilation of     │   │ ↑ Capillary      │  │ ↓ Albumin   │   │ Altered     │
  │ lymph channels  │   │ filtration       │  │ synthesis   │   │ metabolism  │
  │ draining liver  │   │ pressure         │  └─────────────┘   └─────────────┘
  └─────────────────┘   └──────────────────┘        │
          │                                          ▼
          ▼                                 ┌─────────────────┐  ┌──────────────┐
  ┌─────────────────┐                       │ ↓ Capillary     │  │ Peripheral   │
  │ Leakage of      │                       │ oncotic         │  │ arterial     │
  │ lymph into      │                       │ pressure        │  │ vasodilation │
  │ abdominal cavity│                       └─────────────────┘  └──────────────┘
  └─────────────────┘                              │                    │
                                                   ▼                    ▼
  ┌───────────────┐                       ┌─────────────────┐   ┌──────────────┐
  │ Bacterial     │                       │ ↓ Effective     │   │ ↑ Renin,     │
  │ peritonitis   │                       │ plasma volume   │──▶│ aldosterone, │
  └───────────────┘                       └─────────────────┘   │ and          │
          │                                        │            │ antidiuretic │
          ▼                                        ▼            │ hormone      │
  ┌───────────┐  ┌──────────┐   ┌─────────────────────────────┐ └──────────────┘
  │ ↑ Capillary│ │ Loss of  │   │ Leakage of plasma out of    │        │
  │ permeability│▶│ plasma  │   │ vascular space              │        ▼
  └───────────┘  └──────────┘   └─────────────────────────────┘ ┌──────────────┐
                     │                                          │ ↑ Renal      │
                     ▼          ┌──────────┐                    │ absorption   │
                                │ Ascites  │◀───────────────────│ of sodium    │
                                └──────────┘                    │ and water    │
                                                                └──────────────┘
```

FIG. 44-7 Mechanisms for development of ascites.

TABLE 44-9	FACTORS INVOLVED IN ASCITES
Factor	**Mechanism**
Portal hypertension	Increase in resistance of blood flow through liver.
Increased flow of hepatic lymph	Leaking of protein-rich lymph from surface of cirrhotic liver. Intrahepatic blockage of lymph channels.
Decreased serum colloidal oncotic pressure	Impairment of liver synthesis of albumin. Loss of albumin into peritoneal cavity.
Hyperaldosteronism	Increase in aldosterone secretion stimulated by decreased renal blood flow. Decreased liver metabolism of aldosterone.
Impaired water excretion	Reduction in renal blood flow and high serum levels of antidiuretic hormone (ADH).

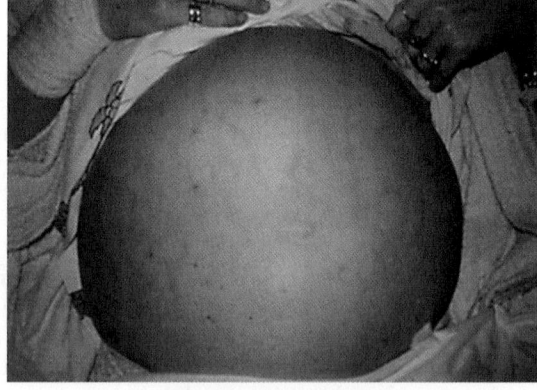

FIG. 44-8 Gross ascites.

A second mechanism of ascites formation is hypoalbuminemia resulting from the liver's inability to synthesize albumin. The hypoalbuminemia results in decreased colloidal oncotic pressure. A third mechanism is hyperaldosteronism, which occurs when aldosterone is not metabolized by damaged hepatocytes. The increased level of aldosterone causes increased sodium reabsorption by the renal tubules. This retention of sodium, combined with an increase in antidiuretic hormone, causes additional water retention. Because of edema formation, there is decreased intravascular volume and, subsequently, decreased renal blood flow and glomerular filtration.

Ascites is manifested by abdominal distention with weight gain (Fig. 44-8). If the ascites is severe, the umbilicus may be everted. Abdominal striae with distended abdominal wall veins may be present. The patient has signs of dehydration (e.g., dry tongue and skin, sunken eyeballs, muscle weakness) and a decrease in urine output. Hypokalemia is common and is due to an excessive loss of potassium caused by hyperaldosteronism. Low potassium levels can also result from diuretic therapy used to treat the ascites.

Because of alterations in immune function associated with cirrhosis, patients with ascites are at risk for *spontaneous bacterial peritonitis* (SBP). SBP is a bacterial infection of the ascites fluid. This occurs in approximately 15% to 25% of hospitalized patients with cirrhosis and ascites and is particularly common after variceal hemorrhage.[20] The bacteria most frequently found are gram-negative enteric pathogens such as *Escherichia coli*.

Hepatic Encephalopathy. Hepatic encephalopathy is a neuropsychiatric manifestation of liver disease. The pathogenesis is multifactorial and includes the neurotoxic effects of ammonia, abnormal neurotransmission, astrocyte swelling, and inflammatory cytokines. A major source of ammonia is the bacterial and enzymatic deamination of amino acids in the intestines. The ammonia that results from this deamination process normally goes to the liver via the portal circulation and is converted to urea, which is then excreted by the kidneys. When blood is shunted past the liver via the collateral vessels or the liver is unable to convert ammonia to urea, the levels of ammonia in the systemic circulation increase. The ammonia crosses the blood-brain barrier and produces neurologic toxic manifestations. Factors that increase ammonia in the circulation may precipitate hepatic encephalopathy (Table 44-10).

Hepatic encephalopathy can occur after placement of transjugular intrahepatic portosystemic shunt (TIPS), which is used to treat portal hypertension.[21]

Clinical manifestations of encephalopathy are changes in neurologic and mental responsiveness; impaired consciousness; and inappropriate behavior, ranging from sleep disturbances to lethargy to deep coma.[21] Changes may occur suddenly because of an increase in ammonia in response to bleeding varices or infection or gradually as blood ammonia levels slowly increase. A grading system is often used to classify the stages of hepatic encephalopathy (Table 44-11).

A characteristic manifestation of hepatic encephalopathy is asterixis (flapping tremors). This may take several forms, with the most common involving the arms and hands. When asked to hold the arms and hands stretched out, the patient is unable to hold this position and performs a series of rapid flexion and extension movements of the hands. Impairments in writing involve difficulty in moving the pen or pencil from left to right and *apraxia* (the inability to construct simple figures). Other signs include hyperventilation, hypothermia, and grimacing and grasping reflexes.

Fetor hepaticus (musty, sweet odor of the patient's breath) occurs in some patients with encephalopathy. This odor is from the accumulation of digestive by-products that the liver is unable to degrade.

Hepatorenal Syndrome. Hepatorenal syndrome can occur in patients with decompensated cirrhosis. It is a type of renal failure with advancing azotemia, oliguria, and intractable ascites. In this syndrome the kidneys have no structural abnormality. The etiology is complex, but the final common pathway is likely to be portal hypertension along with liver decompensation resulting in splanchnic and systemic vasodilation and decreased arterial blood volume. As a result, renal vasoconstriction occurs, and renal failure follows. This renal failure can be reversed by liver transplantation. In the patient with cirrhosis, hepatorenal syndrome frequently follows diuretic therapy, GI hemorrhage, or paracentesis.

Diagnostic Studies

Patients with cirrhosis have abnormalities in most of the liver function studies. Enzyme levels, including alkaline phosphatase, AST, ALT, and γ-glutamyl transpeptidase (GGT), are initially elevated because of their release from damaged liver cells. However, in end-stage liver disease AST and ALT levels may be normal. Patients with cirrhosis have decreased total protein, decreased albumin, increased serum bilirubin, and increased globulin levels. Fat metabolism abnormalities are reflected by decreased cholesterol levels. The prothrombin time is prolonged, and bilirubin metabolism is altered (see Table 44-3). A liver ultrasound may be used to assess the severity of cirrhosis. A liver biopsy may be done to identify liver cell changes and

TABLE 44-10	FACTORS PRECIPITATING HEPATIC ENCEPHALOPATHY
Factor	**Mechanism**
GI hemorrhage	Increase in ammonia in GI tract.
Constipation	Increase in ammonia from bacterial action on feces.
Hypokalemia	Potassium is needed by brain to metabolize ammonia.
Hypovolemia	Increase in blood ammonia because of hepatic hypoxia. Impairment of cerebral, hepatic, and renal function because of decreased blood flow.
Infection	Increase in catabolism and increase in cerebral sensitivity to toxins.
Cerebral depressants (e.g., opioids)	Decrease in metabolism by liver, causing higher drug levels and cerebral depression.
Metabolic alkalosis	Facilitation of transport of ammonia across blood-brain barrier. Increase in renal production of ammonia.
Paracentesis	Loss of sodium and potassium ions. Decrease in blood volume.
Dehydration	Potentiation of ammonia toxicity.
Increased metabolism	Increase in workload of liver.
Uremia (renal failure)	Retention of nitrogenous metabolites.

TABLE 44-11	GRADING SCALE FOR HEPATIC ENCEPHALOPATHY		
Grade	**Level of Consciousness**	**Intellectual Function**	**Neurologic Findings**
0	Insomnia, sleep disturbances	Subtle change in computational skills	Impaired handwriting, tremor
1	Lack of awareness, personality change	Short attention span, mild confusion, depression	Incoordination, asterixis
2	Lethargy, drowsiness, inappropriate behavior	Disoriented	Asterixis, abnormal reflexes
3	Asleep, rousable	Loss of meaningful conversation, marked confusion, incomprehensible speech	Asterixis, abnormal reflexes
4	Not rousable	Absent	Decerebrate May be responsive to painful stimuli

TABLE 44-12   **COLLABORATIVE CARE**

Cirrhosis of the Liver

Diagnostic
- History and physical examination
- Liver function studies
- Liver biopsy (percutaneous needle)
- Upper endoscopy (esophagogastroduodenoscopy)
- CT scan, multiphase
- Liver ultrasound (e.g., FibroScan for stiffness)
- Serum electrolytes
- Prothrombin time
- Serum albumin
- Complete blood count

Collaborative Therapy
Conservative Therapy
- Rest
- Administration of B-complex vitamins
- Avoidance of alcohol
- Minimization or avoidance of aspirin, acetaminophen, and NSAIDs

Ascites
- Low-sodium diet
- Diuretics
- Paracentesis (if indicated)

Esophageal and Gastric Varices
- Drug therapy
  - Nonselective β-blocker (e.g., propranolol [Inderal])
  - octreotide (Sandostatin)
  - vasopressin (Pitressin)
- Endoscopic band ligation or sclerotherapy
- Balloon tamponade
- Transjugular intrahepatic portosystemic shunt (TIPS)

Hepatic Encephalopathy
- Antibiotics (rifaximin [Xifaxan])
- lactulose (Cephulac)

alterations in the lobular structure. Differential analysis of ascitic fluid may help confirm the cause of cirrhosis.

Collaborative Care

The goal of treatment is to slow the progress of cirrhosis and prevent and treat any complications. Collaborative care measures are listed in Table 44-12. Management of specific problems associated with cirrhosis is described next.

Ascites. Management of ascites focuses on sodium restriction, diuretics, and fluid removal. The amount of sodium restriction is based on the degree of ascites. Initially the patient may be encouraged to limit sodium intake to 2 g/day.[22] Patients with severe ascites may need to restrict their sodium intake to 250 to 500 mg/day. Very low sodium intake can result in reduced nutritional intake and subsequent problems associated with malnutrition. The patient is usually not on restricted fluids unless severe ascites develops. Accurately assess and monitor fluid and electrolyte balance. Albumin infusion may be used to help maintain intravascular volume and adequate urine output by increasing plasma colloid osmotic pressure.

Diuretic therapy is an important part of management. Often a combination of drugs that work at multiple sites in the nephron is more effective. Spironolactone (Aldactone) is an effective diuretic, even in patients with severe sodium retention. Spironolactone is an antagonist of aldosterone and is potassium

sparing. Other potassium-sparing diuretics include amiloride (Midamor) and triamterene (Dyrenium). A high-potency loop diuretic, such as furosemide (Lasix), is frequently used in combination with a potassium-sparing drug.

Tolvaptan (Samsca), a vasopressin-receptor antagonist, is used to correct hyponatremia in patients with cirrhosis. It causes an increase in water excretion, resulting in an increase in serum sodium concentrations.[23]

A **paracentesis** (needle puncture of the abdominal cavity) may be performed to remove ascitic fluid or to test the fluid for infection (spontaneous bacterial peritonitis). However, this procedure is reserved for the patient with impaired respiration or abdominal pain caused by severe ascites. It is only a temporary measure because the fluid tends to reaccumulate.

TIPS (discussed later in this section) is used to alleviate ascites that does not respond to diuretics. Peritoneovenous shunt is a surgical procedure that provides continuous reinfusion of ascitic fluid into the venous system. Its use has almost been eliminated because of the high rate of complications.

Esophageal and Gastric Varices. The main therapeutic goal for esophageal and gastric varices is to prevent bleeding and hemorrhage. The patient who has esophageal varices should avoid ingesting alcohol, aspirin, and nonsteroidal antiinflammatory drugs (NSAIDs).

All patients with cirrhosis should have an upper endoscopy (esophagogastroduodenoscopy [EGD]) to screen for varices. The diagnosis of esophageal or gastric variceal bleeding needs to be made by endoscopic examination as soon as possible. Patients with varices at risk of bleeding are started on a nonselective β-blocker (nadolol [Corgard] or propranolol [Inderal]) to reduce the incidence of hemorrhage. β-Blockers decrease high portal pressure.

When variceal bleeding occurs, the first step is to stabilize the patient and manage the airway. IV therapy is initiated and may include administration of blood products. Management that involves a combination of drug therapy and endoscopic therapy is more successful than either approach alone.

Drug therapy for bleeding varices may include the somatostatin analog octreotide (Sandostatin) or vasopressin (VP). The main goal of drug therapy is to stop bleeding so that treatment measures can be initiated. IV administration of VP produces vasoconstriction of the splanchnic arterial bed, decreases portal blood flow, and decreases portal hypertension. However, VP has many side effects, including decreased coronary blood flow, dysrhythmias, and increased BP. Because of this, IV nitroglycerin is often given in combination with VP. The nitroglycerin reduces the adverse effects of the VP while enhancing its beneficial effect. VP should be avoided or used cautiously in the older adult because of the risk of cardiac ischemia.

At the time of endoscopy, band ligation or sclerotherapy may be used to prevent rebleeding. Endoscopic variceal ligation (EVL, or "banding") is performed by placing a small rubber band (elastic O-ring) around the base of the *varix* (enlarged vein). Sclerotherapy involves injection of a sclerosant solution into the varices through an injection needle that is placed through the endoscope.

Balloon tamponade may be used in patients with acute esophageal or gastric variceal hemorrhage that cannot be controlled on initial endoscopy. Balloon tamponade controls the hemorrhage by mechanical compression of the varices. Different types of tubes are available. The Sengstaken-Blakemore tube has two balloons, gastric and esophageal, with three lumens: one for the gastric balloon, one for the esophageal balloon, and one for gastric aspiration (see eFig. 44-1 on the website for this chapter). Two other types of balloons are the Minnesota tube (a modified Sengstaken-Blakemore tube with an esophageal suction port above the esophageal balloon) and the Linton-Nachlas tube.

SAFETY ALERT
- Label each lumen to avoid confusion.
- Deflate balloons for 5 min every 8-12 hr per institutional policy to prevent tissue necrosis.

Supportive measures during an acute variceal bleed include administration of fresh frozen plasma and packed RBCs, vitamin K, and proton pump inhibitors (e.g., pantoprazole [Protonix]). Lactulose (Cephulac) and rifaximin (Xifaxan) may be administered to prevent hepatic encephalopathy from breakdown of blood and the release of ammonia in the intestine. Antibiotics are given to prevent bacterial infection.

Because of the high incidence of recurrent bleeding with each bleeding episode, continued therapy is necessary. Long-term management of patients who have had an episode of bleeding includes nonselective β-blockers, repeated band ligation of the varices, and portosystemic shunts in patients who develop recurrent bleeding.

Shunting Procedures. Nonsurgical and surgical methods of shunting blood away from the varices are available. Shunting procedures tend to be used more after a second major bleeding episode than during an initial bleeding episode. *Transjugular intrahepatic portosystemic shunt (TIPS)* is a nonsurgical procedure in which a tract (shunt) between the systemic and portal venous systems is created to redirect portal blood flow (see eFig. 44-2 on the website for this chapter). A catheter is placed in the jugular vein and then threaded through the superior and inferior vena cava to the hepatic vein. The wall of the hepatic vein is punctured, and the catheter is directed to the portal vein. Stents are positioned along the passageway, overlapping in the liver tissue and extending into both veins.

This procedure reduces portal venous pressure and decompresses the varices, thus controlling bleeding. TIPS does not interfere with a future liver transplantation. Limitations of the procedure include the increased risk of hepatic encephalopathy and stenosis of the stent. TIPS is contraindicated in patients with severe hepatic encephalopathy, hepatocellular carcinoma, severe hepatorenal syndrome, and portal vein thrombosis.

Various surgical shunting procedures may be used to decrease portal hypertension by diverting some of the portal blood flow while allowing adequate liver perfusion. Currently, the surgical shunts most commonly used are the portacaval shunt and the distal splenorenal shunt (Fig. 44-9).

Hepatic Encephalopathy. The goal of management of hepatic encephalopathy is the reduction of ammonia formation. Ammonia formation in the intestines is reduced with lactulose, a drug that traps ammonia in the gut. It can be given orally, as an enema, or through a nasogastric (NG) tube. The laxative effect of the drug expels the ammonia from the colon. Antibiotics such as rifaximin may also be given, particularly in patients who do not respond to lactulose. Constipation should be prevented.

Control of hepatic encephalopathy also involves treatment of precipitating causes (see Table 44-10). This includes controlling GI bleeding and removing the blood from the GI tract to decrease the protein in the intestine.

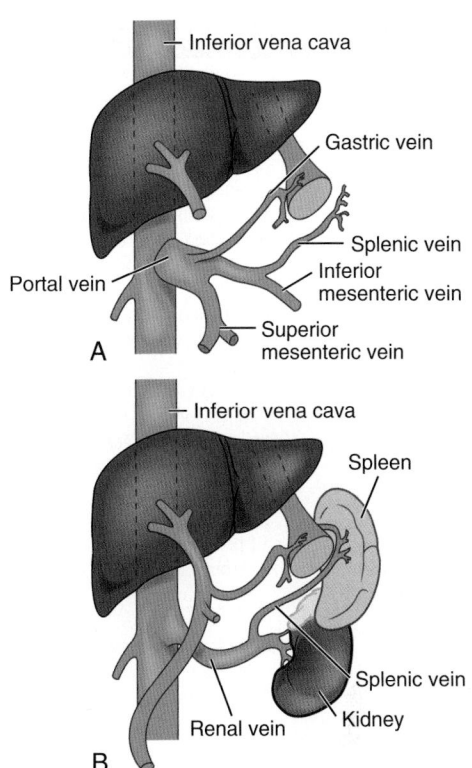

FIG. 44-9 Portosystemic shunts. **A,** Portacaval shunt. The portal vein is anastomosed to the inferior vena cava, diverting blood from the portal vein to the systemic circulation. **B,** Distal splenorenal shunt. The splenic vein is anastomosed to the renal vein. The portal venous flow remains intact while esophageal varices are selectively decompressed. (The short gastric veins are decompressed.) The spleen conducts blood from the high pressure of the esophageal and gastric varices to the low-pressure renal vein.

Drug Therapy. There is no specific drug therapy for cirrhosis. However, a number of drugs are used to treat symptoms and complications of advanced liver disease (Table 44-13).

Nutritional Therapy. The diet for the patient who has cirrhosis without complications is high in calories (3000 cal/day) with high carbohydrate content and moderate to low levels of fat. Protein restriction may be appropriate in some patients immediately after a severe flare of symptoms (i.e., episodic hepatic encephalopathy). However, protein restriction is rarely justified in patients with cirrhosis and persistent hepatic encephalopathy. Malnutrition is a more serious clinical problem than hepatic encephalopathy for many of these patients.[24]

A patient with alcoholic cirrhosis frequently has protein-calorie malnutrition. Enteral formula supplements containing protein from branched-chain amino acids that are metabolized by the muscles may be recommended. These supplements provide protein that is more easily metabolized by the liver. Parenteral nutrition or enteral nutrition therapy may be required.

The patient with ascites and edema is on a low-sodium diet. The degree of sodium restriction depends on the patient's condition. The patient needs instruction regarding the degree of restriction. Table salt is a well-known source of sodium, but sodium is also present in baking soda and baking powder. Foods that are high in sodium content include canned soups and vegetables, many frozen foods, salted snacks (e.g., potato chips), nuts, smoked meats and fish, crackers, breads, olives, pickles, ketchup, and beer. Advise the patient to read labels. The patient and the caregiver may need assistance in making the diet

TABLE 44-13 DRUG THERAPY

Cirrhosis

Drug	Mechanism of Action
vasopressin (Pitressin) octreotide (Sandostatin)	Hemostasis and control of bleeding in esophageal and gastric varices, constriction of splanchnic arterial bed
propranolol (Inderal) nadolol (Corgard)	Reduction of portal venous pressure, reduction of esophageal varices bleeding
lactulose (Cephulac)	Acidification of feces in bowel and trapping of ammonia, causing its elimination in feces
rifaximin (Xifaxan) neomycin sulfate	Decrease in bacterial flora, decreased formation of ammonia
magnesium sulfate	Magnesium replacement, hypomagnesemia possible with liver dysfunction
Vitamin K	Correction of clotting abnormalities from decreased levels of this vitamin
Proton pump inhibitors (e.g., pantoprazole [Protonix])	Decrease in gastric acidity
Diuretics	
• spironolactone (Aldactone)	Blocks action of aldosterone, potassium sparing
• furosemide (Lasix)	Acts on distal tubule and loop of Henle to decrease reabsorption of sodium and water

more palatable by using seasonings such as garlic, parsley, onion, lemon juice, and spices.

NURSING MANAGEMENT
CIRRHOSIS

NURSING ASSESSMENT

Subjective and objective data that should be obtained from an individual with cirrhosis are presented in Table 44-14.

NURSING DIAGNOSES

Nursing diagnoses for the patient with cirrhosis include, but are not limited to, the following:

- Imbalanced nutrition: less than body requirements *related to* anorexia, nausea, and impaired utilization and storage of nutrients
- Impaired skin integrity *related to* peripheral edema, ascites, and pruritus
- Excess fluid volume *related to* portal hypertension and hyperaldosteronism
- Ineffective self-health management *related to* ineffective coping and abuse of alcohol

Additional information on nursing diagnoses for the patient with cirrhosis is presented in eNursing Care Plan 44-2 (available on the website for this chapter).

PLANNING

The overall goals are that the patient with cirrhosis will (1) have relief of discomfort, (2) have minimal to no complications (ascites, esophageal varices, hepatic encephalopathy), and (3) return to as normal a lifestyle as possible.

NURSING IMPLEMENTATION

HEALTH PROMOTION. Common risk factors for cirrhosis include alcoholism, malnutrition, viral hepatitis, biliary obstruction, obesity, and right-sided heart failure. Prevention and early

TABLE 44-14 NURSING ASSESSMENT

Cirrhosis

Subjective Data
Important Health Information
Past health history: Previous viral, toxic, or idiopathic hepatitis; NASH, chronic biliary obstruction and infection; severe right-sided heart failure
Medications: Adverse reaction to any medication; use of anticoagulants, aspirin, NSAIDs, acetaminophen

Functional Health Patterns
Health perception–health management: Chronic alcoholism; weakness, fatigue
Nutritional-metabolic: Anorexia, weight loss, dyspepsia, nausea and vomiting; gingival bleeding
Elimination: Dark urine, decreased urine output; light-colored or black stools, flatulence, change in bowel habits; dry, yellow skin, bruising
Cognitive-perceptual: Dull, right upper quadrant or epigastric pain; numbness, tingling of extremities; pruritus
Sexuality-reproductive: Impotence, amenorrhea

Objective Data
General
Fever, cachexia, wasting of extremities

Integumentary
Icteric sclera, jaundice, petechiae, ecchymoses, spider angiomas, palmar erythema, alopecia, loss of axillary and pubic hair, peripheral edema

Respiratory
Shallow, rapid respirations, epistaxis

Gastrointestinal
Abdominal distention, ascites, distended abdominal wall veins, palpable liver and spleen, foul breath; hematemesis; black, tarry stools; hemorrhoids

Neurologic
Altered mentation, asterixis

Reproductive
Gynecomastia and testicular atrophy (men), impotence (men), loss of libido (men and women), amenorrhea or heavy menstrual bleeding (women)

Possible Diagnostic Findings
Anemia, thrombocytopenia; leukopenia; ↓ serum albumin, potassium; abnormal liver function studies; ↑ INR, ↓ platelets, ↑ ammonia, and ↑ bilirubin levels; abnormal abdominal ultrasound or MRI

INR, International normalized ratio; *NASH*, nonalcoholic steatohepatitis.

treatment of cirrhosis focus on reducing or eliminating these risk factors. Alcoholism must be treated. Urge patients to avoid alcohol ingestion, and support their efforts. (The treatment of alcohol dependence is discussed in Chapter 11.)

Adequate nutrition, especially for the alcoholic and other individuals at risk for cirrhosis, is essential to promote liver regeneration. Identify and treat acute hepatitis early so that it does not progress to chronic hepatitis and cirrhosis. Bariatric surgery for morbidly obese individuals has been shown to reduce the incidence of liver disease.[25]

ACUTE INTERVENTION. Nursing care for the patient with cirrhosis focuses on conserving the patient's strength while maintaining muscle strength and tone (see eNursing Care Plan 44-2 on the website for this chapter). When the patient requires complete bed rest, implement measures to prevent pneumonia, thromboembolic problems, and pressure ulcers. Modify the activity and rest schedule according to signs of clinical improvement (e.g., decreasing jaundice, improvement in liver function studies).

Anorexia, nausea and vomiting, pressure from ascites, and poor eating habits all interfere with adequate intake of nutrients. Oral hygiene before meals may improve the patient's taste sensation. Make between-meal snacks available so the patient can eat them at times when he or she can best tolerate them. Provide food preferences whenever possible. Explain the reason for any dietary restrictions to the patient and caregiver.

Nursing assessment and care should include the patient's physiologic response to cirrhosis. Is jaundice present? Where is it observed—sclera, skin, hard palate? What is the progression of jaundice? If the jaundice is accompanied by pruritus, carry out measures to relieve itching. Cholestyramine or hydroxyzine (Atarax) may be ordered to help relieve the pruritus. Other measures to alleviate pruritus include baking soda or Alpha Keri baths, lotions containing calamine, antihistamines, soft or old linens, and control of the temperature (not too hot and not too cold). Keep the patient's nails short and clean. Teach patients to rub with their knuckles rather than scratch with their nails when they cannot resist scratching.

Note the color of urine and stools. When jaundice is present, the urine is often dark brown and foamy when shaken. The stool is gray or tan.

Edema and ascites are frequent manifestations of cirrhosis and require nursing assessments and interventions. Accurate calculation and recording of intake and output, daily weights, and measurements of extremities and abdominal girth help in the ongoing assessment of the location and extent of the edema. Mark the abdomen with a permanent marker so the girth is measured at the same location each time.

Immediately before a paracentesis have the patient void to prevent a puncture of the bladder. When a paracentesis is done, the patient sits on the side of the bed or is placed in high Fowler's position. After the procedure, monitor for hypovolemia and electrolyte imbalances and check the dressing for bleeding and leakage.

Dyspnea is a frequent problem for the patient with severe ascites and can lead to pleural effusions. A semi-Fowler's or Fowler's position allows for maximal respiratory efficiency. Use pillows to support the arms and chest to increase the patient's comfort and ability to breathe.

Meticulous skin care is essential because the edematous tissues are subject to breakdown. Use an alternating-air pressure mattress or other special mattress. A turning schedule (minimum of every 2 hours) must be adhered to rigidly. Support the abdomen with pillows. If the abdomen is taut, cleanse it gently. The patient tends to move little because of abdominal discomfort and dyspnea. Range-of-motion exercises are helpful. Implement measures such as coughing and deep breathing to prevent respiratory problems. The lower extremities may be elevated. If scrotal edema is present, a scrotal support provides some comfort.

When the patient is taking diuretics, monitor the serum levels of sodium, potassium, chloride, and bicarbonate. Monitor renal function (blood urea nitrogen [BUN], serum creatinine) routinely and with any change in the diuretic dosage. Observe for signs of fluid and electrolyte imbalance, especially hypokalemia. Hypokalemia may be manifested by cardiac dysrhythmias, hypotension, tachycardia, and generalized muscle weakness. Water excess is manifested by muscle cramping, weakness, lethargy, and confusion.

Observe for and provide nursing care for any hematologic problems (bleeding tendencies, anemia, increased susceptibility to infection) (see eNursing Care Plan 44-2 on the website for this chapter).

Assess the patient's response to altered body image resulting from jaundice, spider angiomas, palmar erythema, ascites, and gynecomastia. The patient may experience anxiety and embarrassment about these changes. Explain these phenomena and be a supportive listener. Provide nursing care with concern and warmth to help the patient maintain self-esteem.

Bleeding Varices. If the patient has esophageal or gastric varices, observe for any signs of bleeding from the varices, such as hematemesis and melena. If hematemesis occurs, assess the patient for hemorrhage, call the physician, and be ready to assist with treatment used to control the bleeding. The patient will be admitted to the intensive care unit (ICU). The patient's airway must be maintained.

Balloon tamponade may be used in patients who have bleeding that is unresponsive to band ligation or sclerotherapy. When balloon tamponade is used, the initial nursing task is to explain the use of the tube and how it will be inserted. Check the balloons for patency. It is usually the physician's responsibility to insert the tube by either the nose or the mouth (see eFig. 44-1). Then the gastric balloon is inflated with approximately 250 mL of air, and the tube is retracted until resistance (lower esophageal sphincter) is felt. The tube is secured by placement of a piece of sponge or foam rubber at the nostrils (nasal cuff). For continued bleeding, the esophageal balloon is then inflated. A sphygmomanometer is used to measure and maintain the

ETHICAL/LEGAL DILEMMAS
Rationing

Situation
T.H., a 43-yr-old patient with cirrhosis of the liver, is frequently admitted to the hospital. She has been told that her continued drinking will inevitably lead to her death. Now she has been admitted for gastrointestinal bleeding and needs blood transfusions. She has a rare blood type, and it is frequently difficult to get compatible blood. Should you call an ethics consultation?

Ethical/Legal Points for Consideration
- *Rationing*, or the controlled distribution of scarce resources, is a difficult ethical problem. The needs of an individual patient or group of patients are weighed against the needs of many patients, who may have a greater chance of recovery, and the availability of the needed resources.
- Health interests can supercede the interests or rights of an individual. For example, in anticipation of an anthrax attack, the government could confiscate all relevant antibiotics and restrict their use to treatment of the disease.
- Two individual rights that must be considered with regard to rationing are the constitutional right to privacy and the right to consent to or refuse medical procedures and therapy.
- The competent adult is the only person who may consent to or refuse treatment for his or her health care problems.
- In the situation of T.H., if she consents to a blood transfusion, the ability of an intervening party to refuse that treatment would be permitted only given substantial intervening circumstances, and not as a threat to compel compliant behavior in the future.

Discussion Questions
1. What are your feelings about patients with diseases, such as substance abuse, that have a behavioral component? Do these patients deserve aggressive treatment?
2. How would you proceed to make a decision in T.H.'s case? Would you request an ethics committee consultation?

Applying the Evidence

You have been assigned to care for M.K., a 58-yr-old Hispanic man, who is being admitted with alcohol-related cirrhosis. As a part of his admission assessment, you ask about his current use of alcohol. He tells you that he has been "drinking more" since he lost his job. His admission blood alcohol concentration was 295 mg/dL. You ask if he has ever tried to stop drinking. He tells you many times, but "it never lasts." When asked if he has ever been to Alcoholics Anonymous (AA), he states that that "scene" is not for him. M.K. tells you that he knows he will not live very long and he sees no reason to stop drinking at this point.

Best Available Evidence	Clinician Expertise	Patient Preferences and Values
Although treatment strategies for alcohol dependency include inpatient and outpatient treatment programs for the individual, often they are not effective. Another approach is family therapy, which has been shown to decrease the incidence of alcohol-related disease and inpatient hospital stays.	Abstinence from the use of alcohol is critical in the treatment of cirrhosis. You have known many patients who have attended AA and are "recovering alcoholics." You also know that the family is an essential part of the effectiveness of treatment. You ask M.K. if you could meet with him and his family to discuss treatment options.	M.K. is not motivated to consider any treatment approaches for alcohol dependency. M.K. prefers to continue to use alcohol and he tells you that he knows the consequences.

Your Decision and Action

You acknowledge M.K.'s comments about his continued use of alcohol at this time but reassess his decision throughout his hospitalization. You also plan a meeting with key family members to discuss the issue. Based on the results of meeting with the family, you will try to set up a meeting with M.K., the family, and an appropriate therapist.

Reference for Evidence

Meads C, Ting S, Dretzke J, et al: A systematic review of the clinical and cost-effectiveness of psychological therapy involving family and friends in alcohol misuse or dependence, *Database Abstracts Rev Effects* 3, 2012.

desired pressure at 20 to 40 mm Hg. The position of the balloons is verified by x-ray.

Nursing care includes monitoring for complications of rupture or erosion of the esophagus, regurgitation and aspiration of gastric contents, and occlusion of the airway by the balloon. If the gastric balloon breaks or is deflated, the esophageal balloon will slip upward, obstructing the airway and causing asphyxiation. If this happens, cut the tube or deflate the esophageal balloon. Keep scissors at the bedside. Minimize regurgitation by oral and pharyngeal suctioning and by keeping the patient in a semi-Fowler's position.

The patient is unable to swallow saliva because of the inflated esophageal balloon occluding the esophagus. Encourage the patient to expectorate, and provide an emesis basin and tissues. Frequent oral and nasal care provides relief from the taste of blood and irritation from mouth breathing.

Hepatic Encephalopathy. Nursing care of the patient with hepatic encephalopathy focuses on maintaining a safe environment, sustaining life, and assisting with measures to reduce the formation of ammonia. Assess (1) the patient's level of responsiveness (e.g., reflexes, pupillary reactions, orientation), (2) sensory and motor abnormalities (e.g., hyperreflexia, asterixis, motor coordination), (3) fluid and electrolyte imbalances, (4) acid-base imbalances, and (5) the effect of treatment measures.

Assess the neurologic status, including an exact description of the patient's behavior, at least every 2 hours. Plan your care of the patient with neurologic problems based on the severity of the encephalopathy.

Institute measures to prevent constipation to reduce ammonia production. Give drugs, laxatives, and enemas as ordered. Encourage fluids, if not contraindicated. Any GI bleeding may worsen encephalopathy. Assess the patient taking lactulose for diarrhea and excessive fluid and electrolyte losses.

Control factors known to precipitate encephalopathy as much as possible, including anything that may cause constipation (e.g., dehydration, opioid medications).

AMBULATORY AND HOME CARE. The patient with cirrhosis may be faced with a prolonged course and the possibility of life-threatening problems and complications. The patient and caregiver need to understand the importance of continual health care and medical supervision. Supportive measures include proper diet, rest, avoidance of potentially hepatotoxic OTC drugs such as acetaminophen, and abstinence from alcohol.[25] Abstinence from alcohol is important and results in improvement in most patients. However, some patients find abstinence difficult. Explore your own attitude regarding the patient whose cirrhosis is attributed to alcohol abuse. Provide care without rejection or moralizing. Treat the patient with a caring attitude (see Chapter 11).

Cirrhosis is a chronic disease. The patient is affected not only physically but also psychologically, socially, and economically. Major lifestyle changes may be required, especially if alcohol abuse is the primary etiologic factor. Provide information regarding community support programs, such as Alcoholics Anonymous, for help with alcohol abuse.

When you know a patient's diagnosis is cirrhosis, do not assume the cause is excess alcohol intake. Because cirrhosis has many different causes, it is important for you to find out the primary etiology before jumping to conclusions about the patient.

Teach the patient and caregiver about manifestations of complications and when to seek medical attention. Explain both verbally and in writing information about fluid or possible dietary changes (Table 44-15). Include instructions about adequate rest periods, how to detect early signs of complications, skin care, drug therapy precautions, observation for bleeding, and protection from infection. Counseling information regarding sexual problems may be needed. Referral to a community or home health nurse may be helpful to ensure patient adherence to prescribed therapy. Home care for the patient with cirrhosis should emphasize helping the patient maintain the highest level of wellness possible and initiate and maintain necessary lifestyle changes.

EVALUATION

Expected outcomes are that the patient with cirrhosis will
- Maintain food and fluid intake adequate to meet nutritional needs
- Maintain skin integrity with relief of edema and pruritus
- Experience normalization of fluid balance as a result of medical and nursing interventions
- Acknowledge and get treatment for a substance abuse problem

TABLE 44-15   **PATIENT & CAREGIVER TEACHING GUIDE**
Cirrhosis
When teaching the patient and caregiver about management of cirrhosis, do the following. 1. Explain that cirrhosis is a chronic illness and the importance of continual health care. 2. Teach the symptoms of complications and when to seek medical attention to enable prompt treatment of complications. 3. Teach the patient to avoid potentially hepatotoxic over-the-counter drugs (see Table 39-6) because the diseased liver is unable to metabolize these drugs. 4. Encourage abstinence from alcohol because continued use of alcohol will increase the risk of liver complications. 5. Instruct the patient to avoid aspirin and NSAIDs to prevent hemorrhage when esophageal or gastric varices are present. 6. Teach the patient to avoid activities that increase portal pressure, such as straining at stool, coughing, sneezing, and retching and vomiting. These activities may increase the risk of variceal hemorrhage in patients with portal hypertension and varices.

Additional information on expected outcomes for the patient with cirrhosis is presented in eNursing Care Plan 44-2 (available on the website for this chapter).

ACUTE LIVER FAILURE

Acute liver failure, or *fulminant hepatic failure,* is a clinical syndrome characterized by severe impairment of liver function associated with hepatic encephalopathy. The most common cause is drugs, usually acetaminophen in combination with alcohol.[26] People who abuse alcohol are particularly susceptible to detrimental effects of acetaminophen on the liver. Other drugs that can cause acute liver failure include isoniazid, halothane, sulfa-containing drugs, and NSAIDs. Drugs can cause liver cell failure by disrupting essential intracellular processes or causing an accumulation of toxic metabolic products.

Viral hepatitis, in particular HBV, is the second most common cause of acute liver failure. Hepatitis A is a less common cause.

Acute liver failure is characterized by the rapid onset of severe liver dysfunction in someone with no prior history of liver disease. Although the disease can run its course over 8 weeks, it can last as long as 26 weeks. With improved intensive care, the prognosis is much better now than in the past, with survival rates of approximately 60%.[27]

Clinical Manifestations and Diagnostic Studies

Manifestations include jaundice, coagulation abnormalities, and encephalopathy. In acute liver failure, changes in mentation are the first clinical sign. Patients are susceptible to a wide variety of complications, including cerebral edema, renal failure, hypoglycemia, metabolic acidosis, sepsis, and multiorgan failure.

Serum bilirubin is elevated, and the prothrombin time is prolonged. Liver enzyme levels (AST, ALT) are often markedly elevated. Additional laboratory tests include blood chemistries (especially glucose, since hypoglycemia may be present and require correction), complete blood counts (CBCs), acetaminophen level and screening for other drugs and toxins, viral hepatitis serologies (especially HAV and HBV), serum ceruloplasmin (enzyme synthesized in liver) levels, α_1-antitrypsin levels, iron levels, and autoantibodies (antinuclear and anti–smooth muscle antibodies). Plasma ammonia levels may also be obtained.

CT or magnetic resonance imaging (MRI) is helpful in providing information about the liver size and contour, presence of ascites, tumors, and patency of the blood vessels.

NURSING AND COLLABORATIVE MANAGEMENT ACUTE LIVER FAILURE

Since acute liver failure may progress rapidly, with hour-by-hour changes in consciousness, early transfer to the ICU is preferred once the diagnosis is made. Planning for transfer to a transplant center should begin in patients with grade 1 or 2 encephalopathy because they may worsen rapidly. Early transfer is important because the risks involved with patient transport may increase or even preclude transfer once stage 3 or 4 encephalopathy develops (see Table 44-11).

Renal failure is a frequent complication in patients with liver failure and may be due to dehydration, hepatorenal syndrome, or acute tubular necrosis. The frequency of renal failure may be even greater with acetaminophen overdose or other toxins, where direct renal toxicity occurs. Although few patients die of renal failure alone, it often increases the mortality risk and may worsen the prognosis. Protect renal function by maintaining adequate fluid balance, avoiding nephrotoxic agents (e.g., aminoglycosides, NSAIDs), and promptly identifying and treating infection.

Liver transplantation is the treatment of choice for and increases survival rates in patients with acute liver failure. Cerebral edema, cerebellar herniation, and brainstem compression are the most common causes of death. Treatment of cerebral edema is described in Chapter 57. Monitoring and management of hemodynamic and renal function, as well as glucose, electrolytes, and acid-base status, are critical. Conduct frequent neurologic evaluations for signs of elevated intracranial pressure. Position the patient with the head elevated at 30 degrees. Avoid patient stimulation. Maneuvers that cause straining or Valsalva-like movements may increase intracranial pressure (ICP).

Avoid the use of any sedatives because of their effects on mental status. Only minimal doses of benzodiazepines should be used due to their delayed metabolism by the failing liver. ICP monitoring is discussed in Chapter 57. Additional measures include padding bedrails to avoid injury from possible seizures, closely observing the patient to prevent injuries, monitoring intake and output for renal function, and providing good skin and oral care to avoid breakdown and infection.

Alterations in level of consciousness may compromise nutritional intake. Factors such as coagulation problems may influence whether enteral nutrition is initiated. An NG tube may be irritating to the nasal and esophageal mucosa, thus causing bleeding.[28]

LIVER CANCER (HEPATOCELLULAR CANCER)

Primary liver cancer (hepatocellular carcinoma [HCC] or malignant hepatoma) is the fifth most common cancer and second most common cause of cancer death worldwide.[29] It is the most common cause of death in patients with cirrhosis. The incidence of HCC is rising in the United States because of the large number of patients infected with chronic hepatitis C. Cirrhosis caused by hepatitis C is the most common cause of HCC in the United States, followed by alcoholic cirrhosis.[30] Other

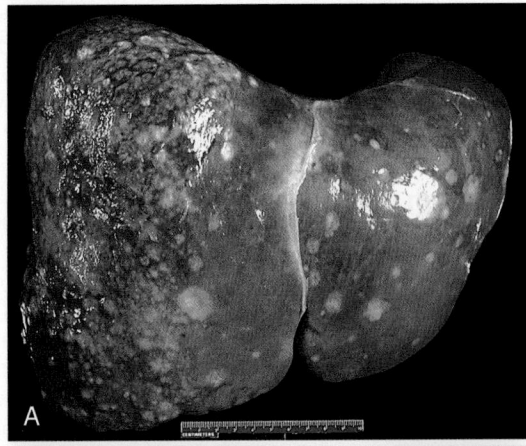

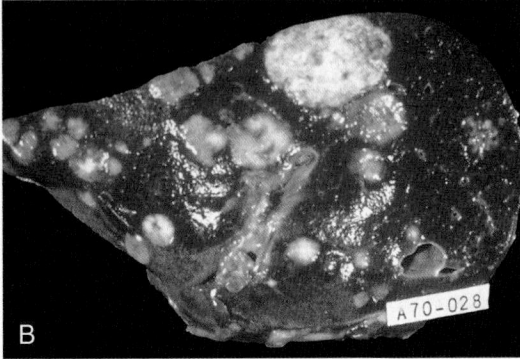

FIG. 44-10 Multiple hepatic metastases from a primary colon cancer. **A,** Gross specimen showing outside of liver. **B,** Liver section showing metastatic lesions.

primary liver tumors are cholangiomas or bile duct cancers (cholangiocarcinoma).

Metastatic carcinoma of the liver is more common than primary carcinoma (Fig. 44-10). The liver is a common site of metastatic growth because of its high rate of blood flow and extensive capillary network. Cancer cells in other parts of the body are commonly carried to the liver via the portal circulation.

In liver cancer, lesions may be singular or numerous and nodular or diffusely spread over the entire liver. Some tumors infiltrate other organs such as the gallbladder or move into the peritoneum or the diaphragm. Primary liver tumors commonly metastasize to the lung.

Clinical Manifestations and Diagnostic Studies

Liver cancer can be difficult to diagnose and differentiate from cirrhosis. They have similar clinical manifestations (e.g., hepatomegaly, splenomegaly, jaundice, weight loss, peripheral edema, ascites, portal hypertension). Other common manifestations of liver cancer include dull abdominal pain in the epigastric or right upper quadrant region, anorexia, nausea and vomiting, and increased abdominal girth. Patients with advanced HCC can have pulmonary emboli and portal vein thrombosis.

Tests used to screen and diagnose liver cancer are ultrasound, CT, and MRI. A percutaneous biopsy is performed when the results of diagnostic imaging studies are inconclusive or tissue is needed to guide treatment. Risks of biopsy include bleeding and potential tumor cell spread. Serum α-fetoprotein (AFP) levels are elevated in approximately 60% of patients with HCC. The level of elevation may not correlate with the clinical

features of HCC (e.g., stage or prognosis). (AFP is discussed in Chapter 16.)

NURSING AND COLLABORATIVE MANAGEMENT LIVER CANCER

Prevention of liver cancer focuses on identifying and treating chronic hepatitis B and C viral infections. Treatment of chronic alcohol ingestion may also lower the risk of liver cancer. Screening for at-risk patients usually involves a combination of serum AFP and either CT, MRI, or ultrasound imaging of the liver, usually obtained every 6 to 12 months.

Treatment of liver cancer depends on the size and number of tumors, any spreading beyond the liver, and the patient's age and overall health. In general, the management is similar to that for cirrhosis. Surgical excision (partial hepatectomy) is performed when there is no evidence of invasion of hepatic blood vessels. Surgical resection is possible in only about 15% of patients because the cancer is usually too advanced when the patient is diagnosed. However, surgical interventions offer the best chance for cure of HCC. Liver transplantation is performed when the tumor is localized. Other treatment options are radiofrequency ablation, chemoembolization, and alcohol injection.

In *radiofrequency ablation* (RFA), a thin needle is inserted into the core of the tumor. Then electrical energy is used to create heat in a specific location for a limited time. The end result is destruction of tumor cells. This procedure can be done percutaneously, laparoscopically, or through an open incision. RFA can be used to treat tumors that are less than 5 cm in size and for palliative purposes. Complications are not common but can include infection, bleeding, dysrhythmias, and skin burn.

Chemoembolization (sometimes called transarterial chemoembolization [TACE]) is a minimally invasive procedure frequently performed in the interventional radiology department. A catheter is placed in the arteries to the tumor and an embolic agent is administered, mixed with one or more chemotherapy agents. The embolic agent reduces the blood supply, thus allowing greater exposure of liver cells to the chemotherapy drugs.

With the technique of alcohol injection, surgeons or interventional radiologists identify (with the use of ultrasound) the location of the liver tumor(s). They insert a needle into the tumor and inject a liquid containing a high concentration of alcohol. The concentrated alcohol kills cells, mostly liver cancer cells. This form of treatment is most effective in treating small liver tumors (less than 3 cm).

Systemic chemotherapy is not used for patients with HCC because of the poor response rates. Sorafenib (Nexavar), a targeted therapy, is used to treat metastatic liver cancer. It inhibits new blood vessel growth to tumors (see Table 16-13).

Nursing intervention for the patient with liver cancer focuses on keeping the patient as comfortable as possible. Because this patient manifests the same problems as any patient with advanced liver disease, the nursing interventions discussed for cirrhosis of the liver apply. (See Chapter 16 for care of the patient with cancer.)

The prognosis for patients with liver cancer is poor. The cancer grows rapidly, and death may occur within 6 to 12 months as a result of hepatic encephalopathy or massive blood loss from GI bleeding.

LIVER TRANSPLANTATION

Liver transplantation has become a practical therapeutic option for many people with end-stage liver disease or localized HCC. Liver disease related to chronic viral hepatitis is the leading indication for liver transplantation. Other indications include congenital biliary abnormalities (biliary atresia), inborn errors of metabolism, liver cancer, sclerosing cholangitis, acute liver failure, and chronic end-stage liver disease. Liver transplants are not recommended for the patient with widespread malignant disease. Currently about 17,000 people are waiting for liver transplants. However, only 6000 transplants are performed annually.[31]

Liver transplant candidates must go through a rigorous pre-surgery screening. This is done to confirm the diagnosis of end-stage liver disease and to assess for other co-morbid conditions (e.g., cardiovascular disease, chronic kidney disease) that may affect the patient's surgical outcome. The evaluation includes physical examination, laboratory tests (CBC, liver function tests), cardiac and pulmonary evaluations, endoscopy, CT scan, and psychologic testing. Potential recipients receive counseling regarding cigarette smoking and alcohol abstinence. Contraindications for liver transplant include severe extrahepatic disease, advanced hepatocellular carcinoma or other cancer, ongoing drug or alcohol abuse, and inability to comprehend or comply with the rigorous posttransplant course.

Liver transplantation is performed using both deceased (cadaver) and live donor livers. (See Chapter 14 for a general discussion of organ transplants.) The live donor liver transplant was developed initially for children whose parents wanted to serve as donors. Today, some liver transplant centers are performing live liver transplant procedures for adults. In this procedure, the living person donates a portion of his or her liver to another. However, live liver donation poses potential risks to the donor, including biliary problems, hepatic artery thrombosis, wound infection, postoperative ileus, and pneumothorax.

Because of the scarcity of available livers, a donor liver may be divided into two parts (split liver transplant) and implanted into two recipients. The decision to use a split donor liver is based on the donor's size and health. The recipients of the split liver generally are smaller than the donor. The success rate associated with split liver transplantation is somewhat lower than that associated with whole organ transplantation because of complications.

Postoperative complications of liver transplant include bleeding, infection, and rejection. However, the liver is subject to a less aggressive immunologic attack than other organs such as the kidneys. (Transplants and immunosuppressive therapy are discussed in Chapter 14.)

Immunosuppressive therapy generally involves a combination of corticosteroids (prednisone), a calcineurin inhibitor (cyclosporine or tacrolimus), and an antiproliferative agent (e.g., azathioprine). (Immunosuppressive therapy is presented in Table 14-16.) Tacrolimus appears to be superior to cyclosporine in liver transplantation and is being used in many centers. Standard regimens often change during the course of a liver transplant recipient's life. In addition, corticosteroid withdrawal, which has been shown to be relatively safe in liver transplant recipients, has been done in some centers.

Approximately 78% of patients survive more than 5 years after liver transplant. Long-term survival depends on the cause of liver failure (e.g., localized liver cancer, chronic hepatitis B or C, biliary disease). Patients who have liver disease secondary to viral hepatitis often experience reinfection of the transplanted liver with hepatitis B or C. For patients with HBV, treatment after surgery with IV HBIG and one of the nucleoside or nucleotide analogs (used to treat HBV infection) has reduced the rates of reinfection of the transplanted liver.

Patients with HCV have lower survival rates than other patient groups. Factors that may contribute to recurrent HCV include the donor's advanced age, HCV genotype 1, high HCV RNA levels before the transplant, and co-infection with other viruses (e.g., cytomegalovirus). Although the recurrence of HCV is nearly universal after liver transplantation, avoidance of changes in immunosuppressive regimen helps to prevent clinically aggressive disease. Because of adverse effects associated with its use, antiviral therapy for hepatitis C after transplant is initiated on an individual basis.

The patient who has had a liver transplant requires highly skilled nursing care, either in an ICU or in some other specialized unit. Postoperative nursing care includes assessing neurologic status; monitoring for signs of hemorrhage; preventing pulmonary complications; monitoring drainage, electrolyte levels, and urine output; and monitoring for signs and symptoms of infection and rejection. Common respiratory problems are pneumonia, atelectasis, and pleural effusions. To prevent these complications, encourage the patient to use measures such as coughing, deep breathing, incentive spirometry, and repositioning. Measure the drainage from the Jackson-Pratt drain, NG tube, and T tube, and note the color and consistency of the drainage.

The first 2 months after the surgery are critical for monitoring for infection. Infection can be viral, fungal, or bacterial. Fever may be the only sign of infection. Emotional support and teaching for the patient and caregiver are essential.

GERONTOLOGIC CONSIDERATIONS

LIVER DISEASE IN THE OLDER ADULT

The incidence of liver disease increases with age. With aging, the liver's size and metabolism of drugs decrease, and hepatobiliary function is altered. The liver has a decreased ability to respond to injury, particularly to regenerate after injury.[32] Transplanted livers take longer to regenerate in the older adult compared with the younger adult.

Older adults are particularly vulnerable to drug-induced liver injury. This is due to several factors, including increased use of prescription and OTC drugs, which can lead to drug interactions and potential drug toxicity. Age-related decreases in liver function caused by decreased liver blood flow and enzyme activity result in decreased drug metabolism. In addition, with aging the liver is less able to recover from drug-induced injury.

A growing number of older adults have chronic hepatitis C and subsequent cirrhosis. HCV and elevated liver enzymes may be found during a routine health assessment. Because older adults have more co-morbid conditions, liver transplant following liver failure may not be an option.

Lifetime health behaviors may also influence the development of chronic liver disease in the older adult. Chronic alcohol abuse and obesity can contribute to cirrhosis, fatty liver inflammation (NASH), and subsequent liver failure. Because of co-morbid cardiovascular and pulmonary diseases, the older adult is less able to tolerate variceal bleeding. In the older adult

PATHOPHYSIOLOGY MAP

Etiologic factors		Activation of pancreatic enzymes		Autodigestive effects of pancreatic enzymes

Etiologic factors
- Alcoholism
- Biliary tract disease
- Trauma
- Infection
- Drugs
- Postoperative GI surgery
- Unknown

Activation of pancreatic enzymes

Injury to pancreatic cells

Autodigestive effects of pancreatic enzymes

Trypsin
- Edema
- Necrosis
- Hemorrhage

Elastase
- Hemorrhage

Phospholipase A and lipase
- Fat necrosis

Kallikrein
- Edema
- Vascular permeability
- Smooth muscle contraction
- Shock

FIG. 44-11 Pathogenic process of acute pancreatitis.

with liver disease, hepatic encephalopathy may be misdiagnosed as dementia.

DISORDERS OF THE PANCREAS

ACUTE PANCREATITIS

Acute pancreatitis is an acute inflammation of the pancreas. The degree of inflammation varies from mild edema to severe hemorrhagic necrosis. Acute pancreatitis is most common in middle-aged men and women. On an annual basis, approximately 210,000 persons are admitted to the hospital with acute pancreatitis. It affects women and men equally. The rate of pancreatitis in African Americans is three times higher than in whites.

Etiology and Pathophysiology

Many factors can cause injury to the pancreas. In the United States the most common cause is gallbladder disease (gallstones), which is more common in women. The second most common cause is chronic alcohol intake, which is more common in men.

Smoking is an independent risk factor for acute pancreatitis. Biliary sludge or microlithiasis, which is a mixture of cholesterol crystals and calcium salts, is found in 20% to 40% of patients with acute pancreatitis. The formation of biliary sludge is seen in patients with bile stasis. Acute pancreatitis attacks are also associated with hypertriglyceridemia (serum levels over 1000 mg/dL). Other less common causes of acute pancreatitis include trauma (postsurgical, abdominal), viral infections (mumps, coxsackievirus B, HIV), penetrating duodenal ulcer, cysts, abscesses, cystic fibrosis, Kaposi sarcoma, certain drugs (corticosteroids, thiazide diuretics, oral contraceptives, sulfonamides, NSAIDs), metabolic disorders (hyperparathyroidism, renal failure), and vascular diseases.[33]

Pancreatitis may occur after surgical procedures on the pancreas, stomach, duodenum, or biliary tract. Pancreatitis can also develop following endoscopic retrograde cholangiopancreatography (ERCP). In some cases the cause is unknown (idiopathic).

The most common pathogenic mechanism is autodigestion of the pancreas (Fig. 44-11). The etiologic factors injure pancreatic cells or activate the pancreatic enzymes in the pancreas rather than in the intestine. This may be due to reflux of bile

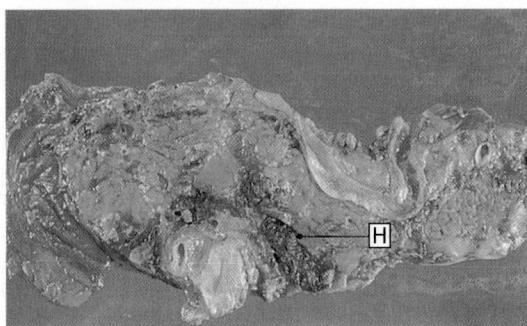

FIG. 44-12 In acute pancreatitis, the pancreas appears edematous and is commonly hemorrhagic *(H).*

acids into the pancreatic ducts through an open or distended sphincter of Oddi. This reflux may be caused by blockage created by gallstones. Obstruction of pancreatic ducts results in pancreatic ischemia.

Trypsinogen is an inactive proteolytic enzyme produced by the pancreas. It is released into the small intestine via the pancreatic duct. In the intestine it is activated to trypsin by enterokinase. Normally, trypsin inhibitors in the pancreas and plasma bind and inactivate any trypsin that is inadvertently produced. In pancreatitis, activated trypsin in the pancreas can digest the pancreas and produce bleeding.

The exact mechanism by which chronic alcohol intake predisposes a person to pancreatitis is not known. It is thought that alcohol increases the production of the digestive enzymes in the pancreas. Approximately 5% to 10% of alcohol abusers develop pancreatitis. This suggests that environmental (high-fat diet, smoking) and genetic factors may also contribute.

The pathophysiologic involvement of acute pancreatitis is classified as either *mild pancreatitis* (also known as edematous or interstitial pancreatitis) or *severe pancreatitis* (also called *necrotizing pancreatitis*) (Fig. 44-12). In severe pancreatitis, approximately half the patients have permanent decreases in endocrine and exocrine function. Patients with severe pancreatitis are also at high risk of developing pancreatic necrosis, organ failure, and septic complications, resulting in a 25% mortality rate.[33,34]

Clinical Manifestations

Abdominal pain is the predominant manifestation of acute pancreatitis. The pain is due to distention of the pancreas, peritoneal irritation, and obstruction of the biliary tract. The pain is usually located in the left upper quadrant, but it may be in the midepigastrium. It commonly radiates to the back because of the retroperitoneal location of the pancreas. The pain has a sudden onset and is described as severe, deep, piercing, and continuous or steady. The pain is aggravated by eating and frequently has its onset when the patient is recumbent. It is not relieved by vomiting. The pain may be accompanied by flushing, cyanosis, and dyspnea. The patient may assume various positions involving flexion of the spine in an attempt to relieve the severe pain. Other manifestations of acute pancreatitis include nausea and vomiting, low-grade fever, leukocytosis, hypotension, tachycardia, and jaundice.

Abdominal tenderness with muscle guarding is common. Bowel sounds may be decreased or absent. Paralytic ileus may occur and causes marked abdominal distention. The lungs are frequently involved, with crackles present. Intravascular damage from circulating trypsin may cause areas of cyanosis or greenish to yellow-brown discoloration of the abdominal wall. Other areas of ecchymoses are the flanks (*Grey Turner's spots* or *sign,* a bluish flank discoloration) and the periumbilical area (*Cullen's sign,* a bluish periumbilical discoloration). These result from seepage of blood-stained exudate from the pancreas and may occur in severe cases.

Shock may occur because of hemorrhage into the pancreas, toxemia from the activated pancreatic enzymes, or hypovolemia as a result of fluid shift into the retroperitoneal space (massive fluid shifts).

Complications

The severity of the disease varies according to the extent of pancreatic destruction. Some patients recover completely, others have recurring attacks, and others develop chronic pancreatitis. Acute pancreatitis can be life threatening.

Two significant local complications of acute pancreatitis are pseudocyst and abscess. A pancreatic pseudocyst is an accumulation of fluid, pancreatic enzymes, tissue debris, and inflammatory exudates surrounded by a wall. Manifestations of pseudocyst are abdominal pain, palpable epigastric mass, nausea, vomiting, and anorexia. The serum amylase level frequently remains elevated. CT, MRI, and endoscopic ultrasound (EUS) may be used in the detection of a pseudocyst. The cysts usually resolve spontaneously within a few weeks but may perforate, causing peritonitis, or rupture into the stomach or the duodenum. Treatment options include surgical drainage, percutaneous catheter placement and drainage, and endoscopic drainage.

A *pancreatic abscess* is a collection of pus. It results from extensive necrosis in the pancreas. It may become infected or perforate into adjacent organs. Manifestations of an abscess include upper abdominal pain, abdominal mass, high fever, and leukocytosis. Pancreatic abscesses require prompt surgical drainage to prevent sepsis.

The main systemic complications of acute pancreatitis are pulmonary (pleural effusion, atelectasis, pneumonia, and acute respiratory distress syndrome [ARDS]) and cardiovascular (hypotension) complications and tetany caused by hypocalcemia. The pulmonary complications are likely due to the passage of exudate containing pancreatic enzymes from the peritoneal cavity through transdiaphragmatic lymph channels. Enzyme-induced inflammation of the diaphragm occurs with the end result being atelectasis caused by reduced diaphragm movement. Trypsin can activate prothrombin and plasminogen,

TABLE 44-16 DIAGNOSTIC STUDIES

Acute Pancreatitis

Laboratory Test	Abnormal Finding
Serum amylase	↑
Serum lipase	↑
Urinary amylase	↑
Blood glucose	↑
Serum calcium	↓
Serum triglycerides	↑

increasing the patient's risk for intravascular thrombi, pulmonary emboli, and disseminated intravascular coagulation. When hypocalcemia occurs, it is a sign of severe disease. It is due in part to the combining of calcium and fatty acids during fat necrosis. The exact mechanisms of how or why hypocalcemia occurs are not well understood.

Patients with severe acute pancreatitis are at risk for abdominal compartment syndrome as a result of intraabdominal hypertension and edema. Abdominal compartment syndrome is discussed in Chapter 43.

Diagnostic Studies

The primary diagnostic tests for acute pancreatitis are serum amylase and lipase (Table 44-16). The serum amylase level is usually elevated early and remains elevated for 24 to 72 hours. Serum lipase level, which is also elevated in acute pancreatitis, is an important test because other disorders (e.g., mumps, cerebral trauma, renal transplantation) may increase serum amylase levels. Other findings include an increase in liver enzymes, triglycerides, glucose, and bilirubin and a decrease in calcium.

Diagnostic evaluation of acute pancreatitis is also directed at determining the cause. An abdominal ultrasound, x-ray, or contrast-enhanced CT scan can be used to identify pancreatic problems. CT scan is the best imaging test for pancreatitis and related complications such as pseudocysts and abscesses. ERCP is used (although ERCP can cause acute pancreatitis), along with EUS, magnetic resonance cholangiopancreatography (MRCP), and angiography. Chest x-rays may show pulmonary changes, including atelectasis and pleural effusions.

Collaborative Care

Goals of collaborative care for acute pancreatitis include (1) relief of pain; (2) prevention or alleviation of shock; (3) reduction of pancreatic secretions; (4) correction of fluid and electrolyte imbalances; (5) prevention or treatment of infections; and (6) removal of the precipitating cause, if possible (Table 44-17).

Conservative Therapy. Treatment is primarily focused on supportive care, including aggressive hydration, pain management, management of metabolic complications, and minimization of pancreatic stimulation. Treatment and control of pain are very important. IV morphine may be used. Pain medications may be combined with an antispasmodic agent. However, atropine and other anticholinergic drugs should be avoided when paralytic ileus is present because they can decrease GI mobility, thus contributing to the problem. Other medications that relax smooth muscles (spasmolytics), such as nitroglycerin or papaverine, may be used. Supplemental oxygen is provided to maintain oxygen saturation greater than 95%. In patients with severe pancreatitis, serum glucose levels are closely monitored for hyperglycemia.

TABLE 44-17   COLLABORATIVE CARE

Acute Pancreatitis

Diagnostic
- History and physical examination
- Serum amylase
- Serum lipase
- Blood glucose
- Serum calcium
- Serum triglycerides
- Flat plate of the abdomen
- Abdominal ultrasound
- Endoscopic ultrasound (EUS)
- Contrast-enhanced CT of pancreas
- Magnetic resonance cholangiopancreatography (MRCP)
- Endoscopic retrograde cholangiopancreatography (ERCP)
- Chest x-ray

Collaborative Therapy
- Pain medication (e.g., morphine)
- NPO with NG tube to suction
- Albumin (if shock present)
- IV calcium gluconate (10%) (if tetany present)
- Lactated Ringer's solution
- Proton pump inhibitor (e.g., omeprazole [Prilosec])
- Antibiotics (if necrotizing pancreatitis)

TABLE 44-18   DRUG THERAPY

Acute and Chronic Pancreatitis

Drug	Mechanism of Action
Acute Pancreatitis	
morphine	Relief of pain
Antispasmodics (e.g., dicyclomine [Bentyl])	↓ Vagal stimulation, motility, pancreatic outflow (↓ volume and concentration of bicarbonate and enzyme secretion) Contraindicated in paralytic ileus
Carbonic anhydrase inhibitor (acetazolamide [Diamox])	↓ Volume and bicarbonate concentration of pancreatic secretion
Antacids	Neutralization of gastric hydrochloric (HCl) acid secretion ↓ Production and secretion of pancreatic enzymes and bicarbonate
Proton pump inhibitors (omeprazole [Prilosec])	↓ HCl acid secretion (HCl acid stimulates pancreatic activity)
Chronic Pancreatitis	
Pancreatic enzyme products (pancrelipase [Pancrease, Zenpep, Creon, Viokase])	Replacement therapy for pancreatic enzymes
Insulin	Treatment for diabetes mellitus or hyperglycemia, if needed

If shock is present, blood volume replacements are used. Plasma or plasma volume expanders such as dextran or albumin may be given. Fluid and electrolyte imbalances are corrected with lactated Ringer's solution or other electrolyte solutions. Central venous pressure readings may be used to assist in determining fluid replacement requirements. Vasoactive drugs such as dopamine (Intropin) may be used to increase systemic vascular resistance in patients with ongoing hypotension.

It is important to reduce or suppress pancreatic enzymes to decrease stimulation of the pancreas and allow it to rest. This is accomplished in several ways. First, the patient is NPO (taking nothing by mouth). Second, NG suction may be used to reduce vomiting and gastric distention and to prevent gastric acidic contents from entering the duodenum. In addition, certain drugs may be used to suppress gastric acid secretion (Table 44-18). With resolution of the pancreatitis, the patient resumes oral intake. For the patient with severe acute pancreatitis who does not resume oral intake, enteral nutrition support may be initiated.

The inflamed and necrotic pancreatic tissue is a good medium for bacterial growth. In patients with acute necrotizing pancreatitis, infection is the leading cause of morbidity and mortality. Therefore it is important to prevent infections. Because many of the organisms come from the intestine, enteral feeding reduces the risk of necrotizing pancreatitis. Monitor the patient closely so that antibiotic therapy can be instituted early if necrosis and infection occur. Endoscopic- or CT-guided percutaneous aspiration with Gram stain and culture may be performed.

Surgical Therapy. When the acute pancreatitis is related to gallstones, an urgent ERCP plus endoscopic *sphincterotomy* (severing of the muscle layers of the sphincter of Oddi) may be done. This may be followed by laparoscopic cholecystectomy to reduce the potential for recurrence. Surgical intervention may also be indicated when the diagnosis is uncertain and for patients who do not respond to conservative therapy. Those with severe acute pancreatitis may require drainage of necrotic fluid collections. This is done either surgically, under CT guid-

ance, or endoscopically. Percutaneous drainage of a pseudocyst can be performed, and a drainage tube is left in place.

Drug Therapy. Several different drugs are used to prevent and treat problems associated with pancreatitis (see Table 44-18). Currently there are no drugs that cure pancreatitis.

Nutritional Therapy. Initially the patient with acute pancreatitis is on NPO status to reduce pancreatic secretion. Depending on the severity of the pancreatitis, enteral feedings via nasojejunal tube are initiated. Because of infection risk, parenteral nutrition is reserved for patients who cannot tolerate enteral nutrition (see Chapter 40). If IV lipids are ordered, blood triglyceride levels need to be monitored. In cases of moderate to severe pancreatitis, the patient may require enteral feeding via a jejunal feeding tube. When food is allowed, small, frequent feedings are given. The diet is usually high in carbohydrate content because that is the least stimulating to the exocrine portion of the pancreas. Suspect intolerance to oral foods when the patient reports pain, has increasing abdominal girth, or has elevations in serum amylase and lipase levels. The patient needs to abstain from alcohol. Supplemental fat-soluble vitamins may be given.

NURSING MANAGEMENT
ACUTE PANCREATITIS

NURSING ASSESSMENT

Subjective and objective data that should be obtained from a person with acute pancreatitis are presented in Table 44-19.

NURSING DIAGNOSES

Nursing diagnoses for the patient with acute pancreatitis may include, but are not limited to, the following:
- Acute pain *related to* distention of pancreas, peritoneal irritation, obstruction of biliary tract, and ineffective pain and comfort measures
- Deficient fluid volume *related to* nausea, vomiting, restricted oral intake, and fluid shift into the retroperitoneal space

---

TABLE 44-19 NURSING ASSESSMENT

Acute Pancreatitis

Subjective Data

Important Health Information

Past health history: Biliary tract disease, alcohol use, abdominal trauma, duodenal ulcers, infection, metabolic disorders

Medications: Thiazides, nonsteroidal antiinflammatory drugs

Surgery or other treatments: Surgical procedures on the pancreas, stomach, duodenum, or biliary tract; endoscopic retrograde cholangiopancreatography (ERCP)

Functional Health Patterns

Health perception–health management: Alcohol abuse; fatigue

Nutritional-metabolic: Nausea and vomiting; anorexia

Activity-exercise: Dyspnea

Cognitive-perceptual: Severe midepigastric or left upper quadrant pain that may radiate to the back, aggravated by food and alcohol intake and unrelieved by vomiting

Objective Data

General

Restlessness, anxiety, low-grade fever

Integumentary

Flushing, diaphoresis, discoloration of abdomen and flanks, cyanosis, jaundice; decreased skin turgor, dry mucous membranes

Respiratory

Tachypnea, basilar crackles

Cardiovascular

Tachycardia, hypotension

Gastrointestinal

Abdominal distention, tenderness, and muscle guarding; diminished bowel sounds

Possible Diagnostic Findings

↑ Serum amylase and lipase, leukocytosis, hyperglycemia, hypocalcemia, abnormal ultrasound and CT scans of pancreas, abnormal ERCP or MRCP

- Imbalanced nutrition: less than body requirements *related to* anorexia, dietary restrictions, nausea, loss of nutrients from vomiting, and impaired digestion
- Ineffective self-health management *related to* lack of knowledge of preventive measures, diet restrictions, alcohol restriction intake, and follow-up care

Additional information on nursing diagnoses for the patient with acute pancreatitis is presented in eNursing Care Plan 44-3 (available on the website for this chapter).

PLANNING

The overall goals are that the patient with acute pancreatitis will have (1) relief of pain, (2) normal fluid and electrolyte balance, (3) minimal to no complications, and (4) no recurrent attacks.

NURSING IMPLEMENTATION

HEALTH PROMOTION. The major factors involved in health promotion are (1) assessment of the patient for predisposing and etiologic factors and (2) encouragement of early treatment of these factors to prevent acute pancreatitis. Encourage early diagnosis and treatment of biliary tract disease, such as cholelithiasis. Encourage the patient to eliminate alcohol intake, especially if he or she has had any previous episodes of pancre-

atitis. Attacks of pancreatitis become milder or disappear with the discontinuance of alcohol use.

ACUTE INTERVENTION. During the acute phase, it is important to monitor vital signs. Hemodynamic stability may be compromised by hypotension, fever, and tachypnea. Monitor the response to IV fluids. Also closely monitor fluid and electrolyte balance. Frequent vomiting, along with gastric suction, may result in decreased chloride, sodium, and potassium levels.

Respiratory failure may develop in the patient with severe acute pancreatitis. Assess respiratory function (e.g., lung sounds, oxygen saturation levels). If ARDS develops, the patient may require intubation and mechanical ventilatory support.

SAFETY ALERT
- Assess for respiratory distress in the patient with severe acute pancreatitis.
- Listen to lung sounds and monitor O_2 saturation on a regular basis.

Because hypocalcemia can also occur, observe for symptoms of tetany, such as jerking, irritability, and muscular twitching. Numbness or tingling around the lips and in the fingers is an early indicator of hypocalcemia. Assess the patient for a positive Chvostek's sign or Trousseau's sign (see Fig. 17-15). Calcium gluconate (as ordered) should be given to treat symptomatic hypocalcemia. Hypomagnesemia may also develop, necessitating the monitoring of serum magnesium levels.

Because abdominal pain is a prominent symptom of pancreatitis, a major focus of your care is the relief of pain (see eNursing Care Plan 44-3). Pain and restlessness can increase the metabolic rate and subsequent stimulation of pancreatic enzymes. In addition, acute pain can contribute to hemodynamic instability. Morphine may be used for pain relief. Assess and document the duration of pain relief. Measures such as comfortable positioning, frequent changes in position, and relief of nausea and vomiting assist in reducing the restlessness that usually accompanies the pain. Assuming positions that flex the trunk and draw the knees up to the abdomen may decrease pain. A side-lying position with the head elevated 45 degrees decreases tension on the abdomen and may help ease the pain.

For the patient who is on NPO status or has an NG tube, provide frequent oral and nasal care to relieve the dryness of the mouth and nose. Oral care is essential to prevent parotitis. If the patient is taking anticholinergics to decrease GI secretions, the mouth will be especially dry. If the patient is taking antacids to neutralize gastric acid secretion, they should be sipped slowly or inserted in the NG tube.

Observe for fever and other manifestations of infection in the patient with acute pancreatitis. Respiratory tract infections are common because the retroperitoneal fluid raises the diaphragm, which causes the patient to take shallow, guarded abdominal breaths. Measures to prevent respiratory tract infections include turning, coughing, deep breathing, and assuming a semi-Fowler's position.

Other important assessments are observation for signs of paralytic ileus, renal failure, and mental changes. Determine the blood glucose level to assess damage to the β cells of the islets of Langerhans in the pancreas.

After pancreatic surgery, the patient may require special wound care for an anastomotic leak or a fistula. To prevent skin irritation, use skin barriers (e.g., Stomahesive, Karaya Paste, or Colly-Seel), pouching, and drains. In addition to protecting the skin, pouching also permits a more accurate determination of fluid and electrolyte losses and increases patient comfort.

Sterile pouching systems are available. Consult with a clinical specialist or wound, ostomy, and continence (WOC) nurse, if available.

AMBULATORY AND HOME CARE. After acute pancreatitis, the patient may require home care follow-up. Because of loss of physical and muscle strength, physical therapy may be needed. Continued care to prevent infection and detect any complications is important. Counseling regarding abstinence from alcohol is important to prevent the patient from experiencing future attacks of acute pancreatitis and development of chronic pancreatitis. Because cigarettes can stimulate the pancreas, smoking should be avoided.

Dietary teaching should include restriction of fats because they stimulate the secretion of cholecystokinin, which then stimulates the pancreas. Carbohydrates are less stimulating to the pancreas and are encouraged. Instruct the patient to avoid crash dieting and bingeing because they can precipitate attacks.

Instruct the patient and the caregiver to recognize and report symptoms of infection, diabetes mellitus, or steatorrhea (foul-smelling, frothy stools). These changes indicate possible ongoing destruction of pancreatic tissue. Teach the patient and caregiver about the prescribed regimen, including the importance of taking the required medications and following the recommended diet.

▌EVALUATION

The expected outcomes are that the patient with acute pancreatitis will

- Have adequate pain control
- Maintain adequate fluid balance
- Be knowledgeable about treatment regimen to restore health
- Get help for alcohol dependence (if appropriate)

CHRONIC PANCREATITIS

Chronic pancreatitis is a continuous, prolonged, inflammatory, and fibrosing process of the pancreas. The pancreas is progressively destroyed as it is replaced by fibrotic tissue. Strictures and calcifications may also occur in the pancreas.

Etiology and Pathophysiology

Chronic pancreatitis can be due to alcohol abuse; obstruction caused by cholelithiasis (gallstones), tumor, pseudocysts, or trauma; and systemic diseases (e.g., systemic lupus erythematosus), autoimmune pancreatitis, and cystic fibrosis. Some patients may not have an identifiable risk factor (idiopathic pancreatitis). Chronic pancreatitis may follow acute pancreatitis, but it may also occur in the absence of any history of an acute condition.

The most common cause of obstructive pancreatitis is inflammation of the sphincter of Oddi associated with cholelithiasis. Cancer of the ampulla of Vater, duodenum, or pancreas can also cause this type of chronic pancreatitis.

In nonobstructive pancreatitis there is inflammation and sclerosis, mainly in the head of the pancreas and around the pancreatic duct. This type of chronic pancreatitis is the most common form. In the United States, chronic pancreatitis is found almost exclusively in individuals who abuse alcohol. A genetic factor may predispose a person who drinks to the direct toxic effect of the alcohol on the pancreas.

Clinical Manifestations

As with acute pancreatitis, a major manifestation of chronic pancreatitis is abdominal pain. The patient may have episodes of acute pain, but it usually is chronic (recurrent attacks at intervals of months or years). The attacks may become more and more frequent until they are almost constant, or they may diminish as pancreatic fibrosis develops. The pain is located in the same areas as in acute pancreatitis, but is usually described as a heavy, gnawing feeling or sometimes as burning and cramplike. The pain is not relieved with food or antacids.

Other clinical manifestations include symptoms of pancreatic insufficiency, including malabsorption with weight loss, constipation, mild jaundice with dark urine, steatorrhea, and diabetes mellitus. The steatorrhea may become severe, with voluminous, foul-smelling, fatty stools. Urine and stool may be frothy. Some abdominal tenderness may be present.

Chronic pancreatitis is also associated with a variety of complications, including pseudocyst formation, bile duct or duodenal obstruction, pancreatic ascites or pleural effusion, splenic vein thrombosis, pseudoaneurysms, and pancreatic cancer.

Diagnostic Studies

Confirming the diagnosis of chronic pancreatitis can be challenging. The diagnosis is based on the patient's signs and symptoms, laboratory studies, and imaging. In chronic pancreatitis the levels of serum amylase and lipase may be elevated slightly or not at all, depending on the degree of pancreatic fibrosis. Serum bilirubin and alkaline phosphatase levels may be increased. There is usually mild leukocytosis and an elevated sedimentation rate.

ERCP is used to visualize the pancreatic and common bile ducts. Imaging studies such as CT, MRI, MRCP, abdominal ultrasound, and EUS are useful in patients with chronic pancreatitis. These procedures show a variety of changes, including calcifications, ductal dilation, pseudocysts, and pancreatic enlargement.

Stool samples are examined for fecal fat content. Deficiencies of fat-soluble vitamins and cobalamin, glucose intolerance, and possibly diabetes may also be found in those with chronic pancreatitis. A secretin stimulation test may be used to assess the degree of pancreatic function (see Chapter 39).

Collaborative Care

When the patient with chronic pancreatitis experiences an acute attack, the therapy is identical to that for acute pancreatitis. At other times the focus is on prevention of further attacks, relief of pain, and control of pancreatic exocrine and endocrine insufficiency. It sometimes takes frequent doses of analgesics (morphine or fentanyl patch [Duragesic]) to relieve the pain if dietary measures and enzyme replacement are not effective.

Diet, pancreatic enzyme replacement, and control of diabetes are ways to control the pancreatic insufficiency. Small, bland, frequent meals that are low in fat content are recommended to decrease pancreatic stimulation. Smoking is associated with accelerated progression of chronic pancreatitis. Teach the patient not to consume alcohol and caffeinated beverages.

Pancreatic enzyme products (PEPs) such as pancrelipase (Pancrease, Zenpep, Creon, Viokase) contain amylase, lipase, and trypsin and are used to replace the deficient pancreatic enzymes. They are usually enteric coated to prevent their breakdown or inactivation by gastric acid. Bile salts are sometimes given to facilitate the absorption of the fat-soluble vitamins (A,

D, E, and K) and prevent further fat loss. If diabetes develops, it is controlled with insulin or oral hypoglycemic agents. Acid-neutralizing drugs (e.g., antacids) and acid-inhibiting drugs (e.g., H_2-receptor blockers, proton pump inhibitors) may be given to decrease hydrochloric acid (HCl) secretion but have little overall effect on patient outcomes. Antidepressants, such as nortriptyline (Aventyl), have been shown to reduce the neuropathic pain associated with chronic pancreatitis.

Treatment of chronic pancreatitis sometimes requires endoscopic therapy or surgery. When biliary disease is present or obstruction or pseudocyst develops, surgery may be indicated. Surgical procedures can divert bile flow or relieve ductal obstruction. A choledochojejunostomy diverts bile around the ampulla of Vater, where there may be spasm or hypertrophy of the sphincter. In this procedure the common bile duct is anastomosed into the jejunum. Another type of surgical diverting procedure is the Roux-en-Y pancreatojejunostomy, in which the pancreatic duct is opened and an anastomosis is made with the jejunum. Pancreatic drainage procedures can relieve ductal obstruction and are often done with ERCP. Some patients may undergo ERCP with sphincterotomy and/or stent placement at the site of obstruction. These patients require follow-up procedures such as ERCP to either exchange or remove the stent.

NURSING MANAGEMENT
CHRONIC PANCREATITIS

Except during an acute episode, nursing management focuses on chronic care and health promotion. Instruct the patient to take measures to prevent further attacks. Dietary control, along with consistency of other treatment measures, such as taking pancreatic enzymes, is essential. The enzymes are usually taken with meals or a snack. Observe the patient's stools for steatorrhea to help determine the effectiveness of the enzymes. Instruct the patient and the caregiver to observe the stools.

If diabetes has developed, instruct the patient regarding testing of blood glucose levels and drug therapy (see Chapter 49). Ensure that the patient who is taking antisecretory agents or antacids takes them as ordered to control gastric acidity. Antacids should be taken after meals and at bedtime.

The patient must avoid alcohol and may need assistance with this problem. If the patient is dependent on alcohol, referral to other agencies or resources may be necessary (see Chapter 11).

PANCREATIC CANCER

Annually in the United States an estimated 42,500 people are diagnosed with pancreatic cancer, and 35,300 people die from pancreatic cancer.[34] It is the fourth leading cause of death from cancer in the United States. The risk increases with age, with the peak incidence occurring between 65 and 80 years of age.

Most pancreatic tumors are adenocarcinomas originating from the epithelium of the ductal system. More than half of the tumors occur in the head of the pancreas. As the tumor grows, the common bile duct becomes obstructed, and obstructive jaundice develops. Tumors starting in the body or the tail often remain silent until their growth is advanced. The majority of cancers have metastasized at the time of diagnosis. The signs and symptoms of pancreatic cancer are often similar to those of chronic pancreatitis. The prognosis of a patient with cancer of the pancreas is poor. The majority of patients die within 5 to 12

months of the initial diagnosis, and the 5-year survival rate is less than 5%.

Etiology and Pathophysiology

The cause of pancreatic cancer remains unknown. Risk factors for pancreatic cancer include chronic pancreatitis, diabetes mellitus, age, cigarette smoking, family history of pancreatic cancer, high-fat diet, and exposure to chemicals such as benzidine. African Americans have a higher incidence of pancreatic cancer than whites. The most firmly established environmental risk factor is cigarette smoking. Smokers are two to three times more likely to develop pancreatic cancer than nonsmokers. The risk is related to both the duration and amount of cigarettes smoked.

Clinical Manifestations

Common manifestations of pancreatic cancer include abdominal pain (dull, aching), anorexia, rapid and progressive weight loss, nausea, and jaundice. The most common manifestations of cancer of the head of the pancreas are pain, jaundice, and weight loss. Pruritus may accompany obstructive jaundice. In general, pain is common and is related to the location of malignancy. Extreme, unrelenting pain is related to extension of the cancer into the retroperitoneal tissues and nerve plexuses. The pain is frequently located in the upper abdomen or left hypochondrium and often radiates to the back. It is commonly related to eating, and it also occurs at night. Weight loss is due to poor digestion and absorption caused by lack of digestive enzymes from the pancreas.

Diagnostic Studies

Abdominal ultrasound or EUS, spiral CT scan, ERCP, MRI, and MRCP are the most commonly used diagnostic imaging techniques for pancreatic diseases, including cancer. EUS involves imaging the pancreas with the use of an endoscope positioned in the stomach and the duodenum. EUS also allows for fine-needle aspiration of the tumor. CT scan is often the initial study and provides information on metastasis and vascular involvement. ERCP allows visualization of the pancreatic duct and the biliary system. When ERCP is used, pancreatic secretions and tissue can be collected for analysis of different tumor markers. MRI and MRCP may also be used for diagnosing and staging pancreatic cancer. A positron emission tomography (PET) scan or PET/CT scan may also be obtained but usually does not provide additional clinical information.

Tumor markers are used both for establishing the diagnosis of pancreatic adenocarcinoma and for monitoring the response to treatment. Cancer-associated antigen 19-9 (CA 19-9) is elevated in pancreatic cancer and is the most commonly used tumor marker. CA 19-9 can also be elevated in gallbladder cancer or in benign conditions such as acute and chronic pancreatitis, hepatitis, and biliary obstruction.

Collaborative Care

Surgery provides the most effective treatment of cancer of the pancreas. Only 15% to 20% of patients have resectable tumors. The classic surgery is a *radical pancreaticoduodenectomy,* or *Whipple procedure* (Fig. 44-13). This procedure involves resection of the proximal pancreas (proximal pancreatectomy), adjoining duodenum (duodenectomy), distal portion of the stomach (partial gastrectomy), and distal segment of the common bile duct. An anastomosis of the pancreatic duct, common

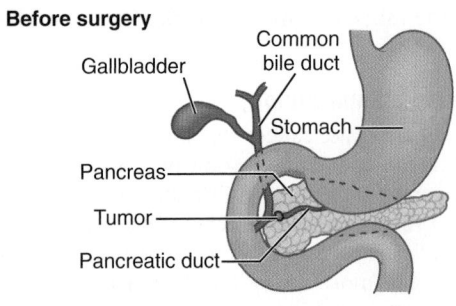

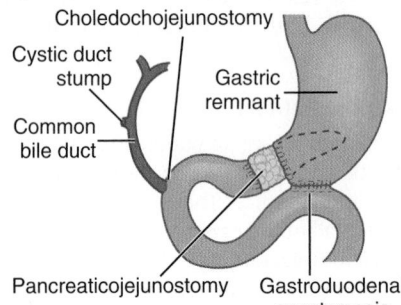

FIG. 44-13 Whipple procedure or radical pancreaticoduodenectomy. This surgical procedure involves resection of the proximal pancreas, adjoining duodenum, distal portion of the stomach, and distal portion of the common bile duct. An anastomosis of the pancreatic duct, common bile duct, and stomach to the jejunum is done.

bile duct, and stomach to the jejunum is done. A total pancreatectomy is performed in some institutions. Sometimes a simple bypass procedure, such as a cholecystojejunostomy to relieve biliary obstruction, may be used as a palliative measure. Some surgeons suggest a more radical resection, such as a total pancreaticoduodenectomy with splenectomy. Endoscopically placed biliary stents can be used as a palliative measure when tumors compress the bile duct.

Radiation therapy alone has little effect on survival, but may be effective for pain relief. External radiation is usually used, but implantation of internal radiation seeds into the tumor has also been used. The current role of chemotherapy in pancreatic cancer is limited. Chemotherapy usually consists of fluorouracil (5-FU) and gemcitabine (Gemzar) either alone or in combination with agents such as capecitabine (Xeloda) or erlotinib (Tarceva). Erlotinib is a targeted therapy (see Table 16-13).

NURSING MANAGEMENT
PANCREATIC CANCER

Because the patient with pancreatic cancer has many of the same problems as the patient with pancreatitis, nursing care includes many of the same measures (see sections on acute and chronic pancreatitis). Provide symptomatic and supportive nursing care. This includes administration of medications and comfort measures to relieve pain. Psychologic support is essential, especially during times of anxiety or depression.

Adequate nutrition is an important part of the nursing care plan. Frequent and supplemental feedings may be necessary. Measures to stimulate the appetite as much as possible and to overcome anorexia, nausea, and vomiting should be included in the nursing care. Because bleeding can result from impaired vitamin K production, assess for bleeding from body orifices

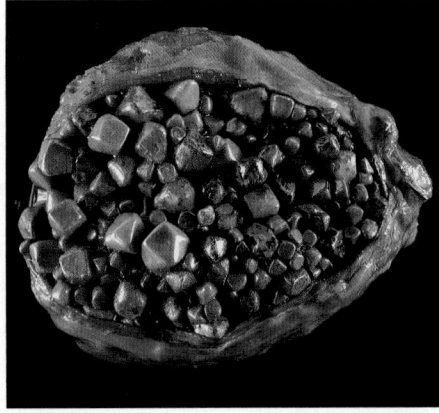

FIG. 44-14 Cholesterol gallstones in a gallbladder that was removed.

and mucous membranes. If the patient is undergoing radiation therapy, observe for adverse reactions, such as anorexia, nausea, vomiting, and skin irritation.

The prognosis for a patient with pancreatic cancer is poor. A significant component of the nursing care is helping the patient and caregiver through the grieving process. Chapter 10 provides information on palliative and end-of-life care.

DISORDERS OF THE BILIARY TRACT

CHOLELITHIASIS AND CHOLECYSTITIS

The most common disorder of the biliary system is cholelithiasis (stones in the gallbladder) (Fig. 44-14 and eFig. 44-3 on the website for this chapter). The stones may be lodged in the neck of the gallbladder or in the cystic duct. Cholecystitis (inflammation of the gallbladder) is usually associated with cholelithiasis. Cholecystitis may be acute or chronic. Cholelithiasis and cholecystitis usually occur together.

Gallbladder disease is a common health problem in the United States. Approximately 8% to 10% of American adults have cholelithiasis. The actual number is not known because many persons with stones are asymptomatic. *Cholecystectomy* (removal of the gallbladder) ranks among the most common surgical procedures performed in the United States.

The incidence of cholelithiasis is higher in women, especially multiparous women, and persons over 40 years of age. Postmenopausal women on estrogen therapy are at somewhat greater risk of having gallbladder disease than are women who are taking birth control pills. Oral contraceptives affect cholesterol production and increase the likelihood of gallbladder cholesterol saturation. Other factors that increase the occurrence of gallbladder disease are a sedentary lifestyle, a familial tendency, and obesity. Obesity causes increased secretion of cholesterol in bile.

Gallbladder disease is more common in Asian Americans and African Americans than in whites. The incidence is especially high in the Native American population, particularly in the Navajo and Pima tribes.

Etiology and Pathophysiology

Cholelithiasis. The cause of gallstones is unknown. Cholelithiasis develops when the balance that keeps cholesterol, bile salts, and calcium in solution is altered so that these substances precipitate. Conditions that upset this balance include infection

GENDER DIFFERENCES

Cholelithiasis

Men	Women
• Incidence of cholelithiasis is lower in men than in women.	• Pregnancy is the greatest risk factor for increased prevalence in women.
• Gender differences in incidence decrease after age 50.	• Obesity increases the risk, especially for women.

TABLE 44-20 MANIFESTATIONS OF OBSTRUCTED BILE FLOW

Manifestation	Etiology
Obstructive jaundice	No bile flow into duodenum
Dark amber urine, which foams when shaken	Soluble bilirubin in urine
No urobilinogen in urine	No bilirubin reaching small intestine to be converted to urobilinogen
Clay-colored stools	Same as above
Pruritus	Deposition of bile salts in skin tissues
Intolerance for fatty foods (nausea, sensation of fullness, anorexia)	No bile in small intestine for fat digestion
Bleeding tendencies	Lack of or decreased absorption of vitamin K, resulting in decreased production of prothrombin
Steatorrhea	No bile salts in duodenum, preventing fat emulsion and digestion

and disturbances in the metabolism of cholesterol. In patients with cholelithiasis, the bile secreted by the liver is supersaturated with cholesterol (lithogenic bile). The bile in the gallbladder also becomes supersaturated with cholesterol. When bile is supersaturated with cholesterol, precipitation of cholesterol occurs.

Other components of bile that precipitate into stones are bile salts, bilirubin, calcium, and protein. Mixed cholesterol stones, which are predominantly cholesterol, are the most common gallstones.

Changes in the composition of bile are probably significant in the formation of gallstones. Stasis of bile leads to progression of the supersaturation and changes in the chemical composition of the bile (biliary sludge). Immobility, pregnancy, and inflammatory or obstructive lesions of the biliary system decrease bile flow. Hormonal factors during pregnancy may cause delayed emptying of the gallbladder, resulting in stasis of bile.

The stones may remain in the gallbladder or migrate to the cystic duct or the common bile duct. They cause pain as they pass through the ducts, and they may lodge in the ducts and produce an obstruction. Small stones are more likely to move into a duct and cause obstruction. Table 44-20 depicts the changes and manifestations that occur when the stones obstruct the common bile duct. If the blockage occurs in the cystic duct, the bile can continue to flow into the duodenum directly from the liver. However, when the bile in the gallbladder cannot escape, this stasis of bile may lead to cholecystitis.

Cholecystitis. Cholecystitis is most commonly associated with obstruction caused by gallstones or biliary sludge. Cholecystitis in the absence of obstruction (*acalculous cholecystitis*) occurs most frequently in older adults and in patients who are critically ill. Acalculous cholecystitis is also associated with pro-

longed immobility and fasting, prolonged parenteral nutrition, and diabetes mellitus. Bacteria reaching the gallbladder via the vascular or lymphatic route, or chemical irritants in the bile, can also produce cholecystitis. *E. coli*, streptococci, and salmonellae are common causative bacteria. Other etiologic factors include adhesions, neoplasms, anesthesia, and opioids.

Inflammation is the major pathophysiologic condition and may be confined to the mucous lining or involve the entire wall of the gallbladder. During an acute attack of cholecystitis, the gallbladder is edematous and hyperemic, and it may be distended with bile or pus. The cystic duct is also involved and may become occluded. The wall of the gallbladder becomes scarred after an acute attack. Decreased functioning occurs if large amounts of tissue are fibrosed.

Clinical Manifestations

Cholelithiasis may produce severe symptoms or none at all. Many patients have "silent cholelithiasis." The severity of symptoms depends on whether the stones are stationary or mobile and whether obstruction is present. When a stone is lodged in the ducts or when stones are moving through the ducts, spasms may result. The gallbladder spasms occur in response to the stone. This sometimes produces severe pain, which is termed *biliary colic* even though the pain is rarely colicky. The pain is more often steady. The pain can be excruciating and accompanied by tachycardia, diaphoresis, and prostration. The severe pain may last up to an hour, and when it subsides, there is residual tenderness in the right upper quadrant. The attacks of pain frequently occur 3 to 6 hours after a high-fat meal or when the patient lies down. When total obstruction occurs, symptoms related to bile blockage are manifested (see Table 44-20).

Manifestations of cholecystitis vary from indigestion to moderate to severe pain, fever, and jaundice. Initial symptoms of acute cholecystitis include indigestion and pain and tenderness in the right upper quadrant, which may be referred to the right shoulder and scapula. The pain may be acute and be accompanied by nausea and vomiting, restlessness, and diaphoresis. Manifestations of inflammation include leukocytosis and fever. Physical findings include right upper quadrant tenderness and abdominal rigidity. Manifestations of chronic cholecystitis include a history of fat intolerance, dyspepsia, heartburn, and flatulence.

Complications. Complications of cholelithiasis and cholecystitis include gangrenous cholecystitis, subphrenic abscess, pancreatitis, *cholangitis* (inflammation of biliary ducts), biliary cirrhosis, fistulas, and rupture of the gallbladder, which can produce bile peritonitis. In older patients and those with diabetes, gangrenous cholecystitis and bile peritonitis are the most common complications of cholecystitis. *Choledocholithiasis* (stone in the common bile duct) may occur, producing symptoms of obstruction.

Diagnostic Studies

Ultrasonography is commonly used to diagnose gallstones (see Table 39-12). It is especially useful for patients with jaundice (because it does not depend on liver function) and for patients who are allergic to contrast medium. ERCP allows for visualization of the gallbladder, the cystic duct, the common hepatic duct, and the common bile duct. Bile taken during ERCP is sent for culture to identify possible infecting organisms.

Percutaneous transhepatic cholangiography is the insertion of a needle directly into the gallbladder duct followed by injection of contrast materials. It is generally done after ultrasonography indicates a bile duct blockage.

Laboratory tests reveal an increased white blood cell (WBC) count as a result of inflammation. Both direct and indirect bilirubin levels are elevated, as is the urinary bilirubin level if an obstructive process is present (see Table 44-3). If the common bile duct is obstructed, no bilirubin will reach the small intestine to be converted to urobilinogen. Serum enzymes, such as alkaline phosphatase, ALT, and AST, may be elevated. Serum amylase is increased if there is pancreatic involvement.

Collaborative Care

Once gallstones become symptomatic, definitive surgical intervention with cholecystectomy is usually indicated. However, in some cases, conservative therapy may be considered.

Conservative Therapy

Cholelithiasis. The treatment of gallstones depends on the stage of disease. Bile acids (cholesterol solvents) such as ursodeoxycholic acid (ursodiol) and chenodeoxycholic acid (chenodiol) are used to dissolve stones. However, the gallstones may recur. Gallstones are not usually treated with drugs because of the high use and success of laparoscopic cholecystectomy.

ERCP with endoscopic sphincterotomy (papillotomy) may be used for stone removal (Fig. 44-15). ERCP allows for visualization of the biliary system, dilation (balloon sphincteroplasty), and placement of stents and sphincterotomy if warranted. Special catheters with wire baskets or inflatable balloon tip may be used for stone removal.[34] The endoscope is passed to the duodenum. With an electrodiathermy knife attached to the endoscope, the stone is commonly left in the duodenum to pass naturally in the stool. When a stent is placed, it is generally removed or changed after a few months.

Extracorporeal shock-wave lithotripsy (ESWL) is an alternative treatment employed when stones cannot be removed by endoscopic approaches. In ESWL a lithotriptor uses high-energy shock waves to disintegrate gallstones once they have been located by ultrasound. It usually takes 1 to 2 hours to disintegrate the stones. After they are broken up, the fragments pass through the common bile duct and into the small intestine. Usually ESWL and oral dissolution therapy are used together.

Cholecystitis. During an acute episode of cholecystitis, treatment focuses on pain control, control of possible infection with antibiotics, and maintenance of fluid and electrolyte balance (Table 44-21). Treatment is mainly supportive and symptomatic. If nausea and vomiting are severe, NG tube insertion and gastric decompression may be used to prevent further gallbladder stimulation. A cholecystostomy may be used to drain purulent material from the obstructed gallbladder. NSAIDs (e.g., ketorolac [Toradol]) are given for pain management. Anticholinergics may be administered to decrease secretion and counteract smooth muscle spasms.

Surgical Therapy. Laparoscopic cholecystectomy is the treatment of choice for symptomatic cholelithiasis. Approximately 90% of cholecystectomies are done laparoscopically. In this procedure, the gallbladder is removed through one to four small punctures in the abdomen. A laparoscope, which has a camera attached, and grasping forceps are inserted into the abdomen through the punctures. (The incision sites may vary.) Using closed-circuit monitors to view the abdominal cavity, the surgeon retracts and dissects the gallbladder and removes it with grasping forceps. This is a safe procedure with minimal morbidity.

Most patients have minimal postoperative pain and are discharged the day of surgery or the day after. They are usually able to resume normal activities and return to work within 1 week. The main complication is injury to the common bile duct. The

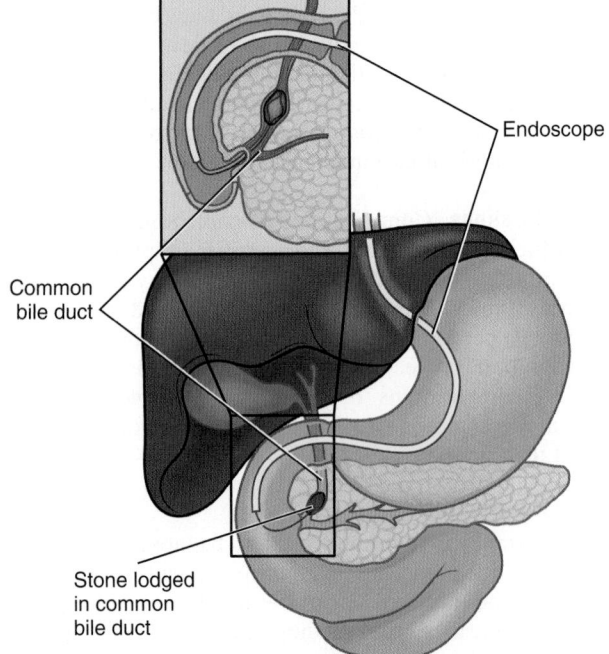

FIG. 44-15 During endoscopic sphincterotomy, an endoscope is advanced through the mouth and stomach until its tip sits in the duodenum opposite the common bile duct. *Inset,* After widening the duct mouth by incising the sphincter muscle, the physician advances a basket attachment into the duct and snags the stone.

Labels on figure: Endoscope; Common bile duct; Stone lodged in common bile duct

TABLE 44-21	**COLLABORATIVE CARE**

Cholelithiasis and Acute Cholecystitis

Diagnostic
- History and physical examination
- Ultrasound
- Endoscopic retrograde cholangiopancreatography (ERCP)
- Percutaneous transhepatic cholangiography
- Liver function studies
- White blood cell count
- Serum bilirubin

Collaborative Therapy
Conservative Therapy
- IV fluid
- NPO with NG tube, later progressing to low-fat diet
- Antiemetics
- Analgesics
- Fat-soluble vitamins (A, D, E, and K)
- Anticholinergics (antispasmodics)
- Antibiotics (for secondary infection)
- Transhepatic biliary catheter
- ERCP with sphincterotomy (papillotomy)
- Extracorporeal shock-wave lithotripsy

Dissolution Therapy
- ursodeoxycholic acid (ursodiol [Actigall])

Surgical Therapy
- Laparoscopic cholecystectomy
- Incisional (open) cholecystectomy

few contraindications to laparoscopic cholecystectomy include peritonitis, cholangitis, gangrene or perforation of the gallbladder, portal hypertension, and serious bleeding disorders.

On selected patients an incisional (open) cholecystectomy may be performed. This involves removal of the gallbladder through a right subcostal incision. A T tube may be inserted into the common bile duct during surgery when a common bile duct exploration is part of the surgical procedure (Fig. 44-16). This ensures patency of the duct until the edema produced by the trauma of exploring and probing the duct has subsided. It also allows the excess bile to drain while the small intestine is adjusting to receiving a continuous flow of bile.

Transhepatic Biliary Catheter. The transhepatic biliary catheter can be used preoperatively in biliary obstruction and in hepatic dysfunction secondary to obstructive jaundice. It can also be inserted for palliative care when inoperable liver, pancreatic, or bile duct carcinoma obstructs bile flow. The catheter is used when endoscopic drainage has been unsuccessful. The catheter is inserted percutaneously and allows for decompression of obstructed extrahepatic bile ducts so that bile can flow freely. After insertion, the catheter is connected to a drainage bag. The skin around the catheter insertion site is cleansed daily with an antiseptic. Observe for bile leakage at the insertion site. The patient may be discharged with it in place.

Drug Therapy. The most common drugs used in the treatment of gallbladder disease are analgesics, anticholinergics (antispasmodics), fat-soluble vitamins, and bile salts. Morphine may be used initially for pain management. NSAIDs (e.g., ketorolac) have also been shown to be helpful in pain management. Anticholinergics such as atropine and other antispasmodics may be used to relax the smooth muscle and decrease ductal tone.

If the patient has chronic gallbladder disease or any biliary tract obstruction, fat-soluble vitamins (A, D, E, and K) may need to be given. Bile salts may be administered to facilitate digestion and vitamin absorption.

Cholestyramine may provide relief from pruritus. Cholestyramine is a resin that binds bile salts in the intestine, increasing their excretion in the feces. It is administered in powder form, mixed with milk or juice. Side effects include nausea, vomiting, diarrhea or constipation, and skin reactions.

Nutritional Therapy. People have fewer problems if they eat smaller, more frequent meals with some fat at each meal to promote gallbladder emptying. If obesity is a problem, a reduced-calorie diet is indicated. The diet should be low in saturated fats (e.g., butter, shortening, lard) and high in fiber and calcium. Rapid weight loss should be avoided because it can promote gallstone formation.

After a laparoscopic cholecystectomy, instruct the patient to have liquids for the rest of the day and eat light meals for a few days. If an incisional cholecystectomy is done, the patient will progress from liquids to a regular diet once bowel sounds have returned. The amount of fat in the postoperative diet depends on the patient's tolerance of fat. A low-fat diet may be helpful if the flow of bile is reduced (usually only in the early postoperative period) or if the patient is overweight. Sometimes the patient is instructed to restrict fats for 4 to 6 weeks. Otherwise, no special dietary instructions are needed other than to eat nutritious meals and avoid excessive fat intake.

NURSING MANAGEMENT
GALLBLADDER DISEASE

NURSING ASSESSMENT

Subjective and objective data that should be obtained from a person with gallbladder disease are presented in Table 44-22.

TABLE 44-22   NURSING ASSESSMENT
Cholecystitis or Cholelithiasis

Subjective Data
Important Health Information
Past health history: Obesity, multiparity, infection, cancer, extensive fasting, pregnancy
Medications: Estrogen or oral contraceptives
Surgery or other treatments: Previous abdominal surgery

Functional Health Patterns
Health perception–health management: Positive family history; sedentary lifestyle
Nutritional-metabolic: Weight loss, anorexia; indigestion, fat intolerance, nausea and vomiting, dyspepsia; chills
Elimination: Clay-colored stools, steatorrhea, flatulence; dark urine
Cognitive-perceptual: Moderate to severe pain in right upper quadrant that may radiate to the back or scapula; pruritus

Objective Data
General
Fever, restlessness

Integumentary
Jaundice, icteric sclera; diaphoresis

Respiratory
Tachypnea, splinting during respirations

Cardiovascular
Tachycardia

Gastrointestinal
Palpable gallbladder, abdominal guarding and distention

Possible Diagnostic Findings
↑ Serum liver enzymes, alkaline phosphatase, and bilirubin; absence of urobilinogen in urine, ↑ urinary bilirubin; leukocytosis, abnormal gallbladder ultrasound

---

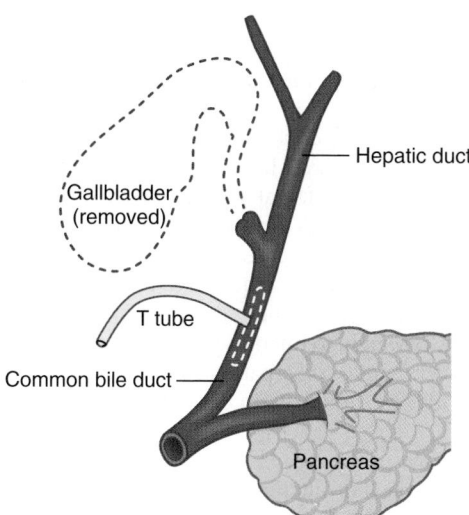

Hepatic duct

Gallbladder
(removed)

T tube

Common bile duct

Pancreas

FIG. 44-16 Placement of T tube. *Dotted lines* indicate parts removed.

NURSING DIAGNOSES

Nursing diagnoses for the patient with gallbladder disease treated surgically include, but are not limited to, the following:

- Acute pain *related to* surgical procedure
- Ineffective self-health management *related to* lack of knowledge of diet and postoperative management

PLANNING

The overall goals are that the patient with gallbladder disease will have (1) relief of pain and discomfort, (2) no complications postoperatively, and (3) no recurrent attacks of cholecystitis or cholelithiasis.

NURSING IMPLEMENTATION

HEALTH PROMOTION. Be aware of predisposing factors for gallbladder disease in general health screening. Teach patients from ethnic groups in which the disease is more common, such as Native Americans, the initial manifestations and to see their health care provider if these manifestations occur. Patients with chronic cholecystitis may not have acute symptoms and may not seek help until jaundice and biliary obstruction occur. Earlier detection in these patients is beneficial so that they can be managed with a low-fat diet and monitored more closely.

ACUTE INTERVENTION. Nursing goals for the patient undergoing conservative therapy include treating pain, relieving nausea and vomiting, providing comfort and emotional support, maintaining fluid and electrolyte balance and nutrition, making accurate assessments to ensure effective treatment, and observing for complications.

The patient with acute cholecystitis or cholelithiasis frequently has severe pain. Give the drugs ordered to relieve the pain as required, before it becomes more severe. Assess what drugs relieve the pain and how much medication is required. Observe for side effects of the drugs as part of the continued assessment. Nursing comfort measures, such as a clean bed, comfortable positioning, and oral care, are appropriate.

Some patients have more severe nausea and vomiting than others. For these patients, it may be necessary to insert an NG tube and use gastric decompression. Eliminating intake of food and fluids also prevents further stimulation of the gallbladder. Oral hygiene, care of nares, accurate intake and output measurements, and maintenance of suction should be a part of the nursing care plan for this patient. For patients with less severe nausea and vomiting, antiemetics are usually adequate. When the patient is vomiting, provide comfort measures such as frequent mouth rinses. Remove any vomitus immediately from the patient's view.

If pruritus occurs with jaundice, measures to relieve itching are necessary (see earlier discussion on p. 1025 and eNCP 44-1).

Assess for progression of the symptoms and development of complications. Observe for signs of obstruction of the ducts by stones. These include jaundice; clay-colored stools; dark, foamy urine; steatorrhea; fever; and increased WBC count.

When manifestations of obstruction are present (see Table 44-20), bleeding may result from decreased prothrombin production. Common sites to observe for bleeding are the mucous membranes of the mouth, nose, gingivae, and injection sites. If injections are given, use a small-gauge needle and apply gentle pressure after the injection. Know the patient's prothrombin time and use it as a guide in the assessment process.

Assessment for infections includes monitoring vital signs. A temperature elevation with chills and jaundice may indicate choledocholithiasis.

Your care of the patient after ERCP with papillotomy includes assessment to detect complications such as pancreatitis, perforation, infection, and bleeding. Monitor the patient's vital signs. Abdominal pain and fever may indicate pancreatitis. The patient should be on bed rest for several hours and should be NPO until the gag reflex returns. Teach the patient the need for follow-up if the stent is to be removed or changed.

Postoperative Care. Postoperative nursing care after a laparoscopic cholecystectomy includes monitoring for complications such as bleeding, making the patient comfortable, and preparing the patient for discharge. A common postoperative problem is referred pain to the shoulder because of the carbon dioxide that is used to inflate the abdominal cavity during surgery. It may not be released or absorbed by the body. The carbon dioxide can irritate the phrenic nerve and the diaphragm, causing some difficulty in breathing. Placing the patient in the Sims' position (on left side with right knee flexed) helps move the gas pocket away from the diaphragm. Encourage deep breathing along with movement and ambulation. The pain can usually be relieved by NSAIDs or codeine. The patient is allowed clear liquids and can walk to the bathroom to void. Most patients go home the same day.

Postoperative nursing care for incisional cholecystectomy focuses on adequate ventilation and prevention of respiratory complications. Other nursing care is the same as general postoperative nursing care (see Chapter 20).

If the patient has a T tube (see Fig. 44-16), you need to maintain bile drainage and observe for T-tube functioning and drainage. The T tube is connected to a closed gravity drainage system. If the Penrose or Jackson-Pratt drain or the T tube is draining large amounts, it is helpful to use a sterile pouching system to protect the skin.

AMBULATORY AND HOME CARE. When the patient has conservative therapy, nursing management depends on the patient's symptoms and on whether surgical intervention is planned. Dietary teaching is usually necessary. The diet is usually low in fat, and sometimes a weight-reduction diet is also recommended. The patient may need to take fat-soluble vitamin supplements. Instruct the patient on observations that indicate obstruction (e.g., stool and urine changes, jaundice, pruritus). Explain the importance of continued health care follow-up.

The patient who undergoes a laparoscopic cholecystectomy is discharged soon after the surgery, so home care and teaching are important (Table 44-23).

After an incisional cholecystectomy, the patient is usually discharged in 2 or 3 days. Instruct the patient to avoid heavy lifting for 4 to 6 weeks. Usual sexual activities, including intercourse, can be resumed as soon as the patient feels ready, unless otherwise instructed by the health care provider.

Sometimes the patient is required to remain on a low-fat diet for 4 to 6 weeks. If so, an individualized dietary teaching plan is necessary. A weight-reduction program may be helpful if the patient is overweight. Most patients tolerate a regular diet with no difficulties but should avoid excessive fats.

EVALUATION

The overall expected outcomes are that the patient with gallbladder disease will

- Appear comfortable and verbalize pain relief
- Verbalize knowledge of activity level and dietary restrictions

GALLBLADDER CANCER

Primary cancer of the gallbladder is uncommon. The majority of gallbladder carcinomas are adenocarcinomas. Annually an estimated 9810 new cases of gallbladder cancer occur with an

TABLE 44-23	PATIENT & CAREGIVER TEACHING GUIDE

Postoperative Laparoscopic Cholecystectomy

Include the following instructions in the patient's postoperative teaching plan.
1. Remove the bandages on the puncture site the day after surgery and you can shower.
2. Notify your surgeon if any of the following signs and symptoms occurs:
   - Redness, swelling, bile-colored drainage or pus from any incision
   - Severe abdominal pain, nausea, vomiting, fever, chills
3. You can gradually resume normal activities.
4. Return to work within 1 wk of surgery.
5. You can resume your usual diet, but a low-fat diet is usually better tolerated for several weeks after surgery.

estimated 3200 deaths. A relationship exists between cancer of the gallbladder and chronic cholecystitis and cholelithiasis.

The early symptoms of carcinoma of the gallbladder are insidious and are similar to those of chronic cholecystitis and cholelithiasis, which makes the diagnosis difficult. Later symptoms are usually those of biliary obstruction. Gallbladder cancer is twice as common in women as in men.[35]

Diagnosis and staging of gallbladder cancer are done using EUS, abdominal ultrasound, CT, MRI, and/or MRCP. Unfortunately, gallbladder cancer often is not detected until the disease is advanced. When it is found early, surgery can be curative. Several factors influence successful surgical outcomes, including the depth of cancer invasion, extent of liver involvement, venous or lymphatic invasion, and lymph node metastasis. Extended cholecystectomy with lymph node dissection has improved the outcomes for patients with gallbladder cancer.

When surgery is not an option, endoscopic stenting of the biliary tree can be done to reduce obstructive jaundice. Adjuvant therapies, including radiation therapy and chemotherapy, may be used depending on the disease state. Overall, cancer of the gallbladder has a poor prognosis.

Nursing management involves palliative care with special attention to nutrition, hydration, skin care, and pain relief. Nursing care measures used for patients with cholecystitis and cholelithiasis are frequently applied, as well as nursing care measures for the patient with cancer (see Chapter 16).

CASE STUDY

Cirrhosis of the Liver

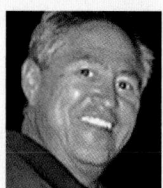

Patient Profile
M.B. is a 55-yr-old Native American man admitted with a diagnosis of cirrhosis of the liver. He has been vomiting for 2 days and noticed blood in the toilet when he vomits.

Subjective Data
- Has had cirrhosis for 12 yr
- Acknowledges that he had been drinking heavily for 20 yr but has been sober for the past 2 yr
- Complains of anorexia, nausea, and abdominal discomfort

Objective Data
Physical Examination
- Thin and malnourished
- Has moderate ascites
- Has jaundice of sclera and skin
- Has 4+ pitting edema of the lower extremities
- Liver and spleen are palpable

Laboratory Values
- Total bilirubin: 15 mg/dL (257 mmol/L)
- AST: 190 U/L (3.2 µkat/L)
- ALT: 210 U/L (3.5 µkat/L)
- ECG is at right:

Discussion Questions
1. What are possible causes of cirrhosis? What type of cirrhosis does M.B. probably have?

2. Describe the pathophysiologic changes that occur in the liver as cirrhosis develops.
3. List M.B.'s clinical manifestations of liver failure. For each manifestation, explain the pathophysiologic basis.
4. Explain the significance of the results of his laboratory values and ECG findings.
5. If M.B. begins to manifest signs and symptoms of hepatic encephalopathy, what would you monitor? What measures should be instituted to control or decrease the encephalopathy?
6. What are possible causes of his gastrointestinal bleeding?
7. **Priority Decision:** Based on the assessment data, what are the priority nursing diagnoses? Are there any collaborative problems?
8. **Priority Decision:** What are the priority nursing interventions for the patient at this stage of his illness?
9. **Evidence-Based Practice:** M.B. discusses his prognosis with you. He says, "There is no hope. I might as well keep drinking." How would you respond to his question?

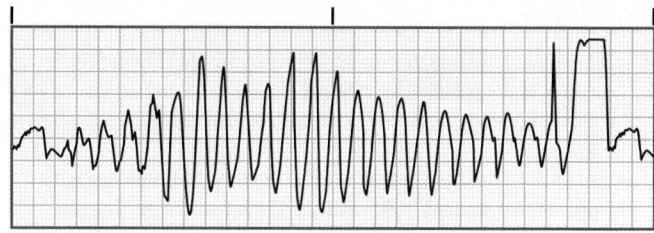

BRIDGE TO NCLEX EXAMINATION

The number of the question corresponds to the same-numbered outcome at the beginning of the chapter.

1. A patient with hepatitis A is in the acute phase. The nurse plans care for the patient based on the knowledge that
   a. pruritus is a common problem with jaundice in this phase.
   b. the patient is most likely to transmit the disease during this phase.
   c. gastrointestinal symptoms are not as severe in hepatitis A as they are in hepatitis B.
   d. extrahepatic manifestations of glomerulonephritis and polyarteritis are common in this phase.

2. A patient with acute hepatitis B is being discharged in 2 days. In the discharge teaching plan the nurse should include instructions to
   a. avoid alcohol for the first 3 weeks.
   b. use a condom during sexual intercourse.
   c. have family members get an injection of immunoglobulin.
   d. follow a low-protein, moderate-carbohydrate, moderate-fat diet.

3. A patient has been told that she has elevated liver enzymes caused by nonalcoholic fatty liver disease (NAFLD). The nursing teaching plan should include
   a. having genetic testing done.
   b. recommending a heart-healthy diet.
   c. the necessity to reduce weight rapidly.
   d. avoiding alcohol until liver enzymes return to normal.

4. The patient with advanced cirrhosis asks why his abdomen is so swollen. The nurse's response is based on the knowledge that
   a. a lack of clotting factors promotes the collection of blood in the abdominal cavity.
   b. portal hypertension and hypoalbuminemia cause a fluid shift into the peritoneal space.
   c. decreased peristalsis in the GI tract contributes to gas formation and distention of the bowel.
   d. bile salts in the blood irritate the peritoneal membranes, causing edema and pocketing of fluid.

5. In planning care for a patient with metastatic liver cancer, the nurse should include interventions that
   a. focus primarily on symptomatic and comfort measures.
   b. reassure the patient that chemotherapy offers a good prognosis.
   c. promote the patient's confidence that surgical excision of the tumor will be successful.
   d. provide information necessary for the patient to make decisions regarding liver transplantation.

6. Nursing management of the patient with acute pancreatitis includes (select all that apply)
   a. checking for signs of hypocalcemia.
   b. providing a diet low in carbohydrates.
   c. giving insulin based on a sliding scale.
   d. observing stools for signs of steatorrhea.
   e. monitoring for infection, particularly respiratory tract infection.

7. A patient with pancreatic cancer is admitted to the hospital for evaluation of possible treatment options. The patient asks the nurse to explain the Whipple procedure that the surgeon has described. The explanation includes the information that a Whipple procedure involves
   a. creating a bypass around the obstruction caused by the tumor by joining the gallbladder to the jejunum.
   b. resection of the entire pancreas and the distal portion of the stomach, with anastomosis of the common bile duct and the stomach into the duodenum.
   c. removal of part of the pancreas, part of the stomach, the duodenum, and the gallbladder, with joining of the pancreatic duct, the common bile duct, and the stomach into the jejunum.
   d. radical removal of the pancreas, the duodenum, and the spleen, and attachment of the stomach to the jejunum, which requires oral supplementation of pancreatic digestive enzymes and insulin replacement therapy.

8. The nursing management of the patient with cholecystitis associated with cholelithiasis is based on the knowledge that
   a. shock-wave therapy should be tried initially.
   b. once gallstones are removed, they tend not to recur.
   c. the disorder can be successfully treated with oral bile salts that dissolve gallstones.
   d. laparoscopic cholecystectomy is the treatment of choice in most patients who are symptomatic.

9. Teaching in relation to home management after a laparoscopic cholecystectomy should include
   a. keeping the bandages on the puncture sites for 48 hours.
   b. reporting any bile-colored drainage or pus from any incision.
   c. using over-the-counter antiemetics if nausea and vomiting occur.
   d. emptying and measuring the contents of the bile bag from the T tube every day.

1. a, 2. b, 3. b, 4. b, 5. a, 6. a, e, 7. c, 8. d, 9. b

ⓔvolve

For rationales to these answers and even more NCLEX review questions, visit *http://evolve.elsevier.com/Lewis/medsurg*.

REFERENCES

1. Centers for Disease Control and Prevention: Viral hepatitis statistics and surveillance—United States, 2010. Retrieved from *www.cdc.gov/hepatitis/Statistics/2010Surveillance/index.htm*.
2. Centers for Disease Control and Prevention: National hepatitis C prevention strategy 2001: a comprehensive strategy for the prevention and control of hepatitis C virus infection and its consequences. Retrieved from *www.cdc.gov/hepatitis/HCV/Strategy/PDFs/NatHepCPrevStrategy.pdf*.
3. Ly KN, Xing J, Klevens RM, et al: The increasing burden of mortality from viral hepatitis in the United States between 1999 and 2007, *Ann Intern Med* 156:271, 2012.
4. Edey M, Barraclough K, Johnson DW: Review article: hepatitis B and dialysis, *Nephrology (Carlton)* 15:137, 2010.
5. Ghany MG, Strader DB, Thomas DL, et al: Diagnosis, management, and treatment of hepatitis C: an update, *Hepatology* 49:1335, 2009.
6. Chevaliez S, Rodriguez C, Pawlotsky JM: New virologic tools for management of chronic hepatitis B and C, *Gastroenterology* 142:1303, 2012.

7. Estrabaud E, Vidaud M, Marcellin P, et al: Genomics and HCV infection: progression of fibrosis and treatment response, *J Hepatol* 57(5):1110, 2012.

8. Stevenson M, Lloyd-Jones M, Morgan MY, et al: Non-invasive diagnostic assessment tools for the detection of liver fibrosis in patients with suspected alcohol-related liver disease: a systematic review and economic evaluation, *Health Technol Assess* 16:1, 2012.

9. Lee H, Park W, Yang JH, et al: Management of hepatitis B virus infection, *Gastroenterol Nurs* 33:120, 2010.

10. Kwon H, Lok AS: Hepatitis B therapy, *Nat Rev Gastroenterol Hepatol* 8:275, 2011.

*11. Poordad F, Dieterich D: Treating hepatitis C: current standard of care and emerging direct-acting antiviral agents, *J Viral Hepat* 19:449, 2012.

12. Rosedale MT, Strauss SM: Depression, interferon therapy, hepatitis C, and substance use: potential treatments and areas for research, *J Am Psychiatr Nurses Assoc* 17:205, 2011.

*13. Centers for Disease Control and Prevention: Advisory Committee for Immunization Practices recommendations. Retrieved from *www.cdc.gov/vaccines/pubs/acip-list.htm*.

14. Centers for Disease Control and Prevention: *CDC announces first ever National Hepatitis Testing Day and proposes that all baby boomers be tested once for hepatitis C (press release)*, May 2012. Retrieved from *www.cdc.gov/nchhstp/newsroom/HepTestingRecsPressRelease2012.html*.

15. Boesecke C, Vogel M: HIV and hepatitis C co-infection: acute HCV therapy, *Curr Opin HIV AIDS* 6:459, 2011.

*16. Ghany MG, Nelson DR, Strader DB, et al: An update on treatment of genotype 1 chronic hepatitis C virus infection: 2011 practice guideline by the American Association for the Study of Liver Diseases, *Hepatology* 54:1433, 2011.

17. Sedky K, Nazir R, Joshi A, et al: Which psychotropic medications induce hepatotoxicity? *Gen Hosp Psychiatry* 34:53, 2012.

18. National Digestive Diseases Information Clearinghouse: Wilson disease, May 2009. Retrieved from *www.digestive.niddk.nih.gov/ddiseases/pubs/wilson*.

19. National Digestive Diseases Information Clearinghouse: Nonalcoholic steatohepatitis, November 2006. Retrieved from *www.digestive.niddk.nih.gov/ddiseases/pubs/nash*.

20. Bajaj JS, O'Leary JG, Reddy KR, et al: Second infections independently increase mortality in hospitalized cirrhotic patients: the NACSELD experience, *Hepatology* 56:2328, 2012.

21. Riggio O, Nardelli S, Moscucci F, et al: Hepatic encephalopathy after transjugular intrahepatic portosystemic shunt, *Clin Liver Dis* 16:133, 2012.

22. Kashani A, Landaverde C, Medici V, et al: Fluid retention in cirrhosis: pathophysiology and management, *QJM* 101:71, 2008.

23. Habib S, Boyer TD: Vasopressin V2-receptor antagonists in patients with cirrhosis, ascites and hyponatremia, *Therap Adv Gastroenterol* 5:189, 2012.

24. Tsien CD, McCullough AJ, Dasarathy S: Late evening snack: exploiting a period of anabolic opportunity in cirrhosis, *J Gastroenterol Hepatol* 27:430, 2012.

25. Page Acnp-Bc J: Nonalcoholic fatty liver disease: the hepatic metabolic syndrome, *J Am Acad Nurse Pract* 24:345, 2012.

*26. Lee WM, Stravitz TR, Larson AM: Introduction to the Revised American Association for the Study of Liver Diseases position paper on acute liver failure 2011. Retrieved from *www.aasld.org/practiceguidelines/Documents/AcuteLiverFailureUpdate2011.pdf*.

27. Sood GK: Acute liver failure. Retrieved from *http://emedicine.medscape.com/article/177354-overview#aw2aab6b2b5aa*.

28. Fisher EM, Brown DK: Hepatorenal syndrome: beyond liver failure, *AACN Adv Crit Care* 21:165, 2010.

29. Jemal A, Bray F, Center MM, et al: Global cancer statistics, *CA Cancer J Clin* 61:69, 2011.

30. Forner A, Llovet JM, Bruix J: Hepatocellular carcinoma, *Lancet* 379:1245, 2012.

31. American Liver Foundation: More about organ donation. Retrieved from *www.liverfoundation.org/patients/organdonor/about*.

32. Carrion AF, Martin P: Viral hepatitis in the elderly, *Am J Gastroenterol* 107:691, 2012.

33. National Digestive Disease Information Clearinghouse: Pancreatitis. Retrieved from *www.digestive.niddk.nih.gov/ddiseases/pubs/pancreatitis*.

34. Bruesehoff MP: Understanding endoscopic retrograde cholangiopancreatography, *OR Nurse* 6:40, 2012.

35. American Cancer Society: Gallbladder cancer. Retrieved from *www.cancer.org/Cancer/GallbladderCancer/DetailedGuide/gallbladder-risk-factors*.

RESOURCES

American Association for the Study of Liver Diseases (AASLD)
www.aasld.org

American Gastroenterological Association
www.gastro.org

American Liver Foundation
www.liverfoundation.org

American Pancreatic Association
www.american-pancreatic-association.org

National Pancreas Foundation
www.pancreasfoundation.org

Pancreatic Cancer Action Network
www.pancan.org

*Evidence-based information for clinical practice.

CASE STUDY
Managing Multiple Patients

Introduction
You are working on the medical-surgical unit and have been assigned to care for the following five patients. You have one LPN who is assigned to help you and a UAP who is assigned to assist you and another RN.

Patients

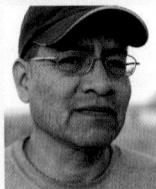

iStockphoto/Thinkstock

L.C. is a 58-year-old Native American man admitted from the emergency department (ED) with acute abdominal pain. A CBC showed a Hgb of 9.0 g/dL and Hct of 26%. The WBC count is normal. A CT scan and colonoscopy indicated two medium-sized tumors in the transverse colon. A hemicolectomy was performed. The adenocarcinoma had spread to the muscle of the colon wall and there were two positive lymph nodes.

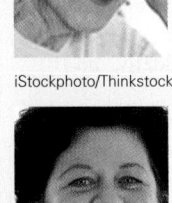

iStockphoto/Thinkstock

M.S. is a 70-year-old white woman who was recently admitted to the unit with generalized weakness and malnutrition. She is 5 feet 4 inches tall and weighs 100 lb, with a 30-lb weight loss in past 2 months. Her PMH includes a recent thrombotic stroke with hemiparesis and dysphagia. She has had nothing by mouth for the past 24 hours and just started enteral nutrition via PEG tube.

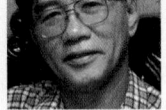
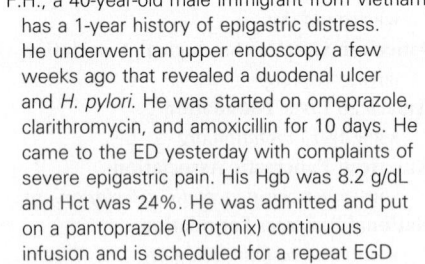

Hemera/Thinkstock

S.R. is a 48-year-old white woman admitted with complaints of chest pain and shortness of breath. She has a history of type 2 diabetes mellitus, hypertension, and osteoarthritis. She is 5 feet 4 inches tall and weighs 210 lb. Her most recent BP was 160/110 mm Hg. Her morning laboratory results reveal elevations in fasting blood glucose, total cholesterol, LDL cholesterol, and triglycerides. Her HDL cholesterol is low. Her cardiac enzymes and ECG are all within normal limits. She is scheduled to undergo a cardiac stress test at 10 AM.

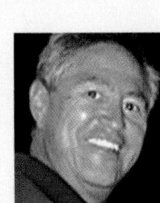

iStockphoto/Thinkstock

F.H., a 40-year-old male immigrant from Vietnam, has a 1-year history of epigastric distress. He underwent an upper endoscopy a few weeks ago that revealed a duodenal ulcer and *H. pylori*. He was started on omeprazole, clarithromycin, and amoxicillin for 10 days. He came to the ED yesterday with complaints of severe epigastric pain. His Hgb was 8.2 g/dL and Hct was 24%. He was admitted and put on a pantoprazole (Protonix) continuous infusion and is scheduled for a repeat EGD today.

M.B. is a 55-year-old Native American man admitted with a diagnosis of upper GI bleeding. He has been vomiting for 2 days and noticed blood in the toilet when he vomits. He has had cirrhosis for 12 years and admits to drinking heavily for 20 years but has been sober for the past 2 years. He currently complains of anorexia, nausea, and abdominal discomfort. He is thin and malnourished, has moderate ascites, jaundice of sclera and skin, 4+ pitting edema of the lower extremities, and palpable liver and spleen. His bilirubin, serum ammonia level, and liver enzymes are all elevated. His morning laboratory test results demonstrate a Hct of 20% and Hgb of 6.8 g/dL.

Management Discussion Questions
1. ***Priority Decision:*** After receiving report, which patient should you see first? Provide a rationale for your decision.
2. ***Delegation Decision:*** Which tasks could you delegate to the LPN *(select all that apply)*?
   a. Assess L.C.'s pain level and bowel sounds.
   b. Administer oral medications to S.R. with a sip of water.
   c. Provide enteral tube feeding for M.S. if gastric residual <500 mL.
   d. Call M.B.'s health care provider regarding the morning laboratory results.
   e. Because she understands Vietnamese, teach F.H.'s wife about his disease.
3. ***Priority and Delegation Decision:*** As you are assessing M.B., the LPN informs you that F.H. just vomited a large amount of bright red blood. What initial action would be most appropriate?
   a. Have the LPN administer an antiemetic to F.H.
   b. Ask the LPN to notify F.H.'s health care provider.
   c. Leave M.B.'s room to perform a focused assessment on F.H.
   d. Ask the UAP to obtain a unit of packed red blood cells from the blood bank.

Case Study Progression
When you enter F.H.'s room, he tells you that his pain actually feels somewhat relieved since he vomited. However, you note that his skin is cool and clammy, his BP is 90/54 mm Hg, and his heart rate is 116 bpm. You notify his health care provider.

4. Which interventions would you expect the health care provider to order for F.H. *(select all that apply)*?
   a. Stat hemoglobin and hematocrit
   b. Emergent endoscopic and endotherapy
   c. Discontinue the pantoprazole (Protonix) infusion
   d. Start a second IV site and administer 500 mL normal saline over 30 minutes
5. ***Priority Decision:*** After administering a bolus feeding of enteral nutrition to M.S., it would be most important to
   a. assess for gastric residual.
   b. obtain an abdominal x-ray.
   c. keep head of bed elevated 30-45 degrees.
   d. record the total amount of fluid administered.
6. Which intervention to treat ascites might you expect the health care provider to order for M.B. *(select all that apply)*?
   a. Paracentesis
   b. Diuretic therapy
   c. 2 g sodium diet
   d. 1800 mL/day fluid restriction
   e. Shunt insertion from peritoneum to heart
7. ***Management Decision:*** As you enter the nurse's station, you overhear derogatory comments made by the UAP to the LPN about S.R.'s weight. Which response would be most appropriate?
   a. Report the incident to charge nurse for follow-up.
   b. Talk to the UAP to discuss possible HIPAA violation.
   c. Talk to S.R. to assess impact of UAP's bias on her self-image.
   d. Provide education to help staff members recognize obesity as a disease process.

SECTION 9

Problems of Urinary Function

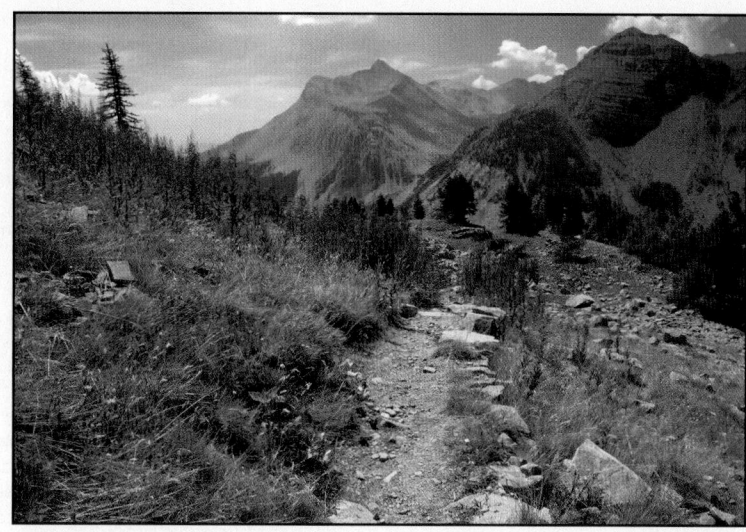

Hemera/Thinkstock

The road to success is always under construction.
Lily Tomlin

45

Bones can break, muscles can atrophy, glands can loaf,
even the brain can go to sleep without immediate danger to survival.
But should the kidneys fail . . . neither bone, muscle, gland,
nor brain could carry on.
Homer Smith

Nursing Assessment
Urinary System

Betty Jean Reid Czarapata

⊖volve WEBSITE

http://evolve.elsevier.com/Lewis/medsurg

- NCLEX Review Questions
- Key Points
- Pre-Test
- Answer Guidelines for Case Study in this chapter
- Rationales for Bridge to NCLEX Examination Questions
- Concept Map Creator

- Glossary
- Videos
  - Physical Examination: Abdomen: Inspection, Auscultation, and Percussion
  - Physical Examination: Abdomen: Palpation
- Content Updates

LEARNING OUTCOMES

1. Differentiate among the anatomic location and functions of the kidneys, ureters, bladder, and urethra.
2. Explain the physiologic events involved in the formation and passage of urine from glomerular filtration to voiding.
3. Select significant subjective and objective data related to the urinary system that should be obtained from a patient.
4. Link the age-related changes of the urinary system to the differences in assessment findings.
5. Select appropriate techniques to use in the physical assessment of the urinary system.
6. Differentiate normal from abnormal findings of a physical assessment of the urinary system.
7. Describe the purpose, significance of results, and nursing responsibilities related to diagnostic studies of the urinary system.
8. Differentiate the normal from the abnormal findings of a urinalysis.

KEY TERMS

costovertebral angle (CVA), p. 1054
creatinine, Table 45-8, p. 1057
cystometrogram, Table 45-8, p. 1060
cystoscopy, Table 45-8, p. 1060

glomerular filtration rate (GFR), p. 1048
glomerulus, p. 1047
intravenous pyelogram (IVP), Table 45-8, p. 1058

nephron, p. 1047
renal biopsy, Table 45-8, p. 1061

Adequate kidney function is essential to the maintenance of a healthy body. If a person has complete kidney failure and treatment is not provided, death is inevitable. This chapter discusses the structures and functions, assessment, and diagnostic studies of the urinary system.

STRUCTURES AND FUNCTIONS OF URINARY SYSTEM

The *upper urinary system* consists of two kidneys and two ureters. The *lower urinary system* consists of a urinary bladder and a urethra (Fig. 45-1). Urine is formed in the kidneys, drains through the ureters to be stored in the bladder, and then passes from the body through the urethra.

Kidneys

The kidneys are the principal organs of the urinary system. The primary functions of the kidneys are to (1) regulate the volume and composition of extracellular fluid (ECF) and (2) excrete waste products from the body. The kidneys also function to control blood pressure, produce erythropoietin, activate vitamin D, and regulate acid-base balance.

Macrostructure. The paired kidneys are bean-shaped organs located retroperitoneally (behind the peritoneum) on either side of the vertebral column at about the level of the twelfth thoracic (T12) vertebra to the third lumbar (L3) vertebra. Each kidney weighs 4 to 6 oz (113 to 170 g) and is about 5 in (12.5 cm) long. The right kidney, positioned at the level of the twelfth rib, is lower than the left. An adrenal gland lies on top of each kidney.

Reviewed by Barbara S. Broome, RN, PhD, FAAN, Associate Dean and Chair, Community/Mental Health, University of South Alabama, College of Nursing, Mobile, Alabama; Marci Langenkamp, RN, MS, Assistant Professor of Nursing, Edison Community College, Piqua, Ohio; and Phyllis A. Matthews, RN, MS, ANCP-BC, CUNP, Urology Nurse Practitioner, Denver VA Medical Center, Denver, Colorado.

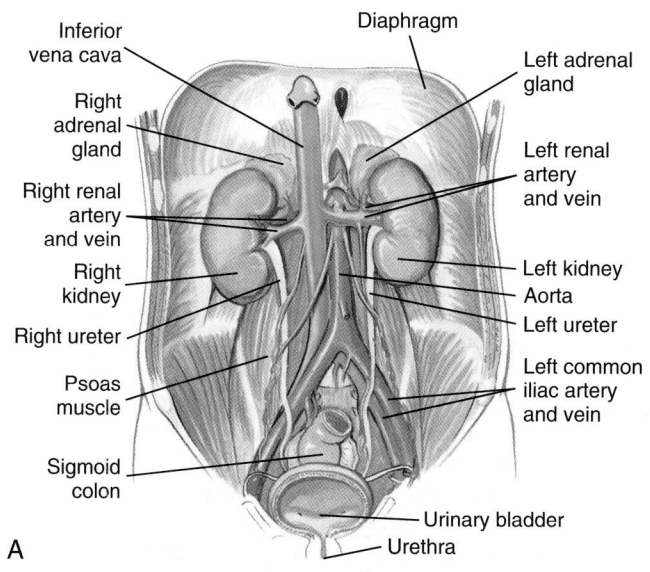

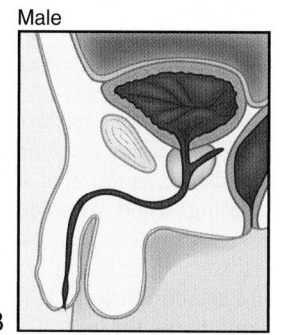
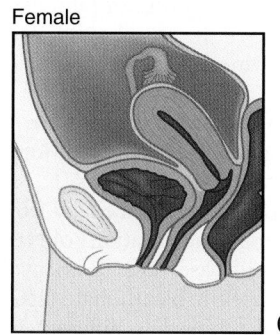

FIG. 45-1 Organs of the urinary system. **A,** Upper urinary tract in relation to other anatomic structures. **B,** Male urethra in relation to other pelvic structures. **C,** Female urethra.

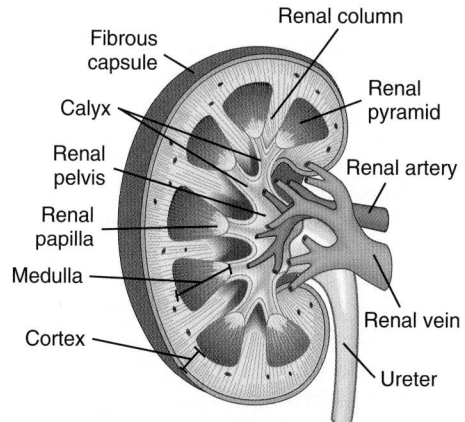

FIG. 45-2 Longitudinal section of the kidney.

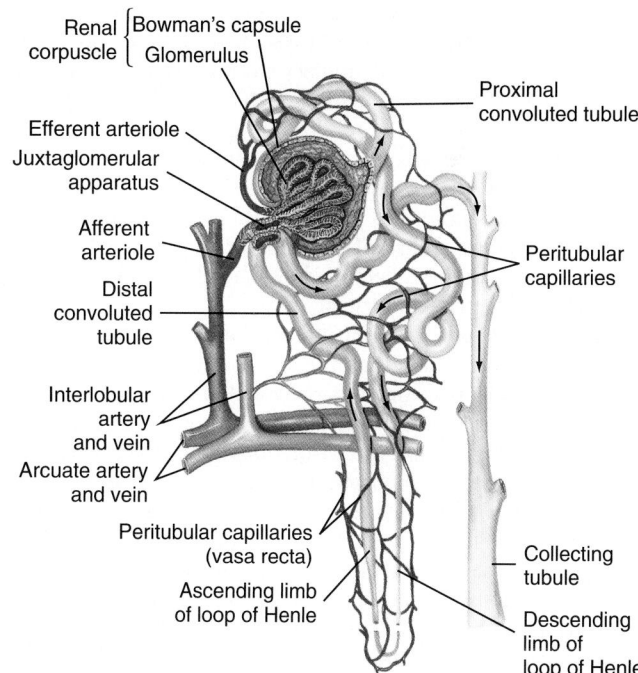

FIG. 45-3 The nephron is the basic functional unit of the kidney. This illustration of a single nephron unit also shows the surrounding blood vessels.

Each kidney is surrounded by a considerable amount of fat and connective tissue that cushions, supports, and maintains its position. A thin, smooth layer of fibrous membrane called the *capsule* covers the surface of each kidney. The capsule protects the kidney and serves as a shock absorber when this area is traumatized from a sudden force or strike. The *hilus* on the medial side of the kidney serves as the entry site for the renal artery and nerves, and as the exit site for the renal vein and ureter.

The parenchyma (actual tissue) of the kidney can be visualized on a longitudinal section of the kidney (Fig. 45-2). The outer layer is the *cortex,* and the inner layer is the *medulla.* The medulla consists of a number of pyramids. The apices (tops) of these pyramids are called *papillae,* through which urine passes to enter the calyces. The minor calyces widen and merge to form major calyces, which form a funnel-shaped sac called the *renal pelvis.* The minor and major calyces transport urine to the renal pelvis, from which it drains through the ureter to the bladder. The renal pelvis can store a small volume of urine (3 to 5 mL).

Microstructure. The nephron is the functional unit of the kidney. Each kidney contains approximately 1 million nephrons. Each nephron is composed of the glomerulus, Bowman's capsule, and a tubular system. The tubular system consists of the proximal convoluted tubule, loop of Henle, distal convoluted tubule, and collecting tubules (Fig. 45-3). The glomerulus, Bowman's capsule, proximal tubule, and distal tubule are located

in the cortex of the kidney. The loop of Henle and collecting tubules are located in the medulla. Several collecting tubules join to form a single collecting duct. The collecting ducts eventually merge into a pyramid that empties via the papilla into a minor calyx.

Blood Supply. Blood flow to the kidneys, approximately 1200 mL/min, accounts for 20% to 25% of the cardiac output. Blood reaches the kidneys via the renal artery, which arises from the aorta and enters the kidney through the hilus. The renal artery divides into secondary branches and then into still smaller branches, each of which forms an afferent arteriole. The afferent arteriole divides into a capillary network, the glomerulus, which is a tuft of up to 50 capillaries (see Fig. 45-3). The capillaries of the glomerulus unite in the efferent arteriole. This efferent arteriole splits to form a capillary network, the peritubular capillaries, which surround the tubular system. All peritubular capillaries drain into the venous system; the renal vein empties into the inferior vena cava.

Physiology of Urine Formation. Urine formation is the outcome of a complex, multistep process of filtration, reabsorption, secretion, and excretion of water, electrolytes, and metabolic waste products. Although urine formation is the result of this process, the primary functions of the kidneys are to filter the blood and maintain the body's internal homeostasis.

Glomerular Function. Urine formation begins at the glomerulus, where blood is filtered. The glomerulus is a semipermeable membrane that allows filtration (see Fig. 45-3). The hydrostatic pressure of the blood within the glomerular capillaries causes a portion of blood to be filtered across the semipermeable membrane into Bowman's capsule, where the filtered portion of the blood (the glomerular filtrate) begins to pass down to the tubule. Filtration is more rapid in the glomerulus than in ordinary tissue capillaries because the glomerular membrane is porous. The ultrafiltrate is similar in composition to blood except that it lacks blood cells, platelets, and large plasma proteins. Under normal conditions, the capillary pores are too small to allow the loss of these large blood components. In many kidney diseases, capillary permeability is increased, which permits plasma proteins and blood cells to pass into the urine.

The amount of blood filtered each minute by the glomeruli is expressed as the glomerular filtration rate (GFR). The normal GFR is about 125 mL/min. The peritubular capillary network reabsorbs most of the glomerular filtrate before it reaches the end of the collecting duct. Therefore only 1 mL/min (on average) is excreted as urine.

Tubular Function. Since the glomerular membrane is a selective filtration membrane that filters primarily by size, provision is made for the reabsorption of essential materials and the excretion of nonessential ones (Table 45-1). The tubules and collecting ducts carry out these functions by means of reabsorption and secretion. *Reabsorption* is the passage of a substance from the lumen of the tubules through the tubule cells and into the capillaries. This process involves both active and passive transport mechanisms. Tubular *secretion* is the passage of a substance from the capillaries through the tubular cells into the lumen of the tubule. Reabsorption and secretion cause numerous changes in the composition of the glomerular filtrate as it moves through the entire length of the tubule.

In the proximal convoluted tubule, about 80% of the electrolytes are reabsorbed. Normally, all the glucose, amino acids, and small proteins are reabsorbed. Although most reabsorption occurs by active transport, hydrogen ions (H^+) and creatinine are secreted into the filtrate.

As reabsorption continues in the loop of Henle, water is conserved, which is important for concentrating the filtrate. The descending loop is permeable to water and moderately permeable to sodium, urea, and other solutes. In the ascending limb, chloride ions (Cl^-) are actively reabsorbed, followed by passive reabsorption of sodium ions (Na^+). About 25% of the filtered sodium is reabsorbed in the ascending limb.

Two important functions of the distal convoluted tubules are final regulation of water balance and acid-base balance. Antidiuretic hormone (ADH) is required for water reabsorption in the kidney and is important in water balance. ADH makes the distal convoluted tubules and the collecting ducts permeable to water. This allows water to be reabsorbed into the peritubular capillaries and eventually returned to the circulation.

Decreases in plasma osmolality are detected in the anterior hypothalamus by osmoreceptors. These osmoreceptors send neural input to *superoptic nuclei cells* in the hypothalamus. These superoptic nuclei cells have neuronal axons that terminate in the posterior pituitary gland and act to inhibit secretion of ADH. In the absence of ADH, the tubules are essentially impermeable to water. Thus any water in the tubules leaves the body as urine.

Aldosterone (released from the adrenal cortex) acts on the distal tubule to cause reabsorption of Na^+ and water. In exchange for Na^+, potassium ions (K^+) are excreted. The secretion of aldosterone is influenced by both circulating blood volume and plasma concentrations of Na^+ and K^+.

Acid-base regulation involves reabsorbing and conserving most of the bicarbonate (HCO_3^-) and secreting excess H^+. The distal tubule has different ways to maintain the pH of ECF within a range of 7.35 to 7.45 (see Chapter 17).

Myocyte cells in the right atrium secrete a hormone, atrial natriuretic peptide (ANP), in response to atrial distention, which is a result of an increase in plasma volume. ANP acts on the kidneys to increase sodium excretion. At the same time ANP inhibits renin, ADH, and the action of angiotensin II on the adrenal glands, thereby suppressing aldosterone secretion. These combined effects of ANP result in the production of a large volume of dilute urine. Furthermore, secretion of ANP causes relaxation of the afferent arteriole, thus increasing the GFR.

The renal tubules are also involved in calcium balance. Parathyroid hormone (PTH) is released from the parathyroid gland in response to low serum calcium levels. PTH maintains serum calcium levels by causing increased tubular reabsorption of calcium ions (Ca^{2+}) and decreased tubular reabsorption of phosphate ions (PO_4^{2-}). In kidney disease the effects of PTH may have a major effect on bone metabolism.

Vitamin D is a hormone that can be obtained in the diet or synthesized by the action of ultraviolet radiation on cholesterol in the skin. These forms of vitamin D are inactive and require two more steps to become metabolically active. The first step in activation occurs in the liver; the second step occurs in the kidneys. Active vitamin D is essential for the absorption of calcium from the gastrointestinal (GI) tract. The patient with kidney failure (also called renal failure) has a deficiency of the active metabolite of vitamin D and manifests problems of altered calcium and phosphate balance (see Chapter 47).

In summary, the basic function of nephrons is to cleanse blood plasma of unnecessary substances. After the glomerulus

TABLE 45-1	FUNCTIONS OF NEPHRON SEGMENTS
Component	**Function**
Glomerulus	Selective filtration.
Proximal tubule	Reabsorption of 80% of electrolytes and water, glucose, amino acids, HCO_3^-. Secretion of H^+ and creatinine.
Loop of Henle	Reabsorption of Na^+ and Cl^- in ascending limb and water in descending loop. Concentration of filtrate.
Distal tubule	Secretion of K^+, H^+, ammonia. Reabsorption of water (regulated by ADH) and HCO_3^-. Regulation of Ca^{2+} and PO_4^{2-} by parathyroid hormone. Regulation of Na^+ and K^+ by aldosterone.
Collecting duct	Reabsorption of water (ADH required).

ADH, Antidiuretic hormone.

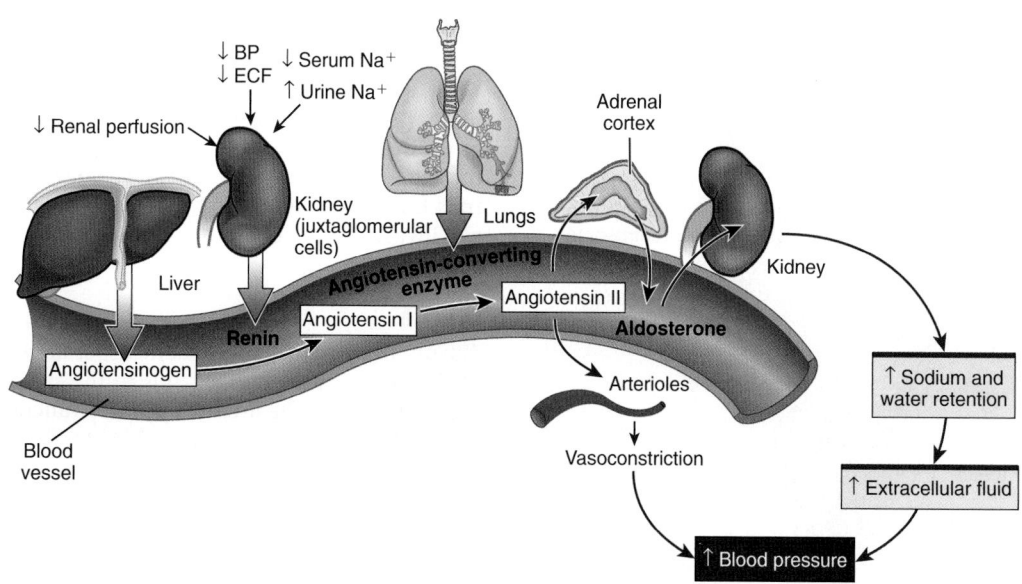

FIG. 45-4 Renin-angiotensin-aldosterone system.

has filtered the blood, the tubules select the unwanted from the wanted portions of tubular fluid. Essential constituents are returned to the blood, and dispensable substances pass into urine.

Other Functions of Kidneys. The kidneys perform vital functions through participation in red blood cell (RBC) production and blood pressure regulation. Erythropoietin is a hormone produced in the kidneys and secreted in response to hypoxia and decreased renal blood flow. Erythropoietin stimulates RBC production in the bone marrow. A deficiency of erythropoietin occurs in kidney failure, leading to anemia.

Renin is important in the regulation of blood pressure. Renin is produced and secreted by the kidney's juxtaglomerular cells (Fig. 45-4). Renin is released into the bloodstream in response to decreased renal perfusion, decreased arterial blood pressure, decreased ECF, decreased serum Na^+ concentration, and increased urinary Na^+ concentration. The plasma protein angiotensinogen (from the liver) is activated to angiotensin I by renin. Angiotensin I is subsequently converted to angiotensin II by angiotensin-converting enzyme (ACE). ACE is located on the inner surface of all blood vessels, with particularly high levels in the vessels of the lungs. Angiotensin II stimulates the release of aldosterone from the adrenal cortex, which causes Na^+ and water retention, leading to increased ECF volume. Angiotensin II also causes increased peripheral vasoconstriction. Release of renin is inhibited by an elevation in blood pressure. Excessive renin production caused by impaired renal perfusion may be a contributing factor in the etiology of hypertension (see Chapters 33 and 47).

Most body tissues synthesize prostaglandins (PGs) from the precursor, arachidonic acid, in response to appropriate stimuli. (See Chapter 12 and Fig. 12-2 for a more detailed discussion of PGs.) In the kidney, PG synthesis (primarily PGE_2 and PGI_2) occurs primarily in the medulla. These PGs have a vasodilating action, thus increasing renal blood flow, and promote Na^+ excretion. They counteract the vasoconstrictor effect of substances such as angiotensin and norepinephrine. Renal PGs may have a systemic effect in lowering blood pressure by decreasing systemic vascular resistance. The significance of renal PGs is related to the kidneys' role in causing hypertension. In renal failure with a loss of functioning tissue, these renal vasodilator factors are also lost, which may contribute to hypertension (see Chapter 47).

Ureters

The ureters are tubes that carry urine from the renal pelvis to the bladder (see Fig. 45-1). Arranged in a meshlike outer layer, circular and longitudinal smooth muscle fibers contract to promote the peristaltic, one-way flow of urine through the ureters. Distention, neurologic and endocrine influences, and drugs can affect these muscle contractions. Each ureter is approximately 10 to 12 in (25 to 30.5 cm) long and 0.08 to 0.3 in (0.2 to 0.8 cm) in diameter.

The narrow area where each ureter joins the renal pelvis is termed the *ureteropelvic junction* (UPJ). Subsequently, the ureters insert into either side of the bladder base at the *ureterovesical junctions* (UVJs). Ureteral lumens are narrowest at the UVJs. These junctions, the UPJ and UVJ, are often sites of obstruction. The narrow ureteral lumens can be easily obstructed internally (e.g., urinary calculi) or externally (e.g., tumors, adhesions, inflammation). Sympathetic and parasympathetic nerves, along with the vascular supply, surround the mucosal lining of the ureters. Stimulation of these nerves during passage of a stone or clot may cause acute, severe pain, termed *renal colic*.

Because the renal pelvis holds only 3 to 5 mL of urine, kidney damage can result from a backflow of more than that amount of urine. The UVJ relies on the ureter's angle of bladder penetration and muscle fiber attachments with the bladder to prevent the backflow *(reflux)* of urine and ascending infection. The distal ureter enters the bladder laterally at its base, courses along obliquely through the bladder wall for about 1.5 cm, and intermingles with muscle fibers of the bladder base. Circular and longitudinal bladder muscle fibers adjacent to the imbedded ureter help secure it. When bladder pressure rises (e.g., during voiding or coughing), muscle fibers that the ureter shares with the bladder base contract first, promoting ureteral lumen closure. Next, the bladder contracts against its base, ensuring UVJ closure and prevention of urine reflux through the junction.

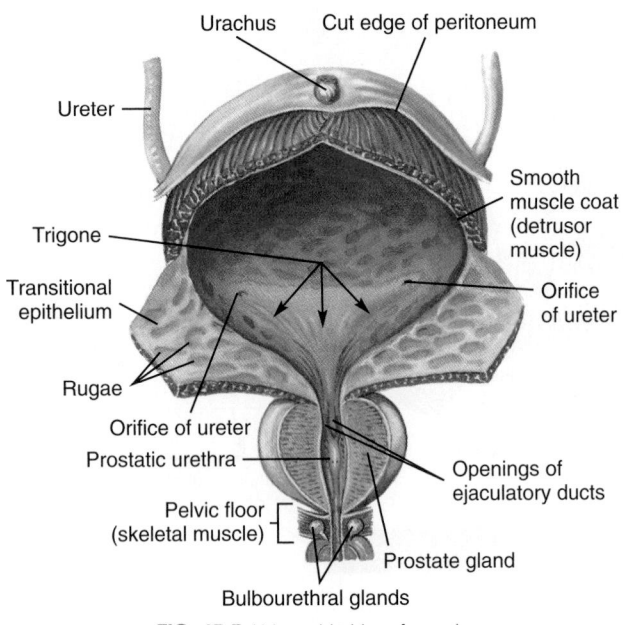

Urachus — Cut edge of peritoneum

Ureter —

Trigone —

Transitional epithelium —

Rugae —

Orifice of ureter —

Prostatic urethra —

Pelvic floor (skeletal muscle)

Bulbourethral glands

Smooth muscle coat (detrusor muscle)

Orifice of ureter

Openings of ejaculatory ducts

Prostate gland

FIG. 45-5 Urinary bladder of a male.

Bladder

The urinary bladder is a stretchable (able to fill at relatively low pressures) organ positioned behind the symphysis pubis and anterior to the vagina and rectum (Fig. 45-5). Its primary functions are to serve as a reservoir for urine and to eliminate waste products from the body. Normal adult urine output is approximately 1500 mL/day, which varies with food and fluid intake. The volume of urine produced at night is less than half of that formed during the day because of hormonal influences (e.g., ADH). This diurnal pattern of urination is normal. Typically, an individual will urinate five or six times during the day and occasionally at night.

The *trigone* is the triangular area formed by the two ureteral openings and the bladder neck at the base of the bladder. The trigone is affixed to the pelvis by many ligaments and does not change its shape during bladder filling or emptying. The bladder muscle *(detrusor)* is composed of layers of intertwined smooth muscle fibers capable of considerable distention during bladder filling and contraction during emptying. It is attached to the abdominal wall by an umbilical ligament, the *urachus.* As a result of this attachment, as the bladder fills, it rises toward the umbilicus. The dome and the anterior and lateral aspects of the bladder expand and contract.

On average, 200 to 250 mL of urine in the bladder cause moderate distention and the urge to urinate. When the quantity of urine reaches approximately 400 to 600 mL, the person feels uncomfortable. Bladder capacity varies with the individual, but generally ranges from 600 to 1000 mL. Evacuation of urine is termed *urination, micturition,* or *voiding.*

The bladder has the same mucosal lining as that of the renal pelvises, ureters, and bladder neck. The bladder is lined by transitional cell epithelium and is referred to as the *urothelium.* The urothelium is unique to the urinary tract. Transitional cell epithelium is resistant to absorption of urine. Therefore urinary wastes produced by the kidneys do not leak out of the urinary system after they leave the kidneys. Microscopically, transitional cell epithelium is several cells deep. However, as urine enters the bladder, these cells stretch out to only a few cells deep to accommodate filling. As the bladder empties, the urothelium resumes its multicellular layer formation.

Transitional cell tumors occurring in one section of the urinary tract can easily metastasize to other urinary tract areas given that the mucosal lining throughout the urinary tract is the same. Malignant cells may move down from upper urinary tract tumors and embed in the bladder, or large bladder tumors can invade the ureter. Tumor recurrence within the bladder is common.

Urethra

The urethra is a small tube that incorporates the smooth muscle of the bladder neck and extends to the striated muscle of the external meatus. The urethra's primary function is to serve as a conduit for urine from the bladder to the outside the body during voiding and to control voiding.

The female urethra is 1 to 2 in (2.5 to 5 cm) long and lies behind the symphysis pubis but anterior to the vagina (see Fig. 45-1, *C*). The male urethra, which is about 8 to 10 in (20 to 25 cm) long, originates at the bladder neck and extends the length of the penis (see Fig. 45-1, *B*).

Urethrovesical Unit

Together, the bladder, urethra, and pelvic floor muscles form what is called the urethrovesical unit. Voluntary control of this unit is defined as *continence.* Stimulating and inhibiting impulses are sent from the brain through the thoracolumbar (T11 to L2) and sacral (S2 to S4) areas of the spinal cord to control voiding. Distention of the bladder stimulates stretch receptors within the bladder wall. Impulses are transmitted to the sacral spinal cord and then to the brain, causing a desire to urinate. If the time to void is not appropriate, inhibitor impulses in the brain are stimulated and transmitted back through the thoracolumbar and sacral nerves innervating the bladder. In a coordinated fashion, the detrusor muscle accommodates to the pressure (does not contract) while the sphincter and pelvic floor muscles tighten (contract) to resist bladder pressure. If voiding is appropriate, cerebral inhibition is voluntarily suppressed, and impulses are transmitted via the spinal cord for the bladder neck, sphincter, and pelvic floor muscles to relax and for the bladder to contract. The sphincter closes and the detrusor muscle relaxes when the bladder is empty.

Any disease or trauma that affects the function of the brain, spinal cord, or nerves that directly innervate the bladder, bladder neck, external sphincter, or pelvic floor can affect bladder function. These conditions include diabetes mellitus, multiple sclerosis, paraplegia, and tetraplegia (quadriplegia). Drugs affecting nerve transmission also can affect bladder function.

GERONTOLOGIC CONSIDERATIONS

EFFECTS OF AGING ON URINARY SYSTEM

Anatomic changes in the aging kidney include a 20% to 30% decrease in size and weight between ages 30 and 90 years. By the seventh decade of life, 30% to 50% of glomeruli have lost their function. Atherosclerosis accelerates the decrease of renal size with age. Despite these changes, older individuals maintain body fluid homeostasis unless they encounter diseases or other physiologic stressors.[1]

Physiologic changes in the aging kidney include decreased renal blood flow, due in part to atherosclerosis, resulting in a

TABLE 45-2   GERONTOLOGIC ASSESSMENT DIFFERENCES

Urinary System

Gerontologic Changes	Differences in Assessment Findings
Kidney	
• ↓ Amount of renal tissue	• Less palpable
• ↓ Number of nephrons and renal blood vessels; thickened basement membrane of Bowman's capsule and glomeruli	• ↓ Creatinine clearance, ↑ BUN level, ↑ serum creatinine
• ↓ Function of loop of Henle and tubules	• Alterations in drug excretion, nocturia, loss of normal diurnal excretory pattern because of ↓ ability to concentrate urine; less concentrated urine
Ureter, Bladder, and Urethra	
• ↓ Elasticity and muscle tone	• Palpable bladder after urination because of retention
• Weakening of urinary sphincter	• Stress incontinence (especially during Valsalva maneuver), dribbling of urine after urination
• ↓ Bladder capacity and sensory receptors	• Frequency, urgency, nocturia, overflow incontinence
• Estrogen deficiency leading to thin, dry vaginal tissue	• Stress or overactive bladder, dysuria
• ↑ Prevalence of unstable bladder contractions	• Overactive bladder
• Prostatic enlargement	• Hesitancy, frequency, urgency, nocturia, straining to urinate, retention, dribbling

FOCUSED ASSESSMENT

Urinary System

Use this checklist to ensure that the key assessment steps have been done.

Subjective
Ask the patient about any of the following and note responses.

Painful urination	Y	N
Changes in color of urine (blood, cloudy)	Y	N
Change in characteristics of urination (diminished, excessive)	Y	N
Problems with frequent nighttime urination (nocturia)	Y	N

Objective: Diagnostic
Check the following laboratory results for critical values.

Blood urea nitrogen	✓
Serum creatinine	✓
Urinalysis	✓
Urine culture and sensitivity	✓

Objective: Physical Examination
Inspect

Abdomen	
Urinary meatus for inflammation or discharge	✓

Palpate

Abdomen for bladder distention, masses, or tenderness	✓

Percuss

Costovertebral angle for tenderness	✓

Auscultate

Renal arteries for bruits	✓

decreased GFR. Alterations in hormone levels, including ADH, aldosterone, and ANP, result in decreased urinary concentrating ability and alterations in the excretion of water, sodium, potassium, and acid. Under normal conditions, the aging kidney is able to maintain homeostasis. However, after abrupt changes in blood volume, acid load, or other insults, the kidney may not be able to function effectively because much of its renal reserve has been lost.

Physiologic changes also occur in the aging urethra and bladder. The female urethra, bladder, vagina, and pelvic floor undergo a loss of elasticity and muscle support. Consequently, older women are more prone to bladder infections and incontinence.

The prostate surrounds the proximal urethra. As men age, the prostate enlarges and may affect urinary patterns, causing hesitancy, retention, slow stream, and bladder infections.[2]

Constipation, a complaint often expressed by older adults, can also affect urination. Partial urethral obstruction may occur because of the rectum's close proximity to the urethra.

Age-related changes in the urinary system and differences in assessment findings are presented in Table 45-2.

ASSESSMENT OF URINARY SYSTEM

Subjective Data

Important Health Information

Past Health History. Question the patient about the presence or history of diseases that are related to renal or other urologic problems. Some of these diseases are hypertension, diabetes

CASE STUDY

Patient Introduction

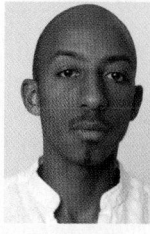
iStockphoto/Thinkstock

A.K. is a 28-yr-old African American man who comes to the emergency department (ED) in acute distress with complaints of severe abdominal pain. The pain began about 6 hr ago after he finished a 10-mile run as part of his training for a marathon. He says that the pain has steadily increased, he is nauseated, and his urine is a dark, smoky color.

Critical Thinking
As you read through this assessment chapter, think about A.K.'s symptoms with the following questions in mind:

1. What are the possible causes of A.K.'s abdominal pain, nausea, and urine color?
2. What would be your priority assessment of A.K.?
3. What questions would you ask A.K.?
4. What should be included in the physical assessment? What would you be looking for?
5. What diagnostic studies might you expect to be ordered?

evolve Answers available at *http://evolve.elsevier.com/Lewis/medsurg*.

mellitus, gout and other metabolic problems, connective tissue disorders (e.g., systemic lupus erythematosus, systemic sclerosis [scleroderma]), skin or upper respiratory tract infections of streptococcal origin, tuberculosis, viral hepatitis, congenital disorders, neurologic conditions (e.g., stroke, back injury), or trauma. Note specific urinary problems such as cancer, infections, benign prostatic hyperplasia, and calculi.

TABLE 45-3	POTENTIALLY NEPHROTOXIC AGENTS	
Antibiotics	**Other Drugs**	**Other Agents**
amikacin (Amikin)	captopril (Capoten)	Gold
amphotericin B	cimetidine (Tagamet)	Heavy metals
bacitracin	cisplatin (Platinol)	
cephalosporins	cocaine	
gentamicin	cyclosporine	
kanamycin	ethylene glycol	
neomycin	heroin	
polymyxin B	lithium	
streptomycin	methotrexate	
sulfonamides	nitrosoureas (e.g., carmustine)	
tobramycin (Nebcin)	Nonsteroidal antiinflammatory drugs (e.g., ibuprofen, indomethacin)	
vancomycin	phenacetin	
	quinine	
	rifampin	
	Salicylates (large quantities)	

Medications. An assessment of the patient's current and past use of medications is important. This should include over-the-counter drugs, prescription medications, and herbs. Drugs affect the urinary tract in several ways. Many drugs are known to be nephrotoxic (Table 45-3). Certain drugs may alter the quantity and character of urine output (e.g., diuretics). A number of drugs such as phenazopyridine (Pyridium) and nitrofurantoin (Macrodantin) change the color of urine. Anticoagulants may cause hematuria. Many antidepressants, calcium channel blockers, antihistamines, and drugs used for neurologic and musculoskeletal disorders affect the ability of the bladder or sphincter to contract or relax normally.

Surgery or Other Treatments. Ask the patient about previous hospitalizations related to renal or urologic diseases and all urinary problems during past pregnancies. Inquire about the duration, severity, and patient's perception of any problem and its treatment. Document past surgeries, particularly pelvic surgeries, or urinary tract instrumentation (e.g., catheterization). Ask the patient about any radiation or chemotherapy treatment for cancer.

Functional Health Patterns. Key questions to ask a patient with problems related to the renal system are listed in Table 45-4.

TABLE 45-4	HEALTH HISTORY

Urinary System

Health Perception–Health Management
- How is your energy level compared with 1 yr ago?
- Do you notice any visual changes?*
- Have you ever smoked? If yes, how many packs per day?

Nutritional-Metabolic
- How is your appetite?
- Has your weight changed over the past yr?*
- Do you take vitamins, herbs, or any other supplements?*
- How much and what kinds of fluids do you drink daily?
- How many dairy products and how much meat do you eat?
- Do you drink coffee? Colas? Tea?
- Do you eat chocolate?
- Do you spice your food heavily?*

Elimination
- Are you able to sit through a 2-hr meeting or ride in a car for 2 hr without urinating?
- Do you awaken at night with the desire to urinate? If so, how many times does this occur during an average night?
- Do you ever notice blood in your urine?* If so, at what point in the urination does it occur?
- Do you ever pass urine when you do not intend to? When?
- Do you use special devices or supplies for urine elimination or control?*
- How often do you move your bowels?
- Do you ever experience constipation?
- Do you frequently experience diarrhea? Do you ever have problems controlling your bowels? If so, do you have problems controlling the passage of gas? Watery or liquid stool? Solid stool?

Activity-Exercise
- Have you noticed any changes in your ability to do your usual daily activities?*
- Do certain activities aggravate your urinary problem?*
- Has your urinary problem caused you to alter or stop any activity or exercise?*
- Do you require assistance in moving or getting to the bathroom?*

Sleep-Rest
- Do you awaken at night from an urge to urinate?*
- Do you awaken at night from pain or other problems and urinate as a matter of routine before returning to sleep?*
- Do you experience daytime sleepiness and fatigue as a result of nighttime urination?*

Cognitive-Perceptual
- Do you ever have pain when you urinate?* If so, where is the pain?

Self-Perception–Self-Concept
- How does your urinary problem make you feel about yourself?
- Do you perceive your body differently since you have developed a urinary problem?

Role-Relationship
- Does your urinary problem interfere with your relationships with family or friends?*
- Has your urinary problem caused a change in your job status or affected your ability to carry out job-related responsibilities?*

Sexuality-Reproductive
- Has your urinary problem caused any change in your sexual pleasure or performance?*
- Do you have hygiene problems related to sexual activities that cause you concern?*

Coping–Stress Tolerance
- Do you feel able to manage the problems associated with your urinary problem? If not, explain.
- What strategies are you using to cope with your urinary problem?

Values-Beliefs
- Has your present illness affected your belief system?*
- Are your treatment decisions related to your urinary problem in conflict with your value system?*

*If yes, describe.

Health Perception–Health Management Pattern. Ask about the patient's general health, particularly when a disorder affecting the kidneys is suspected. Abnormal kidney function may be suggested by changes in weight or appetite; excess thirst; fluid retention; and complaints of headache, pruritus, blurred vision, or "feeling tired all the time." Similarly, an older patient may report malaise and nonlocalized abdominal discomfort as the only symptoms of a urinary tract infection (UTI). Family members may report disorientation or increased confusion that may be a sign of UTI in older adults.

Take an occupational history because exposure to certain chemicals can affect the kidneys and urinary system. Phenol and ethylene glycol are examples of nephrotoxic chemicals. Aromatic amines and some organic chemicals may increase the risk of bladder cancers. Textile workers, painters, hairdressers, and industrial workers have a high incidence of bladder tumors.

Get a smoking history. Cigarette smoking is a major risk factor for bladder cancer. Tumors occur more frequently in cigarette smokers than in nonsmokers.

Obtain information about places where a patient has lived. It has been shown that persons living in certain parts of the United States (Great Lakes, Southwest, Southeast) have a higher than normal incidence of urinary calculi, possibly caused by the higher mineral content of the soil and water. A person living in Middle Eastern countries or Africa can acquire certain parasites that can cause cystitis or bladder cancer.

GENETIC RISK ALERT
- Polycystic kidney disease and congenital urinary tract abnormalities (e.g., Alport syndrome [congenital nephritis]) are genetic disorders.
- A family history of certain renal or urologic problems increases the likelihood of similar problems occurring in the patient.
- Ask about family members who have had any of the diseases that the patient mentions in the past health history.

Nutritional-Metabolic Pattern. The usual quantity and types of fluid a patient drinks are important in relation to urinary tract disease. Dehydration may contribute to UTIs, calculi formation, and kidney failure. Large intake of particular foods, such as dairy products or foods high in proteins, may also lead to calculi formation. Asparagus may cause the urine to smell musty, and red urine caused by beet ingestion may be mistaken for bloody urine. Caffeine, alcohol, carbonated beverages, some artificial sweeteners, or spicy foods often aggravate urinary inflammatory diseases. Green tea and some herbal teas also cause diuresis. An unexplained weight gain may be the result of fluid retention secondary to a renal problem. Anorexia, nausea, and vomiting can dramatically affect fluid status and require careful assessment. Obtain information on vitamin and mineral supplements and herbal therapies. The patient may not think of these supplements and therapies when listing over-the-counter drugs.

Elimination Pattern. Questions about urine elimination patterns are the cornerstone of the health history in the patient with a lower urinary tract disorder. This line of inquiry begins with a question of how the patient manages urine elimination. Most patients eliminate urine by spontaneous voiding. Therefore ask about daytime (diurnal) voiding frequency and the frequency of nocturia. Pelvic organ prolapse, particularly advanced anterior vaginal prolapse, may cause suprapubic pressure, frequency, urgency, and incontinence secondary to urinary retention. Query patients about additional bothersome lower urinary tract symptoms, including urgency, incontinence, or urinary retention. Table 45-5 lists some of the common manifestations of urinary tract disorders.

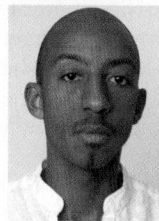

iStockphoto/Thinkstock

A focused subjective assessment of A.K. revealed the following information:

PMH: History of one isolated incidence of possible gout 6 yr ago. He stopped drinking alcohol with no further occurrence. Appendectomy 12 yr ago.

Medications: None.

Health Perception–Health Management: A.K. states that he is usually healthy. He does not smoke or drink alcohol. He has never experienced this type of pain before. Describes the pain as being sharp and colicky (coming in waves). Rates the pain as 9 on a scale of 0-10.

Nutritional-Metabolic: A.K. is currently on a high-protein diet as he trains for the marathon. He eats a lot of chicken, beef, and seafood. He drinks milk-based protein shakes and water after exercising but admits that he does not think he drinks enough to replace fluid loss in perspiration. He drinks coffee for energy but denies eating chocolate or other sweets. He also avoids sodas.

Elimination: Denies any history of difficulty with urination or constipation or diarrhea. This is the first time he has ever noticed a change of color in his urine.

Activity-Exercise: Prides himself in his ability to exercise and run without difficulty.

Sleep-Rest: Does not awaken at night to urinate.

Cognitive-Perceptual: Denies pain on urination.

Self-Perception–Self-Concept: Believes he is able to monitor self and maintain healthy lifestyle.

Coping–Stress Tolerance: Worried that this pain may interfere with his marathon training.

TABLE 45-5	MANIFESTATIONS OF URINARY SYSTEM DISORDERS				
	Specific Manifestations Related to Urinary System				
General Manifestations	**Edema**	**Pain**	**Patterns of Urination**	**Urine Output**	**Urine Composition**
Fatigue	Facial (periorbital)	Dysuria	Frequency	Anuria	Concentrated
Headaches	Ankle	Flank or	Urgency	Oliguria	Dilute
Blurred vision	Ascites	costovertebral	Hesitancy of stream	Polyuria	Hematuria
Elevated blood pressure	Anasarca	angle	Change in stream		Pyuria
Anorexia	Sacral	Groin	Retention		Color (red, brown,
Nausea and vomiting		Suprapubic	Dysuria		yellowish green)
Chills			Nocturia		
Itching			Incontinence		
Excessive thirst			Stress incontinence		
Change in body weight			Dribbling		
Cognitive changes					

Changes in the color and appearance of urine are often significant and should be evaluated. If blood is visible in the urine, determine if it occurs at the beginning of, throughout, or at the end of urination.

Investigate bowel function. Problems with fecal incontinence may signal neurologic causes for bladder problems because of shared nerve pathways. Constipation and fecal impaction can partially obstruct the urethra, causing inadequate bladder emptying, overflow incontinence, and infection.

Determine the patient's method of handling a urinary problem. A patient may already be using a catheter or collection device. Sometimes a patient has to assume a particular position to urinate or perform maneuvers such as pressing on the lower abdomen (Credé's method) or straining (Valsalva maneuver) to empty the bladder.

Activity-Exercise Pattern. Assess the patient's level of activity. A sedentary person is more likely to have stasis of urine than an active individual and thus can be predisposed to infection and calculi. Demineralization of bones in an individual with limited physical activity can cause increased urine calcium precipitation.

An active person may find that increasing activity aggravates the urinary problem. The patient who has had prostate surgery or who has weakened pelvic floor muscles may leak urine when attempting particular activities such as running. Some men develop chronic inflammatory prostatitis or epididymitis after heavy lifting or long-distance driving.

Sleep-Rest Pattern. Nocturia is a common and a particularly bothersome lower urinary tract symptom that often leads to sleep deprivation, daytime sleepiness, and fatigue. It occurs in multiple disorders affecting the lower urinary tract, including urinary incontinence, urinary retention, and interstitial cystitis. Nocturia also may be related to polyuria secondary to kidney disease, poorly controlled diabetes mellitus, alcoholism, excessive fluid intake, or obstructive sleep apnea.[3]

When assessing nocturia, determine whether the need to urinate causes the person to arise from sleep or whether pain or some other symptom interrupts sleep and the person urinates as a matter of habit before returning to bed. Up to one episode of nocturia is considered normal in younger adults, and up to two episodes are acceptable among adults ages 65 years or older. If the older adult has more than two voidings during the night, assess the amount and timing of fluid intake. This information will help determine whether further investigation is needed.

Cognitive-Perceptual Pattern. Level of mobility, visual acuity, and dexterity are important factors to determine for a patient with urologic problems when managing his or her own care at home, particularly when urine retention or incontinence is a problem. Determine if the patient is alert, is able to understand instructions, and can recall the instructions when necessary.

If urinary incontinence is present, elicit a thorough history of the problem to help determine the type of incontinence. Document what the patient has previously tried to manage the problem. Incontinence is a distressing problem and calls for great sensitivity on your part to obtain accurate information.

A frequent symptom of renal and urologic problems is pain, including dysuria, groin pain, costovertebral pain, and suprapubic pain. Assess pain and document the location, character, and duration. The absence of pain when other urinary symptoms exist is also significant. Many urinary tract tumors are painless in the early stages.

Self-Perception–Self-Concept Pattern. Problems associated with the urinary system, such as incontinence, urinary diversion procedures, and chronic fatigue (may indicate anemia), can result in loss of self-esteem and a negative body image.

Role-Relationship Pattern. Urinary problems can affect many aspects of a person's life, including the ability to work and relationships with others. These factors have important implications for future treatment and management of the patient's condition.

Urinary system problems may be serious enough to cause problems in job-related and social situations. Chronic dialysis therapy often makes regular employment or full-time homemaking difficult. Concurrent poor health and negative body image can seriously alter existing roles.

Sexuality-Reproductive Pattern. Question the patient about the effect of a renal or urologic problem on her or his sexual patterns and satisfaction. Problems related to personal hygiene and fatigue can seriously affect a sexual relationship. Although urinary incontinence is not directly associated with sexual dysfunction, it often has a devastating effect on self-esteem and social and intimate relationships. Counseling of both the patient and partner may be indicated.

Objective Data
Physical Examination
Inspection. Assess for changes in the following:

Skin: Pallor, yellow-gray cast, excoriations, changes in turgor, bruises, texture (e.g., rough, dry skin) (see Table 23-6 for assessment of dark-skinned individuals)

Mouth: Stomatitis, ammonia breath odor

Face and extremities: Generalized edema, peripheral edema, bladder distention, masses, enlarged kidneys

Abdomen: Skin changes described earlier, striae, abdominal contour for midline mass in lower abdomen (may indicate urinary retention) or unilateral mass (occasionally seen in adult, indicating enlargement of one or both kidneys from large tumor or polycystic kidney)

Weight: Weight gain secondary to edema; weight loss and muscle wasting in kidney failure

General state of health: Fatigue, lethargy, and diminished alertness

Palpation. The kidneys are posterior organs protected by the abdominal organs, the ribs, and the heavy back muscles. A landmark useful in locating the kidneys is the costovertebral angle (CVA) formed by the rib cage and the vertebral column. The normal-sized left kidney is rarely palpable because the spleen lies directly on top of it. Occasionally the lower pole of the right kidney is palpable.

To palpate the right kidney, place your left (anterior) hand behind and support the patient's right side between the rib cage and the iliac crest (Fig. 45-6). Elevate the right flank with the left hand. Use your right hand to palpate deeply for the right kidney. The lower pole of the right kidney may be felt as a smooth, rounded mass that descends on inspiration. If the kidney is palpable, note its size, contour, and tenderness. Kidney enlargement is suggestive of neoplasm or other serious renal pathologic conditions.

The urinary bladder is normally not palpable unless it is distended with urine. If the bladder is full, it may be felt as a smooth, round, firm organ and is sensitive to palpation.

Percussion. Tenderness in the flank area may be detected by fist percussion (*kidney punch*). This technique is performed by

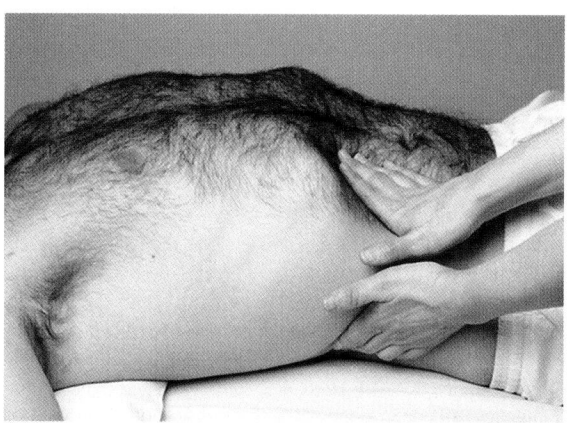

FIG. 45-6 Palpating the right kidney.

| TABLE 45-6 | NORMAL PHYSICAL ASSESSMENT OF URINARY SYSTEM |

- No costovertebral angle tenderness
- Nonpalpable kidney and bladder
- No palpable masses

striking the fist of one hand against the dorsal surface of the other hand, which is placed flat along the posterior CVA margin (Fig. 45-7). Normally a firm blow in the flank area should not elicit pain. If CVA tenderness and pain are present, it may indicate a kidney infection or polycystic kidney disease.

A bladder is not normally percussible until it contains 150 mL of urine. If the bladder is full, dullness is heard above the symphysis pubis. A distended bladder may be percussed as high as the umbilicus.

Auscultation. The bell of the stethoscope may be used to auscultate over both CVAs and in the upper abdominal quadrants. With this technique, auscultate the abdominal aorta and renal arteries for a *bruit* (an abnormal murmur), which indicates impaired blood flow to the kidneys. Use the diaphragm of the stethoscope to auscultate the bowels, since they may also affect the urinary system.

Table 45-6 shows how to record the normal physical assessment findings of the urinary system. Table 45-7 presents assessment abnormalities of the urinary system. Assessment

findings may vary in the older adult. Table 45-2 shows the age-related changes in the urinary system and differences in assessment findings. Use a *focused assessment* to evaluate the status of previously identified urinary system problems and to monitor for signs of new problems (see Table 3-6). A focused assessment of the urinary system is presented in the box on p. 1051.

DIAGNOSTIC STUDIES OF URINARY SYSTEM

Numerous diagnostic studies are available to locate and assess problems of the urinary system. Tables 45-8 and 45-9 describe the most common studies, and select studies are described in more detail in the following text.

The accuracy of these diagnostic studies is influenced by (1) adherence to the proper procedures; and (2) the patient's cooperation in terms of fluid restriction, urine specimen collection, study preparations procedures, ability to remain positioned on examination table, or following of other instructions.

Many radiologic studies require the use of a bowel preparation the evening before the study to clear the lower GI tract of feces and flatus. Because the kidneys lie in a retroperitoneal location, the contents of the colon may obstruct visualization of the urinary tract. If the bowel preparation fails to adequately evacuate the lower tract, the study may be unsuccessful and have to be rescheduled. Commonly used bowel preparations include enemas, castor oil, magnesium citrate, and bisacodyl (Dulcolax) tablets or suppositories. Some bowel preparations, such as magnesium citrate and Fleet enema, are contraindicated because magnesium cannot be excreted by the kidneys in patients with kidney failure (see Chapter 47).

When a patient has had diagnostic studies on consecutive days, it is important to prevent dehydration. Often the patient takes nothing by mouth (NPO) after midnight, spends an

Text continued on p. 1061

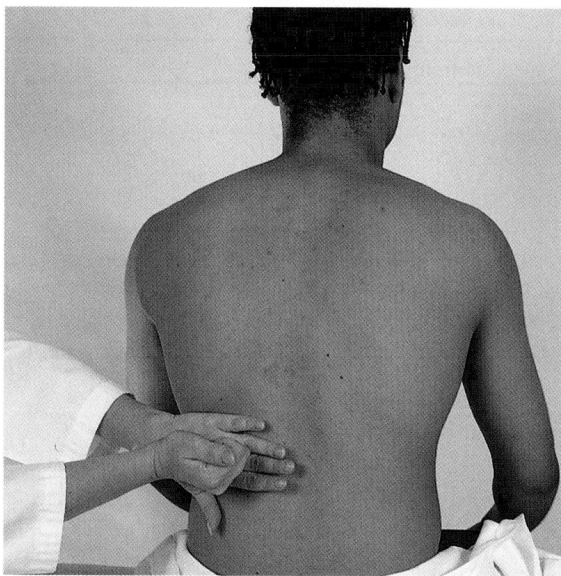

FIG. 45-7 Indirect fist percussion of the costovertebral angle (CVA). To assess the kidney, place one hand over the twelfth rib at the CVA on the back. Thump that hand with the ulnar edge of the other fist. (From Jarvis C: *Physical examination and health assessment,* ed 6, St Louis, 2012, Saunders.)

CASE STUDY—cont'd

Objective Data: Physical Examination

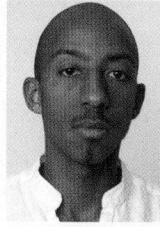

iStockphoto/Thinkstock

A focused assessment of A.K. reveals the following:

A.K. is lying on the ED stretcher with his knees bent and drawn to his abdominal area. He appears restless and keeps moving from back to side in an effort to reduce his discomfort. Vital signs as follows: BP 156/70, apical pulse 108, respiratory rate 24, temperature 37.4° C, O_2 saturation 96% on room air. Awake, alert, and oriented × 3. Lungs clear to auscultation. Apical pulse regular. Abdomen nondistended with + bowel sounds in all 4 quadrants. No rebound tenderness. Positive costovertebral tenderness. Voiding small amounts of dark, smoky urine.

As you continue to read this chapter, consider diagnostic studies you would anticipate being performed for A.K.

TABLE 45-7 ASSESSMENT ABNORMALITIES

Urinary System

Finding	Description	Possible Etiology and Significance
Anuria	Technically no urination (24-hr urine output <100 mL)	Acute kidney injury, end-stage kidney disease, bilateral ureteral obstruction
Burning on urination	Stinging pain in urethral area	Urethral irritation, urinary tract infection
Dysuria	Painful or difficult urination	Sign of urinary tract infection, interstitial cystitis, and wide variety of pathologic conditions
Enuresis	Involuntary nocturnal urination	Symptomatic of lower urinary tract disorder
Frequency	Increased incidence of urination	Acutely inflamed bladder, retention with overflow, excess fluid intake, intake of bladder irritants
	Blood in the urine	Cancer of genitourinary tract, blood dyscrasias, kidney disease, urinary tract infection, stones in kidney or ureter, medications (anticoagulants)
Hesitancy	Delay or difficulty in initiating urination	Partial urethral obstruction, benign prostatic hyperplasia
Incontinence	Inability to voluntarily control discharge of urine	Neurogenic bladder, bladder infection, injury to external sphincter
Nocturia	Frequency of urination at night	Kidney disease with impaired concentrating ability, bladder obstruction, heart failure, diabetes mellitus, finding after renal transplant, excessive evening and nighttime fluid intake
Oliguria	Diminished amount of urine in a given time (24-hr urine output of 100-400 mL)	Severe dehydration, shock, transfusion reaction, kidney disease, end-stage kidney disease
Pain	Suprapubic pain (related to bladder), urethral pain (irritation of bladder neck), flank (CVA) pain	Infection, urinary retention, foreign body in urinary tract, urethritis, pyelonephritis, renal colic or stones
Pneumaturia	Passage of urine containing gas	Fistula connections between bowel and bladder, gas-forming urinary tract infections
Polyuria	Large volume of urine in a given time	Diabetes mellitus, diabetes insipidus, chronic kidney disease, diuretics, excess fluid intake, obstructive sleep apnea
Retention	Inability to urinate even though bladder contains excessive amount of urine	Finding after pelvic surgery, childbirth, catheter removal, anesthesia; urethral stricture or obstruction; neurogenic bladder
Stress incontinence	Involuntary urination with increased pressure (sneezing or coughing)	Weakness of sphincter control, lack of estrogen, urinary retention

CVA, Costovertebral angle.

TABLE 45-8 DIAGNOSTIC STUDIES

Urinary System

Study	Description and Purpose	Nursing Responsibility
Urine Studies		
Urinalysis	General examination of urine to establish baseline information or provide data to establish a tentative diagnosis and determine whether further studies are needed (see Table 45-9).	Try to obtain first urinated morning specimen. Ensure specimen is examined within 1 hr of urinating. Before collecting, wash perineal area (if soiled with menses or fecal material).
Creatinine clearance	Creatinine is a waste product of protein breakdown (primarily body muscle mass). Clearance of creatinine by kidney approximates the GFR. Creatinine clearance is calculated as follows: $$\text{Creatinine clearance} = \frac{\text{Urine creatinine (mg/dL)} \times \text{Urine volume (mL/min)}}{\text{Serum creatinine (mg/dL)}}$$ *Reference interval:* 70-135 mL/min/1.73 m² (corrected for body surface area).	Collect 24-hr urine specimen. Discard first urination when test is started. Save urine from all subsequent urinations for 24 hr. Instruct patient to urinate at end of 24 hr and add specimen to collection. Ensure that serum creatinine is determined during 24-hr period.
Composite urine collection	Measures specific components, such as electrolytes, glucose, protein, 17-ketosteroids, catecholamines, creatinine, and minerals. Composite urine specimens are collected over a period ranging from 2 to 24 hr.	Instruct the patient to urinate and discard this first urine specimen. Note this time as the start of the test. Save all urine from subsequent urinations in a container for designated period. At end of period, ask patient to urinate, and this urine is added to container. Remind patient to save all urine during study period. Specimens may have to be refrigerated, or preservatives may have to be added to container used for collecting urine.

GFR, Glomerular filtration rate.

TABLE 45-8   DIAGNOSTIC STUDIES—cont'd

Urinary System

Study	Description and Purpose	Nursing Responsibility
Urine culture ("clean catch," "midstream")	Confirms suspected urinary tract infection and identifies causative organisms. *Normally*, bladder is sterile, but urethra contains bacteria and a few WBCs. *Reference interval:* If properly collected, stored, and handled: <10^3 organisms/mL usually indicates no infection. 10^3-10^5/mL is usually not diagnostic and test may have to be repeated. >10^5/mL indicates infection.	Use sterile container for collection of urine. Touch only outside of container. For women, separate labia with one hand and clean meatus with other hand, using at least three sponges (saturated with cleansing solution) in a front-to-back motion. For men, retract foreskin (if present) and cleanse glans with at least three cleansing sponges. After cleaning, instruct patient to start urinating and then continue voiding in sterile container. (The initial voided urine flushes out most contaminants in the urethra and perineal area.) Catheterization may be needed if patient is unable to cooperate with procedure.
Concentration test	Evaluates renal concentration ability. Measured by specific gravity readings. *Reference interval:* 1.003-1.030.	Instruct patient to fast after given time in evening (in usual procedure). Collect three urine specimens at hourly intervals in morning.
Residual urine	Determines amount of urine left in bladder after urinating. Finding may be abnormal in problems with bladder innervation, sphincter impairment, BPH, or urethral strictures. *Reference interval:* ≤50 mL urine (increases with age).	Immediately after patient urinates, catheterize patient or use bladder ultrasound equipment. If a large amount of residual urine is obtained, health care provider may want catheter left in bladder.
Protein determination		
• Dipstick (Albustix, Combistix)	Test detects protein (primarily albumin) in urine. *Reference interval:* 0-trace.	Dip end of stick in urine and read result by comparison with color chart on label as directed. Grading is from 0 to 4+. Interpret with caution. Positive result may not indicate significant proteinuria. Some medications may give false-positive readings.
• Quantitative protein test	A 24-hr collection gives a more accurate indication of amount of protein in urine. Persistent proteinuria usually indicates glomerular kidney disease. *Reference interval:* <150 mg/24 hr (mainly albumin).	Perform 24-hr urine collection as above.
Urine cytologic study	Identifies abnormal cellular structures that occur with bladder cancer. Also used to follow the progress of bladder cancer after treatment.	Obtain specimens by voiding, catheterization, or bladder irrigation. Do not use morning's first voided specimen because epithelial cells may change in appearance in urine held in bladder overnight. As with urinalysis, the specimen should be fresh or brought to laboratory within the hour. An alcohol-based fixative is then added to preserve the cellular structure.
Blood Studies		
Blood urea nitrogen (BUN)	Used to detect renal problems. Concentration of urea in blood is regulated by rate at which kidney excretes urea. *Reference interval:* 6-20 mg/dL (2.1-7.1 mmol/L).	When interpreting BUN, be aware that nonrenal factors may cause increase (e.g., rapid cell destruction from infections, fever, GI bleeding, trauma, athletic activity and excessive muscle breakdown, corticosteroid therapy).
Creatinine	More reliable than BUN as a determinant of renal function. Creatinine is end product of muscle and protein metabolism and is released at a constant rate. *Reference interval:* 0.6-1.3 mg/dL (53-115 μmol/L).	Explain test and watch for postpuncture bleeding.
BUN/creatinine ratio	An increased ratio may be due to conditions that decrease blood flow to kidneys (e.g., heart failure, dehydration), GI bleeding, or increased dietary protein. A decreased ratio may occur with liver disease (due to decreased urea formation) and malnutrition. *Reference interval:* 12:1 to 20:1.	
Uric acid	Used as screening test primarily for disorders of purine metabolism but can also indicate kidney disease. Values depend on renal function, rate of purine metabolism, and dietary intake of food rich in purines. *Female:* 2.3-6.6 mg/dL (137-393 μmol/L). *Male:* 4.4-7.6 mg/dL (262-452 μmol/L).	Explain test and watch for postpuncture bleeding.
Sodium	Main extracellular electrolyte determining blood volume. Usually values stay within normal range until late stages of renal failure. *Reference interval:* 135-145 mEq/L (135-145 mmol/L).	Explain test and watch for postpuncture bleeding.

BPH, Benign prostatic hyperplasia.

Continued

TABLE 45-8   DIAGNOSTIC STUDIES—cont'd

Urinary System

Study	Description and Purpose	Nursing Responsibility
Blood Studies—cont'd		
Potassium	Kidneys are responsible for excreting majority of body's potassium. In kidney disease, K+ determinations are critical because K+ is one of the first electrolytes to become abnormal. Elevated K+ levels >6 mEq/L can lead to muscle weakness and cardiac dysrhythmias. *Reference interval:* 3.5-5.0 mEq/L (3.5-5.0 mmol/L).	Explain test and watch for postpuncture bleeding.
Calcium (total)	Main mineral in bone and aids in muscle contraction, neurotransmission, and clotting. In kidney disease, decreased reabsorption of Ca^{2+} leads to renal osteodystrophy. *Reference interval:* 8.6-10.2 mg/dL (2.15-2.55 mmol/L).	Explain test and watch for postpuncture bleeding.
Phosphorus	Phosphorus balance is inversely related to Ca^{2+} balance. In kidney disease, phosphorus levels are elevated because the kidney is the primary excretory organ. *Reference interval:* 2.4-4.4 mg/dL (0.78-1.42 mmol/L).	Explain test and watch for postpuncture bleeding.
Bicarbonate	Most patients in renal failure have metabolic acidosis and low serum HCO$_3^-$ levels. *Reference interval:* 22-26 mEq/L (22-26 mmol/L).	Explain test and watch for postpuncture bleeding.
Radiologic Procedures		
Kidneys, ureters, bladder (KUB)	X-ray examination of abdomen and pelvis delineates size, shape, and position of kidneys. Radiopaque stones and foreign bodies can be seen.	Perform bowel preparation (if ordered).
Intravenous pyelogram (IVP)	Visualizes urinary tract after IV injection of contrast media. Presence, position, size, and shape of kidneys, ureters, and bladder can be evaluated. Cysts, tumors, lesions, and obstructions cause a distortion in normal appearance of these structures. Patient with significantly decreased renal function should not have IVP because contrast media can be nephrotoxic and worsen renal function.*	Evening before procedure, give cathartic or enema to empty colon of feces and gas. Before procedure, assess patient for iodine sensitivity to avoid anaphylactic reaction. Inform patient that procedure involves lying on table and having serial x-rays taken. Advise patient that during injection of contrast material, warmth, a flushed face, and a salty taste may be experienced. After procedure, force fluids (if permitted) to flush out contrast media.
Renal arteriogram (angiogram)	Visualizes renal blood vessels. Can assist in diagnosing renal artery stenosis (Fig. 45-8), additional or missing renal blood vessels, and renovascular hypertension. Can assist in differentiating between a renal cyst and a renal tumor. Also included in workup of a potential renal transplant donor. A catheter is inserted into the femoral artery and passed up the aorta to the level of the renal arteries (Fig. 45-9). Contrast media is injected to outline the renal blood supply.*	*Before procedure:* Prepare patient the prior evening by giving cathartic or enema. Before injection of contrast material, assess for iodine sensitivity. The patient may experience a transient warm feeling along the course of the blood vessel when contrast media is injected. *After procedure:* Place a pressure dressing over femoral artery injection site. Observe site for bleeding. Have patient maintain bed rest with affected leg straight. Take peripheral pulses in the involved leg every 30-60 min to detect occlusion of blood flow caused by a thrombus. Observe for complications, including thrombus, embolus, local inflammation, hematoma.

*N-acetylcysteine (Mucomyst), a renal vasodilator and antioxidant, is sometimes administered to reduce the incidence of contrast-induced nephropathy; can be given by oral or IV route.

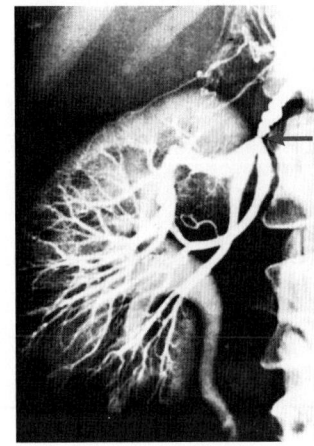

FIG. 45-8 Renal arteriogram showing stenosis of the right renal artery *(arrow)*.

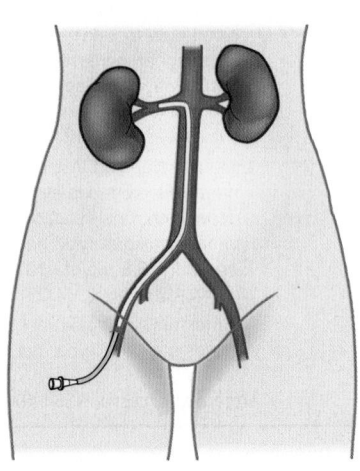

FIG. 45-9 Catheter insertion for a renal arteriogram.

TABLE 45-8 DIAGNOSTIC STUDIES—cont'd

Urinary System

Study	Description and Purpose	Nursing Responsibility
Antegrade pyelogram (nephrostogram)	Evaluates upper urinary tract when patient has allergy to contrast media, decreased renal function, or abnormalities that prevent passage of a ureteral catheter. Contrast media may be injected percutaneously into renal pelvis or via a nephrostomy tube that is already in place when determining tube function or ureteral integrity after trauma or surgery.*	Explain procedure and prepare patient as for IVP. Watch for signs of complications (e.g., hematuria, infection, hematoma).
Retrograde pyelogram	X-ray of urinary tract taken after injection of contrast material into kidneys. It may be done if an IVP does not visualize the urinary tract or if patient is allergic to contrast media or has decreased renal function. A cystoscope is inserted and ureteral catheters are inserted through it into renal pelvis. Contrast media is injected through catheters.*	Prepare patient as for IVP. Inform patient that pain may be experienced from distention of pelvis and discomfort from cystoscope. Inform patient that anesthesia may be given for procedure. Complications are similar to those for cystoscopy (see cystoscopy later in table).
Renal ultrasound	Used to detect renal or perirenal masses, differential diagnosis of renal cysts, solid masses, and identification of obstructions. Small external ultrasound probe is placed on patient's skin. Conductive gel is applied to skin. Noninvasive procedure involves passing sound waves into body structures and recording images as they are reflected back. Computer interprets tissue density based on sound waves and displays it in picture form. It can be used safely in patients with renal failure.	Explain procedure to patient. Because radiation exposure is avoided, a number of images can be obtained and repeat studies can be done over a brief period. Images can be obtained from both prone and supine positions. A bowel preparation is not required.
Computed tomography (CT) scan (CT urogram)	Provides excellent visualization of kidneys. Kidney size can be evaluated. Tumors, abscesses, suprarenal masses (e.g., adrenal tumors, pheochromocytomas), and obstructions can be detected. Advantage of CT over ultrasound is its ability to distinguish subtle differences in density. Use of IV-administered contrast media during CT accentuates density of renal tissue and helps differentiate masses.*	Explain procedure to patient. Ask patient about iodine sensitivity. Instruct the patient to lie still during the procedure while the machine takes precise transaxial images. Sedation may be required if patient is unable to cooperate.
Magnetic resonance imaging (MRI)	Useful for visualization of kidneys. Not proven useful for detecting urinary calculi or calcified tumors. Computer-generated films rely on radiofrequency waves and alteration in magnetic field.	Explain procedure to patient. Have patient remove all metal objects. Patients with a history of claustrophobia may need to be sedated. Contraindications: presence of implanted magnetic clips or prosthesis and pacemakers.
Magnetic resonance angiography	Allows visualization of renal vasculature. Gadolinium-enhanced studies allow visualization of the renal artery.	Same as above. Does not require femoral artery puncture.
Cystogram	Visualizes bladder and evaluates vesicoureteral reflux. Also evaluates patients with neurogenic bladder and recurrent urinary tract infections. Can also delineate abnormalities of the bladder (e.g., diverticula, calculi, tumors). Contrast media is instilled into bladder via cystoscope or catheter.	Explain procedure to patient. If done via cystoscope, follow nursing care related to cystoscopy.
Urethrogram	Similar to a cystogram. Contrast media is injected retrograde into the urethra to identify strictures, diverticula, or other urethral pathologic conditions. When urethral trauma is suspected, a urethrogram is done before catheterization.	Explain procedure to patient.
Voiding cystourethrogram (VCUG)	Voiding study of the bladder opening (bladder neck) and urethra. The bladder is filled with contrast media. Fluoroscopic films are taken to visualize the bladder and urethra. After urination, another film is taken to assess for residual urine. Can detect abnormalities of the lower urinary tract, urethral stenosis, bladder neck obstruction, and prostatic enlargement.	Explain procedure to patient.
Loopogram	Detects obstructions, anastomotic leaks, stones, reflux, and other uropathologic features when patient has a urinary pouch or ileal conduit. Because urinary diversions are created with bowel, there is risk of absorption of contrast media.	Explain procedure to patient. Closely monitor patient for reactions to the contrast media.

*N-acetylcysteine (Mucomyst), a renal vasodilator and antioxidant, is sometimes administered to reduce the incidence of contrast-induced nephropathy; can be given by oral or IV route.

Continued

TABLE 45-8 DIAGNOSTIC STUDIES—cont'd

Urinary System

Study	Description and Purpose	Nursing Responsibility
Endoscopy		
Cystoscopy	Inspects interior of bladder with a tubular lighted scope (cystoscope) (Fig. 45-10). Can be used to insert ureteral catheters, remove calculi, obtain biopsy specimens of bladder lesions, and treat bleeding lesions. Lithotomy position is used. Procedure may be done using local or general anesthesia, depending on patient's needs and condition. Complications include urinary retention, urinary tract hemorrhage, bladder infection, and perforation of the bladder.	*Before procedure:* Force fluids or give IV fluids if general anesthesia is to be used. Ensure consent form is signed. Explain procedure to patient. Give preoperative medication. *After procedure:* Explain that burning on urination, pink-tinged urine, and urinary frequency are expected effects. Observe for bright red bleeding, which is not normal. Do not let patient walk alone immediately after procedure because orthostatic hypotension may occur. Offer warm sitz baths, heat, mild analgesics to relieve discomfort.
Urodynamic Studies		
Urine flow study (uroflow)	Measures urine volume in a single voiding expelled in a period of time. Used to (1) assess the degree of outflow obstruction caused by such conditions as BPH or stricture, (2) assess bladder or sphincter dysfunction effects on voiding, and (3) evaluate effects of treatment for lower urinary tract problems. Graphic displays can illustrate straining and intermittent flow patterns or other abnormal voiding disorders. *Normal maximum flow rate:* men: 20-25 mL/sec; women: 25-30 mL/sec. Volume voided and the patient's age can affect the flow rate.	Explain procedure to patient. Ask the patient to start the test with a comfortably full bladder, urinate into a special container, and try to empty completely. Measure residual urine volume immediately after a urinary flow study because this will help identify the degree of chronic urinary retention that is often associated with abnormal flow patterns.
Cystometrogram	Evaluates bladder's capacity to contract and expel urine. Involves insertion of catheter and instillation of water or saline solution into bladder. Measurements of pressure exerted against bladder wall are recorded. If abdominal pressure is measured, a second tube is inserted into the rectum or vagina. This tube is attached to a small fluid-filled balloon to allow pressure recording.	Explain procedure to patient. During the infusion, ask patient about sensations of bladder filling, usually including the first desire (urge) to urinate, a strong desire to urinate, and perception of bladder fullness. Observe patient for manifestations of urinary tract infection after procedure.
Sphincter electromyography (EMG)	Recording of electrical activity created when nervous system stimulates muscle tissue. By placing needles, percutaneous wires, or patches near the urethra, the clinician can assess the pelvic floor muscle activity. During the cystometrogram, sphincter EMG is used to identify voluntary pelvic floor muscle contractions and the response of these muscles to bladder filling, coughing, and other provocative maneuvers.	Explain procedure to patient.
Voiding pressure flow study	Combines a urinary flow rate, cystometric pressures (intravesical, abdominal, and detrusor pressures), and a sphincter EMG for detailed evaluation of micturition. It is completed by assisting the patient to a specialized toilet to urinate while the various pressure tubes and EMG apparatus remain in place.	Explain procedure to patient.
Videourodynamics	Combination of cystometrogram, sphincter EMG, and/or urinary flow study with anatomic imaging of the lower urinary tract, typically via fluoroscopy. Used in selected cases to identify an obstructive lesion and characterize anatomic changes in the bladder and lower urinary tract.	Explain procedure to patient.

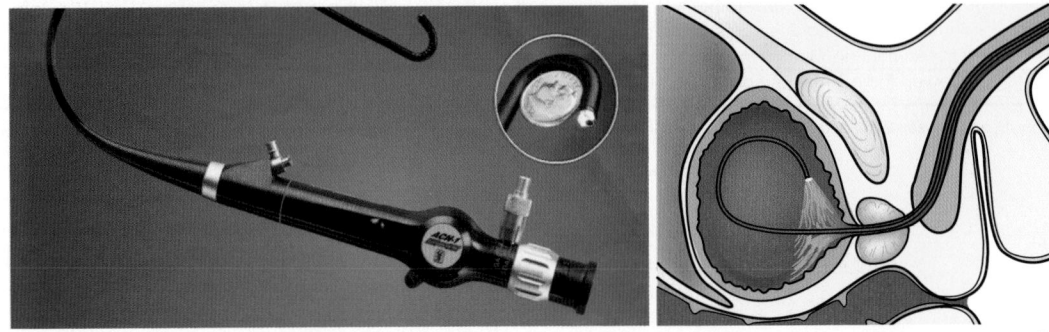

A   B

FIG. 45-10 Cystoscopic examination of the bladder in a man. **A,** Flexible cystonephroscope. **B,** Scope inserted into bladder.

TABLE 45-8 DIAGNOSTIC STUDIES—cont'd

Urinary System

Study	Description and Purpose	Nursing Responsibility
Radionuclide cystography (RNC)	Detects and grades vesicoureteral reflux. Similar to VCUG with a small dose of radioisotope tracer instilled into the bladder via urethral catheter. More sensitive than VCUG, and radiation dose is 1/1000 that of the VCUG.	Explain procedure to patient as in VCUG.
Whitaker study	Measures the pressure differential between the renal pelvis and the bladder. Ureteral obstruction can be assessed. Percutaneous access is gained to the renal pelvis by placing a catheter in the renal pelvis. A catheter is also placed in the bladder. Fluid is perfused through the percutaneous tube or needle at a rate of 10 mL/min. Pressure data are then collected. Pressure measurements are combined with fluoroscopic imaging to identify the level of obstruction.	Explain procedure to patient.
Renal Scan	Evaluates anatomic structures, perfusion, and function of kidneys. Radioactive isotopes are injected IV. Radiation detector probes are placed over kidney, and scintillation counter monitors radioactive material in kidney. Radioisotope distribution in kidney is scanned and mapped. Shows location, size, and shape of kidney and, in general, assesses blood flow, glomerular filtration, tubular function, and urinary excretion. Abscesses, cysts, and tumors may appear as cold spots because of nonfunctioning tissue. Also monitors function of a transplanted kidney.	Requires no dietary or activity restriction. Inform patient that no pain or discomfort should be felt during test.
Renal Biopsy	Obtains renal tissue for examination to determine type of kidney disease or to follow progress of kidney disease. Technique is usually done as a skin (percutaneous) biopsy through needle insertion into lower lobe of kidney. Can be performed with CT or ultrasound guidance. Absolute contraindications are bleeding disorders, single kidney, and uncontrolled hypertension. Relative contraindications include suspected renal infection, hydronephrosis, and possible vascular lesions.	Type and crossmatch patient for blood. Ensure consent form is signed. *Before procedure:* Ascertain coagulation status through patient history, medication history, CBC, hematocrit, prothrombin time, and bleeding and clotting time. Patient should not be taking aspirin or warfarin (Coumadin). *After procedure:* Apply pressure dressing and keep patient on affected side for 30-60 min. Bed rest for 24 hr. Vital signs every 5-10 min, first hour. Assess for flank pain, hypotension, decreasing hematocrit, ↑ temperature, chills, urinary frequency, dysuria, and serial urine specimens (gross or microscopic hematuria). Urine dipstick can be used to test for bleeding in urine. Inspect biopsy site for bleeding. Instruct patient to avoid lifting heavy objects for 5-7 days and to not take anticoagulant drugs until allowed by health care provider.

extended time in the x-ray department, is too tired to eat, sleeps the rest of the day, and is NPO after midnight again because of studies scheduled for the next day. Severe dehydration, especially in a diabetic, debilitated, or older patient, may lead to acute kidney injury. When a patient is scheduled for diagnostic studies, ensure that the patient is properly hydrated and given adequate nourishment between studies. Also check with the health care provider regarding insulin dosage for diabetic patients who are placed on NPO status.

Urine Studies

Urinalysis. *Urinalysis* (see Tables 45-8 and 45-9) is one of the first studies done to evaluate disorders of the urinary tract. Results from the urinalysis may indicate possible abnormalities, suggest the need for further studies, or provide evidence of progression in a previously diagnosed disorder.

Although a specimen may be collected at any time of the day for a routine urinalysis, it is best to obtain the first specimen urinated in the morning. This concentrated specimen is more likely to contain abnormal constituents if they are present in the urine. The specimen should be examined within 1 hour of urinating. Otherwise, bacteria multiply rapidly, RBCs hemolyze, *casts* (molds of renal tubules) disintegrate, and the urine becomes alkaline as a result of urea-splitting bacteria. If it is not possible to send the specimen to the laboratory immediately, refrigerate it. However, to obtain the best results, coordinate specimen collection with routine laboratory hours.

Creatinine Clearance. A common test used to analyze urinary system disorders is creatinine clearance. Creatinine is a waste product produced by muscle breakdown. Urinary excretion of creatinine is a measure of the amount of active muscle tissue in the body, not of body weight. Therefore individuals with larger muscle mass have higher values.[4] Because almost all creatinine in the blood is normally excreted by the kidneys, creatinine clearance is the most accurate indicator of renal function. The result of a creatinine clearance test closely approxi-

TABLE 45-9   DIAGNOSTIC STUDIES

Urinalysis

Test	Normal	Abnormal Finding	Possible Etiology and Significance
Color	Amber yellow	Dark, smoky color Yellow-brown to olive green Orange-red or orange-brown Cloudiness of freshly voided urine Colorless urine	Hematuria. Excessive bilirubin. phenazopyridine (Pyridium). Infection. Excessive fluid intake, kidney disease, or diabetes insipidus.
Odor	Aromatic	Ammonia-like odor Unpleasant odor	Urine allowed to stand. Urinary tract infection.
Protein	Random protein (dipstick): 0-trace 24-hr protein (quantitative): <150 mg/day	Persistent proteinuria	Characteristic of acute and chronic kidney disease, especially involving glomeruli. Heart failure. In absence of disease: high-protein diet, strenuous exercise, dehydration, fever, emotional stress, contamination by vaginal secretions.
Glucose	None	Glycosuria	Diabetes mellitus, low renal threshold for glucose reabsorption (if blood glucose level is normal). Pituitary disorders.
Ketones	None	Present	Altered carbohydrate and fat metabolism in diabetes mellitus and starvation; dehydration, vomiting, severe diarrhea.
Bilirubin	None	Present	Liver disorders. May appear before jaundice is visible (see Chapter 44).
Specific gravity	1.003-1.030 Maximum concentrating ability of kidney in morning urine (1.025-1.030)	Low High Fixed at about 1.010	Dilute urine, excessive diuresis, diabetes insipidus. Dehydration, albuminuria, glycosuria. Renal inability to concentrate urine; end-stage kidney disease.
Osmolality	300-1300 mOsm/kg (300-1300 mmol/kg)	<300 mOsm/kg >1300 mOsm/kg	Tubular dysfunction. Kidney lost ability to concentrate or dilute urine (not part of routine urinalysis).
pH	4.0-8.0 (average, 6.0)	>8.0 <4.0	Urinary tract infection. Urine allowed to stand at room temperature (bacteria decompose urea to ammonia). Respiratory or metabolic acidosis.
RBCs	0-4/hpf	>4/hpf	Calculi, cystitis, neoplasm, glomerulonephritis, tuberculosis, kidney biopsy, trauma.
WBCs	0-5/hpf	>5/hpf	Urinary tract infection or inflammation.
Casts	None Occasional hyaline	Present	Molds of the renal tubules that may contain protein, WBCs, RBCs, or bacteria. Noncellular casts (hyaline in appearance) occasionally found in normal urine.
Culture for organisms	No organisms in bladder <10⁴ organisms/mL result of normal urethral flora	Bacteria counts >10⁵/mL	Urinary tract infection; most common organisms are *Escherichia coli*, enterococci, *Klebsiella*, *Proteus*, and streptococci.

hpf, High-powered field.

mates that of the GFR. A blood specimen for serum creatinine determination should be obtained during the period of urine collection.

Creatinine levels remain remarkably constant for each person because they are not significantly affected by protein ingestion, muscular exercise, water intake, or rate of urine production. Normal creatinine clearance values range from 70 to 135 mL/min (see Table 45-8). After age 40, the creatinine clearance rate decreases at a rate of about 1 mL/min/yr.

Urodynamic Studies

Urodynamic studies measure urinary tract function. Urodynamic tests study the storage of urine within the bladder and the flow of urine through the urinary tract to the outside of the body.[5-7] A combination of techniques may be used for a detailed assessment of urinary function (see Table 45-8).

CASE STUDY—cont'd

Objective Data: Diagnostic Studies

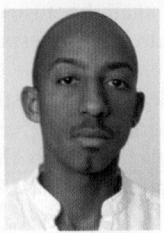

iStockphoto/Thinkstock

The health care provider orders the following initial diagnostic studies for A.K.:
- CBC, basic metabolic panel (electrolytes, BUN, creatinine)
- Urinalysis, culture if indicated
- Renal ultrasound

Although A.K.'s laboratory results are all within normal limits, his renal ultrasound identifies calculi in the left ureter. There is no hydronephrosis at present. The health care provider prescribes parenteral opioids for pain management and admits A.K. to a medical unit for further observation.

BRIDGE TO NCLEX EXAMINATION

The number of the question corresponds to the same-numbered outcome at the beginning of the chapter.

1. A renal stone in the pelvis of the kidney will alter the function of the kidney by interfering with
   a. the structural support of the kidney.
   b. regulation of the concentration of urine.
   c. the entry and exit of blood vessels at the kidney.
   d. collection and drainage of urine from the kidney.

2. A patient with kidney disease has oliguria and a creatinine clearance of 40 mL/min. These findings most directly reflect abnormal function of
   a. tubular secretion.
   b. glomerular filtration.
   c. capillary permeability.
   d. concentration of filtrate.

3. The nurse identifies a risk for urinary calculi in a patient who relates a past health history that includes
   a. hyperaldosteronism.
   b. serotonin deficiency.
   c. adrenal insufficiency.
   d. hyperparathyroidism.

4. Diminished ability to concentrate urine, associated with aging of the urinary system, is attributed to
   a. a decrease in bladder sensory receptors.
   b. a decrease in the number of functioning nephrons.
   c. decreased function of the loop of Henle and tubules.
   d. thickening of the basement membrane of Bowman's capsule.

5. During physical assessment of the urinary system, the nurse
   a. palpates an empty bladder as a small nodule.
   b. auscultates over each CVA to detect impaired renal blood flow.
   c. finds a dull percussion sound when 100 mL of urine is present in the bladder.
   d. palpates above the symphysis pubis to determine the level of urine in the bladder.

6. Normal findings expected by the nurse on physical assessment of the urinary system include *(select all that apply)*
   a. nonpalpable left kidney.
   b. auscultation of renal artery bruit.
   c. CVA tenderness elicited by a kidney punch.
   d. no CVA tenderness elicited by a kidney punch.
   e. palpable bladder to the level of the pubic symphysis.

7. A diagnostic study that indicates renal blood flow, glomerular filtration, tubular function, and excretion is a(n)
   a. IVP.
   b. VCUG.
   c. renal scan.
   d. loopogram.

8. On reading the urinalysis results of a dehydrated patient, the nurse would expect to find
   a. a pH of 8.4.
   b. RBCs of 4/hpf.
   c. color: yellow, cloudy.
   d. specific gravity of 1.035.

1. d, 2. b, 3. d, 4. c, 5. b, 6. a, d, 7. c, 8. d

ℯvolve

For rationales to these answers and even more NCLEX review questions, visit *http://evolve.elsevier.com/Lewis/medsurg*.

REFERENCES

1. Nguyen TV, Goldfarb DS: The older adult patient and kidney function, *Consult Pharm* 27(6):431, 2012.
2. van Doorn B, Bosch JL: Nocturia in older men, *Maturitas* 71(1):8, 2012.
3. Cornu JN, Abrams P, Chapple CR, et al: Contemporary assessment of nocturia: definition, epidemiology, pathophysiology, and management—a systematic review and meta-analysis, *Eur Urol* 62(5):877, 2012.
4. Lascano ME, Poggio ED: Kidney function assessment by creatinine-based estimation equations. Retrieved from *www.clevelandclinicmeded.com/medicalpubs/diseasemanagement/nephrology/kidney-function*.
5. Gray M: Traces: making sense of urodynamics testing, part 9: evaluation of sensations detrusor response to bladder filling, *Urol Nurs* 32(1):21, 2012.
6. Farag FF, Heesakkers JP: Non-invasive techniques in the diagnosis of bladder storage disorders, *Neurourol Urodyn* 30(8):1422, 2011.
7. Al Afraa T, Mahfouz W, Campeau L, et al: Normal lower urinary tract assessment in women, part I: uroflowmetry and post-void residual, pad tests, and bladder diaries, *Int Urogynecol J* 23(6):681, 2012.

RESOURCES

Resources for this chapter are listed in Chapter 46 on p. 1100 and Chapter 47 on p. 1131.

46

*Tears shed for self are tears of weakness, but
tears shed for others are a sign of strength.*
Billy Graham

Nursing Management
Renal and Urologic Problems

Betty Jean Reid Czarapata

℮volve WEBSITE

http://evolve.elsevier.com/Lewis/medsurg

- NCLEX Review Questions
- Key Points
- Pre-Test
- Answer Guidelines for Case Study on p. 1098
- Rationales for Bridge to NCLEX Examination Questions

- Case Studies
  - Patient With Bladder Cancer and Urinary Diversion
  - Patient With Glomerulonephritis and Kidney Disease
- Nursing Care Plans (Customizable)
  - eNCP 46-1: Patient With a Urinary Tract Infection
  - eNCP 46-2: Patient With Urinary Tract Calculi

- eNCP 46-3: Patient With an Ileal Conduit
- Concept Map Creator
- Glossary
- Content Updates

eTables
- eTable 46-1: Staging of Kidney Cancer
- eTable 46-2: Staging of Bladder Cancer

LEARNING OUTCOMES

1. Differentiate the pathophysiology, clinical manifestations, collaborative care, and drug therapy of cystitis, urethritis, and pyelonephritis.
2. Explain the nursing management of urinary tract infections.
3. Describe the immunologic mechanisms involved in glomerulonephritis.
4. Differentiate the clinical manifestations and nursing and collaborative management of acute poststreptococcal glomerulonephritis, Goodpasture syndrome, and chronic glomerulonephritis.
5. Describe the common causes, clinical manifestations, collaborative care, and nursing management of nephrotic syndrome.

6. Compare and contrast the etiology, clinical manifestations, collaborative care, and nursing management of various types of urinary calculi.
7. Differentiate the common causes and management of renal trauma, renal vascular problems, and hereditary kidney diseases.
8. Describe the clinical manifestations and nursing and collaborative management of kidney cancer and bladder cancer.
9. Describe the common causes and management of urinary incontinence and urinary retention.
10. Differentiate among urethral, ureteral, suprapubic, and nephrostomy catheters with regard to indications for use and nursing responsibilities.
11. Explain the nursing management of the patient undergoing nephrectomy or urinary diversion surgery.

KEY TERMS

calculus, p. 1077
cystitis, p. 1065
glomerulonephritis, p. 1073
Goodpasture syndrome, p. 1074
hydronephrosis, p. 1076

hydroureter, p. 1076
ileal conduit, p. 1095
interstitial cystitis (IC), p. 1071
lithotripsy, p. 1079
nephrolithiasis, p. 1076
nephrosclerosis, p. 1082

nephrotic syndrome, p. 1075
polycystic kidney disease (PKD), p. 1082
pyelonephritis, p. 1065
renal artery stenosis, p. 1082
stricture, p. 1081

urethritis, p. 1065
urinary incontinence (UI), p. 1086
urinary retention, p. 1090
urosepsis, p. 1065

Renal and urologic disorders encompass a wide spectrum of problems. The diverse causes of these disorders may involve infectious, immunologic, obstructive, metabolic, collagen-vascular, traumatic, congenital, neoplastic, and neurologic mechanisms. This chapter discusses specific disorders of the upper urinary tract (kidneys and ureter) and lower urinary tract (bladder and urethra). Acute kidney injury and chronic kidney disease are discussed in Chapter 47.

INFECTIOUS AND INFLAMMATORY DISORDERS OF URINARY SYSTEM

URINARY TRACT INFECTION

Urinary tract infections (UTIs) are the most common bacterial infection in women. During their lifetime, at least 20% of women develop at least one UTI.[1] More than 100,000 people

Reviewed by Barbara S. Broome, RN, PhD, FAAN, Associate Dean and Chair, Community/Mental Health, University of South Alabama, College of Nursing, Mobile, Alabama; Marci Langenkamp, RN, MS, Assistant Professor of Nursing, Edison Community College, Piqua, Ohio; and Phyllis A. Matthews, RN, MS, ANCP-BC, CUNP, Urology Nurse Practitioner, Denver VA Medical Center, Denver, Colorado.

TABLE 46-1	CAUSES OF URINARY TRACT INFECTIONS

- *Escherichia coli**
- *Enterococcus*
- *Klebsiella*
- *Enterobacter*
- *Proteus*
- *Pseudomonas*
- *Staphylococcus*
- *Serratia*
- *Candida albicans†*

*Causative microorganism for urinary tract infection (UTI) in 80% of cases without urinary tract structural abnormalities or calculi.
†Typically identified as the causative microorganism for UTI associated with the use of broad-spectrum antibiotic therapy or in patients with an indwelling catheter.

🌐 CULTURAL & ETHNIC HEALTH DISPARITIES
Urologic Disorders

- Urinary tract calculi are more common among whites than African Americans.
- Uric acid stones are more common in Jewish men.
- Bladder cancer has a higher incidence among white men than African American men.
- In all ethnic groups, bladder cancer affects men about three times more often than women.
- Urinary incontinence is underreported because culturally it is seen as a social hygiene problem causing patient embarrassment.

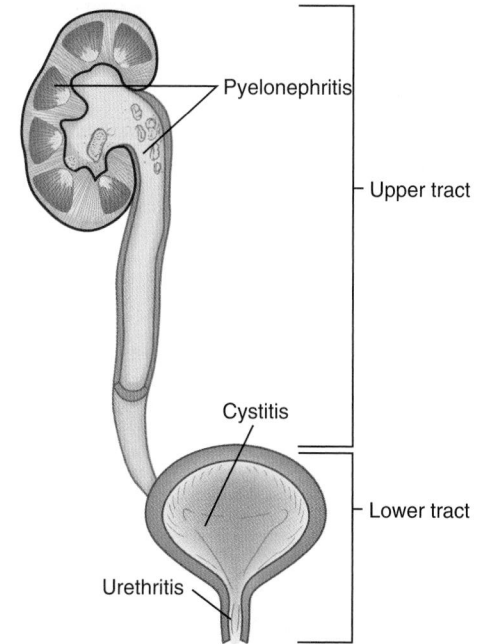

FIG. 46-1 Sites of infectious processes in the upper and lower urinary tracts.

are hospitalized annually for UTIs. More than 15% of patients who develop gram-negative bacteremia die, and one third of these cases are caused by bacterial infections originating in the urinary tract.[2]

Inflammation of the urinary tract may be caused by a variety of disorders, but bacterial infection is by far the most common. The bladder and its contents are free from bacteria in the majority of healthy persons. Nevertheless, a minority of otherwise healthy individuals have some bacteria colonizing the bladder. This condition is called *asymptomatic bacteriuria* and does not justify screening or treatment except in pregnant women.

Escherichia coli is the most common pathogen causing a UTI (Table 46-1) and is primarily seen in women. Bacterial counts of 10^5 colony-forming units per milliliter (CFU/mL) or higher typically indicate a clinically significant UTI. However, counts as low as 10^2 to 10^3 CFU/mL in a person with signs and symptoms are indicative of UTI.

Although fungal and parasitic infections may also cause UTIs, this is uncommon. UTIs from these causes are sometimes found in patients who are immunosuppressed, have diabetes mellitus, or have undergone multiple courses of antibiotic therapy. These types of UTIs may also be found in persons who live in or have traveled to certain developing countries.

Classification of Urinary Tract Infection

A UTI can be broadly classified as an upper or lower UTI according to its location within the urinary system (Fig. 46-1). Infection of the upper urinary tract (involving the renal parenchyma, pelvis, and ureters) typically causes fever, chills, and flank pain, whereas a UTI confined to the lower urinary tract does not usually have systemic manifestations. Specific terms are used to further delineate the location of a UTI. For example, pyelonephritis implies inflammation (usually caused by infection) of the renal parenchyma and collecting system, cystitis indicates inflammation of the bladder, and urethritis means inflammation of the urethra. Urosepsis is a UTI that has spread

systemically and is a life-threatening condition requiring emergency treatment.

Classifying a UTI as complicated or uncomplicated is also useful. *Uncomplicated* UTIs occur in an otherwise normal urinary tract and usually involve only the bladder. *Complicated* UTIs include those infections with coexisting obstruction, stones, or catheters; diabetes or neurologic diseases; or pregnancy-induced changes. The term also applies to a recurrent infection. The individual with a complicated infection is at risk for pyelonephritis, urosepsis, and renal damage.

Etiology and Pathophysiology

The urinary tract above the urethra is normally sterile. Several mechanical and physiologic defense mechanisms assist in maintaining sterility and preventing UTIs. These defenses include normal voiding with complete emptying of the bladder, ureterovesical junction competence, and ureteral peristaltic activity that propels urine toward the bladder. Antibacterial characteristics of urine are maintained by an acidic pH (less than 6.0), high urea concentration, and abundant glycoproteins that interfere with the growth of bacteria. An alteration in any of these defense mechanisms increases the risk for a UTI (Table 46-2).

The organisms that usually cause UTIs are introduced via the ascending route from the urethra and originate in the perineum. Most infections are caused by gram-negative bacilli normally found in the gastrointestinal (GI) tract, although gram-positive organisms such as streptococci, enterococci, and *Staphylococcus saprophyticus* can also cause UTIs.

A common factor contributing to ascending infection is urologic instrumentation (e.g., catheterization, cystoscopic examinations).[3] Instrumentation allows bacteria that are normally present at the opening of the urethra to enter into the urethra or bladder. Sexual intercourse promotes "milking" of bacteria from the vagina and perineum and may cause minor urethral trauma that predisposes women to UTIs.

Rarely do UTIs result from a hematogenous route, where blood-borne bacteria secondarily invade the kidneys, ureters,

TABLE 46-2	RISK FACTORS FOR URINARY TRACT INFECTIONS

Factors Increasing Urinary Stasis
- Intrinsic obstruction (stone, tumor of urinary tract, urethral stricture, BPH)
- Extrinsic obstruction (tumor, fibrosis compressing urinary tract)
- Urinary retention (including neurogenic bladder and low bladder wall compliance)
- Renal impairment

Foreign Bodies
- Urinary tract calculi
- Catheters (indwelling, external condom catheter, ureteral stent, nephrostomy tube, intermittent catheterization)
- Urinary tract instrumentation (cystoscopy, urodynamics)

Anatomic Factors
- Congenital defects leading to obstruction or urinary stasis
- Fistula (abnormal opening) exposing urinary stream to skin, vagina, or fecal stream
- Shorter female urethra and colonization from normal vaginal flora
- Obesity

Factors Compromising Immune Response
- Aging
- Human immunodeficiency virus infection
- Diabetes mellitus

Functional Disorders
- Constipation
- Voiding dysfunction with detrusor sphincter dyssynergia

Other Factors
- Pregnancy
- Hypoestrogenic state (menopause)
- Multiple sex partners (women)
- Use of spermicidal agents or contraceptive diaphragm (women)
- Poor personal hygiene
- Habitual delay of urination ("nurse's bladder," "teacher's bladder")

TABLE 46-3	LOWER URINARY TRACT SYMPTOMS (LUTS)

Symptoms	Description
Emptying Symptoms	
Hesitancy	• Difficulty starting urine stream • Delay between initiation of urination (because of urethral sphincter relaxation) and beginning of flow of urine • Diminished urinary stream
Intermittency	• Interruption of urinary stream while voiding
Postvoid dribbling	• Urine loss after completion of voiding
Urinary retention or incomplete emptying	• Inability to empty urine from bladder • Caused by atonic bladder or obstruction of urethra • Can be acute or chronic
Dysuria	• Painful or difficult urination
Storage Symptoms	
Urinary frequency	• >8 times in 24-hr period • Often <200 mL each voiding
Urgency	• Sudden, strong, or intense desire to void immediately • Commonly accompanied by frequency
Incontinence	• Involuntary or accidental urine loss or leakage
Nocturia	• Awakened by urge to void 2 or more times during sleep • May be diurnal or nocturnal depending on sleep schedule
Nocturnal enuresis	• Adults: loss of urine during sleep

or bladder from elsewhere in the body. There must be prior injury to the urinary tract, such as obstruction of the ureter, damage caused by stones, or renal scars, for a kidney infection to occur from hematogenous transmission.

An important source of UTIs is health care–associated infections (HAIs), previously called *nosocomial* infections, which account for 31% of all HAIs.[2,4] The cause of HAIs is often *E. coli* and, less frequently, *Pseudomonas* organisms. Catheter-acquired urinary tract infections (CAUTIs) are the most common HAIs and are caused by development of bacterial biofilms that are found on the catheter's inner surface. Most often these infections are underrecognized and undertreated, leading to complications such as renal abscesses, epididymitis, periurethral gland infections, and bacteremia.

Clinical Manifestations

Lower urinary tract symptoms (LUTS) are experienced in patients who have UTIs of the upper urinary tract, as well as those confined to the lower tract. Symptoms are related to either bladder storage or bladder emptying. These symptoms are presented in Table 46-3.

These symptoms include dysuria, frequent urination (more than every 2 hours), urgency, and suprapubic discomfort or pressure. The urine may contain grossly visible blood (hematuria) or sediment, giving it a cloudy appearance. Flank pain, chills, and fever indicate an infection involving the upper

urinary tract (pyelonephritis). People with significant bacteriuria may have no symptoms or may have nonspecific symptoms such as fatigue or anorexia.

Remember that these symptoms, considered characteristic of a UTI, are often absent in older adults. Older adults tend to experience nonlocalized abdominal discomfort rather than dysuria and suprapubic pain. In addition, they may have cognitive impairment or generalized clinical deterioration. Because older adults are less likely to experience a fever with a UTI, the value of body temperature as an indicator of a UTI is unreliable.

Multiple factors may produce LUTS similar to the symptoms of a UTI. For example, patients with bladder tumors or those receiving intravesical chemotherapy or pelvic radiation usually experience urinary frequency, urgency, and dysuria. Interstitial cystitis/painful bladder syndrome (discussed on p. 1071) also produces urinary symptoms that are similar to and sometimes confused with a UTI.

Diagnostic Studies

In a patient suspected of having a UTI, initially obtain a dipstick urinalysis to identify the presence of nitrites (indicating bacteriuria), white blood cells (WBCs), and leukocyte esterase (an enzyme present in WBCs indicating pyuria). These findings can be confirmed by microscopic urinalysis. After confirmation of bacteriuria and pyuria, a urine culture may be obtained. A urine culture is indicated in complicated or HAI UTIs, persistent bacteriuria, or frequently recurring UTIs (more than two or three episodes per year). Urine may also be cultured when the infection is unresponsive to empiric therapy or the diagnosis is questionable.[5]

A voided midstream technique *(clean-catch urine sample)* is preferred for obtaining a urine culture in most circumstances. For women, teach them to spread the labia and wipe the periurethral area from front to back using a moistened, clean gauze sponge (no antiseptic is used because it could contaminate the specimen and cause false positives). Then tell them to keep the labia spread, start voiding, and collect the specimen 1 to 2 seconds after voiding starts. For men, instruct them to wipe the glans penis around the urethra and collect the specimen 1 to 2 seconds after voiding begins.

Refrigerate urine immediately on collection. The urine should be cultured within 24 hours of refrigeration. A specimen obtained by catheterization provides more accurate results than a clean-catch specimen. When an adequate clean-catch specimen cannot be readily obtained, a catheterization may be necessary.

A urine culture is accompanied by *sensitivity testing* to determine the bacteria's susceptibility to a variety of antibiotic drugs. The results of this test allow the health care provider to select an antibiotic known to be capable of destroying the bacteria causing a UTI in a specific patient.

Imaging studies of the urinary tract are indicated in selected cases. A computed tomography (CT) urogram or ultrasound may be obtained when obstruction of the urinary system is suspected or UTIs recur.

Collaborative Care

Once a UTI has been diagnosed, appropriate antimicrobial therapy is initiated. An antibiotic may be selected based on the health care provider's best judgment *(empiric therapy)* or the results of sensitivity testing.[6] The collaborative care and drug therapy of UTIs are summarized in Table 46-4. Uncomplicated cystitis can be treated by a short-term course of antibiotics, typically for 1 to 3 days. In contrast, complicated UTIs require longer-term treatment, lasting 7 to 14 days or longer.[7,8]

Many residents of long-term care facilities, especially women, have chronic asymptomatic bacteriuria. However, usually only symptomatic UTIs are treated.

First-choice drugs to empirically treat uncomplicated or initial UTIs are trimethoprim/sulfamethoxazole (TMP/SMX) (Bactrim, Septra), nitrofurantoin (Macrodantin), and fosfomycin (Monurol). TMP/SMX has the advantages of being relatively inexpensive and being taken twice daily. A disadvantage is *E. coli* resistance to TMP/SMX, which is an increasing problem in the United States. Nitrofurantoin is normally given three or four times daily, but a long-acting preparation (Macrobid) is available that is taken twice daily.

Other antibiotics that may be used to treat uncomplicated UTI include ampicillin, amoxicillin, and cephalosporins. The fluoroquinolones are used to treat complicated UTIs. These drugs include ciprofloxacin (Cipro), levofloxacin (Levaquin), norfloxacin (Noroxin), ofloxacin (Floxin), and gatifloxacin (Tequin). In patients with UTIs secondary to fungi, amphotericin or fluconazole (Diflucan) is the preferred therapy.

DRUG ALERT: Nitrofurantoin (Furadantin, Macrodantin)
- Avoid sunlight. Use sunscreen, and wear protective clothing.
- Notify health care provider immediately if fever, chills, cough, chest pain, dyspnea, rash, or numbness or tingling of fingers or toes develops.

A urinary analgesic such as oral phenazopyridine (Azo-Standard, Pyridium) may relieve discomfort caused by severe

---

TABLE 46-4 COLLABORATIVE CARE

Urinary Tract Infection

Diagnostic
- History and physical examination
- Urinalysis (obtain midstream, "clean-catch" voided specimen)
- Urine for culture and sensitivity (if indicated)
- Imaging studies of urinary tract (if indicated)
  - CT urogram
  - Intravenous pyelogram (IVP)
  - CT/IVP
  - Cystoscopy
  - Ultrasound

Collaborative Therapy
Uncomplicated UTI
- Antibiotics
  - trimethoprim/sulfamethoxazole (Bactrim, Septra)
  - trimethoprim alone in patients with sulfa allergy
  - nitrofurantoin (Macrodantin, Macrobid)
  - fosfomycin (Monurol)
- Patient teaching
- Adequate fluid intake (six 8-oz glasses/day)

Recurrent, Uncomplicated UTI
- Repeat urinalysis
- Urine culture and sensitivity testing
- Imaging study of urinary tract (if indicated)
- Antibiotic: trimethoprim/sulfamethoxazole, nitrofurantoin
- Sensitivity-guided antibiotic therapy: ampicillin, amoxicillin, first-generation cephalosporin, fluoroquinolones
- Consider 3- to 6-mo trial of suppressive or prophylactic antibiotic regimen
- Consider postcoital antibiotic prophylaxis: trimethoprim/sulfamethoxazole, nitrofurantoin, cephalexin
- Adequate fluid intake (six 8-oz glasses/day)
- Repeat patient teaching

---

dysuria. Phenazopyridine is an azo dye excreted in urine, where it exerts a topical analgesic effect on the urinary tract mucosa.

Prophylactic or *suppressive antibiotics* are sometimes given to patients who have repeated UTIs. A low dose of TMP/SMX, nitrofurantoin, or another antibiotic may be taken daily to prevent recurring UTIs, or a single dose may be taken before an event likely to provoke a UTI, such as sexual intercourse. Although suppressive therapy is often effective on a short-term basis, this strategy is limited because of the risk of antibiotic resistance, which ultimately leads to breakthrough infections with increasingly virulent pathogens.

NURSING MANAGEMENT
URINARY TRACT INFECTION

NURSING ASSESSMENT

Subjective and objective data that should be obtained from a patient with a UTI are presented in Table 46-5.

NURSING DIAGNOSES

Nursing diagnoses for the patient with a UTI may include, but are not limited to, the following:
- Impaired urinary elimination *related to* the effects of UTI
- Readiness for enhanced self-health management

Additional information on nursing diagnoses for the patient with a UTI is presented in eNursing Care Plan 46-1 (on the website for this chapter).

TABLE 46-5 NURSING ASSESSMENT

Urinary Tract Infection

Subjective Data
Important Health Information
Past health history: Previous urinary tract infections; urinary calculi, stasis, reflux, strictures, or retention; neurogenic bladder; pregnancy; benign prostatic hyperplasia; sexually transmitted infection; bladder cancer
Medications: Antibiotics, anticholinergics, antispasmodics
Surgery or other treatments: Recent urologic instrumentation (catheterization, cystoscopy, surgery)

Functional Health Patterns
Health perception–health management: Urinary hygiene practices; lassitude, malaise
Nutritional-metabolic: Nausea, vomiting, anorexia; chills
Elimination: Urinary frequency, urgency, hesitancy; dysuria, nocturia
Cognitive-perceptual: Suprapubic or low back pain, costovertebral tenderness; bladder spasms, dysuria, burning on urination
Sexuality-reproductive: Multiple sex partners (women), use of spermicidal agents or contraceptive diaphragm (women)

Objective Data
General
Fever, chills, dysuria
Atypical presentation in older adults: afebrile, absence of dysuria, loss of appetite, altered mental status

Urinary
Hematuria; cloudy, foul-smelling urine; tender, enlarged kidney

Possible Diagnostic Findings
Leukocytosis; UA positive for bacteria, pyuria, RBCs, WBCs, and nitrites; positive urine culture; IVP, CT scan, US, VCUG, and cystoscopy indicating urinary tract abnormalities

IVP, Intravenous pyelogram; *VCUG,* voiding cystourethrogram.

PLANNING

The overall goals are that the patient with a UTI will have (1) relief from bothersome LUTS, (2) prevention of upper urinary tract involvement, and (3) prevention of recurrence.

NURSING IMPLEMENTATION

HEALTH PROMOTION. It is important to recognize individuals who are at risk for a UTI. These people include debilitated persons, older adults, patients who are immunocompromised (e.g., cancer, human immunodeficiency virus [HIV], diabetes mellitus), and patients treated with immunosuppressive drugs or corticosteroids. Health promotion activities, particularly for these individuals, can help decrease the frequency of infections and provide for early detection of infection. Health promotion activities include teaching preventive measures such as (1) emptying the bladder regularly and completely, (2) evacuating the bowel regularly, (3) wiping the perineal area from front to back after urination and defecation, and (4) drinking an adequate amount of liquid each day.

To estimate the amount of fluid intake a person should have in 24 hours, take the person's weight in pounds and divide that number in half. The result is the number of ounces of fluid a person should have per day. Thus a 150-pound person would require 75 oz/day. The person will obtain about 20% of this fluid from food, which leaves 60 oz (1775 mL) obtained by drinking, or just over seven 8-oz glasses of fluid.

Daily intake of cranberry juice or cranberry tablets or capsules may reduce the number of UTIs (see Evidence-Based

EVIDENCE-BASED PRACTICE

Translating Research Into Practice

Do Cranberry Products Prevent Urinary Tract Infections?

Clinical Question
Among adults and children (P), what is the effect of cranberry-containing products (I) vs. placebo vs. nonplacebo control (C) in preventing urinary tract infections (O)?

Best Available Evidence
Systematic review of randomized controlled trials (RCTs)

Critical Appraisal and Synthesis of Evidence
- Thirteen RCTs (*n* = 1616) of patients at high risk for recurrent urinary tract infections (UTIs), including women, older adults, patients with neuropathic bladder, and pregnant women. Children were also studied.
- Cranberry products were juice, capsules, or tablets given for 6 mo in most cases.
- Cranberry-containing products had a positive effect in preventing symptomatic UTIs.
- These products showed greater effect in women (especially those with recurrent UTIs), children, cranberry juice drinkers, and those taking the products more than twice daily.

Conclusion
- Cranberry-containing products can prevent UTIs.
- Cranberry juice was more effective than cranberry capsules. This may be due to increased hydration from the juice.

Implications for Nursing Practice
- Inform patients who are at an increased risk for recurrent UTIs that cranberry products have a protective effect in reducing UTIs.
- Cranberry juice works by preventing the attachment of bacteria to the epithelial cells in the bladder wall.
- Emphasize the importance of adequate fluid intake, including drinking cranberry juice.

Reference for Evidence
Wang C, Fang C, Chen N, et al: Cranberry-containing products for prevention of urinary tract infections in susceptible populations: a systematic review and meta-analysis of randomized controlled trials, *Arch Intern Med* 172:988, 2012.

P, Patient population of interest; *I,* intervention or area of interest; *C,* comparison of interest or comparison group; *O,* outcomes of interest (see p. 12).

Practice box). It is thought that enzymes found in cranberries inhibit attachment of urinary pathogens (especially *E. coli*) to the bladder wall.[9]

All patients undergoing instrumentation of the urinary tract are at risk for developing an HAI UTI. You have a major role in the prevention of these infections.[10-12] Avoidance of unnecessary catheterization and early removal of indwelling catheters are the most effective means for reducing HAI UTIs. Always follow aseptic technique during these procedures. Wash your hands before and after contact with each patient.[13] Wear gloves for care involving the urinary system. When a catheter has been inserted, use special measures, as explained in the section on urethral catheterization later in this chapter on p. 1092.

Routine and thorough perineal hygiene is important for all hospitalized patients, especially when a bedpan is used, after a bowel movement, or if fecal incontinence is present. Answer call lights quickly and offer the bedpan or urinal to bedridden patients at frequent intervals. These measures can prevent incontinence and decrease the number of incontinent episodes.

ACUTE INTERVENTION. Acute intervention for a patient with a UTI includes ensuring adequate fluid intake if it is not contraindicated. Maintaining adequate fluid intake may be difficult because of the patient's perception that fluid intake will worsen the discomfort and urinary frequency associated with a UTI. Tell patients that fluids will increase frequency of urination at first but will also dilute the urine, making the bladder less irritable. Fluids will help flush out bacteria before they have a chance to colonize in the bladder. Caffeine, alcohol, citrus juices, chocolate, and highly spiced foods or beverages should be avoided because they are potential bladder irritants.

Application of local heat to the suprapubic area or lower back may relieve the discomfort associated with a UTI. Advise the patient to apply a heating pad (turned to its lowest setting) against the back or suprapubic area. A warm shower or sitting in a tub of warm water filled above the waist can also provide temporary relief.

Instruct the patient about the prescribed drug therapy, including side effects. Emphasize the importance of taking the full course of antibiotics. Often patients stop antibiotic therapy once symptoms disappear. This can lead to inadequate treatment and recurrence of infection or bacterial resistance to antibiotics.

Sometimes a second drug or a reduced dosage of drug is ordered after the initial course to suppress bacterial growth in patients susceptible to recurrent UTI. Instruct the patient to monitor for signs of improvement (e.g., cloudy urine becomes clear) and a decrease in or cessation of symptoms. Teach patients to promptly report any of the following to their health care provider: (1) persistence of bothersome LUTS beyond the antibiotic treatment course, (2) onset of flank pain, or (3) fever.

AMBULATORY AND HOME CARE. Home care for the patient with a UTI should emphasize the importance of adhering to the drug regimen. Your responsibility is to teach the patient and caregiver about the need for ongoing care (Table 46-6). This includes taking antimicrobial drugs as ordered, maintaining adequate daily fluid intake, voiding regularly (approximately every 3 to 4 hours), urinating before and after intercourse, and temporarily discontinuing the use of a diaphragm.

TABLE 46-6 PATIENT & CAREGIVER TEACHING GUIDE

Urinary Tract Infection

When teaching a patient and caregiver measures to prevent a recurrence of a urinary tract infection (UTI), include the following.

1. Take all antibiotics as prescribed. Symptoms may improve after 1-2 days of therapy, but organisms may still be present.
2. Practice appropriate hygiene, including the following:
   - Carefully clean the perineal region by separating the labia when cleansing.
   - Wipe from front to back after urinating.
   - Cleanse with warm soapy water after each bowel movement.
3. Empty the bladder before and after sexual intercourse.
4. Urinate regularly, approximately every 3-4 hr during the day.
5. Maintain adequate fluid intake.
6. Avoid vaginal douches and harsh soaps, bubble baths, powders, and sprays in the perineal area.
7. Report to the health care provider symptoms or signs of recurrent UTI (e.g., fever, cloudy urine, pain on urination, urgency, frequency).
8. Consider drinking unsweetened cranberry juice (8 oz three times a day) or taking cranberry extract tablets 300-400 mg/day for UTI prevention.

If treatment is complete and the symptoms are still present, instruct the patient to get follow-up care. Recurrent symptoms because of bacterial persistence or inadequate treatment typically occur within 1 to 2 weeks after completion of therapy. If the patient has followed the treatment regimen, a relapse indicates the need for further evaluation.[14]

EVALUATION

The expected outcomes are that the patient with a UTI will
- Experience normal urinary elimination patterns
- Report relief of bothersome urinary tract symptoms
- Verbalize knowledge of treatment regimen

Additional information on the expected outcomes for the patient with a UTI is presented in eNursing Care Plan 46-1 (on the website for this chapter).

ACUTE PYELONEPHRITIS

Etiology and Pathophysiology

Pyelonephritis is an inflammation of the renal parenchyma (Fig. 46-2) and collecting system (including the renal pelvis). The most common cause is bacterial infection, but fungi, protozoa, or viruses can also infect the kidney.

Urosepsis is a systemic infection arising from a urologic source. Its prompt diagnosis and effective treatment are critical because it can lead to septic shock and death in 15% of cases unless promptly eradicated. Septic shock is the outcome of unresolved bacteremia involving a gram-negative organism. (Septic shock is discussed in Chapter 67.)

Pyelonephritis usually begins with colonization and infection of the lower urinary tract via the ascending urethral route. Bacteria normally found in the intestinal tract, such as *E. coli* or *Proteus, Klebsiella,* or *Enterobacter* species, frequently cause pyelonephritis. A preexisting factor is often present such as *vesicoureteral reflux* (retrograde, or backward, movement of urine from lower to upper urinary tract) or dysfunction of the lower urinary tract (e.g., obstruction from benign prostatic hyperplasia [BPH], a stricture, a urinary stone). For residents of long-term care facilities, urinary tract catheterization is a common cause of pyelonephritis and urosepsis.

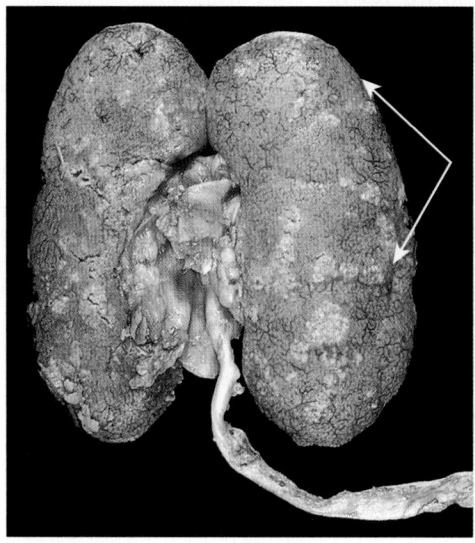

FIG. 46-2 Acute pyelonephritis. Cortical surface shows grayish white areas of inflammation and abscess formation *(arrows)*.

Acute pyelonephritis commonly starts in the renal medulla and spreads to the adjacent cortex. One of the most important risk factors for acute pyelonephritis is pregnancy-induced physiologic changes in the urinary system. Recurring episodes of pyelonephritis, especially in the presence of obstructive abnormalities, can lead to *chronic pyelonephritis* (discussed below).

Clinical Manifestations and Diagnostic Studies

The clinical manifestations of acute pyelonephritis vary from mild fatigue to the sudden onset of chills; fever; vomiting; malaise; flank pain; and the LUTS characteristic of cystitis, including dysuria, urgency, and frequency. *Costovertebral tenderness* to percussion (costovertebral angle [CVA] pain) is typically present on the affected side. Although the clinical manifestations may subside within a few days, even without specific therapy, bacteriuria and pyuria usually persist.

Urinalysis results indicate pyuria, bacteriuria, and varying degrees of hematuria. WBC casts may be found in the urine, indicating involvement of the renal parenchyma. A complete blood count shows leukocytosis and a shift to the left with an increase in bands (immature neutrophils). Urine cultures must be obtained when pyelonephritis is suspected. In patients with more severe illness who are hospitalized, blood cultures are usually obtained as well.

Ultrasonography of the urinary system may be performed to identify anatomic abnormalities, hydronephrosis, renal abscesses, or an obstructing stone. CT urograms are also used to assess for signs of infection in the kidney and complications of pyelonephritis, such as impaired renal function, scarring, chronic pyelonephritis, or abscesses.

Collaborative Care

The diagnostic tests and collaborative therapy of acute pyelonephritis are summarized in Table 46-7. Patients with severe infections or complicating factors such as nausea and vomiting with dehydration require hospitalization.

The patient with mild symptoms may be treated as an outpatient with antibiotics for 14 to 21 days (see Table 46-7). Parenteral antibiotics are often given initially in the hospital to rapidly establish high serum and urinary drug levels. When initial treatment resolves acute symptoms and the patient is able to tolerate oral fluids and drugs, the person may be discharged on a regimen of oral antibiotics for an additional 14 to 21 days. Symptoms and signs typically improve or resolve within 48 to 72 hours after starting therapy.

Relapses may be treated with a 6-week course of antibiotics. Antibiotic prophylaxis may also be used for recurrent infections. The effectiveness of therapy is evaluated based on the presence or absence of bacterial growth on urine culture.

Urosepsis is characterized by bacteriuria and bacteremia (bacteria in blood). Close observation and vital sign monitoring are essential. Prompt recognition and treatment of septic shock may prevent irreversible damage or death.

NURSING MANAGEMENT
ACUTE PYELONEPHRITIS

NURSING ASSESSMENT

Subjective and objective data that should be obtained from a patient with pyelonephritis are similar to those for the patient with a UTI (see Table 46-5).

TABLE 46-7   COLLABORATIVE CARE

Acute Pyelonephritis

Diagnostic
- History and physical examination
- Urinalysis
- Urine for culture and sensitivity
- Imaging studies: ultrasound (initially), CT scan, IVP, CT/IVP, VCUG, radionuclide imaging
- CBC count with WBC differential
- Blood culture (if bacteremia is suspected)
- Percussion for flank (costovertebral angle [CVA]) pain

Collaborative Therapy
Mild Symptoms (Uncomplicated Infection)
- Outpatient management or short hospitalization
  - Empirically selected broad-spectrum antibiotics: ampicillin, vancomycin combined with an aminoglycoside (e.g., tobramycin [Nebcin], gentamicin [Garamycin])
  - Switch to sensitivity-guided therapy: trimethoprim/sulfamethoxazole (Bactrim, Septra) when results of urine and blood culture are available
- Fluoroquinolones: ciprofloxacin (Cipro), ofloxacin (Floxin), norfloxacin (Noroxin), gatifloxacin (Tequin)
- Adequate fluid intake
- Nonsteroidal antiinflammatory drugs (NSAIDs) or antipyretic drugs
- Follow-up urine culture and imaging studies

Severe Symptoms
- Hospitalization
- Parenteral antibiotics
  - Empirically selected broad-spectrum antibiotics: ampicillin, vancomycin combined with an aminoglycoside (e.g., tobramycin, gentamicin)
  - Switch to sensitivity-guided antibiotic therapy when results of urine and blood culture are available
- Oral antibiotics when patient tolerates oral intake
- Adequate fluid intake (parenteral initially; switch to oral fluids as nausea, vomiting, and dehydration subside)
- NSAIDs or antipyretic drugs to reverse fever and relieve discomfort
- Urinary analgesics (as above)
- Follow-up urine culture and imaging studies

IVP, Intravenous pyelogram; *VCUG,* voiding cystourethrogram.

NURSING DIAGNOSES

Nursing diagnoses for the patient with pyelonephritis include, but are not limited to, those for the patient with a UTI (see p. 1067).

PLANNING

The overall goals are that the patient with pyelonephritis will have (1) normal renal function, (2) normal body temperature, (3) no complications, (4) relief of pain, and (5) no recurrence of symptoms.

NURSING IMPLEMENTATION

Health promotion and maintenance measures are similar to those for cystitis (see p. 1072). Early treatment for cystitis can prevent ascending infections. Because patients with structural abnormalities of the urinary tract are at high risk for infection, stress the need for regular medical care.

Nursing interventions vary depending on the severity of symptoms. These interventions include teaching the patient about the disease process with emphasis on (1) continuing medications as prescribed, (2) having a follow-up urine culture, and (3) recognizing manifestations of recurrence or relapse (see

Table 46-6). In addition to antibiotic therapy, encourage the patient to drink at least eight glasses of fluid every day, even after the infection has been treated. Rest will increase patient comfort. The patient who has frequent relapses or reinfections may be treated with long-term, low-dose antibiotics. Making certain the patient understands the rationale for therapy is important to increase adherence.

EVALUATION

The expected outcomes for the patient with pyelonephritis are the same as for UTI (see p. 1069).

CHRONIC PYELONEPHRITIS

In *chronic pyelonephritis* the kidneys become small, atrophic, and shrunken and lose function due to fibrosis (scarring). Chronic pyelonephritis is usually the result of recurring infections involving the upper urinary tract. However, it may also occur in the absence of an existing infection, recent infection, or history of UTIs.

Radiologic imaging and a biopsy, rather than clinical features, are used to confirm the diagnosis of chronic pyelonephritis. Imaging studies reveal a small, fibrotic kidney. The collecting system may be small or hydronephrotic. Biopsy results indicate the loss of functioning nephrons, infiltration of the parenchyma with inflammatory cells, and fibrosis.

The level of renal function in chronic pyelonephritis depends on whether one or both kidneys are affected, the extent of scarring, and the presence of coexisting infection. Chronic pyelonephritis often progresses to end-stage kidney (renal) disease (ESKD) even if the underlying infection is successfully treated. Nursing and collaborative management of the patient with chronic kidney disease is discussed in Chapter 47.

URETHRITIS

Urethritis is an inflammation of the urethra. Causes of urethritis include a bacterial or viral infection, *Trichomonas* and monilial infection (especially in women), chlamydial infection, and gonorrhea (especially in men).

In men the causes of urethritis are usually sexually transmitted. Purulent discharge usually indicates a gonococcal urethritis, whereas a clear discharge typically signifies a nongonococcal urethritis. (Sexually transmitted infections are discussed in Chapter 53.) Urethritis also produces bothersome LUTS, including dysuria, urgency, and frequent urination, similar to those seen with cystitis.

In women, urethritis is difficult to diagnose. It frequently produces bothersome LUTS, but urethral discharge may not be present.

Treatment of urethritis is based on identifying and treating the cause and providing symptomatic relief. Drugs used for bacterial infections include TMP/SMX and nitrofurantoin. Metronidazole (Flagyl) and clotrimazole (Mycelex) may be used for treating *Trichomonas* infection. Drugs such as nystatin (Mycostatin) or fluconazole may be prescribed for monilial infections. In chlamydial infections, doxycycline (Vibramycin) may be used. Women with negative urine cultures and no pyuria usually do not respond to antibiotics.

Warm sitz baths may temporarily relieve bothersome symptoms. Instruct the patient to avoid using vaginal deodorant sprays, properly cleanse the perineal area after bowel movements and urination, and avoid sexual intercourse until symptoms subside. Teach patients with sexually transmitted urethritis to refer their sex partners for evaluation and testing if they had sexual contact in the 60 days preceding the onset of the patient's symptoms or diagnosis.

URETHRAL DIVERTICULA

Urethral diverticula are localized outpouchings of the urethra. Most often they result from enlargement of obstructed periurethral glands. In women, who have a higher incidence than men, the diverticula protrude into the anterior vaginal wall. The rare cases reported in males generally have been associated with lower urinary tract congenital anomalies or surgical trauma.

The periurethral glands are found along the entire length of the urethra, with the majority draining into the distal third of the urethra. Skene's glands are the largest of these glands. Causes of urethral diverticuli include urethral trauma from childbearing, urethral instrumentation, urethral dilation, and infection with gonococcal organisms.

Symptoms include dysuria, postvoid dribbling, frequent urination (more often than every 2 hours), urgency, suprapubic discomfort or pressure, dyspareunia, and a feeling of incomplete bladder emptying. Urinary incontinence is frequently present. However, many women have no symptoms.

The urine may contain gross blood (hematuria) or sediment, which gives it a cloudy appearance. An anterior vaginal wall mass may be felt on physical examination. When palpated, the mass is often quite tender and expresses purulent discharge through the urethra.

Radiographic studies such as voiding cystourethrography (VCUG) can be used to confirm the diagnosis. Additional studies include ultrasound and magnetic resonance imaging (MRI) to determine the size of the diverticulum in relation to the urethral lumen.

Surgical options include transurethral incision of the diverticular neck, marsupialization (creation of a permanent opening) of the diverticular sac into the vagina (often referred to as a Spence procedure), and surgical excision. Stress urinary incontinence is a potential complication of the surgery.

INTERSTITIAL CYSTITIS/ PAINFUL BLADDER SYNDROME

Interstitial cystitis (IC) is a chronic, painful inflammatory disease of the bladder characterized by symptoms of urgency, frequency, and pain in the bladder and/or pelvis. *Painful bladder syndrome* (PBS) is suprapubic pain related to bladder filling. The term *IC/PBS* refers to cases of urinary pain that cannot be attributed to other causes such as infection or urinary calculi.

IC/PBS is more common in women than men. It affects about 3.3 million women and 1.6 million men.[15]

The etiology of IC/PBS remains unknown and is likely multifactorial. Possible causes include neurogenic hypersensitivity of the lower urinary tract, alterations in mast cells in the muscle and/or mucosal layers of the bladder, infection with an unusual organism (e.g., slow-growing virus), or production of a toxic substance in the urine.[16]

The bladder wall may be irritated and inflamed, and can become scarred. *Glomerulations* (superficial ulcerations with pinpoint bleeding) often occur on the bladder wall.

Clinical Manifestations and Diagnostic Studies

The two primary clinical manifestations of IC/PBS are pain and bothersome LUTS (e.g., frequency, urgency). The pain is usually located in the suprapubic area but may involve the vagina, labia, or entire perineal region, including the rectum and anus. The pain varies from moderate to severe and is exacerbated by bladder filling, postponed urination, physical exertion, pressure against the suprapubic area, certain foods, or emotional distress. The pain is transiently relieved by urination. Bothersome LUTS are similar to a UTI, and the condition is often misdiagnosed as a recurring or chronic UTI or, in men, chronic prostatitis.

The patient experiences periods of remission and exacerbation of the pain and bothersome voiding symptoms. Women often report that pain occurs premenstrually and is aggravated by sexual intercourse or emotional stress. Some patients experience symptoms that disappear altogether after a period of weeks to months, whereas others have persistent symptoms over months to years.

IC/PBS is a diagnosis of exclusion.[17] A careful history and physical examination are necessary to rule out other disorders that produce similar symptoms, such as UTI or endometriosis. Urine cultures do not find any bacteria or other organisms in the urine. Furthermore, people with IC/PBS do not respond to antibiotic therapy. Cystoscopic examination may reveal a small bladder capacity and glomerulations, but these findings are frequently not present in patients with IC/PBS.

Collaborative Care

Because the etiology of IC/PBS is unknown, no single treatment consistently reverses or relieves symptoms. Various therapies have been effective, including nutritional and drug therapy.[18,19] Surgical therapy is rarely indicated.

Elimination of foods and beverages that are likely to irritate the bladder may provide some relief from symptoms. Typical bladder irritants include caffeine; alcohol; citrus products; aged cheeses; nuts; foods containing vinegar, curries, or hot peppers; and foods or beverages, including fruits (cranberries), likely to lower urinary pH. Recipes and menus for a well-balanced diet that is specifically designed to avoid bladder-irritating foods and beverages are available at the website for the Interstitial Cystitis Association (www.ichelp.org).

Advise patients that an over-the-counter (OTC) dietary supplement called calcium glycerophosphate (Prelief) alkalinizes the urine and can provide relief from the irritating effects of certain foods. This agent may be particularly helpful when dining away from home, where the patient has less control over food preparation.

Because stress can exacerbate or cause flare-ups of IC/PBS symptoms, stress management techniques such as relaxation breathing and imagery (see Chapter 7) may be helpful. Using lubrication or altering positions may decrease pain associated with sexual intercourse.

Two tricyclic antidepressants, amitriptyline (Elavil) and nortriptyline (Aventyl), are used to reduce the burning pain and urinary frequency. Pentosan (Elmiron) is the only oral agent approved for the treatment of patients with symptoms of IC. It enhances the protective effects of the glycosaminoglycan layer of the bladder, and is thought to relieve pain associated with IC/PBS by reducing the irritative effects of urine on the bladder wall. These drugs are used to provide relief over time (weeks to months), but do not provide the immediate relief that may be needed for an acute exacerbation of symptoms. A short course of opioid analgesics may be used for immediate relief.

Dimethyl sulfoxide (DMSO) can be directly instilled into the bladder through a small catheter. This drug desensitizes pain receptors in the bladder wall. Heparin and hyaluronic acid also may be instilled into the bladder to relieve IC/PBS symptoms. Like pentosan, they are thought to enhance the protective properties of the glycosaminoglycan layer of the bladder. Instillations are often administered with lidocaine, which rapidly desensitizes the bladder wall, helping the patient tolerate instillation of additional heparin or hyaluronic acid and providing transient relief from pain.

Several surgical procedures can be used to relieve severe, debilitating pain. Surgical urinary diversion, such as an ileal conduit, is used when other measures fail. Unfortunately, some patients have reported pain within the urinary diversion, possibly indicating that some factor in the urine may contribute to IC/PBS in certain cases.

NURSING MANAGEMENT INTERSTITIAL CYSTITIS/ PAINFUL BLADDER SYNDROME

Assess the characteristics of the pain associated with IC/PBS. Ask the patient about specific dietary or lifestyle factors that exacerbate or alleviate pain, and assess the intensity of the pain. Instruct the patient to keep a bladder log or voiding diary over a period of at least 3 days to determine voiding frequency and patterns of nocturia. Keeping a pain record at the same time may be useful.

A UTI may occur during the course of IC/PBS management because of diagnostic instrumentation and frequent bladder instillations. A UTI is likely to produce an acute exacerbation of bothersome LUTS and urinary frequency, as well as dysuria (not typically associated with IC/PBS) and odorous urine, possibly with hematuria.

Instruct the patient to maintain good nutrition, particularly in light of the broad dietary restrictions often necessary to control IC-related pain. Advise the patient to take a multivitamin containing no more than the recommended dietary allowance for essential vitamins and to avoid high-potency vitamins because they may irritate the bladder. Advise the patient to avoid clothing that creates suprapubic pressure, including pants with tight belts or restrictive waistlines.

Written educational materials about diet, ways to cope with the need for frequent urination, and strategies for coping with the emotional burden of IC/PBS are available from the Interstitial Cystitis Association (www.ichelp.com). Reassurance that IC/PBS is a real condition experienced by others and that it can be treated may relieve the anxiety, anger, guilt, and frustration related to experiences of chronic pain and voiding dysfunction in the absence of a clear-cut diagnosis and treatment strategy.

RENAL TUBERCULOSIS

Renal tuberculosis (TB) is rarely a primary lesion. It is usually secondary to TB of the lung. In a small percentage of patients with pulmonary TB, the tubercle bacilli reach the kidneys via the bloodstream. Onset occurs 5 to 8 years after the primary lung infection.[20] When the kidney is initially infected with bacilli, the patient is often asymptomatic. Sometimes the patient complains of fatigue and develops a low-grade fever. As the lesions ulcerate, infection descends to the bladder and other genitourinary organs. Then the patient experiences cystitis, frequent urination, burning on voiding, and epididymitis (in men).

Symptoms of a UTI are the first manifestations in the majority of patients with renal TB. Renal lesions may calcify as they heal. Infrequently, renal colic, lumbar and iliac pain, and hematuria may be present.

Tuberculin skin test results are positive in most patients, but this finding only indicates that the person has had previous inhalation of mycobacteria rather than active disease. A diagnosis of renal TB is based on finding tubercle bacilli in the urine.

Radiographic tests that may be done include CT urogram, CT/intravenous pyelogram (IVP), and voiding cystourethrogram (VCUG). These studies help determine the extent and severity of the disease.

Long-term complications of renal TB depend on the duration of the disease. Scarring of the renal parenchyma and the development of ureteral strictures occur. The earlier treatment is initiated, the less likely renal failure will develop. The patient may require long-term urologic follow-up. Nursing and collaborative management for the patient with TB is discussed in Chapter 28.

IMMUNOLOGIC DISORDERS OF KIDNEY

GLOMERULONEPHRITIS

Immunologic processes involving the urinary tract predominantly affect the renal glomerulus. The disease process results in glomerulonephritis (inflammation of the glomeruli), which affects both kidneys equally and is the third leading cause of ESKD in the United States. Although the glomerulus is the primary site of inflammation, tubular, interstitial, and vascular changes also occur.

A variety of conditions can cause glomerulonephritis, ranging from kidney infections to systemic diseases (Table 46-8). Glomerulonephritis can be acute or chronic. With *acute glomerulonephritis,* symptoms come on suddenly and may be temporary or reversible. An example of this is acute poststreptococcal glomerulonephritis (discussed in the next section).

TABLE 46-8 CAUSES OR RISK FACTORS FOR GLOMERULONEPHRITIS

Cause or Risk Factor	Description	Cause or Risk Factor	Description
Infections		**IgA nephropathy**	• Results from deposits of immunoglobulin A (IgA) in the glomeruli.
Poststreptococcal glomerulonephritis	• GN may develop 1-2 wk after a streptococcal throat infection or, rarely, a skin infection (impetigo). • Antibodies (Ab) to strep antigen (Ag) develop and the Ag-Ab deposit in the glomeruli, causing inflammation.		• Characterized by recurrent episodes of hematuria.
		Vasculitis	
		Polyarteritis	• Autoimmune disease that affects small and medium blood vessels. • Can affect any organ but common in heart, kidneys, and intestines.
Infective endocarditis	• Bacteria can cause an infection of one or more of the heart valves (see Chapter 37). • People at risk include those with a heart defect, such as a damaged or artificial heart valve. • Bacterial endocarditis is associated with GN, but the exact cause is not known.	**Wegener's granulomatosis**	• Form of vasculitis affecting small and medium blood vessels. • Most commonly affects kidneys, lungs, and upper respiratory tract.
		Conditions Causing Scarring of Glomeruli	
Viral infections	• Viral infections can trigger GN. • Common viruses include human immunodeficiency virus (HIV) and hepatitis B and hepatitis C viruses.	**Diabetic nephropathy**	• Primary cause of end-stage kidney disease in the United States (see Chapter 47). • Microvascular changes of diffuse glomerulosclerosis involving thickening of the glomerular basement membrane.
Immune Diseases		**Hypertension**	• Nephrosclerosis is a complication of hypertension. • GN can also cause hypertension.
Systemic lupus erythematosus (SLE)	• Autoimmune disorder characterized by the involvement of several tissues and organs, particularly joints, skin, and kidneys (see Chapter 65). • GN frequently occurs in SLE and has a poor prognosis.	**Focal segmental glomerulosclerosis**	• Characterized by scattered scarring of some of the glomeruli. • May result from another disease or occur for unknown reasons.
Scleroderma	• Disease of unknown etiology characterized by widespread alterations of connective tissue and by vascular lesions in many organs (see Chapter 65). • In the kidney, vascular lesions are associated with fibrosis. Severity of renal involvement varies.	**Other Causes**	
		Amyloidosis	• Caused by infiltration of tissues with amyloid (hyaline substance). • Hyaline bodies consist largely of protein. • Kidney involvement is common, and proteinuria is often the first clinical manifestation.
Goodpasture syndrome	• Autoimmune disorder that causes lung and kidney disease. • Causes bleeding into the lungs and GN.	**Illegal drug use**	• People who use these drugs are at increased risk for GN.

GN, Glomerulonephritis.

Chronic glomerulonephritis is slowly progressive glomerulonephritis generally leading to irreversible renal failure (discussed later in this chapter).

Acute Poststreptococcal Glomerulonephritis

Acute poststreptococcal glomerulonephritis (APSGN) is a common type of acute glomerulonephritis. It is most common in children and young adults, but all age-groups can be affected. APSGN develops 5 to 21 days after an infection of the tonsils, pharynx, or skin (e.g., streptococcal sore throat, impetigo) by nephrotoxic strains of group A β-hemolytic streptococci. The person produces antibodies to the streptococcal antigen. Although the specific mechanism is not known, tissue injury occurs as the antigen-antibody complexes are deposited in the glomeruli, complement is activated (see Chapter 12), and inflammation results.

The clinical manifestations of APSGN include generalized body edema, hypertension, oliguria, hematuria with a smoky or rusty appearance, and proteinuria. Fluid retention occurs as a result of decreased glomerular filtration. Initially edema appears in low-pressure tissues, such as those around the eyes (periorbital edema), but later it progresses to involve the total body as ascites or peripheral edema in the legs. Smoky urine indicates bleeding in the upper urinary tract. The degree of proteinuria varies with the severity of the glomerulonephropathy. Hypertension primarily results from increased extracellular fluid volume. The patient with APSGN may have abdominal or flank pain. At times the patient has no symptoms, with the problem found on routine urinalysis.

More than 95% of patients with APSGN recover completely or improve rapidly with conservative management. Accurate recognition and assessment are critical, since chronic glomerulonephritis develops in 5% to 15% of the affected persons, and irreversible renal failure occurs in 1% of patients.[21]

The diagnosis of APSGN is based on a complete history and physical examination. An immune response to the streptococci is often demonstrated by assessment of antistreptolysin-O (ASO) titers. The finding of decreased complement components (especially C3 and CH50) indicates an immune-mediated response. A renal biopsy may be done to confirm the disease.

Dipstick urinalysis and urine sediment microscopy reveal erythrocytes in significant numbers. Erythrocyte casts are highly suggestive of APSGN. Proteinuria may range from mild to severe. Blood tests include blood urea nitrogen (BUN) and serum creatinine to assess the extent of renal impairment.

NURSING AND COLLABORATIVE MANAGEMENT ACUTE POSTSTREPTOCOCCAL GLOMERULONEPHRITIS

The management of APSGN focuses on symptomatic relief. Rest is recommended until the signs of glomerular inflammation (proteinuria, hematuria) and hypertension subside. Edema is treated by restricting sodium and fluid intake and by administrating diuretics. Severe hypertension is treated with antihypertensive drugs. Dietary protein intake may be restricted if there is evidence of an increase in nitrogenous wastes (e.g., elevated BUN). The dietary protein restriction varies with the degree of proteinuria. Low-protein, low-sodium, fluid-restricted diets are discussed in Chapter 47.

Antibiotics should be given only if the streptococcal infection is still present. Corticosteroids and cytotoxic drugs have not been shown to be of value in the treatment of APSGN.

One of the most important ways to prevent APSGN is to encourage early diagnosis and treatment of sore throats and skin lesions. If streptococci are found in the culture, treatment with appropriate antibiotic therapy (usually penicillin) is essential. Encourage the patient to take the full course of antibiotics to ensure that the bacteria have been eradicated. Good personal hygiene is an important factor in preventing the spread of cutaneous streptococcal infections.

In most cases, recovery from the acute glomerulonephritis is complete. However, if progressive involvement occurs and chronic glomerulonephritis develops, ESKD results.

Goodpasture Syndrome

Goodpasture syndrome is an autoimmune disease characterized by circulating antibodies against glomerular and alveolar basement membrane. Damage to the kidneys and lungs results when binding of the antibody causes an inflammatory reaction mediated by complement activation (see Chapter 12).

Goodpasture syndrome is a rare disease that is mostly found in young male smokers. The clinical manifestations include flu-like symptoms with pulmonary symptoms such as cough, mild shortness of breath, hemoptysis, crackles, rhonchi, and pulmonary insufficiency. Renal involvement causes hematuria, weakness, pallor, anemia, and renal failure. Pulmonary hemorrhage usually occurs and may precede glomerular abnormalities by weeks or months.

Current management includes corticosteroids, immunosuppressive drugs (e.g., cyclophosphamide [Cytoxan], azathioprine [Imuran]), plasmapheresis (see Chapter 14), and dialysis. Plasmapheresis removes the circulating anti–glomerular basement membrane (GBM) antibodies, and immunosuppressive therapy inhibits further antibody production. Renal transplantation can be attempted after the circulating anti-GBM antibody titer decreases. Although the disease may recur in the transplanted kidney, this is not a contraindication to transplantation.

Nursing management appropriate for a critically ill patient who is experiencing acute kidney injury (see Chapter 47) and respiratory distress (see Chapter 68) is instituted. Death is often secondary to hemorrhage in the lungs and respiratory failure.

Rapidly Progressive Glomerulonephritis

Rapidly progressive glomerulonephritis (RPGN) is a type of glomerular disease characterized by rapid, progressive loss of renal function over days to weeks. In contrast, chronic glomerulonephritis develops insidiously and progresses over many years. The manifestations of RPGN are hypertension, edema, proteinuria, hematuria, and red blood cell (RBC) casts.

RPGN can occur in a variety of situations: (1) as a complication of inflammatory or infectious disease (e.g., APSGN), (2) as a complication of a systemic disease (e.g., systemic lupus erythematosus), (3) as an idiopathic disease, or (4) with the use of certain drugs (e.g., penicillamine).

Treatment is directed toward correction of fluid overload, hypertension, uremia, and inflammatory injury to the kidney. Treatment includes corticosteroids, cytotoxic agents, and plasmapheresis. Dialysis therapy and transplantation are used as maintenance therapy for the patient with RPGN. After kidney transplantation, RPGN may recur.

Chronic Glomerulonephritis

Chronic glomerulonephritis is a syndrome that reflects the end stage of glomerular inflammatory disease. Most types of glomerulonephritis and nephrotic syndrome can eventually lead to chronic glomerulonephritis. Some people who develop chronic glomerulonephritis have no history of kidney disease. Frequently the cause of chronic glomerulonephritis is not found. Infrequently, it is an inherited disorder (e.g., Alport syndrome [see p. 1083]).

With chronic glomerulonephritis, symptoms develop slowly over time. Patients are often unaware that progressive kidney impairment is occurring. They do not realize that they have severe kidney impairment until a diagnostic evaluation is done. Chronic glomerulonephritis is often discovered coincidentally with the finding of an abnormality on a urinalysis or elevated blood pressure (BP).

The syndrome is characterized by proteinuria, hematuria, and the slow development of uremia (see Chapter 47) as a result of decreasing renal function. Chronic glomerulonephritis progresses insidiously toward renal failure in 2 to 30 years.

Clinical manifestations of glomerulonephritis include varying degrees of hematuria (ranging from microscopic to gross) and urinary excretion of various formed elements, including RBCs, WBCs, and casts. Proteinuria and elevated BUN and serum creatinine levels are other findings. Sometimes fatigue may be a presenting symptom.

The patient's history provides important information related to glomerulonephritis. Assess exposure to drugs, immunizations, microbial infections, and viral infections such as hepatitis. Also evaluate the patient for more generalized conditions involving immune disorders, such as systemic lupus erythematosus and scleroderma. Commonly the patient has no recollection or history of any renal problems.

Ultrasound and CT scanning are generally preferred as diagnostic measures. However, a renal biopsy may be performed to determine the exact cause of the glomerulonephritis.

Treatment is supportive and symptomatic. Management of chronic kidney disease is discussed in Chapter 47.

NEPHROTIC SYNDROME

Nephrotic syndrome results when the glomerulus is excessively permeable to plasma protein, causing proteinuria that leads to low plasma albumin and tissue edema.

Etiology and Clinical Manifestations

Some of the common causes of nephrotic syndrome are listed in Table 46-9. About one third of patients with nephrotic syndrome have a systemic disease such as diabetes or systemic lupus erythematosus.

The characteristic manifestations of nephrotic syndrome include peripheral edema, massive proteinuria, hypertension, hyperlipidemia, and hypoalbuminemia. Characteristic laboratory findings include decreased serum albumin, decreased total serum protein, and elevated serum cholesterol. The increased glomerular membrane permeability found in nephrotic syndrome is responsible for the massive excretion of protein in the urine. This results in decreased serum protein and subsequent edema formation. Ascites and *anasarca* (massive generalized edema) develop if there is severe hypoalbuminemia.[22]

The diminished plasma oncotic pressure from the decreased serum proteins stimulates hepatic lipoprotein synthesis, which results in hyperlipidemia. Initially, cholesterol and low-density lipoproteins are elevated. Later the triglyceride level is also

TABLE 46-9	**CAUSES OF NEPHROTIC SYNDROME**
Primary Glomerular Disease • Membranous proliferative glomerulonephritis • Primary nephrotic syndrome • Focal glomerulonephritis • Inherited nephrotic disease **Extrarenal Causes** **Multisystem Disease** • Systemic lupus erythematosus • Diabetes mellitus • Amyloidosis **Infections** • Bacterial (streptococcal, syphilis) • Viral (hepatitis, human immunodeficiency virus) • Protozoal (malaria)	**Neoplasms** • Hodgkin's lymphoma • Solid tumors of lungs, colon, stomach, breast • Leukemias **Allergens** • Bee sting • Pollen **Drugs** • penicillamine • Nonsteroidal antiinflammatory drugs (NSAIDs) • captopril (Capoten) • heroin

increased. Fat bodies (fatty casts) commonly appear in the urine.

Immune responses, both humoral and cellular, are altered in nephrotic syndrome. As a result, infection is a primary cause of morbidity and mortality. Calcium and skeletal abnormalities may occur, including hypocalcemia, blunted calcium response to parathyroid hormone, hyperparathyroidism, and osteomalacia.

With nephrotic proteinuria, hypercoagulability results from the urinary loss of anticoagulant proteins. Hypercoagulability with thromboembolism is a serious complication of nephrotic syndrome. The renal vein is the most common site for thrombus formation. Pulmonary emboli occur in about 40% of nephrotic patients with thrombosis.

NURSING AND COLLABORATIVE MANAGEMENT NEPHROTIC SYNDROME

Specific treatment of nephrotic syndrome depends on the cause. The goals are to cure or control the primary disease and relieve the symptoms. Corticosteroids and cyclophosphamide may be used for the treatment of nephrotic syndrome. Prednisone has been effective to varying degrees for some causes of nephrotic syndrome (e.g., membranous glomerulonephritis, lupus nephritis). Management of diabetes and treatment of edema are measures used for nephrotic syndrome related to diabetes.

Management of the edema includes the cautious use of angiotensin-converting enzyme inhibitors; nonsteroidal antiinflammatory drugs (NSAIDs); and a low-sodium (2 to 3 g/day), moderate-protein (1 to 2 g/kg/day) diet. If urine protein losses are high (more than 10 g/day), additional protein may be recommended.

Dietary salt restrictions are a key to managing edema. Some individuals may need thiazide or loop diuretics.

The treatment of hyperlipidemia includes lipid-lowering agents, such as colestipol (Colestid) and lovastatin (Mevacor) (see Table 34-5). If thrombosis is detected, anticoagulant therapy may be needed.

A major nursing intervention for a patient with nephrotic syndrome focuses on the management of edema. Assess the edema by weighing the patient daily, accurately recording intake and output, and measuring abdominal girth or extremity size. Compare this information on a daily basis to assess the effectiveness of treatment. Clean the edematous skin carefully. Avoid trauma to the skin. Monitor the effectiveness of diuretic therapy.

Patients with nephrotic syndrome are usually anorexic and have the potential to become malnourished from the excessive loss of protein in the urine. Serve small, frequent meals in a pleasant setting to encourage better dietary intake.

Because the patient with nephrotic syndrome is susceptible to infection, teach the patient to avoid exposure to persons with known infections. Support for the patient, in terms of coping with an altered body image, is essential because of the embarrassment and shame often associated with the edematous appearance.

OBSTRUCTIVE UROPATHIES

Urinary obstruction refers to any anatomic or functional condition that blocks or impedes the flow of urine (Fig. 46-3). It may be congenital or acquired. Damaging effects from urinary tract obstruction affect the system above the level of the obstruction. The severity of these effects depends on the location, duration of obstruction, amount of pressure or dilation, and presence of urinary stasis or infection. Infection increases the risk of irreversible damage.

When obstruction occurs at the level of the bladder neck or prostate, significant bladder changes can occur. Detrusor muscle fibers *hypertrophy* (increase in size) to contract harder to push urine out a narrower pathway. Over a long period, the detrusor loses its ability to compensate for this resistance, eventually leading to large residual urine volume in the bladder.

When *bladder outlet obstruction* is present, pressure increases during bladder filling or storage and can be transmitted to the ureter. This pressure leads to *reflux* (a backflow of urine), hydro-ureter (ureteral dilation and distention), vesicoureteral reflux (backflow, or backward movement, of urine from the lower to upper urinary tract), and hydronephrosis (dilation or enlargement of the renal pelvises and calyces) (Fig. 46-4). Chronic pyelonephritis and renal atrophy may develop. If only one kidney is obstructed, the other kidney may try to compensate by hypertrophy.

Partial obstruction may occur in the ureter or at the ureteropelvic junction (UPJ). If the pressure remains low or moderate, the kidney may continue to dilate with no noticeable loss of function. The risk of pyelonephritis is increased because of urinary stasis and reflux. If only one kidney is involved and the other kidney is functioning, the patient may be asymptomatic.

If both kidneys or only one functioning kidney is involved (e.g., if the patient has only one kidney), alterations in renal function (e.g., increased BUN or serum creatinine levels) are found. Progressive obstruction can lead to renal failure. Treatment requires location and relief of the blockage. This can include insertion of a tube (e.g., urethral or ureteral), surgical correction of the primary problem, or diversion of the urinary stream above the level of blockage.

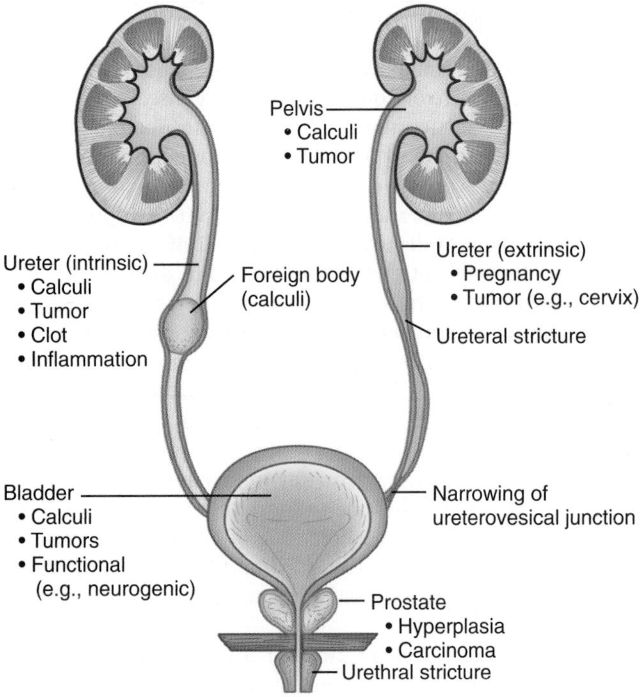

URINARY TRACT CALCULI

Each year an estimated 1 million to 2 million people in the United States have nephrolithiasis (kidney stone disease). In the United States the incidence of urinary stone disease is highest in the Southeast and Southwest, followed by the Midwest. Except for struvite (magnesium ammonium phosphate) stones associated with UTI, stone disorders are more common in men than in women. The majority of patients are between 20 and 55 years of age.[4]

Stone formation is more frequent in whites than in African Americans. The incidence is also higher in persons with a family history of stone formation. Stones can recur in up to 50% of patients. Stone formation occurs more often in the summer months, thus supporting the role of dehydration in this process.

Etiology and Pathophysiology

Many factors are involved in the incidence and type of stone formation, including metabolic, dietary, genetic, climatic, life-

FIG. 46-3 Sites and causes of upper and lower urinary tract obstruction.

Pelvis
• Calculi
• Tumor

Ureter (intrinsic)
• Calculi
• Tumor
• Clot
• Inflammation

Foreign body (calculi)

Ureter (extrinsic)
• Pregnancy
• Tumor (e.g., cervix)

Ureteral stricture

Bladder
• Calculi
• Tumors
• Functional (e.g., neurogenic)

Narrowing of ureterovesical junction

Prostate
• Hyperplasia
• Carcinoma

Urethral stricture

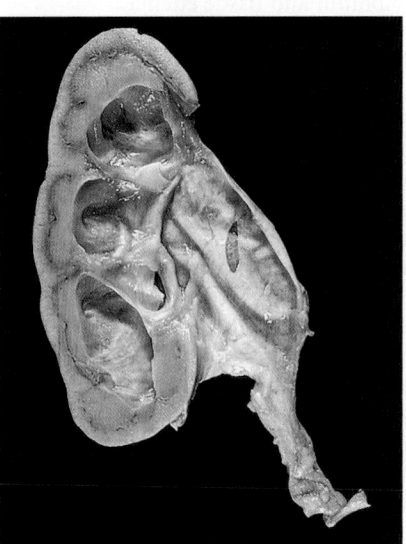

FIG. 46-4 Hydronephrosis of the kidney. Note the marked dilation of the pelvis and calyces and thinning of the renal parenchyma.

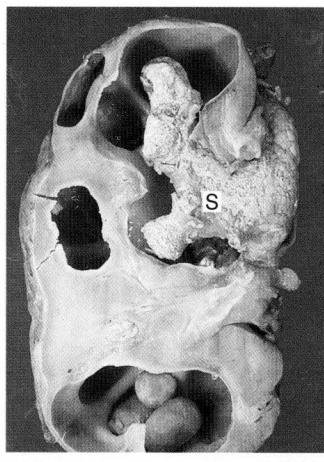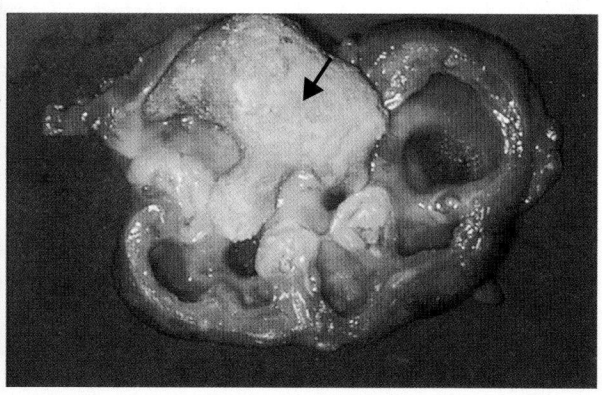

FIG. 46-5 A, Renal staghorn calculus. The renal pelvis is filled with a large calculus that is shaped to its contours, resembling the horns of a stag *(S).* **B,** Imbedded staghorn calculus *(arrow)* in hydronephrotic, infected, nonfunctioning kidney.

style, and occupational influences (Table 46-10). Although many theories have been proposed, no single theory can account for stone formation in all cases. Crystals, when in a supersaturated concentration, can precipitate and unite to form a stone. Keeping urine dilute and free flowing reduces the risk of recurrent stone formation in many individuals. A mucoprotein is formed in the kidneys as a matrix for the stone. Urinary pH, solute load, and inhibitors in the urine affect the formation of stones. The higher the pH (alkaline), the less soluble are calcium and phosphate. The lower the pH (acidic), the less soluble are uric acid and cystine. When a substance is not very soluble in fluid, it is more likely to precipitate out of solution.[23]

GENDER DIFFERENCES

Urinary Tract Calculi

Men	Women
• Urinary calculi disorders (except for struvite stones) are more common in men.	• Struvite stones associated with urinary tract infection are more common in women than in men.

TABLE 46-10	**RISK FACTORS FOR URINARY TRACT CALCULI**

Metabolic
• Abnormalities that result in increased urine levels of calcium, oxaluric acid, uric acid, or citric acid

Climate
• Warm climates that cause increased fluid loss, low urine volume, and increased solute concentration in urine

Diet
• Large intake of dietary proteins that increases uric acid excretion
• Excessive amounts of tea or fruit juices that elevate urinary oxalate level
• Large intake of calcium and oxalate
• Low fluid intake that increases urinary concentration

Genetic Factors
• Family history of stone formation, cystinuria, gout, or renal acidosis
• Lifestyle
• Sedentary occupation, immobility

Other important factors in the development of stones include obstruction with urinary stasis and UTI with urea-splitting bacteria (e.g., *Proteus, Klebsiella, Pseudomonas,* and some species of staphylococci). These bacteria cause the urine to become alkaline and contribute to the formation of struvite stones. Infected stones, entrapped in the kidney (Fig. 46-5), may assume a staghorn configuration as the stone branches to occupy a large portion of the collecting system. These stones can lead to a renal infection, hydronephrosis, and loss of kidney function. Genetic factors may also contribute to urine stone formation. Cystinuria, an autosomal recessive disorder, is characterized by a markedly increased excretion of cystine.

Types of Urinary Calculi

The term calculus refers to the stone, and *lithiasis* refers to stone formation. The five major categories of stones are (1) calcium phosphate, (2) calcium oxalate, (3) uric acid, (4) cystine, and (5) struvite (magnesium ammonium phosphate) (Table 46-11). Although calcium stones are the most common, stone composition may be mixed. Calculi can be found in various locations in the urinary tract (see Figs. 46-3 and 46-5).

Clinical Manifestations

The first symptom of a kidney stone is usually severe pain that begins suddenly. Typically, a person feels a sharp pain in the flank area, back, or lower abdomen. People describe the pain as the most excruciating that a person can endure. *Renal colic* is the term used for the sharp, severe pain, which results from the stretching, dilation, and spasm of the ureter in response to the obstructing stone. Nausea and vomiting may occur due to the severe pain.[24]

Urinary stones cause clinical manifestations when they obstruct urinary flow. Common sites of obstruction are at the UPJ (where the renal pelvis narrows into the ureter) and at the ureterovesical junction (UVJ). The type of pain is determined by the location of the stone. If the stone is nonobstructing, pain may be absent. If the obstruction is in a calyx or at the UPJ, the patient may experience dull costovertebral flank pain or renal colic. Pain resulting from the passage of a calculus down the ureter is intense and colicky.

Patients with renal colic have a hard time being still. They go from walking to sitting to lying down, and then they

TABLE 46-11	TYPES OF URINARY TRACT CALCULI	
Characteristics	**Predisposing Factors**	**Treatment**
Calcium Oxalate* Small, often possible to get trapped in ureter. More frequent in men than in women. *Incidence: 35%-40%*	Idiopathic hypercalciuria, hyperoxaluria, independent of urinary pH, family history	Increase hydration. Reduce dietary oxalate.† Give thiazide diuretics. Give cellulose phosphate to chelate calcium and prevent GI absorption. Give potassium citrate to maintain alkaline urine. Give cholestyramine to bind oxalate. Give calcium lactate to precipitate oxalate in GI tract. Reduce daily sodium intake.
Calcium Phosphate Mixed stones (typically), with struvite or oxalate stones. *Incidence: 8%-10%*	Alkaline urine, primary hyperparathyroidism	Treat underlying causes and other stones.
Struvite (Magnesium Ammonium Phosphate) Three or four times as common in women as men. Always associated with urinary tract infections. Large staghorn type (usually) (see Fig. 46-5). *Incidence: 10%-15%*	Urinary tract infections (usually *Proteus*)	Administer antimicrobial agents, acetohydroxamic acid. Use surgical intervention to remove stone. Take measures to acidify urine.
Uric Acid Predominant in men, high incidence in Jewish men. *Incidence: 5%-8%*	Gout, acidic urine, inherited condition	Reduce urinary concentration of uric acid. Alkalinize urine with potassium citrate. Administer allopurinol. Reduce dietary purines.†
Cystine Genetic autosomal recessive defect. Defective absorption of cystine in GI tract and kidney, excess concentrations causing stone formation. *Incidence: 1%-2%*	Acidic urine	Increase hydration. Give α-penicillamine and tiopronin to prevent cystine crystallization. Give potassium citrate to maintain alkaline urine.

*Calcium stones can exist as calcium oxalate, calcium phosphate, or a mixture of both. Calcium stones account for the majority of all stones.
†See Table 43-12: Causes of Peritonitis.

repeat the process. Some people refer to this as the *kidney stone dance.*

The patient may be in mild shock with cool, moist skin. As a stone nears the UVJ, pain moves around toward the abdomen and down toward the lower quadrant. Men may experience testicular pain, whereas women may complain of labial pain. Both men and women may experience pain in the groin. The patient may also have manifestations of UTI with dysuria, fever, and chills.

Diagnostic Studies

Noncontrast spiral CT, also called a CT/KUB (kidneys, ureters, bladder), is the diagnostic study commonly used in patients with renal colic. It is quick and noninvasive and requires no IV contrast. In some situations, ultrasound and IVP are used. A complete urinalysis helps confirm the diagnosis of a urinary stone by assessing for hematuria, crystalluria, and urinary pH.

Retrieval and analysis of the stones are important in the diagnosis of the underlying problem contributing to stone formation. The patient's serum calcium, phosphorus, sodium, potassium, bicarbonate, uric acid, BUN, and creatinine levels are also measured. A careful history should include any previous episodes of stone formation, prescribed and OTC medications, dietary supplements, and family history of urinary calculi. Measurement of urine pH is useful in the diagnosis of struvite stones and renal tubular acidosis (tendency to alkaline or high pH) and uric acid stones (tendency to acidic or low pH). Patients who are recurrent stone formers should undergo a 24-hour urinary measurement of calcium, phosphorus, magnesium, sodium, oxalate, citrate, sulfate, potassium, uric acid, and total volume.

Collaborative Care

Evaluation and management of a patient with renal calculi consist of two concurrent approaches. The first approach is directed toward management of the acute attack by treating the pain, infection, and/or obstruction. Administer opioids to relieve renal colic pain. Most stones are 4 mm or less in size and will probably pass spontaneously. However, it may take weeks for a stone to pass.

Tamsulosin (Flomax) or terazosin (Hytrin), α-adrenergic blockers that relax the smooth muscle in the ureter, can be used to facilitate stone passage. These drugs are also used to relax the muscle tissue in the prostate in men with BPH.

The second approach is directed toward evaluation of the cause of the stone formation and the prevention of further stone development. Obtain information from the patient, including a family history of stone formation; geographic residence; nutritional assessment, including the intake of vitamins A and D; activity pattern (active or sedentary); history of prolonged illness with immobilization or dehydration; and any history of disease or surgery involving the GI or genitourinary tract.

Therapy for active stone formers requires a comprehensive management approach, with the primary emphasis on teaching. Adequate hydration, dietary sodium restrictions, dietary changes, and drugs are employed to minimize urinary stone formation (see Table 46-11). Various drugs are prescribed, depending on the specific problem underlying the stone formation. These drugs prevent stone formation in various ways, including altering urine pH, preventing excessive urinary excretion of a substance, or correcting a primary disease (e.g., hyperparathyroidism).

Treatment of struvite stones requires control of infection. This may be difficult if the stone remains in place. In addition

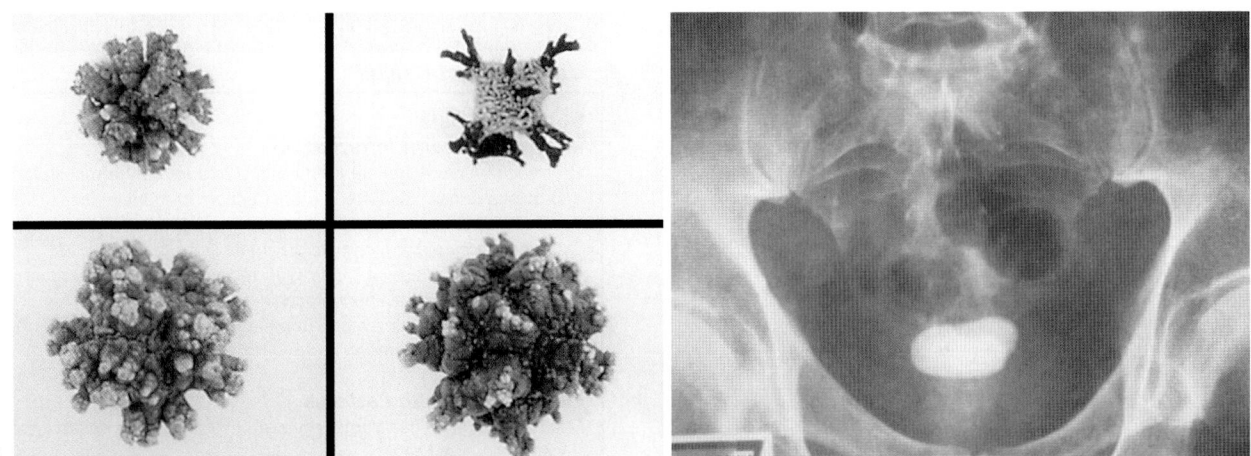

FIG. 46-6 **A,** Calcium oxalate stones. **B,** Plain abdominal x-ray showing large bladder calculus.

to antibiotics, acetohydroxamic acid may be used to treat kidney infections that result in the continual formation of struvite stones. Acetohydroxamic acid inhibits the chemical action caused by the persistent bacteria and thus retards struvite stone formation. The stone may have to be removed surgically if the infection cannot be controlled.

Indications for endourologic, lithotripsy, or open surgical stone removal include the following: (1) stones too large for spontaneous passage (usually greater than 7 mm); (2) stones associated with bacteriuria or symptomatic infection; (3) stones causing impaired renal function; (4) stones causing persistent pain, nausea, or paralytic ileus; (5) inability of patient to be treated medically; and (6) patient with only one kidney.

Endourologic Procedures. If the stone is located in the bladder, a cystoscopy is done to remove small stones. For large stones (Fig. 46-6), a *cystolitholapaxy* is done. In this procedure, large stones are broken up with an instrument called a lithotrite (stone crusher). The bladder is then irrigated and the crushed stones washed out. A *cystoscopic lithotripsy* uses an ultrasonic lithotrite to pulverize (break up) stones. Complications associated with these cystoscopic procedures include hemorrhage, retained stone fragments, and infection.

Flexible *ureteroscopes,* inserted via a cystoscope, can be used to remove stones from the renal pelvis and upper urinary tract. Ultrasonic, laser, or electrohydraulic lithotripsy may be used in conjunction with the ureteroscope to pulverize the stone.

In *percutaneous nephrolithotomy,* a nephroscope is inserted into the kidney pelvis through a track (using a sheath) in the skin. The track is created in the patient's back. The kidney stones can be fragmented using ultrasound, electrohydraulic, or laser lithotripsy. The stone fragments are removed, and the pelvis is irrigated. A percutaneous nephrostomy tube is usually left in place to make sure that the ureter is not obstructed. Complications include bleeding, injury to adjacent structures, and infection.

Lithotripsy. Lithotripsy is a procedure used to eliminate calculi from the urinary tract. Lithotripsy techniques include (1) laser lithotripsy, (2) extracorporeal shock-wave lithotripsy (ESWL), (3) percutaneous ultrasonic lithotripsy, and (4) electrohydraulic lithotripsy. *Laser lithotripsy* is used to fragment ureteral and large bladder stones (bladder stones are described above). To access ureteral stones, a ureteroscope is used to get close to the stone. A small fiber is inserted up the endoscope so that the tip (which emits the laser energy) can come in contact

with the stone. A holmium laser in direct contact with the stone is commonly used. The intense energy breaks the stone into small pieces, which can be extracted or flushed out. Because of the type of laser energy, no other tissue is affected. This minimally invasive treatment usually requires general anesthesia.[25]

In *extracorporeal shock-wave lithotripsy (ESWL),* a noninvasive procedure, the patient is anesthetized (spinal or general) to ensure that he or she maintains the same position during the procedure. Fluoroscopy or ultrasound is used to focus the lithotripter on the affected kidney, and a high-voltage spark generator produces high-energy acoustic shock waves that shatter the stone without damaging the surrounding tissues. The stone is broken into fine sand *(steinstrasse)* and excreted in the urine.

In *percutaneous ultrasonic lithotripsy* an ultrasonic probe is placed in the renal pelvis via a percutaneous nephroscope inserted through a small incision in the flank, and is then positioned against the stone. The patient is given general or spinal anesthesia for this procedure. The probe produces ultrasonic waves, which break the stone into sandlike particles.

In *electrohydraulic lithotripsy* the probe is positioned directly on a stone, but it breaks the stone into small fragments that are removed by forceps or by suction. A continuous saline irrigation flushes out the stone particles, and all of the outflow drainage is strained so that the particles can be analyzed. The calculi can also be removed by basket extraction. Complications are rare but they include hemorrhage, sepsis, and abscess formation. Postoperatively, the patient usually complains of moderate to severe colicky pain. The first few times that the patient urinates, the urine is bright red. As the bleeding subsides, the urine becomes dark red or a smoky color. Antibiotics are usually administered after the procedure to reduce the risk of infection.

Hematuria is common after lithotripsy procedures. A self-retaining ureteral stent is often placed after the procedure to facilitate passage of sand (shattered stone) and prevent sand buildup within the ureter, which might lead to obstruction. The stent is typically removed within 2 weeks following lithotripsy. If a stone is large or positioned in the mid or distal ureter, additional treatment, such as surgery, may be necessary.

Surgical Therapy. A small group of patients require open surgical procedures. The primary indications for surgery include pain, infection, and obstruction. The type of open surgery performed depends on the location of the stone. A *nephrolithotomy* is an incision into the kidney to remove a stone. A *pyelolithot-*

TABLE 46-12   **NUTRITIONAL THERAPY**
Urinary Tract Calculi
Depending on the type of calculi, modify the diet to decrease foods that are high in the substance that is the cause of the calculi. Listed below are foods that are moderate or high in purine, calcium, or oxalate content. **Purine*** *High:* Sardines, herring, mussels, liver, kidney, goose, venison, meat soups, sweetbreads *Moderate:* Chicken, salmon, crab, veal, mutton, bacon, pork, beef, ham **Calcium** *High:* Milk, cheese, ice cream, yogurt, sauces containing milk; all beans (except green beans), lentils; fish with fine bones (e.g., sardines, kippers, herring, salmon); dried fruits, nuts; Ovaltine, chocolate, cocoa **Oxalate** *High:* Dark roughage, spinach, rhubarb, asparagus, cabbage, tomatoes, beets, nuts, celery, parsley, runner beans; chocolate, cocoa, instant coffee, Ovaltine, tea; Worcestershire sauce

*Uric acid is a waste product from purine in food.

omy is an incision into the renal pelvis for stone removal. If the stone is located within the ureter, a *ureterolithotomy* is performed. A *cystotomy* may be indicated for bladder calculi. For open surgery on the kidney or ureter, a flank incision directly below the diaphragm and across the side is usually preferred. The most common complications after surgical procedures for stone removal are related to hemorrhage.

Nutritional Therapy. To manage an obstructing stone, have the patient drink adequate fluids to avoid dehydration. Forcing excessive fluids is not advised, since this has not proved effective in facilitating spontaneous passage (excretion) of stones via the urine. Forcing fluids may also increase the pain or precipitate the development of renal colic.

After an episode of urolithiasis, encourage a high fluid intake (approximately 3 L/day) to produce a urine output of at least 2 L/day. High urine output prevents supersaturation of minerals (i.e., dilutes the concentration of urine) and promotes excretion of minerals within the urine, thus preventing stone formation. Increasing the fluid intake is particularly important for patients at risk for dehydration, including those who (1) are active in sports, (2) live in a dry climate, (3) perform physical exercise, (4) have a family history of stone formation, or (5) work outside or in an occupation that requires a great deal of physical activity. Water is the preferred fluid. Limit consumption of colas, coffee, and tea because high intake of these beverages tends to increase the risk of recurring urinary calculi.

A low-sodium diet is recommended, since high-sodium intake increases calcium excretion in the urine. Foods high in calcium, oxalate, and purines are presented in Table 46-12.

NURSING MANAGEMENT
URINARY TRACT CALCULI

NURSING ASSESSMENT

Subjective and objective data that should be obtained from a patient with urinary tract calculi are presented in Table 46-13.

TABLE 46-13   **NURSING ASSESSMENT**
Urinary Tract Calculi
Subjective Data **Important Health Information** *Past health history:* Recent or chronic UTI; bed rest; immobilization; previous urinary tract stones, obstruction, or kidney disease with urinary stasis; gout; benign prostatic hyperplasia (BPH); hyperparathyroidism, chronic diarrhea *Medications:* Prior use of medication for prevention of stones or treatment of UTI; allopurinol, analgesics, loop diuretics *Surgery or other treatments:* External urinary diversion, long-term indwelling urinary catheter ***Functional Health Patterns*** *Health perception–health management:* Family history of renal calculi; sedentary lifestyle *Nutritional-metabolic:* Nausea, vomiting; dietary intake of purines, excessive calcium ingestion, salt excess, oxalates, phosphates; low fluid intake; chills *Elimination:* Decreased urine output, urinary urgency, frequency, feeling of bladder fullness *Cognitive-perceptual:* Acute, severe, colicky pain in flank, back, abdomen, groin, or genitalia; burning on urination, dysuria; anxiety **Objective Data** **General** Guarding, back pain, fever, dehydration ***Integumentary*** Warm, flushed skin or pallor with cool, moist skin (mild shock) ***Gastrointestinal*** Abdominal distention, absence of bowel sounds ***Urinary*** Oliguria, hematuria, tenderness on palpation of renal areas, passage of stone or stones ***Possible Diagnostic Findings*** ↑ BUN and serum creatinine levels; RBCs, WBCs, pyuria, crystals, casts, minerals, bacteria on urinalysis; ↑ uric acid, calcium, phosphorus, oxalate, or cystine values on 24-hr urine sample; calculi or anatomic changes on IVP or KUB x-ray; direct visualization of obstruction on cystoureteroscopy

IVP, Intravenous pyelogram; *KUB,* kidneys, ureters, bladder; *UTI,* urinary tract infection.

NURSING DIAGNOSES

Nursing diagnoses for the patient with urinary tract calculi include, but are not limited to, the following:

- Impaired urinary elimination *related to* trauma or obstruction of ureters or urethra
- Acute pain *related to* effects of stones and inadequate pain control or comfort measures
- Deficient knowledge *related to* unfamiliarity with information resources and lack of experience with urinary stones

Additional information on nursing diagnoses for the patient with urinary tract calculi is presented in eNursing Care Plan 46-2 (on the website for this chapter).

PLANNING

The overall goals are that the patient with urinary tract calculi will have (1) relief of pain, (2) no urinary tract obstruction, and (3) knowledge of ways to prevent recurrence of stones.

NURSING IMPLEMENTATION

Most people who have had urinary stones can lower their risk of recurrence by changing their lifestyle and dietary habits. Adequate fluid intake is important to produce a urine output of approximately 2 L/day. Consult with the health care provider about recommendations for fluid intake in a given patient. The moderately active, ambulatory person should drink about 3 L/day. Fluid intake needs to be higher in the active patient who works outdoors or who regularly engages in athletic activities. In contrast, fluid intake is less for the sedentary or immobile person. Preventive measures related to the person who is on bed rest or is relatively immobile for a prolonged time include maintaining an adequate fluid intake, turning the patient every 2 hours, and helping the patient sit or stand, if possible, to maximize urinary flow.

Additional preventive measures focus on reducing metabolic or secondary risk factors. For example, dietary restriction of purines may be helpful for the patient at risk for developing uric acid stones. Teach the patient the dosage, scheduling, and potential side effects of drugs used to reduce the risk of stone formation (see Table 46-11). Some patients may be taught to self-monitor urinary pH or urine output.

Pain management and patient comfort are primary nursing responsibilities when managing an obstructing stone and renal colic (see eNursing Care Plan 46-2). To ensure that any spontaneously passed stones are retrieved, strain all urine voided by the patient using a gauze or a urine strainer. Encourage ambulation to promote movement of the stone from the upper to the lower urinary tract. To ensure safety, tell the patient not to walk unattended while experiencing acute renal colic, particularly if opioid analgesics are being given.

EVALUATION

The expected outcomes are that the patient with urinary calculi will

- Maintain free flow of urine with minimal hematuria
- Report satisfactory pain relief
- Verbalize understanding of disease process and measures to prevent recurrence

Additional information on expected outcomes for the patient with urinary calculi is presented in eNursing Care Plan 46-2 (on the website for this chapter).

STRICTURES

A stricture is a narrowing of the lumen of the ureter or urethra.

Ureteral Strictures

Ureteral strictures can affect the entire length of the ureter, from the UPJ to the UVJ. These strictures are usually an unintended result of surgical intervention or secondary to adhesions or scar formation, or they may be due to extrinsic factors such as large tumors in the peritoneal cavity. Depending on its severity, ureteral obstruction can threaten the function of the kidney.

Clinical manifestations of a ureteral stricture include mild to moderate colic. This pain may be moderate to severe in intensity if the patient consumes a large volume of fluids (such as alcohol) over a brief period. Infection is unusual unless a calculus or foreign object such as a stent or nephrostomy tube is present.

The discomfort and obstruction of a ureteral stricture may be temporarily bypassed by placing a stent using endoscopy or by diverting urinary flow via a nephrostomy tube inserted into the renal pelvis of the affected kidney. Definitive correction requires dilation with a balloon or catheter. If the stricture is severe or recurs after initial balloon or catheter dilation, it is surgically incised using an endoscopic procedure *(endoureterotomy)*. In selected cases an open surgical approach may be required to excise the stenotic area and reanastomose the ureter to the contralateral ureter *(ureteroureterostomy)* or to the renal pelvis. Alternatively, distal ureteral strictures may be treated by a *ureteroneocystostomy* (reimplantation of the ureter into the bladder wall).

Urethral Strictures

A *urethral stricture* is the result of fibrosis or inflammation of the urethral lumen. Causes of urethral strictures include trauma, urethritis (particularly after gonococcal infection), surgical intervention or repeated catheterizations (iatrogenic), or a congenital defect of the urethra. Once the process of inflammation and fibrosis begins, the lumen of the urethra narrows, and its compliance (ability to close or open in response to bladder filling or micturition) is compromised. Meatal stenosis, a narrowing of the urethral opening, is also common.

Clinical manifestations associated with a urethral stricture include a diminished force of the urinary stream, straining to void, sprayed stream, postvoid dribbling, or a split urine stream. The patient may report feelings of incomplete bladder emptying with urinary frequency and nocturia. Moderate to severe obstruction of the bladder outlet may lead to acute urinary retention. The patient may report a history of urethritis, difficulty with insertion of a urinary catheter, or trauma involving the penis or the perineum. However, many patients are unable to recall any such events, thus leading to a diagnosis of an idiopathic stricture. A history of UTI is common, particularly if the stricture involves the distal urethra. Retrograde urethrography (RUG) and VCUG are used to identify stricture length, location, and caliber.

Initial management of a stricture is focused on dilation. A metal instrument (urethral sound) may be placed, or a series of progressively large stents (filiforms and followers) can be placed into the urethra to expand its lumen in a stepwise fashion. Although this process is initially successful, stenosis frequently recurs. Recurrences may be managed by teaching the patient to repeatedly dilate the urethra by self-catheterization using a soft (coudé-tip, red rubber) catheter every few days. Alternatively, an endoscopic or open surgical procedure *(urethroplasty)* may be a more definitive therapy for an obstructive urethral stricture. Shorter strictures may be treated by resection of the fibrotic area followed by reanastomosis of the urethra. Longer strictures may require the use of a skin flap as a substitute urethral segment.

RENAL TRAUMA

Renal trauma can be blunt or penetrating. *Blunt trauma* is the most common cause. Injury to the kidney should be considered in sports injuries, motor vehicle collisions, and falls. Renal trauma is especially likely when the patient injures the abdomen, flank, or back. *Penetrating injuries* may result from violent encounters (e.g., gunshot or stabbing incidents). The majority of incidents occur in men younger than 30 years of age.

Clinical findings include a history of trauma to the area of the kidneys. Gross or microscopic hematuria may be present.

Diagnostic studies include urinalysis, ultrasound, CT, or MRI evaluation. Renal arteriography may also be used. Both the injured kidney and the uninvolved kidney should be evaluated. The severity of renal trauma depends on the extent of the injury. Treatments range from bed rest, fluids, and analgesia to exploratory surgery and repair or nephrectomy.

Nursing interventions depend on the type of renal trauma and the extent of any associated injuries. Interventions related to renal trauma include the following: (1) assess the cardiovascular status and monitor for shock, especially in a penetrating injury; (2) ensure adequate fluid intake and monitor intake and output; (3) provide for pain relief and comfort measures; and (4) assess for hematuria and myoglobinuria.

RENAL VASCULAR PROBLEMS

Vascular problems involving the kidney include (1) nephrosclerosis, (2) renal artery stenosis, and (3) renal vein thrombosis.

NEPHROSCLEROSIS

Nephrosclerosis is sclerosis of the small arteries and arterioles of the kidney. The decreased blood flow results in ischemia and necrosis of parts of the kidney. *Benign nephrosclerosis,* which usually occurs in adults 30 to 50 years of age, is caused by vascular changes resulting from hypertension and from the atherosclerosis process. Atherosclerotic vascular changes account for most of the loss of renal function associated with aging. The degree of nephrosclerosis is directly related to the severity of hypertension. In the early stages, the patient with benign nephrosclerosis may have normal renal function, with the only detectable abnormality being hypertension.

Accelerated nephrosclerosis (malignant nephrosclerosis) is associated with malignant hypertension, which is characterized by a sharp increase in BP with a diastolic pressure greater than 130 mm Hg. The patient is usually a young adult, with a male-to-female predominance of 2:1. Renal insufficiency progresses rapidly.

Treatment for benign nephrosclerosis is the same as that for essential hypertension (see Chapter 33). Malignant nephrosclerosis is treated with aggressive antihypertensive therapy (see Chapter 33). The availability and use of antihypertensive drugs have improved the prognosis for patients with benign and malignant nephrosclerosis. Kidney disease, and subsequent renal failure, is a major complication of hypertension. The prognosis for a patient with untreated or refractory malignant hypertension is poor, with the major cause of death related to renal failure.

RENAL ARTERY STENOSIS

Renal artery stenosis is a partial occlusion of one or both renal arteries and their major branches. It can be due to atherosclerotic narrowing or fibromuscular hyperplasia. Renal artery stenosis, which accounts for 1% to 2% of all cases of hypertension, is a cause of secondary hypertension.

When hypertension develops rather abruptly, renal artery stenosis should be considered as a possible cause, especially in patients under 30 or over 50 years of age and in patients with no family history of hypertension. This contrasts with the age distribution for primary hypertension, which is 30 to 50 years of age. Diagnostic tests used to assess for renal artery stenosis include a renal ultrasound, CT scan, MRI scan, and renal arteriogram (the best diagnostic tool).

The goals of therapy are to control the BP and restore perfusion to the kidney. Percutaneous transluminal renal angioplasty is the procedure of choice, especially in older patients who are poor surgical risks. Surgical revascularization of the kidney is indicated when decreased blood flow causes renal ischemia or when renovascular hypertension is present. Revascularization of the kidney may result in the patient becoming normotensive. The surgical procedure usually involves anastomoses between the kidney and another major artery, usually the splenic artery or aorta. In selected cases of unilateral renal involvement, unilateral nephrectomy may be indicated.

RENAL VEIN THROMBOSIS

Renal vein thrombosis may occur unilaterally or bilaterally. Causes include trauma, extrinsic compression (e.g., tumor, aortic aneurysm), renal cell cancer, pregnancy, contraceptive use, and nephrotic syndrome.

The patient has symptoms of flank pain, hematuria, or fever or has nephrotic syndrome. Anticoagulation (e.g., heparin, warfarin [Coumadin]) is important to treat the high incidence of pulmonary emboli. Corticosteroids may be used for the patient with nephrotic syndrome. Surgical thrombectomy may be performed instead of or along with anticoagulation.

HEREDITARY KIDNEY DISEASES

Hereditary kidney (or renal) diseases involve developmental abnormalities of the renal parenchyma. Most inherited structural abnormalities are cystic. However, cysts may also develop as a result of obstructive uropathies, metabolic problems, or neurologic diseases. Cysts may be evaluated to rule out tumors.

POLYCYSTIC KIDNEY DISEASE

Polycystic kidney disease (PKD) is the most common life-threatening genetic disease in the world, affecting 600,000 people in the United States. PKD accounts for 10% to 15% of chronic kidney disease.[26]

Genetic Link

PKD has two hereditary forms: it may be manifested in childhood or adulthood. The childhood form of PKD is a rare autosomal recessive disorder that is often rapidly progressive (see the Genetics in Clinical Practice box). The adult form of PKD is an autosomal dominant disorder (see Figs. 13-4 and 13-5). If one parent has the disease, there is a 50% chance that the disease will pass to the child.

Adult PKD is latent for many years and is usually manifested between 30 and 40 years of age. It involves both kidneys and occurs in both men and women. The cortex and the medulla are filled with large, thin-walled cysts that are several millimeters to several centimeters in diameter (Fig. 46-7). The cysts enlarge and destroy surrounding tissue by compression. The cysts are filled with fluid and may contain blood or pus. PKD kidneys examined during autopsy appear as if they are filled with golf balls.

Early in the disease patients are generally asymptomatic. Symptoms appear when the cysts begin to enlarge. Often the first manifestations of PKD are hypertension; hematuria (from

GENETICS IN CLINICAL PRACTICE

Polycystic Kidney Disease (PKD)

	Adult	Child
Genetic basis	• Autosomal dominant	• Autosomal recessive
Incidence	• 1 in 400-1000	• 1 in 10,000-20,000
Gene location	• *PKD1* gene on chromosome 16 and *PKD2* gene on chromosome 4 • Genes code for polycystins (proteins that promote normal kidney development and function) • Mutations in genes lead to formation of thousands of cysts that disrupt the normal function of kidneys and other organs	• Polycystic kidney and hepatic disease *(PKHD1)* gene on chromosome 6 • Gene codes for fibrocystin • Mutations in gene leads to cyst formation
Genetic testing	• DNA testing available	• DNA testing available*
Age of onset	• Ages 30-40	• Infancy or childhood
Clinical implications	• Multisystem involvement • Systemic hypertension occurs in 60%-80% of patients • Increased risk for cerebral aneurysms • Families at risk should be screened	• Up to 30%-50% of affected newborns die shortly after birth • If infant survives the newborn period, chances of survival are good, but about one third need dialysis or transplantation by age 10 yr

*Genetic testing is also available on fertilized embryos before implantation. This allows embryos free of the disorder to be placed into the uterus.

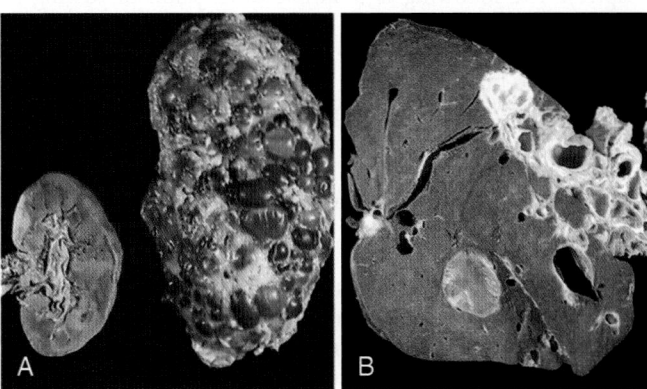

FIG. 46-7 A, Comparison of polycystic kidney with normal kidney. **B,** Cysts in the liver.

rupture of cysts); or a feeling of heaviness in the back, side, or abdomen. However, the first manifestations can also be a UTI or urinary calculi. Chronic pain is one of the most common problems experienced by individuals with PKD. The pain can be constant and severe. Bilateral, enlarged kidneys are often palpable on physical examination. Many people have no symptoms, and the disease is not diagnosed.

PKD can also affect the liver (liver cysts [see Fig. 46-7]), heart (abnormal heart valves), blood vessels (aneurysms), and intestines (diverticulosis). The most serious complication is a cerebral aneurysm, which can rupture.

Diagnosis is based on clinical manifestations, family history, ultrasound (best screening measure), or CT scan. The disease usually progresses from loss of kidney function to ESKD by age 60 in 50% of patients.[27]

NURSING AND COLLABORATIVE MANAGEMENT
POLYCYSTIC KIDNEY DISEASE

There is no specific treatment for PKD. A major aim of treatment is to prevent or treat infections of the urinary tract. Nephrectomy may be necessary if pain, bleeding, or infection becomes a chronic, serious problem. Dialysis and kidney transplant may be needed to treat ESKD (see Chapter 47).

When the patient begins to experience progressive renal failure, the interventions depend on the remaining renal function. Nursing measures are those used for management of ESKD. They include diet modification, fluid restriction, drugs (e.g., antihypertensives), and assistance for the patient and family in coping with the chronic disease process and financial concerns.

The patient who has adult PKD often has children by the time the disease is diagnosed. The patient needs appropriate counseling regarding plans for having more children. In addition, genetic counseling should be provided for the children.

MEDULLARY CYSTIC DISEASE

Medullary cystic disease is a hereditary disorder that occurs in two forms. The *autosomal recessive form* is associated with renal failure before age 20. The *autosomal dominant form* is associated with renal failure after age 20.

Most cysts are located in the medulla. The kidneys are asymmetric in shape and are significantly scarred. Defects in the kidneys' concentrating ability result in polyuria. Other clinical manifestations include hypertension, progressive renal failure, severe anemia, and metabolic acidosis. Genetic counseling may be helpful in family planning. Treatment measures are those related to ESKD (see Chapter 47).

ALPORT SYNDROME

Alport syndrome, also known as *chronic hereditary nephritis,* has two forms: (1) classic Alport syndrome, which is inherited as a sex-linked disorder with hematuria, sensorineural deafness, and deformities of the anterior surface of the lens; and (2) nonclassic Alport syndrome, which is inherited as an autosomal disorder that causes hematuria but not deafness or lens deformities.

Men are affected earlier and more severely than women. The disease is often diagnosed in the first decade of life. The basic defect is a mutation in a gene for collagen that results in altered synthesis of the GBM. Most commonly the patient has hematuria and progressive uremia. Treatment is supportive. Corticosteroids and cytotoxic drugs are not effective. The disease does not recur after kidney transplantation.

URINARY TRACT TUMORS

KIDNEY CANCER

Kidney cancers arise from the cortex or pelvis (and calyces). Tumors from these areas may be benign or malignant. However, malignant tumors are more common. In the United States, about 65,000 new cases of kidney cancer are diagnosed each year and about 13,570 people die from kidney cancer. The incidence of kidney cancer is increasing, but the reason for this is not known.[28]

Renal cell carcinoma (adenocarcinoma) is the most common type of kidney cancer (Fig. 46-8). This type of tumor occurs twice as often in men as in women and is typically discovered when the person is 50 to 70 years of age. Cigarette smoking is the most significant risk factor for the development of renal cell carcinoma. An increased incidence has also been found in first-degree relatives of people who have or had renal cell carcinoma. Other risk factors include obesity; hypertension; and exposure to asbestos, cadmium, and gasoline. Risk for kidney cancer is also increased in individuals who have acquired cystic disease of the kidney associated with ESKD (see Chapter 47).[29]

Clinical Manifestations and Diagnostic Studies

Kidney cancer has no characteristic early symptoms, so many patients go undiagnosed until the disease has significantly progressed. Kidney tumors can cause symptoms by compressing, stretching, or invading structures near or within the kidney. The most common presenting manifestations are hematuria, flank pain, and a palpable mass in the flank or abdomen. Other clinical manifestations include weight loss, fever, hypertension, and anemia.

About 30% of patients have metastasis at the time of diagnosis. Local extension of kidney cancer into the renal vein and vena cava is common (see Fig. 46-8). The most common sites of metastases include lungs, liver, and long bones. Many kidney cancers are diagnosed as incidental findings on imaging studies used to evaluate symptoms for unrelated conditions.

CT scan is commonly used in the diagnosis and can detect small kidney tumors. Ultrasound examinations have improved the ability to differentiate between a solid mass tumor and a cyst. This is significant because the majority of masses detected on imaging are cysts. Angiography, biopsy, and MRI are also used in the diagnosis of renal tumors. Radionuclide isotope scanning is used to detect metastases.

NURSING AND COLLABORATIVE MANAGEMENT KIDNEY CANCER

Preventive measures, such as quitting smoking, maintaining a healthy weight, controlling BP, and reducing or avoiding exposure to toxins, can help reduce the incidence of kidney cancer. Patients in high-risk groups should be aware of their increased risk for kidney cancer. Teach them about early symptoms (e.g., hematuria, hypertension). A cure for kidney cancer is possible when it is detected early and treated.

Collaborative care of the patient with kidney cancer is presented in Table 46-14. Staging of renal carcinoma provides a basis for determining treatment options. A detailed listing of staging is presented in eTable 46-1 (on the website for this chapter). The following is a simple description of staging of kidney cancer:

Stage I: The tumor can be up to 7 cm in diameter but is confined to the kidney.

Stage II: The tumor is larger than a stage I tumor, but is still confined to the kidney.

Stage III: The tumor extends beyond the kidney to the surrounding tissue and may also have spread to a nearby lymph node.

Stage IV: Cancer spreads outside the kidney to multiple lymph nodes or to distant parts of the body, such as bones, brain, liver, or lung.

The treatment of choice for some renal cancers is a partial nephrectomy (for smaller tumors) or a radical nephrectomy (for larger tumors). Radical nephrectomy involves removal of the kidney, adrenal gland, surrounding fascia, part of the ureter, and draining lymph nodes. Nephrectomy can be performed by a conventional (open) approach or laparoscopically (see discussion of nephrectomy on p. 1095). Radiation therapy is used palliatively in inoperable cases and when there is metastasis to bone or lungs.

Other treatment options include cryoablation (freezing technique) and radiofrequency ablation (destroying tumor by using radiofrequency heat). These procedures can be used when surgery is not an option (e.g., patient has co-morbid conditions).

Chemotherapy is used as a treatment in metastatic disease. These drugs include 5-fluorouracil (5-FU), floxuridine (FUDR),

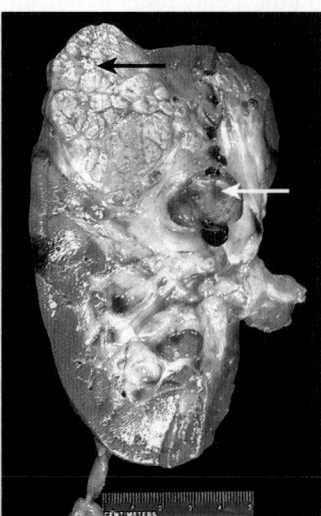

FIG. 46-8 Cross section of kidney with renal cell carcinoma. The carcinoma *(black arrow)* is on the pole of the kidney. Note that the renal vein is involved and thrombosed *(white arrow).*

TABLE 46-14 **COLLABORATIVE CARE**
Renal Cell Carcinoma

Diagnostic	Collaborative Therapy
• History and physical examination	• Surgical treatment
	• Partial nephrectomy
• Urinalysis	• Radical nephrectomy
• Ultrasound	• Ablation
• CT scan	• Cryoablation
• MRI	• Radiofrequency ablation
• Renal biopsy	• Radiation therapy
• Renal scan	• Chemotherapy
• Angiography	• Biologic therapy
	• Targeted therapy

and gemcitabine (Gemzar). However, renal cell carcinoma is refractory to most chemotherapy drugs.

Biologic therapy, including α-interferon and interleukin-2 (IL-2), is another treatment in metastatic disease. (The use of α-interferon and IL-2 is discussed in Chapter 16.)

Targeted therapy is the preferred treatment for metastatic kidney cancer. Kinase inhibitors, one class of targeted therapies, block certain proteins (kinases) that play a role in tumor growth and cancer progression. Kinase inhibitors include sunitinib (Sutent), sorafenib (Nexavar), and axitinib (Inlyta). Bevacizumab (Avastin) and pazopanib (Votrient) inhibit the formation of new blood vessel growth to the tumor. Temsirolimus (Torisel) and everolimus (Afinitor) inhibit a specific protein known as the mammalian target of rapamycin (mTOR). These drugs are presented in Table 16-13, and the mechanisms of action are shown in Fig. 16-16.

The diagnosis of cancer is a shock. In kidney cancer the disease can already be metastasized by the time a person is diagnosed. (The nursing care of the patient with cancer is discussed in Chapter 16.)

BLADDER CANCER

About 73,000 new cases of bladder cancer are diagnosed annually, and about 15,000 deaths related to bladder cancer occur every year.[28] Bladder cancer accounts for nearly 1 in every 20 cancers diagnosed in the United States. The most frequent malignant tumor of the urinary tract is transitional cell carcinoma of the bladder. Most bladder tumors are papillomatous growths within the bladder (Fig. 46-9).

Cancer of the bladder is most common between ages 60 and 70 years and is at least three times more common in men than in women. Risk factors for bladder cancer include cigarette smoking, exposure to dyes used in the rubber and other industries, and chronic abuse of phenacetin-containing analgesics. Phenacetin, once a popular analgesic, has been removed from the market. Women treated with radiation for cervical cancer, patients who received cyclophosphamide, and patients who take the diabetes drug pioglitazone (Actos) also have an increased risk for bladder cancer.

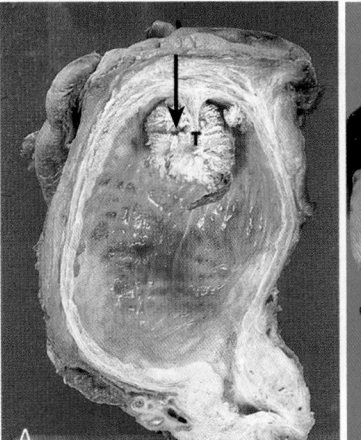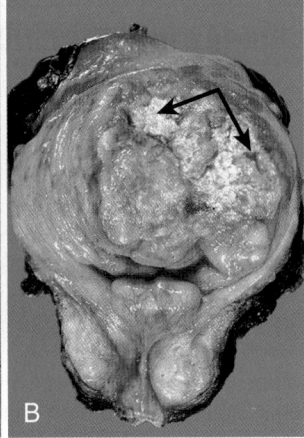

FIG. 46-9 A, Papillary transitional cell carcinoma *(T)* seen arising from the dome of the bladder as a cauliflower-like lesion *(arrow).* **B,** Opened bladder showing bladder cancer at an advanced stage. Yellow areas represent ulcerations and necrosis *(arrows).*

Individuals with chronic, recurrent renal calculi (often bladder) and chronic lower UTIs have an increased risk of squamous cell cancer of the bladder. Patients who have indwelling catheters for long periods are also at an increased risk to develop bladder cancer.

Clinical Manifestations and Diagnostic Studies

Microscopic or gross, painless hematuria (chronic or intermittent) is the most common clinical manifestation of bladder cancer. Bladder irritability with dysuria, frequency, and urgency may also occur. When cancer is suspected, obtain urine specimens to identify any neoplastic or atypical cells. Exfoliated cells from the bladder's epithelial surface can be detected in voided specimens. Other urine tests assess for specific factors associated with bladder cancer, such as bladder tumor antigens.

Bladder cancers can be detected using CT, ultrasound, or MRI. The presence of cancer is confirmed by cystoscopy and biopsy. Cystoscopy with biopsy is the most reliable test for detecting bladder tumors.

NURSING AND COLLABORATIVE MANAGEMENT BLADDER CANCER

The majority of bladder cancers are diagnosed at an early stage when the cancer is treatable. Before a treatment regimen is started, bladder cancers are graded based on the cell type and staged based on the extent and invasiveness of the cancer. A grading system is used to classify the malignant potential of tumor cells, using a scale from well differentiated (closely resembling the normal tissue) to undifferentiated (poorly differentiated) (see p. 254 in Chapter 16).

The clinical staging of bladder cancer is determined by the depth of invasion of the bladder wall and surrounding tissue. Staging of bladder cancer is presented in detail in eTable 46-2 (on the website for this chapter). The following is a simple description of staging of bladder cancer:

Stage I: Cancer is in the inner lining of the bladder but has not invaded the bladder muscle wall.

Stage II: Cancer has invaded the bladder wall but is still confined to bladder.

Stage III: Cancer has spread through the bladder wall to surrounding tissue. It may also have spread to the prostate in men or the uterus or vagina in women.

Stage IV: Cancer has spread to the lymph nodes and other organs, such as lungs, bones, or liver.

Eighty percent of bladder tumors are *superficial*, meaning they do not invade the bladder wall. Low-grade, low-stage bladder cancers are the most responsive to treatment, which includes instillation of intravesical chemotherapy. Although patients with superficial tumors are more easily cured, periodic surveillance is important, since two thirds of patients have tumor recurrence within 5 years and nearly 95% have recurrence by 15 years.

Collaborative care of bladder cancer includes surgery, radiation, chemotherapy, and intravesical therapy (Table 46-15).

SURGICAL THERAPY

Surgical therapies include a variety of procedures. *Transurethral resection of the bladder tumor* (TURBT) is used for superficial lesions of the bladder's inner lining. A wire loop inserted through the cystoscope is used to cauterize (with electric current or laser) and kill the cancer cells. This procedure is also used to

TABLE 46-15　COLLABORATIVE CARE

Bladder Cancer

Diagnostic	Collaborative Therapy
• History and physical examination • Urinalysis • Urine cytology studies • Intravenous pyelogram (IVP) • Cystoscopy with biopsy • Ultrasound • CT scan	• Surgical treatment 　• Transurethral resection with fulguration 　• Laser photocoagulation 　• Open loop resection with fulguration 　• Cystectomy (segmental, partial, or radical) • Radiation therapy • Intravesical immunotherapy 　• Bacille Calmette-Guérin (BCG) 　• α-interferon (Roferon-A, Intron A) • Intravesical chemotherapy 　• thiotepa (Thioplex) 　• valrubicin (Valstar) • Systemic chemotherapy

control bleeding in the patient who is a poor operative risk or who has advanced tumors. The primary disadvantage of this approach is destruction of the tumor so pathologic evaluation for grading and staging cannot be completed.

A *segmental cystectomy (partial cystectomy)* is used to treat larger tumors or those that only involve one area of the bladder. A portion of the bladder wall containing the tumor is removed along with a margin of normal tissue.

When the tumor is invasive or involves the trigone (the area where the ureters insert into the bladder) and the patient is free from metastasis beyond the pelvic area, a radical cystectomy is the treatment of choice. A *radical cystectomy* involves removal of the bladder, prostate, and seminal vesicles in men and the bladder, uterus, cervix, urethra, and ovaries in women. After a radical cystectomy, a new way needs to be created for urine to leave the body. This surgical technique is called a urinary diversion (discussed on p. 1095 later in this chapter).

Postoperative instructions for any of these surgical procedures include drinking a large volume of fluid for the first week after the procedure. Teach the patient to self-monitor the color and consistency of the urine. The urine is pink for the first several days after the procedure, but it should not be bright red or contain blood clots. Approximately 7 to 10 days after tumor resection, the patient may observe dark red or rust-colored flecks in the urine. These may be from the healing tumor resection site.

Administer opioid analgesics for a brief period after the procedure, along with stool softeners. Also help the patient and family cope with fears about cancer, surgery, and sexuality. Emphasize the importance of regular follow-up care. Follow-up cystoscopies are required on a regular basis after surgery for bladder cancer.

RADIATION THERAPY AND CHEMOTHERAPY

Radiation therapy can be used in combination with cystectomy or as the primary therapy when the cancer is inoperable or the patient refuses surgery. Chemotherapy drugs used in treating invasive bladder cancer include cisplatin (Platinol), vinblastine (Velban), doxorubicin (Adriamycin), and methotrexate.

INTRAVESICAL THERAPY

Chemotherapy with local instillation of chemotherapeutic or immune-stimulating agents can be delivered directly into the

GENDER DIFFERENCES

Urinary Incontinence

Men	Women
• Urinary incontinence is a common manifestation of benign prostatic hyperplasia and prostate cancer in men. • Urinary incontinence in men most often is overflow incontinence caused by urinary retention.	• Prevalence of urinary incontinence is higher in women than men. • Women more frequently experience stress and urge incontinence than men.

bladder by a urethral catheter.[30] *Intravesical therapy* is usually initiated at weekly intervals for 6 to 12 weeks. The chemotherapy drug is instilled directly into the patient's bladder and retained for about 2 hours. The patient's bladder must be empty before instillation. Change the patient's position every 15 minutes for maximum contact in all areas of the bladder. Maintenance therapy after the initial induction regimen may be beneficial.

Bacille Calmette-Guérin (BCG), a weakened strain of *Mycobacterium bovis,* is the treatment of choice for carcinoma in situ. BCG stimulates the immune system rather than acting directly on cancer cells in the bladder. When BCG fails, α-interferon in addition to BCG may be used. Other treatments that can be used when BCG fails include thiotepa (Thioplex), an alkylating agent, and valrubicin (Valstar), a chemotherapy antibiotic.

Most patients have irritative voiding symptoms and hemorrhagic cystitis after intravesical therapy. Thiotepa can significantly reduce WBC and platelet counts in some individuals when absorbed into the circulation from the bladder wall. BCG may cause flu-like symptoms, increased urinary frequency, hematuria, or systemic infection. Other side effects of chemotherapy (e.g., nausea, vomiting, hair loss) are not experienced with intravesical chemotherapy.

Encourage patients to increase their daily fluid intake and to quit smoking. Assess the patient for secondary UTI, and stress the need for routine urologic follow-up. The patient may have fears or concerns about sexual activity or bladder function that need to be addressed. Because of the high rate of disease recurrence and progression in bladder cancer, follow-up studies are very important.

BLADDER DYSFUNCTION

URINARY INCONTINENCE

Urinary incontinence (UI) is an involuntary leakage of urine. Approximately 17 million people in the United States suffer from UI. The prevalence is 30% to 40% among young adult to middle-aged women, and increases to 30% to 50% in older women. In contrast, the incidence of UI in men tends to be considerably lower, ranging from 1% to 5% in young adult men and increasing to 9% to 34% in older men.[31] Although incontinence is more prevalent among older women and older men, it is not a natural consequence of aging. UI has traditionally been viewed as a social or hygienic problem, but it also has a major effect on quality of life and contributes to serious health problems, especially in older adults.

Etiology and Pathophysiology

UI occurs when bladder pressure exceeds urethral closure pressure. Anything that interferes with bladder or urethral sphincter

TABLE 46-16 DRUG THERAPY

Drugs Affecting Lower Urinary Tract Function

Drug	Effect
Alcohol	Polyuria, frequency, urgency, sedation, delirium
α-Adrenergic receptor agonists: pseudoephedrine (Sudafed), ephedrine	Urethral constriction and urinary retention (males)
α-Adrenergic receptor antagonists: prazosin (Minipress), terazosin (Hytrin), doxazosin (Cardura)	Urethral relaxation and stress urinary incontinence in females
ACE inhibitors: captopril (Capoten), lisinopril (Zestril), enalapril (Vasotec)	Cough triggering stress urinary incontinence
Anticholinergics: H₁-antihistamines, antiparkinsonian agents	Urinary retention, overflow incontinence, fecal impaction
Tricyclic antidepressants	Anticholinergic effect, α-adrenergic receptor antagonist effect
β-Adrenergic receptor antagonists: propranolol (Inderal), metoprolol (Toprol, Lopressor), atenolol (Tenormin)	Urinary retention
Calcium channel blockers: verapamil (Calan), diltiazem (Cardizem), nifedipine (Procardia)	Urinary retention, fecal impaction
Opioids	Urinary retention, fecal impaction, sedation, delirium
Sedative-hypnotics	Sedation, delirium, muscle relaxation
Diuretics: loop diuretics such as furosemide (Lasix)	Polyuria, frequency, urgency
Methylxanthines (caffeine, theophylline)	Polyuria, bladder irritation
Antiseizure agents: thioridazine (Mellaril), chlorpromazine (Thorazine)	Anticholinergic effect, sedation

ACE, Angiotensin-converting enzyme.

COMPLEMENTARY & ALTERNATIVE THERAPIES

Biofeedback

Scientific Evidence

Biofeedback has been shown to be helpful in treating a variety of medical conditions: urinary incontinence, asthma, Raynaud's disease, irritable bowel syndrome, hot flashes, nausea and vomiting associated with chemotherapy, headaches, hypertension, and seizure disorders.*

Nursing Implications

- Feedback from monitoring equipment can teach patients to control certain involuntary body responses, such as urinary incontinence.
- Although biofeedback is considered safe, patients should consult a qualified professional before using biofeedback.

*Based on a systematic review of scientific literature. Retrieved from *www.naturalstandard.com.*

voiding diary documenting the timing of urinations, episodes of urinary leakage, and frequency of nocturia for a period of 1 to 7 days. This record can be kept by nursing staff if the person is in an inpatient or long-term care facility.

A urinalysis is used to identify possible factors contributing to transient UI (e.g., UTI, diabetes mellitus). Measure postvoid residual (PVR) urine in the patient undergoing evaluation for UI. The PVR volume is obtained by asking the patient to urinate, followed by catheterization or use of a bladder ultrasound within a relatively brief period (preferably 10 to 20 minutes).

Urodynamic testing is indicated in selected cases of UI. Imaging studies of the upper urinary tract (e.g., ultrasound) are obtained when UI is associated with UTIs or evidence of upper urinary tract involvement.

Collaborative Care

An estimated 80% of incontinence can be cured or significantly improved.[32] Transient, reversible factors are corrected initially, followed by management of the type of UI (see Table 46-17). In general, less invasive treatments are attempted before more invasive methods (e.g., surgery). Nevertheless, the choice of the initial treatment is individualized, based on patient preference, the type and severity of UI, and associated anatomic defects.

Several behavioral therapies may be used to improve UI (Table 46-18). Pelvic floor muscle training (Kegel exercises) is used to manage stress, urge, or mixed UI (Table 46-19). Biofeedback is used to help the patient identify, isolate, contract, and relax the pelvic muscles (see the Complementary & Alternative Therapies box on this page).

Drug Therapy. Drug therapy varies according to the UI type (Table 46-20 on p. 1091). In stress UI, drugs have a limited role in the management. α-Adrenergic agonists can be used to increase bladder sphincter tone and urethral resistance, but have limited benefit.

In urge and reflex UI, drugs play a key management role. Anticholinergic drugs and muscarinic receptor antagonists relax the bladder muscle and inhibit overactive detrusor contractions. Several preparations of these drugs are available, including immediate and extended-release tolterodine (Detrol, Detrol LA); immediate, extended-release, and transdermal oxybutynin (Ditropan XL, Oxytrol Transdermal System [also available over-the-counter]); twice-daily trospium chloride (Sanctura); extended-release solifenacin (VESIcare); darifenacin (Enablex); and fesoterodine (Toviaz). Side effects of these drugs include dry mouth, dry eyes, constipation, blurred vision, and somnolence.

control can result in UI. Using the acronym *DRIP,* the causes can include *D:* delirium, dehydration, depression; *R:* restricted mobility, rectal impaction; *I:* infection, inflammation, impaction; and *P:* polyuria, polypharmacy. (Table 46-16 lists drugs that can affect the lower urinary tract.) Patients may have more than one type of incontinence (Table 46-17).

Diagnostic Studies

The basic evaluation for UI includes a focused history, a physical assessment, and a bladder log or voiding record whenever possible. Obtain information on the onset of UI, factors that provoke urinary leakage, and associated conditions. Pay special attention to factors known to produce transient UI, particularly when the onset of urine loss is relatively sudden. Begin the physical examination with an assessment of general health and functional issues associated with urination, including mobility, dexterity, and cognitive function.

A pelvic examination includes careful inspection of the perineal skin for signs of erosion or rashes related to UI and existence of pelvic organ prolapse. Also evaluate local innervation and pelvic floor muscle strength, including a digital examination of the pelvic floor muscle to determine weakness or tension. Whenever possible, ask the patient to keep a bladder log or

TABLE 46-17	TYPES OF URINARY INCONTINENCE	
Description	**Causes**	**Treatment**
Stress Incontinence* Sudden increase in intraabdominal pressure causes involuntary passage of urine. Can occur during coughing, laughing, sneezing, or physical activities such as heavy lifting, exercising. Leakage usually is in small amounts and may not be daily.	Found most commonly in women with relaxed pelvic floor musculature (from delivery, use of instrumentation during vaginal delivery, or multiple pregnancies). Structures of the female urethra atrophy when estrogen decreases. Prostate surgery for BPH or prostate cancer.	Pelvic floor muscle exercises (e.g., Kegel exercises), weight loss if patient is obese, cessation of smoking, topical estrogen products, external condom catheters or penile clamp in men, surgery Urethral inserts, patches, or bladder neck support devices (e.g., incontinence pessary) to correct underlying problem
Urge Incontinence* Condition occurs randomly when involuntary urination is preceded by urinary urgency. Seen with overactive bladder symptoms of urgency and frequency. Leakage is periodic but frequent and usually in large amounts. Nocturnal frequency and incontinence are common.	Condition is caused by uncontrolled contraction or overactivity of detrusor muscle. Bladder escapes central inhibition and contracts reflexively. Conditions include: • Central nervous system disorders (e.g., cerebrovascular disease, Alzheimer's disease, brain tumor, Parkinson's disease) • Bladder disorders (e.g., carcinoma in situ, radiation effects, interstitial cystitis) • Interference with spinal inhibitory pathways (e.g., malignant growth in spinal cord, spondylosis) • Bladder outlet obstruction or conditions of unknown etiology	Treatment of underlying cause Biobehavioral interventions, including bladder retraining with urge suppression, decrease in dietary irritants, bowel regularity, and pelvic floor muscle exercises Anticholinergic drugs (e.g., oxybutynin [Ditropan XL, Oxytrol], tolterodine [Detrol, Detrol LA], trospium chloride [Sanctura], solifenacin [VESIcare], and darifenacin [Enablex]); imipramine (Tofranil) at bedtime; calcium channel blockers Containment devices (e.g., external condom catheters) Vaginal estrogen creams Absorbent products
Overflow Incontinence Condition occurs when the pressure of urine in overfull bladder overcomes sphincter control. Leakage of small amounts of urine is frequent throughout the day and night. Urination may also occur frequently in small amounts. Bladder remains distended and is usually palpable.	Disorder is caused by bladder or urethral outlet obstruction (bladder neck obstruction, urethral stricture, pelvic organ prolapse) or by underactive detrusor muscle caused by myogenic or neurogenic factors (e.g., herniated disc, diabetic neuropathy). May also occur after anesthesia and surgery (e.g., hemorrhoidectomy, herniorrhaphy, cystoscopy). Neurogenic bladder (flaccid type).	Urinary catheterization to decompress bladder Implementation of Credé or Valsalva maneuver α-Adrenergic blocker (doxazosin [Cardura], terazosin [Hytrin], tamsulosin [Flomax], alfuzosin [Uroxatral]) 5α-Reductase inhibitors (e.g., finasteride [Proscar]) to decrease outlet resistance bethanechol (Urecholine) to enhance bladder contractions Intravaginal device such as a pessary to support prolapse Intermittent catheterization Surgery to correct underlying problem
Reflex Incontinence Condition occurs when no warning or stress precedes periodic involuntary urination. Urination is frequent, is moderate in volume, and occurs equally during the day and night.	Spinal cord lesion above S2 interferes with central nervous system inhibition. Disorder results in detrusor hyperreflexia and interferes with pathways coordinating detrusor contraction and sphincter relaxation.	Treatment of underlying cause Bladder decompression to prevent ureteral reflux and hydronephrosis Intermittent self-catheterization diazepam (Valium) or baclofen (Lioresal) to relax external sphincter Prophylactic antibiotics Surgical sphincterotomy
Incontinence After Trauma or Surgery In women, vesicovaginal or urethrovaginal fistula may occur. In men, alteration in continence control involves proximal urethral sphincter (bladder neck and prostatic urethra) and distal urethral sphincter (external striated muscle).	Fistulas may occur during pregnancy, after delivery of baby, as a result of hysterectomy or invasive cancer of cervix, or after radiation therapy. Incontinence is a postoperative complication of transurethral, perineal, or retropubic prostatectomy.	Surgery to correct fistula Urinary diversion surgery to bypass urethra and bladder External condom catheter Penile clamp Placement of artificial implantable sphincter
Functional Incontinence Loss of urine resulting from cognitive, functional, or environmental factors.	Older adults often have problems that affect balance and mobility.	Modifications of environment or care plan that facilitates regular, easy access to toilet and promotes patient safety (e.g., better lighting, removal of scatter rugs, ambulatory assistance equipment, clothing alterations, timed voiding, different toileting equipment)

*Patients can have a combination of stress and urge incontinence, referred to as mixed incontinence.

Botox (onabotulinumtoxin A) can be used in the treatment of UI as a result of detrusor overactivity. Botox is injected into the bladder, resulting in relaxation of the bladder, an increase in its storage capacity, and a decrease in UI.

DRUG ALERT: Tolterodine (Detrol)
- Overdosage can result in severe anticholinergic effects.
- These effects include GI cramping, diaphoresis, blurred vision, and urinary urgency.

Surgical Therapy. Surgical techniques also vary depending on the type of UI. Surgical correction of stress UI is aimed at making the urinary structures more receptive to intraabdominal pressure and augmenting the urethral resistance of the internal sphincter. It may involve repositioning the urethra and/or creating a backboard of support to stabilize the urethra and bladder neck and make them more receptive to changes in intraabdominal pressure. Another technique for stress UI augments the urethral resistance of the intrinsic sphincter with a sling or periurethral injectables.

Retropubic colposuspension and pubovaginal sling placement appear to be most effective. Typically, both procedures are performed through low transverse incisions. Complications specific to the retropubic suspensions include postoperative voiding dysfunction, urgency, and vaginal prolapse.

Placement of a suburethral sling, using the person's own fascia, cadaveric fascia, or a synthetic material, is also used to correct stress UI in women. Complications include vascular and bowel injury, urinary retention, mesh or sling erosion, infection, urgency, and bladder perforation. Suburethral slings have success rates comparable to those of colposuspensions or slings and are associated with shorter recovery periods. An artificial urethral sphincter can be used in men with intrinsic sphincter deficiency and severe stress UI.

Alternatively, one of several bulking agents can be injected underneath the mucosa of the urethra to correct stress UI in women or men. Bulking agents include glutaraldehyde cross-linked bovine collagen (GAX collagen), small silicone beads (Durasphere), or polytetrafluoroethylene (Teflon). Because of the risk of migration of Teflon particles, GAX collagen or Durasphere injections are most commonly used today. Although treatment with suburethral compounds avoids the risk associated with open surgery, reinjection is typically required after several years.

Injecting autologous stem cells into the rhabdosphincter and urethral submucosa of women is a recent experimental therapy for stress UI. This technique increases urethral closure pressure and periurethral electromyography activity. However, the injection requires use of transurethral ultrasonography for correct placement of the stem cells.[33]

NURSING MANAGEMENT
URINARY INCONTINENCE

It is important to recognize both the physical and the emotional problems associated with UI. Maintain and enhance the patient's dignity, privacy, and feelings of self-worth. This is a two-step approach: (1) containment devices to manage existing urinary leakage and (2) a definitive plan to reduce or resolve the factors leading to UI.

Management options are reviewed in Tables 46-18 and 46-19. They include lifestyle interventions such as teaching the patient about consumption of an adequate volume of fluids and reduction or elimination of bladder irritants (particularly

TABLE 46-18 INTERVENTIONS FOR URINARY INCONTINENCE

Intervention	Description
Lifestyle Modifications	Self-management strategies to reduce or eliminate risk factors, including the following: • Smoking cessation • Weight reduction • Good bowel regimen • Reduction of bladder irritants (e.g., caffeine, aspartame artificial sweetener, citrus juices) • Fluid modifications for those with urge incontinence
Scheduled Voiding Regimens	
Timed voiding	Toileting on a fixed schedule (typically every 2-3 hr during waking hours).
Habit retraining	Scheduled toileting with adjustments of voiding intervals (longer or shorter) based on the individual's voiding pattern.
Prompted voiding	Scheduled toileting that requires prompts to void from a caregiver (typically every 3 hr). Used in conjunction with operant conditioning techniques to reward individuals for maintaining continence and appropriate toileting.
Bladder retraining and urge-suppression strategies	Scheduled toileting with progressive voiding intervals. Includes teaching of urge-control strategies using relaxation and distraction techniques, self-monitoring, reinforcement techniques, and other strategies such as conscious contraction of pelvic floor muscles.
Pelvic Floor Muscle Rehabilitation	
Pelvic floor muscle (Kegel) exercises or training	See Table 46-19.
Vaginal weight training	Active retention of increasing vaginal weights at least twice a day. Typically used in combination with pelvic floor muscle exercises.
Biofeedback	See Complementary & Alternative Therapies box on p. 1087.
Electrical stimulation	Application of low-voltage electric current to sacral and pudendal afferent fibers through vaginal, anal, or surface electrodes. Used to inhibit bladder overactivity and improve awareness, contractility, and efficiency of pelvic muscle contraction.
Anti-Incontinence Devices	
Intravaginal support devices (pessaries and bladder neck support prostheses)	Devices support bladder neck, relieve minor pelvic organ prolapse, and change pressure transmission to the urethra.
Intraurethral occlusive device (urethral plug)	Single-use device that is worn in the urethra to provide mechanical obstruction to prevent urine leakage. Removed for voiding.
Penile compression device	Mechanical fixed compression applied to the penis to prevent any flow or leakage via the urethra. Must be released hourly to void.
Containment Devices	
External collection devices	External catheter (condom) systems (e.g., penile sheaths) direct urine into a drainage bag. Most commonly used by men.
Absorbent products	Variety of reusable and disposable pads and undergarment systems.

TABLE 46-19   PATIENT TEACHING GUIDE

Pelvic Floor Muscle (Kegel) Exercises

Include the following instructions when teaching the patient to perform Kegel exercises.

What Is the Pelvic Floor Muscle?

- Your pelvic floor muscle provides support for your bladder and rectum and, in women, the vagina and the uterus.
- If it weakens or is damaged, it cannot support these organs and their position can change.
- This causes problems with the normal bladder and rectal function.
- If you have a weak pelvic floor muscle, you might want to do special exercises to make the muscle stronger, prevent unwanted urine leakage, and lessen urinary urgency.

Finding the Pelvic Floor Muscle

- Without tensing the muscles of your leg, buttocks, or abdomen, imagine that you are trying to control the passing of gas or pinching off a stool.
- Or imagine you are in an elevator full of people and you feel the urge to pass gas. What do you do?
- You tighten or pull in the ring of muscle around your rectum—your pelvic floor muscle.
- You should feel a lifting sensation in the area around the vagina or a pulling in of your rectum.

How to Do the Exercises

There are two different kinds of exercises—short squeezes and long squeezes.

1. To do the *short squeezes*, tighten your pelvic floor muscle quickly, squeeze hard for 2 sec, and then relax the muscle. Also, when you have strong urinary urges, try to tighten your pelvic floor muscle quickly and hard several times in a row until the urge passes.
2. To do the *long squeezes*, tighten the muscle for 5-10 sec before you relax.

Do both of these exercises 40-50 times each day.

When to Do These Exercises

- You can do these exercises anytime and anywhere.
- You can do these exercises in any position, but sitting or lying down may be the easiest.

How Long Does It Take Before I Notice a Change?

After 4-6 wk of doing these exercises, you should start to see less urine leakage and urinary urgency.

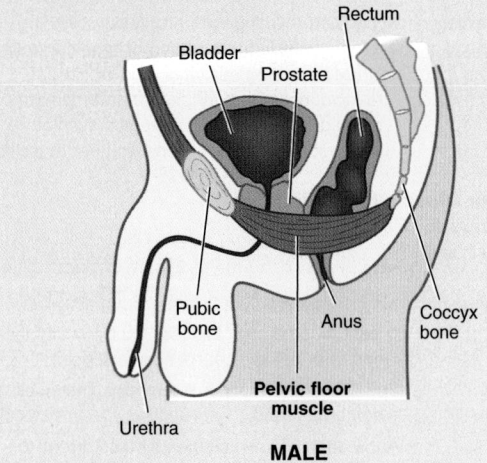

MALE

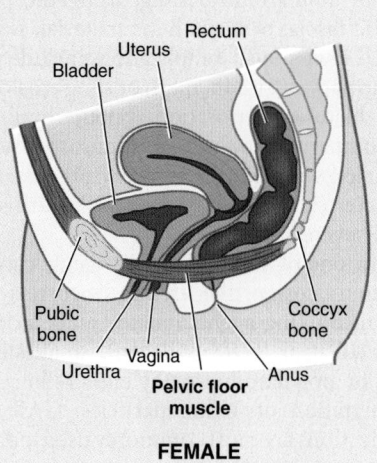

FEMALE

Courtesy Diane Newman.

caffeine and alcohol) from the diet. Advise the patient to maintain a regular, flexible schedule of urination (usually every 2 to 3 hours while awake). Advise patients to quit smoking because this habit increases the risk of stress UI. Counsel patients about the relationship among constipation, UI, and urinary retention. Aggressive management of constipation is recommended, beginning with ensuring adequate fluid intake, increasing dietary fiber, lightly exercising, and judiciously using stool softeners. (The management of constipation is discussed in Chapter 43.)

Behavioral treatments include scheduled voiding regimens (timed voiding, habit training, and prompted voiding), bladder retraining, and pelvic floor muscle training. Assess strategies that the patient uses to contain UI and offer alternative devices when indicated. When attempting to manage UI, many women use feminine hygiene pads, and many men and women use household products such as rags, paper towels, or folded toilet tissue. Unfortunately, none of these products is adequately designed to wick urine away from the skin, prevent soiling of clothing, and reduce or eliminate odor.

Instead, provide information on products specifically designed to contain urine. For example, patients with mild to moderate UI often benefit from incontinent pads containing superabsorbent material, designed to absorb many times its weight in water. Patients with higher-volume urine loss or those with both urinary and fecal incontinence may benefit from disposable or reusable incontinence protective underwear, briefs, or pad/pant systems.

In inpatient or long-term care facilities, nursing management of UI includes maximizing toilet access. This assistance may take the form of offering the urinal or bedpan or assisting the patient to the bathroom every 2 to 3 hours or at scheduled times. Ensure that toilets are accessible to patients and provide privacy to allow effective urine elimination.

URINARY RETENTION

Urinary retention is the inability to empty the bladder when a person voids (micturition) or the accumulation of urine in the bladder because of an inability to urinate. In certain cases, it is

TABLE 46-20 DRUG THERAPY
Voiding Dysfunction*

Class and Mechanism of Action	Drug
Muscarinic Receptor Antagonists and Anticholinergics	
Reduce overactive bladder contractions in urge urinary incontinence and overactive bladder	oxybutynin (Ditropan IR, Ditropan XL, Oxytrol Transdermal System)
	tolterodine (Detrol, Detrol LA)
	trospium chloride (Sanctura)
	solifenacin (VESIcare)
	darifenacin (Enablex)
	hyoscyamine (Levsin, Levbid)
	dicyclomine (Bentyl)
	flavoxate (Urispas)
	propantheline (Pro-Banthine)
	fesoterodine (Toviaz)
α-Adrenergic Antagonists	
Reduce urethral sphincter resistance to urinary outflow	doxazosin (Cardura)
	terazosin (Hytrin)
	tamsulosin (Flomax)
	alfuzosin (Uroxatral)
5α-Reductase Inhibitors	
Androgen suppression that results in epithelial atrophy and a decrease in total prostate size	finasteride (Proscar)
	dutasteride (Avodart)
α-Adrenergic Agonists	
Increase urethral resistance	phenylpropanolamine
	pseudoephedrine
β$_3$-Adrenergic Agonist	
Improves the bladder's storage capacity by relaxing the bladder muscle during filling	mirabegron (Myrbetriq)
Tricyclic Antidepressants	
Reduce sensory urgency and burning pain of interstitial cystitis	imipramine (Tofranil)
	amitriptyline (Elavil)
Reduce overactive bladder contractions	
Calcium Channel Blockers	
Reduce smooth muscle contraction strength	nifedipine (Adalat)
	diltiazem (Cardizem)
May reduce burning pain of interstitial cystitis	verapamil (Calan, Isoptin)
Hormone Therapy	
Local application reduces urethral irritation and increases host defenses against UTI	estrogen cream (Premarin, Estrace)
	estrogen vaginal ring (Estring)
	estrogen vaginal tablets (Vagifem)

*The type of drug therapy depends on the type of incontinence.

DELEGATION DECISIONS
Caring for the Incontinent Patient

All members of the health care team are responsible for decreasing the risk for incontinence and preventing complications such as skin breakdown in patients who are experiencing incontinence.

Role of Registered Nurse (RN)
- Assess for risk factors for incontinence or urinary retention.
- Determine type of incontinence that patient is experiencing.
- Develop plan of care to decrease incontinence.
- Teach patient ways to decrease incontinence such as pelvic floor muscle (Kegel) exercises.
- Assist patient in choosing appropriate products to contain urine.

Role of Licensed Practical/Vocational Nurse (LPN/LVN)
- Use bladder scanner to estimate the postvoid residual volume (PVR).
- Catheterize patient and measure PVR.
- Administer medications to decrease incontinence or urinary retention.

Role of Unlicensed Assistive Personnel (UAP)
- Assist incontinent patient to commode or bedpan at regular intervals.
- Clean patient and provide skin care.
- Notify RN about new-onset incontinence in a previously continent patient.

further evaluation. Even smaller volumes may justify further evaluation when the patient has recurring UTIs or lower urinary tract symptoms suggestive of UTI.

Etiology and Pathophysiology
Urinary retention is caused by two different dysfunctions of the urinary system: bladder outlet obstruction and deficient detrusor (bladder muscle) contraction strength. *Bladder outlet obstruction* leads to urinary retention when the blockage is so severe that the bladder can no longer evacuate its contents despite a detrusor contraction. A common cause of obstruction in men is an enlarged prostate.

Deficient detrusor contraction strength leads to urinary retention when the muscle is no longer able to contract with enough force or for a sufficient time to completely empty the bladder. Common causes of deficient detrusor contraction strength are neurologic diseases affecting sacral segments 2, 3, and 4; long-standing diabetes mellitus; overdistention; chronic alcoholism; and drugs (e.g., anticholinergic drugs).

Diagnostic Studies
The diagnostic studies for urinary retention are the same as the ones for UI (see pp. 1066-1067).

Collaborative Care
Behavioral therapies that were described for UI may also be used in the management of urinary retention. Scheduled toileting and double voiding may be effective in chronic urinary retention with moderate PVR volumes. *Double voiding* is an attempt to maximize bladder evacuation. The patient is asked to urinate, sit on the toilet for 3 to 4 minutes, and urinate again before exiting the bathroom.

For acute or chronic urinary retention, catheterization may be required. Intermittent catheterization allows the patient to remain free of an indwelling catheter with its associated risk of UTI and urethral irritation. In some situations, an indwelling catheter is preferred (e.g., if the patient is unwilling or unable

associated with urinary leakage or postvoid dribbling, called *overflow UI*. *Acute urinary retention* is the total inability to pass urine via micturition. It is a medical emergency. *Chronic urinary retention* is an incomplete bladder emptying despite urination. The postvoid residual (PVR) volumes in patients with chronic urinary retention vary widely. Normal PVR is between 50 and 75 mL. Findings over 100 mL indicate the need to repeat the measurement. An abnormal PVR in the older patient of more than 200 mL obtained on two separate occasions requires

to perform intermittent catheterization). An indwelling catheter is also used when urethral obstruction makes intermittent catheterization uncomfortable or infeasible.

Drug Therapy. Several drugs may be administered to promote bladder evacuation. For the patient with obstruction at the level of the bladder neck, an α-adrenergic blocker may be prescribed. These drugs relax the smooth muscle of the bladder neck, the prostatic urethra, and possibly the rhabdosphincter, diminishing urethral resistance. Examples of α-adrenergic blocking agents are listed in Table 46-20. They are indicated in patients with BPH, bladder neck dyssynergia (muscle incoordination), or detrusor sphincter dyssynergia.

Surgical Therapy. Surgical interventions are used to manage urinary retention caused by obstruction. Transurethral or open surgical techniques are used to treat benign or malignant prostatic enlargement, bladder neck contracture, urethral strictures, or dyssynergia of the bladder neck. Pelvic reconstruction using an abdominal or transvaginal approach can correct bladder outlet obstruction in women with severe pelvic organ prolapse.

Unfortunately, surgery has a minimal role in the management of urinary retention caused by deficient detrusor contraction strength. Attempts to create a bladder stimulator (implanted device capable of stimulating micturition) have proved largely unsuccessful because of the difficulty in achieving a coordinated detrusor contraction associated with pelvic muscle and striated sphincter relaxation.

NURSING MANAGEMENT
URINARY RETENTION

Acute urinary retention is a medical emergency that requires prompt recognition and bladder drainage. Insert a catheter (as ordered) unless otherwise directed. Use a catheter with a retention balloon in anticipation of the need for an indwelling catheter.

Teach the patient with acute urinary retention (and the patient predisposed to these episodes) strategies to minimize risk, including avoiding intake of large volumes of fluid over a brief period. Instead, advise the patient to drink small amounts throughout the day. In addition, instruct the patient (if chilled) to warm up before attempting to urinate and to avoid excessive alcohol intake because it leads to polyuria and a diminished awareness of the need to urinate until the bladder is distended.

Advise the patient who is unable to urinate to drink a cup of coffee or brewed caffeinated tea to create or maximize urinary urgency. Tell patients that sitting in a tub of warm water or taking a warm shower may also help them urinate. If these measures do not lead to successful urination, advise the patient to seek immediate care.

Patients with chronic urinary retention may be managed by behavioral methods, indwelling or intermittent catheterization, surgery, or drugs. Scheduled toileting and double voiding are the primary behavioral interventions used for chronic retention. Scheduled toileting is used to reduce rather than expand bladder capacity. In this case, ask the patient to void every 3 to 4 hours regardless of the desire to urinate. This intervention is particularly useful in the patient with chronic overdistention, diabetes mellitus, or chronic alcoholism characterized by a large bladder capacity and diminished or delayed sensations of bladder filling and urgency.

TABLE 46-21 INDICATIONS FOR URINARY CATHETERIZATION

Indwelling Catheter
- Relief of urinary retention caused by lower urinary tract obstruction, paralysis, or inability to void
- Bladder decompression preoperatively and operatively for lower abdominal or pelvic surgery
- Facilitation of surgical repair of urethra and surrounding structures
- Splinting of ureters or urethra to facilitate healing after surgery or other trauma in area
- Accurate measurement of urine output in critically ill patient
- Contamination of stage III or IV pressure ulcers with urine that has impeded healing, despite appropriate personal care for the incontinence
- Terminal illness or severe impairment, which makes positioning or clothing changes uncomfortable, or which is associated with intractable pain

Intermittent (Straight, In and Out) Catheter
- Study of anatomic structures of urinary system
- Urodynamic testing
- Collection of sterile urine sample in selected situations
- Instillation of medications into bladder
- Measurement of residual urine after urination (postvoid residual [PVR]) if portable ultrasound not available

CATHETERIZATION

INDICATIONS FOR AND COMPLICATIONS OF CATHETERIZATION

Indications for short-term urinary catheterization are listed in Table 46-21. Two unacceptable reasons for catheterization are (1) routine acquisition of a urine specimen for laboratory analysis and (2) convenience of the nursing staff or the patient's family. The risks of HAI are too high to allow catheterization of a patient for the convenience of hospital personnel or family members.

Complications that are seen more frequently with long-term use (more than 30 days) of indwelling catheters include HAIs, bladder spasms, periurethral abscess, pain, urosepsis, UTIs, urethral trauma or erosion, fistula or stricture formation, and stones. Catheterization for sterile urine specimens may occasionally be necessary when patients have a history of complicated UTI. A catheter should be the final resort to provide the patient with a dry environment to prevent skin breakdown and protect dressings or skin lesions.

Urinary catheterization is commonly used in the management of the hospitalized patient. However, it is not without serious complications. The urinary tract is the most common site of HAIs. Urinary catheterization is a major cause of UTIs. Scrupulous aseptic technique is mandatory when a urinary catheter is inserted. After insertion, maintenance and protection of the closed drainage system are major nursing responsibilities. Do not routinely irrigate the catheter; this should be done only if ordered.

While the patient has a catheter in place, maintain patency of the catheter, manage fluid intake, provide for the patient's comfort and safety, and prevent infection. Address the psychologic implications of urinary drainage. Patient concerns can include embarrassment related to exposure of the body, an altered body image, and fear that care of the catheter will result in increased dependency.

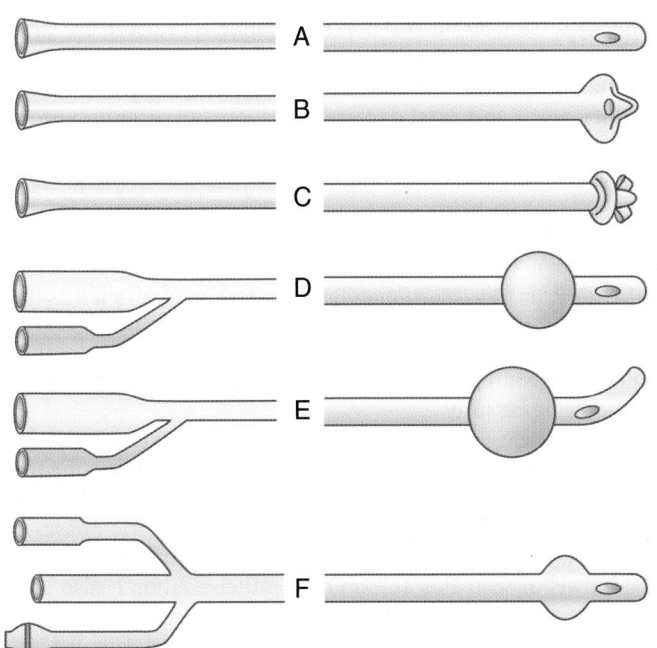

FIG. 46-10 Types of urinary catheters. **A,** Simple urethral catheter. **B,** Mushroom-tip de Pezzer catheter (can be for suprapubic catheterization). **C,** Wing-tip Malecot catheter. **D,** Indwelling urethral catheter with inflated balloon. **E,** Indwelling Tiemann catheter with coudé-tip–inflated balloon. **F,** Three-way indwelling catheter (third lumen can be used for irrigation).

CATHETER CONSTRUCTION

Catheter materials include Teflon-coated latex, silicone elastomer, and hydrogel-coated silicone. Catheters coated with silver or antimicrobial agents may prevent UTIs.

Catheters vary in construction materials, tip shape (Fig. 46-10), and size of the lumen. A coudé-tip catheter is commonly used in men. Catheters are sized according to the French scale. Each French unit (F) equals 0.33 mm of diameter. The diameter listed is the internal diameter of the catheter. The size used varies with the patient's size and the purpose of catheterization. In women, urethral catheter sizes 14F to 16F are the most common. In men, sizes 14F to 18F are used. Balloon sizes are either 5 or 30 mL. The primary problem resulting from too large a catheter is tissue erosion secondary to excessive pressure on the meatus or urethra.

TYPES OF CATHETERS

Four routes are used for urinary tract catheterization: urethral, ureteral, suprapubic, and via a nephrostomy tube.

Urethral Catheters

Urethral catheterization, the most common route of catheterization, involves the insertion of a catheter through the external meatus into the urethra, past the internal sphincter, and into the bladder. Consider the following principles in the management of the patient with an indwelling urethral catheter:

- Teach catheter care to the catheterized patient, particularly one who is ambulatory.
- Use a sterile, closed drainage system in short-term catheterization. Do not disconnect the distal urinary catheter and the proximal drainage tube except for necessary catheter irrigation. Maintain unobstructed downhill flow.

Empty the collecting bag regularly, and keep it below the level of the bladder. Replace a poorly functioning catheter.

- Provide perineal care (once or twice a day and when necessary), including cleaning the meatus-catheter junction with soap and water. Do not use lotion or powder near the catheter.
- Anchor catheters using some type of securement device. It is recommended that the catheter be anchored to the upper thigh in women and to the lower abdomen in men to prevent catheter movement and urethral tension.
- Use sterile technique whenever the collecting system is open. If frequent irrigations are necessary in short-term catheterization to maintain catheter patency, a triple-lumen catheter may be preferable, permitting continuous irrigations within a closed system.
- Aspirate small volumes of urine for culture from the catheter sampling port by means of a sterile syringe and a needle. First prepare the puncture site with a tincture of iodine or alcohol solution.
- When the patient is catheterized for less than 2 weeks, routine catheter change is not necessary. For long-term use of an indwelling catheter, replace the catheter based on patient assessment and not on a routine changing schedule.
- With long-term use of a catheter, a leg bag may be used. If the collection bag is reused, wash it in soap and water and rinse thoroughly. When it is not reused immediately, fill it with ½ cup of vinegar and drain. The vinegar is effective against *Pseudomonas* and other organisms and eliminates odors.
- Remove the catheter as early as possible. Intermittent catheterization and external catheters are alternatives that may be associated with fewer cases of bacteriuria and UTI than chronic indwelling urethral catheters.

Ureteral Catheters

The *ureteral catheter* is placed through the ureters into the renal pelvis. The catheter is inserted either (1) by being threaded up the urethra and bladder to the ureters under cystoscopic observation or (2) by surgical insertion through the abdominal wall into the ureters. The ureteral catheter is used after surgery to splint the ureters and to prevent them from being obstructed by edema. Record the urine volume from the ureteral catheter separately from that of other urinary catheters.

The patient is often kept on bed rest while a ureteral catheter is in place until specific orders indicate that ambulation is permitted. The self-retaining ureteral catheter is often inserted after a lithotripsy procedure or when ureteral obstruction from adjacent tumors or fibrosis threatens renal function. The double-J ureteral catheter is frequently used and allows the patient to ambulate. One end coils up in the kidney pelvis, while the other coils in the bladder.

Check the placement of the ureteral catheter frequently, and avoid tension on the catheter. The catheter drains urine from the renal pelvis, which has a capacity of 3 to 5 mL. If the volume of urine in the renal pelvis increases, tissue damage to the pelvis will result from pressure. Do not clamp the ureteral catheter. If the physician orders irrigation of the ureteral catheter, use strict aseptic technique. If the output is decreased, notify the physician immediately. Check the drainage often (at least every 1 or 2 hours). It is normal for some urine to drain around the ureteral catheter into the bladder. Accurately record the urine output from both the ureters and the urethral catheter. Sometimes a ureteral catheter may be used as a stent and is not expected to drain. It is important to check with the physician as to the type of catheter and what to expect.

Suprapubic Catheters

Suprapubic catheterization is the simplest and oldest method of urinary diversion. The two methods of insertion of a suprapubic catheter into the bladder are (1) through a small incision in the abdominal wall and (2) by the use of a trocar. A suprapubic catheter is placed while the patient is under general anesthesia for another surgical procedure or at the bedside with a local anesthetic. The catheter may be sutured into place. Tape the catheter to prevent dislodgment. The care of the tube and catheter is similar to that of the urethral catheter. A pectin-base skin barrier (e.g., Stomahesive) is effective in protecting the skin around the insertion site from breakdown.

The suprapubic catheter is used in temporary situations such as bladder, prostate, and urethral surgery. The suprapubic catheter is also used on a long-term basis in selected patients.

A suprapubic catheter is prone to poor drainage because of mechanical obstruction of the catheter tip by the bladder wall, sediment, and clots. To ensure patency of the tube (1) prevent tube kinking by coiling the excess tubing and maintaining gravity drainage, (2) have the patient turn from side to side, and (3) milk the tube. If these measures are not effective, obtain a physician order to irrigate the catheter using sterile technique.

If the patient experiences bladder spasms that are difficult to control, urinary leakage may result. Oxybutynin or other oral antispasmodics or belladonna and opium (B&O) suppositories may be prescribed to decrease bladder spasms.

Nephrostomy Tubes

The *nephrostomy tube* (catheter) is inserted on a temporary basis to preserve renal function when a ureter is completely obstructed. The tube is inserted through a small flank incision directly into the pelvis of the kidney and attached to connecting tubing for closed drainage. The principle is the same as with the ureteral catheter—that is, the catheter should never be kinked, compressed, or clamped. If the patient complains of excessive pain in the area or if there is excessive drainage around the tube,

check the catheter for patency. If irrigation is ordered, use strict aseptic technique. Gently instill no more than 5 mL of sterile saline solution at one time to prevent overdistention of the kidney pelvis and renal damage. Infection and secondary stone formation are complications associated with the insertion of a nephrostomy tube.

Intermittent Catheterization

An alternative approach to a long-term indwelling catheter is *intermittent catheterization,* often referred to as "straight" catheterization or "in-and-out" catheterization. The main goal of intermittent catheterization is to prevent urinary retention, stasis, and compromised blood supply to the bladder caused by prolonged pressure.

It is being used with increasing frequency in conditions such as neurogenic bladder (e.g., spinal cord injuries, chronic neurologic diseases) or bladder outlet obstruction in men. This type of catheterization is used in the oliguric and anuric phases of acute kidney injury to reduce the possibility of infection from an indwelling catheter. Intermittent catheterization is also used postoperatively after a surgical procedure to treat UI.

The technique consists of inserting a urethral catheter into the bladder every 3 to 5 hours. Some patients perform intermittent catheterization only once or twice a day to measure residual urine and to ensure an empty bladder.

The techniques and protocols for intermittent catheterization vary. Catheters can be sterile (single use) or clean (multiple use). Catheters can be coated (prelubricated) or uncoated. Available data on intermittent catheterization do not provide convincing evidence that any specific technique (sterile or clean), catheter type (coated or uncoated), method (single-use or multiple-use), person (self or other), or strategy is better than any other for all clinical settings.[34]

The design of single-use, self-lubricating, silicone-coated (closed-sterile) systems is useful for patients who have recurrent UTIs or need to catheterize while at work or during travel. Instruct patients to wash and rinse the catheter and their hands with soap and water before and after catheterization. Lubricant is necessary for men and may make catheterization more comfortable for women. The catheter may be inserted by the patient, caregiver, or health care provider.

Sterile technique is used for catheterization in the hospital or long-term care facility. For home care, a clean technique that includes good hand washing with soap and water is used. Teach the patient to observe for signs of UTI so that treatment can be instituted early. If indicated, some patients are placed on a regimen of prophylactic antibiotics. Urethral damage from intermittent catheterization in men is similar to problems seen with indwelling catheterization. Complications include urethritis, urethral sphincter damage (especially if there is a forceful catheterization against a closed sphincter), urethral stricture, and creation of a false passage.

SURGERY OF THE URINARY TRACT

RENAL AND URETERAL SURGERY

The most common indications for nephrectomy are a renal tumor, polycystic kidneys that are bleeding or severely infected, massive traumatic injury to the kidney, and the elective removal of a kidney from a donor to be transplanted. Surgery involving the ureters and kidneys is most commonly performed to remove calculi that become obstructive, correct congenital anomalies, and divert urine when necessary.

Surgical Procedure

Nephrectomy can be performed by a conventional (open) approach or laparoscopically. In the open approach an incision of about 6 to 10 in is made through several layers of muscle. The incision can be made in the flank or abdominal area.

Laparoscopic Nephrectomy. *Laparoscopic nephrectomy* can be performed in selected situations to remove a diseased kidney. Laparoscopic nephrectomy can also be used to obtain a kidney from a living donor to be transplanted into a person with ESKD. A laparoscopic nephrectomy is performed using five puncture sites. One incision is to view the kidney, and another is to dissect it. The laparoscope contains a miniature camera so that the surgeons can watch what they are doing on a video monitor. Once dissected, the kidney is maneuvered into a nylon impermeable sack and then safely removed from the patient. Compared with conventional nephrectomy, the laparoscopic approach is less painful, involves a shorter hospital stay, and has a much faster recovery.

Preoperative Management

The basic needs of the patient undergoing renal and ureteral surgery are similar to those of any patient who experiences surgery (see Chapters 18 through 20). In addition, it is important preoperatively to ensure adequate fluid intake and a normal electrolyte balance. Tell the patient that, if there is a flank incision, surgery will require a hyperextended, side-lying position. This position frequently causes the patient to experience muscle aches after surgery. If a nephrectomy is planned, it is important that the patient have one working kidney to maintain normal renal function.

Postoperative Management

Specific postoperative needs of a patient are related to urine output, respiratory status, and abdominal distention.

Urine Output. In the immediate postoperative period, measure and record the urine output at least every 1 or 2 hours. Measure drainage from the various catheters and record it separately. Do not clamp or irrigate the catheter or tube without a specific order. The total urine output should be at least 0.5 mL/kg/hr. It is important to assess for urine drainage on the dressing and to estimate this amount. Observe and monitor the color and consistency of urine. Urine with increased amounts of mucus, blood, or sediment may occlude the drainage tubing or catheter.

Weigh the patient daily using the same scale, and have the patient wear similar clothing and dressings each time. A significant change in daily weight can indicate retention of fluids, which places the patient at cardiovascular risk for developing heart failure. Retention of fluids can increase the work required of the remaining kidney to perform its functions.

Respiratory Status. A nephrectomy can be performed through a flank incision just below the diaphragm. Postoperatively, it is important to ensure adequate ventilation. The patient is often reluctant to turn, cough, and deep breathe because of the incisional pain. Give adequate pain medication to ensure the patient's comfort and ability to perform coughing and deep-breathing exercises. Frequently, additional respiratory devices such as an incentive spirometer are used every 2 hours while the patient is awake. In addition, early and frequent ambulation assists in maintaining adequate respiratory function.

Abdominal Distention. Abdominal distention is present to some degree in most patients who have had surgery on their kidneys or ureters. It is most commonly due to paralytic ileus caused by manipulation and compression of the bowel during surgery. Oral intake is restricted until bowel sounds are present (usually 24 to 48 hours after surgery). IV fluids are given until the patient can take oral fluids. Progression to a regular diet follows.

URINARY DIVERSION

Urinary diversion may be performed with or without cystectomy. Urinary diversion procedures are performed to treat cancer of the bladder, neurogenic bladder, congenital anomalies, strictures, trauma to the bladder, and chronic infections with deterioration of renal function. Numerous urinary diversion techniques and bladder substitutes are possible, including an incontinent urinary diversion, a continent urinary diversion catheterized by the patient, or an orthotopic bladder so that the patient voids urethrally.[35] Types of surgical procedures for urinary diversion are presented in Table 46-22 and Fig. 46-11.

Incontinent Urinary Diversion

Incontinent urinary diversion is diversion to the skin, requiring an appliance. The simplest form is the cutaneous ureterostomy, but scarring and strictures of the ureter have led to the use of ileal or colonic conduits. The most commonly performed incontinent urinary diversion procedure is the ileal conduit (ileal loop). In this procedure a 6- to 8-in (15- to 20-cm) segment of the ileum is converted into a conduit for urinary drainage. The colon (colon conduit) can be used instead of the ileum. The ureters are anastomosed into one end of the conduit, and the other end of the bowel is brought out through the abdominal wall to form a stoma (Fig. 46-12). Although the segment of bowel remains supported by the mesentery, it is completely isolated from the intestinal tract. The bowel is anastomosed and continues to function normally.

Because there is no valve and no voluntary control over the stoma, drops of urine flow from the stoma every few seconds, requiring a permanent external collecting device. The visible stoma and the need for external collection devices are disadvantages of this procedure. The lifelong need to care for and deal with the stoma and collection devices may be psychologically difficult. These problems have led to the increasing use of continent diversions and orthotopic bladder substitutes.

Continent Urinary Diversions

A *continent urinary diversion* is an intraabdominal urinary reservoir that can be catheterized or that has an outlet controlled by the anal sphincter. Continent diversions are internal pouches created similarly to the ileal conduit. Reservoirs are constructed from the ileum, ileocecal segment, or colon. Large segments of bowel are altered to prevent peristaltic action. A continence mechanism is formed between this large, low-pressure reservoir and the stoma by intussuscepting a portion of bowel. In this way, a patient does not leak involuntarily. The patient with a continent reservoir needs to self-catheterize every 4 to 6 hours but does not need to wear external attachments. Patients may wear a small bandage on the stoma to collect any mucous drainage or excess drainage. Examples of continent diversions are the Kock (Fig. 46-13), Mainz, Indiana, and Florida pouches. The main difference among the various diversions is the segment of

TABLE 46-22   URINARY DIVERSION SURGERY

Description	Advantages	Disadvantages	Special Considerations
Ileal Conduit Ureters are implanted into part of ileum or colon that has been resected from intestinal tract. Abdominal stoma is created.	Relatively good urine flow with few physiologic alterations.	External appliance necessary to continually collect urine.	Surgical procedure is complex. Postoperative complications may be increased. Reabsorption of urea by ileum occurs. Meticulous attention is necessary to care for stoma and collecting device.
Cutaneous Ureterostomy Ureters are excised from bladder and brought through abdominal wall, and stoma is created. Ureteral stomas may be created from both ureters, or ureters may be brought together and one stoma created.	No need for major surgery as required with ileal conduit.	External appliance necessary because of continuous urine drainage. Possibility of stricture or stenosis of small stoma.	Periodic catheterizations may be required to dilate stomas to maintain patency.
Nephrostomy Catheter is inserted into pelvis of kidney. Procedure may be done to one or both kidneys and may be temporary or permanent. It is most frequently done in advanced disease as palliative procedure.	No need for major surgery.	High risk of renal infection. Predisposition to calculus formation from catheter.	Nephrostomy tube may have to be changed every month. Never clamp the catheter.

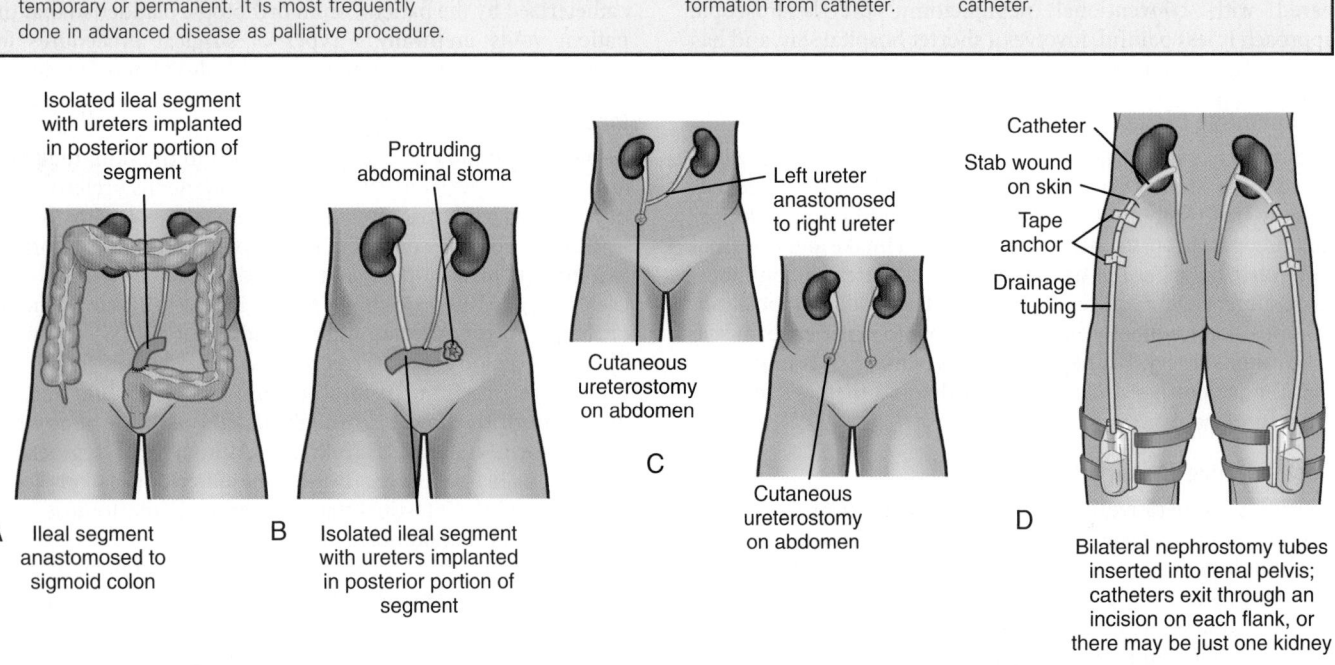

FIG. 46-11 Methods of urinary diversion. **A,** Ureteroileosigmoidostomy. **B,** Ileal loop (ileal conduit). **C,** Ureterostomy (transcutaneous ureterostomy and bilateral cutaneous ureterostomies). **D,** Nephrostomy.

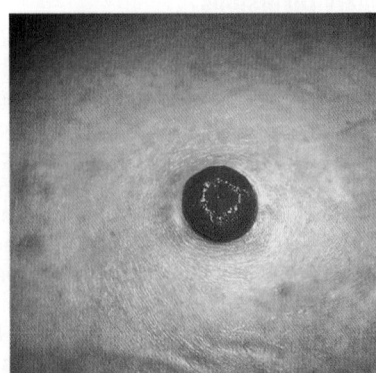

FIG. 46-12 Urinary stoma. Symmetric, no skin breakdown, protrudes about 1.5 cm. Mucosa is healthy red. This configuration is flat when the patient is upright or supine.

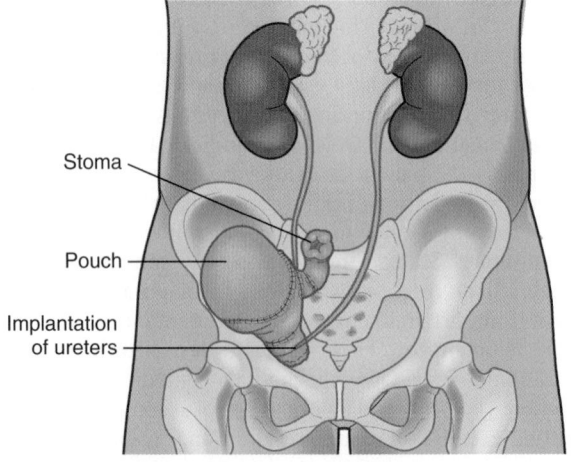

FIG. 46-13 Creation of a Kock pouch with implantation of ureters into one intussuscepted portion of the pouch and creation of a stoma with the other intussuscepted portion.

bowel used. For example, the Indiana pouch uses the right colon as a reservoir and has become a popular form of continent urinary diversion.

Orthotopic Bladder Reconstruction

Orthotopic bladder reconstruction, or orthotopic neobladder, is the construction of a new bladder in the bladder's normal anatomic position, with discharge of urine through the urethra. The reconstruction or neobladder can be derived from various segments of the intestines to create a low-pressure reservoir. An isolated segment of the distal ileum is often preferred. Various procedures include the hemi-Kock pouch, the Studer pouch, and the W-shaped ileoneobladder. In these procedures the bowel is surgically reshaped to become a neobladder. The ureters and urethra are sutured into the neobladder.

Orthotopic bladder reconstruction has become a more viable option for both men and women if cancer does not involve the bladder neck or urethra. Ideal candidates for this procedure have normal renal and liver function, longer than 1- to 2-year life expectancy, adequate motor skills, and no history of inflammatory bowel disease or colon cancer. Obese patients and those with inflammatory bowel disease are not good candidates for this procedure. The advantage of orthotopic bladder substitution is that it allows for natural micturition. Incontinence is a possible problem with this technique, and intermittent catheterization may be required.

NURSING MANAGEMENT URINARY DIVERSION

PREOPERATIVE MANAGEMENT

Teaching is important for the patient awaiting cystectomy and urinary diversion surgery. Assess the patient's ability and readiness to learn before initiating a teaching program. If the patient is not ready to learn, modify the teaching plan. The patient's anxiety and fear may be decreased by providing more information. However, the anxiety and fear may also interfere with learning. Involve the patient's caregiver and family in the teaching process.

Discuss the psychosocial aspects of living with a stoma (including clothing, changes in body image and sexuality, exercise, and odor). This may allay some fears. Teach the patient with a continent diversion (e.g., Indiana pouch) to catheterize at least every 6 hours and irrigate the pouch daily. The patient with an orthotopic neobladder may have problems with incontinence. Discuss the patient's concerns about sexual activities. A wound, ostomy, and continence (WOC) nurse should be involved in the preoperative phase of the patient's care. A visit from an ostomate or WOC nurse can be helpful. Additional interventions are presented in eNursing Care Plan 46-3 for the patient with an ileal conduit (on the website for this chapter).

POSTOPERATIVE MANAGEMENT

Plan the nursing interventions during the postoperative period (see eNursing Care Plan 46-3 for care after an ileal conduit) to prevent surgical complications such as postoperative atelectasis and shock (see Chapter 20). After pelvic surgery, there is an increased incidence of thrombophlebitis, small bowel obstruction, and UTI. With removal of part of the bowel, the incidence of paralytic ileus and small bowel obstruction is increased, the patient is kept on NPO status, and a nasogastric tube is necessary for a few days.

Prevent injury to the stoma and maintain urine output. Advise the patient that mucus in the urine is a normal occurrence. The mucus is secreted by the mucosa of the intestine (which is used to create the ileal conduit) in response to the irritating effect of urine. Encourage a high fluid intake to "flush" the ileal conduit or continent diversion.

When an ileal conduit is created, provide meticulous care for the skin around the stoma. Alkaline encrustations with dermatitis may occur when alkaline urine comes in contact with exposed skin (Fig. 46-14). The urine is kept acidic to prevent alkaline encrustations. Other common peristomal skin problems include yeast infections, product allergies, and shearing-effect excoriations. Changing appliances (pouches) is described in Table 46-23. A properly fitting appliance is essential to prevent skin problems. The appliance should be about 0.1 in (0.2 cm) larger than the stoma. It is normal for the stoma to shrink within the first few weeks after surgery.

Patients with a neobladder may have postoperative urinary retention and require catheterization. It may take up to 6 months for them to regain bladder control. Patients empty their neo-

---

TABLE 46-23 PATIENT & CAREGIVER TEACHING GUIDE

Ileal Conduit Appliances

Include the following instructions when teaching a patient or a caregiver how to change an ileal conduit appliance.

Temporary Appliance
1. Cut hole in pouch to fit over stoma (pouch ⅛ in [3.2 mm] larger than stoma).
2. Remove old pouch.
3. Clean area gently and remove old adhesive.
4. Wash area with warm water.
5. Place wick (rolled-up 4 × 4-in pad) over stoma to keep area dry during rest of procedure.
6. Dry skin around stoma.
7. Apply tincture of benzoin or other skin protectant around stoma to area where pouch will be placed.
8. Apply pouch by first smoothing its edges toward side and lower portion of body.
9. Remove wick and complete application of bag.
10. If patient is usually in bed, apply bag so that it lies toward side of body.
11. If patient is ambulatory, apply bag so that it lies vertically.
12. Connect drainage tubing to pouch.
13. Keep drainage pouch on same side of bed as stoma.

Permanent Appliance*
1. Keep appliance in place for 2-14 days.
2. Change appliance when fluid intake has been restricted for several hours.
3. Sit or stand in front of mirror.
4. Moisten edge of faceplate with adhesive solvent and gently remove.
5. Clean skin with adhesive solvent.
6. Wash skin with warm water (may be done while showering).
7. Dry skin and inspect.
8. Place wick (rolled-up 4 × 4-in pad) over stoma to keep skin free of urine.
9. Apply skin cement to faceplate and skin.
10. Place appliance over stoma.
11. Wash removed appliance with soap and lukewarm water; soak in distilled vinegar; rinse with lukewarm water and air dry.

*Many disposable appliances with self-adhesive backing are used as permanent appliances.

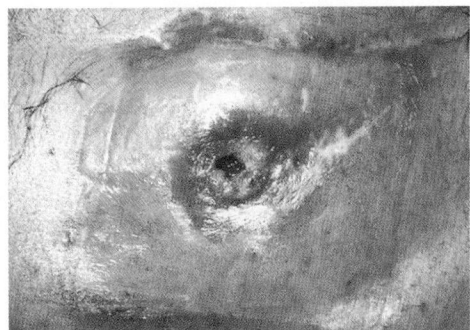

FIG. 46-14 Ammonia salt encrustation secondary to alkaline urine.

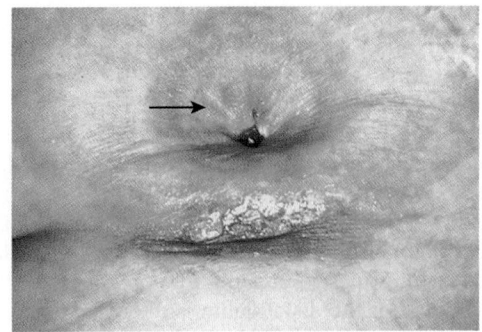

FIG. 46-15 Retracted urinary stoma with pressure sore from faceplate above stoma *(arrow).*

bladders by relaxing their outlet sphincter muscles and bearing down with their abdominal muscles. Since there is no longer neurologic feedback between the reservoir and the brain, the patient should not expect a normal desire to void. To avoid bladder overdistention, patients should void at least every 2 to 4 hours, sit during voiding, and practice pelvic floor muscle relaxation to aid voiding. Follow-up x-ray studies include a "pouchogram" 3 to 4 weeks after surgery to assess for healing.

Acceptance of the surgery and of alterations in body image is needed to ensure the patient's best adjustment. Meeting and sharing feelings with similar patients can enhance a patient's adjustment to a urinary diversion. Patient concerns include fear that the stoma will be offensive to others and will interfere with sexual, personal, professional, and recreational activities. Advise the patient that few activities will be restricted as a result of the urinary diversion.

Discharge planning after an ileal conduit includes teaching the patient symptoms of obstruction or infection and care of the ostomy. The patient with an ileal conduit is fitted for a permanent appliance 7 to 10 days after surgery and may need to be refitted at a later time, depending on the degree of stoma healing and shrinkage.

Appliances are made of a variety of products, including natural and synthetic rubbers, plastics, and metals. Most appliances have a faceplate that adheres to the skin, a collecting pouch, and an opening to drain the pouch. The faceplate may be secured to the skin with glues, adhesives, or adherent synthetic wafers. Some appliances do not require adhesives, but their design relies on pressure to keep the pouch in place. If improperly fitted or applied, the faceplate may cause skin problems (Fig. 46-15). Inform the patient and caregiver about where to purchase supplies, emergency telephone numbers, location of ostomy clubs, and follow-up visits with a WOC nurse. Physician follow-up is imperative to monitor the patient's recovery, detect any complications, and assess renal function.

CASE STUDY

Urinary Tract Infection

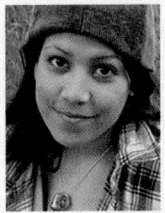

iStockphoto/Thinkstock

Patient Profile
S.U., a 38-yr-old Hispanic woman, was seen in the nurse practitioner's office for a history of painful, frequent urination.

Subjective Data
- Has a history of painful, frequent urination with passage of small volumes of urine for 3 days
- Had intermittent fever, chills, and back pain during these 3 days
- Was frightened when she saw blood in her urine
- Reports this is her third attack of painful urination and back pain in 4 mo
- Is anxious because her father died of kidney cancer
- Remembers having many UTIs as a child
- Has had four pregnancies with difficult vaginal deliveries

Objective Data
Physical Examination
- Complains of bilateral flank pain and abdominal tenderness to palpation
- Temperature is 100.4° F (38° C)

Diagnostic Studies
- Urinalysis: pyuria and hematuria
- Follow-up studies to be done

Discussion Questions
1. What are the most common organisms that cause UTIs?
2. What additional information do you or the nurse practitioner need from S.U.?
3. What factors predispose a patient to a UTI?
4. What is the difference between upper and lower UTIs?
5. *Priority Decision:* What are the priority nursing interventions for S.U.?
6. Why might S.U. be having recurrent bouts of UTIs? What other diagnostic tests may be indicated?
7. *Evidence-Based Practice:* S.U. wants to know what she can do to prevent another UTI. What are you going to tell her?
8. *Priority Decision:* Based on the data presented, write one or more appropriate nursing diagnoses. Are there any collaborative problems?

ⓔvolve Answers available at *http://evolve.elsevier.com/Lewis/medsurg.*

■ BRIDGE TO NCLEX EXAMINATION

The number of the question corresponds to the same-numbered outcome at the beginning of the chapter.

1. In teaching a patient with pyelonephritis about the disorder, the nurse informs the patient that the organisms that cause pyelonephritis most commonly reach the kidneys through
   a. the bloodstream.
   b. the lymphatic system.
   c. a descending infection.
   d. an ascending infection.

2. The nurse teaches the female patient who has frequent UTIs that she should
   a. take tub baths with bubble bath.
   b. urinate before and after sexual intercourse.
   c. take prophylactic sulfonamides for the rest of her life.
   d. restrict fluid intake to prevent the need for frequent voiding.

3. The immunologic mechanisms involved in acute poststreptococcal glomerulonephritis include
   a. tubular blocking by precipitates of bacteria and antibody reactions.
   b. deposition of immune complexes and complement along the GBM.
   c. thickening of the GBM from autoimmune microangiopathic changes.
   d. destruction of glomeruli by proteolytic enzymes contained in the GBM.

4. One of the nurse's most important roles in relation to acute poststreptococcal glomerulonephritis is to
   a. promote early diagnosis and treatment of sore throats and skin lesions.
   b. encourage patients to obtain antibiotic therapy for upper respiratory tract infections.
   c. teach patients with APSGN that long-term prophylactic antibiotic therapy is necessary to prevent recurrence.
   d. monitor patients for respiratory symptoms that indicate the disease is affecting the alveolar basement membrane.

5. The edema that occurs in nephrotic syndrome is due to
   a. increased hydrostatic pressure caused by sodium retention.
   b. decreased aldosterone secretion from adrenal insufficiency.
   c. increased fluid retention caused by decreased glomerular filtration.
   d. decreased colloidal osmotic pressure caused by loss of serum albumin.

6. A patient is admitted to the hospital with severe renal colic. The nurse's first priority in management of the patient is to
   a. administer opioids as prescribed.
   b. obtain supplies for straining all urine.
   c. encourage fluid intake of 3 to 4 L/day.
   d. keep the patient NPO in preparation for surgery.

7. The nurse recommends genetic counseling for the children of a patient with
   a. nephrotic syndrome.
   b. chronic pyelonephritis.
   c. malignant nephrosclerosis.
   d. adult-onset polycystic kidney disease.

8. The nurse identifies a risk factor for kidney and bladder cancer in a patient who relates a history of
   a. aspirin use.
   b. tobacco use.
   c. chronic alcohol abuse.
   d. use of artificial sweeteners.

9. In planning nursing interventions to increase bladder control in the patient with urinary incontinence, the nurse includes
   a. teaching the patient to use Kegel exercises.
   b. clamping and releasing a catheter to increase bladder tone.
   c. teaching the patient biofeedback mechanisms to suppress the urge to void.
   d. counseling the patient concerning choice of incontinence containment device.

10. A patient with a ureterolithotomy returns from surgery with a nephrostomy tube in place. Postoperative nursing care of the patient includes
    a. encouraging the patient to drink fruit juices and milk.
    b. encouraging fluids of at least 2 to 3 L/day after nausea has subsided.
    c. irrigating the nephrostomy tube with 10 mL of normal saline solution as needed.
    d. notifying the physician if nephrostomy tube drainage is more than 30 mL/hr.

11. A patient has had a cystectomy and ileal conduit diversion performed. Four days postoperatively, mucous shreds are seen in the drainage bag. The nurse should
    a. notify the physician.
    b. notify the charge nurse.
    c. irrigate the drainage tube.
    d. chart it as a normal observation.

1. d, 2. b, 3. b, 4. a, 5. d, 6. a, 7. d, 8. b, 9. a, 10. b, 11. d

ⓔvolve

For rationales to these answers and even more NCLEX review questions, visit *http://evolve.elsevier.com/Lewis/medsurg*.

REFERENCES

1. Brusch JL, Bavaro MF, Cunha BA, et al: Cystitis in females. Retrieved from *http://emedicine.medscape.com/article/233101-overview*.
2. Urinary tract infections—adults. Retrieved from *www.ncbi.nlm.nih.gov/pubmedhealth/PMH0001549*.
3. Tambyah PA, Oon J: Catheter-associated urinary tract infection, *Curr Opin Infect Dis* 25(4):365, 2012.
4. National Kidney and Urologic Diseases Information Clearinghouse: Kidney and urologic diseases statistics for the United States. Retrieved from *http://kidney.niddk.nih.gov/kudiseases/pubs/pdf/KUStatistics.pdf*.
*5. Dason S, Dason JT, Kapoor A: Guidelines for the diagnosis and management of recurrent urinary tract infection in women, *Can Urol Assoc J* 5(5):316, 2011.
6. Denes E, Prouzergue J, Ducroix-Roubertou S, et al: Antibiotic prescription by general practitioners for urinary tract infections in outpatients, *Eur J Clin Microbiol Infect Dis* 31(11):3079, 2012.

*Evidence-based information for clinical practice.

7. Hooton TM: Clinical practice: uncomplicated urinary tract infection, *N Engl J Med* 366(11):1028, 2012.

8. Colgan R, Williams M: Diagnosis and treatment of acute uncomplicated cystitis, *Am Fam Physician* 84(7):771, 2011.

*9. Wang C, Fang C, Chen N, et al: Cranberry-containing products for prevention of urinary tract infections in susceptible populations: a systematic review and meta-analysis of randomized controlled trials, *Arch Intern Med* 172:988, 2012.

10. Wenger JE: Reducing rates of catheter-associated urinary tract infection, *Am J Nurs* 110:40, 2010.

11. Dumont C, Wakeman J: Preventing catheter-associated UTIs: survey report, *Nursing* 40(12):24, 2010.

12. Oman KS, Makic MB, Fink R, et al: Nurse-directed interventions to reduce catheter-associated urinary tract infections, *Am J Infect Control* 40(6):548, 2012.

13. Conner BT: Reducing catheter-associated urinary tract infections, *Am Nurse Today* 7:16, 2012.

*14. Nosseir SB, Lind LR, Winkler HA: Recurrent uncomplicated urinary tract infections in women: a review, *J Womens Health* 21(3):347, 2012.

15. National Kidney and Urologic Diseases Information Clearinghouse: Interstitial cystitis/painful bladder syndrome. Retrieved from *http://kidney.niddk.nih.gov/kudiseases/pubs/interstitialcystitis*.

16. Gish BA: Interstitial cystitis/bladder pain syndrome: symptoms, screening, and treatment, *Nurs Womens Health* 15(6):496, 2011.

*17. Hanno P, Burks D, Clemens J, et al: AUA guideline for the diagnosis and treatment of interstitial cystitis/bladder pain syndrome, *J Urol* 185:2162, 2011.

18. Gish BA: Interstitial cystitis/bladder pain syndrome: symptoms, screening and treatment, *Nurs Womens Health* 15(6):496, 2011.

19. Quillin RB, Erickson DR: Management of interstitial cystitis/bladder pain syndrome: a urology perspective, *Urol Clin North Am* 39(3):389, 2012.

20. Soliman MS: Tuberculosis of the genitourinary system. Retrieved from *http://emedicine.medscape.com/article/450651-overview*.

21. Ralph AP, Carapetis JR: Group A streptococcal diseases and their global burden, *Curr Top Microbiol Immunol* 368:1, 2013.

22. Siddall EC, Radhakrishnan J: The pathophysiology of edema formation in the nephrotic syndrome, *Kidney Int* 82(6):635, 2012.

23. Worcester EM, Coe FL: Calcium kidney stones, *N Engl J Med* 363:954, 2010.

24. Stoller ML: Urinary stone disease: symptoms and signs at presentation. Retrieved from *www.urologytoday.net/article/urinary-stone-disease-symptoms-signs-at-presentation*.

*25. Aboumarzouk OM, Kata SG, Keeley FX, et al: Extracorporeal shock wave lithotripsy (ESWL) versus ureteroscopic management for ureteric calculi, *Cochrane Database Syst Rev* 5:CD006029, 2012.

*26. Chandok N: Polycystic liver disease: a clinical review, *Ann Hepatol* 11(6):819, 2012.

*27. Steinman TI: Polycystic kidney disease: a 2011 update, *Curr Opin Nephrol Hypertens* 21(2):189, 2012.

28. American Cancer Society: Cancer facts and figures. Retrieved from *www.cancer.org/research/cancerfactsfigures/index*.

29. Patel C, Ahmed A, Ellsworth P: Renal cell carcinoma: a reappraisal, *Urol Nurs* 32(4):182, 2012.

*30. Houghton BB, Chalasani V, Hayne D, et al: Intravesical chemotherapy plus bacille Calmette-Guérin in non-muscle invasive bladder cancer: a systematic review with meta-analysis, *BJU Int* 111:977, 2013.

31. Schultz JM: Urinary incontinence, *Nursing* 40:33, 2010.

32. Schultz JM: Rethink urinary continence, *Nursing* 42:32, 2012.

33. Stem cell therapy: a future treatment of stress urinary incontinence. Retrieved from *www.medscape.com/viewarticle/735539*.

*34. Newman DK, Willson M: Review of intermittent catheterization and current best practices. Retrieved from *www.medscape.com/viewarticle/745908_7*.

35. Hautmann RE, Abol-Enein H, Davidsson T, et al: ICUD-EAU International Consultation on Bladder Cancer 2012: urinary diversion, *Eur Urol* 63(1):67. 2013.

RESOURCES

American Association of Kidney Patients
www.aakp.org
American Nephrology Nurses' Association
www.annanurse.org
American Urological Association
www.auanet.org
Interstitial Cystitis Association
www.ichelp.org
National Association for Continence (NAFC)
www.nafc.org
National Kidney Foundation
www.kidney.org
National Kidney and Urologic Diseases Information Clearinghouse
www.kidney.niddk.nih.gov
PKD Foundation
www.pkdcure.org
Society of Urologic Nurses and Associates
www.suna.org
United Ostomy Associations of America
www.ostomy.org
Wound, Ostomy, and Continence Nurses Society
www.wocn.org
Also see Resources for Chapter 47 on p. 1131.

Everywhere you go, take a smile with you.
Sasha Azevedo

Nursing Management

Acute Kidney Injury and Chronic Kidney Disease

Carol Headley

LEARNING OUTCOMES

1. Differentiate between acute kidney injury and chronic kidney disease.
2. Identify criteria used in the classification of acute kidney injury using the acronym RIFLE (*R*isk, *I*njury, *F*ailure, *L*oss, *E*nd-stage kidney disease).
3. Describe the clinical course of acute kidney injury.
4. Explain the collaborative care and nursing management of a patient with acute kidney injury.
5. Define *chronic kidney disease* and delineate its five stages based on the glomerular filtration rate.
6. Select risk factors that contribute to the development of chronic kidney disease.
7. Summarize the significance of cardiovascular disease in individuals with chronic kidney disease.
8. Explain the conservative collaborative care for and the related nursing management of the patient with chronic kidney disease.
9. Differentiate among renal replacement therapy options for individuals with end-stage kidney disease.
10. Compare and contrast nursing interventions for individuals on peritoneal dialysis and hemodialysis.
11. Discuss the role of nurses in the management of individuals who receive a kidney transplant.

KEY TERMS

acute kidney injury (AKI), p. 1101
acute tubular necrosis (ATN), p. 1103
arteriovenous fistula (AVF), p. 1120
arteriovenous grafts (AVGs), p. 1120
automated peritoneal dialysis (APD), p. 1119
azotemia, p. 1102

chronic kidney disease (CKD), p. 1107
CKD mineral and bone disorder (CKD-MBD), p. 1110
continuous ambulatory peritoneal dialysis (CAPD), p. 1119
continuous renal replacement therapy (CRRT), p. 1123

dialysis, p. 1117
end-stage kidney (renal) disease (ESKD), p. 1107
hemodialysis (HD), p. 1117
oliguria, p. 1103
peritoneal dialysis (PD), p. 1117
uremia, p. 1108

Kidney failure (also called *renal failure*) is the partial or complete impairment of kidney function. It results in an inability to excrete metabolic waste products and water, and it contributes to disturbances of all body systems. Kidney disease can be classified as acute or chronic (Table 47-1). Acute kidney injury (AKI) has a rapid onset. Chronic kidney disease (CKD) is linked with the development of cardiovascular (CV) disease.

ACUTE KIDNEY INJURY

Acute kidney injury (AKI), previously known as *acute kidney failure,* is the term used to encompass the entire range of the syndrome, ranging from a slight deterioration in kidney function to severe impairment. AKI is characterized by a rapid loss of kidney function. This loss is accompanied by a rise in serum

Reviewed by Kay Helzer, RN, MSN, Former Renal/Pancreas Transplant Coordinator, Banner Good Samaritan Medical Center, Phoenix, Arizona; and Marci Langenkamp, RN, MS, Assistant Professor of Nursing, Edison Community College, Piqua, Ohio.

creatinine and/or a reduction in urine output. The severity of dysfunction can range from a small increase in serum creatinine or reduction in urine output to the development of azotemia (an accumulation of nitrogenous waste products [urea nitrogen, creatinine] in the blood).

Although AKI is potentially reversible, it has a high mortality rate.[1] AKI usually affects people with other life-threatening conditions[2] (Table 47-2). Most commonly, AKI follows severe, prolonged hypotension or hypovolemia or exposure to a nephrotoxic agent.

AKI can develop over hours or days with progressive elevations of blood urea nitrogen (BUN), creatinine, and potassium with or without a reduction in urine output. Hospitalized patients develop AKI at a high rate (1 in 5) and have a high mortality rate. When AKI develops in patients in intensive care units (ICUs), the mortality rate can be as high as 70% to 80%.[3-5]

Etiology and Pathophysiology

The causes of AKI, which are multiple and complex, are categorized as prerenal, intrarenal (or intrinsic), and postrenal causes (see Table 47-2).

Prerenal. *Prerenal* causes of AKI are factors external to the kidneys. These factors reduce systemic circulation, causing a reduction in renal blood flow. The decrease in blood flow leads to decreased glomerular perfusion and filtration of the kidneys. Although kidney tubular and glomerular function is preserved, glomerular filtration is reduced as a result of decreased perfusion.

It is important to distinguish prerenal oliguria from the oliguria of intrarenal AKI. In prerenal oliguria there is no damage to the kidney tissue (parenchyma). The oliguria is caused by a decrease in circulating blood volume (e.g., severe dehydration, heart failure [HF], decreased cardiac output) and is readily reversible with appropriate treatment. With a decrease in circulating blood volume, autoregulatory mechanisms that increase angiotensin II, aldosterone, norepinephrine, and antidiuretic hormone attempt to preserve blood flow to essential organs. Prerenal azotemia results in a reduction in the excretion of sodium (less than 20 mEq/L), increased sodium and water retention, and decreased urine output.

Prerenal conditions can lead to intrarenal disease if renal ischemia is prolonged. Prerenal conditions account for many cases of intrarenal AKI. If decreased perfusion persists for an extended time, the kidneys lose their ability to compensate and damage to kidney parenchyma occurs (intrarenal damage).

Intrarenal. *Intrarenal* causes of AKI (see Table 47-2) include conditions that cause direct damage to the kidney tissue, resulting in impaired nephron function. The damage from intrarenal causes usually results from prolonged ischemia, nephrotoxins

TABLE 47-1	COMPARISON OF ACUTE KIDNEY INJURY AND CHRONIC KIDNEY DISEASE	
	Acute Kidney Injury	**Chronic Kidney Disease**
Onset	Sudden	Gradual, often over many years
Most common cause	Acute tubular necrosis	Diabetic nephropathy
Diagnostic criteria	Acute reduction in urine output and/or Elevation in serum creatinine	GFR <60 mL/min/1.73m² for >3 mo and/or Kidney damage >3 mo
Reversibility	Potentially	Progressive and irreversible
Primary cause of death	Infection	Cardiovascular disease

GFR, Glomerular filtration rate.

TABLE 47-2	COMMON CAUSES OF ACUTE KIDNEY INJURY	
Prerenal	**Intrarenal**	**Postrenal**
Hypovolemia • Dehydration • Hemorrhage • GI losses (diarrhea, vomiting) • Excessive diuresis • Hypoalbuminemia • Burns **Decreased Cardiac Output** • Cardiac dysrhythmias • Cardiogenic shock • Heart failure • Myocardial infarction **Decreased Peripheral Vascular Resistance** • Anaphylaxis • Neurologic injury • Septic shock **Decreased Renovascular Blood Flow** • Bilateral renal vein thrombosis • Embolism • Hepatorenal syndrome • Renal artery thrombosis	**Nephrotoxic Injury** • Drugs: aminoglycosides (gentamicin, amikacin), amphotericin B • Contrast media • Hemolytic blood transfusion reaction • Severe crush injury • Chemical exposure: ethylene glycol, lead, arsenic, carbon tetrachloride **Interstitial Nephritis** • Allergies: antibiotics (sulfonamides, rifampin), nonsteroidal antiinflammatory drugs, ACE inhibitors • Infections: bacterial (acute pyelonephritis), viral (CMV), fungal (candidiasis) **Other Causes** • Prolonged prerenal ischemia • Acute glomerulonephritis • Thrombotic disorders • Toxemia of pregnancy • Malignant hypertension • Systemic lupus erythematosus	• Benign prostatic hyperplasia • Bladder cancer • Calculi formation • Neuromuscular disorders • Prostate cancer • Spinal cord disease • Strictures • Trauma (back, pelvis, perineum)

ACE, Angiotensin-converting enzyme; *CMV*, cytomegalovirus.

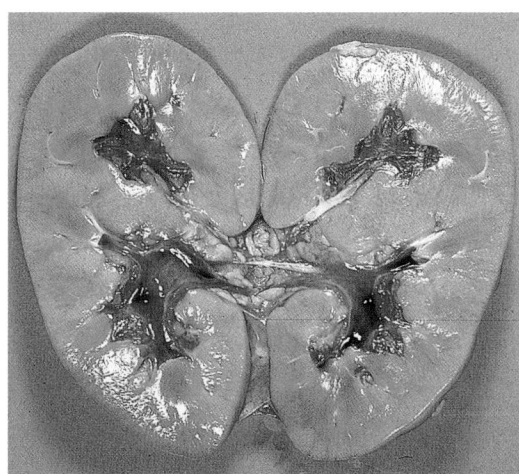

FIG. 47-1 Acute tubular necrosis. The kidneys are swollen and pale.

TABLE 47-3	RIFLE CLASSIFICATION FOR STAGING ACUTE KIDNEY INJURY	
Stage	**GFR Criteria**	**Urine Output Criteria**
Risk	Serum creatinine increased × 1.5 OR GFR decreased by 25%	Urine output <0.5 mL/kg/hr for 6 hr
Injury	Serum creatinine increased × 2 OR GFR decreased by 50%	Urine output <0.5 mL/kg/hr for 12 hr
Failure	Serum creatinine increased × 3 OR GFR decreased by 75% OR Serum creatinine >4 mg/dL with acute rise ≥0.5 mg/dL	Urine output <0.3 mL/kg/hr for 24 hr (oliguria) OR Anuria for 12 hr
Loss	Persistent acute kidney failure; complete loss of kidney function >4 wk	—
End-stage kidney disease	Complete loss of kidney function >3 mo	—

GFR, Glomerular filtration rate.

(e.g., aminoglycoside antibiotics, contrast media), hemoglobin released from hemolyzed red blood cells (RBCs), or myoglobin released from necrotic muscle cells.

Nephrotoxins can cause obstruction of intrarenal structures by crystallizing or by causing damage to the epithelial cells of the tubules. Hemoglobin and myoglobin can block the tubules and cause renal vasoconstriction. Diseases of the kidney such as acute glomerulonephritis and systemic lupus erythematosus may also cause AKI.

Acute tubular necrosis (ATN) is the most common intrarenal cause of AKI and is primarily the result of ischemia, nephrotoxins, or sepsis (Fig. 47-1). Ischemic and nephrotoxic ATN is responsible for 90% of intrarenal AKI cases.[6,7] Severe kidney ischemia causes a disruption in the basement membrane and patchy destruction of the tubular epithelium. Nephrotoxic agents cause necrosis of tubular epithelial cells, which slough off and plug the tubules. ATN is potentially reversible if the basement membrane is not destroyed and the tubular epithelium regenerates.

ATN is the most common cause of AKI for hospitalized patients. Risks associated with development of ATN while in the hospital include major surgery, shock, sepsis, blood transfusion reaction, muscle injury from trauma, prolonged hypotension, and nephrotoxic agents (see Table 47-2).

Postrenal. *Postrenal* causes of AKI involve mechanical obstruction in the outflow of urine. As the flow of urine is obstructed, urine refluxes into the renal pelvis, impairing kidney function. The most common causes are benign prostatic hyperplasia, prostate cancer, calculi, trauma, and extrarenal tumors. Bilateral ureteral obstruction leads to *hydronephrosis* (kidney dilation), increase in hydrostatic pressure, and tubular blockage, resulting in a progressive decline in kidney function. If bilateral obstruction is relieved within 48 hours of onset, complete recovery is likely. After 12 weeks, recovery is unlikely. Prolonged obstruction can lead to tubular atrophy and irreversible kidney fibrosis. Postrenal causes of AKI account for less than 10% of AKI cases.[7,8]

Clinical Manifestations

Prerenal and postrenal AKI that has not caused intrarenal damage usually resolves quickly with treatment of the cause. However, when parenchymal damage occurs due to either prerenal or postrenal causes, or when parenchymal damage occurs directly as with intrarenal causes, AKI has a prolonged course.

Clinically, AKI may progress through phases: oliguric, diuretic, and recovery. When a patient does not recover from AKI, then CKD may develop.

The RIFLE classification is used to describe the stages of AKI (Table 47-3). *Risk,* the first stage of AKI, is followed by *Injury,* which is the second stage. Then AKI increases in severity to the final or third stage, *Failure.* The two outcome variables are *Loss* and *End-stage kidney disease.* (See eTable 47-2 for a case study showing how RIFLE classification is used.)

Oliguric Phase. Manifestations of AKI are presented in eTable 47-1 (available on the website for this chapter). The most common manifestations are discussed in this section.

Urinary Changes. The most common initial manifestation of AKI is oliguria, a reduction in urine output to less than 400 mL/ day. Nonoliguria AKI indicates a urine output greater than 400 mL/day. Oliguria usually occurs within 1 to 7 days of the injury to the kidneys. If the cause is ischemia, oliguria often occurs within 24 hours. In contrast, when nephrotoxic drugs are involved, the onset may be delayed for as long as 1 week. The oliguric phase lasts on average about 10 to 14 days but can last months in some cases. The longer the oliguric phase lasts, the poorer the prognosis for complete recovery of kidney function.[1]

About 50% of patients will not be oliguric, making the initial diagnosis more difficult.[5] Changes in urine output generally do not correspond to changes in glomerular filtration rate (GFR). However, changes in urine output are often helpful in differentiating the etiology of AKI. For example, anuria is usually seen with urinary tract obstruction, oliguria is commonly seen with prerenal etiologies, and nonoliguric AKI is seen with acute interstitial nephritis and ATN.[8]

A urinalysis may show casts, RBCs, and white blood cells (WBCs). The casts are formed from mucoprotein impressions of the necrotic renal tubular epithelial cells, which detach or slough into the tubules. In addition, a urinalysis may show a specific gravity fixed at around 1.010 and urine osmolality at about 300 mOsm/kg (300 mmol/kg). This is the same specific gravity and osmolality of plasma, thus reflecting tubular damage with a loss of concentrating ability by the kidney. Proteinuria may be present if kidney failure is related to glomerular membrane dysfunction.

Fluid Volume. Hypovolemia (volume depletion) has the potential to exacerbate all forms of AKI. The reversal of hypovolemia with fluid replacement is often sufficient to treat many forms of AKI, especially prerenal causes.

When urine output decreases, fluid retention occurs. The severity of the symptoms depends on the extent of the fluid overload. In the case of reduced urine output (anuria and oliguria), the neck veins may become distended with a bounding pulse. Edema and hypertension may develop. Fluid overload can eventually lead to HF, pulmonary edema, and pericardial and pleural effusions.

Metabolic Acidosis. In kidney failure the kidneys cannot synthesize ammonia (needed for hydrogen ion excretion) or excrete acid products of metabolism. The serum bicarbonate level decreases because bicarbonate is depleted in buffering hydrogen ions. In addition, defective reabsorption and regeneration of bicarbonate occur. With development of severe acidosis, the patient may develop Kussmaul respirations (rapid, deep respirations) in an effort to compensate by increasing the exhalation of carbon dioxide.

Sodium Balance. Damaged tubules cannot conserve sodium. Consequently, the urinary excretion of sodium may increase, resulting in normal or below-normal levels of serum sodium. Excessive intake of sodium should be avoided because it can lead to volume expansion, hypertension, and HF. Uncontrolled hyponatremia or water excess can lead to cerebral edema.

Potassium Excess. The kidneys normally excrete 80% to 90% of the body's potassium. In AKI the serum potassium level increases because the kidney's normal ability to excrete potassium is impaired. Hyperkalemia is more of a risk if AKI is caused by massive tissue trauma because the damaged cells release additional potassium into the extracellular fluid. Additionally, bleeding and blood transfusions may cause cellular destruction, releasing more potassium into the extracellular fluid. Last, acidosis worsens hyperkalemia as hydrogen ions enter the cells and potassium is driven out of the cells into the extracellular fluid.

Even though patients with hyperkalemia are usually asymptomatic, some patients may complain of weakness with severe hyperkalemia. Acute or rapid development of hyperkalemia may result in clinical signs that are apparent on electrocardiogram (ECG). These changes include peaked T waves, widening of the QRS complex, and ST segment depression. Progressive changes in the ECG that are related to increasing potassium levels are depicted in Fig. 17-14. Because cardiac muscle is intolerant of acute increases in potassium, treatment is essential whenever hyperkalemia develops.[9]

Hematologic Disorders. Several hematologic disorders are seen in patients with AKI. Hospital-acquired AKI often occurs in patients who have multiorgan failure. Leukocytosis is often present with AKI. The most common cause of death in AKI is infection. The most common sites of infection are the urinary and respiratory systems. A complete blood count with evidence of eosinophilia suggests an allergic response and possibly interstitial nephritis, polyarteritis nodosa, or atheroemboli.

Waste Product Accumulation. The kidneys are the primary excretory organs for urea (an end product of protein metabolism) and creatinine (an end product of endogenous muscle metabolism). BUN and serum creatinine levels are elevated in kidney failure. An elevated BUN level must be interpreted

with caution because it can also be caused by dehydration; corticosteroids; or catabolism resulting from infections, fever, severe injury, or GI bleeding. The best serum indicator of AKI is creatinine because it is not significantly altered by other factors.

Neurologic Disorders. Neurologic changes can occur as the nitrogenous waste products accumulate in the brain and other nervous tissue. The manifestations can be as mild as fatigue and difficulty concentrating, and then escalate to seizures, stupor, and coma. *Asterixis* (flapping tremor when the wrist is extended) is most common with liver failure, but has been known to occur with advanced and severe kidney dysfunction. The flapping resembles a bird flapping its wings when the hands and wrists are extended outward.

Diuretic Phase. During the diuretic phase of AKI, daily urine output is usually around 1 to 3 L, but may reach 5 L or more. Although urine output is increasing, the nephrons are still not fully functional. The high urine volume is caused by osmotic diuresis from the high urea concentration in the glomerular filtrate and the inability of the tubules to concentrate the urine. In this phase the kidneys have recovered their ability to excrete wastes, but not to concentrate the urine. Hypovolemia and hypotension can occur from massive fluid losses. Patients who develop an oliguric phase will have greater diuresis than patients without oliguria.

Because of the large losses of fluid and electrolytes, the patient must be monitored for hyponatremia, hypokalemia, and dehydration. The diuretic phase may last 1 to 3 weeks. Near the end of this phase, the patient's acid-base, electrolyte, and waste product (BUN, creatinine) values begin to normalize.

Recovery Phase. The recovery phase begins when the GFR increases, allowing the BUN and serum creatinine levels to plateau and then decrease. Although the major improvements occur in the first 1 to 2 weeks of this phase, kidney function may take up to 12 months to stabilize.

The outcome of AKI is influenced by the patient's overall health, the severity of kidney failure, and the number and type of complications. Some individuals do not recover and progress to end-stage kidney disease. The older adult is less likely to have a complete recovery of kidney function. Most patients who recover achieve clinically normal kidney function with no complications (e.g., hypertension). Some scar tissue remains, but loss of function is not clinically significant.

Diagnostic Studies

A thorough history is essential for diagnosing the etiology of AKI. Consider prerenal causes when there is a history of dehydration, blood loss, or severe heart disease. Suspect intrarenal causes if the patient has been exposed to potentially nephrotoxic drugs or has a recent history of a blood transfusion or radiologic study using contrast media. Postrenal causes are suggested by a history of changes in the urinary stream, stones, benign prostatic hyperplasia, or cancer of the bladder or prostate.

Although changes in urine output and serum creatinine occur relatively late in the course of AKI, there are no better criteria for a diagnosis of AKI. An increase in serum creatinine may not be evident until there is a loss of more than 50% of kidney function. The rate of increase in serum creatinine is also important as a diagnostic indicator and in determining the severity of injury.

Urinalysis is an important diagnostic test. Urine sediment containing abundant cells, casts, or proteins suggests intrarenal disorders. The urine osmolality, sodium content, and specific gravity help in differentiating the causes of AKI. Urine sediment may be normal in both prerenal and postrenal AKI. In intrarenal problems, hematuria, pyuria, and crystals may be seen.

To establish a diagnosis of AKI, other testing may be required. A kidney ultrasound is often the first test done, since it provides imaging without exposure to potentially nephrotoxic contrast agents. It is useful for evaluating for possible kidney disease and obstruction of the urinary collection system. A renal scan can assess abnormalities in kidney blood flow, tubular function, and the collecting system. A computed tomography (CT) scan can identify lesions, masses, obstructions, and vascular anomalies. A renal biopsy is considered the best method for confirming intrarenal causes of AKI.

Obtaining a magnetic resonance imaging (MRI) or magnetic resonance angiography (MRA) study with the contrast media gadolinium is not advised in patients with kidney failure unless there is a significant reason to do these tests or unless the ultrasound or CT will not provide the information needed. Administration of gadolinium has been associated with the development of a devastating and potentially lethal disorder, *nephrogenic systemic fibrosis,* in patients with kidney failure. The disease is characterized by skin hyperpigmentation and induration and joint contractures. However, the fibrosis can also develop in other organs.

In patients with normal kidney function, administration of contrast media poses minimal risk. In patients with kidney failure, *contrast-induced nephropathy* (CIN) can occur when contrast media for diagnostic studies causes nephrotoxic injury. The best way to avoid CIN is to avoid exposure to contrast media by using other diagnostic tests such as ultrasound. If contrast media must be administered to a high-risk patient, the patient needs to have optimal hydration and a low dose of the contrast agent. Treatment to prevent CIN remains controversial. Optimal hydration is the goal, but debate continues on whether a bicarbonate or sodium chloride solution with or without the

prophylactic administration of *N*-acetylcysteine (Mucomyst) is beneficial.

Collaborative Care

Because AKI is potentially reversible, the primary goals of treatment are to eliminate the cause, manage the signs and symptoms, and prevent complications while the kidneys recover[2] (Table 47-4). The first step is to determine if there is adequate intravascular volume and cardiac output to ensure adequate perfusion of the kidneys. Diuretic therapy is often administered but not recommended in high doses. Diuretic therapy usually includes loop diuretics (e.g., furosemide [Lasix], bumetanide [Bumex]) or an osmotic diuretic (e.g., mannitol). If AKI is already established, forcing fluids and diuretics will not be effective and may, in fact, be harmful.

Closely monitor fluid intake during the oliguric phase of AKI. The general rule for calculating the fluid restriction is to add all losses for the previous 24 hours (e.g., urine, diarrhea, emesis, blood) plus 600 mL for insensible losses (e.g., respiration, diaphoresis). For example, if a patient excreted 300 mL of urine on Tuesday with no other losses, the fluid allocation on Wednesday would be 900 mL.

Hyperkalemia is one of the most serious complications in AKI because it can cause life-threatening cardiac dysrhythmias. The various therapies used to treat elevated potassium levels are listed in Table 47-5. Both insulin and sodium bicarbonate serve as a temporary measure for treatment of hyperkalemia by promoting a shift of potassium into the cells, but potassium will eventually be released. Calcium gluconate raises the threshold at which dysrhythmias occur, temporarily stabilizing the myocardium. Only sodium polystyrene sulfonate (Kayexalate) and

---

TABLE 47-4 COLLABORATIVE CARE

Acute Kidney Injury

Diagnostic
- History and physical examination
- Identification of precipitating cause
- Serum creatinine and BUN levels
- Serum electrolytes
- Urinalysis
- Renal ultrasound
- Renal scan
- CT scan

Collaborative Therapy
- Treatment of precipitating cause
- Fluid restriction (600 mL plus previous 24-hr fluid loss)
- Nutritional therapy
  - Adequate protein intake (0.6-2 g/kg/day) depending on degree of catabolism
  - Potassium restriction
  - Phosphate restriction
  - Sodium restriction
- Measures to lower potassium (if elevated) (see Table 47-5)
- Calcium supplements or phosphate-binding agents
- Enteral nutrition
- Parenteral nutrition
- Initiation of dialysis (if necessary)
- Continuous renal replacement therapy (if necessary)

TABLE 47-5 THERAPIES FOR ELEVATED POTASSIUM LEVELS

Regular Insulin IV
- Potassium moves into cells when insulin is given.
- IV glucose is given concurrently to prevent hypoglycemia.
- When effects of insulin diminish, potassium shifts back out of cells.

Sodium Bicarbonate
- Therapy can correct acidosis and cause a shift of potassium into cells.

Calcium Gluconate IV
- Generally used in advanced cardiac toxicity (with evidence of hyperkalemic ECG changes).
- Calcium raises the threshold for excitation, resulting in dysrhythmias.

Hemodialysis
- Most effective therapy to remove potassium.
- Works within a short time.

Sodium Polystyrene Sulfonate (Kayexalate)
- Cation-exchange resin is administered by mouth or retention enema.
- When resin is in the bowel, potassium is exchanged for sodium.
- Therapy removes 1 mEq of potassium per gram of drug.
- It is mixed in water with sorbitol to produce osmotic diarrhea, allowing for evacuation of potassium-rich stool from body.

Dietary Restriction
- Potassium intake is limited to 40 mEq/day.
- Primarily used to prevent recurrent elevation; not used for acute elevation.

dialysis actually remove potassium from the body. Never give this drug to a patient with a paralytic ileus because bowel necrosis can occur.

Conservative therapy may be all that is necessary until kidney function improves. Controversy exists about the timing of renal replacement therapy (RRT) in AKI.[10] The most common indications for RRT in AKI are (1) volume overload, resulting in compromised cardiac and/or pulmonary status; (2) elevated serum potassium level; (3) metabolic acidosis (serum bicarbonate level less than 15 mEq/L [15 mmol/L]); (4) BUN level greater than 120 mg/dL (43 mmol/L); (5) significant change in mental status; and (6) pericarditis, pericardial effusion, or cardiac tamponade. Although laboratory values provide rough parameters, the best guide to treatment is good clinical assessment.

If RRT is required, many options are available, but there is no consensus regarding the best approach.[10] Even though peritoneal dialysis (PD) is considered a viable option for RRT, it is not frequently used. Intermittent hemodialysis (HD) (e.g., at intervals of 4 hours either daily, every other day, or 3 or 4 times per week) and *continuous renal replacement therapy* (CRRT) have both been used effectively.

CRRT is provided continuously over approximately 24 hours through cannulation of an artery and vein or cannulation of two veins. CRRT has much slower blood flow rates compared with intermittent HD.

HD is the method of choice when rapid changes are required in a short time. It is technically more complicated because specialized staff and equipment and a vascular access are required. It also requires anticoagulation therapy to prevent the patient's blood from clotting when the blood contacts the foreign material in the extracorporeal dialysis circuit. Rapid fluid shifts during HD may cause hypotension.

RRT and CRRT are discussed later in this chapter on pp. 1123-1124.

Nutritional Therapy. The challenge of nutritional management in AKI is to provide adequate calories to prevent catabolism despite the restrictions required to prevent electrolyte and fluid disorders and azotemia. A primary nutritional goal in AKI is to maintain adequate caloric intake (providing 30 to 35 kcal/kg and 0.8 to 1.0 g of protein per kilogram of desired body weight) to prevent the further breakdown of body protein for energy purposes. Adequate energy should be primarily from carbohydrate and fat sources to prevent ketosis from endogenous fat breakdown and gluconeogenesis from muscle protein breakdown. Supplementation of essential amino acids can be given.

Potassium and sodium are regulated in accordance with plasma levels. Sodium is restricted as needed to prevent edema, hypertension, and HF. Dietary fat intake is increased so that the patient receives at least 30% to 40% of total calories from fat. Fat emulsion IV infusions given as a nutritional supplement provide a good source of nonprotein calories (see Chapter 40).

If a patient cannot maintain adequate oral intake, enteral nutrition is the preferred route for nutritional support (see Chapter 40). When the gastrointestinal (GI) tract is not functional, parenteral nutrition is necessary to provide adequate nutrition. The patient treated with parenteral nutrition may need daily HD or CRRT to remove the excess fluid. Concentrated formulas of parenteral nutrition are available to minimize fluid volume.

NURSING MANAGEMENT ACUTE KIDNEY INJURY

NURSING ASSESSMENT

Monitor vital signs and fluid intake and output. Daily monitoring of a patient's urine output has prognostic implications and is crucial for determining therapy and daily fluid volume replacement. Examine the urine for color, specific gravity, glucose, protein, blood, and sediment. Assess the patient's general appearance, including skin color, edema, neck vein distention, and bruises.

If a patient is receiving dialysis, observe the access site for inflammation and exudate. Evaluate the patient's mental status and level of consciousness. Examine the oral mucosa for dryness and inflammation. Auscultate the lungs for crackles and rhonchi or diminished breath sounds. Monitor the heart for an S_3 gallop, murmurs, or a pericardial friction rub. Assess ECG readings for dysrhythmias. Review laboratory values and diagnostic test results. All of the previous data are essential for developing a collaborative plan of care.

NURSING DIAGNOSES

Nursing diagnoses and a potential complication for the patient with AKI include, but are not limited to, the following:

- Excess fluid volume *related to* kidney failure and fluid retention
- Risk for infection *related to* invasive lines, uremic toxins, and altered immune responses secondary to kidney failure
- Fatigue *related to* anemia, metabolic acidosis, and uremic toxins
- Anxiety *related to* disease processes, therapeutic interventions, and uncertainty of prognosis
- Potential complication: dysrhythmias *related to* electrolyte imbalances

PLANNING

The overall goals are that the patient with AKI will (1) completely recover without any loss of kidney function, (2) maintain normal fluid and electrolyte balance, (3) have decreased anxiety, and (4) adhere to and understand the need for careful follow-up care.

NURSING IMPLEMENTATION

HEALTH PROMOTION. Prevention and early recognition of AKI are the most important components of care.[11] Prevention is primarily directed toward identifying and monitoring high-risk populations, controlling exposure to nephrotoxic drugs and industrial chemicals, and preventing prolonged episodes of hypotension and hypovolemia. In the hospital the factors that increase the risk for developing AKI are preexisting CKD, older age, massive trauma, major surgical procedures, extensive burns, cardiac failure, sepsis, or obstetric complications.

Careful monitoring of intake and output and fluid and electrolyte balance is essential. Assess and record extrarenal losses of fluid from vomiting, diarrhea, hemorrhage, and increased insensible losses. Prompt replacement of significant fluid losses helps prevent ischemic tubular damage associated with trauma, burns, and extensive surgery. Intake and output records and the patient's weight provide valuable indicators of fluid volume status. Aggressive diuretic therapy for the patient with fluid overload from any cause can lead to a reduction in renal blood flow.[12]

The individual who is taking drugs that are potentially nephrotoxic (see Table 45-3) must have his or her kidney function monitored. Nephrotoxic drugs should be used sparingly in the high-risk patient. When these drugs must be used, they should be given in the smallest effective doses for the shortest possible periods. Caution the patient about abuse of over-the-counter analgesics (especially nonsteroidal antiinflammatory drugs [NSAIDs]) because some of these may worsen kidney function in the patient with mild CKD.

Angiotensin-converting enzyme (ACE) inhibitors can also decrease perfusion pressure and cause hyperkalemia. If other measures such as diet modification, diuretics, and sodium bicarbonate cannot control the hyperkalemia, ACE inhibitors may need to be reduced or eliminated. However, ACE inhibitors are frequently used to prevent proteinuria and progression of kidney disease, especially in diabetic patients.[13]

ACUTE INTERVENTION. The patient with AKI is critically ill and suffers from the effects of not only kidney disease but also co-morbid diseases or conditions (e.g., diabetes, CV disease). Focus on the patient holistically, since he or she will have many physical and emotional needs. Usually the changes caused by AKI arise suddenly. Both the patient and caregiver need assistance in understanding that the whole body's functioning can be disrupted by kidney failure.

You have an important role in managing fluid and electrolyte balance during the oliguric and diuretic phases. Observe and record accurate intake and output. Take daily weights with the same scale at the same time each day to detect excessive gains or losses of body fluid (1 kg is equivalent to 1000 mL of fluid). Assess for the common signs and symptoms of hypervolemia (in the oliguric phase) or hypovolemia (in the diuretic phase), potassium and sodium disturbances, and other electrolyte imbalances that may occur in AKI (see Chapter 17).

Because infection is the leading cause of death in AKI, meticulous aseptic technique is critical. Protect the patient from other individuals with infectious diseases. Be alert for local manifestations of infection (e.g., swelling, redness, pain), as well as systemic manifestations (e.g., fever, malaise, leukocytosis), but realize that the temperature may not always be elevated. Patients with kidney failure have a blunted febrile response to an infection (e.g., pneumonia). If antibiotics are used to treat an infection, the type, frequency, and dosage must be carefully considered because the kidneys are the primary route of excretion for many antibiotics. Dosages need to be considered in light of the patient's level of kidney function if the drug is primarily eliminated by the kidneys. Nephrotoxic drugs (see Table 45-3) should be used judiciously.

Perform skin care and take measures to prevent pressure ulcers because the patient usually develops edema and decreased muscle tone. Mouth care is important to prevent stomatitis, which develops when ammonia (produced by bacterial breakdown of urea) in saliva irritates the mucous membranes.

INFORMATICS IN PRACTICE

Computer Monitoring of Antibiotic Safety

- Many patients receiving antibiotic therapy are at risk for kidney failure.
- Set the computer to alert you about elevated creatinine levels and, if possible, send you a text message.
- With earlier notification of the health care provider, medications can be stopped or doses adjusted and the patient's kidney function preserved.

AMBULATORY AND HOME CARE. Recovery from AKI is highly variable and depends on other organ system failures, the patient's general condition and age, the length of the oliguric phase, and the severity of nephron damage. Protein and potassium intake should be regulated in accordance with kidney function. Follow-up care and regular evaluation of kidney function are necessary. Teach the patient the signs and symptoms of recurrent kidney disease. Emphasize measures to prevent the recurrence of AKI.

The long-term convalescence of 3 to 12 months may cause psychosocial and financial hardships for both the patient and the family. Make appropriate referrals for counseling. If the kidneys do not recover, the patient will need to transition to life on chronic dialysis or possible future transplantation.

EVALUATION

The expected outcomes are that the patient with AKI will
- Regain and maintain normal fluid and electrolyte balance
- Adhere to the treatment regimen
- Experience no complications
- Have a complete recovery

GERONTOLOGIC CONSIDERATIONS

ACUTE KIDNEY INJURY

Older adults are at risk for the same causes of AKI as younger adults. However, they are more susceptible to AKI. Dehydration is a predisposing factor and tends to occur much more frequently in older adults. Dehydration is associated with polypharmacy (diuretics, laxatives, and drugs that suppress appetite or consciousness), acute febrile illnesses, and immobility from being bedridden.

In addition to dehydration, other common causes of AKI in the older adult include hypotension, diuretic therapy, aminoglycoside therapy, obstructive disorders (e.g., prostatic hyperplasia), surgery, infection, and contrast media.

In older adults, impaired function of other organ systems from CV disease or diabetes mellitus can increase the risk of developing AKI. The aging kidney is less able to compensate for changes in fluid volume, solute load, and cardiac output. Mortality rates are similar for older patients and younger patients. However, patients over 65 years of age are less likely to recover from AKI. Despite this, a patient's chronologic age should not be factored into the decision about whether to institute RRT.[9,10]

CHRONIC KIDNEY DISEASE

Chronic kidney disease (CKD) involves progressive, irreversible loss of kidney function. The Kidney Disease Outcomes Quality Initiative (KDOQI) of the National Kidney Foundation defines CKD as either the presence of kidney damage or a decreased GFR less than 60 mL/min/1.73 m^2 for longer than 3 months. The classification of CKD is presented in Table 47-6. The last stage of kidney failure, end-stage kidney (renal) disease (ESKD), occurs when the GFR is less than 15 mL/min. At this point, RRT (dialysis or transplantation) is required to maintain life.

Although CKD has many different causes, the leading causes are diabetes (about 50%) and hypertension (about 25%). Less common etiologies include glomerulonephritis, cystic diseases, and urologic diseases.[14] (Diseases of the renal system that affect the kidney are discussed in Chapter 46.) CKD is much more

TABLE 47-6	STAGES OF CHRONIC KIDNEY DISEASE	
Description	**GFR (mL/ min/1.73 m²)**	**Clinical Action Plan**
Stage 1 Kidney damage with normal or ↑ GFR	≥90	Diagnosis and treatment CVD risk reduction Slow progression
Stage 2 Kidney damage with mild ↓ GFR	60-89	Estimation of progression
Stage 3 Moderate ↓ GFR	30-59	Evaluation and treatment of complications
Stage 4 Severe ↓ GFR	15-29	Preparation for renal replacement therapy (dialysis, kidney transplant)
Stage 5 Kidney failure	<15 (or dialysis)	Renal replacement therapy (if uremia present and patient desires treatment)

Source: National Kidney Foundation. *www.kidney.org/kidneydisease/aboutckd.cfm.*

⊕ CULTURAL & ETHNIC HEALTH DISPARITIES
Chronic Kidney Disease

- Chronic kidney disease (CKD) has a high incidence in minority populations, especially African Americans and Native Americans.
- Hypertension and diabetes mellitus are also more common in African Americans and Native Americans.

African Americans
- The risk of CKD as a complication of hypertension is significantly increased in African Americans.
- African Americans have the highest rate of CKD, nearly four times that of whites.

Native Americans
- Native Americans have a rate of CKD twice that of whites.
- The rate of CKD is six times higher among Native Americans with diabetes than among other ethnic groups with diabetes.

Hispanics
- The rate of CKD in Hispanics is 1.5 times higher than in non-Hispanic whites.

common than AKI (see Table 47-1). The increasing prevalence of CKD has been partially attributed to the increase in risk factors, including an aging population, rise in rates of obesity, and increased incidence of diabetes and hypertension.[14,15]

More than 26 million American adults have CKD, and a million more are at increased risk. One of every nine Americans has CKD. Over half a million Americans are receiving treatment (dialysis, transplant) for ESKD. Despite all the technologic advances in life-sustaining treatment with dialysis, patients with ESKD have a high mortality rate. As the stage of kidney disease progresses, the mortality rate also increases. Mortality rates are as high as 19% to 24% for individuals with stage 5 CKD on dialysis. About 20% of patients with ESKD receiving dialysis die each year.[14]

Because the kidneys are highly adaptive, kidney disease is often not recognized until there has been considerable loss of nephrons. Because patients with CKD are frequently asymptomatic, CKD is underdiagnosed and undertreated. It has been estimated that about 70% of people with CKD are unaware that they have the disease.[14]

The prognosis and course of CKD are highly variable depending on the etiology, patient's condition and age, and adequacy of health care follow-up. Some individuals live normal, active lives with compensated kidney failure, whereas others may rapidly progress to ESKD (stage 5). Since 1972, the United States has covered the majority of the costs of providing dialysis for those eligible for Medicare benefits. Under Title XVIII of the Social Security Act, ESKD was recognized as a disability. As such, more than 90% of individuals of any age who have ESKD are eligible for financial assistance for treatment through Medicare. Medicare pays for 80% of eligible charges, with the remaining being paid for by state or private insurance or out of pocket.[14]

Clinical Manifestations

As kidney function deteriorates, every body system becomes affected. The clinical manifestations are a result of retained sub-stances, including urea, creatinine, phenols, hormones, electrolytes, and water. Uremia is a syndrome in which kidney function declines to the point that symptoms may develop in multiple body systems (Fig. 47-2). It often occurs when the GFR is 10 mL/min or less.

The manifestations of uremia vary among patients according to the cause of the kidney disease, co-morbid conditions, age, and degree of adherence to the prescribed medical regimen. Many patients are tolerant of the changes because they occur gradually.

Urinary System. In the early stages of CKD, patients usually do not report any change in urine output. Since diabetes is the primary cause of CKD, polyuria may be present, but not necessarily as a consequence of kidney disease. Because most people continue to have sufficient urine output, it is often difficult to convince them that they have kidney disease. As CKD progresses, patients have increasing difficulty with fluid retention and require diuretic therapy. After a period on dialysis, patients may develop anuria.

Metabolic Disturbances

Waste Product Accumulation. As the GFR decreases, the BUN and serum creatinine levels increase. The BUN is increased not only by kidney failure, but also by protein intake, fever, corticosteroids, and catabolism. For this reason, serum creatinine clearance determinations (calculated GFR) are considered more accurate indicators of kidney function than BUN or creatinine. Significant elevations in BUN contribute to development of nausea, vomiting, lethargy, fatigue, impaired thought processes, and headaches.

Altered Carbohydrate Metabolism. Defective carbohydrate metabolism is caused by impaired glucose metabolism, resulting from cellular insensitivity to the normal action of insulin. Mild to moderate hyperglycemia and hyperinsulinemia may occur. Insulin and glucose metabolism may improve (but not to normal values) after the initiation of dialysis.

Patients with diabetes who develop uremia may require less insulin than before the onset of CKD. This is because insulin, which depends on the kidneys for excretion, remains in circulation longer. As a result, a number of patients who required insulin before starting dialysis will be able to discontinue insulin therapy when they start dialysis and their kidney disease pro-

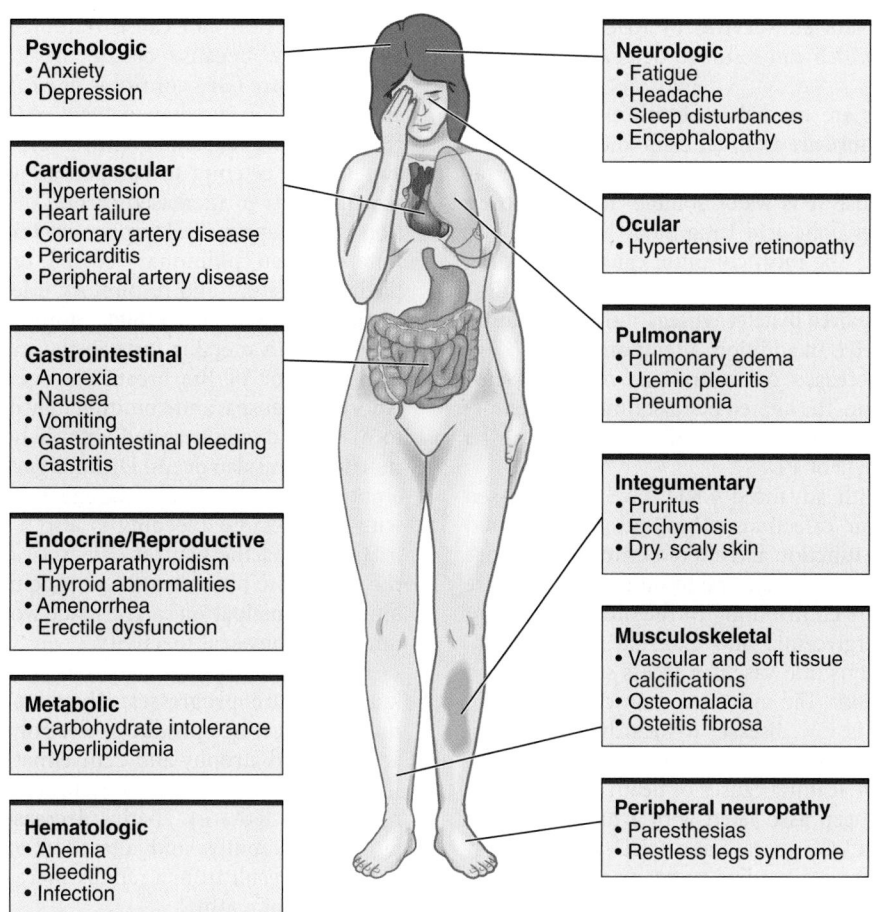

Psychologic
• Anxiety
• Depression

Cardiovascular
• Hypertension
• Heart failure
• Coronary artery disease
• Pericarditis
• Peripheral artery disease

Gastrointestinal
• Anorexia
• Nausea
• Vomiting
• Gastrointestinal bleeding
• Gastritis

Endocrine/Reproductive
• Hyperparathyroidism
• Thyroid abnormalities
• Amenorrhea
• Erectile dysfunction

Metabolic
• Carbohydrate intolerance
• Hyperlipidemia

Hematologic
• Anemia
• Bleeding
• Infection

Neurologic
• Fatigue
• Headache
• Sleep disturbances
• Encephalopathy

Ocular
• Hypertensive retinopathy

Pulmonary
• Pulmonary edema
• Uremic pleuritis
• Pneumonia

Integumentary
• Pruritus
• Ecchymosis
• Dry, scaly skin

Musculoskeletal
• Vascular and soft tissue
  calcifications
• Osteomalacia
• Osteitis fibrosa

Peripheral neuropathy
• Paresthesias
• Restless legs syndrome

FIG. 47-2 Possible clinical manifestations of chronic kidney disease.

gresses. The insulin dosing must be individualized and glucose levels monitored carefully.

Elevated Triglycerides. Hyperinsulinemia stimulates hepatic production of triglycerides. Almost all patients with uremia develop dyslipidemia, with increased very-low-density lipoproteins (VLDLs), increased low-density lipoproteins (LDLs), and decreased high-density lipoproteins (HDLs). The altered lipid metabolism is related to decreased levels of the enzyme lipoprotein lipase, which is important in the breakdown of lipoproteins. Most patients with CKD die from CV disease.[15]

Electrolyte and Acid-Base Imbalances

Potassium. Hyperkalemia is a serious electrolyte disorder associated with kidney disease. Fatal dysrhythmias have been reported when the serum potassium level reaches 7 to 8 mEq/L (7 to 8 mmol/L). Hyperkalemia results from the decreased excretion of potassium by the kidneys, the breakdown of cellular protein, bleeding, and metabolic acidosis. Potassium may also come from the food consumed, dietary supplements, drugs, and IV infusions.

Sodium. Sodium may be elevated, normal, or low in kidney failure. Because of impaired sodium excretion, sodium along with water is retained. If large quantities of water are retained, dilutional hyponatremia occurs. Sodium retention can contribute to edema, hypertension, and HF. Sodium intake must be individually determined but is generally restricted to 2 g/day.

Calcium and Phosphate. Calcium and phosphate alterations are discussed in the section on the musculoskeletal system on p. 1110.

Magnesium. Magnesium is primarily excreted by the kidneys. Hypermagnesemia is generally not a problem unless the

patient is ingesting magnesium (e.g., milk of magnesia, magnesium citrate, antacids containing magnesium). Clinical manifestations of hypermagnesemia can include absence of reflexes, decreased mental status, cardiac dysrhythmias, hypotension, and respiratory failure.

Metabolic Acidosis. Metabolic acidosis results from the kidneys' impaired ability to excrete the acid load (primarily ammonia) and from defective reabsorption and regeneration of bicarbonate. The average adult produces 80 to 90 mEq of acid per day. This acid is normally buffered by bicarbonate. In kidney failure, plasma bicarbonate, which is an indirect measure of acidosis, usually falls to a new steady state at around 16 to 20 mEq/L (16 to 20 mmol/L). The decrease in plasma bicarbonate reflects its use in buffering metabolic acids. The bicarbonate level generally does not progress below this level because hydrogen ion production is usually balanced by buffering from demineralization of the bone (the phosphate buffering system).

Hematologic System

Anemia. A normocytic, normochromic anemia is associated with CKD. The anemia is due to decreased production of the hormone erythropoietin by the kidneys. Erythropoietin normally stimulates precursor cells in the bone marrow to produce RBCs (erythropoiesis). Other factors contributing to anemia are nutritional deficiencies, decreased RBC life span, increased hemolysis of RBCs, frequent blood samplings, and bleeding from the GI tract. For patients receiving maintenance hemodialysis (HD), blood loss in the dialyzer may also contribute to the anemic state. Elevated levels of parathyroid hormone (PTH) (produced to compensate for low serum calcium levels) can inhibit erythropoiesis, shorten survival of RBCs, and cause bone marrow fibrosis, which can result in decreased numbers of hematopoietic cells.

Sufficient iron stores are needed for erythropoiesis. Many patients with kidney failure are iron deficient and require oral iron supplements. Folic acid, which is essential for RBC maturation, is dialyzable because it is water soluble. It needs to be supplemented in the diet (folic acid 1 mg/day).

Bleeding Tendencies. The most common cause of bleeding in uremia is a qualitative defect in platelet function. This dysfunction is caused by impaired platelet aggregation and impaired release of platelet factor III. In addition, alterations in the coagulation system with increased concentrations of both factor VIII and fibrinogen occur. The altered platelet function, hemorrhagic tendencies, and GI bleeding susceptibility can usually be corrected with regular HD or PD.

Infection. Patients with advanced CKD have an increased susceptibility to infection. Infectious complications are caused by changes in leukocyte function and altered immune response and function. Both cellular and humoral immune responses are suppressed. Other factors contributing to the increased risk of infection include hyperglycemia and external trauma (e.g., catheters, needle insertions into vascular access sites).

Cardiovascular System. The most common cause of death in patients with CKD is CV disease. Myocardial infarction, ischemic heart disease, peripheral arterial disease, HF, cardiomyopathy, and stroke are leading causes of death. Even a slight reduction in GFR has been associated with a higher risk for coronary artery disease.[15] CV disease and CKD are so closely linked that if patients develop cardiac events (e.g., myocardial infarction, HF), evaluation of kidney function is recommended.

Traditional CV risk factors such as hypertension and elevated lipids are common in CKD patients. However, CV disease may also be related to nontraditional CV risk factors such as vascular calcification and arterial stiffness, which are major contributors to CV disease in patients with CKD. The calcium deposits in the vascular medial layer are associated with stiffening of the blood vessels. The mechanisms involved are multifactorial. They include (1) vascular smooth muscle cells changing into chondrocytes or osteoblast-like cells, (2) high total body amount of calcium and phosphate resulting from abnormal bone metabolism, (3) impaired renal excretion, and (4) drug therapies to treat the bone disease (e.g., calcium phosphate binders).[16]

Hypertension is highly prevalent in patients with CKD because hypertension is both a cause and a consequence of CKD. Hypertension is aggravated by sodium retention and increased extracellular fluid volume.[17] In some individuals, increased renin production contributes to hypertension (see Fig. 45-4).

Hypertension and diabetes mellitus are contributing risk factors for vascular complications. The vascular changes from long-standing hypertension and the accelerated atherosclerosis contribute to the higher rate of CV disease in CKD. Left ventricular hypertrophy (LVH) is present in about 75% of patients receiving dialysis. Long-standing hypertension, extracellular fluid volume overload, and anemia contribute to development of LVH that may eventually lead to cardiomyopathy and HF.

Patients with CKD are susceptible to cardiac dysrhythmias that result from hyperkalemia and decreased coronary artery perfusion. Uremic pericarditis can develop and occasionally progresses to pericardial effusion and cardiac tamponade. Pericarditis is typically manifested by a friction rub, chest pain, and low-grade fever.

Hypertension can cause retinopathy, encephalopathy, and nephropathy. Because of the many effects of hypertension, blood pressure (BP) control is one of the most important therapeutic goals in the management of CKD.

Respiratory System. With severe acidosis, the respiratory system may attempt to compensate with Kussmaul breathing, which results in increased carbon dioxide removal by exhalation (see Chapter 17). Dyspnea may occur as a manifestation of fluid overload, pulmonary edema, uremic pleuritis (pleurisy), pleural effusions, and respiratory infections (e.g., pneumonia).

Gastrointestinal System. Stomatitis with exudates and ulcerations, a metallic taste in the mouth, and *uremic fetor* (a urinous odor of the breath) are commonly found in CKD. Anorexia, nausea, and vomiting may develop if CKD progresses to ESKD and is not treated with dialysis. Weight loss and malnutrition may also occur. Diabetic *gastroparesis* (delayed gastric emptying) can compound the effects of malnutrition for patients with diabetes. GI bleeding is also a risk because of mucosal irritation and the platelet defect. Constipation may be due to the ingestion of iron salts or calcium-containing phosphate binders. Constipation can be made worse by limitations on fluid intake and physical inactivity.

Neurologic System. Neurologic changes are expected as kidney failure progresses. They are the result of increased nitrogenous waste products, electrolyte imbalances, metabolic acidosis, and atrophy and demyelination of nerve fibers.

The central nervous system (CNS) becomes depressed, resulting in lethargy, apathy, decreased ability to concentrate, fatigue, irritability, and altered mental ability. Seizures and coma may result from a rapidly increasing BUN and hypertensive encephalopathy.

Peripheral neuropathy is initially manifested by a slowing of nerve conduction to the extremities. Individuals with advanced stage 5 CKD may complain of restless legs syndrome (see Chapter 59), described as "bugs crawling inside the leg." Paresthesias are most often experienced in the feet and legs and may be described by the patient as a burning sensation. Eventually, motor involvement may lead to bilateral footdrop, muscular weakness and atrophy, and loss of deep tendon reflexes. Muscle twitching, jerking, *asterixis* (hand-flapping tremor), and nocturnal leg cramps also occur. In patients with diabetes, uremic neuropathy is compounded by the neuropathy associated with diabetes mellitus.

Dialysis should improve general CNS manifestations and may slow or halt the progression of neuropathies. However, motor neuropathy may not be reversible. The treatment for neurologic problems is dialysis or transplantation. Altered mental status, a late manifestation of CKD stage 5, is rarely seen unless the patient has chosen to forgo RRT.

Musculoskeletal System. CKD mineral and bone disorder (CKD-MBD) develops as a systemic disorder of mineral and bone metabolism caused by progressive deterioration in kidney function (Fig. 47-3). As kidney function deteriorates, less vitamin D is converted to its active form, resulting in decreased serum levels. Activated vitamin D is necessary to optimize absorption of calcium from the GI tract; thus low levels of active vitamin D result in decreased serum calcium levels.[18]

Normally serum calcium levels are tightly regulated. PTH is the primary regulator of serum calcium levels. When hypocalcemia occurs, the parathyroid gland secretes PTH, which stimulates bone demineralization, thereby releasing calcium from the bones. Phosphate is released as well, leading to elevated

PATHOPHYSIOLOGY MAP

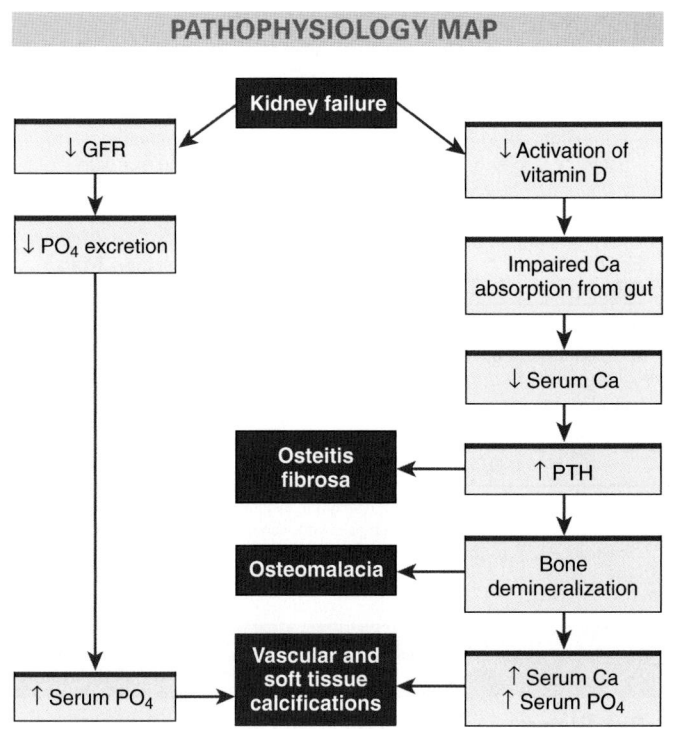

FIG. 47-3 Mechanisms of chronic kidney disease mineral and bone disorder (CKD-MBD). *GFR,* Glomerular filtration rate; *PTH,* parathyroid hormone.

serum phosphate levels. Hyperphosphatemia also results from decreased phosphate excretion by the kidneys. Hyperphosphatemia decreases serum calcium levels and further reduces the kidneys' ability to activate vitamin D.

Low serum calcium, elevated phosphate, and decreased vitamin D contribute to the stimulation of the parathyroid gland and excretion of PTH. The PTH acts on the bone to increase remodeling and increase serum calcium levels. The accelerated rate of bone remodeling causes a weakened bone matrix and places the patient at a higher risk for fractures.

Normally plasma calcium is found ionized or free (physiologically active form) or bound to protein. In kidney failure, it is unusual for hypocalcemia to be symptomatic. The reason for this is that, in the acidotic state associated with renal failure, more calcium is in the ionized form than is bound to protein. However, a low ionized calcium level can lead to tetany (see Chapter 17).

CKD-MBD is a common complication of CKD and results in both skeletal complications and extraskeletal complications (vascular and soft tissue complications). Skeletal complications include *osteomalacia,* which results from demineralization from slow bone turnover and defective mineralization of newly formed bone, and *osteitis fibrosa,* a decalcification of the bone and replacement of bone tissue with fibrous tissue.

Extraskeletal complications result from vascular calcifications. As previously mentioned, vascular calcifications are a significant contributing factor to CV disease. "Uremic red eye" is caused by the irritation from calcium deposits in the eye. Intracardiac calcifications can disrupt the conduction system and cause cardiac arrest. CKD-MBD contributes significantly to a patient's increased morbidity and mortality risks.[18]

Integumentary System. Pruritus is more prevalent in patients receiving dialysis than in the earlier stages of CKD. A small percentage of patients develop refractory pruritus that can have a devastating impact on their well-being and quality of life. Pruritus has multiple causes, including dry skin, calcium-phosphate deposition in the skin, and sensory neuropathy. The itching may be so intense that it can lead to bleeding or infection secondary to scratching. Uremic frost is an extremely rare condition in which urea crystallizes on the skin; this is usually seen only when BUN levels are extremely elevated (e.g., over 200 mg/dL).

Reproductive System. Both men and women can experience infertility and a decreased libido. Women usually have decreased levels of estrogen, progesterone, and luteinizing hormone, causing anovulation and menstrual changes (usually amenorrhea). Menses and ovulation may return after dialysis is started. Men experience loss of testicular consistency, decreased testosterone levels, and low sperm counts.

Sexual dysfunction may also be caused by anemia, which causes fatigue and decreased libido. In addition, peripheral neuropathy can cause impotence in men and anorgasmy in women. Additional factors that may cause changes in sexual function are psychologic problems (e.g., anxiety, depression), physical stress, and side effects of drugs.

Sexual function may improve with maintenance dialysis and may become normal with successful transplantation. Patients that become pregnant while receiving dialysis have been able to carry a fetus to term, but there is significant risk to the mother and infant. Pregnancy in patients with a kidney transplant is more common, but there is still considerable risk to both the mother and fetus.

Psychologic Changes. Personality and behavioral changes, emotional lability, withdrawal, and depression are commonly observed in patients with CKD. Fatigue and lethargy contribute to the feeling of illness. The changes in body image caused by edema, integumentary disturbances, and access devices (e.g., fistulas, catheters) may lead to anxiety and depression. Decreased ability to concentrate and slowed mental activity can give the appearance of dullness and disinterest in the environment. The patient must also deal with significant changes in lifestyle, occupation, family responsibilities, and financial status. Long-term survival depends on medications, dietary restrictions, dialysis, and possibly transplantation. The patient also grieves the loss of kidney function. This can be a prolonged process for some individuals.

Diagnostic Studies

Because persistent proteinuria is usually the first indication of kidney damage, screening for CKD involves a dipstick evaluation of protein in the urine or evaluation for microalbuminuria, which is not detected with routine urinalysis. Patients with diabetes need to have examination of their urine for microalbuminuria if none is detected on routine urinalysis.

A person with persistent proteinuria (1+ protein on standard dipstick testing two or more times over a 3-month period) should have further assessment of risk factors and a diagnostic workup with blood and urine tests to evaluate for CKD. A urine test for albumin-to-creatinine ratio provides an accurate estimate of the protein and albumin excretion rate. A ratio greater than 300 mg albumin per 1 g creatinine signals CKD.

A urinalysis can detect RBCs, WBCs, protein, casts, and glucose. An ultrasound of the kidneys is usually done to detect any obstructions and to determine the size of the kidneys. Other diagnostic studies (Table 47-7) help establish the diagnosis and

TABLE 47-7   COLLABORATIVE CARE

Chronic Kidney Disease

Diagnostic
- History and physical examination
- Identification of reversible kidney disease
- Renal ultrasound
- Renal scan
- CT scan
- Renal biopsy
- BUN, serum creatinine, and creatinine clearance levels
- Serum electrolytes
- Lipid profile
- Protein-to-creatinine ratio in first morning voided specimen
- Urinalysis
- Hematocrit and hemoglobin levels

Collaborative Therapy
- Correction of extracellular fluid volume overload or deficit
- Nutritional therapy*
- Erythropoietin therapy
- Calcium supplementation, phosphate binders, or both
- Antihypertensive therapy
- Angiotensin-converting enzyme (ACE) inhibitors or angiotensin receptor blockers (ARBs)
- Measures to treat hyperlipidemia
- Measures to lower potassium†
- Adjustment of drug dosages to degree of renal function
- Renal replacement therapy (dialysis, kidney transplant)

*See Tables 47-10 and 47-11.
†See Table 47-5.

cause of CKD. A kidney biopsy may be necessary to provide a definitive diagnosis.

Many consider serum creatinine the best indicator of kidney function, but in reality serum creatinine alone poorly reflects kidney function. GFR is the preferred measure to determine kidney function. Several GFR calculators are available. The two equations used most frequently to estimate GFR are the Cockcroft-Gault formula and the Modification of Diet in Renal Disease (MDRD) Study equation (Table 47-8). The National Kidney Foundation KDOQI guidelines recommend the MDRD Study equation to estimate GFR.[19]

Collaborative Care

The overall goals of CKD therapy are to preserve existing kidney function, reduce the risks of CV disease, prevent complications, and provide for the patient's comfort (Table 47-9). For many, early recognition, diagnosis, and treatment can deter the progression of kidney disease. It is important that patients with CKD receive appropriate follow-up and referral to a nephrologist early in the course of the disease. Every effort is made to detect and treat potentially reversible causes of kidney failure (e.g., HF, dehydration, infections, nephrotoxins, urinary tract obstruction, glomerulonephritis, renal artery stenosis).

Patients with CKD have a high incidence of CV complications. A higher percentage of patients will die from CV disease than live to need dialysis. When a patient is diagnosed as having CKD, therapy is aimed at treating the CV disease in addition to slowing the progression of kidney disease (see Table 47-7).

A focus on stages 1 through 4 (see Table 47-6) before the need for dialysis (stage 5) includes the control of hypertension, hyperparathyroid disease, anemia, hyperglycemia, and dyslipidemia. The following section focuses primarily on the drug and nutritional aspects of care.

TABLE 47-8   INDICATORS OF KIDNEY FUNCTION

This example shows why serum creatinine is a poor indicator of kidney function. Calculation of GFR is considered the best index to estimate kidney function as indicated by the following example.

Estimation of GFR	Type of Patient	
	76-Yr-Old African American Woman (Weight 56 kg)	28-Yr-Old African American Man (Weight 74 kg)
Serum creatinine	1.4 mg/dL	1.4 mg/dL
GFR, estimated by the Cockcroft-Gault formula*	30.2 mL/min	82.2 mL/min
GFR, estimated by MDRD equation†	47 mL/min/1.73 m^2	64 mL/min/1.73 m^2

*Cockcroft-Gault GFR = (140 − Age) × (Weight in kilograms) × (0.85 if female)/(72 × Cr).
†GFR as estimated by MDRD equation calculator can be accessed at *www.mdrd.com*.
Cr, Creatinine; *GFR*, glomerular filtration rate; *MDRD*, modification of diet in renal disease.

TABLE 47-9   RISK FACTORS FOR CHRONIC KIDNEY DISEASE

Risk Factors	Prevention and Management
Diabetes	Achieve optimal glycemic control.
Hypertension	Maintain BP in normal range with angiotensin-converting enzyme (ACE) inhibitors or angiotensin receptor blockers (ARBs).
Age >60 yr	Prevent insult or kidney injury.
Cardiovascular disease	Institute aggressive risk factor reduction.
Family history of CKD	Teach about increased risk and assist with appropriate screening (BP measurement, urinalysis).
Exposure to nephrotoxic drugs	Limit exposure and give sodium bicarbonate as treatment.
Ethnic minority (e.g., African American, Native American)	Teach about increased risk and assist with appropriate screening (BP measurement, urinalysis).

Drug Therapy

Hyperkalemia. Multiple strategies are used to manage hyperkalemia (see Table 47-5). Every effort is made to control hyperkalemia with the restriction of high-potassium foods and drugs. Acute hyperkalemia may require treatment with IV glucose and insulin or IV 10% calcium gluconate. Sodium polystyrene sulfonate, a cation-exchange resin, is commonly used to lower potassium levels in stage 4 and can be administered on an outpatient basis.

Tell the patient to expect some diarrhea because this preparation contains sorbitol, a sugar alcohol that has an osmotic laxative action and ensures evacuation of the potassium from the bowel. Never give sodium polystyrene sulfonate to a patient with a hypoactive bowel (paralytic ileus) because fluid shifts could lead to bowel necrosis. As sodium polystyrene sulfonate exchanges sodium ions for potassium ions, observe the patient for sodium and water retention. If changes appear in the ECG such as peaked T waves and widened QRS complexes, dialysis may be required to remove excess potassium.

Hypertension. For some, the progression of CKD can be delayed by controlling hypertension. (Control and treatment of

Translating Research Into Practice

Can Exercise Improve Physical Fitness in Chronic Kidney Disease?

Clinical Question

For adults with chronic kidney disease (P), what is the effect of exercise (I) on physical fitness and functioning (O)?

Best Available Evidence

Systematic review of randomized controlled trials (RCTs)

Critical Appraisal and Synthesis of Evidence

- Forty-five RCTs (n = 1863) of adults with chronic kidney disease (CKD) or kidney transplant. Physical exercise interventions lasted at least 8 wk. Most common intervention was aerobic exercise.
- Fitness and cardiovascular parameters were measured.
- Regular exercise improved muscle strength, walking ability, blood pressure and heart rate, and quality of life.
- Exercise did not significantly affect total cholesterol or triglyceride levels.

Conclusion

- Exercise significantly improved physical fitness (aerobic capacity).

Implications for Nursing Practice

- Encourage regular aerobic exercise to counter muscle strength loss in patients with CKD.
- Maintain contact with patient to promote and encourage adherence to recommended exercise.

Reference for Evidence

Heiwe S, Jacobson SH: Exercise training for adults with chronic kidney disease, *Cochrane Database Syst Rev* 10:CD003236, 2011.

P, Patient population of interest; *I,* intervention or area of interest; *O,* outcomes of interest (see p. 12).

hypertension are discussed in Chapter 33.) It is recommended that the target BP be less than 130/80 mm Hg for patients with CKD and 125/75 mm Hg for patients with significant proteinuria.[17] Treatment of hypertension includes (1) weight loss (if obese), (2) therapeutic lifestyle changes (e.g., exercise, avoidance of alcohol, smoking cessation), (3) diet recommendations (DASH Diet; see eTable 33-1), and (4) administration of antihypertensive drugs. Most patients require two or more drugs to reach target BP.

The antihypertensive drugs most commonly used are diuretics, calcium channel blockers, ACE inhibitors, and angiotensin receptor blocker (ARB) agents. Prescribed medications depend on whether the patient with CKD has diabetes or not. The ACE inhibitors and ARBs are used with diabetics and those with nondiabetic proteinuria because they decrease proteinuria and possibly delay the progression of CKD. However, they must be used cautiously in patients with ESKD because they can further decrease the GFR and increase serum potassium levels.

Periodically measure the BP with the patient in the supine, sitting, and standing positions to monitor the effect of antihypertensive drugs. Teach the patient and caregiver how to monitor the BP at home and what readings require immediate intervention. BP control is essential to slow atherosclerotic changes that could further impair kidney function.

CKD-MBD. Interventions for CKD-MBD include limiting dietary phosphorus, administering phosphate binders, supplementing vitamin D, and controlling hyperparathyroidism.[18] Phosphate intake is not usually restricted until the patient requires RRT. At that time, phosphate is usually limited to about 1 g/day, but dietary control alone is usually inadequate.

Phosphate binders include calcium-based binders: calcium acetate (PhosLo) and calcium carbonate (Caltrate). They bind phosphate in the bowel and are then excreted in the stool. The administration of calcium may increase the calcium load and place the patient at increased risk for vascular calcifications. Therefore, when calcium levels are increased or there is evidence of existing vascular or soft tissue calcifications, consider changing to noncalcium-based phosphate binders, such as lanthanum carbonate (Fosrenol) and sevelamer carbonate (Renvela).

To be most effective, administer phosphate binders with each meal. Constipation is a frequent side effect of phosphate binders and may necessitate the use of stool softeners.

Because bone disease (osteomalacia) is associated with excessive aluminum, aluminum preparations should be used with caution in patients with kidney failure. Do not use magnesium-containing antacids (e.g., Maalox, Mylanta) because magnesium depends on the kidneys for excretion.

Hypocalcemia is a problem in the later stages of CKD because of the inability of the GI tract to absorb calcium in the absence of active vitamin D. If hypocalcemia persists even if the serum phosphate levels are normal, then supplemental calcium and vitamin D should be given. Assess vitamin D levels to determine the need for supplementation. If the levels are low (serum values less than 30 ng/mL), vitamin D supplementation is recommended in the form of cholecalciferol.

Treatment of secondary hyperparathyroidism in ESKD patients requires the activated form of vitamin D because the kidneys no longer possess the ability to activate vitamin D. Active vitamin D is available as oral or IV calcitriol (Rocaltrol, Calcijex), IV paricalcitol (Zemplar), or oral or IV doxercalciferol (Hectorol), and can reduce the elevated levels of PTH.

Hypercalcemia may occur with calcium and vitamin D supplementation. If hypercalcemia occurs, then reduce or discontinue vitamin D and calcium-based phosphate binders. Noncalcium-based phosphate binders can be substituted.

Cinacalcet (Sensipar), a calcimimetic agent, is used to control secondary hyperparathyroidism. Calcimimetics mimic calcium and increase the sensitivity of the calcium receptors in the parathyroid glands. As a result, the parathyroid glands detect calcium at lower serum levels and decrease PTH secretion.

If hyperparathyroid disease becomes severe despite medical management, a subtotal or total parathyroidectomy may be performed to decrease the synthesis and secretion of PTH. In most cases, a total parathyroidectomy is performed, and some parathyroid tissue is transplanted into the forearm. The transplanted cells produce PTH as needed. If production of PTH becomes excessive, some of the cells can be removed from the forearm.

It is difficult to determine what type of bone disease a patient might have by just looking at the serum levels of calcium, phosphorus, PTH, and alkaline phosphatase. The gold standard for diagnosis is a bone biopsy.

Anemia. The most important cause of anemia is a decreased production of erythropoietin. Exogenous erythropoietin (EPO) is used in the treatment. It is available as epoetin alfa (Epogen, Procrit), which can be administered IV or subcutaneously, usually two or three times per week. Darbepoetin alfa (Aranesp) is longer acting and can be administered weekly or biweekly.

A significant increase in hemoglobin and hematocrit levels is usually not seen for 2 to 3 weeks. Higher hemoglobin levels (more than 12 g/dL) and higher doses of EPO are associated with a higher rate of thromboembolic events and increased risk of death from serious CV events (heart attack, HF, stroke). The recommendation is to use the lowest possible dose of EPO to treat anemia. Furthermore, treatment of CKD-related anemia should be individualized with the goal being to reduce the need for blood transfusions. There is no target hemoglobin or widely accepted EPO dosing strategy.[20] Teach people who are prescribed EPO about the risks and benefits and allow them to make an informed decision regarding their individual treatment.

If EPO is used in the management of anemia, recognize that uncontrolled hypertension is a contraindication and that EPO may exacerbate an individual's hypertension. The underlying mechanism is related to the hemodynamic changes (e.g., increased whole blood viscosity) that occur as the anemia is corrected.

Another side effect of EPO therapy is the development of iron deficiency from the increased demand for iron to support erythropoiesis. Iron supplementation is recommended if the plasma ferritin concentrations fall below 100 ng/mL. Some studies have supported the use of parenteral iron with a much higher ferritin value (e.g., 800 ng/mL) in order to optimize treatment. Most CKD patients receive iron supplementation either by mouth or parenterally. Nonadherence may be an issue with oral supplementation because iron has GI side effects such as gastric irritation and constipation. Orally administered iron should not be taken at the same time as phosphate binders because calcium binds the iron, preventing its absorption. Tell the patient that iron may make the stool dark in color.

Most patients receiving HD are prescribed IV iron sucrose injection (Venofer) or sodium ferric gluconate complex in sucrose injection (Ferrlecit). Supplemental folic acid (1 mg/day) is usually given because it is needed for RBC formation and is removed by dialysis.

Blood transfusions should be avoided in treating anemia unless the patient experiences an acute blood loss or has symptomatic anemia (i.e., dyspnea, excess fatigue, tachycardia, palpitations, chest pain). Undesirable effects of transfusions are the increased sensitization and development of antibodies, thus making it more difficult to find a compatible donor for transplantation. Multiple blood transfusions may lead to iron overload because each unit of blood contains about 250 mg of iron.

Dyslipidemia. Dyslipidemia, a known traditional risk factor for CV disease, is a common problem in CKD. Statins (HMG-CoA reductase inhibitors), such as atorvastatin (Lipitor), are used to lower LDL cholesterol levels (see Table 34-5). Evidence supports the use of statins in patients with CKD (especially patients with diabetes) not yet on dialysis. However, simvastatin has been associated with a higher rate of myopathy. It is recommended that patients who develop myopathy on simvastatin be switched to atorvastatin, which has minimal renal clearance and less chance of causing myopathy. The effectiveness of statins in patients on dialysis is still being studied. Fibrates (fibric acid derivatives), such as gemfibrozil (Lopid), are used to lower triglyceride levels (see Table 34-5) and can also increase HDLs. Specific drugs of these classes that are used depend on the individual patient response and physician recommendation.

Complications of Drug Therapy. Many drugs are partially or totally excreted by the kidneys. Delayed and decreased elimination leads to an accumulation of drugs and the potential for drug toxicity. Drug doses and frequency of administration must be adjusted based on the severity of the kidney disease. Increased sensitivity may result as drug levels increase in the blood and tissues. Drugs of particular concern include digoxin, diabetic agents (metformin, glyburide), antibiotics (e.g., vancomycin, gentamicin), and opioid medications.

Nutritional Therapy

Protein Restriction. The current diet is designed to be as normal as possible to maintain good nutrition (Table 47-10). Calorie-protein malnutrition is a potential and serious problem that results from altered metabolism, anemia, proteinuria, anorexia, and nausea. Additional factors leading to malnutrition include depression and complex diets that restrict protein, phosphorus, potassium, and sodium. Frequent monitoring of laboratory parameters, especially serum albumin, prealbumin (may be a better indicator of recent or current nutritional status than albumin), and ferritin, and anthropometric measurements are necessary to evaluate nutritional status. All patients with CKD should be referred to a dietitian for nutritional education and guidance.

For the patient who is undergoing dialysis, protein is not routinely restricted (see Table 47-10). The beneficial role of protein restriction in CKD stages 1 through 4 as a means to reduce the decline in kidney function is being studied.

Historically, dietary counseling often encouraged a restriction of protein for individuals with CKD. Despite some evidence that protein restriction has benefits, many patients find it difficult to adhere to these diets. For CKD stages 1 through 4, many clinicians just encourage a diet with normal protein

TABLE 47-10   NUTRITIONAL THERAPY

Chronic Kidney Disease*

	Pre–End-Stage Kidney Disease	Hemodialysis	Peritoneal Dialysis
Fluid allowance	As desired or depends on urine output	Urine output plus 600-1000 mL	Unrestricted if weight and blood pressure controlled and residual renal function
Calories	30-35 kcal/kg/day	30-35 kcal/kg/day	25-35 kcal/kg/day (includes calories from dialysate glucose absorption)
Protein	Individualized or 0.6-1.0 g/kg/day (low protein)	1.2 g/kg/day	1.2-1.3 g/kg/day
Sodium	Individualized or 1-3 g/day	Individualized or 2-3 g/day	Individualized or 2-4 g/day
Potassium	Individualized based on laboratory values	Individualized or about 2-4 g/day	Usually not restricted
Phosphorus	Individualized or 1.0-1.8 g/day	Individualized or about 0.6-1.2 g/day	Individualized or about 0.6-1.2 g/day
Calcium	About 1000-1500 mg/day	Individualized	Individualized
Iron	Supplement recommended if receiving erythropoietin	Supplement recommended if receiving erythropoietin	Supplement recommended if receiving erythropoietin

*Diets must be individualized in accordance with needs.

intake. However, teach patients to avoid high-protein diets and supplements because they may overstress the diseased kidneys.

Dietary protein guidelines for PD differ from those for HD because of protein loss in the dialysate. During PD, protein intake must be high enough to compensate for the losses so that the nitrogen balance is maintained. The recommended protein intake is at least 1.2 g/kg of ideal body weight (IBW) per day; this can be increased depending on the patient's individual needs.

For patients with malnutrition or inadequate caloric or protein intake, commercially prepared products that are high in protein but low in sodium and potassium are available (e.g., Nepro, Amin-Aid).[21] As an alternative, liquid or powder breakfast drinks may be purchased at the grocery store.

Water Restriction. Water and any other fluids are not routinely restricted in patients with CKD stages 1 to 5 who are not receiving HD. In an effort to reduce fluid retention, diuretics are often used. Patients on HD have a more restricted fluid intake than patients receiving PD. For those receiving HD, as their urine output diminishes, fluids are restricted. Recommended fluid intake depends on the daily urine output. Generally, 600 mL (from insensible loss) plus an amount equal to the previous day's urine output is allowed for a patient receiving HD.

Foods that are liquid at room temperature (e.g., gelatin, ice cream) should be counted as fluid intake. The fluid allotment should be spaced throughout the day so that the patient does not become thirsty. Patients are advised to limit fluid intake so that weight gains are no more than 1 to 3 kg between dialyses (termed *interdialytic weight gain*).

Sodium and Potassium Restriction. Patients with CKD are advised to restrict sodium. Sodium-restricted diets may vary from 2 to 4 g/day. Do not equate sodium and salt because the sodium content in 1 g of sodium chloride is equivalent to 400 mg of sodium. Instruct the patient to avoid high-sodium foods such as cured meats, pickled foods, canned soups and stews, frankfurters, cold cuts, soy sauce, and salad dressings (see Chapter 35, Table 35-8). Potassium restriction depends on the kidneys' ability to excrete potassium. Most salt substitutes should be avoided if patients have been instructed to restrict potassium because they contain potassium chloride.

Dietary restrictions for potassium range from about 2 to 3 g (39 mg = 1 mEq). Teach patients receiving HD which foods are high in potassium and to avoid them (Table 47-11).

Patients using PD do not usually need potassium restrictions and may even be prescribed oral potassium supplementation because of the loss of potassium with dialysis exchanges.

Phosphate Restriction. As kidney function deteriorates, phosphate elimination by the kidneys is diminished and the patient begins to develop hyperphosphatemia. By the time a patient reaches ESKD, phosphate should be limited to approximately 1 g/day. Foods that are high in phosphate include meat, dairy products (e.g., milk, ice cream, cheese, yogurt), and foods containing dairy products (e.g., pudding). Many foods that are high in phosphate are also high in protein. Since patients on dialysis are encouraged to eat a diet containing protein, phosphate binders are essential to control phosphate.

NURSING MANAGEMENT
CHRONIC KIDNEY DISEASE

NURSING ASSESSMENT

Obtain a complete history of any existing kidney disease or family history of kidney disease. Some kidney disorders,

TABLE 47-11   **NUTRITIONAL THERAPY**
High-Potassium Foods

Fruits	Vegetables	Other Foods
• Apricot, raw (medium)	• Baked beans	• Bran or bran products
• Avocado (¼ whole)	• Butternut squash	• Chocolate (1.5-2 oz)
• Banana (½ whole)	• Refried beans	• Granola
• Cantaloupe	• Black beans	• Milk, all types (1 cup)
• Dried fruits	• Broccoli, cooked	• Nutritional supplements (use only under the direction of physician or dietitian)
• Grapefruit juice	• Carrots, raw	
• Honeydew	• Greens, except kale	
• Orange (medium)	• Mushrooms, canned	• Nuts and seeds (1 oz)
• Orange juice	• Potatoes, white and sweet	• Peanut butter (2 tbs)
• Prunes	• Spinach, cooked	• Salt substitutes, Lite Salt
• Raisins	• Tomatoes or tomato products	• Salt-free broth
	• Vegetable juices	• Yogurt

Source: National Kidney Foundation: Potassium and your CKD diet. *www.kidney.org/atoz/content/potassium.cfm*
*Contain at least 200 mg/portion. Portion = ½ cup unless otherwise noted.

including Alport syndrome and polycystic kidney disease, have a genetic basis. Other disorders that can lead to CKD are diabetes mellitus, hypertension, and systemic lupus erythematosus.

Because many drugs are potentially nephrotoxic, ask the patient about both current and past use of prescription and over-the-counter drugs and herbal preparations. Decongestants and antihistamines that contain pseudoephedrine and phenylephrine cause vasoconstriction and lead to an increase in BP. Also assess the use of antacids. Magnesium and aluminum from antacids can accumulate in the body because they cannot be excreted. Some antacids contain high levels of salt, contributing to hypertension. In addition, antacids may interfere with absorption of other medications.

NSAIDs (aspirin, ibuprofen, naproxen) can contribute to the development of AKI and progression of CKD, especially when taken in higher doses than recommended. Analgesics in combination and in large quantities have been associated with the development of kidney failure. If taken as prescribed for short periods, these analgesics are usually considered safe.

Assess the patient's dietary habits and discuss any problems regarding intake. Measure the height and weight, and evaluate any recent weight changes.

Recognize that CKD is a lifelong illness. The chronicity of kidney disease and the long-term treatment affect virtually every area of a person's life, including family relationships, social and work activities, self-image, and emotional state. Assess the patient's support systems. The choice of treatment modality may be related to support systems available.

NURSING DIAGNOSES

Nursing diagnoses for CKD may include, but are not limited to, the following:

- Excess fluid volume *related to* impaired kidney function
- Risk for electrolyte imbalance *related to* impaired kidney function resulting in hyperkalemia, hypocalcemia, hyperphosphatemia, and altered vitamin D metabolism
- Imbalanced nutrition: less than body requirements *related to* restricted intake of nutrients (especially protein), nausea, vomiting, anorexia, and stomatitis

Additional information on nursing diagnoses is presented in eNursing Care Plan 47-1 (available on the website for this chapter).

PLANNING

The overall goals are that a patient with CKD will (1) demonstrate knowledge of and ability to comply with the therapeutic regimen, (2) participate in decision making for the plan of care and future treatment modality, (3) demonstrate effective coping strategies, and (4) continue with activities of daily living within physiologic limitations.

NURSING IMPLEMENTATION

HEALTH PROMOTION. Identify individuals at risk for CKD. These include people who have been diagnosed with diabetes or hypertension and people with a history (or a family history) of kidney disease and repeated urinary tract infections. These individuals should have regular checkups along with calculation of the estimated GFR and a routine urinalysis.

People with diabetes need to have their urine checked for microalbuminuria if routine urinalysis is negative for protein. Advise patients with diabetes to report any changes in urine appearance (color, odor), frequency, or volume to the health care provider. If a patient needs a potentially nephrotoxic drug, it is important to monitor kidney function with serum creatinine and BUN.

Individuals identified as at risk need to take measures to prevent or delay the progression of CKD. Most important are measures to reduce the risk or progression of CV disease. These include glycemic control for patients with diabetes (see Chapter 49); BP control; and lifestyle modifications, including smoking cessation.

ACUTE INTERVENTION. Most of the care of the patient with CKD occurs on an outpatient basis. In-hospital care is required for management of complications and for kidney transplantation (if applicable).

AMBULATORY AND HOME CARE. Teach the patient and caregiver about the diet, drugs, and follow-up medical care (Table 47-12). The patient needs to understand the drugs and the common side effects. Because patients with CKD take many medications, a pillbox organizer or a list of the drugs and the times of administration that can be posted in the home may be helpful. Instruct the patient to avoid certain over-the-counter drugs such as NSAIDs and aluminum- and magnesium-based laxatives and antacids. Any over-the-counter medications need to be considered as a risk, since even acetaminophen taken in large doses can be toxic to the kidneys.

Teach the patient to take daily BPs and identify signs and symptoms of fluid overload, hyperkalemia, and other electrolyte

imbalances. The dietitian should meet with the patient and caregiver on a regular basis for diet planning. A diet history and consideration of cultural variations facilitate diet planning and adherence.

Motivate patients to the highest level of self-management that is possible for them to achieve. The length of time that a patient can receive conservative medical management for CKD is highly variable. It depends on the rate of progression to kidney failure and the presence of other co-morbid conditions. Specific nursing management of the patient with CKD is presented in eNursing Care Plan 47-1.

Preferably, if the patient is considered a candidate for kidney transplantation, the evaluation can be accomplished before initiation of dialysis. In the best of circumstances, patients can receive a transplant before ever having to start dialysis. Even though transplantation offers the best therapeutic management for patients with kidney failure, the critical shortage of donor organs has limited this treatment option.

Most patients require dialysis, either peritoneal dialysis (PD) or hemodialysis (HD). The majority of patients in the United States choose HD. Clearly explain to the patient and caregiver what is involved in dialysis, transplantation, and even the option for palliative care. Discuss the opportunity for home HD.

Provide information about the treatment options so the patient can be involved in the decision-making process and be given a sense of control over life-altering decisions. Inform the patient that if dialysis is chosen, the option of transplantation still remains. Let the patient know that if a transplanted organ fails, the patient can return to dialysis. Counsel the patient that retransplantation may also be an option.

It is important to respect the patient's choice to not receive treatment.[22] Many times, patients themselves initiate the

---

HEALTHY PEOPLE

Prevention and Detection of Chronic Kidney Disease

- Early detection and treatment are the primary methods for reducing chronic kidney disease.
- Monitor blood pressure to detect elevations so treatment can be started early.
- Treat hypertension appropriately and aggressively, since it is the second leading cause of chronic kidney disease.
- Ensure proper diagnosis and treatment of diabetes mellitus, since it is the leading cause of chronic kidney disease.

TABLE 47-12   PATIENT & CAREGIVER TEACHING GUIDE

Chronic Kidney Disease

Include the following information in the teaching plan for the patient and caregiver.

1. Necessary dietary (protein, sodium, potassium, phosphate) and fluid restrictions.
2. Difficulties in modifying diet and fluid intake.
3. Signs and symptoms of electrolyte imbalance, especially high potassium.
4. Alternative ways of reducing thirst, such as sucking on ice cubes, lemon, or hard candy.
5. Rationales for prescribed drugs and common side effects.
   Examples:
   - Phosphate binders (including calcium supplements used as phosphate barriers) should be taken with meals.
   - Calcium supplements prescribed to treat hypocalcemia directly should be taken on an empty stomach (but not at the same time as iron supplements).
   - Iron supplements should be taken between meals.
6. The importance of reporting any of the following:
   - Weight gain >4 lb (2 kg)
   - Increasing BP
   - Shortness of breath
   - Edema
   - Increasing fatigue or weakness
   - Confusion or lethargy
7. Need for support and encouragement. Share concerns about lifestyle changes, living with a chronic illness, and decisions about type of dialysis or transplantation.

conversation about palliative care. Focus the discussion on moving from the curative approach to promotion of comfort care and consideration of hospice care. Listen to the patient and caregiver, allowing them to do most of the talking, and pay special attention to their hopes and fears. (Palliative and end-of-life care is discussed in Chapter 10.)

EVALUATION

The expected outcomes are that the patient with CKD will maintain

- Fluid and electrolyte levels within normal ranges
- An acceptable weight with no more than a 10% weight loss

Additional information on expected outcomes is presented in eNursing Care Plan 47-1 (available on the website).

DIALYSIS

Dialysis is the movement of fluid and molecules across a semipermeable membrane from one compartment to another. Clinically, dialysis is a technique in which substances move from the blood through a semipermeable membrane and into a dialysis solution *(dialysate)*. It is used to correct fluid and electrolyte imbalances and to remove waste products in kidney failure. It can also be used to treat drug overdoses.

The two methods of dialysis available are peritoneal dialysis (PD) and hemodialysis (HD) (Table 47-13). In PD the peritoneal membrane acts as the semipermeable membrane. In HD an artificial membrane (usually made of cellulose-based or synthetic materials) is used as the semipermeable membrane and is in contact with the patient's blood.

Dialysis is begun when the patient's uremia can no longer be adequately treated with conservative medical management. Generally dialysis is initiated when the GFR is less than 15 mL/min/1.73 m². This criterion can vary widely in different clinical situations, and the physician determines when to start dialysis based on the patient's clinical status. Certain uremic complications, including encephalopathy, neuropathies, uncontrolled hyperkalemia, pericarditis, and accelerated hypertension, indicate a need for immediate dialysis.

Most patients with ESKD are treated with dialysis because (1) there is a lack of donated organs, (2) some patients are physically or mentally unsuitable for transplantation, or (3) some patients do not want transplants. An increasing number of individuals, including older adults and those with complex medical problems, are receiving maintenance dialysis. A patient's chronologic age is not a factor in determining candidacy for dialysis. Factors that are important are the patient's ability to cope and the existing support system.

General Principles of Dialysis

Solutes and water move across the semipermeable membrane from the blood to the dialysate or from the dialysate to the blood in accordance with concentration gradients. The principles of diffusion, osmosis, and ultrafiltration are involved in dialysis (Fig. 47-4). *Diffusion* is the movement of solutes from an area of greater concentration to an area of lesser concentration. In kidney failure, urea, creatinine, uric acid, and electrolytes (potassium, phosphate) move from the blood to the dialysate with the net effect of lowering their concentration in the blood. RBCs, WBCs, and plasma proteins are too large to diffuse through the pores of the membrane. Small-molecular-weight substances can pass from the dialysate into a patient's blood, so the purity of the water used for dialysis is monitored and controlled.

Osmosis is the movement of fluid from an area of lesser concentration to an area of greater concentration of solutes. Glucose is added to the dialysate and creates an osmotic gradient across the membrane, pulling excess fluid from the blood.

TABLE 47-13	COMPARISON OF PERITONEAL DIALYSIS AND HEMODIALYSIS	
Advantages	**Disadvantages**	

Peritoneal Dialysis (PD)

Advantages	Disadvantages
• Immediate initiation in almost any hospital • Less complicated than hemodialysis • Portable system with CAPD • Fewer dietary restrictions • Relatively short training time • Usable in patient with vascular access problems • Less cardiovascular stress • Home dialysis possible • Preferable for diabetic patient	• Bacterial or chemical peritonitis • Protein loss into dialysate • Exit site and tunnel infections • Self-image problems with catheter placement • Hyperglycemia • Surgery for catheter placement • Contraindicated in patient with multiple abdominal surgeries, trauma, unrepaired hernia • Requires completion of education program • Catheter can migrate • Best instituted with willing partner

Hemodialysis (HD)

Advantages	Disadvantages
• Rapid fluid removal • Rapid removal of urea and creatinine • Effective potassium removal • Less protein loss • Lowering of serum triglycerides • Home dialysis possible • Temporary access can be placed at bedside	• Vascular access problems • Dietary and fluid restrictions • Heparinization may be necessary • Extensive equipment necessary • Hypotension during dialysis • Added blood loss that contributes to anemia • Specially trained personnel necessary • Surgery for permanent access placement • Self-image problems with permanent access

CAPD, Continuous ambulatory peritoneal dialysis.

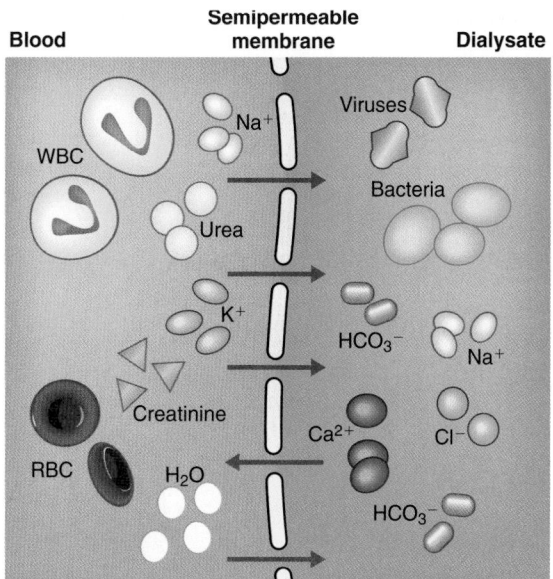

FIG. 47-4 Osmosis and diffusion across a semipermeable membrane.

Excess fluid is removed by creating a pressure differential between the blood and the dialysate solution. *Ultrafiltration* (water and fluid removal) results when there is an osmotic gradient or pressure gradient across the membrane. In PD, excess fluid is removed by increasing the osmolality of the dialysate (osmotic gradient) with the addition of glucose. In HD, the gradient is created by increasing pressure in the blood compartment (positive pressure) or decreasing pressure in the dialysate compartment (negative pressure). Extracellular fluid moves into the dialysate because of the pressure gradient. The excess fluid is removed by creating a pressure differential between the blood and the dialysate solution with a combination of positive pressure in the blood compartment or negative pressure in the dialysate compartment.

PERITONEAL DIALYSIS

Although PD was first used in 1923, it did not come into widespread use for chronic treatment until the 1970s with the development of soft, pliable peritoneal solution bags and the introduction of the concept of continuous PD. In the United States, approximately 12% of patients receiving dialysis treatments are on PD.

Catheter Placement

Peritoneal access is obtained by inserting a catheter through the anterior abdominal wall (Fig. 47-5). The catheter is about 60 cm long and has one or two Dacron cuffs on its subcutaneous and peritoneal portions. The cuffs act as anchors and prevent the migration of microorganisms down the shaft from the skin. Within a few weeks, fibrous tissue grows into the Dacron cuff, holding the catheter in place and preventing bacterial penetration into the peritoneal cavity. The tip of the catheter rests in the peritoneal cavity and has many perforations spaced along the distal end of the tubing to allow fluid to flow in and out of the catheter.

The technique for catheter placement varies. Although it is possible to place a permanent catheter in the peritoneal cavity at the bedside with a trocar, it is usually done via surgery so that its placement can be directly visualized, minimizing potential complications. Preparation of the patient for catheter insertion includes emptying the bladder and bowel, weighing the patient,

and obtaining a signed consent form. After placement, PD may be initiated immediately with low volume exchanges, or delayed for 2 weeks pending healing and sealing of the exit site. Once the catheter incision site is healed, the patient may shower and then pat the catheter and exit site dry.

Daily catheter care varies. Some patients just wash with soap and water and go without a dressing (Fig. 47-6), whereas others require daily dressing changes. Teach all patients to examine their catheter site for signs of infection. Showering is preferred to bathing.[23]

Dialysis Solutions and Cycles

PD is accomplished by putting dialysis solution into the peritoneal space. The three phases of the PD cycle are inflow (fill), dwell (equilibration), and drain. The three phases are called an *exchange*. During *inflow,* a prescribed amount of solution, usually 2 L, is infused through an established catheter over about 10 minutes. The flow rate may be decreased if the patient has pain. After the solution has been infused, the inflow clamp is closed before air enters the tubing.

The next part of the cycle is the *dwell* phase, or equilibration, during which diffusion and osmosis occur between the patient's blood and the peritoneal cavity. The duration of the dwell time can last from 20 or 30 minutes to 8 or more hours, depending on the method of PD.

Drain time takes 15 to 30 minutes and may be facilitated by gently massaging the abdomen or changing position. The cycle starts again with the infusion of another 2 L of solution. For manual PD, a period of about 30 to 50 minutes is required to complete an exchange.

Dialysis solutions vary, and the choice of the exchange volume is primarily determined by the size of the peritoneal cavity. A larger person may tolerate a 3-L exchange volume without any difficulty, whereas an average-size person usually tolerates a 2-L exchange. Smaller exchange volumes are used for patients with a smaller body, pulmonary compromise (the added pressure of the large volume may precipitate respiratory difficulty), or inguinal hernias.

Ultrafiltration (fluid removal) during PD depends on osmotic forces, with glucose being the most effective osmotic agent currently available. Dextrose remains the most commonly used osmotic agent in PD solutions. It is relatively safe and inexpensive, but has been associated with high rates of peritoneal glucose absorption leading to problems with hypertriglyceridemia, hyperglycemia, and long-term peritoneal membrane dysfunction.

Alternatives to dextrose PD solution include icodextrin and amino acid solutions. Icodextrin is a commercially available

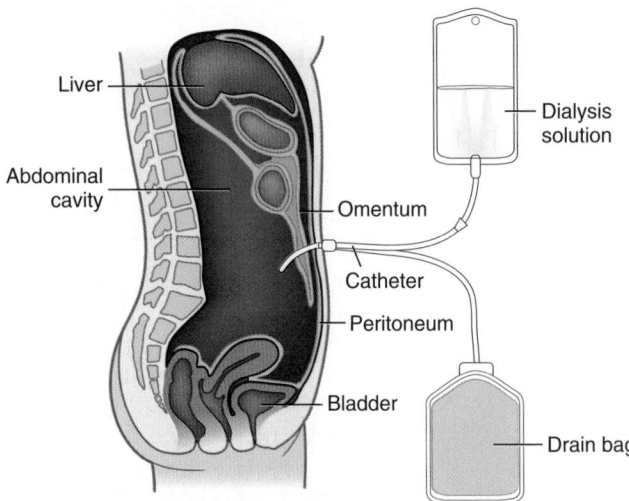

FIG. 47-5 Peritoneal dialysis showing peritoneal catheter inserted into peritoneal cavity.

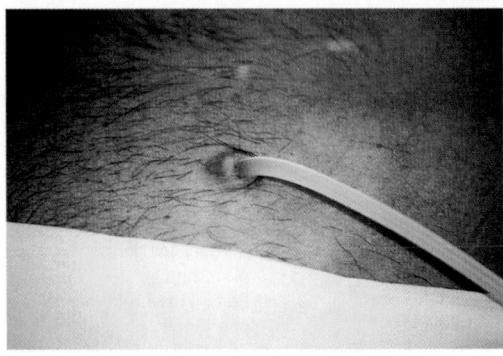

FIG. 47-6 Peritoneal catheter exit site.

isoosmolar preparation and induces ultrafiltration by its oncotic effect. Amino acid PD solutions are also available and primarily used for patients requiring nutritional supplementation.

Peritoneal Dialysis Systems

Automated Peritoneal Dialysis. Automated peritoneal dialysis (APD) is the most popular form of PD because it allows patients to do dialysis while they sleep. An automated device called a cycler is used to deliver the dialysate for APD (Fig. 47-7). The automated cycler times and controls the fill, dwell, and drain phases. The machine cycles four or more exchanges per night with 1 to 2 hours per exchange. Alarms and monitors are built into the system to make it safe for the patient to sleep while dialyzing. The patient disconnects from the machine in the morning and usually leaves fluid in the abdomen during the day.

It is difficult to achieve the required solute and fluid clearance solely with nighttime APD. Therefore one or two daytime manual exchanges may also be prescribed to ensure adequate dialysis. Cyclers are about the size of a DVD player and have longer tubing to allow greater mobility.

Continuous Ambulatory Peritoneal Dialysis. Continuous ambulatory peritoneal dialysis (CAPD) is done while the patient is awake during the day. Exchanges are carried out manually by exchanging 1.5 to 3 L of peritoneal dialysate at least four times daily, with dwell times averaging 4 hours. For example, one schedule exchanges at 7 AM, 12 noon, 5 PM, and 10 PM. In this procedure, the person instills 2 to 3 L of dialysate from a collapsible plastic bag into the peritoneal cavity through a disposable plastic tube.

In CAPD the bag and line can be disconnected after the instillation of the fluid. After the equilibration period, the line is reconnected to the catheter, the dialysate (effluent) is drained from the peritoneal cavity, and a new 2- to 3-L bag of dialysate solution is infused. In PD it is critical to maintain aseptic technique to avoid peritonitis. Several tubing connections and devices are commercially available to help in maintaining an aseptic system.

Complications of Peritoneal Dialysis

Exit Site Infection. Infection of the peritoneal catheter exit site is most commonly caused by *Staphylococcus aureus* or *Staphylococcus epidermidis* (from skin flora). Clinical manifestations of an exit site infection include redness at the site, ten-

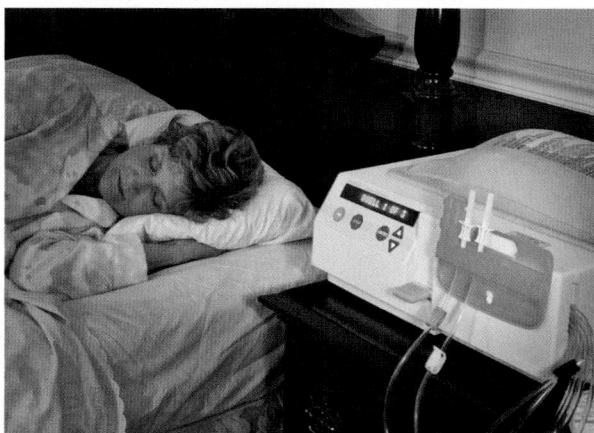

FIG. 47-7 Automated peritoneal dialysis that can be used while the patient is sleeping.

derness, and drainage. Superficial exit site infections caused by these organisms are generally resolved with antibiotic therapy. If not treated immediately, subcutaneous tunnel infections usually progress to abscess formation and may cause peritonitis, necessitating catheter removal.

Peritonitis. Peritonitis results from contamination or from progression of an exit site or tunnel infection. Most frequently peritonitis occurs because of improper technique in making or breaking connections for exchanges. Less commonly, peritonitis results from bacteria in the intestine crossing over into the peritoneal cavity. Peritonitis is usually caused by *S. aureus* or *S. epidermidis.*

The primary clinical manifestations of peritonitis are abdominal pain and cloudy peritoneal effluent with a WBC count greater than 100 cells/µL (more than 50% neutrophils) or demonstration of bacteria in the peritoneal effluent by Gram stain or culture. GI manifestations of peritonitis may include diarrhea, vomiting, abdominal distention, and hyperactive bowel sounds. Fever may or may not be present.

Cultures, Gram stain, and a WBC differential of the peritoneal effluent are used to confirm the diagnosis of peritonitis. Antibiotics can be given orally, IV, or intraperitoneally. In most cases, the patient is treated on an outpatient basis. The formation of adhesions in the peritoneum can result from repeated infections and interferes with the peritoneal membrane's ability to act as a dialyzing surface. Repeated infections may require the removal of the peritoneal catheter and termination of PD.

Hernias. Because of increased intraabdominal pressure secondary to the dialysate infusion, hernias can develop in predisposed individuals such as multiparous women and older men. However, in most situations after hernia repair, PD can be resumed after several days using small dialysate volumes and keeping the patient supine.

Lower Back Problems. Increased intraabdominal pressure can cause or aggravate lower back pain. The lumbosacral curvature is increased by intraperitoneal infusion of dialysate. Orthopedic binders and a regular exercise program for strengthening the back muscles have been beneficial for some patients.

Bleeding. After Tenckhoff catheter placement, it is not uncommon for the PD effluent drained after the first few exchanges to be pink or slightly bloody secondary to the trauma associated with catheter insertion. However, bloody effluent over several days or the new appearance of blood in the effluent can indicate active intraperitoneal bleeding. If this occurs, check the BP and hematocrit. Blood may also be present in the effluent of women who are menstruating or ovulating, and this requires no intervention.

Pulmonary Complications. Atelectasis, pneumonia, and bronchitis may occur from repeated upward displacement of the diaphragm, resulting in decreased lung expansion. The longer the dwell time, the greater the likelihood of pulmonary problems. Frequent repositioning and deep-breathing exercises can help. When the patient is lying in bed, elevate the head of the bed to prevent these problems.

Protein Loss. The peritoneal membrane is permeable to plasma proteins, amino acids, and polypeptides. These substances are lost in the dialysate fluid. The amount of loss is usually about 0.5 g/L of dialysate drainage, but it can be as high as 10 to 20 g/day. This loss may increase to as much as 40 g/day during episodes of peritonitis as the peritoneal membrane becomes more permeable. Unresolved peritonitis is associated with exaggerated protein loss that can result in malnutrition and may indicate the need to terminate PD temporarily or sometimes permanently.

Effectiveness of Chronic Peritoneal Dialysis

Learning the self-management skills required to do PD is usually accomplished in a 3- to 7-day training program. Mortality rates are about equal between in-center HD patients and PD patients for the first few years or possibly even a little lower for patients receiving PD. However, after about 2 years, mortality rates for patients receiving PD are higher, especially for the older person with diabetes and patients with a prior history of CV disease.

The primary advantage of PD is its simplicity and that it is a home-based program, allowing the patient to be in control. There is no need for special water systems, and equipment setup is relatively simple. PD is especially indicated for the individual who has vascular access problems or responds poorly to the hemodynamic stresses of HD.[23]

HEMODIALYSIS

Vascular Access

Obtaining vascular access is one of the most difficult problems associated with HD. To perform HD, a very rapid blood flow is required, and access to a large blood vessel is essential. The types of vascular access include arteriovenous fistulas (AVFs), arteriovenous grafts (AVGs), and temporary vascular access.[24]

Arteriovenous Fistulas and Grafts. A subcutaneous arteriovenous fistula (AVF) is usually created in the forearm or upper arm with an anastomosis between an artery and a vein (usually cephalic or basilic) (Figs. 47-8, *A*, and 47-9). The fistula allows arterial blood to flow through the vein. The vein becomes "arterialized" with a larger caliber and thicker walls. The arterial blood flow is essential to provide the rapid blood flow required for HD. As the arterialized vein matures, it is more amenable to repeated venipunctures. Maturation may take 6 weeks to months. AVF should be placed at least 3 months before the need to initiate HD.

Normally, a *thrill* can be felt by palpating the area of anastomosis, and a *bruit* (rushing sound) can be heard with a stethoscope. The bruit and thrill are created by arterial blood moving at a high velocity through the vein. AVFs are more difficult to create in patients with a history of severe peripheral vascular disease, those with prolonged IV drug use, and obese women. For these individuals, a synthetic graft may be required.

Arteriovenous grafts (AVGs) are made of synthetic materials (polytetrafluoroethylene [PTFE, Teflon]) and form a "bridge" between the arterial and venous blood supplies. Grafts are placed under the skin and are surgically anastomosed between an artery (usually brachial) and a vein (usually antecubital) (Fig. 47-8, *B*). An interval of 2 to 4 weeks is usually necessary to allow the graft to heal, but some centers may use it earlier. Because grafts are made of artificial materials, they are more likely than AVFs to become infected, and they also have a tendency to be thrombogenic. When AVG infections occur, they may require surgical removal, since it is difficult to completely resolve the infection from the synthetic material.

Surgical creation of an arteriovenous access for HD has several risks, including development of distal ischemia (*steal syndrome*) and pain because too much of the arterial blood is being shunted or "stolen" from the distal extremity. Classic manifestations of steal syndrome are pain distal to the access site, numbness or tingling of fingers that may worsen during dialysis, and poor capillary refill. Aneurysms can also develop in the arteriovenous access and can rupture if left untreated.

Never perform BP measurements, insertion of IV lines, and venipuncture in the extremity with the vascular access. These special precautions are taken to prevent infection and clotting of the vascular access.

Temporary Vascular Access. In some situations, when immediate vascular access is required, catheterization of the internal jugular or femoral vein is performed. A flexible Teflon, silicone rubber, or polyurethane catheter is inserted at the bedside into one of these large veins and provides access to the circulation without surgery (Fig. 47-10). The catheters usually have a double external lumen with an internal septum separating the two internal segments. One lumen is used for blood removal and the other for blood return (Fig. 47-11, *A* and *B*). It is now recommended that patients not be discharged from the hospital with a temporary catheter. These catheters have high rates of infection, dislodgment, and malfunction.

Long-term cuffed HD catheters are often used for temporary vascular access. These catheters provide temporary access while the patient is waiting for fistula placement or as long-term access when other forms of access have failed. This type of catheter exits on the upper chest wall and is tunneled subcutaneously to the internal or external jugular vein (Fig. 47-11, *C*). The catheter tip rests in the right atrium. It has one or two

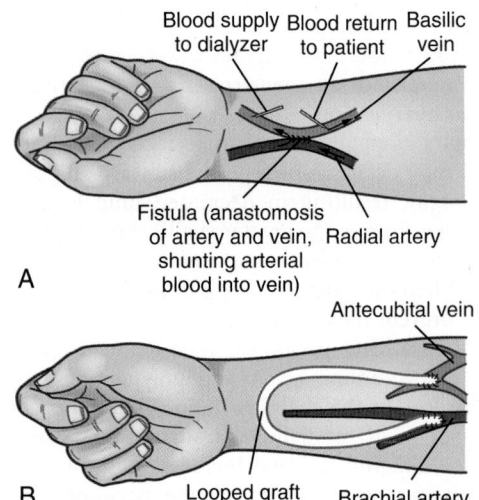

Blood supply to dialyzer · Blood return to patient · Basilic vein

Fistula (anastomosis of artery and vein, shunting arterial blood into vein) · Radial artery

A

Antecubital vein

B   Looped graft · Brachial artery

FIG. 47-8 Vascular access for hemodialysis. **A,** Arteriovenous fistula. **B,** Arteriovenous graft.

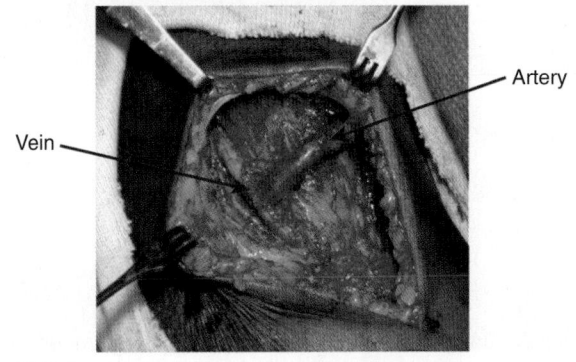

Vein · Artery

FIG. 47-9 Arteriovenous fistula created by anastomosing an artery and a vein.

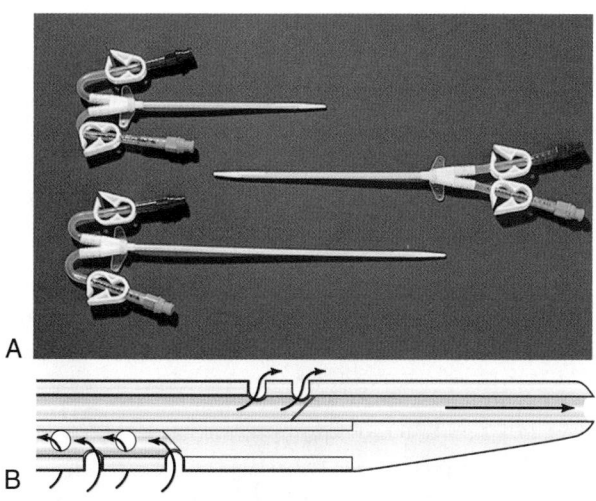

FIG. 47-10 Temporary double-lumen vascular access catheter for acute hemodialysis. **A,** Soft, flexible double-lumen tube is attached to a Y hub. **B,** The distance between the arterial intake lumen and the venous return lumen typically provides recirculation rates of 5% or less.

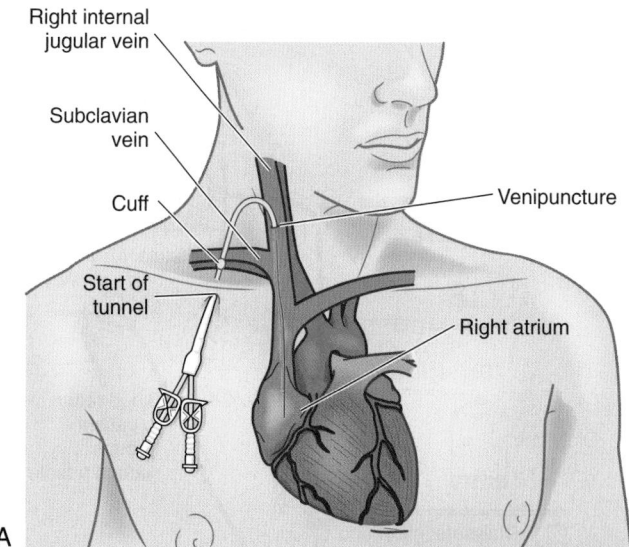

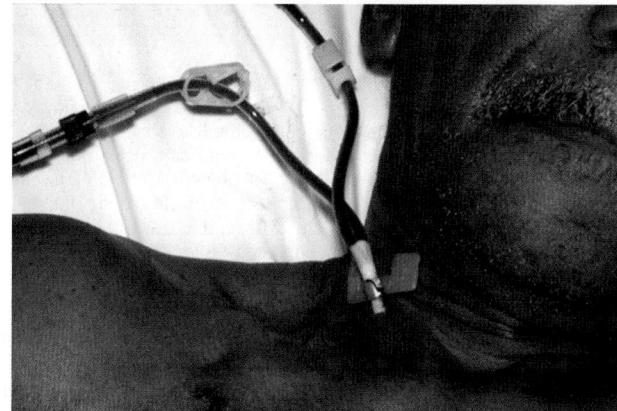

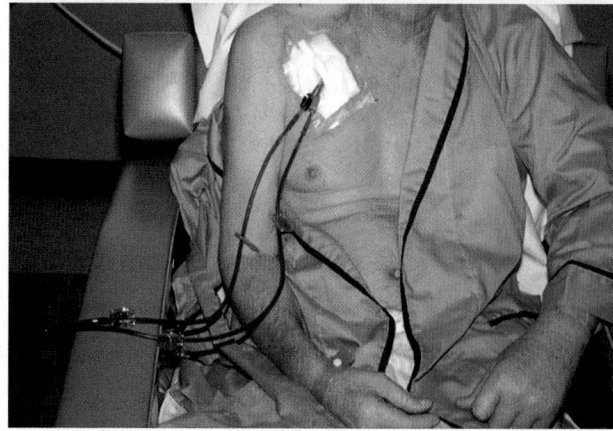

FIG. 47-11 **A,** Right internal jugular placement for a tunneled, cuffed semi-permanent catheter. **B,** Temporary hemodialysis catheter in place. **C,** Long-term cuffed hemodialysis catheter.

subcutaneous Dacron cuffs that prevent infection from tracking along the catheter and anchor the catheter, thus eliminating the need for sutures.

Advance planning is essential for management of the patient with kidney failure who is approaching end-stage disease and the need for dialysis. Enough time is needed for evaluation and consideration of the best arteriovenous access for HD and preparation for PD.

Dialyzers. The HD dialyzer is a long plastic cartridge that contains thousands of parallel hollow tubes or fibers. The fibers are semipermeable membranes made of cellulose-based or other synthetic materials. The blood is pumped into the top of the cartridge and is dispersed into all of the fibers. Dialysis fluid *(dialysate)* is pumped into the bottom of the cartridge and bathes the outside of the fibers. Ultrafiltration, diffusion, and osmosis occur across the pores of this semipermeable membrane. When the dialyzed blood reaches the end of the thousands of semipermeable fibers, it converges into a single tube that returns it to the patient. Dialyzers differ in regard to surface area, membrane composition and thickness, clearance of waste products, and removal of fluid.

Procedure for Hemodialysis

The needles used for HD are large bore, usually 14 to 16 gauge, and are inserted into the fistula or graft to obtain vascular access. One needle is placed to pull blood from the circulation to the HD machine, and the other needle is used to return the dialyzed blood to the patient. The needles are attached via tubing to dialysis lines.

If a patient has a catheter, the two blood lines are attached to the two catheter lumens. The needle closer to the fistula (red catheter lumen) is used to pull blood from the patient and send it to the dialyzer with the assistance of a blood pump. Heparin is added to the blood as it flows into the dialyzer because any time blood contacts a foreign substance, it has a tendency to clot. Blood is returned from the dialyzer to the patient through the second needle (blue catheter lumen).

In addition to the dialyzer, a dialysate delivery and monitoring system is used (Fig. 47-12). This system pumps the dialysate through the dialyzer, countercurrent to the blood flow. Dialysis is terminated by flushing the dialyzer with saline solution to

return the blood in the extracorporeal circuit back to the patient through the vascular access. Then the needles are removed from the patient, and firm pressure is applied to the venipuncture sites until the bleeding stops.

Before beginning treatment, complete an assessment that includes fluid status (weight, BP, peripheral edema, lung and heart sounds), condition of vascular access, temperature, and general skin condition. The difference between the last postdialysis weight and the present predialysis weight determines the ultrafiltration or the amount of weight (from fluid)

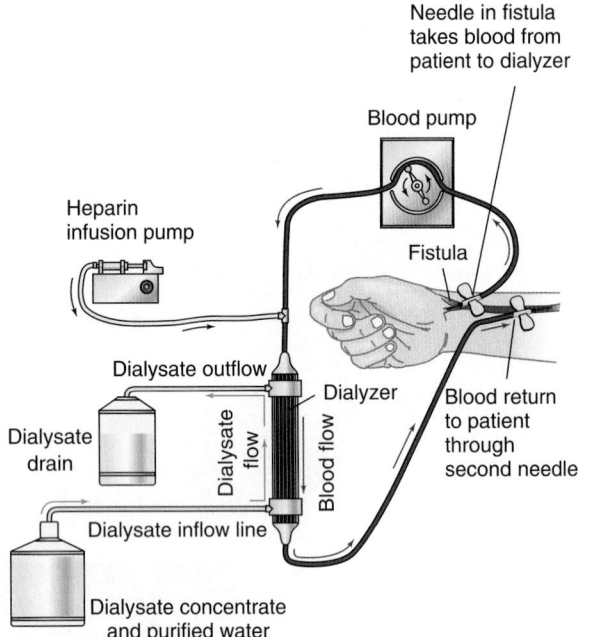

FIG. 47-12 Components of a hemodialysis system. Blood is removed via a needle inserted in a fistula or via catheter lumen. It is propelled to the dialyzer by a blood pump. Heparin is infused either as a bolus predialysis or through a heparin pump continuously to prevent clotting. Dialysate is pumped in and flows in the opposite direction of the blood. The dialyzed blood is returned to the patient through a second needle or catheter lumen. Old dialysate and ultrafiltrate are drained and discarded.

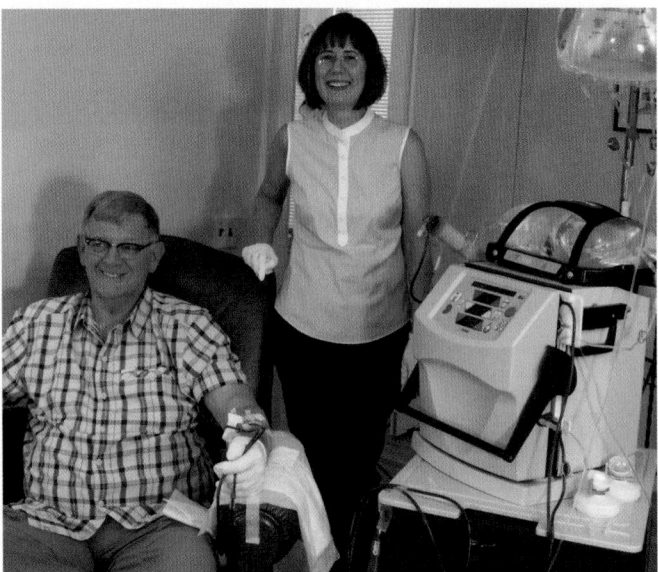

FIG. 47-13 Home hemodialysis is growing in popularity, and machines are more compact.

to be removed. While the patient is on dialysis, take vital signs at least every 30 to 60 minutes because rapid BP changes may occur.

Most maintenance dialysis facilities use reclining chairs that allow for elevation of the feet if hypotension develops. Most people sleep, read, talk, or watch television during dialysis.

Settings and Schedules for Hemodialysis. The majority of HD patients are treated in a community-based center and dialyze for 3 to 4 hours 3 days per week. Other schedule options for HD are short daily HD and long nocturnal HD. In short daily HD, the patient dialyzes for 2½ to 3 hours per session 5 to 6 days per week. Short daily HD is usually done at home.

In-center HD programs have adapted their dialysis schedules so patients can be free during the day. The patient receiving long nocturnal HD has the advantage of sleeping while dialyzing. Each nocturnal treatment lasts 6 to 8 hours, and the patient dialyzes up to six times per week. Patients who choose daily dialysis or nocturnal dialysis tend to feel better, are more in control of their lives, tend to require fewer medications, and have fewer dialysis-related side effects (e.g., hypotension, cramps).

In addition to in-center HD, home HD is available (Fig. 47-13). The option for home HD often depends on a patient's family support. One of the main advantages of home HD is that it allows greater freedom in choosing dialysis times. Daily home HD also offers the potential of significant health benefits. Currently only about 2% of HD patients dialyze at home.

Complications of Hemodialysis

Hypotension. Hypotension that occurs during HD primarily results from rapid removal of vascular volume (hypovolemia), decreased cardiac output, and decreased systemic vascular resistance. The drop in BP during dialysis may precipitate light-

headedness, nausea, vomiting, seizures, vision changes, and chest pain from cardiac ischemia. The usual treatment for hypotension includes decreasing the volume of fluid being removed and infusion of 0.9% saline solution.

Muscle Cramps. The pathogenesis of muscle cramps in HD is poorly understood. Factors associated with the development of muscle cramps include hypotension, hypovolemia, high ultrafiltration rate (large interdialytic weight gain), and low-sodium dialysis solution. Cramps are more frequently seen in the first month after initiation of dialysis than in the subsequent period. Treatment includes reducing the ultrafiltration rate and administering fluids (saline, glucose, mannitol). Hypertonic saline is not recommended, since the sodium load can be problematic. Hypertonic glucose administration is preferred.

Loss of Blood. Blood loss may result from blood not being completely rinsed from the dialyzer, accidental separation of blood tubing, dialysis membrane rupture, or bleeding after the removal of needles at the end of dialysis. If a patient has received too much heparin or has clotting problems, postdialysis bleeding can be significant. It is essential to rinse back all blood, to closely monitor heparinization to avoid excess anticoagulation, and to hold firm but nonocclusive pressure on access sites until the risk of bleeding has passed.

Hepatitis. At one time, hepatitis B had an unusually high prevalence in dialysis patients, but the incidence today is low. Lower transfusion requirements, screening, and recommendations for vaccinations have lowered the incidence. However, outbreaks of hepatitis B still occur, since transmission is attributed to breaks in infection control practices. To prevent transmission, the Centers for Disease Control and Prevention (CDC) has recommended that all patients and personnel in dialysis units receive hepatitis B vaccine.

Currently, hepatitis C virus (HCV) is responsible for the majority of cases of hepatitis in dialysis patients. (Hepatitis is discussed in more detail in Chapter 44.) Approximately 8% to 10% of patients undergoing dialysis in the United States are positive for anti-HCV, which indicates a previous infection. Infection control precautions are mandated in care of the patient with hepatitis C to protect the patient and staff. (Infection control precautions are discussed in Chapter 15.) Currently, no vaccine is available for hepatitis C.[25]

Effectiveness of Hemodialysis

HD is still an imperfect therapy for management of ESKD. It cannot fully replace the normal functions of the kidneys. It can ease many of the symptoms of CKD and, if started early, can prevent certain complications. However, it does not alter the accelerated rate of development of CV disease and the related high mortality rate.

The yearly death rate of patients receiving maintenance dialysis remains high at an estimated 19% to 24%. The majority of deaths are caused by CV disease (stroke or myocardial infarction). Infectious complications are the second leading cause of death.

Individual adaptation to maintenance HD varies considerably. Initially many patients feel positive about the dialysis because it makes them feel better and keeps them alive, but there is often great ambivalence about whether it is worthwhile. Dependence on a machine is a reality. In response to their illness, dialysis patients may be nonadherent or depressed and exhibit suicidal tendencies. The primary nursing goals are to assist the patient in maintaining a healthy self-image and, if possible, rehabilitate with the hopes of returning to work.

CONTINUOUS RENAL REPLACEMENT THERAPY

Continuous renal replacement therapy (CRRT) is an alternative or adjunctive method for treating AKI. It provides a means by which uremic toxins and fluids are removed, while acid-base status and electrolytes are adjusted slowly and continuously in a hemodynamically unstable patient. The patients selected are usually those who do not respond to dietary interventions and drug therapy. The principle of CRRT is to dialyze patients in a more physiologic way over 24 hours, just like the kidneys.

CRRT is contraindicated if a patient has life-threatening manifestations of uremia (hyperkalemia, pericarditis) that require rapid resolution. CRRT can be used in conjunction with HD.

Various types of CRRT are available (Table 47-14). CRRT most commonly uses the venovenous approaches of continuous venovenous hemofiltration (CVVH), continuous venovenous hemodialysis (CVVHD), and continuous venovenous hemodiafiltration (CVVHDF).

Vascular access for CVVH or CVVHD is achieved through the use of a double-lumen catheter (as used in HD [see Fig. 47-10]) placed in the jugular or femoral vein. A blood pump is used to propel the blood through the circuit. A highly permeable, hollow-fiber hemofilter removes plasma water and nonprotein solutes, which are collectively termed *ultrafiltrate*. The ultrafiltration rate (UFR) may range from 0 to 500 mL/hr. Under the influence of hydrostatic pressure and osmotic pressure, water and nonprotein solutes pass out of the filter into the extracapillary space and drain through the ultrafiltrate port into a collection device (drainage bag) (Fig. 47-14). The remaining fluid continues through the filter and returns to the patient via the return port of the double-lumen catheter.

While the ultrafiltrate drains out of the hemofilter, fluid and electrolyte replacements can be infused into the infusion port located after the filter as the blood returns to the patient. This fluid is designed to replace volume and solutes such as sodium, chloride, bicarbonate, and glucose. It also further

TABLE 47-14	CONTINUOUS RENAL REPLACEMENT THERAPIES	
Therapy	**Abbreviation**	**Purpose**
Continuous venovenous hemofiltration	CVVH	Removes both fluid and solutes. Replacement fluid required.
Slow continuous ultrafiltration	SCUF	Simplified version of CVVH. Removes fluid. No fluid replacement required.
Continuous venovenous hemodialysis	CVVHD	Removes both fluids and solutes. Requires both dialysate and replacement fluid.
Continuous venovenous hemodiafiltration	CVVHDF	Removes both fluids and solutes. Requires both dialysate and replacement fluid.

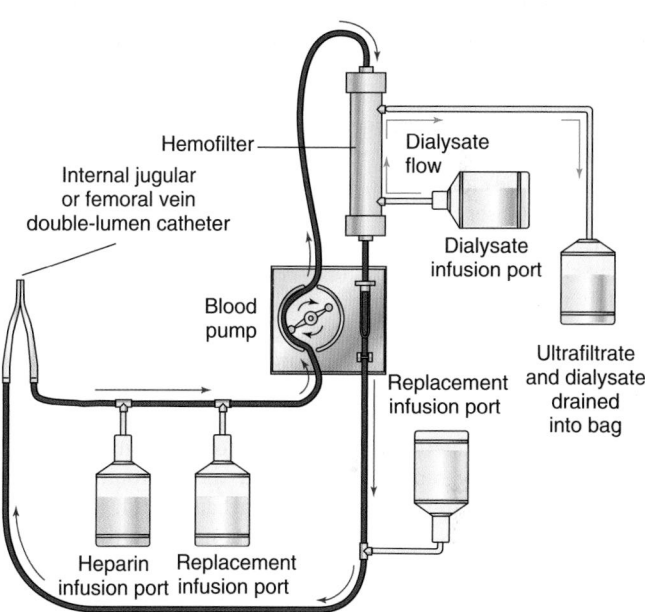

FIG. 47-14 Basic schematic of continuous venovenous therapies. Blood pump is required to pump blood through the circuit. Replacement ports are used for instilling replacement fluids and can be given prefilter or postfilter. Dialysate port is used for infusing dialysis solution. Regardless of modality, ultrafiltrate is drained via the ultrafiltration drain port.

dilutes intravascular fluid, decreasing the concentration of unwanted solutes such as BUN, creatinine, and potassium. The infusion rate of replacement fluid is determined by the degree of fluid and electrolyte imbalance. Replacement fluid may also be infused into the infusion port before the hemofilter. This method allows for greater clearance of urea and can decrease filter clotting.

Anticoagulation is needed to prevent blood clotting during CRRT. Heparin may be infused as a bolus at the initiation of CRRT or through the heparin infusion port before the hemofilter.

Several features of CRRT differ from HD:

- It is continuous rather than intermittent. Large volumes of fluid can be removed over days (24 hours to more than 2 weeks) versus hours (3 to 4 hours).
- Solute removal can occur by *convection* (no dialysate required) in addition to osmosis and diffusion.

- It causes less hemodynamic instability (e.g., hypotension).
- It does not require constant monitoring by a specialized HD nurse but does require a trained ICU nurse.
- It does not require complicated HD equipment, but a blood pump is needed for venovenous therapies.

The type of CRRT can be customized to the patient's needs. Some types involve the introduction of replacement fluids. Large volumes of fluid may be removed hourly (200 to 800 mL), and then a portion of this fluid is replaced. The type of fluid replacement depends on the patient's stability and individual needs. Ultrafiltration and convective losses occur, and solute concentrations in the blood are diluted with the replacement fluid.

The *hemodialysis therapies* (CVVHD and CVVHDF) use dialysate. Dialysis fluid is attached to the distal end of the hemofilter, and the fluid is pumped countercurrent to the blood flow (see Fig. 47-14). As in dialysis, diffusion of solutes and ultrafiltration via hydrostatic pressure and osmosis occur. This is an ideal treatment for a patient who needs both fluid and solute control but cannot tolerate the rapid fluid shifts associated with HD.

CRRT can be continued as long as 30 to 40 days, but the hemofilter should be changed every 24 to 48 hours because of loss of filtration efficiency or potential for clotting. The ultrafiltrate should be clear yellow, and specimens may be obtained for evaluation of serum chemistries. If the ultrafiltrate becomes bloody or blood tinged, a possible rupture in the filter membrane should be suspected, and treatment is suspended immediately to prevent blood loss and infection.

Specific nursing interventions include obtaining weights and monitoring and documenting laboratory values daily to ensure adequate fluid and electrolyte balance. Assessment of hourly intake and output, vital signs, and hemodynamic status is essential. Although reductions in central venous pressure and pulmonary artery pressure are expected, there should be little change in mean arterial pressure or cardiac output. Patency of the CRRT system is assessed and maintained, and the patient's vascular access site is cared for to prevent infection. Treatment is discontinued and the needle(s) removed once the patient's AKI is resolved or there is a decision to withdraw treatment because of patient deterioration.

KIDNEY TRANSPLANTATION

Major progress has been made in kidney transplantation since the first live donor kidney transplant was performed in 1954 in Boston between identical twins. The advances made in organ procurement and preservation, surgical techniques, tissue typing and matching, immunosuppressant therapy, and prevention and treatment of graft rejection have dramatically increased the success of kidney transplantation. (A general discussion of organ transplantation is in Chapter 14, pp. 219-223).

Even though kidney transplantation is by far the best treatment option available to patients with ESKD, fewer than 4% ever receive a transplant. This is because of the high disparity between the supply and demand for kidneys. Every year thousands are waiting for kidney transplantation (more than 93,000 are currently on the list), yet less than one fourth ever receive a kidney. Most die while waiting. Transplantation from a deceased donor usually requires a prolonged waiting period with differences in waiting time depending on age, gender, and race. Average wait times in the United States for a

cadaveric kidney to become available usually ranges from 2 to 5 years.[26]

Kidney transplantation is very successful, with 1-year graft survival rates over 90% for deceased donor transplants and 95% for live donor transplants.[26] An advantage of kidney transplantation when compared with dialysis is that it reverses many of the pathophysiologic changes associated with renal failure. It also eliminates the dependence on dialysis and the accompanying dietary and lifestyle restrictions. Transplantation is also less expensive than dialysis after the first year.

Recipient Selection

Appropriate recipient selection is important for a successful outcome. Candidacy is determined by a variety of medical and psychosocial factors that vary among transplant centers. Some transplant programs exclude patients who are morbidly obese or who continue to smoke (despite smoking cessation interventions). A careful evaluation is completed in an attempt to identify and minimize potential complications after transplantation. Certain patients, particularly those with CV disease and diabetes mellitus, are considered high risk and must be carefully evaluated and then monitored closely after the transplantation. For a small number of patients who are approaching ESKD, a *preemptive transplant* (before dialysis is required) is possible if they have a living donor. This approach is most advantageous for patients with diabetes, who have a much higher mortality rate on dialysis than nondiabetics.

Contraindications to transplantation include disseminated malignancies, refractory or untreated cardiac disease, chronic respiratory failure, extensive vascular disease, chronic infection, and unresolved psychosocial disorders (e.g., nonadherence to medical regimens, alcoholism, drug addiction). At one time, patients diagnosed with human immunodeficiency virus (HIV) infection were denied the opportunity for kidney transplantation. However, centers that have included HIV patients demonstrate graft and patient survival rates for patients with HIV that are comparable to those in the HIV-negative population. The presence of hepatitis B or C is not a contraindication to transplantation.[25]

Surgical procedures may be required before transplantation based on the results of the recipient evaluation. Coronary artery bypass or coronary angioplasty may be indicated for advanced coronary artery disease. Cholecystectomy may be necessary for patients with a history of gallstones, biliary obstruction, or cholecystitis. On rare occasions, bilateral nephrectomies are necessary for patients with refractory hypertension, recurrent urinary tract infections, or grossly enlarged kidneys from polycystic kidney disease. In general, the recipient's own kidneys do not need to be removed before he or she receives a kidney transplant.

Histocompatibility Studies

Histocompatibility studies, including human leukocyte antigen (HLA) testing and crossmatching, are discussed in Chapter 14 on pp. 220-221.

Donor Sources

Kidneys for transplantation may be obtained from compatible blood-type deceased donors, blood relatives, emotionally related (close and distant) living donors (e.g., spouses, distant cousins, etc.), and altruistic living donors who are known (friends) or unknown to the recipient.

ETHICAL/LEGAL DILEMMAS

Allocation of Resources

Situation

T.H., a transplant nurse coordinator, is considering her feelings about two patients who are being evaluated for placement on the deceased (cadaveric) kidney transplant waiting list. One patient is a 40-yr-old African American schoolteacher. She is married and has two children. The other patient is a 22-yr-old unemployed white man. He misses three or four dialysis treatments per month and does not take his antihypertensive medications consistently.

Ethical/Legal Points for Consideration

- The foundation of this conflict resides in the Constitution where the founders made education a free public resource and ignored health care as a right. Health care then became a privilege, a resource to be obtained by persons with the funds to pay for it.
- It took almost 200 yr for health entitlement programs to be developed. Medicare is a federally administered program. Individuals covered by Medicare are protected by Constitutional laws prohibiting discrimination based on race, gender, religion, and ethnic background.
- Medicaid is a federally sponsored program jointly administered by the various states. The states have the right to set coverage eligibility and limits, but may not violate an individual's constitutionally protected rights against discrimination.
- It is highly unlikely that the standard prohibitions against discrimination will change, but it is possible that definitions of unhealthy behavior such as substance abuse, alcoholism, smoking, and obesity might be used to screen out candidates.
- Nurses are concerned about social justice because of their health advocacy role. Today the situation is immensely more complex because of the cost and availability of care.

Discussion Questions

1. What does the 2001 American Nurses Association (ANA) Code of Ethics say about how you as a nurse should view patients?
2. What are your thoughts about which of the patients should receive the next available kidney transplant?

Another option is *paired organ donation* where one donor/recipient pair who are incompatible or poorly matched with each other find another donor/recipient pair with whom they can exchange kidneys. Thus a spouse (person A) who wants to donate a kidney to his wife (person B) but is incompatible is paired with another donor/recipient pair involving a son with ESKD (person C) and his mother (person D). In this example, person A would donate his kidney to person C, and person D would donate her kidney to person B. Paired organ donation is the practice of matching biologically incompatible donor/recipient pairs to permit transplantation of both candidates with a well-matched organ. Expanding the living donor pool is one of the best possibilities for decreasing the size of the waiting list and reducing wait times for people needing a deceased donor.

Live Donors. Live donors undergo an extensive multidisciplinary evaluation to be certain that they are in good health and have no history of disease that would place them at risk for developing kidney failure or operative complications. Psychosocial and financial evaluations are also done. Crossmatches are done at the time of the evaluation and about a week before the transplant to ensure that no antibodies to the donor are present or that the antibody titer is below the allowed level. Advantages of a live donor kidney include better patient and graft survival rates regardless of histocompatibility match, immediate organ availability, immediate function because of minimal *cold time* (kidney out of body and not getting blood supply), and the opportunity to have the recipient in the best possible medical condition because the surgery is elective.

The potential donor sees a nephrologist for a complete history and physical examination and laboratory and diagnostic studies. Laboratory studies include a 24-hour urine study for creatinine clearance and total protein, complete blood count, and chemistry and electrolyte profiles. Hepatitis B and C, HIV, and cytomegalovirus (CMV) testing is done to assess for any transmitted diseases. An ECG and chest x-ray are also done. A renal ultrasound and a renal arteriogram or three-dimensional CT scan is performed to ensure that the blood vessels supplying each kidney are adequate and that there are no anomalies and to determine which kidney will be removed.

A transplant psychologist or social worker determines if the individual is emotionally stable and able to deal with the issues related to organ donation. All donors must be informed about the risks and benefits of donation, the potential short- and long-term complications, and what to expect during the hospitalization and recovery phases. Kidney donation is considered safe without any long-term health consequences. Although the costs of the evaluation and surgery are covered by the recipient's insurance, no compensation is available for lost wages during the posthospitalization recovery period. This period can last 6 weeks or longer.

When there is ABO incompatibility between a donor and recipient, paired donor exchange is a viable alternative. Another option for ABO incompatibility or a positive crossmatch between the donor and recipient is to use plasmapheresis to remove antibodies from the recipient. (Crossmatching is discussed in Chapter 14.) This allows transplant candidates to receive kidneys from live donors with blood types that have traditionally been considered incompatible. After the transplant, the patient undergoes additional plasmapheresis treatments.

Deceased Donors. Deceased (cadaver) kidney donors are relatively healthy individuals who have suffered an irreversible brain injury and are declared brain dead. The most common causes of injury are cerebral trauma from motor vehicle accidents or gunshot wounds, intracerebral or subarachnoid hemorrhage, and anoxic brain damage caused by cardiac arrest. The brain-dead donor must have effective CV function and be supported on a ventilator to preserve the organs. The donor must be free of active IV drug abuse; severe hypertension; longstanding diabetes mellitus; malignancies; sepsis; and communicable diseases, including HIV, hepatitis B and C, syphilis, and tuberculosis.

Even if the donor carried a signed donor card, permission from the donor's legal next of kin is still requested after brain death is determined. That is why it is important for you to talk with your family about your wishes before losing the capacity to convey your desires.

The kidneys are removed and preserved. They can be preserved for up to 72 hours, but most transplant surgeons prefer to transplant kidneys before the cold time (time outside of the body when being transported from the deceased donor to the recipient) reaches 24 hours. Prolonged cold time increases the likelihood that the kidney will not function immediately, and acute tubular necrosis (ATN) may develop.

The United Network for Organ Sharing (UNOS) distributes deceased donor kidneys using an objective computerized point system. The ABO group, HLA typing, age, antibody level, and length of time waiting are entered into the national computer for each candidate. When a donor becomes available, the donor's key information is compared with the data of all patients awaiting transplantation locally and nationwide. Points are given for how close the HLA match is, how long the patient has been waiting, if the antibody level is unusually high, and if the recipient is younger than 19 years old. Extra points are given for high antibody levels because this can severely limit the number of donors with whom the patient will not have a positive crossmatch. The kidney is offered to the recipient with the most points in the local area. If no patients in the local area are suitable, the organ is then offered in the region and then in the nation. When a kidney arrives at the recipient's transplant center, a final crossmatch is done and must be negative for the deceased donor transplantation to proceed. (Crossmatching is discussed in Chapter 14.)

The only exception to the previous plan is if a patient needs an emergency transplant or if a donor and recipient match on all six HLA antigens (zero antigen mismatch). The patient meeting either one of these criteria goes to the top of the list. Emergency transplants are given priority because the patient is facing imminent death if not transplanted (e.g., a patient who had no vascular access sites left and can no longer dialyze). Zero antigen mismatches are given priority because statistically these grafts have better survival rates. If a zero antigen mismatch patient is identified nationally, one of the donor kidneys must be sent to that recipient's transplant center regardless of location.

Surgical Procedure

Live Donor. Living donation accounts for nearly 27% of all kidney transplants in the United States, and most transplant centers regard them as the preferred donation modality. The donor nephrectomy is performed by a urologist or transplant surgeon. The donor's surgery begins 1 to 2 hours before the recipient's surgery. The recipient is surgically prepared for the kidney transplant in a nearby operating room.

Laparoscopic donor nephrectomy is the most common technique for removing a kidney in a living donor. (Laparoscopic nephrectomy is discussed in Chapter 46.) After the kidney has been removed, it is flushed with a chilled, sterile electrolyte solution and prepared for immediate transplant into the recipient. The use of a laparoscopic donor nephrectomy procedure is minimally invasive with fewer risks and shorter recovery time than an open procedure. The laparoscopic approach significantly decreases hospital stay, pain, operative blood loss, debilitation, and length of time off work. For these reasons, the number of people willing to donate a kidney has increased significantly.

For an *open (conventional) nephrectomy,* the donor is placed in the lateral decubitus position on the operating table so that the flank is exposed laterally. An incision is made at the level of the eleventh rib. The rib may have to be removed to provide adequate visualization of the kidney.

Kidney Transplant Recipient. The transplanted kidney is usually placed extraperitoneally in the iliac fossa. The right iliac fossa is preferred to facilitate anastomoses of the blood vessels and ureter and minimize the occurrence of paralytic ileus.

Before any incisions are made, a urinary catheter is placed into the bladder. An antibiotic solution is instilled to distend the bladder and decrease the risk of infection. A crescent-shaped incision is made extending from the iliac crest to the symphysis pubis (Fig. 47-15).

Rapid revascularization is critical to prevent ischemic injury to the kidney. The donor artery is anastomosed to the recipient's internal iliac (hypogastric) or external iliac artery. The donor vein is anastomosed to the recipient's external iliac vein.

When the anastomoses are complete, the clamps are released, and blood flow to the kidney is reestablished. The kidney should become firm and pink. Urine may begin to flow from the ureter immediately.

The donor ureter in most cases is then tunneled through the bladder submucosa before entering the bladder cavity and being sutured in place. This approach is called *ureteroneocystostomy.* This allows the bladder wall to compress the ureter as it contracts for micturition, thereby preventing reflux of urine up the ureter into the transplanted kidney. The transplant surgery takes about 3 to 4 hours.

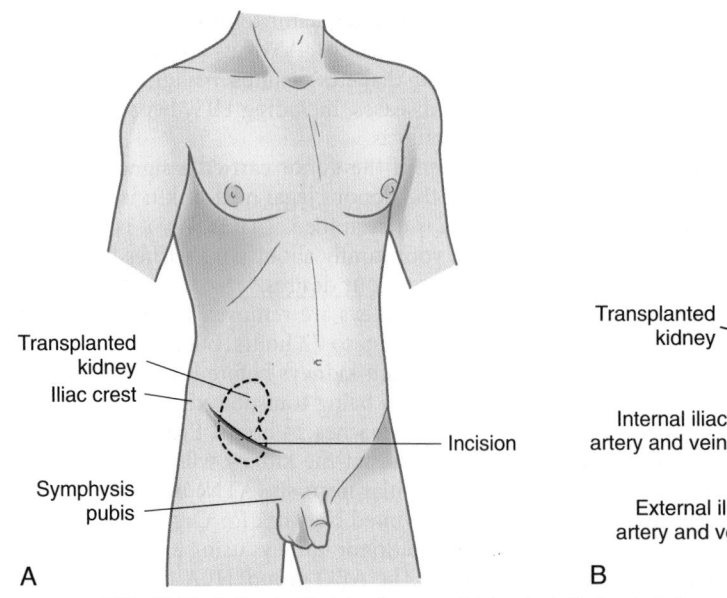

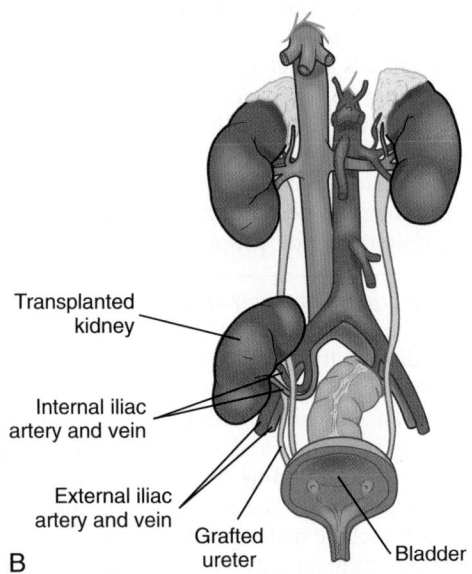

FIG. 47-15 A, Surgical incision for a renal transplant. **B,** Surgical placement of transplanted kidney.

NURSING MANAGEMENT
KIDNEY TRANSPLANT RECIPIENT

PREOPERATIVE CARE

Nursing care of the patient in the preoperative phase includes emotional and physical preparation for surgery. Because the patient and caregiver may have been waiting years for the kidney transplant, a review of the operative procedure and what can be expected in the immediate postoperative recovery period is necessary. Stress that there is a chance the kidney may not function immediately, and dialysis may be required for days to weeks. Review the need for immunosuppressive drugs and measures to prevent infection.

To ensure the patient is in optimal physical condition for surgery, an ECG, chest x-ray, and laboratory studies are ordered. Dialysis may be required before surgery for any significant problems such as fluid overload or hyperkalemia. A patient on PD must empty the peritoneal cavity of all dialysate solution before going to surgery. Because dialysis may be required after transplantation, the patency of the vascular access must be maintained. The vascular access extremity should be labeled "dialysis access, no procedures" to prevent use of the affected extremity for BP measurement, blood drawing, or IV infusions.

POSTOPERATIVE CARE

LIVE DONOR. The usual postoperative care for the donor is similar to that following open (conventional) or laparoscopic nephrectomy (see Chapter 46). Closely monitor renal function to assess for impairment, and monitor the hematocrit to assess for bleeding. Donors experience more pain after an open nephrectomy than a laparoscopic procedure. Generally, all donors have more pain than their recipients do. Donors who have had an open surgical approach are ready to be discharged from the hospital in 4 or 5 days and can usually return to work in 6 to 8 weeks. With a laparoscopic approach, donors are discharged from the hospital in 2 to 4 days and can return to work in 4 to 6 weeks. The donor is seen by the surgeon 1 to 2 weeks after discharge.

Nurses caring for the living donor need to acknowledge the precious gift that this person has given. The donor has taken physical, emotional, and financial risks to assist the recipient. It is vital that the donor not be forgotten postoperatively. The donor will need even more support if the donated organ does not work immediately or for some reason fails.

KIDNEY TRANSPLANT RECIPIENT. The first priority during this period is maintenance of fluid and electrolyte balance. Because close monitoring is required, kidney transplant recipients spend the first 12 to 24 hours in the ICU. Very large volumes of urine may be produced soon after the blood supply to the transplanted kidney is reestablished. This diuresis is due to (1) the new kidney's ability to filter BUN, which acts as an osmotic diuretic; (2) the abundance of fluids administered during the operation; and (3) initial renal tubular dysfunction, which inhibits the kidney from concentrating urine normally. Urine output during this phase may be as high as 1 L/hr and gradually decreases as the BUN and serum creatinine levels return toward normal.

Urine output is replaced with fluids milliliter for milliliter hourly for the first 12 to 24 hours. Central venous pressure readings are essential for monitoring postoperative fluid status. Dehydration must be avoided to prevent subsequent renal hypoperfusion and renal tubular damage. Electrolyte monitor-ing to assess for the hyponatremia and hypokalemia often associated with rapid diuresis is critical. Treatment with potassium supplements or infusion of 0.9% normal saline may be indicated. IV sodium bicarbonate may also be required if the patient develops metabolic acidosis from delayed kidney function.

Acute tubular necrosis (ATN) can occur because of prolonged cold times causing ischemic damage and the use of marginal cadaveric donors (those who are medically suboptimal). While the patient is in ATN, dialysis is required to maintain fluid and electrolyte balance. Some patients have high-output ATN with the ability to excrete fluid but not metabolic wastes or electrolytes. Other patients have oliguric or anuric ATN. These patients are at risk for fluid overload in the immediate postoperative period and must be assessed closely for the need for dialysis. The period of ATN can last anywhere from days to weeks, with gradually improving kidney function. Most patients with ATN are discharged from the hospital on dialysis. This is extremely discouraging for the patient, who needs reassurance that renal function usually improves. Dialysis is discontinued when urine output increases and serum creatinine and BUN begin to normalize.

A sudden decrease in urine output in the early postoperative period is a cause for concern. It may be due to dehydration, rejection, a urine leak, or obstruction. A common cause of early obstruction is a blood clot in the urinary catheter. Catheter patency must be maintained, since the catheter remains in the bladder for 3 to 5 days to allow the ureter-bladder anastomosis to heal. If blood clots are suspected, gentle catheter irrigation (if ordered by the health care provider) can reestablish patency.

With a hospital length of stay averaging 4 to 5 days, discharge planning and teaching needs must be identified and addressed early in the hospital course. Postoperative teaching includes how to recognize signs of rejection, infection, and any complications of surgery. Frequent blood tests and clinic visits help detect rejection early. Patient teaching to ensure a smooth transition from the hospital to the home is an integral part of the nursing care.

Immunosuppressive Therapy

The goal of immunosuppression is to adequately suppress the immune response to prevent rejection of the transplanted kidney while maintaining sufficient immunity to prevent overwhelming infection. Immunosuppressive therapy is discussed in Chapter 14 and in Table 14-16.

Complications of Transplantation

Complications of RRTs, including PD, HD, and kidney transplantation, are compared in Table 47-15.

Rejection. Rejection is one of the major problems following kidney transplantation. Rejection can be hyperacute, acute, or chronic. These types of rejection are discussed in Chapter 14 on p. 221. Patients with chronic rejection should be put on the transplant list in the hope that they can be retransplanted before dialysis is required.

Infection. Infection remains a significant cause of morbidity and mortality after transplantation. The transplant recipient is at risk for infection because of suppression of the body's normal defense mechanisms by surgery, immunosuppressive drugs, and the effects of ESKD. Underlying systemic illness such as diabetes mellitus or systemic lupus erythematosus, malnutrition, and older age can further compound the negative effects on the

TABLE 47-15	**COMPLICATIONS OF DIALYSIS AND TRANSPLANTATION**	
Peritoneal Dialysis (PD)	**Hemodialysis (HD)**	**Transplantation**
• Exit site infection	• Hypotension	• Rejection of transplant
• Peritonitis	• Muscle cramps	• Hyperacute
• Abdominal pain	• Exsanguination	• Acute
• Catheter outflow	• Hepatitis	• Chronic
• Hernias	• Infection, including sepsis	• Susceptibility to infection
• Lower back pain	• Disequilibrium syndrome	• Cardiovascular disease
• Cardiovascular disease	• Cardiovascular disease	• Malignancies
• Pulmonary problems		• Recurrence of kidney disease
• Atelectasis		• Corticosteroid-related complications
• Pneumonia		
• Bronchitis		
• Protein loss		
• Carbohydrate abnormalities		
• Lipid abnormalities		
• Encapsulating sclerosing peritonitis		

immune response. At times the signs and symptoms of infection can be subtle. You need to be astute in your observation and assessment of kidney transplant recipients because prompt diagnosis and treatment of infections will improve patient outcomes.

The most common infections observed in the first month after transplantation are similar to those acquired by any postoperative patient, such as pneumonia, wound infections, IV line and drain infections, and urinary tract infections. Fungal and viral infections are not uncommon because of the patient's immunosuppressed state. Fungal infections include *Candida, Cryptococcus,* and *Aspergillus* organisms and *Pneumocystis jiroveci.* Fungal infections are difficult to treat, require prolonged treatment periods, and often involve the administration of nephrotoxic drugs. Transplant recipients usually receive prophylactic antifungal drugs to prevent these infections, such as clotrimazole (Mycelex), fluconazole (Diflucan), and trimethoprim/sulfamethoxazole (Bactrim).

Viral infections, including CMV, Epstein-Barr virus, herpes simplex virus (HSV), varicella-zoster virus, and polyomavirus (e.g., BK virus), can be primary infections or reactivations of existing disease. Primary infections occur as new infections after transplantation from an exogenous source such as the donated organ or a blood transfusion. Reactivation occurs when a virus exists in a patient and becomes reactivated after transplantation because of immunosuppression.

CMV is one of the most common viral infections. If a recipient has never had CMV and receives an organ from a donor with a history of CMV, antiviral prophylaxis will be administered (e.g., ganciclovir [Cytovene], valganciclovir [Valcyte]). If a primary active CMV infection is diagnosed or there is symptomatic reactivation of CMV, IV ganciclovir is given along with an immune globulin that contains CMV antibodies. To prevent HSV infections, oral acyclovir (Zovirax) is given for several months after the transplant.

Cardiovascular Disease. Transplant recipients have an increased incidence of atherosclerotic vascular disease. CV disease is the leading cause of death after renal transplantation. Hypertension, dyslipidemia, diabetes mellitus, smoking, rejection, infections, and increased homocysteine levels can all

contribute to CV disease. Immunosuppressants can worsen hypertension and dyslipidemia. Teach the patient to control risk factors such as elevated cholesterol, triglycerides, and blood glucose and weight gain. Adherence to the prescribed antihypertensive regimen is essential not only to prevent CV events but also to prevent damage to the new kidney. (Hypertension is discussed in Chapter 33.)

Malignancies. The overall incidence of malignancies in kidney transplant recipients is greater than in the general population, primarily because of immunosuppressive therapy. Not only do immunosuppressants suppress the immune system to prevent rejection, but they also suppress the ability to fight infection and the production of abnormal cells such as cancer cells.[27]

The most common types of cancer after transplant are basal and squamous cell carcinoma of the skin, Hodgkin's and non-Hodgkin's lymphoma, and Kaposi sarcoma. Patients are also at risk for cancers of the liver, stomach, oropharynx, anus, vulva, and penis.

Regular screening for cancer is an important part of the transplant recipient's preventive care. Advise the patient to avoid sun exposure by using protective clothing and sunscreens to minimize the incidence of skin cancers.

Recurrence of Original Kidney Disease. Recurrence of the original disease that destroyed the native kidneys occurs in some kidney transplant recipients. It is most common with certain types of glomerulonephritis, immunoglobulin A (IgA) nephropathy, diabetic nephropathy, and focal segmental sclerosis. Disease recurrence can result in the loss of a functioning kidney transplant. Patients must be advised before transplantation if they have a disease known to recur.

Corticosteroid-Related Complications. Aseptic necrosis of the hips, knees, and other joints can result from chronic corticosteroid therapy and renal osteodystrophy. Other significant problems related to corticosteroids include peptic ulcer disease, glucose intolerance and diabetes, cataracts, dyslipidemia, infections, and malignancies. In the first year after transplantation, corticosteroid doses are usually decreased to 5 to 10 mg/day. The use of tacrolimus and cyclosporine has allowed the corticosteroid doses to be much lower than they were in the past.

Many transplant programs have initiated corticosteroid-free drug regimens because of the problems of long-term corticosteroid use. Other centers withdraw patients from corticosteroids over a short period after transplantation. For patients who remain on corticosteroids, vigilant monitoring for side effects and early treatment are essential.

GERONTOLOGIC CONSIDERATIONS

CHRONIC KIDNEY DISEASE

The incidence of CKD in the United States is increasing most rapidly in older patients. The most common diseases leading to renal failure in older people are hypertension and diabetes.

The care of this older population is particularly challenging, not only because of the normal physiologic changes of aging but also because of the disabilities, chronic diseases, and number of co-morbid conditions that develop.[28] Physiologic changes of clinical importance in the older CKD patient include diminished cardiopulmonary function, bone loss, immunodeficiency, altered protein synthesis, impaired cognition, and altered drug metabolism. Malnutrition is common in these patients for a variety of reasons, including lack of mobility, lack of understanding of basic nutritional requirements, social isolation, physical disability, impaired cognitive function, and malabsorption problems.

When conservative therapy for CKD is no longer effective, the older patient needs to consider the best treatment modality based on his or her physical and emotional health, personal preferences, and availability of support. PD allows the patient to be more mobile and to enjoy an increased sense of control over the illness. PD causes less hemodynamic instability than HD but does require self-care or assistance from another person, which may not always be available.

Most individuals 65 years of age or older select treatment with HD, specifically in-center treatment, because of a lack of assistance in the home and reluctance to manage the technology of dialysis. Establishing vascular access for HD may be a concern for an older patient because of atherosclerotic changes. Although transplantation is an option, older patients are less likely to be considered as candidates. Older adults need to be carefully screened to ensure that the benefits of transplantation outweigh the risks.[29] A living donor is preferable so that there is not a prolonged waiting time.

The most common cause of death in older ESKD patients is CV disease (myocardial infarction, stroke), followed by withdrawal from dialysis. If a competent patient decides to withdraw from dialysis, it is essential to support the patient and family. Ethical issues (see the Ethical/Legal Dilemmas box on this page) to consider in this situation include patient competency, benefit versus burden of treatment, and futility of treatment. Withdrawal from treatment is not a failure if the patient is well informed and comfortable with the decision.[30]

The increasing number of older, debilitated ESKD patients receiving dialysis has raised a number of ethical concerns about the use of scarce resources in a population with a limited life expectancy. Dialysis (especially PD) has been successfully used in older adults. Quality of life is good in many older ESKD patients receiving dialysis. There appears to be no justification for excluding the older adult from dialysis programs. Rationing dialysis based on age alone is not supported based on current outcome and quality-of-life data.

ETHICAL/LEGAL DILEMMAS
Withdrawing Treatment

Situation

L.R., a 70-yr-old patient with diabetes mellitus and end-stage kidney disease, has been on dialysis for 10 yr. He tells you that he wants to discontinue his dialysis. His quality of life has diminished during the past 2 yr since his wife died. He is not a transplant candidate.

Ethical/Legal Points for Consideration

- Informed consent includes the legal right to refuse treatment. However, the right to refuse may be more difficult if (1) it is contrary to the wishes of family and friends, (2) the treatment still appears to have some effectiveness, and (3) the treatment has been in place for some time.
- Quality-of-life decisions often outweigh the benefit against the burden of treatment. When a treatment becomes too burdensome, the patient (if competent) may request to withdraw the treatment.
- It must be determined whether some other treatable problem such as depression may be clouding the patient's judgment.
- Some health care professionals become conflicted when they are asked to withdraw treatment, since they may think they are contributing to the patient's untimely death.
- If a decision is made to withdraw treatment, the health care team, patient, and family should develop an appropriate follow-up plan that includes palliative care and hospice support.

Discussion Questions

1. How should you respond to L.R.'s request?
2. What is the American Nurses Association's position on withdrawing or withholding treatment that no longer benefits the patient or causes suffering?

CASE STUDY
Chronic Kidney Disease

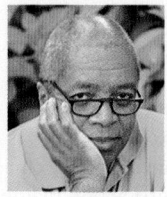
iStockphoto/Thinkstock

Patient Profile

M.B. is a 56-yr-old African American college professor. He is seen by his primary care provider for a routine physical examination. He has not been seen by a physician in a little over a year. He complains of generalized malaise, frequent urination, and "increasing thirst." His medical history is significant for borderline hypertension and dyslipidemia. He also smokes at least one pack of cigarettes per day, and his efforts to quit have been unsuccessful.

Subjective Data

- Family history: father died of a heart attack at age 62, brother had coronary artery bypass graft (CABG) at age 50, mother died from complications of diabetes
- Becomes "winded" when walking from his car to his office at the university
- Wakes up at night to urinate and has more frequent urination
- Increasing thirst

Objective Data
Laboratory Data

- Calculated creatinine clearance using the MDRD equation: 42 mL/min/1.73 m^2

- Serum creatinine 2.5 mg/dL
- BUN 35 mg/dL
- Serum glucose 264 mg/dL
- Hgb 13 g/dL
- Serum cholesterol 236 mg/dL

Physical Examination

- Weight 220 lb, height 5 ft, 11 in
- Blood pressure 168/104 mm Hg

Discussion Questions

1. What do you think caused M.B.'s kidney failure?
2. What stage of chronic kidney disease does he have?
3. What are the most important treatments for M.B.?
4. Identify the abnormal diagnostic study results and why each would occur.
5. *Priority Decision:* What are the priority nursing interventions that would help promote M.B.'s self-management of his disease process?
6. *Priority Decision:* Based on the assessment data provided, what are the priority nursing diagnoses? Are there any collaborative problems?
7. *Evidence-Based Practice:* M.B. tells you that he has not been taking his blood pressure medications regularly. When he asks you how important they are, what will you tell him?

Ⓔvolve Answers available at *http://evolve.elsevier.com/Lewis/medsurg.*

BRIDGE TO NCLEX EXAMINATION

The number of the question corresponds to the same-numbered outcome at the beginning of the chapter.

1. Which descriptions characterize acute kidney injury (select all that apply)?
   a. Primary cause of death is infection.
   b. It almost always affects older people.
   c. Disease course is potentially reversible.
   d. Most common cause is diabetic nephropathy.
   e. Cardiovascular disease is most common cause of death.

2. RIFLE defines three stages of AKI based on changes in
   a. blood pressure and urine osmolality.
   b. fractional excretion of urinary sodium.
   c. estimation of GFR with the MDRD equation.
   d. serum creatinine or urine output from baseline.

3. During the oliguric phase of AKI, the nurse monitors the patient for (select all that apply)
   a. hypotension.
   b. ECG changes.
   c. hypernatremia.
   d. pulmonary edema.
   e. urine with high specific gravity.

4. If a patient is in the diuretic phase of AKI, the nurse must monitor for which serum electrolyte imbalances?
   a. Hyperkalemia and hyponatremia
   b. Hyperkalemia and hypernatremia
   c. Hypokalemia and hyponatremia
   d. Hypokalemia and hypernatremia

5. A patient is admitted to the hospital with chronic kidney disease. The nurse understands that this condition is characterized by
   a. progressive irreversible destruction of the kidneys.
   b. a rapid decrease in urine output with an elevated BUN.
   c. an increasing creatinine clearance with a decrease in urine output.
   d. prostration, somnolence, and confusion with coma and imminent death.

6. Nurses need to teach patients at risk for developing chronic kidney disease. Individuals considered to be at increased risk include (select all that apply)
   a. older African Americans.
   b. patients more than 60 years old.
   c. those with a history of pancreatitis.
   d. those with a history of hypertension.
   e. those with a history of type 2 diabetes.

7. Patients with chronic kidney disease experience an increased incidence of cardiovascular disease related to (select all that apply)
   a. hypertension.
   b. vascular calcifications.
   c. a genetic predisposition.
   d. hyperinsulinemia causing dyslipidemia.
   e. increased high-density lipoprotein levels.

8. Nutritional support and management are essential across the entire continuum of chronic kidney disease. Which statements would be considered true related to nutritional therapy (select all that apply)?
   a. Fluid is not usually restricted for patients receiving peritoneal dialysis.
   b. Sodium and potassium may be restricted in someone with advanced CKD.
   c. Decreased fluid intake and a low potassium diet are hallmarks of the diet for a patient receiving hemodialysis.
   d. Decreased fluid intake and a low potassium diet are hallmarks of the diet for a patient receiving peritoneal dialysis.
   e. Increased fluid intake and a diet with potassium-rich foods are hallmarks of a diet for a patient receiving hemodialysis.

9. An ESKD patient receiving hemodialysis is considering asking a relative to donate a kidney for transplantation. In assisting the patient to make a decision about treatment, the nurse informs the patient that
   a. successful transplantation usually provides better quality of life than that offered by dialysis.
   b. if rejection of the transplanted kidney occurs, no further treatment for the renal failure is available.
   c. hemodialysis replaces the normal functions of the kidneys, and patients do not have to live with the continual fear of rejection.
   d. the immunosuppressive therapy following transplantation makes the person ineligible to receive other forms of treatment if the kidney fails.

10. To assess the patency of a newly placed arteriovenous graft for dialysis, the nurse should (select all that apply)
    a. monitor the BP in the affected arm.
    b. irrigate the graft daily with low-dose heparin.
    c. palpate the area of the graft to feel a normal thrill.
    d. listen with a stethoscope over the graft to detect a bruit.
    e. frequently monitor the pulses and neurovascular status distal to the graft.

11. A major advantage of peritoneal dialysis is
    a. the diet is less restricted and dialysis can be performed at home.
    b. the dialysate is biocompatible and causes no long-term consequences.
    c. high glucose concentrations of the dialysate cause a reduction in appetite, promoting weight loss.
    d. no medications are required because of the enhanced efficiency of the peritoneal membrane in removing toxins.

12. A kidney transplant recipient complains of having fever, chills, and dysuria over the past 2 days. What is the first action that the nurse should take?
    a. Assess temperature and initiate workup to rule out infection.
    b. Reassure the patient that this is common after transplantation.
    c. Provide warm cover for the patient and give 1 g acetaminophen orally.
    d. Notify the nephrologist that the patient has developed symptoms of acute rejection.

1. a, c, 2. d, 3. b, d, 4. c, 5. a, 6. a, b, d, 7. a, b, d, 8. a, b, c, 9. a, 10. c, d, e, 11. a, 12. a

ⓔvolve

For rationales to these answers and even more NCLEX review questions, visit *http://evolve.elsevier.com/Lewis/medsurg*.

REFERENCES

1. Workeneh BT: Acute renal failure. Retrieved from *http://emedicine.medscape.com/article/243492-overview*.

2. Kidney Disease: improving Global Outcomes: clinical practice guidelines on acute kidney injury. Retrieved from *www.kdigo.org*.

*3. Murugan R, Kellum JA: Acute kidney injury: what's the prognosis? *Nat Rev Nephrol* 7(4):209, 2011.

*4. Wang HE, Muntner P, Chertow G, et al: Acute kidney injury and mortality in hospitalized patients, *Am J Neph* 35(4):349, 2012.

5. Singbartl K, Kellum J: AKI in the ICU: definition, epidemiology, risk stratification, and outcomes, *Kidney Int* 81(9):819, 2012.

*6. Wu VC, Wang CH, Wang WJ, et al: Sustained low-efficiency dialysis versus continuous veno-venous hemofiltration for postsurgical acute renal failure, *Am J Surg* 199(4):466, 2010.

7. Davies H, Leslie G: Acute kidney injury and the critically ill patient, *Dimens Crit Nurs* 31(3):135, 2012.

8. Yaklin K: Acute kidney injury: an overview of pathophysiology and treatments, *Nephrol Nurs J* 38(1):13, 2011.

9. Dirkes S: Acute kidney injury: not just acute renal failure anymore? *Crit Care Nurse* 31(1):37, 2011.

10. Ostermann M, Dickie H, Barrett N: Renal replacement therapy in critically ill patients with acute kidney injury: when to start, *Nephrol Dial Transplant* 26(13):1027, 2012.

11. Ali B, Gray-Vickrey P: Limiting the damage from acute kidney injury, *Nursing* 41(3):22, 2011.

12. Kellum J, Lameire N: Clinical practice guidelines for acute kidney injury: KDIGO, *Kidney Int* 2(Suppl 1):1, 2012. Retrieved from *www.kdigo.org/clinical_practice_guidelines/pdf/KDIGO%20AKI%20Guideline.pdf*.

13. Thakar CV, Christianson A, Himmelfarb J, et al: Acute kidney injury episodes and chronic kidney disease risk in diabetes mellitus, *Clin J Am Soc Nephrol* 6(11):2567, 2011.

14. US Renal Data System: *USRDS 2012 annual data report: atlas of end-stage renal disease*, Bethesda, Md, 2012, National Institute of Diabetes and Digestive and Kidney Diseases. Retrieved from *www.usrds.org/adr.aspx*.

15. Foody J, Cleary J, Davis L, et al: Chronic kidney disease and cardiovascular risk: a perfect storm, 2011. Retrieved from *www.aapa.org/uploadedFiles/content/CME/PostTest/W175_176%20CKD%20Mono%20JAPPA.pdf*.

16. US Department of Health and Human Services: ESRD: general information, Centers for Medicare and Medicaid Services. Retrieved from *www.cms.hhs.gov/ESRDGeneralInformation*.

17. National Kidney Foundation: High blood pressure and chronic kidney disease. Retrieved from *www.kidney.org/atoz/pdf/hbpandckd.pdf*.

18. Brancaccio D, Cozzolino M: CKD-MBD: an endless story, *J Nephrol* 24(Suppl 18):42, 2011.

19. National Kidney Foundation Kidney Disease Outcomes Quality Initiative (NKF KDOQI). Retrieved from *www.kidney.org/Professionals/kdoqi*.

20. Hasegawa G, Bragg-Gresham J, Pisoni R, et al: Changes in anemia management and hemoglobin levels following revision of a bundling policy to incorporate recombinant human erythropoietin, *Kidney Inter* 79(3):340, 2011.

21. Aparicio M, Bellizzi V, Chauvea P, et al: Protein-restricted diets plus keto/amino acids: a valid therapeutic approach for chronic kidney disease patients, *J Renal Nutr* 22(2 Suppl):S1, 2012.

22. Holley J: Providing optimal care before and after discontinuation, *Semin Dialy* 25(1):33, 2012.

23. National Kidney and Urologic Diseases Information Clearinghouse: Treatment methods for kidney failure: peritoneal dialysis. Retrieved from *http://kidney.niddk.nih.gov/kudiseases/pubs/peritoneal*.

24. National Kidney and Urologic Diseases Information Clearinghouse: Treatment methods for kidney failure: hemodialysis. Retrieved from *http://kidney.niddk.nih.gov/Kudiseases/pubs/hemodialysis*.

25. Abboud O, Becker G, Bellorin-Font E, et al: KDIGO clinical practice guidelines on hepatitis C in chronic kidney disease acknowledged by ISN. Retrieved from *www.kdigo.org/clinical_practice_guidelines/pdf/ISN_HepC_Commentary.pdf*.

26. United Network for Organ Sharing: *2011 annual report: the US scientific registry of transplant recipients and the organ procurement and transplantation network*, Bethesda, Md, 2011, US Department of Health and Human Services.

27. Danovitch GM: *Handbook of kidney transplantation*, ed 5, Philadelphia, 2010, Lippincott Williams & Wilkins.

28. Bleevins C, Toutman M: Successful aging theory and the patient with chronic renal disease: application in the clinical setting, *Nephrol Nurs J* 38(3):255, 2011.

29. Schaeffner E, Rose C, Gill J: Access to kidney transplantation among the elderly in the United States: a glass half full, not half empty, *Clin J Am Soc Nephrol* 5(11):2109, 2010.

*30. Hopkins DJ, Kott MR, Pirozzi J, et al: End-of-life issues and the patient with renal disease: an evidence-based practice project, *Nephrol Nurs J* 38(1):79, 2011.

RESOURCES

American Association of Kidney Patients (AAKP)
www.aakp.org

American Nephrology Nurses' Association
www.annanurse.org

American Organ Transplant Association
www.a-o-t-a.org

International Society of Nephrology (ISN)
www.theisn.org

International Transplant Nurses Society
www.itns.org

Kidney Transplant/Dialysis Association, Inc.
http://ktda.org

National Kidney Disease Education Program
www.nkdep.nih.gov

National Kidney Foundation
www.kidney.org

RenalWEB Patient Education
www.renalweb.com/topics/patiented/patiented.htm

United Network for Organ Sharing
www.unos.org

United States Renal Data System
www.usrds.org/adr.htm

*Evidence-based information for clinical practice.

CASE STUDY

Managing Multiple Patients

Introduction

You are working on the medical-surgical unit and have been assigned to care for the following four patients. You are also assigned to receive a new admission to the clinical unit. You have one UAP on your team to help you.

Patients

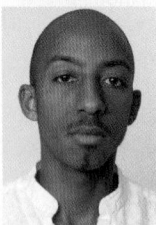

iStockphoto/Thinkstock

A.K., a 28-year-old African American man, was admitted for observation after a renal ultrasound identified calculi in the left ureter. A.K. came to the ED with complaints of sharp, colicky left flank pain for which the health care provider prescribed IV opioids. His last pain medication was given 2 hours ago. His current pain level is 4 on a scale of 1-10. He is voiding dark, smoky colored urine. His vital signs are within normal limits. He has positive costovertebral tenderness.

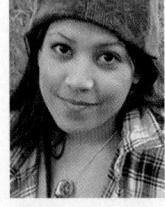

iStockphoto/Thinkstock

S.U., a 38-year-old Hispanic woman, was admitted with acute pyelonephritis following a recent UTI. She complains of bilateral flank pain and has abdominal tenderness to palpation. Her temperature is 100.4° F (38° C). Her urinalysis indicates pyuria and hematuria. Her WBC is elevated at 12,000/μL. Blood culture results are pending. IV antibiotics have been started.

M.B., a 56-year-old African American college professor, was admitted with uncontrolled hypertension. He was recently diagnosed with CKD. He smokes at least one pack of cigarettes per day and is experiencing some nicotine withdrawal symptoms. His BP on admission was 224/102 mm Hg. He is receiving IV metoprolol (Lopressor) 5 mg q4hr prn for SBP >180 mm Hg. His most recent BP 3 hr ago was 174/86 mm Hg.

iStockphoto/Thinkstock

D.M., an 82-year-old woman, was admitted to the ED with severe dehydration, heart failure, and acute kidney injury. Her daughter found her unconscious and lying on the floor. She is confused. Her serum potassium level is 5.7 mEq/L. Her urine output for the past 8 hours was 90 mL.

iStockphoto/Thinkstock

Management Discussion Questions

1. ***Priority Decision:*** After receiving report, which patient should you see first? Second? Provide a rationale for your decision.
2. ***Delegation Decision:*** Which tasks could you delegate to the UAP (select all that apply)?
   a. Obtain vital signs on M.B.
   b. Strain A.K.'s voided urine.
   c. Report D.M.'s potassium level to health care provider.
   d. Assess S.U. for potential side effects of the IV antibiotics.
   e. Measure D.M.'s urine output and report the results to the RN.

3. ***Priority and Delegation Decision:*** As you are assessing D.M., the UAP informs you that M.B.'s blood pressure is 190/86. He is asymptomatic. Additionally, the charge nurse informs you that you will be receiving a patient with heart failure from the ED within the next 10 minutes. Which action would be most appropriate?
   a. Ask the charge nurse to assign the new admission to someone else.
   b. Have the UAP admit the new patient while you administer M.B.'s IV metoprolol.
   c. Call the ED and have them hold the new admission until after you have assessed all your patients.
   d. Ask the charge nurse to administer M.B.'s IV metoprolol while you complete your assessment of D.M.

Case Study Progression

As you complete your assessment of D.M., you notice her apical pulse is irregular. She has +1 pitting edema in her lower extremities. Her blood pressure is 160/90 mmHg, heart rate 88 bpm, and respiratory rate 28/min. Her respirations are deep. You notify her health care provider.

4. Which interventions would you expect the health care provider to order for M.B. *(select all that apply)?*
   a. Administer IV Kayexalate.
   b. Obtain arterial blood gas levels.
   c. Place an indwelling urinary catheter.
   d. Perform continuous cardiac monitoring.
   e. Prepare M.B. for hemodialysis and notify her family.
5. ***Priority Decision:*** Which nursing diagnosis would be of highest priority when planning care for A.K.?
   a. Risk for injury
   b. Impaired comfort
   c. Risk for infection
   d. Ineffective self-health management
6. Which statement would be most appropriate when teaching S.U. about her kidney infection?
   a. "The damage to your kidneys will likely require dialysis."
   b. "Influenza is the most likely cause of your kidney infection."
   c. "You will need to be in the hospital for a 2-week course of IV antibiotics."
   d. "It is very important that you maintain adequate hydration to flush your kidneys."
7. ***Management Decision:*** As the UAP prepares the room for the patient being admitted from the ED, you overhear her telling a co-worker that she has to do all your work for you. What is your best initial action?
   a. Report the incident to the charge nurse for follow-up.
   b. Ask the UAP to discuss her concerns with you in private.
   c. Tell the UAP how much you appreciate and value her input on your team.
   d. Immediately clarify the situation by telling the UAP all the tasks you are completing.

Problems Related to Regulatory and Reproductive Mechanisms

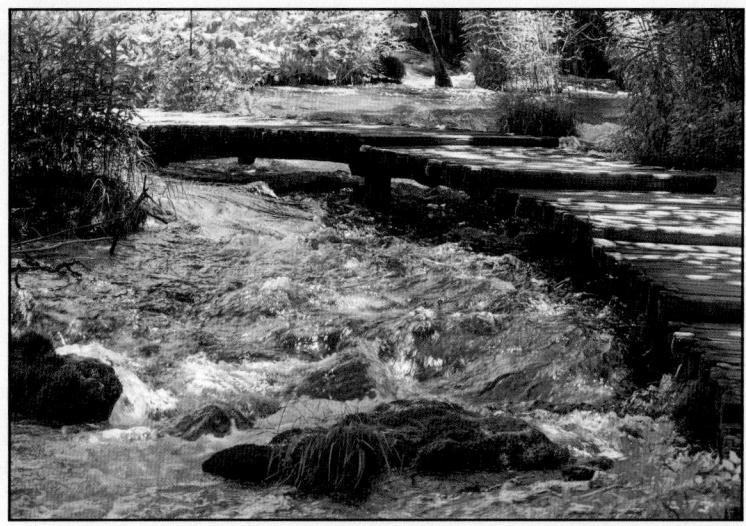

iStockphoto/Thinkstock

We keep moving forward, opening new doors, and doing new things, because we're curious and curiosity keeps leading us down new paths.
Walt Disney

Nobody can go back and start a new
beginning, but anyone can start today and
make a new ending.
Maria Robinson

Nursing Assessment
Endocrine System

Susan C. Landis

⊘volve WEBSITE

LEARNING OUTCOMES

1. Describe the common characteristics and functions of hormones.
2. Identify the locations of the endocrine glands.
3. Describe the functions of hormones secreted by the pituitary, thyroid, parathyroid, and adrenal glands and the pancreas.
4. Describe the locations and roles of hormone receptors.
5. Select the significant subjective and objective assessment data related to the endocrine system that should be obtained from a patient.
6. Link age-related changes in the endocrine system to differences in assessment findings.
7. Differentiate normal from common abnormal findings of a physical assessment of the endocrine system.
8. Describe the purpose, significance of results, and nursing responsibilities related to diagnostic studies of the endocrine system.

KEY TERMS

aldosterone, p. 1140
antidiuretic hormone (ADH), p. 1138
catecholamines, p. 1140
circadian rhythm, p. 1137
corticosteroid, p. 1140
cortisol, p. 1140

glucagon, p. 1140
growth hormone (GH), p. 1138
hormones, p. 1134
insulin, p. 1140
islets of Langerhans, p. 1140
melatonin, p. 1139

negative feedback, p. 1137
positive feedback, p. 1137
thyroxine (T_4), p. 1139
triiodothyronine (T_3), p. 1139
tropic hormones, p. 1138

STRUCTURES AND FUNCTIONS OF ENDOCRINE SYSTEM

Glands

Endocrine glands include the hypothalamus, pituitary, thyroid, parathyroids, adrenals, pancreas, ovaries, testes, and pineal gland (Fig. 48-1). *Exocrine glands* are not part of the endocrine system. They secrete their substances into ducts that then empty into a body cavity or onto a surface. For example, salivary glands produce saliva, which is secreted through salivary ducts into the mouth.

Hormones

Hormones are chemical substances produced in the body that control and regulate the activity of certain target cells or organs. Many are produced in one part of the body and control and regulate the activity of certain cells or organs in another part of the body.

Endocrine glands produce and secrete hormones that travel to affect their specific target tissues. For example, the thyroid gland synthesizes the hormone thyroxine, which affects all body tissues. Some hormones are released directly into the circulation, whereas others may act locally on cells

---

Reviewed by Saundra J. Hendricks, RN, MS, FNP, BC-ADM, Endocrine Nurses Society, Former President, The Methodist Hospital, Department of Medicine, Houston, Texas; Beth Lucasey, RN, MA, Endocrine Nurses Society Board Member, VP Marketing and Communication, TVAX Biomedical, Kansas City, Missouri; Barbara Lukert, MD, Endocrine Nurses Society Advisor, Endocrinologist, University of Kansas Medical Center, Kansas City, Kansas; and Teresa J. Seright, RN, PhD, CCRN, Assistant Professor of Nursing, Montana State University, Bozeman, Montana.

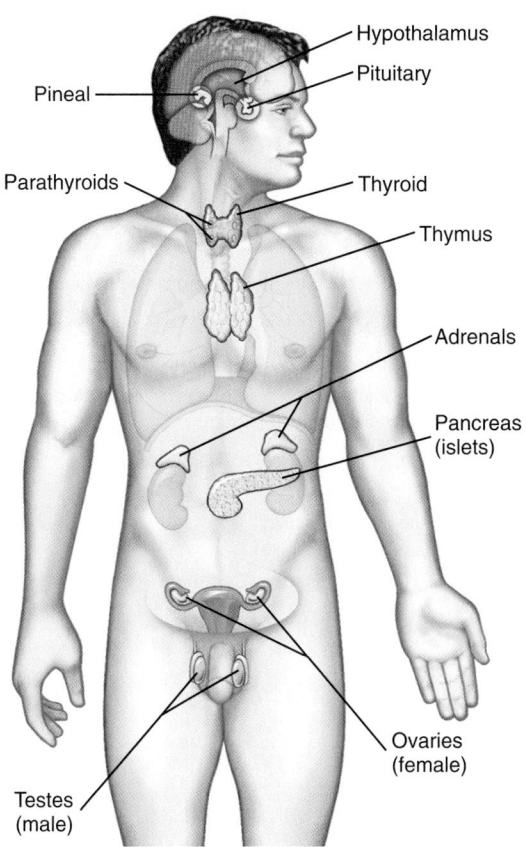

FIG. 48-1 Location of the major endocrine glands. The parathyroid glands lie on the posterior surface of the thyroid gland.

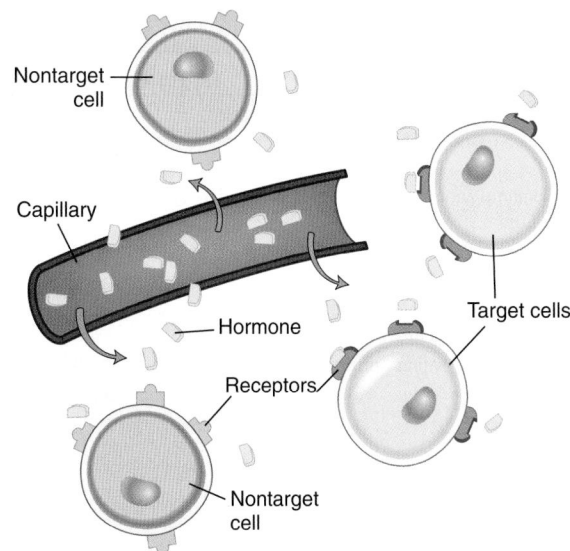

FIG. 48-2 The target cell concept. Hormones act only on cells that have receptors specific to that hormone, since the shape of the receptor determines which hormone can react with it. This is an example of the lock-and-key model of biochemical reactions.

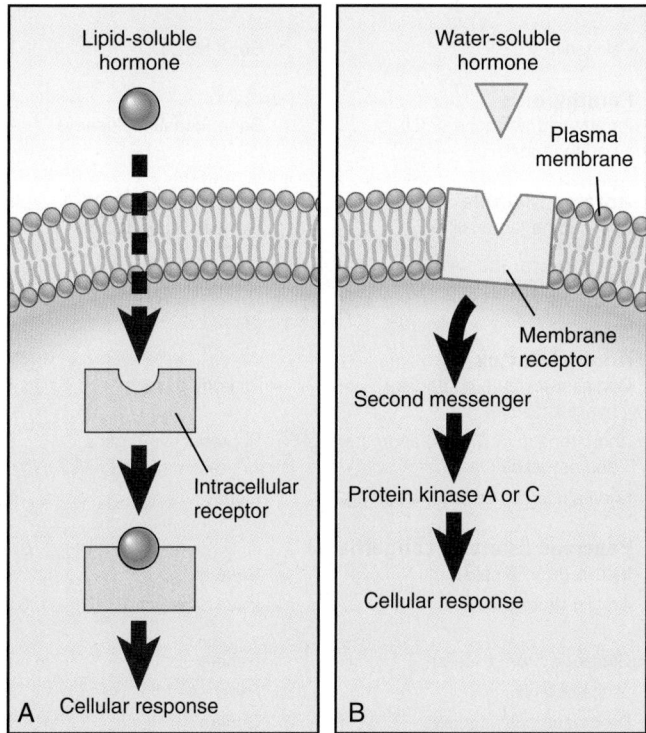

FIG. 48-3 A, Lipid-soluble hormones (e.g., steroid hormones) penetrate the cell membrane and interact with intracellular receptors. **B,** Water-soluble hormones (e.g., protein hormones) bind to receptors located in the cell membrane. The hormone-receptor interaction stimulates various cell responses.

where they are released and never enter the bloodstream. This local effect is called *paracrine action*. The action of sex steroids on the ovary is an example of paracrine action.

Most hormones have common characteristics, including (1) secretion in small amounts at variable but predictable rates; (2) regulation by feedback systems; and (3) binding to specific target cell receptors. Table 48-1 summarizes the major hormones, glands or tissues from which they are synthesized, target organs or tissues, and functions.

In addition to important physiologic activities, hormones help regulate the nervous system. For example, catecholamines are hormones when they are secreted by the adrenal medulla, but act as neurotransmitters when secreted by nerve cells in the brain and peripheral nervous system. When epinephrine, a catecholamine, travels through the blood, it is a hormone and affects target tissues. When it travels across synaptic junctions, it acts as a neurotransmitter.[1]

In addition to the endocrine glands, other body organs may secrete hormones. For example, the kidneys secrete erythropoietin, the heart secretes atrial natriuretic peptide, and the gastrointestinal (GI) tract secretes numerous peptide hormones (e.g., gastrin). These hormones are discussed in their respective assessment chapters.

Hormone Receptors. Hormones exert their effects by recognizing their target tissues and attaching to receptor sites in a "lock-and-key" type of mechanism. Therefore a hormone will act only on cells that have a receptor specific for that hormone (Fig. 48-2).

Lipid-Soluble and Water-Soluble Hormones. Hormones are classified by their chemical structure as either lipid soluble or water soluble. The differences in solubility become important in understanding how the hormone interacts with the target cell.

Lipid-soluble hormones are synthesized from cholesterol and are produced by the adrenal cortex, sex glands, and thyroid.[2] Lipid-soluble hormones (steroids, thyroid) are relatively small molecules that cross the target cell membrane by simple diffusion. Steroid and thyroid hormone receptors are located inside the cell (Fig. 48-3). Lipid-soluble hormones are bound to plasma

TABLE 48-1   ENDOCRINE GLANDS AND HORMONES

Hormones	Target Tissue	Functions
Anterior Pituitary (Adenohypophysis)		
Growth hormone (GH), or somatotropin	All body cells	Promotes protein anabolism (growth, tissue repair) and lipid mobilization and catabolism.
Thyroid-stimulating hormone (TSH), or thyrotropin	Thyroid gland	Stimulates synthesis and release of thyroid hormones, growth and function of thyroid gland.
Adrenocorticotropic hormone (ACTH)	Adrenal cortex	Fosters growth of adrenal cortex. Stimulates secretion of corticosteroids.
Gonadotropic hormones • Follicle-stimulating hormone (FSH) • Luteinizing hormone (LH)*	Reproductive organs	Stimulate sex hormone secretion, reproductive organ growth, reproductive processes.
Melanocyte-stimulating hormone (MSH)	Melanocytes in skin	Increases melanin production in melanocytes to make skin darker.
Prolactin	Ovary and mammary glands in women Testes in men	Stimulates milk production in lactating women. Increases response of follicles to LH and FSH. Stimulates testicular function in men.
Posterior Pituitary (Neurohypophysis)		
Oxytocin	Uterus, mammary glands	Stimulates milk secretion, uterine contractility.
Antidiuretic hormone (ADH), or vasopressin	Renal tubules, vascular smooth muscle	Promotes reabsorption of water, vasoconstriction.
Thyroid		
Thyroxine (T_4)	All body tissues	Precursor to T_3.
Triiodothyronine (T_3)	All body tissues	Regulates metabolic rate of all cells and processes of cell growth and tissue differentiation.
Calcitonin	Bone tissue	Regulates calcium and phosphorus blood levels. Decreases serum Ca^{2+} levels.
Parathyroids		
Parathyroid hormone (PTH), or parathormone	Bone, intestine, kidneys	Regulates calcium and phosphorus blood levels. Promotes bone demineralization and increases intestinal absorption of Ca^{2+}. Increases serum Ca^{2+} levels.
Adrenal Medulla		
Epinephrine (adrenaline)	Sympathetic effectors	Increases in response to stress. Enhances and prolongs effects of sympathetic nervous system.
Norepinephrine (noradrenaline)	Sympathetic effectors	Increases in response to stress. Enhances and prolongs effects of sympathetic nervous system.
Adrenal Cortex		
Corticosteroids (e.g., cortisol, hydrocortisone)	All body tissues	Promote metabolism. Increased in response to stress. Antiinflammatory.
Androgens (e.g., DHEA, androsterone) and estradiol	Reproductive organs	Promote growth spurt in adolescence, secondary sex characteristics, and libido in both sexes.
Mineralocorticoids (e.g., aldosterone)	Kidney	Regulate sodium and potassium balance and thus water balance.
Pancreas (Islets of Langerhans)		
Insulin (from β cells)	General	Promotes movement of glucose out of blood and into cells.
Amylin (from β cells)	Liver, stomach	Decreases gastric motility, glucagon secretion, and endogenous glucose release from liver. Increases satiety.
Glucagon (from α-cells)	General	Stimulates glycogenolysis and gluconeogenesis.
Somatostatin	Pancreas	Inhibits insulin and glucagon secretion.
Pancreatic polypeptide	General	Influences regulation of pancreatic exocrine function and metabolism of absorbed nutrients.
Gonads *Women: Ovaries*		
Estrogen	Reproductive system, breasts	Stimulates development of secondary sex characteristics, preparation of uterus for fertilization and fetal development. Stimulates bone growth.
Progesterone	Reproductive system	Maintains lining of uterus necessary for successful pregnancy.
Men: Testes		
Testosterone	Reproductive system	Stimulates development of secondary sex characteristics, spermatogenesis.

*In men, sometimes referred to as interstitial cell–stimulating hormone (ICSH).
DHEA, Dehydroepiandrosterone.

proteins for transport in the blood. Although lipid-soluble hormones are inactive when bound to plasma proteins, they can be released when appropriate and immediately exert their action at the target tissue.

Water-soluble hormones (insulin, growth hormone [GH], and prolactin) have receptors on or in the cell membrane.[3] Water-soluble hormones circulate freely in the blood to their target tissues, where they act. Water-soluble hormones are not dependent on plasma proteins for transport (see Fig. 48-3).

Regulation of Hormonal Secretion. The regulation of endocrine activity is controlled by specific mechanisms of varying levels of complexity. These mechanisms stimulate or inhibit hormone synthesis and secretion and include feedback, nervous system control, and physiologic rhythms.

Simple Feedback. Negative feedback relies on the blood level of a hormone or other chemical compound regulated by the hormone (e.g., glucose). It is the most common type of endocrine feedback system and results in the gland increasing or decreasing the release of a hormone. Negative feedback is similar to the functioning of a thermostat in which cold air in a room activates the thermostat to release heat, and hot air signals the thermostat to prevent more warm air from entering the room.

The pattern of insulin secretion is a physiologic example of negative feedback between glucose and insulin. Elevated blood glucose levels stimulate the secretion of insulin from the pancreas (see eFig. 48-1 available on the website for this chapter). As blood glucose levels decrease, the stimulus for insulin secretion also decreases. The homeostatic mechanism is considered negative feedback because it reverses the change in blood glucose level. Another example of negative feedback is the relationship between calcium and parathyroid hormone (PTH). Low blood levels of calcium stimulate the parathyroid gland to release PTH, which acts on bone, the intestine, and the kidneys to increase blood calcium levels. The increased blood calcium level then inhibits further PTH release (Fig. 48-4).

Positive feedback is also used to regulate hormone synthesis and release. The female ovarian hormone estradiol operates by this type of feedback. Increased levels of estradiol produced by the follicle during the menstrual cycle result in increased production and release of follicle-stimulating hormone (FSH) by the anterior pituitary. FSH causes further increases in estradiol until the death of the follicle. This results in a drop of FSH serum levels. Thus with this type of feedback, rising hormone levels cause another gland to release a hormone that then stimulates further release of the first hormone. A mechanism for shutting off release of the first hormone (e.g., follicle death) is required or it will continue to be released.

Nervous System Control. In addition to chemical regulation, some endocrine glands are directly affected by the activity of the nervous system. Pain, emotion, sexual excitement, and

stress can stimulate the nervous system to modulate hormone secretion. Neural involvement is initiated by the central nervous system (CNS) and implemented by the sympathetic nervous system (SNS). For example, stress is sensed or perceived by the CNS with subsequent stimulation of the SNS. The SNS secretes catecholamines that increase heart rate and blood pressure to deal with stress more effectively. (Effects of stress are discussed in Chapter 7.)

Rhythms. A common physiologic rhythm is the circadian rhythm. This is an endogenous 24-hour rhythm that can be driven and altered by sleep-wake or dark-light 24-hour (diurnal) cycles. Hormone levels fluctuate predictably during these cycles. For example, cortisol rises early in the day, declines toward evening, and rises again toward the end of sleep to peak by morning (Fig. 48-5). GH, thyroid-stimulating hormone (TSH), and prolactin secretions peak during sleep.

The menstrual cycle is an example of a body rhythm that is longer than 24 hours *(ultradian).* These rhythms must be considered when interpreting laboratory results for hormone levels. (See diagnostic studies section in this chapter and Chapter 51.)

Hypothalamus

Although the pituitary gland has been referred to as the "master gland," most of its functions rely on its interrelationship with the hypothalamus. Two important groups of hormones from the hypothalamus are *releasing* hormones and *inhibiting* hormones. The function of these hormones is to either stimulate the release or inhibit the release of hormones from the anterior pituitary (Table 48-2).

The hypothalamus also contains neurons, which receive input from the CNS, including the brainstem, limbic system, and cerebral cortex. Neurons from the hypothalamus create a circuit to facilitate coordination of the endocrine system and autonomic nervous system (ANS). In addition, the hypothalamus coordinates the expression of complex behavioral responses, such as anger, fear, and pleasure.

Pituitary

The pituitary gland *(hypophysis)* is located in the sella turcica under the hypothalamus at the base of the brain above the sphenoid bone (see Fig. 48-1). The pituitary is connected to the hypothalamus by the infundibular *(hypophyseal)* stalk. This

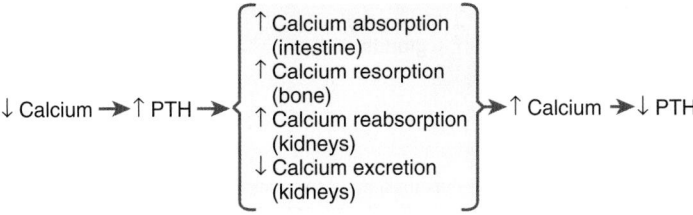

FIG. 48-4 Feedback mechanism between parathyroid hormone *(PTH)* and calcium.

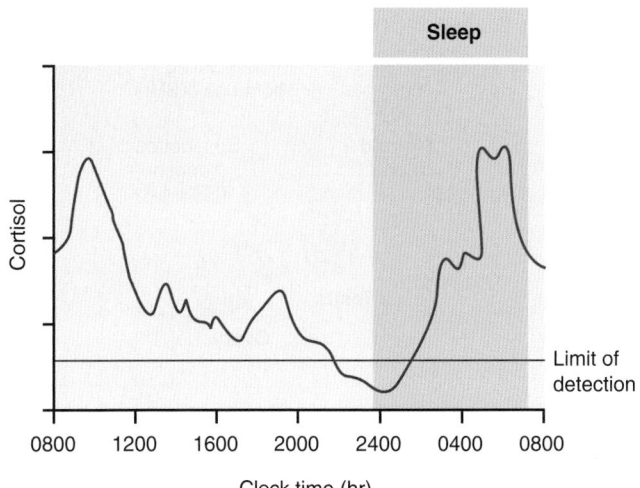

FIG. 48-5 Circadian rhythm of cortisol secretion.

stalk relays information between the hypothalamus and the pituitary. The pituitary consists of two major parts, the anterior lobe *(adenohypophysis)* and the posterior lobe *(neurohypophysis)*. A smaller intermediate lobe produces melanocyte-stimulating hormone.

Anterior Pituitary. The anterior lobe accounts for 80% of the gland by weight and is regulated by the hypothalamus through releasing and inhibiting hormones. These hypothalamic hormones reach the anterior pituitary through a network of capillaries known as the *hypothalamus-hypophyseal portal system.* The releasing and inhibiting hormones in turn affect the secretion of six hormones from the anterior pituitary (Fig. 48-6).

TABLE 48-2   HORMONES OF THE HYPOTHALAMUS

The following hormones from the hypothalamus target the anterior pituitary.

Releasing Hormones
- Corticotropin-releasing hormone (CRH)
- Thyrotropin-releasing hormone (TRH)
- Growth hormone–releasing hormone (GHRH), or somatotropin-releasing hormone
- Gonadotropin-releasing hormone (GnRH)
- Prolactin-releasing factor (PRF)

Inhibiting Hormones
- Somatostatin (inhibits growth hormone release)
- Prolactin-inhibiting factor (PIF)

Several hormones secreted by the anterior pituitary are referred to as tropic hormones. These are hormones that control the secretion of hormones by other glands. Thyroid-stimulating hormone (TSH) stimulates the thyroid gland to secrete thyroid hormones. Adrenocorticotropic hormone (ACTH) stimulates the adrenal cortex to secrete corticosteroids. Follicle-stimulating hormone (FSH) stimulates secretion of estrogen and the development of ova in women and sperm in men. Luteinizing hormone (LH) stimulates ovulation in women and secretion of sex hormones in both men and women. In men LH is sometimes referred to as interstitial cell–stimulating hormone (ICSH).

Growth hormone (GH) affects the growth and development of all body tissues. It also has numerous biologic actions, including a role in protein, fat, and carbohydrate metabolism. Prolactin stimulates breast development necessary for lactation after childbirth. Prolactin is also referred to as a lactogenic hormone.

Posterior Pituitary. The posterior pituitary is composed of nerve tissue and is essentially an extension of the hypothalamus. Communication between the hypothalamus and posterior pituitary occurs through nerve tracts known as the *median eminence.* The hormones secreted by the posterior pituitary, antidiuretic hormone (ADH) and oxytocin, are actually produced in the hypothalamus. These hormones travel down the nerve tracts from the hypothalamus to the posterior pituitary and are stored until their release is triggered by the appropriate stimuli (see Fig. 48-6).

The major physiologic role of ADH (also called arginine vasopressin) is regulation of fluid volume by stimulating

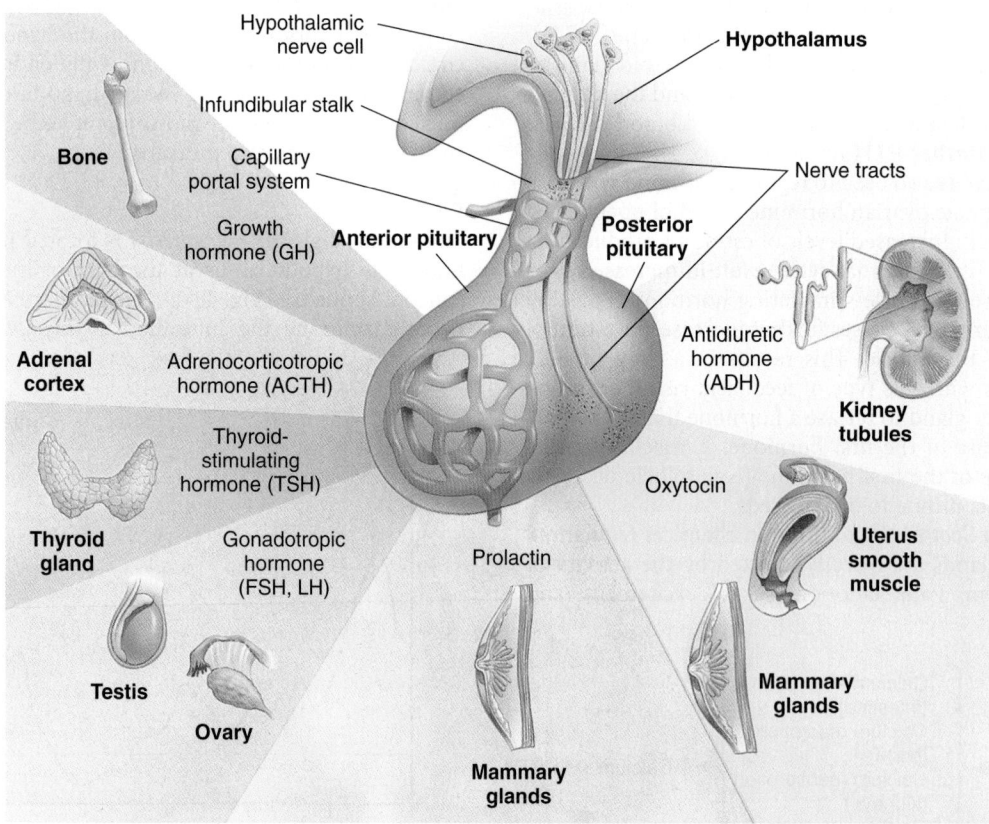

FIG. 48-6 Relationship between the hypothalamus, pituitary, and target organs. The hypothalamus communicates with the anterior pituitary via a capillary system and with the posterior pituitary via nerve tracts. The anterior and posterior pituitary hormones are shown with their target tissues. *FSH,* Follicle-stimulating hormone; *LH,* luteinizing hormone.

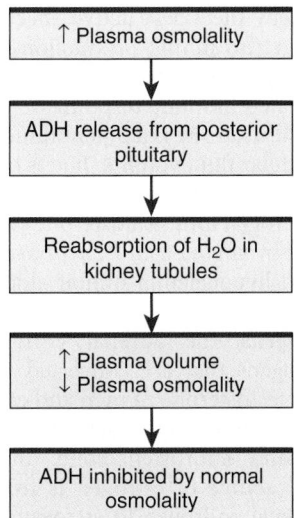

FIG. 48-7 Relationship of plasma osmolality to antidiuretic hormone *(ADH)* release and action.

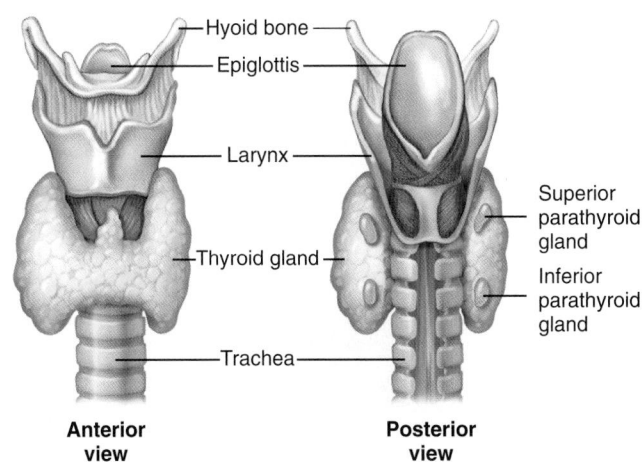

FIG. 48-8 Thyroid and parathyroid glands. Note the surrounding structures.

reabsorption of water in the renal tubules. ADH is also a potent vasoconstrictor. ADH secretion is stimulated by *plasma osmolality* (a measure of solute concentration of circulating blood) and hypovolemia (Fig. 48-7). Plasma osmolality increases when there is a decrease in ECF or an increase in solute concentration. The increased plasma osmolality activates osmoreceptors, which are extremely sensitive, specialized neurons in the hypothalamus. These activated osmoreceptors stimulate ADH release. Volume receptors in large veins, heart atria, and carotid arteries that sense pressure changes also contribute to ADH control. When ADH is released, the renal tubules reabsorb water and the urine becomes more concentrated. When ADH release is inhibited, renal tubules do not reabsorb water, resulting in a more dilute urine excretion.

Oxytocin stimulates ejection of milk into mammary ducts during lactation and contraction of the uterus; it may also affect sperm motility. Oxytocin secretion is increased by stimulation of touch receptors in the nipples of lactating women and vaginal pressure receptors during childbirth.

Pineal Gland

The pineal gland is located in the brain and is composed of photoreceptive cells. The secretion of the hormone melatonin is its primary function. Melatonin secretion is increased in response to exposure to the dark and decreased in response to light. The gland helps to regulate circadian rhythms and the reproductive system at the onset of puberty.

Thyroid Gland

The thyroid gland is located in the anterior portion of the neck in front of the trachea. It consists of two encapsulated lateral lobes connected by a narrow isthmus (Fig. 48-8). The thyroid gland is a highly vascular organ, and its size is regulated by TSH from the anterior pituitary. The three hormones produced and secreted by the thyroid gland are thyroxine (T_4), triiodothyronine (T_3), and calcitonin.

Thyroxine and Triiodothyronine. Thyroxine (T_4) accounts for 90% of thyroid hormone produced by the thyroid gland. However, triiodothyronine (T_3) is much more potent and has greater metabolic effects. About 20% of circulating T_3 is secreted directly by the thyroid gland, and the remainder is obtained by peripheral conversion of T_4. Iodine is necessary for the synthesis of both T_3 and T_4. These two hormones affect metabolic rate, caloric requirements, oxygen consumption, carbohydrate and lipid metabolism, growth and development, brain function, and other nervous system activities. More than 99% of thyroid hormones are bound to plasma proteins, especially thyroxine-binding globulin synthesized by the liver. Only the unbound "free" hormones are biologically active.

Thyroid hormone production and release is stimulated by TSH from the anterior pituitary gland. When circulating levels of thyroid hormone are low, the hypothalamus releases thyrotropin-releasing hormone (TRH), which in turn causes the anterior pituitary to release TSH. High circulating thyroid hormone levels inhibit the secretion of both TRH from the hypothalamus and TSH from the anterior pituitary gland.

Calcitonin. *Calcitonin* is produced by C cells (parafollicular cells) of the thyroid gland in response to high circulating calcium levels. Calcitonin inhibits the transfer of calcium from bone to blood, increases calcium storage in bone, and increases renal excretion of calcium and phosphorus, thereby lowering serum calcium levels. Calcitonin and PTH regulate calcium balance.

Parathyroid Glands

Two pairs of parathyroid glands are usually arranged behind each thyroid lobe (see Fig. 48-8). Although there are usually four glands, their number may range from two to six.

Parathyroid Hormone. The parathyroid glands secrete parathyroid hormone (PTH), also called *parathormone*. Its major role is to regulate the blood level of calcium. PTH acts on bone, the kidneys, and indirectly on the GI tract. PTH stimulates the transfer of calcium from the bone into the blood and inhibits bone formation, resulting in increased serum calcium and phosphate. In the kidney, PTH increases calcium reabsorption and phosphate excretion. In addition, PTH stimulates the renal conversion of vitamin D to its most active form (1,25-dihydroxyvitamin D_3). This active vitamin D promotes absorption of calcium and phosphorus by the GI tract, which ultimately increases bone mineralization. The secretion of PTH is directly regulated by a feedback system. When the serum calcium level is low, PTH secretion increases. When the serum calcium level rises, PTH secretion falls. In addition, high levels of active vitamin D inhibit PTH, and low levels of magnesium stimulate PTH secretion.

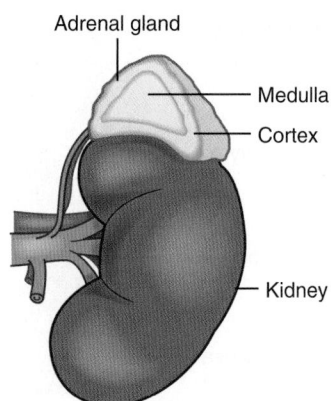

FIG. 48-9 The adrenal gland is composed of the adrenal cortex and the adrenal medulla.

Adrenal Glands

The adrenal glands are small, paired, highly vascularized glands located on the upper portion of each kidney. Each gland consists of two parts, the medulla and the cortex (Fig. 48-9). Each part has distinct functions, and the glands act independently from one another.

Adrenal Medulla. The adrenal medulla is the inner part of the gland and consists of sympathetic postganglionic neurons. The medulla secretes the catecholamines *epinephrine* (adrenaline), *norepinephrine* (noradrenaline), and *dopamine*. Catecholamines are synthesized from the amino acid phenylalanine. Catecholamines, usually considered neurotransmitters, are hormones when secreted by the adrenal medulla because they are released into the circulation. They are an essential part of the body's "fight or flight" response to stress (see Chapter 7).

Adrenal Cortex. The adrenal cortex is the outer part of the adrenal gland. It secretes several steroid hormones, including *glucocorticoids, mineralocorticoids,* and *androgens.* Cholesterol is the precursor for steroid hormone synthesis. Glucocorticoids (e.g., cortisol) are named for their effects on glucose metabolism. Mineralocorticoids (e.g., aldosterone) are essential for the maintenance of fluid and electrolyte balance. The term corticosteroid refers to hormones synthesized by the adrenal cortex excluding androgens.

Cortisol. Cortisol, the most abundant and potent glucocorticoid, is necessary to maintain life and protect the body from stress. Cortisol is secreted in a diurnal pattern (see Fig. 48-5). The major control of cortisol is through a negative feedback mechanism that involves the secretion of corticotropin-releasing hormone (CRH) from the hypothalamus. CRH stimulates the secretion of ACTH by the anterior pituitary.

One major function of cortisol is the regulation of blood glucose concentration through stimulation of hepatic glucose formation *(gluconeogenesis).* Cortisol decreases peripheral glucose use in the fasting state, inhibits protein synthesis, and stimulates the mobilization of glycerol and free fatty acids. Cortisol also helps maintain vascular integrity and fluid volume through its action on mineralocorticoid receptors. Cortisol levels are increased by stress, burns, infection, fever, acute anxiety, and hypoglycemia.

Glucocorticoids inhibit the inflammatory response and are considered antiinflammatory. Cortisol decreases the inflammatory response by stabilizing the membranes of cellular lysosomes and preventing increased capillary permeability. The lysosomal stabilization reduces the release of proteolytic enzymes and thereby their destructive effects on surrounding tissue. Cortisol can also inhibit production of prostaglandins, thromboxanes, and leukotrienes (see Chapter 12, Fig. 12-2) and alter the cell-mediated immune response.

Aldosterone. Aldosterone is a potent mineralocorticoid that maintains extracellular fluid volume. It acts on the renal tubule to promote renal reabsorption of sodium and excretion of potassium and hydrogen ions. Aldosterone synthesis and secretion are stimulated by angiotensin II, hyponatremia, and hyperkalemia. ANP and hypokalemia inhibit aldosterone synthesis and release.

Adrenal Androgens. The adrenal cortex secretes small amounts of androgens that are converted to sex steroids in peripheral tissues: testosterone in men and estrogen in women. The most common adrenal androgens are dehydroepiandrosterone (DHEA) and androstenedione. In postmenopausal women the major source of estrogen is from the peripheral conversion of adrenal androgen to estrogen. Because they are precursors to other sex steroids, their actions are similar to those of testosterone and estrogen.

Pancreas

The pancreas is a long, tapered, lobular, soft gland located behind the stomach and anterior to the first and second lumbar vertebrae. The pancreas has both exocrine and endocrine functions. The hormone-secreting portion of the pancreas is referred to as the islets of Langerhans. The islets account for less than 2% of the gland and consist of four types of hormone-secreting cells: α, β, delta, and F cells. α Cells produce and secrete the hormone glucagon. Insulin and amylin are produced and secreted by β cells. Somatostatin is produced and secreted by the delta cells. Pancreatic polypeptide (PP) is secreted by the F (or PP) cells.

Glucagon. Glucagon is synthesized and released from pancreatic α cells and the gut in response to low levels of blood glucose, protein ingestion, and exercise. Glucagon increases blood glucose by stimulating glycogenolysis, gluconeogenesis, and ketogenesis. Glucagon and insulin function in a reciprocal manner to maintain normal blood glucose levels. In the fasting state, hormones such as catecholamines, cortisol, and glucagon break down stored complex fuels *(catabolism)* to provide glucose as fuel for energy.

Insulin. Insulin is the principal regulator of metabolism and storage of ingested carbohydrates, fats, and proteins. Insulin facilitates glucose transport across cell membranes in most tissues. However, the brain, nerves, lens of the eye, hepatocytes, erythrocytes, and cells in the intestinal mucosa and kidney tubules are not dependent on insulin for glucose uptake. An increased blood glucose level is the major stimulus for insulin synthesis and secretion. Other stimuli to insulin secretion are increased amino acid levels and vagal stimulation. Insulin secretion is usually inhibited by low blood glucose levels, glucagon, somatostatin, hypokalemia, and catecholamines.

A major effect of insulin on glucose metabolism occurs in the liver, where the hormone enhances glucose incorporation into glycogen and triglycerides by altering enzymatic activity and inhibiting gluconeogenesis. After a meal, insulin is responsible for the storage of nutrients *(anabolism).* Another major effect occurs in peripheral tissues, where insulin facilitates glucose transport into cells, transport of amino acids across muscle membranes and their synthesis into protein, and transport of triglycerides into adipose tissue.

GERONTOLOGIC CONSIDERATIONS

EFFECTS OF AGING ON ENDOCRINE SYSTEM

Normal aging has many effects on the endocrine system (Table 48-3). These include (1) decreased hormone production and secretion, (2) altered hormone metabolism and biologic activity, (3) decreased responsiveness of target tissues to hormones, and (4) alterations in circadian rhythms.

Assessment of the effects of aging on the endocrine system may be difficult because the subtle changes of aging may mimic manifestations of endocrine disorders. Endocrine problems may manifest differently in an older adult than in a younger person. Older adults may have multiple co-morbidities and take medications that alter the body's usual response to endocrine dysfunction. Symptoms of endocrine dysfunction such as fatigue, constipation, or mental impairment are often missed because they are attributed solely to aging. For example, the symptoms of thyroid disease may be attributed to aging, resulting in delayed treatment.

It is important to assess renal function (serum creatinine, blood urea nitrogen [BUN]) in the older adult undergoing diagnostic studies with contrast medium. Older adults with renal dysfunction may be more prone to renal failure with the use of contrast medium.[4]

ASSESSMENT OF ENDOCRINE SYSTEM

Endocrine dysfunction may be the result of hypersecretion or hyposecretion of hormones. The onset of symptoms for specific disorders may be insidious and produce subtle or vague symptoms that are attributed to other physiologic and psychologic causes. Consequently, patients with endocrine dysfunction may be labeled as depressed, malingering, apathetic, or neurotic. In other instances, or in late stages of endocrine dysfunction, the patient may be seen with symptoms that are life threatening and demand immediate intervention.

Subjective Data

Information obtained from the patient can provide important clues as to the functioning of the endocrine system. Obtain a thorough history from the patient or a family member if the patient's mental acuity is compromised (Table 48-4).

Important Health Information

Past Health History. Patients with endocrine disorders often are seen with nonspecific complaints. The chief complaint may relate to not just one but a group of symptoms. The most common presenting problems include fatigue, weakness, menstrual problems, and weight changes. It is important to determine if the onset of symptoms has been gradual or sudden and what the patient has done about them.[5]

Because some of the more general signs of dysfunction are the easiest to overlook, you need to evaluate any reported or observed changes in weight, appetite, skin, libido, mental acuity, emotional stability, or energy levels.

TABLE 48-3	GERONTOLOGIC ASSESSMENT DIFFERENCES

Endocrine System

Changes	Clinical Significance
Thyroid Atrophy of thyroid gland. TSH, T$_3$, and T$_4$ secretion are decreased. Increased nodules.	Increased incidence of hypothyroidism with aging. However, most older adults maintain adequate thyroid function. Thyroid hormone replacement dose lower in older adults.
Parathyroid Increased secretion of PTH and increased basal level of PTH.	Increased calcium resorption from bone. Hypercalcemia, hypercalciuria (may reflect defective renal mechanism).
Adrenal Cortex Adrenal cortex becomes more fibrotic and slightly smaller. Decreased metabolism of cortisol. Decreased plasma levels of adrenal androgens and aldosterone.	Decreased metabolic clearance rate for glucocorticoids.
Adrenal Medulla Increased secretion and basal level of norepinephrine. No change in plasma epinephrine levels. Decreased β-adrenergic receptor response to norepinephrine.	Decreased responsiveness to β-adrenergic agonists and receptor blockers. May partly explain increased incidence of hypertension with aging.
Pancreas Increase in fibrosis and fatty deposits in pancreas. Increased glucose intolerance and decreased sensitivity to insulin.	May partly contribute to increased incidence of diabetes mellitus with advanced aging.
Gonads *Women:* Decline in estrogen secretion.	Women experience symptoms associated with menopause and have increased risk for atherosclerosis and osteoporosis.
Men: Decline in testosterone secretion.	Men may or may not experience symptoms.

PTH, Parathyroid hormone; *T$_3$,* triiodothyronine; *T$_4$,* thyroxine; *TSH,* thyroid-stimulating hormone.

CASE STUDY

Patient Introduction

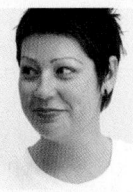

iStockphoto/Thinkstock

L.M. is a 35-yr-old Hispanic woman who comes to the clinic complaining of "just not feeling well." She is accompanied by her female partner, H.H. L.M. states that she has gained a lot of weight despite trying to watch her diet and just seems to be getting more and more tired. H.H. voices concerns about changes in her partner's energy level.

Critical Thinking

As you read through this assessment chapter, think about L.M.'s concerns with the following questions in mind:
1. What are the possible causes of L.M.'s weight gain, fatigue, and irritability?
2. What would be your priority assessment of L.M.?
3. What questions would you ask L.M.?
4. What should be included in the physical assessment? What would you be looking for?
5. What diagnostic studies might you expect to be ordered?

evolve Answers available at *http://evolve.elsevier.com/Lewis/medsurg.*

TABLE 48-4   HEALTH HISTORY

Endocrine System

Health Perception–Health Management
- What is your usual day like?
- Have you noticed any changes in your ability to perform your usual activities compared with last year? Five yr ago?*

Nutritional-Metabolic
- What is your weight and height?
- How much do you want to weigh?
- Have there been any changes in your appetite or weight?*
- Have you noticed any changes in the distribution of the hair anywhere on your body?*
- Have you noticed any changes in the color of your skin, particularly on your face, neck, hands, or body creases?*
- Has the texture of your skin changed? For example, does it seem thicker and drier than it used to?*
- Have you noticed any difficulty swallowing, throat pain, or hoarseness? Is the top button on your shirt or blouse more difficult to button?*
- Do you feel more nervous than you used to? Do you notice your heart pounding or that you sweat when you do not think you should be sweating?
- Do you have difficulty holding things because of shakiness of your hands?*
- Do you feel that most rooms are too hot or too cold? Do you frequently have to put on a sweater, or feel as though you need to open windows when others in the room seem comfortable?*
- Do you have or have you had any wounds that were slow to heal?*

Elimination
- Do you have to get up at night to urinate? If so, how many times? Do you keep water by your bed at night?
- Have you ever had a kidney stone?*
- Describe your usual bowel pattern. Have you noted any bowel changes?*
- Do you use anything, such as laxatives, to help you move your bowels?*

Activity-Exercise
- What is your usual activity pattern during a typical day?
- Do you have a planned exercise program? If yes, what is it and have you had to make any changes in this routine lately? If so, why and what kinds of changes?
- Do you experience fatigue with or without activity?*
- Have you had any trouble with breathing?*

Sleep-Rest
- How many hours do you sleep at night? Do you feel rested on awakening?
- Are you ever awakened by sweating during the night?*
- Do you have nightmares?*

Cognitive-Perceptual
- How is your memory? Have you noticed any changes?*
- Have you experienced any blurring or double vision?*
- When was your last eye examination?

Self-Perception–Self-Concept
- Have you noticed any changes in your physical appearance or size?*
- Are you concerned about your weight?*
- Do you feel you are able to do what you think you should be capable of doing? If not, why not?
- Does your health problem affect how you feel about yourself?*

Role-Relationship
- Do you have a support system or partner? Are you married? Do you have any children? Do you think you are able to take care of your family and home? If no, why not?
- Where do you work? What kind of work do you do? Are you able to do what is expected of you and what you expect of yourself?
- Are you retired? What type of work did you do before you retired? How do you spend your time now that you've retired?

Sexuality-Reproductive
Women
- When did you start to menstruate? Was this earlier or later than other women in your family?
- When was your last menstrual period? Do you have scant, heavy, or irregular menstrual flows?
- How many children have you had? How much did they weigh at birth? Were you told you had diabetes during any pregnancy?*
- Are you menopausal? If so, for how long?
- Are you attempting to get pregnant but cannot?*
- Are you postmenopausal? If so, do you have any bleeding from your uterus?

Men
- Have you noticed any changes in your ability to have an erection?*
- Are you trying to have children but cannot?*

Coping–Stress Tolerance
- What kind of stressors do you have?
- How do you deal with stress or problems?
- What is your support system? To whom do you turn when you have a problem?

Value-Belief
- Do you think medicine should still be taken even though you feel okay?
- Do any of your prescribed therapies cause any conflict in your value-belief system?*

*If yes, describe.

Medications. Ask about the use of all medications (both prescription and over-the-counter drugs), herbs, and dietary supplements. Ask about the reason for taking the drug, the dosage, and the length of time the drug has been taken. In particular, ask about the use of hormone replacements. Knowing that the patient is currently taking hormone replacements such as insulin, thyroid hormone, or corticosteroids (e.g., prednisone) alerts you to possible problems associated with the use of these agents (e.g., corticosteroids may cause increased blood glucose levels and bone loss with long-term use). The side and adverse effects of many nonhormone medications can contribute to problems affecting endocrine function (e.g., many drugs can affect blood glucose levels) (see eTable 49-1).

Surgery or Other Treatments. Inquire about past medical, surgical, and obstetric history, including number of pregnancies and live births. Ask about traumatic events, birth weight, growth patterns, and stages of physical and emotional development. The depth of information required may vary depending on the presenting condition. For example, data regarding past radiation therapy to the head and neck are especially important when thyroid or pituitary dysfunction is suspected.

Functional Health Patterns. Key questions to ask the patient with an endocrine problem are summarized in Table 48-4.

Health Perception–Health Management Pattern. Ask patients what their usual day is like and how they view their general health. Inquire as to how their perceptions compare to their health a year ago. Ask if their health-related concerns are preventing them from completing things they would like to accomplish.

 GENETIC RISK ALERT

Pituitary
- Nephrogenic diabetes insipidus can be inherited as a sex-linked or autosomal disorder.

Thyroid
- Genetics has a role in many cases of hypothyroid and hyperthyroid disorders.
  - Hashimoto's thyroiditis, the most common cause of hypothyroidism, is a chronic autoimmune disorder that has a genetic basis.
  - Graves' disease, a cause of hyperthyroidism, is an autoimmune disease in which genetic factors are involved.

Multiple Endocrine Neoplasia
- Multiple endocrine neoplasia is when two or more different endocrine tumors occur in a person and there is evidence for either a causative mutation or genetic transmission.
- The features of this disorder are relatively consistent within any one family.
- A common endocrine tumor is medullary thyroid carcinoma.
- Some people with this disorder also develop pheochromocytoma.

Diabetes Mellitus
- Genetics has a strong role in the development of type 2 diabetes, and to a lesser extent in type 1 diabetes.

Heredity often plays an important role in the development of endocrine dysfunction. Ask about the occurrence of diabetes mellitus, thyroid disease, and endocrine gland cancers, since these conditions have a familial tendency. A genetic assessment of family members may be appropriate.[5]

Nutritional-Metabolic Pattern. Reported changes in appetite and weight can indicate endocrine dysfunction. Weight loss with increased appetite may indicate hyperthyroidism or diabetes mellitus. Weight gain may indicate hypothyroidism or hypocortisolism. Truncal obesity, purple abdominal striae, and thin extremities occur in patients with hypercortisolism. Obese individuals are more likely to develop type 2 diabetes.

Ask if there have been problems with nausea, vomiting, or diarrhea. Difficulty swallowing or a change in neck size may indicate an enlarged thyroid gland. Increased SNS activity, including nervousness, palpitations, sweating, and tremors, may indicate thyroid dysfunction or a rare tumor of the adrenal medulla *(pheochromocytoma)*. Heat or cold intolerance may indicate hyperthyroidism or hypothyroidism, respectively.

Also ask about changes in the patient's skin, particularly on the face, neck, hands, or body creases. Ask if the patient has noticed any change in the distribution of hair anywhere on the body. Changes in the texture of the skin and whether it seems thicker or drier may indicate endocrine dysfunction. Hair loss can indicate hypopituitarism, hypothyroidism, hyperthyroidism, hypoparathyroidism, or increased testosterone and other androgens. Increased body hair may indicate hypercortisolism. Decreased skin pigmentation can occur in hypopituitarism, hypothyroidism, and hypoparathyroidism, whereas increased skin pigmentation, particularly in sun-exposed areas, can indicate hypocortisolism. A patient with hypothyroidism or excess GH may have skin that feels coarse or leathery. A patient with hyperthyroidism may mention fine, silky hair.

Elimination Pattern. Because maintenance of fluid balance is a major role of the endocrine system, questions related to elimination patterns may uncover endocrine dysfunction. For example, increased thirst and urination can indicate diabetes mellitus (pancreas disorder) or diabetes insipidus (pituitary disorder). Ask about the frequency and consistency of bowel

Subjective Data

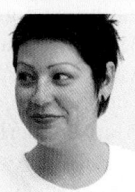

iStockphoto/Thinkstock

A focused subjective assessment of L.M. revealed the following information:

PMH: Denies any medical or surgical history. Has not seen a health care provider (HCP) for 8 yr.

Medications: None.

Health Perception–Health Management: L.M. works as a receptionist for a local law firm and states it is all she can do some days to make it through the workday. She states that she frequently wakes up with a headache and goes to bed with the same headache, describing it as a dull, throbbing ache between her eyes. She definitely does not have the energy she had 5 yr ago or even 6 mo ago. She used to enjoy gardening and going out with their friends but now can barely manage work and coming home.

Nutritional-Metabolic: L.M. reports a steady weight gain over the past 6 mo, mainly in her abdominal area. She feels as if she looks pregnant but knows that is not possible. Her appetite has actually decreased but she has not been able to lose any weight. She says she feels "bloated." She also complains of facial hair growth and has noticed that she bruises easily. Whenever she gets a bug bite, it seems to take forever to heal. L.M. denies difficulty with swallowing, hoarseness, palpitations, or tremors.

Elimination: Denies any changes or difficulty with urination or bowel movements.

Activity-Exercise: L.M. states that she has no ambition to exercise. She is just too tired at the end of the workday and has no energy on the weekends either. She also complains of leg cramps with walking.

Sleep-Rest: Sleeps 10+ hr at night but does not feel rested on awakening.

Cognitive-Perceptual: L.M. is worried she is going crazy. She finds herself easily angered and irritable, frequently snapping at co-workers and her partner. She states this is not her usual self and she at first thought it was because she was dealing with a constant, dull headache. Lately, she has noticed that her vision is blurry and that is making work and life even more difficult and stressful. When asked about her headache, she states it hurts between her eyes. She rates the pain is a 4 on a scale of 0-10 and states that Tylenol or ibuprofen does not alleviate the pain. The pain is typically worse on arising in the morning and slowly decreases during the day.

Self-Perception–Self-Concept: L.M. hates the way she looks. She says when she looks in the mirror, she can't believe what she sees. She feels as if she has aged 10 yr over the past 6 mo and has gained weight in her face, neck, and trunk. She is concerned that her scalp hair is thinning and she is growing a beard. States that she is beginning to wonder if she is "turning into a man!"

Coping–Stress Tolerance: L.M. states that she is finding it more and more difficult to cope with the stresses of her job, her relationship with her partner, and life in general. She believes her emotions are very "raw and labile," totally different from the easy-going, smiling person she had once prided herself in being.

movements. Frequent defecation may indicate hyperthyroidism or autonomic neuropathy of diabetes mellitus. Constipation is also seen in patients with hypothyroidism, hypoparathyroidism, and hypopituitarism.

Activity-Exercise Pattern. Ask about the usual pattern of activity during a typical day and if the patient has had to make any changes in that activity. Inquire how his or her energy levels compared with past levels. Ask if the patient experiences fatigue with or without activity or if he or she has excessive levels of energy on a daily basis.

Sleep-Rest Pattern. Ask the patient how many hours he or she typically sleeps, and if he or she feels rested on awakening.

Inquire if anything prevents the patient from staying asleep such as nocturia (excessive urination at night), which may indicate diabetes. The patient with type 1 diabetes mellitus on a tight glucose control regimen who complains of sweating or nightmares may be experiencing hypoglycemia. Ask the patient about snoring, which could indicate sleep apnea; this is especially common in men with diabetes mellitus.

Cognitive-Perceptual Pattern. A patient with an endocrine dysfunction may manifest apathy or depression. Question both the patient and family to determine if any cognitive changes are present. Memory deficits and an inability to concentrate are common in endocrine disorders. Visual changes such as blurring or double vision could indicate endocrine problems. Headaches may indicate abnormal pituitary growth.

Self-Perception–Self-Concept Pattern. Endocrine disorders may affect the patient's self-perception because of the associated changes in physical appearance. Determine changes in weight, size of hands and facial features, and level of fatigue. The chronic nature of endocrine disorders and lifelong need for therapy can affect the patient's self-perception. Ask patients to describe how the present illness affects how they feel about themselves.

Role-Relationship Pattern. Ask whether there have been any changes in the patient's ability to maintain roles at home, at work, or in the community. Often the patient with an endocrine disorder is unable to sustain life's roles. However, in most cases the patient can be advised that, with adequate management, previous roles can be resumed. This can be reassuring for the patient and family.

Sexuality-Reproductive Pattern. Document the development of abnormal secondary sex characteristics such as facial hair *(hirsutism)* in women. Ask a detailed history of menstruation and pregnancy. Menstrual dysfunction may be seen in disorders of the ovaries and pituitary, thyroid, and adrenal glands. A history of large-birth-weight babies may indicate gestational diabetes, which may put the patient at a higher risk of developing diabetes mellitus. The inability to lactate may indicate a pituitary disorder.

Male sexual dysfunction may take the form of impotence, decreased libido, infertility, or the lack of development of secondary sexual characteristics. Retrograde ejaculation can occur in diabetes mellitus.

Coping–Stress Tolerance Pattern. Because some endocrine conditions are exacerbated by stress, ask patients about their level of stress and usual coping patterns. Patients' perception of the impact of their condition and treatments on their lifestyle is very important.

Value-Belief Pattern. Determining a patient's ability to make lifestyle changes is an important nursing function. Identify the patient's value-belief patterns so you can help to determine appropriate treatment regimens. This is particularly important in a condition such as diabetes mellitus, which may require major lifestyle changes. Other disorders, such as hypothyroidism or hypocortisolism, may be managed with medications but require lifelong monitoring with the health care provider.

Objective Data

Most endocrine glands (with the exception of the thyroid and testes) are inaccessible to direct examination. Assessment can be accomplished using objective data, including physical examination and diagnostic tests. It is imperative that you understand the actions of hormones so that you can assess the function of a gland by monitoring the target tissue.

Physical Examination. Specific clinical findings for the various endocrine problems are discussed in Chapters 49 and 50. Regardless of the type of endocrine dysfunction, the following general examination should be followed.[6]

Take a full set of vital signs at the beginning of the examination. Variations in temperature, tachycardia, bradycardia, hypotension, or hypertension may be seen with a variety of endocrine-related problems.

Assessment of the endocrine system includes a history of growth and development patterns, weight distribution and changes, and comparisons of these factors with normal findings. Body mass index (BMI) is a height-to-weight ratio used to assess nutritional status (see Chapter 41, Fig. 41-2).

Endocrine disorders may cause changes in mental and emotional status. Throughout the examination, assess the patient's orientation, alertness, memory, affect, personality, and anxiety and the appropriateness of his or her behavior.

Integument. Note the color and texture of the skin, hair, and nails. Note the overall skin color as well as pigmentation and possible ecchymosis (bruise). Hyperpigmentation, or "bronzing" of the skin (particularly on knuckles, elbows, knees, genitalia, and palmar creases), is a classic finding in Addison's disease. Palpate the skin for texture and moisture. Examine hair distribution not only on the head but also on the face, trunk, and extremities. Also assess the appearance and texture of the hair. Dull, brittle hair; excessive hair growth; or hair loss may indicate endocrine dysfunction. Assess any wounds and ask how long they have been present.

Head. Inspect the size and contour of the head. Facial features should be symmetric. Hyperreflexia and facial muscle contraction upon percussion of the facial nerve *(Chvostek's sign)* may occur in hypoparathyroidism. Inspect the eyes for position, symmetry, and shape. Large and protruding eyes (exophthalmos) are associated with hyperthyroidism. Assess visual acuity using a Snellen eye chart. Visual field loss may indicate a pituitary tumor. In the mouth, inspect the buccal mucosa, condition of teeth, and tongue size. Note hair distribution on the scalp and face. Hearing loss is common in acromegaly (from excess GH).[7]

Neck. The thyroid gland is not usually visible during inspection. A feature that distinguishes the thyroid from other masses in the neck is its upward movement on swallowing. Inspect the neck while the patient swallows a sip of water. The neck should appear symmetric without lumps or bulging.

If there is no noticeable enlargement of the thyroid gland, perform palpation using either a posterior or anterior approach. Because palpation may trigger the release of thyroid hormones, it should not be attempted by the inexperienced clinician. This is especially true when examining patients with a diagnosis of goiter or hyperthyroidism. Auscultate the lateral lobes of an enlarged thyroid gland with the stethoscope bell to identify a *bruit,* a soft swishing sound that may indicate a goiter or hyperthyroidism.

The thyroid gland is difficult to palpate and requires practice and validation by a more experienced practitioner. For *anterior palpation,* stand in front of the patient, with the patient's neck flexed. Place your thumb horizontally with the upper edge along the lower border of the cricoid cartilage. Then move your thumb over the isthmus as the patient swallows water. Place your fingers laterally to the anterior border of the sternocleidomastoid muscle, and palpate each lateral lobe before and while the patient swallows water.

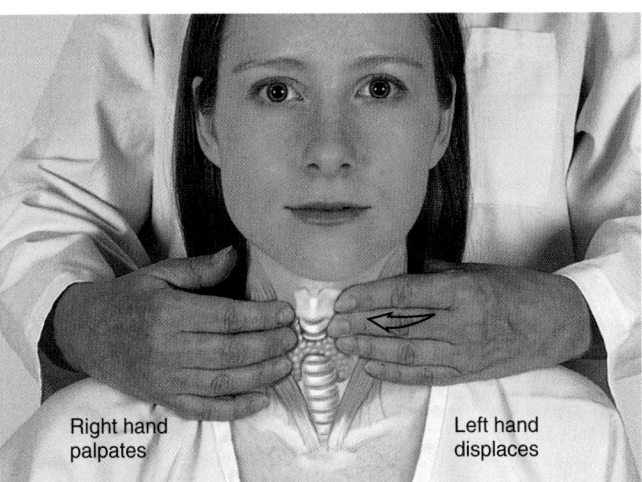

FIG. 48-10 Posterior palpation of the thyroid gland. (From Jarvis C: *Physical examination and health assessment,* ed 6, St Louis, 2012, Saunders.)

Right hand palpates

Left hand displaces

For *posterior palpation,* stand behind the patient (Fig. 48-10). With the thumbs of both hands resting on the nape of the patient's neck, use your index and middle fingers of both hands to feel for the thyroid isthmus and for the anterior surfaces of the lateral lobes. To relax the neck muscles, ask the patient to flex the neck slightly forward and to the right. Displace the thyroid cartilage to the right with your left hand and fingers. Palpate with your right hand after placing the thumb deep and behind the sternocleidomastoid muscle with the index and middle fingers in front of it. Ask the patient to swallow water, and the thyroid will move up.

Repeat this procedure on the left side. Palpate the thyroid for its size, shape, symmetry, and tenderness and for any nodules.

In a normal person, the thyroid is often not palpable. If palpable, it usually feels smooth with a firm consistency, but is not tender with gentle pressure. If nodules, enlargement, asymmetry, or hardness (abnormal findings) are present, refer the patient for further evaluation.

Thorax. Inspect the thorax for shape and characteristics of the skin. Note the presence of breast gynecomastia in men. Auscultate lung sounds and heart sounds, noting any adventitious lung sounds (wheezing, diminished sounds) or extra heart sounds.

CASE STUDY—cont'd

Objective Data: Physical Examination

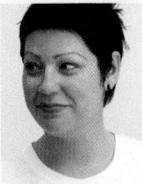

iStockphoto/Thinkstock

A focused assessment of L.M. reveals the following:

L.M. is sitting on the edge of the examination table. She appears somewhat anxious. Her BP is 190/80, heart rate 84, respiratory rate 20, temp 37° C. Her weight is 182 lb, and she is 5 ft, 3 in tall. L.M.'s face is reddened and puffy, and she appears to have a lump on the back of her neck and shoulders. She has some acne on her face, along with some hair growth on her upper lip and chin area. Her abdomen is protruding but her arms and legs are thin. She has +1 edema in her ankles bilaterally. There are several ecchymotic areas on her upper and lower extremities, as well as purple stretch marks on her abdomen.

As you continue to read this chapter, consider diagnostic studies you would anticipate being performed for L.M.

Abdomen. Inspect the contour of the abdomen and note the symmetry and color. Cushing syndrome (hypercortisolism) causes the skin to be fragile, resulting in purple-blue striae across the abdomen. Note general obesity or truncal obesity. Auscultate bowel sounds.

Extremities. Assess the size, shape, symmetry, and general proportion of hands and feet. Inspect the skin for changes in pigmentation, lesions, and edema. Evaluate muscle strength and deep tendon reflexes. In the upper extremities, assess for tremors by placing a piece of paper on the outstretched fingers, palm down. Muscular spasms of the hand elicited on application of an occlusive blood pressure cuff for 3 minutes *(Trousseau's sign)* may be noted in hypoparathyroidism.

Genitalia. Inspect the hair distribution pattern, since it may be altered with hormone irregularities. Normally the shape of pubic hair is a diamond in men and an inverted triangle in women.[6] In men, palpate the testes. In women, note any clitoral enlargement.

Assessment abnormalities related to the endocrine system are presented in Table 48-5. A focused assessment of the endocrine system is presented on in the box above.

DIAGNOSTIC STUDIES OF ENDOCRINE SYSTEM

Diagnostic studies of the endocrine system are presented in Table 48-6. The selection of diagnostic studies is guided by

Text continued on p. 1151

TABLE 48-5 ASSESSMENT ABNORMALITIES

Endocrine System

Finding	Description	Possible Etiology and Significance
Integument		
Hyperpigmentation	Darkening of the skin, particularly in creases and skinfolds	Addison's disease caused by increased secretion of melanocyte-stimulating hormone; acanthosis nigricans
Depigmentation (vitiligo)	Patchy areas of light skin	May be a marker of autoimmune endocrine disorders
Striae	Purplish red marks below the skin surface. Usually seen on abdomen, breasts, and buttocks	Cushing syndrome
Changes in skin texture	Thick, cold, dry skin Thick, leathery, oily skin Warm, smooth, moist skin	Hypothyroidism Growth hormone excess (acromegaly) Hyperthyroidism
Changes in hair distribution	Hair loss Diminished axillary and pubic hair Hirsutism (excessive facial hair on women)	Hypothyroidism, hyperthyroidism, decreased pituitary secretion Cortisol deficiency Cushing syndrome, prolactinoma (a pituitary tumor)
Skin ulceration	Areas of ulcerated skin, most commonly found on legs and feet	Peripheral neuropathy and peripheral vascular disease, which are contributory factors in the development of diabetic foot ulcers
Edema	Generalized edema	Mucopolysaccharide accumulation in tissue in hypothyroidism
Head and Neck		
Visual changes	Decreased visual acuity and/or decreased peripheral vision	Pituitary gland enlargement or tumor leading to pressure on optic nerve
Exophthalmos	Eyeball protrusion from orbits	Occurs in hyperthyroidism as a result of fluid accumulation in eye and retroorbital tissue
Moon face	Periorbital edema and facial fullness	Cushing syndrome as a result of increased cortisol secretion
Myxedema	Puffiness, periorbital edema, masklike affect	Hydrophilic mucopolysaccharides infiltrating dermis in patients with hypothyroidism
Goiter	Generalized enlargement of thyroid gland	Hyperthyroidism, hypothyroidism, iodine deficiency
Thyroid nodule(s)	Localized enlargement of thyroid gland	May be benign or malignant
Cardiovascular		
Chest pain	Angina caused by increased metabolic demands, effusions	Hyperthyroidism, hypothyroidism
Dysrhythmias	Tachycardia, atrial fibrillation	Hypothyroidism or hyperthyroidism, hypoparathyroidism or hyperparathyroidism, pheochromocytoma
Hypertension	Elevated blood pressure caused by increased metabolic demands and catecholamines	Hyperthyroidism, pheochromocytoma, Cushing syndrome
Musculoskeletal		
Changes in muscular strength or muscle mass	Generalized weakness and/or fatigue Decreased muscle mass	Common symptoms associated with many endocrine problems, including pituitary, thyroid, parathyroid, and adrenal dysfunctions Diabetes mellitus, diabetes insipidus Specifically seen in those with growth hormone deficiency and in Cushing syndrome secondary to protein wasting
Enlargement of bones and cartilage	Coarsening of facial features. Increases in size of hands and feet over a period of several years	Gradual enlargement and thickening of bony tissue occurring with growth hormone excess in adults as seen in acromegaly
Nutrition		
Changes in weight	Weight loss	Hyperthyroidism caused by increases in metabolism, type 1 diabetes mellitus, diabetic ketoacidosis
Altered glucose levels	Weight gain Increased serum glucose	Hypothyroidism, Cushing syndrome, type 2 diabetes mellitus Diabetes mellitus, Cushing syndrome, growth hormone excess
Neurologic		
Lethargy	State of mental sluggishness or somnolence	Hypothyroidism
Tetany	Intermittent involuntary muscle spasms usually involving the extremities	Severe hypocalcemia that can occur with hypoparathyroidism
Seizure	Sudden involuntary contraction of muscles	Consequence of a pituitary tumor Fluid and electrolyte imbalance associated with excessive ADH secretion Complications of diabetes mellitus, severe hypothyroidism
Increased deep tendon reflexes	Hyperreflexia	Hyperthyroidism, hypoparathyroidism

TABLE 48-5   ASSESSMENT ABNORMALITIES—cont'd

Endocrine System

Finding	Description	Possible Etiology and Significance
Gastrointestinal		
Constipation	Passage of infrequent hard stools	Hypothyroidism or calcium imbalances caused by hyperparathyroidism
Reproductive		
Changes in reproductive function	Menstrual irregularities, decreased libido, decreased fertility, impotence	Reproductive function is significantly affected by various endocrine abnormalities, including pituitary hypofunction, growth hormone excess, thyroid dysfunction, and adrenocortical dysfunction
Other		
Polyuria	Excessive urine output	Diabetes mellitus (secondary to hyperglycemia) or diabetes insipidus (associated with decreased ADH)
Polydipsia	Excessive thirst	Extreme water losses in diabetes mellitus (with severe hyperglycemia) and diabetes insipidus, dehydration
Decreased urine output	ADH leading to reabsorption of water from kidney tubules	Syndrome of inappropriate antidiuretic hormone (SIADH)
Thermoregulation	Cold insensitivity Heat intolerance	Hypothyroidism caused by a slowing of metabolic processes Hyperthyroidism caused by excessive metabolism

ADH, Antidiuretic hormone.

TABLE 48-6   DIAGNOSTIC STUDIES

Endocrine System

Study	Purpose and Description	Nursing Responsibility
Pituitary Studies		
Blood Studies		
Growth hormone (GH) (somatotropin)	Evaluates GH secretion. Used to identify GH deficiency or GH excess. GH levels are affected by time of day, food intake, and stress. Difficult to interpret significance of isolated GH level. Further evaluation requires stimulation tests (see below). *Men:* <4 ng/mL (<4.0 mcg/L) *Women:* <18 ng/mL (<18 mcg/L) Values >50 ng/mL (>50 mcg/L) suggest acromegaly.	Make sure that patient has been fasting. Emotional and physical stress may alter results. Indicate patient fasting status and recent activity level on the laboratory slip. Send blood sample to laboratory immediately.
Somatomedin C (insulin-like growth factor 1 [IGF-1])	Evaluates GH secretion. Provides a more accurate reflection of mean plasma concentration of GH because it is not subject to circadian rhythm and fluctuations. Low levels indicate GH deficiency. High levels indicate GH excess. *Reference interval:* 135-449 ng/mL	Overnight fasting is preferred but not necessary.
Growth hormone (GH) stimulation	***Insulin tolerance test:*** Regular insulin given IV and blood drawn at –30, 0, 30, 45, 60, and 90 min for measurement of glucose and GH. *Reference interval:* GH >5 mcg/L ***Arginine-GHRH test:*** GHRH bolus followed by 30-min infusion of arginine. *Reference interval:* GH >4.1 mcg/L	Patient must be NPO after midnight. Water is permitted on morning of test. IV access is established for administration of medications and frequent blood sampling. Continually assess for hypoglycemia and hypotension. Keep 50% dextrose and 5% dextrose IV solution at the bedside in case severe hypoglycemia occurs.
Gonadotropins • Follicle-stimulating hormone (FSH) • Luteinizing hormone (LH)	Useful in distinguishing primary gonadal problems from pituitary insufficiency. In women, there are marked differences during menstrual cycle and in postmenopausal period. Levels are low in pituitary insufficiency and high in primary gonadal failure. ***FSH*** *Women:* Follicular phase: 1.37-9.9 mU/mL Ovulatory phase: 6.17-17.2 mU/mL Luteal phase: 1.09-9.2 mU/mL Postmenopause: 19.3-100.6 mU/mL *Men:* 1.42-15.4 mU/mL ***LH*** *Women:* Follicular phase: 1.68-15 IU/L Ovulatory phase: 21.9-56.6 IU/L Postmenopause: 14.2-52.3 IU/L *Men:* 1.24-7.8 IU/L	There is no special preparation of the patient. Only one blood tube is needed for both FSH and LH. Note on the laboratory slip time of menstrual cycle or whether woman is menopausal.

GHRH, Growth hormone–releasing hormone.

Continued

TABLE 48-6 DIAGNOSTIC STUDIES—cont'd

Endocrine System

Study	Purpose and Description	Nursing Responsibility
Pituitary Studies—cont'd **Blood Studies—cont'd**		
Water deprivation (restriction) (ADH stimulation)	Used to differentiate causes of diabetes insipidus (DI), including central DI, nephrogenic DI, and psychogenic polydipsia. ADH (vasopressin) is administered. *Reference interval:* In patients with central DI, urine osmolality increases after ADH. In patients with nephrogenic DI, no or minimal response to ADH.	CAUTION: Patient is NPO for test. Severe dehydration may occur with central or nephrogenic DI during this test. Should be performed only if serum sodium is normal and urine osmolality is <300 mOsm/kg. Obtain baseline weight and urine and plasma osmolality. Assess urine hourly for volume and specific gravity. Send hourly urine samples to laboratory for osmolality determination. Send blood samples for sodium and osmolality every 2 hr. Discontinue test and rehydrate if patient's weight drops >2 kg at any time. Rehydrate with oral fluids. Check orthostatic BP and pulse after rehydration to ensure adequate fluid volume.
Radiologic Studies		
Magnetic resonance imaging (MRI)	Examination of choice for radiologic evaluation of the pituitary gland and hypothalamus. Useful in identifying tumors involving the hypothalamus or pituitary.	Inform patient of the need to lie as still as possible during the test. Explain that tests are painless and noninvasive.
Computed tomography (CT) scan	Used to detect tumor and size of tumor. Oral and/or IV contrast medium may be used.	Inform patient of procedure. Assess renal function before test. Contrast medium may induce renal failure in compromised patients. Patient must lie still during the procedure. If IV contrast is used, check for iodine or shellfish allergy.
Thyroid Studies **Blood Studies**		
Thyroid-stimulating hormone (TSH) (thyrotropin)	Measures levels of TSH. Considered the most sensitive diagnostic test used for evaluating thyroid dysfunction. *Reference interval:* 0.4-4.2 µU/mL (0.4-4.2 mU/L)	Explain blood draw procedure to the patient. No specific preparations are necessary.
Thyroxine (T$_4$), total	Measures total serum level of T$_4$. Useful in evaluating thyroid function and monitoring thyroid therapy. *Reference interval:* 4.6-11.0 mcg/dL (59-142 nmol/L)	See above.
Free thyroxine (FT$_4$)	Measures active component of total T$_4$. Because level remains constant, considered better indicator of thyroid function than total T$_4$. *Reference interval:* 0.8-2.7 ng/dL (10-35 pmol/L)	Instruct patient that FT$_4$ levels may be measured until symptoms of hyperthyroidism have abated and levels have returned to normal.
Triiodothyronine (T$_3$), total	Measures serum levels of T$_3$. Helpful in diagnosing hyperthyroidism if T$_4$ levels are normal. *Ages 20-50:* 70-204 ng/dL (1.08-3.14 nmol/L) *Ages >50:* 40-181 ng/dL (0.62-2.79 nmol/L)	No specific preparation.
Free triiodothyronine (FT$_3$)	Measures active component of total T$_3$. *Reference interval:* 260-480 pg/dL (4.0-7.4 pmol/L)	See above.
T$_3$ uptake (T$_3$ resin uptake)	Indirectly measures binding capacity of thyroid-binding globulin. *Reference interval:* 24%-34%	See above.
Thyroid antibodies (Ab) • Thyroid peroxidase (TPO) Ab • Thyroglobulin Ab • Thyroid-stimulating Ab	Measures levels of thyroid antibodies. Assist in the diagnosis of an autoimmune thyroid disease and separate it from other forms of thyroiditis. One or more antibody tests may be ordered depending on symptoms.	See above.
Thyroglobulin	Identifies functioning thyroid tissue or thyroid cancer cells. Primarily used as a tumor marker for patients being treated for thyroid cancer. *Reference interval:* *Men:* 0.5-53 ng/mL *Women:* 0.5-43 ng/mL	See above.
Radiologic Studies		
Ultrasound	Evaluates thyroid nodule(s) to determine if it is a fluid-filled (cystic) or solid tumor and follows change over time.	Explain that gel and a transducer will be used over the neck. The test lasts 15 min. No fasting or sedation required.

ADH, Antidiuretic hormone.

TABLE 48-6 DIAGNOSTIC STUDIES—cont'd

Endocrine System

Study	Purpose and Description	Nursing Responsibility
Thyroid scan and uptake	*Scan:* Used to evaluate nodules of thyroid. Radioactive isotopes are given orally or IV. Scanner passes over thyroid and makes graphic record of radiation emitted. Normal thyroid scan reveals homogeneous pattern with symmetric lobes. Benign nodules appear as warm spots because they take up radionuclide. Malignant tumors appear as cold spots because they tend not to take up radionuclide. *Radioactive iodine uptake (RAIU):* Provides direct measure of thyroid activity. Evaluates function of thyroid nodules. Patient is given radioactive iodine either orally or IV. The uptake by the thyroid gland is measured with a scanner at several time intervals such as 2-4 hr and at 24 hr. The values of RAIU are expressed in percentage of uptake. *Reference interval:* For 2-4 hr, 3%-19% For 24 hr, 11%-30%	Explain procedure to the patient. Reaction to iodine in allergic patients is rare because amount of iodine in preparation is minimal. Instruct patient to drink increased amount of fluids for 24-48 hr unless contraindicated. Radionuclide will be eliminated 6-24 hr.

Parathyroid Studies
Blood Studies

Study	Purpose and Description	Nursing Responsibility
Parathyroid hormone (PTH)	Measures PTH level in serum. Must be interpreted in terms of concomitantly drawn serum calcium level. *Reference interval:* 50-330 pg/mL (50-330 ng/L)	Fasting specimen preferred. Inform patient that blood sample will be drawn. Keep sample on ice.
Calcium (total)	Used to detect bone and parathyroid disorders. Hypercalcemia can indicate primary hyperparathyroidism, and hypocalcemia can indicate hypoparathyroidism. *Reference interval:* 8.6-10.2 mg/dL (2.15-2.55 mmol/L)	See above.
Calcium (ionized)	Free form of calcium unaffected by variable serum albumin levels. *Reference interval:* 4.64-5.28 mg/dL (1.16-1.32 mmol/L)	See above.
Phosphate	Measures inorganic phosphorus. ↑ Levels indicate primary hypoparathyroidism or secondary causes (e.g., renal failure). ↓ Levels indicate hyperparathyroidism. Phosphorus and calcium levels are inversely related. *Reference interval:* 2.4-4.4 mg/dL (0.78-1.42 mmol/L)	See above.

Radiologic Studies

Study	Purpose and Description	Nursing Responsibility
Parathyroid scan	Uses radioactive isotopes that are taken up by cells in parathyroid glands to obtain an image of the glands and any abnormally active areas. Assists in identifying the number and location of parathyroid glands.	No food, fluid, or medication restrictions before test.

Adrenal Studies
Blood Studies

Study	Purpose and Description	Nursing Responsibility
Cortisol (total)	Measures amount of total cortisol in serum and evaluates status of adrenal cortex function. *Reference interval:* At 8 AM: 5-23 mcg/dL (138-635 nmol/L) At 4 PM: 3-16 mcg/dL (83-441 nmol/L)	Cortisol has diurnal variation; levels are higher in morning than in evening. Sample should be drawn in morning; evening samples may also be ordered. Note if patient does night shift work. Mark time of blood draw on laboratory slip. Stress and excessive physical activity produce elevated results.
Aldosterone	Used to assess for hyperaldosteronism. *Reference interval:* Upright posture: 7-30 ng/dL (0.19-0.83 nmol/L) Supine position: 3-16 ng/dL (0.08-0.44 nmol/L)	Usually morning blood sample is preferred. Inform patient that the required position, supine or sitting/standing, must be maintained for 2 hr before the specimen is drawn.
Adrenocorticotropic hormone (ACTH) (corticotropin)	Measures plasma level of ACTH. Although ACTH is a pituitary hormone, it controls adrenal cortex secretion, thus helping to determine if underproduction or overproduction of cortisol is caused by dysfunction of the adrenal gland or pituitary gland. *Reference interval:* Morning: <120 pg/mL (<26 pmol/L) Evening: <85 pg/mL (<19 pmol/L)	Patient should be NPO after midnight before morning blood draw between 6-8 AM. Diurnal levels correspond with variation of cortisol levels. Levels are higher in morning, lower in evening. ACTH is unstable; use prechilled blood tube and place on ice and send to laboratory immediately.
ACTH stimulation with cosyntropin	Used to evaluate adrenal function. After baseline cortisol sample is drawn, give cosyntropin (synthetic ACTH) by IV bolus. Cortisol samples are drawn 30 and 60 min after bolus. Plasma cortisol at 60 min should increase by >7 mcg/dL from baseline.	Obtain baseline cortisol level at beginning of cosyntropin infusion. Inject cosyntropin with a plastic syringe and collect blood samples in plastic heparinized tubes. Administer test with continuous-infusion method. Monitor site and rate of IV infusion. Ensure sample collection at appropriate times.

Continued

TABLE 48-6   DIAGNOSTIC STUDIES—cont'd

Endocrine System

Study	Purpose and Description	Nursing Responsibility
Adrenal Studies—cont'd		
Blood Studies—cont'd		
ACTH suppression (dexamethasone suppression)	Assesses adrenal function. Especially helpful if hyperactivity (Cushing syndrome) is suspected. *Overnight method:* Dexamethasone (Decadron) 1 mg (low dose) or 4 mg (high dose) is given at 11 PM to suppress secretion of corticotropin-releasing hormone. Plasma cortisol sample is drawn at 8 AM. *Reference interval:* Cortisol level <3 mcg/dL (<0.08 µmol/L) for low dose and <50% of baseline in high dose indicates normal adrenal response.	Ensure that patient has fasted. Inform patient that blood sample will be taken. Observe venipuncture site for bleeding and hematoma formation. Do not test acutely ill patients or those under stress. Stress-stimulated ACTH may override suppression. Screen patient for drugs such as estrogen and corticosteroids that may give false-positive results. Ensure accurate timing of medication and sample collection.
Metanephrine	Screens for pheochromocytoma more accurately than urinary vanillylmandelic acid (VMA) and catecholamine measurements.	Ask about recent history of vigorous exercise, high levels of stress, or starvation (may artificially ↑ levels). Ingestion of caffeine, alcohol, levodopa, lithium, nitroglycerin, acetaminophen, and medications containing epinephrine or norepinephrine can alter test results.
Urine Studies		
17-Ketosteroids	Measures androgen metabolites in urine and evaluates adrenocortical and gonadal function. *Reference interval:* Men: 6-20 mg/day (20-70 µmol/day) Women: 6-17 mg/day (20-60 µmol/day)	Instruct patient regarding 24-hr urine collection. Tell patient that specimen must be kept refrigerated or iced during entire collection period. Determine whether preservative is required.
Cortisol (free)	Measures free (unbound) cortisol. Preferred test to evaluate hypercortisolism. *Reference interval:* 20-90 mcg/24 hr (55-248 nmol/day)	Instruct patient about 24-hr urine collection and avoidance of stressful situations and excessive physical exercise. Some drugs (e.g., reserpine, diuretics, phenothiazines, insulin, amphetamines) may alter results.
Vanillylmandelic acid (VMA)	Measures urinary excretion of catecholamine metabolite. Levels are increased in pheochromocytoma. *Reference interval:* 1.4-6.5 mg/24 hr (7-33 µmol/day)	Keep 24-hr urine collection at pH <3.0 with HCl acid as preservative. Keep on ice. Consult with laboratory or health care provider about patient discontinuing any drugs 3 days before urine collection.
Radiologic Studies		
Computed tomography (CT)	Abdominal CT is radiologic examination of choice for the adrenal gland. Used to detect tumor and size or metastatic spread. Oral and/or IV contrast medium may be used.	Inform patient of procedure. Patient must lie still during the procedure. Assess renal function if IV contrast is used. Check for iodine or shellfish allergy.
Magnetic resonance imaging (MRI)	Same as MRI above.	Same as MRI above.
Pancreatic Studies		
Blood Studies		
Fasting blood glucose (FBG)	Measures circulating glucose level. *Reference interval:* 70-99 mg/dL (3.9-5.5 mmol/L).	Patient should fast 8-12 hr. Water intake is permitted. Many medications may influence results.
Oral glucose tolerance test (OGTT)	Used to evaluate abnormal FBG levels that do not clearly indicate diabetes. Patient drinks 75 g of glucose; samples for glucose are drawn at baseline and at 30, 60, and 120 min. Test takes 2 hr to complete. *Reference interval:* <100 mg/dL (5.5 mmol/L) at baseline, <200 mg/dL (11.1 mmol/L) at 30 and 60 min, and <140 mg/dL (7.8 mmol/L) at 120 min. Values >200 mg/dL (11.1 mmol/L) at 120 min are considered diagnostic for diabetes mellitus.	Perform test on ambulatory patients after fasting 8-12 hr. Many drugs may influence results, including caffeine and smoking. Ensure that patient's diet 3 days before test includes 150-300 g of carbohydrate with intake of at least 1500 cal/day.
Glycosylated hemoglobin (Hb A1C [A1C])	Indicates the amount of glucose linked to hemoglobin. Assesses long-term glycemic control during previous 3 mo. *Reference interval:* 4.0%-6.0% ADA treatment goal <7%	Inform patient that fasting is not necessary and that blood sample will be drawn. Observe venipuncture site for bleeding or hematoma formation.
Urine Studies		
Glucose	Estimate amount of glucose in urine by using an enzymatic method. Dipstick is dipped into the urine and read for color changes after 1 min. *Reference interval:* Negative	Use freshly voided urine. Many drugs alter glucose readings. Errors are great if directions are not followed exactly.

ADA, American Diabetes Association.

TABLE 48-6 DIAGNOSTIC STUDIES—cont'd

Endocrine System

Study	Purpose and Description	Nursing Responsibility
Ketones	Measures amount of acetone (a type of ketone) excreted in urine as result of incomplete fat metabolism. Tested with a dipstick as described above. Positive result can indicate lack of insulin and diabetic acidosis. *Reference interval:* Negative	Use freshly voided urine specimen. Test is often done with glucose test. Directions must be followed exactly. Certain drugs can produce false-positive or false-negative results.
Radiologic Studies Computed tomography (CT)	Abdominal CT is the radiologic examination of choice for pancreas. Used to identify tumors or cysts. Oral and/or IV contrast medium may be ordered.	Inform patient of procedure. Patient must lie still during the procedure. If IV contrast is used, check for iodine and shellfish allergy. Assess renal function if contrast is used.

ADA, American Diabetes Association; *ADH,* antidiuretic hormone; *GHRH,* growth hormone–releasing hormone.

pertinent findings from the history and physical examination. Laboratory studies may include direct measurement of the hormone level, or they may involve an indirect indication of gland function by evaluating blood or urine components affected by the hormone such as glucose or electrolytes.

Hormones with fairly constant basal levels such as T_4 require a single measurement. Note the time of the sample collection on the laboratory slip. Information about night shift work is important for hormones with circadian or sleep-related secretion (e.g., cortisol). Evaluation of other hormones may require multiple blood samplings such as in suppression tests (e.g., dexamethasone) and stimulation tests (e.g., glucose tolerance). In these situations, it is often necessary to obtain IV access to administer the testing medication and fluids and to draw multiple blood samples.

Disorders associated with the pituitary gland can manifest in a wide variety of ways because of the number of hormones produced. Many diagnostic studies evaluate these hormones either directly or indirectly (see Table 48-6).

A number of tests are available to evaluate thyroid function. The most sensitive and accurate laboratory test is measurement of TSH. Thus it is often recommended as a first diagnostic test for evaluation of thyroid function.[8] Common additional tests ordered in the presence of an abnormal TSH level include total T_4, free T_4, and total T_3. Free T_4 is the unbound thyroxine and is a more accurate reflection of thyroid function than total T_4.

The only hormone secreted by the parathyroid glands is PTH. Because PTH regulates serum calcium and phosphate levels, abnormalities in PTH secretion are reflected in these

CASE STUDY—cont'd

Objective Data: Diagnostic Studies

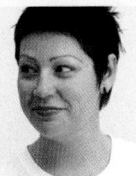

iStockphoto/Thinkstock

The health care provider orders the following initial diagnostic studies to be drawn in the morning after an 8-hr fast:
- CBC, basic metabolic panel (electrolytes, BUN, creatinine)
- Fasting blood glucose (FBG)
- TSH, free T_4
- Plasma cortisol levels
- Plasma ACTH levels

CBC results reveal a WBC of 12,200/μL and a decreased lymphocyte count at 800 cells/μL. The rest of the CBC is within normal limits (WNL). The FBG is 130 mg/dL. The plasma cortisol and ACTH levels are elevated. Thyroid studies are WNL.

levels. For this reason, diagnostic tests for the parathyroid gland typically include PTH, serum calcium, and serum phosphate levels.

Diagnostic tests associated with the adrenal cortex function focus on the three types of hormones secreted: glucocorticoids, mineralocorticoids, and androgens. These hormone levels can be measured both in blood plasma and in urine. The urine studies often require 24-hour urine collection to eliminate the impact of short-term fluctuations in plasma hormone levels.[9]

The tests found in Table 48-6 are used to evaluate the metabolism of glucose. They are important in the diagnosis and management of diabetes mellitus. (Diagnostic studies for diabetes mellitus are also discussed in Chapter 49.)

■ BRIDGE TO NCLEX EXAMINATION

The number of the question corresponds to the same-numbered outcome at the beginning of the chapter.

1. A characteristic common to all hormones is that they
   a. circulate in the blood bound to plasma proteins.
   b. influence cellular activity of specific target tissues.
   c. accelerate the metabolic processes of all body cells.
   d. enter a cell to alter the cell's metabolism or gene expression.

2. A patient is receiving radiation therapy for cancer of the kidney. The nurse monitors the patient for signs and symptoms of damage to the
   a. pancreas.
   b. thyroid gland.
   c. adrenal glands.
   d. posterior pituitary gland.

3. A patient has a serum sodium level of 152 mEq/L (152 mmol/L). The normal hormonal response to this situation is
   a. release of ADH.
   b. release of ACTH.
   c. secretion of aldosterone.
   d. secretion of corticotropin-releasing hormone.

4. All cells in the body are believed to have intracellular receptors for
   a. insulin.
   b. glucagon.
   c. growth hormone.
   d. thyroid hormone.

5. When obtaining subjective data from a patient during assessment of the endocrine system, the nurse asks specifically about
   a. energy level.
   b. intake of vitamin C.
   c. employment history.
   d. frequency of sexual intercourse.

6. Endocrine disorders often go unrecognized in the older adult because
   a. symptoms are often attributed to aging.
   b. older adults rarely have identifiable symptoms.
   c. endocrine disorders are relatively rare in the older adult.
   d. older adults usually have subclinical endocrine disorders that minimize symptoms.

7. An abnormal finding by the nurse during an endocrine assessment would be *(select all that apply)*
   a. blood pressure of 100/70 mm Hg.
   b. excessive facial hair on a woman.
   c. soft, formed stool every other day.
   d. 3-lb weight gain over last 6 months.
   e. hyperpigmented coloration in lower legs.

8. A patient has a total serum calcium level of 3 mg/dL (1.5 mEq/L). If this finding reflects hypoparathyroidism, the nurse would expect further diagnostic testing to reveal
   a. decreased serum PTH.
   b. increased serum ACTH.
   c. increased serum glucose.
   d. decreased serum cortisol levels.

1. b, 2. c, 3. a, 4. d, 5. a, 6. a, 7. b, e, 8. a

⊝volve

For rationales to these answers and even more NCLEX review questions, visit *http://evolve.elsevier.com/Lewis/medsurg*.

REFERENCES

1. Huether SE, McCance KL, editors: *Understanding pathophysiology*, ed 5, St Louis, 2013, Mosby.
2. Brashers VL, Heuther SE: Mechanisms of hormonal regulation. In Heuther SE, McCance KL, editors: *Understanding pathophysiology*, ed 5, St Louis, 2013, Mosby.
3. Eliopoulos C: *Gerontological nursing*, ed 7, Philadelphia, 2010, Lippincott Williams & Wilkins.
4. Clark JJ, Wong LL, Lurie F, et al: Proteinuria as a predictor of renal dysfunction in trauma patients receiving intravenous contrast, *Am Surg* 77:1194, 2011.
5. Kirmani S: Molecular genetic testing in endocrinology: a practical guide, *Endocr Pract* 31:1, 2012.
6. Jarvis C: *Physical examination and health assessment*, ed 6, St Louis, 2012, Saunders.
7. Aydin K, Ozturk B, Turkyilmaz MD, et al: Functional and structural evaluation of hearing loss in acromegaly, *Clin Endocrinol* 76:415, 2012.
8. Mitrou P, Raptis SA, Dimitriadis G: Thyroid disease in older people, *Maturitas* 70:5, 2011.
9. Wilson SF, Giddens JF: Health assessment for nursing practice, ed 5, St Louis, 2012, Mosby.

RESOURCES

Resources for this chapter are listed in Chapter 49 on p. 1188 and Chapter 50 on p. 1217.

*What happens is not as important as how
you react to what happens.*
Thaddeus Golas

Nursing Management
Diabetes Mellitus

Janice Lazear

⊖volve WEBSITE

http://evolve.elsevier.com/Lewis/medsurg

- NCLEX Review Questions
- Key Points
- Pre-Test
- Answer Guidelines for Case Study on p. 1186
- Rationales for Bridge to NCLEX Examination Questions

- Case Studies
  - Patient With Type 1 Diabetes Mellitus and Diabetic Ketoacidosis
  - Patient With Type 2 Diabetes Mellitus and Hyperosmolar Hyperglycemic Syndrome
- Nursing Care Plans (Customizable)
  - eNCP 49-1: Patient With Diabetes Mellitus
- Concept Map Creator

- Concept Map for Case Study on p. 1186
- Glossary
- Content Updates

eFigure
- eFig. 49-1: Create Your Plate Method

eTable
- eTable 49-1: Effect of Drugs on Blood Glucose Levels

LEARNING OUTCOMES

1. Describe the pathophysiology and clinical manifestations of diabetes mellitus.
2. Differentiate between type 1 and type 2 diabetes mellitus.
3. Describe the collaborative care of the patient with diabetes mellitus.
4. Describe the role of nutrition and exercise in the management of diabetes mellitus.
5. Discuss the nursing management of a patient with newly diagnosed diabetes mellitus.
6. Describe the nursing management of the patient with diabetes mellitus in the ambulatory and home care settings.
7. Relate the pathophysiology of acute and chronic complications of diabetes mellitus to the clinical manifestations.
8. Explain the collaborative care and nursing management of the patient with acute and chronic complications of diabetes mellitus.

KEY TERMS

dawn phenomenon, p. 1163
diabetes mellitus (DM), p. 1153
diabetic ketoacidosis (DKA), p. 1176
diabetic nephropathy, p. 1182
diabetic neuropathy, p. 1182
glycemic index (GI), p. 1166

hyperosmolar hyperglycemic syndrome (HHS), p. 1178
impaired fasting glucose (IFG), p. 1156
impaired glucose tolerance (IGT), p. 1156
insulin resistance, p. 1156

intensive insulin therapy, p. 1158
prediabetes, p. 1156
self-monitoring of blood glucose (SMBG), p. 1167
Somogyi effect, p. 1163

This chapter discusses the pathophysiology, clinical manifestations, complications, and collaborative care of diabetes mellitus. The nurse's role in teaching to promote patient management of diet, activities, and drugs for good control of diabetes is emphasized.

DIABETES MELLITUS

Diabetes mellitus (DM) is a chronic multisystem disease related to abnormal insulin production, impaired insulin utilization, or both. Diabetes mellitus is a serious health problem throughout the world, and its prevalence is rapidly increasing. Currently in the United States an estimated 25.8 million people, or 8.3% of the population, have diabetes mellitus, and 79 million more people have prediabetes.[1] Approximately 7 million people with diabetes mellitus have not been diagnosed and are unaware that they have the disease. Diabetes mellitus is the seventh leading cause of death in the United States, but it is likely to be underreported. The annual cost of diabetes exceeds $174 billion, with $116 billion in direct medical costs.[2]

Reviewed by Teressa Sanders Hunter, RN, PhD, Assistant Professor, Langston University, School of Nursing and Health Professions, Langston, Oklahoma; Jane Faith Kapustin, PhD, CRNP, BC-ADM, FAANP, Associate Professor and Assistant Dean for the Master's and DNP Programs and Faculty Practice as Adult NP, Medical Center for Diabetes and Endocrinology, Baltimore, Maryland; Nancy Karnes, RN, MSN, CCRN, CDE, Faculty Nursing Program, Bellevue College, Bellevue, Washington; Lorraine Nowakowski-Grier, MSN, APRN, BC, CDE, Diabetes Nurse Practitioner, Christiana Care Health Services, Newark, Delaware; Susan A. Sandstrom, RN, MSN, BC, CNE, Associate Professor in Nursing (retired), College of Saint Mary, Omaha, Nebraska; and Elaine K. Strouss, RN, MSN, Associate Professor of Nursing, Community College of Beaver County, Monaca, Pennsylvania.

The long-term complications of diabetes make it a devastating disease. Diabetes is the leading cause of adult blindness, end-stage kidney disease, and nontraumatic lower limb amputations. It is also a major contributing factor to heart disease and stroke. Adults with diabetes have heart disease death rates two to four times higher than adults without diabetes. The risk for stroke is also two to four times higher among people with diabetes. In addition, it is estimated that 67% of adults with diabetes have hypertension.[1]

Etiology and Pathophysiology

Current theories link the causes of diabetes, singly or in combination, to genetic, autoimmune, and environmental factors (e.g., virus, obesity). Regardless of its cause, diabetes is primarily a disorder of glucose metabolism related to absent or insufficient insulin supply and/or poor utilization of the insulin that is available.

The American Diabetes Association (ADA) recognizes four different classes of diabetes. The two most common are type 1 and type 2 diabetes mellitus (Table 49-1). The two other classes are gestational diabetes and other specific types of diabetes with various causes.

Normal Insulin Metabolism. Insulin is a hormone produced by the β cells in the islets of Langerhans of the pancreas. Under normal conditions, insulin is continuously released into the bloodstream in small pulsatile increments, with increased release when food is ingested (Fig. 49-1). Insulin lowers blood glucose and facilitates a stable, normal glucose range of approximately 70 to 120 mg/dL (3.9 to 6.66 mmol/L). The average amount of insulin secreted daily by an adult is approximately 40 to 50 U, or 0.6 U/kg of body weight.

Insulin promotes glucose transport from the bloodstream across the cell membrane to the cytoplasm of the cell. The rise in plasma insulin after a meal stimulates storage of glucose as glycogen in liver and muscle, inhibits gluconeogenesis, enhances fat deposition of adipose tissue, and increases protein synthesis. For this reason insulin is an *anabolic,* or storage, hormone. The fall in insulin level during normal overnight fasting facilitates the release of stored glucose from the liver, protein from muscle, and fat from adipose tissue.

Skeletal muscle and adipose tissue have specific receptors for insulin and are considered insulin-dependent tissues. Insulin is required to "unlock" these receptor sites, allowing the transport of glucose into the cells to be used for energy. Other tissues (e.g.,

brain, liver, blood cells) do not directly depend on insulin for glucose transport but require an adequate glucose supply for normal function. Although liver cells are not considered insulin-dependent tissue, insulin receptor sites on the liver facilitate hepatic uptake of glucose and its conversion to glycogen.

Other hormones (glucagon, epinephrine, growth hormone, and cortisol) work to oppose the effects of insulin and are referred to as *counterregulatory hormones.* These hormones increase blood glucose levels by stimulating glucose production and output by the liver and by decreasing the movement of glucose into the cells. The counterregulatory hormones and insulin usually maintain blood glucose levels within the normal range by regulating the release of glucose for energy during food intake and periods of fasting.

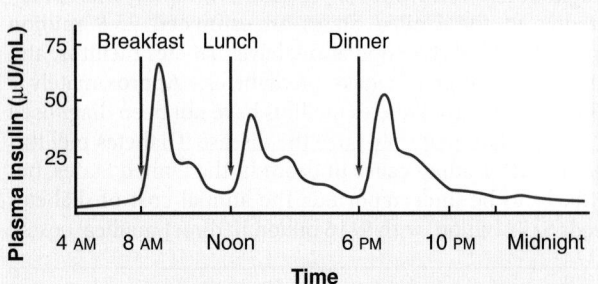

FIG. 49-1 Normal endogenous insulin secretion. In the first hour or two after meals, insulin concentrations rise rapidly in blood and peak at about 1 hour. After meals, insulin concentrations promptly decline toward preprandial values as carbohydrate absorption from the gastrointestinal tract declines. After carbohydrate absorption from the gastrointestinal tract is complete and during the night, insulin concentrations are low and fairly constant, with a slight increase at dawn.

TABLE 49-1	COMPARISON OF TYPE 1 AND TYPE 2 DIABETES MELLITUS	
Factor	**Type 1 Diabetes Mellitus**	**Type 2 Diabetes Mellitus**
Age at onset	More common in young people but can occur at any age.	Usually age 35 yr or older but can occur at any age. Incidence is increasing in children.
Type of onset	Signs and symptoms usually abrupt, but disease process may be present for several years.	Insidious, may go undiagnosed for years.
Prevalence	Accounts for 5%-10% of all types of diabetes.	Accounts for 90%-95% of all types of diabetes.
Environmental factors	Virus, toxins.	Obesity, lack of exercise.
Primary defect	Absent or minimal insulin production.	Insulin resistance, decreased insulin production over time, and alterations in production of adipokines.
Islet cell antibodies	Often present at onset.	Absent.
Endogenous insulin	Absent.	Initially increased in response to insulin resistance. Secretion diminishes over time.
Nutritional status	Thin, normal, or obese.	Frequently overweight or obese. May be normal.
Symptoms	Polydipsia, polyuria, polyphagia, fatigue, weight loss.	Frequently none, fatigue, recurrent infections. May also experience polyuria, polydipsia, and polyphagia.
Ketosis	Prone at onset or during insulin deficiency.	Resistant except during infection or stress.
Nutritional therapy	Essential.	Essential.
Insulin	Required for all.	Required for some. Disease is progressive and insulin treatment may need to be added to treatment regimen.
Vascular and neurologic complications	Frequent.	Frequent.

Insulin is synthesized from a precursor, proinsulin. Enzymes split proinsulin to form insulin and C-peptide, and then the two substances are released in equal amounts. Therefore measuring C-peptide in serum and urine is a useful clinical indicator of pancreatic β cell function.

Type 1 Diabetes Mellitus. *Type 1 diabetes mellitus,* formerly known as juvenile-onset diabetes or insulin-dependent diabetes, accounts for approximately 5% of all people with diabetes. Type 1 diabetes generally affects people under 40 years of age, and 40% develop it before 20 years of age. The incidence of type 1 diabetes has increased 3% to 5% over recent decades, and for unknown reasons it is occurring more frequently in younger children.[3]

Etiology and Pathophysiology. Type 1 diabetes is an immune-mediated disease, caused by autoimmune destruction of the pancreatic β cells, the site of insulin production. This eventually results in a total absence of insulin production. Autoantibodies to the islet cells cause a reduction of 80% to 90% of normal function before hyperglycemia and other manifestations occur (Fig. 49-2). A genetic predisposition and exposure to a virus are factors that may contribute to the pathogenesis of immune-related type 1 diabetes.

Genetic Link

Predisposition to type 1 diabetes is related to human leukocyte antigens (HLAs). (See Chapter 14 for a discussion of HLAs and disease associations.) Theoretically, when an individual with certain HLA types is exposed to a viral infection, the β cells of the pancreas are destroyed, either directly or through an autoimmune process. The HLA types associated with an increased risk for type 1 diabetes include HLA-DR3 and HLA-DR4 (see Genetics in Clinical Practice box).

Idiopathic diabetes is a form of type 1 diabetes that is strongly inherited and not related to autoimmunity. It occurs only in a small number of people with type 1 diabetes, most often of Hispanic, African, or Asian ancestry.[3] Latent autoimmune diabetes in adults (LADA), a slowly progressing autoimmune form of type 1 diabetes, usually occurs in people who are over the age of 35 who are not obese.[4]

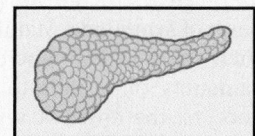

Type 1 Diabetes Mellitus

Pancreas

- Autoimmune destruction of β cells
- Autoantibodies present for months to years before clinical symptoms
- No production of insulin

Type 2 Diabetes Mellitus

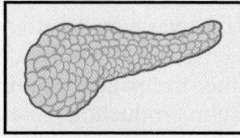

Pancreas

- Defective β cell secretion of insulin
- Insulin resistance stimulates ↑ insulin secretion
- Eventual exhaustion of β cells in many people

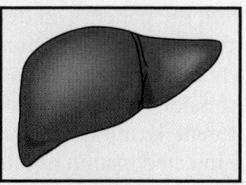

Liver

- Excess glucose production
- Inappropriate regulation of glucose production

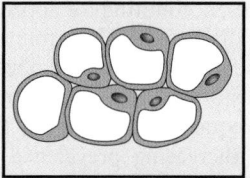

Adipose tissue

- ↓ Adiponectin and ↑ leptin
- Results in altered glucose and fat metabolism

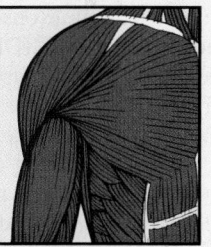

Muscle

- Defective insulin receptors
- Insulin resistance
- Decreased uptake of glucose by cells resulting in hyperglycemia

FIG. 49-2 Altered mechanisms in type 1 and type 2 diabetes mellitus.

GENETICS IN CLINICAL PRACTICE

Types 1 and 2 Diabetes Mellitus

Type 1 Diabetes Mellitus	Type 2 Diabetes Mellitus	Maturity-Onset Diabetes of the Young (MODY)
Genetic Basis		
• Increased susceptibility (40%-50%) when one has specific human leukocyte antigens (HLA-DR3, HLA-DR4). • Polygenic (>40 genes influence susceptibility).	• Polygenic (>25 genes influence susceptibility).	• Autosomal dominant. • Monogenic (single gene). • Caused by mutations in any of six MODY genes (types 1-6). • Mutations in genes lead to β-cell dysfunction.
Risk to Offspring		
• Risk to offspring of diabetic mothers is 1%-4%. • Risk to offspring of diabetic fathers is 5%-6%. • When one identical twin has type 1 diabetes, the other gets the disease about 30%-40% of the time.	• Risk to offspring is 8%-14%. • When one identical twin gets type 2 diabetes, the other gets it about 60%-75% of the time.	• If one parent has MODY, a child has a 50% chance of developing disease. • If one parent has MODY, a child has a 50% chance of being a carrier.
Clinical Implications		
• Disease is a result of complex interaction of genetic, autoimmune, and environmental factors.	• Disease is a result of complex genetic interactions, which are modified by environmental factors such as body weight and exercise.	• MODY accounts for 1% to 5% of people with diabetes. • Characterized by young age of onset (often before age 25). • Not associated with obesity or hypertension. • Treatment varies depending on the genetic mutation that caused MODY.

Onset of Disease. In type 1 diabetes the islet cell autoantibodies responsible for β-cell destruction are present for months to years before the onset of symptoms. Manifestations of type 1 diabetes develop when the person's pancreas can no longer produce sufficient amounts of insulin to maintain normal glucose. Once this occurs, the onset of symptoms is usually rapid, and patients often are initially seen with impending or actual ketoacidosis. The patient usually has a history of recent and sudden weight loss and the classic symptoms of *polydipsia* (excessive thirst), *polyuria* (frequent urination), and *polyphagia* (excessive hunger).

The individual with type 1 diabetes requires insulin from an outside source *(exogenous insulin)* to sustain life. Without insulin, the patient will develop diabetic ketoacidosis (DKA), a life-threatening condition resulting in metabolic acidosis. Newly diagnosed patients with type 1 diabetes may experience a remission, or "honeymoon period," for 3 to 12 months after treatment is initiated. During this time, the patient requires little injected insulin because β-cell insulin production remains sufficient for glucose control. Eventually, as more β cells are destroyed and blood glucose levels increase, the honeymoon period ends and the patient will require insulin on a permanent basis.

Type 2 Diabetes Mellitus. *Type 2 diabetes mellitus* was formerly known as adult-onset diabetes (AODM) or non–insulin-dependent diabetes (NIDDM). Type 2 diabetes mellitus is, by far, the most prevalent type of diabetes, accounting for approximately 90% to 95% of patients with diabetes.[2] Risk factors for developing type 2 diabetes include being overweight or obese, being older, and having a family history of type 2 diabetes. Although the disease is seen less frequently in children, the incidence is increasing due to the increasing prevalence of childhood obesity. Type 2 diabetes is more prevalent in some ethnic populations. African Americans, Asian Americans, Hispanics, Native Hawaiians or other Pacific Islanders, and Native Americans have a higher rate of type 2 diabetes than whites.[4]

Etiology and Pathophysiology. In type 2 diabetes the pancreas usually continues to produce some *endogenous* (self-made) insulin. However, the insulin that is produced is either insufficient for the needs of the body or is poorly used by the tissues, or both. The presence of endogenous insulin is a major distinction between type 1 and type 2 diabetes. (In type 1 diabetes, there is an absence of endogenous insulin.)

Many factors contribute to the development of type 2 diabetes. The most powerful risk factor is obesity, especially abdominal and visceral adiposity.

✇ Genetic Link

Although the genetics of type 2 diabetes is not yet fully understood, it is likely multiple genes are involved. Genetic mutations that lead to insulin resistance and a higher risk for obesity have been found in many people with type 2 diabetes. Individuals with a first-degree relative with the disease are 10 times more likely to develop type 2 diabetes.

Four major metabolic abnormalities have a role in the development of type 2 diabetes (see Fig. 49-2). The first factor is insulin resistance, a condition in which body tissues do not respond to the action of insulin because insulin receptors are unresponsive, are insufficient in number, or both. Most insulin receptors are located on skeletal muscle, fat, and liver cells. When insulin is not properly used, the entry of glucose into the cell is impeded, resulting in hyperglycemia. In the early stages

of insulin resistance, the pancreas responds to high blood glucose by producing greater amounts of insulin (if β-cell function is normal). This creates a temporary state of hyperinsulinemia that coexists with hyperglycemia.

A second factor in the development of type 2 diabetes is a marked decrease in the pancreas's ability to produce insulin, as the β cells become fatigued from the compensatory overproduction of insulin or when β-cell mass is lost. The underlying basis for the failure of β cells to adapt is unknown. It may be linked to the adverse effects of chronic hyperglycemia or high circulating free fatty acids.

A third factor is inappropriate glucose production by the liver. Instead of properly regulating the release of glucose in response to blood levels, the liver does so in a haphazard way that does not correspond to the body's needs at the time.

A fourth factor is altered production of hormones and cytokines by adipose tissue *(adipokines)*. Adipokines secreted by adipose tissue appear to play a role in glucose and fat metabolism and are likely to contribute to the pathophysiology of type 2 diabetes.[5] Adipokines are thought to cause chronic inflammation, a factor involved in insulin resistance, type 2 diabetes, and cardiovascular disease (CVD). The two main adipokines believed to affect insulin sensitivity are adiponectin and leptin.

Individuals with *metabolic syndrome* are at an increased risk for the development of type 2 diabetes. Metabolic syndrome has five components: elevated glucose levels, abdominal obesity, elevated blood pressure (BP), high levels of triglycerides, and decreased levels of high-density lipoproteins (HDLs) (see Table 41-10). An individual with three of the five components is considered to have metabolic syndrome.[6] Overweight individuals with metabolic syndrome can prevent or delay the onset of diabetes through a program of weight loss and regular physical activity. (See Chapter 41 for a discussion of metabolic syndrome.)

Onset of Disease. The disease onset in type 2 diabetes is usually gradual. The person may go for many years with undetected hyperglycemia that might produce few, if any, symptoms. Many people are diagnosed on routine laboratory testing or when they undergo treatment for other conditions, and elevated glucose or glycosylated hemoglobin (A1C or Hb A1C [not commonly used]) levels are found.

Prediabetes. Individuals diagnosed with prediabetes are at increased risk for the development of type 2 diabetes. Prediabetes is defined as impaired glucose tolerance (IGT), impaired fasting glucose (IFG), or both. It is an intermediate stage between normal glucose homeostasis and diabetes where the blood glucose levels are elevated, but not high enough to meet the diagnostic criteria for diabetes. A diagnosis of IGT is made if the 2-hour oral glucose tolerance test (OGTT) values are 140 to 199 mg/dL (7.8 to 11.0 mmol/L).[3] IFG is diagnosed when fasting blood glucose levels are 100 to 125 mg/dL (5.56 to 6.9 mmol/L).

Persons with prediabetes usually do not have symptoms. However, long-term damage to the body, especially the heart and blood vessels, may already be occurring. It is important for you to encourage patients to undergo screening and to provide instruction about managing risk factors for diabetes. Patients with prediabetes can take action to prevent or delay the development of type 2 diabetes. Those with prediabetes should have their blood glucose and A1C tested regularly and monitor for symptoms of diabetes, such as polyuria, polyphagia, and polydipsia. Maintaining a healthy weight, exercising regularly, and eating a healthy diet have all been found to reduce the risk of developing overt diabetes in people with prediabetes.

Gestational Diabetes. *Gestational diabetes* develops during pregnancy and occurs in about 2% to 10% of pregnancies in the United States.[7] Women with gestational diabetes have a higher risk for cesarean delivery, and their babies have increased risk for perinatal death, birth injury, and neonatal complications. Women who are at high risk for gestational diabetes should be screened at the first prenatal visit.[8] Those at high risk include women who are obese, are of advanced maternal age, or have a family history of diabetes. Women with an average risk for gestational diabetes are screened using an OGTT at 24 to 28 weeks of gestation. Most women with gestational diabetes have normal glucose levels within 6 weeks postpartum. Be aware that women with a history of gestational diabetes have a 35% to 60% chance of developing type 2 diabetes within 10 years.[7] Gestational diabetes and management of the pregnant patient with diabetes are specialized areas not covered in detail in this chapter. Consult an obstetric text for more information.

Other Specific Types of Diabetes. Diabetes occurs in some people because of another medical condition or treatment of a medical condition that causes abnormal blood glucose levels. Conditions that may cause diabetes can result from damage to, injury to, interference with, or destruction of the β-cell function in the pancreas. These include Cushing syndrome, hyperthyroidism, recurrent pancreatitis, cystic fibrosis, hemochromatosis, and parenteral nutrition. Commonly used medications that can induce diabetes in some people include corticosteroids (prednisone), thiazides, phenytoin (Dilantin), and atypical antipsychotics (e.g., clozapine [Clozaril]). Diabetes caused by medical conditions or medications can resolve when the underlying condition is treated or the medication discontinued. (Drugs that can alter blood glucose levels are listed in eTable 49-1 available on the website for this chapter.)

Clinical Manifestations

Type 1 Diabetes Mellitus. Because the onset of type 1 diabetes is rapid, the initial manifestations are usually acute. The classic symptoms are *polyuria, polydipsia,* and *polyphagia.* The osmotic effect of glucose produces the manifestations of polydipsia and polyuria. Polyphagia is a consequence of cellular malnourishment when insulin deficiency prevents utilization of glucose for energy. Weight loss may occur because the body cannot get glucose and turns to other energy sources, such as fat and protein. Weakness and fatigue may result because body cells lack needed energy from glucose. Ketoacidosis, a complication most common in those with untreated type 1 diabetes, is associated with additional clinical manifestations and is discussed later in this chapter.

Type 2 Diabetes Mellitus. The clinical manifestations of type 2 diabetes are often nonspecific, although it is possible that an individual with type 2 diabetes will experience some of the classic symptoms associated with type 1 diabetes, including polyuria, polydipsia, and polyphagia. Some of the more common manifestations associated with type 2 diabetes are fatigue, recurrent infections, recurrent vaginal yeast or candidal infections, prolonged wound healing, and visual changes.

Diagnostic Studies

The diagnosis of diabetes mellitus is made through one of the following four methods.

1. A1C of 6.5% or higher.
2. Fasting plasma glucose (FPG) level greater than or equal to 126 mg/dL (7.0 mmol/L). *Fasting* is defined as no caloric intake for at least 8 hours.
3. Two-hour plasma glucose level greater than or equal to 200 mg/dL (11.1 mmol/L) during an OGTT, using a glucose load of 75 g.
4. In a patient with classic symptoms of hyperglycemia (polyuria, polydipsia, unexplained weight loss) or hyperglycemic crisis, a random plasma glucose greater than or equal to 200 mg/dL (11.1 mmol/L).

If a patient is seen with a hyperglycemic crisis or clear symptoms of hyperglycemia (polyuria, polydipsia, polyphagia) with a random plasma glucose greater than or equal to 200 mg/dL, repeat testing is not warranted.[3] Otherwise, criteria 1 through 3 should be confirmed by repeat testing to rule out laboratory error. It is preferable for the repeat test to be the same test used initially. For example, if a random blood glucose test showed an elevated blood glucose, that same test should be used again when the person is retested.

The accuracy of test results depends on adequate patient preparation and attention to the many factors that may influence the test results. For example, factors that can falsely elevate values include recent severe restrictions of dietary carbohydrate, acute illness, medications (e.g., contraceptives, corticosteroids), and restricted activity such as bed rest. A patient with impaired gastrointestinal absorption or one who has recently taken acetaminophen may have false-negative test results.

A1C measures the amount of glycosylated hemoglobin as a percentage of total hemoglobin (e.g., A1C of 6.5% means that 6.5% of the total hemoglobin has glucose attached to it). The amount of hemoglobin that is glycosylated depends on the blood glucose level. When blood glucose levels are elevated over time, the amount of glucose attached to hemoglobin molecules increases. This glucose remains attached to the red blood cell (RBC) for the life of the cell (approximately 120 days). Therefore the A1C test provides a measurement of glycemic control over the previous 2 to 3 months, with increases in the A1C reflecting elevated blood glucose levels. The A1C has several advantages over the FPG, including greater convenience, since fasting is not required.[3] Diseases affecting RBCs (e.g., iron deficiency anemia or sickle cell anemia) can influence the A1C and should be considered when interpreting test results.

A1C results may be reviewed with patients using the same units (mg/dL or mmol/L) that patients see routinely in blood glucose measurements. An *estimated average glucose* (eAG) can be determined from the A1C. The $eAG = 28.7 \times A1C - 46.7$, or the eAG may be obtained by using an online calculator at *http://professional.diabetes.org/glucosecalculator.aspx*. For example, an A1C of 8.0% is equivalent to a glucose level of 183 mg/dL.

All patients with diabetes and prediabetes should have their A1C monitored regularly to determine the success of the current treatment plan and make changes in the plan if glycemic goals are not achieved. The ADA identifies an A1C goal for patients with diabetes of less than 7.0%. The American College of Endocrinology recommends an A1C of less than 6.5%. When the A1C is maintained at near-normal levels, the risk for the development of microvascular and macrovascular complications is greatly reduced. For individuals with prediabetes, monitoring the A1C can detect overt diabetes and provide feedback on efforts to prevent diabetes.

Fructosamine can also be used to assess glucose control. Fructosamine is formed by a chemical reaction of glucose with plasma protein. It reflects glucose control in the previous 1 to 3 weeks. Fructosamine levels may show a change in glucose control before A1C does.

Islet cell autoantibody testing is primarily ordered to help distinguish between autoimmune type 1 diabetes and diabetes from other causes. Autoantibodies can develop to one or several of the autoantigens—GAD65, IA-2, or insulin.

Collaborative Care

The goals of diabetes management are to reduce symptoms, promote well-being, prevent acute complications of hyperglycemia, and prevent or delay the onset and progression of long-term complications. These goals are most likely to be met when the patient is able to maintain blood glucose levels as near to normal as possible. Diabetes is a chronic disease that requires daily decisions about food intake, blood glucose testing, medication, and exercise. Patient teaching, which enables the patient to become the most active participant in his or her own care, is essential to achieve glycemic goals. Nutritional therapy, drug therapy, exercise, and self-monitoring of blood glucose are the tools used in the management of diabetes (Table 49-2).

The three major types of glucose-lowering agents (GLAs) used in the treatment of diabetes are insulin, oral agents (OAs), and noninsulin injectable agents. All individuals with type 1 diabetes require insulin. For some people with type 2 diabetes, a regimen of proper nutrition, regular physical activity, and maintenance of desirable body weight is sufficient to attain optimal blood glucose control. However, eventually most people with type 2 diabetes will require medication management because diabetes is a progressive disease.

TABLE 49-2 COLLABORATIVE CARE

Diabetes Mellitus

Diagnostic
- History and physical examination
- Blood tests, including fasting blood glucose, postprandial blood glucose, A1C, fructosamine, lipid profile, blood urea nitrogen and serum creatinine, electrolytes, islet cell autoantibodies
- Urine for complete urinalysis, microalbuminuria, and acetone (if indicated)
- Blood pressure
- ECG (if indicated)
- Funduscopic examination (dilated eye examination)
- Dental examination
- Neurologic examination, including monofilament test for sensation to lower extremities
- Ankle-brachial index (ABI) (if indicated) (see Table 38-3)
- Foot (podiatric) examination
- Monitoring of weight

Collaborative Therapy
- Patient and caregiver teaching and follow-up programs
- Nutritional therapy (see Table 49-8)
- Exercise therapy (see Tables 49-9 and 49-10)
- Self-monitoring of blood glucose (SMBG) (see Table 49-11)
- Drug therapy
  - Insulin (see Fig. 49-3 and Tables 49-3 and 49-4)
  - Oral and noninsulin injectable agents (see Table 49-7)
  - Enteric-coated aspirin (81-162 mg/day)
  - Angiotensin-converting enzyme (ACE) inhibitors (see Table 33-7)
  - Angiotensin II receptor blockers (ARBs) (see Table 33-7)
  - Antihyperlipidemic drugs (see Table 34-5)

Drug Therapy: Insulin

Exogenous (injected) insulin is needed when a patient has inadequate insulin to meet specific metabolic needs. People with type 1 diabetes require exogenous insulin to survive and may need multiple daily injections of insulin (often four or more) or continuous insulin infusion via an insulin pump to adequately control blood glucose levels. People with type 2 diabetes may require exogenous insulin during periods of severe stress such as illness or surgery. In addition, since type 2 diabetes is a progressive disease, over time the combination of nutritional therapy, exercise, OAs, and noninsulin injectable agents may no longer adequately control blood glucose levels. At that point exogenous insulin would be added as a permanent part of the management plan. People with type 2 diabetes may also need up to four injections per day to adequately control their blood glucose levels. Occasionally insulin pumps are used for patients with type 2 diabetes who have not achieved good glycemic control with other therapies.

Types of Insulin. Today only genetically engineered human insulin made in laboratories is used. The insulin is derived from common bacteria (e.g., *Escherichia coli*) or yeast cells using recombinant deoxyribonucleic acid (DNA) technology (see eFig. 14-1 available on the website for Chapter 14). In the past, insulin was extracted from beef and pork pancreas, but their use was associated with high rates of allergic reactions and complications. These forms of insulin are no longer available.

Insulins differ by their onset, peak action, and duration (Fig. 49-3) and are categorized as rapid-acting, short-acting, intermediate-acting, and long-acting insulin (Table 49-3).

Insulin Regimens. Examples of insulin regimens are presented in Table 49-4. The insulin regimen that most closely mimics endogenous insulin production is the basal-bolus regimen, which uses rapid- or short-acting (bolus) insulin before meals and intermediate- or long-acting (basal) background insulin once or twice a day. The basal-bolus regimen is intensive insulin therapy, consisting of multiple daily insulin injections together with frequent self-monitoring of blood

---

TABLE 49-3 DRUG THERAPY

Types of Insulin

Classification	Examples	Clarity of Solution
Rapid-acting insulin	lispro (Humalog) aspart (NovoLog) glulisine (Apidra)	Clear
Short-acting insulin	regular (Humulin R, Novolin R)	Clear
Intermediate-acting insulin	NPH (Humulin N, Novolin N)	Cloudy
Long-acting insulin	glargine (Lantus) detemir (Levemir)	Clear
Combination therapy (premixed)	NPH/regular 70/30* (Humulin 70/30, Novolin 70/30) NPH/regular 50/50* (Humulin 50/50) lispro protamine/lispro 75/25* (Humalog Mix 75/25) lispro protamine/lispro 50/50* (Humalog Mix 50/50) aspart protamine/aspart 70/30* (NovoLog Mix 70/30)	Cloudy

*These numbers refer to percentages of each type of insulin.

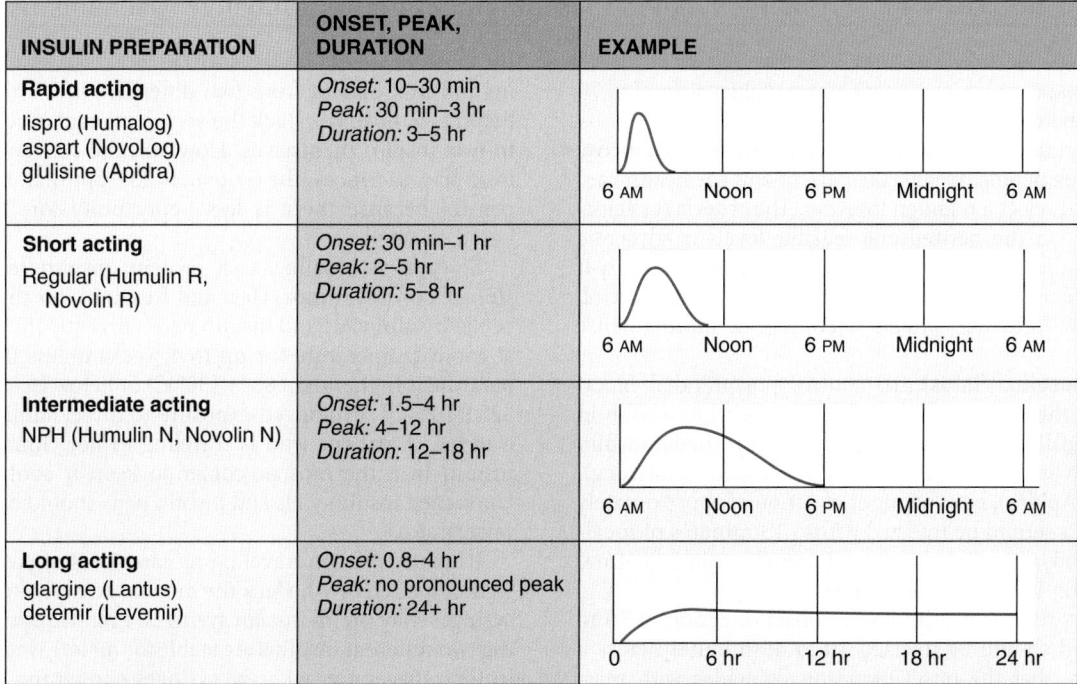

INSULIN PREPARATION	ONSET, PEAK, DURATION	EXAMPLE
Rapid acting lispro (Humalog) aspart (NovoLog) glulisine (Apidra)	*Onset:* 10–30 min *Peak:* 30 min–3 hr *Duration:* 3–5 hr	6 AM　Noon　6 PM　Midnight　6 AM
Short acting Regular (Humulin R, 　Novolin R)	*Onset:* 30 min–1 hr *Peak:* 2–5 hr *Duration:* 5–8 hr	6 AM　Noon　6 PM　Midnight　6 AM
Intermediate acting NPH (Humulin N, Novolin N)	*Onset:* 1.5–4 hr *Peak:* 4–12 hr *Duration:* 12–18 hr	6 AM　Noon　6 PM　Midnight　6 AM
Long acting glargine (Lantus) detemir (Levemir)	*Onset:* 0.8–4 hr *Peak:* no pronounced peak *Duration:* 24+ hr	0　6 hr　12 hr　18 hr　24 hr

FIG. 49-3 Commercially available insulin preparations showing onset, peak, and duration of action. Individual patient responses to each type of insulin are different and affected by many different factors.

TABLE 49-4　DRUG THERAPY

Insulin Regimens

Regimen	Type of Insulin and Frequency	Action Profile	Comments
Once a day Single dose	Intermediate (NPH) *At bedtime*	7 AM　Noon　6 PM　Midnight　7 AM	One injection should provide nighttime coverage.
	OR Long-acting (glargine [Lantus], detemir [Levemir]) *In AM or at bedtime*	7 AM　Noon　6 PM　Midnight　7 AM	One injection will last 24 hr with no peaks and less chance for hypoglycemia. Does not cover postprandial blood glucose levels.
Twice a day Split-mixed dose	NPH and regular or rapid (both regular and rapid are shown on the diagram) *Before breakfast and at dinner*	7 AM　Noon　6 PM　Midnight　7 AM	Two injections provide coverage for 24 hr. Patient must adhere to a set meal plan.
Three times a day Combination of mixed and single dose	NPH and regular or rapid (both regular and rapid are shown on the diagram) *Before breakfast* + Regular or rapid *Before dinner* + NPH *At bedtime*	7 AM　Noon　7 PM 9 PM　Midnight　7 AM	Three injections provide coverage for 24 hr, particularly during early AM hours. Decreased potential for 2-3 AM hypoglycemia.
Basal-bolus Multiple dose	Regular or rapid (both regular and rapid are shown on the diagram) *Before breakfast, lunch, and dinner* + Long-acting (glargine or detemir) *Once a day* OR Regular or rapid (both regular and rapid are shown on the diagram) *Before breakfast, lunch, and dinner* + NPH *Twice a day*	7 AM　Noon　6 PM　Midnight　7 AM 7 AM　Noon　6 PM　Midnight　7 AM	More flexibility is allowed at mealtimes and for amount of food intake. Good postprandial control. Preprandial blood glucose checks and establishing and following individualized algorithms are necessary. Patients with type 1 diabetes require basal insulin to cover 24 hr. Most physiologic approach, except for pump.

─────── Rapid-acting (lispro, aspart, glulisine) insulin.
─────── Short-acting (regular) insulin.
- - - - - - - Intermediate-acting (NPH) or long-acting (glargine, detemir) insulin.

glucose. The goal is to achieve a near-normal glucose level of 70 to 130 mg/dL before meals.

Other, less intense regimens can also give good glucose control for some people. Ideally, the patient and the health care provider should select a regimen together. The criteria for selection are based on the desired and feasible levels of glycemic control and the patient's lifestyle, diet, and activity patterns. If a less intense regimen is not giving the person optimal control, the health care provider should encourage a more intense approach.

Mealtime Insulin (Bolus). To control postprandial blood glucose levels, the timing of rapid- and short-acting insulin in relation to meals is crucial. Rapid-acting synthetic insulin analogs, which include lispro (Humalog), aspart (NovoLog), and glulisine (Apidra), have an onset of action of approximately 15 minutes and should be injected within 15 minutes of mealtime. The rapid-acting analogs most closely mimic natural insulin secretion in response to a meal.

Short-acting regular insulin has an onset of action of 30 to 60 minutes and should be injected 30 to 45 minutes before a meal to ensure that the onset of action coincides with meal absorption. Because timing an injection 30 to 45 minutes before a meal is difficult for people to incorporate into their lifestyles, the flexibility that rapid-acting insulins offer is preferred by those taking insulin with their meals.[9] Short-acting insulin is also more likely to cause hypoglycemia because of a longer duration of action.

Long- or Intermediate-Acting (Basal) Background Insulin. In addition to mealtime insulin, people with type 1 diabetes must also use a long- or intermediate-acting basal (background) insulin to control blood glucose levels in between meals and overnight. Without 24-hour background insulin, people with type 1 diabetes are more prone to developing DKA.

Many people with type 2 diabetes who use oral medications also require insulin to adequately control blood glucose levels. The long-acting insulins, glargine (Lantus) and detemir (Levemir), are often added to the medication regimen. This type of insulin is released steadily and continuously, and for most people do not have a peak of action (see Fig. 49-3). Although they are typically used for once-daily subcutaneous administration, detemir can be given twice daily. Because they lack peak action time, the risk for hypoglycemia from this type of insulin is greatly reduced. Glargine and detemir must not be diluted or mixed with any other insulin or solution in the same syringe. Mealtime insulin may also be added if oral agents and long-acting insulin are not adequate to achieve glycemic goals.

Intermediate-acting insulin (NPH) is also used as a basal insulin. It has a duration of 12 to 18 hours. The disadvantage of NPH is that it has a peak ranging from 4 to 12 hours, which can result in hypoglycemia. NPH is the only basal insulin that can be mixed with short- and rapid-acting insulins. NPH is a cloudy insulin that must be gently agitated before administration.

Combination Insulin Therapy. For those who want to use only one or two injections per day, a short- or rapid-acting insulin is mixed with intermediate-acting insulin in the same syringe. This allows the patient to have both mealtime and basal coverage without having to administer two separate injections. Although this may be more appealing to the patient, most patients achieve better control with basal-bolus therapy. Patients may mix the two types of insulin themselves or may use a commercially premixed formula or pen (see Table 49-3). Premixed formulas offer convenience to patients, who do not have to draw up and mix insulin from two different vials. This is especially helpful to those who lack the visual, manual, or cognitive skills to mix insulin themselves. However, the convenience of these formulas sacrifices the potential for optimal blood glucose control because there is less opportunity for flexible dosing based on need.

Storage of Insulin. As a protein, insulin requires special storage considerations. Heat and freezing alter the insulin molecule. Insulin vials and insulin pens currently in use may be left at room temperature for up to 4 weeks unless the room temperature is higher than 86° F (30° C) or below freezing (less than 32° F [0° C]). Prolonged exposure to direct sunlight should be avoided. A patient who is traveling in hot climates may store insulin in a thermos or cooler to keep it cool (not frozen). Unopened insulin vials and insulin pens should be stored in the refrigerator.

Patients who are traveling or caregivers of patients who are sight impaired or who lack the manual dexterity to fill their own syringes may prefill insulin syringes. Prefilled syringes containing two different insulins are stable for up to 1 week when stored in the refrigerator, whereas syringes containing only one type of insulin are stable up to 30 days.[10]

Syringes should be stored in a vertical position with the needle pointed up to avoid clumping of suspended insulin in the needle. Before injection, gently roll prefilled syringes between the palms 10 to 20 times to warm the insulin and resuspend the particles. Some insulin combinations are not appropriate for prefilling and storage because the mixture can alter the onset, action, and/or peak times of either of the types. Consult a pharmacy reference as needed when mixing and prefilling different types of insulin.

Administration of Insulin. Routine doses of insulin are usually administered by subcutaneous injection. Regular insulin can be given IV when immediate onset of action is desired. Insulin is not taken orally because it is inactivated by gastric juices.

Insulin Injection. The steps in administering a subcutaneous insulin injection are outlined in Table 49-5. Teach this technique to new insulin users and review periodically with long-term users. Never assume that because the patient already uses insulin, he or she knows and practices the correct insulin injection technique. The patient may not have understood prior instructions, or changes in eyesight may result in inaccurate preparation. The patient may not see air bubbles in the syringe or may improperly read the scale on the syringe. The patient receiving mixed insulins in the same syringe needs to learn the proper technique for combining them if commercially prepared premixed insulins are not used (Fig. 49-4).

The speed with which peak serum concentrations are reached varies with the anatomic site for injection. The fastest subcutaneous absorption is from the abdomen, followed by the arm, thigh, and buttock. Although the abdomen is the preferred injection site, other sites are appropriate as well (Fig. 49-5). Caution the patient about injecting into a site that is to be exercised. For example, the patient should not inject insulin into the thigh and then go jogging. Exercise of the injection site, together with the increased body heat and circulation generated by the exercise, may increase the rate of absorption and speed the onset of insulin action.

Teach patients to rotate the injection within one anatomic site, such as the abdomen, for at least 1 week before using a different site, such as the right thigh. This allows for better

TABLE 49-5	**PATIENT & CAREGIVER TEACHING GUIDE**

Insulin Therapy

Include the following instructions when teaching the patient and caregiver about insulin therapy.

1. Wash hands thoroughly.
2. Always inspect insulin bottle before using it. Make sure that it is the proper type and concentration, expiration date has not passed, and top of bottle is in perfect condition. The insulin (except for NPH) should look clear and colorless. Discard if it appears discolored or if you see particles in the solution.
3. If insulin solutions are cloudy (see Table 49-3), gently roll the insulin bottle between the palms of hands to mix the insulin.
4. Select proper injection site (see Fig. 49-5).
5. Cleanse the skin with soap and water or alcohol.
6. Pinch up the skin, and push the needle straight into the pinched-up area (90-degree angle). If you are very thin or using a ⁵⁄₁₆-in needle, you may need to use a 45-degree angle.
7. Push the plunger all the way down, let go of pinched skin, leave needle in place for 5 sec to ensure that all insulin has been injected, and then remove needle.
8. Destroy and dispose of single-use syringe safely.

insulin absorption. It may be helpful to think of the abdomen as a checkerboard, with each ½-in square representing an injection site. Injections are rotated systematically across the board, with each injection site at least ½ to 1 in away from the previous injection site.

Most commercial insulin is available as U100, indicating that 1 mL contains 100 U of insulin. U100 insulin must be used with a U100-marked syringe. Disposable plastic insulin syringes are available in a variety of sizes, including 1.0, 0.5, and 0.3 mL. The 0.5-mL size may be used for doses of 50 U or less, and the 0.3-mL syringe can be used for doses of 30 U or less. The 0.5- and 0.3-mL syringes are in 1-U increments. This provides more accurate delivery when the dose is an odd number. The 1.0-mL syringe is necessary for patients who require more than 50 U of insulin. The 1.0-mL syringe is in 2-U increments. When patients change from a 0.3- or a 0.5-mL to a 1.0-mL syringe, make them aware of the dose increment difference.

Insulin syringe needles come in the following lengths: 6 mm (¼ in), 8 mm (⁵⁄₁₆ in), and 12.7 mm (½ in).[11] Needle gauges also vary among syringes. The needle gauges available are 28, 29, 30, and 31. The higher the gauge number, the smaller the diameter, thus resulting in a more comfortable injection. Only the person using the syringe should recap the needle; never recap a needle used for a patient. The use of an alcohol swab on the site before self-injection is no longer recommended. Routine hygiene such as washing with soap and rinsing with water is adequate. This applies primarily to patient self-injection technique. When injection occurs in a health care facility, policy may dictate site preparation with alcohol to prevent health care–associated infection (HAI). Perform injections at a 45- to 90-degree angle, depending on the thickness of the patient's fat pad.

An insulin pen is a compact portable device loaded with an insulin cartridge that serves the same function as a needle and syringe (Fig. 49-6). Pen needles are available in lengths of 4 mm (⁵⁄₃₂ in), 5 mm (³⁄₁₆ in), 8 mm (⁵⁄₁₆ in), and 12.7 mm (½ in) and in three gauges, 29, 31, and 32. Many patients prefer using insulin pens because of greater convenience and flexibility.[12] They are portable and compact, are more discreet than using a vial and syringe, and provide consistent and accurate dosing.

1 Wash hands.
2 Gently rotate NPH insulin bottle.
3 Wipe off tops of insulin vials with alcohol sponge.
4 Draw back amount of air into the syringe that equals total dose.

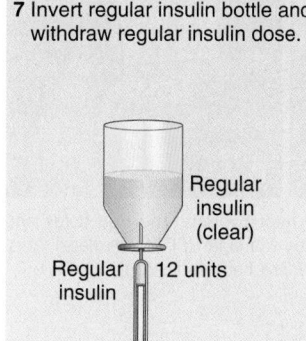
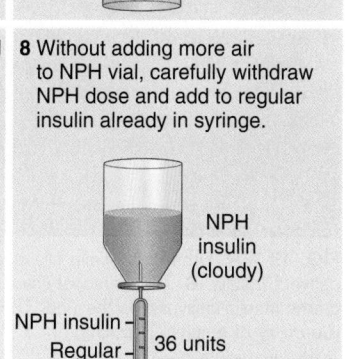

5 Inject air equal to NPH dose into NPH vial. Remove syringe from vial.

36 units

36 U Air NPH insulin (cloudy)

6 Inject air equal to regular dose into regular vial.

12 units

12 U Air Regular insulin (clear)

7 Invert regular insulin bottle and withdraw regular insulin dose.

Regular insulin (clear)

Regular insulin   12 units

8 Without adding more air to NPH vial, carefully withdraw NPH dose and add to regular insulin already in syringe.

NPH insulin (cloudy)

NPH insulin
Regular insulin   36 units
48 units (total dose)

FIG. 49-4 Mixing insulins. This step-order process avoids the problem of contaminating regular insulin with intermediate-acting insulin.

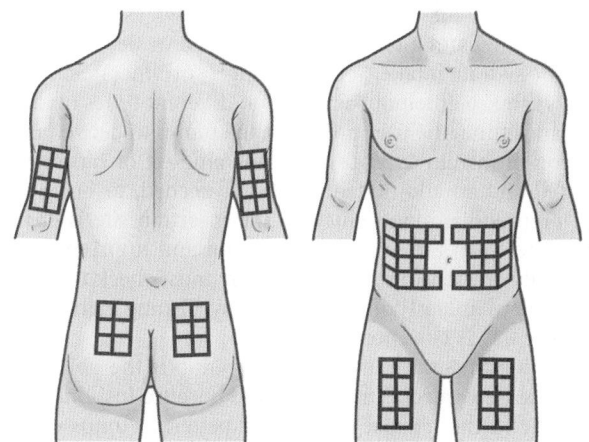

FIG. 49-5 Injection sites for insulin.

For patients with poor vision, the pen is a better option, since they can hear the clicks of the pen as the dose is selected. Insulin pens come packaged with printed instructions, including pictures of the steps to take when using the pen. These instructions are helpful when teaching new users and reviewing technique with current users of a pen.

Insulin Pump. Continuous subcutaneous insulin infusion can be administered using an *insulin pump*, a small battery-operated device that resembles a standard paging device in size

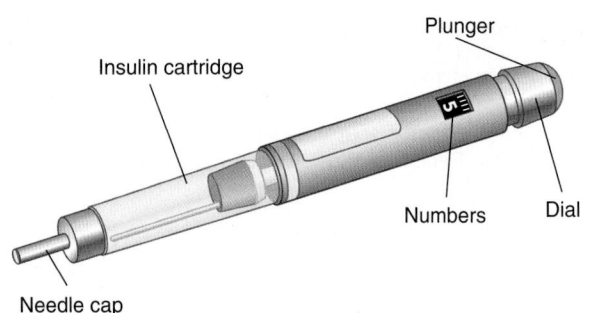

FIG. 49-6 Parts of insulin pen.

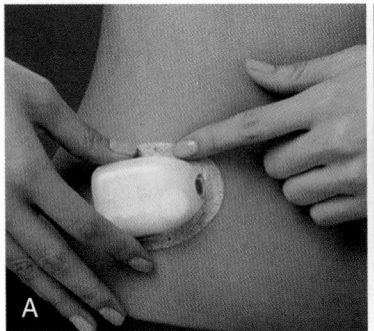
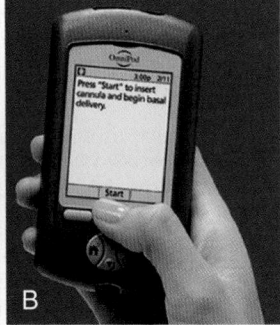

FIG. 49-7 A, OmniPod Insulin Management System. The Pod holds and delivers insulin. **B,** The Personal Diabetes Manager (PDM) wirelessly programs insulin delivery via the Pod. The PDM has a built-in glucose meter. (Courtesy of Insulet Corporation.)

and appearance. Most insulin pumps are worn on the belt or under clothing and loaded with rapid-acting insulin, which is connected via plastic tubing to a catheter inserted into the subcutaneous tissue in the abdominal wall. Insulet Corporation has an insulin pump that is a tubing-free system (Fig. 49-7). All insulin pumps are programmed to deliver a continuous infusion of rapid-acting insulin 24 hours a day, known as the *basal rate.* Basal insulin can be temporarily increased or decreased based on carbohydrate intake, activity changes, or illness. Some individuals require different basal rates at different times of the day.

At mealtime, the user programs the pump to deliver a bolus infusion of insulin appropriate to the amount of carbohydrate ingested and an additional amount, if needed, to bring down high preprandial blood glucose. The insertion site is changed every 2 to 3 days to avoid site infection and to promote good insulin absorption. Insulin pump users must check their blood glucose level at least four times per day. Testing eight times or more per day is common.

A major advantage of the insulin pump is the potential for tight glucose control. This is possible because insulin delivery is similar to the normal physiologic pattern. Pumps offer the benefit of a more normal lifestyle, allowing users more flexibility with meal and activity patterns. Problems and complications of insulin pump therapy are infection at the insertion site, an increased risk for DKA if the insulin infusion is disrupted because of a problem at the infusion site, and the increased cost of the pump and supplies.[13]

Problems With Insulin Therapy. Problems associated with insulin therapy include hypoglycemia, allergic reactions, lipodystrophy, and the Somogyi effect. Hypoglycemia is discussed in detail later in this chapter. (Guidelines for assessing patients treated with insulin and other GLAs are presented in Table 49-6.)

TABLE 49-6	ASSESSING THE PATIENT TREATED WITH GLUCOSE-LOWERING AGENTS
Category	**Assessment**
For Patient With Newly Diagnosed Diabetes or for Reevaluation of Drug Regimen	
Cognitive	• Is patient or caregiver able to understand why insulin or OAs are being used as part of diabetes management?
	• Is patient or caregiver able to understand concepts of asepsis, combining insulins, and side effects of medications?
	• Is patient able to remember to take >1 dose/day?
	• Does patient take medications at right times in relation to meals?
Psychomotor	• Is patient or caregiver physically able to prepare and administer accurate doses of the drugs?
Affective	• What emotions and attitudes are patient and caregiver displaying concerning diagnosis of diabetes and insulin or OA treatment?
For Follow-up of GLA-Treated Patient	
Effectiveness of therapy	• Is patient having symptoms of hyperglycemia?
	• Does blood glucose record show good or poor control?
	• Is A1C consistent with glucose records?
Side effects of therapy	• Is atrophy or hypertrophy present at injection sites?
	• Has patient had hypoglycemic episodes? If so, how often? What time of day? What were the symptoms of hypoglycemia?
	• Are there complaints of nightmares, night sweats, or early morning headaches?
	• Has patient had a skin rash or GI upset since taking OAs?
	• Has patient gained or lost weight?
Self-management behaviors	• If patient is having hyperglycemic or hypoglycemic episodes, how are those episodes managed?
	• Has patient analyzed episodes to determine reason for hyperglycemic or hypoglycemic episodes?
	• How much insulin or OA is patient taking and at what time of day? Is patient adjusting insulin dose? Under what circumstances and by how much?
	• Has exercise pattern changed?
	• Is patient adhering to the meal plan? Are meals taken at times corresponding to peak insulin action?

A1C, Glycosylated hemoglobin; *GLA,* glucose-lowering agent; *OA,* oral agent.

Allergic Reactions. Local inflammatory reactions to insulin may occur, such as itching, erythema, and burning around the injection site. Local reactions may be self-limiting within 1 to 3 months or may improve with a low dose of antihistamine. A true insulin allergy is rare. It is manifested by a systemic response with urticaria and possibly anaphylactic shock. Zinc or protamine used as a preservative in the insulin and the latex or rubber stoppers on the vials have been implicated in allergic reactions.

Lipodystrophy. *Lipodystrophy* (atrophy of subcutaneous tissue) may occur if the same injection sites are used frequently. The use of human insulin has significantly reduced the risk for lipodystrophy. *Hypertrophy,* a thickening of the subcutaneous tissue, eventually regresses if the patient does not use the site for at least 6 months. The use of hypertrophied sites may result in erratic insulin absorption.

Somogyi Effect and Dawn Phenomenon. Hyperglycemia in the morning may be due to the Somogyi effect. A high dose of insulin produces a decline in blood glucose levels during the night. As a result, counterregulatory hormones (e.g., glucagon, epinephrine, growth hormone, cortisol) are released, stimulating lipolysis, gluconeogenesis, and glycogenolysis, which in turn produce rebound hyperglycemia. The danger of this effect is that when blood glucose levels are measured in the morning, hyperglycemia is apparent and the patient (or the health care professional) may increase the insulin dose.

If a patient is experiencing morning hyperglycemia, checking blood glucose levels between 2:00 and 4:00 AM for hypoglycemia will help determine if the cause is the Somogyi effect. The patient may report headaches on awakening and recall having night sweats or nightmares. A bedtime snack, a reduction in the dose of insulin, or both can help to prevent the Somogyi effect.

The dawn phenomenon is also characterized by hyperglycemia that is present on awakening. It has been suggested that two counterregulatory hormones, growth hormone and cortisol, excreted in increased amounts in the early morning hours are responsible. The dawn phenomenon affects a majority of people with diabetes and tends to be most severe when growth hormone is at its peak in adolescence and young adulthood.

Careful assessment is required to document the Somogyi effect or dawn phenomenon because the treatment for each differs. The treatment for Somogyi effect is less insulin. The treatment for dawn phenomenon is an increase in insulin or an adjustment in administration time. Your assessment must include insulin dose, injection sites, and variability in the time of meals or insulin administration. Ask the patient to measure and document bedtime, nighttime (between 2:00 and 4:00 AM), and morning fasting blood glucose levels on several occasions. If the predawn levels are less than 60 mg/dL (3.3 mmol/L) and signs and symptoms of hypoglycemia are present, the insulin dosage should be reduced. If the 2:00 to 4:00 AM blood glucose is high, the insulin dosage should be increased. In addition, counsel the patient on appropriate bedtime snacks.

Drug Therapy: Oral and Noninsulin Injectable Agents

OAs and noninsulin injectable agents work to improve the mechanisms by which the body produces and uses insulin and glucose. These drugs work on three defects of type 2 diabetes: (1) insulin resistance, (2) decreased insulin production, and (3) increased hepatic glucose production. These drugs may be used in combination with agents from other classes or with insulin to achieve blood glucose goals. Oral and noninsulin injectable agents are listed in Table 49-7.

Biguanides. The most widely used oral diabetes agent is metformin, the only medication in the biguanide class available in the United States. Forms of metformin include Glucophage (immediate release), Glucophage XR (extended release), Fortamet (extended release), and Riomet (liquid form of metformin). The primary action of metformin is to reduce glucose production by the liver. It also enhances insulin sensitivity at the tissue level and improves glucose transport into the cells. Additionally, it has beneficial effects on plasma lipids.

Metformin is the first-choice drug for most people with type 2 diabetes.[14] Because it may cause moderate weight loss, met-

formin may be useful for people with type 2 diabetes and prediabetes who are overweight or obese. It is also used in the prevention of type 2 diabetes in those with prediabetes who are less than age 60 and have risk factors such as hypertension or a history of gestational diabetes.

Patients who are undergoing surgery or any radiologic procedures that involve the use of a contrast medium are instructed to temporarily discontinue metformin before surgery or the procedure. They should not resume the metformin until 48 hours afterward, once their serum creatinine has been checked and is normal.[10]

DRUG ALERT: Metformin
- Do not use in patients with kidney disease, liver disease, or heart failure. Lactic acidosis is a rare complication of metformin accumulation.
- IV contrast media that contain iodine pose a risk of acute kidney injury, which could exacerbate metformin-induced lactic acidosis.
- To reduce risk of kidney injury, discontinue metformin a day or two before the procedure.
- May be resumed 48 hours after the procedure assuming kidney function is normal.
- Do not use in people who drink excessive amounts of alcohol.

Sulfonylureas. Sulfonylureas include glipizide (Glucotrol, Glucotrol XL), glyburide (Micronase, DiaBeta, Glynase), and glimepiride (Amaryl). The primary action of the sulfonylureas is to increase insulin production by the pancreas. Therefore hypoglycemia is the major side effect with sulfonylureas.

Meglitinides. Like the sulfonylureas, repaglinide (Prandin) and nateglinide (Starlix) increase insulin production by the pancreas. However, because they are more rapidly absorbed and eliminated than sulfonylureas, they are less likely to cause hypoglycemia. When they are taken just before meals, pancreatic insulin production increases during and after the meal, mimicking the normal response to eating. Instruct patients to take meglitinides any time from 30 minutes before each meal right up to the time of the meal. These drugs should not be taken if a meal is skipped.

α-Glucosidase Inhibitors. Also known as "starch blockers," these drugs work by slowing down the absorption of carbohydrate in the small intestine. Acarbose (Precose) and miglitol (Glyset) are the available drugs in this class. Taken with the first bite of each main meal, they are most effective in lowering postprandial blood glucose. Their effectiveness is measured by checking 2-hour postprandial glucose levels.

Thiazolidinediones. Sometimes referred to as "insulin sensitizers," these agents include pioglitazone (Actos) and rosiglitazone (Avandia). They are most effective for people who have insulin resistance. These agents improve insulin sensitivity, transport, and utilization at target tissues. Because they do not increase insulin production, thiazolidinediones do not cause hypoglycemia when used alone. However, these drugs are rarely used today because of their adverse effects. Rosiglitazone is associated with adverse cardiovascular events (e.g., myocardial infarction) and can be obtained only through restricted access programs. Pioglitazone can worsen heart failure and is associated with an increased risk of bladder cancer.

Dipeptidyl Peptidase-4 (DPP-4) Inhibitors. Incretin hormones are released by the intestines throughout the day, but levels increase in response to a meal. When glucose levels are normal or elevated, incretins increase insulin synthesis and release from the pancreas, as well as decrease hepatic glucose production. The incretin hormones are normally inactivated by dipeptidyl peptidase-4 (DPP-4).

TABLE 49-7   DRUG THERAPY

Oral Agents and Noninsulin Injectable Agents

Type	Mechanism of Action	Side Effects
Oral Agents		
Biguanide		
metformin (Glucophage, Glucophage XR, Riomet, Fortamet, Glumetza)	Decreases rate of hepatic glucose production; augment glucose by tissues, especially muscles.	Diarrhea, lactic acidosis. Needs to be held 1-2 days before IV contrast media given and for 48 hr after.
Sulfonylureas		
glipizide (Glucotrol, Glucotrol XL)	Stimulate release of insulin from pancreatic islets.	Weight gain, hypoglycemia.
glyburide (Micronase, DiaBeta, Glynase PresTab)	Decrease glycogenolysis and gluconeogenesis. Enhance cellular sensitivity to insulin.	
glimepiride (Amaryl)		
Meglitinides		
nateglinide (Starlix)	Stimulate a rapid and short-lived release of insulin from the pancreas.	Weight gain, hypoglycemia.
repaglinide (Prandin)		
α-Glucosidase Inhibitors		
acarbose (Precose)	Delay absorption of glucose from GI tract.	Gas, abdominal pain, diarrhea.
miglitol (Glyset)		
Thiazolidinediones		
pioglitazone (Actos)	Increase glucose uptake in muscle; decrease endogenous glucose production.	Weight gain, edema.
rosiglitazone (Avandia)		*pioglitazone:* increases risk for bladder cancer and exacerbates heart failure.
		rosiglitazone: increases risk for cardiovascular events (e.g., myocardial infarction, stroke).
Dipeptidyl Peptidase-4 (DPP-4) Inhibitors		
linagliptin (Tradjenta)	Enhance activity of incretins, stimulate release of insulin from pancreatic β cells, decrease hepatic glucose production.	Pancreatitis, allergic reactions.
saxagliptin (Onglyza)		
sitagliptin (Januvia)		
alogliptin (Nesina)		
Dopamine Agonist		
bromocriptine (Cycloset)	Activates dopamine receptors in the central nervous system. Unknown how it improves glycemic control.	Orthostatic hypotension.
Combination Therapy		
Glucovance	metformin and glyburide	See side effects for individual drugs.
Metaglip	metformin and glipizide	Same as above.
Avandamet	rosiglitazone and metformin	Same as above.
Duetact	pioglitazone and glimepiride	Same as above.
Actoplus Met, Actoplus Met XR	metformin and pioglitazone	Same as above.
Janumet, Janumet XR	metformin and sitagliptin	Same as above.
Jentadueto	linagliptin and metformin	Same as above.
PrandiMet	metformin and repaglinide	Same as above.
Avandaryl	rosiglitazone and glimepiride	Same as above.
Juvisync	sitagliptin and simvastatin	Same as above.
Kombiglyze	saxagliptin and metformin	Same as above.
Kazano	alogliptin and metformin	Same as above.
Oseni	alogliptin and pioglitazone	Same as above.
Noninsulin Injectable Agents		
Glucagon-Like Peptide-1 (GLP-1) Receptor Agonists*		
exenatide (Byetta)	Stimulate release of insulin, decrease glucagon secretion and gastric emptying; increase satiety.	Nausea, vomiting, hypoglycemia, diarrhea, headache.
exenatide extended-release (Bydureon)		
liraglutide (Victoza)		
Amylin Analog†		
pramlintide (Symlin)	Decreases gastric emptying, glucagon secretion, and endogenous glucose output from liver. Increases satiety.	Hypoglycemia, nausea, vomiting, decreased appetite, headache.

*Administered subcutaneously
†Administered subcutaneously only in abdomen or thigh.

DPP-4 inhibitors (also known as gliptins) include sitagliptin (Januvia), saxagliptin (Onglyza), linagliptin (Tradjenta), and alogliptin (Nesina). DPP-4 inhibitors block the action of the DPP-4 enzyme, which is responsible for inactivating incretin hormones (gastric inhibitory peptide [GIP] and glucagon-like peptide-1 [GLP-1]). The result is an increase in insulin release, decrease in glucagon secretion, and decrease in hepatic glucose production. Since the DPP-4 inhibitors are glucose dependent, they lower the potential for hypoglycemia. The main benefit of these drugs over other medications for diabetes with similar effects is the absence of weight gain as a side effect.

Sodium-Glucose Co-Transporter 2 (SGLT2) Inhibitors. Canagliflozin (Invokana) is the first drug in a new class of drugs known as sodium-glucose co-transporter 2 (SGLT2) inhibitors. It works by blocking the reabsorption of glucose by the kidney, increasing glucose excretion, and lowering blood glucose levels in diabetics.

Dopamine Receptor Agonist. Bromocriptine (Cycloset) is a dopamine receptor agonist that improves glycemic control. The mechanism of action is unknown. Patients with type 2 diabetes are thought to have low levels of dopamine activity in the morning. These low levels of dopamine may interfere with the body's ability to control blood glucose. Bromocriptine increases dopamine receptor activity. It can be used alone or as an add-on to another type 2 diabetes treatment.

Combination Oral Therapy. Many combination drugs are currently available. These drugs combine two different classes of medications to treat diabetes. Examples of these agents are listed in Table 49-7. One advantage of combined therapy is improved patient adherence.

Glucagon-Like Peptide Receptor Agonists. Exenatide (Byetta), exenatide extended-release (Bydureon), and liraglutide (Victoza) simulate GLP-1 (one of the incretin hormones), which is found to be decreased in people with type 2 diabetes. These drugs increase insulin synthesis and release from the pancreas, inhibit glucagon secretion, decrease gastric emptying, and reduce food intake by increasing satiety.

These drugs may be used as monotherapy or adjunct therapy for patients with type 2 diabetes who have not achieved optimal glucose control on OAs. Exenatide and liraglutide are administered using a subcutaneous injection in a prefilled pen. In contrast to exenatide, which is given twice a day, and liraglutide, which is given once daily, Bydureon is given once every 7 days. The delayed gastric emptying that occurs with these medications may affect the absorption of oral medications. Advise patients to take fast-acting oral medications at least 1 hour before injecting exenatide or liraglutide.

DRUG ALERT: Exenatide (Byetta)
- Acute pancreatitis and kidney problems have been associated with its use.

DRUG ALERT: Liraglutide (Victoza)
- Do not use in patients with a personal or family history of medullary thyroid cancer.
- Acute pancreatitis has been associated with its use.

Amylin Analog. Pramlintide (Symlin) is the only available amylin analog. Amylin, a hormone secreted by the β cells of the pancreas in response to food intake, slows gastric emptying, reduces glucagon secretion, and increases satiety.[10] Pramlintide is used in addition to mealtime insulin in patients with type 1 or type 2 diabetes who do not have good glucose control on ideal insulin therapy. It is only used concurrently with insulin and is not a replacement for insulin. Pramlintide is adminis-

tered before major meals subcutaneously into the thigh or abdomen. It cannot be injected into the arm because absorption from this site is too variable. The drug cannot be mixed in the same syringe with insulin.

The concurrent use of pramlintide and insulin increases the risk of severe hypoglycemia during the 3 hours after injection, especially in patients with type 1 diabetes. Instruct patients to eat a meal with at least 250 calories and keep a form of fast-acting glucose on hand in the event that hypoglycemia develops. When pramlintide is used, the bolus dose of insulin should be reduced.

DRUG ALERT: Pramlintide (Symlin)
- Can cause severe hypoglycemia when used with insulin.

Other Drugs Affecting Blood Glucose Levels. Both the patient and the health care provider must be aware of drug interactions that can potentiate hypoglycemic and hyperglycemic effects. For example, β-adrenergic blockers can mask symptoms of hypoglycemia and prolong the hypoglycemic effects of insulin. Thiazide and loop diuretics can potentiate hyperglycemia by inducing potassium loss, although low-dose therapy with a thiazide is usually considered safe. See eTable 49-1 (available on the website) for a list of medications that may influence glycemic control.

Nutritional Therapy

Individualized nutritional therapy, consisting of counseling, education, and ongoing monitoring, is a cornerstone of care for people with diabetes and prediabetes.[15] Adherence to a dietary regimen is challenging for many people. Achieving nutritional goals requires a coordinated team effort that takes into account the person's behavioral, cognitive, socioeconomic, cultural, and religious backgrounds and preferences. Because of these complexities, it is recommended that a dietitian with expertise in diabetes management take the lead. The dietitian should conduct a dietary assessment and develop an individualized food plan. Additional team members may include nurses, certified diabetes educators, clinical nurse specialists, health care providers, and social workers.

Guidelines from the ADA indicate that, within the context of an overall healthy eating plan, a person with diabetes can eat the same foods as a person who does not have diabetes. This means that the same principles of good nutrition that apply to the general population also apply to the person with diabetes. Table 49-8 describes nutritional therapy for patients with diabetes. According to the ADA, the overall goal of nutrition therapy is to assist people with diabetes in making healthy nutritional choices that will lead to improved metabolic control. Additional specific goals include the following:

- Maintain blood glucose levels as near normal as safely possible to prevent or reduce the risk for complications of diabetes.
- Achieve lipid profiles and BP levels that reduce the risk for CVD.
- Prevent or slow the rate of development of chronic complications of diabetes by modifying nutrient intake and lifestyle.
- Address individual nutritional needs while taking into account personal and cultural preferences and respecting the individual's willingness to change eating and dietary habits.
- Maintain the pleasure of eating by allowing as many food choices as appropriate.

TABLE 49-8 NUTRITIONAL THERAPY

Diabetes Mellitus

Component	Recommendations
Total carbohydrate	• Minimum of 130 g/day. • Include carbohydrate from fruits, vegetables, grains, legumes, and low-fat milk. • Monitor by carbohydrate counting, exchange lists, or use of appropriate proportions (eFig. 49-1). • Glycemic index may provide additional benefit. • Sucrose-containing food can be substituted for other carbohydrates in the meal plan. • Fiber intake at 25-30 g/day. • Nonnutritive sweeteners are safe when consumed within FDA daily intake levels.
Protein	• 15%-20% of total calories. • High-protein diets are not recommended for weight loss.
Fat	• Limit saturated fat to <7% of total calories. • *Trans* fat should be minimized. • Dietary cholesterol <200 mg/day. • ≥2 servings of fish per week to provide polyunsaturated fatty acids.
Alcohol	• Limit to moderate amount (maximum 1 drink per day for women and 2 drinks per day for men). • Alcohol should be consumed with food to reduce risk of nocturnal hypoglycemia in those using insulin or insulin secretagogues. • Moderate alcohol consumption has no acute effect on glucose and insulin concentrations, but carbohydrate taken with the alcohol (mixed drink) may raise blood glucose.

Source: American Diabetes Association: Clinical practice recommendations: nutrition recommendations and interventions for diabetes, *Diabetes Care* 31:S61, 2008.

Type 1 Diabetes Mellitus. Meal planning should be based on the individual's usual food intake and preferences and balanced with insulin and exercise patterns. The insulin regimen should be developed with the patient's eating habits and activity pattern in mind. Day-to-day consistency in timing and amount of food eaten is important for those individuals using conventional, fixed insulin regimens. Patients using rapid-acting insulin can adjust the dose before the meal based on the current blood glucose level and the carbohydrate content of the meal. Intensified insulin therapy, such as multiple daily injections or the use of an insulin pump, allows considerable flexibility in food selection and can be adjusted for alterations from usual eating and exercise habits.

Type 2 Diabetes Mellitus. Nutritional therapy in type 2 diabetes should emphasize achieving glucose, lipid, and BP goals. Modest weight loss has been associated with improved insulin resistance. Therefore weight loss is recommended for all individuals with diabetes who are overweight or obese.[15]

No one proven strategy or method can be uniformly recommended. A nutritionally adequate meal plan with appropriate serving sizes, a reduction of saturated and *trans* fats, and low carbohydrates can bring about decreased calorie consumption. Spacing meals is another strategy that spreads nutrient intake throughout the day. A weight loss of 5% to 7% of body weight often improves glycemic control, even if desirable body weight is not achieved. Weight loss is best attempted by a moderate decrease in calories and an increase in caloric expenditure. Regularly exercising and learning new behaviors and attitudes can facilitate long-term lifestyle changes. Monitoring of blood

glucose levels, A1C, lipids, and BP provides feedback on how well the goals of nutritional therapy are being met.

Food Composition. The nutrient balance of a diabetic diet is essential to maintain blood glucose levels. Nutritional energy intake should be balanced with the patient's energy output. Each patient's individual meal plan should be constructed with her or his lifestyle and health goals in mind. The following are general recommendations for nutrient balance.

Carbohydrates. Carbohydrates include sugars, starches, and fiber. Carbohydrates provide important sources of energy, fiber, vitamins, and minerals and are therefore important to all people, including those with diabetes. Foods containing carbohydrates from whole grains, fruits, vegetables, and low-fat milk should be included as part of a healthy meal plan. The recommended dietary allowance for carbohydrates is a minimum of 130 g/day.[15]

Glycemic index (GI) is the term used to describe the rise in blood glucose levels after a person has consumed a carbohydrate-containing food. The GI of foods was developed to compare the postprandial responses to carbohydrate-containing foods. Foods with a high GI raise glucose levels faster and higher than foods with a low GI.

GI of 100 refers to the response to 50 g of glucose or white bread in a normal person without diabetes. All other food with an equivalent carbohydrate value is measured against this standard. For example, the GI of an apple is 52, regular milk 27, baked potato 93, cornflake cereal 119, and baked beans 69. An online calculator for GI is available at *www.glycemicindex.com*. The use of GI may provide a modest additional benefit over consideration of total carbohydrates alone.[15]

With all individuals, dietary fiber should be included as part of a healthy meal plan. There is no evidence that a person with diabetes should consume more fiber than an individual who does not have diabetes. The current recommendation for the general population is 25 to 30 g/day.[15]

Nutritive and nonnutritive sweeteners may be included in a healthy meal plan in moderation. Nonnutritive sweeteners include the sugar substitutes saccharine, aspartame, sucralose, neotame, and acesulfame-K.

Fats. Dietary fat provides energy, carries fat-soluble vitamins, and provides essential fatty acids. The ADA recommends limiting saturated fat to less than 7% of total calories. Less than 200 mg/day of cholesterol and limited *trans* fats are also recommended as part of a healthy meal plan. Decreasing fat and cholesterol intake assists in reducing the risk for CVD.

Protein. The amount of daily protein in the diet for people with diabetes and normal renal function is the same as for the general population. The suggested protein intake is 15% to 20% of the total calories consumed. High-protein diets are not recommended as a weight loss method for people with diabetes.

Alcohol. Alcohol inhibits gluconeogenesis (breakdown of glycogen to glucose) by the liver. This can cause severe hypoglycemia in patients on insulin or oral hypoglycemic medications that increase insulin secretion. Encourage patients to honestly discuss their use of alcohol with their health care providers because its use can make blood glucose more difficult to control.

Moderate alcohol consumption can sometimes be safely incorporated into the meal plan if blood glucose levels are well controlled and if the patient is not on medications that will cause adverse effects. Moderate consumption is defined as one drink per day for women and two drinks per day for men. A patient can reduce the risk for alcohol-induced hypoglycemia by eating carbohydrates when drinking alcohol. To decrease the carbohydrate content, recommend using sugar-free mixes and drinking dry, light wines.

Patient Teaching Related to Nutritional Therapy. Most often the dietitian initially teaches the principles of the nutritional therapy regimen. Whenever possible, work with dietitians as part of an interdisciplinary diabetes care team. Some patients who have limited insurance coverage or live in remote areas do not have access to a dietitian. In these cases, you may need to assume responsibility for teaching basic dietary management to patients with diabetes.

Carbohydrate counting is a meal planning technique used to keep track of the amount of carbohydrates eaten with each meal and per day. Often patients are advised to limit carbohydrates to a predetermined number. The amount of total carbohydrates per day depends on previous glycemic control, age, weight, activity level, patient preference, and prescribed medications. A serving size of carbohydrates is 15 g. Patients usually start with 45 to 60 g of carbohydrate per meal. For some patients, insulin regimens are tailored to the number of carbohydrates that a patient will consume at the meal, with a set number of units of insulin given per gram of carbohydrate (e.g., 1 U/15 g carbohydrate, 2 U/25 g carbohydrate). Teach the patient about the foods that contain carbohydrates, how to read food labels, and appropriate serving sizes.

Diabetes exchange lists are another method for meal planning. Instead of counting carbohydrates, the individual is given a meal plan with specific numbers of helpings from a list of exchanges for each meal and snack. The exchanges are starches, fruits, milk, meat, sweets, fats, and free foods. The patient chooses foods from the various exchanges based on the prescribed meal plan. This method may be easier for some patients than carbohydrate counting. Another advantage is that this approach helps the patient limit portion sizes and overall food intake, an important component of weight management.

MyPlate was developed by the U.S. Department of Agriculture (USDA) to represent national nutritional guidelines. This simple method helps the patient visualize the amount of vegetables, starch, and meat that should fill a 9-in plate. For a person with diabetes, each meal needs to have one half of the plate filled with nonstarchy vegetables, one fourth filled with a starch, and one fourth filled with a protein (see eFig. 49-1 available on the website). A glass of nonfat milk and a small piece of fresh fruit complete the meal.[16]

Whenever possible, include family members and caregivers in nutrition education and counseling, particularly the person who cooks for the household. However, the responsibility for maintaining a diabetic diet should not fall to someone other than the person with diabetes. Reliance on another person to make health decisions interferes with the patient's ability to develop self-care skills, which is essential in the management of diabetes. Foster independence, even in patients with visual or cognitive impairment. It is also important to discuss traditional foods with the patient. To improve adherence, the diet needs to be individualized to take into account the patient's preferences and foods that are culturally appropriate.

Exercise

Regular, consistent exercise is an essential part of diabetes and prediabetes management.[17] The ADA recommends that people with diabetes perform at least 150 min/wk (30 minutes, 5 days/

TABLE 49-9	**ACTIVITIES THAT AFFECT CALORIC EXPENDITURE**	
Light Activity (100-200 kcal/hr)	**Moderate Activity (200-350 kcal/hr)**	**Vigorous Activity (400-900 kcal/hr)**
• Driving a car • Fishing • Light housework • Secretarial work • Teaching • Walking casually	• Active housework • Bicycling (light) • Bowling • Dancing • Gardening • Golf • Roller skating • Walking briskly	• Aerobic exercise • Bicycling (vigorous) • Hard labor • Ice skating • Outdoor sports • Running • Soccer • Tennis • Wood chopping

wk) of a moderate-intensity aerobic physical activity (Table 49-9). The ADA also encourages people with type 2 diabetes to perform resistance training three times a week in the absence of contraindications.[18]

Exercise decreases insulin resistance and can have a direct effect on lowering blood glucose levels. It also contributes to weight loss, which further decreases insulin resistance. The therapeutic benefits of regular physical activity may result in a decreased need for diabetes medications to reach target blood glucose goals. Regular exercise may also help reduce triglyceride and low-density lipoprotein (LDL) cholesterol levels, increase high-density lipoprotein (HDL), reduce BP, and improve circulation.[6]

Any new exercise program for diabetic patients should be started only after medical clearance. Patients should start slowly with gradual progression toward the desired goal. Patients who use insulin, sulfonylureas, or meglitinides are at increased risk for hypoglycemia when they increase physical activity, especially if they exercise at the time of peak drug action or eat too little to maintain adequate blood glucose levels. This can also occur if a normally sedentary patient with diabetes has an unusually active day.

The glucose-lowering effects of exercise can last up to 48 hours after the activity, so it is possible for hypoglycemia to occur long after the activity. It is recommended that patients who use medications that can cause hypoglycemia schedule exercise about 1 hour after a meal or that they have a 10- to 15-g carbohydrate snack and check their blood glucose before exercising. They can eat small carbohydrate snacks every 30 minutes during exercise to prevent hypoglycemia. Patients using medications that place them at risk for hypoglycemia should always carry a fast-acting source of carbohydrate, such as glucose tablets or hard candies, when exercising. Table 49-10 describes exercise guidelines for patients with diabetes.

Although exercise is generally beneficial to blood glucose levels, strenuous activity can be perceived by the body as a stress, causing a release of counterregulatory hormones and a temporary elevation of blood glucose. In a person with type 1 diabetes who is hyperglycemic and ketotic, exercise can worsen these conditions. Therefore vigorous activity should be avoided if the blood glucose level is over 250 mg/dL and ketones are present in the urine. If hyperglycemia is present without ketosis, it is not necessary to postpone exercise.[4]

Monitoring Blood Glucose

Self-monitoring of blood glucose (SMBG) is a critical part of diabetes management. By providing a current blood glucose

| TABLE 49-10 | PATIENT & CAREGIVER TEACHING GUIDE |

Exercise for Patients With Diabetes Mellitus

Include the following information in the exercise teaching plan for the patient and caregiver.

1. Exercise does not have to be vigorous to be effective. The blood glucose–reducing effects of exercise can be attained with activity such as brisk walking.
2. The exercises selected should be enjoyable to foster regularity.
3. It is important to have properly fitting footwear.
4. The exercise session should have a warm-up period and a cool-down period. The exercise program should be started gradually and increased slowly.
5. Exercise is best done after meals, when the blood glucose level is rising.
6. Exercise plans should be individualized and monitored by the health care provider.
7. It is important to self-monitor blood glucose levels before, during, and after exercise to determine the effect exercise has on blood glucose level at particular times of the day.
   - *Before exercise, if blood glucose ≤100 mg/dL,* eat a 15-g carbohydrate snack. After 15 to 30 min, retest blood glucose levels. Do not exercise if <100 mg/dL.
   - *Before exercise, if blood glucose ≥250 mg/dL* in a person with type 1 diabetes and ketones are present, avoid vigorous activity.
8. Delayed exercise-induced hypoglycemia may occur several hours after the completion of exercise.
9. Taking a glucose-lowering medication does not mean that planned or spontaneous exercise cannot occur.
10. It is important to compensate for extensive planned and spontaneous activity by monitoring blood glucose levels to make adjustments in the insulin dose (if taken) and food intake.

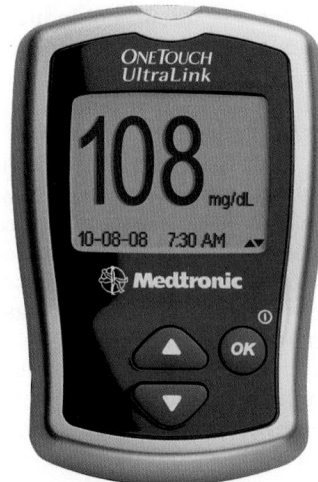

FIG. 49-8 Blood glucose monitors are used to measure blood glucose levels. Medtronic OneTouch UltraLink glucose meter. (Courtesy of Medtronic Diabetes.)

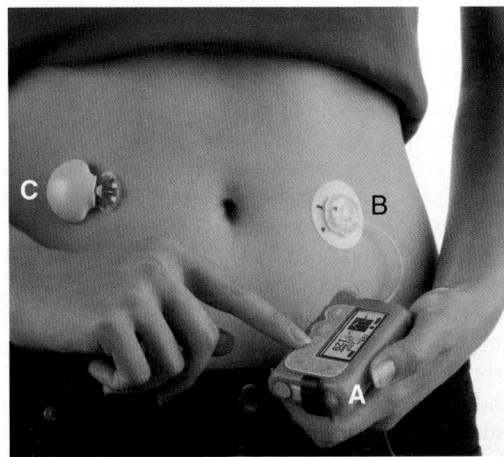

FIG. 49-9 The MiniMed Paradigm® REAL-Time Revel™ Insulin Pump *(A)* delivers insulin through a thin plastic tubing to an infusion set, which has a cannula *(B)* that sits under the skin. Continuous glucose monitoring occurs through a tiny sensor *(C)* inserted under the skin. Sensor data are sent continuously to the insulin pump through wireless technology giving a more complete picture of glucose levels, which can lead to better treatment decisions and better glucose control. (MiniMed Paradigm® REAL-Time Revel™ Insulin Pump manufactured by the diabetes division of Medtronic, Inc.)

reading, SMBG enables the patient to make decisions regarding food intake, activity patterns, and medication dosages. It also produces accurate records of daily glucose fluctuations and trends, and it alerts the patient to acute episodes of hyperglycemia and hypoglycemia. Furthermore, it provides patients with a tool for achieving and maintaining specific glycemic goals. SMBG is recommended for all insulin-treated patients with diabetes. Other patients with diabetes use SMBG to help achieve and maintain glycemic goals and monitor for acute fluctuations in blood glucose.

The frequency of monitoring depends on several factors, including the patient's glycemic goals, type of diabetes, medication regimen, patient's ability to perform the test independently, and patient's willingness to test. Patients who use multiple insulin injections or insulin pumps should monitor their blood glucose four or more times a day. Patients using less frequent insulin injections, noninsulin therapy, or nutritional therapy will monitor as often as needed to achieve their glycemic goals.[10]

Patients who perform SMBG use portable blood glucose monitors (glucometers). A wide variety of blood glucose monitors are available (Fig. 49-8). Disposable lancets are used to obtain a small drop of capillary blood (usually from a finger stick) that is placed onto a reagent strip. After a specified time, the monitor displays a digital reading of the capillary blood glucose value. The technology of SMBG is rapidly changing, with newer and more convenient systems being introduced on an ongoing basis.

Newer systems allow the user to collect blood from alternative sites such as the forearm or palm. Alternate site testing is

not recommended with rapidly changing blood glucose readings, during pregnancy, or when symptoms of low blood glucose are present. The data from some glucose monitors can be uploaded to a computer and e-mailed to health care providers for review, allowing for more frequent and efficient adjustment of the plan of care if needed.

Continuous glucose monitoring (CGM) systems provide another route for monitoring glucose. The CGM systems available include the (1) Dexcom Seven by Dexcom, (2) MiniMed Paradigm® REAL-Time Revel™ by Medtronic (Fig. 49-9), (3) Guardian REAL-Time by Medtronic, and (4) FreeStyle Navigator by Abbott. Using a sensor inserted subcutaneously, the systems display glucose values that are updated every 1 to 5 minutes. The patient inserts the sensor using an automatic insertion device. Data are sent from the sensor to a transmitter, which displays the glucose value on either an insulin pump (MiniMed Paradigm® REAL-Time Revel™ and Guardian REAL-

Time) or a pager-like receiver (Dexcom Seven and FreeStyle Navigator). The glucose monitor can be used without an insulin pump.

CGMs assist the patient and the health care provider in identifying trends and patterns in glucose levels and are useful for the management of insulin therapy or when continuous blood glucose readings are clinically important. The patient is alerted to episodes of hypoglycemia and hyperglycemia, thus allowing corrective action to be quickly taken. These systems still require finger-stick measurements using a blood glucose monitor to calibrate the sensor and to make treatment decisions.

The blood glucose level reported by a laboratory is sometimes higher than the patient's home glucose monitor or the hospital's portable monitor. This is because some home monitors give capillary blood glucose values from whole blood (via finger stick), whereas tests performed in laboratories provide plasma readings. Plasma samples, or venous samples, are approximately 10% to 12% higher. Most current monitors are automatically calibrated to give a "plasma" test result (even though whole blood was used for the sample) so that the home readings can be more readily compared with laboratory values. It is important to read the literature accompanying a monitor to find out if it is displaying values as whole blood or plasma.

Because errors in monitoring technique can cause errors in management strategies, comprehensive patient teaching is essential. Initial instruction should be followed up with regular reassessment. Review the instructions that accompany each product. Teach patients to use and interpret control solutions. Control solution should be used when first using a glucometer, when a new bottle of strips is used, or when there is a reason to believe that the readings are not correct. Table 49-11 lists the steps to include when teaching the patient how to perform SMBG.

People with type 1 diabetes often test their blood glucose before meals. This is because many patients use insulin pumps or multiple daily injections and base the insulin dose on the carbohydrates in a meal or make adjustments if the preprandial

TABLE 49-11   PATIENT & CAREGIVER TEACHING GUIDE

Self-Monitoring of Blood Glucose (SMBG)

Include the following instructions when teaching the patient and caregiver about SMBG.
1. Wash hands in warm water. It is not necessary to clean the site with alcohol, and it may interfere with test results. Finger should be dry before puncturing it.
2. If it is difficult to obtain an adequate drop of blood for testing, warm the hands in warm water or let the arms hang dependently for a few minutes before the finger puncture is made.
3. A penlet lancing device is usually used. Place the lancet in the device, following the instructions that come with it. If the puncture is made on the finger, use the side of the finger pad rather than near the center. Fewer nerve endings are along the side of the finger pad. If an alternative site is used (e.g., forearm), special equipment may be needed. Refer to manufacturer's instructions for alternative site use, except during hypoglycemic episodes.
4. Set penlet device to make a puncture just deep enough to obtain a sufficiently large drop of blood. Unnecessarily deep punctures may cause pain and bruising.
5. Follow instructions on monitor for testing the blood.
6. Record results. Compare with personal target blood glucose goals.

value is above or below target. Testing 2 hours after the first bite of food is taken helps a person see how effectively he or she judged what was eaten or to determine if the bolus insulin dose was adequate for that meal.

Blood glucose testing should be performed whenever hypoglycemia is suspected so that immediate action can be taken. During times of illness, the person should test blood glucose levels at 4-hour intervals to determine the effects of the illness on glucose levels. Teach the patient to test blood glucose before and after exercise to determine the effects of exercise on metabolic control. This is especially important in the patient with type 1 diabetes.

A patient who is visually impaired, cognitively impaired, or limited in manual dexterity needs careful evaluation of the degree to which SMBG can be performed independently. Nurses preparing patients for discharge from the hospital, and nurses working in home health and outpatient settings, may need to identify caregivers who can assume this responsibility. Adaptive devices are available to help patients with certain limitations. These include talking meters and other equipment for the visually impaired.

Bariatric Surgery
Bariatric surgery may be considered for patients with type 2 diabetes who have a body mass index (BMI) greater than 35 kg/m², especially if the diabetes or associated co-morbidities are difficult to control with lifestyle and drug therapy (see Evidence-Based Practice box on p. 1170). Patients with type 2 diabetes who have undergone bariatric surgery need lifelong lifestyle support and monitoring. (Bariatric surgery is discussed in Chapter 41.)

Pancreas Transplantation
Pancreas transplantation can be used as a treatment option for patients with type 1 diabetes. Usually it is done for patients who have end-stage kidney disease and have had or plan to have a kidney transplant. Kidney and pancreas transplants are often performed together, or a pancreas may be transplanted after a kidney transplant. If renal failure is not present, the ADA recommends that pancreas transplantation be considered only for patients who exhibit the following three criteria: (1) a history of frequent, acute, and severe metabolic complications (e.g., hypoglycemia, hyperglycemia, ketoacidosis) requiring medical attention; (2) clinical and emotional problems with the use of exogenous insulin therapy that are so severe as to be incapacitating; and (3) consistent failure of insulin-based management to prevent acute complications.

Successful pancreas transplantation can improve the quality of life for people with diabetes, primarily by eliminating the need for exogenous insulin, frequent blood glucose measurements, and many of the dietary restrictions imposed by the disorder. Transplantation can also eliminate the acute complications commonly experienced by patients with type 1 diabetes (e.g., hypoglycemia, hyperglycemia). However, pancreas transplantation is only partially successful in reversing the long-term renal and neurologic complications of diabetes. The patient will also require lifelong immunosuppression to prevent rejection of the organ. Complications can result from immunosuppressive therapy. (Immunosuppressive therapy is discussed in Chapter 14.)

Pancreatic islet cell transplantation is another potential treatment measure. During this procedure, the islets are harvested

Translating Research Into Practice

Bariatric Surgery for Obese Adults With Type 2 Diabetes

Clinical Question

In severely obese adults (P), how do gastric bypass and biliopancreatic diversion (I) compare with medical therapy (C) for remission from type 2 diabetes mellitus (O)?

Best Available Evidence

Systematic review of randomized controlled trials (RCTs)

Critical Appraisal and Synthesis of Evidence

- Sixty adults with type 2 diabetes for ≥5 yr with a BMI ≥35 kg/m² and Hb A1C ≥7.0%.
- Roux-en-Y gastric bypass (*n* = 20), biliopancreatic diversion (*n* = 20), or medical therapy (*n* = 20).
- At 2 yr, more patients in the gastric bypass and biliopancreatic diversion groups achieved diabetes remission than in the medical therapy group.
- Bypass and biliopancreatic diversion each reduced A1C, glucose levels, and BMI more than medical therapy.

Conclusion

- Bariatric surgery (gastric bypass and biliopancreatic diversion) decreases BMI, improves glycemic control, and increases remission from type 2 diabetes more than medical therapy in severely obese adults.

Implications for Nursing Practice

- In addition to behavioral and medical approaches, bariatric surgery often normalizes blood glucose levels, reduces or avoids the need for drugs, and provides a potentially cost-effective approach to treating the disease.
- Bariatric surgery is an appropriate treatment for people with type 2 diabetes and obesity not achieving recommended treatment targets with medical therapies, especially when there are other major co-morbidities.

Reference for Evidence

Mingrone G, Panunzi S, De Gaetano A, et al: Bariatric surgery versus conventional medical therapy for type 2 diabetes, *N Engl J Med* 366: 1577, 2012.

P, Patient population of interest; *I*, intervention or area of interest; *C*, comparison of interest or comparison group; *O*, outcomes of interest (see p. 12).

Diabetes Mellitus

- The highest incidence of diabetes is among Native Americans and Alaska Natives (16.5% are being treated for diabetes).
- Pima Indians in Arizona have the highest rate of diabetes in the world (50% of adults have diabetes).
- The rates of diabetes are non-Hispanic whites 7.1%, Asian Americans 8.4%, Hispanics 11.8%, and non-Hispanic blacks 12.6%.
- Diabetes is 1.5 times more likely to cause death in Hispanics and 2.2 times more likely to cause death in African Americans than in non-Hispanic whites.
- Complications from diabetes are a major cause of death among Native Americans. Native Americans have a six times higher rate of end-stage kidney disease and a four times higher rate of amputation than other people with diabetes.
- Treatment for end-stage kidney disease for men with diabetes is 1.6 times higher in Hispanics and 2.7 times higher in African Americans compared with non-Hispanic white men.

Explore the influences of culture on food choices and meal planning with the patient as part of the health history. When giving diet instructions, consider the patient's cultural food preferences. Nutritional resources specifically designed for members of different cultural groups are available from the ADA.

NURSING MANAGEMENT
DIABETES MELLITUS

NURSING ASSESSMENT

Table 49-12 provides initial subjective and objective data that should be obtained from a person with diabetes mellitus. After the initial assessment, perform periodic patient assessments on a regular basis.

NURSING DIAGNOSES

Nursing diagnoses related to diabetes mellitus may include, but are not limited to, those found in eNursing Care Plan 49-1.

PLANNING

The overall goals are for the patient with diabetes mellitus to (1) engage in self-care behaviors to actively manage his or her diabetes, (2) experience few or no episodes of acute hyperglycemic or hypoglycemic emergencies, (3) maintain blood glucose levels at normal or near-normal levels, (4) prevent or minimize chronic complications of diabetes, and (5) adjust lifestyle to accommodate the diabetes regimen with a minimum of stress.

NURSING IMPLEMENTATION

HEALTH PROMOTION. Your role in health promotion is to identify, monitor, and teach the patient at risk for diabetes. Obesity is the primary risk factor for type 2 diabetes. The findings from the Diabetes Prevention Program indicated that a modest weight loss of 5% to 7% of body weight and regular exercise of 30 minutes five times a week lowered the risk of developing type 2 diabetes up to 58%.[18]

The ADA recommends routine screening for type 2 diabetes for all adults who are overweight or obese (BMI greater than or equal to 25 kg/m²) or have one or more risk factors. For people who do not have risk factors for diabetes, screening should begin at age 45. Table 49-13 provides criteria to test for prediabetes and diabetes. If results are normal, repeat testing at 3-year

from the pancreas of a deceased organ donor. Most recipients require the use of two or more pancreases. The islets are infused via a catheter through the upper abdomen into the portal vein of the liver. With only the islets transplanted, pain and recovery time are diminished compared with whole pancreas transplants. Currently this procedure is experimental in the United States. Research is continuing to investigate the best ways to implant the islet cells and to prevent their rejection.

CULTURALLY COMPETENT CARE

DIABETES MELLITUS

Because culture can have a strong influence on dietary preferences and meal preparation practices, culturally competent care has special relevance for the patient with diabetes. For example, certain ethnic and cultural groups, such as Hispanics, Native Americans, and African Americans, have a high incidence of diabetes. The increased prevalence can be attributed to genetic predisposition, environmental factors, and dietary choices.

TABLE 49-12   NURSING ASSESSMENT

Diabetes Mellitus

Subjective Data
Important Health Information
Past health history: Mumps, rubella, coxsackievirus or other viral infections; recent trauma, infection, or stress; pregnancy, gave birth to infant >9 lb; chronic pancreatitis; Cushing syndrome; acromegaly; family history of type 1 or type 2 diabetes mellitus
Medications: Use of and adherence to regimen with insulin or OAs; corticosteroids, diuretics, phenytoin (Dilantin)
Surgery or other treatments: Any recent surgery

Functional Health Patterns
Health perception–health management: Positive family history; malaise; date of last eye and dental examination
Nutritional-metabolic: Obesity; weight loss (type 1), weight gain (type 2); thirst, hunger; nausea and vomiting; poor healing (especially involving the feet), adherence to diet in patients with previously diagnosed diabetes
Elimination: Constipation or diarrhea; frequent urination, frequent bladder infections, nocturia, urinary incontinence
Activity-exercise: Muscle weakness, fatigue
Cognitive-perceptual: Abdominal pain; headache; blurred vision; numbness or tingling of extremities; pruritus
Sexuality-reproductive: Erectile dysfunction; frequent vaginal infections; decreased libido
Coping–stress tolerance: Depression, irritability, apathy
Value-belief: Commitment to lifestyle changes involving diet, medication, and activity patterns

Objective Data
Eyes
Soft, sunken eyeballs;* vitreal hemorrhages; cataracts

Integumentary
Dry, warm, inelastic skin; pigmented lesions (on legs); ulcers (especially on feet); loss of hair on toes; acanthosis nigricans

Respiratory
Rapid, deep respirations (Kussmaul respirations)*

Cardiovascular
Hypotension;* weak, rapid pulse*

Gastrointestinal
Dry mouth; vomiting;* fruity breath*

Neurologic
Altered reflexes; restlessness; confusion; stupor; coma

Musculoskeletal
Muscle wasting

Possible Findings
Serum electrolyte abnormalities; fasting blood glucose level ≥126 mg/dL; oral glucose tolerance test >200 mg/dL; random glucose ≥200 mg/dL; leukocytosis; ↑ blood urea nitrogen, creatinine, triglycerides, cholesterol, LDL, VLDL; ↓ HDL; A1C >6.0%; glycosuria; ketonuria; albuminuria; acidosis

*Indicates manifestations of diabetic ketoacidosis.
A1C, Glycosylated hemoglobin; *HDL,* high-density lipoprotein; *LDL,* low-density lipoprotein; *OAs,* oral agents; *VLDL,* very-low-density lipoprotein.

TABLE 49-13   TESTING FOR DIABETES IN ASYMPTOMATIC, UNDIAGNOSED INDIVIDUALS

Who Should Be Tested
1. Testing should be considered in all adults who are overweight (BMI >25 kg/m^2) and have additional risk factors:
   * First-degree relative with diabetes
   * Physically inactive
   * Members of a high-risk ethnic population (e.g., African American, Hispanic, Native American, Asian American, Pacific Islander)
   * Women who delivered a baby weighing >9 lb or were diagnosed with gestational diabetes mellitus
   * Hypertensive (≥140/90 mm Hg) or on therapy for hypertension
   * HDL cholesterol level ≤35 mg/dL (0.90 mmol/L) and/or a triglyceride level ≥250 mg/dL (2.82 mmol/L)
   * Women with polycystic ovary syndrome
   * A1C ≥5.7%, IGT, or IFG on previous testing
   * Other clinical conditions associated with insulin resistance (e.g., severe obesity, acanthosis nigricans)
2. In the absence of the above criteria, testing for diabetes should begin at age 45 yr.
3. If results are normal, testing should be repeated at least at 3-yr intervals, with consideration of more frequent testing depending on initial results and risk status.

What Testing Should Be Used
To test for diabetes or to assess risk of future diabetes, A1C, FPG, or 2-hour OGTT is appropriate.

Source: American Diabetes Association: Clinical practice recommendations: standards of medical care, *Diabetes Care* 36 (Suppl):S11, 2013.
A1C, Glycosylated hemoglobin; *BMI,* body mass index; *FPG,* fasting plasma glucose; *HDL,* high-density lipoprotein; *IFG,* impaired fasting glucose; *IGT,* impaired glucose tolerance; *OGTT,* oral glucose tolerance test.

HEALTHY PEOPLE

Prevention and Early Detection of Diabetes Mellitus

* Increase level of exercise because physical activity reduces the risk of type 2 diabetes.
* Maintain a healthy weight because obesity increases the risk of type 2 diabetes.
* If overweight, lose weight and get on a regular exercise program to reduce the risk of diabetes.
* Use a diet that is low in fat content, total calories, and processed foods and high in whole grains, fruits, and vegetables.
* If overweight and over age 45, get a diabetes screening test done.

intervals.[3] Many factors put an individual at an increased risk for diabetes. These include age, ethnicity (being Native American, Hispanic, African American, Asian, Pacific Islander), obesity, having a baby that weighs more than 9 lb, having gestational diabetes, and a family history of diabetes. A diabetes risk test is available at *www.diabetes.org/risk-test.jsp*. The diabe-tes risk test determines if the person is at risk for prediabetes or diabetes based on the number of risk factors present.

ACUTE INTERVENTION. Acute situations involving the patient with diabetes include hypoglycemia, DKA, and hyperosmolar hyperglycemic syndrome (HHS). Nursing management for these situations is discussed in more detail later in this chapter. Other areas of acute intervention relate to management during stress, such as during acute illness and surgery.

Stress of Acute Illness and Surgery. Both emotional and physical stress can increase the blood glucose level and result in hyperglycemia. Because stress is unavoidable, certain situations may require more intense treatment, such as extra insulin, to maintain glycemic goals and avoid hyperglycemia.

Acute illness, injury, and surgery are situations that may evoke a counterregulatory hormone response, resulting in hyperglycemia. Even common illnesses such as a viral upper respiratory tract infection or the flu can cause this response. When patients with diabetes are ill, they should check blood glucose at least every 4 hours. An acutely ill patient with type 1 diabetes with a blood glucose greater than 240 mg/dL (13.3 mmol/L) should test his or her urine for ketones every 3 to 4 hours.

Patients should report to the health care provider when glucose levels are over 300 mg/dL for two tests in a row or urine ketone levels are moderate to large. A patient with type 1 diabetes may need an increase in insulin to prevent DKA. Insulin therapy may be required for a patient with type 2 diabetes to prevent or treat hyperglycemic symptoms and avoid an acute hyperglycemic emergency. In critically ill patients, insulin therapy may be started if the blood glucose is persistently greater than 180 mg/dL. These patients have a higher targeted blood glucose goal, which is usually 140 to 180 mg/dL.

Food intake is important during times of stress and illness, when the body requires extra energy. If patients are able to eat normally, they should continue with their regular meal plan while increasing the intake of noncaloric fluids, such as water, diet gelatin, and other decaffeinated beverages, and continue taking OAs, noninsulin injectable agents, and insulin as prescribed. When illness causes patients to eat less than normal, they should continue to take OAs, noninsulin injectable agents, and/or insulin as prescribed while supplementing food intake with carbohydrate-containing fluids. Examples include low-sodium soups, juices, and regular decaffeinated soft drinks. It is important to tell the patient to contact a health care provider if the patient is unable to keep down food or fluid.

During the intraoperative period, adjustments in the diabetes regimen can be planned to ensure glycemic control. The patient is given IV fluids and insulin (if needed) immediately before, during, and after surgery when there is no oral intake. The patient with type 2 diabetes who has been on OAs should understand that this is a temporary measure, not a sign of worsening diabetes.

When caring for an unconscious surgical patient receiving insulin, be alert for hypoglycemic signs such as sweating, tachycardia, and tremors. Frequent monitoring of blood glucose will prevent episodes of severe hypoglycemia.

AMBULATORY AND HOME CARE. Successful management of diabetes requires ongoing interaction among the patient, caregiver, and health care team. It is important that a certified diabetes educator (CDE) be involved in the care of the patient and the family. Because diabetes is a complex chronic condition, a great deal of patient contact takes place in outpatient and home settings. The major goal of patient care in these settings is to enable the patient (with the help of a caregiver) to reach an optimal level of independence in self-care activities. Unfortunately, many patients with diabetes face challenges in reaching these goals. Diabetes increases the risk for other chronic conditions that can affect self-care activities. These include visual impairment, lower extremity problems that affect mobility, and other functional limitations related to a stroke.

An important nursing function is to assess the ability of patients and caregivers in performing activities such as SMBG and insulin injection. Assistive devices for self-administration of insulin include syringe magnifiers, vial stabilizers, and dosing aids for the visually impaired. In some cases, referrals are made to help the patient achieve the self-care goal. These may include an occupational therapist, a social worker, a home care nurse, a home health aide, or a dietitian.

A diagnosis of diabetes affects the patient in many profound ways. Self-management of the disease is demanding. Patients with diabetes continually face lifestyle choices that affect the foods they eat, their activities, and demands on their time and energy. The requirements of scheduled meals, SMBG, medication, and insulin management may interfere with the patient's other responsibilities. Any change in the daily routine is difficult. In addition, they face the challenge of preventing or dealing with the devastating complications of diabetes.

Careful assessment of what it means to the patient to have diabetes should be the starting point of teaching. The goals of teaching should be mutually determined by you and the patient, based on individual needs and therapeutic requirements. Identify the patient's support system, and include them in planning, teaching, and counseling. When family members and other individuals close to the patient are included, they can support the patient's self-care behaviors. Additionally, they can provide care if self-care is not possible. Encourage the family and caregivers to provide emotional support and encouragement as the patient deals with the reality of living with a chronic disease.

Insulin Therapy. Nursing responsibilities for the patient receiving insulin include proper administration, assessment of the patient's response to insulin therapy, and teaching the patient about administration and side effects of insulin (see Table 49-5). Table 49-6 lists guidelines for assessing a patient using glucose-lowering agents, including insulin and OAs.

Assessment of the patient who is a new user of insulin must include an evaluation of his or her ability to safely manage this therapy. This includes the ability to understand the interaction of insulin, diet, and activity and to recognize and treat the symptoms of hypoglycemia appropriately. If the patient does not have the cognitive skills to do these things, identify and teach another responsible person. The patient or caregiver must have the cognitive and manual skills needed to prepare and inject insulin. Otherwise, additional resources will be needed to assist the patient. For patients with cognitive, physical, and other barriers, consider referral to a CDE because he or she has the specialized knowledge and skills to promote self-care behaviors for these patients.

Many patients are fearful when they first begin using insulin.[19] Some find it difficult to self-inject because they are afraid of needles or the pain associated with an injection. Others may think that the insulin is not necessary or that they will experience hypoglycemia after an injection. Explore the patient's underlying fears before beginning the teaching. Assessment of the patient's beliefs and concerns regarding starting insulin will guide the teaching, counseling, and plan of care. Having open discussion with patients, providing educational materials and programs, and working with a diabetes educator are all beneficial for patients starting insulin.

Follow-up assessment of the patient who has been using insulin therapy includes an inspection of injection sites for signs of lipodystrophy and other reactions, review of insulin preparation and injection technique, a history pertaining to the occurrence of hypoglycemic episodes, and assessment of the patient's method for handling hypoglycemic episodes. A review of the patient's recorded blood glucose tests is vital in assessing overall glycemic control and making any needed adjustments.

Oral and Noninsulin Injectable Agents. Your responsibilities for the patient taking oral and noninsulin injectable agents are similar to those for the patient taking insulin. Proper administration of these drugs, assessment of the patient's use of and response to these drugs, and teaching the patient and family are all essential nursing actions.

Your assessment is valuable in determining the most appropriate drug for a patient. Factors such as the patient's mental status, eating habits, home environment, attitude toward diabetes, and medication history all play a significant role in determining the most appropriate drug. For example, frail older adults who live alone are at high risk for severe hypoglycemia because low blood glucose is frequently undetected or untreated in this population. This is especially true if the patient has cognitive impairment. In these cases, an OA that does not cause hypoglycemia, or a shorter-acting OA, would be most appropriate.

Patient teaching is essential. Some patients may assume that their diabetes is not a serious condition if they are only taking a pill for glycemic control. Instruct the patient that these agents will help control blood glucose and help prevent serious long- and short-term complications of diabetes. Teach patients that OAs and noninsulin injectable agents are used in addition to diet and activity as therapy for diabetes and the importance of following their meal and activity plans. Patients should not take extra pills if they have overeaten. If the patient uses sulfonylureas and metformin, instruct the patient about prevention, symptom recognition, and management of hypoglycemia.

Personal Hygiene. The potential for infection requires diligent skin and dental hygiene practices. Because of the susceptibility to periodontal disease, encourage daily brushing and flossing in addition to regular visits to the dentist. When having dental work done, the patient should inform the dentist that he or she has diabetes. Teach patients regarding the importance of sharing their diagnosis with dentists and other health care professionals.

Routine care includes regular bathing, with particular emphasis on foot care. Advise patients to inspect their feet daily, avoid going barefoot, and wear shoes that are supportive and comfortable. If cuts, scrapes, or burns occur, they should be treated promptly and monitored carefully. Wash the area and apply a nonabrasive or nonirritating antiseptic ointment. Cover the area with a dry, sterile pad. Patients should notify the health care provider immediately if the injury does not begin to heal within 24 hours or if signs of infection develop.

Medical Identification and Travel. Instruct the patient to carry medical identification at all times indicating that he or she has diabetes. Police, paramedics, and many private citizens are aware of the need to look for this identification when working with sick or unconscious persons. Every person with diabetes should wear a Medic Alert bracelet or necklace. An identification card (Fig. 49-10) can supply valuable information, such as the name of the health care provider; the type of diabetes; and the type and dosage of insulin, noninsulin injectable agents, or OAs.

Travel for a patient with diabetes requires planning. Being sedentary for long periods may raise the person's glucose level. Encourage the patient to get up and walk at least every 2 hours to lower the risk for deep vein thrombosis and to prevent elevation of glucose levels. The patient should have a full set of diabetes care supplies in the carry-on luggage when traveling by plane, train, or bus. This includes blood glucose monitoring equipment, insulin, noninsulin injectable agents, oral medications, and syringes or insulin pens.

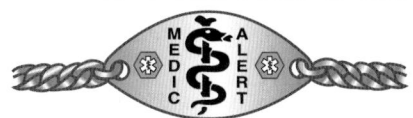

FIG. 49-10 Medical alerts. A patient with diabetes should carry a card and wear a bracelet or necklace that indicates diabetes. If the patient with diabetes is unconscious, these measures will ensure prompt and appropriate attention.

When equipment such as syringes, lancing devices, insulin vials or pens, and insulin pumps are taken onto a commercial airliner, the professional printed pharmaceutical labels should accompany them. A letter from the prescribing health care provider indicating medical necessity may prevent delays at security checkpoints. Notify screeners if an insulin pump is used so they can inspect it while it is on the body, rather than removing it.

For patients who use insulin or OAs that can cause hypoglycemia, snack items and a quick-acting carbohydrate source for treating hypoglycemia should be included in the carry-on luggage. Extra insulin should be available in case a bottle breaks or is lost. For longer trips, the patient should carry a full day's supply of food in the event of canceled flights, delayed meals, or closed restaurants. If the patient is planning a trip out of the country, it is wise to have a letter from the health care provider explaining that the patient has diabetes and requires all the materials, particularly syringes, for ongoing health care.

When travel involves time changes such as traveling coast to coast or across the International Date Line, the patient should contact the health care provider to plan an appropriate insulin schedule. During travel, most patients find it helpful to keep watches set to the time of the city of origin until they reach their destination. The key to travel when taking insulin is to know the type of insulin being taken, its onset of action, the anticipated peak time, and mealtimes.

Patient and Caregiver Teaching. The goals of diabetes self-management education are to match the level of self-management to the patient's individual ability so he or she can become the most active participant possible. Patients who actively manage their diabetes care have better outcomes than those who do not. For this reason, an educational approach that facilitates informed decision making by the patient is advocated. Sometimes this is referred to as the *empowerment approach* to education.

Unfortunately, patients can encounter a variety of physical, psychologic, and emotional barriers when it comes to effectively managing their diabetes. These barriers may include feelings of inadequacy about one's own abilities, unwillingness to make the necessary behavioral changes, ineffective coping strategies, and cognitive deficits. If the patient is not able to manage the disease, a family member may be able to assume part of this role. If the patient or the caregiver cannot make decisions related to diabe-

COMPLEMENTARY & ALTERNATIVE THERAPIES

Herbs and Supplements That May Affect Blood Glucose

Scientific Evidence*
- Herbs and supplements that may lower blood glucose include aloe, α-lipoic acid, cinnamon, chromium, garlic, and ginseng.
- However, many studies have been small and not well designed. Further research is needed.

Nursing Implications
- Teach patients to use herbs and supplements with caution, since they may affect blood glucose.
- Patients with diabetes mellitus should consult their health care provider before using herbs or nutritional supplements.
- Patients who use herbs should monitor their blood glucose levels carefully and regularly.

*Based on a systematic review of scientific literature. Retrieved from *www.naturalstandard.com.*

INFORMATICS IN PRACTICE

Patient Teaching Using Gaming

- Teaching is a critical part of nursing care for patients with diabetes. Put some fun into patient teaching by using gaming applications.
- Try an application with a quiz-show format. The patient answers questions about diabetes and then compares his or her answers in real time to those of other players. The questions (e.g., How does exercise affect insulin?) are written to help the patient learn to manage diabetes on a daily basis.
- Players in online simulations become either a caregiver to or a patient with type 1 diabetes. Players earn rewards by properly managing blood glucose levels.

tes management, consider a referral to a CDE, social worker, or other resources within the community. These resources can assist the patient and the family in outlining a feasible treatment program that meets their capabilities. Patient and health care provider resources are listed at the end of this chapter.

An assessment of the patient's knowledge of diabetes and lifestyle preferences is useful in planning a teaching program. Tables 49-14 and 49-15 present guidelines to use for patient and caregiver teaching. Assess the patient's knowledge base frequently so that gaps in knowledge or incorrect or inaccurate ideas can be corrected.

The ADA offers resources for patients in the form of pamphlets, booklets, books, and a monthly magazine called *Diabetes Forecast.* Affiliates of the ADA are located in all states, and most can be reached by dialing 1-800-DIABETES (800-342-2383). The ADA publishes materials and sponsors conferences for health care professionals concerned with diabetes education, research, and management of patients. The ADA website (*www.diabetes.org*) has extensive information for the public and health care professionals. This organization also recognizes education programs that meet the national standards of diabetes education and can provide a list of these programs. Drug companies manufacturing diabetes-related products also have free educational materials for patients and health care providers.

EVALUATION

The expected outcomes for the patient with diabetes mellitus are addressed in eNursing Care Plan 49-1.

TABLE 49-14 PATIENT & CAREGIVER TEACHING GUIDE

Management of Diabetes Mellitus

Include the following instructions when teaching the patient and caregiver how to manage diabetes mellitus.

Component	What to Teach
Disease Process	• Include an introduction about the pancreas and the islets of Langerhans. • Describe how insulin is made and what affects its production. • Discuss the relationship of insulin and glucose. • Explain the difference between type 1 and type 2 diabetes.
Physical Activity	• Discuss the effect of regular exercise on the management of blood glucose, improvement of cardiovascular function, and general health.
Menu Planning	• Stress the importance of a well-balanced diet as part of a diabetes management plan. • Explain the impact of carbohydrates on the glycemic index and blood glucose levels.
Medication Adherence	• Ensure that the patient understands the proper use of prescribed medication (e.g., insulin [see Table 49-5], OAs, and noninsulin injectables). • Account for a patient's physical limitations or inabilities for self-medication. If necessary, involve the family or the caregiver in proper use of medication. • Discuss all side effects and safety issues regarding medication.
Monitoring Blood glucose	• Teach correct blood glucose monitoring. • Include when blood glucose levels should be checked, how to record them, and how to adjust insulin levels if necessary.
Risk Reduction	• Ensure that the patient understands and appropriately responds to the signs and symptoms of hypoglycemia and hyperglycemia (see Table 49-16). • Stress the importance of proper foot care (see Table 49-21), regular eye examinations, and consistent glucose monitoring. • Inform the patient about the effect that stress can have on blood glucose.
Psychosocial	• Advise the patient of resources that are available to facilitate the adjustment and answer questions about living with a chronic condition such as diabetes (see Resources at end of chapter).

OAs, Oral agents.

ACUTE COMPLICATIONS OF DIABETES MELLITUS

The acute complications of diabetes mellitus arise from events associated with hyperglycemia and hypoglycemia. It is important for the health care provider to distinguish between hyperglycemia and hypoglycemia because hypoglycemia worsens rapidly and constitutes a serious threat if action is not immediately taken. Table 49-16 compares the manifestations, causes, management, and prevention of hyperglycemia and hypoglycemia.

TABLE 49-15   PATIENT & CAREGIVER TEACHING GUIDE

Instructions for Patients With Diabetes Mellitus

Include the following essential instructions for diabetes management.

Do	Do Not
Blood Glucose	
• Monitor your blood glucose at home and record results in a log. • Take your insulin, OA, and/or noninsulin injectable agent as prescribed. • Obtain A1C blood test every 3-6 mo as an indicator of your long-term blood glucose control. • Know the symptoms of hypoglycemia and hyperglycemia. • Carry some form of rapid-acting glucose at all times so you can treat hypoglycemia quickly. • Instruct family members how and when to use glucagon if patient becomes unresponsive because of hypoglycemia.	• Skip doses of your insulin, especially when you are sick. • Run out of insulin. • Ignore the symptoms of hypoglycemia and hyperglycemia.
Exercise	
• Learn how exercise and food affect your blood glucose levels. • Begin an exercise program after approval from health care provider.	• Forget that exercise will lower your blood glucose level.
Diet	
• Have an individualized meal plan created by a dietitian. • Follow your diet, eating regular meals at regular times. • Choose foods low in saturated and *trans* fat. • Limit the amount of alcohol you drink. • Know your cholesterol level.	• Drink excessive amounts of alcohol because this may lead to unpredictable low blood glucose reactions. • Use a fad diet. • Drink regular soda or lots of fruit juice.
Other Guidelines	
• Obtain an annual eye examination by an ophthalmologist. • Obtain annual urine testing for protein. • Examine your feet at home. • Wear comfortable, well-fitting shoes to help prevent foot injury. Break in new shoes gradually. • Always carry identification that says you have diabetes. • Have other medical problems treated, especially high blood pressure and high cholesterol. • Quit cigarette smoking. • Have a yearly influenza vaccination.	• Smoke cigarettes or use nicotine products. • Apply hot or cold directly to your feet. • Go barefoot. • Put oil or lotion between your toes.

A1C, Glycosylated hemoglobin; *OA,* oral agent.

TABLE 49-16   COMPARISON OF HYPERGLYCEMIA AND HYPOGLYCEMIA

Hyperglycemia	Hypoglycemia
Manifestations*	
Elevated blood glucose† Increase in urination Increase in appetite followed by lack of appetite Weakness, fatigue Blurred vision Headache Glycosuria Nausea and vomiting Abdominal cramps Progression to DKA or HHS	Blood glucose <70 mg/dL (3.9 mmol/L) Cold, clammy skin Numbness of fingers, toes, mouth Rapid heartbeat Emotional changes Headache Nervousness, tremors Faintness, dizziness Unsteady gait, slurred speech Hunger Changes in vision Seizures, coma
Causes	
Illness, infection Corticosteroids Too much food Too little or no diabetes medication Inactivity Emotional, physical stress Poor absorption of insulin	Alcohol intake without food Too little food—delayed, omitted, inadequate intake Too much diabetic medication Too much exercise without adequate food intake Diabetes medication or food taken at wrong time Loss of weight without change in medication Use of β-adrenergic blockers interfering with recognition of symptoms
Treatment	
Get medical care Continue diabetes medication as ordered Check blood glucose frequently and check urine for ketones record results Drink fluids at least on an hourly basis Contact health care provider regarding ketonuria	Follow the Rule of 15 (see p. 1179). See Table 49-19 for treatment of hypoglycemia.
Preventive Measures	
Take prescribed dose of medication at proper time Accurately administer insulin, noninsulin injectables, OA Maintain diet Adhere to sick-day rules when ill Check blood for glucose as ordered Wear diabetic identification	Take prescribed dose of medication at proper time. Accurately administer insulin, noninsulin injectables, OA. Ingest all recommended foods at proper time. Provide adequate food intake needed for calories for exercise. Be able to recognize and know symptoms and treat them immediately. Carry simple carbohydrates. Educate family and caregiver about symptoms and treatment. Check blood glucose as ordered. Wear Medic Alert (diabetic) identification.

*There is usually a gradual onset of symptoms in hyperglycemia and a rapid onset in hypoglycemia.

†Specific clinical manifestations related to elevated levels of blood glucose vary according to the patient.

DKA, Diabetic ketoacidosis; *HHS,* hyperosmolar hyperglycemic syndrome; *OA,* oral agent.

DIABETIC KETOACIDOSIS

Etiology and Pathophysiology

Diabetic ketoacidosis (DKA) is caused by a profound deficiency of insulin and is characterized by hyperglycemia, ketosis, acidosis, and dehydration. It is most likely to occur in people with type 1 diabetes but may be seen in people with type 2 diabetes in conditions of severe illness or stress when the pancreas cannot meet the extra demand for insulin. Precipitating factors include illness and infection, inadequate insulin dosage, undiagnosed type 1 diabetes, poor self-management, and neglect.

When the circulating supply of insulin is insufficient, glucose cannot be properly used for energy. The body compensates by breaking down fat stores as a secondary source of fuel (Fig. 49-11). Ketones are acidic by-products of fat metabolism that can cause serious problems when they become excessive in the blood. Ketosis alters the pH balance, causing metabolic acidosis to develop. Ketonuria is a process that occurs when ketone bodies are excreted in the urine. During this process, electrolytes become depleted as cations are eliminated along with the anionic ketones in an attempt to maintain electrical neutrality.

Insulin deficiency impairs protein synthesis and causes excessive protein degradation. This results in nitrogen losses from the tissues. Insulin deficiency also stimulates the production of glucose from amino acids (from proteins) in the liver and leads to further hyperglycemia. Because of the deficiency of insulin, the additional glucose cannot be used and the blood glucose level rises further, adding to the osmotic diuresis.

If not treated, the patient will develop severe depletion of sodium, potassium, chloride, magnesium, and phosphate. Vomiting caused by the acidosis results in more fluid and electrolyte losses. Eventually, hypovolemia followed by shock will ensue. Renal failure, which may eventually occur from hypovolemic shock, causes the retention of ketones and glucose, and the acidosis progresses. Untreated, the patient becomes comatose as a result of dehydration, electrolyte imbalance, and acidosis. If the condition is not treated, death is inevitable.

Clinical Manifestations

Dehydration occurs in DKA with manifestations of poor skin turgor, dry mucous membranes, tachycardia, and orthostatic hypotension. Early symptoms may include lethargy and weakness. As the patient becomes severely dehydrated, the skin becomes dry and loose, and the eyes become soft and sunken. Abdominal pain may be present and accompanied by anorexia, nausea, and vomiting. *Kussmaul respirations* (rapid, deep breathing associated with dyspnea) are the body's attempt to reverse metabolic acidosis through the exhalation of excess carbon dioxide. Acetone is noted on the breath as a sweet, fruity odor. (See Chapter 17 for a discussion of respiratory compensation of metabolic acidosis.) Laboratory findings include a blood glucose level greater than or equal to 250 mg/dL (13.9 mmol/L), arterial blood pH less than 7.30, serum bicarbonate level less than 16 mEq/L (16 mmol/L), and moderate to large ketones in the urine or serum.[10]

Collaborative Care

Before the advent of SMBG, patients with DKA required hospitalization for treatment. Today, hospitalization may not be required. If fluid and electrolyte imbalances are not severe and blood glucose levels can be safely monitored at home, DKA may be managed on an outpatient basis (Table 49-17). Other factors

TABLE 49-17 **COLLABORATIVE CARE**
Diabetic Ketoacidosis (DKA) and Hyperosmolar Hyperglycemic Syndrome (HHS)
Diagnostic • History and physical examination • Blood studies, including immediate blood glucose, complete blood count, pH, ketones, electrolytes, blood urea nitrogen, arterial or venous blood gases • Urinalysis, including specific gravity, glucose, acetone **Collaborative Therapy** • Administration of IV fluids • IV administration of short-acting insulin • Electrolyte replacement • Assessment of mental status • Recording of intake and output • Central venous pressure monitoring (if indicated) • Assessment of blood glucose levels • Assessment of blood and urine for ketones • ECG monitoring • Assessment of cardiovascular and respiratory status

to consider when deciding where the patient is managed include the presence of fever, nausea, vomiting, and diarrhea; altered mental status; the cause of the ketoacidosis; and availability of frequent communication with the health care provider (every few hours). Patients with DKA who have an illness such as pneumonia or a urinary tract infection are usually admitted to the hospital.

DKA is a serious condition that proceeds rapidly and must be treated promptly. Refer to Table 49-18 for the emergency management of a patient with DKA. Because fluid imbalance is potentially life threatening, the initial goal of therapy is to establish IV access and begin fluid and electrolyte replacement. Typically, an infusion of 0.45% or 0.9% NaCl at a rate to restore urine output to 30 to 60 mL/hr and to raise BP constitutes the initial fluid therapy regimen. When blood glucose levels approach 250 mg/dL (13.9 mmol/L), 5% to 10% dextrose is added to the fluid regimen to prevent hypoglycemia and a sudden drop in glucose that can be associated with cerebral edema.[10] Overzealous rehydration, especially with hypotonic IV solutions, can result in cerebral edema.

The aim of fluid and electrolyte therapy is to replace extracellular and intracellular water and to correct deficits of sodium, chloride, bicarbonate, potassium, phosphate, magnesium, and nitrogen. Monitor patients with renal or cardiac compromise for fluid overload. Obtain a serum potassium level before starting insulin. If the patient is hypokalemic, insulin administration will further decrease the potassium levels, making early potassium replacement essential. Although initial serum potassium may be normal or high, levels can rapidly decrease once therapy starts as insulin drives potassium into the cells, leading to life-threatening hypokalemia.

IV insulin administration therapy is directed toward correcting hyperglycemia and hyperketonemia. Insulin is immediately started at 0.1 U/kg/hr by a continuous infusion. It is important to prevent rapid drops in serum glucose to avoid cerebral edema. A blood glucose reduction of 36 to 54 mg/dL/hr (2 to 3 mmol/L/hr) will avoid complications.[10] Insulin allows water and potassium to enter the cell along with glucose and can lead to a depletion of vascular volume and hypokalemia, so monitor the patient's fluid balance and potassium levels.

PATHOPHYSIOLOGY MAP

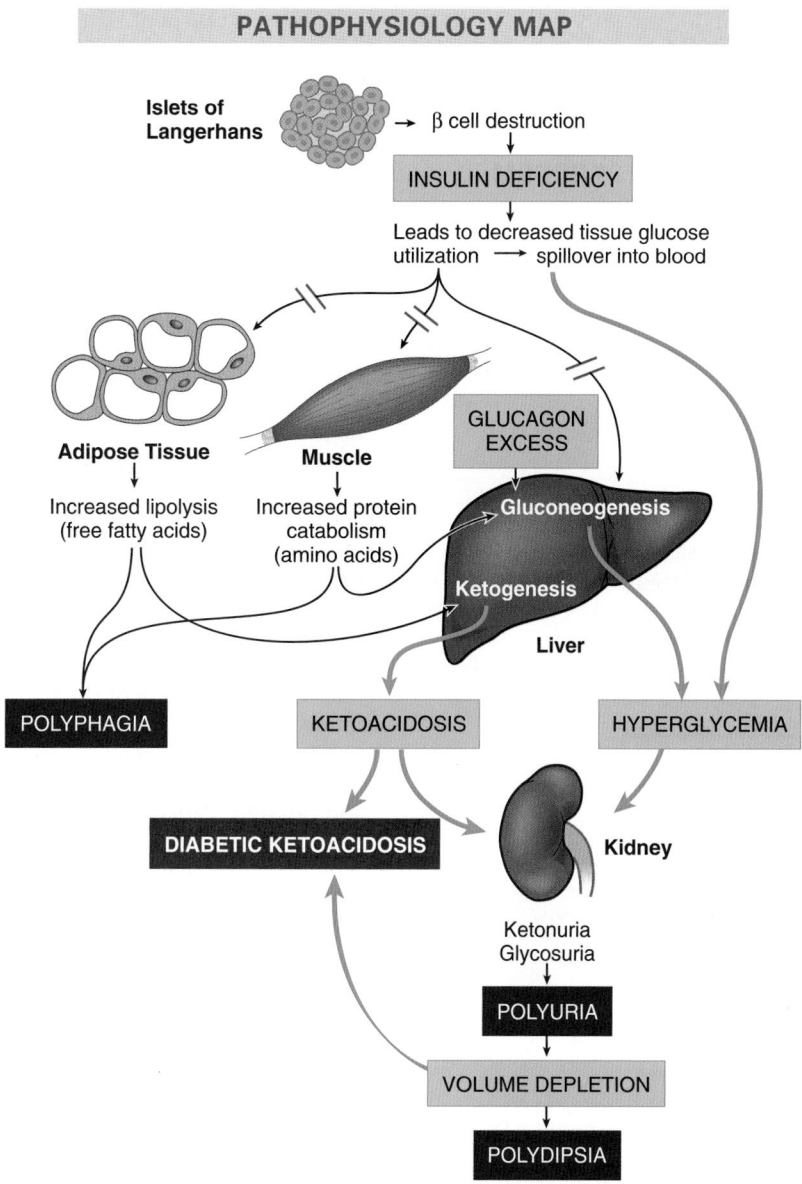

FIG. 49-11 Metabolic events leading to diabetic ketoacidosis.

✚ TABLE 49-18 EMERGENCY MANAGEMENT

Diabetic Ketoacidosis

Etiology	Assessment Findings	Interventions
• Undiagnosed diabetes mellitus • Inadequate treatment of existing diabetes mellitus • Insulin not taken as prescribed • Infection • Change in diet, insulin, or exercise regimen	• Dry mouth • Thirst • Abdominal pain • Nausea and vomiting • Gradually increasing restlessness, confusion, lethargy • Flushed, dry skin • Eyes appearing sunken • Breath odor of ketones • Rapid, weak pulse • Labored breathing (Kussmaul respirations) • Fever • Urinary frequency • Serum glucose >250 mg/dL (13.9 mmol/L) • Glucosuria and ketonuria	**Initial** • Ensure patent airway. • Administer O_2 via nasal cannula or non-rebreather mask. • Establish IV access with large-bore catheter. • Begin fluid resuscitation with 0.9% NaCl solution 1 L/hr until BP stabilized and urine output 30-60 mL/hr. • Begin continuous regular insulin drip 0.1 U/kg/hr. • Identify history of diabetes, time of last food, and time and amount of last insulin injection. **Ongoing Monitoring** • Monitor vital signs, level of consciousness, cardiac rhythm, O_2 saturation, and urine output. • Assess breath sounds for fluid overload. • Monitor serum glucose and serum potassium. • Administer potassium to correct hypokalemia. • Administer sodium bicarbonate if severe acidosis (pH <7.0).

SAFETY ALERT
- Too rapid administration of IV fluids and a rapid lowering of serum glucose can lead to cerebral edema.
- Incorrect fluid replacement, especially with hypotonic fluids, can cause a sudden fall in serum sodium that can cause cerebral edema.

HYPEROSMOLAR HYPERGLYCEMIC SYNDROME

Hyperosmolar hyperglycemic syndrome (HHS) is a life-threatening syndrome that can occur in the patient with diabetes who is able to produce enough insulin to prevent DKA but not enough to prevent severe hyperglycemia, osmotic diuresis, and extracellular fluid depletion (Fig. 49-12). HHS is less common than DKA. It often occurs in patients over 60 years of age with type 2 diabetes.

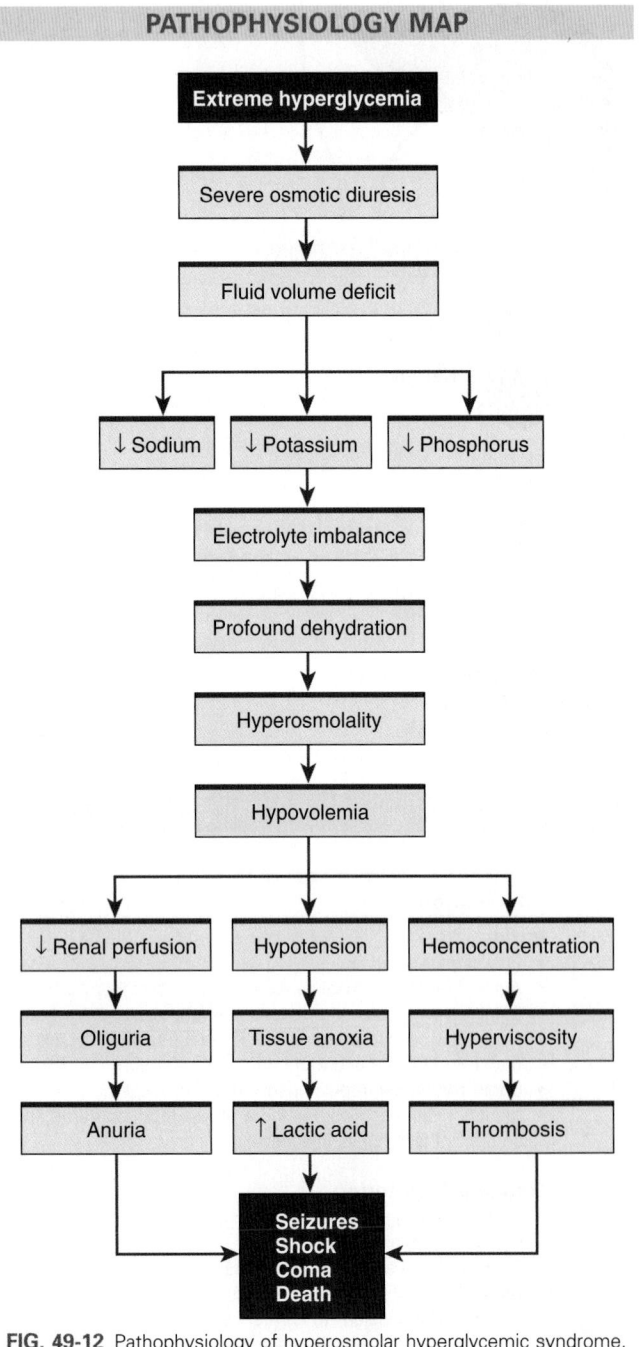

PATHOPHYSIOLOGY MAP

FIG. 49-12 Pathophysiology of hyperosmolar hyperglycemic syndrome.

Common causes of HHS are urinary tract infections, pneumonia, sepsis, any acute illness, and newly diagnosed type 2 diabetes. HHS is often related to impaired thirst sensation and/or a functional inability to replace fluids. There is usually a history of inadequate fluid intake, increasing mental depression, and polyuria.

The main difference between HHS and DKA is that the patient with HHS usually has enough circulating insulin so that ketoacidosis does not occur. Because HHS produces fewer symptoms in the earlier stages, blood glucose levels can climb quite high before the problem is recognized. The higher blood glucose levels increase serum osmolality and produce more severe neurologic manifestations, such as somnolence, coma, seizures, hemiparesis, and aphasia. Since these manifestations resemble a stroke, immediate determination of the glucose level is critical for correct diagnosis and treatment.

Laboratory values in HHS include a blood glucose level greater than 600 mg/dL (33.33 mmol/L) and a marked increase in serum osmolality. Ketone bodies are absent or minimal in both blood and urine.

Collaborative Care

HHS constitutes a medical emergency and has a high mortality rate. The management of DKA and HHS is similar and includes immediate IV administration insulin and either 0.9% or 0.45% NaCl. HHS usually requires greater volumes of fluid replacement (see Table 49-17). This should be accomplished slowly and carefully. Patients with HHS are commonly older and may have cardiac or renal compromise, requiring hemodynamic monitoring to avoid fluid overload during fluid replacement. When blood glucose levels fall to approximately 250 mg/dL (13.9 mmol/L), IV fluids containing glucose are administered to prevent hypoglycemia.

Electrolytes are monitored and replaced as needed. Hypokalemia is not as significant in HHS as it is in DKA, although fluid losses may result in milder potassium deficits that require replacement. Assess vital signs, intake and output, tissue turgor, laboratory values, and cardiac monitoring to check the efficacy of fluid and electrolyte replacement. This includes monitoring serum osmolality and frequently assessing cardiac, renal, and mental status.[10] Once the patient is stabilized, initiate attempts to detect and correct the underlying cause.

NURSING MANAGEMENT
DIABETIC KETOACIDOSIS AND HYPEROSMOLAR HYPERGLYCEMIC SYNDROME

Closely monitor the hospitalized patient with appropriate blood and urine tests. You are responsible for monitoring blood glucose and urine for output and ketones and using laboratory data to determine appropriate patient care.

Monitor the administration of (1) IV fluids to correct dehydration, (2) insulin therapy to reduce blood glucose and serum ketone levels, and (3) electrolytes given to correct electrolyte imbalance. Assess renal status and the cardiopulmonary status related to hydration and electrolyte levels. Monitor the level of consciousness.

Assess for signs of potassium imbalance resulting from hypoinsulinemia and osmotic diuresis (see Chapter 17). When insulin treatment is begun, serum potassium levels may decrease rapidly as potassium moves into the cells once insulin becomes available. This movement of potassium into and out of extracellular fluid influences cardiac functioning. Cardiac monitoring is useful in detecting hyperkalemia and hypokalemia because characteristic changes indicating potassium excess or deficit are observable on electrocardiogram (ECG) tracings (see Fig. 17-14). Assess vital signs often to identify fever, hypovolemic shock, tachycardia, and Kussmaul respirations.

HYPOGLYCEMIA

Hypoglycemia, or low blood glucose, occurs when there is too much insulin in proportion to available glucose in the blood. This causes the blood glucose level to drop to less than 70 mg/dL (3.9 mmol/L). When plasma glucose drops below 70 mg/dL, counterregulatory hormones are released and the autonomic nervous system is activated. Suppression of insulin secretion and production of glucagon and epinephrine provide defense against hypoglycemia. Epinephrine release causes manifestations that include shakiness, palpitations, nervousness, diaphoresis, anxiety, hunger, and pallor. Because the brain requires a constant supply of glucose in sufficient quantities to function properly, hypoglycemia can affect mental functioning. These manifestations are difficulty speaking, visual disturbances, stupor, confusion, and coma. Manifestations of hypoglycemia can mimic alcohol intoxication. Untreated hypoglycemia can progress to loss of consciousness, seizures, coma, and death.

Hypoglycemic unawareness is a condition in which a person does not experience the warning signs and symptoms of hypoglycemia until the glucose levels reach a critical point. Then the person may become incoherent and combative or lose consciousness. This is often related to autonomic neuropathy of diabetes that interferes with the secretion of counterregulatory hormones that produce these symptoms. Patients at risk for hypoglycemic unawareness include those who have had repeated episodes of hypoglycemia, older patients, and patients who use β-adrenergic blockers. Using intensive treatment to get tight blood glucose control in patients who are at risk for hypoglycemic unawareness may not be an appropriate goal because a major drawback is hypoglycemia. These patients are usually managed with blood glucose goals that are somewhat higher than those of patients who are able to detect and manage the onset of hypoglycemia.

Causes of hypoglycemia are often related to a mismatch in the timing of food intake and the peak action of insulin or oral hypoglycemic agents that increase endogenous insulin secretion. The balance between blood glucose and insulin can be disrupted by administering too much insulin or medication, ingesting too little food, delaying the time of eating, and performing unusual amounts of exercise. Hypoglycemia can occur at any time, but most episodes occur when the OA or insulin is at its peak of action or when the patient's daily routine is disrupted without adequate adjustments in diet, medications, and activity. Although hypoglycemia is more common with insulin therapy, it can occur with noninsulin injectable agents and OAs, and it may be severe and persist for an extended time because of the longer duration of action.

Hypoglycemic symptoms may occur when a very high blood glucose level falls too rapidly (e.g., a blood glucose level of 300 mg/dL [16.7 mmol/L] falling quickly to 180 mg/dL [10 mmol/L]). Although the blood glucose level is above normal by definition and measurement, the sudden metabolic shift can evoke hypoglycemic symptoms. Too vigorous management of hyperglycemia with insulin can cause this type of situation.

NURSING AND COLLABORATIVE MANAGEMENT HYPOGLYCEMIA

Hypoglycemia can usually be quickly reversed with effective treatment. At the first sign of hypoglycemia, check the blood glucose if possible. If it is less than 70 mg/dL (3.9 mmol/L), immediately begin treatment for hypoglycemia. If the blood glucose is greater than 70 mg/dL, investigate other possible causes of the signs and symptoms. If the patient has manifestations of hypoglycemia and monitoring equipment is not available or the patient has a history of chronic poor glycemic control, hypoglycemia should be assumed and treatment initiated.

Follow the "Rule of 15" to treat hypoglycemia (Table 49-19). A blood glucose less than 70 mg/dL is treated by ingesting 15 g of a simple (fast-acting) carbohydrate, such as 4 to 6 oz of fruit juice or a regular soft drink. Commercial products such as gels or tablets containing specific amounts of glucose are convenient for carrying in a purse or pocket to be used in such situations. Recheck the blood glucose 15 minutes later. If the value is still less than 70 mg/dL, ingest 15 g more of carbohydrate and recheck the blood glucose in 15 minutes. If no significant improvement occurs after two or three doses of 15 g of simple carbohydrate, contact the health care provider. Because of the potential for rebound hypoglycemia after an acute episode, have the patient ingest a complex carbohydrate after recovery to prevent another hypoglycemic attack.

Avoid treatment with carbohydrates that contain fat, such as candy bars, cookies, whole milk, and ice cream. The fat in those foods will slow the absorption of the glucose and delay the response to treatment. Avoid overtreatment with large quantities of quick-acting carbohydrates so that a rapid fluctuation to hyperglycemia does not occur.

TABLE 49-19   COLLABORATIVE CARE

Hypoglycemia

Diagnostic
- History of hypoglycemic episodes and symptoms.
- Blood glucose—immediately.

Collaborative Therapy
- Determine cause of hypoglycemia (after correction of condition).

Conscious Patient
- Have patient eat or drink 15 g of quick-acting carbohydrate (4-6 oz of regular soda, 8-10 LifeSavers, 1 tbs syrup or honey, 4 tsp jelly, 4-6 oz orange juice, commercial dextrose products [per label instructions]).
- Wait 15 min. Then check blood glucose again.
- If blood glucose is still <70 mg/dL, have patient repeat treatment of 15 g of carbohydrate.
- Once the glucose level is stable and the next meal is more than 1 hr away, give patient additional food of longer-acting combination carbohydrate plus protein or fat (e.g., crackers with peanut butter or cheese) after symptoms subside.
- Immediately notify health care provider or emergency service (if patient outside hospital) if symptoms do not subside after two or three administrations of quick-acting carbohydrate.

Worsening Symptoms or Unconscious Patient
- Subcutaneous or IM injection of 1 mg glucagon. IV administration of 25-50 mL of 50% glucose.

In an acute care setting, patients with hypoglycemia may be treated with 20 to 50 mL of 50% dextrose IV push. Another option, if the patient is not alert enough to swallow and no IV access is available, is to administer 1 mg of glucagon by intramuscular (IM) or subcutaneous injection. An IM injection in a site such as the deltoid muscle will result in a quicker response. Glucagon stimulates a strong hepatic response to convert glycogen to glucose and therefore makes glucose rapidly available. Nausea is a common reaction after glucagon injection. Therefore, to prevent aspiration if vomiting occurs, turn the patient on the side until he or she becomes alert. Patients with minimal glycogen stores will not respond to glucagon. This includes patients with alcohol-related hepatic disease, starvation, and adrenal insufficiency. Teach family members and others likely to be present when a severe hypoglycemic episode occurs when to use and how to inject glucagon.

Once the acute hypoglycemia has been reversed, explore with the patient the reasons why the situation developed. This assessment may indicate the need for additional teaching of the patient and the family to avoid future episodes of hypoglycemia.

CHRONIC COMPLICATIONS OF DIABETES MELLITUS

ANGIOPATHY

Chronic complications of diabetes are primarily those of end-organ disease from damage to blood vessels *(angiopathy)* secondary to chronic hyperglycemia (Fig. 49-13). Angiopathy is one of the leading causes of diabetes-related deaths, with about 68% of deaths caused by CVD and 16% caused by strokes for those ages 65 or older.[2] These chronic blood vessel dysfunctions are divided into two categories: macrovascular complications and microvascular complications.

Several theories exist as to how and why chronic hyperglycemia damages cells and tissues. Possible causes include (1) the accumulation of damaging by-products of glucose metabolism, such as sorbitol, which is associated with damage to nerve cells; (2) the formation of abnormal glucose molecules in the basement membrane of small blood vessels such as those that circulate to the eye and kidney; and (3) a derangement in red blood cell function that leads to a decrease in oxygenation to the tissues.

The Diabetes Control and Complications Trial (DCCT), a landmark study in diabetes management, demonstrated that in patients with type 1 diabetes the risk for microvascular complications could be significantly reduced by keeping blood glucose levels as near to normal as possible for as much of the time as possible *(tight glucose control)*.[20] Subjects who maintained tight glucose control reduced their risk of developing retinopathy and nephropathy, some of the most common microvascular complications. Based on these findings, the ADA issued recommendations for the management of diabetes that included treatment goals to maintain blood glucose levels as near to normal as possible. Specific targets for individual patients must take into account the risk for severe or undetected hypoglycemia as a side effect of tight glucose control.

The United Kingdom Prospective Diabetes Study (UKPDS) demonstrated that intensive treatment of type 2 diabetes significantly lowered the risk for developing diabetes-related eye, kidney, and neurologic problems. The findings from this study included a 25% reduction of microvascular disease and a 16%

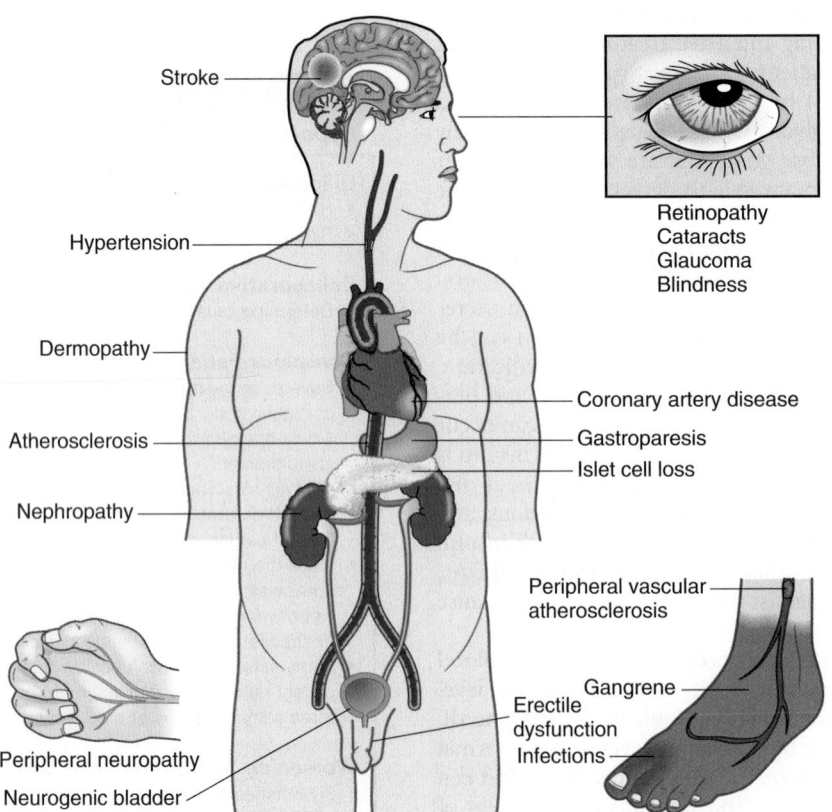

Stroke

Hypertension

Dermopathy

Atherosclerosis

Nephropathy

Peripheral neuropathy

Neurogenic bladder

Retinopathy
Cataracts
Glaucoma
Blindness

Coronary artery disease
Gastroparesis
Islet cell loss

Peripheral vascular atherosclerosis

Gangrene

Erectile dysfunction

Infections

FIG. 49-13 Long-term complications of diabetes mellitus.

reduction in the risk for myocardial infarction in subjects who maintained long-term glycemic control.[21]

Because of the devastating effects of long-term complications, patients with diabetes require scheduled and ongoing monitoring for the detection and prevention of chronic complications. The ADA recommendations for ongoing evaluation are listed in Table 49-20. It is imperative that patients understand the importance of participating in regular follow-up examinations.

Macrovascular Complications

Macrovascular complications are diseases of the large and medium-size blood vessels that occur with greater frequency and with an earlier onset in people with diabetes. Macrovascular diseases include cerebrovascular, cardiovascular, and peripheral vascular disease. Women with diabetes have a four to six times increased risk for CVD, and men with diabetes have a two to three times increased risk for CVD compared with those without diabetes.[4] Patients with diabetes can decrease several risk factors associated with macrovascular complications, such as obesity, smoking, hypertension, high fat intake, and sedentary lifestyle. Smoking, which is detrimental to health in general, is especially injurious to people with diabetes and significantly increases their risk for blood vessel and cardiovascular disease, stroke, and lower extremity amputation. The ADA recommends yearly screening of diabetic patients for CVD risk factors.[10]

Optimizing BP control in patients with diabetes is significant for the prevention of cardiovascular and renal disease. Treating hypertension in diabetic patients results in a decrease in mac-

rovascular and microvascular complications. Hypertension in people with diabetes causes an increase in mortality greater than for those with hypertension without diabetes.[2] A target BP of less than 130/80 mm Hg is recommended for most patients with diabetes.[22]

Patients with diabetes have an increase in lipid abnormalities. This contributes to the increase in CVD seen in this population. The ADA recommends target values of LDL cholesterol less than 100 mg/dL (2.6 mmol/L), triglycerides less than 150 mg/dL (1.7 mmol/L), and HDL cholesterol greater than 40 mg/dL (1.0 mmol/L) in men and greater than 50 mg/dL (1.3 mmol/L) in women.[10] The ADA advocates lifestyle interventions, including nutritional therapy, exercise, weight loss, and smoking cessation to treat hyperlipidemia. Medications (primarily statins) are recommended for those who do not reach lipid goals with lifestyle modifications and for people over 40 years of age with other CVD risk factors regardless of their baseline lipid levels. (Hypertension is discussed in Chapter 33, and coronary artery disease is discussed in Chapter 34.)

Insulin resistance has an important role in the development of CVD and is implicated in the pathogenesis of essential hypertension and dyslipidemia. The role of insulin resistance in the pathogenesis of CVD is not well understood, but it seems to combine with dyslipidemia in contributing to greater risk of CVD in patients with diabetes mellitus. All patients with diabetes should be screened for dyslipidemia at the time diabetes is diagnosed.

Microvascular Complications

Microvascular complications result from thickening of the vessel membranes in the capillaries and arterioles in response to conditions of chronic hyperglycemia. They differ from the macrovascular complications in that they are specific to diabetes. Although microangiopathy can be found throughout the body, the areas most noticeably affected are the eyes (retinopathy), the kidneys (nephropathy), and the skin (dermopathy). Microvascular changes are present in some patients with type 2 diabetes at the time of diagnosis.

DIABETIC RETINOPATHY

Etiology and Pathophysiology

Diabetic retinopathy refers to the process of microvascular damage to the retina as a result of chronic hyperglycemia, nephropathy, and hypertension in patients with diabetes. Diabetic retinopathy is estimated to be the most common cause of new cases of adult blindness.[2]

Retinopathy can be classified as nonproliferative or proliferative. In *nonproliferative retinopathy*, the most common form, partial occlusion of the small blood vessels in the retina causes microaneurysms to develop in the capillary walls. The walls of these microaneurysms are so weak that capillary fluid leaks out, causing retinal edema and eventually hard exudates or intraretinal hemorrhages. Vision may be affected if the macula is involved.

Proliferative retinopathy, the most severe form, involves the retina and the vitreous. When retinal capillaries become occluded, the body compensates by forming new blood vessels to supply the retina with blood, a pathologic process known as *neovascularization*. These new vessels are extremely fragile and hemorrhage easily, producing vitreous contraction. Eventually light is prevented from reaching the retina as the vessels become

TABLE 49-20	MONITORING FOR LONG-TERM COMPLICATIONS OF DIABETES MELLITUS	
Complication	**Type of Examination**	**Frequency**
Retinopathy	• Funduscopic—dilated eye examination • Fundus photography	• Annually
Nephropathy	• Urine for albuminuria • Serum creatinine	• Annually
Neuropathy (foot and lower extremities)	• Visual examination of foot	• Daily by patient • Every visit to health care provider

	• Comprehensive foot:
	  • Visual examination
	  • Sensory examination with monofilament and tuning fork
	  • Palpation (pulses, temperature, callus formation)
		• Annually

Cardiovascular disease	• Risk factor assessment: hypertension, dyslipidemia, smoking, family history of premature coronary artery disease, and presence of microalbuminuria or macroalbuminuria	• At least annually
	• Exercise stress testing (may include stress ECG, stress echocardiogram, stress nuclear imaging)	• As needed based on risk factors

Source: Standards of medical care in diabetes, *Diabetes Care* 36 (Suppl):S11, 2013.

torn and bleed into the vitreous cavity. The patient sees black or red spots or lines. If these new blood vessels pull the retina while the vitreous contracts, causing a tear, partial or complete retinal detachment will occur. If the macula is involved, vision is lost. Without treatment, more than half of patients with proliferative diabetic retinopathy will be blind.

Persons with diabetes are also prone to other visual problems. Glaucoma occurs as a result of the occlusion of the outflow channels secondary to neovascularization. This type of glaucoma is difficult to treat and often results in blindness. Cataracts develop at an earlier age and progress more rapidly in people with diabetes.

Collaborative Care

The earliest and most treatable stages of diabetic retinopathy often produce no changes in the vision. Therefore patients with type 2 diabetes should have a dilated eye examination by an ophthalmologist or a specially trained optometrist at the time of diagnosis and annually thereafter for early detection and treatment. A person with type 1 diabetes should have a dilated eye examination within 5 years after the onset of diabetes and then repeated annually.[10]

The best approach to the management of diabetic eye disease is to prevent it by maintaining good glycemic control and managing hypertension. Laser photocoagulation therapy is indicated to reduce the risk of vision loss in patients with proliferative retinopathy or macular edema and in some cases of nonproliferative retinopathy.[23] Laser photocoagulation destroys the ischemic areas of the retina that produce growth factors that encourage neovascularization. A patient who develops vitreous hemorrhage and retinal detachment of the macula may need to undergo vitrectomy. *Vitrectomy* is the aspiration of blood, membrane, and fibers from the inside of the eye through a small incision just behind the cornea. (Photocoagulation and vitrectomy are discussed in Chapter 22.)

Recent research has identified the importance of vascular endothelial growth factor (VEFG) in the development of diabetic retinopathy. Drugs injected into the eye that block the action of VEGF and reduce inflammation are currently being studied for their effectiveness in treating retinopathy.[23]

NEPHROPATHY

Diabetic nephropathy is a microvascular complication associated with damage to the small blood vessels that supply the glomeruli of the kidney. It is the leading cause of end-stage kidney disease in the United States and is seen in 20% to 40% of people with diabetes. Risk factors for diabetic nephropathy include hypertension, genetic predisposition, smoking, and chronic hyperglycemia. Results of the DCCT and UKPDS research have demonstrated that kidney disease can be significantly reduced when near-normal blood glucose control is maintained.[20,21]

Patients with diabetes are screened for nephropathy annually with a random spot urine collection to assess for albuminuria and measure the albumin-to-creatinine ratio. Serum creatinine is also measured to provide an estimation of the glomerular filtration rate and thus the degree of kidney function.

Patients with diabetes who have microalbuminuria or macroalbuminuria should receive either angiotensin-converting enzyme (ACE) inhibitor drugs (e.g., lisinopril [Prinivil, Zestril]) or angiotensin II receptor antagonists (e.g., losartan [Cozaar]).

Both classifications of these drugs are used to treat hypertension and have been found to delay the progression of nephropathy in patients with diabetes.[10] Hypertension significantly accelerates the progression of nephropathy. Therefore aggressive BP management is indicated for all patients with diabetes. Tight blood glucose control is also critical in the prevention and delay of diabetic nephropathy. (See Chapter 33 for a discussion of hypertension and Chapter 47 for a discussion of renal failure.)

NEUROPATHY

Diabetic neuropathy is nerve damage that occurs because of the metabolic derangements associated with diabetes mellitus. About 60% to 70% of patients with diabetes have some degree of neuropathy.[2] The most common type of neuropathy affecting persons with diabetes is sensory neuropathy. This can lead to the loss of protective sensation in the lower extremities, and, coupled with other factors, significantly increases the risk for complications that result in a lower limb amputation. More than 60% of nontraumatic amputations in the United States occur in people with diabetes.[2] Screening for neuropathy should begin at the time of diagnosis in patients with type 2 diabetes and 5 years after diagnosis in patients with type 1 diabetes.[10]

Etiology and Pathophysiology

The pathophysiologic processes of diabetic neuropathy are not well understood. Several theories exist, including metabolic, vascular, and autoimmune factors. The prevailing theory is that persistent hyperglycemia leads to an accumulation of sorbitol and fructose in the nerves that causes damage by an unknown mechanism. The result is reduced nerve conduction and demyelinization. Ischemic damage by chronic hyperglycemia in blood vessels that supply the peripheral nerves is also implicated in the development of diabetic neuropathy. Neuropathy can precede, accompany, or follow the diagnosis of diabetes.

Classification

The two major categories of diabetic neuropathy are *sensory neuropathy*, which affects the peripheral nervous system, and *autonomic neuropathy*. Each of these types can take on several forms.

Sensory Neuropathy. The most common form of sensory neuropathy is distal symmetric polyneuropathy, which affects the hands and/or feet bilaterally. This is sometimes referred to as *stocking-glove neuropathy*. Characteristics of distal symmetric polyneuropathy include loss of sensation, abnormal sensations, pain, and paresthesias. The pain, which is often described as burning, cramping, crushing, or tearing, is usually worse at night and may occur only at that time. The paresthesias may be associated with tingling, burning, and itching sensations. The patient may report a feeling of walking on pillows or numb feet. At times the skin becomes so sensitive (hyperesthesia) that even light pressure from bed sheets cannot be tolerated. Complete or partial loss of sensitivity to touch and temperature is common. Foot injury and ulcerations can occur without the patient ever having pain (Fig. 49-14). Neuropathy can also cause atrophy of the small muscles of the hands and feet, causing deformity and limiting fine movement.

Control of blood glucose is the only treatment for diabetic neuropathy. It is effective in many, but not all, cases. Drug therapy may be used to treat neuropathic symptoms, particu-

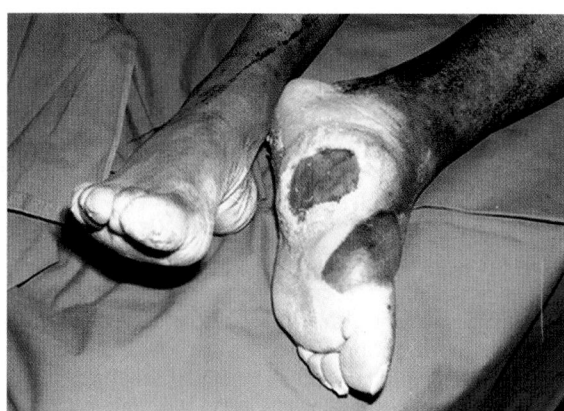

FIG. 49-14 Neuropathy: neurotrophic ulceration.

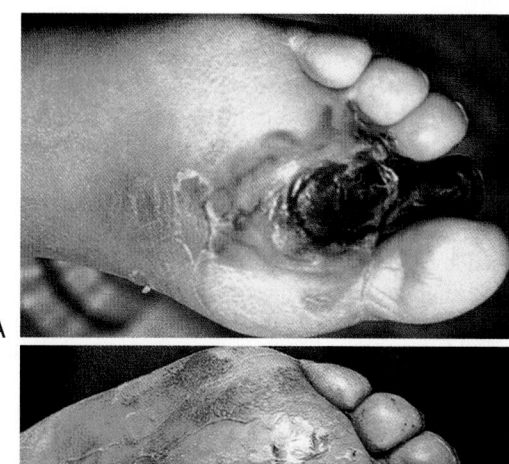

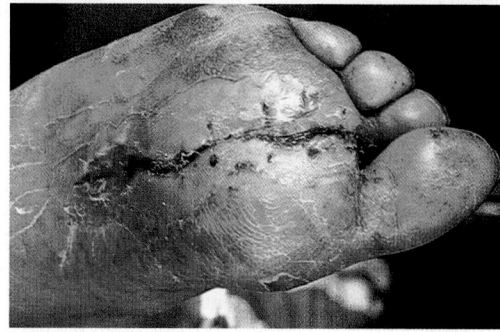

FIG. 49-15 The necrotic toe developed as a complication of diabetes. **A,** Before amputation. **B,** After amputation.

larly pain. Medications commonly used include topical creams (e.g., capsaicin [Zostrix]), tricyclic antidepressants (e.g., amitriptyline [Elavil]), selective serotonin and norepinephrine reuptake inhibitors (e.g., duloxetine [Cymbalta]), and antiseizure medications (e.g., gabapentin [Neurontin], pregabalin [Lyrica]). Capsaicin is a moderately effective topical cream made from chili peppers. It depletes the accumulation of pain-mediating chemicals in the peripheral sensory neurons. The cream is applied three or four times a day. At the start of therapy, symptoms usually increase, followed by relief of pain in 2 to 3 weeks. Tricyclic antidepressants are moderately effective in treating the symptoms of diabetic neuropathy. They work by inhibiting the reuptake of norepinephrine and serotonin, which are neurotransmitters believed to play a role in the transmission of pain through the spinal cord. Duloxetine is thought to relieve pain by increasing the levels of serotonin and norepinephrine, which improves the body's ability to regulate pain. Antiseizure medications decrease the release of neurotransmitters that transmit pain.[24]

Autonomic Neuropathy. Autonomic neuropathy can affect nearly all body systems and lead to hypoglycemic unawareness, bowel incontinence and diarrhea, and urinary retention. *Gastroparesis* (delayed gastric emptying) is a complication of autonomic neuropathy that can produce anorexia, nausea, vomiting, gastroesophageal reflux, and persistent feelings of fullness. Gastroparesis can trigger hypoglycemia by delaying food absorption. Cardiovascular abnormalities associated with autonomic neuropathy are postural hypotension, resting tachycardia, and painless myocardial infarction. Assess patients with diabetes for postural hypotension to determine if they are at risk for falls. Instruct the patient with postural hypotension to change from a lying or sitting position slowly.

Diabetes can affect sexual function in men and women. Erectile dysfunction (ED) in diabetic men is well recognized and common, often being the first manifestation of autonomic neuropathy. ED in diabetes is also associated with other factors, including vascular disease, poor metabolic control, endocrine disorders, psychogenic factors, and medications. Decreased libido is a problem for some women with diabetes. Candidal and nonspecific vaginitis is also common. ED or sexual dysfunction requires sensitive therapeutic counseling for both the patient and the patient's partner. (See Chapter 55 for a further discussion of ED.)

A neurogenic bladder may develop as the sensation in the inner bladder wall decreases, causing urinary retention. A patient with retention has infrequent voiding, difficulty voiding, and a weak stream of urine. Emptying the bladder every 3 hours in a sitting position helps prevent stasis and subsequent infection. Tightening the abdominal muscles during voiding and using the Credé maneuver (mild massage downward over the lower abdomen and bladder) may also help with complete bladder emptying. Cholinergic agonist drugs such as bethanechol (Urecholine) may be used. The patient may also need to learn self-catheterization (see Chapter 46).

COMPLICATIONS OF FEET AND LOWER EXTREMITIES

People with diabetes are at high risk for foot ulcerations and lower extremity amputations.[25] The development of diabetic foot complications can be the result of a combination of microvascular and macrovascular diseases that place the patient at risk for injury and serious infection (Fig. 49-15). Sensory neuropathy and peripheral artery disease (PAD) are risk factors for foot complications. In addition, clotting abnormalities, impaired immune function, and autonomic neuropathy also have a role. Smoking is deleterious to the health of lower extremity blood vessels and increases the risk for amputation.

Sensory neuropathy is a major risk factor for lower extremity amputation in the person with diabetes. *Loss of protective sensation* (LOPS) often prevents the patient from being aware that a foot injury has occurred. Improper footwear and injury from stepping on foreign objects while barefoot are common causes of undetected foot injury in the person with LOPS.[26] Because the primary risk factor for lower extremity amputation is LOPS, annual screening using a *monofilament* is important. This is done by applying a thin, flexible filament to several spots on the plantar surface of the foot and asking the patient to report if it is felt. Insensitivity to a monofilament has been shown to greatly increase the risk for diabetic foot ulcers that can lead to amputation.

PAD increases the risk for amputation by causing a reduction in blood flow to the lower extremities. When blood flow is decreased, oxygen, white blood cells, and vital nutrients are not available to the tissues. Wounds take longer to heal, and the risk for infection increases. Signs of PAD include intermittent claudication, pain at rest, cold feet, loss of hair, delayed capillary filling, and dependent rubor (redness of the skin that occurs when the extremity is in a dependent position). The disease is diagnosed by history, ankle-brachial index (ABI) (see Table 38-3), and angiography. Management includes control or reduction of risk factors, particularly smoking, high cholesterol intake, and hypertension. Bypass or graft surgery is indicated in some patients. (PAD is discussed in Chapter 38.)

If the patient has LOPS or PAD, aggressive measures must be taken to teach the patient how to prevent foot ulcers. These measures include the selection of proper footwear, including prescription shoes. The patient also must carefully avoid injury to the foot, practice diligent skin and nail care, inspect the foot thoroughly each day, and treat small problems promptly.[26] Guidelines for patient teaching are listed in Table 49-21.

Proper care of a diabetic foot ulcer is critical for wound healing. Several forms of treatment can be used. Casting can be done to redistribute the weight on the plantar surface of the foot. Wound control for the ulcer can include debridement, dressings, advanced wound healing products (becaplermin [Regranex]), vacuum-assisted closure, ultrasound, hyperbaric oxygen, and skin grafting.[26]

| TABLE 49-21 | **PATIENT & CAREGIVER TEACHING GUIDE***|

Foot Care

Include the following instructions when teaching the patient and caregiver about diabetic foot care.

1. Wash feet daily with a mild soap and warm water. First test water temperature with hands.
2. Pat feet dry gently, especially between toes.
3. Examine feet daily for cuts, blisters, swelling, and red, tender areas. Do not depend on feeling sores. If eyesight is poor, have others inspect feet.
4. Use lanolin on feet to prevent skin from drying and cracking. Do not apply between toes.
5. Use mild foot powder on sweaty feet.
6. Do not use commercial remedies to remove calluses or corns.
7. Cleanse cuts with warm water and mild soap, covering with clean dressing. Do not use iodine, rubbing alcohol, or strong adhesives.
8. Report skin infections or nonhealing sores to health care provider immediately.
9. Cut toenails evenly with rounded contour of toes. Do not cut down corners. The best time to trim nails is after a shower or bath.
10. Separate overlapping toes with cotton or lamb's wool.
11. Avoid open-toe, open-heel, and high-heel shoes. Leather shoes are preferred to plastic ones. Wear slippers with soles. Do not go barefoot. Shake out shoes before putting on.
12. Wear clean, absorbent (cotton or wool) socks or stockings that have not been mended. Colored socks must be colorfast.
13. Do not wear clothing that leaves impressions, hindering circulation.
14. Do not use hot water bottles or heating pads to warm feet. Wear socks for warmth.
15. Guard against frostbite.
16. Exercise feet daily either by walking or by flexing and extending feet in suspended position. Avoid prolonged sitting, standing, and crossing of legs.

*This teaching guide is also appropriate for patients with peripheral vascular problems.

Neuropathic arthropathy, or *Charcot's foot,* results in ankle and foot changes that ultimately lead to joint dysfunction and footdrop. These changes occur gradually and promote an abnormal distribution of weight over the foot, further increasing the chances of developing a foot ulcer as new pressure points emerge. Foot deformity should be recognized early and proper footwear fitted before ulceration occurs.

INTEGUMENTARY COMPLICATIONS

Up to two thirds of persons with diabetes develop skin problems.[10] Diabetic dermopathy, the most common diabetic skin lesion, is characterized by reddish brown, round or oval patches. They initially are scaly, then they flatten out and become indented. The lesions appear most frequently on the shins, but can also be found on the front of the thighs, forearm, side of the foot, scalp, and trunk.

Acanthosis nigricans is a velvety light brown to black skin thickening, predominantly seen on flexures, axillae, and the neck. *Necrobiosis lipoidica diabeticorum* usually appears as red-yellow lesions, with atrophic skin that becomes shiny and transparent revealing tiny blood vessels under the surface (Fig. 49-16). This condition is uncommon and occurs more frequently in young women. It may appear before other clinical signs or symptoms of diabetes. Because the thin skin is prone to injury, special care must be taken to protect affected areas from injury and ulceration.

INFECTION

A person with diabetes is more susceptible to infections because of a defect in the mobilization of white blood cells and an impaired phagocytosis by neutrophils and monocytes. Recurring or persistent infections such as *Candida albicans,* as well as boils and furuncles, in the undiagnosed patient often lead the health care provider to suspect diabetes. Loss of sensation (neuropathy) may delay the detection of an infection.

Persistent glycosuria may predispose patients to bladder infections, especially patients with a neurogenic bladder.

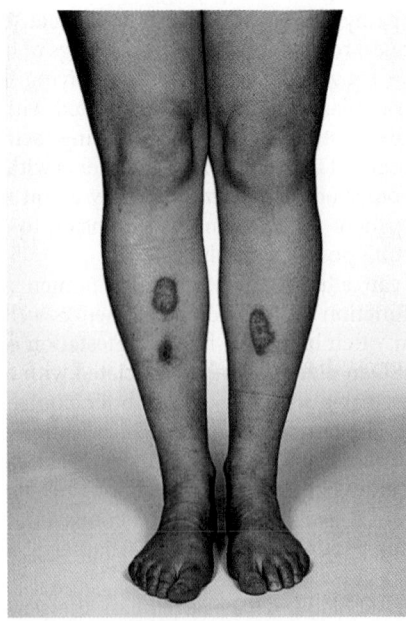

FIG. 49-16 Necrobiosis lipoidica diabeticorum.

Decreased circulation resulting from angiopathy can prevent or delay the immune response. Antibiotic therapy has prevented infection from being a major cause of death in diabetic patients. The treatment of infections must be prompt and vigorous. Teach diabetic patients measures to prevent infection: practicing good hand hygiene, avoiding exposure to individuals who have a communicable illness, and getting an annual influenza vaccine and pneumococcal vaccine (Pneumovax) every 5 years.

PSYCHOLOGIC CONSIDERATIONS

Patients with diabetes have high rates of depression, anxiety, and eating disorders. Depression contributes to poor adherence to diabetes self-care, feelings of helplessness related to chronic illness, and poor outcomes.[10] Assess patients for manifestations of depression.

Persons with type 1 diabetes have an increased risk of developing disordered eating behaviors (DEB).[27] The greatest incidence of eating disorders is seen in females. Adolescent girls

with diabetes are more than twice as likely to develop DEB than those who do not have diabetes.[28] DEBs include anorexia, bulimia, binge eating, excessive restriction of calories, and intense exercise. Patients may intentionally decrease their dose of insulin or omit the dose. This leads to weight loss, hyperglycemia, and glycosuria because the food ingested cannot be used for energy without adequate insulin. Insulin omission and DEBs can have serious consequences, including retinopathy, neuropathy, lipid abnormalities, DKA, and death.[28] Open com-

---

DELEGATION DECISIONS

Caring for the Patient With Diabetes Mellitus

Oral agents (OAs), noninsulin injectable agents, and insulin can be administered by licensed practical/vocational nurses (LPN/LVNs) (and in some states and settings by unlicensed assistive personnel [UAP]) to stable patients. In patients experiencing acute complications of diabetes mellitus (DM), actions such as insulin administration and infusion of IV fluids should be done or directly supervised by a registered nurse (RN).

Role of Registered Nurse (RN)
- Assess for risk factors for prediabetes and type 1 and type 2 DM.
- Teach the patient and caregiver about self-management of DM, including self-monitoring of blood glucose (SMBG), insulin, noninsulin injectables, OAs, nutrition, physical activity, and recognition and management of hypoglycemia.
- Develop a plan to avoid hypoglycemia or hyperglycemia in the patient with DM who is acutely ill or having surgery.
- Assess for acute complications and implement appropriate actions: hypoglycemia, diabetic ketoacidosis (DKA), and hyperosmolar hyperglycemic syndrome (HHS).
- Assess for chronic complications of diabetes, including cardiovascular disease, retinopathy, nephropathy, neuropathy, and diabetic foot complications.
- Teach patient and caregiver about prevention and management of chronic complications of diabetes.

Role of Licensed Practical/Vocational Nurse (LPN/LVN)
- Administer OAs and routinely scheduled insulin regimens.
- Monitor the diabetic patient for symptoms of hypoglycemia, DKA, and HHS.
- In the ambulatory or home setting, monitor patient self-management of insulin, OAs, nutrition, and physical activity.
- Report concerns with patient self-management in the home setting to the RN.

Role of Unlicensed Assistive Personnel (UAP)
- Check capillary blood glucose (CBG) levels (after being trained and evaluated in this procedure) and report values to the RN.
- Report changes in patient vital signs, urine output, behavior, or level of consciousness to the RN.
- In a community or home care setting, administer OAs and insulin to the stable diabetic patient (consider state nurse practice act and agency policy).

ETHICAL/LEGAL DILEMMAS

Durable Power of Attorney for Health Care

Situation
G.V., a 64-yr-old white woman, is admitted to the intensive care unit with heart failure. She has many complications from a long-term history of type 1 diabetes and hypertension, including a right leg above-the-knee amputation and blindness related to diabetic retinopathy. She severed ties with her family 30 yr ago. She has a life partner of 35 yr whom she designated as her proxy in her signed Durable Power of Attorney. She has stated many times that she would rather die than have renal dialysis. She has been sedated and intubated for 3 days. The physician plans to extubate her and resuscitate her so that dialysis can be initiated. Her brother shows up at the hospital and supports the physician's decision. Her partner disagrees with the decision. The physician refuses to recognize her partner as proxy because she is not a blood relative.

Ethical/Legal Points for Consideration
- The Patient Self-Determination Act (1990) requires all health care facilities receiving Medicare and Medicaid funding to make available advance directives allowing individuals to state their preferences or refusals of health care in the event that they are incapable of consenting for themselves.
- Durable Power of Attorney for health care is one type of advance directive in which people, when they are competent, identify someone else to make decisions for them, should they lose their decision-making ability in the future.
- The Living Will, another type of advance directive, permits individuals to state their own preferences and refusals.
- Many health care providers mistakenly think that proxies must be family members or blood relatives. Lesbian, gay, bisexual, and transgender individuals often have difficulty having their partnership recognized as valid, especially if the patient's family disputes their rights.
- Some families are deeply divided on decisions for their loved ones, and sometimes difficulties occur when money and property are also disputed. The passage of time may be an issue where the original documents were executed and then changes occurred (e.g., divorce, death or disability of the proxy, inability to contact the proxy, inability to find a valid original of the advance directive).
- Within your scope of nursing practice, you need to be informed as to decision-making laws and regulations in your own state and make advance directive documents available to patients. In addition, you need to (1) teach patients and their families about advance directives, (2) make sure that health care providers are aware of the presence of advance directives, (3) assist the patient and family in communicating with the health care providers when a "No Code" order is requested, and (4) assist a conflicted family in obtaining appropriate counseling whenever necessary.

Discussion Questions
1. How would you handle a situation in which the family and surrogate decision maker disagree?
2. How can you assess the patient and family's understanding of durable power of attorney and assist them in understanding their role in decision making?
3. What should you do when a physician orders dialysis to be initiated when you know that this goes against the patient's advance directive?

munication is critical to identify these behaviors early. Patients with eating disorders need to be seen by a mental health professional with expertise in eating disorders and an understanding of diabetes management.

GERONTOLOGIC CONSIDERATIONS

DIABETES MELLITUS

Diabetes is present in more than 25% of persons over 65 years of age, with this age-group being the fastest growing segment of the population developing diabetes.[2] Older people with diabetes have higher rates of premature death, functional disability, and coexisting illnesses such as hypertension and stroke than those without diabetes. The prevalence of diabetes increases with age. A major reason for this is that the process of aging is associated with a reduction in β-cell function, decreased insulin sensitivity, and altered carbohydrate metabolism. Aging is also associated with a number of conditions that are more likely to be treated with medications that impair insulin action (e.g., corticosteroids, antihypertensives, phenothiazines). Undiagnosed and untreated diabetes is more common in older adults, partly because many of the normal physiologic changes of aging resemble those of diabetes, such as low energy levels, falls, dizziness, confusion, and chronic urinary tract infections.

Several factors are taken into account when determining glycemic goals for an older adult. One is that hypoglycemic unawareness is more common in older adults, making these patients more likely to suffer adverse consequences from blood glucose–lowering therapy. They may have delayed psychomotor function that could interfere with the ability to treat hypoglycemia. Other factors to consider in establishing glycemic goals for the older patient include the patient's own desire for treatment and coexisting medical problems such as cognitive impairment. Compounding the challenge, diabetes has been found to contribute to a greater rate of decline of cognitive function. Although it is generally agreed that treatment is indicated to prevent acute complications and avoid unpleasant symptoms, strict glycemic control may be difficult to achieve.

Diet and exercise are recommended as therapy for older adult patients with diabetes. This should take into account functional limitations that may interfere with physical activity and the ability to prepare meals. Because of the physiologic changes that occur with aging, the therapeutic outcome for the older adult with diabetes who receives OAs may be altered. Assess renal function and creatinine clearance in patients over 80 years of age taking metformin. Monitor those taking sulfonylurea drugs (e.g., glipizide) for hypoglycemia and renal and liver dysfunction. Insulin therapy may be instituted if OAs are not effective. However, it is important to recognize that older adults are more likely to have limitations in the manual dexterity and visual acuity necessary for accurate insulin administration. Insulin pens may be a safer alternative for older adults.

Base patient teaching on the individual's needs, using a slower pace with simple printed or audio materials in patients with cognitive and functional limitations. Include the family or caregivers in the teaching. The patient education issues for the older patient include those related to altered vision, mobility, cognitive status, and functional ability. Consider the patient's financial and social situation and the effect of multiple medications, eating habits, and quality-of-life issues.

CASE STUDY

Diabetic Ketoacidosis

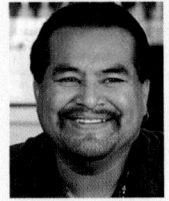

iStockphoto/Thinkstock

Patient Profile

N.B., a 34-yr-old Native American man, was admitted to the emergency department after he was found unconscious by his wife in their home.

Subjective Data (Provided by Wife)

- Was diagnosed with type 1 diabetes mellitus 12 mo ago
- Was taking 50 U/day of insulin: 5 U of lispro insulin with breakfast, 5 U with lunch, and 10 U with dinner plus 30 U of glargine insulin at bedtime
- Has history of gastroenteritis for 1 wk with vomiting and anorexia
- Stopped taking insulin 2 days ago when he was unable to eat

Objective Data

Physical Examination

- Breathing is deep and rapid
- Fruity acetone smell on breath
- Skin flushed and dry

Diagnostic Studies

- Blood glucose level 730 mg/dL (40.5 mmol/L)
- Blood pH 7.26

Discussion Questions

1. Briefly explain the pathophysiology of the development of diabetic ketoacidosis (DKA) in this patient.
2. What clinical manifestations of DKA does this patient exhibit?
3. What factors precipitated this patient's DKA?
4. ***Priority Decision:*** What is the priority nursing intervention for N.B.?
5. What distinguishes this case history from one of hyperosmolar hyperglycemic syndrome (HHS) or hypoglycemia?
6. ***Priority Decision:*** What is the priority teaching that should be done with this patient and his family?
7. What role should N.B.'s wife have in the management of his diabetes?
8. ***Priority Decision:*** Based on the assessment data presented, what are the priority nursing diagnoses? Are there any collaborative problems?
9. ***Evidence-Based Practice:*** N.B.'s wife asks you if she should have given her husband insulin when he got sick. How would you respond?

ⓔvolve Answers and a corresponding concept map are available at *http://evolve.elsevier.com/Lewis/medsurg.*

BRIDGE TO NCLEX EXAMINATION

The number of the question corresponds to the same-numbered outcome at the beginning of the chapter.

1. Polydipsia and polyuria related to diabetes mellitus are primarily due to
   a. the release of ketones from cells during fat metabolism.
   b. fluid shifts resulting from the osmotic effect of hyperglycemia.
   c. damage to the kidneys from exposure to high levels of glucose.
   d. changes in RBCs resulting from attachment of excessive glucose to hemoglobin.

2. Which statement would be correct for a patient with type 2 diabetes who was admitted to the hospital with pneumonia?
   a. The patient must receive insulin therapy to prevent ketoacidosis.
   b. The patient has islet cell antibodies that have destroyed the pancreas's ability to produce insulin.
   c. The patient has minimal or absent endogenous insulin secretion and requires daily insulin injections.
   d. The patient may have sufficient endogenous insulin to prevent ketosis but is at risk for hyperosmolar hyperglycemic syndrome.

3. Analyze the following diagnostic findings for your patient with type 2 diabetes. Which result will need further assessment?
   a. A1C 9%
   b. BP 126/80 mm Hg
   c. FBG 130 mg/dL (7.2 mmol/L)
   d. LDL cholesterol 100 mg/dL (2.6 mmol/L)

4. Which statement by the patient with type 2 diabetes is accurate?
   a. "I am supposed to have a meal or snack if I drink alcohol."
   b. "I am not allowed to eat any sweets because of my diabetes."
   c. "I do not need to watch what I eat because my diabetes is not the bad kind."
   d. "The amount of fat in my diet is not important. Only carbohydrates raise my blood sugar."

5. You are caring for a patient with newly diagnosed type 1 diabetes. What information is essential to include in your patient teaching before discharge from the hospital (select all that apply)?
   a. Insulin administration
   b. Elimination of sugar from diet
   c. Need to reduce physical activity
   d. Use of a portable blood glucose monitor
   e. Hypoglycemia prevention, symptoms, and treatment

6. What is the priority action for the nurse to take if the patient with type 2 diabetes complains of blurred vision and irritability?
   a. Call the physician.
   b. Administer insulin as ordered.
   c. Check the patient's blood glucose level.
   d. Assess for other neurologic symptoms.

7. A diabetic patient has a serum glucose level of 824 mg/dL (45.7 mmol/L) and is unresponsive. After assessing the patient, the nurse suspects diabetic ketoacidosis rather than hyperosmolar hyperglycemic syndrome based on the finding of
   a. polyuria.
   b. severe dehydration.
   c. rapid, deep respirations.
   d. decreased serum potassium.

8. Which are appropriate therapies for patients with diabetes mellitus (select all that apply)?
   a. Use of statins to treat dyslipidemia
   b. Use of diuretics to treat nephropathy
   c. Use of ACE inhibitors to treat nephropathy
   d. Use of serotonin agonists to decrease appetite
   e. Use of laser photocoagulation to treat retinopathy

1. b, 2. d, 3. a, 4. a, 5. a, d, e, 6. c, 7. c, 8. a, c, e

ℯvolve

For rationales to these answers and even more NCLEX review questions, visit *http://evolve.elsevier.com/Lewis/medsurg*.

REFERENCES

1. American Diabetes Association: Total prevalence of diabetes and prediabetes. Retrieved from *www.diabetes.org*.
2. Centers for Disease Control and Prevention: National diabetes fact sheet, 2011. Retrieved from *www.cdc.gov/diabetes/pubs/pdf/ndfs_2011.pdf*.
3. American Diabetes Association: Diagnosis and classification of diabetes mellitus, *Diabetes Care* 36 (Suppl):S67, 2013.
4. Centers for Disease Control and Prevention: Diabetes public health resource: groups especially affected, 2012. Retrieved from *www.cdc.gov/diabetes/consumer/groups.htm*.
5. McKenny R, Short D: Tipping the balance: the pathophysiology of obesity and type 2 diabetes mellitus, *Surg Clin North Am* 91:1139, 2011.
*6. Grundy S: Prediabetes, metabolic syndrome, and cardiovascular disease, *J Am Coll Cardiol* 14:635, 2012.

7. National Diabetes Information Clearinghouse: National diabetes statistics, 2011. Retrieved from *http://diabetes.niddk.nih.gov/dm/pubs/statistics*.
*8. HAPO Study Cooperative Research Group: Hyperglycemia and adverse pregnancy outcomes, *N Engl J Med* 358:1991, 2008. (Classic)
*9. Spollett G: Insulin initiation in type 2 diabetes: what are the treatment regimen options and how can we best help patients feel empowered? *JAANP* 24:249, 2012.
10. American Association of Diabetes Educators: *The art and science of self-management education desk reference*, ed 2, Chicago, 2011, The Association.
11. BD Diabetes: Syringe and needle sizes. Retrieved from *www.bd.com/us/diabetes/page.aspx?cat=7001&id=7253*.
12. Magwire M: Addressing barriers to insulin therapy: the role of insulin pens, *Am J Therap* 18:392, 2011.
13. Pickup J: Insulin-pump therapy for type 1 diabetes mellitus, *N Engl J Med* 366:1616, 2012.

*Evidence-based information for clinical practice.

14. Levesque C: Medical management of type 2 diabetes, *J Nurse Pract* 7:492, 2011.

15. American Diabetes Association: Nutrition recommendations and interventions for diabetes, *Diabetes Care* 31:S61, 2008. (Classic)

16. American Diabetes Association: Food and fitness: create your plate. Retrieved from *www.diabetes.org/food-and-fitness/food/planning-meals/create-your-plate*.

17. US Department of Health and Human Services: A report of the surgeon general physical activity and health executive summary. Retrieved from *www.cdc.gov/nccdphp/sgr/index.htm*.

*18. Diabetes Control and Complications Trial Research Group: The effect of intensive treatment of diabetes on the development and progression of long-term complications in insulin-dependent diabetes mellitus, *N Engl J Med* 329:977, 1993. (Classic)

*19. Wang H, Yeh M: Psychological resistance to insulin therapy in adults with type 2 diabetes: mixed-method systematic review, *J Adv Nurs* 68:43, 2012.

20. Boucher J, Hurrell D: Cardiovascular disease and diabetes, *Diabetes Spectrum* 21:154, 2008. (Classic)

*21. UK Prospective Diabetes Study (UKPDS) Group: Intensive blood-glucose control with sulphonylureas or insulin compared with conventional treatment and risk of complications in patients with type 2 diabetes, *Lancet* 352:837, 1998. (Classic)

22. National High Blood Pressure Education Coordinating Committee: The seventh report of the Joint National Committee on Prevention, Detection, Evaluation, and Treatment of High Blood Pressure: the JNC report, *JAMA* 289:2560, 2003. (Classic)

23. Antonetti D, Klein R, Gardner T: Diabetic retinopathy, *N Engl J Med* 366:1227, 2012.

24. Callaghan B, Cheng H, Stables C, et al: Diabetic neuropathy: clinical manifestations and current treatments, *Lancet Neuro* 11:521, 2012.

25. Lipsky B, Berendt A, Cornia P, et al: Infectious Diseases Society of America clinical practice guideline for the diagnosis and treatment of diabetic foot infections, *CID* 54:E132, 2012.

26. Alexiadou K, Doupis J: Management of diabetic foot ulcers, *Diabetes Ther* 3:1, 2012.

27. Young-Hyman D, Davis C: Disordered eating behaviors in individuals with diabetes: importance of context, evaluation and classification, *Diabetes Care* 33:683, 2010.

*28. Jaser S, Yates H, Dumser S, et al: Risk behaviors in adolescents with type 1 diabetes, *Diabetes Educ* 37:756, 2011.

RESOURCES

American Association of Diabetes Educators
www.diabeteseducator.org
American Diabetes Association
www.diabetes.org
Diabetes Monitor
www.diabetesmonitor.com
Diabetes at Work
www.diabetesatwork.org
National Diabetes Education Program
www.ndep.nih.gov
National Diabetes Education Program's Better Diabetes Care
www.betterdiabetescare.nih.gov
National Diabetes Information Clearinghouse
www.diabetes.niddk.nih.gov

The worst thing that can happen to you may be the best thing for you, if you don't let it get the best of you.
Will Rogers

Nursing Management
Endocrine Problems

Katherine A. Kelly

⊜volve WEBSITE

LEARNING OUTCOMES

1. Explain the pathophysiology, clinical manifestations, collaborative care, and nursing management of the patient with an imbalance of hormones produced by the anterior pituitary gland.
2. Describe the pathophysiology, clinical manifestations, collaborative care, and nursing management of the patient with an imbalance of hormones produced by the posterior pituitary gland.
3. Explain the pathophysiology, clinical manifestations, collaborative care, and nursing management of the patient with thyroid dysfunction.
4. Describe the pathophysiology, clinical manifestations, collaborative care, and nursing management of the patient with an imbalance of the hormone produced by the parathyroid glands.

5. Identify the pathophysiology, clinical manifestations, collaborative care, and nursing management of the patient with an imbalance of hormones produced by the adrenal cortex.
6. Describe the pathophysiology, clinical manifestations, collaborative care, and nursing management of the patient with an excess of hormones produced by the adrenal medulla.
7. List the side effects of corticosteroid therapy.
8. Describe common nursing assessments, interventions, rationales, and expected outcomes related to patient teaching for management of chronic endocrine problems.

KEY TERMS

acromegaly, p. 1190
Addison's disease, p. 1211
Cushing syndrome, p. 1207
diabetes insipidus (DI), p. 1194
exophthalmos, p. 1197
goiter, p. 1195
Graves' disease, p. 1196

hyperaldosteronism, p. 1214
hyperparathyroidism, p. 1205
hyperthyroidism, p. 1196
hypoparathyroidism, p. 1206
hypopituitarism, p. 1192
hypothyroidism, p. 1201
myxedema, p. 1202

pheochromocytoma, p. 1214
syndrome of inappropriate antidiuretic hormone (SIADH), p. 1193
thyroid cancer, p. 1204
thyroiditis, p. 1196
thyrotoxicosis, p. 1197

Reviewed by Dorothy (Dottie) M. Mathers, RN, DNP, CNE, Professor, School of Health Sciences, Pennsylvania College of Technology, Williamsport, Pennsylvania; Teresa J. Seright, RN, PhD, CCRN, Assistant Professor of Nursing, Montana State University, Bozeman, Montana; Daryle Wane, PhD, ARNP, FNP-BC, Professor of Nursing, Generic Program Track Coordinator, Pasco-Hernando Community College, New Port Richey, Florida; Saundra J. Hendricks, RN, MS, FNP, BC-ADM, Department of Medicine, Endocrine Division, The Methodist Hospital, Houston, Texas; Beth Lucasy, RN, MA, VP Marketing and Communications, TVAX Biomedical, Kansas City, Missouri; and Barbara Lukert, MD, Endocrinologist, University of Kansas Medical Center, Kansas City, Kansas.

The endocrine system is made up of a number of organs and glands that are involved in the synthesis and secretion of hormones that affect every body system. Because these hormones have such a wide range of action, endocrine problems are associated with a variety of clinical manifestations. Many aspects of a person's life are affected when an endocrine problem is present.

DISORDERS OF ANTERIOR PITUITARY GLAND

ACROMEGALY

Acromegaly is a rare condition characterized by an overproduction of growth hormone (GH). Approximately six out of every 1 million adults in the United States are diagnosed annually.[1] Both genders are affected equally. The mean age at the time of diagnosis is 40 to 45 years old.

Etiology and Pathophysiology

Acromegaly most often occurs as a result of a benign pituitary tumor (adenoma). The excessive secretion of GH results in an overgrowth of soft tissues and bones in the hands, feet, and face. Because the problem develops after epiphyseal closure, the bones of the arms and legs do not grow longer.

Clinical Manifestations

The changes resulting from excess GH can occur over a number of years and may go unnoticed by family and friends. Patients experience enlargement of hands and feet with joint pain that can range from mild to crippling. Carpal tunnel syndrome may be present. Thickening and enlargement of the bony and soft tissues on the face, feet, and head occur (Fig. 50-1).

Enlargement of the tongue results in speech difficulties, and the voice deepens because of hypertrophy of the vocal cords. Sleep apnea may occur because of upper airway narrowing and obstruction from increased amounts of pharyngeal soft tissues. The skin becomes thick, leathery, and oily. Persons with acromegaly may experience peripheral neuropathy and proximal muscle weakness. Women may develop menstrual disturbances.

Visual changes may occur due to pressure on the optic nerve from a pituitary adenoma. Headaches are common. Since GH antagonizes the action of insulin leading to hyperglycemia,

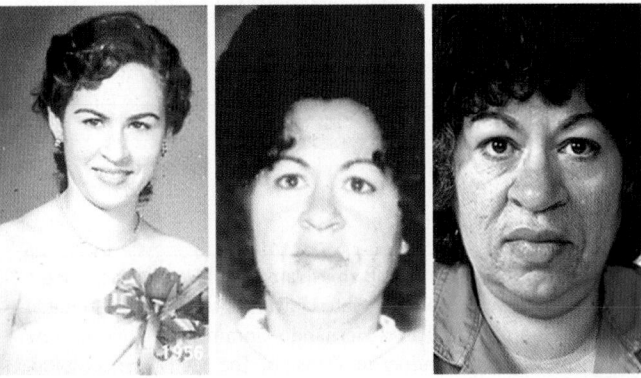

FIG. 50-1 Progressive development of facial changes associated with acromegaly.

glucose intolerance and manifestations of diabetes mellitus may occur, including *polydipsia* (increased thirst) and *polyuria* (increased urination).[2] Because GH mobilizes stored fat for energy, it increases free fatty acid levels in the blood and predisposes the patient to atherosclerosis.

The life expectancy of patients with acromegaly is reduced by 5 to 10 years. They are more likely to succumb to cardiac and respiratory diseases, diabetes mellitus, and colorectal cancer.[3] Even when patients are cured or acromegaly is well controlled, manifestations such as joint pain and deformities often remain.

Diagnostic Studies

In addition to the history and physical examination, a diagnosis of acromegaly requires evaluation of plasma insulin-like growth factor 1 (IGF-1) levels and GH response to an oral glucose tolerance test (OGTT). The peripheral actions of GH are mediated by IGF-1. As GH levels rise, so do IGF-1 levels. However, GH is released in a pulsatile fashion, requiring several samples to obtain an accurate measure. Serum IGF-1 levels are more constant, providing a more reliable diagnostic measure of acromegaly.

OGTT is a specific test for acromegaly. Because GH secretion is normally inhibited by glucose, measurement of glucose nonsuppressibility is useful. Two baseline GH levels are obtained before ingestion of 75 or 100 g of oral glucose, and additional GH measurements are made at 30, 60, 90, and 120 minutes. Normally, GH concentration falls during an OGTT. In acromegaly GH levels do not fall, and in some cases GH concentration rises.

Magnetic resonance imaging (MRI) and a high-resolution computed tomography (CT) scan with contrast media are used to detect pituitary tumors. A complete ophthalmologic examination, including visual fields, is done because a tumor may cause pressure on the optic chiasm or optic nerves.

Collaborative Care

The patient's prognosis depends on the age at onset, age when treatment started, and tumor size. The overall goal is to return the patient's GH levels to normal. Treatment consists of surgery, radiation therapy, drug therapy, or a combination of these therapies. With treatment, bone growth can be stopped and tissue hypertrophy reversed. However, sleep apnea and diabetic and cardiac complications may persist.

Surgical Therapy. Surgery (hypophysectomy) is the treatment of choice because it offers the best chance for a cure, especially for smaller pituitary adenomas. Most surgeries are done by an endoscopic *transsphenoidal* approach (Fig. 50-2).

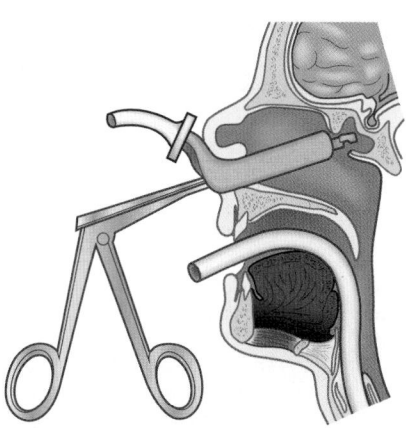

FIG. 50-2 Surgery on the pituitary gland is most commonly performed with the transsphenoidal approach. An incision is made in the inner aspect of the upper lip and gingiva. The sella turcica is entered through the floor of the nose and sphenoid sinuses.

Surgery produces an immediate reduction in GH levels followed by a drop in IGF-1 levels within a few weeks. When the entire pituitary gland is removed, there is permanent loss of all pituitary hormones. Rather than replacing the pituitary (tropic) hormones, which requires parenteral administration, the essential hormones produced by target organs (glucocorticoids, thyroid hormone, and sex hormones) are given. Hormone therapy continues throughout life. Patients with larger tumors or those with GH levels greater than 45 ng/mL may require adjuvant radiation or drug therapy.

Radiation Therapy. Radiation therapy is used when surgery has failed to produce a cure or when patients are poor candidates for surgery. Radiation therapy is usually offered in combination with drugs that reduce GH levels. However, the full effects may not be noted for months to years. Radiation can also be used to reduce the size of a tumor before surgery. Radiation therapy may lead to hypopituitarism, which then requires lifelong hormone replacement therapy.

Stereotactic radiosurgery (gamma knife surgery, proton beam, linear accelerator) may be used for small, surgically inaccessible pituitary tumors or in place of conventional radiation (see Chapter 57). This procedure consists of radiation delivered to one site from multiple angles.

Drug Therapy. Drugs are most commonly used in patients who have had an inadequate response to surgery and/or in combination with radiation therapy. The primary drug used for acromegaly is octreotide (Sandostatin), a somatostatin analog that reduces GH levels to normal in many patients. Octreotide is given by subcutaneous injection three times a week. Two long-acting analogs, octreotide (Sandostatin LAR) and lanreotide SR (Somatuline Depot), are available as intramuscular (IM) injections given every 4 weeks. GH levels are measured every 2 weeks to guide drug dosing, and then every 6 months until the desired response is obtained.

Dopamine agonists (e.g., bromocriptine [Parlodel], pergolide [Permax], cabergoline [Dostinex]) may be given alone or added to somatostatin analogs if complete remission has not been achieved after surgery. These drugs reduce the secretion of GH from the tumor.

GH antagonists (e.g., pegvisomant [Somavert]) reduce the effect of GH in the body by blocking the hepatic production of IGF-1. With the use of drug therapy, most patients achieve normal IGF-1 levels with symptom improvement.[2]

NURSING MANAGEMENT
ACROMEGALY

NURSING ASSESSMENT

Assess the patient for signs and symptoms of abnormal tissue growth and evaluate changes in physical size. It is important to question patients about increases in hat, glove, and shoe sizes. Older photographs are helpful to evaluate any changes (see Fig. 50-1). Because physical changes occur slowly and over a long period, the individual may not even be aware of any changes.

NURSING IMPLEMENTATION

Postoperative care after a transsphenoidal hypophysectomy includes elevating the head of the patient's bed at all times to a 30-degree angle. This elevation avoids pressure on the sella turcica and decreases headaches, a frequent postoperative problem. Monitor the pupillary response, speech patterns, and extremity strength to detect neurologic complications. Perform mouth care every 4 hours to keep the surgical area clean and free of debris. Avoid tooth brushing for at least 10 days to protect the suture line. Observe the patient for any signs of bleeding, since hemorrhage may be a complication, particularly when larger tumors are removed by this approach.

Instruct the patient to avoid vigorous coughing, sneezing, and straining at stool (Valsalva maneuver) to prevent cerebrospinal fluid (CSF) leakage. Notify the surgeon, and send any clear nasal drainage to the laboratory to be tested for glucose. A glucose level greater than 30 mg/dL (1.67 mmol/L) indicates CSF leakage from an open connection to the brain. If this happens, the patient is at increased risk for meningitis. Complaints of persistent and severe generalized or supraorbital headache may indicate CSF leakage into the sinuses. A CSF leak usually resolves within 72 hours when treated with head elevation and bed rest. If the leak persists, daily spinal taps may be done to reduce pressure to below-normal levels.

If stereotactic radiosurgery is used, the patient is usually moved from the specialized radiation center to the neurosurgical nursing unit for overnight observation. The patient will be in a stereotactic head frame. Carefully monitor vital signs, neurologic status, and fluid volume status. Possible complications of sterotactic surgery include increased headaches, seizures, nausea, and vomiting. Perform pin-site care according to institutional policy. Instruct family members on pin-site care if the patient is discharged with pins in place.

Observe the patient for transient diabetes insipidus (DI). This may occur because of the loss of antidiuretic hormone (ADH), which is stored in the posterior lobe of the pituitary gland, or cerebral edema related to manipulation of the pituitary during surgery. To assess for DI, closely monitor urine output and serum and urine osmolarity. Clinical manifestations and treatment of DI are discussed in more detail later in this chapter.

If a hypophysectomy is performed or the pituitary gland is damaged, hormone therapy will be necessary. ADH, cortisol, and thyroid hormone replacement will be needed. Surgery may result in permanent loss or deficiencies in follicle-stimulating hormone (FSH) and luteinizing hormone (LH). This can lead to decreased fertility. Assist the patient in working through the grieving process associated with these losses.

If hormones are prescribed, teach the patient about the need for lifelong therapy. Serial photographs to show improvement may be helpful. Patients with acromegaly are at higher risk for colon polyps and colorectal cancer and should have a screening colonoscopy every 3 to 4 years.

EXCESSES OF OTHER TROPIC HORMONES

In addition to GH, the pituitary also secretes prolactin, adrenocorticotropic hormone (ACTH), thyroid-stimulating hormone (TSH), and ADH. An excess of any of these hormones (discussed later in the chapter) can cause significant disturbances in metabolism and general health.

Prolactinomas are among the most common type of pituitary adenomas.[4] Women with prolactinomas frequently experience galactorrhea, anovulation, infertility, oligomenorrhea or amenorrhea, decreased libido, and hirsutism. In men, impotence and decreased sperm density and libido may result. Compression of the optic chiasm can cause visual problems and signs of increased intracranial pressure, including headache, nausea, and vomiting. Because prolactinomas do not typically progress in size, drug therapy is usually the first-line treatment. The dopamine agonists cabergoline and bromocriptine have successfully been used to treat prolactinomas. Surgery may be done depending on the extent and size of the tumor. Radiation therapy may be used to reduce the risk of tumor recurrence for patients with large tumors.

HYPOFUNCTION OF PITUITARY GLAND

Hypopituitarism is a rare disorder that involves a decrease in one or more of the pituitary hormones. The anterior pituitary gland secretes ACTH, TSH, FSH, LH, GH, and prolactin. The posterior pituitary gland secretes ADH and oxytocin. A deficiency of only one pituitary hormone is referred to as *selective hypopituitarism*. Total failure of the pituitary gland results in deficiency of all pituitary hormones—a condition referred to as *panhypopituitarism*. The most common hormone deficiencies associated with hypopituitarism involve GH and gonadotropins (i.e., LH, FSH).

Etiology and Pathophysiology

The usual cause of pituitary hypofunction is a pituitary tumor. Autoimmune disorders, infections, pituitary infarction (Sheehan syndrome), or destruction of the pituitary gland (from trauma, radiation, or surgical procedures) can also cause hypopituitarism. African Americans have a higher incidence of pituitary adenomas than other ethnic groups.[5]

Anterior pituitary hormone deficiencies can lead to end-organ failure. Deficiencies of TSH and ACTH are life threatening. ACTH deficiency can lead to acute adrenal insufficiency and shock. Hypovolemic shock is due to sodium and water depletion. (Acute adrenal insufficiency is discussed later in this chapter on pp. 1211-1212.)

Clinical Manifestations and Diagnostic Studies

The manifestations associated with pituitary hypofunction vary with the type and degree of dysfunction. Early manifestations associated with a space-occupying lesion include headaches, visual changes (decreased visual acuity or decreased peripheral vision), loss of smell, nausea and vomiting, and seizures. Manifestations associated with hyposecretion of the target glands vary widely (Table 50-1).

In addition to a history and physical examination, diagnostic studies such as MRI and CT are used to identify a pituitary

TABLE 50-1	CLINICAL MANIFESTATIONS OF HYPOPITUITARISM
Hormone Deficiency	**Manifestations**
Growth hormone (GH)	Subtle, nonspecific findings. Truncal obesity, decreased muscle mass and strength, weakness, fatigue, depression or flat affect.
Follicle-stimulating hormone (FSH) and luteinizing hormone (LH)	*Women:* Menstrual irregularities, loss of libido, changes in secondary sex characteristics such as decreased breast size. *Men:* Testicular atrophy, diminished spermatogenesis, loss of libido, impotence, decreased facial hair and muscle mass.
Thyroid-stimulating hormone (TSH)	Mild form of primary hypothyroidism: fatigue, cold intolerance, constipation, lethargy, weight gain.
Adrenocorticotropic hormone (ACTH)	Involves a deficiency of cortisol: weakness, fatigue, headache, dry and pale skin, diminished axillary and pubic hair, lowered resistance to infection, fasting hypoglycemia.

tumor. Laboratory tests for diagnosing hypopituitarism vary widely, but generally involve the direct measurement of pituitary hormones (e.g., TSH) or an indirect determination of the target organ hormones (e.g., triiodothyronine [T_3], thyroxine [T_4]). (See Chapter 48 for more information regarding diagnostic studies.)

NURSING AND COLLABORATIVE MANAGEMENT HYPOPITUITARISM

The treatment for hypopituitarism often consists of surgery or radiation therapy followed by lifelong hormone therapy. Surgery and radiation therapy for pituitary tumors are discussed earlier in this chapter on pp. 1190 and 1191. Appropriate hormone therapy is used (e.g., GH, corticosteroids, thyroid hormone, sex hormones). Hormone therapies for thyroid hormone and corticosteroids are discussed later in this chapter on pp. 1202 and 1213.

Somatropin (Omnitrope, Genotropin, Humatrope), which is recombinant human GH, is used for long-term hormone therapy in adults with GH deficiency. These patients respond well to GH replacement and experience increased energy, increased lean body mass, a feeling of well-being, and improved body image. Mild to moderate side effects of GH include fluid retention with swelling in the feet and hands, myalgia, joint pain, and headache. GH is given daily as a subcutaneous injection (preferably in the evening). The dosing is variable because it is adjusted based on symptoms, IGF-1 levels, and the development of adverse effects.

Although gonadal deficiency is not life threatening, hormone therapy is offered to improve sexual function and general well-being. This therapy is contraindicated in individuals with certain medical conditions, such as breast cancer, phlebitis, and pulmonary embolism in women and prostate cancer in men. Estrogen and progesterone replacement therapy may be indicated for hypogonadal women to treat hot flashes, vaginal dryness, and decreased libido. Hormone therapy for women is discussed in Chapter 54. Testosterone is used to treat men with gonadotropin deficiency. The benefits achieved with testoster-

PATHOPHYSIOLOGY MAP

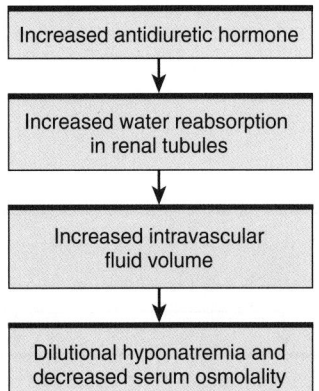

FIG. 50-3 Pathophysiology of syndrome of inappropriate antidiuretic hormone (SIADH).

one therapy include a return of male secondary sex characteristics; improvement in libido; and increased muscle mass, bone mass, and bone density. Hormone therapy for men is discussed in Chapter 55.

DISORDERS OF POSTERIOR PITUITARY GLAND

The hormones secreted by the posterior pituitary, antidiuretic hormone (ADH) and oxytocin, are produced in the hypothalamus and then transported and stored in the posterior pituitary gland. ADH, also referred to as *arginine vasopressin* (AVP) or vasopressin, plays a major role in the regulation of water balance and osmolarity (see Chapter 48).

The two primary problems associated with ADH secretion are a result of either overproduction or underproduction of ADH. Overproduction or oversecretion of ADH results in a condition known as syndrome of inappropriate antidiuretic hormone (SIADH). Underproduction or undersecretion of ADH results in a condition referred to as *diabetes insipidus* (DI).

SYNDROME OF INAPPROPRIATE ANTIDIURETIC HORMONE

Etiology and Pathophysiology
SIADH results from abnormally high production or sustained secretion of ADH. In SIADH, ADH is released despite normal or low plasma osmolarity (Fig. 50-3). This disorder is characterized by fluid retention, serum hypoosmolality, dilutional hyponatremia, hypochloremia, concentrated urine in the presence of normal or increased intravascular volume, and normal renal function.

This syndrome occurs more commonly in older adults. SIADH has various causes (Table 50-2). The most common cause is malignancy, especially small cell lung cancer. Although SIADH tends to be self-limiting when it is caused by head trauma or drugs, it is chronic when associated with tumors or metabolic diseases.

Clinical Manifestations and Diagnostic Studies
ADH increases the permeability of the renal distal tubule and collecting duct, which leads to the reabsorption of water

TABLE 50-2	CAUSES OF SYNDROME OF INAPPROPRIATE ANTIDIURETIC HORMONE
Malignant Tumors • Small cell lung cancer • Pancreatic cancer • Lymphoid cancers (Hodgkin's lymphoma, non-Hodgkin's lymphoma, lymphocytic leukemia) • Thymus cancer • Prostate cancer • Colorectal cancer **Central Nervous System Disorders** • Head injury (skull fracture, subdural hematoma, subarachnoid hemorrhage) • Stroke • Brain tumors • Infection (encephalitis, meningitis) • Cerebral atrophy • Guillain-Barré syndrome • Systemic lupus erythematosus	**Drug Therapy** • carbamazepine (Tegretol) • chlorpropamide (Diabinese) • General anesthesia agents • Opioids • oxytocin • Thiazide diuretics • SSRI antidepressants • Tricyclic antidepressants • Chemotherapy drugs (vincristine [Oncovin], vinblastine [Velban], cyclophosphamide [Cytoxan]) **Miscellaneous Conditions** • Hypothyroidism • Lung infection (pneumonia, tuberculosis, lung abscess) • Chronic obstructive pulmonary disease • Positive pressure mechanical ventilation • HIV • Adrenal insufficiency

SIADH, Syndrome of inappropriate antidiuretic hormone; *SSRI*, selective serotonin reuptake inhibitor.

into the circulation. Consequently, extracellular fluid volume expands, plasma osmolality declines, glomerular filtration rate increases, and sodium levels decline (dilutional hyponatremia).[6] Hyponatremia causes muscle cramping, pain, and weakness. Initially, the patient displays thirst, dyspnea on exertion, and fatigue.

The patient with SIADH experiences low urine output and increased body weight. As the serum sodium level falls (usually below 120 mEq/L [120 mmol/L]), manifestations become more severe and include vomiting, abdominal cramps, muscle twitching, and seizures. As plasma osmolality and serum sodium levels continue to decline, cerebral edema may occur, which leads to lethargy, confusion, headache, seizures, and coma.

The diagnosis of SIADH is made by simultaneous measurements of urine and serum osmolality. Dilutional hyponatremia is indicated by a serum sodium less than 134 mEq/L, serum osmolality less than 280 mOsm/kg (280 mmol/kg), and a urine specific gravity greater than 1.025. A serum osmolality much lower than the urine osmolality indicates the inappropriate excretion of concentrated urine in the presence of dilute serum.

NURSING AND COLLABORATIVE MANAGEMENT SYNDROME OF INAPPROPRIATE ANTIDIURETIC HORMONE

In your assessment of individuals at risk and those who have confirmed SIADH, be alert for low urine output with a high specific gravity, a sudden weight gain without edema, or a decreased serum sodium level. Monitor intake and output, vital signs, and heart and lung sounds. Observe for signs of hyponatremia, including seizures, nausea and vomiting, muscle cramping, and decreased neurologic function.

Once SIADH is diagnosed, treatment is directed at the underlying cause. Medications that stimulate the release of

ADH should be avoided or discontinued (see Table 50-2). If symptoms are mild and serum sodium is greater than 125 mEq/L (125 mmol/L), the only treatment may be a fluid restriction of 800 to 1000 mL/day. This restriction should result in gradual reductions in weight, a progressive rise in serum sodium concentration and osmolality, and symptomatic improvement.

In the acute care setting restrict the patient's total fluid intake to no more than 1000 mL/day (including that taken with medications) and obtain daily weights. Position the head of the bed flat or elevated no more than 10 degrees to enhance venous return to the heart and increase left atrial filling pressure, thereby reducing the release of ADH. Frequent turning, positioning, and range-of-motion exercise (if patient is bedridden) are important to maintain skin integrity and joint mobility. Protect the patient from injury (e.g., assist with ambulation, bed alarm) because of the potential for alterations in mental status. Implement seizure precautions. Provide the patient with frequent oral care and distractions to decrease discomfort related to thirst from the fluid restrictions.

In cases of severe hyponatremia (less than 120 mEq/L), especially in the presence of neurologic manifestations such as seizures, IV hypertonic saline solution (3% to 5%) may be slowly administered. A loop diuretic such as furosemide (Lasix) may be used to promote diuresis, but only if the serum sodium is at least 125 mEq/L (125 mmol/L) because it may promote a further loss of sodium. Because furosemide increases potassium, calcium, and magnesium losses, supplements may be needed. A fluid restriction of 500 mL/day may be indicated for those with severe hyponatremia.

Vasopressin receptor antagonists, tolvaptan (Samsca) and conivaptan (Vaprisol), are used to treat euvolemia-hyponatremia in hospitalized patients. These medications should be initiated in a closely monitored setting to prevent rapid correction of serum sodium.

Assist the patient with chronic SIADH in self-management of the treatment regimen. In chronic SIADH, a fluid restriction of 800 to 1000 mL/day is recommended. Because this degree of restriction may be difficult, demeclocycline (Declomycin) may be administered. This drug blocks the effect of ADH on the renal tubules, resulting in a more dilute urine. The use of ice chips or sugarless chewing gum helps to decrease thirst. Have the patient weigh daily to monitor changes in fluid balance. Teach the patient to supplement the diet with sodium and potassium, especially if loop diuretics are also prescribed. Solutions of these electrolytes must be well diluted to prevent gastrointestinal (GI) irritation or damage. They are best taken at mealtime to allow mixing with and dilution by food. Teach the patient the symptoms of fluid and electrolyte imbalances, especially those involving sodium and potassium (see Chapter 17).

DIABETES INSIPIDUS

Etiology and Pathophysiology

Diabetes insipidus (DI) is caused by a deficiency of production or secretion of ADH or a decreased renal response to ADH. The decrease in ADH results in fluid and electrolyte imbalances caused by increased urine output and increased plasma osmolality (Fig. 50-4). Depending on the cause, DI may be transient or a chronic, lifelong condition.

There are several types of DI (Table 50-3). Central DI is the most common form.

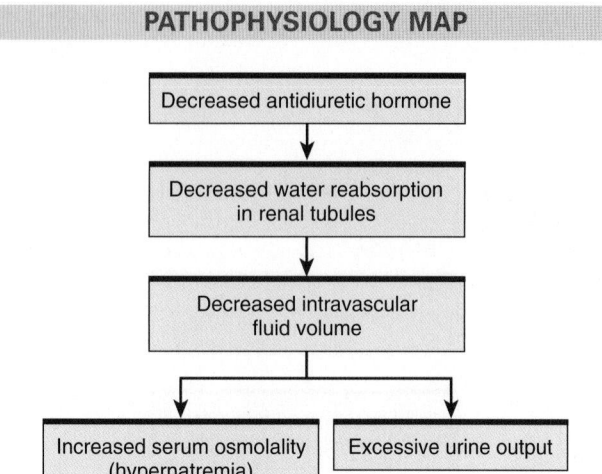

FIG. 50-4 Pathophysiology of diabetes insipidus (DI).

TABLE 50-3	**TYPES OF DIABETES INSIPIDUS**
Type	**Etiology**
Central (neurogenic) DI	Results from an interference with ADH synthesis, transport, or release *Examples:* Brain tumor, head injury, brain surgery, CNS infections
Nephrogenic DI	Results from inadequate renal response to ADH despite presence of adequate ADH *Examples:* Drug therapy (especially lithium), renal damage, hereditary renal disease
Primary DI	Results from excessive water intake *Examples:* Structural lesion in thirst center, psychologic disorder

Clinical Manifestations

DI is characterized by polydipsia and polyuria.[6] The primary characteristic is the excretion of large quantities of urine (2 to 20 L/day) with a very low specific gravity (less than 1.005) and urine osmolality of less than 100 mOsm/kg (100 mmol/kg). Serum osmolality is elevated (usually greater than 295 mOsm/kg [295 mmol/kg]) because of hypernatremia caused by pure water loss in the kidneys. Most patients compensate for fluid loss by drinking large amounts of water so that serum osmolality remains normal or is moderately elevated. The patient may be fatigued from nocturia and experience generalized weakness.

The onset of central DI is usually acute and accompanied by excessive fluid loss. After intracranial surgery, central DI has a triphasic pattern: the acute phase with an abrupt onset of polyuria, an interphase in which urine volume normalizes, and a third phase in which central DI is permanent. The third phase occurs within 10 to 14 days postoperatively. Central DI that results from head trauma is often self-limiting and improves with treatment of the underlying problem. DI following cranial surgery is more likely to be permanent. Although the clinical manifestations of nephrogenic DI are similar to those of central DI, the onset and amount of fluid loss are less dramatic.

If oral fluid intake cannot keep up with urinary losses, severe dehydration results. This is manifested by poor tissue turgor, hypotension, tachycardia, and hypovolemic shock. In addition, the patient may show central nervous system (CNS) manifestations, ranging from irritability and mental dullness to coma, related to increasing serum osmolality and hypernatremia.

Diagnostic Studies

Patients with DI excrete dilute urine at a rate greater than 200 mL/hr with a specific gravity of less than 1.005. Identification of central DI requires a water deprivation test. Before the test, body weight, and urine osmolality, volume, and specific gravity are measured. The patient is deprived of water for 8 to 12 hours, and then given desmopressin acetate (DDAVP) subcutaneously or nasally. Patients with central DI exhibit a dramatic increase in urine osmolality, from 100 to 600 mOsm/kg, and a significant decrease in urine volume. The patient with nephrogenic DI will not be able to increase urine osmolality to greater than 300 mOsm/kg.

Another test to differentiate central DI from nephrogenic DI is to measure the level of ADH after an analog of ADH (e.g., desmopressin) is given. If the cause is central DI, the kidneys will respond to the hormone by concentrating urine. If the kidneys do not respond in this way, then the cause is nephrogenic.

NURSING AND COLLABORATIVE MANAGEMENT DIABETES INSIPIDUS

Nursing management of the patient with DI includes early detection, maintenance of adequate hydration, and patient teaching for long-term management. A therapeutic goal is maintenance of fluid and electrolyte balance.

For central DI, fluid and hormone therapy is the cornerstone of treatment. Fluids are replaced orally or IV, depending on the patient's condition and ability to drink copious amounts of fluids. In acute DI, IV hypotonic saline or dextrose 5% in water (D_5W) is given and titrated to replace urine output. If IV glucose solutions are used, monitor serum glucose levels because hyperglycemia and glycosuria can lead to osmotic diuresis, which increases the fluid volume deficit. Monitoring of blood pressure (BP), heart rate, and urine output and specific gravity is essential and may be required hourly in the patient who is acutely ill. Monitor the level of consciousness and for signs of acute dehydration by assessing alertness, response to stimuli, mucous membranes, tachycardia, and skin turgor. Maintain an accurate record of intake and output and daily weights to determine fluid volume status. Adjustments in fluid replacement should be made accordingly.

DDAVP, an analog of ADH, is the hormone replacement of choice for central DI. Other ADH replacement drugs include aqueous vasopressin (Pitressin) or lysine vasopressin (Diapid). DDAVP can be given orally, IV, subcutaneously, or as a nasal spray. Assess the response to DDAVP (e.g., weight gain, headache, depression, restlessness, hyponatremia). Monitor pulse, BP, level of consciousness, fluid intake and output, and urine specific gravity. Teach the patient about the need for close follow-up. Chlorpropamide (Diabinese) and carbamazepine (Tegretol) are used to help decrease thirst associated with central DI.

Because the kidney is unable to respond to ADH in nephrogenic DI, hormone therapy has little effect. Instead, the treatment includes dietary measures (low-sodium diet) and thiazide diuretics (e.g., hydrochlorothiazide [HydroDIURIL], chlorothiazide [Diuril]), which may reduce flow to the ADH-sensitive distal nephrons. Limiting sodium intake to no more than 3 g/

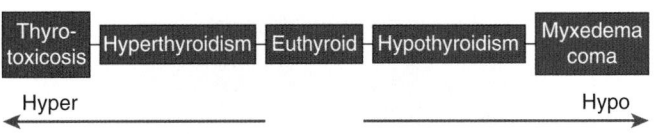

FIG. 50-5 Continuum of thyroid dysfunction.

day often helps decrease urine output. When a low-sodium diet and thiazide drugs are not effective, indomethacin (Indocin) may be prescribed. Indomethacin, a nonsteroidal antiinflammatory drug (NSAID), helps increase renal responsiveness to ADH.

DISORDERS OF THYROID GLAND

Alterations in thyroid function are among the most common endocrine disorders. The thyroid hormones, thyroxine (T_4) and triiodothyronine (T_3), regulate energy metabolism and growth and development. Disorders of the thyroid gland include goiter, benign and malignant nodules, inflammation, hyperthyroidism, and hypothyroidism (Fig. 50-5).

GOITER

A **goiter** is an enlarged thyroid gland. In a person with a goiter the thyroid cells are stimulated to grow, which may result in an overactive thyroid (hyperthyroidism) or an underactive thyroid (hypothyroidism). The most common cause of goiter worldwide is a lack of iodine in the diet. In the United States, where most people use iodized salt, goiter is more often due to the overproduction or underproduction of thyroid hormones or to nodules that develop in the gland itself. *Goitrogens* (foods or drugs that contain thyroid-inhibiting substances) can cause goiter[7] (Table 50-4).

A nontoxic goiter is a diffuse enlargement of the thyroid gland that does not result from a malignancy or inflammatory process. Normal levels of thyroid hormone are associated with this type of goiter. *Nodular goiters* are thyroid hormone–secreting nodules that function independent of TSH stimulation. There may be multiple nodules (multinodular goiter) or a single nodule (solitary autonomous nodule). The nodules are usually benign follicular adenomas. If these nodules are associated with hyperthyroidism, they are termed *toxic nodular goiters*. This type of goiter is commonly found in patients with Graves' disease (Fig. 50-6). Toxic nodular goiters occur equally in men and women. Although they can appear at any age, the frequency is greatest in people over 40 years of age.

TABLE 50-4	**GOITROGENS**	
Thyroid Inhibitors		**Foods***
• propylthiouracil (PTU)		• Broccoli
• methimazole (Tapazole)		• Brussels sprouts
• Iodine in large doses		• Cabbage
		• Cauliflower
Other Drugs		• Kale
• Sulfonamides		• Mustard
• Salicylates		• Peanuts
• *p*-Aminosalicylic acid		• Turnips
• lithium		
• amiodarone (Cordarone)		

*List is not all-inclusive.

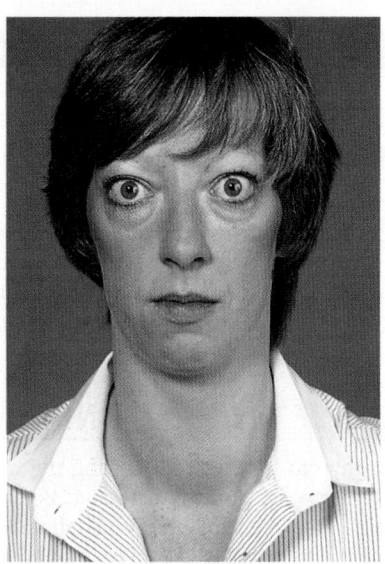

FIG. 50-6 Exophthalmos and goiter of Graves' disease.

In a person with a goiter, TSH and T_4 levels are measured to determine whether a goiter is associated with normal thyroid function, hyperthyroidism, or hypothyroidism. Thyroid antibodies (e.g., thyroid peroxidase [TPO] antibody) are measured to assess for *thyroiditis* (inflammation of the thyroid). Treatment with thyroid hormone may prevent further thyroid enlargement. Surgery is used to remove large goiters. Goiter as a clinical manifestation of thyroid disorders is further discussed in the following sections.

THYROIDITIS

Thyroiditis, an inflammation of the thyroid gland, is a frequent cause of goiter. *Subacute granulomatous thyroiditis* is thought to be caused by a viral infection. *Acute thyroiditis* is due to bacterial or fungal infection. Subacute and acute forms of thyroiditis have an abrupt onset. The patient complains of pain localized in the thyroid or radiating to the throat, ears, or jaw.[8] Other systemic manifestations include fever, chills, sweats, and fatigue.

Hashimoto's thyroiditis (chronic autoimmune thyroiditis) results in hypothyroidism caused by the destruction of thyroid tissue by antibodies. It is the most common cause of hypothyroid goiters in the United States. Factors placing an individual at higher risk include female gender, a positive family history, older age, and white ethnicity. The goiter, which is the hallmark of Hashimoto's thyroiditis, may develop gradually or rapidly (see eFig. 50-1 available on the website for this chapter). If the thyroid gland enlarges rapidly, structures in the neck (e.g., trachea and laryngeal nerves) may become compressed, thus changing the voice and affecting breathing.

Silent, painless thyroiditis, which may be early Hashimoto's thyroiditis, can occur in postpartum women. This condition, which is usually seen in the first 6 months after delivery, may be due to an autoimmune reaction to fetal cells in the mother's thyroid gland.

T_4 and T_3 levels are initially elevated in subacute, acute, and silent thyroiditis but become depressed with time. In chronic Hashimoto's thyroiditis, thyroid hormone levels are usually low and the TSH level is high. Suppression of radioactive iodine uptake (RAIU) is seen in subacute and silent thyroiditis. Antithyroid antibodies are present in Hashimoto's thyroiditis.

Recovery from acute or subacute thyroiditis may be complete in weeks or months without any treatment. If the thyroiditis is bacterial in origin, treatment may include specific antibiotics or surgical drainage. In the subacute and acute forms, NSAIDs (aspirin or naproxen [Aleve]) are used to relieve symptoms. With more severe pain, corticosteroids (e.g., prednisone up to 40 mg/day) are used to relieve discomfort. This treatment may be required for several months and then should be withdrawn gradually.[9] Propranolol (Inderal) or atenolol (Tenormin) may be used to treat the cardiovascular symptoms related to a hyperthyroid condition. Thyroid hormone therapy is indicated if the patient is hypothyroid.

Nursing care of the patient with thyroiditis includes patient teaching regarding the disease process and course of treatment. Stress the importance of not abruptly discontinuing medications. Instruct the patient to remain under close health care supervision so that progress can be monitored. In addition, teach the patient to report to the health care provider any change in symptoms, such as difficulty breathing or swallowing, swelling to face and extremities, or rapid weight gain or loss.

The patient with Hashimoto's thyroiditis is at risk for other autoimmune diseases such as Addison's disease, pernicious anemia, or Graves' disease. Teach the patient the signs and symptoms of these disorders, particularly Addison's disease. Instruct the patient receiving thyroid hormone about the expected side effects of these drugs and measures to manage them (see p. 1202).

HYPERTHYROIDISM

Hyperthyroidism is hyperactivity of the thyroid gland with sustained increase in synthesis and release of thyroid hormones. Hyperthyroidism occurs in women more than men, with the highest frequency in persons 20 to 40 years old. The most common form of hyperthyroidism is Graves' disease. Other causes include toxic nodular goiter, thyroiditis, excess iodine intake, pituitary tumors, and thyroid cancer.

The term *thyrotoxicosis* refers to the physiologic effects or clinical syndrome of hypermetabolism that results from excess circulating levels of T_4, T_3, or both.[10] Hyperthyroidism and thyrotoxicosis usually occur together, as seen in Graves' disease.

Etiology and Pathophysiology

Graves' Disease. Graves' disease is an autoimmune disease of unknown etiology characterized by diffuse thyroid enlargement and excessive thyroid hormone secretion. Graves' disease accounts for up to 80% of the cases of hyperthyroidism. Women are five times more likely than men to develop Graves' disease. Precipitating factors such as insufficient iodine supply, infection, and stressful life events may interact with genetic factors to cause Graves' disease. Cigarette smoking increases the risk of Graves' disease and the development of eye problems associated with the disease.[11]

In Graves' disease the patient develops antibodies to the TSH receptor. These antibodies attach to the receptors and stimulate the thyroid gland to release T_3, T_4, or both. The excessive release of thyroid hormones leads to the clinical manifestations associated with thyrotoxicosis. The disease is characterized by remissions and exacerbations, with or without treatment. It may progress to destruction of the thyroid tissue, causing hypothyroidism.

TABLE 50-5 CLINICAL MANIFESTATIONS OF THYROID DYSFUNCTION

Hyperfunction	Hypofunction	Hyperfunction	Hypofunction
Cardiovascular System		**Musculoskeletal System**	
• Systolic hypertension	• Increased capillary fragility	• Fatigue	• Fatigue
• Increased rate and force of cardiac contractions	• Decreased rate and force of contractions	• Muscle weakness	• Weakness
• Bounding, rapid pulse	• Varied changes in blood pressure	• Proximal muscle wasting	• Muscular aches and pains
• Increased cardiac output	• Cardiac hypertrophy	• Dependent edema	• Slow movements
• Cardiac hypertrophy	• Distant heart sounds	• Osteoporosis	• Arthralgia
• Systolic murmurs	• Anemia		
• Dysrhythmias	• Tendency to develop heart failure, angina, myocardial infarction	**Nervous System**	
• Palpitations		• Difficulty focusing eyes	• Apathy
• Atrial fibrillation (more common in the older adult)		• Nervousness	• Lethargy
• Angina		• Fine tremor (of fingers and tongue)	• Fatigue
		• Insomnia	• Forgetfulness
Respiratory System		• Lability of mood, delirium	• Slowed mental processes
• Increased respiratory rate	• Dyspnea	• Restlessness	• Hoarseness
• Dyspnea on mild exertion	• Decreased breathing capacity	• Personality changes of irritability, agitation	• Slow, slurred speech
		• Exhaustion	• Prolonged relaxation of deep tendon muscles
Gastrointestinal System		• Hyperactive deep-tendon reflexes	• Stupor, coma
• Increased appetite, thirst	• Decreased appetite	• Depression, fatigue, apathy (in the older adult)	• Paresthesias
• Weight loss	• Nausea and vomiting	• Lack of ability to concentrate	• Anxiety, depression
• Increased peristalsis	• Weight gain	• Stupor, coma	
• Diarrhea, frequent defecation	• Constipation		
• Increased bowel sounds	• Distended abdomen	**Reproductive System**	
• Splenomegaly	• Enlarged, scaly tongue	• Menstrual irregularities	• Prolonged menstrual periods or amenorrhea
• Hepatomegaly	• Celiac disease	• Amenorrhea	
		• Decreased libido	• Decreased libido
Integumentary System		• Impotence in men	• Infertility
• Warm, smooth, moist skin	• Dry, thick, inelastic, cold skin	• Gynecomastia in men	
• Thin, brittle nails detached from nail bed (onycholysis)	• Thick, brittle nails	• Decreased fertility	
• Hair loss (may be patchy)	• Dry, sparse, coarse hair	**Other**	
• Clubbing of fingers (thyroid acropachy) (see Fig. 50-7)	• Poor turgor of mucosa	• Intolerance to heat	• Increased susceptibility to infection
• Palmar erythema	• Generalized interstitial edema	• Elevated basal temperature	• Increased sensitivity to opioids, barbiturates, anesthesia
• Fine silky hair	• Puffy face	• Lid lag, stare	
• Premature graying (in men)	• Decreased sweating	• Eyelid retraction	• Intolerance to cold
• Diaphoresis	• Pallor	• Exophthalmos	• Decreased hearing
• Vitiligo		• Goiter (see Fig. 50-6)	• Sleepiness
• Pretibial myxedema (infiltrative dermopathy)		• Rapid speech	• Goiter

Clinical Manifestations

Clinical manifestations of hyperthyroidism are related to the effect of excess circulating thyroid hormone. It directly increases metabolism and tissue sensitivity to stimulation by the sympathetic nervous system.

Palpation of the thyroid gland may reveal a goiter. When the thyroid gland is excessively large, a goiter may be noted on inspection. Auscultation of the thyroid gland may reveal bruits, a reflection of increased blood supply. Another common finding is *ophthalmopathy,* a term used to describe abnormal eye appearance or function. A classic finding in Graves' disease is exophthalmos, a protrusion of the eyeballs from the orbits that is usually bilateral (see Fig. 50-6). Exophthalmos results from increased fat deposits and fluid (edema) in the orbital tissues and ocular muscles. The increased pressure forces the eyeballs outward. The upper lids are usually retracted and elevated, with the sclera visible above the iris. When the eyelids do not close completely, the exposed corneal surfaces become dry and irritated. Serious consequences, such as corneal ulcers and eventual loss of vision, can occur. The changes in the ocular muscles result in muscle weakness, causing diplopia.

Other manifestations of thyroid hyperfunction are summarized in Table 50-5. Abnormal laboratory findings are listed in Table 50-6. A patient in the early stages of hyperthyroidism may exhibit only weight loss and increased nervousness. *Acropachy* (clubbing of the digits) may occur with advanced disease (Fig. 50-7). Manifestations (e.g., palpitations, tremors, weight loss) in older adults with hyperthyroidism do not differ significantly from those of younger adults (Table 50-7). In older patients with reports of confusion and agitation, dementia may be suspected and delay the diagnosis.

Complications

Thyrotoxicosis (also called *thyrotoxic crisis* or *thyroid storm*) is an acute, severe, and rare condition that occurs when excessive amounts of thyroid hormones are released into the circulation. Although it is considered a life-threatening emergency, death is rare when treatment is initiated early. Thyrotoxicosis is thought to result from stressors (e.g., infection, trauma, surgery) in a patient with preexisting hyperthyroidism, either diagnosed or undiagnosed. Patients particularly prone to thyrotoxicosis are those having a thyroidectomy, since manipulation of the

TABLE 50-6	**LABORATORY RESULTS FOR HYPERTHYROID AND HYPOTHYROID PATIENTS**		
		Hypothyroid	
Test	**Hyperthyroid**	**Primary**	**Secondary**
Thyroid-stimulating hormone (TSH)	↓	↑	↓
T₄ (thyroxine)	↑	↓	↓
Total cholesterol	N	↑	↑
Low-density lipoproteins (LDLs)	↓	↑	↑
Triglycerides	N	↑	↑
Creatine kinase (CK)	N	↑	↑
Basal metabolic rate (BMR)	↑	↓	↓
Thyroid peroxidase (TPO) antibody	N	+ (in autoimmune hypothyroidism)	N

N, Normal; *+,* positive.

hyperactive thyroid gland results in an increase in hormones released.[11]

In thyrotoxicosis, all the symptoms of hyperthyroidism are prominent and severe. Manifestations include severe tachycardia, heart failure, shock, hyperthermia (up to 105.3° F [40.7° C]), restlessness, irritability, seizures, abdominal pain, vomiting, diarrhea, delirium, and coma. Treatment is aimed at reducing circulating thyroid hormone levels and the clinical manifestations with appropriate drug therapy. Supportive therapy is directed at managing respiratory distress, reducing fever, replacing fluid, and eliminating or managing the initiating stressor(s).

Diagnostic Studies

The two primary laboratory findings used to confirm the diagnosis of hyperthyroidism are decreased TSH levels and elevated free thyroxine (free T₄) levels. Total T₃ and T₄ levels may also

TABLE 50-7	**COMPARISON OF HYPERTHYROIDISM IN YOUNGER AND OLDER ADULTS**	
	Younger Adult	**Older Adult**
Common causes	Graves' disease in >90% of cases	Graves' disease or toxic nodular goiter
Common symptoms	Nervousness, irritability, weight loss, heat intolerance, warm moist skin	Anorexia, weight loss, apathy, lassitude, depression, confusion
Goiter	Present in >90% of cases	Present in about 50% of cases
Ophthalmopathy	Exophthalmos (see Fig. 50-6) present in 20%-40% of cases	Exophthalmos less common
Cardiac features	Tachycardia and palpitations common, but without heart failure	Angina, dysrhythmia (especially atrial fibrillation), heart failure may occur

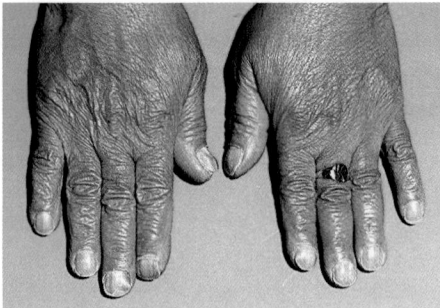

FIG. 50-7 Thyroid acropachy. Digital clubbing and swelling of fingers.

be assessed, but they are not as definitive. Total T₃ and T₄ determine both free and bound (to protein) hormone levels. The free hormone is the only biologically active form of these hormones.

The RAIU test is used to differentiate Graves' disease from other forms of thyroiditis. The patient with Graves' disease shows a diffuse, homogeneous uptake of 35% to 95%, whereas the patient with thyroiditis shows an uptake of less than 2%. The person with a nodular goiter has an uptake in the high normal range.

Collaborative Care

The goal of management of hyperthyroidism is to block the adverse effects of excessive thyroid hormone, suppress oversecretion of thyroid hormone, and prevent complications. There are several treatment options, including antithyroid medications, radioactive iodine therapy, and surgical intervention (Table 50-8). The choice of treatment is influenced by the patient's age and preferences, coexistence of other diseases, and pregnancy status.

Drug Therapy. Drugs used in the treatment of hyperthyroidism include antithyroid drugs, iodine, and β-adrenergic blockers. These drugs are useful in the treatment of thyrotoxic states, but they are not considered curative. Radiation therapy or surgery may ultimately be required.

Antithyroid Drugs. The first-line antithyroid drugs are propylthiouracil (PTU) and methimazole (Tapazole).[12] These drugs

TABLE 50-8	**COLLABORATIVE CARE**

Hyperthyroidism

Diagnostic
- History and physical examination
- Ophthalmologic examination
- ECG
- Laboratory tests
  - TSH levels, serum free T₄
  - Thyroid antibodies (e.g., thyroid peroxidase [TPO] antibody)
  - Total serum T₃ and T₄
- Radioactive iodine uptake (RAIU)

Collaborative Therapy
Drug Therapy
- Antithyroid drugs
  - methimazole (Tapazole)
  - propylthiouracil (PTU)
- Iodine (Lugol's solution, SSKI)
- β-Adrenergic receptor blockers
  - propranolol (Inderal)
  - atenolol (Tenormin) or metoprolol (Toprol)

Radiation Therapy
- Radioactive iodine

Surgical Therapy
- Subtotal thyroidectomy

Nutritional Therapy
- High-calorie, high-protein diet
- Frequent meals

SSKI, Saturated solution of potassium iodine; *TSH,* thyroid-stimulating hormone.

inhibit the synthesis of thyroid hormones. Indications for the use of antithyroid drugs include Graves' disease in the young patient, hyperthyroidism during pregnancy, and the need to achieve a euthyroid state before surgery or radiation therapy. PTU is generally used for patients who are in their first trimester of pregnancy, have an adverse reaction to methimazole, or require a rapid reduction in symptoms. PTU is also considered first line in thyrotoxicosis, since it also blocks the peripheral conversion of T_4 to T_3. The advantage of PTU is that it achieves the therapeutic goal of being euthyroid more quickly, but it must be taken three times per day. In contrast, methimazole is given in a single daily dose.

Individuals vary, but improvement usually begins 1 to 2 weeks after the start of drug therapy. Good results are usually seen within 4 to 8 weeks. Therapy is usually continued for 6 to 15 months to allow for spontaneous remission, which occurs in 20% to 40% of patients. Emphasize to the patient the importance of adherence to the drug regimen. Abrupt discontinuation of drug therapy can result in a return of hyperthyroidism.

Iodine. Iodine is used with other antithyroid drugs to prepare the patient for thyroidectomy or for treatment of thyrotoxicosis. The administration of iodine in large doses rapidly inhibits synthesis of T_3 and T_4 and blocks the release of these hormones into circulation. It also decreases the vascularity of the thyroid gland, making surgery safer and easier. The maximal effect of iodine is usually seen within 1 to 2 weeks. Because of a reduction in the therapeutic effect, long-term iodine therapy is not effective in controlling hyperthyroidism. Iodine is available in the form of saturated solution of potassium iodine (SSKI) and Lugol's solution.

β-Adrenergic Blockers. β-Adrenergic blockers are used for symptomatic relief of thyrotoxicosis. These drugs block the effects of sympathetic nervous stimulation, thereby decreasing tachycardia, nervousness, irritability, and tremors. Propranolol is usually administered with other antithyroid agents. Atenolol is the preferred β-adrenergic blocker for use in the hyperthyroid patient with asthma or heart disease.

Radioactive Iodine Therapy. Radioactive iodine (RAI) therapy is the treatment of choice for most nonpregnant adults. RAI damages or destroys thyroid tissue, thus limiting thyroid hormone secretion. RAI has a delayed response, and the maximum effect may not be seen for up to 3 months. For this reason, the patient is usually treated with antithyroid drugs and propranolol before and for 3 months after the initiation of RAI until the effects of radiation become apparent. Although RAI is usually effective, it has a high incidence of posttreatment hypothyroidism (80% of adequately treated persons), resulting in the need for lifelong thyroid hormone therapy. Teach the patient and the family about the symptoms of hypothyroidism and to seek medical help if these symptoms occur.

RAI therapy is usually administered on an outpatient basis. A pregnancy test is done before initiation of therapy on all women who experience menstrual cycles. Instruct the patient that radiation thyroiditis and parotiditis are possible and may cause dryness and irritation of the mouth and throat. Relief may be obtained with frequent sips of water, ice chips, or a salt and soda gargle three or four times per day. This gargle is made by dissolving 1 tsp of salt and 1 tsp of baking soda in 2 cups of warm water. The discomfort should subside in 3 to 4 days. A mixture of antacid (Mylanta or Maalox), diphenhydramine (Benadryl), and viscous lidocaine can be used to swish and spit, increasing patient comfort when eating. To limit radiation

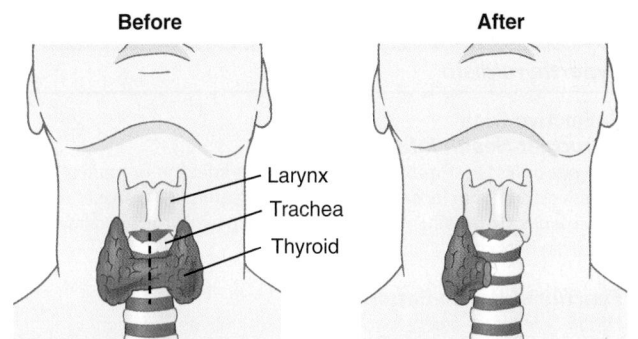

Before   **After**

Larynx
Trachea
Thyroid

FIG. 50-8 Subtotal thyroidectomy. Part of the thyroid gland is removed.

exposure to others, instruct the patient receiving RAI on the importance of home precautions, including (1) using private toilet facilities if possible and flushing two or three times after each use; (2) separately laundering towels, bed linens, and clothes daily at home; (3) not preparing food for others that requires prolonged handling with bare hands; and (4) avoiding being close to pregnant women or children for 7 days after therapy.

Surgical Therapy. Thyroidectomy is indicated for individuals who have (1) a large goiter causing tracheal compression, (2) been unresponsive to antithyroid therapy, or (3) thyroid cancer (Fig. 50-8). Additionally, surgery may be done when an individual is not a candidate for RAI. One advantage that thyroidectomy has over RAI is a more rapid reduction in T_3 and T_4 levels. A *subtotal thyroidectomy* is often the preferred surgical procedure and involves the removal of a significant portion (90%) of the thyroid gland.

An endoscopic thyroidectomy is a minimally invasive procedure. Several small incisions are made, and a scope is inserted. Instruments are passed through the scope to remove thyroid tissue or nodules. Endoscopic thyroidectomy is an appropriate procedure for patients with small nodules (less than 3 cm) and no evidence of malignancy. Advantages of endoscopic thyroidectomy over open thyroidectomy include less scarring, less pain, and a faster return to normal activity.

Nutritional Therapy. With the increased metabolic rate in hyperthyroid patients, there is a high potential for the patient to have a nutritional deficit. A high-calorie diet (4000 to 5000 cal/day) may be ordered to satisfy hunger, prevent tissue breakdown, and decrease weight loss. This can be accomplished with six full meals a day and snacks high in protein, carbohydrates, minerals, and vitamins. The protein content should be 1 to 2 g/kg of ideal body weight. Increase carbohydrate intake to compensate for increased metabolism. Carbohydrates provide energy and decrease the use of body-stored protein. Teach the patient to avoid highly seasoned and high-fiber foods because these foods can further stimulate the already hyperactive GI tract. Instruct the patient to avoid caffeine-containing liquids such as coffee, tea, and cola to decrease the restlessness and sleep disturbances associated with these fluids. Refer the patient to a dietitian for help in meeting individual nutritional needs.

NURSING MANAGEMENT
HYPERTHYROIDISM

NURSING ASSESSMENT

Subjective and objective data that should be obtained from an individual with hyperthyroidism are presented in Table 50-9.

TABLE 50-9 NURSING ASSESSMENT

Hyperthyroidism

Subjective Data
Important Health Information
Past health history: Preexisting goiter; recent infection or trauma, immigration from iodine-deficient area, autoimmune disease
Medications: Thyroid hormones, herbal therapies that may contain thyroid hormone

Functional Health Patterns
Health perception–health management: Positive family history of thyroid or autoimmune disorders
Nutritional-metabolic: Iodine intake; weight loss; increased appetite, thirst; nausea, vomiting
Elimination: Diarrhea; polyuria; sweating
Activity-exercise: Dyspnea on exertion; palpitations; muscle weakness, fatigue
Sleep-rest: Insomnia
Cognitive-perceptual: Chest pain; nervousness; heat intolerance; pruritus
Sexuality-reproductive: Decreased libido; impotence; gynecomastia (in men); amenorrhea (in women)
Coping–stress tolerance: Emotional lability, irritability, restlessness, personality changes, delirium

Objective Data
General Observation
Agitation, rapid speech and body movements; anxiety, restlessness, hyperthermia, enlarged or nodular thyroid gland

Eyes
Exophthalmos, eyelid retraction; infrequent blinking

Integumentary
Warm, diaphoretic, velvety skin; thin, loose nails; fine, silky hair and hair loss; palmar erythema; clubbing; white pigmentation of skin (vitiligo), diffuse edema of legs and feet

Respiratory
Tachypnea, dyspnea on exertion

Cardiovascular
Tachycardia, bounding pulse, systolic murmurs, dysrhythmias, hypertension, bruit over the thyroid gland

Gastrointestinal
Increased bowel sounds; increased appetite, diarrhea, weight loss, hepatosplenomegaly

Neurologic
Hyperreflexia; diplopia; fine tremors of hands, tongue, eyelids

Musculoskeletal
Muscle wasting

Reproductive
Menstrual irregularities, infertility; impotence, gynecomastia in men

Possible Diagnostic Findings
↑ T_3, ↑ T_4; ↑ T_3 resin uptake; ↓ or undetectable TSH; chest x-ray showing enlarged heart; ECG findings of tachycardia, atrial fibrillation

TSH, Thyroid-stimulating hormone.

NURSING DIAGNOSES

Nursing diagnoses for the patient with hyperthyroidism include, but are not limited to, the following:

- Activity intolerance *related to* fatigue and heat intolerance
- Imbalanced nutrition: less than body requirements *related to* hypermetabolism and inadequate food intake

Additional information on nursing diagnoses is presented in eNursing Care Plan 50-1 for the patient with hyperthyroidism (available on the website for this chapter).

PLANNING

The overall goals are that the patient with hyperthyroidism will (1) experience relief of symptoms, (2) have no serious complications related to the disease or treatment, (3) maintain nutritional balance, and (4) cooperate with the therapeutic plan.

NURSING IMPLEMENTATION

ACUTE INTERVENTION. Individuals who have hyperthyroidism are usually treated in an outpatient setting. However, patients who develop acute thyrotoxicosis or those who undergo thyroidectomy require hospitalization and acute care.

Acute Thyrotoxicosis. Acute thyrotoxicosis is a systemic syndrome that requires aggressive treatment, often in an intensive care unit. Administer medications (previously discussed) that block thyroid hormone production and the sympathetic nervous system. Provide supportive therapy, including monitoring for cardiac dysrhythmias and decompensation, ensuring adequate oxygenation, and administering IV fluids to replace fluid and electrolyte losses. This is especially important in the patient who experiences fluid losses due to vomiting and diarrhea.

Ensuring adequate rest may be a challenge because of the patient's irritability and restlessness. Provide a calm, quiet room because increased metabolism and sensitivity of the sympathetic nervous system causes sleep disturbances. Other interventions may include (1) placing the patient in a cool room away from very ill patients and noisy, high-traffic areas; (2) using light bed coverings and changing the linen frequently if the patient is diaphoretic; and (3) encouraging and assisting with exercise involving large muscle groups (tremors can interfere with small-muscle coordination) to allow the release of nervous tension and restlessness. It is important to establish a supportive, trusting relationship to facilitate coping by a patient who is irritable, restless, and anxious.

If exophthalmos is present, there is a potential for corneal injury related to irritation and dryness. The patient may have orbital pain. Nursing interventions to relieve eye discomfort and prevent corneal ulceration include applying artificial tears to soothe and moisten conjunctival membranes. Salt restriction may help reduce periorbital edema. Elevate the patient's head to promote fluid drainage from the periorbital area. The patient should sit upright as much as possible.

Dark glasses reduce glare and prevent irritation from smoke, air currents, dust, and dirt. If the eyelids cannot be closed, lightly tape them shut for sleep. To maintain flexibility, teach the patient to exercise the intraocular muscles several times a day by turning the eyes in the complete range of motion. Good grooming can help reduce the loss of self-esteem from an altered body image. If the exophthalmos is severe, treatment options include corticosteroids, radiation of retroorbital tissues, orbital decompression, or corrective lid or muscle surgery.

Thyroid Surgery. When subtotal thyroidectomy is the treatment of choice, the patient must be adequately prepared to avoid postoperative complications. Before surgery, antithyroid drugs, iodine, and β-adrenergic blockers may be administered to achieve a euthyroid state. Iodine reduces vascularization of the thyroid gland, reducing the risk of hemorrhage. Iodine is mixed with water or juice, sipped through a straw, and administered after meals. Assess the patient for signs of iodine toxicity such as swelling of the buccal mucosa and other mucous membranes, excessive salivation, nausea and vomiting, and skin reactions. If toxicity occurs, discontinue iodine administration and notify the health care provider.

Preoperatively, teach the patient about comfort and safety measures. Teach the patient the importance of performing leg exercises. Instruct the patient in how to support the head manually while turning in bed, since this maneuver minimizes stress on the suture line after surgery. The patient should practice range-of-motion exercises of the neck. Explain routine postoperative care such as IV infusions. Tell the patient that talking is likely to be difficult for a short time after surgery.

Postoperative Care. Postoperative complications include hypothyroidism, damage to or inadvertent removal of parathyroid glands causing hypoparathyroidism and hypocalcemia, hemorrhage, injury to the recurrent or superior laryngeal nerve, thyrotoxicosis, and infection.[13] Recurrent laryngeal nerve damage leads to vocal cord paralysis. If both cords are paralyzed, spastic airway obstruction will occur, requiring an immediate tracheostomy.

SAFETY ALERT
- Although not common, airway obstruction after thyroid surgery is an emergency situation.
- Oxygen, suction equipment, and a tracheostomy tray should be readily available in the patient's room.

Respiration may also become difficult because of excess swelling of the neck tissues, hemorrhage, and hematoma formation. *Laryngeal stridor* (harsh, vibratory sound) may occur during inspiration and expiration as a result of edema of the laryngeal nerve. Laryngeal stridor may also be related to tetany, which occurs if the parathyroid glands are removed or damaged during surgery, leading to hypocalcemia. To treat tetany, IV calcium salts (e.g., calcium gluconate, calcium gluceptate) should be available.

Important nursing interventions after a thyroidectomy include the following:
- Assess the patient every 2 hours for 24 hours for signs of hemorrhage or tracheal compression such as irregular breathing, neck swelling, frequent swallowing, sensations of fullness at the incision site, choking, and blood on the anterior or posterior dressings.
- Place the patient in a semi-Fowler's position and support the patient's head with pillows. Avoid flexion of the neck and any tension on the suture lines.[13]
- Monitor vital signs and calcium levels. Complete the initial assessment by checking for signs of tetany secondary to hypoparathyroidism (e.g., tingling in toes, fingers, around the mouth; muscular twitching; apprehension) and by evaluating difficulty in speaking and hoarseness. Monitor Trousseau's sign and Chvostek's sign (see Chapter 17, Fig. 17-15). Expect some hoarseness for 3 or 4 days after surgery because of edema.
- Control postoperative pain by giving medication.

If postoperative recovery is uneventful, the patient ambulates within hours after surgery, is permitted to take fluid as soon as tolerated, and eats a soft diet the day after surgery.

The appearance of the incision may be distressing to the patient. Reassure the patient that the scar will fade in color and eventually look like a normal neck wrinkle. A scarf, jewelry, a high collar, or other covering can effectively camouflage the scar.

AMBULATORY AND HOME CARE. The patient, caregiver, and family need to be aware that thyroid hormone balance should be monitored periodically. Most patients experience a period of relative hypothyroidism soon after surgery because of the substantial reduction in the size of the thyroid. However, the remaining tissue usually hypertrophies over time and recovers the capacity to produce hormones. The administration of thyroid hormone is avoided because the exogenous hormone inhibits pituitary production of TSH and delays or prevents the restoration of normal gland function and tissue regeneration.

To prevent weight gain, caloric intake must be reduced substantially below the amount that was required before surgery. Adequate iodine is necessary to promote thyroid function, but excesses can inhibit the thyroid gland. Seafood once or twice a week or normal use of iodized salt should provide sufficient iodine intake. Encourage regular exercise to stimulate the thyroid gland. Teach the patient to avoid high environmental temperatures because they inhibit thyroid regeneration.

Regular follow-up care is necessary. The patient should see the health care provider biweekly for a month and then at least semiannually to assess thyroid function. If a complete thyroidectomy has been performed, instruct the patient about the need for lifelong thyroid hormone replacement. Teach the patient the signs and symptoms of progressive thyroid failure and to seek medical care if these develop. Hypothyroidism is relatively easy to manage with oral administration of thyroid replacement.

▌EVALUATION
The expected outcomes are that the patient with hyperthyroidism will
- Experience relief of symptoms
- Have no serious complications related to the disease or treatment
- Cooperate with the therapeutic plan

Additional information on expected outcomes is presented in eNursing Care Plan 50-1 for the patient with hyperthyroidism (available on the website for this chapter).

HYPOTHYROIDISM

Hypothyroidism is a deficiency of thyroid hormone that causes a general slowing of the metabolic rate. About 4% of the U.S. population has mild hypothyroidism, with about 0.3% having more severe disease.[14] Hypothyroidism is more common in women than men.

Etiology and Pathophysiology

Hypothyroidism can be classified as primary or secondary. *Primary hypothyroidism* is caused by destruction of thyroid tissue or defective hormone synthesis. *Secondary hypothyroidism* is caused by pituitary disease with decreased TSH secretion or hypothalamic dysfunction with decreased thyrotropin-releasing hormone (TRH) secretion. Hypothyroidism may also be transient and related to thyroiditis or discontinuance of thyroid hormone therapy.

Iodine deficiency is the most common cause of hypothyroidism worldwide. In the United States, the most common cause of primary hypothyroidism is atrophy of the thyroid gland. This atrophy is the end result of Hashimoto's thyroiditis or Graves' disease. These autoimmune diseases destroy the thyroid gland. Hypothyroidism may also develop due to treatment for hyperthyroidism, specifically the surgical removal of the thyroid gland or RAI therapy. Drugs such as amiodarone (Cordarone) (contains iodine) and lithium (blocks hormone production) can cause hypothyroidism.

Hypothyroidism that develops in infancy (*cretinism*) is caused by thyroid hormone deficiencies during fetal or early neonatal life. All infants in the United States are screened for decreased thyroid function at birth.

Clinical Manifestations

Regardless of the cause, hypothyroidism has common features. It has systemic effects characterized by a slowing of body processes. Manifestations vary depending on the severity and the duration of thyroid deficiency, as well as the patient's age at the onset of the deficiency. The onset of symptoms may occur over months to years unless hypothyroidism occurs after a thyroidectomy, after thyroid ablation, or during treatment with antithyroid drugs.

The patient is often fatigued and lethargic and experiences personality and mental changes, including impaired memory, slowed speech, decreased initiative, and somnolence. Many individuals with hypothyroidism appear depressed. Weight gain is most likely a result of a decreased metabolic rate.

Hypothyroidism is associated with decreased cardiac contractility and decreased cardiac output. Thus the patient may experience low exercise tolerance and shortness of breath on exertion. Hypothyroidism may cause significant cardiovascular problems, especially in a person with previous cardiovascular disorders.

Anemia is a common feature of hypothyroidism. Erythropoietin levels may be low or normal. Because the metabolic rate is lower, oxygen demand is reduced. Other hematologic problems are related to cobalamin, iron, and folate deficiencies. The patient may bruise easily. Increased serum cholesterol and triglyceride levels and the accumulation of mucopolysaccharides in the intima of small blood vessels can result in coronary atherosclerosis.

Patients with severe, long-standing hypothyroidism may display myxedema, which alters the physical appearance of the skin and subcutaneous tissues with puffiness, facial and periorbital edema, and a masklike affect. Myxedema occurs due to the accumulation of hydrophilic mucopolysaccharides in the dermis and other tissues (Fig. 50-9). Individuals with hypothyroidism may describe an altered self-image related to their disabilities and altered appearance. Other manifestations of hypothyroidism are summarized in Table 50-5.

In the older adult the typical manifestations of hypothyroidism (including fatigue, cold and dry skin, hoarseness, hair loss,

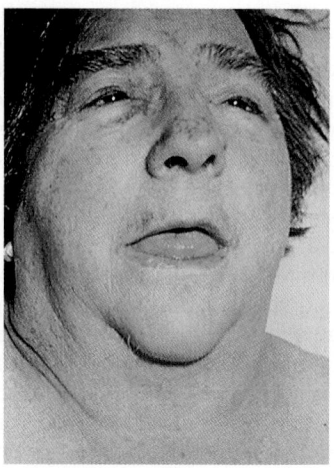

FIG. 50-9 Common features of myxedema. Dull, puffy skin; coarse, sparse hair; periorbital edema; and prominent tongue.

TABLE 50-10   **COLLABORATIVE CARE**
Hypothyroidism

Diagnostic	**Collaborative Therapy**
• History and physical examination	• Thyroid hormone replacement (e.g., levothyroxine)
• Serum TSH and free T_4	• Monitor thyroid hormone levels and adjust dosage (if needed)
• Total serum T_3 and T_4	• Nutritional therapy to promote weight loss
• Thyroid peroxidase (TPO) antibodies	• Patient and caregiver teaching (see Table 50-11)

TSH, Thyroid-stimulating hormone.

constipation, and cold intolerance) may be attributed to normal aging. For this reason, the patient's symptoms may not raise suspicion of an underlying condition. Older adults who have confusion, lethargy, and depression should be evaluated for thyroid disease.

Complications

The mental sluggishness, drowsiness, and lethargy of hypothyroidism may progress gradually or suddenly to a notable impairment of consciousness or coma. This situation, termed *myxedema coma,* is a medical emergency. Myxedema coma can be precipitated by infection, drugs (especially opioids, tranquilizers, and barbiturates), exposure to cold, and trauma.[14] It is characterized by subnormal temperature, hypotension, and hypoventilation. Cardiovascular collapse can result from hypoventilation, hyponatremia, hypoglycemia, and lactic acidosis. For the patient to survive a myxedema coma, vital functions must be supported and IV thyroid hormone replacement administered.

Diagnostic Studies

The most common and reliable laboratory tests for thyroid function are TSH and free T_4. These values, correlated with symptoms gathered from the history and physical examination, confirm the diagnosis of hypothyroidism. Serum TSH levels help determine the cause of hypothyroidism. Serum TSH is high when the defect is in the thyroid and low when it is in the pituitary or the hypothalamus. The presence of thyroid antibodies suggests an autoimmune origin of the hypothyroidism. Other abnormal laboratory findings are elevated cholesterol and triglycerides, anemia, and increased creatine kinase (see Table 50-6).

Collaborative Care

The treatment goal for a patient with hypothyroidism is restoration of a euthyroid state as safely and rapidly as possible with hormone therapy (Table 50-10). A low-calorie diet is also indicated to promote weight loss or prevent weight gain.

Levothyroxine (Synthroid) is the drug of choice to treat hypothyroidism. In the young and otherwise healthy patient, the maintenance replacement dosage is adjusted according to the patient's response and laboratory findings. When thyroid hormone therapy is initiated, the initial dosages are low to avoid increases in resting heart rate and BP. In the patient with compromised cardiac status, careful monitoring is needed when starting and adjusting the dosage because the usual dose may increase myocardial oxygen demand.[15] The increased oxygen demand may cause angina and cardiac dysrhythmias.

DRUG ALERT: Levothyroxine (Synthroid)
- Carefully monitor patients with cardiovascular disease who take this drug.
- Monitor heart rate and report pulse greater than 100 beats/min or an irregular heartbeat.
- Promptly report chest pain, weight loss, nervousness, tremors, and/or insomnia.

In a patient without side effects, the dose is increased at 4- to 6-week intervals. It may take up to 8 weeks before the full effect of hormone therapy is seen, It is important that the patient regularly take replacement medication. Lifelong thyroid therapy is usually required.

Liotrix is a synthetic mix of levothyroxine (T_4) and liothyronine (T_3) in a 4:1 combination. Levothyroxine has a peak of action of 1 to 3 weeks. In contrast, liotrix has a faster onset of action with a peak of 2 to 3 days. Liotrix can be used in acutely ill individuals with hypothyroidism.

NURSING MANAGEMENT HYPOTHYROIDISM

NURSING ASSESSMENT

Careful assessment may reveal early and subtle changes in a patient suspected of having hypothyroidism. Note any previous history of hyperthyroidism and treatment with antithyroid medications, radioactive iodine, or surgery. Ask the patient about prescribed iodine-containing medications (see Table 50-4) and any changes in appetite, weight, activity level, speech, memory, and skin such as increased dryness or thickening. Assess for cold intolerance, constipation, and signs of depression. Further assessment should focus on heart rate, tenderness over the thyroid gland, and edema in the extremities and face.

NURSING DIAGNOSES

Nursing diagnoses for the patient with hypothyroidism may include, but are not limited to, the following:
- Imbalanced nutrition: more than body requirements *related to* calorie intake in excess of metabolic rate
- Constipation *related to* GI hypomotility
- Impaired memory *related to* hypometabolism

Additional information on nursing diagnoses is presented in the eNursing Care Plan 50-2 for the patient with hypothyroidism (available on the website for this chapter).

PLANNING

The overall goals are that the patient with hypothyroidism will (1) experience relief of symptoms, (2) maintain a euthyroid state, (3) maintain a positive self-image, and (4) comply with lifelong thyroid therapy.

NURSING IMPLEMENTATION

HEALTH PROMOTION. Currently no consensus exists regarding thyroid function screening. Although hypothyroidism is relatively common, particularly among women over age 50, there does not appear to be strong justification for screening the general population.[16] High-risk populations should be screened for subclinical (asymptomatic) thyroid disease. High-risk individuals include those with a family history of thyroid disease, those with a history of neck radiation, women over 50 years old, and postpartum women.

ACUTE INTERVENTION. Most individuals with hypothyroidism are treated on an outpatient basis. The patient who develops myxedema coma requires acute nursing care, often in an inten-

sive care setting. Mechanical respiratory support and cardiac monitoring are frequently necessary.

Administer thyroid hormone therapy and all other medications IV because paralytic ileus may be present in myxedema coma. Monitor the core temperature because hypothermia often occurs in myxedema coma. Use soap gently and moisturize frequently to prevent skin breakdown. Frequent changes in patient positioning and a low-pressure mattress can also assist in maintaining skin integrity.

Monitor the patient's progress by assessing vital signs, body weight, fluid intake and output, and visible edema. Cardiac assessment is especially important because the cardiovascular response to hormone therapy determines the medication regimen. Note energy level and mental alertness, which should increase within 2 to 14 days and continue to improve steadily to normal levels. The patient's neurologic status and free T_4 levels are used to determine continuing treatment.

AMBULATORY AND HOME CARE. Patient teaching is essential for the patient with hypothyroidism and the caregiver (Table 50-11). Initially the hypothyroid patient may have difficulty processing complex instructions. It is important to provide written instructions, repeat the information often, and assess the patient's comprehension level.

Stress the need for receiving lifelong drug therapy and avoiding abrupt discontinuation of drugs. Instruct the patient in expected and unexpected side effects. In the teaching plan include the signs and symptoms of hypothyroidism or hyperthyroidism that indicate hormone imbalance. Clearly define toxic symptoms. Table 50-5 lists manifestations of hyperthyroidism, which are the same as the toxic manifestations of thyroid hormone replacement.

Teach the patient to immediately contact a health care provider if manifestations of overdose occur, such as orthopnea, dyspnea, rapid pulse, palpitations, chest pain, nervousness, or insomnia. The patient with diabetes mellitus should test his or

---

TABLE 50-11 PATIENT & CAREGIVER TEACHING GUIDE

Hypothyroidism

Include the following instructions when teaching the patient and caregiver about management of hypothyroidism.

1. Discuss the importance of thyroid hormone therapy.
   - Need for lifelong therapy
   - Taking thyroid hormone in the morning before food
   - Need for regular follow-up care
2. Caution the patient not to switch brands of the hormone unless prescribed, since the bioavailability of thyroid hormones may differ.
3. Emphasize the need for a comfortable, warm environment because of intolerance to cold.
4. Teach measures to prevent skin breakdown. Soap should be used sparingly and lotion applied to skin.
5. Caution the patient, especially if an older adult, to avoid sedatives. If they must be used, suggest that the lowest dose be used. Caregiver should closely monitor mental status, level of consciousness, and respirations.
6. Discuss with the patient and the caregiver measures to minimize constipation, including
   - Gradual increase in activity and exercise
   - Increased fiber in diet
   - Use of stool softeners
   - Regular bowel elimination time
7. Tell patient to avoid using enemas because they produce vagal stimulation, which can be hazardous if cardiac disease is present.

her capillary blood glucose at least daily because the return to the euthyroid state frequently increases insulin requirements. In addition, thyroid drugs potentiate the effects of anticoagulants and decrease the effect of digitalis compounds. Instruct the patient about the toxic signs and symptoms of these medications and the need to remain under close medical observation until stable.

With treatment, striking transformations occur in both appearance and mental function. Most adults return to a normal state. Cardiovascular conditions and (occasionally) psychosis may persist despite corrections of the hormonal imbalance. Relapses occur if treatment is interrupted.

EVALUATION

The expected outcomes are that the patient with hypothyroidism will

- Have relief from symptoms
- Maintain a euthyroid state as evidenced by normal thyroid hormone and TSH levels
- Avoid complications of therapy
- Adhere to lifelong therapy

Additional information on expected outcomes is presented in the eNursing Care Plan 50-2 for the patient with hypothyroidism (available on the website for this chapter).

THYROID NODULES AND CANCER

A *thyroid nodule* (growth in the thyroid gland) may be benign or malignant (thyroid cancer). More than 95% of all thyroid gland nodules are benign. A person's chance of getting a thyroid nodule increases with age. Benign nodules are usually not dangerous, but they can cause tracheal compression if they become too large.

Thyroid cancer is the most common form of an endocrine system cancer. An estimated 56,460 new cases of thyroid cancer are diagnosed annually.[17] The incidence of thyroid cancer has risen significantly in the past 25 years. Thyroid cancer affects more women, and the incidence is higher in Asian Americans.[18]

Radiation exposure significantly increases the risk for thyroid cancer. Adults at higher risk for thyroid cancer include those who were given radiation treatment during childhood for lymphoma, Wilms' tumor, and neuroblastoma. Having a personal or family history of goiter also increases a person's risk.

Types of Thyroid Cancer

The four main types of thyroid cancer are papillary, follicular, medullary, and anaplastic. *Papillary* thyroid cancer is the most common type, accounting for about 70% to 80% of all thyroid cancers. Papillary cancer tends to grow slowly and spreads initially to lymph nodes in the neck.

Follicular thyroid cancer makes up about 15% of all thyroid cancers. It tends to occur in older patients. Follicular cancer first metastasizes into the cervical lymph nodes, then spreads to the neck, lungs, and bones.

Medullary thyroid cancer, which accounts for up to 10% of all thyroid cancers, is more likely to occur in families and to be associated with other endocrine problems. It is diagnosed by genetic testing for a proto-oncogene called *RET*. Medullary thyroid cancer is a type of multiple endocrine neoplasia (see discussion at right). This type of cancer is often poorly differentiated and associated with early metastasis.

Anaplastic thyroid cancer, which is found in less than 2% of patients with thyroid cancer, is the most advanced and aggressive thyroid cancer. It is the least likely to respond to treatment and has a poor prognosis.

Clinical Manifestations and Diagnostic Studies

The primary manifestation of thyroid cancer is a painless, palpable nodule or nodules in an enlarged thyroid gland. Patients or health care providers discover most of these nodules during a routine palpation of the neck. Physical examination may reveal firm, palpable, cervical masses that are suggestive of lymph node metastasis. Hemoptysis and airway obstruction may occur if the trachea is involved.

Nodular enlargement of the thyroid gland or palpation of a mass requires further evaluation. Ultrasound is often the first test used. Follow-up testing may involve CT, MRI, positron emission tomography (PET), and ultrasound-guided fine-needle aspiration (FNA). FNA is indicated when a tissue sample for pathologic examination is necessary. A thyroid scan may also be done to evaluate for possible malignancy. The scan shows whether nodules on the thyroid are "hot" or "cold." Tumors that take up radioactive iodine are called "hot" nodules and are nearly always benign. If the nodule does not take up the radioactive iodine, it appears as "cold" and has a higher risk of being malignant (see eFig. 50-2, available on the website for this chapter).

Elevations in serum calcitonin are associated with medullary thyroid cancer. In papillary and follicular cancers, serum thyroglobulin is elevated. In families with a history of medullary thyroid cancer, encourage family members to get genetic testing done and have thyroid screening on a regular basis.

NURSING AND COLLABORATIVE MANAGEMENT THYROID CANCER

Surgical removal of the tumor is usually indicated for thyroid cancer.[19] Surgical procedures may range from unilateral total lobectomy to near-total thyroidectomy with bilateral lobectomy. Lymph nodes in the neck may be removed with surgery to determine if the cancer has spread. RAI may be given to some patients to destroy any remaining cancer cells after surgery. RAI therapy has been shown to improve survival rates in patients with papillary and follicular thyroid cancer. External beam radiation may be given as palliative treatment for patients with metastatic thyroid cancer.

Many thyroid cancers are TSH dependent, and thyroid hormone therapy in high doses is often prescribed to inhibit pituitary secretion of TSH. Chemotherapy including doxorubicin (Adriamycin), and cyclophosphamide (Cytoxan) may be used for advanced disease. Vandetanib (Caprelsa) and cabozantinib (Cometriq) are targeted therapies used for medullary thyroid cancer that has metastasized. These drugs inhibit tyrosine kinases, which are enzymes that are involved in growth of cancer cells.

Nursing care for the patient with thyroid cancer is similar to that of a patient undergoing thyroidectomy (see p. 1199). Because of the surgical site location and the potential for hypocalcemia, the patient requires frequent postoperative assessment. Assess the patient for airway obstruction, bleeding, and tetany, since the parathyroid gland may have been disturbed or removed during surgery.

MULTIPLE ENDOCRINE NEOPLASIA

Multiple endocrine neoplasia is an inherited condition characterized by hormone-secreting tumors.[20] Multiple endocrine neoplasia is caused by the mutation of one of two genes, *MEN1* or *RET,* that normally control cell growth. Tumors may develop in childhood or later in life.

The two major types of multiple endocrine neoplasia are type 1 and type 2. Both types are commonly inherited as autosomal dominant disorders. Persons with type 1 commonly show signs of parathyroid gland hyperactivity (hyperparathyroidism). Other signs may include hyperactivity of the pituitary gland (prolactinoma) and pancreas (gastrinomas). In most cases the tumors are initially benign, and some tumors later become malignant. Persons with type 2 neoplasia often have clinical manifestations of medullary thyroid carcinoma. They may also develop pheochromocytoma (tumor of the adrenal glands). (Pheochromocytoma is discussed later in this chapter on pp. 1214-1215.)

Treatment of the tumor(s) may include conservative management (watchful waiting), medication to block the effects of excess hormone, and surgical removal of the gland and/or tumor. It is important for patients to have regular screening visits with their health care provider so that new tumors may be detected early and existing tumors carefully monitored.

DISORDERS OF PARATHYROID GLANDS

HYPERPARATHYROIDISM

Etiology and Pathophysiology

Hyperparathyroidism is a condition involving an increased secretion of parathyroid hormone (PTH). PTH helps regulate serum calcium and phosphate levels by stimulating bone resorp-

tion of calcium, renal tubular reabsorption of calcium, and activation of vitamin D. Thus oversecretion of PTH is associated with increased serum calcium levels. Hyperparathyroidism affects approximately 1% of the U.S. population and is more common in women than in men.

Hyperparathyroidism is classified as primary, secondary, or tertiary. *Primary hyperparathyroidism* is due to an increased secretion of PTH leading to disorders of calcium, phosphate, and bone metabolism. The most common cause is a benign tumor (adenoma) in the parathyroid gland. Patients who have previously undergone head and neck radiation may have an increased risk of developing a parathyroid adenoma. Long-term lithium therapy has also been associated with primary hyperparathyroidism. The peak incidence of primary hyperparathyroidism is in the 40s and 50s.

Secondary hyperparathyroidism appears to be a compensatory response to conditions that induce or cause hypocalcemia, the main stimulus of PTH secretion. These conditions include vitamin D deficiencies, malabsorption, chronic kidney disease, and hyperphosphatemia.

Tertiary hyperparathyroidism occurs when there is hyperplasia of the parathyroid glands and a loss of negative feedback from circulating calcium levels. Thus there is autonomous secretion of PTH, even with normal calcium levels. This condition is seen in patients who have had a kidney transplant after a long period of dialysis treatment for chronic kidney disease (see Chapter 47).

Excessive levels of circulating PTH usually lead to hypercalcemia and hypophosphatemia. Multiple body systems are affected (Table 50-12). Decreased bone density can occur

TABLE 50-12	CLINICAL MANIFESTATIONS OF PARATHYROID DYSFUNCTION		
Hyperfunction	**Hypofunction**	**Hyperfunction**	**Hypofunction**
Cardiovascular		**Visual**	
• Dysrhythmias	• Decreased contractility of heart muscle	• Corneal calcification on slit-lamp examination	• Eye changes, including lenticular opacities, cataracts, papilledema
• Shortened QT interval on ECG	• Decreased cardiac output		
• Hypertension	• Prolongation of QT and ST intervals on ECG	**Gastrointestinal**	
	• Dysrhythmias	• Vague abdominal pain	• Abdominal cramps
		• Anorexia	• Fecal incontinence (in older adult)
Neurologic		• Nausea and vomiting	• Malabsorption
• Personality disturbances	• Personality changes	• Constipation	
• Emotional irritability	• Psychiatric manifestations of depression, anxiety, psychosis	• Pancreatitis	
• Memory impairment	• Irritability	• Peptic ulcer disease	
• Psychosis, depression	• Memory impairment	• Cholelithiasis	
• Delirium, confusion, coma	• Headache, increased intracranial pressure	• Weight loss	
• Poor coordination	• Seizures	**Integumentary**	
• Hyperactive deep-tendon reflexes	• Positive Chvostek's sign or Trousseau's phenomenon (see Fig. 17-15)	• Skin necrosis	• Dry, scaly skin
• Abnormalities of gait	• Tremor	• Moist skin	• Hair loss on scalp and body
• Psychomotor retardation	• Paresthesias of lips, hands, feet		• Brittle nails, transverse ridging
• Headache	• Hyperactive deep-tendon reflexes		• Changes in developing teeth, lack of tooth enamel
• Paresthesias	• Disorientation, confusion (in older adult)	**Musculoskeletal**	
		• Skeletal pain	• Fatigue
		• Backache	• Weakness
		• Weakness, fatigue	• Painful muscle cramps
		• Pain on weight bearing	• Skeletal x-ray changes, osteosclerosis
		• Osteoporosis	• Soft tissue calcification
Renal		• Pathologic fractures of long bones	• Difficulty walking
• Hypercalciuria	• Urinary frequency	• Compression fractures of spine	
• Kidney stones (nephrolithiasis)	• Urinary incontinence	• Decreased muscle tone, muscle atrophy	
• Urinary tract infections			
• Polyuria			

because of the effect of PTH on osteoclastic (bone resorption) and osteoblastic (bone formation) activity. In the kidneys the excess calcium cannot be reabsorbed, leading to increased levels of calcium in the urine (hypercalciuria). This urinary calcium, along with a large amount of urinary phosphate, can lead to calculi formation.

Clinical Manifestations and Complications

Clinical manifestations range from the asymptomatic individual (diagnosed through testing for unrelated problems) to the patient with overt symptoms.[21] The manifestations are associated with hypercalcemia (see Table 50-12). Muscle weakness, loss of appetite, constipation, fatigue, emotional disorders, and shortened attention span are often noted. Other signs of hyperparathyroidism include osteoporosis, fractures, and kidney stones (nephrolithiasis). Neuromuscular abnormalities are characterized by muscle weakness, particularly in the proximal muscles of the lower extremities. Serious complications of hyperparathyroidism are renal failure; pancreatitis; cardiac changes; and long bone, rib, and vertebral fractures.

Diagnostic Studies

PTH levels are elevated in patients with hyperparathyroidism. Serum calcium levels usually exceed 10 mg/dL (2.50 mmol/L). Because of its inverse relation with calcium, the serum phosphorus level is usually less than 3 mg/dL (0.1 mmol/L). Hypercalcemia in asymptomatic cases is often identified through a routine chemistry panel.

Elevations in other laboratory tests include urine calcium, serum chloride, uric acid, creatinine, amylase (if pancreatitis is present), and alkaline phosphatase (in the presence of bone disease). Bone density measurements may be used to detect bone loss. Conversely, individuals found to have bone loss on a screening dual-energy x-ray absorptiometry (DEXA) scan should be tested for hypercalcemia. MRI, CT, and/or ultrasound may be used for localization of an adenoma.

Collaborative Care

The goal of treatment is to relieve symptoms and prevent complications caused by excess PTH. The choice of therapy depends on the urgency of the clinical situation, the degree of hypercalcemia, and the underlying cause of the disorder.

Surgical Therapy. The most effective treatment of primary and secondary hyperparathyroidism is surgical intervention. Surgery involves partial or complete removal of the parathyroid glands. The most commonly used procedure involves endoscopy and is done on an outpatient basis. Criteria for surgery include elevated serum calcium levels (more than 1 mg/dL above the upper limit of normal), hypercalciuria (greater than 400 mg/day), markedly reduced bone mineral density, overt symptoms (e.g., neuromuscular effects, nephrolithiasis), or those under age 50. Parathyroidectomy leads to a rapid reduction of high calcium levels.

Patients who have multiple parathyroid glands removed may undergo autotransplantation of normal parathyroid tissue in the forearm or near the sternocleidomastoid muscle. This allows PTH secretion to continue with normalization of calcium levels. If autotransplantation is not possible or if it fails, the patient will need to take calcium supplements for life.

Nonsurgical Therapy. A conservative approach is often used in patients who are asymptomatic or have mild symptoms of hyperparathyroidism. Ongoing care includes an annual examination with measurements of serum PTH, calcium, phosphorus, alkaline phosphatase, creatinine and blood urea nitrogen (BUN) (to assess renal function), and urinary calcium excretion. X-rays and DEXA are done to assess for metabolic bone loss. Continued ambulation and the avoidance of immobility are important aspects of management. Dietary measures include high fluid and moderate calcium intake.

Several drugs help lower calcium levels, but they do not treat the underlying problem. Bisphosphonates (e.g., alendronate [Fosamax]) inhibit osteoclastic bone resorption, normalizing serum calcium levels and improving bone mineral density. IV bisphosphonates (e.g., pamidronate [Aredia]) can rapidly lower serum calcium in patients with dangerously elevated levels. Phosphorus is usually supplemented unless contraindicated in a person with an increased risk for urinary calculi formation. Phosphates should be used only if the patient has normal renal function and low serum phosphate levels. Loop diuretics may be given to increase the urinary excretion of calcium.

Calcimimetic agents (e.g., cinacalcet [Sensipar]) increase the sensitivity of the calcium receptor on the parathyroid gland, resulting in decreased PTH secretion and calcium blood levels. Drugs in this class are given for secondary hyperparathyroidism in individuals with chronic kidney disease on dialysis and for patients with parathyroid cancer. Cinacalcet remains under investigation for use in primary hyperparathyroidism.

NURSING MANAGEMENT HYPERPARATHYROIDISM

Nursing care for the patient after a parathyroidectomy is similar to that for a patient after thyroidectomy. The major postoperative complications are associated with hemorrhage and fluid and electrolyte disturbances. *Tetany,* a condition of neuromuscular hyperexcitability associated with sudden decrease in calcium levels, is another concern. It is usually apparent early in the postoperative period but may develop over several days. Mild tetany, characterized by unpleasant tingling of the hands and around the mouth, may be present but should decrease over time. If tetany becomes more severe (e.g., muscular spasms or laryngospasms), IV calcium may be given. IV calcium gluconate or gluceptate should be readily available for patients after parathyroidectomy in the event that acute tetany occurs.

Monitor intake and output to evaluate fluid status. Assess calcium, potassium, phosphate, and magnesium levels frequently, as well as Chvostek's and Trousseau's signs (see Fig. 17-15). Encourage mobility to promote bone calcification.

If surgery is not performed, treatment to relieve symptoms and prevent complications is initiated. Assist the patient with hyperparathyroidism to adapt the meal plan to his or her lifestyle. A referral to a dietitian may be useful. Because immobility can aggravate the bone loss, emphasize the importance of an exercise program. Encourage the patient to keep the regular follow-up appointments. Instruct the patient regarding the symptoms of hypocalcemia or hypercalcemia, and to report them should they occur. Hypocalcemia and hypercalcemia are discussed in Chapter 17.

HYPOPARATHYROIDISM

Hypoparathyroidism is an uncommon condition associated with inadequate circulating PTH. It is characterized by hypocalcemia resulting from a lack of PTH to maintain serum calcium levels. PTH resistance at the cellular level may also occur *(pseudohypoparathyroidism)*. This is caused by a genetic defect resulting in hypocalcemia in spite of normal or high PTH levels and is often associated with hypothyroidism and hypogonadism.

The most common cause of hypoparathyroidism is iatrogenic. This may include accidental removal of the parathyroid glands or damage to the vascular supply of the glands during neck surgery (e.g., thyroidectomy).[22] Idiopathic hypoparathyroidism resulting from the absence, fatty replacement, or atrophy of the glands is a rare disease that usually occurs early in life and may be associated with other endocrine disorders. Affected patients may have antiparathyroid antibodies. Severe hypomagnesemia (e.g., malnutrition, chronic alcoholism, renal failure) also leads to a suppression of PTH secretion. Other causes of parathyroid deficiency include tumors and heavy metal poisoning.

The clinical features of acute hypoparathyroidism are due to hypocalcemia (see Table 50-12). Sudden decreases in calcium concentration cause tetany, characterized by tingling of the lips and stiffness in the extremities. Painful tonic spasms of smooth and skeletal muscles can cause dysphagia and laryngospasms, which compromise breathing. Lethargy, anxiety, and personality changes may occur. Abnormal laboratory findings include decreased serum calcium and PTH levels and increased serum phosphate levels.

NURSING AND COLLABORATIVE MANAGEMENT HYPOPARATHYROIDISM

Treatment goals for the patient with hypoparathyroidism are to treat acute complications such as tetany, maintain normal serum calcium levels, and prevent long-term complications. Emergency treatment of tetany after surgery requires the administration of IV calcium.

Give IV calcium chloride, calcium gluconate, or calcium gluceptate slowly. Use ECG monitoring during calcium administration because high serum calcium blood levels can cause hypotension, serious cardiac dysrhythmias, or cardiac arrest. The patient who takes digoxin is particularly vulnerable. IV calcium chloride can cause venous irritation and inflammation, and extravasation may cause cellulitis, necrosis, and tissue sloughing. It is important to assess IV patency before administering calcium chloride.

Rebreathing may partially alleviate acute neuromuscular symptoms associated with hypocalcemia such as generalized muscle cramps or mild tetany. Instruct the patient (if cooperative) to breathe in and out of a paper bag or breathing mask. This reduces carbon dioxide excretion from the lungs, increases carbonic acid levels in the blood, and lowers the pH. A lower pH (acidic environment) enhances calcium ionization, which causes more total body calcium to be available in the active form. This will temporarily relieve the manifestations of hypocalcemia.

The patient with hypoparathyroidism needs instruction in the management of long-term drug and nutritional therapy. PTH replacement is not recommended because of the expense and need for parenteral administration. Oral calcium supplements of at least 1.5 to 3 g/day in divided doses are usually prescribed. Hypomagnesemia needs to be corrected in some patients before the hypocalcemia can be treated.

Vitamin D is used in hypocalcemia to enhance intestinal calcium absorption. Vitamin D (e.g., dihydrotachysterol [Hytak-erol], 1,25-dihydroxycholecalciferol, or calcitriol [Rocaltrol]) raises calcium levels rapidly and is quickly metabolized. Rapid metabolism is desired because vitamin D is a fat-soluble vitamin and toxicity can cause irreversible renal impairment. A high-calcium meal plan includes foods such as dark green vegetables, soybeans, and tofu. Tell the patient to avoid foods containing oxalic acid (e.g., spinach, rhubarb) because they inhibit the absorption of calcium. Instruct the patient about the need for follow-up care, including monitoring of calcium levels three or four times a year.

DISORDERS OF ADRENAL CORTEX

Adrenal cortex steroid hormones have three main classifications: glucocorticoids, mineralocorticoids, and androgens. Glucocorticoids regulate metabolism, increase blood glucose levels, and are critical in the physiologic stress response. The primary glucocorticoid is cortisol. Mineralocorticoids regulate sodium and potassium balance. The primary mineralocorticoid is aldosterone. Androgens contribute to growth and development in both genders and to sexual activity in adult women. The term *corticosteroid* refers to any one of these three types of hormones produced by the adrenal cortex.

CUSHING SYNDROME

Etiology and Pathophysiology

Cushing syndrome is a clinical condition that results from chronic exposure to excess corticosteroids, particularly glucocorticoids.[23] Several conditions can cause Cushing syndrome. The most common cause is iatrogenic administration of exogenous corticosteroids (e.g., prednisone). Approximately 85% of the cases of endogenous Cushing syndrome are due to an ACTH-secreting pituitary adenoma (Cushing disease). Other causes of Cushing syndrome include adrenal tumors and ectopic ACTH production by tumors (usually of the lung or pancreas) outside of the hypothalamic-pituitary-adrenal axis. Cushing disease and primary adrenal tumors are more common in women in the 20- to 40-year-old age-group. Ectopic ACTH production is more common in men.

Clinical Manifestations

Manifestations of Cushing syndrome can be seen in most body systems and are related to excess levels of corticosteroids (Table 50-13). Although signs of glucocorticoid excess usually predominate, symptoms of mineralocorticoid and androgen excess may also be seen.

Corticosteroid excess causes pronounced changes in physical appearance (Fig. 50-10). Weight gain, the most common feature, results from the accumulation of adipose tissue in the trunk, face, and cervical spine area (Fig. 50-11). Hyperglycemia occurs because of glucose intolerance (associated with cortisol-induced insulin resistance) and increased gluconeogenesis by the liver. Muscle wasting causes weakness, especially in the extremities. A loss of bone matrix leads to osteoporosis and back pain. The loss of collagen makes the skin weaker and thinner and more easily bruised. Catabolic processes lead to a delay in wound healing. Irritability, anxiety, euphoria, and occasionally psychosis may also occur.

Mineralocorticoid excess may cause hypertension (secondary to fluid retention), whereas adrenal androgen excess may cause severe acne, virilization in women, and feminization in

TABLE 50-13 **CLINICAL MANIFESTATIONS OF ADRENOCORTICAL DYSFUNCTION**

System	Hyperfunction (Cushing Syndrome)	Hypofunction (Addison's Disease)
Glucocorticoids		
General appearance	Truncal obesity, thin extremities, rounding of face (moon face), fat deposits on back of neck and shoulders (buffalo hump) (see Fig. 50-11).	Weight loss, emaciation.
Integumentary	Thin, fragile skin, purplish red striae (see Fig. 50-12). Petechial hemorrhages, bruises. Florid cheeks (plethora), acne, poor wound healing.	Bronzed or smoky hyperpigmentation of face, neck, hands (especially creases) (see Fig. 50-13), buccal membranes, nipples, genitalia, and scars (if pituitary function normal). Vitiligo, alopecia.
Cardiovascular	Hypervolemia, hypertension, edema of lower extremities.	Hypotension, tendency to develop refractory shock, vasodilation.
Gastrointestinal	Increase in secretion of pepsin and HCl acid, risk of peptic ulcer disease, anorexia.	Anorexia, nausea and vomiting, cramping abdominal pain, diarrhea.
Renal/urinary	Glycosuria, hypercalciuria, risk for kidney stones.	
Musculoskeletal	Muscle wasting in extremities, fatigue, osteoporosis, awkward gait, back pain, weakness, fractures.	Fatigue.
Immune	Inhibition of immune response, suppression of allergic response.	Tendency for coexisting autoimmune diseases.
Metabolic	Hyperglycemia, negative nitrogen balance, dyslipidemia.	Hyponatremia, insulin sensitivity, fever.
Emotional	Euphoria, irritability, depression, insomnia.	Depression, exhaustion or irritability, confusion, delusions.
Mineralocorticoids		
Fluid and electrolytes	Marked sodium and water retention, edema, marked hypokalemia, alkalosis.	Sodium loss, decreased volume of extracellular fluid, hyperkalemia, salt craving.
Cardiovascular	Hypertension, hypervolemia.	Hypovolemia, tendency toward shock, decreased cardiac output.
Androgens		
Integumentary	Hirsutism, acne, hyperpigmentation.	Decreased axillary and pubic hair (in women).
Reproductive	Menstrual irregularities and enlargement of clitoris (in women), gynecomastia and testicular atrophy (in men).	No effect in men, decreased libido in women.
Musculoskeletal	Muscle wasting and weakness.	Decrease in muscle size and tone.

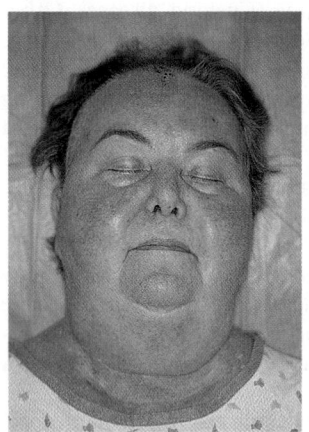

FIG. 50-10 Cushing syndrome. Facies include a rounded face ("moon face") with thin, reddened skin. Hirsutism may also be present.

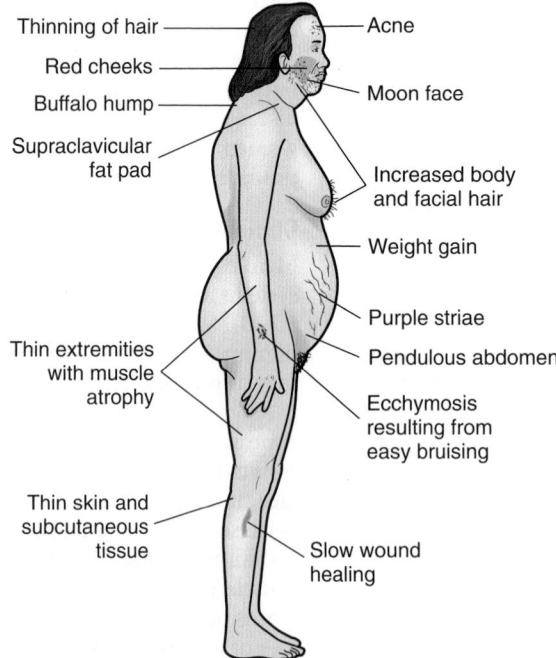

Thinning of hair
Red cheeks
Buffalo hump
Supraclavicular fat pad
Acne
Moon face
Increased body and facial hair
Weight gain
Thin extremities with muscle atrophy
Purple striae
Pendulous abdomen
Ecchymosis resulting from easy bruising
Thin skin and subcutaneous tissue
Slow wound healing

FIG. 50-11 Common characteristics of Cushing syndrome.

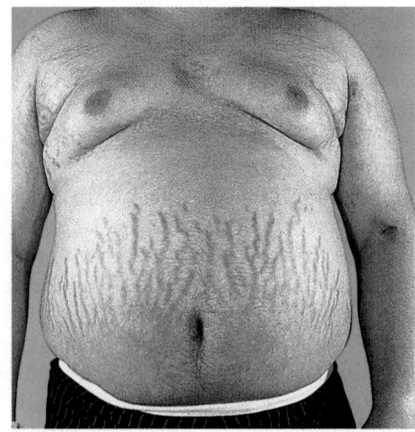

FIG. 50-12 Cushing syndrome. Truncal obesity; broad, purple striae; and easy bruising (left antecubital fossa).

men. Menstrual disorders and hirsutism in women and gynecomastia and impotence in men are seen more commonly in adrenal carcinomas.

The first indication of Cushing syndrome may be the clinical presentation, including (1) centripetal (truncal) obesity or generalized obesity; (2) *"moon face"* (fullness of the face) with facial plethora; (3) purplish red striae (usually depressed below the skin surface) on the abdomen, breast, or buttocks (Fig. 50-12); (4) hirsutism in women; (5) menstrual disorders in women; (6) hypertension; and (7) unexplained hypokalemia.

Diagnostic Studies

Plasma cortisol (the primary glucocorticoid) levels may be elevated, with loss of diurnal variation. When Cushing syndrome is suspected, a 24-hour urine collection for free cortisol is done. Urine cortisol levels higher than the normal range of 80 to 120 mcg/24 hr indicate Cushing syndrome. If results are borderline, a low-dose dexamethasone suppression test is done. False-positive results can occur in patients with depression and those taking certain medications, including phenytoin (Dilantin) and rifampicin (rifampin [Rifadin]). Urine levels of 17-ketosteroids may be elevated.[24] A CT scan and MRI of the pituitary and adrenal glands may be done.

Plasma ACTH levels may be low, normal, or elevated depending on the underlying cause of Cushing syndrome. High or normal ACTH levels indicate Cushing disease, whereas low or undetectable levels indicate an adrenal or medication etiology. Other findings on diagnostic tests associated with, but not diagnostic of, Cushing syndrome include leukocytosis, lymphopenia, eosinopenia, hyperglycemia, glycosuria, hypercalciuria, and osteoporosis. Hypokalemia and alkalosis are seen in ectopic ACTH syndrome and adrenal carcinoma.

Collaborative Care

The primary goal of treatment for Cushing syndrome is to normalize hormone secretion. The specific treatment depends on the underlying cause (Table 50-14). If the underlying cause is a pituitary adenoma, the standard treatment is surgical removal of the pituitary tumor using the transsphenoidal approach.[25] (The transsphenoidal approach is discussed earlier in this chapter on pp. 1190-1191.) Radiation therapy may also be used for patients who are not good surgical candidates.

Adrenalectomy is indicated for Cushing syndrome caused by adrenal tumors or hyperplasia. Occasionally, bilateral adrenalectomy is necessary. Laparoscopic adrenalectomy is used unless a malignant adrenal tumor is suspected. An open surgical adrenalectomy is usually performed for adrenal cancer.

Patients with ectopic ACTH-secreting tumors are best managed by locating and removing the tumor (usually lung or pancreas). This is usually possible when the tumor is benign. When a tumor is malignant and it has already metastasized, surgical removal may not be possible or successful.

When the patient is a poor candidate for surgery or prior surgery has failed, then drug therapy may be attempted. The goal of drug therapy is to suppress the synthesis and secretion of cortisol from the adrenal gland *(medical adrenalectomy)*. Drugs used include ketoconazole (Nizoral), aminoglutethimide (Cytadren), and mitotane (Lysodren). These are used cautiously because they are often toxic at the dosages needed to reduce cortisol secretion. Hydrocortisone or prednisone may be needed to avoid adrenal insufficiency. Mifepristone (Korlym) may be used to control hyperglycemia in patients with endogenous Cushing syndrome who have type 2 diabetes.

TABLE 50-14 COLLABORATIVE CARE

Cushing Syndrome

Diagnostic
- History and physical examination
- Mental status examination
- Plasma cortisol levels for diurnal variations
- Plasma ACTH levels
- Complete blood count (CBC) with WBC differential
- Blood chemistries for sodium, potassium, glucose
- Dexamethasone suppression test
- 24-hr urine for free cortisol and 17-ketosteroids
- CT scan, MRI

Collaborative Therapy*
Pituitary Adenoma
- Transsphenoidal resection
- Radiation therapy

Adrenocortical Adenoma, Carcinoma, or Hyperplasia
- Adrenalectomy (open or laparoscopic)
- Drug therapy (e.g., ketoconazole [Nizoral], aminoglutethimide [Cytadren], mitotane [Lysodren], mifepristone [Korlym])

Ectopic ACTH-Secreting Tumor
- Treatment of the tumor (surgical removal or radiation)

Exogenous Corticosteroid Therapy
- Discontinue or alter the dose of exogenous corticosteroids

*Treatment is based on underlying cause.
ACTH, Adrenocorticotropic hormone.

If Cushing syndrome has developed during the course of prolonged administration of corticosteroids (e.g., prednisone), the following alternatives may be tried: (1) gradual discontinuance of corticosteroid therapy, (2) reduction of the corticosteroid dose, and (3) conversion to an alternate-day regimen. Gradual tapering of the corticosteroids is necessary to avoid potentially life-threatening adrenal insufficiency. In an alternate-day regimen, twice the daily dosage of a shorter-acting corticosteroid is given every other morning to minimize hypothalamic-pituitary-adrenal suppression, growth suppression, and altered appearance. This regimen is not used when the corticosteroids are given as hormone therapy.

NURSING MANAGEMENT CUSHING SYNDROME

NURSING ASSESSMENT

Subjective and objective data that should be obtained from a patient with Cushing syndrome are presented in Table 50-15.

NURSING DIAGNOSES

Nursing diagnoses for the patient with Cushing syndrome may include, but are not limited to, the following:

- Risk for infection *related to* lowered resistance to stress and suppression of immune system
- Imbalanced nutrition: more than body requirements *related to* increased appetite, high caloric content of foods, and inactivity
- Disturbed body image *related to* change in appearance from disease process
- Impaired skin integrity *related to* excess corticosteroids, immobility, and altered skin fragility

Additional information on nursing diagnoses is presented in eNursing Care Plan 50-3 for the patient with Cushing syndrome (available on the website for this chapter).

TABLE 50-15 NURSING ASSESSMENT

Cushing Syndrome

Subjective Data
Important Health Information
Past health history: Pituitary tumor (Cushing disease); adrenal, pancreatic, or pulmonary neoplasms; GI bleeding; frequent infections
Medications: Corticosteroids

Functional Health Patterns
Health perception–health management: Malaise
Nutritional-metabolic: Weight gain, anorexia; prolonged wound healing, easy bruising
Elimination: Polyuria
Activity-exercise: Weakness, fatigue
Sleep: Insomnia, poor sleep quality
Cognitive-perceptual: Headache; back, joint, bone, and rib pain; poor concentration and memory
Self-perception–self-concept: Negative feelings regarding changes in personal appearance
Sexuality-reproductive: Amenorrhea, impotence, decreased libido
Coping–stress tolerance: Anxiety, mood disturbances, emotional lability, psychosis

Objective Data
General
Truncal obesity, supraclavicular fat pads, buffalo hump, moon face

Integumentary
Plethora; hirsutism of body and face, thinning of head hair; thin, friable skin; acne; petechiae; purpura; hyperpigmentation; purplish red striae on breasts, buttocks, and abdomen; edema of lower extremities

Cardiovascular
Hypertension

Musculoskeletal
Muscle wasting, thin extremities, awkward gait

Reproductive
Gynecomastia, testicular atrophy (in men), enlarged clitoris (in women)

Possible Diagnostic Findings
Hypokalemia, hyperglycemia, dyslipidemia; polycythemia, granulocytosis, lymphocytopenia, eosinopenia; ↑ plasma cortisol; high, low, or normal ACTH levels; abnormal dexamethasone suppression test; ↑ urine free cortisol, 17-ketosteroids; glycosuria, hypercalciuria; osteoporosis on x-ray

ACTH, Adrenocorticotropic hormone.

PLANNING

The overall goals are that the patient with Cushing syndrome will (1) experience relief of symptoms, (2) avoid serious complications, (3) maintain a positive self-image, and (4) actively participate in the therapeutic plan.

NURSING IMPLEMENTATION

HEALTH PROMOTION. Health promotion is focused on identifying patients at risk for Cushing syndrome. Patients receiving long-term, exogenous corticosteroids for a variety of diseases are at risk. Patient teaching related to using medications and monitoring side effects is an important preventive measure.

ACUTE INTERVENTION. The patient with Cushing syndrome is seriously ill. Because the therapy has many side effects, assessment focuses on signs and symptoms of hormone and drug toxicity and complicating conditions (e.g., cardiovascular disease, diabetes mellitus, infection). Assess and monitor vital signs, daily weight, glucose, and possible infection. Because signs and symptoms of inflammation (e.g., fever, redness) may be minimal or absent, assess for pain, loss of function, and purulent drainage. Monitor for signs and symptoms of abnormal thromboembolic events such as pulmonary emboli (e.g., sudden chest pain, dyspnea, tachypnea).

Another important focus of nursing care is emotional support. Changes in appearance such as centripetal obesity, multiple bruises, hirsutism in women, and gynecomastia in men can be distressing. The patient may feel unattractive, repulsive, or unwanted. You can help by remaining sensitive to the patient's feelings and offering respect and unconditional acceptance. Reassure the patient that the physical changes and much of the emotional lability will resolve when hormone levels return to normal.

If treatment involves surgical removal of a pituitary adenoma, an adrenal tumor, or one or both adrenal glands, nursing care will also focus on preoperative and postoperative care.

Preoperative Care. Before surgery the patient should be brought to optimal physical condition. Hypertension and hyperglycemia must be controlled, and hypokalemia must be corrected with diet and potassium supplements. A high-protein diet helps correct the protein depletion. Preoperative teaching depends on the type of surgical approach planned (hypophysectomy or adrenalectomy) and should include information regarding the anticipated postoperative care. Preoperative management for the patient undergoing a hypophysectomy is discussed earlier in this chapter on pp. 1190-1191.

Postoperative Care. Surgery on the adrenal glands poses greater risks than other operations. Because the adrenal glands are vascular, the risk of hemorrhage is increased. In the postoperative period (for both laparoscopic and open adrenalectomy), patients may have a nasogastric tube, a urinary catheter, IV therapy, central venous pressure monitoring, and leg sequential compression devices to prevent emboli.

Manipulation of glandular tissue during surgery may release large amounts of hormones into the circulation, producing marked fluctuations in the metabolic processes affected by these hormones. Postoperatively, BP, fluid balance, and electrolyte levels may be unstable due to these hormone fluctuations.

High doses of corticosteroids (e.g., hydrocortisone [Solu-Cortef]) are administered IV during surgery and for several days afterward to ensure adequate responses to the stress of the procedure. If large amounts of endogenous hormone have been released into the systemic circulation during surgery, the patient is likely to develop hypertension, increasing the risk of hemorrhage. High levels of corticosteroids increase susceptibility to infection and delay wound healing.

The critical period for circulatory instability ranges from 24 to 48 hours after surgery. During this time you must constantly be alert for signs of corticosteroid imbalance. Report any rapid or significant changes in BP, respirations, or heart rate. Monitor fluid intake and output carefully and assess for potential imbalances. IV corticosteroids are given, and the dosage and flow rate are adjusted to the patient's clinical manifestations and fluid and electrolyte balance. Oral doses are given as tolerated. After IV corticosteroids are withdrawn, keep the IV line open for quick administration of corticosteroids or vasopressors. Obtain morning urine samples (collected at the same time each morning) for cortisol measurement to evaluate the surgery's effectiveness.

If corticosteroid dosage is tapered too rapidly after surgery, acute adrenal insufficiency may develop. Vomiting, increased weakness, dehydration, and hypotension may indicate hypocortisolism. In addition, the patient may complain of painful joints, pruritus, or peeling skin and may experience severe emotional disturbances. Report these signs and symptoms so that drug doses can be adjusted as necessary.

After surgery the patient is usually maintained on bed rest until the BP stabilizes. Be alert for subtle signs of postoperative infection because the usual inflammatory responses are suppressed. To prevent infection, provide meticulous care when changing the dressing and during any other procedures that involve access to body cavities, circulation, or areas under the skin. eNursing Care Plan 50-3 for the patient with Cushing syndrome is available on the website for this chapter.

AMBULATORY AND HOME CARE. Discharge instructions are based on the patient's lack of endogenous corticosteroids and resulting inability to physiologically react to stressors. Consider a home health nurse referral, especially for older adults, because of the need for ongoing evaluation and teaching. Instruct the patient to wear a Medic Alert bracelet at all times and carry medical identification and instructions in a wallet or purse. Teach the patient to avoid exposure to extreme temperatures, infections, and emotional disturbances. Stress may produce or precipitate acute adrenal insufficiency because the remaining adrenal tissue cannot meet an increased hormonal demand. Teach patients to adjust their corticosteroid replacement therapy in accordance with their stress levels. Consult with the patient's health care provider to determine the parameters for dosage changes if this plan is feasible. If the patient cannot adjust his or her own medication or if weakness, fainting, fever, or nausea and vomiting occur, the patient should contact the health care provider for a possible adjustment in corticosteroid dosage. Many patients require lifetime replacement therapy. However, patients should be prepared for it to take several months to adjust the hormone dose satisfactorily.

EVALUATION

The expected outcomes are that the patient with Cushing syndrome will
- Experience no signs or symptoms of infection
- Attain weight appropriate for height
- Verbalize acceptance of appearance and treatment regimen
- Demonstrate healing of skin and maintenance of intact skin

Additional information on expected outcomes is presented in eNursing Care Plan 50-3 for the patient with Cushing syndrome (available on the website for this chapter).

ADRENOCORTICAL INSUFFICIENCY

Etiology and Pathophysiology

Adrenocortical insufficiency (hypofunction of the adrenal cortex) may be from a primary cause (Addison's disease) or a secondary cause (lack of pituitary ACTH secretion). In Addison's disease, all three classes of adrenal corticosteroids (glucocorticoids, mineralocorticoids, and androgens) are reduced. In secondary adrenocortical insufficiency, corticosteroids and androgens are deficient but mineralocorticoids rarely are. ACTH deficiency may be caused by pituitary disease or suppression of the hypothalamic-pituitary axis because of the administration of exogenous corticosteroids.

The most common cause of Addison's disease in the United States is an autoimmune response.[26] Adrenal tissue is destroyed by antibodies against the patient's own adrenal cortex. Often, other endocrine conditions are present and Addison's disease is considered a component of *autoimmune polyglandular syndrome.* This rare syndrome is caused by a mutation in a gene that helps to regulate the immune system. The condition is inherited as an autosomal recessive trait. Addison's disease, if caused by an autoimmune response, is most common in white females.

Although tuberculosis causes Addison's disease worldwide, it is now an uncommon cause in the United States. Other causes include infarction, fungal infections (e.g., histoplasmosis), acquired immunodeficiency syndrome (AIDS), and metastatic cancer. Iatrogenic Addison's disease may be due to adrenal hemorrhage, often related to anticoagulant therapy, chemotherapy, ketoconazole therapy for AIDS, or bilateral adrenalectomy. Adrenal insufficiency most often occurs in adults younger than 60 years of age and affects both genders equally.

Clinical Manifestations

Because manifestations do not tend to become evident until 90% of the adrenal cortex is destroyed, the disease is often advanced before it is diagnosed. The manifestations have a slow (insidious) onset and include progressive weakness, fatigue, weight loss, and anorexia as primary features. Increased ACTH causes the striking feature of a bronze-colored skin hyperpigmentation. It is seen primarily in sun-exposed areas of the body; at pressure points; over joints; and in the creases, especially palmar creases (Fig. 50-13). The changes in the skin are most likely due to increased secretion of β-lipotropin (which contains melanocyte-stimulating hormone [MSH]). This tropic hormone is increased because of decreased negative feedback and subsequent low corticosteroid levels. Other manifestations of adrenal insufficiency are orthostatic hypotension, hyponatremia, salt craving, hyperkalemia, nausea and vomiting, and diarrhea. Irritability and depression may also occur in primary adrenal hypofunction.

Patients with secondary adrenocortical hypofunction may have many signs and symptoms similar to those of patients with Addison's disease. However, they usually do not have hyperpigmented skin because ACTH levels are low.

Complications

Patients with adrenocortical insufficiency are at risk for acute adrenal insufficiency *(addisonian crisis),* a life-threatening

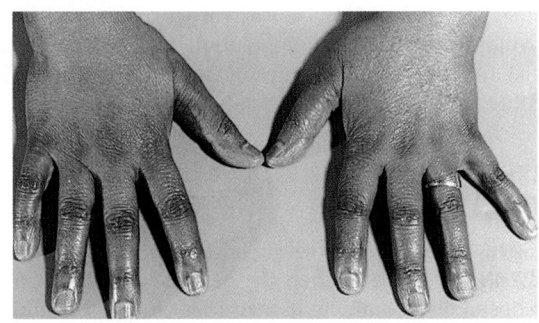

FIG. 50-13 Hyperpigmentation typically seen in Addison's disease.

emergency caused by insufficient adrenocortical hormones or a sudden sharp decrease in these hormones. Addisonian crisis is triggered by (1) stress (e.g., from infection, surgery, psychologic distress), (2) the sudden withdrawal of corticosteroid hormone therapy (which is often done by a patient who lacks knowledge of the importance of this therapy), (3) adrenal surgery, or (4) sudden pituitary gland destruction.

During acute adrenal insufficiency, the patient exhibits severe manifestations of glucocorticoid and mineralocorticoid deficiencies, including hypotension (particularly postural), tachycardia, dehydration, hyponatremia, hyperkalemia, hypoglycemia, fever, weakness, and confusion. Hypotension may lead to shock. Circulatory collapse associated with adrenal insufficiency is often unresponsive to the usual treatment (vasopressors and fluid replacement). GI manifestations include severe vomiting, diarrhea, and pain in the abdomen. Pain may occur in the lower back or the legs.

Diagnostic Studies

Adrenal insufficiency is characterized by depressed serum and urinary cortisol levels. ACTH levels are increased in primary adrenal insufficiency and decreased in secondary disease. Primary adrenal insufficiency is confirmed when cortisol levels fail to rise over basal levels with an ACTH stimulation test. A positive response to ACTH stimulation test indicates a functioning adrenal gland and points to a probable diagnosis of secondary adrenocortical insufficiency related to the pituitary gland. Urine levels of free cortisol are low, as is the urine level of aldosterone.

Other abnormal laboratory findings in some cases include hyperkalemia, hypochloremia, hyponatremia, hypoglycemia, anemia, and increased BUN levels.[25] An ECG may show low voltage and peaked T waves caused by hyperkalemia. CT scans and MRI may be used to identify causes other than autoimmune, including tumors, fungal infections, tuberculosis, or adrenal calcification.

Collaborative Care

Treatment of adrenocortical insufficiency is focused on management of the underlying cause when possible. The mainstay of treatment for the adrenocortical insufficiency is hormone therapy (Table 50-16). Hydrocortisone, the most commonly used form of hormone therapy, has both glucocorticoid and mineralocorticoid properties. During stressful situations the glucocorticoid dosage is increased to prevent addisonian crisis. Mineralocorticoid replacement with fludrocortisone (Florinef) is administered daily. Increased salt needs to be added in the diet.

Addisonian crisis is a life-threatening emergency requiring aggressive management. Treatment must be directed toward shock management and high-dose hydrocortisone replacement. Large volumes of 0.9% saline solution and 5% dextrose are administered to reverse hypotension and electrolyte imbalances until BP returns to normal.

NURSING MANAGEMENT
ADDISON'S DISEASE

NURSING IMPLEMENTATION

ACUTE INTERVENTION. When the patient with Addison's disease is hospitalized, nursing management focuses on monitoring the patient while correcting fluid and electrolyte balance.

TABLE 50-16   **COLLABORATIVE CARE**

Addison's Disease

Diagnostic
- History and physical examination
- Serum cortisol
- Serum ACTH
- Urine cortisol and aldosterone
- Serum electrolytes
- ACTH-stimulation test
- CT scan, MRI

Collaborative Therapy
- Daily glucocorticoid (e.g., hydrocortisone) replacement (two thirds on awakening in morning, one third in late afternoon)*
- Daily mineralocorticoid (fludrocortisone [Florinef]) in morning*
- Salt additives for excess heat or humidity
- Increased doses of cortisol for stress situations (e.g., surgery, hospitalization)

*For conditions of normal daily stress in individuals with usual daytime activity.
ACTH, Adrenocorticotropic hormone.

Assess vital signs and signs of fluid volume deficit and electrolyte imbalance. Monitor trends in serum glucose, sodium, and potassium. Establish baseline data regarding mental status, vital signs, and weight. Obtain a complete medication history to determine drugs that can potentially interact with corticosteroids. These drugs include oral hypoglycemics, cardiac glycosides, oral contraceptives, anticoagulants, and NSAIDs.

Note changes in BP, weight gain, weakness, or other manifestations of Cushing syndrome. In addition, protect against exposure to infection and assist with daily hygiene. Protect the patient from noise, light, and environmental temperature extremes. The patient cannot cope with these stresses because of the inability to produce corticosteroids.

AMBULATORY AND HOME CARE. You have an important role in the long-term management of Addison's disease. The serious nature of the disease and the need for lifelong hormone therapy necessitate a comprehensive teaching plan. Table 50-17 outlines the major areas to include in your teaching plan.

Glucocorticoids are usually given in divided doses, two thirds in the morning and one third in the afternoon. Mineralocorticoids are given once daily, preferably in the morning. This dosage schedule reflects normal circadian rhythm in endogenous hormone secretion and decreases the side effects associated with corticosteroid therapy. Help the patient maintain hormone balance while managing the medication regimen.

The patient with Addison's disease is unable to tolerate physical or emotional stress without additional exogenous corticosteroids. Long-term care revolves around recognizing the need for extra medication and techniques for stress management. Examples of situations requiring corticosteroid adjustment are fever, influenza, extraction of teeth, and rigorous physical activity such as playing tennis on a hot day or running a marathon. If vomiting or diarrhea occurs, as may happen with influenza, notify the health care provider immediately because electrolyte replacement and parenteral administration of cortisol may be necessary. Overall, patients who take their medications consistently can anticipate a normal life expectancy.

Teach the patient about the signs and symptoms of corticosteroid deficiency and excess (Cushing syndrome) and to report these signs to their health care provider so the dose can be adjusted. It is critical that the patient wear an identification

TABLE 50-17 PATIENT & CAREGIVER TEACHING GUIDE

Addison's Disease

Include the following information in the teaching plan for Addison's disease.

1. Names, dosages, and actions of drugs
2. Symptoms of overdosage and underdosage
3. Conditions requiring increased medication (e.g., trauma, infection, surgery, emotional crisis)
4. Course of action to take relative to changes in medication
   - Increase in dose of corticosteroid
   - Administration of large dose of corticosteroid intramuscularly, including demonstration and return demonstration
   - Consultation with health care provider
5. Prevention of infection and need for prompt and vigorous treatment of existing infections
6. Need for lifelong replacement therapy
7. Need for lifelong medical supervision
8. Need for medical identification device
9. Prevention of falls
10. Adverse effects of corticosteroid therapy and prevention techniques
11. Special instruction for patients who are diabetics and management of blood glucose when taking corticosteroids

TABLE 50-18 DRUG THERAPY

Diseases and Disorders Treated With Corticosteroids

Hormone Therapy
Adrenal insufficiency
Congenital adrenal hyperplasia

Therapeutic Effect
Allergic Reactions
- Anaphylaxis
- Bee stings
- Contact dermatitis
- Drug reactions
- Serum sickness
- Urticaria

Collagen Diseases
- Giant cell arteritis
- Mixed connective tissue disorders
- Polymyositis
- Polyarteritis nodosa
- Rheumatoid arthritis
- Systemic lupus erythematosus

Neurologic Diseases
- Prevention of cerebral edema and increased intracranial pressure
- Head trauma

Gastrointestinal Diseases
- Inflammatory bowel disease
- Celiac disease

Endocrine Diseases
- Hypercalcemia
- Hashimoto's thyroiditis
- Thyrotoxicosis

Liver Diseases
- Alcoholic hepatitis
- Autoimmune hepatitis

Pulmonary Diseases
- Aspiration pneumonia
- Asthma
- Chronic obstructive pulmonary disease

Other Diseases or Disorders
- Skin diseases
- Malignancies, leukemia, lymphoma
- Immunosuppression
- Inflammation
- Nephrotic syndrome

bracelet (Medic Alert) and carry a wallet card stating the patient has Addison's disease so that appropriate therapy can be initiated in case of an emergency. Provide verbal instruction and handouts about other medications that can cause a need to increase (e.g., phenytoin, barbiturates, rifampin, antacids) or decrease (e.g., estrogen) glucocorticoid dosage. Instruct patients using mineralocorticoid therapy (fludrocortisone) how to take their BP, increase salt intake, and report any significant changes to their health care provider.

The patient should carry an emergency kit at all times with 100 mg of IM hydrocortisone, syringes, and instructions for use. Instruct the patient and significant others in how to give an IM injection in case the hormone therapy cannot be taken orally. Have the patient verbalize instructions and practice IM injections with saline. Provide written instructions on when the dose should be changed.[27]

CORTICOSTEROID THERAPY

Corticosteroids are used to relieve the signs and symptoms associated with many diseases (Table 50-18). Corticosteroids are effective in treating many diseases and disorders. However, the long-term administration of corticosteroids in therapeutic doses often leads to serious complications and side effects (Table 50-19). For this reason, corticosteroid therapy is not recommended for minor chronic conditions. Therapy should be reserved for diseases that have a risk of death or permanent loss of function, and for conditions in which short-term therapy is likely to produce remission or recovery. The potential benefits of treatment must always be weighed against the risks.

A beneficial effect of corticosteroids in one situation may be a harmful one in another. For example, decreasing inflammation in arthritis is an important therapeutic effect, but increasing the risk for infection is a harmful effect. Suppression of inflammation and the immune response may help save lives in persons with anaphylaxis and in those receiving an organ transplant, but it can reactivate latent tuberculosis and greatly reduces resistance to other infections and cancers. The vasopressive

effect of corticosteroids is critical in enabling a person to function in stressful situations, but can produce hypertension when used for drug therapy. Effects and side effects related to corticosteroid therapy are listed in Table 50-19.

DRUG ALERT: Corticosteroids
- Instruct the patient not to abruptly discontinue these drugs.
- Monitor the patient for signs of infection.
- Instruct patients with diabetes to closely monitor blood glucose.

Patients receive corticosteroid therapy for many reasons (see Table 50-18). Detailed instruction is necessary to ensure patient

TABLE 50-19 DRUG THERAPY

Effects and Side Effects of Corticosteroids

- Hypokalemia may develop.
- Patient is predisposed to peptic ulcer disease.
- Skeletal muscle atrophy and weakness occur.
- Mood and behavior changes may be observed.
- Glucose intolerance predisposes patient to diabetes mellitus.
- Fat from extremities is redistributed to trunk and face.
- Hypocalcemia related to anti–vitamin D effect may occur.
- Healing is delayed, with increased risk for wound dehiscence.
- Susceptibility to infection is increased. Infection develops more rapidly and spreads more widely.
- Manifestations of inflammation, including redness, tenderness, heat, swelling, and local edema, are suppressed.
- Pituitary ACTH synthesis is suppressed. Corticosteroid deficiency is likely if hormones are withdrawn abruptly. Taper corticosteroid doses.
- Blood pressure increases because of excess blood volume and potentiation of vasoconstrictor effects. Hypertension predisposes patient to heart failure.
- Protein depletion decreases bone formation, density, and strength, leading to predisposition to pathologic fractures, especially compression fractures of the vertebrae (osteoporosis).

ACTH, Adrenocorticotropic hormone.

adherence. When corticosteroids are used as nonreplacement therapies, they are taken once daily or once every other day. They should be taken early in the morning with food to decrease gastric irritation. Because exogenous corticosteroid administration may suppress endogenous ACTH and therefore endogenous cortisol (suppression is time and dose dependent), emphasize the danger of abrupt cessation of corticosteroid therapy to patients and caregivers. Corticosteroids taken for longer than 1 week will suppress adrenal production, and oral corticosteroids must be tapered. Ensure that increased doses of corticosteroids are prescribed in acute care or home care settings in situations of physical or emotional stress.

Corticosteroid-induced osteoporosis is an important concern for patients who receive corticosteroid treatment for prolonged periods (longer than 3 months).[28] Therapies to reduce the resorption of bone may include increased calcium intake, vitamin D supplementation, bisphosphonates (e.g., alendronate), and a low-impact exercise program. Further instruction and interventions to minimize the side effects and complications of corticosteroid therapy are presented in Table 50-20.

HYPERALDOSTERONISM

Hyperaldosteronism (Conn's syndrome) is characterized by excessive aldosterone secretion. The main effects of aldosterone are (1) sodium retention and (2) potassium and hydrogen ion excretion. Thus the hallmark of this disease is hypertension with hypokalemic alkalosis. *Primary hyperaldosteronism* (PA) is most commonly caused by a small solitary adrenocortical adenoma. Occasionally multiple lesions are involved and are associated with bilateral adrenal hyperplasia. PA affects women more than men and usually occurs between 30 and 60 years of age. A genetic link has been identified in some patients.[29] Up to 2%

TABLE 50-20	PATIENT & CAREGIVER TEACHING GUIDE

Corticosteroid Therapy

Include the following instructions when teaching the patient and caregiver to manage corticosteroid therapy.

1. Plan a diet high in protein, calcium (at least 1500 mg/day) and potassium but low in fat and concentrated simple carbohydrates such as sugar, honey, syrups, and candy.
2. Identify measures to ensure adequate rest and sleep, such as daily naps and avoidance of caffeine late in the day.
3. Develop and maintain an exercise program to help maintain bone integrity.
4. Recognize edema and ways to restrict sodium intake to <2000 mg/day if edema occurs.
5. Monitor glucose levels and recognize symptoms of hyperglycemia (e.g., polydipsia, polyuria, blurred vision). Report hyperglycemic symptoms or capillary glucose levels >120 mg/dL (10 mmol/L).
6. Notify health care provider if experiencing heartburn after meals or epigastric pain that is not relieved by antacids.
7. See an eye specialist yearly to assess for cataracts.
8. Use safety measures such as getting up slowly from bed or a chair and use good lighting to avoid accidental injury.
9. Maintain good hygiene practices and avoid contact with persons with colds or other contagious illnesses to prevent infection.
10. Inform all health care providers about long-term corticosteroid use.
11. Recognize need for increased doses of corticosteroids in times of physical and emotional stress.
12. Never abruptly stop the corticosteroids because this could lead to addisonian crisis and possibly death.

---

of all cases of hypertension are caused by PA. *Secondary hyperaldosteronism* occurs in response to a nonadrenal cause of elevated aldosterone levels such as renal artery stenosis, renin-secreting tumors, and chronic kidney disease.

Elevated levels of aldosterone are associated with sodium retention and excretion of potassium. Sodium retention leads to hypernatremia, hypertension, and headache. Edema does not usually occur because the rate of sodium excretion increases, which prevents more severe sodium retention. The potassium wasting leads to hypokalemia, which causes generalized muscle weakness, fatigue, cardiac dysrhythmias, glucose intolerance, and metabolic alkalosis that may lead to tetany.

Hyperaldosteronism should be suspected in all hypertensive patients with hypokalemia who are not being treated with diuretics. PA is associated with elevated plasma aldosterone levels, elevated sodium levels, decreased serum potassium levels, and decreased plasma renin activity. Adenomas are localized by means of a CT scan or an MRI.[30] If a tumor is not found, plasma 18-hydroxycorticosterone is measured after overnight bed rest. A level greater than 50 ng/dL indicates an adenoma.

NURSING AND COLLABORATIVE MANAGEMENT PRIMARY HYPERALDOSTERONISM

The preferred treatment for PA is surgical removal of the adenoma (adrenalectomy). A laparoscopic approach is most often used. Before surgery, patients should be treated with potassium-sparing diuretics (spironolactone [Aldactone], eplerenone [Inspra]) and antihypertensive agents to normalize serum potassium levels and BP. Spironolactone and eplerenone block the binding of aldosterone to the mineralocorticoid receptor in the terminal distal tubules and collecting ducts of the kidney, thus increasing the excretion of sodium and water and the retention of potassium. Oral potassium supplements and sodium restrictions may also be necessary. However, potassium supplementation and a potassium-sparing diuretic should not be started simultaneously because of the danger of hyperkalemia. Teach patients taking eplerenone to avoid grapefruit juice.

Patients with bilateral adrenal hyperplasia are treated with a potassium-sparing diuretic (e.g., spironolactone, amiloride [Midamor]) or aminoglutethimide, which blocks aldosterone synthesis. Calcium channel blockers may also be used to control BP. Dexamethasone may be used to decrease adrenal hyperplasia.

Nursing care includes careful assessment for signs of fluid and electrolyte balance (especially potassium) and cardiovascular status. Monitor BP frequently before and after surgery because unilateral adrenalectomy is successful in controlling hypertension in only 80% of patients with an adenoma. Instruct patients receiving maintenance therapy with spironolactone or amiloride about the possible side effects of gynecomastia, impotence, and menstrual disorders, as well as the signs and symptoms of hypokalemia and hyperkalemia. Teach patients how to monitor their own BP and the need for frequent monitoring. Stress the need for continued health supervision.

DISORDERS OF ADRENAL MEDULLA

PHEOCHROMOCYTOMA

Pheochromocytoma, which is a rare condition caused by a tumor in the adrenal medulla affecting the chromaffin cells, results in an excess production of catecholamines (epinephrine, norepinephrine). The most dangerous immediate effect of the disease is severe hypertension.[31] If left untreated, it may lead to hypertensive encephalopathy, diabetes mellitus, cardiomyopathy, and death. It is most commonly seen in young to middle-aged adults. Pheochromocytoma may be inherited in persons with multiple endocrine neoplasia.

The most striking clinical features of pheochromocytoma are severe, episodic hypertension accompanied by the classic manifestations of severe, pounding headache; tachycardia with palpitations; profuse sweating; and unexplained abdominal or chest pain. Attacks may be provoked by many medications, including antihypertensives, opioids, radiologic contrast media, and tricyclic antidepressants. The attacks may last from a few minutes to several hours.

Although pheochromocytoma is associated with a number of symptoms, the diagnosis is often missed. Pheochromocytoma is an uncommon cause of hypertension, accounting for only 0.1% of all cases. Consider this condition in patients who do not respond to traditional hypertensive treatments.

The simplest and most reliable diagnostic test for pheochromocytoma is measurement of urinary fractionated metanephrines (catecholamine metabolites) and fractionated catecholamines and creatinine, usually done as a 24-hour urine collection. Values are elevated in at least 95% of persons with pheochromocytoma. Serum catecholamines may be elevated during an "attack." CT scans and MRI are used for diagnosing tumors. Avoid palpating the abdomen of a patient with suspected pheochromocytoma, since it may cause the sudden release of catecholamines and severe hypertension.

NURSING AND COLLABORATIVE MANAGEMENT PHEOCHROMOCYTOMA

The primary treatment of pheochromocytoma is surgical removal of the tumor. Treatment with α- and β-adrenergic receptor blockers is required preoperatively to control BP and prevent an intraoperative hypertensive crisis. The α-adrenergic receptor blocker phenoxybenzamine (Dibenzyline) is given 7 to 10 days preoperatively to reduce BP and alleviate other symptoms of catecholamine excess. After adequate α-adrenergic blockade, β-adrenergic receptor blockers (e.g., propranolol) are used to decrease tachycardia and other dysrhythmias. If β-blockers are started too early, unopposed α-adrenergic stimulation could precipitate a hypertensive crisis. They can also cause orthostatic hypotension. Advise the patient to make postural changes cautiously.

Surgery is most commonly done using a laparoscopic approach. Removal of the adrenal tumor usually cures the hypertension, but hypertension persists in approximately 10% to 30% of patients. If surgery is not an option, metyrosine (Demser) is used to decrease catecholamine production by the tumor.

Case finding is an important nursing role. Any patient with hypertension accompanied by symptoms of sympathoadrenal stimulation should be referred to a health care provider for definitive diagnosis. Assess the patient for the classic triad of symptoms of pheochromocytoma (severe pounding headache, tachycardia, and profuse sweating). Monitor the BP immediately if the patient is experiencing an "attack."

Attempt to make the patient with pheochromocytoma as comfortable as possible. Monitor blood glucose levels to assess for diabetes mellitus. Patients need rest, nourishing food, and emotional support during this period. Preoperative and postoperative care is similar to that for any patient undergoing adrenalectomy except that BP fluctuations from catecholamine excesses tend to be severe and must be carefully monitored. Emphasize the importance of follow-up and routine BP monitoring because hypertension may persist even when the tumor is removed. If metyrosine is being used, instruct the patient to rise slowly and hold onto a secure object, since this drug can cause orthostatic hypotension.

CASE STUDY

Graves' Disease

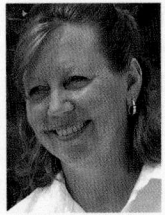

Jupiterimages/Photos. com/Thinkstock

Patient Profile

R.D., a 47-yr-old white woman, was admitted to the hospital with a high fever. Unable to find a source of infection, the health care provider does an endocrine workup. R.D. is diagnosed with Graves' disease.

Subjective Data
- Reports recent job loss because she is no longer able to tolerate work-related stress
- Reports symptoms including fatigue, unintentional weight loss, insomnia, palpitations, and heat intolerance

Objective Data
Physical Examination
- Fever of 104° F (40° C)
- BP of 150/80 mm Hg, pulse of 116 beats/min, and respiratory rate of 26 breaths/min
- Hot, moist skin
- Fine tremors of the hands
- 4+ deep tendon reflexes and muscle strength of 1 to 2 out of 5

Collaborative Care
- Subtotal thyroidectomy planned for 2 mo later
- Started on propylthiouracil (PTU) and propranolol (Inderal)

Discussion Questions
1. What is the etiology of R.D.'s symptoms?
2. What diagnostic studies would be important in evaluating R.D.'s condition? What results would establish the diagnosis of Graves' disease?
3. Why was surgery delayed?
4. What is the purpose of drug therapy for R.D.?
5. *Priority Decision:* What are the patient's priority teaching needs? What teaching strategies would you use if R.D. could not read?
6. What are the nursing interventions for successful long-term management of R.D. after the subtotal thyroidectomy?
7. *Priority Decision:* Based on the assessment data presented, what are the priority nursing diagnoses pertinent to this patient while hospitalized? Are there any collaborative problems?
8. *Evidence-Based Practice:* Why is R.D. counseled to give up her long-standing cigarette smoking habit?

BRIDGE TO NCLEX EXAMINATION

The number of the question corresponds to the same-numbered outcome at the beginning of the chapter.

1. After a hypophysectomy for acromegaly, postoperative nursing care should focus on
   a. frequent monitoring of serum and urine osmolarity.
   b. parenteral administration of a GH-receptor antagonist.
   c. keeping the patient in a recumbent position at all times.
   d. patient teaching regarding the need for lifelong hormone therapy.

2. A patient with a head injury develops SIADH. Manifestations the nurse would expect to find include
   a. hypernatremia and edema.
   b. muscle spasticity and hypertension.
   c. low urine output and hyponatremia.
   d. weight gain and decreased glomerular filtration rate.

3. The health care provider prescribes levothyroxine (Synthroid) for a patient with hypothyroidism. After teaching regarding this drug, the nurse determines that further instruction is needed when the patient says
   a. "I can expect the medication dose may need to be adjusted."
   b. "I only need to take this drug until my symptoms are improved."
   c. "I can expect to return to normal function with the use of this drug."
   d. "I will report any chest pain or difficulty breathing to the doctor right away."

4. After thyroid surgery, the nurse suspects damage or removal of the parathyroid glands when the patient develops
   a. muscle weakness and weight loss.
   b. hyperthermia and severe tachycardia.
   c. hypertension and difficulty swallowing.
   d. laryngospasms and tingling in the hands and feet.

5. Important nursing intervention(s) when caring for a patient with Cushing syndrome include (select all that apply)
   a. restricting protein intake.
   b. monitoring blood glucose levels.
   c. observing for signs of hypotension.
   d. administering medication in equal doses.
   e. protecting patient from exposure to infection.

6. An important preoperative nursing intervention before an adrenalectomy for hyperaldosteronism is to
   a. monitor blood glucose levels.
   b. restrict fluid and sodium intake.
   c. administer potassium-sparing diuretics.
   d. advise the patient to make postural changes slowly.

7. To control the side effects of corticosteroid therapy, the nurse teaches the patient who is taking corticosteroids to
   a. increase calcium intake to 1500 mg/day.
   b. perform glucose monitoring for hypoglycemia.
   c. obtain immunizations due to high risk of infections.
   d. avoid abrupt position changes because of orthostatic hypotension.

8. The nurse teaches the patient that the best time to take corticosteroids for replacement purposes is
   a. once a day at bedtime.
   b. every other day on awakening.
   c. on arising and in the late afternoon.
   d. at consistent intervals every 6 to 8 hours.

1. a, 2. c, 3. b, 4. d, 5. b, e, 6. c, 7. a, 8. c

ⓔvolve

For rationales to these answers and even more NCLEX review questions, visit *http://evolve.elsevier.com/Lewis/medsurg.*

REFERENCES

1. National Library of Medicine: Acromegaly. Retrieved from *www.ncbi.nlm.nih.gov/pubmedhealth/PMH0001364.*

2. Jones R, Brashers V, Huether S: Alterations of hormonal regulation. In Huether S, McCance K, editors: *Understanding pathophysiology*, ed 5, St Louis, 2012, Mosby.

3. Miller RE, Learned-Miller EG, Trainer P, et al: Early diagnosis of acromegaly: computers versus clinicians, *Clin Endocrinol* 75:226, 2011.

4. Pituitary Network Association. Pituitary disorders: prolactinomas. Retrieved from *www.pituitary.org/disorders/prolactinomas.*

5. McDowell B, Wallace R, Carnahan R, et al: Demographic differences in incidence for pituitary adenoma, *Pituitary* 14:23, 2011.

6. John C, Day MW: Central neurogenic diabetes insipidus, syndrome of inappropriate secretion of antidiuretic hormone, and cerebral salt-wasting syndrome in traumatic brain injury, *Crit Care Nurse* 32:e1, 2012.

7. Medeiros-Neto G, Camargo R, Tomimori E: Approach to and treatment of goiters, *Med Clin North Am* 96:351, 2012.

8. Samuels MH: Subacute, silent, and postpartum thyroiditis, *Med Clin North Am* 96:223, 2012.

9. Li Y, Nishihara E, Kakudo K: Hashimoto's thyroiditis: old concepts and new insights, *Curr Opin Rheumatol* 23:102, 2011.

10. Seigel S, Hodak S: Thyrotoxicosis, *Med Clin North Am* 96:175, 2012.

11. Bahn R, Burch H, Cooper D, et al: Hyperthyroidism and other causes of thyrotoxicosis: management guidelines of the American Thyroid Association and American Association of Clinical Endocrinologists, *Endocr Pract* 17:456 , 2011.

12. Kim M, Ladenson P: Thyroid. In Goldman L, Schafer A, editors: *Goldman: Goldman's Cecil medicine*, ed 24, Philadelphia, 2011, Saunders.

13. Furtado L: Thyroidectomy: postoperative care and common complications, *Nurs Stand* 25:43, 2011.

14. Brent G, Davie T: Hypothyroidism and thyroiditis. In Kronenberg HM, Melmed S, Polonsky KS, et al, editors: *Williams textbook of endocrinology*, ed 12, Philadelphia, 2011, Saunders.

15. Almandoz JP: Hypothyroidism: etiology, diagnosis, and management, *Med Clin North Am* 96:203, 2012.

*16. U.S. Preventive Services Task Force: Screening for thyroid disease: systematic evidence review. Retrieved from *www.ahrq.gov/clinic.*

*Evidence-based information for clinical practice.

17. National Cancer Institute: Thyroid cancer. Retrieved from *www.cancer.gov/cancertopics/types/thyroid.*

18. Popoveniuc G, Jonklaas J: Thyroid nodules, *Med Clin North Am* 96:329, 2012.

19. American Cancer Society: Detailed guide: thyroid cancer. Retrieved from *www.cancer.org.*

20. National Institutes of Health: Genetics home reference: multiple endocrine neoplasia. Retrieved from *ghr.nlm.nih.gov/condition/ multiple-endocrine-neoplasia.*

21. Mayo Clinic: Hyperparathyroidism. Retrieved from *www.mayoclinic.com/health/hyperparathyroidism.*

22. Khan MI: Medical management of postsurgical hypoparathyroidism, *Endocr Pract* 17(Suppl 1):18, 2011.

23. Guaraldi F, Salvatori R: Cushing syndrome: maybe not so uncommon of an endocrine disease, *J Am Board Family Med* 25:199, 2012.

24. Pagana KD, Pagana TJ: *Mosby's diagnostic and laboratory test reference*, ed 10, St Louis, 2011, Mosby.

25. Hunt D: Is it Addison's disease or Cushing syndrome? *Am Nurse Today* 7:8, 2012.

26. Bratland E, Husebye E: Cellular immunity and immunopathology in autoimmune Addison's disease, *Molec Cell Endocrinol* 336:180, 2011.

27. National Institute of Diabetes and Digestive and Kidney Diseases: Addison's disease: adrenal insufficiency. Retrieved from *endocrine.niddk.nih.gov/pubs/addison.*

28. Arthritis Foundation: Controlling bone loss when taking steroids. Retrieved from *www.arthritis.org/control-bone-loss -steroids.php.*

29. American Urological Association Foundation: Primary hyperaldosteronism (Conn's syndrome). Retrieved from *www.urologyhealth.org/urology.*

30. Hyperaldosteronism: primary. From F Ferri, editor: *Ferri's clinical advisor*, Mosby, 2013, Mosby.

31. Zuber S: Hypertension in pheochromocytoma: characteristics and treatment, *Endocrinol Metab Clin North Am* 40:295, 2011.

RESOURCES

American Association of Clinical Endocrinologists (AACE)
www.aace.com
American Thyroid Association
www.thyroid.org
Endocrine Nurses Society (ENS)
www.endo-nurses.org
Endocrine Society
www.endo-society.org
Pituitary Network Association
www.pituitary.org
Thyroid Federation International
www.thyroid-fed.org

51

Happiness resides not in possessions and not in gold.
The feeling of happiness dwells in the soul.
Democritus, 420 BC

Nursing Assessment
Reproductive System

Catherine (Kate) Lein

⊖volve WEBSITE

http://evolve.elsevier.com/Lewis/medsurg

- NCLEX Review Questions
- Key Points
- Pre-Test
- Answer Guidelines for Case Study in this chapter
- Rationales for Bridge to NCLEX Examination Questions
- Concept Map Creator
- Glossary
- Animations
  - Lymphatic Drainage of Breast
  - The Menstrual Cycle

- Videos
  - Inspection and Palpation: Standing Position (Male)—1
  - Inspection and Palpation: Standing Position (Male)—2
  - Inspection: External Genitalia (Female)
  - Inspection: Female Breasts—Sitting Position
  - Inspection: Speculum Examination (Female)
  - Palpation: Bimanual Examination (Female)
  - Palpation: Female Breasts—Supine Position

- Palpation: Inguinal Hernia Evaluation (Male)
- Physical Examination: Abdominal Reflexes, Abdominal Muscles, and Inguinal Area
- Physical Examination: Breasts
- Physical Examination: Breasts and Heart
- Physical Examination: Genitalia and Rectum (Female)
- Physical Examination: Rectum and Prostate Gland (Male)
- Content Updates

LEARNING OUTCOMES

1. Describe the structures and functions of the male and female reproductive systems.
2. Summarize the functions of the major hormones essential for the functioning of the male and female reproductive systems.
3. Explain the physiologic changes during the stages of sexual response for both a man and a woman.
4. Link the age-related changes of the male and female reproductive systems to the differences in assessment findings.
5. Select the significant subjective and objective data related to the male and female reproductive systems and information about sexual function that should be obtained from a patient.

6. Select the appropriate techniques to use in the physical assessment of the male and female reproductive systems.
7. Differentiate normal from common abnormal findings of a physical assessment of the male and female reproductive systems.
8. Describe the purpose, significance of results, and nursing responsibilities related to diagnostic studies of the male and female reproductive systems.

KEY TERMS

amenorrhea, p. 1224
clitoris, p. 1221
ductus deferens, p. 1219
dyspareunia, p. 1228

epididymis, p. 1219
gonads, p. 1218
menarche, p. 1223
menopause, p. 1224

menstrual cycle, p. 1223
mons pubis, p. 1221
nulliparous, p. 1220
spermatogenesis, p. 1219

STRUCTURES AND FUNCTIONS OF MALE AND FEMALE REPRODUCTIVE SYSTEMS

The reproductive system of both males and females consists of primary (or essential) organs and secondary (or accessory) organs. The primary reproductive organs are referred to as gonads. The female gonads are the ovaries; the male gonads are the testes. The main responsibility of the gonads is secretion of hormones and production of gametes (ova and sperm).

Secondary (or accessory) organs are responsible for (1) transporting and nourishing the ova and sperm and (2) preserving and protecting the fertilized eggs.

Male Reproductive System

The three primary roles of the male reproductive system are (1) production and transportation of sperm, (2) deposition of sperm in the female reproductive tract, and (3) secretion of hormones. The primary reproductive organs in the male are

Reviewed by Brenda Pavill, RN, PhD, FNP, Associate Professor–Nursing, Misericordia University, Dallas, Pennsylvania.

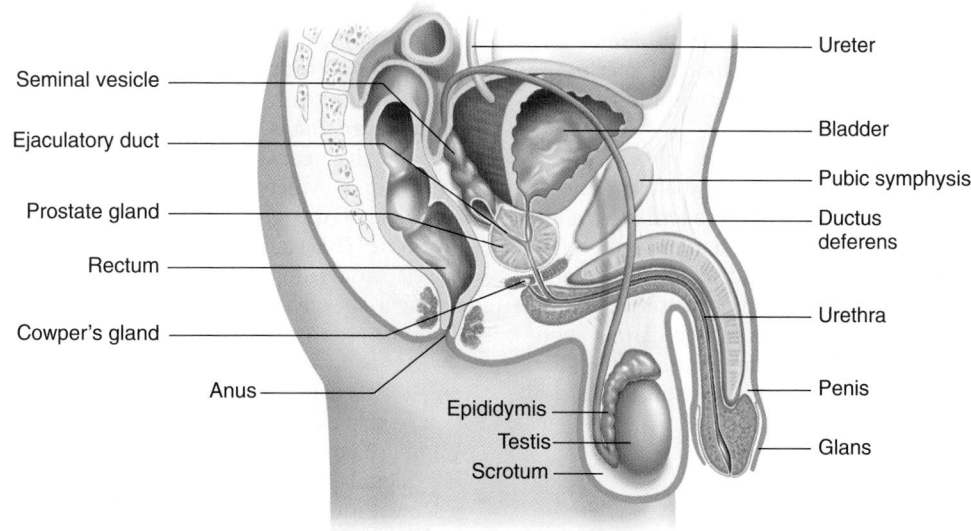

FIG. 51-1 Male reproductive tract.

the testes. Secondary reproductive organs include ducts (epididymis, ductus deferens, ejaculatory duct, and urethra), sex glands (prostate gland, Cowper's glands, and seminal vesicles), and the external genitalia (scrotum and penis)[1] (Fig. 51-1).

Testes. The paired testes are ovoid, smooth, firm organs measuring 1.4 to 2.2 in (3.5 to 5.6 cm) long and 0.8 to 1.2 in (2 to 3 cm) wide. They are within the scrotum, which is a loose protective sac composed of a thin outer layer of skin over a tough connective tissue layer. Within the testes, coiled structures known as seminiferous tubules form *spermatozoa* (immature sperm). The process of sperm production is called **spermatogenesis.** Interstitial cells of the testes lie between the seminiferous tubules and produce the male sex hormone testosterone.

Ducts. Sperm formed in the seminiferous tubules move through a series of ducts. These ducts transport the sperm from the testes to the outside of the body. As sperm exit the testes, they enter and pass through the epididymis, ductus deferens, ejaculatory duct, and urethra.

The **epididymis** is a comma-shaped structure located on the posterosuperior aspect of each testis within the scrotum (see Figs. 51-1 and 51-2). It is a very long, tightly coiled structure that measures about 20 ft in length.[1] The epididymis transports the sperm as they mature. Sperm exit the epididymis through a long, thick tube known as the ductus deferens.

The **ductus deferens** (also known as the *vas deferens*) is continuous with the epididymis within the scrotal sac. It travels upward through the scrotum and continues through the inguinal ring into the abdominal cavity. The spermatic cord is composed of a connective tissue sheath that encloses the ductus deferens, arteries, veins, nerves, and lymph vessels as it ascends up through the inguinal canal (see Fig. 51-2). In the abdominal cavity, the ductus deferens travels up, over, and behind the bladder. Posterior to the bladder the ductus deferens joins the seminal vesicle to form the ejaculatory duct (see Fig. 51-1).

The ejaculatory duct passes downward through the prostate gland, connecting with the urethra. The urethra extends from the bladder, through the prostate, and ends in a slitlike opening (the meatus) on the ventral side of the *glans,* the tip of the penis.

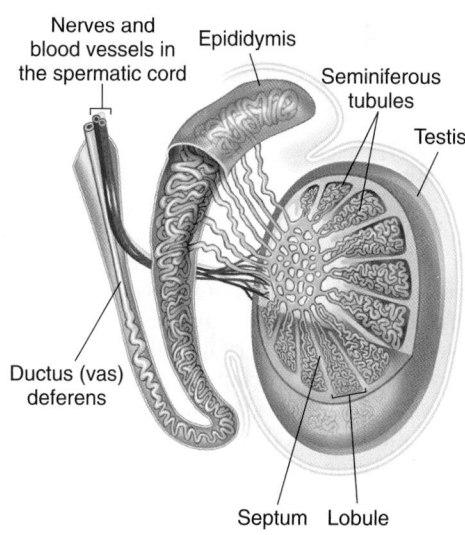

FIG. 51-2 Seminiferous tubules, testis, epididymis, and ductus (vas) deferens in the male.

During the process of ejaculation, sperm travels through the urethra and out of the penis.

Glands. The seminal vesicles, the prostate gland, and Cowper's (bulbourethral) glands are the accessory glands of the male reproductive system. These glands produce and secrete seminal fluid (semen), which surrounds the sperm and forms the *ejaculate.*

The seminal vesicles lie posterior to the bladder and between the rectum and bladder. The ducts of the seminal vesicles fuse with the ductus deferens to form the ejaculatory ducts that enter the prostate gland. The prostate gland lies beneath the bladder. Its posterior surface is in contact with the rectal wall. The prostate normally measures 0.8 in (2 cm) wide and 1.2 in (3 cm) long and is divided into the right and left lateral lobes and an anteroposterior median lobe. Cowper's glands lie on each side of the urethra and slightly posterior to it, just below the prostate. The ducts of these glands enter directly into the urethra.

Secretions from the seminal vesicles, prostate, and Cowper's glands make up most of the fluid in the ejaculate. These various secretions serve as a medium for the transport of sperm and create an alkaline, nutritious environment that promotes sperm motility and survival.

External Genitalia. The external genitalia consist of the penis and the scrotum. The penis consists of a shaft, and the tip is known as the glans. The glans is covered by a fold of skin, the prepuce (or foreskin), that forms at the junction of the glans and the shaft of the penis. In circumcised males the prepuce has been removed. The shaft of the penis consists of erectile tissue composed of the corpus cavernosum, the corpus spongiosum (the fibrous sheath that encases the erectile tissue), and the urethra. The skin covering the penis is thin, loose, and hairless.

Female Reproductive System

The three primary roles of the female reproductive system are (1) production of ova (eggs), (2) secretion of hormones, and (3) protection and facilitation of the development of the fetus in a pregnant female. Like the male, the female has primary and secondary reproductive organs. The primary reproductive organs in the female are the paired ovaries. Secondary reproductive organs include the ducts (fallopian tubes), uterus, vagina, sex glands (Bartholin's glands and breasts), and external genitalia (vulva).

Pelvic Organs

Ovaries. The ovaries are located on either side of the uterus, just behind and below the fallopian (uterine) tubes (Fig. 51-3). The almond-shaped ovaries are firm and solid, approximately 0.6 in (1.5 cm) wide and 1.2 in (3 cm) long. Their functions include ovulation and secretion of the two major reproductive hormones, estrogen and progesterone.

The outer zone of the ovary contains follicles with germ cells, or *oocytes.* Each follicle contains a primordial (immature) oocyte surrounded by granulosa and theca cells. These two layers protect and nourish the oocyte until the follicle reaches maturity and ovulation occurs. However, not all follicles reach maturity. In a process termed *atresia,* most of the primordial follicles become smaller and are reabsorbed by the body. Thus the number of follicles declines from 2 million to 4 million at birth to approximately 300,000 to 400,000 at menarche. Fewer than 500 oocytes are actually released by ovulation during the reproductive years of the normal healthy woman.

Fallopian Tubes. Normally, each month during a woman's reproductive years, one ovarian follicle reaches maturity, and the ovum is ovulated, or expelled, from the ovary through the stimulus of the gonadotropic hormones, follicle-stimulating hormone (FSH) and luteinizing hormone (LH). The ovum then travels up a fallopian tube where fertilization by sperm may occur, if sperm are present. An ovum can be fertilized up to 72 hours after its release.

The distal ends of the fallopian tubes consist of fingerlike projections called *fimbriae* that "massage" the ovaries at ovulation to help extract the mature ovum. The tubes, which average 4.8 in (12 cm) in length, extend from the fimbriae to the superior lateral borders of the uterus. Fertilization usually takes place within the outer one third of the fallopian tubes.

Uterus. The uterus is a pear-shaped, hollow, muscular organ (see Fig. 51-3). It is located between the bladder and the rectum. In the mature **nulliparous** (never pregnant) woman, the uterus is approximately 2.4 to 3.2 in (6 to 8 cm) long and 1.6 in (4 cm) wide. The uterine walls consist of an outer serosal layer, the *perimetrium;* a middle muscular layer, the *myometrium;* and an inner mucosal layer, the *endometrium.*

The uterus consists of the fundus, body (or corpus), and cervix (see Fig. 51-3). The body makes up about 80% of the uterus and connects with the cervix at the isthmus, or neck. The cervix is the lower portion of the uterus that projects into the anterior wall of the vaginal canal. It makes up about 15% to 20% of the uterus in the nulliparous female. The cervix consists of the *ectocervix,* the outer portion that protrudes into the vagina, and the *endocervix,* the canal in the opening of the cervix. The ectocervix is covered with squamous epithelial cells, which give it a smooth, pinkish appearance. The endocervix contains a lining of columnar epithelial cells, which give it a rough, reddened appearance. The junction at which the two types of epithelial cells meet is termed the *squamocolumnar junction* and contains the optimal types of cells needed for an accurate Papanicolaou (Pap) test to screen for cervical cancer.

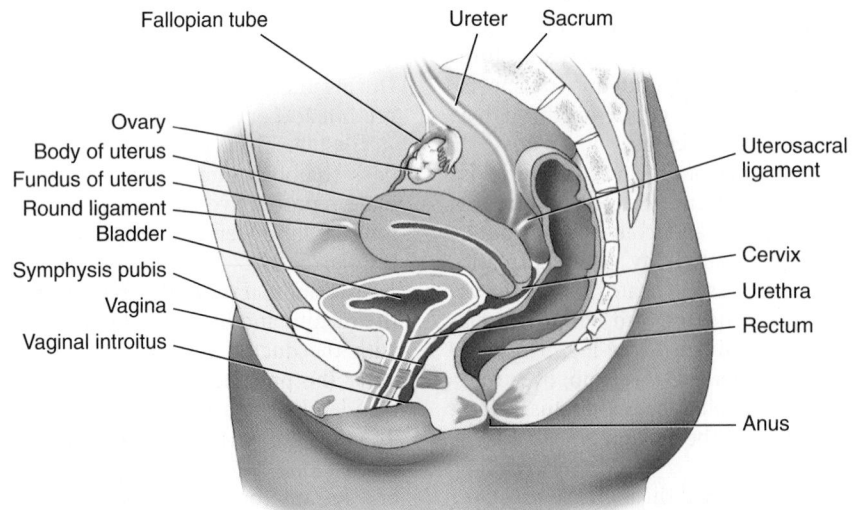

FIG. 51-3 Female reproductive tract.

The cervical canal is 0.8 to 1.6 in (2 to 4 cm) long and is relatively tightly closed. However, the cervix allows sperm to enter the uterus and also allows menses to be expelled. The columnar epithelium, under hormonal influence, provides elasticity during labor for the cervix to stretch to allow passage of a fetus during the birth process. The entrance of sperm into the uterus is facilitated by mucus produced by the cervix under the influence of estrogen. Under normal conditions, the cervical mucus becomes watery, stretchy, and more abundant at ovulation. The postovulatory cervical mucus, under the influence of progesterone, is thick and inhibits sperm passage.

Vagina. The vagina is a tubular structure 3 to 4 in (7.6 to 10 cm) long that is lined with squamous epithelium. The secretions of the vagina consist of cervical mucus, desquamated epithelium, and, during sexual stimulation, a watery secretion. These fluids help protect against vaginal infection. The muscular and erectile tissue of the vaginal walls allows enough dilation and contraction to accommodate the passage of the fetus during labor, as well as penetration of the penis during intercourse. The anterior vaginal wall lies along the urethra and bladder. The posterior vaginal wall is adjacent to the rectum.

Pelvis. The female pelvis consists of four bones (two pelvic bones, sacrum, coccyx) held together by several strong ligaments. The sections of these bones that lie below the iliopectineal line are important during birth and are often a factor determining the ability of a woman to deliver a child vaginally.

External Genitalia. The external portion of the female reproductive system (Fig. 51-4), commonly called the *vulva,* consists of the mons pubis, labia majora, labia minora, clitoris, urethral meatus, Skene's glands, vaginal introitus (opening), and Bartholin's glands.

The mons pubis is a fatty layer lying over the pubic bone. It is covered with coarse hair that lies in a triangular pattern. (The male hair pattern is diamond shaped.) The labia majora are folds of adipose tissue that form the outer borders of the vulva. The hairless labia minora form the borders of the vaginal orifice and extend anteriorly to enclose the clitoris.

The *vestibule* is a boat-shaped fossa between the labia minora, extending from the clitoris at the anterior end to the vaginal opening at the posterior end. The perineum is the area between the vagina and the anus. The vaginal introitus is surrounded by thin membranous tissue called the *hymen.* In the adult woman the hymen usually appears as folds or hymenal tags and separates the external genitalia from the vagina. At the posterior aspect of the vagina, a tense band of mucous membrane connecting the posterior ends of the labia minora is referred to as the *posterior fourchette.*

The clitoris is erectile tissue that becomes engorged during sexual excitation. It lies anterior to the urethral meatus and the vaginal orifice and is usually covered by the prepuce. Clitoral stimulation is an important part of sexual activity for many women.

Ducts of the Skene's glands lie alongside the urinary meatus and are thought to help lubricate the urinary meatus.[2] The Bartholin's glands, located at the posterior and lateral aspects of the vaginal orifice, secrete a thin, mucoid material believed to contribute slightly to lubrication during sexual intercourse. These glands are not usually palpable unless sebaceous-like cysts form or they are swollen in the presence of an infection, such as a sexually transmitted infection (STI).

Breasts. The breasts are a secondary sex characteristic that develops during puberty in response to estrogen and progesterone. Cyclic hormonal changes lead to regular changes in breast tissue to prepare it for lactation when fertilization and pregnancy occur.

The breasts extend from the second to the sixth ribs, with the tail reaching the axilla (Fig. 51-5). The fully mature breast is dome shaped and contains a pigmented center termed the *areola.* The areolar region contains Montgomery's tubercles, which are similar to sebaceous glands and assist in lubricating the nipple. During lactation, the alveoli secrete milk. The milk then flows into a ductal system and is transported to the lactiferous sinuses. The nipple contains 15 to 20 tiny openings through which the milk flows during breastfeeding. The fibrous and fatty tissue that supports and separates the channels of the mammary duct system is primarily responsible for the varying sizes and shapes of the breasts in different individuals.

The breast has a rich lymphatic network that drains into axillary and clavicular channels (see Fig. 52-5). Superficial

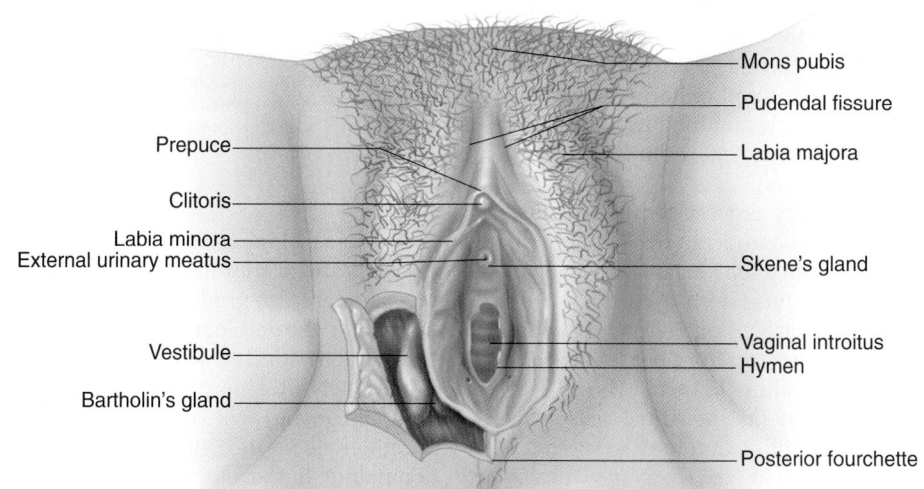

FIG. 51-4 External female genitalia.

Prepuce — Clitoris — Labia minora — External urinary meatus — Vestibule — Bartholin's gland

Mons pubis — Pudendal fissure — Labia majora — Skene's gland — Vaginal introitus — Hymen — Posterior fourchette

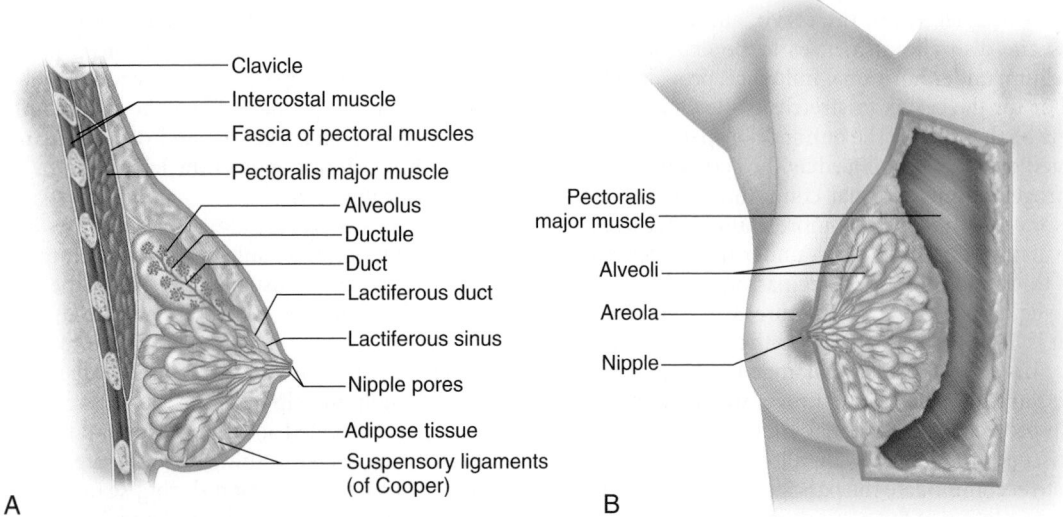

FIG. 51-5 The lactating female breast. **A,** Glandular structures are anchored to the overlying skin and the pectoralis muscle by suspensory ligaments of Cooper. Each lobule of glandular tissue is drained by a lactiferous duct that eventually opens through the nipple. **B,** Anterior view of a lactating breast. In nonlactating breasts, glandular tissue is less evident with adipose tissue comprising most of the breast.

lymph nodes are located in the axilla and are accessible to examination. This system is often responsible for the metastasis of a malignant tumor from the breast to other parts of the body.

Neuroendocrine Regulation of Reproductive System

The hypothalamus, pituitary gland, and gonads secrete numerous hormones (Fig. 51-6). (Endocrine hormones are discussed in Chapter 48.) These hormones regulate the processes of ovulation, spermatogenesis (formation of sperm), and fertilization and the formation and function of the secondary sex characteristics. The hypothalamus secretes gonadotropin-releasing hormone (GnRH), which stimulates the anterior pituitary gland to secrete its hormones, including FSH and LH. LH in males is sometimes called interstitial cell–stimulating hormone (ICSH). The gonadal hormones are estrogen, progesterone, and testosterone.

In women, FSH production by the anterior pituitary stimulates the growth and maturity of the ovarian follicles necessary for ovulation.[3] The mature follicle produces estrogen, which in turn suppresses the release of FSH. Another hormone, inhibin, is also secreted by the ovarian follicle and inhibits both GnRH and FSH secretion. In men, FSH stimulates the seminiferous tubules to produce sperm.

LH contributes to the ovulatory process because it causes follicles to complete maturation and undergo ovulation. It also affects the development of a ruptured follicle (area where ovum exited during ovulation), which turns into a corpus luteum from which progesterone is secreted. Progesterone maintains the rich vascular state of the uterus (secretory phase) in preparation for fertilization and implantation. In men, LH (or ICSH) triggers testosterone production by the interstitial cells of the testes and thus is essential for the full maturation of sperm.

Prolactin has no known function in men. In women, prolactin stimulates the development and growth of the mammary glands. During lactation, it initiates and maintains milk production.

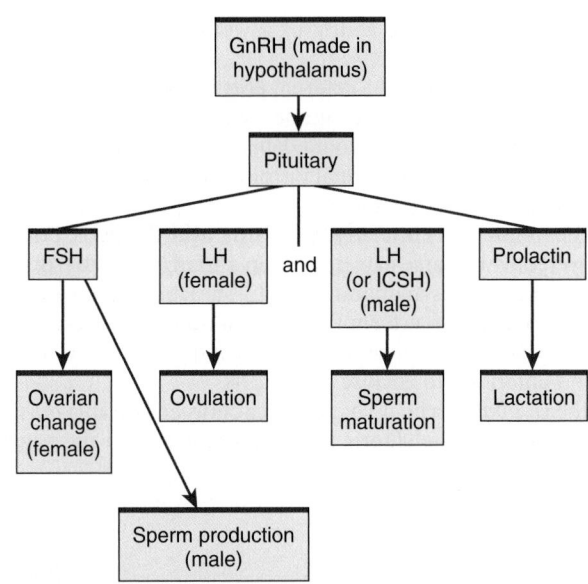

FIG. 51-6 Hypothalamic-pituitary-gonadal axis. Only the major pituitary hormone actions are depicted. *FSH,* Follicle-stimulating hormone; *GnRH,* gonadotropin-releasing hormone; *ICSH,* interstitial cell–stimulating hormone; *LH,* luteinizing hormone.

The gonadal hormones, estrogen and progesterone, are produced by the ovaries in women. Small amounts of an estrogen precursor are also produced in the adrenal cortices. Estrogen is essential to the development and maintenance of the secondary sex characteristics, the proliferative phase of the menstrual cycle immediately after menstruation, and the uterine changes essential to pregnancy. The role and importance of estrogen in men are not well understood. In men, estrogen is produced predominantly in the adrenal cortex.

Progesterone plays a major role in the menstrual cycle but most specifically in the secretory phase. Like estrogen, progesterone is involved in the bodily changes associated with preg-

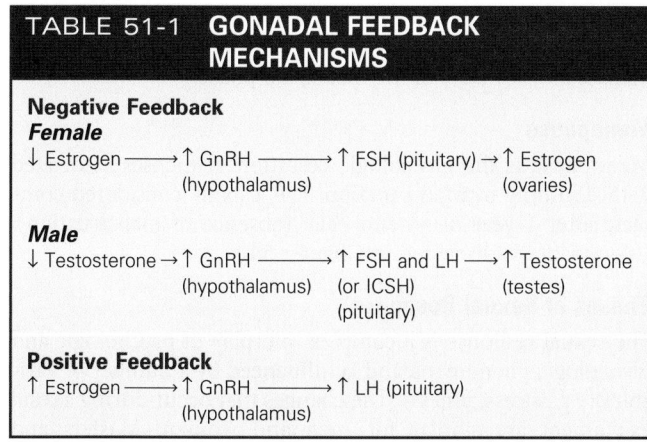

TABLE 51-1	GONADAL FEEDBACK MECHANISMS

Negative Feedback
Female
↓ Estrogen ⟶ ↑ GnRH ⟶ ↑ FSH (pituitary) → ↑ Estrogen
　　　　　　(hypothalamus)　　　　　　　　　　　　(ovaries)

Male
↓ Testosterone → ↑ GnRH ⟶ ↑ FSH and LH ⟶ ↑ Testosterone
　　　　　　　(hypothalamus)　(or ICSH)　　　　　(testes)
　　　　　　　　　　　　　　(pituitary)

Positive Feedback
↑ Estrogen ⟶ ↑ GnRH ⟶ ↑ LH (pituitary)
　　　　　　(hypothalamus)

FSH, Follicle-stimulating hormone; *GnRH*, gonadotropin-releasing hormone; *ICSH*, interstitial cell–stimulating hormone; *LH*, luteinizing hormone.

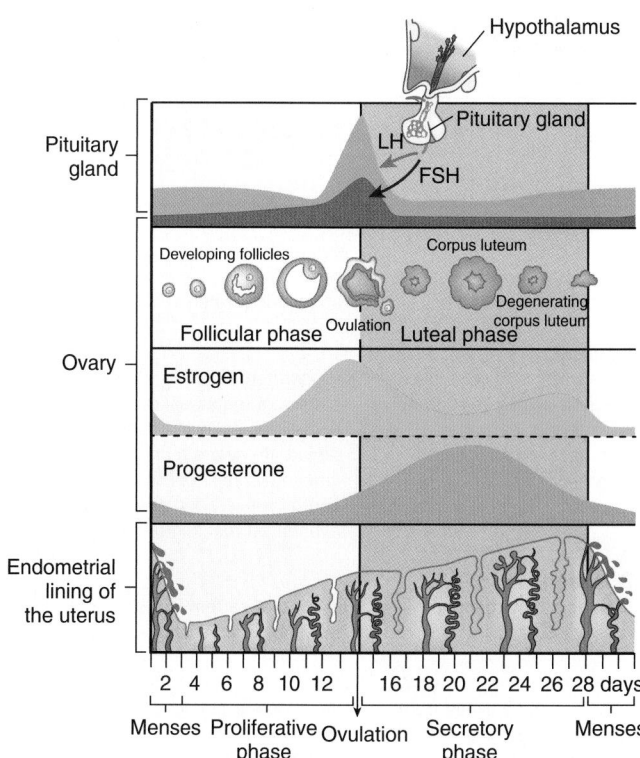

FIG. 51-7 Events of the menstrual cycle. The lines depict the changes in blood hormone levels, the development of the follicles, and the changes in the endometrium during the cycle. *FSH*, Follicle-stimulating hormone; *LH*, luteinizing hormone.

nancy. Adequate progesterone is necessary to maintain an implanted egg.

In men, the major gonadal hormone is testosterone, which is produced by the testes. Testosterone is responsible for the development and maintenance of secondary sex characteristics, as well as for adequate spermatogenesis. In women, androgens are produced in small amounts by the adrenal glands and ovaries.

The circulating levels of gonadal hormones are controlled primarily by a *negative feedback process*. Receptors within the hypothalamus and pituitary are sensitive to the circulating blood levels of the hormones (Table 51-1). Increased levels of hormones stimulate a hypothalamic response to decrease the high circulating levels. Likewise, low circulating levels provoke a hypothalamic response that increases the low circulating levels. For example, if the circulating level of testosterone in men is low, the hypothalamus is stimulated to secrete GnRH. This triggers the anterior pituitary to secrete greater amounts of FSH and LH, which in turn causes an increase in the production of testosterone. The high level of testosterone signals a decrease in the production of GnRH and thus of FSH and LH.

In women, however, there is a slight variation. The circulating levels are controlled through a combination of both a negative and a positive feedback system. A *negative feedback control* mechanism exists similar to that described above. When circulating estrogen levels are low, the hypothalamus is stimulated to increase its production of GnRH. GnRH stimulates the pituitary to secrete greater amounts of FSH and LH, resulting in higher levels of estrogen production by the ovaries. Reciprocally higher levels of circulating estrogen result in a decreasing secretion of GnRH and thus a decrease in the secretion of FSH by the pituitary.

Women also have a *positive feedback control* mechanism. Thus with increasing levels of circulating estrogen, a greater level of GnRH is produced, resulting in an increased level of LH from the pituitary. Likewise, lowered levels of estrogen result in a lowered level of LH.

Menarche

Menarche is the first episode of menstrual bleeding, indicating that a girl has reached puberty. Menarche usually occurs at approximately 12 to 13 years of age but can occur as early as 10 years of age in some individuals. Menstrual cycles are often irregular for the first 1 to 2 years after menarche because of *anovulatory cycles* (cycles without ovulation).

Menstrual Cycle

The major functions of the ovaries are ovulation and the secretion of hormones. These functions are accomplished during the normal menstrual cycle, a monthly process mediated by the hormonal activity of the hypothalamus, pituitary gland, and ovaries. Menstruation occurs during each month in which an egg is not fertilized (Fig. 51-7). The endometrial cycle is divided into three phases labeled in relation to uterine and ovarian changes: (1) the *proliferative*, or *follicular, phase*; (2) the *secretory*, or *luteal, phase*; and (3) the *menstrual*, or *ischemic, phase*. The length of the menstrual cycle ranges from 21 to 35 days, with an average of 28 days.[4]

The menstrual cycle begins on the first day of menstruation, which usually lasts 4 to 6 days. Table 51-2 includes characteristics of the menstrual cycle and related teaching. During menstruation, estrogen and progesterone levels are low, but FSH levels begin to increase. During the follicular phase, a single follicle matures fully under the stimulation of FSH. (The mechanism that ensures that usually only one follicle reaches maturity is not known.) The mature follicle stimulates estrogen production, causing a negative feedback with resulting decreased FSH secretion.

Although the initial stage of follicular maturation is stimulated by FSH, complete maturation and ovulation occur only in the presence of LH. When estrogen levels peak on about the twelfth day of the cycle, there is a surge of LH, which triggers ovulation a day or two later. After ovulation (maturation and

TABLE 51-2   PATIENT TEACHING GUIDE

Characteristics of Menstruation

Include the following information when teaching the patient about menstruation.

Characteristic	Teaching
Menarche Occurs between ages 10 and 16 yr. Average age at onset is 12-13 yr.	See health care provider regarding possible endocrine or developmental abnormality when delayed.
Interval Usually is 21-35 days, but regular cycles as short as 17 days or as long as 45 days are considered normal if pattern is consistent for individual.	Keep written record to identify own pattern of menstrual cycle. Expect some irregularity in perimenopausal period. Be aware that drugs (phenothiazines, opioids, contraceptives) and stressful life events can result in missed periods.
Duration Menstrual flow generally lasts 2-8 days.	Realize that pattern is fairly constant but that wide variations do exist.
Amount Menstrual flow varies from 20-80 mL per menses; average is 30 mL. Amount varies among women and in the same woman at different times. It is usually heaviest first 2 days.	Count pads or tampons used per day. The average tampon or pad, when completely saturated, absorbs 20-30 mL. Very heavy flow is indicated by complete soaking of two pads in 1-2 hr. Flow increases and then gradually decreases in perimenopausal period. IUD or drugs such as anticoagulants and thiazides can produce heavy menses.
Composition Menstrual discharge is mixture of endometrium, blood, mucus, and vaginal cells. It is dark red and less viscous than blood and usually does not clot.	Clots indicate heavy flow or vaginal pooling.

IUD, Intrauterine device.

release of an ovum), LH promotes the development of the corpus luteum.

The fully developed corpus luteum continues to secrete estrogen and initiates progesterone secretion. If fertilization occurs, high levels of estrogen and progesterone continue to be secreted because of the continued activity of the corpus luteum from stimulation by human chorionic gonadotropin (hCG). If fertilization does not take place, menstruation occurs because of a decrease in estrogen production and progesterone withdrawal.

During the *follicular phase,* the endometrial lining of the uterus also undergoes change. As more estrogen is produced, the endometrial lining undergoes proliferative changes, including an increase in the length of blood vessels and glandular tissue.

With ovulation and the resulting increased levels of progesterone, the *luteal* (or *secretory*) *phase* begins. If the corpus luteum regresses (when fertilization does not occur) and estrogen and progesterone levels fall, the endometrial lining can no longer be supported. As a result, the blood vessels contract, and tissue begins to slough (fall away). This sloughing results in the menses and the start of the menstrual phase.[4]

Menopause

Menopause is the physiologic cessation of menses associated with declining ovarian function. It is usually considered complete after 1 year of amenorrhea (absence of menstruation). (Menopause is discussed in Chapter 54.)

Phases of Sexual Response

The sexual response is a complex interplay of psychologic and physiologic phenomena and is influenced by a number of variables (e.g., stress, illness). The changes that occur during sexual excitement are similar for men and women. Masters and Johnson described the sexual response in terms of the excitement, plateau, orgasmic, and resolution phases.[5]

Male Sexual Response. The penis and the urethra are essential to the transport of sperm into the vagina and the cervix during intercourse. This transport is facilitated by penile erection in response to sexual stimulation during the *excitement phase.* Erection results from the filling of the large venous sinuses within the erectile tissue of the penis. In the flaccid state the sinuses hold only a small amount of blood, but during the erection stage they are congested with blood. Because the penis is richly endowed with sympathetic, parasympathetic, and pudendal nerve endings, it is readily stimulated to erection. The loose skin of the penis becomes taut as a result of the venous congestion. This erectile tautness allows for easy insertion into the vagina.

As the man reaches the *plateau phase,* the erection is maintained, and the penis increases in diameter as a result of a slight increase in vasocongestion. Testicle size also increases. Sometimes the glans penis becomes more reddish purple.

The subsequent contraction of the penile and urethral musculature during the *orgasmic phase* propels the sperm outward through the meatus. In this process, termed *ejaculation,* sperm are released into the ductus deferens during contractions. Sperm advance through the urethra, where fluids from the prostate and seminal vesicles are added to the ejaculate. The sperm continue their path through the urethra, receiving a small amount of fluid from the Cowper's glands, and are finally ejaculated through the urinary meatus. *Orgasm* is characterized by the rapid release of the vasocongestion and muscular tension (myotonia) that have developed. The rapid release of muscular tension (through rhythmic contractions) occurs primarily in the penis, prostate gland, and seminal vesicles. After ejaculation, a man enters the *resolution phase.* The penis undergoes involution, gradually returning to its unstimulated, flaccid state.

Female Sexual Response. The changes that occur in a woman during sexual excitation are similar to those in a man. In response to stimulation, the clitoris becomes congested and vaginal lubrication increases from secretions from the cervix, Bartholin's glands, and vaginal walls. This initial response is the excitation phase.

As excitation is maintained in the plateau phase, the vagina expands and the uterus is elevated. In the orgasmic phase, contractions occur in the uterus from the fundus to the lower uterine segment. There is a slight relaxation of the cervical os, which helps the entrance of the sperm, and rhythmic contractions of the vagina. Muscular tension is rapidly released through rhythmic contractions in the clitoris, vagina, and uterus. This phase is followed by a resolution phase in which these organs return to their preexcitation state. However, women do not have to go through the resolution (refractory) recovery state before they can be orgasmic again. They can be multiorgasmic without resolution between orgasms.

GERONTOLOGIC CONSIDERATIONS

EFFECTS OF AGING ON REPRODUCTIVE SYSTEMS

With advancing age, changes occur in the male and female reproductive systems (Table 51-3). In women many of these changes are related to the altered estrogen production that is associated with menopause.[6] A reduction in circulating estrogen along with an increase in androgens in postmenopausal women is associated with breast and genital atrophy, reduction in bone mass, and increased rate of atherosclerosis. Vaginal dryness may occur, which can lead to urogenital atrophy and changes in the composition of vaginal secretions.

A gradual testosterone decline in older men occurs. Manifestations of hormonal decline in men can be physical, psychologic, or sexual. Some of the changes include an increase in prostate size and a decrease in testosterone level, sperm production, muscle tone of the scrotum, and size and firmness of the testicles. Erectile dysfunction and sexual dysfunction occur in some men as a result of these changes.[7]

Gradual changes resulting from advancing age occur in the sexual responses of men and women. The cumulative effects of these changes, as well as the negative social attitude toward sexuality in older adults, can affect the sexual practices of older adults. You have an important role in providing accurate and unbiased information about sexuality and age. Emphasize the normalcy of sexual activity in older adults.

ASSESSMENT OF MALE AND FEMALE REPRODUCTIVE SYSTEMS

Subjective Data

Important Health Information. In addition to general health information, elicit information specifically relating to the reproductive system. Reproduction and sexual issues are often considered extremely personal and private. Develop trust with the patient to elicit such information. A professional demeanor is important when taking a reproductive or sexual history. Be sensitive, use gender-neutral terms when asking about partners, and maintain an awareness of a patient's culture and beliefs. Begin with the least sensitive information (e.g., menstrual history) before asking questions about more sensitive issues such as sexual practices or STIs.

Past Health History. The past health history should include information about major illnesses, hospitalizations, immunizations, and surgeries. Inquire about any infections involving the reproductive system, including STIs. Also take a complete obstetric and gynecologic history from the female patient.

Common pediatric illnesses that affect reproductive function are mumps and rubella. The occurrence of mumps in young men has been associated with an increase in sterility. Bilateral testicular atrophy may occur secondary to mumps-related orchitis. In the health history ask male patients if they have had mumps, been immunized with the mumps vaccine, or have any indications of sterility.

TABLE 51-3 GERONTOLOGIC ASSESSMENT DIFFERENCES

Reproductive Systems

Changes	Differences in Assessment Findings
Male	
Penis	
Decreased subcutaneous fat, decreased skin turgor	Easily retractable foreskin (if uncircumcised). Decrease in size. Fewer sustained erections.
Testes	
Decreased testosterone production	Decrease in size. Change in position (lower).
Prostate	
Benign hyperplasia	Enlargement.
Breasts	
Enlargement	Gynecomastia (abnormal enlargement).
Female	
Breasts	
Decreased subcutaneous fat, increased fibrous tissue, decreased skin turgor	Less resilient, looser, more pendulous tissue. Decreased size. Duct around nipple may feel like stringy strand.
Vulva	
Decreased skin turgor	Atrophy. Decreased amount of pubic hair; decreased size of clitoris and labia.
Vagina	
Atrophy of tissue, decreased muscle tone, alkaline pH	Pale and dry mucosa. Relaxation of outlet, mucosa thins, vagina narrower and shorter, increased potential for infection.
Urethra	
Decreased muscle tone	Cystocele (protrusion of bladder through vaginal wall).
Uterus	
Decreased thickness of myometrium	Decrease in size, uterine prolapse.
Ovaries	
Decreased ovarian function	Nonpalpable ovaries, decreased size.

GENDER DIFFERENCES

Effects of Aging on Sexual Function

Men	Women
• Increased stimulation necessary for erection	• Decreased vaginal lubrication
• Decreased force of ejaculation	• Decreased sensitivity with labia shrinking and more clitoris exposed
• Decreased ability to attain or sustain erection	• Difficulty in maintaining arousal
• Decreased size and rigidity of the penis at full erection	• Difficulty in achieving orgasm after stimulation
• Decreased libido and interest in sex	• Decreased libido and interest in sex

Rubella is of primary concern to women of childbearing age. If rubella occurs during the first 3 months of pregnancy, the possibility of congenital anomalies is increased. For this reason, you should encourage immunization for all women of childbearing age who have not been immunized for rubella or have not already had the disease. (Rubella immunity can be determined by antibody titers.) However, women should not be immunized if they are already pregnant.[8] Advise women not to conceive for at least 3 months after immunization.

Question the patient regarding current health status and any acute or chronic health problems. Problems in other body systems are often related to problems with the reproductive system. Ask questions relating to possible endocrine disorders, particularly diabetes mellitus (DM), hypothyroidism, and hyperthyroidism, because these disorders directly interfere with women's menstrual cycles and with sexual performance. Men who have DM may experience erectile dysfunction and retrograde ejaculation. In women with uncontrolled DM, pregnancy may have significant health risks. Many other chronic illnesses such as cardiovascular disease, respiratory disorders, anemia, cancer, and kidney and urinary tract disorders may affect the reproductive system and sexual functioning.

Determine if the patient has a history of a stroke. In men, strokes may cause physiologic or psychologic erectile dysfunction. Men who have suffered a myocardial infarction (MI) may experience erectile dysfunction because of fear that sexual activity could precipitate another MI. Women share this concern, both as partners of someone who has had an MI and as patients recovering from an MI. Although most patients have concerns about sexual activity after an MI, many are not comfortable expressing these fears to the nurse. Be sensitive to this concern. In women, a history of cardiovascular disease (e.g., hypertension, thrombophlebitis, angina) is associated with a higher incidence of morbidity and mortality with pregnancy or the use of oral contraceptives.

Medications. Document all prescription and over-the-counter medications that the patient is taking, including the reason for the medication, the dosage, and the length of time that the medication has been taken. Ask the patient about the use of herbal products and dietary supplements.

Particularly relevant in the assessment of the reproductive system is the use of diuretics (sometimes prescribed for premenstrual edema), psychotropic agents (which may interfere with sexual performance), and antihypertensives (some of which may cause erectile dysfunction). Patients who use drugs such as amlodipine (Norvasc), lisinopril (Prinivil), propranolol (Inderal), and clonidine (Catapres) must be closely assessed for these problems.[9] Also note the use of drugs such as alcohol, marijuana, barbiturates, amphetamines, or phencyclidine hydrochloride (PCP [also called "angel dust"]), which can have serious behavioral or physiologic effects on the reproductive system.

In women, document the use of oral contraceptives or other hormone therapy (HT). The long-term use of both estrogen and progesterone in HT appears to increase the risk of blood clots, cardiovascular disease, stroke, and breast cancer in postmenopausal women.[10] The short-term use of HT appears to be appropriate for women experiencing moderate to severe menopausal symptoms. Women who use tobacco have a much higher risk of clotting disorders. (HT is discussed in Chapter 54.)

A history of cholecystitis and hepatitis is important because these conditions may be contraindications for the use of oral contraceptives. Cholecystitis is often aggravated by oral contraceptives, and chronic active inflammation of the liver generally precludes the use of estrogen products because they are metabolized by the liver. Chronic obstructive pulmonary disease may be a contraindication to oral contraceptive use because progesterone thickens respiratory secretions.

Surgery or Other Treatments. Note any surgical procedures in the health history. Surgical procedures involving the reproductive system are listed in Table 51-4. Also document any therapeutic or spontaneous abortions.

TABLE 51-4	SURGERIES OF THE REPRODUCTIVE SYSTEMS
Surgery	**Description**
Male	
Herniorrhaphy	Repair of hernia
Orchiectomy	Removal of one or both testes
Prostatectomy	Removal of prostate gland
Repair of testicular torsion	Correction of axial rotation of spermatic cord, which cuts off blood supply to the testicle, the epididymis, and other structures
Varicocelectomy	Repair of varicose vein of scrotum
Vasectomy	Removal of part of ductus (vas) deference. Can be an elective procedure for sterilization or contraception
Female	
Cryosurgery	Use of subfreezing temperature to destroy tissue, especially in treatment of abnormal cells
Dilation and curettage	Dilation of cervix and scraping of endometrium, performed to diagnose disease of uterus, correct heavy or prolonged vaginal bleeding, or empty uterus of products of conception. Also used in the treatment of infertility to correlate state of endometrium and time of cycle
Hysterectomy	Removal of uterus
Mastectomy	Removal of one or both breasts
Oophorectomy	Removal of one or both ovaries
Repair of cystocele	Correction of protrusion of urinary bladder through vaginal wall
Repair of rectocele	Correction of protrusion of rectum into vagina
Salpingectomy	Removal of one or both fallopian tubes
Tubal sterilization	Ligation of fallopian tubes

CASE STUDY

Patient Introduction

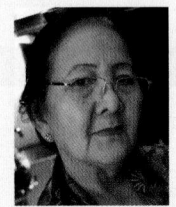

iStockphoto/Thinkstock

A.K. is a 68-yr-old Asian American woman who comes to the breast center because she found a large lump in her right breast while showering. She is somewhat anxious, stating "My breasts are typically lumpy, but this feels different!"

Critical Thinking

As you read through this chapter, think about A.K.'s concerns with the following questions in mind:

1. What are the possible causes for a lump in A.K.'s breast?
2. What would be your priority assessment of A.K.?
3. What questions would you ask A.K.?
4. What should be included in the physical assessment? What would you be looking for?
5. What diagnostic studies might you expect to be ordered?

Functional Health Patterns. The key questions to ask a patient with a reproductive problem are presented in Table 51-5.

Health Perception–Health Management Pattern. Two of the primary focuses of this health pattern are the patient's perception of his or her own health and measures that the patient takes to maintain health. Specifically, ask about self-examination practices and screenings. Mammography (based on current guidelines [see Chapter 52]), Pap tests, and breast self-examinations (BSEs) are integral to a woman's health. Testicular self-examination (TSE) should be practiced by all men, starting in adolescence (see Table 55-9). Starting at age 50, men should discuss with their health care provider the risks and benefits of annual prostate cancer screening with specific antigen (PSA) blood testing and a digital rectal examination (DRE)[11] (see Chapter 55). Men at high risk for prostate cancer (i.e., African Americans, men with prostate cancer in first-degree relatives) should begin these discussions earlier with their provider.

🧬 GENETIC RISK ALERT
- Breast, ovarian, uterine, and prostate cancer have known genetic risk factors.
- Having a first-degree relative with any of these cancers significantly increases the risk of cancer for the patient.
- The risk increases if several family members have been affected with these cancers over succeeding generations.
- Individuals with a known hereditary predisposition to breast or ovarian cancer can use this information to make informed decisions about how to minimize their risks.

Family history is also an important component of this health pattern. Inquire about a history of cancer, particularly cancer of the reproductive organs. Determine if the patient has a familial tendency for diabetes mellitus, hypothyroidism, hyperthyroidism, hypertension, stroke, angina, MI, endocrine disorders, or anemia.

Assessment of the reproductive system is incomplete without knowledge of the patient's lifestyle choices. Determine whether a woman uses cigarettes, alcohol, caffeine, or other drugs

---

TABLE 51-5 HEALTH HISTORY

Reproductive System

Health Perception–Health Management
- How would you describe your overall health?
- *Women:* Explain how you examine your breasts. Have you had a Pap test or mammogram recently? If so, what were the results and dates of these tests?
- *Men:* Explain how you examine your testes. Have you had a prostate examination recently? If so, what were the results and date of this examination?
- Describe the health of your family members. Any history of breast, uterine, ovarian, or prostate cancer?
- Do you use tobacco products, alcohol, or drugs?*

Nutritional-Metabolic
- Describe what you usually eat and drink.
- Have you experienced any changes in weight?*
- How do you feel about your current weight?
- Do you take any nutritional supplements such as calcium or vitamins?*
- Do you have any dietary restrictions?*

Elimination
- Do you experience problems with urination (e.g., pain, burning, dribbling, incontinence, frequency)?*
- Have you had bladder infections? If so, when? How often?
- Do you experience problems with bowel movements?* Do you use laxatives?*

Activity-Exercise
- What activities do you typically do each day?
- Do you have enough energy for your desired activities?
- Can you dress yourself? Feed yourself? Walk without help?

Sleep-Rest
- How many hours do you typically sleep each night?
- Do you feel rested after sleep?
- Do you experience any problems associated with sleeping?*

Cognitive-Perceptual
- Are you able to read and write?
- Do you experience problems with dizziness?*
- Do you experience pain? If yes, where?
- Do you experience pain during sexual activity or intercourse?*

Self-Perception–Self-Concept
- How would you describe yourself?
- Have there been any recent changes that have made you feel differently about yourself?*
- Are you experiencing any problems that are affecting your sexuality?*

Role-Relationship
- Describe your living arrangements. Who do you live with?
- Do you have a significant other? If yes, is this relationship satisfying?
- Are you experiencing any role-related problems in your family?* At work?*
- What are the relationships among your family members?

Sexuality-Reproductive
- Are you sexually active? If so, how many partners do you have?
- What kind of sex do you engage in (e.g., oral, vaginal, rectal)?
- How do you protect yourself against sexually transmitted infections and unwanted pregnancy?
- Are you satisfied with your present means of sexual expression? If no, explain.
- Have you experienced any recent changes in your sexual practices?*
- *Women:* Date of last menstruation, description of menstrual flow, problems with menstruation, age of menarche, age of menopause.
- *Women:* Pregnancy history—number of times pregnant, number of living children, number of miscarriages or abortions.

Coping–Stress Tolerance
- Have there been any major changes in your life within the past couple of years?*
- What is stressful in your life right now?
- How do you handle health problems when they occur?

Value-Belief
- What beliefs do you have about your health and illnesses?
- Do you use home remedies?*
- Is religion an important part of your life?*
- Do you think that any of your personal beliefs or values may be compromised because of your treatment?*

*If yes, describe.

because these substances can be detrimental to both mother and fetus. Cigarette smoking may delay conception and can also increase the risk of morbidity in women using oral contraceptives. Smoking in women is also associated with early menopause. These substances may also adversely affect the sperm count in men and cause erectile dysfunction or decreased libido.

Also document if the patient is allergic to sulfonamides, penicillin, rubber, or latex. Sulfonamides and penicillin are used frequently in the treatment of reproductive and genitourinary problems such as vaginitis and gonorrhea. Rubber and latex are commonly used in diaphragms and condoms. An allergy to these substances precludes their use as contraceptive methods.

Nutritional-Metabolic Pattern. Anemia is a common problem in women in their reproductive years, particularly during pregnancy and the postpartum period. Evaluate the adequacy of the diet with this condition in mind.

Take a thorough nutritional and psychologic history to assess for the presence of an eating disorder. Anorexia nervosa can cause amenorrhea and subsequent problems, such as osteoporosis, that are related to menopause. Obesity can be related to polycystic ovarian syndrome and may be a precursor to type 2 diabetes.

From early adolescence, counsel women regarding adequate calcium and vitamin D intake to prevent osteoporosis. Estimate the patient's daily calcium intake to determine whether supplementation is needed. Evaluate folic acid intake for women in their reproductive years because a deficiency can result in spina bifida and other neural tube defects in the fetus.[12]

Elimination Pattern. Many gynecologic problems can result in genitourinary problems. Stress and urge incontinence is common in older women because of relaxation of the pelvic musculature caused by multiple births or advancing age. Vaginal infections predispose patients to chronic or recurrent urinary tract infections. Metastasis of malignant tumors of the reproductive system to the genitourinary system is possible because of their proximity. Benign prostatic hyperplasia is a common problem of older men. It can alter normal urination, causing retention and difficulty in initiating the urinary stream.

Activity-Exercise Pattern. Record the amount, type, and intensity of activity and exercise. Lack of stress on bones secondary to lack of exercise is an important factor in the development of osteoporosis. Weight-bearing exercise decreases the risk of osteoporosis in women. Women who engage in excessive exercise may experience amenorrhea, which may result from decreased estrogen related to a low percentage of body fat (estrogen is stored in fat cells).[13] Anemia can result in fatigue and activity intolerance and can interfere with satisfactory performance of the activities of daily living.

Sleep-Rest Pattern. Sleep patterns may be affected during the postpartum period and also while raising young children. Hot flashes and sweating that are often present during perimenopause can cause serious sleep interruption when the woman awakens in a drenching sweat. The need to change her nightgown and bedding further disrupts her sleep. Insomnia is also a common complaint of perimenopausal women. Daytime fatigue often results from such sleep disruptions. In men, sleep disturbances may be caused by frequent urination at night associated with prostate enlargement or HT for prostate cancer.

Cognitive-Perceptual Pattern. Pelvic pain is associated with various gynecologic disorders such as pelvic inflammatory disease, ovarian cysts, and endometriosis. Dyspareunia (painful intercourse) can be particularly problematic for women. The pain associated with intercourse can create a reluctance to participate in sexual activity and strain relationships with sexual partners. Refer women with dyspareunia to their health care providers.

Self-Perception–Self-Concept Pattern. Changes that occur with aging, such as pendulous breasts and vaginal dryness in women and decreased size of the penis in men, may lead to emotional distress. The subtle changes associated with sexuality and advancing age may alter the self-concept of many persons.

Role-Relationship Pattern. Obtain information regarding the family structure and occupation. Question the patient regarding recent changes in work-related relationships or family conflict. Determine the patient's role in the family as a starting point in determining family dynamics.

Roles and relationships are affected by changes within the family. The addition of a new baby may change family dynamics. Role-relationship patterns change as children begin their careers and move away from home. Another change occurs when people retire.

Sexuality-Reproductive Pattern. The extent and depth of the interview about a patient's sexuality depend primarily on the interviewer's expertise and on the patient's needs and willingness. Before taking a sexual history, assess your comfort with your own sexuality, because any discomfort in questioning becomes obvious to the patient. Carry out interviews in an environment that provides reassurance, confidentiality, and a nonjudgmental attitude. Begin with the least sensitive areas of questioning and then move to more sensitive areas.

For women, obtain a menstrual and an obstetric history. The menstrual history includes the first day of the last menstrual period, description of menstrual flow, age of menarche, and, if applicable, age at menopause. Menstrual history data are used in the detection of pregnancy, infertility, and numerous other gynecologic problems. Have the patient explicitly describe changes in the usual menstrual pattern to determine whether the change is transient and unimportant or connected with a more serious gynecologic problem. *Metrorrhagia* (spotting or bleeding between menstruations), *menorrhagia* (excessive menstrual bleeding), *amenorrhea* (lack of menstruation), and *postcoital bleeding* are examples of such problems.

Identify changes in menstrual patterns associated with the use of contraceptive pills, intrauterine devices (IUDs), birth control patches, vaginal rings, subdermal progesterone-only implants (Implanon, Nextplanon), or medroxyprogesterone (Depo-Provera) injections. Contraceptive pills usually decrease the amount and duration of flow, whereas some IUDs may cause an increase in the amount and duration. Some IUDs also increase the severity of dysmenorrhea. However, newer IUDs contain progestin and may be therapeutic.

The obstetric history includes the number of pregnancies, full-term births, preterm births, and live births. Also include information about any ectopic pregnancies or abortions, either spontaneous or therapeutic. Document any problems that occurred with pregnancy.

A sexual history should include information regarding sexual activity, beliefs, and practices. Explore sexual preference (heterosexual, homosexual, bisexual), the frequency and type of sexual activity (penile-vaginal, penile-rectal, recipient rectal, oral), and the number of partners and protective measures against STIs and pregnancy. Determine the patient's knowledge

TABLE 51-6 SEXUAL HISTORY FORMAT

1. Are you currently in a relationship that involves sexual intercourse? If yes, do you have one or multiple partners?
2. How frequently do you engage in sexual activities? Are you and your partner(s) satisfied with the sexual relationship?
3. How many sexual partners have you had in the past 6 mo?
4. Do you prefer relationships with men, women, or both? (Inquire whether the patient is in a significant relationship.)
5. Has your sex life changed during the past year? If yes, how?
6. Have you ever had a sexually transmitted infection? If yes, what?
7. What are you doing to protect yourself from sexually transmitted infections? If protection is used, what type? Do you use protection every time you have intercourse?
8. Are you currently using any birth control measures? If yes, what type? How long have you been using this product? How effective do you think this has been?
9. Have you ever been in a relationship with anyone who hurt you? Have you ever been forced into sexual acts as a child or an adult?
10. How often have you experienced erectile dysfunction (male) or difficulty with vaginal lubrication (female) or pain with intercourse?

CASE STUDY—cont'd

Subjective Data

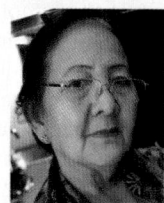

iStockphoto/Thinkstock

A focused assessment of A.K. revealed the following information:

PMH: Type 2 diabetes for 5 yr, hypertension, stress incontinence, osteoarthritis. No surgical history.

Medications: metformin (Glucophage) 500 mg PO bid for the past 4 yr, estrogen/medroxyprogesterone (Prempro) 0.3 mg/1.5 mg/day PO for the past 14 yr, lisinopril (Prinivil) 10 mg/day PO for past 3 yr.

Health Perception–Health Management: A.K. has no personal history of breast cancer, but she does have a family history of breast cancer. Her mother was diagnosed at age 60 and her sister at age 40. She is afraid that she may now have cancer. Her last mammogram and clinical breast examination were 2 yr ago. She does not smoke but does enjoy one to two glasses of wine with her dinner every evening.

Nutritional-Metabolic: A.K. is 5 ft, 2 in tall and weighs 166 lb. She reports gaining most of her weight after menopause. She tries to eat a well-balanced meal and watch her carbohydrate intake because of her diabetes.

Elimination: Denies any changes or difficulty with urination or bowel movements except for stress incontinence when she coughs or laughs. States she always wears a panty liner "just in case."

Activity-Exercise: Does not routinely exercise. Occasionally takes a walk around the block with her husband. Otherwise her life is fairly sedentary.

Cognitive-Perceptual: Denies breast pain.

Sexuality-Reproductive: Had onset of menarche at age 11, menopause at age 53. Has two daughters (34 and 32) and a son (30).

---

of safe sexual practices. A history of multiple sex partners and unprotected sex increases the risk of contracting an STI. For a woman, this can increase the risk of pelvic inflammatory disease, which can compromise her ability to become pregnant.

Table 51-6 outlines specific questions for a sexual history. Only a skilled interviewer should approach some of these questions, and then only with discretion and sensitivity to cultural differences.

Ask both men and women about their general satisfaction with sexuality. The patient's satisfaction with the opportunities for sexual gratification is important information. Question the patient about sexual beliefs and practices and whether orgasm is achieved. Explore any unexplained change in sexual practices or performance. Problems of the reproductive system can cause physiologic or psychologic problems that can lead to painful intercourse, erectile dysfunction, sexual dysfunction, or infertility. Try to determine both the cause and the effect of such problems.

Coping–Stress Tolerance Pattern. The stress related to situations such as pregnancy or menopause increases dependence on support systems. Determine who the support people are in the patient's life. The diagnosis of an STI can cause stress for the patient and the partner. Explore ways to manage this stress.

Value-Belief Pattern. Sexual and reproductive functioning is closely related to cultural, religious, moral, and ethical values. Be aware of your own beliefs in these areas, and recognize and sensitively react to the patient's personal beliefs associated with reproductive and sexuality issues.

Objective Data

Physical Examination: Male. The examination of the male external genitalia includes inspection and palpation. An examination may be performed with the patient lying or standing. The standing position is generally preferred. Sit in front of the standing patient. Use gloves during examination of the male genitalia.

Pubis. Observe the distribution and general characteristics of the pubic hair and the skin. Normally, the hair is in a diamond-shaped pattern and coarser than scalp hair. The absence of hair is not a normal finding unless the man is shaving

or waxing the pubic hair. Carefully assess the skin for irritation and inflammation.

Penis. Note the size and skin texture of the penis and any lesions, scars, or swelling. Also note the location of the urethral meatus and the presence or absence of a foreskin. If present, the foreskin should be retracted to note any redness, discharge, irritation, or swelling. Replace the foreskin over the glans after observation. Then compress the glans to note any discharge and its amount, color, and odor if present. Palpate the penile shaft for tenderness or masses and observe the ventral and dorsal aspects.

Scrotum and Testes. This part of the examination is usually not performed by the nurse generalist. The nurse with advanced skills starts by performing a complete skin examination by lifting each testis to inspect all sides of the scrotal sac. Palpate the scrotum to note changes in consistency or any masses. Note if the testes are descended. The left testis usually hangs lower than the right. An undescended testis is a major risk factor for testicular cancer and a potential cause of male infertility.[14]

Inguinal Region and Spermatic Cord. This part of the examination is usually not performed by the nurse generalist. The examiner with advanced skills first inspects the skin overlying the inguinal regions for rashes or lesions. Then ask the patient to bear down or cough. While he is straining, inspect the inguinal area for a bulge. No bulging should be seen.

Examination of the inguinal area continues with palpation. Palpate the right and left inguinal rings using the index or middle finger. Insert the finger into the lower aspect of the scrotum and follow the spermatic cord upward through the triangular, slitlike opening of the inguinal ring. At this point, ask the patient to bear down and cough. Determine whether the strain produces a bulging of the intestines through the ring, indicating a hernia, a condition that requires follow-up. Also palpate the inguinal lymph nodes. Enlargement of the lymph nodes *(lymphadenopathy)* could suggest a pelvic organ infection or malignancy.

Anus and Prostate. Inspect the anal sphincter and perineal regions for lesions, masses, and hemorrhoids. A DRE is required for all men who have symptoms of prostate trouble, such as difficulty initiating urination and the urge to void frequently. This examination should be performed by the health care provider annually for all men 50 years of age and older.

Physical Examination: Female. Physical examination of women often begins with inspection and palpation of the breasts and axillae and then proceeds to the abdomen and genitalia. Examination of the abdomen provides an opportunity to detect pain or any masses that may involve the genitourinary system. Abdominal examination is discussed in Chapter 39.

Breasts. First examine the breasts by visual inspection. With the patient seated, observe the breasts for symmetry, size, shape, skin color, vascular patterns, dimpling, and unusual lesions. Ask the patient to put her arms at her sides, arms overhead, lean forward, and press hands on hips. Observe for any abnormalities during these maneuvers. Palpate the axillae and the clavicular areas for enlarged lymph nodes.

After the patient assumes a supine position, place a pillow under her back on the side to be examined. Ask the patient to put her arm above and behind her head. These maneuvers flatten breast tissue and make palpation easier. Then palpate the breast in a systematic fashion, preferably using a vertical line (see Fig. 52-1). Use the distal finger pads for palpation. Include the axillary tail of Spence in the examination. This area of the breast lies adjacent to the upper outer quadrant, which is where most breast malignancies develop (see Fig. 52-1). Finally, palpate the area around the areolae for masses. Compress the nipple to detect any discharge or masses. Document the color, consistency, and odor of any discharge.

External Genitalia. Use gloves for examination of the external genitalia. Inspect the mons pubis, labia majora, labia minora, posterior fourchette, perineum, and anal region for characteristics of skin, hair distribution, and contour. Note any lesions, inflammation, swelling, and discharge. Separate the labia to fully inspect the clitoris, urethral meatus, and vaginal orifice.

Internal Pelvic Examination. This part of the examination is usually not performed by the nurse generalist. During the speculum examination, the examiner observes the walls of the vagina and the cervix for inflammation, discharge, polyps, and suspicious growths. During this examination, it is possible to obtain a Pap test and collect cells for culture and microscopic examination. After the speculum examination, a bimanual examination is performed to assess the size, shape, and consistency of the uterus and ovaries. The tubes are not normally palpable.

Parts of the pelvic and bimanual examinations are not included in this text, since they are considered advanced skills and are not usually within the scope of the nurse generalist.

Table 51-7 provides an example of a recording format for the physical assessment findings for the male and female reproductive systems. Tables 51-8 through 51-10 summarize assessment abnormalities of the breasts, female reproductive system, and male reproductive system, respectively.

CASE STUDY—cont'd
Objective Data: Physical Examination

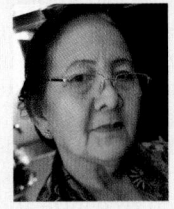

Focused assessment of A.K. reveals the following: A palpable, firm, fixed, 1.5-cm mass in upper, outer quadrant of right breast. No dimpling, redness, or swelling noted. No masses palpated in left breast. No lymphadenopathy noted.

As you continue to read this chapter, consider diagnostic studies you would anticipate being performed for A.K.

iStockphoto/Thinkstock

A *focused assessment* is used to evaluate the status of previously identified reproductive problems and to monitor for signs of new problems (see Table 3-6). A focused assessment of the reproductive system is presented in the box above.

DIAGNOSTIC STUDIES OF REPRODUCTIVE SYSTEMS

The most commonly used diagnostic studies in the assessment of the reproductive systems are summarized in Table 51-11 on p. 1233, and select studies are described in more detail below.

Urine Studies

Pregnancy Testing. Pregnancy is generally validated by measuring human chorionic gonadotropin (hCG) in the urine.[15] A solution containing monoclonal antibodies specific for hCG is mixed with a small amount of urine. The presence of hCG causes a change in color of the tested urine.

Home pregnancy test kits use the same assay principle. Positive results are based on the presence of hCG in urine. Some tests can detect pregnancy as early as the first day after a missed menstrual period. These tests are 98% accurate if the test is performed exactly per instructions. A second test is recommended within a week if the first test is negative (assuming menses has not yet occurred).

Hormone Studies. Although estrogen studies are performed on urine, the results are often inaccurate because of variable estrogen levels during the normal cycle and the difficulty in estimating the day of the cycle in women with irregular menses. Adrenal androgens are precursors of estrogens and can be measured in the urine of both men and women. For more information on hormone studies, see Chapter 48.

Blood Studies

Hormone Studies. Serum assays for hCG can detect pregnancy before a woman misses her menstrual period. The prolactin assay is used primarily in the workup of a patient with amenorrhea. High levels of prolactin are normally associated with low levels of estrogen, such as those that occur during lactation. However, the same finding can occur with pituitary adenomas, especially with otherwise unexplained galactorrhea (excessive secretion of breast milk). Serum progesterone and estradiol are sometimes measured to assess ovarian function, particularly for amenorrhea. In addition, hormonal blood studies are essential components of a fertility workup.

Tumor Markers. Biologic tumor markers are used to assess for malignant disease and to monitor therapy (marker levels

TABLE 51-7	NORMAL PHYSICAL ASSESSMENT OF REPRODUCTIVE SYSTEM	
Male	**Female**
Breasts	
Nipples soft. No lumps, nodules, swelling, or enlarged tissue noted.	Symmetric without dimpling. Nipples soft. No drainage, retraction, or lesions noted. No masses or tenderness. No lymphadenopathy.
External Genitalia	
Diamond-shaped hair distribution. No penile lesions or discharge noted. Scrotum symmetric, no masses, descended testes. No inguinal hernia.	Triangular hair distribution. Genitalia dark pink, no lesions, redness, swelling, or inflammation in perineal region. No vaginal discharge noted. No tenderness with palpation of Skene's ducts and Bartholin's glands.
Anus	
No hemorrhoids, fissures, or lesions noted.	No hemorrhoids, fissures, or lesions noted.

TABLE 51-8 ASSESSMENT ABNORMALITIES

Breast

Finding	Description	Possible Etiology and Significance
Nipple inversion or retraction	Recent onset, erythematous, pain, unilateral.	Abscess, inflammation, cancer.
	Recent onset (usually within past year), unilateral presentation, lack of tenderness.	Neoplasm.
Nipple secretions		
• Galactorrhea (female)	Milky, no relationship to lactation, unilateral or bilateral, intermittent or consistent presentation.	Drug therapy, particularly phenothiazines, tricyclic antidepressants, methyldopa. Hypofunction or hyperfunction of thyroid or adrenal glands. Tumors of hypothalamus or pituitary gland. Excessive estrogen. Prolonged suckling or breast foreplay.
• Galactorrhea (male)	Milky, bilateral presentation.	Chorioepithelioma of testes, manifestation of pituitary tumor.
• Purulent	Gray-green or yellow color. Frequent unilateral presentation. Association with pain, erythema, induration, nipple inversion.	Puerperal (after birth) mastitis (inflammatory condition of breast) or abscess.
	Same as above but usually without nipple inversion.	Infected sebaceous cyst.
• Serous discharge	Clear appearance, unilateral or bilateral, intermittent or consistent presentation.	Intraductal papilloma.
• Dark green or multicolored discharge	Thick, sticky, and frequently bilateral.	Ductal ectasia (dilation of mammary ducts).
• Serosanguineous or bloody drainage	Unilateral presentation.	Papillomatosis (widespread development of nipple-like growths), intraductal papilloma, carcinoma (male and female).
Scaling or irritation of nipple	Unilateral or bilateral presentation, crusting, possible ulceration.	Paget's disease, eczema, infection.
Nodules, lumps, or masses	Multiple, bilateral, well-delineated, soft or firm, mobile cysts. Pain. Premenstrual occurrence.	Fibrocystic changes.
	Rubbery consistency, fluid-filled interior, pain.	Ductal ectasia.
	Soft, mobile, well-delineated cyst, absence of pain.	Lipoma, fibroadenoma.
	Erythema, tenderness, induration.	Infected sebaceous cysts, abscesses.
	Usually singular, hard, irregularly shaped, poorly delineated, nonmobile.	Neoplasm.
Dimpling of breast	Unilateral, recent onset, no pain.	Neoplasm.

TABLE 51-9 **ASSESSMENT ABNORMALITIES**

Female Reproductive System

Finding and Description	Possible Etiology and Significance
Vulvar Discharge	
White, thick, curdy, frequent itching and inflammation, lack of odor or yeast-like smell	Candidiasis (*Candida* or yeast infection), vaginitis
Thin gray or white, copious flow, malodorous or fishy, vulvar irritation	Bacterial vaginosis infection
Frothy green or yellow color; malodorous	*Trichomonas vaginalis*
Bloody discharge	*Chlamydia trachomatis* or *Neisseria gonorrhoeae* infection, menstruation, trauma, cancer
Vulvar Erythema	
Bright or beefy red color, itching	*Candida albicans*, allergy, chemical vaginitis
Reddened base, painful vesicles or ulcerations	Genital herpes
Macules or papules, itching	Chancroid (STI), contact dermatitis, scabies, pediculosis
Vulvar Growths	
Soft, fleshy growth, nontender	Condyloma acuminatum
Flat and warty appearance, nontender	Condyloma latum
Same as either of above, possible pain	Neoplasm
Reddened base, vesicles, and small erosions; pain	Lymphogranuloma venereum, genital herpes, chancroid
Indurated, firm ulcers, no pain	Chancre (syphilis), granuloma inguinale
Abdominal Pain or Tenderness	
Intermittent or consistent tenderness in right or left lower quadrant	Salpingitis (infection of fallopian tube), ectopic pregnancy, ruptured ovarian cyst, PID, tubal or ovarian abscess
Periumbilical location, consistent occurrence	Cystitis, endometritis (inflammation of endometrium), ectopic pregnancy
Abnormal Vaginal Bleeding	
Unusual and inappropriate uterine bleeding	Dysfunctional uterine bleeding, usually anovulatory bleeding, menorrhagia (heavy menstrual bleeding), metrorrhagia (irregular, frequent bleeding), postmenopausal bleeding

PID, Pelvic inflammatory disease.

TABLE 51-10 **ASSESSMENT ABNORMALITIES**

Male Reproductive System

Finding and Description	Possible Etiology and Significance
Penile Growths or Masses	
Indurated, smooth, disklike appearance; absence of pain; singular presentation	Chancre
Papular to irregularly shaped ulceration with pus, lack of induration	Chancroid
Ulceration with induration and nodularity	Cancer
Flat, wartlike nodule	Condyloma latum
Elevated, fleshy, moist, elongated projections with single or multiple projections	Condyloma acuminatum
Localized swelling with retracted, tight foreskin	Paraphimosis (inability to replace foreskin to its normal position after retraction), trauma
Vesicles, Erosions, or Ulcers	
Painful, erythematous base. Vesicular or small erosions	Genital herpes, balanitis (inflammation of glans penis), chancroid
Painless, singular, small erosion with eventual lymphadenopathy	Lymphogranuloma venereum, cancer
Scrotal Masses	
Localized swelling with tenderness, unilateral or bilateral presentation	Epididymitis (inflammation of epididymis), testicular torsion, orchitis (mumps)
Swelling, tenderness	Incarcerated hernia
Swelling without pain. Unilateral or bilateral presentation. Translucent, cordlike or wormlike appearance	Hydrocele (accumulation of fluid in outer covering of testes), spermatocele (firm, sperm-containing cyst of epididymis), varicocele (dilation of veins that drain testes), hematocele (accumulation of blood within scrotum)
Firm, nodular testes or epididymis. Frequent unilateral presentation	Tuberculosis, cancer
Penile Discharge	
Clear to purulent color, minimal to copious flow	Urethritis or gonorrhea, *Chlamydia trachomatis* infection, trauma
Penile or Scrotal Erythema	
Macules and papules	Scabies, pediculosis
Inguinal Masses	
Bulging unilateral presentation during straining	Inguinal hernia
1- to 3-cm nodules	Lymphadenopathy

rise as disease progresses and fall with disease regression). α-Fetoprotein (AFP), hCG, and CA-125 are sometimes used as tumor markers for reproductive system malignancies. A specific tumor antigen such as PSA is another type of tumor marker, frequently used for prostate cancer.

Serology Tests for Syphilis. The Venereal Disease Research Laboratory (VDRL) test and the rapid plasma reagin (RPR) test detect the presence of antibodies in the serum of patients infected with syphilis. These tests are inexpensive and reliable but have high levels of false-positive results. The fluorescent treponemal antibody absorption (FTA-Abs) test is highly reliable and should be used after a positive VDRL or RPR.

Cultures and Smears

Cultures and smears are most frequently used in the diagnosis of STIs. Specimens for cultures and smears are commonly taken from the vagina, endocervix, and rectum for females and the urethra and rectum for males. For a culture, the specimen is placed on a special culture medium. A smear involves rubbing the specimen on a slide for direct examination. Gram stain smears have been shown to be effective in the diagnosis of *Chlamydia* infection. A nucleic acid amplification test (NAAT)

Text continued on p. 1236

TABLE 51-11 DIAGNOSTIC STUDIES

Male and Female Reproductive Systems

Study	Description and Purpose	Nursing Responsibility
Urine Studies		
Human chorionic gonadotropin (hCG)	Detects pregnancy. Also detects hydatidiform mole and chorioepithelioma (in men and women). *Males and nonpregnant females:* Negative	Obtain menstrual history from patient, including birth control methods. Determine presence or absence of presumptive signs of pregnancy (e.g., breast changes, increased whitish vaginal discharge).
Testosterone	Detects tumors and developmental anomalies of the testes. *Female:* 2-12 mcg/24 hr (6.9-41.6 nmol/24 hr) *Male:* 40-135 mcg/24 hr (139-469 nmol/24 hr)	Instruct patient to collect 24-hr urine specimen and to keep refrigerated.
Follicle-stimulating hormone (FSH)	Indicates gonadal failure because of pituitary dysfunction. *Female:* Follicular phase: 2-15 U/24 hr Midcycle: 8-60 U/24 hr Luteal phase: 2-10 U/24 hr Postmenopause: 35-100 U/24 hr *Male:* 3-11 U/24 hr	Instruct patient to collect 24-hr urine specimen. Indicate phase of menstrual cycle, if menopausal, and if on oral contraceptives or hormones.
Blood Studies		
Prolactin	Detects pituitary dysfunction that can cause amenorrhea. *Female:* 3.8-23.2 ng/mL (3.8-23.2 mg/L) *Male:* 3.0-14.7 ng/mL (3.0-14.7 mg/L)	Observe venipuncture site for bleeding or hematoma formation.
Prostate-specific antigen (PSA)	Detects prostate cancer. Also a sensitive test for monitoring response to therapy. *Reference interval:* <4 ng/mL (<4 mcg/L)	No food or fluid restrictions. Collect 5 mL blood. Observe venipuncture site for bleeding.
hCG	Detects pregnancy. Can also be used as a tumor marker for testicular malignancy. Also used to detect hydatidiform mole. *Males and nonpregnant females:* <5 mIU/mL (<5 IU/L)	Find out where patient is in her menstrual cycle, whether she has missed menses, and if so, how late she is.
Testosterone	Determines whether elevated androgens are due to testicular, adrenal, or ovarian dysfunction or pituitary tumors. Serum testosterone also drawn to assess male infertility and tumors of testicle or ovary. *Male:* 280-1100 ng/dL (10.4-38.17 nmol/L) *Female:* 15-70 ng/dL (0.52-2.43 nmol/L)	Collect health history to eliminate potential sources of interference with accuracy of results (e.g., use of corticosteroids or barbiturates, hypothyroidism or hyperthyroidism).
Progesterone	Determines cause of infertility, monitors success of drugs for infertility or the effect of treatment with progesterone, determines whether ovulation is occurring, and diagnoses problems with the adrenal glands and some types of cancer. *Female:* Follicular phase: 15-70 ng/dL (0.5-2.2 nmol/L) Luteal phase: 200-2500 ng/dL (6.4-79.5 nmol/L) Postmenopause: <40 ng/dL (1.28 nmol/L) *Male:* 13-97 ng/dL (0.4-3.1 nmol/L)	Observe venipuncture site for bleeding or hematoma formation. Include information about last menstrual period and trimester of pregnancy because progesterone levels vary with gestation.
Estradiol	Measures ovarian function. Useful in assessing estrogen-secreting tumors and states of precocious female puberty. May be used to confirm perimenopausal status. Increased serum estradiol levels in men may be indicative of testicular tumors. *Female:* Follicular phase: 20-150 pg/mL (73-1285 pmol/L) Luteal phase: 30-450 pg/mL (110-1652 pmol/L) Postmenopause: ≤20 pg/mL (≤73 pmol/L) *Male:* 10-50 pg/mL (37-184 pmol/L)	Observe venipuncture site for bleeding or hematoma formation.
FSH	Indicates gonadal failure due to pituitary dysfunction. Used to validate menopausal status. *Female:* Follicular phase: 1.37-9.9 mU/mL Ovulatory phase: 6.17-17.2 mU/mL Luteal phase: 1.09-9.2 mU/mL Postmenopause: 19.3-100.6 mU/mL *Male:* 1.42-15.4 mU/mL	No food or fluid restrictions required. State phase of menstrual cycle, if menopausal, or if on oral contraceptive or hormones.
Venereal Disease Research Laboratory (VDRL) (flocculation)	Nonspecific antibody tests used to screen for syphilis. Positive readings can be made within 1-2 wk after appearance of primary lesion (chancre) or 4-15 wk after initial infection. *Reference interval:* Negative or nonreactive	Observe venipuncture site for bleeding or hematoma formation.
Rapid plasma reagin (RPR) (agglutination)	Nonspecific antibody test used to screen for syphilis. *Reference interval:* Negative or nonreactive	Obtain data to identify conditions such as hepatitis, pregnancy, and autoimmune diseases that may interfere with accuracy of results.

Continued

TABLE 51-11   DIAGNOSTIC STUDIES—cont'd

Male and Female Reproductive Systems

Study	Description and Purpose	Nursing Responsibility
Blood Studies—cont'd		
Fluorescent treponemal antibody absorption (FTA-Abs)	Detects syphilis antibodies. Also detects early syphilis with great accuracy. Usually performed if results of VDRL and RPR are questionable. *Reference interval:* Negative or nonreactive	Inform patient that blood sample will be drawn. Observe venipuncture site for bleeding or hematoma formation.
Cultures and Smears		
Dark-field microscopy	Direct examination of specimen obtained from potential syphilitic lesion (chancre) is performed to detect *Treponema pallidum.*	Avoid direct skin contact with open lesion.
Wet mounts	Direct microscopic examination of specimen of vaginal discharge is performed immediately after collection. Determines presence or absence and number of *Trichomonas* organisms, bacteria, white and red blood cells, and candidal buds or hyphae. Other clues or causes of inflammation or infection may be determined.	Explain procedure and purpose to patient. Instruct patient not to douche before examination. Prepare for collection of specimens (glass slide, 10%-20% potassium hydroxide [KOH] solution, sodium chloride [NaCl] solution, and cotton-tipped applicators).
Cultures	Specimens of vaginal, urethral, or cervical discharge are cultured to assess for gonorrhea or *Chlamydia* organisms. Rectal and throat cultures may also be taken, depending on data obtained from sexual history.	Obtain specific contact and sexual history, including oral and rectal intercourse. Instruct against douching before examination. Obtain urethral specimen from men before they void. Instruct sexually active women with multiple partners to have at least a yearly culture for gonorrhea and *Chlamydia*. Instruct sexually active men to have any discharge evaluated immediately to rule out gonorrhea strains that do not cause classic symptoms of dysuria.
Gram stain	Used for rapid detection of gonorrhea. Presence of gram-negative intracellular diplococci generally warrants treatment. Not highly accurate for women. Also a valid alternative for *Chlamydia* testing.	Same as above.
Cytologic Studies		
Papanicolaou (Pap) test	Microscopic study of exfoliated cells via special staining and fixation technique to detect abnormal cells. Most commonly studies cells obtained directly from the endocervix and ectocervix.	Instruct sexually active women to have Pap test according to American Cancer Society guidelines *(www.cancer.org)*. Instruct patient not to douche for at least 24 hr before examination. Collect careful menstrual and gynecologic history.
Nipple discharge test	Cytologic study of nipple discharge.	Indicate if patient is taking hormonal preparations or other drugs, is breastfeeding, or has a history of amenorrhea. Instruct patient that nipple discharge should always be evaluated.
Radiologic Studies		
Mammography • Screening • Diagnostic	X-ray image of breast tissue on radiographic film is used to assess breast tissue. Detects benign and malignant masses. Performed when patient has suspicious clinical symptoms or abnormality found on screening mammogram. Additional views of affected breast are taken.	Instruct patient about the examination and American Cancer Society recommendations for screening (see Chapter 52).
Ultrasound (abdominal and transvaginal)	Measures and records high-frequency sound waves as they pass through tissues of variable density. In women, useful in detecting masses >3 cm, such as ectopic pregnancy, IUD, ovarian cyst, and hydatidiform mole. In men, used to detect testicular torsion or masses.	Instruct patient that a full bladder may be required depending on reason for the study.
Ultrasound-guided biopsy	Use of ultrasound guidance while performing a biopsy. Ultrasound is used to direct the biopsy needle into the region of interest and obtain a sample of tissue. Removal of small tissue sample to diagnose infection, inflammation, or mass.	Inform patient of purpose for this procedure. It is usually done as an outpatient procedure.
Computed tomography (CT) of pelvis	Detects tumors within the pelvis.	Inform patient of procedure. Patient must lie still during the procedure. If IV contrast medium is used, check for iodine allergy.
Magnetic resonance imaging (MRI)	Radio waves and magnetic field are used to view soft tissue. Useful after an abnormal mammogram or for breast dysplasia. Also used to diagnose abnormalities in the female and male reproductive systems.	Screen patient for metal parts and pacemaker. Inform patient the procedure is painless. Patient must lie still during the procedure.

TABLE 51-11 DIAGNOSTIC STUDIES—cont'd

Male and Female Reproductive Systems

Study	Description and Purpose	Nursing Responsibility
Invasive Procedures		
Breast biopsy	Histologic examination of excised breast tissue, obtained either by needle aspiration or excisional biopsy.	*Before biopsy:* Instruct patient about operative procedures and sedation. *After biopsy:* Perform wound care and instruct patient about breast self-examination.
Hysteroscopy	Allows visualization of uterine lining through insertion of scope through cervix. Used mainly to diagnose and treat abnormal bleeding such as polyps and fibroids. Biopsy may be taken during procedure.	Explain purpose and method of procedure and that it may be done in the physician's office. Inform patient that mild cramping and slight bloody discharge after procedure is normal.
Hysterosalpingogram	Involves instillation of contrast media through cervix into uterine cavity and subsequently through the fallopian tubes. X-ray images taken to detect abnormalities of uterus and its adnexa (ovaries and tubes) as contrast progresses through them. Test may be most useful in diagnostic assessment of fertility (e.g., to detect adhesions near ovary, an abnormal uterine shape, blockage of tubal pathways).	Inform patient about procedure and that it may be fairly uncomfortable. Ask about iodine allergy.
Colposcopy	Direct visualization of cervix with binocular microscope that allows magnification and study of cellular dysplasia and cervix abnormalities. Used as follow-up for abnormal Pap test and for examination of women exposed to DES in utero. Biopsy of cervix may be taken during examination. Valuable in decreasing number of false-negative cervical biopsies.	Instruct patient about this outpatient procedure. Inform patient that this examination is similar to speculum examination.
Conization	Cone-shaped sample of squamocolumnar tissue of cervix is removed for direct study.	Explain purpose and method of procedure and that it requires use of surgical facilities and anesthesia. Instruct patient to avoid sexual intercourse and tampons for about 3-4 wk. Also discuss necessity for 3-wk follow-up.
Loop electrosurgical excision procedure (LEEP)	Excision of cervical tissue via an electrosurgical instrument. Diagnoses and treats cervical dysplasia. Minimizes amount of tissue removed, preserves childbearing ability.	Explain purpose and method of procedure and that it may be done in the physician's office. Patient may feel slight tingling or abdominal cramping during procedure. Discharge, bleeding, and cramping may occur for 1-3 days after procedure.
Culdotomy, culdoscopy, and culdocentesis	*Culdotomy* is an incision made through posterior fornix of cul-de-sac and allows visualization of peritoneal cavity (i.e., uterus, tubes, and ovaries). *Culdoscopy* can then be used to closely study these structures. This technique is valuable in fertility evaluations. Withdrawal of fluid *(culdocentesis)* allows examination of fluid.	Explain purpose and method of procedure. Prepare patient for vaginal operation with preoperative instruction and sedation. Perform assessment of bleeding and discomfort after surgery.
Laparoscopy (peritoneoscopy)	Allows visualization of pelvic structures via fiberoptic scopes inserted through small abdominal incisions. Instillation of CO_2 into cavity improves visualization. Used in diagnostic assessment of uterus, tubes, and ovaries (Fig. 51-8). Can be used in conjunction with tubal sterilization.	Before surgery, instruct patient about procedure, prepare abdomen, and reassure patient about sedation. Inform patient of probability of shoulder pain because of air in the abdomen.
Dilation and curettage (D&C)	Operative procedure dilates cervix and allows curetting of endometrial lining. Used in assessment of abnormal bleeding and cytologic evaluation of lining.	Before surgery, instruct patient about procedure and sedation. Perform postoperative assessment of degree of bleeding (frequent pad check during first 24 hr).
Fertility Studies		
Semen analysis	Semen is assessed for volume (2-5 mL), viscosity, sperm count (>20 million/mL), sperm motility (60% motile), and percent of abnormal sperm (60% with normal structure).	Instruct patient to bring in fresh specimen within 2 hr after ejaculation.
Basal body temperature assessment	Measurement indirectly indicates whether ovulation has occurred. (Temperature rises at ovulation and remains elevated during secretory phase of normal menstrual cycle.)	Instruct woman to take temperature using special basal temperature thermometer (calibrated in tenths of degrees) every morning before getting out of bed. Instruct to record temperature on graph.
Huhner, Sims-Huhner, test	Mucus sample of cervix is examined within 2-8 hr after intercourse. Total number of sperm is assessed in relation to number of live sperm. Used to determine whether cervical mucus is "hostile" to passage of sperm from vagina into uterus.	Instruct couples to have intercourse at estimated time of ovulation and be present for test within 2-8 hr after intercourse.
Endometrial biopsy	Small curette is used to obtain piece of endometrial lining to assess endometrial changes common to progesterone secretion after ovulation. Also used to assess abnormal menstrual or postmenopausal uterine bleeding.	Tell patient test must be performed postovulation. Explain that procedure should cause only short period of uterine cramping and light, bloody vaginal discharge for about 24 hr.
Hysterosalpingogram	Same as operative procedures.	Same as operative procedures.
Serum progesterone	Same as blood studies.	Same as blood studies.

DES, Diethylstilbestrol; *IUD,* intrauterine device.

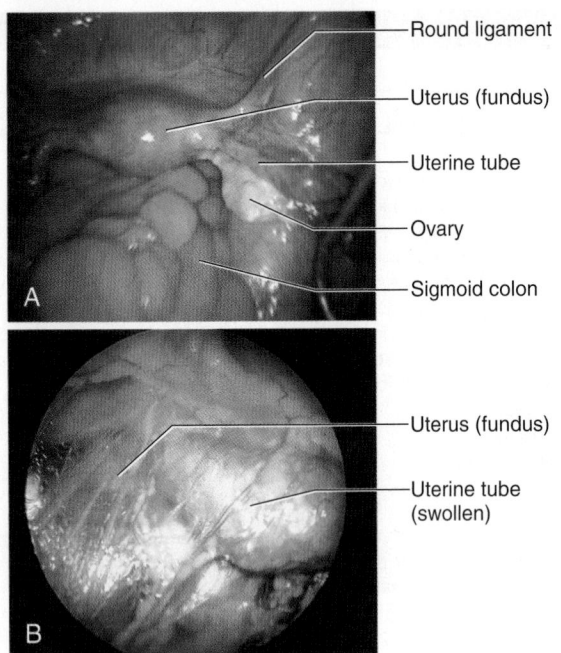

Round ligament
Uterus (fundus)
Uterine tube
Ovary
Sigmoid colon

A

Uterus (fundus)
Uterine tube (swollen)

B

FIG. 51-8 Laparoscopic views of the female pelvis. **A,** Normal image. **B,** Pelvic inflammatory disease. Note reddish inflammatory membrane covering and fixing the ovary and uterus to the surrounding structures.

can screen for both gonorrhea and *Chlamydia* from a wide variety of samples, including vaginal, endocervical, urinary, and urethral specimens. Dark-field microscopy involves the direct examination of a specimen obtained from a chancre for the diagnosis of syphilis.

Objective Data: Diagnostic Studies

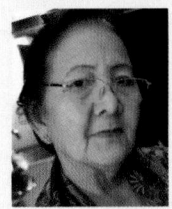

iStockphoto/Thinkstock

The breast specialist orders the following for A.K.:
• Digital mammography
• Ultrasound of breasts
• MRI of breasts

The mammography reveals an increased density on the right breast. The ultrasound identifies the mass as solid and not fluid filled. The MRI confirms the presence of a suspicious mass in the right breast.

The health care provider schedules A.K. for a fine-needle aspiration (FNA) biopsy. The results of the ultrasound-guided FNA biopsy reveal an adenocarcinoma.

Radiologic Studies

Mammography. Mammography, one of the most frequently used diagnostic tools to assess the reproductive system, is used to detect breast masses. Mammography and screening guidelines for mammography are discussed in Chapter 52.

Ultrasound. Ultrasound has many applications for diagnostic studies. Pelvic ultrasound is used to obtain images of the pelvic organs. Transvaginal ultrasound is used to visualize the female genital tract. These types of ultrasound are also used to detect pregnancy in the uterus, ectopic pregnancy, ovarian cysts, and other pelvic masses.

Breast ultrasound is useful in the detection of fluid-filled masses. In men, ultrasound is used to detect testicular masses and testicular torsion. Transrectal ultrasound (TRUS) is useful for diagnosing prostate tumors.

▌ BRIDGE TO NCLEX EXAMINATION

The number of the question corresponds to the same-numbered outcome at the beginning of the chapter.

1. A normal male reproductive function that may be altered in a patient who undergoes a prostatectomy is
   a. sperm production.
   b. production of testosterone.
   c. production of seminal fluid.
   d. release of sperm from the epididymis.

2. Estrogen production by a mature ovarian follicle causes
   a. decreased secretion of FSH and LH.
   b. increased production of GnRH and FSH.
   c. release of GnRH and increased secretion of LH.
   d. decreased release of FSH and decreased progesterone production.

3. Female orgasm is the result of (select all that apply)
   a. constriction of the cervical os.
   b. uterine and vaginal contractions.
   c. vaginal enlargement and uterine elevation.
   d. clitoral swelling and increased vaginal lubrication.
   e. rapid release of muscular tension in the reproductive structures.

4. An age-related finding noted by the nurse during the assessment of the older woman's reproductive system is
   a. dyspareunia.
   b. vaginal dryness.
   c. nipple retraction.
   d. increased sensitivity of labia.

5. Significant information about a patient's past health history related to the reproductive system should include
   a. extent of sexual activity.
   b. general satisfaction with sexuality.
   c. previous sexually transmitted infections.
   d. self-image and relationships with others.

6. To evaluate the female patient's breasts, the nurse would use the examination technique of (select all that apply)
   a. palpation.
   b. inspection.
   c. percussion.
   d. auscultation.

7. An abnormal finding noted during physical assessment of the male reproductive system is
   a. descended testes.
   b. symmetric scrotum.
   c. slight clear urethral discharge.
   d. the glans covered with prepuce.

8. The nurse is caring for a patient scheduled for an endometrial biopsy who is having difficulty becoming pregnant. The nurse explains to the woman that
   a. the outpatient procedure is usually done preovulation.
   b. bleeding and discharge are common 2 to 4 days after the procedure.
   c. a small sample of tissue is obtained to diagnose and treat cervical dysplasia.
   d. common changes in endometrial cells in relation to progesterone levels will be assessed.

1. c, 2. c, 3. b, c, 4. b, 5. c, 6. a, b, 7. c, 8. d

⊖volve

For rationales to these answers and even more NCLEX review questions, visit *http://evolve.elsevier.com/Lewis/medsurg.*

REFERENCES

1. Thibodeau G, Patton K: *Structure and function of the body,* ed 14, St Louis, 2012, Mosby.
2. McCance K, Huether S: *Pathophysiology: the biologic basis for disease in adults and children,* ed 6, St Louis, 2010, Mosby.
3. Bulun S: Physiology and pathology of the female reproductive axis. In Melmed S, Polonsky K, Larsen PR, et al, editors: *Williams textbook of endocrinology,* ed 12, St Louis, 2011, Saunders.
4. Rebar R, Erickson G: Reproductive endocrinology and infertility. In Goldman C, Schafer A, editors: *Goldman's Cecil medicine,* ed 24, St Louis, 2011, Saunders.
5. Masters WH, Johnson E: *Human sexual response,* Boston, 1966, Little Brown. (Classic)
6. Mayo Clinic: Menopause. Retrieved from *www.mayoclinic.com/health/menopause.*
7. Laborde E, Brannigan R: Androgen deficiency in the aging male: the tip of the iceberg? *Urol Times* 39:44, 2011.
8. National Institute of Child Health and Human Development: Care before and during pregnancy: prenatal care. Retrieved from *www.nichd.nih.gov/womenshealth.*
9. Saunders 2014 drug reference, St Louis, 2014, Saunders.
10. National Institutes of Health, Women's Health Initiative: Facts about postmenopausal hormonal therapy. Retrieved from *www.nhlbi.nih.gov/health/women.*
11. American Cancer Society: Prostate cancer: early detection. Retrieved from *www.cancer.org.*
*12. Sumar N, McLaren L: Impact on social inequalities of population strategies of prevention for folate intake in women of childbearing age, *Am J Public Health* 101:1218, 2011.
13. Zach K, Smith Machin A, Hoch A: Advances in management of the female athlete triad and eating disorders, *Clin Sports Med* 30:551, 2011.
14. Zoltick B: Shedding light on testicular cancer, *Nurse Pract* 36:32, 2011.
15. US Department of Health and Human Services, Office on Women's Health: Pregnancy tests fact sheet. Retrieved from *www.womenshealth.gov/publications/our-publications/fact-sheet/pregnancy-tests.cfm.*

RESOURCES

Resources for this chapter are listed in Chapter 54 on p. 1306 and Chapter 55 on p. 1332.

*Evidence-based information for clinical practice.

What you leave behind is not what is engraved in stone monuments, but what is woven into the lives of others.
Pericles

Nursing Management
Breast Disorders

Deborah Hamolsky

LEARNING OUTCOMES

1. Summarize screening guidelines for the early detection of breast cancer.
2. Describe accurate clinical breast examination techniques, including inspection and palpation.
3. Explain the types, causes, clinical manifestations, and nursing and collaborative management of common benign breast disorders.
4. Assess the risk factors for breast cancer.
5. Describe the pathophysiology and clinical manifestations of breast cancer.
6. Describe the collaborative care and nursing management of breast cancer.
7. Specify the physical and psychologic preoperative and postoperative aspects of nursing management for the patient undergoing a mastectomy.
8. Explain the indications for reconstructive breast surgery, types and complications of reconstructive breast surgery, and nursing management after reconstructive breast surgery.

KEY TERMS

ductal ectasia, p. 1242
fibroadenoma, p. 1242
fibrocystic changes, p. 1241
galactorrhea, p. 1242

gynecomastia, p. 1242
intraductal papilloma, p. 1242
lumpectomy, p. 1247
lymphedema, p. 1249

mammoplasty, p. 1256
mastalgia, p. 1240
mastitis, p. 1240
Paget's disease, p. 1245

Breast disorders are a significant health concern for women. Whether the actual diagnosis is a benign condition or a malignancy, the initial discovery of a lump or change in the breast often triggers intense feelings of anxiety, fear, and denial.

The most frequently encountered breast disorders in women are fibrocystic changes, fibroadenoma, intraductal papilloma, ductal ectasia, and breast cancer. In a woman's lifetime there is a 1 in 8 chance she will be diagnosed with breast cancer.[1] In men, gynecomastia is the most common breast disorder.

ASSESSMENT OF BREAST DISORDERS

Breast Cancer Screening Guidelines

Screening guidelines for the early detection of breast cancer include the following:[2-5]

- Yearly mammograms starting at age 40 and continuing for as long as a woman is in good health. A controversial recommended change is that women at normal risk for breast cancer should begin annual screening at age 50 and stop screening at age 75.[6]

Reviewed by Carole Martz, RN, MS, AOCN, CBCN, Clinical Coordinator, Living in the Future Cancer Survivorship Program, Northshore University Health System, Highland Park Hospital, Highland Park, Illinois; Shannon T. Harrington, RN, PhD, Nursing Lecturer, School of Nursing, Old Dominion University, Norfolk, Virginia; Mary Scheid, RN, MSN, OCN, CBCN, Breast Health Nurse, NCMC Breast Center, North Colorado Medical Center, Greeley, Colorado; and Mary Blessing, RN, MSN, Director, Academic RN Residency Program, University of New Mexico Hospitals, Albuquerque, New Mexico.

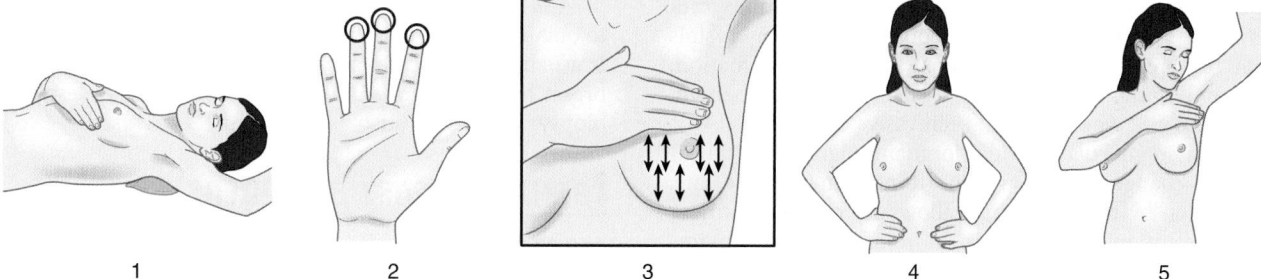

1   2   3   4   5

FIG. 52-1 Breast self-examination and patient instruction. *1,* Lie down and place your left arm behind your head. Lying down spreads breast tissue evenly and thinly over the chest wall, making it easier to feel the tissue. *2,* Use finger pads of three middle fingers on your right hand to feel for lumps in left breast. Use overlapping dime-sized circular motions to feel the breast tissue. Use three different levels of pressure to feel the breast tissue. Light pressure to feel tissue closest to the skin; medium pressure to feel a little deeper; and firm pressure to feel tissue closest to the chest and ribs. A firm ridge in the lower curve of each breast is normal. *3,* The up-and-down (vertical) pattern is recommended for examining the entire breast. Move around the breast in an up-and-down pattern starting at an imaginary line straight down your side from the underarm (including the tail of Spence, which is the triangular breast tissue projecting into the axilla), and moving across the breast to the middle of the sternum. Examine the entire breast going down until you feel only ribs and up to the neck or clavicle. Repeat procedure while examining your right breast. *4,* Stand in front of a mirror. Place your hands firmly on your hips, which will tighten the pectoralis muscles. Look at your breasts for size, shape, redness, scaliness, or dimpling of the breast skin or nipple. *5,* Examine each underarm while standing or sitting with arm slightly raised. Check for any lump, hard knot, or thickening of tissue.

- Clinical breast examination (CBE) preferably at least every 3 years for women in their 20s and 30s, and every year for women beginning at age 40.[7]
- Women should report any breast changes promptly to their health care provider. Breast self-examination (BSE) is an option for women starting at age 20.
- Women at increased risk (family history, genetic link, past breast cancer) should talk with their health care provider about the benefits and limitations of starting mammography screening earlier, having additional tests (e.g., breast ultrasound or magnetic resonance imaging [MRI]), or having more frequent examinations.

In recent years there has been some controversy regarding the value of BSE and its role in reducing mortality rates from breast cancer in women. While the benefit of BSE in reducing breast cancer deaths continues to be reviewed, BSE remains a useful technique in helping women develop awareness of how their breasts normally look and feel. Teach women beginning at age 20 the benefits and limitations of BSE and the importance of reporting breast changes (e.g., nipple discharge, a lump) to their health care provider.[8]

When teaching the woman about BSE, include information related to potential benefits, limitations, and harm (chance of a false-positive test result). Allow time for questions about the procedure and a return demonstration. At every periodic health examination, ask the woman who is performing BSE to demonstrate her technique. For women who choose to do BSE, the technique has recently been revised (Fig. 52-1).

BSE is recommended on a monthly schedule. For women who are having regular menstrual periods, this would be right after menstruation when breasts are less lumpy and tender. If menses are irregular or a woman is postmenopausal, advise choosing the same day each month. For women taking oral contraceptives, the first day of a new package may be a helpful reminder.

Diagnostic Studies

Radiologic Studies. Several techniques can be used to screen for breast disease or to help diagnose a suspicious

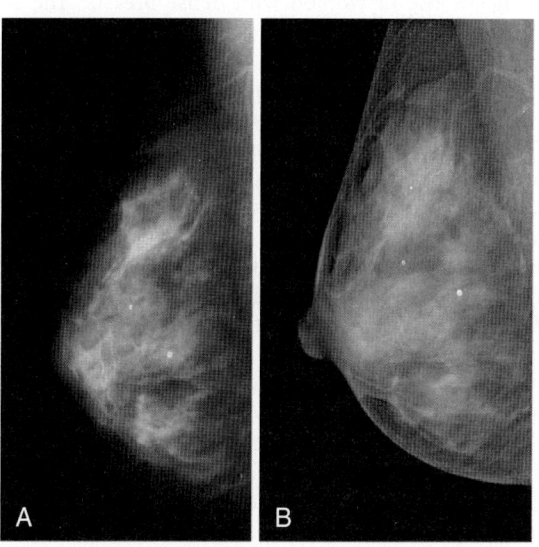

FIG. 52-2 Screening mammogram showing dense breast tissue and benign, scattered microcalcifications of a 57-year-old. **A,** Using conventional x-rays. **B,** Using digital x-rays.

physical finding. *Mammography* is a method used to visualize the breast's internal structure using x-rays (Fig. 52-2). This generally well-tolerated procedure can detect suspicious lumps that cannot be felt. Mammography has significantly improved the early and accurate detection of breast malignancies. Improved imaging technology has also reduced the radiation dose from mammography.

Digital mammography is a technique in which x-ray images are digitally coded into a computer (see Fig. 52-2). It is not clear whether mammogram interpretation has improved with the aid of a computer. The associated costs of using computer-aided detection may also outweigh the benefits.[9]

Three-dimensional (3D) mammography, a new type of mammogram that produces a 3D image of the breast, provides a clearer view of overlapping breast tissue structures. 3-D images help to accurately detect and diagnose breast cancer.

Calcifications are the most easily recognized mammogram abnormality (see Fig. 52-2). These deposits of calcium crystals form in the breast for many reasons, such as inflammation, trauma, and aging. Although most calcifications are benign, they may also be associated with preinvasive cancer.

A comparison of current and prior mammograms may show early tissue changes. Because some tumors metastasize late, early detection by mammography allows for earlier treatment and the prevention of metastasis. In younger women, mammography is less sensitive because of the greater density of breast tissue, resulting in more false-negative results.

About 10% to 15% of all breast cancers cannot be seen on mammography and are detected by palpation or additional diagnostic studies, including ultrasound and MRI. If the clinical findings are suspicious and the mammogram is normal, an ultrasound or MRI may be used. Based on these additional findings, a biopsy may be done.

Ultrasound is used in conjunction with mammography. It may be used to differentiate a solid mass from a cystic mass, to evaluate a mass in a pregnant or lactating woman, or to locate and biopsy a suspicious lesion.

The somo-v ABUS is an ultrasound device for breast cancer screening for use in women with dense breasts. The somo-v ABUS scans a woman's breast, capturing multiple ultrasound images that can be reviewed in 3D. This device is used along with standard mammography in women with a negative mammogram and no breast cancer symptoms.

MRI is recommended as a sensitive screening tool for women who are at high risk for breast cancer, whose mammography or ultrasound is suspicious for malignancy, or who have previously had an occult breast cancer detected by mammogram.

Biopsies. A definitive diagnosis of a suspicious area is made by analyzing biopsied tissue. Biopsy techniques include *fine-needle aspiration* (FNA), core (core needle), vacuum-assisted, and surgical biopsies.

FNA biopsy is performed by inserting a needle into a lesion to sample fluid from a breast cyst, remove cells from intercellular spaces, or sample cells from a solid mass. Before the procedure, the breast area is first locally anesthetized. Then the needle is placed into the breast, and fluid and cells are aspirated into a syringe. Three or four passes are usually made. If the results are negative with a suspicious lesion, an additional biopsy may be necessary. Inform patients that biopsy results are usually available in 1 to 3 days.

A *core (core needle) biopsy* involves removing small samples of breast tissue using a hollow "core" needle. For palpable lesions, this is accomplished by fixing the lesion with one hand and performing a needle biopsy with the other. In the case of nonpalpable lesions, *stereotactic mammography, ultrasound,* or MRI image guidance is used. Stereotactic mammography uses computers to pinpoint the exact location of a breast mass based on mammograms. With ultrasound, the radiologist or surgeon watches the needle on the ultrasound monitor to help guide it to the area of concern. Because a core biopsy removes more tissue than an FNA, it is more accurate.

Vacuum-assisted biopsy is a version of core biopsy that uses a vacuum technique to help collect the tissue sample. In core biopsy, several separate needle insertions are used to acquire multiple samples. During vacuum-assisted biopsy, the needle is inserted only once into the breast, and the needle can be rotated, which allows for multiple samples through a single needle insertion.

A *surgical biopsy* is used to remove a breast mass or lump or to obtain a sample of breast tissue for analysis. A surgical biopsy is usually performed in an operating room. Ten years ago, most breast biopsies were surgical procedures. Today less invasive biopsy procedures, such as core biopsies, are used.

BENIGN BREAST DISORDERS

MASTALGIA

Mastalgia (breast pain) is the most common breast-related complaint in women.[10] The most common form is *cyclic mastalgia,* which coincides with the menstrual cycle. It is described as diffuse breast tenderness or heaviness. Breast pain may last 2 or 3 days or most of the month. The pain is related to hormonal sensitivity. The symptoms often decrease with menopause.

Noncyclic mastalgia has no relationship to the menstrual cycle and can continue into menopause. It may be constant or intermittent throughout the month and last for several years. Symptoms include a burning, aching, or soreness in the breast. The pain may be from trauma, fat necrosis, ductal ectasia, costochrondritis, or arthritic pain in the chest or neck radiating to the breast.

Mammography and targeted ultrasound are frequently done to exclude cancer and provide information on the etiology of mastalgia. Some relief for cyclic pain may occur by reducing intake of caffeine and dietary fat; taking vitamins E, A, and B complex and gamma-linolenic acid (evening primrose oil); and continually wearing a support bra. Compresses, ice, analgesics, and antiinflammatory drugs may also help. Helpful drugs include oral contraceptives and danazol (Danocrine). The androgenic side effects of danazol (acne, edema, hirsutism) may make this therapy unacceptable for many women.

BREAST INFECTIONS

Mastitis

Mastitis is an inflammatory condition of the breast that occurs most frequently in lactating women (Table 52-1). *Lactational mastitis* manifests as a localized area that is erythematous, painful, and tender to palpation. Fever is often present. The infection develops when organisms (usually staphylococci) gain access to the breast through a cracked nipple. In its early stages, mastitis can be cured with antibiotics. Breastfeeding should continue unless an abscess is forming or purulent drainage is noted. The mother may wish to use a nipple shield or to hand-express milk from the involved breast until the pain subsides. The woman should see her health care provider promptly to begin a course of antibiotic therapy. Any breast that remains red, tender, and not responsive to antibiotics requires follow-up care and evaluation for inflammatory breast cancer.[11]

Lactational Breast Abscess

If lactational mastitis persists after several days of antibiotic therapy, a lactational breast abscess may have developed. In this condition, the skin may become red and edematous over the involved breast, often with a corresponding palpable mass, and the patient may have a fever. Antibiotics alone are insufficient treatment for a breast abscess. Ultrasound-guided drainage of the abscess or surgical incision and drainage are necessary. The drainage is cultured, sensitivities are obtained, and therapy with

TABLE 52-1 **BENIGN BREAST DISORDERS***

Disorder	Risk Factors	Clinical Manifestations
Lactational mastitis	Occurs in up to 10% of postpartum lactating mothers (both primipara and multipara), usually 2-4 wk after birth.	Warm to touch, indurated, painful, often unilateral, most commonly caused by *Staphylococcus aureus.*
Fibrocystic changes	Most common between ages 35 and 50.	Not usually discrete masses—nodularity instead. Usually accompanied by cyclic pain and tenderness. Mass(es) often cyclic in occurrence (movable, soft).
Cysts	Most common over age 35. Incidence decreases after menopause. Develop in one out of every 14 women.	Palpable fluid-filled mass (movable, soft). Multiple cysts can occur and recur. Rarely associated with breast cancer.
Fibroadenoma	Commonly occurs in 10% of all women ages 15-40.	Palpable mass (firm, movable), usually 2-3 cm in size, rarely associated with breast cancer.
Fat necrosis	Many women report previous history of trauma to breast.	Usually a hard, tender, mobile, indurated mass with irregular borders.
Ductal ectasia	Perimenopausal woman—most common in women in their 50s, previous lactation, inverted nipples.	Fixation of nipple, usually accompanied by nipple discharge of thick gray material. Often associated with breast pain.

*This list is not inclusive; other benign breast disorders are discussed in the text.

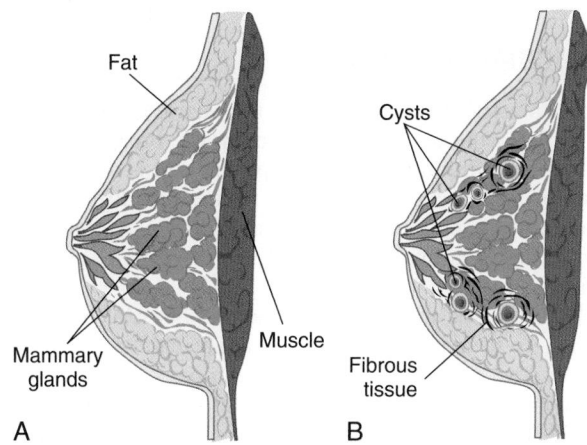

FIG. 52-3 A, Normal breast tissue. **B,** Fibrocystic breast tissue.

an appropriate antibiotic is begun. Breastfeeding can continue in most cases with ongoing treatment of the abscess.

FIBROCYSTIC CHANGES

Fibrocystic changes in the breast are a benign condition characterized by changes in breast tissue[12] (Fig. 52-3). The changes include the development of excess fibrous tissue, hyperplasia of the epithelial lining of the mammary ducts, proliferation of mammary ducts, and cyst formation. Fibrocystic changes are thought to be due to a heightened responsiveness of breast tissue to circulating estrogen and progesterone. These changes produce pain related to nerve irritation from edema in the connective tissue and to fibrosis that pinches the nerve. Fibrocystic changes are the most common breast disorder.

The use of the term *fibrocystic disease* is incorrect because the cluster of problems is actually an exaggerated response to hormonal influence. The terms *fibrocystic condition* or *fibrocystic complex* are more accurate.

Fibrocystic changes alone are not associated with increased breast cancer risk. Masses or nodularities can appear in both breasts. They are often found in the upper, outer quadrants and usually occur bilaterally.

Fibrocystic changes occur most frequently in women between 35 and 50 years of age but often begin as early as 20 years of age. Pain and nodularity often increase over time but tend to subside after menopause unless high doses of estrogen replace-

ment are used. Fibrocystic changes most commonly occur in women with premenstrual abnormalities, nulliparous women, women with a history of spontaneous abortion, nonusers of oral contraceptives, and women with early menarche and late menopause. Symptoms related to fibrocystic changes often worsen in the premenstrual phase and subside after menstruation.

Manifestations of fibrocystic breast changes include one or more palpable lumps that are often round, well delineated, and freely movable within the breast (see Table 52-1). Discomfort ranging from tenderness to pain may also occur. The lump is usually observed to increase in size and perhaps in tenderness before menstruation. Cysts may enlarge or shrink rapidly. Nipple discharge associated with fibrocystic breasts is often milky, watery-milky, yellow, or green.

Mammography may be helpful in distinguishing fibrocystic changes from breast cancer. However, in some women the breast tissue is so dense that it is difficult to obtain a mammogram. In these situations, ultrasound may be more useful in differentiating a cystic mass from a solid mass.

NURSING AND COLLABORATIVE MANAGEMENT
FIBROCYSTIC CHANGES

With the initial discovery of a discrete mass in the breast by a woman or her health care provider, aspiration or surgical biopsy may be indicated. If the nodularity is recurrent, a wait of 7 to 10 days may be planned in order to note any changes that may be related to the menstrual cycle. With large or frequent cysts, surgical removal may be favored over repeated aspiration. An excisional biopsy may be done if (1) no fluid is found on aspiration, (2) the fluid that is found is hemorrhagic, or (3) a residual mass remains after fluid aspiration. The biopsy is usually performed in an outpatient surgery unit.

Biopsies in women with fibrocystic disease may be indicated if these women have an increased risk for breast cancer. Atypical hyperplasia discovered by breast biopsy increases a woman's risk of developing breast cancer later in life.

Encourage the woman with cystic changes to maintain regular follow-up care. Also teach her BSE to self-monitor changes. Severe fibrocystic changes may make palpation of the breast more difficult. Teach her to report any changes in symptoms or changes found during the BSE so they can be evaluated.

Treatment for a fibrocystic condition is similar to that described earlier for mastalgia. Teach the woman with fibrocystic breasts that she may expect a recurrence of the cysts in one or both breasts until menopause and that the cysts may enlarge or become painful just before menstruation. Additionally, reassure her that the cysts do not "turn into" cancer. Advise her that any new lump that does not respond in a cyclic manner over 1 to 2 weeks should be examined by her health care provider.

FIBROADENOMA

Fibroadenoma is a common cause of discrete benign breast lumps in young women. It generally occurs in women between 15 and 40 years of age. It is the most frequent cause of breast masses in women under 25 years of age.

The possible cause of fibroadenoma may be increased estrogen sensitivity in a localized area of the breast. Fibroadenomas are usually small (but can be large [2 to 3 cm]), painless, round, well delineated, and very mobile. They may be soft but are usually solid, firm, and rubbery in consistency. There is no accompanying retraction or nipple discharge. The lump is often painless. The fibroadenoma may appear as a single unilateral mass, although multiple bilateral fibroadenomas have been reported. Growth is slow and often ceases when the size reaches 2 to 3 cm. Size is not affected by menstruation. However, pregnancy can stimulate dramatic growth.

Fibroadenomas are easily detected by physical examination and may be visible on mammography and ultrasound. However, definitive diagnosis requires FNA, core, or surgical biopsy and tissue examination by a pathologist to exclude other tumors. Treatment of fibroadenomas can include observation with regular monitoring after a malignancy has been ruled out, or surgical excision. In women over 35 years of age, all new lesions should be evaluated by breast ultrasound and possible biopsy.

As an alternative to surgery, tumor removal can be done using *cryoablation*. In this procedure, a cryoprobe is inserted into the tumor using ultrasound guidance. Extremely cold gas is piped into the tumor. The frozen tumor dies and gradually shrinks.

NIPPLE DISCHARGE

Nipple discharge may occur spontaneously or as a result of nipple manipulation. A milky secretion is due to inappropriate lactation (termed galactorrhea) and may be a result of problems such as drug therapy, endocrine problems, and neurologic disorders. Nipple discharge may also be idiopathic (no known cause).

Secretions can also be serous, grossly bloody, or brown to green.[13] These secretions may be caused by either benign or malignant disease. A cytology slide may be made of the secretion to determine the specific disease. Diseases associated with nipple discharge include malignancies, cystic disease, intraductal papilloma, and ductal ectasia. Treatment depends on identification of the cause. In most cases, nipple discharge is not related to malignancy.

Intraductal Papilloma

An intraductal papilloma is a benign, soft, wartlike growth found in the mammary ducts. It is usually unilateral. Typically, the nipple has a bloody discharge that can be intermittent or spontaneous. Most intraductal papillomas are beneath the areola, and they may be difficult to palpate. They are usually found in women 40 to 60 years of age. A single duct or several ducts may be involved. Treatment includes excision of the papilloma and the involved duct or duct system. Papillomas may be associated with an increased risk of cancer.

Ductal Ectasia

Ductal ectasia (duct dilation) is a benign breast disease of perimenopausal and postmenopausal women involving the ducts in the subareolar area. It usually involves several bilateral ducts. Multicolored, sticky nipple discharge is the primary symptom. Ductal ectasia is initially painless but may progress to burning, itching, and pain around the nipple, as well as swelling in the areolar area. Inflammatory signs are often present, the nipple may retract, and the discharge may become bloody in more advanced disease. Ductal ectasia is not associated with malignancy. If an abscess develops, warm compresses and antibiotics are usually effective treatments. Therapy consists of close follow-up examinations or surgical excision of the involved ducts.

GYNECOMASTIA IN MEN

Gynecomastia, a transient, noninflammatory enlargement of one or both breasts, is the most common breast problem in men. The condition is usually temporary and benign. Gynecomastia in itself is not a risk factor for breast cancer. The most common cause of gynecomastia is a disturbance of the normal ratio of active androgen to estrogen in plasma or within the breast itself.

Gynecomastia may also be a manifestation of other problems. It is seen in developmental abnormalities of the male reproductive organs. It may also accompany diseases such as testicular tumors, adrenal cancer, pituitary adenomas, hyperthyroidism, and liver disease.[14] Gynecomastia may occur as a side effect of drug therapy, particularly with estrogens and androgens, digitalis, isoniazid (INH), ranitidine (Zantac), and spironolactone (Aldactone). The use of heroin and marijuana can also cause gynecomastia.

Senescent Gynecomastia

Senescent gynecomastia occurs in many older men. A probable cause is the elevation in plasma estrogen in older adult men as the result of increased conversion of androgens to estrogens in peripheral circulation. Although initially unilateral, the tender, firm, centrally located enlargement may become bilateral. When gynecomastia is characterized by a discrete, circumscribed mass, it must be biopsied to differentiate it from the rarer breast cancer in males. Senescent hyperplasia requires no treatment and generally regresses within 6 to 12 months.

GERONTOLOGIC CONSIDERATIONS

AGE-RELATED BREAST CHANGES

The loss of subcutaneous fat and structural support and the atrophy of mammary glands often result in pendulous breasts in the postmenopausal woman. Encourage older women to wear a well-fitting bra. Adequate support can improve physical appearance and reduce pain in the back, shoulders, and neck. It can also prevent *intertrigo* (dermatitis caused by friction between opposing surfaces of skin). Sagging breasts can be surgically lifted (mastopexy). This procedure can be done in conjunction with breast reconstruction after a mastectomy is performed.

The decrease in glandular tissue in older women makes a breast mass easier to palpate. This decreased density is likely a result of age-related decreases in estrogen. Rib margins may be palpable in a thin woman and can be confused with a mass. That is why it is so important that women become familiar with their own breasts and what is normal for them. Because the incidence of breast cancer increases with age, encourage older women to continue BSE, to have annual mammograms and CBEs, and to have any breast mass evaluated by their health care provider.

BREAST CANCER

Breast cancer is the most common malignancy in American women except for skin cancer. It is second only to lung cancer as the leading cause of death from cancer in women. In the United States more than 230,480 new cases of invasive breast cancer and more than 57,650 cases of in situ breast cancer are diagnosed annually.[1] About 2140 of those new cases are diagnosed in men. Approximately 39,920 deaths (39,510 women and 410 men) occur each year related to breast cancer.

The incidence of breast cancer is slowly decreasing, with a slight drop in the number of deaths related to breast cancer. This decline may be the result of the decreased use of hormone therapy after menopause.[2] Approximately 2.6 million women are alive in the United States today who are breast cancer survivors.

Patients diagnosed with localized breast cancer with no axillary node involvement have a 5-year survival rate of 98%. Conversely, only 23% of patients diagnosed with advanced-stage breast cancer with metastases to distant sites will survive 5 years or more.[1,2]

Etiology and Risk Factors

Although the etiology is not completely understood, a number of risk factors are related to breast cancer (Table 52-2). Risk factors appear to be cumulative and interacting. Therefore the presence of multiple risk factors may greatly increase the overall risk, especially for people with a positive family history.

Risk Factors for Women. The risk factors most associated with breast cancer include female gender and advancing age. Women are at far greater risk than men, with 99% of breast cancers occurring in women. Increasing age also increases the risk of developing breast cancer. The incidence of breast cancer in women under 25 years of age is very low and increases gradually until age 60. After age 60, the incidence increases dramatically.

Hormonal regulation of the breast is related to the development of breast cancer, but the mechanisms are poorly understood. The hormones estrogen and progesterone may act as tumor promoters to stimulate breast cancer growth if malignant changes in the cells have already occurred. The Women's Health Initiative study showed that the use of combined hormone therapy (estrogen plus progesterone) increases the risk of breast cancer and also the risk of having a larger, more advanced breast cancer at diagnosis.[15] The use of estrogen therapy alone for longer than 10 years (for women with a prior hysterectomy) increases a woman's long-term risk for breast cancer. A link may exist between recent oral contraceptive use and increased risk of breast cancer for younger women.[16]

Modifiable risk factors include excess weight gain during adulthood, sedentary lifestyle, smoking, dietary fat intake, obesity, and alcohol intake.[10] Environmental factors such as radiation exposure may also play a role.

TABLE 52-2   RISK FACTORS FOR BREAST CANCER

Risk Factor	Comments
Female	Women account for 99% of breast cancer cases.
Age ≥50 yr	Majority of breast cancers are found in postmenopausal women. After age 60, increase in incidence.
Hormone use	Use of estrogen and/or progesterone as hormone therapy, especially in postmenopausal women.
Family history	Breast cancer in a first-degree relative, particularly when premenopausal or bilateral, increases risk.
Genetic factors	Gene mutations (BRCA1 or BRCA2) play a role in 5%-10% of breast cancer cases.
Personal history of breast cancer, colon cancer, endometrial cancer, ovarian cancer	Personal history significantly increases risk of breast cancer, risk of cancer in other breast, and recurrence.
Early menarche (before age 12), late menopause (after age 55)	A long menstrual history increases the risk of breast cancer.
First full-term pregnancy after age 30, nulliparity	Prolonged exposure to unopposed estrogen increases risk for breast cancer.
Benign breast disease with atypical epithelial hyperplasia, lobular carcinoma in situ	Atypical changes in breast biopsy increase the risk of breast cancer.
Dense breast tissue	Mammograms harder to read and interpret. Dense tissue may be associated with more aggressive tumors.
Weight gain and obesity after menopause	Fat cells store estrogen, which increases the likelihood of developing breast cancer.
Exposure to ionizing radiation	Radiation damages DNA (e.g., prior treatment for Hodgkin's lymphoma).
Alcohol consumption	Women who drink ≥1 alcoholic beverage per day have an increased risk of breast cancer.
Physical inactivity	Breast cancer risk is decreased in physically active women.

Genetic Link

Family history of breast cancer is an important risk factor, especially if the involved family member also had ovarian cancer, was premenopausal, had bilateral breast cancer, or is a first-degree relative (i.e., mother, sister, daughter). Having any first-degree relative with breast cancer increases a woman's risk of breast cancer 1.5 to 3 times, depending on age. A breast cancer risk assessment tool for health care providers is available through the National Cancer Institute (see Resources at the end of this chapter). About 5% to 10% of all breast cancers are hereditary. This means that specific genetic abnormalities that contribute to the development of breast cancer have been inherited (passed from parent to child). Most inherited cases of breast cancer are associated with mutations in two genes: BRCA1 and BRCA2 (BRCA stands for BReast CAncer). Everyone has BRCA genes. The BRCA1 gene, located on chromosome 17, is a tumor suppressor gene that inhibits tumor development when func-

GENETICS IN CLINICAL PRACTICE

Breast Cancer

Genetic Basis
- Mutations occur in *BRCA1* and/or *BRCA2* genes.
- Normally these genes are tumor suppressor genes involved in DNA repair.
- Transmission is autosomal dominant.

Incidence
- Approximately 5% to 10% of breast cancers are related to *BRCA1* and *BRCA2* gene mutations.
- Women with *BRCA1* and *BRCA2* gene mutations have a 40% to 80% lifetime risk of developing breast cancer.
- *BRCA1* and *BRCA2* gene mutations are associated with early-onset breast cancer that is more likely to involve both breasts.
- Men with mutations in *BRCA1* and *BRCA2* have an increased risk of breast cancer and prostate cancer.
- Family history of both breast and ovarian cancer increases the risk of having a *BRCA* mutation.

Genetic Testing
- DNA testing is available for *BRCA1* and *BRCA2* gene mutations.

Clinical Implications
- Most breast cancers (about 90%-95%) are not inherited. They are associated with genetic changes that occur after a person is born (somatic mutations). There is no risk of passing on the mutated gene to children.
- Bilateral oophorectomy and/or bilateral mastectomy reduces the risk of breast cancer in women with *BRCA1* and *BRCA2* mutations.
- Mutations in the *BRCA1* and *BRCA2* genes increase the risk of ovarian cancer.
- Genetic counseling and testing for *BRCA* mutations should be considered for women whose personal or family history puts them at high risk for a genetic predisposition to breast cancer.

BRCA, BReast CAncer.

tioning normally. Women who have *BRCA1* mutations have a 40% to 80% lifetime chance of developing breast cancer. The *BRCA2* gene, located on chromosome 11, is another tumor suppressor gene. Women with a mutation of this gene have a similar risk of breast cancer.

Mutations in *BRCA* genes may cause as many as 10% to 40% of all inherited breast cancers. As many as 1 in 200 to 400 women in the United States may be carriers for these genetic abnormalities. Women with *BRCA* mutations are also at higher risk for developing ovarian, colon, pancreatic, and uterine cancers.[17]

In addition to *BRCA* gene mutations, many other abnormal genes have been identified that increase a person's risk of developing breast cancer. These include the tumor suppressor gene *p53* (which inhibits tumor development when functioning normally), *ATM* (which helps to repair damaged deoxyribonucleic acid [DNA]), and *CHEK2* (which stops tumor growth).

Most people who develop breast cancer do not inherit an abnormal breast cancer gene, and they do not have a family history of breast cancer. Ongoing research continues to investigate the role of genes in the development of breast cancer.

Risk Factors for Men. Predisposing risk factors for breast cancer in men include hyperestrogenism, a family history of breast cancer, and radiation exposure. A thorough examination of the male breast should be a routine part of a physical examination. Men in *BRCA*-positive families may consider genetic testing. Men with an abnormal *BRCA* gene also have an increased risk of developing prostate cancer.

TABLE 52-3 TYPES OF BREAST CANCER

Type	Frequency of Occurrence
Noninvasive	20%
• Ductal carcinoma in situ	
Invasive/Infiltrating Ductal Carcinoma	70%-75%
• Medullary	
• Tubular	
• Colloid (mucinous)	
• Inflammatory	
• Paget's disease	
Invasive/Infiltrating Lobular Carcinoma	5%-10%

Prophylactic Oophorectomy and Mastectomy. In women with *BRCA1* or *BRCA2* mutations, prophylactic bilateral oophorectomy can decrease the risk of breast cancer and ovarian cancer. Removing the ovaries lowers the risk of breast cancer because the ovaries are the main source of estrogen in a premenopausal woman. Removing the ovaries does not reduce the risk of breast cancer in postmenopausal women because the ovaries are not the main producers of estrogen in these women. A woman who has a high risk of developing breast cancer (i.e., related to factors such as family history and prior tissue biopsies) may choose (in consultation with her physician and genetic counselor) to undergo prophylactic bilateral mastectomy.

Younger women with hereditary (non-*BRCA*) early-stage, estrogen receptor–negative breast cancer may have a higher risk of developing a secondary primary breast cancer in the unaffected (contralateral) breast.[18] These women may also choose to have the unaffected breast removed prophylactically at the time of initial surgery for breast cancer or at a later time.

Pathophysiology

The main components of the breast are lobules (milk-producing glands) and ducts (milk passages that connect the lobules and the nipple). In general, breast cancer arises from the epithelial lining of the ducts *(ductal carcinoma)* or from the epithelium of the lobules *(lobular carcinoma)*. Breast cancers may be *in situ* (within the duct) or invasive (arising from the duct and invading through the wall of the duct).

Metastatic breast cancer is breast cancer that has spread to other organs, with the most common sites being bone, liver, lung, and brain. Cancer growth rates can range from slow to rapid. Factors that affect cancer prognosis are tumor size, axillary node involvement (the more nodes involved, the worse the prognosis), tumor differentiation, estrogen and progesterone receptor status, and *human epidermal growth factor receptor 2* (HER-2) status. HER-2 is a protein that helps regulate cell growth. It is overexpressed in about 25% of patients with breast cancer.[19,20]

Types of Breast Cancer

Breast cancer can be classified as noninvasive or invasive, and ductal or lobular (Table 52-3).

Noninvasive Breast Cancer. An estimated 20% of all diagnosed breast cancers are noninvasive. These intraductal cancers include *ductal carcinoma in situ* (DCIS) and *lobular carcinoma in situ* (LCIS). DCIS tends to be unilateral and may progress to invasive breast cancer if left untreated.

Although the management of DCIS can be controversial, patients should discuss treatment options with their health care provider, including breast-conserving treatment (lumpectomy), mastectomy with breast reconstruction, radiation therapy, and/or hormone therapy (tamoxifen [Nolvadex], anastrozole [Arimidex]).

The term *lobular carcinoma in situ* is somewhat misleading. Although LCIS is a risk factor for developing breast cancer, it is not known to be a premalignant lesion. No surgical or radiation treatment is indicated for LCIS. Hormone therapy may be used as a preventive measure to reduce breast cancer risk for some patients.

Invasive (Infiltrating) Ductal Carcinoma. *Invasive (infiltrating) ductal carcinoma* is the most common type of breast cancer. It starts in the milk duct and then breaks through the wall of the duct, invading the surrounding tissue. From there it may metastasize to other parts of the body.

Types of invasive (infiltrating) ductal carcinoma include *medullary carcinoma,* which accounts for 15% of all breast cancers. It most frequently occurs in women in their late 40s and 50s, manifesting with cells that resemble the medulla of the brain. *Tubular carcinoma* accounts for about 2% of all breast cancers. This type of breast cancer is usually found in women over 50. It has an excellent prognosis. *Colloid (mucinous) carcinoma* accounts for about 1% to 2% of all breast cancer. These tumors, which produce mucus, usually have a favorable prognosis.

Inflammatory Breast Cancer. *Inflammatory breast cancer* is an aggressive and fast-growing breast cancer with a high risk for metastasis. The lymph channels in the skin of the breast become blocked by cancer cells. Because of skin involvement, the breast looks red, feels warm, and has a thickened appearance that is often described as resembling an orange peel *(peau d'orange).*[21] Sometimes the breast develops ridges and small bumps that look like hives. A breast mass may or may not be present.

Paget's Disease. Paget's disease is a rare breast malignancy characterized by a persistent lesion of the nipple and areola with or without a mass. (This is different from Paget's disease of the bone, which is discussed in Chapter 64.) Most women with Paget's disease have underlying ductal carcinoma. Only in rare cases is the cancer confined to the nipple itself.

Itching, burning, bloody nipple discharge with superficial skin erosion and ulceration may be present. Diagnosis of Paget's disease is confirmed by pathologic examination of the lesion. Nipple changes are often diagnosed as an infection or dermatitis, which can lead to treatment delays.

The treatment of Paget's disease is surgical removal of the involved tissue (central lumpectomy or mastectomy). Radiation therapy may also be used after surgery. The prognosis is good when the cancer is confined to the nipple. The nursing care for the patient with Paget's disease is the same as the care for a patient with breast cancer.

Invasive (Infiltrating) Lobular Carcinoma. *Invasive (infiltrating) lobular carcinoma* begins in the lobules (milk-producing glands) of the breast. The cancer cells can break out of the lobule and have the potential to metastasize to other areas of the body. Invasive lobular carcinoma is a type of breast cancer that usually appears as a subtle thickening in the upper outer quadrant of the breast. Often positive for estrogen and progesterone receptors, these tumors respond well to hormone therapy.

Clinical Manifestations

Breast cancer is usually detected as a lump or thickening in the breast or mammographic abnormality. It occurs most often in

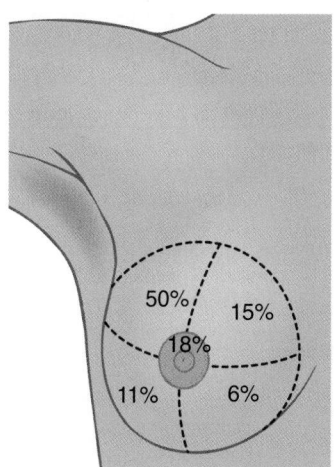

FIG. 52-4 Distribution of where breast cancer occurs.

the upper, outer quadrant of the breast, which is the location of most of the glandular tissue (Fig. 52-4). Breast cancers vary in their growth rate. If palpable, breast cancer is characteristically hard and may be irregularly shaped, poorly delineated, nonmobile, and nontender.

A small percentage of breast cancers cause nipple discharge. The discharge is usually unilateral and may be clear or bloody. Nipple retraction may occur. Peau d'orange may occur due to plugging of the dermal lymphatics. In large cancers, infiltration, induration, and dimpling (pulling in) of the overlying skin may also occur.

Complications

The main complication of breast cancer is recurrence (Table 52-4). Recurrence may be *local* or *regional* (skin or soft tissue near the mastectomy site, axillary or internal mammary lymph nodes) or *distant* (most commonly involving bone, lung, brain, and liver). However, metastatic disease can be found in any site in the body.

Widely disseminated or metastatic disease involves the growth of colonies of cancerous breast cells in parts of the body distant from the breast. Metastases primarily occur through the lymphatics, usually those of the axilla (Fig. 52-5). However, the cancer can spread to other parts of the body without invading the axillary nodes even when the primary breast tumor is small. Even in patients who do not have lymph node involvement (node-negative breast cancer), there is a possibility of distant metastasis.

Diagnostic Studies

In addition to radiologic and biopsy studies used to diagnose breast cancer (see earlier discussion in this chapter on pp. 1239-1240), other tests are used to predict the risk of local or systemic recurrence. These tests include axillary lymph node status, tumor size, estrogen and progesterone receptor status, cell-proliferative indices, and genomic assays.

Axillary lymph node involvement is one of the most important prognostic factors in breast cancer. *Axillary lymph nodes* are often examined to determine if cancer has spread to the axilla on the side of the breast cancer. The more nodes involved, the greater the risk of recurrence.

Lymphatic mapping and *sentinel lymph node dissection* (SLND) help the surgeon identify the lymph node(s) that drain first from the tumor site *(sentinel node).* An SLND is less inva-

TABLE 52-4   SITES OF BREAST CANCER RECURRENCE AND METASTASIS

Site	Clinical Manifestations
Local Recurrence	
Skin, chest wall	Firm, discrete nodules. Occasionally pruritic, usually painless, commonly in or near a scar.
Regional Recurrence	
Lymph nodes	Enlarged nodes in axilla or supraclavicular area, usually nontender.
Distant Metastasis	
Skeletal	Localized pain of gradually increasing intensity, percussion tenderness at involved sites, pathologic fracture caused by involvement of bone cortex.
Spinal cord	Progressive back pain, localized and radiating. Change in bladder or bowel function. Loss of sensation in lower extremities.
Brain	Headache described as "different," unilateral sensory loss, focal muscular weakness, hemiparesis, incoordination (ataxia), nausea and vomiting unrelated to medication, cognitive changes.
Pulmonary (including lung nodules and pleural effusions)	Shortness of breath, tachypnea, nonproductive cough (not present in all patients).
Liver	Abdominal distention. Right lower quadrant abdominal pain sometimes with radiation to scapular area. Nausea and vomiting, anorexia, weight loss. Weakness and fatigue. Hepatomegaly, ascites, jaundice. Peripheral edema. Elevated liver enzymes.
Bone marrow	Anemia, infection, increased bleeding, bruising, petechiae. Weakness, fatigue, mild confusion, light-headedness. Dyspnea.

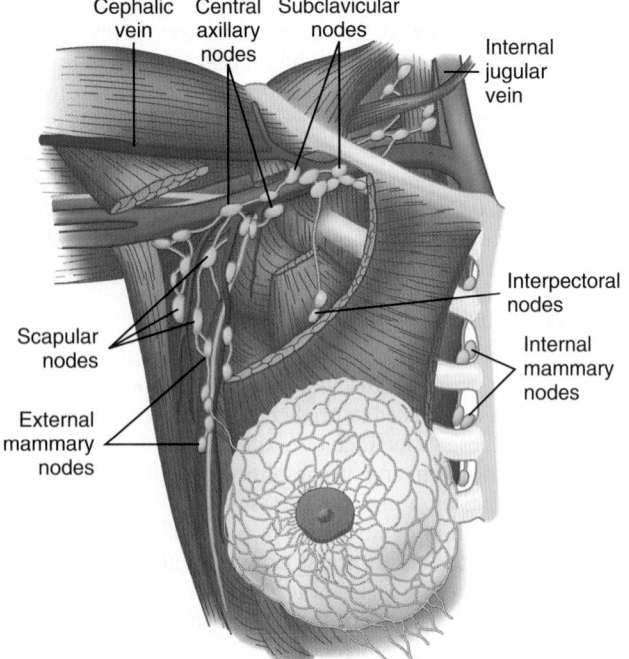

FIG. 52-5 Lymph nodes and drainage in the axilla. The sentinel lymph node is usually found in the external mammary nodes. A complete axillary dissection would remove all nodes.

sive than an axillary lymph node dissection (ALND). In SLND a radioisotope and/or blue dye is injected into the affected breast, and intraoperatively it is determined in which sentinel lymph nodes (SLNs) the radioisotope or dye is located. A local incision is made in the axilla, and the surgeon dissects the blue-stained or radioactive SLNs. Generally, with an SLND, one to four axillary lymph nodes are removed. The nodes may be sent for pathologic analysis. If the SLNs are negative, no further axillary surgery is required. If the SLNs are positive, a complete axillary dissection may be done, depending on the patient's clinical situation. SLND is associated with lower morbidity rates and greater accuracy compared with complete ALND.

Tumor size is a prognostic variable: the larger the tumor, the poorer the prognosis. The wide variety of biologic types of breast cancer explains the variability of disease behavior. In general, the more well differentiated (like the original cell type) the tumor, the less aggressive it is. The cells of poorly differentiated (unlike the original cell type) tumors appear morphologically disorganized, and they are more aggressive.

Estrogen and progesterone receptor status is another diagnostic test useful for decisions about both treatment and prognosis.[12] Receptor-positive tumors (1) commonly show histologic evidence of being well differentiated, (2) frequently have a *diploid* (more normal) DNA content and low proliferative indices, (3) have a lower chance for recurrence, and (4) are frequently hormone dependent and responsive to hormone therapy. Receptor-negative tumors (1) are often poorly differentiated histologically, (2) have a high incidence of *aneuploidy* (abnormally high or low DNA content) and higher proliferative indices, (3) frequently recur, and (4) are usually unresponsive to hormone therapy.

Ploidy status correlates with tumor aggressiveness. Diploid tumors have been shown to have a significantly lower risk of recurrence than aneuploid tumors.

Cell-proliferative indices indirectly measure the rate of tumor cell proliferation. The percentage of tumor cells in the synthesis (S) phase of the cell cycle (see Chapter 16, Fig. 16-1) is another important prognostic indicator. Patients with cells that have high S-phase fractions have a higher risk for recurrence and earlier cancer death.

Another prognostic indicator is the marker HER-2. Overexpression of this receptor has been associated with unusually aggressive tumor growth, a greater risk for recurrence, and a poorer prognosis in breast cancer.[20] About 25% of metastatic breast cancers produce excessive HER-2. The presence of this marker assists in the selection and sequence of drug therapy and predicts the patient's response to treatment.

A patient whose breast cancer tests negative for all three receptors (estrogen, progesterone, and HER-2) has *triple-negative breast cancer.*[22] This subtype of breast cancer accounts for approximately 10% to 20% of cases. The incidence of triple-negative breast cancer is higher in Hispanics, African Americans, younger women, and women with a *BRCA1* mutation. These patients tend to have more aggressive tumors with a poorer prognosis.

A *genomic assay* is a test that uses a sample of the breast cancer tissue to analyze the activity of a group of genes. Knowing whether certain genes are present or absent, or overly active or not active enough, can provide information about the risk of recurrence and the likely benefit of chemotherapy or hormone therapy. Two genomic assays are currently in use for breast cancer: Oncotype DX and MammaPrint. These tests are typically reserved for patients who (1) have early-stage breast cancer with no to few lymph nodes involved; and (2), in the case of Oncotype DX, have estrogen receptor–positive breast cancer that can be treated with hormone therapy.

Cancer markers for breast cancer include CA 15-3 and CA 27-29. These proteins are produced by the *MUC1* gene. Breast cancer cells shed copies of these proteins into the bloodstream. These markers are not specific or sensitive enough to be used as a screening tool to detect early breast cancer. Although not recommended at this time, these markers may be used to monitor a patient's response to treatment of invasive breast cancer and detect recurrence of the disease.

Collaborative Care

A wide range of treatment options is available to the patient and health care providers making critical decisions about how to treat breast cancer (Table 52-5). Prognostic factors are considered when treatment decisions are made. The therapeutic regimen is often determined by the clinical stage and biology of the cancer.

Staging of Breast Cancer. The most widely accepted staging method for breast cancer is the TNM system.[23] This system uses tumor size (T), nodal involvement (N), and presence of metastasis (M) to determine the stage of disease. The stage of a breast cancer describes its size and the extent to which it has spread (Table 52-6).

The stages range from 0 to IV, with stage 0 being in situ cancer with no lymph node involvement and no metastasis. Further classification within these stages depends on tumor size and the number of lymph nodes involved. Stage IV indicates metastatic spread, regardless of tumor size or lymph node involvement. The presence or absence of malignant cells in lymph nodes remains a powerful prognostic factor related to local recurrence or metastasis after primary therapy.

Surgical Therapy. Surgery is considered the primary treatment for breast cancer. Table 52-7 describes the most common surgical procedures used to treat breast cancer. The most common surgical options for resectable breast cancer are (1) breast conservation surgery (lumpectomy) and (2) modified radical mastectomy. Most women diagnosed with early-stage breast cancer (tumors smaller than 4 to 5 cm) are candidates for either treatment choice. The overall survival rate with lumpectomy and radiation is about the same as that with modified radical mastectomy.

Breast-Conserving Surgery. Breast-conserving surgery (also called lumpectomy or partial mastectomy) usually involves removal of the entire tumor along with a margin of normal surrounding tissue (Fig. 52-6, *A*). After surgery, radiation therapy is delivered to the entire breast, ending with a boost to

---

TABLE 52-5 COLLABORATIVE CARE

Breast Cancer

Diagnostic
Prediagnosis
- Health history, including risk factors
- Physical examination, including breast and lymph nodes
- Mammography
- Ultrasound
- Breast MRI (if indicated)
- Biopsy

Postdiagnosis
- Lymphatic mapping and sentinel lymph node dissection (SLND)
- Estrogen and progesterone receptor status
- Cell-proliferative indices
- HER-2 marker
- Genetic assays (MammaPrint and Oncotype DX)

Staging
- Complete blood count, platelet count
- Calcium and phosphorus levels
- Liver function tests
- Chest x-ray
- Bone scan (if indicated)
- CT scan of chest, abdomen, pelvis (if indicated)
- MRI (if indicated)
- PET/CT scan (if indicated)

Collaborative Therapy
Surgery
- Breast-conserving surgery (lumpectomy) with SLND and biopsy and/or axillary lymph node dissection
- Modified radical mastectomy (may include immediate or delayed reconstruction)

Radiation Therapy
- Primary radiation therapy
- Brachytherapy
- Palliative radiation therapy

Drug Therapy (see Table 52-8)
- Chemotherapy
- Hormone therapy
- Biologic and targeted therapy
- Chemotherapy
- Hormone therapy
- Biologic and targeted therapy

HER-2, Human epidermal growth factor receptor 2; *PET,* positron emission tomography.

TABLE 52-6 STAGING OF BREAST CANCER

Stage	Tumor Size	Lymph Node Involvement	Metastasis
0	TIS*	No	No
I	<2 cm	No	No
II			
A	No evidence of tumor ranging to 5 cm	No, or 1-3 axillary nodes and/or internal mammary nodes	No
B	Ranging from 2 to >5 cm	No, or 1-3 axillary nodes and/or internal mammary nodes	No
III			
A	No evidence of tumor ranging to >5 cm	Yes, 4-9 axillary nodes and/or internal mammary nodes	No
B	Any size with extension to chest wall or skin	Yes, 4-9 axillary nodes and/or internal mammary nodes	No
C	Any size	Yes, ≥10 axillary nodes, internal mammary nodes, or infraclavicular nodes	No
IV	Any size	Any type of nodal involvement	Yes

Modified from American Joint Committee on Cancer: AJCC cancer staging manual, ed 7. Retrieved from *www.cancerstaging.org/staging/changes2010.*
**TIS,* Tumor in situ.

TABLE 52-7   **SURGICAL PROCEDURES FOR BREAST CANCER**

Procedure	Side Effects	Complications	Patient Issues
Breast-Conserving Surgery (Lumpectomy) With Radiation Therapy			
Wide excision of tumor, sentinel lymph node dissection (SLND) and/or axillary lymph node dissection (ALND). Radiation therapy.	Breast soreness Breast edema Skin reactions Arm swelling Sensory changes in breast and arm	*Short-term:* Moist desquamation,* hematoma, seroma, infection *Long-term:* Fibrosis, lymphedema,† myositis, pneumonitis,* rib fractures*	Prolonged treatment* Impaired arm mobility† Change in texture and sensitivity of breast
Modified Radical Mastectomy			
Removal of breast, preservation of pectoralis muscle. SLND and/or ALND.	Chest wall tightness, scar Phantom breast sensations Lymphedema Sensory changes Impaired range of motion	*Short-term:* Skin flap necrosis, seroma, hematoma, infection *Long-term:* Sensory loss, muscle weakness, lymphedema	Loss of breast Incision Body image Need for prosthesis Impaired arm mobility
Tissue Expansion and Breast Implants			
Expander used to slowly stretch tissue. Saline gradually injected into reservoir over weeks to months. Insertion of implant under musculofascial layer of chest wall.	Discomfort Chest wall tightness	*Short-term:* Skin flap necrosis, wound separation, seroma, hematoma, infection *Long-term:* Capsular contractions, displacement of implant	Altered body image Prolonged physician visits to expand implants Potential additional surgeries for nipple construction, symmetry
Breast Reconstruction Tissue Flap Procedures ***Transverse Rectus Abdominis Musculocutaneous (TRAM) Flap***			
Musculocutaneous flap (muscle, skin, fat, blood supply) is transposed from abdomen to the mastectomy site. May be done concurrently with mastectomy.	Pain related to two surgical sites and extensive surgery	*Short-term:* Delayed wound healing, infection, skin flap necrosis, abdominal hernia, hematoma	Prolonged postoperative recovery
Deep Inferior Epigastric Artery Perforator (DIEP) Flap			
Free flap that transfers skin and fat from the abdomen to the chest. Differs from TRAM flap because no muscle is moved.	Requires more time in surgery than TRAM flap Pain related to two surgical sites	If procedure fails, tissue flap may die and have to be completely removed If tissue dies, new reconstruction may not be done for 6-12 mo	Patients may experience less pain and restriction of movement than with a TRAM flap.

*Specific to radiation therapy.
†If ALND (less likely with SLND).

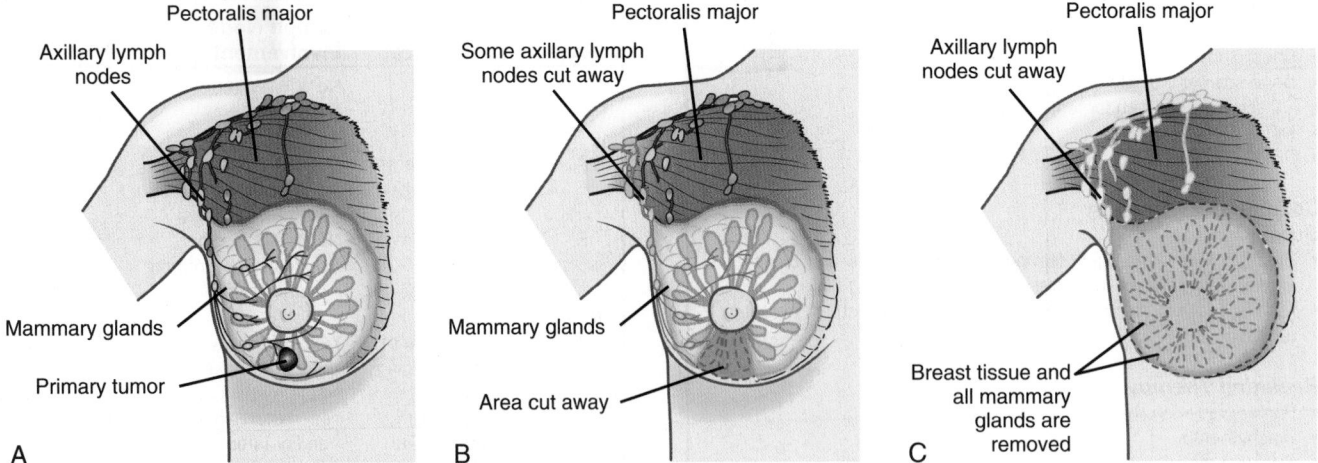

FIG. 52-6 Breast cancer surgery. **A,** Preoperative. **B,** Lumpectomy. **C,** Modified radical mastectomy.

the tumor bed. If evidence exists that the risk for recurrence is high, chemotherapy may be administered before radiation therapy. Contraindications to breast-conserving surgery include the following: breast size is too small in relation to the tumor size to yield an acceptable cosmetic result, masses and calcifications are multifocal (within the same breast quadrant), masses are multicentric (in more than one quadrant), and diffuse cal-

cifications occur in more than one quadrant. Contraindications to radiation therapy (e.g., active lupus or prior radiation therapy in the radiation field) may make mastectomy a better surgical option.

One of the main advantages of breast-conserving surgery and radiation is that it preserves the breast, including the nipple. The goal of the combined surgery and radiation is to maximize

EVIDENCE-BASED PRACTICE

Applying the Evidence

M.S. is a 53-yr-old woman who was diagnosed with breast cancer 2 wk ago. She is recovering from a lumpectomy with negative lymph nodes. Her physician has recommended adjuvant therapy with radiation.

Best Available Evidence	Clinician Expertise	Patient Preferences and Values
The addition of radiation therapy to lumpectomy reduces the risk of local cancer recurrence.	Radiation is recommended even with negative lymph nodes after a lumpectomy. Many patients have minimal or no side effects from radiation therapy. The most common ones are fatigue, malaise, skin reactions, and ulcers or irritation of the skin.	She tells you that she is not sure if she wants to have the radiation treatment because she is afraid of the side effects.

Your Decision and Action

Review the possible side effects and how they can be managed. Then explain the risks of not taking the radiation treatment, which can include recurrence. She tells you that she will discuss it with her husband and possibly reconsider. You understand her concerns and inform the physician of her indecisiveness.

Reference for Evidence

National Cancer Institute: Breast cancer treatment: stage I, II, IIIA, and operable IIIC breast cancer. Retrieved from *www.cancer.gov/cancertopics/pdq/treatment/breast/healthprofessional/page6.*

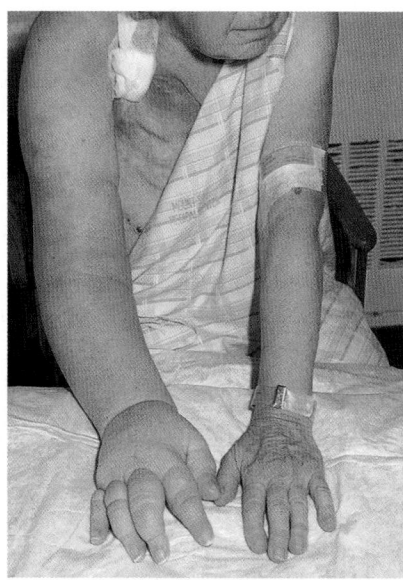

FIG. 52-7 Lymphedema. Accumulation of fluid in the tissue after excision of lymph nodes.

the benefits of both cancer treatment and cosmetic outcome while minimizing risks. Disadvantages of this surgery include the increased cost of the surgery plus radiation over surgery alone and the possible side effects of radiation.

Axillary Lymph Node Dissection. Axillary lymph node dissection (ALND) on the same side as the breast cancer is often performed when breast-conserving surgery is done. A typical ALND generally involves the removal of 12 to 20 nodes. Recently, sentinel lymph node dissection (SLND) has become the standard of care, with ALND reserved for patients when clinically indicated (evidence of disease in the axilla) (see Fig. 52-5). Examination of the lymph nodes provides prognostic information and helps determine further treatment (chemotherapy, hormone therapy, or both).

Lymphedema (accumulation of lymph in soft tissue) can occur as a result of the excision or radiation of lymph nodes[24] (Fig. 52-7). When the axillary nodes cannot return lymph fluid to the central circulation, the fluid accumulates in the arm, hand, or breast, causing obstructive pressure on the veins and venous return. The patient may experience heaviness, pain, impaired motor function in the arm, and numbness and paresthesia of the fingers. Fever and a red, painful rash may also be present with infection of the affected arm. These symptoms may indicate the beginning or worsening of lymphedema. Cellulitis and progressive fibrosis of the skin can result from lymphedema. (See further discussion on lymphedema later in this chapter on p. 1254.)

Modified Radical Mastectomy. A *modified radical mastectomy* includes removal of the breast and axillary lymph nodes, but it preserves the pectoralis major muscle (Fig. 52-6, *B*). This surgery would be selected over breast-conserving surgery if the tumor were too large to excise with good margins and attain a

reasonable cosmetic result. Some patients may select this surgical procedure over lumpectomy when presented with a choice.

When a modified radical mastectomy is performed, the patient has the option of breast reconstruction. If the patient chooses to have reconstructive surgery, it can be performed immediately after the mastectomy, or it can be delayed until postoperative recovery is complete.

Postmastectomy Pain Syndrome. *Postmastectomy pain syndrome* can occur in patients after a mastectomy or an axillary node dissection. Common symptoms include chest and upper arm pain, tingling down the arm, numbness, shooting or pricking pain, and unbearable itching that persist beyond the normal 3-month healing time. The most common theory for the onset of this syndrome is injury to intercostobrachial nerves, which are sensory nerves that exit the chest wall muscles and provide sensation to the shoulder and the upper arm.

Treatments include nonsteroidal antiinflammatory drugs, antidepressants, topical lidocaine patches, EMLA (local anesthetics: lidocaine and prilocaine), and antiseizure drugs (e.g., gabapentin [Neurontin]). Other possible treatment modalities include imagery, biofeedback, physical therapy to prevent "frozen shoulder" syndrome as a result of inadequate movement, and psychologic counseling with a therapist trained in the management of chronic pain syndromes.

Radiation Therapy. Radiation therapy is one form of *adjuvant (additional)* therapy that can be used after surgery. Radiation therapy may be used for breast cancer as treatment to (1) prevent local breast cancer recurrences after breast-conserving surgery; (2) prevent local and nodal recurrences after mastectomy; or (3) relieve pain caused by local, regional, or distant recurrence.

Primary Radiation Therapy. When radiation therapy is a primary treatment, it is usually performed after excision of the breast mass. The decision to use radiation therapy after mastectomy is based on the probability that local residual cancer cells are present. The possible presence of residual cells is related to tumor size and biology and number of involved lymph nodes.

In traditional whole breast (and regional lymph nodes in some cases) radiation treatment, the area is radiated 5 days per week over the course of about 5 to 7 weeks. An external beam of radiation is used to deliver an approximate total dose of 45 to 50 Gy (4500 to 5000 cGy or rads). A "boost" is a dose of radiation delivered to the area in which the original tumor was located. It can be given by external beam and adds five to eight more treatments to the total number given.

Studies are examining whether whole breast radiation over 3 weeks and accelerated partial-breast radiation (radiation to area surrounding the tumor site) over 7 days are safe and effective alternatives to traditional radiation. In both these approaches, larger radiation doses are used for each treatment session.[25]

Fatigue, skin changes, and breast edema may be temporary side effects of external beam radiation therapy. Radiation of the axilla and/or supraclavicular nodes may be indicated when lymph nodes are involved to decrease the risk of axillary recurrence. Radiating a localized area will not prevent distant metastasis. Chemotherapy may be used in select cases (e.g., local recurrence after mastectomy). (Nursing management of the patient receiving radiation therapy is discussed in Chapter 16.)

Brachytherapy. Brachytherapy (internal radiation) is used for partial-breast radiation as an alternative to traditional external radiation treatment for early-stage breast cancer. Radiation is delivered directly into the cavity left after a tumor is surgically removed by a lumpectomy. This approach is a minimally invasive way to deliver radiation. Because the radiation is concentrated and focused on the area with the highest risk for tumor recurrence, internal radiation only requires 5 days. Traditional external radiation treatments can take 5 to 7 weeks. Internal radiation therapy is primarily delivered using a multicatheter method or balloon-catheter system.

In the *multicatheter method* (e.g., SAVI) many very small catheters are placed in the breast at the site of the tumor. The SAVI is inserted through a small incision, and the catheter bundle expands uniformly. The ends of the catheters stick out through little holes in the skin. Small radioactive seeds are placed in the catheters. The seeds are left in place just long enough to deliver the radiation dose (e.g., 5 to 10 minutes). The tiny radioactive seeds are inserted only during treatment and then removed. The radiation does not remain in the body between treatments or after the final treatment is over.

In the *balloon-catheter system,* the balloon is placed where the tumor is located. The balloon is filled with fluid to keep it in place. Radioactive seeds are inserted (Fig. 52-8). Radiation is emitted by a tiny radioactive seed attached by a wire on the way to an afterloader, a computer-controlled machine. The seed travels through the MammoSite applicator into the inflated balloon. As with the multicatheter system, the radiation does not remain in the body between treatments or after the final treatment is over. Once the final session is completed, the balloon is deflated and the system is removed.

Internal radiation may also be used as a boost therapy in conjunction with external radiation. The long-term effectiveness and safety of brachytherapy is currently under investigation.[25]

Palliative Radiation Therapy. In addition to reducing the primary tumor mass with a resultant decrease in pain, radiation therapy is also used to treat symptomatic metastatic lesions in such sites as bone, soft tissue organs, brain, and chest. Radiation therapy often relieves pain and is successful in controlling recurrent or metastatic disease.

Drug Therapy. Drug therapy, another type of adjuvant therapy, is used to destroy tumor cells that may have spread to

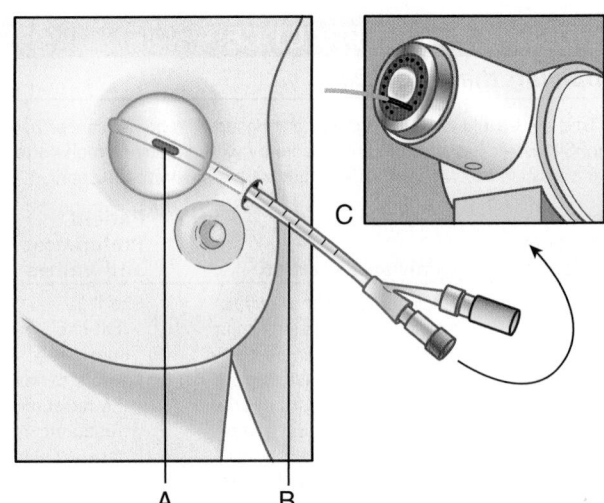

FIG. 52-8 High-dose brachytherapy for breast cancer. The MammoSite system involves the insertion of a single small balloon catheter *(B)* at the time of the lumpectomy or shortly thereafter into the tumor resection cavity (the space that is left after the surgeon removes the tumor). A tiny radioactive seed *(A)* is inserted into the balloon, connected to a machine called an afterloader *(C)*, and delivers the radiation therapy.

distant sites. Drug therapy can decrease the rate of recurrence and increase the length of survival. Because of the risk for recurrent disease, nearly all women with evidence of node involvement, particularly those who are hormone receptor negative, will have some type of drug therapy. Some women, particularly those with a larger or more aggressive tumor, are known to be at higher risk for recurrent or metastatic disease. These women may be recommended for systemic therapy even when there is no evidence of node involvement. Weighing the risks and benefits of drug therapy is a complex process.

Chemotherapy. Chemotherapy refers to the use of cytotoxic drugs to destroy cancer cells. Many breast cancers are responsive to chemotherapy. In some patients, chemotherapy is given preoperatively. Preoperative *(neoadjuvant)* chemotherapy may decrease the size of the primary tumor, with the goal of less extensive surgery.

The use of combinations of drugs is usually superior to the use of a single drug. The benefit of combination treatment results from the use of drugs that have different mechanisms of action and work at different parts of the cell cycle. The more common combination-therapy protocols are (1) CMF—cyclophosphamide (Cytoxan), methotrexate, and 5-fluorouracil (5-FU); (2) AC—doxorubicin (Adriamycin) and cyclophosphamide, with or without the addition of a taxane such as paclitaxel (Taxol) or docetaxel (Taxotere); or (3) CEF or CAF—cyclophosphamide, epirubicin (Ellence) or doxorubicin (Adriamycin), and 5-FU.

DRUG ALERT: Doxorubicin (Adriamycin)
- Monitor for signs of cardiotoxicity and heart failure (e.g., new onset of shortness of breath, pedal edema, decreased activity tolerance, dysrhythmias, ECG changes).
- Instruct patient not to have immunizations without physician's approval.
- Instruct patient to avoid contact with those who recently received live virus vaccine.

Docetaxel, capecitabine (Xeloda), ixabepilone (Ixempra), and an albumin-bound form of paclitaxel (Abraxane) are used in women whose metastatic breast cancer has not responded to standard chemotherapy. Vinorelbine (Navelbine), used to treat metastatic breast cancer, is better tolerated with fewer and milder side effects than other chemotherapy drugs. Eribulin mesylate (Halaven), a microtubule inhibitor, may be used in treating metastatic breast cancer in patients who have received at least two prior chemotherapy regimens.[26]

Because healthy cells are also affected by chemotherapy, a variety of side effects accompany this treatment modality. The incidence and severity of common side effects are influenced by the specific drug combination, drug schedule, and dosage. The most common side effects involve rapidly dividing cells in the gastrointestinal tract (nausea, anorexia, weight loss), bone marrow (anemia), and hair follicles (alopecia [hair loss]).

Cognitive changes during and after treatment, especially with chemotherapy, have been reported in patients with cancer. This phenomenon, called *"chemobrain,"* may affect up to 83% of breast cancer survivors.[27] These changes include difficulties in concentration, memory, focus, and attention. It is not clear if chemobrain is related to specific cancer treatments or is an overall systemic reaction.[28]

Hormone Therapy. Estrogen can promote the growth of breast cancer cells if the cells are estrogen receptor positive. Hormone therapy can block the effect and source of estrogen, thus promoting tumor regression. Hormone therapy may be used as an adjuvant to primary treatment or in patients with recurrent or metastatic cancer.

Both estrogen and progesterone receptor status assays have been developed to identify women whose breast cancers are likely to respond to hormone therapy. These assays reliably predict whether hormone therapy is a treatment option. Chances of tumor regression are significantly greater in women whose tumors contain estrogen and progesterone receptors.

Hormone therapy can (1) block estrogen receptors or (2) suppress estrogen synthesis by inhibiting aromatase, an enzyme needed for estrogen synthesis (Table 52-8). Antiestrogens include tamoxifen, toremifene (Fareston), and fulvestrant (Faslodex).

Estrogen Receptor Blockers. Tamoxifen has been the hormonal agent of choice in estrogen receptor–positive women with all stages of breast cancer over the past 30 years. It is commonly used in early-stage or advanced breast cancer and to treat recurrent disease. Tamoxifen may also be used in high-risk premenopausal and postmenopausal women to prevent breast cancer. Side effects of tamoxifen may include hot flashes, mood swings, vaginal discharge and dryness, and other effects commonly associated with decreased estrogen. It also increases the risk of blood clots, cataracts, stroke, and endometrial cancer in postmenopausal women. Treatment with tamoxifen is generally prescribed for 5 years.

DRUG ALERT: Tamoxifen (Nolvadex)
- Irregular vaginal bleeding or spotting may occur.
- Decreased visual acuity, corneal opacity, and retinopathy can occur in women receiving high doses (240-320 mg/day for >17 mo). These problems may be irreversible.
- Instruct patient to immediately report decreased visual acuity.
- Monitor for signs of deep vein thrombosis, pulmonary embolism, and stroke, including shortness of breath, leg cramps, and weakness.

Toremifene is an antiestrogen agent similar to tamoxifen. It is indicated in the treatment of metastatic breast cancer in postmenopausal women. Fulvestrant may be given to women with advanced breast cancer who no longer respond to tamoxifen. Fulvestrant is given intramuscularly on a monthly basis.

TABLE 52-8 DRUG THERAPY

Breast Cancer

Drug Class	Mechanism of Action	Indications
Hormone Therapy		
Estrogen Receptor Blockers		
tamoxifen (Nolvadex)	Blocks estrogen receptors (ERs)	ER-positive breast cancer in premenopausal and postmenopausal women. Used as a preventive measure in high-risk premenopausal and postmenopausal women
toremifene (Fareston)	Blocks ERs	ER-positive breast cancer in postmenopausal women only
fulvestrant (Faslodex)	Blocks ERs	ER-positive breast cancer in postmenopausal women only
Aromatase Inhibitors		
anastrozole (Arimidex) letrozole (Femara) exemestane (Aromasin)	Prevents production of estrogen by inhibiting aromatase	ER-positive breast cancer in postmenopausal women only
Estrogen Receptor Modulator		
raloxifene (Evista)	In breast blocks the effect of estrogen. In bone promotes effect of estrogen and prevents bone loss	Postmenopausal women
Biologic and Targeted Therapy		
trastuzumab (Herceptin) pertuzumab (Perjeta)	Blocks HER-2 receptor	ER-positive breast cancer in postmenopausal women only
lapatinib (Tykerb)	Inhibits HER-2 tyrosine kinase and EGFR tyrosine kinase	ER-positive breast cancer in postmenopausal women only

EGFR, Epidermal growth factor receptor; *HER-2,* human epidermal growth factor receptor 2.

Common side effects include injection site pain, fatigue, hot flashes, and nausea.

Aromatase Inhibitors. Aromatase inhibitor drugs interfere with the enzyme aromatase, which is needed for the synthesis of estrogen. These drugs, including anastrozole, letrozole (Femara), and exemestane (Aromasin), are used in the treatment of breast cancer in postmenopausal women. Aromatase inhibitors do not block the production of estrogen by the ovaries. Thus they are of little benefit and may be harmful in premenopausal women.

Clinical trials have demonstrated greater disease-free survival when these drugs are given after tamoxifen treatment has ended. They also appear to be more effective than tamoxifen in preventing breast cancer recurrence and possibly more effective in preventing contralateral disease (disease in the other breast).[29]

Aromatase inhibitors have different side effects than tamoxifen. They rarely cause blood clots, and they do not cause endometrial cancer. Because they block the production of estrogen in postmenopausal women, osteoporosis and bone fractures may occur. These drugs have been associated with night sweats, nausea, arthralgias, and myalgias.

Estrogen Receptor Modulator and Others. Raloxifene (Evista) is a selective estrogen receptor modulator that produces both estrogen-agonistic effects on bone and estrogen-antagonistic effects on breast tissue. (Raloxifene is discussed in the section on osteoporosis in Chapter 64.)

Additional drugs that may be used to suppress hormone-dependent breast tumors include megestrol acetate (Megace), diethylstilbestrol (DES), and fluoxymesterone (Halotestin).

Biologic and Targeted Therapy. Trastuzumab (Herceptin) is a monoclonal antibody to HER-2. After the antibody attaches to the antigen, it is taken into the cells and eventually kills them.[20] It can be used alone or in combination with chemotherapy agents such as docetaxel or paclitaxel to treat patients whose tumors overexpress HER-2. Additional genetic testing (e.g., SPoT-Light test) may offer information on which patients are good candidates for treatment with trastuzumab.

> **DRUG ALERT: Trastuzumab (Herceptin)**
> * Use with caution in women with preexisting heart disease.
> * Monitor for signs of ventricular dysfunction and heart failure.

Ado-trastuzumab emtansine (Kadcyla) is trastuzumab connected to a chemotherapy drug called DM1. This antibody-drug combination is a new kind of targeted cancer drug that can attach to certain types of cancer cells and deliver the chemotherapy directly to them.

Pertuzumab (Perjeta) is a new anti-HER-2 therapy that is used for patients who have not received prior treatment for metastatic breast cancer with an anti-HER-2 agent or chemotherapy. Pertuzumab is combined with trastuzumab and docetaxel.

Lapatinib (Tykerb) works inside the cell by blocking the function of the HER-2 protein. It may be used in combination with capecitabine for patients with advanced metastatic disease who are HER-2 positive. The combination treatment is indicated for women who have become resistant to other cancer drugs.

Advanced breast cancer in postmenopausal women who are estrogen and progesterone receptor positive and HER-2 positive may be treated with lapatinib in combination with letrozole. Everolimus (Afinitor) is used in combination with exemestane to treat postmenopausal women with advanced hormone-receptor positive, HER-2-negative breast cancer. The drug combination is intended for use in women with recurrence or progression of their cancer after treatment with letrozole or anastrozole.

Denosumab (Prolia, Xgeva), a monoclonal antibody, may be used to increase bone mass in patients at high risk of fracture from aromatase inhibitor therapy. It is also given to prevent fractures in patients with metastasis to the bone. (The use of biologic and targeted therapies is discussed in Chapter 16.)

Follow-up and Survivorship Care. After treatment for breast cancer, the patient will have ongoing survivorship care. Recommended follow-up examinations generally occur every 3 to 6 months for the first 5 years, and then annually thereafter. Survivorship care plans summarize a patient's care and care plan for ongoing surveillance.[30] In addition, advise women to perform monthly BSE and self–chest wall examination, and report any changes to their health care provider. Local recurrence of breast cancer is usually at the surgical site. The woman should have appropriate breast imaging done at regular inter-

vals (usually 6 months to 1 year) as determined by her risk of recurrence and breast cancer history.

CULTURALLY COMPETENT CARE

BREAST CANCER

Differences exist in the incidence, mortality rates, and relevant care issues among diverse ethnic groups related to breast cancer (see Cultural & Ethnic Health Disparities box on the facing page). In addition, cultural differences may involve gender roles, health beliefs, religion, and family structure. Other differences may be due to dietary factors and disparities related to access to and use of CBEs and screening mammograms.

Cultural values strongly influence how women respond to and cope with breast cancer and treatment. Health beliefs and behaviors are influenced by diverse cultural norms.[31] Breast cancer screening, diagnosis, and treatment are affected by the cultural values and meanings (body image, sexuality, modesty, motherhood) attached to the breasts. Women may delay screening or treatment for varying reasons, including an acceptance of disease as inevitable fate or "God's will," a mistrust of Western medicine, lack of health care benefits, fear, modesty, or the stigma of a cancer diagnosis.

🌐 CULTURAL & ETHNIC HEALTH DISPARITIES

Breast Cancer

- White women have a higher incidence of breast cancer than other ethnic groups.
- African American women have lower survival rates from breast cancer than white women, even when diagnosed at an early stage.
- Triple-negative breast cancer (negative for estrogen, progesterone, and HER-2 receptors) has a higher incidence in Hispanic and African American women.
- Breast cancer incidence and mortality rates are lower among Hispanic and Asian/Pacific Islander women than among white and African American women.
- Breast cancer is the most commonly diagnosed cancer among Hispanic women.
- Hispanic women, especially Mexican Americans, have the lowest rate of cancer screening of any ethnic group.
- Hispanic and African American women are more likely to be diagnosed at a later stage of breast cancer than white women.

HER-2, Human epidermal growth factor receptor 2.

NURSING MANAGEMENT
BREAST CANCER

NURSING ASSESSMENT

Many factors need to be considered when you assess a patient with a breast problem. The history of the breast disorder assists in establishing the diagnosis. Investigate the presence of nipple discharge, pain, rate of growth of the lump, breast asymmetry, and correlation with the menstrual cycle.

Carefully document the size and location of the lump or lumps. Assess the physical characteristics of the lesion, such as consistency, mobility, and shape. If nipple discharge is present, note the color and consistency and whether it occurs from one or both breasts.

Subjective and objective data that should be obtained from an individual suspected of having or diagnosed with breast cancer are presented in Table 52-9.

NURSING DIAGNOSES

Nursing diagnoses related to the care of a patient diagnosed with breast cancer vary. After diagnosis and before a treatment plan has been selected, the following nursing diagnoses would apply:

- Decisional conflict *related to* lack of knowledge about treatment options and their effects
- Fear and/or anxiety *related to* diagnosis of breast cancer
- Disturbed body image *related to* physical and emotional effects of treatment modalities

If a mastectomy or lumpectomy is planned, the nursing diagnoses may include, but are not limited to, those presented in eNursing Care Plan 52-1 (available on the website for this chapter).

PLANNING

The overall goals are that the patient with breast cancer will (1) actively participate in the decision-making process related to treatment, (2) adhere to the therapeutic plan, (3) communicate about and manage the side effects of adjuvant therapy, and (4) access and benefit from the support provided by significant others and health care providers.

TABLE 52-9 NURSING ASSESSMENT

Breast Cancer

Subjective Data
Important Health Information
Past health history: Benign breast disease with atypical changes; previous unilateral breast cancer; menstrual history (early menarche with late menopause); pregnancy history (nulliparity or first full-term pregnancy after age 30); previous endometrial, ovarian, or colon cancer; hyperestrogenism and testicular atrophy (in men)
Medications: Hormones, especially as postmenopausal hormone therapy and in oral contraceptives, infertility treatments
Surgery or other treatments: Exposure to therapeutic radiation (e.g., Hodgkin's lymphoma or thyroid radiation)

Functional Health Patterns
Health perception–health management: Family history of breast cancer (especially mother or sister, young age at diagnosis); history of abnormal mammogram or atypical prior biopsy; palpable change found on BSE; frequent alcohol use
Nutritional-metabolic: Obesity; unexplained severe weight loss (possible indicator of metastasis)
Cognitive-perceptual: Changes in cognition, headache, bone pain (possible indicators of metastasis)
Sexuality-reproductive: Unilateral nipple discharge (clear, milky, or bloody); change in breast contour, size, or symmetry
Coping–stress tolerance: Psychologic stress
Self-perception–self-concept: Anxiety regarding threat to self-esteem
Physical activity: Level of usual activity

Objective Data
General
Axillary and supraclavicular lymphadenopathy

Integumentary
Hard, irregular, nonmobile breast lump most often in upper, outer sector, possibly fixated to fascia or chest wall; thickening of breast; nipple inversion or retraction, erosion; edema ("peau d'orange"), erythema, induration, infiltration, or dimpling (in later stages); firm, discrete nodules at mastectomy site (possible indicator of local recurrence); peripheral edema (possible indicator of metastasis)

Respiratory
Pleural effusions (possible indicator of metastasis)

Gastrointestinal
Hepatomegaly, jaundice; ascites (possible indicators of liver metastasis)

Possible Diagnostic Findings
Finding of mass or change in tissue on breast examination; abnormal mammogram, ultrasound, or breast MRI; positive results of FNA or surgical biopsy or similar results with a needle biopsy

BSE, Breast self-examination; *FNA*, fine-needle aspiration.

NURSING IMPLEMENTATION

HEALTH PROMOTION. Review the risk factors in Table 52-2. A person can reduce her risk factors by maintaining a healthy weight, exercising regularly, limiting alcohol, eating nutritious food, and never smoking (or quitting if she does smoke).

It is important for you to encourage people to adhere to the breast cancer screening guidelines presented on pp. 1238-1239. If a person is at high risk, she needs to develop an individualized plan with the health care provider. Early detection can decrease the morbidity and mortality associated with breast cancer.

Along with these lifestyle choices, there are other risk-reduction options for women at high risk. Genetic testing for *BRCA* gene mutations is available. People with a strong family history of breast cancer should talk with their health care provider about the possibility of genetic testing. Routine screening for genetic abnormalities in women without evidence of a strong family history of breast cancer is not warranted.

In women with an abnormal *BRCA1* or *BRCA2* gene, prophylactic oophorectomy may reduce their risk of developing breast cancer. In deciding whether and when to undergo this surgical procedure, women should receive counseling about the risks and benefits of prophylactic oophorectomy, including fertility issues.

Prophylactic surgery decisions require a great deal of thought, patience, and discussion with the health care provider, genetic counselor, and family. Patients need to consider these options and make decisions with which they feel comfortable. Removing both breasts and ovaries at a young age does not eliminate the risk of breast cancer. A small risk exists that cancer can develop in the areas where the breasts used to be. Close follow-up is necessary, even after prophylactic surgery.

ACUTE INTERVENTION. The times of waiting for the initial biopsy results and waiting for the care provider to make treatment recommendations are difficult for the woman and her family.[32] Even after the health care provider has discussed treatment options, the woman often relies on you to clarify and expand on these options. During this stressful time, the woman may not be coping effectively. Appropriate nursing interventions are to explore the woman's usual decision-making processes, help her evaluate the advantages and disadvantages of the options, provide information relevant to the decision, clarify unresolved issues with the health care provider, and support the patient and family once the decision is made.

Regardless of the surgery planned, provide the patient with sufficient information to ensure informed consent. Some patients seek extensive, detailed information to maintain a sense of control, whereas others avoid information to decrease anxiety and fear. Be sensitive to the individual's need for and preferred type of information. These include (1) preoperative instructions on pain control and what to expect after surgery (e.g., reporting of complications, dressing and drain care, turning, coughing, deep breathing); (2) a review of mobility restrictions and postoperative exercises; and (3) explanation of the recovery period from the time of surgery until the first postoperative visit.

The woman who has breast-conserving surgery usually has an uncomplicated postoperative course with variable pain intensity. Pain primarily depends on the extent of the lymph node dissection performed. If an ALND has been done or if a woman had a mastectomy, drains are generally left in place and patients are discharged home with them. Teach the patient and the family, with a return demonstration, how to manage the drains at home.

Restoring arm function on the affected side after mastectomy and ALND is a key nursing goal. In the hospital, place the woman in a semi-Fowler's position with the arm on the affected side elevated on a pillow. Flexing and extending the fingers should begin in the recovery room with progressive increases in activity encouraged. Postoperative arm and shoulder exercises are instituted gradually (Fig. 52-9). These exercises are designed to prevent contractures and muscle shortening, maintain muscle tone, and improve lymph and blood circulation. The difficulty and pain encountered in performing what used to be simple tasks included in the exercise program may cause frustration and depression. The goal of all exercise is a gradual return to full range of motion within 4 to 6 weeks.

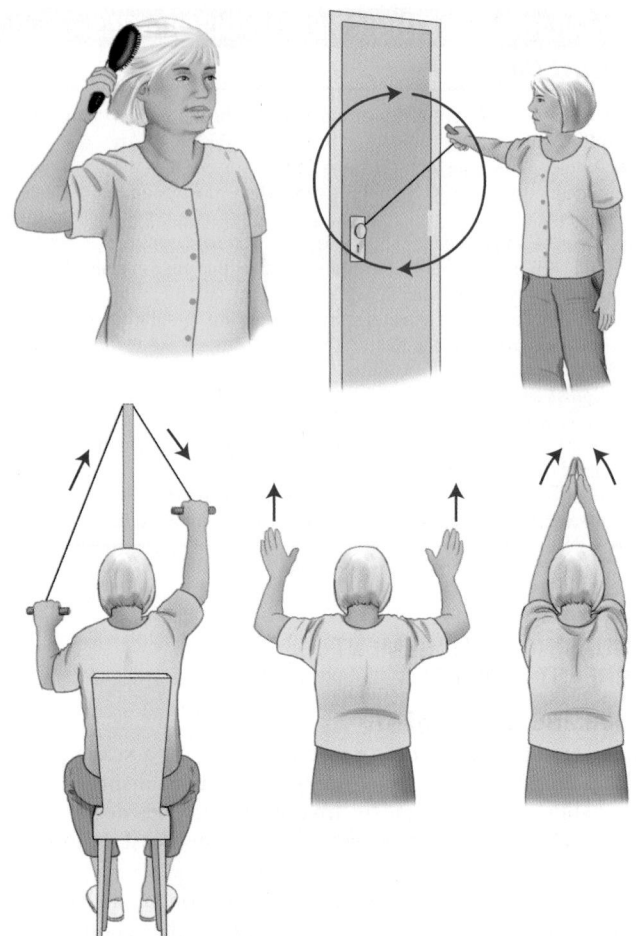

FIG. 52-9 Postoperative exercises for the patient with a mastectomy or lumpectomy with axillary lymph node dissection.

Postoperative discomfort can be minimized by administering analgesics regularly when the patient is in pain and about 30 minutes before initiating exercises. When the patient is able to shower, the warm water on the involved shoulder often relaxes the muscle and reduces joint stiffness. Application of ice, except where contraindicated with plastic surgery procedures, can reduce swelling, inflammation, and pain.

The incidence of arm lymphedema ranges from 2% to 65%, and it can develop 1 to 5 years after surgery.[33] Women who are overweight or obese have a higher risk of developing lymphedema. Teach the woman measures to prevent and reduce lymphedema, including no blood pressure readings, venipunctures, or injections on the affected arm. The affected arm should not be dependent for long periods, and caution should be used to prevent infection, burns, or compromised circulation on the affected side.

If trauma to the arm occurs, the area should be washed thoroughly with soap and water and observed. A topical antibiotic ointment and a bandage or other sterile dressing may be applied.

When the patient's lymphedema is acute (see Fig. 52-7), complete decongestive therapy may be recommended. This therapy consists of a massage-like technique to mobilize the subcutaneous accumulation of fluid. This may then be followed by use of compression bandaging and an intermittent pneumatic compression sleeve. The sleeve applies mechanical massage to the arm and facilitates lymph drainage up toward the heart. Elevation of the arm so that it is level with the heart, diuretics, and isometric exercises may be used to reduce the fluid volume in the arm. To maintain maximum volume reduction, the patient may need to wear a fitted compression sleeve during waking hours and preventively during air travel.

Emotional and Psychologic Care. Throughout history, the female breast has been regarded as a symbol of beauty, femininity, sexuality, and motherhood. The potential loss of a breast, or part of a breast, may be devastating for many women because of the significant psychologic, social, sexual, and body image implications associated with it.

From the time of diagnosis through treatment, survivorship, or metastatic disease, the woman may exhibit signs of distress or tension (e.g., tachycardia, increased muscle tension, sleep disturbances, restlessness, changes in appetite or mood). Assess the woman's body language and affect during periods of high stress and indecision so that appropriate interventions, including referral to a mental health provider, can be initiated.

Remain sensitive to the complex psychologic impact that a diagnosis of cancer and subsequent breast surgery can have on a woman and her family. A relationship in which the woman can express her feelings is therapeutic. With an accepting attitude and the offer of resources, you can help with the feelings of fear, anger, anxiety, and depression. Help to meet the woman's psychologic needs by

- Providing a safe environment for the expression of the full range of feelings.
- Helping her identify sources of support and strength, such as her partner, family, and spiritual or religious practices.
- Encouraging her to identify and learn individual coping strengths.
- Promoting communication between the patient and her family or friends.
- Providing accurate and complete answers to questions about her disease; treatment options; and reproductive, fertility, or lactation issues (if appropriate).
- Making resources available for mental health counseling.
- Offering information about local and national community resources. Referring her to peer support resources, such as Reach to Recovery or local breast cancer organizations, is invaluable. The Reach to Recovery program of the American Cancer Society is a rehabilitation program to help meet the psychologic, physical, and cosmetic needs of women who have had breast surgery. The American Cancer Society and the National Cancer Institute can provide excellent materials to assist you in meeting the special needs of women with breast cancer.

AMBULATORY AND HOME CARE. Explain the specific follow-up plan to the patient and emphasize the importance of ongoing monitoring and self-care. Immediately after surgery, advise the patient to report to the health care provider symptoms such as fever, inflammation at the surgical site, erythema, postoperative constipation, and unusual swelling. Other changes to report are new back pain, weakness, shortness of breath, and change in mental status, including confusion.

For women who have had a mastectomy without breast reconstruction, a variety of products are available. These include garments such as camisoles with soft breast prosthetic inserts or a fitted prosthesis with bra. Should the woman choose a breast prosthesis, a certified fitter can help her select a comfortable, more permanent weighted prosthesis and bra, generally at

---

COMPLEMENTARY & ALTERNATIVE THERAPIES
Imagery

Imagery is the use of one's mind to generate images that have a calming effect on the body

Scientific Evidence*
- Good evidence for decreasing cancer pain and postoperative pain.
- Good evidence for treatment of migraine or tension headache in conjunction with standard medical care.

Nursing Implications
- Used by nurses to help patients promote relaxation, decrease stress, and manage pain.
- Should be used as a supplemental technique, not a replacement for medical care.

*Based on a systematic review of scientific literature. Retrieved from *www. naturalstandard.com*.

---

4 to 8 weeks postoperatively. Your role is to present the choices and resources without judgment.

How the loss of part or all of the breast and cancer affect the woman's sexual identity, body image, and relationships can vary. If you are comfortable, initiate a discussion of sexuality by inviting questions about relationships or intimacy concerns. Often the husband, sexual partner, or family members need help dealing with their emotional reactions to the diagnosis and surgery before they can provide effective support for the patient. There are no physical reasons why a mastectomy would prevent sexual satisfaction. The woman taking hormone therapy may have a decreased sexual drive or vaginal dryness. She may need to use lubrication to prevent discomfort during intercourse. Concerns about sexuality are not well addressed by many health care providers.[34] If difficulty in adjustment or other problems develop, counseling may be necessary to deal with the emotional component of a mastectomy and the diagnosis of cancer.

Depression and anxiety may occur with the continued stress and uncertainty of a cancer diagnosis. A woman's self-esteem and identity may also be threatened. The support of family and friends and participation in a cancer support group are important aspects of care that may improve the patient's quality of life.

EVALUATION
The expected outcomes for the patient after a mastectomy or lumpectomy are presented in eNursing Care Plan 52-1 (available on the website for this chapter).

GERONTOLOGIC CONSIDERATIONS

BREAST CANCER
A major risk for breast cancer is increasing age, and more than half of all breast cancers are diagnosed in women who are age 65 or older. Older women are less likely to have mammograms. Screening and treatment decisions for breast cancer should be based on a woman's general health status rather than biologic age, since health status has a greater influence on tolerance to treatment and long-term prognosis. In addition to medical co-morbidities and life expectancy, treatment decisions for the older woman with breast cancer should be based on an assessment of nutritional and functional status; vision, gait, and balance; and the presence of delirium, dementia, or depression.

Breast cancer treatment is similar for older and younger patients, including the use of surgery, radiation therapy, and drug therapy. For healthy older women, breast cancer survival rates are similar to those of younger women when matched by cancer stage.

MAMMOPLASTY

Mammoplasty is the surgical change in the size or shape of the breast. It may be done electively for cosmetic purposes to either enlarge or reduce the size of the breasts. It may also be done to reconstruct the breast after a mastectomy.

A professional, nonjudgmental attitude and clear information about surgical breast options is most useful for women engaged in decision making about mammoplasty. The desire to change the appearance of the breasts has special significance for each woman as she attempts to alter or recreate her body image. Be aware of the cultural value the woman places on the breast. Help the patient set realistic expectations about what mammoplasty can accomplish and about possible complications (e.g., hematoma formation, hemorrhage, infection). If an implant is involved, capsular contracture and loss of the implant are possible.

Breast Reconstruction

Breast reconstructive surgery is done to achieve symmetry and to restore or preserve body image. It may be done simultaneously with a mastectomy or some time afterward. The timing of reconstructive surgery is individualized based on the patient's physical and psychologic needs. Breast reconstruction is also safe and effective for older women.[35]

Indications. The main indication for breast reconstruction is to improve a woman's self-image, regain a sense of normalcy,

and assist in coping with the loss of the breast. Current reconstruction techniques cannot restore lactation, nipple sensation, or erectility. Although the breast will not fully resemble its premastectomy appearance, the reconstructed appearance usually represents an improvement over the mastectomy scar (Fig. 52-10). The contour of the breast is restored without the use of an external prosthesis.

Types of Reconstruction

Breast Implants and Tissue Expansion. A tissue expander can be used to stretch the skin and the muscle at the mastectomy site before inserting permanent implants (Fig. 52-11). The use of tissue expanders and breast implants is the most common breast reconstruction technique currently used. Placement of the expander may be immediate or delayed. The tissue expander is placed in a pocket under the pectoralis muscle, which protects the implant and provides soft tissue coverage. The tissue expander is minimally inflated and then gradually filled by weekly injections of sterile water or saline solution. This procedure stretches the skin and muscle and can be painful. A small magnet is embedded in most expanders to help locate the port where the fluid is injected. Therefore a woman should not have an MRI with a magnet in place. In a second procedure, the expander is surgically removed and a permanent implant is inserted. Some expanders are designed to remain in place and become the implant, eliminating the need for a second surgical procedure. Tissue expansion does not work well in individuals with extensive scar tissue from surgery or radiation therapy.

The body's natural response to the presence of a foreign substance is the formation of a fibrous capsule around the implant. If excessive capsular formation occurs as a result of infection, hematoma, trauma, or reaction to a foreign body, a

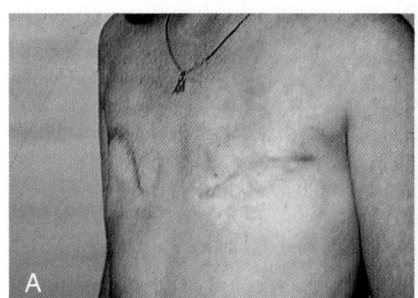 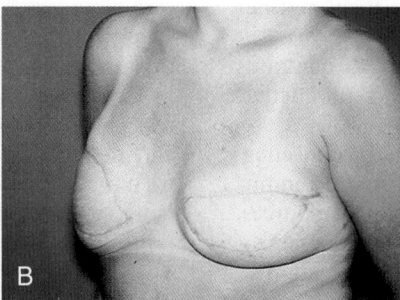 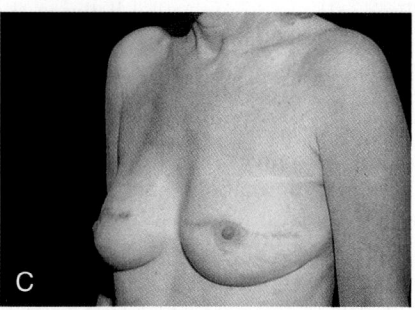

FIG. 52-10 A, Appearance of chest after bilateral mastectomy. **B,** Postoperative breast reconstruction before nipple-areolar reconstruction. **C,** Postoperative breast reconstruction after nipple-areolar reconstruction.

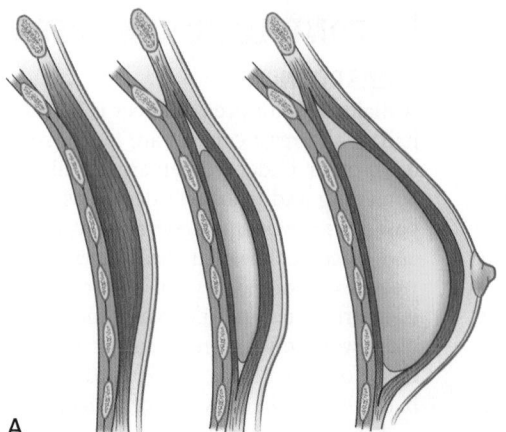 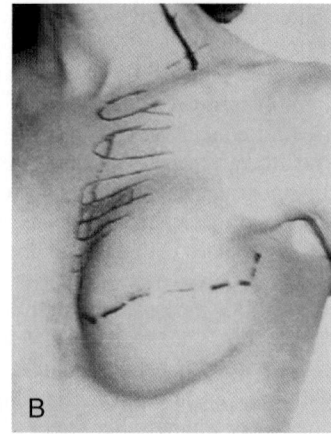

FIG. 52-11 A, Tissue expander with gradual expansion. **B,** Tissue expander in place after mastectomy.

contracture can develop, resulting in deformity. Although surgeons differ in their approaches to the prevention of contracture formation, gentle manual massage around the implant is routine. Other adverse outcomes include wrinkling, scarring, asymmetry, pain, and infection at the incision site.[36]

Tissue Flap Procedures. Another choice for breast reconstruction is the use of autologous tissue to recreate a breast mound. If insufficient muscle is left after mastectomy or if the chest wall has been radiated, the person's own tissue may be used to repair the soft tissue defects. Musculocutaneous flaps are most often taken from the back (latissimus dorsi muscle) or the abdomen (transverse rectus abdominis muscle). In the latissimus dorsi musculocutaneous flap, a block of skin and muscle from the patient's back is used to replace tissue removed during mastectomy. A small implant may be needed beneath the flap to gain reasonable breast shape and size. A disadvantage of this technique is an additional scar on the back.

The *transverse rectus abdominis musculocutaneous (TRAM) flap* is a frequently used flap operation. The rectus abdominis muscles are paired flat muscles running from the rib cage down to the pubic bone. Arteries running inside the muscles provide branches at many levels, and these branches supply the fat and skin across a large expanse of the abdomen. With this technique, the surgeon elevates a large block of tissue from the lower abdominal area, but leaves it attached to the rectus muscle (Fig. 52-12). This tissue is then tunneled or placed as "free flaps" under the skin up to the area where the breast will be reconstructed. Then it is molded and fashioned to form a breast. The abdominal incision is closed, giving the patient a result that is similar to having an abdominoplasty ("tummy tuck"). This surgical procedure can last 6 to 8 hours with recovery taking 6 to 8 weeks. Some patients have reported pain and fatigue for up to 3 months. Complications include bleeding, seroma, hernia, infection, and low back pain. An implant may be used in addition to the flap if the flap does not provide the desired cosmetic result alone.

A *deep inferior epigastric artery perforator (DIEP) flap* is a version of the free flap that does not use muscle tissue. With the DIEP flap, only the skin and fat are taken from the same lower abdominal area as the TRAM flap. Patients may experience less pain and restriction of movement with this procedure.

Total skin-sparing mastectomy is the preservation of the skin of the nipple and areola with the removal of underlying breast tissue. It can be done at the same time as immediate breast reconstructive surgery.

Nipple-Areolar Reconstruction. Many patients undergoing breast reconstruction also have nipple-areolar reconstruction. Nipple reconstruction gives the reconstructed breast a much more natural appearance (Fig. 52-10, *C*). Nipple-areolar reconstruction is usually done a few months after breast reconstruction. Tissue to construct a nipple may be taken from the opposite breast or from a small flap of tissue on the reconstructed breast mound. The areola may be grafted from the labia, skin in the area of the groin, or lower abdominal skin, or it may be tattooed with a permanent pigmented dye. In some patients, a small implant may be placed under the completed nipple-areolar reconstruction to add additional projection.

Breast Augmentation

In augmentation mammoplasty (the procedure to enlarge the breasts), an implant is placed in a surgically created pocket between the capsule of the breast and the pectoral fascia, or ideally under the pectoralis muscle. Most implants are silicone envelopes filled with a fluid such as dextran, saline, or silicone. Implants filled with silicone gel most closely resemble the human breast. The U.S. Food and Drug Administration (FDA) has approved the use of silicone gel implants for breast augmentation and reconstruction.[36] Studies continue to collect data on the safety and effectiveness of these implants.

Saline-filled implants are often used in the United States. The silicone shells are filled with normal saline. This implant has an outer shell of silicone that is filled with highly refined soybean oil.

Breast Reduction

For some women, large breasts can be a source of physical and psychologic discomfort. They can interfere with normal daily activities such as walking, using a computer, and driving a car. The weight of large breasts can lead to back, shoulder, and neck problems, including degenerative nerve changes. Overly large breasts can interfere with self-esteem, self-image, and comfort in wearing some clothing. Reduction in the size of the breasts

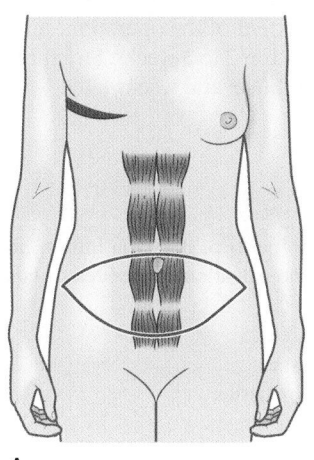 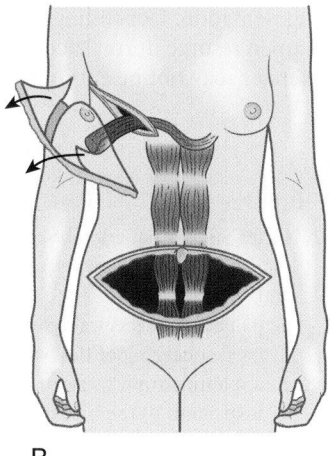 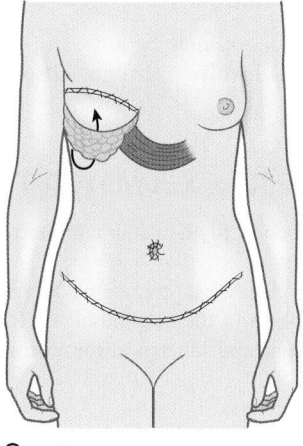 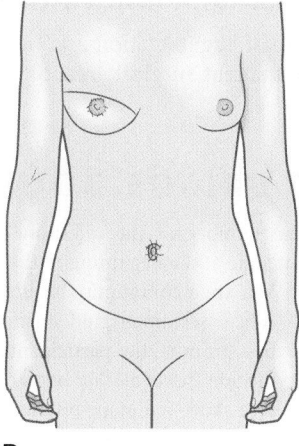

A   B   C   D

FIG. 52-12 Transverse rectus abdominis musculocutaneous (TRAM) flap. **A,** TRAM flap is planned. **B,** The abdominal tissue, while attached to the rectus muscle, nerve, and blood supply, is tunneled through the abdomen to the chest. **C,** The flap is trimmed to shape the breast. The lower abdominal incision is closed. **D,** Nipple and areola are reconstructed after the breast is healed.

CASE STUDY

Breast Cancer

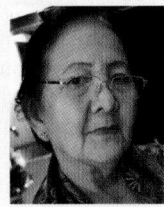

iStockphoto/Thinkstock

Patient Profile

A.K., a 68-year-old married Asian American woman, has been diagnosed with breast cancer (see Chapter 51 case study on p. 1226). She is scheduled for surgery in the morning for a lumpectomy and sentinel lymph node dissection with possible axillary dissection.

Collaborative Care
Preoperative

• When she is seen in the preoperative clinic 1 week before surgery, she is crying uncontrollably and says, "My husband does not want to look at me anymore. He is afraid of what I am going to look like with a flat chest."
• She says, "I cannot sleep and I just pace the floor at night."
• Expresses concern that her two daughters (34 and 32) and their daughters are going to get "this horrible disease."

Operative Procedure

• A lumpectomy and sentinel lymph node dissection are performed.
• A.K. has cancer cells in her sentinel lymph node.
• Axillary node dissection is then done involving the removal of 12 to 20 nodes.

Postoperative

• Does not want to leave hospital. She wants to stay in bed.
• Fever with swelling and restricted range of motion in right arm.
• Pain not controlled well with pain medication.

Follow-up Findings and Treatment

• Two positive lymph nodes are found.
• Scheduled for outpatient chemotherapy followed by external beam radiation.

Discussion Questions

1. What in A.K.'s breast cancer experience with her family members (see assessment case study in Chapter 51 on p. 1229) might influence her coping response?
2. What information would you provide to A.K. about her surgery?
3. What complication did she develop after her surgery?
4. Which common postoperative exercises will A.K. need to practice after her surgery?
5. **Delegation Decision:** Which of the following personnel should provide this instruction to A.K.: registered nurse, licensed practical/vocational nurse, unlicensed assistive personnel?
6. What community resources are available to help A.K. and her family adjust to the change in her body and to cope with the diagnosis of cancer? How can you access these resources?
7. What information is important for you to provide to A.K. about her radiation treatment and chemotherapy?
8. **Priority Decision:** Based on the assessment data, what are the priority nursing diagnoses? Are there any collaborative problems?
9. What information is important for you to provide to A.K. and her daughters? What early detection measures are important for them to know?
10. **Evidence-Based Practice:** A.K. wants to know what the psychologic benefit may be for her daughters if they decide on a breast cancer genetic risk assessment.

⊝volve Answers and a corresponding concept map available at *http://evolve.elsevier.com/Lewis/medsurg.*

can have positive effects on the patient's psychologic and physical health.

Reduction mammoplasty is performed by resecting wedges of tissue from the upper and lower quadrants of the breast. The excess skin is removed, and the areola and nipple are relocated on the breast. Lactation can usually be accomplished if massive amounts of tissue are not removed and the nipples are left connected during surgery.

NURSING MANAGEMENT
BREAST AUGMENTATION AND REDUCTION

Breast augmentation and breast reduction may be done in the outpatient surgical area, or they may involve overnight hospi-

talization. General anesthesia is used. Drains are generally placed in the surgical site to prevent hematoma formation and then removed 2 or 3 days after surgery or when drainage is under 20 to 30 mL/day. The drainage must be examined for color and odor to detect postoperative infection or hemorrhage. Also monitor the woman's temperature. Dressings should be changed as necessary using sterile technique. After surgery, assure the woman that the breast's appearance will improve when healing is completed. Depending on physician preference, the patient may be instructed to wear a bra that provides good support continuously for 2 or 3 days after breast reduction or augmentation. Depending on the extent of the operation, most women resume normal activities within 2 to 3 weeks. Strenuous exercise may not be appropriate until several weeks later.

BRIDGE TO NCLEX EXAMINATION

The number of the question corresponds to the same-numbered outcome at the beginning of the chapter.

1. You are a community health nurse planning a program on breast cancer screening guidelines for women in the neighborhood. To best promote the participants' learning and adherence, you would include *(select all that apply)*
   a. a short audiotape on the BSE procedure.
   b. a packet of articles from the medical literature.
   c. written guidelines for mammography and CBE.
   d. a discussion of the value of early breast cancer detection.
   e. community resources where they can obtain an ultrasound and MRI.

2. In teaching a patient who wants to perform BSE, you inform her that the technique involves both the palpation of the breast tissue and
   a. palpation of cervical lymph nodes.
   b. hard squeezing of the breast tissue.
   c. a mammogram to evaluate breast tissue.
   d. inspection of the breasts for any changes.

3. You are caring for a young woman who has painful fibrocystic breast changes. Management of this patient would include
   a. scheduling a biopsy to rule out malignant changes.
   b. teaching that symptoms will probably subside if she stops using oral contraceptives.
   c. preparing her for surgical removal of the lumps, since they will become larger and more painful.
   d. explaining that restrictions of coffee and chocolate and supplements of vitamin E may relieve some discomfort.

4. When discussing risk factors for breast cancer with a group of women, you emphasize that the greatest known risk factor for breast cancer is
   a. being a woman over age 60.
   b. experiencing menstruation for 30 years or more.
   c. using hormone therapy for 5 years for menopausal symptoms.
   d. having a paternal grandmother with postmenopausal breast cancer.

5. A patient with breast cancer has a lumpectomy with sentinel lymph node dissection that is positive for cancer. You explain that, of the other tests done to determine the risk for cancer recurrence or spread, the results that support the more favorable prognosis are *(select all that apply)*
   a. well-differentiated tumor.
   b. estrogen receptor–positive tumor.
   c. overexpression of HER-2 cell marker.
   d. involvement of two to four axillary nodes.
   e. aneuploidy status from cell proliferation studies.

6. A modified radical mastectomy has been scheduled for your patient with breast cancer. Postoperatively, to restore arm function on the affected side, you would
   a. apply heating pads or blankets to increase circulation.
   b. place daily ice packs to minimize the risk of lymphedema.
   c. teach passive exercises with the affected arm in a dependent position.
   d. emphasize regular exercises for the affected shoulder to increase range of motion.

7. Preoperatively, to meet the psychologic needs of a woman scheduled for a modified radical mastectomy, you would
   a. discuss the limitations of breast reconstruction.
   b. include her significant other in all conversations.
   c. promote an environment for expression of feelings.
   d. explain the importance of regular follow-up screening.

8. To prevent capsular formation after breast reconstruction with implants, teach the patient to
   a. gently massage the area around the implant.
   b. bind the breasts tightly with elastic bandages.
   c. exercise the arm on the affected side to promote drainage.
   d. avoid strenuous exercise until the implant has healed.

1. c, d, 2. d, 3. d, 4. a, 5. a, b, 6. d, 7. c, 8. a

evolve

For rationales to these answers and even more NCLEX review questions, visit *http://evolve.elsevier.com/Lewis/medsurg*.

REFERENCES

1. Jemal A, Siegel R, Naishadham D, et al: Cancer statistics 2012, *CA Cancer J Clin* 62:10, 2012.
2. American Cancer Society: Cancer facts and figures 2012. Retrieved from *www.cancer.org*.
3. American Cancer Society: Guidelines for the early detection of cancer. Retrieved from *www.cancer.org*.
*4. National Cancer Institute: Breast cancer screening (PDQ) summary of the evidence. Retrieved from *www.cancer.gov/cancertopics/pdq/screening/breast/healthprofessional*.
5. NCCN Clinical Practice Guidelines in Oncology: Breast cancer. Retrieved from *www.nccn.org*.
6. US Preventive Services Task Force: Screening for breast cancer. Retrieved from *www.uspreventiveservicestaskforce.org/uspstf/uspsbrca.htm*.
7. American Cancer Society: How to examine your breasts. Retrieved from *www.cancer.org/Cancer/BreastCancer/MoreInformation/BreastCancerEarlyDetection/breast-cancer-early-detection-acs-recs-bse*.
8. American Cancer Society: Recommendations for early breast cancer detection in women without breast symptoms. Retrieved from *www.cancer.org*.
*9. Fenton J, Abraham L, Taplin S, et al: Effectiveness of computer-aided detection in community mammography practice, *J Natl Cancer Inst* 103:1152, 2011.
10. Katz V, Dotters D: Breast diseases: diagnosis and treatment of benign and malignant disease. In Lentz G, Lobo R, Gershenson D, et al, editors: *Lentz comprehensive gynecology*, ed 6, St Louis, 2012, Mosby.
11. Robertson F, Bondy M, Yang W, et al: Inflammatory breast cancer, *CA Cancer J Clin* 60:351, 2011.
12. Lewis J, Borgan P: Breast disease. In Bope E, Kellerman R, editors: *Conn's current therapy*, St Louis, 2012, Saunders.
13. Seow J, Metcalf C, Wylie E: Nipple discharge in a screening programme: imaging findings with pathological correlation, *J Med Imaging Radiat Oncol* 55:577, 2011.
14. Ikard RW, Vavra D, Forbes RC, et al: Management of senescent gynecomastia in the Veterans Health Administration, *Breast J* 17:160, 2011.
*15. National Institutes of Health: Women's Health Initiative study. Retrieved from *www.nhlbi.nih.gov/whi*.
16. National Cancer Institute: Oral contraceptives and cancer risk. Retrieved from *www.cancer.gov/cancertopics/factsheet/Risk/oral-contraceptives*.
17. National Cancer Institute: *BRCA1* and *BRCA2*: cancer risk and genetic testing. Retrieved from *www.cancer.gov/cancertopics/factsheet/Risk/BRCA*.
*18. Bedrosian I, Hu C, Chang G: Population-based study of contralateral prophylactic mastectomy and survival outcomes of breast cancer patients, *J Natl Cancer Inst* 102:401, 2010.
*19. Slamon D, Eiermann W, Robert N, et al: Adjuvant trastuzumab in HER-2 positive breast cancer, *N Engl J Med* 365:1273, 2011.
20. Gradishar W: HER-therapy: an abundance of riches, *N Engl J Med* 366:176, 2012.
21. Morris L: Targeting the red-hot danger of inflammatory breast cancer, *Nursing* 40:58, 2010.
22. Lee E, McKean-Cowdin R, Ma H, et al: Characteristics of triple-negative breast cancer in patients with a *BRCA1* mutation: results from a population-based study of young women, *J Clin Oncol* 29:4373, 2011.
23. American Joint Committee on Cancer: *AJCC cancer staging manual*, ed 7. Retrieved from *www.cancerstaging.org/staging/changes2010f*.

*Evidence-based information for clinical practice.

*24. Sherman K, Koelmeyer L: The role of information sources and objective risk status on lymphedema risk-minimization behaviors in women recently diagnosed with breast cancer, *Oncol Nurs Forum* 38:66, 2011.

25. National Cancer Institute: A closer look: studies raise concerns about partial-breast radiation therapy, *NCI Cancer Bull*, January 10, 2012. Retrieved from *www.cancer.gov/ncicancerbulletin/01012*.

26. US Food and Drug Administration: FDA approves new treatment option for late-stage breast cancer. Retrieved from *www.fda.gov/NewsEvents/Newsroom/PressAnnouncements/ucm233863.htm*.

*27. Myers J: Chemotherapy-related cognitive impairment: the breast cancer experience, *Oncol Nurs Forum* 39:69, 2012.

28. National Cancer Institute: Chemotherapy associated with microscopic changes in the brain, *NCI Cancer Bull*, January 10, 2012. Retrieved from *www.cancer.gov/ncicancerbulletin/01012*.

29. National Cancer Institute: Study of raloxifene and tamoxifen (STAR) trial. Retrieved from *www.cancer.gov/clinicaltrials/noteworthy-trials/star/Page1*.

30. Memorial Sloan-Kettering Cancer Center: Survivorship care plan. Retrieved from *www.mskcc.org/cancer-care/survivorship/survivorship-care-plan*.

31. Goel M, Gracia G, Baker D: Development and pilot testing of a culturally sensitive multimedia program to improve breast cancer screening in Latina women, *Patient Educ Couns* 84:128, 2011.

*32. Lacovara J, Arzouman J, Kim C, et al: Are patients with breast cancer satisfied with their decision-making? *Clin J Oncol Nurs* 15:320, 2011.

*33. Cemal Y, Pusic A, Mehrara B: Preventative measures for lymphedema: separating fact from fiction, *J Am Coll Surg* 213:543, 2011.

34. Hill E, Sandbo S, Abramsohn E, et al: Assessing gynecologic and breast cancer survivors' sexual health care needs, *Cancer* 117:2643, 2010.

35. Johns Hopkins Medicine: Breast reconstruction improves well-being and quality of life, *HealthAfter50* 24:1, 2012.

36. US Food and Drug Administration: Breast implants. Retrieved from *www.fda.gov/MedicalDevices/ProductsandMedicalProcedures/ImplantsandProsthetics/BreastImplants/default.htm*.

RESOURCES

American Cancer Society
www.cancer.org/cancer/breastcancer/index
CancerCare
www.cancercare.org
Inflammatory Breast Cancer Research Foundation
www.ibcresearch.org
Livestrong
www.livestrong.org
Living Beyond Breast Cancer
www.lbbc.org
National Breast Cancer Coalition
www.natlbcc.org
National Cancer Institute
www.cancer.gov/cancertopics/types/breast
www.cancer.gov/bcrisktool/about-tool.aspx
National Coalition for Cancer Survivorship (NCCS)
www.canceradvocacy.org
National Lymphedema Network (NLN)
www.lymphnet.org
OncoLink (cancer information site)
www.oncolink.upenn.edu
Oncology Nursing Society
www.ons.org
Sisters Network (national African American breast cancer survivor group)
www.sistersnetworkinc.org
Susan G. Komen for the Cure
www.komen.org
Triple Negative Breast Cancer Foundation
www.tnbcfoundation.org
Young Survivor Coalition
www.youngsurvivor.org
Y-ME National Breast Cancer Organization (Y-ME)
http://en.wikipedia.org/wiki/Y-ME_National_Breast_Cancer_Organization

The doors we open and close each day decide the lives we live.
Flora Whittemore

Nursing Management
Sexually Transmitted Infections

Kay Jarrell

evolve WEBSITE

http://evolve.elsevier.com/Lewis/medsurg

- NCLEX Review Questions
- Key Points
- Pre-Test

- Answer Guidelines for Case Study on p. 1274
- Rationales for Bridge to NCLEX Examination Questions

- Concept Map Creator
- Glossary
- Content Updates

LEARNING OUTCOMES

1. Assess the factors contributing to the high incidence of sexually transmitted infections (STIs).
2. Describe the etiology, clinical manifestations, complications, and diagnostic abnormalities of gonorrhea, syphilis, chlamydial infections, genital herpes, and genital warts.
3. Compare and contrast primary genital herpes with recurrent genital herpes.
4. Explain the collaborative care and drug therapy of gonorrhea, syphilis, chlamydial infections, genital herpes, and genital warts.
5. Integrate the nursing assessment and nursing diagnoses for patients who have an STI.
6. Summarize the nursing role in the prevention and control of STIs.
7. Describe the nursing management of patients with STIs.

KEY TERMS

chancre, Table 53-3, p. 1265
chlamydial infections, p. 1266
genital herpes, p. 1267

genital warts, p. 1269
gonorrhea, p. 1262

sexually transmitted infections (STIs), p. 1261
syphilis, p. 1264

Sexually transmitted infections (STIs) are infectious diseases that are commonly acquired through sexual contact (Table 53-1). They may also be contracted by other routes such as through blood, blood products, perinatal transmission, and autoinoculation. STI is becoming the more common term used for sexually transmitted disease.

Most infections start as lesions on the genitalia and other sexually exposed mucous membranes. Wide dissemination to other areas of the body can then occur. A latent or subclinical phase is present with all STIs. This can lead to a long-term persistent infection and the transmission of disease from an asymptomatic (but infected) person to another person. Having one STI increases the risk of acquiring another. A person can have different STIs at the same time.

In the United States all cases of gonorrhea and syphilis, and in most states chlamydial infection, must be reported to the state or local public health authorities for purposes of surveillance and partner notification. In spite of this requirement, many cases of these infections go unreported. An estimated 65 million Americans are currently infected with one or more STI. Every year an additional 19 million Americans are newly infected with an STI. About 50% of these new cases are in persons 15 to 24 years old.[1]

The most commonly diagnosed STIs are discussed in this chapter. Human immunodeficiency virus (HIV) infection is discussed in Chapter 15. Hepatitis B and C infections are discussed in Chapter 44.

Factors Affecting Incidence of Sexually Transmitted Infections

Many factors contribute to the current STI rates. Earlier reproductive maturity and increased longevity have resulted in a longer sexual life span. The increase in the total population has resulted in an increase in the number of susceptible hosts. Other factors include greater sexual freedom, lack of barrier methods (e.g., condoms) during sexual activity, and the media's increased emphasis on sexuality. Substance abuse contributes to unsafe sexual practices. In addition, increased

Reviewed by Suzanne L. Jed, MSN, FNP-BC, Instructor of Clinical Family Medicine, Keck School of Medicine, University of Southern California, Los Angeles, California; and Danette Y. Wall, ACRN, MSN, MBA/HCM, ISO9001 Lead Auditor, Regional Nurse, Department of Veterans Affairs–Veterans Health Administration, Tampa, Florida.

TABLE 53-1	CAUSES OF SEXUALLY TRANSMITTED INFECTIONS

Sexually Transmitted Infection	Cause
Bacterial	
Gonorrhea	*Neisseria gonorrhoeae*
Syphilis	*Treponema pallidum*
Nongonococcal urethritis (NGU), cervicitis, lymphogranuloma venereum	*Chlamydia trachomatis*
Viral	
Genital herpes	Herpes simplex virus (HSV)
Genital warts. Cervical, vulvar, vaginal, penile, anal, and oropharyngeal cancers	Human papillomavirus (HPV)
Human immunodeficiency virus (HIV) infection, acquired immunodeficiency syndrome (AIDS)	HIV virus (see Chapter 15)
Hepatitis B and C	Hepatitis B and C viruses (see Chapter 44)
Encephalitis, esophagitis, retinitis, pneumonitis in immunocompromised patients	Cytomegalovirus (CMV)

leisure time, more national and international travel, and urbanization have brought together people with varying social behaviors and value systems.

Changes in the methods of contraception are also reflected in the incidence of STIs. The condom is considered to be the best form of protection (other than abstinence) against STIs. Although condom use has increased, condoms are still not used frequently in the general population.[2] Commonly used oral contraceptives cause the secretions of the cervix and the vagina to become more alkaline. This change produces a more favorable environment for the growth of organisms that cause STIs at these sites. Women who take oral contraceptives may have a lower risk of pelvic inflammatory disease (PID) as a result of the ability of the cervical mucus to act as a barrier against bacteria. However, the proliferation of *Chlamydia* organisms, the leading cause of nongonococcal PID, may be enhanced by oral contraceptive use.

Whether or not intrauterine device (IUD) users are at increased risk of PID is controversial, but it is clear that IUDs confer no protection against STIs. Long-acting contraceptives such as medroxyprogesterone (Depo-Provera) also offer no protection against STIs. Although these methods do not prevent transmission from partner to partner, they do prevent pregnancy and, therefore, transmission of the infection to the fetus.

BACTERIAL INFECTIONS

GONORRHEA

Gonorrhea is the second most frequently reported STI in the United States (chlamydial infections are the most common). In 2009 the gonorrhea rates were the lowest since recording of rates began. Since that time gonorrhea rates have increased slightly. A total of 309,341 cases of gonorrhea have been reported in the United States.[3] Gonorrhea rates are highest in adolescents of all racial and ethnic groups and among African Americans. Most states have enacted laws that permit examination and treatment of minors without parental consent.

Etiology and Pathophysiology

Gonorrhea is caused by *Neisseria gonorrhoeae*, a gram-negative diplococcus. The infection is spread by direct physical contact with an infected host, usually during sexual activity (vaginal, oral, or anal). Mucosal tissues in the genitalia (urethra in men, cervix in women), rectum, and oropharynx are especially sensitive to gonococcal infection. The delicate gonococcus is easily killed by drying, heating, or washing with an antiseptic solution. Consequently, indirect transmission by instruments or linens is rare.

The incubation period is 3 to 8 days. The infection confers no immunity to subsequent reinfection. Gonococcal infection elicits an inflammatory response, which, if left untreated, leads to the formation of fibrous tissue and adhesions. This fibrous scarring is responsible for many complications in women such as strictures and tubal abnormalities, which can lead to tubal pregnancy, chronic pelvic pain, and infertility.

Clinical Manifestations

Men. The initial site of infection in men is usually the urethra. Symptoms of urethritis consist of dysuria and profuse, purulent urethral discharge developing 2 to 5 days after infection (Fig. 53-1). Painful or swollen testicles may also occur. Men generally seek medical evaluation early in the infection because their symptoms are usually obvious and distressing. It is unusual for men with gonorrhea to be asymptomatic.[4]

Women. Many women who contract gonorrhea are asymptomatic or have minor symptoms that are often overlooked, making it possible for them to remain a source of infection. A few women may complain of vaginal discharge, dysuria, or frequency of urination. Changes in menstruation may be a symptom, but the women often disregard these changes. After the incubation period, redness and swelling occur at the site of

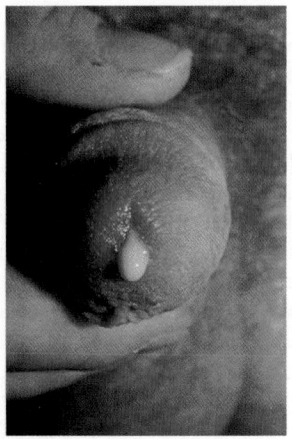

FIG. 53-1 Profuse, purulent drainage in a patient with gonorrhea.

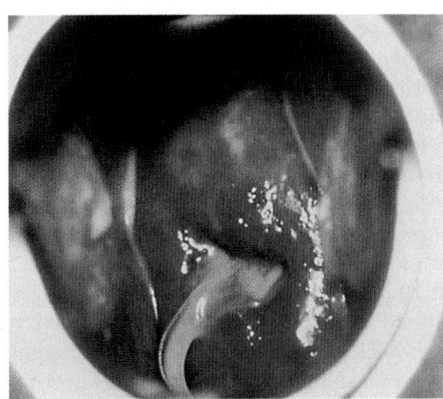

FIG. 53-2 Endocervical gonorrhea. Cervical redness and edema with discharge.

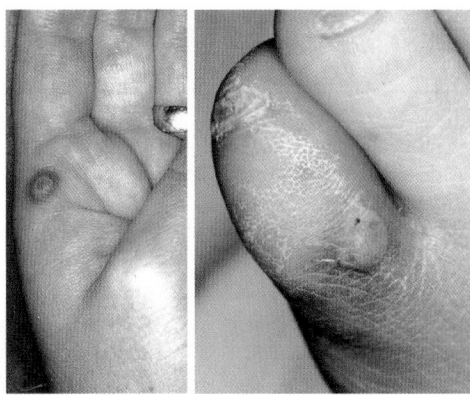

FIG. 53-3 Skin lesions with disseminated gonococcal infection. **A,** On the hand. **B,** On the fifth toe.

contact, which is usually the cervix or urethra (Fig. 53-2). A greenish yellow purulent exudate often develops with a potential for abscess formation. The infection may remain local or can spread by direct tissue extension to the uterus, fallopian tubes, and ovaries. Although the vulva and vagina are uncommon sites for a gonorrheal infection, they may become involved when little or no estrogen is present, as in prepubertal girls and postmenopausal women. Because the vagina acts as a natural reservoir for infectious secretions, transmission is often more efficient from men to women than it is from women to men.

General. Anorectal gonorrhea may be present, usually as a result of anal intercourse. Symptoms may include mucopurulent anal discharge, bleeding, and tenesmus.[5] Most patients with anorectal infections and infections in the throat have few symptoms. A small percentage of individuals develop gonococcal pharyngitis from orogenital sexual contact. When the gonococcus can be demonstrated by a laboratory culture, individuals of either gender are infectious to their sexual partners.

Complications

Because men often seek treatment early in the course of the infection, they are less likely to develop complications. The complications that do occur in men are prostatitis, urethral strictures, and sterility from orchitis or epididymitis. Because women who are asymptomatic seldom seek treatment, complications are more common and usually constitute the reason for seeking medical attention. PID, Bartholin's abscess, ectopic pregnancy, and infertility are the main complications of gonorrhea in women. A small percentage of infected persons, mainly women, may develop a disseminated gonococcal infection (DGI). In DGI the appearance of skin lesions, fever, arthralgia, arthritis, or endocarditis usually causes the patient to seek medical help (Fig. 53-3).

Neonates can develop a gonococcal infection during delivery from an infected mother. Untreated infected infants develop permanent blindness. Almost all states have a health department regulation or law requiring the use of a prophylactic drug such as erythromycin ophthalmic ointment or silver nitrate aqueous solution in the eyes of all newborns. Therefore gonorrheal eye infections in newborns (*ophthalmia neonatorum*) are relatively rare today.

Diagnostic Studies

For men, a presumptive diagnosis of gonorrhea is made if there is a history of sexual contact with a new or infected partner

GENDER DIFFERENCES
Sexually Transmitted Infections

Men	Women
• Syphilis more common, especially in men who have sex with men	• Chlamydial infection three times more common
• More likely to be symptomatic	• Gonorrhea more common
• Easier to diagnose because of less complex anatomy	• HSV-2 more common
	• Have more frequent and serious complications related to STIs (e.g., pelvic inflammatory disease)

HSV-2, Herpes simplex type 2.

followed within a few days by a urethral discharge. Typical clinical manifestations, combined with a positive finding on a Gram-stained smear of the purulent discharge from the penis, give an almost certain diagnosis. A culture of the discharge is indicated for men whose smears are negative in the presence of strong clinical evidence. The nucleic acid amplification test (NAAT) (using ligase or polymerase chain reaction) is a nonculture test with sensitivity similar to culture tests for *N. gonorrhoeae*. It can be done on a wide variety of samples, including vaginal, endocervical, urethral, and urine specimens.[6]

For women, making a diagnosis of gonorrhea on the basis of symptoms is difficult because most women are symptom free or have complaints that may be confused with other conditions. Smears and purulent discharge do not establish a diagnosis of gonorrhea because the female genitourinary tract normally harbors a large number of organisms that resemble *N. gonorrhoeae*. A culture must be performed to confirm the diagnosis. Although the cervix is the most common site of sampling, specimens for culture may also be taken from the urethra, anus, or oropharynx. A urine specimen can reveal gonorrhea if it is present in the cervix or urethra.

Collaborative Care

Drug Therapy. Because of a short incubation period and high infectivity, treatment is generally instituted without awaiting culture results. The treatment of gonorrhea in the early stage is curative with a cephalosporin antibiotic. Treatment for gonorrhea is an intramuscular (IM) dose of ceftriaxone (Rocephin) or cefixime (Suprax) orally (Table 53-2).

Over the years, *N. gonorrhoeae* has developed a resistance to multiple classes of antimicrobial drugs, including fluoroquinolones (ciprofloxacin [Cipro], ofloxacin [Floxin], levofloxacin

TABLE 53-2   COLLABORATIVE CARE

Gonorrhea

Diagnostic

History and physical examination

Gram-stained smears of urethral or endocervical exudate

Culture for *Neisseria gonorrhoeae*

Nucleic acid amplification test (NAAT) to detect *N. gonorrhoeae*

Testing for other STIs (syphilis, HIV, chlamydial infection)

Collaborative Therapy

Uncomplicated gonorrhea: ceftriaxone (Rocephin) IM or cefixime (Suprax) orally

If chlamydial infection is not ruled out: azithromycin (Zithromax) or doxycycline (Vibramycin)

Treatment of sexual contacts

Instruction on abstinence from sexual intercourse and alcohol during treatment

Reexamination if symptoms persist or recur after completion of treatment

Source: Centers for Disease Control and Prevention: Sexually transmitted diseases treatment guidelines, 2010. Retrieved from *www.cdc.gov/STD/treatment*.

[Levaquin]) and tetracyclines (doxycycline [Vibramycin]). Gonococcal resistance to cephalosporin has recently been reported.[7]

The high frequency (up to 20% in men and 40% in women) of coexisting chlamydial and gonococcal infections has led to the addition of azithromycin (Zithromax) or doxycycline to the treatment regimen. Patients with coexisting syphilis are likely to be treated with the same drugs used for gonorrhea.

DRUG ALERT: Doxycycline (Vibramycin)
- Patients on this drug should avoid unnecessary exposure to sunlight.
- Do not take with antacids, iron products, or dairy products.

All sexual contacts of patients with gonorrhea must be evaluated and treated to prevent reinfection after resumption of sexual relations. The "ping-pong" effect of reexposure, treatment, and reinfection can end only when infected partners are treated simultaneously. Additionally, counsel the patient to abstain from sexual intercourse and alcohol during treatment. Sexual intercourse allows the infection to spread and can delay complete healing. Alcohol has an irritant effect on the healing urethral walls. Caution men against squeezing the penis to look for further discharge. Reinfection, rather than treatment failure, is the main cause of infections after treatment has ended.

SYPHILIS

The incidence of syphilis reported in the United States in 2000 was at its lowest rate since reporting started in 1941. During the past decade, syphilis rates increased until 2010 when the rate slightly decreased.[1] Many new cases of syphilis are being seen in men who have sex with men.

Etiology and Pathophysiology

Syphilis is caused by *Treponema pallidum*, a spirochete. This bacterium is thought to enter the body through very small breaks in the skin or mucous membranes. Its entry is facilitated by the minor abrasions that often occur during sexual intercourse. Syphilis is a complex disease in which many organs and tissues of the body can become infected by *T. pallidum*. The infection causes the production of antibodies that also react with normal tissues.

After a short period of protection, antibody levels decrease and a person is susceptible to reinfection. Not all people who are exposed to syphilis acquire the infection, since about one third become infected after intercourse with an infected person. In addition to sexual contact, syphilis may be spread through contact with infectious lesions and sharing of needles among IV drug users.

T. pallidum is extremely fragile and easily destroyed by drying, heating, or washing. The incubation period for syphilis ranges from 10 to 90 days (average 21 days). Congenital syphilis is transmitted from an infected mother to the fetus in utero after the tenth week of pregnancy. An infected pregnant woman has a high risk of a stillbirth or a baby dying shortly after birth.[8] Pregnant women need to be tested for syphilis at their first prenatal visit. Some states require all women to be screened at delivery.

Persons at high risk for acquiring syphilis are also at an increased risk for acquiring HIV infection. Often, both infections are present. Syphilitic lesions (chancres) on the genitalia enhance HIV transmission. Patients with HIV and syphilis appear to be at greatest risk for clinically significant central nervous system (CNS) involvement and may require more intensive treatment than do other patients with syphilis. Therefore the evaluation of all patients with syphilis should also include testing for HIV (with the patient's consent). Conversely, HIV patients should be tested at least annually for syphilis.

Clinical Manifestations

Syphilis has a variety of signs and symptoms that can mimic a number of other diseases. Consequently, compared with other STIs, it is more difficult to recognize syphilis. If it is not treated, specific clinical stages are characteristic of the progression of the disease (Table 53-3).

Complications

Complications of the disease occur mostly in late syphilis. The gummas of benign late syphilis may produce irreparable damage to bone, liver, or skin. In cardiovascular syphilis, the resulting aneurysm may press on structures such as the intercostal nerves, causing pain. The possibility of a rupture exists as the aneurysm increases in size. Scarring of the aortic valve results in aortic valve insufficiency and eventually heart failure.

Neurosyphilis causes degeneration of the brain with mental deterioration. Problems related to sensory nerve involvement are a result of *tabes dorsalis* (progressive locomotor ataxia). There may be sudden attacks of pain anywhere in the body, which can confuse the diagnosis with other conditions. Loss of vision and sense of position in the feet and legs can also occur. Walking may become even more difficult as joint stability is lost. (Late syphilis is also discussed in Chapter 59.)

Diagnostic Studies

The first step in diagnosis is to obtain a detailed and accurate sexual history. Asking if the patient has sex with men, women, or both can be more effective than asking directly about sexual orientation, since some men do not identify themselves as gay or homosexual. In addition, inquire about vaginal, oral, or anal sex. A physical examination should be done to identify any suspicious lesions or other significant signs and symptoms. Since syphilis is "the great imitator" of other conditions, it is easily missed. Oral sex is an important transmission route that is sometimes overlooked.

TABLE 53-3 STAGES OF SYPHILIS

Manifestations	Communicability
Primary	
Chancre (painless indurated lesion of penis, vulva, lips, mouth, vagina, and rectum) (Fig. 53-4) occurs 10 to 90 days after inoculation.	Exudate from chancre highly infectious; blood is infectious.
Regional lymphadenopathy (draining of the microorganisms into the lymph nodes).	Most infectious stage, but transmission can occur at any stage if there are moist lesions.
Genital ulcers.	
Duration of stage: 3-8 wk	
Secondary	
Occurs a few weeks after chancre appears.	Exudate from skin and mucous membrane lesions highly infectious.
Systemic manifestations: flu-like symptoms (e.g., malaise, fever, sore throat, headaches, fatigue, arthralgia, headache, generalized adenopathy).	
Cutaneous lesions bilateral. Symmetric rash that begins on the trunk and involves the palms and soles. Mucous patches in the mouth (Fig. 53-5), tongue, or cervix. *Condylomata lata* (moist, weeping papules) in the anal and genital area.	
Weight loss, alopecia.	
Duration of stage: 1-2 yr	
Latent	
Absence of signs or symptoms.	Noninfectious after 4 yr. Possible placental transmission.
Diagnosis based on positive specific treponemal antibody test together with normal CSF and absence of clinical manifestations.	Almost 25% of persons with latent syphilis develop late syphilis, in some cases many years later.
Duration of stage: Throughout life or progression to late stage	
Late (tertiary)*	
Appearance 3-20 yr after initial infection.	Noninfectious.
Gummas (chronic, destructive lesions affecting any organ of body, especially skin, bone, liver, mucous membranes) (Fig. 53-6).	Spinal fluid possibly containing organism.
Cardiovascular: Aneurysms, heart valve insufficiency, heart failure, aortitis.	
Neurosyphilis: General paresis (personality changes from minor to psychotic, tremors, physical and mental deterioration), tabes dorsalis (ataxia, areflexia, paresthesias, lightning pains, damaged joints), speech disturbances.	
Duration of stage: Chronic (without treatment), possibly fatal	

*Several forms such as cardiovascular syphilis and neurosyphilis occur together in approximately 25% of untreated cases.

CSF, Cerebrospinal fluid.

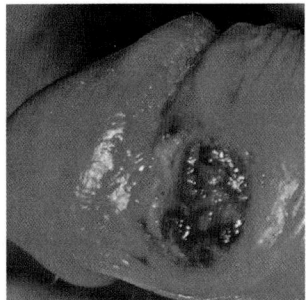

FIG. 53-4 Primary syphilis chancre.

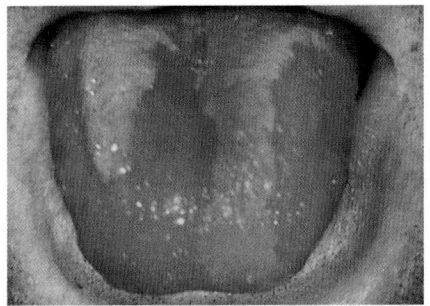

FIG. 53-5 Secondary syphilis. Mucous patch in the mouth.

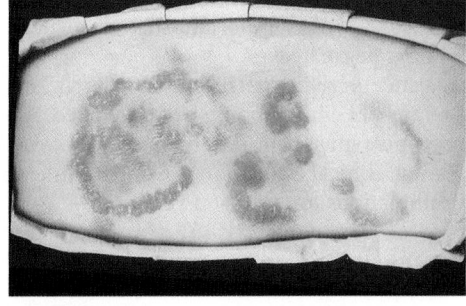

FIG. 53-6 Destructive skin gummas associated with tertiary syphilis.

Diagnostic studies for syphilis are presented in Table 53-4. The presence of spirochetes on dark-field microscopy and direct fluorescent antibody (DFA) tests of lesion exudate or tissue can confirm a clinical diagnosis of syphilis. However, syphilis is more commonly diagnosed by a serologic test.[4] Tests for syphilis may be classified as those performed for screening and those performed for confirmation of a positive screening test. Nonspecific antitreponemal antibodies can be detected by tests such as the Venereal Disease Research Laboratory (VDRL) test and the rapid plasma reagin (RPR) test. These nontreponemal tests are suitable for screening purposes, and usually become positive 10 to 14 days after the appearance of a chancre. The fluorescent treponemal antibody absorption (FTA-Abs) test and the *T. pallidum* particle agglutination (TP-PA) test detect specific antitreponemal antibodies and are used for confirming the diagnosis.

False-negative and false-positive test results do occur with the nontreponemal tests (VDRL, RPR). A false-negative result may be obtained during primary syphilis if the test is done before the individual has had time to produce antibodies. A false-positive finding may occur if patients have other diseases or conditions such as hepatitis, infectious mononucleosis, collagen diseases (e.g., systemic lupus erythematosus), pregnancy, or aging. Positive nontreponemal test results should be confirmed by more specific treponemal tests to rule out other causes. In the cerebrospinal fluid (CSF), changes such as increased white blood cell count, increased total protein, and a positive treponemal antibody test are diagnostic of neurosyphilis.

TABLE 53-4 COLLABORATIVE CARE

Syphilis

Diagnostic
- History and physical examination
- Dark-field microscopy
- Nontreponemal and/or treponemal serologic testing
- Testing for other STIs (HIV, gonorrhea, chlamydial infection)

Collaborative Therapy
- Antibiotic therapy
  - penicillin G benzathine (Bicillin) or aqueous procaine penicillin G
  - doxycycline (Vibramycin) or tetracycline (when penicillin is contraindicated)
- Confidential counseling and testing for HIV infection
- Surveillance
  - Repeat of nontreponemal tests at 6 and 12 mo
  - Examination of cerebrospinal fluid at 1 yr*

*If treatment involves alternative antibiotics or treatment failure has occurred.

If treatment with antibiotics is initiated early in the course of the disease on the basis of the history and the symptoms, the serologic testing may not indicate syphilis. Once a person has positive serologic findings for syphilis, indicating the presence of antibodies, these findings may remain positive for an indefinite period in spite of successful treatment.

Collaborative Care

Table 53-4 describes collaborative care of syphilis. Specific management is based on the symptoms.

Drug Therapy. Management of syphilis is aimed at eradicating all syphilitic organisms. Penicillin G benzathine (Bicillin) or aqueous procaine penicillin G is the treatment of choice for all stages of syphilis.[9] When penicillin is contraindicated, doxycycline or tetracycline may be used. However, treatment cannot reverse damage that is already present in the late stage of the disease. It is also important that all sexual contacts in the last 90 days be treated.

Patients having persistent or recurring symptoms after drug therapy has ended should be reevaluated. All patients with neurosyphilis must be carefully monitored, with periodic serologic testing, clinical evaluation at 6-month intervals, and repeat CSF examinations for at least 3 years.

CHLAMYDIAL INFECTIONS

Chlamydial infections are the most commonly reported STI in the United States. Infection rates have increased over the past 20 years, with more than 1.3 million cases reported in 2010.[1] This increase may be due in part to better and more intensive screening for the infection. Underreporting is significant because many people are asymptomatic and do not seek testing.

The incidence of chlamydia is higher in women than men, which may be because more women are screened for this infection. Women younger than 25 years old are five times more likely to have a chlamydial infection than women over age 30. Women infected with *Chlamydia* may also be at high risk for acquiring HIV from an infected partner.

Etiology and Pathophysiology

Chlamydial infections are caused by *Chlamydia trachomatis,* a gram-negative bacterium. *Chlamydia* can be transmitted during

TABLE 53-5 RISK FACTORS FOR CHLAMYDIAL INFECTION

- Women and adolescents
- New or multiple sexual partners
- Sexual partners who have had multiple partners
- History of STIs and cervical ectopy
- Coexisting STIs
- Inconsistent or incorrect use of condom

Modified from Centers for Disease Control and Prevention: CDC fact sheet: chlamydia. Retrieved from *www.cdc.gov/std/Chlamydia/STD fact.*

EVIDENCE-BASED PRACTICE

Translating Research Into Practice

What Strategies Improve Screening Rates for Repeat Chlamydial Infections?

Clinical Question

In patients with repeat chlamydial infections (P), what is the effect of reminders and mailed screening kits (I) versus no intervention (C) on rescreening rates (O)?

Best Available Evidence

Systematic review of randomized controlled trials (RCTs) and observational studies

Critical Appraisal and Synthesis of Evidence
- Eight trials (n = 25 to 5863/trial) compared patient rescreening rates for repeat chlamydial infections.
- Interventions were mailed screening kits, motivational interviewing, financial incentives, and reminders.
- Rescreening occurred 3 wk to 12 mo after the initial chlamydial infection.
- Mailed screening kits for sample self-collection and phone call, postcard, and e-mail reminders significantly increased rescreening rates.

Conclusion
- Mailed screening kits, reminders, and a combination of both methods increased rescreening rates.

Implications for Nursing Practice
- Repeat chlamydial infections are common and increase the risk of complications.
- Remind patient of importance of rescreening.
- To increase rescreening rates, tailor interventions to meet patient needs and preferences.
- Text message and automated phone calling reminders may also be effective.

Reference for Evidence

Guy R, Hocking J, Low N, et al: Interventions to increase rescreening for repeat chlamydial infection, *Sex Trans Dis* 2:136, 2012.

P, Patient population of interest; *I,* intervention or area of interest; *C,* comparison of interest or comparison group; *O,* outcomes of interest (see p. 12).

vaginal, anal, or oral sex. Numerous different serotypes, or strains, of *C. trachomatis* cause urogenital infections (e.g., nongonococcal urethritis [NGU] in men and cervicitis in women), ocular trachoma, and lymphogranuloma venereum. Risk factors for chlamydial infection are presented in Table 53-5. As with gonorrhea, chlamydial infections result in a superficial mucosal infection that can become more invasive.

Clinical Manifestations

Chlamydial infection is known as a silent disease because symptoms may be absent or minor in most infected women and in

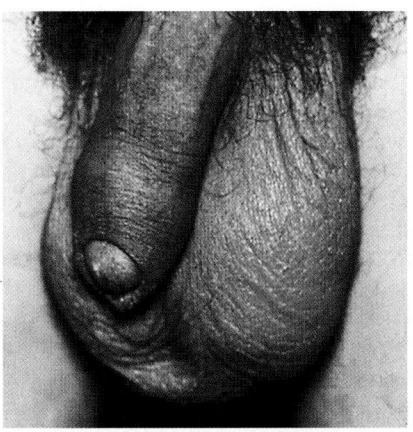

FIG. 53-7 Chlamydial epididymitis. Red, swollen scrotum.

TABLE 53-6 **COLLABORATIVE CARE**
Chlamydial Infection
Diagnostic
• History and physical examination
• Nucleic acid amplification test (NAAT)
• Direct fluorescent antibody (DFA) test
• Enzyme immunoassay (EIA)
• Testing for other STIs (gonorrhea, HIV, syphilis)
Collaborative Therapy
• doxycycline (Vibramycin) or azithromycin (Zithromax)
• Alternative regimen: erythromycin, ofloxacin (Floxin), or levofloxacin (Levaquin)
• Instruction on abstinence from sexual intercourse for 7 days after completing treatment
• Treatment of all sexual partners

many men.[10] In men, signs and symptoms include urethritis (dysuria, urethral discharge), proctitis (rectal discharge and pain during defecation), and epididymitis (unilateral scrotal pain, swelling, tenderness, fever) (Fig. 53-7).

In women, signs and symptoms include cervicitis (mucopurulent discharge, hypertrophic ectopy [area that is edematous and bleeds easily]), urethritis (dysuria, frequent urination, pyuria), bartholinitis (purulent exudate), dyspareunia (pain with intercourse), and menstrual abnormalities.

Because chlamydial infections are closely associated with gonococcal infections, clinical differentiation may be difficult. In men, urethritis, epididymitis, and proctitis may occur with both infections. In women, bartholinitis, cervicitis, and salpingitis (inflammation of the fallopian tube) can occur in both chlamydial and gonococcal infections. Therefore both infections are usually treated concurrently even without diagnostic proof. The incubation period of 1 to 3 weeks for chlamydial infection is longer than that for gonorrhea, and the symptoms are often milder.

Complications

Complications often develop from poorly managed, inaccurately diagnosed, or undiagnosed chlamydial infections. The infection is often not diagnosed until complications appear.

In men, epididymitis can lead to rare complications, including abscess, sepsis, infertility, and reactive arthritis (a systemic condition accompanied by skin lesions and inflammation of the eye and urethra).

In women, chlamydial infections can cause fallopian tube damage, a leading cause of ectopic pregnancy and infertility. Complications from chlamydial infections in women may result in PID, which can lead to chronic pelvic pain.[11] PID can also cause nausea, vomiting, fever, malaise, and abnormal vaginal bleeding.

Diagnostic Studies

Chlamydial infections in men and women can be diagnosed by testing urine or collecting swab specimens from the endocervix or vagina (women) or urethra (men). Rectal swab specimens are tested in persons engaging in anal sex. Table 53-6 outlines collaborative care for chlamydial infections.

Cell culture can be used to detect *Chlamydia* organisms. The most common diagnostic tests include the NAAT, DFA test, and enzyme immunoassay (EIA). These tests do not require special handling of specimens and are easier to perform than cell cultures. Amplification tests are the most sensitive diagnostic methods available and require fewer organisms. In addition, these tests can be used with urine samples rather than urethral and cervical swabs.

Collaborative Care

The Centers for Disease Control and Prevention (CDC) recommends that all sexually active women 25 years of age or younger be routinely screened for *Chlamydia*.[9] The CDC further recommends annual screening of all women older than 25 years of age with one or more risk factors for the infection (see Table 53-5).

Drug Therapy. To avoid complications from chlamydial infection, treatment should not be delayed. Doxycycline or azithromycin is used to treat patients and their partners. Treatment of pregnant women usually prevents transmission to the fetus. Patients treated for chlamydial infections should abstain from sexual intercourse for 7 days after treatment and until all sexual partners have completed a full course of treatment. Follow-up care includes advising the patient to return if symptoms persist or recur, treating sexual partners, and encouraging condom use during all sexual contacts.

The high incidence of recurrence may be due to failure to treat the sexual partners of infected people. Because of the high prevalence of asymptomatic infections, screening of high-risk populations is needed to identify those who are infected.

VIRAL INFECTIONS

GENITAL HERPES

Genital herpes is caused by herpes simplex virus (HSV). It is not a reportable infection in most states. Its true incidence is difficult to determine because most people have few to no symptoms. In the United States at least 50 million people are infected with HSV type 2. In people ages 14 to 49 approximately one out of six have genital herpes.[12]

Etiology and Pathophysiology

HSV enters through the mucous membranes or breaks in the skin during contact with an infected person. The virus then reproduces inside the cell and spreads to the surrounding cells. The virus next enters the peripheral or autonomic nerve endings and ascends to the sensory or autonomic nerve ganglion, where it often becomes dormant. Viral reactivation (recurrence) may occur when the virus descends to the initial site of infection, either the mucous membranes or skin. When a person is infected with HSV, the virus usually persists within the individual for life. Transmission of HSV occurs through direct contact with skin or mucous membranes when an infected individual is symptomatic or through asymptomatic viral shedding.

Two different strains of HSV cause infection. In general, HSV type 1 (HSV-1) causes infection above the waist, involving the gingivae, the dermis, the upper respiratory tract, and the CNS. HSV type 2 (HSV-2) most frequently infects the genital tract and the perineum (i.e., locations below the waist). However, either strain can cause infection on the mouth or the genitalia. Although the majority of genital herpes cases are from HSV-2 infection, the incidence of anogenital herpes from HSV-1 is increasing among young women and men who have sex with men.

Clinical Manifestations

Primary Episode. In the *primary (initial) episode* of genital herpes the patient may complain of burning, itching, or tingling at the site of inoculation. Multiple small, vesicular, and sometimes painless lesions may appear on the inner thigh, penis, scrotum, vulva, perineum, perianal region, vagina, or cervix.[13] The vesicles contain large quantities of infectious viral particles (Fig. 53-8). The lesions rupture and form shallow, moist ulcerations. Finally, crusting and epithelialization of the erosions occur. Primary infections tend to be associated with local inflammation and pain, accompanied by systemic manifestations of fever, headache, malaise, myalgia, and regional lymphadenopathy.

Urination may be painful from the urine touching active lesions. Urinary retention may occur as a result of HSV urethritis or cystitis. A purulent vaginal discharge may develop with HSV cervicitis.

Primary lesions are generally present for 17 to 20 days, but new lesions sometimes continue to develop for 6 weeks. The duration of symptoms is longer and the frequency of complications is greater in women. The lesions heal spontaneously unless secondary infection occurs.

Recurrent Episodes. *Recurrent genital herpes* occurs in about 50% to 80% of individuals during the year following the primary episode. Common trigger factors include stress, fatigue, sunburn, general illness, immunosuppression, and menses. Many patients can predict a recurrence by noticing the prodromal symptoms of tingling, burning, and itching at the site where the lesions will eventually appear.[13]

The symptoms of recurrent episodes are less severe, and the lesions usually heal within 8 to 12 days. With time, the recurrent lesions generally occur less frequently. In extreme cases this can indicate immunosuppression and may signal a need to test for HIV.

Complications

Autoinoculation of the virus to extragenital sites such as the fingers and lips ("cold sores") may occur (Fig. 53-9). Although most infections are relatively benign, complications of genital herpes may involve the CNS, causing aseptic meningitis and lower motor neuron damage. Neuron damage may result in atonic bladder, impotence, and constipation. Immunocompromised patients (e.g., HIV-infected patients) should be monitored closely for treatment failure and a slower healing time of HSV lesions.

Women with a primary episode of HSV near the time of delivery have the highest risk of transmitting genital herpes to the neonate. An active genital lesion at the time of delivery is usually an indication for cesarean delivery.[9] Acyclovir (Zovirax) may be given to pregnant women who are at least at 36 weeks of gestation to prevent neonatal transmission.[14]

Diagnostic Studies and Collaborative Care

A diagnosis of genital herpes is usually based on the patient's symptoms and history. Highly accurate serologic tests are available for the diagnosis of HSV-1 and HSV-2. These type-specific immunoassays test for antibodies to HSV. A viral culture of the active lesion can also be used to isolate the virus.

Encourage symptomatic treatment such as using good genital hygiene and wearing loose-fitting cotton undergarments. The lesions should be kept clean and dry. To ensure complete drying of the perineal area, women may use a hair dryer set on a cool setting. Frequent sitz baths may soothe the area and reduce inflammation. Drying agents such as colloidal oatmeal (Aveeno) and aluminum salts (Burow's solution) may

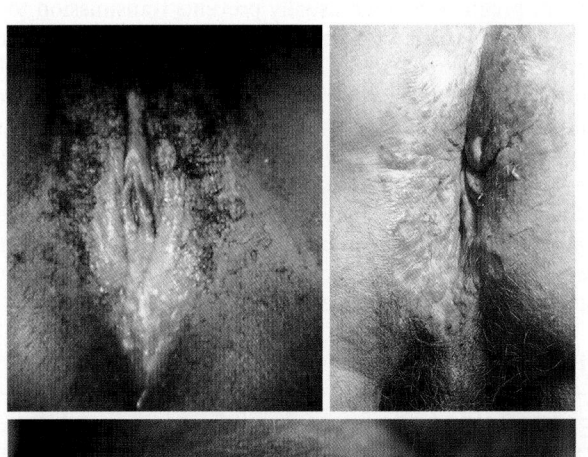

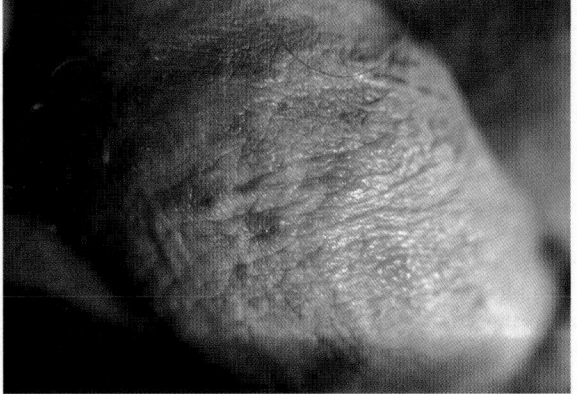

FIG. 53-8 Unruptured vesicles of herpes simplex virus type 2 (HSV-2). **A,** Vulvar area. **B,** Perianal area. **C,** Penile herpes simplex, ulcerative stage.

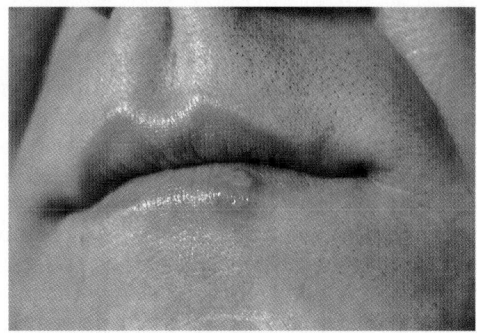

FIG. 53-9 Autoinoculation of herpes simplex virus (HSV) to the lips.

provide some relief from the burning and itching. Techniques to reduce pain on urination include pouring a pitcher of water onto the perineal area while voiding to dilute the urine, and voiding in a warm tub of water or shower. Pain may require a local anesthetic such as lidocaine (Xylocaine) or systemic analgesics such as codeine and aspirin.

Sexual transmission of HSV can occur during asymptomatic periods, and the use of barrier methods, especially condoms, should be encouraged. When lesions are present, the patient should avoid sexual activity altogether because even barrier protection is not satisfactory in eliminating infection transmission.

Drug Therapy. Treatment of HSV infection should be started before diagnostic results are available because early treatment reduces transmission and duration of the ulcers. Three antiviral agents are available for the treatment of HSV: acyclovir, valacyclovir (Valtrex), and famciclovir (Famvir). These drugs inhibit herpetic viral replication and are prescribed for primary and recurrent infections (Table 53-7). Acyclovir, valacyclovir, and famciclovir are also used to suppress frequent recurrences (six or more episodes per year).

Although not a cure, these drugs shorten the duration of viral shedding and the healing time of genital lesions and reduce outbreaks by 75%.[9] Continued use of oral acyclovir as suppressive therapy for up to 6 years is safe and effective for persons with frequent or severe recurrences. Adverse reactions are mild and include headache, occasional nausea and vomiting, and diarrhea. Acyclovir ointment has no clinical benefit in the treatment of recurrent lesions, either in speed of healing or in resolution of pain, and is not commonly recommended.

IV acyclovir is reserved for severe or life-threatening infections in which hospitalization is required for the treatment of disseminated infections, CNS infections (meningitis), or pneumonitis. Nephrotoxicity has been observed with high-dose IV use. Clinical trials are examining the effectiveness of a vaccine for HSV-2.[15]

TABLE 53-7 COLLABORATIVE CARE

Genital Herpes

Diagnostic
- History and physical examination
- Antibody assay for HSV type
- Viral isolation by tissue culture

Collaborative Therapy
Primary (Initial) Infection
- acyclovir (Zovirax), famciclovir (Famvir), or valacyclovir (Valtrex)

Recurrent Episodic Infection
- acyclovir, famciclovir, or valacyclovir
- Identify triggering factors
- Yearly Pap test
- Abstinence from sexual contact while lesions are present
- Symptomatic care
- Confidential counseling and testing for HIV

Suppressive Therapy
- acyclovir, famciclovir, or valacyclovir

Severe Infection
- acyclovir IV until clinical improvement, followed by oral antiviral therapy

Modified from Centers for Disease Control and Prevention: STD treatment guidelines. Retrieved from *www.cdc.gov/STD/treatment.*

GENITAL WARTS

Genital warts (*Condylomata acuminata*) are caused by the human papillomavirus (HPV). HPV is a highly contagious STI seen frequently in sexually active young adults. There are more than 100 types of papillomaviruses, many of which are sexually transmitted. Ninety percent of genital warts are caused by HPV types 6 and 11. Although genital warts are not malignant, other HPV types (e.g., types 16 and 18) are oncogenic and associated with cervical, vaginal, vulvar, anal, and penile cancers.[16] In most states, genital warts are not a reportable infection.

Minor trauma during intercourse can cause abrasions that allow HPV to enter the body. The epithelial cells infected with HPV undergo transformation and proliferation to form a warty growth. The incubation period of the virus is generally 3 to 4 months, but may be longer.

Clinical Manifestations and Complications
Most individuals who have HPV infection do not know that they are infected because symptoms are often not present. Genital warts are discrete single or multiple papillary growths that are white to gray and pink-flesh colored. They may grow and coalesce to form large, cauliflower-like masses. Most patients have 1 to 10 genital warts.

In men the warts may occur on the penis and scrotum, around the anus, or in the urethra. In women the warts may be located on the inner thighs, vulva, vagina, or cervix and in the perianal area (Fig. 53-10). There are usually no other signs or symptoms. Itching may occur with anogenital warts. Bleeding on defecation may occur with anal warts.

During pregnancy, genital warts tend to grow rapidly and increase in size. An infected mother may transmit the condition to her newborn. Cesarean delivery is not routinely indicated unless the birth canal becomes blocked by massive warts.

Diagnostic Studies and Collaborative Care
Up to two thirds of the early lesions caused by HPV are undetectable by visual examination. A diagnosis of genital warts can be made on the basis of the gross appearance of the lesions. Warts may be confused with condylomata lata of secondary syphilis, carcinoma, or benign neoplasms. Serologic and cytologic testing should be done to rule out these conditions. HPV deoxyribonucleic acid (DNA) tests help determine if women with abnormal Papanicolaou (Pap) test results need further follow-up. Currently, HPV cannot be confirmed by culture.

Prevention of genital warts is hampered by the high proportion of asymptomatic infections and lack of curative treatment. The primary goal when treating visible genital warts is the removal of symptomatic warts.

Treatment consists of chemical or ablative (removal with laser or electrocautery) methods. One common treatment is the use of 80% to 90% trichloroacetic acid (TCA) or bichloroacetic acid (BCA) applied directly to the wart surface. Petroleum jelly is applied to the surrounding normal skin to minimize irritation before a small amount of TCA is applied to the wart with a cotton swab. A sharp stinging pain is often felt with initial acid contact, but this quickly subsides. TCA is not washed off after treatment.

Podophyllin resin (10% to 25%), a cytotoxic agent, is recommended therapy for small external genital warts. When podophyllin is used, it is applied carefully to each wart, avoiding normal tissue, and is then thoroughly washed off in 1 to 4 hours. This substance encourages the sloughing of skin containing

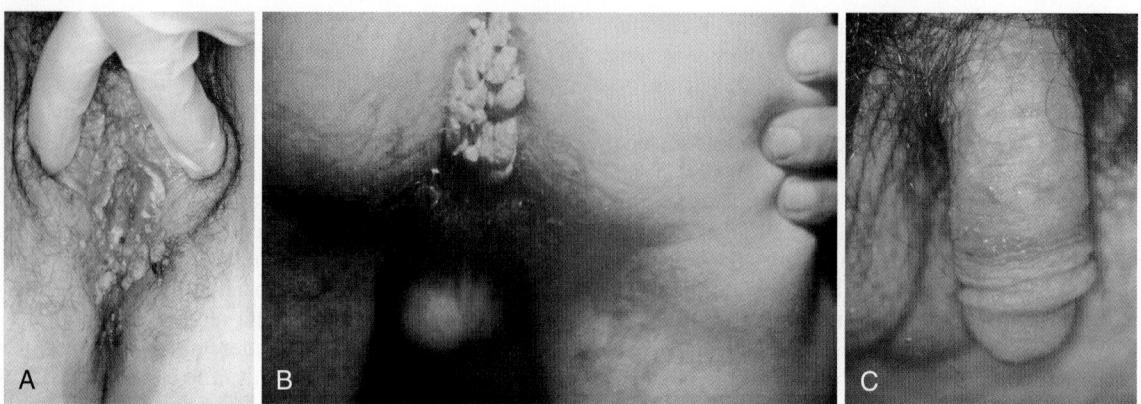

FIG. 53-10 Genital warts. **A,** Severe vulvar warts. **B,** Perineal wart. **C,** Multiple genital warts of the glans penis.

viral particles. Podophyllin has local (e.g., pain, burning) and systemic (e.g., nausea, dizziness, leukopenia, respiratory distress) toxic symptoms. In general, warts located on moist surfaces respond better to topical treatment (e.g., TCA, podophyllin) than do warts on drier surfaces.

Patient-managed treatment is also an option. Podofilox (5%) liquid and gel are available by prescription (Condylox and Condylox Gel). The patient applies the solution or gel for 3 successive days followed by 4 days of no treatment. Treatment can be repeated for up to 4 weeks or until the lesions resolve. Imiquimod (5%) cream (Aldara) is an immune response modifier that is applied once daily at bedtime, three times a week for up to 16 weeks.

The removal of warts may or may not decrease infectivity. Genital warts are difficult to treat and often require multiple office visits.[17] The therapy should be modified if a patient has not improved after three treatments or if the warts have not completely disappeared after six treatments.

If the warts do not regress with any of these therapies, treatments such as cryotherapy with liquid nitrogen, electrocautery, laser therapy, intralesional use of α-interferon, and surgical excision may be indicated. Because treatment does not destroy the virus, merely the infected tissue, recurrences and reinfection are possible, and careful long-term follow-up is advised.

HPV Vaccines. Vaccines are available to protect against HPV types 6, 11, 16, and 18 (Gardasil) and HPV types 16 and 18 (Cervarix). The vaccine is given in three IM doses over a 6-month period and has few side effects.

For females, either Gardasil or Cervarix vaccine is recommended at age 11 or 12 years. It may be given to girls starting at age 9. The vaccine is also recommended for females 13 through 26 years of age who did not get all three doses when they were younger.

For males, Gardasil vaccine is recommended at ages 11 or 12 years. It may be given to boys starting at age 9. This vaccine is recommended for males 13 through 21 years of age who have not completed the three-dose series. This vaccine may be given to men 22 through 26 years of age who have not completed the three-dose series. It is recommended for men through age 26 who have sex with men or whose immune system is weakened because of HIV infection, other illness, or medications.[18]

Because of reported cases of syncope (fainting) during vaccine administration, the patient should remain seated or lying down and be closely observed for 15 minutes after vac-cination. These vaccines do not treat active HPV infection. Ideally, individuals should receive the vaccine before the start of sexual activity, but those who are active or even infected still get protection from the HPV types not already acquired. HPV vaccine reduces the risk of anal cancer and may also protect against oropharynx cancer.[19]

NURSING MANAGEMENT
SEXUALLY TRANSMITTED INFECTIONS

NURSING ASSESSMENT
Subjective and objective data that should be obtained from a person with an STI are presented in Table 53-8.

NURSING DIAGNOSES
Nursing diagnoses for the patient with an STI include, but are not limited to, the following:
- Risk for infection *related to* lack of knowledge about mode of transmission, inadequate personal and genital hygiene, and failure to practice precautionary measures
- Anxiety *related to* impact of the condition on relationships, disease outcome, and lack of knowledge of disease
- Ineffective health maintenance *related to* lack of knowledge about disease process, inadequate follow-up measures, and possibility of reinfection

PLANNING
The overall goals are that the patient with an STI will (1) demonstrate understanding of the mode of transmission of STIs and the risk posed by STIs, (2) complete treatment and return for appropriate follow-up, (3) notify or assist in notification of sexual contacts about their need for testing and treatment, (4) abstain from intercourse until infection is resolved, and (5) demonstrate knowledge of safer sex practices.

NURSING IMPLEMENTATION
HEALTH PROMOTION. Many approaches to stopping the spread of STIs have been advocated and have met with varying degrees of success. Be prepared to discuss "safe" sex practices with all patients, not only those who are perceived to be at risk. These practices include abstinence, monogamy, avoidance of certain high-risk sexual practices, and use of condoms and other barriers to limit contact with potentially infectious body fluids or lesions. Sexual abstinence is a certain method of avoiding all

EVIDENCE-BASED PRACTICE

Applying the Evidence

F.C. is a 19-yr-old man who is being seen in the health care center for signs and symptoms of a urinary tract infection. When asked, he shares with you that he is sexually active. After reviewing his health history, you learn that he has not received the human papillomavirus (HPV) vaccine. You discuss the risks and benefits of the vaccine and suggest that he consider getting it.

Best Available Evidence	Clinician Expertise	Patient Preferences and Values
Males ages 9-26 can get vaccinated with Gardasil to reduce the incidence of anogenital HPV infections, which are caused by HPV types 6, 11, 16, or 18. Gardasil protects against the two HPV types (6 and 11) that cause 90% of genital warts.	Approximately 90% of anal cancers have been linked to HPV infection. Males may be unaware of the expanded recommendations for Gardasil, which was originally approved to prevent cervical, vulvar, and vaginal cancer caused by HPV types 6, 11, 16, and 18 in females ages 9 through 26.	F.C. states that he never has unprotected sex and does not like injections.

Your Decision and Action

After listening carefully, F.C. decides to talk to a few of his friends before making a decision about the vaccine. He tells you that he had no idea that he could get HPV infections. If he decides to get the vaccine, he will be back. You document your discussion in his chart.

Reference for Evidence

Advisory Committee on Immunization Practices: Recommendations on the use of quadrivalent human papillomavirus vaccine in males—advisory committee on immunization practices (ACIP) 2011, Centers for Disease Control and Prevention. Retrieved from *www.cdc.gov/mmwr/preview/mmwrhtml/mm6050a3.htm.*

HEALTHY PEOPLE

Health Impact of Responsible Sexual Behavior

- Greatly reduces the risk of contracting sexually transmitted infections, including infection from human immunodeficiency virus, gonorrhea, chlamydial infection, syphilis, and herpes
- Greatly reduces the risk of spreading viruses such as human papillomavirus that could potentially cause cervical, vulvar, vaginal, penile, anal, and oropharyngeal cancers

TABLE 53-8 NURSING ASSESSMENT

Sexually Transmitted Infections

Subjective Data
Important Health Information
Past health history: Contact with individuals with STIs, multiple sexual partners
Medications: Oral contraceptives; allergy to any antibiotics, especially penicillin

Functional Health Patterns
Health perception–health management: Shared needles during IV drug use; malaise
Nutritional-metabolic: Nausea, vomiting, anorexia; pharyngitis, oral lesions, itching at infected site; chills; alopecia
Elimination: Dysuria, urinary frequency, retention; urethral discharge; tenesmus, proctitis
Cognitive-perceptual: Arthralgia; headache; painful, burning lesions
Sexuality-reproductive: Dyspareunia; vaginal discharge, menstrual abnormalities; genital or perianal lesions

Objective Data
General
Fever, lymphadenopathy (generalized or inguinal)

Integumentary
Syphilis: Primary: Painless, indurated genital, oral, or perianal lesions
  Secondary: Bilateral, symmetric rash on palms, soles, or entire body; mucous patches on mouth or tongue; alopecia
Genital herpes: Painful genital or anal vesicular lesions
Genital warts: Single or multiple gray or white genital or anal warts (possibly becoming massive)

Gastrointestinal
Purulent rectal discharge (indicator of gonorrhea), rectal lesions, proctitis

Urinary
Urethral discharge, erythema

Reproductive
Cervical discharge, lesions, inflamed Bartholin's glands

Possible Diagnostic Findings
Gonorrhea: Positive Gram stain, smears, cultures, and DNA amplification for *Neisseria gonorrhoeae*
Syphilis: Positive findings on VDRL and RPR, spirochetes on dark-field microscopy
Chlamydia: Positive culture or DNA amplification for *Chlamydia*
Genital herpes: Positive HSV-1 or HSV-2 antibody titer; positive tissue culture for HSV-1 or HSV-2

DNA, Deoxyribonucleic acid; *HSV-1,* herpes simplex virus type 1; *HSV-2,* herpes simplex virus type 2; *RPR,* rapid plasma reagin; *STIs,* sexually transmitted infections; *VDRL,* Venereal Disease Research Laboratory.

STIs, but few people consider this a feasible alternative to sexual expression. Limiting sexual intimacies outside of a well-established monogamous relationship can reduce the risk of contracting an STI. A teaching guide for the patient with an STI is presented in Table 53-9.

All sexually active women should be screened for cervical cancer using a Pap test. Women with a history of STIs are at greater risk for cervical cancer. Anal Pap tests should also be done for all individuals who are recipients of anal sex. (Pap tests are discussed in Chapter 54.)

Measures to Prevent Infection. An inspection of the sexual partner's genitalia before coitus is recommended. Discharge, sores, blisters, or rash should be viewed with concern. A patient who is aware of specific signs and symptoms of infection can intelligently make the decision to continue the sexual interaction with modifications or elect not to have sexual relations. The patient should remember that, when engaging in sex, he or she is exposed to the infections of everyone with whom the partner has ever had sex.

Tell men that some protection is provided if they void immediately after intercourse and wash their genitalia and the adjacent areas with soap and water. Women may also benefit from postcoital voiding and washing. However, emphasize that these practices do not provide adequate protection against STIs after exposure to infection.

Spermicidal jellies and creams have not been shown to reduce the risk of contracting STIs.[20] These same barriers may serve as supplementary lubrication, thereby decreasing irritation and friction. They also reduce the chance that a minor laceration could serve as the entry point for an infectious organism.

TABLE 53-9   PATIENT TEACHING GUIDE

Sexually Transmitted Infections

When teaching the patient with sexually transmitted infections:
1. Explain precautions to take such as
   - voiding and washing genitalia and surrounding area after coitus to flush out some organisms and reduce the occurrence of infection
   - using condoms
   - being monogamous
   - asking potential partners about sexual history
   - avoiding sex with partners who use IV drugs or who have visible oral, inguinal, genital, perineal, or anal lesions
2. Explain the importance of taking all antibiotics and/or antiviral agents as prescribed. Symptoms will improve after 1-2 days of therapy, but organisms may still be present.
3. Teach patient about the need for treatment of sexual partners to prevent transmission of infection.
4. Instruct patient to abstain from sexual intercourse during treatment and to use condoms when sexual activity is resumed to prevent spread of infection and reinfection.
5. Explain the importance of follow-up examination and reculture at least once after treatment if appropriate to confirm complete cure and prevent relapse.
6. Allow patient and partner to verbalize concerns to clarify areas that need explanation.
7. Instruct patient about symptoms of complications and need to report problems to ensure proper follow-up and early treatment of reinfection.
8. Inform patient regarding state of infectivity to prevent a false sense of security, which might result in careless sexual practices and poor personal hygiene.

Proper use of a condom provides a highly effective mechanical barrier to infection. The condom should be undamaged and correctly in place throughout all phases of sexual activity. A deterrent to barrier usage is alcohol and drug use. Use of barrier contraceptives requires planning and motivation, both of which are impaired with alcohol or drug ingestion. Give specific verbal and written instructions on the proper use of condoms (see eTable 15-4 available at the website for Chapter 15). Partners should discuss any objections to condom usage, such as interference with spontaneity and the presence of a barrier. Information about the mechanics of sexual arousal and incorporating a condom into lovemaking can help in overcoming the individual's or partner's resistance to its use. Female condoms are lubricated polyurethane sheaths designed for vaginal use but are considerably more expensive than male condoms (see eTable 15-5 available at the website for Chapter 15).

Among couples with one infected partner, consistent and scrupulous condom use can reduce transmission to the uninfected partner. Unprotected anal intercourse and other high-risk behaviors should be eliminated, and condoms should be used if sexual contact continues.

Initiate a discussion to assess the risk for contracting an STI. Questions to ask include number of partners, type of birth control used, use of condoms, history of an STI, use of IV drugs, and sexual preference. Instead of asking if a patient is homosexual or asking only about sexual preference, it can be more revealing to ask, "Do you have sex with men or women or both?" Some men who have sex with men do not identify themselves as homosexual or bisexual, which is a major contributor to infection of wives and female or male partners. Although the majority of STIs are transmitted between men having sex with men and heterosexual contact, it is possible to transmit an STI between women.[21]

Plan teaching based on the response to these questions. Interpersonal skills necessary for this interview include respect, compassion, and a nonjudgmental attitude. Tailor your counseling to the individual. Do not assume that older people are not at risk, since an increasing number of older people are becoming infected.

Screening Programs. Screening programs can help prevent certain STIs. For many years, there have been various screening programs to identify cases of syphilis. Many institutions offer voluntary prenatal HIV and syphilis testing and counseling for pregnant women.

Screening programs have been developed and implemented for detection of gonorrhea and chlamydial infection. These programs are targeted to women because women are more likely to have asymptomatic gonorrhea and thereby serve as sources of infection. Routine gonorrheal and chlamydial testing during pelvic examinations and prenatal visits are a major part of these programs. Mass application of screening programs for genital chlamydial infections, genital herpes, and HPV infections (warts) may also be possible with the advent of rapid, cost-effective tests.

Case Finding. Interviewing and case finding are other methods used to control STIs. These activities are directed toward locating and examining all contacts of each known patient with an STI as soon after sexual exposure as possible so that effective treatment can be initiated. Trained interviewers may often find cases even if they are supplied with only limited information. The caseworkers, who are often nurses, are aware of the social implications of these diseases and the need for discretion. Sexual contacts are often not informed about the origin of the information naming them as a contact so that greater cooperation and privacy are ensured.

Partner notification and treatment impose a heavy burden on public health departments and, as a result, the notification often becomes the responsibility of the infected partner. The infected partner may choose not to inform sexual partners, and the partners may choose not to seek treatment. *Expedited partner therapy* (EPT) is a safe, effective tool for treating STIs that allows a health care provider to provide prescriptions or medications to a patient to take to his or her partner, without examining the partner. EPT has been shown to be useful in ensuring partner treatment among men and reducing repeat infections among women.[22] Several states have adopted legislation to allow health care providers to dispense antibiotic therapy for sex partners of individuals with chlamydial infection or gonorrhea. The legality of treating without evaluating the patient is uncertain in some states, and it is illegal in others.

Educational and Research Programs. Actively encourage your community to provide better education about STIs for its citizens. Teenagers, who are known to have a high incidence of infection, should be a prime target for such educational programs. STI rates are also rising in older adults.[23] Older adults are less likely to use condoms and in general have a harder time initiating discussion of sexual health issues.

Knowledge and understanding can decrease the STI epidemic. The HPV vaccine that protects against genital warts and cervical cancer should be encouraged before the start of sexual activity. Accurate and current information may help reduce parental fears related to the vaccine. Consider stressing the prevention of cancer as a reason for the vaccine, which may be more productive and less controversial, thus making the parent and adolescent more receptive. Efforts are being made to develop vaccines for syphilis, gonorrhea, genital herpes, and HIV. Many clinicians view the development of effective vaccines as a prerequisite for the eradication of STIs.

ACUTE INTERVENTION

Psychologic Support. The diagnosis of an STI may be met with a variety of emotions, such as shame, guilt, anger, and a desire for vengeance. Provide counseling and encourage the patient to verbalize feelings. Couples in marital or committed relationships are confronted with an added problem when an STI is diagnosed, and they must face the implication of sexual activity outside the relationship. The acute problem raises other concerns about their relationship and may serve as an incentive for further problem solving. The couple needs support and counseling. A referral for professional counseling to explore the ramifications of an STI in their relationship may be indicated.

A patient who has genital herpes is faced with the fact that repeated infections can occur and that no cure is available. This can be frustrating and disruptive to the patient's physical, emotional, social, and sexual life. Help the patient identify and avoid any factors that may precipitate the condition. Inform the patient that the frequency and severity of recurrences will probably decrease over time.

HPV infections involve a prolonged course of treatment. The patient can become frustrated and distressed because of frequent office visits, associated costs, potential for unpleasant side effects as a result of treatment, and effects of the infection on future health and sexual relationships. Support and a willingness to listen to the patient's concerns are needed. Support groups are also available.

Follow-up. If you work in public health facilities, clinics, or other outpatient settings, you are more likely to care for a patient with an STI than if you work in a hospital setting. Whatever the setting, as a nurse you are in a position to explain and interpret treatment measures such as the purpose and possible side effects of prescribed drugs and the need for follow-up care.

Frequently, single-dose treatment for gonorrhea, chlamydial infection, and syphilis helps prevent the problems associated with nonadherence with drug therapy. Give special instructions to the patient requiring multiple-dose therapy to complete the prescribed regimen. Also inform the patient about problems resulting from nonadherence. All patients should return to the treatment center for a repeat culture from the infected sites or for serologic testing at designated times to determine the effectiveness of the treatment. Explaining to the patient that cures are not always obtained on the first treatment can reinforce the need for a follow-up visit. Also advise the patient to inform sexual partners of the need for testing and treatment, regardless of whether they are free of symptoms or experiencing symptoms.

Hygiene Measures. Emphasize to the patient with an STI the importance of certain hygiene measures. An important component is frequent hand washing and bathing. Bathing and cleaning of the involved areas can provide local comfort and prevent secondary infection. Because douching may spread the infection or undermine local immune responses, it is contraindicated. The synthetic materials used in most undergarments frequently increase or exacerbate local irritations by trapping moisture. Cotton undergarments provide better absorption and are cooler and more comfortable for the patient with an STI.

Sexual Activity. Sexual abstinence is indicated during the communicable phase of the infection. If sexual activity occurs before treatment has been completed, emphasize to the patient

---

ETHICAL/LEGAL DILEMMAS
Confidentiality and HIPAA

Situation

P.H., a 22-yr-old woman, is informed of the positive results of a test for chlamydial infection. You advise her to tell her sexual partners that she has this disease. She refuses to tell her boyfriend because he will know that she has had sex with another partner. You later learn that the nursing student who was in the clinic for the day, who is a friend of the boyfriend, hinted to him that he should have STI testing.

Ethical/Legal Points for Consideration

- Each state has requirements for reporting communicable diseases and other health-related data. Inform the patient of the reporting requirements for communicable diseases.
- Nurses and other health care professionals have both a legal and an ethical obligation to maintain confidentiality of patient information. The Health Insurance Portability and Accountability Act (HIPAA) ensures the privacy of personal health information.
- Your primary obligation is to the patient seeking care. Patient teaching is one way to establish a partnership with this woman. Share information about the effects of the disease if it is not treated, the consequences of reinfection, and the effect of the disease on others who may not know that they are infected. Then encourage the patient to inform her partners of the diagnosis for the good of everyone.

Discussion Questions

1. What are your state's requirements for reportable conditions?
2. In your opinion, what is the best way to balance the needs of an individual patient with those of the general public?
3. What are the risks to the institution for the breach of confidentiality and HIPAA?

---

the importance of using condoms to help prevent the spread of infection and reinfection. Also encourage condom usage after treatment to prevent future exposure to infection. The patient can also choose to relate to a partner in an intimate way that avoids both coitus and oral-genital contact. Note that even single-dose treatments can take up to 1 week to be effective and thus the patient is infectious during this period.

AMBULATORY AND HOME CARE. Because many STIs are cured with a single dose or short course of antibiotic therapy, many persons are casual about the outcome of these infections. The consequences of this attitude can include delays in treatment, nonadherence with instructions, and subsequent development of complications. The complications are serious and costly. They can result in disfigurement and destruction of important tissues and organs.

Surgery and prolonged therapy are indicated for many patients with infection-related complications. Major surgical procedures such as resection of an aneurysm or aortic valve replacement may be necessary to treat cardiovascular problems caused by syphilis. Pelvic surgery and procedures to correct fertility problems secondary to an STI may include lysis of adhesions, dilation of strictures, reconstructive tuboplasty, and in vitro fertilization.

EVALUATION

Expected outcomes for the patient with an STI are that the patient will

- Describe modes of transmission
- Use appropriate hygienic measures
- Experience no reinfection
- Demonstrate compliance with follow-up protocol

CASE STUDY

Gonorrhea and Chlamydial Infection

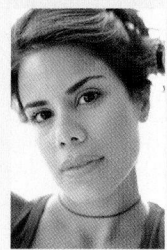

Eyecandy Images/
Thinkstock

Patient Profile

C.R. is a 24-yr-old Hispanic woman who is seen at the outpatient clinic with complaints of a purulent yellow-white discharge and frequent urination over the past 2 wk. She is sexually active with a new partner after breaking up with a long-term boyfriend. She was treated in the past for *Chlamydia* at age 20.

Subjective Data

- Her sexual partner does not use a condom or spermicide with intercourse
- Her last menstrual period was 3 wk ago
- Her sexual partner was recently treated for epididymitis
- Appears very nervous

Objective Data

- Cervical ectopy noted during Pap test
- Mucopurulent cervical discharge
- Urine pregnancy test is negative
- Nucleic acid amplification test is positive for *Neisseria gonorrhoeae* and *Chlamydia trachomatis*

Collaborative Care

- ceftriaxone 250 mg IM once
- doxycycline 100 mg bid for 7 days

Discussion Questions

1. What were C.R.'s risk factors for acquiring gonorrhea and chlamydial infection?
2. What complications could occur if C.R.'s infections are not treated?
3. *Priority Decision:* What is the priority of care for C.R.?
4. What instructions should C.R. receive to ensure successful treatment? To prevent reinfection? To prevent further transmission of the infection?
5. *Delegation Decision:* Which nursing personnel should be responsible for teaching C.R. what she needs to know about other sexually transmitted infections (STIs): registered nurse, licensed practical/vocational nurse, unlicensed assistive personnel?
6. What impact is her diagnosis likely to have on C.R.'s self-image? On her relationship with her sexual partner?
7. *Priority Decision:* Based on the assessment data presented, what are the priority nursing diagnoses? Are there any collaborative problems?
8. *Evidence-Based Practice:* C.R. mentions she is using the spermicide nonoynol-9 (N-9) to protect herself against STIs. Would you advise her to continue to use it?

ⓔvolve Answers available at *http://evolve.elsevier.com/Lewis/medsurg.*

BRIDGE TO NCLEX EXAMINATION

The number of the question corresponds to the same-numbered outcome at the beginning of the chapter.

1. The individual with the lowest risk for sexually transmitted pelvic inflammatory disease is a woman who uses
   a. oral contraceptives.
   b. barrier methods of contraception.
   c. an intrauterine device for contraception.
   d. a Norplant implant or injectable Depo-Provera for contraception.

2. The nurse is obtaining a subjective data assessment from a woman reported as a sexual contact of a man with chlamydial infection. The nurse understands that symptoms of chlamydial infection in women
   a. are frequently absent.
   b. are similar to those of genital herpes.
   c. include a macular palmar rash in the later stages.
   d. may involve chancres inside the vagina that are not visible.

3. A primary HSV infection differs from recurrent HSV episodes in that (select all that apply)
   a. only primary infections are sexually transmitted.
   b. symptoms are less severe during recurrent episodes.
   c. transmission of the virus to a fetus is less likely during primary infection.
   d. systemic manifestations such as fever and myalgia are more common in primary infection.
   e. lesions from recurrent HSV are more likely to transmit the virus than lesions from primary HSV.

4. Explain to the patient with gonorrhea that treatment will include both ceftriaxone and doxycycline because
   a. most patients need both drugs to eradicate the organism.
   b. coverage with more than one antibiotic will prevent reinfection.
   c. no single agent successfully eradicates both primary and recurrent infections.
   d. the high rate of coexisting chlamydial infection and gonorrhea indicates coverage with both drugs.

5. In assessing patients for STIs, the nurse needs to know that many STIs can be asymptomatic. Which STIs can be asymptomatic (select all that apply)?
   a. Syphilis
   b. Gonorrhea
   c. Genital warts
   d. Genital herpes
   e. Chlamydial infection

6. To prevent the infection and transmission of STIs, the nurse's teaching plan would include an explanation of
   a. the appropriate use of oral contraceptives.
   b. sexual positions that can be used to avoid infection.
   c. the necessity of annual Pap tests for patients with HPV.
   d. sexual practices that are considered high-risk behaviors.

7. Provide emotional support to a patient with an STI by
   a. offering information on how safer sexual practices can prevent STIs.
   b. showing concern when listening to the patient who expresses negative feelings.
   c. reassuring the patient that the disease is highly curable with appropriate treatment.
   d. helping the patient who received an STI from his or her sexual partner in forgiving the partner.

1. b, 2. a, 3. b, 4. d, 5. a, b, c, d, 6. d, 7. b

⊖volve

For rationales to these answers and even more NCLEX review questions, visit *http://evolve.elsevier.com/Lewis/medsurg*.

REFERENCES

1. Centers for Disease Control and Prevention: STD trends in the United States: 2010 national data for gonorrhea, *Chlamydia,* and syphilis. Retrieved from *www.cdc.gov/std/stats10/trends.htm*.

*2. Reece M, Herbenick D, Schick V, et al: Condom use rates in a national probability sample of males and females ages 14 to 94 in the United States, *J Sex Med* 7(Suppl 5):266, 2010.

3. Centers for Disease Control and Prevention: 2010 Sexually transmitted disease surveillance: gonorrhea. Retrieved from *www.cdc.gov/std/stats10/gonorrhea.htm*.

4. Brill J: Sexually transmitted infections in men, *Prim Care* 37:509, 2010.

5. Knox T, Wanke C: Gastrointestinal manifestations of HIV and AIDS: anorectal diseases. In Goldman L, Schafer A, editors: *Goldman's Cecil medicine,* ed 24, Philadelphia, 2011, Saunders.

6. Borhart J, Birnbaumer D: Emergency department management of sexually transmitted infections, *Emerg Med Clin North Am* 29:587, 2011.

7. Centers for Disease Control and Prevention: Cephalosporin susceptibility among *Neisseria gonorrhoeae* isolates—United States, 2000-2010, *MMWR* 60:873, 2011.

*8. Hawkes S, Matin N, Broutet N, et al: Effectiveness of interventions to improve screening for syphilis in pregnancy: a systematic review and meta-analysis, *Lancet Infect Dis* 11:684, 2011.

9. Centers for Disease Control and Prevention: Sexually transmitted diseases treatment guidelines 2010, *MMWR* 59(#RR-12):1-110, 2010.

10. Champion J, Collins J: Reducing STIs: screening, treatment, and counseling, *Nurse Pract* 37:40, 2012.

11. Haggerty C, Gottlieb S, Taylor B, et al: Risk of sequelae after *Chlamydia trachomatis* genital infection in women, *J Infect Dis* 202(Suppl 2):S134, 2010.

12. Centers for Disease Control and Prevention: Genital herpes: CDC fact sheet. Retrieved from *www.cdc.gov/std/stats10/trends.htm*.

13. Roett M, Mayor M, Uduhiri K: Diagnosis and management of genital ulcers, *Am Fam Physician* 85:254, 2012.

14. Su C, McKay B: Treatment of HSV infection in late pregnancy, *Am Fam Physician* 85:390, 2012.

15. Johnston C, Koelle DM, Wald A: HSV-2: in pursuit of a vaccine, *J Clin Invest* 121:4600, 2011.

16. Hariri S, Unger ER, Sternberg M, et al: Prevalence of genital human papillomavirus among females in the United States: the national health and nutrition examination survey, 2003-2006, *J Infect Dis* 204:566, 2011.

17. American Academy of Dermatology: Genital warts. Retrieved from *www.aad.org/skin-conditions/dermatology-a-to-z/genital-warts*.

18. Centers for Disease Control and Prevention: HPV vaccine (Gardasil): what you need to know. Retrieved from *www.cdc.gov/vaccines/pubs/vis/downloads/vis-hpv-gardasil.pdf*.

19. Palefsky J, Giuliano A, Goldstone S, et al: HPV vaccine against anal HPV infection and anal intraepithelial neoplasia, *N Engl J Med* 365:1576, 2011.

*20. Wilkinson D, Ramjee G, Tholandi M, et al: Nonoxynol-9 for preventing vaginal acquisition of HIV infection by women from men, *Cochrane Database Syst Rev* 4:CD003936, 2002 (republished online 2009, 2012).

21. Ripley V: Promoting sexual health in women who have sex with women, *Nurs Stand* 25:41, 2011.

22. Centers for Disease Control and Prevention: *Expedited partner therapy in the management of sexually transmitted diseases,* Atlanta, 2006, US Department of Health and Human Services. Retrieved from *www.cdc.gov/std/treatment/eptfinalreport2006.pdf*.

23. Jeffers L, DiBartolo M: Raising health care provider awareness of sexually transmitted disease in patients over age 50, *MEDSURG Nurs* 20:285, 2011.

*Evidenced-based information for clinical practice.

RESOURCES

American Social Health Association
www.ashastd.org
(for teens) *www.iwannaknow.org/teens/index.html*
Centers for Disease Control and Prevention, STD/HIV/AIDS
www.cdc.gov/std
Sexuality Information and Education Council of the United States
www.siecus.org

54

What we have once enjoyed we can never lose.
All that we love deeply becomes a part of us.
Helen Keller

Nursing Management
Female Reproductive Problems

Nancy MacMullen and Laura Dulski

LEARNING OUTCOMES

1. Summarize the etiologies of infertility and the strategies for diagnosis and treatment of the infertile woman.
2. Describe the etiology, clinical manifestations, and nursing and collaborative management of menstrual problems and abnormal vaginal bleeding.
3. Identify the risk factors, clinical manifestations, and collaborative care of ectopic pregnancy.
4. Describe the changes related to menopause and the nursing and collaborative management of the patient with menopausal symptoms.
5. Differentiate among the common problems that affect the vulva, vagina, and cervix and the related nursing and collaborative management.
6. Describe the assessment, collaborative care, and nursing management of women with pelvic inflammatory disease and endometriosis.
7. Explain the clinical manifestations, diagnostic studies, collaborative care, and surgical therapy for cervical, endometrial, ovarian, and vulvar cancers.
8. Summarize the preoperative and postoperative nursing management for the patient requiring surgery of the female reproductive system.
9. Differentiate among the common problems that occur with cystoceles, rectoceles, and fistulas and the related nursing and collaborative management.
10. Summarize the clinical manifestations of sexual assault and the appropriate nursing and collaborative management of the patient who has been sexually assaulted.

KEY TERMS

abortion, p. 1278
amenorrhea, p. 1280
cystocele, p. 1300
dysmenorrhea, p. 1280
ectopic pregnancy, p. 1282

endometriosis, p. 1289
hysterectomy, p. 1282
infertility, p. 1276
leiomyomas, p. 1290
menopause, p. 1283

pelvic inflammatory disease
  (PID), p. 1287
perimenopause, p. 1283
premenstrual syndrome
  (PMS), p. 1279

rectocele, p. 1300
sexual assault, p. 1301
uterine prolapse, p. 1300

INFERTILITY

Infertility is the inability to conceive after at least 1 year of regular unprotected intercourse.[1] Approximately 15% of couples in North America are infertile. Understandably, infertility can be both a physical and an emotional crisis.

Etiology and Pathophysiology

Infertility may be caused by either female or male or combined factors. (Conditions that cause male infertility are discussed in Chapter 55.) In some cases, the cause of infertility may not be identified.

The factors usually causing female infertility include problems with ovulation (anovulation or inadequate corpus luteum), tubal obstruction or dysfunction (endometriosis or damage from pelvic infection), and uterine or cervical factors (fibroid tumors or structural anomalies). Risk factors for infertility include tobacco and illicit drug use and being obese or thin. In women the risk for infertility starts about age 30 and increases after age 40.[2]

Reviewed by Brenda Pavill, RN, PhD, FNP, Associate Professor–Nursing, Misericordia University, Dallas, Pennsylvania; and Beth Perry Black, RN, PhD, Professor of Nursing, UNC at Chapel Hill School of Nursing, UNC School of Nursing, Chapel Hill, North Carolina.

TABLE 54-1 COLLABORATIVE CARE

Infertility

Diagnostic
- History and physical examination of both partners, including psychosocial functioning
- Review of menstrual and gynecologic history
- Assessment of possible sexually transmitted infections
- Hormone levels
  - Serum hormone levels (e.g., FSH, LH, prolactin)
  - Urinary LH
- Pap test
- Ovulatory study
- Tubal patency study
  - Hysterosalpingogram
- Postcoital test
  - Cervical mucus
  - Sperm penetration assay
  - Semen analysis
- Pelvic ultrasound
- Genetic screening

Collaborative Therapy
- Hormone therapy
- Drug therapy (see Table 54-2)
- Intrauterine insemination
- Assisted reproductive technologies (ARTs)

FSH, Follicle-stimulating hormone; *LH,* luteinizing hormone.

TABLE 54-2 DRUG THERAPY

Infertility

Drug	Mechanism of Action
Selective Estrogen Receptor Modulator	
clomiphene (Clomid, Serophene)	Stimulates hypothalamus to ↑ production of GnRH, which ↑ release of LH and FSH. End result is stimulation of ovulation.
Menotropins (Human Menopausal Gonadotropin)	
Pergonal Repronex Humegon	Product made of FSH and LH to promote the development and maturation of follicles in the ovaries.
Follicle-Stimulating Hormone Agonists	
urofollitropin (Fertinex, Bravelle) follitropin (Gonal-f, Follistim)	Stimulate follicle growth and maturation by mimicking the body's natural FSH.
GnRH Antagonists	
cetrorelix (Cetrotide) ganirelix (Antagon)	Prevent premature LH surges and premature ovulation in women undergoing ovarian stimulation.
GnRH Agonists	
leuprolide (Lupron) nafarelin (Synarel)	Suppress release of LH and FSH with continuous use. May also be used in the treatment of endometriosis.
Human Chorionic Gonadotropin (hCG)	
Pregnyl Profasi Novarel	Induces ovulation by stimulating the release of eggs from follicles.

FSH, Follicle-stimulating hormone; *GnRH,* gonadotropin-releasing hormone; *LH,* luteinizing hormone.

Diagnostic Studies

A detailed history and a general physical examination of the woman and her partner provide the basis for selecting diagnostic studies (Table 54-1). The possibility of medical, genetic, or gynecologic diseases is explored before tests are performed to determine problems affecting general health and fertility. These tests include hormone levels, ovulatory studies, tubal patency studies, and postcoital studies. Other screening tests for infertility include semen analysis and pelvic ultrasound.

Ovulatory Studies. A basal body temperature record is kept to determine whether there is regular ovulation. The woman is instructed to take and graph her temperature, referred to as basal body temperature, on awakening before any activity. As ovulation approaches, the production of estrogen increases, which may cause a drop in temperature of about 2° F. When ovulation occurs, progesterone is produced, causing a rise in temperature. Thus a temperature graph helps detect ovulation and suggests the timing of intercourse if pregnancy is desired. Ovulation prediction kits are now available for use by women at home. Other tests for ovulation include cervical and vaginal smears, endometrial biopsy, and plasma progesterone levels.

Tubal Patency Studies. Tubal factors (occlusion or deformity) are most commonly assessed using a hysterosalpingogram. This procedure consists of the radiographic visualization of the uterus and fallopian tubes by injecting a radiopaque dye through the cervix. Tubal patency, shape, position, and any distortions of the endometrial cavity can be determined. Laparoscopy may be used when hysterosalpingogram is contraindicated or other pelvic pathologic conditions appear likely.

Postcoital Studies. A postcoital test can determine whether the cervical environment is favorable for the sperm. The couple is asked to have intercourse about the time ovulation is expected and 2 to 12 hours before the office visit. Douching or bathing should be avoided before the test. The cervical and vaginal secretions are aspirated and examined for the number and motility of sperm present.

NURSING AND COLLABORATIVE MANAGEMENT INFERTILITY

The management of infertility problems depends on the cause. If infertility is secondary to an alteration in ovarian function, supplemental hormone therapy to restore and maintain ovulation may be used. Drug therapy to treat infertility is presented in Table 54-2. Chronic cervicitis and inadequate estrogenic stimulation are cervical factors causing infertility. Antibiotic therapy is indicated for cervicitis. Inadequate estrogenic stimulation is treated using estrogen.

When a couple has not succeeded in conceiving while under infertility management, an option is intrauterine insemination with sperm from the partner or a donor. If this technique does not succeed, assisted reproductive technologies (ARTs) may be used. ARTs include in vitro fertilization (IVF), gamete intrafallopian transfer (GIFT), zygote intrafallopian transfer (ZIFT), donor gametes, and embryo cryopreservation. IVF is the removal of mature oocytes from the woman's ovarian follicle via laparoscopy, followed by in vitro fertilization of the ova with the partner's sperm. When fertilization and cleavage have occurred, the resulting embryos are transferred into the woman's uterus. The procedure requires 2 to 3 days to complete and is used in cases of fallopian tube obstruction, diminished sperm count, and unexplained infertility. Frequently, multiple attempts are needed for successful implantation. IVF is financially costly and emotionally stressful.[3]

Assist women experiencing infertility by providing information about the physiology of reproduction and the infertility evaluation, and by addressing the psychologic and social distress that can accompany infertility. Reducing psychologic stress can improve the emotional climate, making it more conducive to achieving a pregnancy.

Teaching and providing emotional support are major responsibilities throughout infertility testing and treatment. Feelings of anger, frustration, grief, and helplessness may heighten as additional diagnostic tests are performed. Infertility can generate great tension in a marriage as the couple exhausts financial and emotional resources. Few insurance carriers cover the high cost of infertility testing and treatment. Encourage couples to participate in a support group for infertile couples, as well as individual therapy.

ABORTION

An abortion is the loss or termination of a pregnancy before the fetus has developed to a state of viability (ability to survive outside the uterus). Abortions are classified as *spontaneous* (those occurring naturally) or *induced* (those occurring as a result of mechanical or medical intervention). *Miscarriage* is the common term for the unintended loss of a pregnancy.

Spontaneous Abortion

Spontaneous abortion is the natural loss of pregnancy before 20 weeks of gestation. Fetal chromosomal anomalies may account for many miscarriages before 8 weeks of gestation. Other causes of spontaneous abortions include endocrine abnormalities, maternal infection, acquired anatomic abnormalities (e.g., uterine fibroids, endometriosis), immunologic factors, and environmental factors. About 10% to 15% of all pregnancies end as a result of spontaneous abortion.

Uterine cramping coupled with vaginal bleeding often indicates a spontaneous abortion. Serial measurements of serum β-human chorionic gonadotropin (β-hCG) hormone and vaginal ultrasound examination of the pelvis are the most reliable indicators of viability of the pregnancy.

Treatment to prevent a possible spontaneous abortion is limited. Although bed rest and avoidance of vaginal intercourse are often recommended, there is no evidence that these measures improve the outcome. The woman is advised to report any bleeding to her health care provider. Most women proceed to abortion regardless of treatment. If the products of conception do not pass completely or bleeding becomes excessive, a *dilation and curettage* (D&C) procedure is generally performed.[4] The D&C involves dilating the cervix and scraping the endometrium of the uterus to empty the contents of the uterus.

Women who are experiencing bleeding and cramping during pregnancy may be admitted to the hospital. Vital signs and estimated blood loss are monitored. Women are distressed and experience both physical and emotional pain. Arrange for someone to stay with the patient, since emotional support is important. Be aware of the grieving process that results from the loss of a pregnancy.

Induced Abortion

Induced abortion is an intentional or elective termination of a pregnancy. Induced abortion is done for personal reasons (at the request of the woman) and for medical reasons. Several techniques are used to induce abortion, including menstrual extraction, suction curettage, dilation and evacuation (D&E), and drug therapy (Table 54-3). Deciding on which technique to use to terminate a pregnancy depends on the gestational age (length of the pregnancy) and the woman's condition. Suction curettage may be performed up to 14 weeks of gestation and accounts for more than 90% of abortion procedures.

Drug therapy is another method to induce abortion (medical abortion) early in pregnancy. These agents must be given within the first 49 days of pregnancy (day 1 being the first day of the last menstrual period).

Once the decision is made to have an abortion, the woman and her significant others need support and acceptance.

TABLE 54-3 METHODS FOR INDUCING ABORTION

Method	Length of Pregnancy	Description
Early Abortion		
Menstrual extraction	Usually up to 2 wk after first missed period	Catheter is inserted through cervix into uterus, and suction is applied. Endometrium and contents of uterus are aspirated.
Suction aspiration (curettage)	Up to 14 wk	Cervix is usually dilated, uterine aspirator is introduced, and suction is applied, removing endometrial tissue and implanted pregnancy.
Dilation and evacuation (D&E)	10-16 wk (approximate)	Cervix is dilated, and products of conception are removed by vacuum cannula and use of other instruments as needed.
mifepristone (Mifeprex, RU-486) with misoprostol (Cytotec)	Up to 7 wk	Mifepristone is administered orally. Misoprostol (prostaglandin) is administered orally or intravaginally 2 days later.
methotrexate with misoprostol	Up to 7 wk	Methotrexate is administered intramuscularly. Misoprostol is given intravaginally 5-7 days later.
Late Abortion *Instillation of Drugs*		
Hypertonic saline solution	After 16 wk	About 200 mL of amniotic fluid is withdrawn, with similar amount of 20% normal saline solution injected. Uterus is irritated and begins to contract within 12-36 hr. Contractions may be assisted with IV oxytocin.
Prostaglandins • carboprost (Hemabate) • dinoprostone (Prostin E2, Cervidil)	After 16 wk	Amniocentesis is done, and prostaglandin is inserted into amniotic sac, resulting in stimulation of smooth muscle of uterus. Expulsion of uterine contents occurs within 24 hr.
Hysterotomy	16-20 wk	Miniature cesarean delivery is performed. Incision is made into uterus and contents are removed.

Prepare the patient for what to expect both emotionally and physically. Grief and sadness are normal emotions after an abortion. The patient needs to understand the procedure, including instructions for preprocedure and postprocedure care. Your caring attitude can be a positive factor in the patient's experience.

After the procedure, teach the patient the signs and symptoms of possible complications, such as abnormal vaginal bleeding, severe abdominal cramping, fever, and foul-smelling drainage. Also stress to the patient to avoid intercourse and vaginal insertions until reexamination, which needs to be in 2 weeks. Contraception can be started the day of the procedure or during the patient's return visit in accordance with her needs and desires.

PROBLEMS RELATED TO MENSTRUATION

The normal menstrual cycle is discussed in Chapter 51. The hormonal changes related to the menstrual cycle are shown in Fig. 51-7. Menstruation may be irregular during the first few years after menarche and the years preceding menopause. Once established, a woman's menstrual cycles usually have a predictable pattern. However, considerable normal variation exists among women in cycle length and in duration, amount, and character of the menstrual flow (see Table 51-2).

PREMENSTRUAL SYNDROME

Premenstrual syndrome (PMS) is a symptom complex related to the luteal phase of the menstrual cycle. The symptoms can be severe enough to impair interpersonal relationships or interfere with usual activities. Because many symptoms may be associated with PMS, it is difficult to define. However, PMS symptoms always occur cyclically during the luteal phase before the onset of menstruation and are not present at other times of the month. About 40% of all women have been significantly affected by PMS during their lifetime.[5]

Etiology and Pathophysiology

The etiology and pathophysiology of PMS are not well understood. It may have a biologic trigger with compounding psychosocial factors. Neurotransmitters, such as serotonin, could also be involved. Some women may have a genetic predisposition to PMS. Other proposed causes of PMS include hormone imbalance and nutritional deficiencies. *Premenstrual dysphoric disorder* (PMDD) is the term applied when women with PMS have a severe mood disorder.

Clinical Manifestations

PMS is extremely variable in its clinical manifestations between women and, for an individual woman, from one cycle to another. Common physical symptoms include breast discomfort, peripheral edema, abdominal bloating, sensation of weight gain, episodes of binge eating, and migraine headache. Abdominal bloating and breast swelling are caused by fluid shifts because total body weight does not generally change. Anxiety, depression, irritability, and mood swings are some of the emotional symptoms that women may experience.

Diagnostic Studies and Collaborative Care

PMS can be diagnosed only when other possible causes for the symptoms have been ruled out. A focused health history and

---

TABLE 54-4   COLLABORATIVE CARE

Premenstrual Syndrome (PMS)

Diagnostic
- History and physical examination
- Symptom diary

Collaborative Therapy
- Stress management and relaxation therapy
- Nutritional therapy
- Aerobic exercise
- Drug therapy
  - Diuretics
  - Prostaglandin inhibitors (e.g., ibuprofen [Advil, Motrin])
  - Selective serotonin reuptake inhibitors (e.g., sertraline [Zoloft])
  - Combined oral contraceptives

---

physical examination are done to identify any underlying conditions such as thyroid dysfunction, uterine fibroids, or depression that may account for the symptoms. No definitive diagnostic test is available for PMS. When PMS or PMDD is a possible diagnosis, a woman is given a symptom diary to record her symptoms prospectively for two or three menstrual cycles. Diagnosis is based on an evaluation of the woman's symptoms.

Nondrug and drug strategies can relieve some PMS symptoms (Table 54-4). However, no single treatment is available. The goal of treatment is to reduce the severity of symptoms and enhance the woman's sense of control and quality of life.

Several conservative approaches to managing PMS symptoms are considered helpful, including stress management, diet changes, exercise, education, and counseling. Techniques for stress reduction include yoga, meditation, and biofeedback. To decrease autonomic nervous system arousal, women should avoid caffeine, reduce dietary intake of refined carbohydrates, exercise on a regular basis, and practice relaxation techniques. Eating complex carbohydrates with high fiber, foods rich in vitamin B$_6$, and sources of tryptophan (dairy and poultry) are thought to promote serotonin production, which improves the symptoms. Vitamin B$_6$ may be found in such foods as pork, milk, and legumes.

Exercise results in a release of endorphins, leading to mood elevation. Aerobic exercise can also have a relaxing effect. Because fatigue tends to exaggerate the symptoms of PMS, adequate rest in the premenstrual period is a priority.

Explanations about PMS help the woman understand the complexity of the disorder and ways that she can regain a sense of control. Assure the patient that her symptoms are real, PMS exists, and she is not "crazy." Acknowledgment that she has PMS can itself be therapeutic. Teaching the woman's partner about the nature of PMS helps the partner better understand PMS and its effects.

Drug Therapy. Drug therapy is considered when symptoms persist or interfere with daily functioning. Currently no single drug can treat all the symptoms associated with PMS. One therapy may be tried for a time; if no improvement is noted, another approach is tried. Many treatments are symptom specific. For fluid retention, diuretics such as spironolactone (Aldactone) are used. For reducing cramping pain, backache, and migraine headache, prostaglandin inhibitors such as ibuprofen (Motrin, Advil) are used. To improve negative mood, vitamin B$_6$ supplementation (50 mg/day) may be used. Calcium and magnesium supplementation may also be effective in alleviating psychologic and physiologic symptoms. For anxiety, buspirone

(BuSpar) taken during the luteal phase has helped some women. Women with PMDD may benefit from antidepressants, including fluoxetine (Prozac, Sarafem) and tricyclic antidepressants (e.g., amitriptyline [Elavil]).

Selective serotonin reuptake inhibitors (SSRIs) (e.g., sertraline [Zoloft]) have provided significant relief to women with severe PMS. Other treatments include oral contraceptives containing estrogen and progesterone. Evening primrose oil may help in reducing menstrual cramping for some women.

> **DRUG ALERT: Oral Contraceptives (Both Estrogen and Progesterone)**
> - May increase the risk of cervical, liver, and perhaps breast cancer
> - May elevate blood pressure and cholesterol (related to estrogen)
> - Increase risk of cardiac disease if patient is also smoking
> - May impair effectiveness of concurrent use of antibiotics
> - Are contraindicated in patients with migraine headaches and depression

DYSMENORRHEA

Dysmenorrhea is abdominal cramping pain or discomfort associated with menstrual flow. The degree of pain and discomfort varies with the individual. The two types of dysmenorrhea are *primary* (no pathologic condition exists) and *secondary* (pelvic disease is the underlying cause).[5] Dysmenorrhea is one of the most common gynecologic problems.

Etiology and Pathophysiology

Primary dysmenorrhea is not a disease. It is caused by an excess of prostaglandin $F_{2\alpha}$ ($PGF_{2\alpha}$) and/or an increased sensitivity to it. Stimulation of the endometrium by estrogen, followed by progesterone, results in a dramatic increase in prostaglandin production by the endometrium. With the onset of menses, degeneration of the endometrium releases prostaglandin. Locally, prostaglandins increase myometrial contractions and constriction of small endometrial blood vessels. This causes tissue ischemia and increased sensitization of the pain receptors, resulting in menstrual pain. Primary dysmenorrhea begins in the first few years after menarche, typically with the onset of regular ovulatory cycles.

Secondary dysmenorrhea is usually acquired after adolescence, occurring most commonly at 30 to 40 years of age. Common pelvic conditions that cause secondary dysmenorrhea include endometriosis, chronic pelvic inflammatory disease, and uterine fibroids. Because secondary dysmenorrhea can be caused by many conditions, symptoms vary. However, painful menses is present in all situations.

Clinical Manifestations

Primary dysmenorrhea starts 12 to 24 hours before the onset of menses. The pain is most severe the first day of menses and rarely lasts more than 2 days. Characteristic manifestations include lower abdominal pain that is colicky in nature, frequently radiating to the lower back and upper thighs. The abdominal pain is often accompanied by nausea, diarrhea, fatigue, and headache.

Secondary dysmenorrhea usually occurs after the woman has experienced problem-free periods for some time. The pain, which may be unilateral, is generally more constant and continues longer than in primary dysmenorrhea. Depending on the cause, symptoms such as *dyspareunia* (painful intercourse), painful defecation, or irregular bleeding may occur at times other than menstruation.

NURSING AND COLLABORATIVE MANAGEMENT DYSMENORRHEA

Evaluation begins with distinguishing primary from secondary dysmenorrhea. Obtain a complete health history with special attention to menstrual and gynecologic history. A pelvic examination is performed by the health care provider. The probable diagnosis is primary dysmenorrhea if the history reveals an onset shortly after menarche, symptoms are associated only with menses, and the pelvic examination is normal. If a specific cause of dysmenorrhea is evident, the diagnosis is secondary dysmenorrhea.

Treatment for primary dysmenorrhea includes heat, exercise, and drug therapy. Heat is applied to the lower abdomen or back. Regular exercise is beneficial because it may reduce endometrial hyperplasia and subsequent prostaglandin production. Primary drug therapy is nonsteroidal antiinflammatory drugs (NSAIDs) such as naproxen (Naprosyn), which has antiprostaglandin activity. NSAIDs should be started at the first sign of menses and continued every 4 to 8 hours to maintain a sufficient level of the drug to inhibit prostaglandin synthesis for the usual duration of discomfort.

Oral contraceptives may also be used. They decrease dysmenorrhea by reducing endometrial hyperplasia. Acupuncture and transcutaneous nerve stimulation may be used for women who have inadequate relief from medications or who prefer not to take medications. Patients who are unresponsive to these treatments should be evaluated for chronic pelvic pain (discussed later in this chapter on p. 1289).

Treatment of secondary dysmenorrhea depends on the cause. Some individuals with secondary dysmenorrhea are helped by the approaches used for primary dysmenorrhea.

Instruct women on why dysmenorrhea occurs and how to treat it. This will provide women with a foundation for coping with this common problem and increase feelings of control and self-reliance.

Women often ask what can be done for minor discomforts associated with menstrual cycles. Advise women that during acute pain, relief may be obtained by applying heat to the abdomen or back and taking NSAIDs for analgesia. Also suggest noninvasive pain-relieving practices such as relaxation breathing and guided imagery.

Other health care measures to reduce the discomfort of dysmenorrhea include regular exercise and proper nutritional habits. Avoiding constipation, maintaining good body mechanics, and eliminating stress and fatigue, particularly before menstrual periods, can also decrease discomfort. Staying active and interested in activities may also help.

ABNORMAL VAGINAL BLEEDING

Abnormal vaginal or uterine bleeding is a common gynecologic concern. Abnormalities include *oligomenorrhea* (long intervals between menses, generally greater than 35 days), amenorrhea (absence of menstruation), *menorrhagia* (excessive or prolonged menstrual bleeding), and *metrorrhagia* (irregular bleeding or bleeding between menses). The cause of abnormal bleeding may vary from anovulatory menstrual cycles to more serious conditions such as ectopic pregnancy or endometrial cancer.

The woman's age provides direction for identifying the cause of bleeding. For example, a postmenopausal woman with abnormal bleeding must always be evaluated for endometrial cancer but does not need to be evaluated for possible pregnancy. For a 20-year-old woman with abnormal bleeding, the possibility of pregnancy must always be considered, and endometrial cancer would be unlikely.

Abnormal bleeding may be caused by dysfunction of the hypothalamic-pituitary-ovarian axis such as a pituitary adenoma. Another possible cause is infection. Changes in lifestyle such as marriage, recent moves, a death in the family, financial stress, and other emotional crises can also cause irregular bleeding. Because psychologic factors can influence endocrine function, they should be considered when the patient is evaluated.

Types of Irregular Bleeding

Oligomenorrhea and Amenorrhea. Anovulation is the most common reason for missing menses once pregnancy has been ruled out. Additional causes of amenorrhea are listed in Table 54-5. *Primary amenorrhea* refers to the failure of menstrual cycles to begin by age 16 years or by age 14 years if secondary sex characteristics are present. *Secondary amenorrhea* refers to the cessation of menstrual cycles once they had been established.

Ovulation is often erratic for several years after menarche and before menopause. Thus oligomenorrhea due to anovulation is common for women at the beginning and end of menstruation. In anovulatory cycles the corpus luteum that produces progesterone does not form. This may result in a situation referred to as *unopposed estrogen.* When unopposed by progesterone, estrogen can cause excessive buildup of the endometrium. Persistent overgrowth of the endometrium increases a woman's risk for endometrial cancer. To reduce this risk, progesterone or oral contraceptives are prescribed to ensure that the patient's endometrial lining is shed at least four to six times per year.

Menorrhagia. The excessive bleeding associated with menorrhagia can be characterized as an increased duration (more than 7 days), increased amount (more than 80 mL), or both. Anovulatory uterine bleeding is the most common cause of menorrhagia. An unopposed estrogen state continues to build up the endometrium until it becomes unstable, resulting in menorrhagia. For young women with excessive bleeding, clotting disorders must be considered. Uterine fibroids (also called *leiomyomas*) and endometrial polyps are common causes of menorrhagia for women in their childbearing years.[6]

TABLE 54-5	**CAUSES OF AMENORRHEA**
Natural Amenorrhea	**Hormonal Imbalance**
• Pregnancy	• Polycystic ovary syndrome
• Breastfeeding	• Pituitary tumors
• Menopause	• Premature menopause
Medications	**Structural Problems**
• Antipsychotics	• Uterine scarring
• Chemotherapy	• Structural abnormalities of vagina
• Antidepressants	• Damage to ovaries or uterus from radiation
Lifestyle	
• Stress	
• Excessive exercise	
• Low body weight	
• Acute and chronic illness	

Metrorrhagia. Metrorrhagia, also referred to as *spotting* or *breakthrough bleeding,* is bleeding between menstrual periods. For all reproductive-age women, pregnancy complications such as spontaneous abortion or ectopic pregnancy must be considered as a possible cause. Other causes include cervical or endometrial polyps, infection, and cancer. Spotting is common during the first three cycles of oral contraceptives. If spotting continues beyond that, a different pill formulation can be prescribed once other causes of metrorrhagia have been ruled out. Spotting with long-acting progestin therapy (e.g., Mirena intrauterine device [IUD]) or progestin-only pills (medroxyprogesterone [Depo-Provera, Provera]) is also common. For postmenopausal women, endometrial cancer must be considered whenever spotting is experienced. In postmenopausal women, exogenous estrogen administration during hormone therapy is a common cause of metrorrhagia.

Diagnostic Studies and Collaborative Care

Because abnormal vaginal bleeding has multiple causes, the diagnostic and collaborative care varies. A health history and physical examination directed at the most likely causes of vaginal bleeding for the woman's age-group is the first step. These findings provide the basis for selecting laboratory tests and diagnostic procedures. Treatment depends on the etiology of the problem (e.g., menorrhagia, amenorrhea), degree of threat to the patient's health, and whether children are desired in the future.

Combined oral contraceptives may be prescribed for a woman with amenorrhea to ensure regular shedding of the endometrium if she also wants contraception. Tranexamic acid (Lysteda) may be used to treat heavy menstrual bleeding. This drug stabilizes a protein that helps blood to clot. Side effects may include headache, back pain, abdominal pain, muscle and joint pain, anemia, and fatigue. Women using hormonal contraception should take tranexamic acid only if they have a strong medical need, since there is an increased risk of blood clots and stroke. Estradiol valerate/dienogest (Natazia) may be given to women with heavy menstrual bleeding who desire an oral contraceptive to prevent pregnancy.

The treatment goal for women with menorrhagia is to minimize further blood loss. If menorrhagia is the result of anovulatory cycles, the endometrium must be stabilized by a combination of oral estrogen and progesterone.

Balloon thermotherapy is a technique for menorrhagia that involves the introduction of a soft, flexible balloon into the uterus. The balloon is then inflated with sterile fluid (Fig. 54-1). The fluid in the balloon is heated and maintained for 8 minutes, thus causing ablation (removal) of the uterine lining. When the treatment is completed, the fluid is withdrawn from the balloon and the catheter is removed from the uterus. The uterine lining sloughs off in the next 7 to 10 days. Uterine balloon thermotherapy is contraindicated for women who desire to maintain their fertility and for women with any suspected uterine abnormalities such as fibroids, suspected endometrial cancer, prior cesarean delivery, or myomectomy. With severe bleeding, hospitalization is indicated. All patients with menorrhagia should be evaluated for anemia and treated as indicated.

Surgical Therapy. Surgery may be indicated depending on the underlying cause of the abnormal vaginal bleeding. D&C is used only in cases of acute excess bleeding or for older women when endometrial biopsy and ultrasonography have not pro-

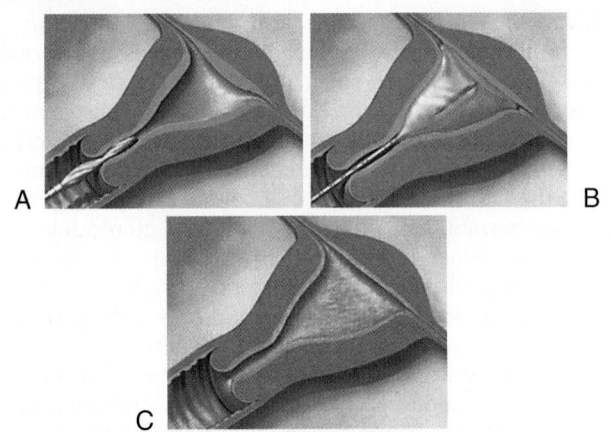

C

FIG. 54-1 Balloon thermotherapy for treatment of menorrhagia. **A,** Balloon-tipped catheter is inserted into the uterus through the vagina and the cervix. **B,** The balloon is inflated with a sterile fluid that expands to fit the size and shape of the uterus. The fluid is heated to 188° F (87° C) and maintained for 8 minutes while the uterine lining is treated. **C,** Fluid is withdrawn from the balloon and the catheter is removed. (Courtesy Ethicon, Inc, Cornelia, Ga.)

vided the necessary diagnostic information. Endometrial ablation for menorrhagia may be done by laser, thermal balloon, cryotherapy, or microwave energy for patients who do not want to have children.

If menorrhagia is caused by uterine fibroids, a hysterectomy (surgical removal of the uterus) may be performed. A *myomectomy* (removal of fibroids without removal of the uterus) may be performed if the patient wants to preserve her uterus. The myomectomy is done via laparotomy, laparoscopy, or hysteroscopy. Hormonal regimens and embolization of the blood vessels supplying the fibroid tumor are other treatment options.

NURSING MANAGEMENT
ABNORMAL VAGINAL BLEEDING

Teaching women about the characteristics of the menstrual cycle will enable them to identify normal variations. Table 51-2 includes characteristics of the menstrual cycle and related patient teaching. This knowledge can decrease apprehension and dispel misconceptions about the menstrual cycle. If the patient's menstrual cycle pattern does not fall within the normal range, urge her to discuss this with her health care provider.

The selection of internal or external sanitary protection is a matter of personal preference. Tampons are convenient and make menstrual hygiene easier, whereas pads may provide better protection. Using a combination of tampons and pads and avoiding prolonged use of superabsorbent tampons may decrease the risk of *toxic shock syndrome* (TSS). TSS is an acute life-threatening condition caused by a toxin from *Staphylococcus aureus*. TSS causes high fever, vomiting, diarrhea, weakness, myalgia, and a sunburn-like rash.[7]

Whenever excessive, the amount of the vaginal bleeding should be assessed as accurately as possible. The patient should record and report the number and size of pads or tampons used and the degree of saturation. The patient's fatigue level, along with variations in blood pressure and pulse, should be monitored because anemia and hypovolemia may be present. For the patient requiring a surgical procedure, provide the appropriate preoperative and postoperative care.

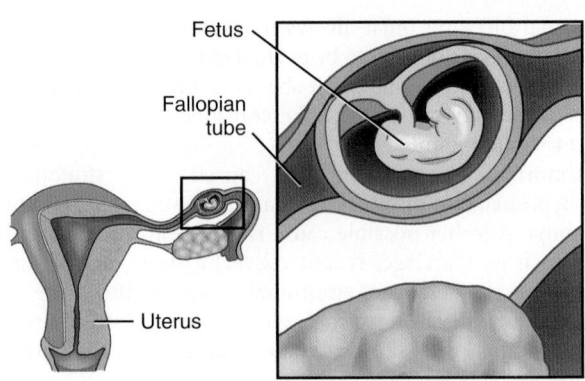

FIG. 54-2 Ectopic pregnancy occurring in the fallopian tube.

ECTOPIC PREGNANCY

An ectopic pregnancy is the implantation of the fertilized ovum anywhere outside the uterine cavity. Approximately 3% of all pregnancies are ectopic, and approximately 98% of these occur in the fallopian tube[8] (Fig. 54-2). The remaining 2% to 3% may be ovarian, abdominal, or cervical. Ectopic pregnancy is a life-threatening condition. Earlier identification has contributed to decreased mortality rates.

Etiology and Pathophysiology

Any blockage of the fallopian tube or reduction of tubal peristalsis that impedes or delays the zygote passing to the uterine cavity can result in tubal implantation. After implantation, the growth of the gestational sac expands the tubal wall. Eventually the tube ruptures, causing acute peritoneal symptoms. Less acute symptoms usually begin within 6 to 8 weeks after the last normal menstrual period and weeks before rupture would occur.

Risk factors for ectopic pregnancy include a history of pelvic inflammatory disease, prior ectopic pregnancy, current progestin-releasing IUD, progestin-only birth control failure, and prior pelvic or tubal surgery. Additional risk factors for ectopic pregnancy include procedures used in infertility treatment, including IVF, embryo transfer, and ovulation induction.

Clinical Manifestations

The classic manifestations of ectopic pregnancy are abdominal or pelvic pain, missed menses, and irregular vaginal bleeding. Other manifestations include morning sickness, breast tenderness, gastrointestinal disturbance, malaise, and syncope. Pain is almost always present and is caused by distention of the fallopian tube. It may start unilaterally and then spread to become bilateral. The character of the pain varies among women and can be colicky or vague. If tubal rupture occurs, the pain is intense and may be referred to the shoulder as a result of irritation of the diaphragm by blood released into the abdominal cavity. Symptom severity does not necessarily correlate with the extent of external bleeding present. With rupture, the risk of hemorrhage and hypovolemic shock is present. Suspected rupture is treated as an emergency.

The vaginal bleeding that may accompany ectopic pregnancy is usually described as spotting. However, bleeding may be heavier and can be confused with menses.

Diagnostic Studies

Ectopic pregnancy can be a diagnostic challenge because of its similarity to other pelvic and abdominal disorders, such as salpingitis, spontaneous abortion, ruptured ovarian cyst, appendicitis, and peritonitis. A serum (radioimmunoassay) pregnancy test should be performed. If the test is negative, an ectopic pregnancy is not likely. If ectopic pregnancy cannot be excluded by the pregnancy test, further evaluation is warranted. If the patient is in stable condition, a combination of serial measurements of serum β-hCG and vaginal ultrasonography is used.[9] Absence of a normal intrauterine pregnancy means that the diagnosis is probably a spontaneous abortion or an ectopic pregnancy. With a spontaneous abortion, serial serum β-hCG levels will decrease over time. A complete blood count is obtained when there is any concern regarding the amount of blood loss or if surgery is contemplated.

NURSING AND COLLABORATIVE MANAGEMENT ECTOPIC PREGNANCY

Surgery remains the primary approach for treating ectopic pregnancies and should be performed immediately. However, medical management with methotrexate (Folex) is being used with increasing success in patients who are hemodynamically stable and have a mass less than 3 cm in size.[10] A conservative surgical approach limits damage to the reproductive system as much as possible. Removal of the fetus from the tube is preferred to removing the tube. Laparoscopy is preferable to laparotomy because it decreases blood loss and the length of the hospital stay (Fig. 54-3). If the tube ruptures, conservative surgical approaches may not be possible. The patient may need a blood transfusion and supplemental IV fluid therapy to relieve shock and restore a satisfactory blood volume for safe anesthesia and surgery. The use of laparoscopy has resulted in fewer repeated ectopic pregnancies and a higher rate of future successful pregnancies.

Nursing care depends on the patient's condition. Before the diagnosis has been confirmed, be alert to patient signs of increasing pain and vaginal bleeding, which may indicate that the tube has ruptured. Monitor vital signs closely and observe for signs of shock. Give explanations and prepare the patient for diagnostic procedures when appropriate. Preparation of the patient for abdominal surgery may follow rapidly. Provide reassurance and support for the surgery to the patient and her family. Postoperatively, the patient may express a fear of future ectopic pregnancies and have many questions about the impact of this experience on her fertility.

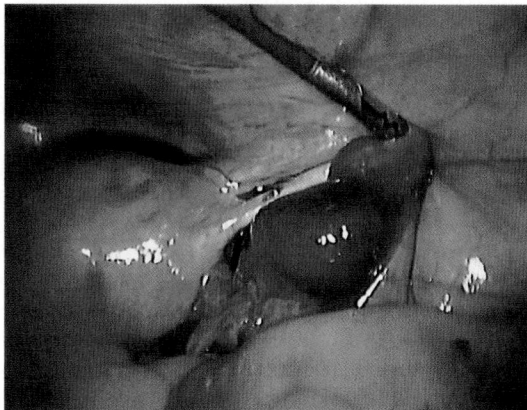

FIG. 54-3 Laparoscopic treatment of ectopic pregnancy in the right fallopian tube.

PERIMENOPAUSE AND POSTMENOPAUSE

Perimenopause is a normal life transition that begins with the first signs of change in menstrual cycles and ends after cessation of menses.[11] Menopause is the physiologic cessation of menses associated with declining ovarian function. It is usually considered complete after 1 year of *amenorrhea* (absence of menstruation). Menopause starts gradually and is usually associated with changes in menstruation, including menstrual flows that are increased, decreased, or irregular. Eventually complete cessation of menses occurs. *Postmenopause* is a term that refers to the time in a woman's life after menopause.

The age at which menopause occurs ranges from 44 to 55 years, with an average age of 51 years. Menopause may occur earlier due to illness, surgical removal of the uterus or both ovaries, side effects of radiation therapy or chemotherapy, or drugs. The age at which menopause occurs is not affected by age at menarche, physical characteristics, number of pregnancies, date of last pregnancy, or oral contraceptive use. However, genetic factors, autoimmune conditions, cigarette smoking, and racial or ethnic factors are related to an earlier age at menopause.

Changes within the ovary start the cascade of events that finally result in menopause. The regression of the follicles within each ovary begins at puberty and accelerates after age 35. With age, fewer follicles remain that are responsive to follicle-stimulating hormone (FSH). FSH normally stimulates the dominant follicle to secrete estrogen. When the follicles can no longer respond to FSH, the production of estrogen and progesterone from the ovary declines. However, perimenopausal women can get pregnant until menopause has occurred, since many women have long anovulatory cycles interspersed with shorter, ovulatory cycles.

With decreased ovarian function, decreased levels of estrogen cause a gradual increase in FSH and luteinizing hormone (LH) as a result of the negative feedback process. By the time menopause occurs, there is a 10- to 20-fold increase in FSH. The elevated FSH level may take several years to return to the premenopausal level. The reduced estrogen level also causes a decrease in the frequency of ovulation and results in changes in the reproductive organs and tissues (e.g., atrophy of vaginal tissue).

Clinical Manifestations

Clinical manifestations of perimenopause and postmenopause are presented in Table 54-6. Perimenopause is a time of erratic hormonal fluctuation. Irregular vaginal bleeding is common.

TABLE 54-6	MANIFESTATIONS OF PERIMENOPAUSE AND POSTMENOPAUSE
Perimenopause	**Postmenopause**
• Irregular menses	• Cessation of menses
• Occasional vasomotor symptoms	• Vasomotor instability (hot flashes and night sweats)
• Atrophy of genitourinary tissue with decreased support	• Atrophy of genitourinary tissue (e.g., vaginal epithelium)
• Stress and urge incontinence	• Stress and urge incontinence
• Osteoporosis	• Breast tenderness
• Mood changes	

TABLE 54-7	**MANIFESTATIONS OF ESTROGEN DEFICIENCY**

Vasomotor
- Hot flashes
- Night sweats

Genitourinary
- Atrophic vaginitis
- Dyspareunia secondary to poor lubrication
- Incontinence

Psychologic
- Emotional lability
- Change in sleep pattern
- Decreased REM sleep

Musculoskeletal
- Increased fracture rate, especially vertebral bodies but also humerus, distal radius, and upper femur

Cardiovascular
- Decreased high-density lipoproteins (HDLs)
- Increased low-density lipoproteins (LDLs)

Other
- Diminished collagen content of skin
- Breast tissue changes

REM, Rapid eye movement.

With decreasing estrogen, hot flashes and other symptoms begin. The signs and symptoms of diminished estrogen are listed in Table 54-7. The loss of estrogen plays a significant role in the cause of age-related alterations. Changes most critical to a woman's well-being are the increased risks for coronary artery disease (CAD) and osteoporosis (secondary to bone density loss). Other changes include a redistribution of fat, a tendency to gain weight more easily, muscle and joint pain, loss of skin elasticity, changes in hair amount and distribution, and atrophy of external genitalia and breast tissue.

Hallmarks of perimenopause include *vasomotor instability* (hot flashes) and irregular menses. A hot flash (occurs in up to 80% of all women) is described as a sudden sensation of intense heat along with perspiration and flushing.[12] These sensations may last from several seconds to 5 minutes and occur most often at night, thereby disturbing sleep. The cause of hot flashes, or vasomotor instability, is not clearly understood. It has been theorized that temperature regulators in the brain are in proximity to the area where gonadotropin-releasing hormone (GnRH) is released. The lowered estrogen levels are correlated with dilation of cutaneous blood vessels, resulting in hot flashes and increased sweating. The more sudden the withdrawal of estrogen (e.g., surgical removal of the ovaries), the more likely the symptoms will be severe if no hormone replacement is provided. Symptoms usually subside over time and typically last from 5 to 10 years with or without treatment.[13] Hot flashes can be triggered by stress and situations that affect body temperature, such as eating a hot meal, hot weather, or warm clothing. Women who smoke are at higher risk for hot flashes because smoking affects estrogen metabolism. African American women report the highest incidence of hot flashes, whereas Asian American women report the lowest number.[13]

Atrophic vaginal changes secondary to decreased estrogen include thinning of the vaginal mucosa and disappearance of rugae. Vaginal secretions also decrease and become more alkaline. As a result of these changes, the vagina is easily traumatized and more susceptible to infection, including a higher risk for human immunodeficiency virus (HIV) infection if exposed. *Dyspareunia* (painful intercourse) may also occur. This can lead to unnecessary and premature cessation of sexual activity. Dryness is a problem that can be corrected with water-soluble lubricants or, if needed, with hormonal creams or systemic hormone therapy.

Atrophic changes in the lower urinary tract also occur with a decrease in estrogen. Bladder capacity decreases, and the bladder and urethral tissue lose tone. These changes can cause symptoms that mimic a bladder infection (e.g., dysuria, urgency, frequency) when no infection is present.

Whether decreasing estrogen causes the psychologic changes associated with perimenopause is unclear. Depression, irritability, and cognitive problems, which are often attributed to menopause, could result from life stressors or sleep deprivation from hot flashes. Depressive symptoms appear to improve when hormone levels stabilize.

Collaborative Care

The diagnosis of perimenopause should be made only after careful consideration of other possible causes for the woman's symptoms. Depression, thyroid dysfunction, anemia, or anxiety can cause the same symptoms. Review a woman's history of menstrual patterns as part of establishing the diagnosis. Because of the hormonal fluctuations that occur before menopause, routine testing of the serum FSH level to establish a diagnosis is not indicated.

Drug Therapy. Hormone therapy (HT) was once standard therapy in the United States for treating menopausal symptoms. HT includes estrogen for women without a uterus or estrogen and progesterone for women with a uterus. Findings from the Women's Health Initiative (WHI) clinical trials changed this practice.[14] The data showed that women who had taken estrogen plus progestin (Prempro) had an increased risk of breast cancer, stroke, heart disease, and emboli. However, these women had fewer hip fractures and a lower risk of developing colorectal cancer. Women who took only estrogen (Premarin) had an increased risk of stroke and emboli. However, these women had decreased risk for fractures with no increased risk for heart disease or breast or colorectal cancer. A recent systematic review has updated and validated the results of the WHI trials.[15]

If women wish to consider taking HT for the short-term treatment (4 to 5 years) of menopausal symptoms, the risks and benefits of therapy (e.g., minimizes bone loss, hot flashes, vaginal atrophic changes) should be considered carefully. The woman and her health care provider should thoroughly discuss the decision to take HT, and which ones to take. If a woman chooses to use HT, the lowest effective dose should be used. The age that a woman starts HT may determine her risk of heart disease. The risk appears to increase the further a woman moves away from menopause.

The side effects of estrogen include nausea, fluid retention, headache, and breast enlargement. Side effects of progesterone include increased appetite, weight gain, irritability, depression, spotting, and breast tenderness. A commonly used estrogen preparation is 0.625 mg of conjugated estrogen (Premarin) daily. For symptom relief, a higher dose may be needed. To receive the protective benefit of progesterone, 5 to 10 mg of medroxyprogesterone is indicated for 12 days of each month on a cyclic regimen, or 2.5 mg on a continuous regimen. If the estrogen is increased for symptom relief, the progesterone should also be increased. Other forms of progesterone include norethindrone (Aygestin) and micronized progesterone creams, dermal patches, gels, and lotions; rings placed around the cervix; and subcutaneous pellets. Vaginal creams are especially useful for urogenital symptoms (e.g., dryness). Transdermal estrogen (skin patch or spray [EvaMist]) has the advantage of bypassing the liver, but the disadvantage of causing skin irritation.

SSRI antidepressants, including paroxetine (Paxil), fluoxetine, and venlafaxine (Effexor), are an effective alternative to HT in reducing hot flashes. This effect is noted even if the user is not depressed. The mechanism of action is unknown. Clonidine (Catapres), an antihypertensive drug, and gabapentin (Neurontin), an antiseizure drug, have also been shown to relieve hot flashes.

Selective estrogen receptor modulators (SERMs), such as raloxifene (Evista), are also used to treat menopausal problems. These drugs have some of the positive benefits of estrogen, such as preventing bone loss, without the negative effects such as endometrial hyperplasia. Raloxifene competes with estrogen for estrogen receptor sites.[16] It decreases bone loss and serum cholesterol with minimal effects on breast and uterine tissue.

Bisphosphonates, including alendronate (Fosamax) and risedronate (Actonel), are also used to decrease the risk for osteoporosis in postmenopausal women. These drugs enhance bone mineral density by suppressing resorption. SERMs and bisphosphonates are discussed further in Chapter 64 with respect to their role in the management of osteoporosis.

Nonhormonal Therapy. Because of the risks associated with HT, many women try other therapies to relieve menopausal symptoms. Paroxetine (Brisdelle) is a newer nonhormonal treatment that may be used for moderate to severe hot flashes associated with menopause. This drug is a selective serotonin reuptake inhibitor.

Hot flash frequency and severity can be reduced through measures that lead to a decrease in heat production and an increase in heat loss. Keeping a cool environment and limiting caffeine and alcohol intake lower heat production. Relaxation techniques (e.g., relaxation breathing, imagery) may also help. To promote heat loss at night when hot flashes can disrupt sleep, increase air circulation in the room and avoid bedding that traps the heat (e.g., heavy quilts). Loose-fitting clothes do not retain body heat, whereas clothes with tight necks and wrists do. Cool cloths applied to flushed areas also aid in heat loss.

Daily intake of vitamin E in doses up to 800 IU may also help reduce hot flashes in some women. Changing sleep patterns may be helped by avoiding alcohol and controlling hot flashes. Relaxation techniques can promote a better night's sleep by decreasing anxiety. A regular moderate program (three to four times per week) of aerobic and weight-bearing exercises can slow the process of bone loss and a tendency toward weight gain.

Nutritional Therapy. Good nutrition can decrease the risk of cardiovascular disease and osteoporosis in addition to assisting with vasomotor symptoms. A daily intake of about 30 cal/kg of body weight is recommended. A decrease in metabolic rate and careless eating habits can cause the weight gain and fatigue often attributed to menopause. An adequate intake of calcium and vitamin D helps maintain healthy bones and counteracts loss of bone density. Postmenopausal women not receiving supplemental estrogen should have a daily calcium intake of at least 1500 mg, whereas those taking estrogen replacement need at least 1000 mg/day. Calcium supplements are best absorbed when taken with meals. Either dietary calcium or calcium supplements may be used (see Tables 64-14 and 64-15).

COMPLEMENTARY & ALTERNATIVE THERAPIES
Herbs and Supplements for Menopause

Herb	Scientific Evidence	Nursing Implications
Black cohosh	Mixed evidence for use in the treatment of menopausal symptoms*	• Generally well tolerated in recommended doses for up to 6 mo. • Should not be used in people with a liver disorder.
Soy	Mixed evidence for treatment of menopausal symptoms*	• Women with a history of breast, ovarian, or uterine cancer or endometriosis should consult their health care provider before using soy or soy products. • Soy may interact with warfarin. Patients taking warfarin should consult their health care provider before using soy or soy products.

*In general, the evidence for use of these herbs as treatments for menopause symptoms is limited by a lack of well-designed, controlled trials (www. naturalstandard.com).

The diet should be high in complex carbohydrates and vitamin B complex, especially B_6. Phytoestrogens (soy, tofu, chickpeas, sunflower seeds) have been used to reduce menopausal symptoms. Herbal remedies, such as black cohosh, have become popular in treating menopausal symptoms (see Complementary & Alternative Therapies box above). Consultation with an experienced herbal practitioner is recommended before initiating therapy.

NURSING MANAGEMENT
PERIMENOPAUSE AND POSTMENOPAUSE

Foster a positive image of perimenopause as a time of vitality and attractiveness. Perimenopause can provide women with a renewed incentive to enhance self-care and well-being. Provide teaching and reassurance to perimenopausal women who experience difficulty in managing their symptoms. Tell them that symptoms are normal and often are temporary. Discuss nondrug approaches to managing symptoms.

Dry skin can be improved by the use of moisturizing soaps and body lotions. Kegel exercises may help decrease stress incontinence (see Table 46-19). Sexual function can continue with little change in the vast majority of postmenopausal women. Cessation of menstruation and ability to bear children should not be equated with cessation of sexual capability. For some women, menopause may be liberating.

Femininity and libido do not disappear with menopause. A water-soluble lubricant (e.g., Replens, Astroglide, K-Y jelly) is often effective in managing atrophic changes in vaginal epithelium. An active sex life helps increase lubrication and maintains the pliability of vaginal tissues. Provide the patient with an opportunity to candidly discuss concerns related to sexual functioning.

CULTURALLY COMPETENT CARE
MENOPAUSE

Although all women experience menopause, the perception of menopause varies by culture. Ethnic groups have different traditions and beliefs regarding menopause, including the use of complementary and alternative therapies to manage symptoms.[17] Be aware of the attitudes and beliefs regarding menopause among women from various ethnic and cultural backgrounds. In many cultures, menopause is considered a normal part of aging, and little emphasis is placed on the physical and emotional symptoms that accompany the loss of fertility. In cultures where older adults are revered, menopause may be seen as a liberating transition to a state of being a "wise woman."

American culture generally has a negative attitude toward aging and places a high value on youth. Menopause is often considered a disorder that requires treatment. Menopausal symptoms may be viewed as troublesome, with a strong need to treat hot flashes and mood swings. Numerous substances, from HT to herbal preparations, are often used to treat menopausal symptoms.

Menopause is a milestone in a woman's life that is embedded in her own personality and her culture. Approaching the menopausal woman with this understanding is important to provide culturally competent care.

CONDITIONS OF VULVA, VAGINA, AND CERVIX

Etiology and Pathophysiology

Infection and inflammation of the vagina, cervix, and vulva commonly occur when the natural defenses of the acid vaginal secretions (maintained by sufficient estrogen levels) and the presence of *Lactobacillus* are disrupted. The woman's resistance may also be decreased as a result of aging, poor nutrition, and drugs that alter the bacterial flora or mucosa. Organisms gain entrance to the areas through contaminated hands, clothing, douching, and intercourse. Table 54-8 presents the causes, manifestations, diagnostic methods, and collaborative care of common infections and inflammations.

Most lower genital tract infections are related to sexual intercourse. Intercourse can transmit organisms, injure tissues, and alter the acid-base balance of the vagina. Vulvar infections caused by viruses such as herpes and genital warts can be sexually transmitted when no lesions are apparent. Oral contraceptives, antibiotics, and corticosteroids may produce changes in the vaginal pH and trigger an overgrowth of the organisms present. For example, *Candida albicans* may be present in small numbers in the vagina. An overgrowth of this organism causes vulvovaginitis.

Clinical Manifestations

Abnormal vaginal discharge and reddened vulvar lesions are common clinical manifestations. In addition to a thick white curdlike discharge, women with vulvovaginal candidiasis (VVC) often experience intense itching and dysuria, which is the result of urine coming into contact with fissures and irritated areas on the vulva. The hallmark of bacterial vaginosis is the fishy odor of the discharge. Women with cervicitis may notice spotting after intercourse.

Common vulvar lesions include herpes infection and genital warts. Initial or primary herpes infections may be extremely painful. Herpes begins as a small vesicle followed by a superficial red ulcer. Most herpes lesions are painful. Genital warts, caused by the human papillomavirus (HPV), vary in appearance. Irregularly shaped "cauliflower" lesions are common. Genital warts are painless unless traumatized. (Herpes infection and genital warts are discussed in Chapter 53.)

Postmenopausal women may develop gynecologic problems such as *lichen sclerosis*.[18] This chronic inflammatory condition is associated with intense itching in the genital skin area (e.g., labia minora, clitoris). The lesions are white with a "tissue

TABLE 54-8   INFECTIONS OF THE LOWER GENITAL TRACT

Infection and Etiology	Manifestations and Diagnostic Methods	Drug Therapy
Vulvovaginal Candidiasis (VVC) (Monilial Vaginitis)		
Candida albicans (fungus)	Commonly found in mouth, gastrointestinal tract, and vagina. Pruritus, thick white curdlike discharge. KOH microscopic examination: pseudohyphae, pH 4.0-4.7.	Antifungal agents (e.g., miconazole [Monistat], clotrimazole [Gyne-Lotrimin, Mycelex] [available over the counter, in cream or suppository]) Fluconazole (Diflucan).
Trichomonas Vaginitis		
Trichomonas vaginalis (protozoa)	Sexually transmitted. Pruritus, frothy greenish or gray discharge. Hemorrhagic spots on cervix or vaginal walls. Saline microscopic examination: swimming trichomonads, pH >4.5.	Metronidazole (Flagyl) for patient and partner.
Bacterial Vaginosis		
Gardnerella vaginalis *Corynebacterium vaginale*	Mode of transmission unclear. Watery discharge with fishy odor. May or may not have other symptoms. Saline microscopic examination: epithelial cells, pH >4.5.	Oral or vaginal metronidazole (Flagyl) or clindamycin (Clindesse). Examine and treat partner. Lactobacillus acidophilus taken orally by diet (e.g., yogurt, fermented soy products) or supplements can decrease unwanted vaginal bacteria.
Cervicitis		
Chlamydia trachomatis	Sexually transmitted; mucopurulent discharge with postcoital spotting from cervical inflammation. Culture for *Chlamydia* and *Neisseria gonorrhoeae*.	Azithromycin (Zithromax). Treat patient and partner.
Severe Recurrent Vaginitis		
C. albicans (most often)	May be indication of HIV infection. All women who are unresponsive to first-line treatment should be offered HIV testing.	Drug appropriate to opportunistic organism.

KOH, Potassium hydroxide.

paper" appearance initially, although scratching produces changes in the appearance. The cause is unknown. High-potency topical corticosteroid ointment such as clobetasol (Temovate) helps relieve itching.

Collaborative Care

Evaluate genital problems by taking a history, performing a physical examination, and obtaining the appropriate laboratory and diagnostic studies. Because many problems relate to sexual activity, a sexual history is essential. The nature of the problem determines the extent of the evaluation. When ulcerative lesions are present, do a culture for herpes and a blood test for syphilis. Genital warts are usually identified by their clinical appearance. Vulvar dystrophies may be examined via colposcopy with a biopsy taken for diagnosis.

Problems involving vaginal discharge are evaluated by microscopy and cultures. The most common vaginal conditions (i.e., bacterial vaginosis, VVC, and trichomoniasis) are diagnosed by a procedure called a *wet mount*. The findings characteristic of each condition are shown in Table 54-8. To assess for cervicitis, endocervical cultures are obtained for chlamydial infection and gonorrhea. If purulent discharge is observed coming from the cervix, a sample of endocervical cells may be taken to conduct a Gram stain. The Gram-stained slide is examined with a microscope to identify white blood cells and gram-negative diplococci (indicative of gonorrhea). (Sexually transmitted infections [STIs] are discussed in Chapter 53.)

Drug therapy is based on the diagnosis (see Table 54-8). Antibiotics taken as directed will cure bacterial infections. Treatment duration and medications vary with specific STIs. Teach patients how to properly take their medications and to follow up to verify a cure. Partners should be treated so that reinfection does not occur.

Women with vaginal conditions or cervical infection should abstain from intercourse for at least 1 week. Douching should be avoided because it has been adversely linked to pelvic inflammatory disease, STIs, and ectopic pregnancy. Sexual partners must be evaluated and treated if the patient is diagnosed with trichomoniasis, chlamydial infection, gonorrhea, syphilis, or HIV.

Treatment of vulvar dystrophies is symptomatic because no cures are available. Treatment involves controlling the itching and hence the scratching. Interrupting the "itch-scratch cycle" prevents further secondary damage to the skin.

NURSING MANAGEMENT
CONDITIONS OF VULVA, VAGINA, AND CERVIX

Teach women about common genital conditions and how to reduce their risks. Recognize symptoms that indicate a problem, and help women seek care in a timely manner. Discussing problems that concern the patient's genitalia or sexual intercourse is frequently difficult. Use a nonjudgmental attitude to make women feel more comfortable while empowering them to ask questions.

When a woman is diagnosed with a genital condition, ensure that she fully understands the directions for treatment. Taking the full course of medication is especially important to decrease the chance of relapse. Because genitalia are such a private area, the use of graphs and models is especially helpful for patient teaching. When a woman is using a vaginal medication for the first time, show her the applicator and how to fill it. Also

teach where and how the applicator should be inserted using visual aids or models. Vaginal creams should be inserted before going to bed so that the medication will remain in the vagina for a long period. Women using vaginal creams or suppositories may wish to use panty liners during the day when the residual medication may drain out.

PELVIC INFLAMMATORY DISEASE

Pelvic inflammatory disease (PID) is an infectious condition of the pelvic cavity that may involve the fallopian tubes (salpingitis), ovaries (oophoritis), and pelvic peritoneum (peritonitis). A tubo-ovarian abscess may also form (Fig. 54-4). In the United States it is estimated that 1 million women experience an acute episode of PID annually.[19] PID is referred to as "silent" when women do not perceive any symptoms. Other women with PID are in acute distress. PID may also be a cause of chronic pelvic pain (discussed on p. 1289).

Etiology and Pathophysiology

PID is often the result of untreated cervicitis. The organism infecting the cervix ascends higher into the uterus, fallopian tubes, ovaries, and peritoneal cavity. *Chlamydia trachomatis* and *Neisseria gonorrhoeae* are the most common causative organisms of PID. These organisms, as well as anaerobes, mycoplasma, streptococci, and enteric gram-negative rods, gain entrance during sexual intercourse or after pregnancy termination, pelvic surgery, or childbirth. It is important to remember that not all cases of PID are the result of an STI.

Women at increased risk for chlamydial infections (those younger than 24 years of age, who have multiple sex partners, or who have a new sex partner) should be routinely tested for chlamydia. Chlamydial infections can be asymptomatic and unknowingly transmitted during intercourse. Silent PID is a major cause of female infertility.

Clinical Manifestations

Women with PID usually go to a health care provider because they are experiencing lower abdominal pain. The pain typically starts gradually and then becomes constant. The intensity may vary from mild to severe. Movement such as walking can increase the pain. The pain is also frequently associated with intercourse. Spotting after intercourse and purulent cervical or

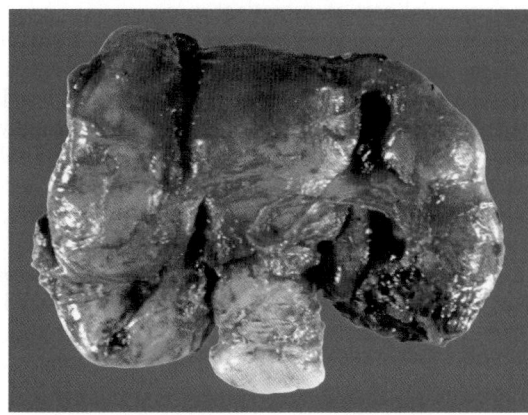

FIG. 54-4 Pelvic inflammatory disease. Acute infection of the fallopian tubes and the ovaries. The tubes and the ovaries have become an inflamed mass attached to the uterus. A tubo-ovarian abscess is also present.

vaginal discharge may also be noted. Fever and chills may be present. Women with less acute symptoms often notice increased cramping pain with menses, irregular bleeding, and some pain with intercourse. Women who have mild symptoms may go untreated either because they did not seek care or the health care provider misdiagnosed their complaints.

A pelvic examination assists in the diagnosis of PID. Women with PID have lower abdominal tenderness, adnexal tenderness, and positive cervical motion tenderness. Additional criteria useful for diagnosis may include fever and abnormal discharge (vaginal or cervical). Cultures for *N. gonorrhoeae* and *C. trachomatis* are also obtained, and a pregnancy test is done to rule out an ectopic pregnancy. Drug therapy begins when minimal diagnostic criteria are met. Thus treatment is not delayed for culture results. When the patient's pain or obesity compromises the pelvic examination and a tubo-ovarian abscess may be present, a vaginal ultrasound is indicated.

Complications

Immediate complications of PID include septic shock and *Fitz-Hugh-Curtis syndrome*, which occurs when PID spreads to the liver and causes acute perihepatitis. The patient has symptoms of right upper quadrant pain, but liver function tests are normal. Tubo-ovarian abscesses may "leak" or rupture, resulting in pelvic or generalized peritonitis. As the general circulation is flooded with bacterial endotoxins from the infected areas, septic shock may result. Embolisms may occur as the result of thrombophlebitis of the pelvic veins.

PID can cause adhesions and strictures in the fallopian tubes. Ectopic pregnancy may result when a tube is partially obstructed because the sperm can pass through the stricture, but the fertilized ovum cannot reach the uterus. After one episode of PID, the risk of having an ectopic pregnancy increases 10-fold. Further damage can obstruct the fallopian tubes and cause infertility.

Collaborative Care

PID is usually treated on an outpatient basis. The patient is given a combination of antibiotics such as cefoxitin (Mefoxin) and doxycycline (Vibramycin) to provide broad coverage against the causative organisms.[19] With effective antibiotic therapy, the pain should subside. The patient must have no intercourse for 3 weeks. Her partner(s) must be examined and treated. An important part of care is physical rest and oral fluids. Reevaluation in 48 to 72 hours, even if symptoms are improving, is an essential part of outpatient care.

If outpatient treatment is unsuccessful or if the patient is acutely ill or in severe pain, admission to the hospital is indicated. If a tubo-ovarian abscess is present, hospitalization is also indicated. Maximum doses of parenteral antibiotics are given in the hospital. Corticosteroids may be added to the antibiotic regimen to reduce inflammation, allowing for faster recovery and optimizing the chances for subsequent fertility. Application of heat to the lower abdomen or sitz baths may improve circulation and decrease pain. Bed rest in a semi-Fowler's position promotes drainage of the pelvic cavity by gravity and may prevent the development of abscesses high in the abdomen. Analgesics to relieve pain and IV fluids to prevent dehydration are also used.

Surgery is indicated for abscesses that fail to resolve with IV antibiotics. The abscess may be drained by laparoscopy or laparotomy. In extreme cases of infection or severe chronic pelvic pain, a hysterectomy may be performed. When surgery is necessary, the capacity for childbearing is preserved whenever possible.

NURSING MANAGEMENT
PELVIC INFLAMMATORY DISEASE

Subjective and objective data that should be obtained from the woman with PID are presented in Table 54-9. Prevention, early recognition, and prompt treatment of vaginal and cervical infections can help prevent PID and its serious complications. Provide accurate information about factors that place a woman at increased risk for PID. Urge women to seek medical attention for any unusual vaginal discharge or possible infection of their reproductive organs. Inform patients that not all discharge indicates infection, but that early diagnosis and treatment of an infection, if present, can prevent serious complications. Teach patients methods to decrease the risk of getting STIs and to recognize the signs of infection in their partner(s).

The patient may feel guilty about having PID, especially if it is associated with an STI. She may also be concerned about the complications associated with PID, such as adhesions and strictures of the fallopian tubes, infertility, and the increased incidence of ectopic pregnancy. Discuss with the patient her feelings and concerns to help her cope with them more effectively.

For patients requiring hospitalization, you have an important role in implementing drug therapy, monitoring the patient's health status, and providing symptom relief and patient teaching. Record vital signs and the character, amount, color, and odor of the vaginal discharge. Explain the need for limiting

---

TABLE 54-9   NURSING ASSESSMENT

Pelvic Inflammatory Disease

Subjective Data
Important Health Information
Past health history: Use of IUD; previous PID, gonorrhea, or chlamydial infection; multiple sexual partners; exposure to partner with urethritis; infertility
Medications: Use of and allergy to any antibiotics
Surgery or other treatments: Recent abortion or pelvic surgery

Functional Health Patterns
Health perception–health management: Malaise
Nutritional-metabolic: Nausea, vomiting; chills, fever
Elimination: Urinary frequency, urgency
Cognitive-perceptual: Lower abdominal and pelvic pain; low back pain; onset of pain just after a menstrual cycle; dysmenorrhea, dyspareunia, dysuria, vulvar pruritus
Sexuality-reproductive: Abnormal vaginal bleeding and menstrual irregularity; vaginal discharge

Objective Data
Reproductive
Mucopurulent cervicitis, vulvar maceration, vaginal discharge (heavy and purulent to thin and mucoid), tenderness on motion of cervix and uterus; presence of inflammatory masses on palpation

Possible Diagnostic Findings
Leukocytosis; ↑ erythrocyte sedimentation rate; positive culture of secretions or endocervical fluid; pelvic inflammation and positive endometrial biopsy on laparoscopic examination; abscess or inflammation on ultrasonography

IUD, Intrauterine device; *PID,* pelvic inflammatory disease.

activity, being in a semi-Fowler's position, and increasing fluid intake. Assess the degree of abdominal pain to determine the effectiveness of drug therapy.

CHRONIC PELVIC PAIN

Chronic pelvic pain refers to pain in the pelvic region (below the umbilicus and between the hips) that lasts 6 months or longer.[20] It accounts for 10% of all visits to gynecologists and is the reason for 20% to 30% of all laparoscopies. Up to one third of women who have PID have chronic pelvic pain.[21]

The cause of chronic pelvic pain is often hard to find. Many different conditions can cause pelvic pain. Gynecologic etiologies include dysmenorrhea, endometriosis, PID, ovarian cysts, uterine fibroids, pelvic adhesions, and ectopic pregnancies. Abdominal etiologies include irritable bowel syndrome, interstitial cystitis, appendicitis, and colitis. Psychologic factors (e.g., depression, chronic stress, history of sexual or physical abuse) may increase the risk of developing chronic pelvic pain. Emotional distress makes pain worse, and living with chronic pain contributes to emotional distress.

Chronic pelvic pain has many different clinical manifestations, including severe and steady pain, intermittent pain, dull and achy pain, pelvic pressure or heaviness, and sharp pain or cramping. In addition, pain may occur during intercourse or while having a bowel movement.

Determining the cause of chronic pelvic pain often involves a process of elimination. In addition to a detailed history and physical examination (including a pelvic examination), the patient may be asked to keep a journal of the onset of symptoms and any precipitating factors.

Diagnostic tests may include cultures from cervix or vagina (used to detect STIs), ultrasound, computed tomography (CT) scan, or magnetic resonance imaging (MRI) to detect abnormal structures or growths. Laparoscopy may be used to visualize the pelvic organs. This procedure is especially useful in detecting endometriosis and chronic PID.

If the cause of chronic pelvic pain is found, treatment focuses on that cause. If no cause can be found, treatment involves managing the pain. Over-the-counter pain medications (e.g., aspirin, ibuprofen, acetaminophen) may provide some relief. Sometimes stronger pain drugs may be needed. Birth control pills or other hormonal medications may help relieve cyclic pelvic pain related to menstrual cycles. If an infection is the source of the problem, antibiotics are used.

Tricyclic antidepressants (e.g., amitriptyline, nortriptyline [Pamelor]) have pain-relieving and antidepressant effects. These drugs may help improve chronic pelvic pain even in women who do not have depression. The patient may be encouraged to get counseling for any emotional issues.

Laparoscopic surgery may be used to remove pelvic adhesions or endometrial tissue. As a last resort, a hysterectomy may be done.

ENDOMETRIOSIS

Endometriosis is the presence of normal endometrial tissue in sites outside the endometrial cavity.[22] The most frequent sites are in or near the ovaries, uterosacral ligaments, and uterovesical peritoneum (Fig. 54-5). However, endometrial tissues can be in many other locations such as stomach, lungs, intestines, and spleen. The tissue responds to the hormones of the ovarian

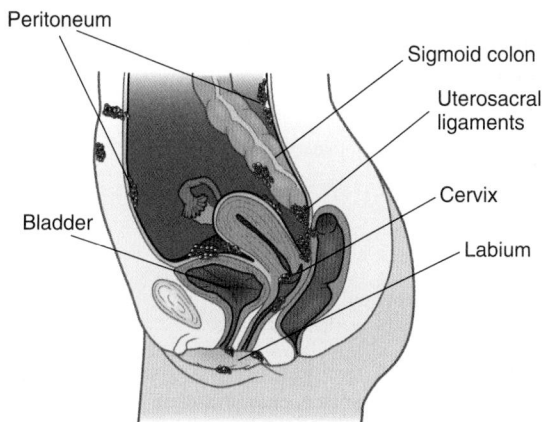

FIG. 54-5 Common sites of endometriosis.

cycle and undergoes a "mini-menstrual cycle" similar to the uterine endometrium.

The typical patient with endometriosis is in her late twenties or early thirties and has never had a full-term pregnancy. Although it is not a life-threatening condition, endometriosis can cause considerable pain. It is also a common cause of infertility and increases the risk of ovarian cancer. Endometriosis is one of the most common gynecologic problems, affecting more than 5.5 million women in North America.[23]

Etiology and Pathophysiology

Although the etiology of endometriosis is poorly understood, many theories have been proposed. A widely held view is that retrograde menstrual flow passes through the fallopian tubes carrying viable endometrial tissues into the pelvis. The tissue attaches to various sites (see Fig. 54-5). Another theory suggests that undifferentiated embryonic peritoneal cavity cells remain dormant in the pelvic tissue until the ovaries produce sufficient hormones to stimulate their growth. Other proposed causes include a genetic predisposition and altered immune function.

Clinical Manifestations

Patients with endometriosis have a wide range of clinical manifestations and severity. The magnitude of a woman's symptoms does not necessarily correlate with the clinical extent of her endometriosis. Dysmenorrhea after years of relatively pain-free menses and infertility may serve as clues to the presence of endometriosis. The most common manifestations are secondary dysmenorrhea, infertility, pelvic pain, dyspareunia, and irregular bleeding. Less common manifestations include backache, painful bowel movements, and dysuria. With menopause, estrogen is no longer produced in the ovaries, and the symptoms may disappear.

When the ectopic endometrial tissues "menstruate," the blood collects in cystlike nodules that have a characteristic bluish black color. When a cyst ruptures, the pain may be acute, and the resulting irritation promotes the formation of adhesions, which attach and fix the affected area to another pelvic structure. Endometrial lesions may become severe enough to cause a bowel obstruction or painful micturition.

Collaborative Care

Endometriosis may be suspected based on a woman's history of the characteristic symptoms and the health care provider's palpation of firm nodular lumps in the adnexa on bimanual

TABLE 54-10 COLLABORATIVE CARE

Endometriosis

Diagnostic
- History and physical examination
- Pelvic examination
- Laparoscopy
- Pelvic ultrasound
- MRI

Collaborative Therapy
- Conservative therapy (watch and wait)

Drug Therapy
- Nonsteroidal antiinflammatory drugs (NSAIDs)
- Oral contraceptives
- danazol (Danocrine)
- GnRH agonists (e.g., leuprolide [Lupron])

Surgical Therapy
- Laparotomy to remove implanted tissue and adhesions
- Total abdominal hysterectomy and bilateral salpingo-oophorectomy (TAH-BSO)

GnRH, Gonadotropin-releasing hormone; *MRI,* magnetic resonance imaging.

examination. However, laparoscopy is necessary for a definitive diagnosis. The treatment of endometriosis is influenced by the patient's age, desire for pregnancy, symptom severity, and extent and location of the disease. When symptoms are not disruptive, a "watch and wait" approach is used (Table 54-10). When endometriosis is identified as a probable cause of infertility, therapy proceeds more rapidly.

Drug Therapy. Drug therapy is used to reduce symptoms. Pain may be relieved with NSAIDs such as ibuprofen and diclofenac (Voltaren). Drugs to inhibit estrogen production by the ovary are often used to shrink the endometrial tissue. These drugs imitate a state of pregnancy or menopause. Continuous use (for 9 months) of combined oral contraceptives causes regression of endometrial tissue. Ovulation is suppressed by progestin agents such as medroxyprogesterone. Another approach to hormonal treatment is danazol (Danocrine), a synthetic androgen that inhibits the anterior pituitary. This drug causes atrophy of ectopic endometrial tissue. Subjective relief of symptoms is noted within 6 weeks of danazol use. The side effects of weight gain, acne, hot flashes, and hirsutism and the expense of this drug restrict its use.

Another class of drugs used is GnRH agonists (e.g., leuprolide [Lupron], nafarelin [Synarel]). These drugs result in amenorrhea. Side effects are usually the same as those of menopause (hot flashes, vaginal dryness, emotional lability). Loss of bone density has also been reported in women who remain on the therapy longer than 6 months. Endometriosis is controlled but not cured by HT. Persistent lesions give rise to subsequent recurrences once the menstrual cycle is reestablished.

DRUG ALERT: Leuprolide (Lupron)
- Assess patient for pregnancy before initiating therapy.
- Monitor patient for dysrhythmias, palpitations.
- Instruct patient to use nonhormonal contraceptive measures during therapy.

Surgical Therapy. The only cure for endometriosis is surgical removal of all the endometrial implants. Surgical therapy may be conservative or definitive. Conservative surgery is done to confirm the diagnosis or to remove implants. It involves removal or destruction of endometrial implants and lysing or excision of adhesions by means of laparoscopic laser surgery or laparotomy. GnRH agonist therapy (e.g., leuprolide) can be administered for 4 to 6 months to reduce the size of the lesions before surgery. By reducing the extent of the surgery, this preoperative drug treatment helps reduce the development of adhesions that may further threaten fertility. Definitive surgery involves removal of the uterus, fallopian tubes, ovaries, and as many endometrial implants as possible.

For women wishing to get pregnant, conservative surgical therapy is used to remove implants blocking the fallopian tube. Adhesions are removed from the tubes, ovaries, and pelvic structures. Efforts are made to conserve all tissues necessary to maintain fertility.

The individual woman should be actively involved in making the decision about preserving part or all of her ovaries, if surgically possible. Explore her feelings about maintaining her ovarian function. The health care provider should assess the woman's risk for ovarian cancer and provide this information for her consideration.

NURSING MANAGEMENT ENDOMETRIOSIS

Teach and reassure the patient that endometriosis is not life threatening. This may permit her to accept a conservative and progressive treatment approach. When the symptoms are less severe, teach about nondrug comfort measures that may be helpful. Assist patients in understanding the drugs that have been ordered to treat their condition. Explain the action and possible side effects of the prescribed drug. Psychologic support may be needed for women experiencing severe disabling pain, sexual difficulties secondary to dyspareunia, and infertility.

If conservative surgery is the treatment selected, care is similar to the general preoperative and postoperative care of a patient undergoing laparotomy (see Chapter 43, p. 971). If definitive surgery is planned, the care is similar to that for the patient undergoing an abdominal hysterectomy (see eNursing Care Plan 54-1 on the website for this chapter). Know the extent of the procedure so that appropriate preoperative teaching can be done.

BENIGN TUMORS OF THE FEMALE REPRODUCTIVE SYSTEM

LEIOMYOMAS

Etiology and Pathophysiology

Leiomyomas (uterine fibroids) are benign smooth-muscle tumors that occur within the uterus. Leiomyomas are common benign tumors of the female genital tract (Fig. 54-6). By 50 years of age, 60% of all women will have had at least one uterine leiomyoma.[24] The cause of leiomyomas is unknown. They appear to depend on ovarian hormones because they grow slowly during the reproductive years and undergo atrophy after menopause.

Clinical Manifestations

The majority of women with leiomyomas do not have any symptoms. When present, the most common symptoms include abnormal uterine bleeding, pain, and symptoms associated with pelvic pressure. Increased bleeding is associated with increased

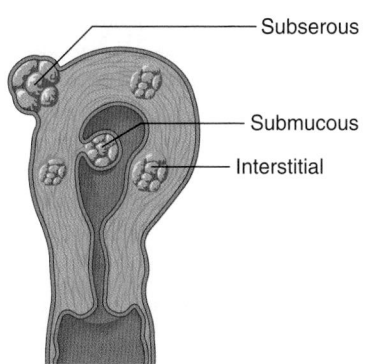

FIG. 54-6 Leiomyomas. Uterine section showing whorl-like appearance and locations of leiomyomas.

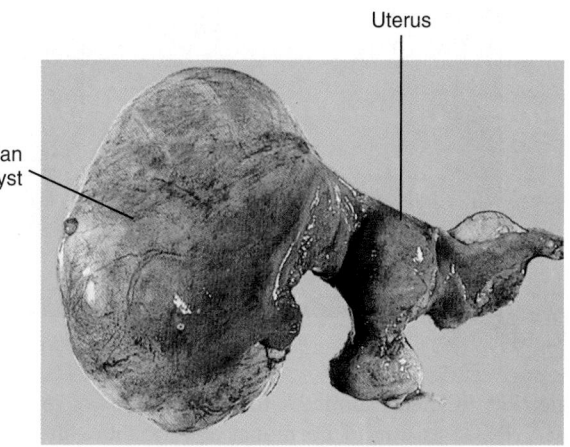

FIG. 54-7 Large ovarian cyst.

endometrial surface area caused by leiomyomas. Pain occurs with infection or twisting of the pedicle from which the tumor is growing. Devascularization and blood vessel compression may also contribute to pain. Pressure on surrounding organs may result in rectal, bladder, and lower abdominal discomfort. Large tumors may cause a general enlargement of the lower abdomen. These tumors are sometimes associated with miscarriage and infertility.

Collaborative Care

Clinical diagnosis is based on the characteristic pelvic findings of an enlarged uterus distorted by nodular masses. Treatment depends on the symptoms, the patient's age, her desire to bear children, and the location and size of the tumors. If the symptoms are minimal, the health care provider may elect to follow the patient closely for a time.

Persistent heavy menstrual bleeding causing anemia and large or rapidly growing tumors are indications for surgery. The leiomyomas are removed by hysterectomy or by myomectomy for women who wish to have children. In this case, only the fibroids are removed to preserve the uterus. Small tumors may be removed using a hysteroscope and laser resection instruments.

Uterine artery embolization is an increasingly used alternative treatment for uterine fibroids.[25] Embolic material (small plastic or gelatin beads) is injected into the uterine artery and carried to the fibroid branches.

Cryosurgery is another option. In cases of large leiomyomas, a GnRH agonist (e.g., leuprolide) may be used preoperatively to shrink the tumor. However, the risks and benefits of this drug should be fully discussed, including the potential for irreversible loss of bone mass. The treatment should not be used on women planning to have children.

Another treatment option uses MRI-guided focused ultrasound to target and destroy uterine fibroids. Treatment requires repeated targeting and heating of the fibroid tissue while the patient lies inside the MRI machine. The procedure can last as long as 3 hours.

CERVICAL POLYPS

Cervical polyps are benign pedunculated lesions that generally arise from the endocervical mucosa and are seen protruding through the cervical os during a speculum examination. Polyps are a characteristic bright cherry-red and are soft and fragile in consistency. They are generally small, measuring less than 3 cm in length, and may be single or multiple. Their cause is unknown.

Symptoms are usually not present, but metrorrhagia and bleeding after straining for a bowel movement and coitus can occur. Polyps are prone to infection. When the polyp is small, it can be excised in an outpatient procedure. If the point of attachment of the polyp cannot be identified and is not accessible to cautery, a polypectomy is performed in an operating room. All tissue removed is sent for pathologic review because polyps occasionally undergo malignant changes.

BENIGN OVARIAN TUMORS

There are many different types of benign tumors. The cause of most of them is unknown. They can be divided into cysts and neoplasms. *Cysts* are usually soft, are surrounded by a thin capsule, and may be detected during the reproductive years. Follicle and corpus luteum cysts are common ovarian cysts (Fig. 54-7). Multiple small ovarian follicles may occur in a condition called *polycystic ovary syndrome* (PCOS) (discussed in the next section). Epithelial ovarian neoplasms may be cystic or solid, and small or extremely large. Cystic teratomas, or dermoid cysts, originate from germ cells and can contain bits of any type of body tissue, such as hair or teeth.

Ovarian masses are often asymptomatic until they are large enough to cause pressure in the pelvis. Constipation, menstrual irregularities, urinary frequency, a full feeling in the abdomen, anorexia, an increase in abdominal girth, and peripheral edema may occur, depending on the tumor's size and location. Pelvic pain may be present if the tumor is growing rapidly. Severe pain results when the cyst twists on its pedicle (ovarian torsion).

In some cases, an ovarian cyst can rupture. A ruptured ovarian cyst is not only extremely painful, but it can lead to serious complications, such as hemorrhage and infection.

Pelvic examination reveals a mass or an enlarged ovary that demands further investigation. If the mass is cystic and smaller than 8 cm, the patient is asked to return for reexamination in 4 to 6 weeks. If the mass is cystic and greater than 8 cm or is solid, laparoscopic surgery or laparotomy is performed. Immediate surgery is necessary if ovarian torsion occurs, causing the ovary to rotate and cutting off circulation. Surgical techniques are used to save as much of the ovary as possible.

Polycystic Ovary Syndrome

Polycystic ovary syndrome (PCOS) is a chronic disorder in which many benign cysts form on the ovaries. It most commonly occurs in women under 30 years old and is a cause of

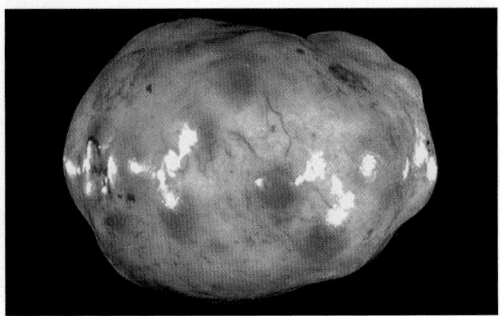

FIG. 54-8 Polycystic ovary syndrome. Multiple fluid-filled cysts in the ovary.

infertility. It affects about 3% to 7% of women of reproductive age.[26] PCOS is due to hormonal abnormalities in which the ovaries produce estrogen and excess testosterone but not progesterone. Fluid-filled cysts develop from mature ovarian follicles that fail to rupture (thereby releasing an egg) each month (Fig. 54-8). This problem affects both ovaries.

Classic manifestations include irregular menstrual periods, amenorrhea, hirsutism, and obesity. Of these manifestations, obesity in particular has been associated with severe symptoms such as excess androgens, oligorrhea, amenorrhea, and infertility. Many women start with normal menstrual periods, which after 1 to 2 years become irregular and then infrequent. If PCOS is left untreated, cardiovascular disease and abnormal insulin resistance with type 2 diabetes mellitus may develop.[27,28]

Pelvic ultrasound reveals enlarged ovaries with multiple small cysts. Successful management includes early diagnosis and treatment to improve quality of life and decrease the risk of complications. Oral contraceptives are useful in regulating menstrual cycles. Hirsutism may be treated with spironolactone. Hyperandrogenism can be treated with flutamide (Eulexin) and a GnRH agonist such as leuprolide. Metformin (Glucophage) reduces hyperinsulinemia and has been shown to improve hyperandrogenism and restore ovulation. For women wishing to become pregnant, fertility drugs (e.g., clomiphene [Clomid]) may be used to induce ovulation. If all other treatments are unsuccessful, a hysterectomy with bilateral salpingectomy and oophorectomy may be performed.

> **DRUG ALERT: Clomiphene (Clomid)**
> Instruct the patient to notify her physician immediately if
> • Lower abdominal pain occurs.
> • Pregnancy is suspected.

Teach the patient the importance of weight management and exercise to decrease insulin resistance. Obesity exacerbates the problems related to PCOS. Monitor lipid profile and fasting glucose levels. Hirsutism is cosmetically distressing for many women. Support the patient as she explores measures to remove unwanted hair (e.g., depilating agents, electrolysis). Stress the importance of regular follow-up care to monitor the effectiveness of therapy and to detect any complications.

CANCERS OF THE FEMALE REPRODUCTIVE SYSTEM

CERVICAL CANCER

Approximately 12,000 women in the United States are diagnosed with cervical cancer and 4200 women die from cervical cancer annually.[29] Noninvasive cervical cancer (in situ) is about

four times more common than invasive cervical cancer. The mortality rate for cervical cancer in the United States is twice as high for African American women as it is for white women. An increased risk of cervical cancer is associated with low socioeconomic status, early sexual activity (before 17 years of age), multiple sexual partners, infection with HPV, immunosuppression, and smoking.

The number of deaths from cervical cancer in the United States has fallen steadily over the past 50 years because of better and earlier diagnosis with the widespread use of the Papanicolaou (Pap) test. In addition to cancer, the Pap test screens for precancerous changes. Treatment of precancerous lesions can prevent progression to cervical cancer.

Etiology and Pathophysiology

The progression from normal cervical cells to dysplasia and then to invasive cervical cancer appears to be related to repeated injuries to the cervix. The progression occurs slowly over years. A strong relationship exists between dysplasia and HPV infections. HPV types 16 and 18 together cause about 70% of cervical cancers. Cancer rates are expected to decline further with vaccines (e.g., Gardasil, Cervarix) now being used for the prevention of HPV.[30]

Clinical Manifestations

Precancerous changes are asymptomatic. This highlights the importance of routine screening. The peak incidence of noninvasive cervical cancer is in women in their early thirties. The average age for women with invasive cervical cancer is 50 (Fig. 54-9). Early cervical cancer is generally asymptomatic, but leukorrhea and intermenstrual bleeding eventually occur. The discharge is usually thin and watery but becomes dark and foul smelling as the disease advances, suggesting an infection. The vaginal bleeding is initially only spotting. As the tumor enlarges, bleeding becomes heavier and more frequent. Pain is a late symptom and is followed by weight loss, anemia, and cachexia.

Diagnostic Studies

The American Cancer Society recommends the following guidelines for annual Pap testing:[31]
• Begin testing at age 21 regardless of when a woman becomes sexually active.

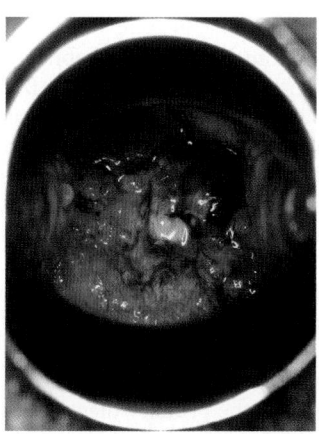

FIG. 54-9 Cervical cancer. View through a speculum inserted into the vagina.

Stage	Extent	Treatment
0	In situ	Cervical conization, hysterectomy, cryosurgery, laser surgery
I	Confinement to cervix	Radiation, radical hysterectomy
II	Spread beyond cervix to upper two thirds of vagina but not to tissues around uterus	Radiation, cisplatin-based chemotherapy, radical hysterectomy
III	Spread to pelvic wall, involvement of lower third of vagina, and/or has caused kidney problems	Radiation, cisplatin-based chemotherapy
IV	Spread to other parts of the body such as bladder, rectum, liver, lungs, and bones	Radiation, surgery (e.g., pelvic exenteration), cisplatin-based chemotherapy

TABLE 54-11 **STAGING AND TREATMENT OF CERVICAL CANCER**

Modified from National Cancer Institute: Cancer cervical treatment: stages of cervical cancer. Retrieved from *www.cancer.gov/cancertopics/pdq/treatment/cervical/Patient/page2.*

• Women ages 21 to 65 years old should be screened with the Pap test every 3 years.
• Women who have had a total hysterectomy (uterus and cervix removed) for reasons not related to cervical cancer do not need to be tested.
• Women 65 and older should no longer be screened after having two or three consecutive negative Pap tests within the last 2 years.

Women with a history of cervical cancer should continue with screening as recommended by their health care provider for at least 20 years. A woman who has been vaccinated against HPV needs to continue following the screening guidelines for her age-group.

The two types of HPV that have been associated with most cases of cervical cancer (types 16 and 18) can be identified through deoxyribonucleic acid (DNA) testing. HPV DNA tests help determine if women with abnormal Pap test results need further follow-up. Women ages 30 to 65 who have the HPV DNA test and the Pap test (co-testing) can be screened every 5 years rather than every 3 years.

Pap tests are less than 100% accurate in screening for cervical cell abnormalities. Problems occur with both false-positive and false-negative reports. ThinPrep, a liquid-based technique for Pap tests, has reduced the number of inaccurate test results.

The finding of an abnormal Pap test indicates the need for follow-up. Women with minor changes may be followed with a repeated Pap test in 4 to 6 months for 2 years. Up to 80% may revert to normal spontaneously. Women with more prominent changes receive additional procedures, such as colposcopy and biopsy, before a definitive diagnosis can be made. Colposcopy helps identify possible epithelial abnormalities and suggests areas for biopsy. Biopsies are sent for pathologic evaluation. Colposcopy and biopsy have improved diagnosis and allow more focused treatments.

The type and extent of the biopsy vary with the abnormality seen. A punch biopsy may be done on an outpatient basis with a special punch biopsy forceps. The excision of a cone-shaped section of the cervix may be used for both diagnosis and treatment. Conization is accomplished using one of several techniques, depending on the health care provider's experience and the availability of equipment. *Cryotherapy* (freezing) and laser cone vaporization destroy the tissue. Laser cone excision and the *loop electrosurgery excision procedure*

(LEEP) remove the identified tissue and allow for histologic examination to ensure that all microinvasive tissue has been removed. These can be performed as outpatient procedures with mild analgesics or sedation. Complications of these procedures include excessive bleeding and possible cervical stenosis after healing.

Collaborative Care

Vaccines against HPV reduce the incidence of both cervical-related neoplasia and cervical cancer due to infection from HPV types 16 and 18. Vaccination against HPV is recommended for females and males beginning at ages 11 or 12 years. (Vaccines are discussed further in Chapter 53, p. 1270.)

The treatment of cervical cancer is guided by the stage of the tumor and the patient's age and general state of health (Table 54-11). There are four procedures in which fertility can be preserved. Conization may be the only type of therapy needed for noninvasive cervical cancer if analysis of removed tissue demonstrates that a wide area of normal tissue surrounds the excised tissue. Laser treatments can be used in which a directed infrared beam is employed to destroy abnormal tissue. Cautery and cryosurgery may also be used.

Invasive cancer of the cervix is treated with surgery, radiation, and chemotherapy as single treatments or in combination. Surgical procedures include hysterectomy, radical hysterectomy (involving adjacent structures), and, rarely, pelvic exenteration. (Surgical therapy is discussed on p. 1297.) Radiation may be by external (e.g., cobalt) or internal implants (e.g., cesium, radium). Standard radiation treatment is 4 to 6 weeks of external radiation followed by one or two treatments with internal implants (brachytherapy). (Radiation therapy is discussed in Chapter 16.) Cisplatin-based chemotherapy regimens benefit patients with cancer spread beyond the cervix.

ENDOMETRIAL CANCER

Cancer of the endometrium is the most common gynecologic malignancy. Approximately 47,000 newly diagnosed cases of

EVIDENCE-BASED PRACTICE
Applying the Evidence

H.K. is a 33-yr-old African American woman who had a tubal ligation in the outpatient surgery unit. As you prepare her for discharge, you remind her that she needs to have regular Pap tests to screen for cervical cancer. She expresses concern over the expense of this procedure. She tells you that her health care insurance will not pay for diagnostic tests, and she does not remember when she last had a Pap test done.

Best Available Evidence	Clinician Expertise	Patient Preferences and Values
For women after age 30 who have had three normal Pap tests, the American Cancer Society recommends screening every 2-3 yr.	You know that the incidence and death rate of cervical cancer is twice as high for African Americans as for whites.	H.K. is concerned about the costs related to her current procedure and future Pap tests. She adds that no one in her family has ever had cervical cancer.

Your Action and Decision
As her nurse, you explain the American Cancer Society recommendations and her increased risk for cervical cancer. She tells you that she understands and will schedule a follow-up appointment, but unless the cost of the Pap test is reasonable, she will probably not be able to get yearly Pap tests unless her health care plan improves.

Reference for Evidence
American Cancer Society: American Cancer Society guidelines for the early detection of cancer. Retrieved from *www.cancer.org/Healthy/FindCancerEarly/CancerScreeningGuidelines*.

endometrial cancer and 8000 deaths occur annually. Endometrial cancer has a relatively low mortality rate, since most cases are diagnosed early. The survival rate is over 95% if the cancer has not spread at the time of diagnosis.

Etiology and Pathophysiology

The major risk factor for endometrial cancer is estrogen, especially unopposed estrogen.[32] Additional risk factors include increasing age, nulliparity, late menopause, obesity, smoking, diabetes mellitus, and a personal or family history of hereditary nonpolyposis colorectal cancer (HNPCC) (see the Genetics in Clinical Practice box for HNPCC in Chapter 43 on p. 986). Obesity is a risk factor because adipose cells store estrogen, thus increasing endogenous estrogen. Pregnancy and oral contraceptives are protective factors.

Endometrial cancer arises from the lining of the endometrium. Most tumors are adenocarcinomas. The precursor may be a hyperplastic state that progresses to invasive carcinoma. Hyperplasia occurs when estrogen is not counteracted by progesterone. The cancer directly extends into the cervix and through the uterine serosa. As invasion of the myometrium occurs, regional lymph nodes, including the paravaginal and para-aortic, become involved. Hematogenous metastases develop concurrently. The usual sites of metastases are lung, bone, liver, and eventually the brain. Malignant cells can be found in the peritoneal cavity, probably after transport through the fallopian tubes.

Prognostic factors include histologic differentiation, myometrial invasion, peritoneal cytology, lymph node and adnexal metastases, and tumor size. Endometrial cancer grows slowly, metastasizes late, and is curable with therapy if diagnosed early.

Clinical Manifestations

The first sign of endometrial cancer is abnormal uterine bleeding, usually in postmenopausal women. Because perimenopausal women have sporadic periods for a time, it is important that this sign not be ignored or attributed to menopause.

Pain occurs late in the disease process. Other manifestations that may arise are related to metastasis to other organs. Metastatic spread occurs in a characteristic pattern. Spread to the pelvic and para-aortic nodes is common. When distant metastasis occurs, it most commonly involves the lungs, liver, bones, brain, and vagina.

Collaborative Care

Endometrial biopsy is the primary diagnostic test for endometrial cancer. Endometrial biopsy is done on an outpatient basis. Any abnormal or unexpected bleeding in a postmenopausal woman requires obtaining a tissue sample to exclude endometrial cancer. For women who have or are at risk of developing HNPCC, the American Cancer Society recommends annual screening with endometrial biopsy beginning at 35 years of age. The Pap test is not a reliable diagnostic tool for endometrial cancer, but it can rule out cervical cancer.

Most cases of endometrial cancer are diagnosed at an early stage when surgery alone may result in cure. Treatment of endometrial cancer is a total hysterectomy and bilateral salpingo-oophorectomy with lymph node biopsies. The lack of estrogen and progesterone receptors is a poor prognostic indicator. Surgery may be followed by radiation, either to the pelvis or the abdomen externally or intravaginally, to decrease local recurrence.

No tumor markers with high sensitivity and high specificity for endometrial cancer are known at present, although CA-125 is often used in clinical practice. CA-125 has been used in surveillance of advanced endometrial cancer. In patients who have increased CA-125 values pretreatment, this test might prove useful in posttreatment surveillance.

Treatment of advanced or recurrent disease is difficult. Progesterone HT (e.g., megestrol [Megace]) can be used when the progesterone receptor status is positive and the tumor is well differentiated.[32] Tamoxifen (Nolvadex), either alone or in combination with progesterone therapy, is also effective in women with advanced or recurrent endometrial cancer. Chemotherapy is considered when progesterone therapy is unsuccessful. Agents used include doxorubicin (Adriamycin), cisplatin (Platinol), 5-fluorouracil (5-FU), carboplatin (Paraplatin), and paclitaxel (Taxol).

OVARIAN CANCER

Ovarian cancer is a malignant tumor of the ovaries. About 22,280 new cases of ovarian cancer are diagnosed in the United States each year, and about 15,000 women die from the disease annually. It is the fifth leading cause of cancer deaths in women in the United States. Most women with ovarian cancer have advanced disease at diagnosis.[33] It occurs most frequently in women between 55 and 65 years of age. White women are at greater risk for ovarian cancer than African American women.

Etiology and Pathophysiology
Genetic Link

The cause of ovarian cancer is not known. Women who have mutations of the *BRCA* genes have an increased susceptibility

🧬 GENETICS IN CLINICAL PRACTICE

Ovarian Cancer

Genetic Basis
- Mutations in *BRCA1* and/or *BRCA2* genes.
- Normally these genes are tumor suppressor genes involved in DNA repair.
- Autosomal dominant transmission.
- Mutations passed down from either mother or father.

Incidence
- About 10% of cases of ovarian cancer are related to hereditary factors.
- Women with *BRCA1* mutations have a 25%-40% lifetime risk of developing ovarian cancer.
- Women with *BRCA2* mutations have a 10%-20% lifetime risk of developing ovarian cancer.
- Family history of both breast and ovarian cancer increases the risk of having a *BRCA* mutation.
- *BRCA* mutations occur in 10%-20% of patients with ovarian cancer who have no family history of breast or ovarian cancer.

Genetic Testing
- DNA testing is available for *BRCA1* and *BRCA2* genetic mutations.

Clinical Implications
- Bilateral oophorectomy reduces the risk of ovarian cancer in women with *BRCA1* and *BRCA2* mutations.
- Genetic counseling and testing for *BRCA* mutations should be considered for women whose personal or family history puts them at high risk for a genetic predisposition to ovarian cancer.

TABLE 54-12   COLLABORATIVE CARE

Ovarian Cancer

Diagnostic
- History and physical examination
- Pelvic examination
- Abdominal and transvaginal ultrasound
- CA-125 level
- Laparotomy for diagnostic staging

Collaborative Therapy
- Surgery
  - Abdominal hysterectomy and bilateral salpingo-oophorectomy with pelvic lymph node biopsies
  - Debulking for advanced disease
- Chemotherapy
  - Adjuvant and palliative
- Radiation therapy
  - Adjuvant and palliative

to ovarian cancer. The *BRCA* genes are tumor suppressor genes that inhibit tumor growth when functioning normally. When they mutate, they lose their tumor suppressor ability. This results in an increased risk for women to develop ovarian or breast cancer (see the Genetics in Clinical Practice box).

The major risk factor for ovarian cancer is family history (one or more first-degree relatives). A family history of breast or colon cancer is also a risk factor. Other risk factors include a personal history of breast or colon cancer and HNPCC (see the Genetics in Clinical Practice box on HNPCC in Chapter 43 on p. 986).

Women who have never been pregnant (nulliparity) are also at higher risk. Other risk factors include increasing age, high-fat diet, increased number of ovulatory cycles (usually associated with early menarche and late menopause), HT, and possibly the use of infertility drugs.

Breastfeeding, multiple pregnancies, oral contraceptive use (more than 5 years), and early age at first birth seem to reduce the risk of ovarian cancer. These factors may have a protective effect because they reduce the number of ovulatory cycles, and thus reduce the exposure to estrogen.

About 90% of ovarian cancers are epithelial carcinomas that arise from malignant transformation of the surface epithelial cells. Germ cell tumors account for another 10%. Histologic grading is an important prognostic determinant. Tumor cells are graded according to the level of differentiation, ranging from well differentiated (grade I) to poorly differentiated (grade III) to undifferentiated (grade IV). Grade IV cells carry a poorer prognosis than the other grades.

Intraperitoneal dissemination is a common characteristic of ovarian cancer. It metastasizes to the uterus, bladder, bowel, and omentum. In advanced disease, it can spread to the stomach, colon, liver, and other parts of the body.

Clinical Manifestations

Symptoms are vague in the early stages. An accumulation of fluid initially causes abdominal enlargement. Nonspecific symptoms that warrant further evaluation include pelvic or abdominal pain, bloating, urinary urgency or frequency, and difficulty eating or feeling full quickly.[33] Women who have one or more of these symptoms, especially if they are new, persistent (occur at least 12 days per month), or worsening, need to see their health care provider. Vaginal bleeding rarely occurs, and pain is not an early symptom. Later signs are increased abdominal girth, unexplained weight loss or gain, and menstrual changes.

Diagnostic Studies

No screening test exists for ovarian cancer. Because early ovarian cancer has vague symptoms, yearly bimanual pelvic examinations should be performed to identify an ovarian mass (Table 54-12). Postmenopausal women should not have palpable ovaries, so a mass of any size should be suspected as possible ovarian cancer. An abdominal or a transvaginal ultrasound can be done to detect ovarian masses. An exploratory laparotomy may be used to establish the diagnosis and stage the disease.

A test called OVA1 can help detect whether a pelvic mass is benign or malignant before it is surgically removed. OVA1 uses a blood sample to test for levels of five biomarkers that change due to ovarian cancer. It is not intended for ovarian cancer screening or for a definitive diagnosis of ovarian cancer.

For women with a high risk for ovarian cancer, screening using a combination of the tumor marker (CA-125) and ultrasound is often recommended in addition to a yearly pelvic examination. CA-125 is positive in 80% of women with epithelial ovarian cancer and is used to monitor the course of the disease. However, levels of CA-125 may be elevated with other malignancies (e.g., pancreatic cancer) or with benign conditions such as fibroids or endometriosis. A large recent clinical trial has reported that screening by CA-125 and ultrasound did not result in fewer deaths from ovarian cancer.[34] Currently only 20% of ovarian cancers are diagnosed at an early stage.

Collaborative Care

Women identified as being at high risk based on family and health history may require counseling regarding options such as prophylactic oophorectomy and oral contraceptives. It is important to note that although oophorectomy significantly reduces the risk of ovarian cancer, it does not completely eliminate the possibility of the disease.

Ovarian cancer staging is critical for guiding treatment decisions. Stage I describes disease limited to the ovaries; stage II, disease limited to the pelvis; stage III, disease limited to the abdominal cavity; and stage IV, distant metastatic disease. The overall survival rate is 90% with early disease, 36% with local spread, and 20% with distant metastases.

Most patients with ovarian cancer have widespread disease at presentation. The initial treatment for all stages of ovarian cancer is surgery, which is usually a total abdominal hysterectomy and bilateral salpingo-oophorectomy with omentectomy and removal of as much of the tumor as possible (i.e., tumor debulking). Surgery facilitates chemotherapy by reducing the number of cells that the chemotherapy has to kill.

Depending on the differentiation of the cells and the stage of cancer, other treatment options include intraperitoneal and systemic chemotherapy, intraperitoneal instillation of radioisotopes, and external abdominal and pelvic radiation therapy. If a patient is clinically free of symptoms after completing treatment, a "second-look" surgical procedure is often performed to determine whether there is any evidence of disease. If no disease is found, the patient is monitored for recurrent disease.

Chemotherapy usually consists of a combination of a platinum compound, such as cisplatin or carboplatin, and a taxane, such as paclitaxel or docetaxel (Taxotere). The typical course of chemotherapy involves three to six cycles. A cycle is a schedule that allows regular doses of a drug, followed by a rest period.

Other chemotherapy drugs used include altretamine (Hexalen), topotecan (Hycamtin), etoposide (VePesid), gemcitabine (Gemzar), and oxaliplatin (Eloxatin). These drugs may be used to treat recurrent disease or as a palliative measure to shrink the tumor to relieve pressure and pain.

VAGINAL CANCER

Primary vaginal cancers are rare, with about 2680 new cases reported annually. The peak incidence is between ages 50 and 70. Vaginal tumors are usually secondary sites or metastases of other cancers such as cervical or endometrial carcinomas. The most common type of vaginal cancer is squamous cell carcinoma. Intrauterine exposure to diethylstilbestrol (DES) places a woman at risk for clear cell adenocarcinoma of the vagina.

Treatment of vaginal cancer depends on the type of cells involved, the stage of the disease, and the size and location of the tumor. Squamous cell carcinomas can be treated with both surgery and radiation.

VULVAR CANCER

Cancer of the vulva is relatively rare, with about 4490 new cases reported annually. Similar to cervical cancer, preinvasive lesions referred to as vulvar intraepithelial neoplasia (VIN) precede invasive vulvar cancer. The invasive form occurs mainly in women over 60 years of age, with the highest incidence being in women in their seventies.

Patients with vulvar neoplasia may have symptoms of vulvar itching or burning, pain, bleeding, or discharge. Women who are immunosuppressed and/or have diabetes mellitus, hypertension, or chronic vulvar dystrophies are at a higher risk for developing vulvar cancers. Several subtypes of HPV have been identified in some but not all vulvar cancers. Vaccines (Gardasil, Cervarix) are now available to protect against some vaginal and vulvar cancers that are caused by these HPV subtypes. (Vaccines for HPV are discussed in Chapter 53, p. 1270.)

Diagnosis of vulvar cancer is based on physical examination, colposcopy, and biopsy results of the suspicious lesion. VIN can be treated topically with imiquimod cream (Aldara) or surgery.

Laser therapy may be used to kill cancer cells. Surgery is the most common treatment for cancer of the vulva. The goal of surgery is to remove all the cancer without any loss of the woman's sexual function. A local excision with removal of the lesion and surrounding tissue may be done. For more extensive lesions, vulvectomy may be done (various types of vulvectomies are presented in Table 54-13). If the cancer is

TABLE 54-13	SURGICAL PROCEDURES INVOLVING THE FEMALE REPRODUCTIVE SYSTEM
Type of Surgery	**Description**
Abdominal Hysterectomy	
Total hysterectomy	Uterus and cervix removed using large abdominal incision (bikini cut).
Total abdominal hysterectomy and bilateral salpingo-oophorectomy (TAH-BSO)	Uterus, cervix, fallopian tubes, and ovaries removed using large abdominal incision.
Radical hysterectomy	Panhysterectomy, partial vaginectomy, and dissection of lymph nodes in pelvis.
Vaginal Hysterectomy	Uterus and cervix removed through a cut in the top of vagina.
Laparoscopic Hysterectomy	Laparoscope (video camera and small surgical instruments).
Laparoscopic-assisted vaginal hysterectomy (LAVH)	Incision made at top of vagina. Uterus and cervix removed through the vagina. Laparoscope inserted into abdomen to assist in the procedure.
Laparoscopic supracervical hysterectomy	Uterus removed using only laparoscopic instruments. Cervix is left intact.
Robotic-Assisted Surgery	Robot (special machine) used to do surgery through small abdominal incisions. Most often used when a patient has cancer or is very overweight and vaginal surgery is not safe.
Vulvectomy	Surgical procedure to remove part or all of the vulva.
Skinning vulvectomy	Removal of top layer of vulvar skin where the cancer is found. Skin grafts from other parts of the body may be needed to cover the area.
Simple vulvectomy	Entire vulva is removed
Radical vulvectomy	Entire vulva, including clitoris, labia majora and minora, and nearby tissue, is removed. Nearby lymph nodes may also be removed.
Vaginectomy	Removal of vagina.
Pelvic Exenteration	Radical hysterectomy, total vaginectomy, removal of bladder with diversion of urinary system and resection of colon and rectum with colostomy.

extensive, a pelvic exenteration may be done. As adjuvant measures, the patient may have *chemotherapy* or *radiation therapy* after surgery.

SURGICAL PROCEDURES: FEMALE REPRODUCTIVE SYSTEM

A variety of surgical procedures are performed when benign or malignant tumors of the genital tract are found (see Table 54-13). A *hysterectomy* (removal of the uterus) is performed for excision of cancerous tumors of the female reproductive system. A hysterectomy may be done abdominally, vaginally, or laparoscopically. The abdominal route is used when large tumors are present and the pelvic cavity is to be explored or when the tubes and ovaries are to be removed at the same time (Fig. 54-10). The abdominal route can present more postoperative problems because it involves an incision and the opening of the abdominal cavity.

A vaginal route is often used when vaginal repair is done in addition to removal of the uterus. In both vaginal and abdominal hysterectomies, the ligaments that support the uterus are attached to the vaginal cuff to maintain the normal depth of the vagina. Laparoscopic procedures have the advantage of quicker recovery time and fewer complications.[35]

Depending on the findings and reason for the hysterectomy, the cervix may be left in place and not removed. Preserving the cervix may decrease the risk of pelvic floor prolapse and urinary incontinence. The patient needs to continue to get Pap tests if the cervix is left in place or the surgery was done to treat cancer.

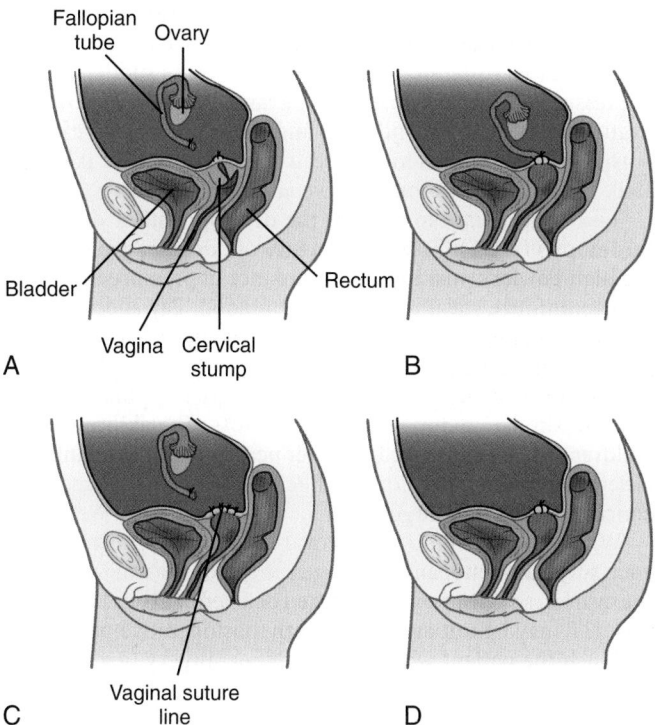

FIG. 54-10 A, Cross section of subtotal hysterectomy. Note that cervical stump, fallopian tubes, and ovaries remain. **B,** Cross section of total hysterectomy. Note that fallopian tubes and ovaries remain. **C,** Cross section of vaginal hysterectomy. Note that fallopian tubes and ovaries remain. **D,** Total hysterectomy, salpingectomy, and oophorectomy. Note that uterus, fallopian tubes, and ovaries are completely removed.

RADIATION THERAPY: CANCERS OF FEMALE REPRODUCTIVE SYSTEM

Radiation is used to cure or control or as a palliative measure for cancers of the female reproductive system, either alone or in combination with other treatments. The goal of radiation therapy is to deliver a specific amount of high-energy (or ionizing) radiation to the cancer with minimal damage to the normal surrounding tissue. Radiation therapy may be external or internal (brachytherapy).

External Radiation Therapy

With external radiation therapy, a source outside of the body delivers electromagnetic radiation in the form of waves. (External radiation therapy and related nursing care are discussed in Chapter 16.)

Brachytherapy

Brachytherapy allows the radiation to be placed internally near or into the tumor. This method can deliver a high dose of radiation directly to the tumor.[36] The dose decreases sharply farther away from the source, causing less damage to the surrounding normal tissue. A variety of forms are used to deliver the therapy, including wires, capsules, needles, tubes, and seeds. Brachytherapy is used in the management of cervical and endometrial cancer because of the accessibility of these body parts and the favorable results obtained. Radium and cesium are two commonly used isotopes.

To prepare the patient for the treatment, give a cleansing enema to prevent straining at stool, which could cause displacement of the isotope. Insert an indwelling catheter to prevent a distended bladder from coming into contact with the radioactive source.

A variety of applicators have been developed for intrauterine treatment. Applicators are inserted into the endometrial cavity and vagina in the operating room. When the applicator contains the radioactive material, this is known as *preloading*. In *afterloading* the applicator is implanted in the operating room but is not loaded with the radioactive material until its correct placement is verified and the patient has returned to her room.

Radiation exposure to the patient is precisely controlled. The radiation exposure to the physician and other personnel involved in the implantation is reduced when the afterload technique is used. The applicator is secured with vaginal packing and is left in place for 24 to 72 hours.

During treatment the patient is placed in a lead-lined private room and is on absolute bed rest. She may be turned from side to side. The presence of an intrauterine applicator produces uterine contractions that may require analgesics. The destruction of cells results in a foul-smelling vaginal discharge, and a deodorizer is helpful. Nausea, vomiting, diarrhea, and malaise may develop as a systemic reaction to the radiation.

At the end of the prescribed period of radiation, the radioactive material and the catheter are removed. The patient is allowed off bed rest and is discharged from the hospital when stable. Late complications that may arise include fistulas (vesicovaginal, ureterovaginal), cystitis, phlebitis, hemorrhage, and fibrosis. If fibrosis occurs, the vaginal wall becomes smaller in diameter and shorter. Dilation of the vagina through intercourse or the use of sequentially sized dilators may be indicated. The patient is urged to report any unusual symptoms or complaints to her physician. (Brachytherapy and related nursing care are discussed in Chapter 16.)

NURSING MANAGEMENT
CANCERS OF FEMALE REPRODUCTIVE SYSTEM

NURSING ASSESSMENT
Malignant tumors of the female reproductive system can be found in the cervix, endometrium, ovaries, vagina, and vulva. A patient with any of these malignant tumors may experience a variety of clinical manifestations, including leukorrhea, irregular vaginal bleeding, vaginal discharge, abdominal pain and pressure, bowel and bladder dysfunction, and vulvar itching and burning. Assessment for these signs and symptoms is an important nursing responsibility.

NURSING DIAGNOSES
Nursing diagnoses for the female patient with cancer of the reproductive system include, but are not limited to, the following:

- Anxiety *related to* threat of a malignancy and lack of knowledge about the disease process and prognosis
- Acute pain *related to* pressure secondary to an enlarging tumor
- Disturbed body image *related to* loss of body part and loss of good health
- Ineffective sexuality pattern *related to* physiologic limitations and fatigue
- Grieving *related to* poor prognosis of advanced disease

PLANNING
The overall goals are that the patient with cancer of the female reproductive system will (1) actively participate in treatment decisions, (2) achieve satisfactory pain and symptom management, (3) recognize and report problems promptly, (4) maintain preferred lifestyle as long as possible, and (5) continue to practice cancer detection strategies.

NURSING IMPLEMENTATION
HEALTH PROMOTION. Through your contact with women in a variety of settings, teach women the importance of routine screening for cancers of the reproductive system. Cancer can be prevented when screening reveals precancerous conditions of the vulva, cervix, endometrium, and, rarely, the ovaries. Also, routine screening increases the chance that a cancer will be found in an early stage. When cancer is identified early, treatment can be more conservative and the woman's prognosis improves. A yearly pelvic examination and Pap test (as indicated) allow the health care provider to detect lesions on the vulva or any uterine or ovarian irregularities and screen for cervical cancer. Encourage women to view routine cancer screening and vaccination against cervical cancer as important self-care activities.

Teaching women about risk factors for cancers of the reproductive system is also important. Limiting sexual activity during adolescence, using condoms, having fewer sexual partners, and not smoking reduce the risk of cervical cancer. When high-risk behaviors are identified, assist women in modifying their lifestyles to decrease risk.

ACUTE INTERVENTION RELATED TO SURGERY. All patients experience a degree of anxiety when contemplating surgery, but the prospect of major gynecologic surgery increases these concerns.

Some women may experience guilt, anger, or embarrassment. Still others may focus on the effect the surgery will have on their reproductive and sexual functions. Some women view the whole process as annoying, whereas others are relieved by the thought of no longer having menstrual periods or becoming pregnant. Try to understand the patient's fears and concerns. Each patient needs to be assessed as an individual. Be willing to listen, since this can provide considerable psychologic support.

Preoperatively, prepare the patient physically for surgery with the standard perineal or abdominal preparation. A vaginal douche and enemas may be given (based on the surgeon's preference). The bladder should be emptied before the patient is sent to the operating room. An indwelling catheter is commonly inserted preoperatively. (See Chapter 18 for discussion of general preoperative patient care.)

Hysterectomy. Postoperatively, the patient who has had an abdominal hysterectomy will have an abdominal dressing. Observe the dressing frequently for any sign of bleeding during the first 8 hours after surgery. (See eNursing Care Plan 54-1 for care of the patient after a total abdominal hysterectomy.)

The patient who has had a vaginal hysterectomy will have a perineal pad. A moderate amount of serosanguineous drainage on the perineal pad is expected. The patient may experience urinary retention postoperatively because of temporary bladder atony resulting from edema or nerve trauma. At times an indwelling catheter is used for 1 to 2 days postoperatively to maintain constant drainage of the bladder and prevent strain on the suture line. If an indwelling catheter is not used, catheterization may be necessary if the patient has not urinated for 8 hours postoperatively. If residual urine is suspected after the removal of an indwelling catheter, catheterization is done to prevent bladder infection caused by pooling of urine. Accidental ligation of a ureter is a serious surgical complication. Report any complaint of backache or decreased urine output to the surgeon.

Abdominal distention may develop from the sudden release of pressure on the intestines when a large tumor is removed or from paralytic ileus secondary to anesthesia and pressure on the bowel. Food and fluids may be restricted if the patient is nauseated. Ambulation will help relieve abdominal flatus.

Take special care to prevent the development of deep vein thrombosis (DVT). Frequent changes of position, avoidance of the high Fowler's position, and avoidance of pressure under the knees minimize stasis and pooling of blood. Pay special attention to patients with varicosities. Encourage leg exercises to promote circulation.

The loss of the uterus may bring about grief response in some women, similar to any great personal loss. The ability to bear children may be associated with her perception of womanhood. Grief from this loss is normal. Elicit the woman's feelings and concerns about her surgery.

When surgery removes the ovaries as well, women experience surgical menopause. Estrogen is no longer available from the ovaries, so symptoms of estrogen deficiency arise. To counter this, HT may be initiated in the early postoperative period.

Teach the patient what to expect after surgery (e.g., she will not menstruate). Instructions should include specific activity restrictions. Intercourse should be avoided until the wound is healed (about 4 to 6 weeks). However, intercourse is not contraindicated once healing is complete. If a vaginal hysterectomy is performed, inform the patient that she may have a temporary loss of vaginal sensation. Reassure her that the sensation will return in several months.

Physical restrictions are limited for a short time. Heavy lifting should be avoided for 2 months. Teach her to avoid activities that may increase pelvic congestion, such as dancing and walking swiftly, for several months. However, activities such as swimming may be both physically and mentally helpful. Assure her that once healing is complete, all previous activity can be resumed.

Many women report a decrease in the quality of their sex lives after cancer treatment.[37] Provide information on what to expect related to their sexual functioning before the treatment and reinforce it afterward.

Salpingectomy and Oophorectomy. Postoperative care of the woman who has undergone removal of a fallopian tube (salpingectomy) or an ovary (oophorectomy) is similar to that for any patient having abdominal surgery. However, if a large ovarian cyst was removed, she may have abdominal distention caused by the sudden release of pressure in the intestines. An abdominal binder may provide relief until the distention subsides.

When both ovaries are removed (bilateral oophorectomy), surgical menopause results. The symptoms are similar to those of regular menopause but may be more severe because of the sudden withdrawal of hormones. Attempts may be made to leave at least a portion of an ovary.

Vulvectomy. Although cancer of the vulva is relatively uncommon, it is important to recognize the extent of the vulvectomy and the significant effect it is likely to have on the patient's life. Having an honest, open attitude with the patient and her partner preoperatively can be most helpful in the postoperative period.

After a vulvectomy (see Table 54-13), the patient has a wound in the perineal area extending to the groin. The wound may be covered or left exposed and frequently has drains attached to portable suction (e.g., Hemovac, Jackson-Pratt). A heavy pressure dressing is often in place for the first 24 to 48 hours. The wound is cleaned with normal saline solution or an antiseptic twice daily. Solutions can be applied with an aseptic bulb syringe or a Waterpik machine. Wound care must be meticulous to prevent infection, which results in delayed healing.

Special attention to bowel and bladder care is needed. A low-residue diet and stool softeners prevent straining and wound contamination. An indwelling catheter is used to provide urinary drainage. Be careful not to dislodge the catheter because extensive edema makes its reinsertion difficult. Heavy, taut sutures are often used to close the wounds, resulting in severe discomfort. In other instances, the wound may be allowed to heal by granulation. Analgesics may be required to control pain. Carefully position the patient using strategically placed pillows to provide comfort. Anticoagulant therapy to prevent DVTs is common.

Because the surgery causes mutilation of the perineal area and the healing process is slow, the patient is likely to become discouraged. Provide opportunities for the patient to express her feelings and concerns about the operation. Teach the patient specific instructions in self-care before discharge. Instruct her to report any unusual odor, fresh bleeding, breakdown of incision, or perineal pain. Home care nursing can benefit the patient during her adjustment period.

Sexual function is often retained. Whether clitoral sensation is retained may be critical to some women, particularly if it was a primary source of orgasmic satisfaction. Discussing alternative methods of achieving sexual satisfaction may be indicated.

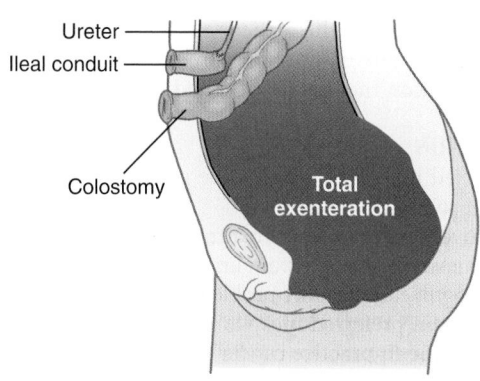

FIG. 54-11 Total exenteration is removal of all pelvic organs with creation of an ileal conduit and a colostomy.

Pelvic Exenteration. When other forms of therapy fail to control the spread of cancer and no metastases have been found outside of the pelvis, pelvic exenteration may be performed. This radical surgery usually involves removal of the uterus, ovaries, fallopian tubes, vagina, bladder, urethra, and pelvic lymph nodes (Fig. 54-11). In some situations, the descending colon, rectum, and anal canal may also be removed. Candidates for this procedure are selected on the basis of their likelihood of surviving the surgery and their ability to adjust to and accept the resulting limitations.

Postoperative care is similar to that of a patient who has had a radical hysterectomy, an abdominal perineal resection, and an ileostomy or a colostomy. The physical, emotional, and social adjustments to life required by the woman and her family are great. There are urinary or fecal diversions in the abdominal wall, a reconstructed vagina, and the onset of menopausal symptoms.

Assess the patient's physical and emotional adjustment to the changes in body image produced by the surgery and her ability to carry out any treatment measures. The patient's rehabilitative process should keep pace with her acceptance of the situation. Much understanding and support are needed from the nursing staff during a long recovery period. Gently encourage the patient to regain her independence. She needs to verbalize her feelings about her altered body structure. Including the family in the plan of care is important. Careful follow-up monitoring is needed so that early recurrence of the cancer can be identified and treated.

ACUTE INTERVENTION WITH RADIATION THERAPY. Instruct the patient who is to receive external radiation to urinate immediately before the treatment to minimize radiation exposure to the bladder. Advise her about radiation side effects, including enteritis and cystitis. These are natural reactions to radiation therapy and do not indicate an overdose. Fully inform the patient of the possible side effects and measures that can be used to reduce their impact.

Nursing management of the patient receiving internal radiation therapy requires special considerations. Do not stay in the immediate area any longer than is necessary to give proper care and attention. No individual nurse should take care of the patient for more than 30 minutes per day. Stay at the foot of the bed or at the entrance to the room to minimize radiation exposure. Instruct visitors to stay 6 ft away from the bed and limit visits to less than 3 hr/day. Efficient organization of nursing care is essential so that you do not stay in the patient's immediate area any longer than is necessary. Fully explain the reasons for these precautions to the patient and her visitors. (A more detailed discussion of nursing care of the patient receiving internal radiation therapy is presented in Chapter 16.)

EVALUATION

The expected outcomes are that the patient with cancer of the female reproductive system will
- Actively participate in treatment decisions
- Achieve satisfactory pain and symptom management
- Recognize and report problems promptly
- Maintain preferred lifestyle as long as possible
- Continue to practice cancer detection strategies

PROBLEMS WITH PELVIC SUPPORT

The most commonly occurring problems with pelvic support are uterine prolapse, cystocele, and rectocele. Although vaginal birth increases the risk for these problems, these conditions can occur in women who have never experienced childbirth. Obesity, chronic coughing, and straining during bowel movements can increase the likelihood of these problems. The decreased estrogen that normally accompanies perimenopause also reduces some connective tissue support.

UTERINE PROLAPSE

Uterine prolapse is the downward displacement of the uterus into the vaginal canal[38] (Fig. 54-12). Prolapse is rated by degrees. In first-degree prolapse the cervix rests in the lower part of the vagina. Second-degree prolapse means the cervix is at the vaginal opening. Third-degree prolapse means the uterus protrudes through the introitus.

Symptoms vary with the degree of prolapse. The patient may describe a feeling of "something coming down." She may have dyspareunia, a dragging or heavy feeling in the pelvis, backache, and bowel or bladder problems if cystocele or rectocele is also present. Stress incontinence is a common and troubling problem. When third-degree uterine prolapse occurs, the

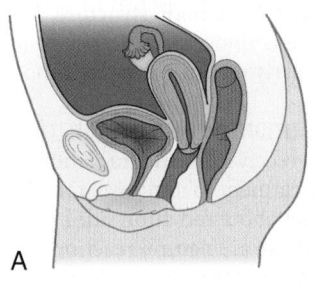
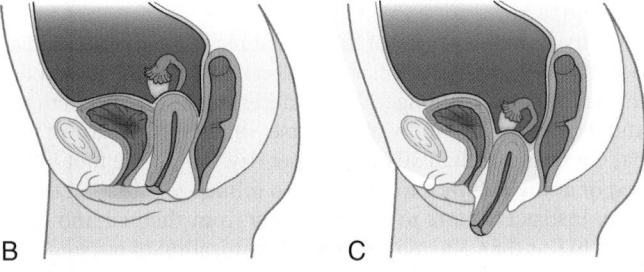

FIG. 54-12 Uterine prolapse. **A,** First-degree prolapse. **B,** Second-degree prolapse. **C,** Third-degree prolapse.

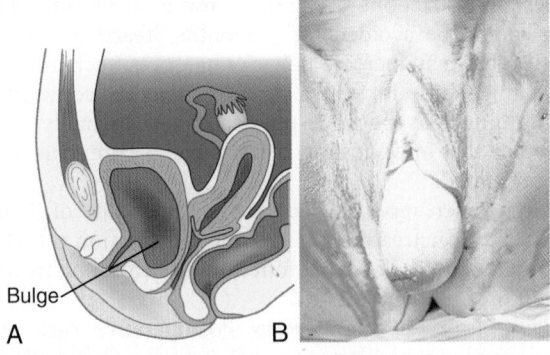

FIG. 54-13 A, Cystocele. **B,** Bladder has prolapsed into the vagina, causing a uterine prolapse.

protruding cervix and vaginal walls are subjected to constant irritation, and tissue changes may occur.

Therapy depends on the degree of prolapse and how much the woman's daily activities have been affected. Pelvic muscle strengthening exercises (Kegel exercises) may be effective for some women (see Table 46-19). If not, a pessary may be used. A *pessary* is a device that is placed in the vagina to help support the uterus. A wide variety of shapes exist, including rings, arches, and balls. Most are made of plastic or wire coated with plastic. When a woman first receives a pessary, she needs instructions for its cleaning and follow-up. Pessaries that are left in place for long periods are associated with erosion, fistulas, and vaginal carcinoma.

If more conservative measures are not successful, surgery is indicated. Surgery generally involves a vaginal hysterectomy with anterior and posterior repair of the vagina and the underlying fascia.

CYSTOCELE AND RECTOCELE

Cystocele occurs when support between the vagina and bladder is weakened (Fig. 54-13). Similarly, a **rectocele** results from weakening between the vagina and rectum (Fig. 54-14). Cystocele and rectocele are common problems, and in many women they are asymptomatic. With large cystoceles, complete emptying of the bladder can be difficult, predisposing women to bladder infections. A woman with a large rectocele may not be able to completely empty her rectum when defecating unless she helps push the stool out by putting her fingers in her vagina.

As with uterine prolapse, Kegel exercises (see Table 46-19) may be used to strengthen the weakened perineal muscles if the cystocele or rectocele is not too problematic. A pessary may be helpful for cystoceles. Surgery designed to tighten the vaginal

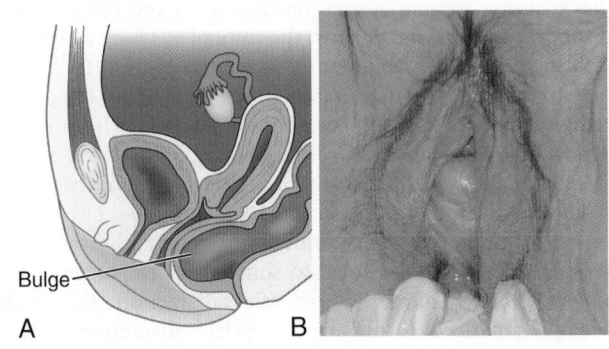

FIG. 54-14 A, Rectocele. **B,** Rectum has prolapsed into the vagina.

wall is generally the method of treatment. A cystocele is corrected with a procedure called an anterior colporrhaphy, whereas a posterior colporrhaphy is done for a rectocele. If further surgery is needed to relieve stress incontinence, procedures to support the urethra and restore the proper angle between the urethra and the posterior bladder wall are used.

NURSING MANAGEMENT
PROBLEMS WITH PELVIC SUPPORT

Assist women in avoiding or decreasing problems with pelvic support by teaching them how to do Kegel exercises. Women of all ages may benefit from these exercises. Instruct the patient to pull in or contract her muscles as if she were trying to stop the flow of urine. She should hold the contraction for several seconds and then relax. Sets of 5 to 10 contractions each should be done several times daily.

If vaginal surgery is necessary, the preoperative preparation usually includes a cleansing douche the morning of surgery. A cathartic and a cleansing enema are usually given when a rectocele repair is scheduled. A perineal shave may be done.

In the postoperative period the goals of care are to prevent wound infection and pressure on the vaginal suture line. This necessitates perineal care at least twice a day and after each urination or defecation. Apply an ice pack locally to help relieve the initial perineal discomfort and swelling. A disposable glove filled with ice and covered with a cloth works well. Later, sitz baths may be used.

After an anterior colporrhaphy, an indwelling catheter is usually left in the bladder for 4 days to allow the local edema to subside. The catheter keeps the bladder empty, preventing strain on the sutures. Twice-daily catheter care with an antiseptic is generally done. After posterior colporrhaphy, straining at stool is avoided by means of a low-residue diet and the prevention of constipation. A stool softener is usually given each night.

Review discharge instructions before the patient leaves the hospital. These include the use of douches or a mild laxative as needed; restrictions on heavy lifting and prolonged standing, walking, or sitting; and avoidance of intercourse until the physician gives permission. There may be a temporary loss of vaginal sensation, which can last for several months.

FISTULA

A *fistula* is an abnormal opening between internal organs or between an organ and the exterior of the body (Fig. 54-15).

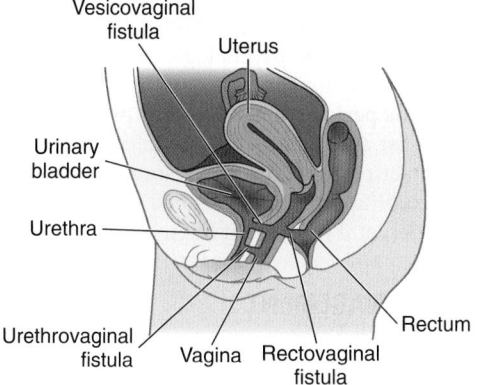

FIG. 54-15 Common fistulas involving the vagina.

Gynecologic procedures cause most urinary tract fistulas. Other causes include injury during childbirth and disease processes, such as cancer. Fistulas may develop between the vagina and the bladder, urethra, ureter, or rectum. When *vesicovaginal* fistulas (between the bladder and the vagina) develop, some urine leaks into the vagina, whereas with *rectovaginal* fistulas (between the rectum and the vagina), flatus and feces escape into the vagina. In both instances, excoriation and irritation of the vaginal and vulvar tissues occur and may lead to severe infections. In addition to wetness, offensive odors may develop, causing embarrassment and severely limiting socialization.

Because small fistulas may heal spontaneously within a matter of months, treatment may not be needed. If the fistula does not heal, surgical excision is required. Inflammation and tissue edema must be eliminated before surgery is attempted, which may involve a wait of up to 6 months. The fistulectomy may result in the patient's having an ileal conduit or temporary colostomy.

NURSING MANAGEMENT
FISTULAS

Perineal hygiene is of great importance both preoperatively and postoperatively. Cleanse the perineum every 4 hours. Warm sitz baths should be taken three times daily if possible. Change perineal pads frequently. Encourage the patient to maintain an adequate fluid intake. Encouragement and reassurance are needed to help the patient cope with her problems.

Postoperatively, emphasize the avoidance of stress on the repaired areas and prevention of infection. Take care so that the indwelling catheter, usually in place for 7 to 10 days, is draining at all times. Urge oral fluids to provide for internal catheter irrigation. Use minimal pressure and strict asepsis if catheter irrigation becomes necessary. The first stool after bowel surgery may be purposely delayed to prevent contamination of the wound. Later, give stool softeners or mild laxatives. (See Chapter 46 for care of a patient with an ileal conduit and Chapter 43 for care of a patient with a colostomy.) Surgical repair of fistulas is not always effective, even in the best conditions. Therefore supportive nursing care for the patient and her significant others is especially important.

SEXUAL ASSAULT

Sexual assault is the forcible perpetration of a sexual act on a person without his or her consent. It can include any of the following actions: sodomy (anal or oral copulation with a person of the same or opposite sex), forced vaginal intercourse, assault with a foreign object, and serial battery.

Sexual assault may be committed by a stranger or by an intimate partner. Intimate partner violence (IPV) is a major health problem in the United States.[39] Survivors can suffer physical trauma and mental health consequences. Pregnancy, STIs, and gynecologic problems can result from IPV. More than half of all female rape victims were raped by an intimate partner. Female victims of IPV frequently report chronic pain, sleep disturbances, poor physical health, and activity limitations.

Clinical Manifestations

Physical. Many women who seek help immediately after the assault will not have any evidence of physical trauma. Evidence of trauma may be limited because women do not resist for fear

✚ TABLE 54-14 EMERGENCY MANAGEMENT

Sexual Assault

Etiology	Assessment Findings	Interventions
• Sexual molestation • Sodomy • Assault involving genitalia (male or female) without consent	• Emotional or physical manifestations of shock • Hysteria • Crying • Anger • Silence • Decreased level of consciousness • Hyperventilation • Oral, vaginal, and rectal injuries • Extragenital injuries • Pain in genital or extragenital area	**Initial** • Treat shock and other urgent medical problems (e.g., head injury, hemorrhage, wounds, fractures). • Assess emotional state. • Contact support person (i.e., social worker, rape advocate, sexual assault nurse examiner). • Do *not* clean the patient until all evidence is collected. Make sure the patient does not wash, douche, urinate, brush teeth, or gargle. • Place sheet on floor. Then have patient stand on sheet to remove clothing. Place sheet with clothing in paper bag. • Obtain forensic evidence per local protocol (e.g., body hair, nail scrapings, tissue, dried semen, vaginal washing, blood samples). • Maintain chain of evidence for all legal specimens. Clearly label evidence and keep in locked cabinet until given to law enforcement agency. • Obtain baseline HIV, syphilis, and other STI screening. • Determine method of contraception, date of last menstrual period, and date of last tetanus immunization. • Consider tetanus prophylaxis if lacerations contain soil or dirt. • Vaccinate against hepatitis B if not already done. **Ongoing Monitoring** • Monitor vital signs and emotional status. • Provide clothing as needed. • Counsel patient regarding confidential HIV and STI testing.

HIV, Human immunodeficiency virus; *STI,* sexually transmitted infection.

of physical danger and injury. When present, physical injuries may include bruising and lacerations to the perineum, hymen, vulva, vagina, cervix, and anus. Fractures, subdural hematomas, cerebral concussions, and intraabdominal injuries may result in the need for hospitalization. Sexual assault also places women at risk for STIs and pregnancy.

Psychologic. Immediately after the assault, women may show shock, numbness, denial, or withdrawal. Some women may seem unnaturally calm; others may cry or express anger. Feelings of humiliation, degradation, embarrassment, anger, self-blame, and fear of another assault are commonly expressed. These symptoms usually decrease after 2 weeks, and victims may appear to have adjusted. Yet any time from 2 to 3 weeks to months or years after the assault, symptoms may return and become more severe. *Rape trauma syndrome* is a classification of posttraumatic stress disorder. Flashbacks, intrusive recall, sleep disturbances, gastrointestinal symptoms, and numbing of feelings are common initial symptoms. Women feel embarrassment, self-blame, and powerlessness. Later symptoms include mood swings, irritability, and anger. Feelings of despair, shame, and hopelessness are often the cause of the anger. These feelings may be internalized and lead to depression. Suicidal ideations may also occur.

Collaborative Care

In the acute care of an assault survivor, ensuring the woman's emotional and physical safety has the highest priority. Table 54-14 outlines the emergency management of the patient who has been sexually assaulted. Most emergency departments (EDs) have identified personnel who have received special training to work with women who have been assaulted.

Many crime-fighting or victim advocate agencies within communities have implemented the position of the sexual assault nurse examiner (SANE).[40] The SANE is a registered nurse who is certified to provide care to victims of sexual assault, while ensuring evidence is safeguarded. Special procedures are followed in taking the history and conducting the examination to preserve all evidence in case of future prosecution.

When the survivor of an assault is admitted to the ED or clinic, a specific chain of events occurs (Table 54-15). A signed informed consent is obtained from the woman before any data are collected. All materials gathered are well documented, labeled, and given to the appropriate person, such as the pathologist or a police officer. The materials are handled by as few people as possible, and signatures of all responsible for keeping and handling the data are obtained. Many items can be used as evidence if the victim chooses to file a complaint. Consequently, the integrity of the material must be maintained. Your involvement in the medicolegal process depends on the policies of the individual institution and state law.

A gynecologic and sexual history and an account of the assault (who, what, when, and where), as well as a general physical and pelvic examination, add further information about the incident. Laboratory tests are done primarily to look for sperm in the vagina and to identify any existing STIs or pregnancy.

Follow-up physical and psychologic care is essential. Women should return weekly for the first month after the assault. This includes the time period when a woman's psychologic reactions may be the most severe. Provide the telephone numbers and names of contact persons for local resources for sexual assault survivors, including rape crisis centers, legal and law enforcement authorities, and human services.

▌ NURSING MANAGEMENT
▌ SEXUAL ASSAULT

Assist all women in becoming aware of prevention tactics (Table 54-16). Also encourage women to learn some basic techniques

TABLE 54-15 EVALUATION OF ALLEGED SEXUAL ASSAULT

1. Medicolegal
- Valid written consent for examination, photographs, laboratory tests, release of information, and laboratory samples
- Appropriate "chain of evidence" documentation

2. History
- History of assault (who, what, when, where)
- Penetration, ejaculation, extragenital acts
- Activities since assault (e.g., changed clothes, bathed, douched)
- Inquire about safety
- Menstrual and contraceptive history
- Medical history
- Emotional status
- Current symptoms

3. General Physical Examination
- Vital signs and general appearance
- Extragenital trauma—mouth, breasts, neck
- Cuts, bruises, scratches (photographs taken)

4. Pelvic Examination
- Vulvar trauma, erythema; hymen, anal, and rectal status
- Matted hairs or free hairs
- Vaginal examination with unlubricated speculum for discharge, blood, lacerations
- Uterine size
- Adnexa, especially hematomas

5. Laboratory Samples
- Vaginal vault content sampling
- Vaginal smears—microscope evaluation for trichomonads and semen
- Oral or rectal swabs and smears, if indicated
- Blood samples—VDRL serology, pregnancy test; serologic testing for HIV and hepatitis B infection
- Freeze serum sample for later testing
- Cultures—cervix and other areas (if indicated) for gonorrhea and chlamydial infection
- Fingernail scrapings
- Pubic hair scrapings
- Clipping of matted pubic hairs

6. Treatment
- Care of injuries and emotional trauma
- Prophylaxis for STIs, tetanus, and hepatitis B (see appropriate chapters)
- If appropriate, consider levonorgestrel (Plan-B One-Step) emergency contraceptive pill up to 72 hr after assault; follow-up for pregnancy test in 2-3 wk
- Testing for HIV, syphilis, and hepatitis B may be done at 6-8 wk
- Protection of legal rights
- Recommendation of continued follow-up and services of rape crisis center

VDRL, Venereal Disease Research Laboratory.

TABLE 54-16 PATIENT TEACHING GUIDE

Sexual Assault Prevention

Include the following instructions when teaching measures to prevent sexual assault.

1. Be proactive and take a self-defense class.
2. Be aware of date-rape drugs (e.g., GHB, Rohypnol, Ketamine). Never leave your beverage unattended when socializing.
3. Place and maintain lights at all entrances to your home.
4. Keep your doors locked and do not open them to a stranger. Ask for identification if a service person comes to the door.
5. Do not advertise that you live alone. List only your initials with your last name in the telephone directory or on the mailbox. Never reveal to a caller that you are home alone.
6. Avoid walking alone in deserted areas. Walk to the parking lot with a friend; be sure you see each other leave.
7. Have your keys ready as you approach your car or home.
8. Keep all doors locked and the windows up when driving.
9. Never get on an elevator with a suspicious person. Pretend you have forgotten something and get off.
10. Say what you mean in social situations. Be sure your voice and body language reflect your response.
11. Proceed with caution in online correspondence.
12. Carry a loud whistle and use it when you think you are in danger.
13. Yell "Fire!" if you are attacked and run toward a lighted area.

may be inconsistent, confused, and inappropriate. Maintain a nonjudgmental attitude.

The patient usually has many feelings and thoughts about the assault and generally wants to talk about them to an interested listener. Talking may help the patient feel better and gain understanding of her reactions to the incident. When you listen carefully, the patient feels that she is not alone and is better able to gain control over the situation.

Assess the patient's stress level before preparing her for the various procedures that will follow. Let her know what to expect and what is expected of her, as well as why the particular procedure must be done. Because the pelvic examination may trigger a flashback of the attack, answer all related questions before the examination and be a supportive presence during the examination.

After the examination, consider the patient's physical comfort needs. She will need a change of clothing because her original garments may be torn or soiled, or kept as evidence. Most women who have been sexually assaulted feel dirty and need a place to wash and to use a mouthwash, especially if oral sex was involved. Food and drink may also provide comfort to the victim.

Discuss the possibility of pregnancy and offer the patient an emergency contraception pill. Taking a single tablet of levonorgestrel (Plan-B One-Step) within 72 hours after unprotected sexual intercourse reduces the risk of pregnancy. Levonorgestrel is generally effective and safe, and it will not affect an existing pregnancy. Mifepristone (RU-486) is approved for use in early abortions in the United States but not for emergency contraception.

Many sexual assault survivors are unaware of the availability of financial compensation (a law in most states) and appreciate information about the application process. This compensation is to assist them in paying for emergency services and for emotional injuries that may temporarily interfere with their ability to work.

When the patient is discharged, make certain the patient has transportation home. If friends or family members are not

of self-defense. Local high schools and the YWCA usually have self-defense classes for formal instruction. Practicing the various techniques with a friend strengthens a woman's confidence in her ability to fight back. Learning self-defense can make the woman less vulnerable and more self-reliant.

When a sexual assault survivor is brought to the clinic or ED, a quiet, private area should be used for the initial assessment and the examinations that follow. Do not leave the patient alone. Whenever possible, the same nurse should remain with her throughout her stay and provide needed emotional support. The patient's actions and words as she describes the incident

CASE STUDY

Uterine Prolapse and Vaginal Hysterectomy

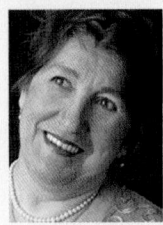

Jupiterimages/
Photos.com/
Thinkstock

Patient Profile

N.B. is a 65-yr-old white woman who has developed lower pelvic discomfort and stress incontinence. She has type 2 diabetes and hypertension. N.B. is the mother of three children. A second-degree uterine prolapse is diagnosed. N.B. was treated conservatively with a pessary, but her symptoms did not improve. She comes to the hospital for a vaginal hysterectomy and anteroposterior repair.

Subjective Data

- Was initially reluctant about surgery
- Concerned about her dyspareunia and her husband's reaction to the surgery
- Concerned she may have uterine cancer
- States she has stress incontinence and pelvic discomfort

Objective Data

Physical Examination

- Second-degree uterine prolapse on vaginal examination
- BP 150/100 mm Hg, pulse 110 beats/min, respirations 20 breaths/min

Laboratory Studies

- Hemoglobin 10 g/dL (0.10 g/L)
- Hemoglobin A1C 9%

Postoperative Status

- Returned to room with indwelling urinary catheter in place
- Vaginal packing in place
- Sequential compression devices on lower extremities
- Patient-controlled analgesia (PCA) pump for pain management

Discussion Questions

1. What are the common causes of uterine prolapse?
2. N.B. asks you about the effect of the surgery on her sexuality. How would you respond?
3. *Priority Decision:* What are priorities of care for N.B.?
4. What possible complications (including reasons for their development) can occur after a vaginal hysterectomy?
5. *Delegation Decision:* Which nursing personnel should be responsible for teaching N.B. related to her diabetes and hypertension: registered nurse, licensed practical/vocational nurse, unlicensed assistive personnel? What should she be taught?
6. *Priority Decision:* Based on the assessment data presented, what are the priority nursing diagnoses? Are there any collaborative problems?

evolve Answers available at *http://evolve.elsevier.com/Lewis/medsurg.*

---

available, the hospital or clinic should make arrangements with an appropriate community resource. The patient should not be sent home alone. The victim's partner and family have tremendous potential as both a negative and positive influence. If the partner is the perpetrator of the assault, consultation with the risk management department and law enforcement is necessary to protect the woman.

Many communities today have crisis centers. These public service organizations have trained professional and nonprofessional volunteers who provide an emotional support system on request. Their programs provide advocacy to ensure dignified treatment throughout the medical and police procedures, short-term counseling for the woman and her family, and court assistance and public education on rape-related issues.

BRIDGE TO NCLEX EXAMINATION

The number of the question corresponds to the same-numbered outcome at the beginning of the chapter.

1. In telling a patient with infertility what she and her partner can expect, the nurse explains that
   a. ovulatory studies can help determine tube patency.
   b. a hysterosalpingogram is a common diagnostic study.
   c. the cause will remain unexplained for 40% of couples.
   d. if postcoital studies are normal, infection tests will be done.

2. An appropriate question to ask the patient with painful menstruation to differentiate primary from secondary dysmenorrhea is
   a. "Does your pain become worse with activity or overexertion?"
   b. "Have you had a recent personal crisis or change in your lifestyle?"
   c. "Is your pain relieved by nonsteroidal antiinflammatory medications?"
   d. "When in your menstrual history did the pain with your period begin?"

3. The nurse should advise the woman recovering from surgical treatment of an ectopic pregnancy that
   a. she has an increased risk for salpingitis.
   b. bed rest must be maintained for 12 hours to assist in healing.
   c. having one ectopic pregnancy increases her risk for another.
   d. intrauterine devices and infertility treatments should be avoided.

4. To prevent or decrease age-related changes that occur after menopause in a patient who chooses not to take hormone therapy, the most important self-care measure to teach is
   a. maintaining usual sexual activity.
   b. increasing the intake of dairy products.
   c. performing regular aerobic, weight-bearing exercise.
   d. taking vitamin E and B-complex vitamin supplements.

5. The patient's thick, white, and curdlike vaginal discharge and vulvar pruritus are most consistent with
   a. trichomoniasis.
   b. monilial vaginitis.
   c. bacterial vaginosis.
   d. chlamydial cervicitis.

6. In caring for a patient with pelvic inflammatory disease, the nurse should place her in semi-Fowler's position. The rationale for this measure is to
   a. relieve severe pain.
   b. promote drainage to prevent abscesses.
   c. improve circulation and promote healing.
   d. prevent complication of bowel obstruction.

7. Nursing responsibilities related to the patient receiving brachytherapy for endometrial cancer include
   a. maintaining absolute bed rest.
   b. keeping the patient in high Fowler's position.
   c. allowing visitors if they stay 3 ft (1 m) from the bed.
   d. limiting direct nurse-to-patient contact to 30 minutes per shift.

8. Postoperative goals in caring for the patient who has undergone an abdominal hysterectomy include (select all that apply)
   a. monitoring urine output.
   b. changing position frequently.
   c. restricting all food for 24 hours.
   d. observing perineal pad for bleeding.
   e. encouraging leg exercises to promote circulation.

9. Postoperative nursing care for the woman with a gynecologic fistula includes (select all that apply)
   a. ambulation.
   b. bladder training.
   c. warm sitz baths.
   d. perineal hygiene.
   e. use of stool softeners.

10. The first nursing intervention for the patient who has been sexually assaulted is to
    a. treat urgent medical problems.
    b. contact support person for the patient.
    c. provide supplies for the patient to cleanse self.
    d. document bruises and lacerations of the perineum and the cervix.

1. b, 2. d, 3. c, 4. c, 5. b, 6. b, 7. a, 8. a, b, e, 9. c, d, 10. a

⊜volve

For rationales to these answers and even more NCLEX review questions, visit *http://evolve.elsevier.com/Lewis/medsurg.*

REFERENCES

1. Sabanegh E, Agarwal A: Definition and demographics of infertility. In Wien A, editor-in-chief: *Campbell-Walsh urology,* ed 10, St Louis, 2011, Saunders.

2. Schmidt L, Sobotka T, Bentzen B, et al: Demographic and medical consequences of the postponement of parenthood, *Hum Reprod Update* 18:29, 2012.

*3. Nachtigall R, MacDougall K, Davis A, et al: Expensive but worth it: older parents' attitudes and opinions about the costs and insurance coverage for in vitro fertilization, *Fertil Steril* 97:82, 2012.

4. Williams D, Pridjian G: Obstetrics. In Rakel R, Rakel D, editors: *Textbook of family medicine,* ed 8, St Louis, 2011, Saunders.

5. Lentz G: Premenstrual syndrome and premenstrual dysphoric disorder. In Lentz G, Lobo R, Gershenson D, et al, editors: *Comprehensive gynecology,* ed 6, St Louis, 2013, Mosby.

6. Mayo Clinic: Menorrhagia (heavy menstrual bleeding). Retrieved from *www.mayoclinic.com/health/menorrhagia.*

7. Centers for Disease Control and Prevention: Toxic shock syndrome. Retrieved from *www.cdc.gov/ncidod/dbmd/diseaseinfo/toxicshock_t.htm.*

8. McQueen A: Ectopic pregnancy: risk factors, diagnostic procedures and treatment, *Nurs Stand* 25:49, 2011.

9. Givens M, Lipscomb G: Diagnosis of ectopic pregnancy, *Clin Obstet Gynecol* 55:387, 2012.

10. Sitka C: Methotrexate: the pharmacology behind medical treatment for ectopic pregnancy, *Clin Obstet Gynecol* 55:433, 2012.

11. Harvard Medical School: Perimenopause: rocky road to menopause, Harvard Health Publications. Retrieved from *www.health.harvard.edu/newsweek/Perimenopause_Rocky_road_to_menopause.htm.*

12. University of California–Berkeley: When a flush is not a winning hand, *Wellness Letter* 27:4, 2011. Retrieved from *www.wellnessletter.com/ucberkeley.*

13. Roush K: Managing menopausal symptoms, *Am J Nurs* 112:28, 2012.

*14. Women's Health Initiative Study: Findings from the WHI post-menopausal hormone therapy trials, Department of Health and Human Services. Retrieved from *www.nhlbi.nih.gov/whi.*

*15. Nelson HD, Walker M, Zakher B, et al: *Menopausal hormone therapy for the primary prevention of chronic conditions: a systematic review to update the U.S. Preventive Services Task Force Recommendations,* AHRQ Pub No 12-05168-EF-1, Washington, DC, 2012, Agency for Healthcare Research and Quality, Department of Health and Human Services.

16. American Cancer Society: Tamoxifen and raloxifene. Retrieved from *www.cancer.org/Cancer/BreastCancer/MoreInformation/MedicinestoReduceBreastCancer.*

17. Im E, Ko Y, Hwang H, et al: "Symptom-specific or holistic": menopausal symptom management, *Health Care Women Int* 33:575, 2012.

18. Stiles M, Redmer J, Paddock E, et al: Gynecologic issues in geriatric women, *J Women's Health* 21:4, 2012.

19. Centers for Disease Control and Prevention: Pelvic inflammatory disease fact sheet. Retrieved from *www.cdc.gov/std/PID/STDFact-PID.htm.*

20. Shin J, Howard F: Management of chronic pelvic pain, *Curr Pain Headache Rep* 15:377, 2011.

21. Apte G, Nelson P, Brisme JM: Chronic female pelvic pain, part 1: clinical pathoanatomy and examination of the pelvic region, *Pain Pract* 12:88, 2012.

22. Donegan C: Caring for women with endometriosis, *Pract Nurse* 42:24, 2012.

23. Cleveland Clinic: Facts about endometriosis. Retrieved from *www.my.clevelandclinic.org/disorders/Endometriosis/hic_Facts_About_Endometriosis.*

24. Munro M: Uterine leiomyomas, current concepts: pathogenesis, impact on reproductive health, and medical, procedural, and surgical management, *Obstet Gynecol Clin North Am* 38:703, 2011.

*25. Gupta J, Sinha A, Lumsden M, et al: Uterine artery embolization for symptomatic uterine fibroids, *Cochrane Database Syst Rev* 5:CD005073, 2012.

*Evidence-based information for clinical practice.

26. Lobo R: Hyperandrogenism. In Lentz G, Lobo R, Gershenson D, et al, editors: *Comprehensive gynecology*, ed 6, St Louis, 2013, Mosby.

*27. Toulis K, Goulis D, Mintziori G, et al: Meta-analysis of cardiovascular disease risk markers in women with polycystic ovary syndrome, *Hum Reprod Update* 17:741, 2011.

28. Androgen Excess and PCOS Society: Polycystic ovary syndrome. Retrieved from *www.ae-society.org/poly_syndrome*.

29. American Cancer Society: *Cancer facts and figures 2012*, Atlanta, 2012, The Society. Retrieved from *www.cancer.org*.

30. National Institutes of Health. National Cancer Institute: Snapshot of cervical cancer. Retrieved from *www.cancer.gov/aboutnci/servingpeople/snapshots/cervical.pdf*.

31. American Cancer Society: American Cancer Society guidelines for the early detection of cancer. Retrieved from *www.cancer.org/Healthy/FindCancerEarly/CancerScreeningGuidelines*.

32. Arora V, Quinn M: Endometrial cancer, *Best Pract Res Clin Obstet Gynaecol* 26:31, 2012.

33. Jelovac D, Armstrong D: Recent progress in the diagnosis and treatment of ovarian cancer, *CA Cancer J Clin* 61:183, 2011.

34. Buys S, Partridge E, Black A, et al: Effect of screening on ovarian cancer mortality: the prostate, lung, colorectal and ovarian (PLCO) cancer screening randomized controlled trial, *JAMA* 305:229, 2011.

35. Koehler C, Gottschalk E, Chiantera V, et al: From laparoscopic assisted radical vaginal hysterectomy to vaginal assisted laparoscopic radical hysterectomy, *BJOG Int J Obstet Gynaecol* 119:254, 2012.

36. Viswanathan A: Advances in the use of radiation for gynecologic cancers, *Hematol Oncol Clin North Am* 26:15, 2012.

*37. Lara L, deAndrade J, Consolo F, et al: Women's poorer satisfaction with their sex lives following gynecological cancer treatment, *Clin J Oncology Nurs* 16:273, 2011.

38. Prasad A, Alvero R: Uterine prolapse. In Ferri F, editor: *Ferri's clinical advisor 2013*, Philadelphia, 2011, Mosby.

39. Cronholm PF, Fogarty CT, Ambuel B, et al: Intimate partner violence, *Am Fam Physician* 83:1165, 2011.

40. Georgia Network to End Sexual Assault: Basic SANE training. Retrieved from *www.gnesa.org*.

RESOURCES

American Congress of Obstetricians and Gynecologists
www.acog.org

American Urological Association
www.auanet.org

Hysterectomy Educational Resources and Services (HERS) Foundation
www.hersfoundation.com

North American Menopause Society
www.menopause.org

Sexuality Information and Education Council of the United States (SIECUS)
www.siecus.org

Only a life lived for others is a life worthwhile.
Albert Einstein

Nursing Management
Male Reproductive Problems

Shannon Ruff Dirksen

evolve WEBSITE

LEARNING OUTCOMES

1. Describe the pathophysiology, clinical manifestations, and collaborative care of benign prostatic hyperplasia.
2. Describe the nursing management of benign prostatic hyperplasia.
3. Describe the pathophysiology, clinical manifestations, and collaborative care of prostate cancer.
4. Explain the nursing management of prostate cancer.
5. Specify the pathophysiology, clinical manifestations, and nursing and collaborative management of prostatitis and problems of the penis and scrotum.
6. Explain the clinical manifestations and collaborative care of testicular cancer.
7. Describe the pathophysiology, clinical manifestations, and nursing and collaborative management of problems related to male sexual function.
8. Summarize the psychologic and emotional implications related to male reproductive problems.

KEY TERMS

This chapter discusses problems of the male reproductive system. These involve a variety of structures, including the prostate, penis, urethra, ejaculatory duct, scrotum, testes, epididymis, ductus (vas) deferens, and rectum (Fig. 55-1).

PROBLEMS OF THE PROSTATE GLAND

BENIGN PROSTATIC HYPERPLASIA

Benign prostatic hyperplasia (BPH) is a benign enlargement of the prostate gland. It is the most common urologic problem in male adults. About 50% of all men in their lifetime will develop BPH. Of these men, almost half of them will have bothersome lower urinary tract symptoms.[1] Research is not clear about whether having BPH leads to an increased risk of developing prostate cancer.[2,3]

Etiology and Pathophysiology

Although the cause of BPH is not completely understood, it is thought that BPH results from hormonal changes associated with the aging process.[1] One possible cause is excessive accumulation of dihydroxytestosterone (DHT) (the principal intraprostatic androgen) in the prostate cells. This can stimulate cell growth and an overgrowth of prostate tissue. Older

Reviewed by Debra Backus, RN, PhD, CNE, NEA-BC, Associate Professor of Nursing, State University of New York, Canton, New York; and David J. Derrico, RN, MSN, Assistant Clinical Professor, University of Florida, Gainesville, Florida.

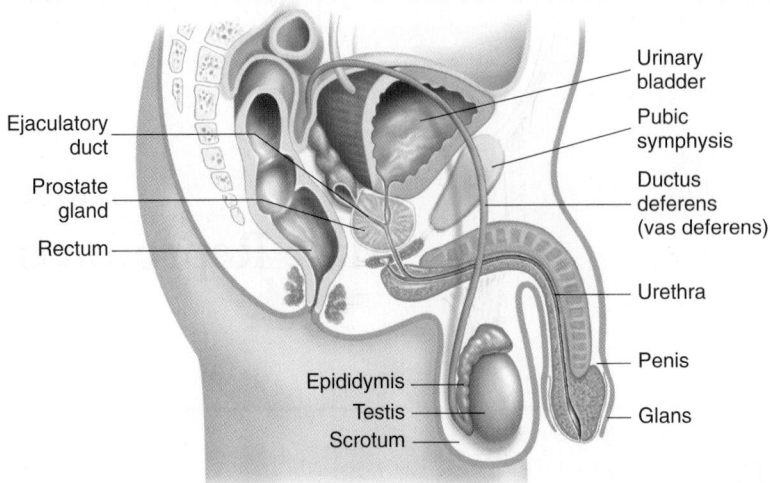

FIG. 55-1 Areas of the male reproductive system in which problems are likely to develop.

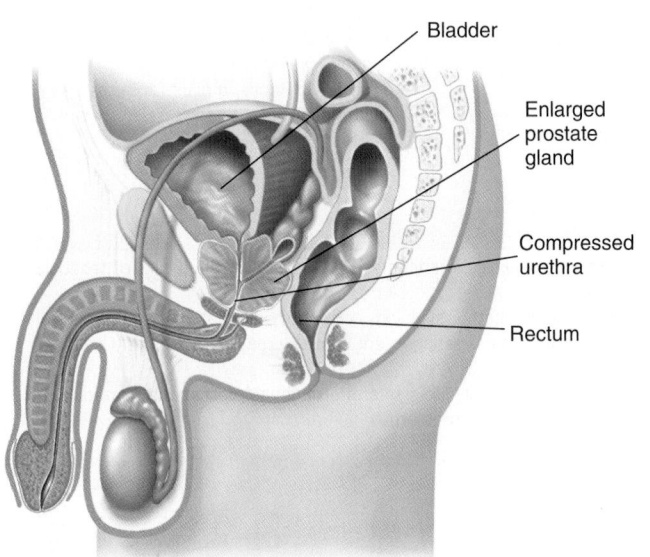

FIG. 55-2 Benign prostatic hyperplasia. The enlarged prostate compresses the urethra.

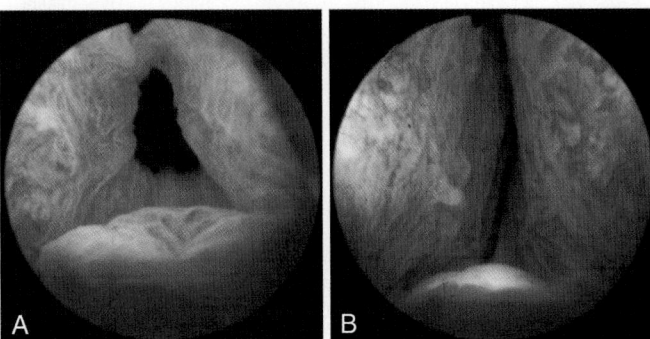

FIG. 55-3 Views of the prostate by cystoscopy. **A,** Normal appearance. **B,** Moderate benign prostatic hyperplasia with urethral obstruction.

men have a decrease in the blood's testosterone level, but continue to produce and accumulate high levels of DHT in the prostate.

Another possible cause is an increased proportion of estrogen (as compared to testosterone) in the blood. Throughout their lives, men produce both testosterone and small amounts of estrogen. As men age, the amount of active testosterone in the blood decreases, leaving a higher proportion of estrogen. A higher amount of estrogen within the gland increases the activity of substances (e.g., DHT) that promote cell growth.

Typically BPH develops in the inner part of the prostate. (Prostate cancer is most likely to develop in the outer part.) This enlargement gradually compresses the urethra, eventually leading to partial or complete obstruction (Fig. 55-2). The compression of the urethra ultimately leads to the development of clinical symptoms. There is no direct relationship between the size of the prostate and the severity of symptoms or degree of obstruction. The location of the enlargement is most significant in the development of obstructive symptoms (Fig. 55-3). For example, it is possible for mild hyperplasia to cause severe

obstruction, or for extreme hyperplasia to cause few obstructive symptoms.

Risk factors for BPH include aging, obesity (in particular increased waist circumference), lack of physical activity, alcohol consumption, erectile dysfunction, smoking, and diabetes.[4] A positive family history of BPH in first-degree relatives may also be a risk factor.

Clinical Manifestations

Manifestations of BPH are mainly associated with symptoms of the lower urinary tract.[5] The patient's symptoms are usually gradual in onset and may not be noticed until prostatic enlargement has been present for some time. Early symptoms are often minimal because the bladder can compensate for a small amount of resistance to urine flow. The symptoms gradually worsen as the degree of urethral obstruction increases.

Symptoms can be divided into two groups: irritative and obstructive. *Irritative symptoms,* which include nocturia, urinary frequency, urgency, dysuria, bladder pain, and incontinence, are associated with inflammation or infection. Nocturia is often the first symptom that the patient notices.[5]

Obstructive symptoms caused by prostate enlargement include a decrease in the caliber and force of the urinary stream, difficulty in initiating voiding, intermittency (stopping and starting stream several times while voiding), and dribbling at the end of urination. These symptoms are due to urinary retention.

TABLE 55-1 AUA SYMPTOM INDEX TO DETERMINE SEVERITY OF PROSTATIC PROBLEMS

Questions	AUA Symptom Score* (circle one number on each line)					
	Not At All	Less Than 1 Time in 5	Less Than Half the Time	About Half the Time	More Than Half the Time	Almost Always
Over the past month						
1. How often do you have the sensation that your bladder is not completely empty after you finish urinating?	0	1	2	3	4	5
2. How often do you have to urinate again, less than 2 hr after you finish urinating?	0	1	2	3	4	5
3. How often do you stop and start again several times when you urinate?	0	1	2	3	4	5
4. How often do you find it difficult to postpone urination?	0	1	2	3	4	5
5. How often do you have a weak urinary stream?	0	1	2	3	4	5
6. How often do you have to push or strain to begin urination?	0	1	2	3	4	5
7. How many times do you usually get up to urinate from the time you go to bed at night until the time you get up in the morning?	0 (None)	1 (1 time)	2 (2 times)	3 (3 times)	4 (4 times)	5 (5 times or more)
Sum of circled numbers (AUA Symptom Score): _____ *						

Source: Barry MJ, Fowler FJ, O'Leary MP, et al: The American Urological Association symptom index for benign prostatic hyperplasia, *J Urol* 148:1549, 1992. Used with permission.
*Score is interpreted as follows: 0-7, mild; 8-19, moderate; 20-35, severe.
AUA, American Urological Association.

The American Urological Association (AUA) symptom index for BPH (Table 55-1) is a widely used tool to assess voiding symptoms associated with obstruction. Although this tool is not diagnostic, it helps determine the extent of symptoms.[6] Higher scores on this tool indicate greater symptom severity.

Complications

Complications of urinary obstruction are relatively uncommon in BPH. Acute urinary retention is a complication that is manifested by the sudden and painful inability to urinate. Treatment involves the insertion of a catheter to drain the bladder. Surgery may also be indicated.

Another complication is urinary tract infection (UTI) and potentially sepsis secondary to UTI. Incomplete bladder emptying (associated with partial obstruction) results in residual urine, which provides a favorable environment for bacterial growth. Calculi may develop in the bladder because of the alkalinization of the residual urine. Bladder stones are more common in men with BPH, although the risk of renal calculi is not significantly increased. Additional complications include renal failure caused by *hydronephrosis* (distention of pelvis and calyces of kidney by urine that cannot flow through the ureter to the bladder), pyelonephritis, and bladder damage if treatment for acute urinary retention is delayed.

Diagnostic Studies

The primary methods used to diagnose BPH include a history and physical examination. (Diagnostic studies are outlined in Table 55-2.) The prostate can be palpated by digital rectal examination (DRE) to estimate its size, symmetry, and consistency. In BPH, the prostate is symmetrically enlarged, firm, and smooth.

Additional diagnostic tests may be indicated, depending on the type and severity of symptoms and clinical findings. A urinalysis with culture is routinely done to identify any infection. Bacteria, white blood cells (WBCs), or microscopic hematuria indicate infection or inflammation.

A prostate-specific antigen (PSA) blood test may be done to rule out prostate cancer. However, PSA levels may be slightly

TABLE 55-2 COLLABORATIVE CARE

Benign Prostatic Hyperplasia

Diagnostic
- History and physical examination
- Digital rectal examination (DRE)
- Urinalysis with culture
- Prostate-specific antigen (PSA)
- Serum creatinine
- Postvoid residual
- Transrectal ultrasound (TRUS)
- Uroflowmetry
- Cystoscopy

Collaborative Therapy
Active Surveillance
Drug Therapy
- 5α-Reductase inhibitors (e.g., finasteride [Proscar], dutasteride [Avodart], dutasteride plus tamsulosin [Jalyn])
- α-Adrenergic receptor blockers (e.g., silodosin [Rapaflo], alfuzosin [Uroxatral], doxazosin [Cardura], prazosin [Minipress], terazosin [Hytrin], tamsulosin [Flomax])
- Erectogenic drugs (e.g., tadalafil [Cialis])

Minimally Invasive Therapy*
- Transurethral microwave thermotherapy (TUMT)
- Transurethral needle ablation (TUNA)
- Laser prostatectomy
- Transurethral electrovaporization of the prostate (TUVP)
- Intraprostatic urethral stents

Invasive (Surgery) Therapy*
- Transurethral resection of the prostate (TURP)
- Transurethral incision of the prostate (TUIP)
- Open prostatectomy

*See Table 55-3.

elevated in patients with BPH. Serum creatinine levels may be ordered to rule out renal insufficiency. Because symptoms of BPH are similar to those of a neurogenic bladder, a neurologic examination may also be performed.

In patients with an abnormal DRE and elevated PSA, a transrectal ultrasound (TRUS) scan is typically indicated. This examination allows for accurate assessment of prostate size and is helpful in differentiating BPH from prostate cancer. Biopsies can be taken during the ultrasound procedure. Uroflowmetry, a study that measures the volume of urine expelled from the bladder per second, is helpful in determining the extent of urethral blockage and thus the type of treatment needed. Postvoid residual urine volume is often measured to determine the degree of urine flow obstruction. Cystoscopy, a procedure allowing internal visualization of the urethra and bladder, is performed if the diagnosis is uncertain and in patients scheduled for prostatectomy.

Collaborative Care

The goals of collaborative care are to (1) restore bladder drainage, (2) relieve the patient's symptoms, and (3) prevent or treat the complications of BPH. Treatment is generally based on the degree to which the symptoms bother the patient or the presence of complications, rather than the size of the prostate. Alternatives to surgical intervention for some patients now include drug therapy and minimally invasive procedures.

The most conservative treatment that may be recommended for some patients with BPH is referred to as *active surveillance,* or *watchful waiting.*[7] When the patient has no symptoms or only mild ones (AUA symptom scores of 0 to 7), a wait-and-see approach is taken. Because some patients have symptoms that disappear, a conservative approach has value. Making dietary changes (decreasing intake of caffeine, artificial sweeteners, and spicy or acidic foods), avoiding medications such as decongestants and anticholinergics, and restricting evening fluid intake may improve symptoms.

A timed voiding schedule may reduce or eliminate symptoms, thus negating the need for further intervention. If the patient begins to have signs or symptoms that indicate an increase in obstruction, further treatment is indicated.

Drug Therapy. Drugs that have been used to treat BPH with variable degrees of success include 5α-reductase inhibitors and α-adrenergic receptor blockers. Combination therapy using both types of these drugs has been shown to be more effective in reducing symptoms than using one drug alone.

5α-Reductase Inhibitors. These drugs work by reducing the size of the prostate gland. Finasteride (Proscar) blocks the enzyme 5α-reductase, which is necessary for the conversion of testosterone to DHT, the principal intraprostatic androgen. This drug results in regression of hyperplastic tissue through suppression of androgens. Finasteride is an appropriate treatment option for individuals who have a moderate to severe symptom score on the AUA symptom index (see Table 55-1). Although more than 50% of men who are treated with the drug show symptom improvement, it takes about 6 months to be effective. Furthermore, the drug must be taken on a continuous basis to maintain therapeutic results. Serum PSA levels are decreased by almost 50% when taking finasteride. Therefore PSA levels should be doubled when comparing the patient's current levels to premedication levels.

Dutasteride (Avodart) has the same effect on prostatic tissue as finasteride and is a dual inhibitor of 5α-reductase type 1 and 2 isoenzymes. (Finasteride inhibits only the type 2 isoenzyme.) The combination of a 5α-reductase inhibitor (dutasteride) and an α-adrenergic receptor blocker (tamsulosin) is now available in a single oral medication (Jalyn).

In addition to decreasing the symptoms of BPH, finasteride, dutasteride, and Jalyn (finasteride plus tamsulosin) may also

lower the risk of prostate cancer.[8] However, the use of these drugs in prevention of prostate cancer has not been advised because of the increased risk of developing aggressive prostate cancer. Patients with an increased PSA level while taking these medications should be referred to their health care provider. The need for regular prostate cancer screening should also be discussed with the provider.

> **DRUG ALERT: Finasteride (Proscar)**
> - Patient should be aware of the increased risk of orthostatic hypotension with concomitant use of erectile dysfunction drugs.
> - Women who may be or are pregnant should not handle tablets due to potential risk to male fetus (anomaly).

α-Adrenergic Receptor Blockers. α-Adrenergic receptor blockers are another drug treatment option for BPH. These agents selectively block α1-adrenergic receptors, which are abundant in the prostate and are increased in hyperplastic prostate tissue. Although α-adrenergic blockers are more commonly used for treatment of hypertension, these drugs promote smooth muscle relaxation in the prostate, facilitating urinary flow through the urethra. These agents demonstrate a 50% to 60% efficacy in improvement of symptoms, which occurs within 2 to 3 weeks.

Several α-adrenergic blockers are currently in use, including silodosin (Rapaflo), alfuzosin (Uroxatral), doxazosin (Cardura), prazosin (Minipress), terazosin (Hytrin), and tamsulosin (Flomax). Note that although these drugs offer symptomatic relief of BPH, they do not treat hyperplasia.

Erectogenic Drugs. Tadalafil (Cialis) has been used in men who have symptoms of BPH alone or in combination with erectile dysfunction (ED). The drug has shown to be effective in reducing symptoms for both these conditions (see erectile dysfunction later in this chapter).[9]

Herbal Therapy. Herbal extracts have been used in the management of lower urinary symptoms associated with BPH. In particular, some patients take plant extracts such as saw palmetto *(Serenoa repens).* However, research indicates that saw palmetto has no benefit over a placebo.[10,11] In a limited number of small trials, herbal preparations such as saxifrage, betasitosterol, *Pygeum africanum,* and Cernilton have shown some success in reducing the symptoms of BPH. Advise patients to tell their health care provider about all herbal supplements that they use.

Minimally Invasive Therapy. Minimally invasive therapies are becoming more common as an alternative to watchful waiting and invasive treatment (Table 55-3). They generally do not require hospitalization or catheterization and are associated with few adverse events. Many minimally invasive therapies have outcomes comparable to those of invasive techniques.[12]

Transurethral Microwave Thermotherapy. *Transurethral microwave thermotherapy* (TUMT) is an outpatient procedure that involves the delivery of microwaves directly to the prostate through a transurethral probe to raise the temperature of the prostate tissue to about 113° F (45° C). The heat causes death of tissue, thus relieving the obstruction. A rectal temperature probe is used during the procedure to ensure that the temperature is kept below 110° F (43.5° C) to prevent rectal tissue damage. The procedure takes about 90 minutes.

Postoperative urinary retention is a common complication. Thus the patient is generally sent home with an indwelling catheter for 2 to 7 days to maintain urinary flow and to facilitate the passing of small clots or necrotic tissue. Antibiotics, pain medication, and bladder antispasmodic medications are used to

TABLE 55-3   TREATMENT FOR BENIGN PROSTATIC HYPERPLASIA

Description	Advantages	Disadvantages
Minimally Invasive		
Transurethral Microwave Thermotherapy (TUMT)		
Use of microwave radiating heat to produce coagulative necrosis of the prostate.	Outpatient procedure Erectile dysfunction, urinary incontinence, and retrograde ejaculation are rare	Potential for damage to surrounding tissue Urinary catheter needed after procedure
Transurethral Needle Ablation (TUNA)		
Low-wave radiofrequency used to heat the prostate, causing necrosis.	Outpatient procedure Erectile dysfunction, urinary incontinence, and retrograde ejaculation are rare Precise delivery of heat to desired area Very little pain experienced	Urinary retention common Irritative voiding symptoms Hematuria
Laser Prostatectomy		
Procedure uses a laser beam to cut or destroy part of the prostate. Different techniques are available: • Visual laser ablation of prostate (VLAP) • Contact laser • Photovaporization of prostate (PVP) • Interstitial laser coagulation (ILC)	Short procedure Comparable results to TURP Minimal bleeding Fast recovery time Rapid symptom improvement Very effective	Catheter (up to 7 days) needed after procedure due to edema and urinary retention Delayed sloughing of tissue Takes several weeks to reach optimal effect Retrograde ejaculation
Transurethral Electrovaporization of Prostate (TUVP)		
Electrosurgical vaporization and desiccation are used together to destroy prostatic tissue.	Minimal risks Minimal bleeding and sloughing	Retrograde ejaculation Intermittent hematuria
Intraprostatic Urethral Stents		
Insertion of self-expandable metallic stent into the urethra where enlarged area of prostate occurs.	Safe and effective Low risk	Stent may move Long-term effect is unknown
Invasive (Surgery)		
Transurethral Resection of Prostate (TURP)		
Use of excision and cauterization to remove prostate tissue cystoscopically. Remains the standard for treatment of BPH.	Erectile dysfunction unlikely	Bleeding Retrograde ejaculation
Transurethral Incision of Prostate (TUIP)		
Involves transurethral incisions into prostatic tissue to relieve obstruction. Effective for men with small to moderate prostates.	Outpatient procedure Minimal complications Low occurrence of erectile dysfunction or retrograde ejaculation	Urinary catheter needed after procedure
Open Prostatectomy		
Surgery of choice for men with large prostates, bladder damage, or other complicating factors. Involves external incision with two possible approaches (see Fig. 55-6).	Complete visualization of prostate and surrounding tissue	Erectile dysfunction Bleeding Postoperative pain Risk of infection

treat and prevent postprocedure problems. The procedure is not appropriate for men with rectal problems. Anticoagulant therapy should be stopped 10 days before treatment. Mild side effects include occasional problems of bladder spasm, hematuria, dysuria, and retention.

Transurethral Needle Ablation. *Transurethral needle ablation* (TUNA) is another procedure that increases the temperature of prostate tissue, thus causing localized necrosis. TUNA differs from TUMT in that low-wave radiofrequency is used to heat the prostate. Only prostate tissue in direct contact with the needle is affected, thus allowing greater precision in removal of the target tissue. The extent of tissue removed by this process is determined by the amount of tissue contact (needle length), amount of energy delivered, and duration of treatment. The majority of the patients undergoing TUNA have an improvement in symptoms.

This procedure is performed in an outpatient unit or physician's office using local anesthesia and IV or oral sedation. The TUNA procedure lasts approximately 30 minutes. The patient typically experiences little pain with an early return to regular activities. Complications include urinary retention, UTI, and irritative voiding symptoms (e.g., frequency, urgency, dysuria). Some patients require a urinary catheter for a short time. Patients often have hematuria for up to a week.

Laser Prostatectomy. The use of laser therapy through visual or ultrasound guidance is an effective alternative to transurethral resection of the prostate (TURP) in treating BPH. The laser beam is delivered transurethrally through a fiber instrument and is used for cutting, coagulation, and vaporization of prostatic tissue. There are a variety of laser procedures using different sources, wavelengths, and delivery systems. Retreatment rates are comparable to those of a TURP.[13]

One common procedure is *visual laser ablation of the prostate* (VLAP), which uses the laser beam to produce deep coagulation necrosis. The affected prostate tissue gradually sloughs in the urinary stream. It takes several weeks before the patient reaches optimal results after this type of laser therapy. At the completion of VLAP, a urinary catheter is inserted to allow for drainage.

Contact laser techniques involve the direct contact of the laser with the prostate tissue, producing an immediate vaporization of the tissue. Blood vessels near the laser tip are immediately cauterized. Thus bleeding during the procedure is rare. A three-way catheter with slow-drip irrigation is placed immediately after the procedure for a short time. Typically the catheter is removed within 6 to 8 hours after the procedure. Advantages of this procedure over TURP include minimal bleeding both during and after the procedure, faster recovery time, and ability to perform the surgery on patients taking anticoagulants.

Photovaporization of the prostate (PVP) uses a high-power green laser light to vaporize prostate tissue. Improvements in urine flow and symptoms are almost immediate after the procedure. Bleeding is minimal, and a catheter is usually inserted for 24 to 48 hours afterward. PVP works well for larger prostate glands.

Another approach to laser prostatectomy is *interstitial laser coagulation* (ILC). The prostate is viewed through a cystoscope. A laser is used to quickly treat precise areas of the enlarged prostate by placement of interstitial light guides directly into the prostate tissue.

Intraprostatic Urethral Stents. Symptoms from obstruction in patients who are poor surgical candidates can be relieved with intraprostatic urethral stents. The stents are placed directly into the prostatic tissue. Complications include chronic pain, infection, and encrustation. The long-term effects are not known.

Invasive Therapy (Surgery). Invasive treatment of symptomatic BPH involves surgery. The choice of the treatment approach depends on the size and location of the prostatic enlargement and patient factors such as age and surgical risk. Invasive treatments are summarized in Table 55-3.

Invasive therapy is indicated when the decrease in urine flow is sufficient to cause discomfort, persistent residual urine, acute urinary retention because of obstruction with no reversible precipitating cause, or hydronephrosis. Intermittent catheterization or insertion of an indwelling catheter can temporarily reduce symptoms and bypass the obstruction. However, avoid long-term catheter use because of the increased risk of infection.

Transurethral Resection of the Prostate. Transurethral resection of the prostate (TURP) is a surgical procedure involving the removal of prostate tissue using a resectoscope inserted through the urethra. TURP has long been considered the gold standard for surgical treatments of obstructing BPH. Although this procedure remains the most common operation performed, the number of TURP procedures done in recent years has declined due to the development of less invasive technologies.[12]

TURP is performed under a spinal or general anesthetic and requires a 1- to 2-day hospital stay. No external surgical incision is made. A resectoscope is inserted through the urethra to excise and cauterize obstructing prostatic tissue (Fig. 55-4). A large three-way indwelling catheter with a 30-mL balloon is inserted into the bladder after the procedure to provide hemostasis and to facilitate urinary drainage. The bladder is irrigated, either

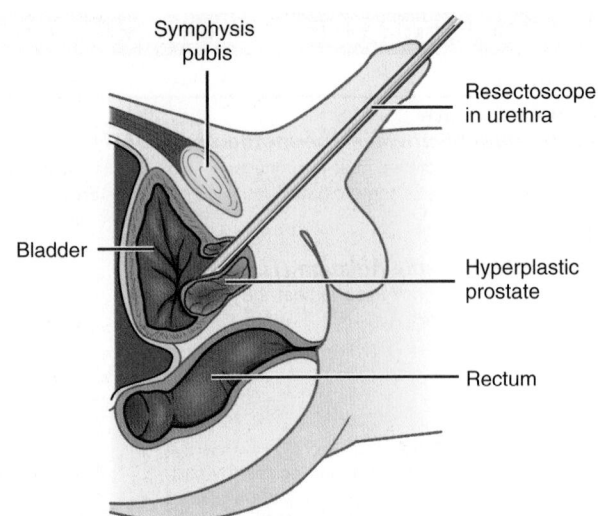

FIG. 55-4 Transurethral resection of the prostate.

continuously or intermittently, usually for the first 24 hours to prevent obstruction from mucus and blood clots.

The outcome for 80% to 90% of patients is excellent, with marked improvements in symptoms and urinary flow rates. Quality of life is also improved. TURP is a surgical procedure with a relatively low risk. Postoperative complications include bleeding, clot retention, and dilutional hyponatremia associated with irrigation. Because bleeding is a common complication, patients taking aspirin, warfarin (Coumadin), or other anticoagulants must discontinue these medications several days before surgery.

Transurethral Incision of the Prostate. Transurethral incision of the prostate (TUIP) is a surgical procedure done under local anesthesia for men with moderate to severe symptoms. Several small incisions are made into the prostate gland to expand the urethra, which relieves pressure on the urethra and improves urine flow. TUIP is an option for patients with a small or moderately enlarged prostate gland. TUIP has similar patient outcomes to TURP in relieving symptoms.

NURSING MANAGEMENT
BENIGN PROSTATIC HYPERPLASIA

Because you will be most directly involved in care of patients with BPH having invasive therapies, the focus of nursing management in this section is on preoperative and postoperative care.

NURSING ASSESSMENT

Subjective and objective data that should be obtained from a patient with BPH are presented in Table 55-4.

NURSING DIAGNOSES

Nursing diagnoses for the patient with BPH preoperatively may include, but are not limited to, the following:

- Acute pain *related to* bladder distention secondary to enlarged prostate
- Risk for infection *related to* an indwelling catheter, urinary stasis, or environmental pathogens

Nursing diagnoses for the patient with BPH who has invasive therapy (surgery) are presented in eNursing Care Plan 55-1 (available on the website for this chapter).

TABLE 55-4 NURSING ASSESSMENT

Benign Prostatic Hyperplasia

Subjective Data
Important Health Information
Medications: Estrogen or testosterone supplementation
Surgery or other treatments: Previous treatment for BPH

Functional Health Patterns
Health perception–health management: Knowledge of the condition
Nutritional-metabolic: Voluntary fluid restriction
Elimination: Urinary urgency, diminution in caliber and force of urinary stream; hesitancy in initiating voiding; postvoid dribbling; urinary retention; incontinence
Sleep: Nocturia
Cognitive-perceptual: Dysuria, sensation of incomplete voiding; bladder discomfort
Sexuality-reproductive: Anxiety about sexual dysfunction

Objective Data
General
Older adult male

Urinary
Distended bladder on palpation; smooth, firm, elastic enlargement of prostate on rectal examination

Possible Diagnostic Findings
Enlarged prostate on ultrasonography; vesicle neck obstruction on cystoscopy; residual urine with postvoiding catheterization; white blood cells, bacteria, or microscopic hematuria with infection; ↑ serum creatinine levels with renal involvement

PLANNING

The overall preoperative goals for the patient having invasive procedures are to have (1) restoration of urinary drainage; (2) treatment of any UTI; and (3) understanding of the upcoming procedure, implications for sexual function, and urinary control. The overall postoperative goals are to have (1) no complications, (2) restoration of urinary control, (3) complete bladder emptying, and (4) satisfying sexual expression.

NURSING IMPLEMENTATION

HEALTH PROMOTION. The cause of BPH is largely attributed to the aging process.[14] Health promotion focuses on early detection and treatment. The American Cancer Society, along with the AUA, recommends a yearly medical history and DRE for men over 50 years of age in an effort to detect prostate problems early. When symptoms of prostatic hyperplasia are present, further diagnostic screening may be necessary (see Table 55-2).

Some men find that the ingestion of alcohol and caffeine tends to increase prostatic symptoms because the diuretic effect increases bladder distention. Compounds found in common cough and cold remedies such as pseudoephedrine (in Sudafed) and phenylephrine (in Allerest PE and Coricidin D) often worsen the symptoms of BPH. These drugs are α-adrenergic agonists that cause smooth muscle contraction. If this happens, the patient should avoid these drugs.

Advise patients with obstructive symptoms to urinate every 2 to 3 hours and when they first feeling the urge. This will minimize urinary stasis and acute urinary retention. Fluid intake should be maintained at a normal level to avoid dehydration or fluid overload. The patient may believe that if he restricts his fluid intake, symptoms will be less severe, but this only increases the chances of an infection. However, if the patient increases his intake too rapidly, bladder distention can develop because of the prostatic obstruction.

ACUTE INTERVENTION. The following discussion focuses on preoperative and postoperative care for the patient undergoing a TURP.

Preoperative Care. Urinary drainage must be restored before surgery. Prostatic obstruction may result in acute retention or inability to void. A urethral catheter such as a coudé (curved-tip) catheter may be needed to restore drainage. In many health care settings, 10 mL of sterile 2% lidocaine gel is injected into the urethra before insertion of the catheter. The lidocaine gel not only acts as a lubricant, but also provides local anesthesia and helps open the urethral lumen. If a sizable obstruction of the urethra exists, the urologist may insert a filiform catheter with sufficient rigidity to pass the obstruction. Aseptic technique is important at all times to avoid introducing bacteria into the bladder. (Urinary catheters are discussed in Chapter 46.)

Antibiotics are usually administered before any invasive procedure. Any infection of the urinary tract must be treated before surgery. Restoring urinary drainage and encouraging a high fluid intake (2 to 3 L/day unless contraindicated) are also helpful in managing the infection.

Patients are often concerned about the impact of the impending surgery on sexual function. Provide an opportunity for the patient and the partner to express their concerns. Inform the patient that surgery may affect sexual function. The ejaculate may be decreased in amount or be totally absent. Most types of prostatic surgery result in some degree of retrograde ejaculation. This may decrease orgasmic sensations felt during ejaculation. Retrograde ejaculation is not harmful because the semen is eliminated during the next urination.

Postoperative Care. The main complications after surgery are hemorrhage, bladder spasms, urinary incontinence, and infection. The plan of care should be adjusted to the type of surgery, the reasons for surgery, and the patient's response to surgery.

After surgery the patient will have a standard catheter or a triple-lumen catheter. Bladder irrigation is typically done to remove clotted blood from the bladder and ensure drainage of urine. The bladder is irrigated either manually on an intermittent basis or more commonly as continuous bladder irrigation (CBI) with sterile normal saline solution or another prescribed solution. If the bladder is manually irrigated (if ordered), instill 50 mL of irrigating solution and then withdraw with a syringe to remove clots that may be in the bladder and catheter. Painful bladder spasms often occur as a result of manual irrigation.

With CBI, irrigating solution is continuously infused and drained from the bladder. The rate of infusion is based on the color of drainage. Ideally the urine drainage should be light pink without clots. Continuously monitor the inflow and outflow of the irrigant. If outflow is less than inflow, assess the catheter patency for kinks or clots. If the outflow is blocked and patency cannot be reestablished by manual irrigation, stop the CBI and notify the physician.

Use careful aseptic technique when irrigating the bladder because bacteria can easily be introduced into the urinary tract. To prevent urethral irritation and minimize the risk of bladder infection, secure the catheter to the leg with tape or a catheter strap. The catheter should be connected to a closed-drainage system. Do not disconnect unless it is being removed, changed, or irrigated. Proper care of the catheter is important. On a daily basis, cleanse the secretions that accumulate around the meatus with soap and water.

Blood clots are expected after prostate surgery for the first 24 to 36 hours. However, large amounts of bright red blood in the urine can indicate hemorrhage. Postoperative hemorrhage may occur from displacement of the catheter, dislodgment of a large clot, or increases in abdominal pressure.

Release or displacement of the catheter dislodges the balloon that provides counterpressure on the operative site. Traction on the catheter may be applied to provide counterpressure (tamponade) on the bleeding site in the prostate, thereby decreasing bleeding. Such traction can result in local necrosis if pressure is applied for too long. Therefore pressure should be relieved on a scheduled basis by qualified personnel. Activities that increase abdominal pressure, such as sitting or walking for prolonged periods and straining to have a bowel movement (Valsalva maneuver), should be avoided in the postoperative recovery period.

Bladder spasms are a distressing complication for the patient after transurethral procedures. They occur as a result of irritation of the bladder mucosa from the insertion of the resectoscope, presence of a catheter, or clots leading to obstruction of the catheter. Instruct the patient not to urinate around the catheter because this increases the likelihood of spasm. If bladder spasms develop, check the catheter for clots. If present, remove the clots by irrigation so that urine can flow freely. Belladonna and opium suppositories or other antispasmodics (e.g., oxybutynin [Ditropan]), along with relaxation techniques, are used to relieve the pain and decrease spasm.

The catheter is often removed 2 to 4 days after surgery. The patient should urinate within 6 hours after catheter removal. If he cannot, reinsert a catheter for a day or two. If the problem continues, instruct the patient to perform clean intermittent self-catheterization (see Chapter 46).

Sphincter tone may be poor immediately after catheter removal, resulting in urinary incontinence or dribbling. This is a common but distressing situation for the patient. Sphincter tone can be strengthened by having the patient practice Kegel exercises (pelvic floor muscle technique) 10 to 20 times per hour while awake. (Kegel exercises are discussed in Table 46-19.) Encourage the patient to practice starting and stopping the stream several times during urination. This facilitates learning the pelvic floor exercises.

It usually takes several weeks to achieve urinary continence. In some instances, control of urine may never be fully regained. Continence can improve for up to 12 months. If continence has not been achieved by that time, refer the patient to a continence clinic. A variety of methods, including biofeedback, have been used to achieve positive results.

You can also instruct the patient to use a penile clamp, a condom catheter, or incontinence pads or briefs to avoid embarrassment from dribbling. In severe cases, an occlusive cuff that serves as an artificial sphincter can be surgically implanted to restore continence. Assist the patient in finding ways to manage the problem that allow him to continue socializing and interacting with others.

Observe the patient for signs of postoperative infection. If an external wound is present (from an open prostatectomy), assess the area for redness, heat, swelling, and purulent drainage. Special care must be taken if a perineal incision is present because of the proximity of the anus. Avoid rectal procedures, such as taking rectal temperatures and administering enemas. The insertion of well-lubricated belladonna and opium suppositories is acceptable.

Dietary intervention and stool softeners are important in the postoperative period to prevent the patient from straining while having bowel movements. Straining increases the intraabdominal pressure, which can lead to bleeding at the operative site. A diet high in fiber facilitates the passage of stool.

AMBULATORY AND HOME CARE. Discharge planning and home care issues are important aspects of care after prostate surgery. Instructions include (1) caring for an indwelling catheter (if one is left in place); (2) managing urinary incontinence; (3) maintaining adequate oral fluid intake; (4) observing for signs and symptoms of urinary tract and wound infection; (5) preventing constipation; (6) avoiding heavy lifting (more than 10 lb [4.5 kg]); and (7) refraining from driving or intercourse after surgery as directed by the physician.

The patient may experience a change in sexual function after surgery. Many men experience *retrograde ejaculation* because of trauma to the internal urethral sphincter. Semen is discharged into the bladder at orgasm and may produce cloudy urine when the patient urinates after orgasm. ED may occur if the nerves are cut or damaged during surgery. The patient may experience anxiety over the change because of a perceived loss of his sex role, self-esteem, or quality of sexual interaction with his partner.

Discuss these changes with the patient and his partner and allow them to ask questions and express their concerns. Sexual counseling and treatment options may be necessary if ED becomes a chronic or permanent problem. (ED is discussed later in this chapter.)

Point out that although some patients experience concerns regarding change in sexual function, this is not a universal concern. Recovery depends on the type of surgery performed and the interval of time between when symptoms first appeared and the date of surgery. It may take up to 1 year for complete sexual function to return.

The bladder may take up to 2 months to return to its normal capacity. Instruct the patient to drink at least 2 to 3 L of fluid per day and urinate every 2 to 3 hours to flush the urinary tract. Teach the patient to avoid or limit the amounts of bladder irritants such as caffeine products, citrus juices, and alcohol. Because the patient may experience incontinence or dribbling, he may incorrectly believe that decreasing fluid intake will relieve this problem.

Urethral strictures may result from instrumentation or catheterization. Treatment may include teaching the patient intermittent clean self-catheterization or having a urethral dilation.

Advise the patient to continue having a yearly DRE if he has had any procedure other than complete removal of the prostate. Hyperplasia or cancer can occur in the remaining prostatic tissue.

EVALUATION

The expected outcomes are that the patient with BPH who has surgery will

- Report satisfactory pain control
- Report improved urinary function with no pain or incontinence

Additional information on expected outcomes for the patient with BPH is presented in eNursing Care Plan 55-1.

PROSTATE CANCER

Prostate cancer is a malignant tumor of the prostate gland. It is estimated that 241,740 new cases of prostate cancer are diagnosed and 28,170 men die annually from the disease in the United States.[15] One of every six men will develop prostate cancer at some point during his life. Prostate cancer is the most common cancer among men, excluding skin cancer. It is the second leading cause of cancer death in men (exceeded only by lung cancer). The majority (more than 60%) of cases occur in men over age 65. However, many cases occur in younger men who sometimes have a more aggressive type of cancer. Almost 2.8 million men in the United States are survivors of prostate cancer.[16]

Etiology and Pathophysiology

Prostate cancer is an androgen-dependent adenocarcinoma that is usually slow growing. It can spread by three routes: direct extension, through the lymph system, or through the bloodstream. Spread by direct extension involves the seminal vesicles, urethral mucosa, bladder wall, and external sphincter. The cancer later spreads through the lymphatic system to the regional lymph nodes. The bloodstream seems to be the mode of spread to pelvic bones, head of the femur, lower lumbar spine, liver, and lungs.

Age, ethnicity, and family history are known risk factors for prostate cancer. (Additional information on ethnicity is presented in the Cultural & Ethnic Health Disparities box on this page.) The incidence of prostate cancer rises markedly after age 50 with a median age at diagnosis of 67 years old.[16] The incidence of prostate cancer worldwide is higher in African Americans than in any other ethnic group (except Jamaican men of African descent).[15] The reasons for the higher rate are unknown. In addition, African American men are likely to have more aggressive tumors at diagnosis and have higher mortality rates from prostate cancer. Differences in survival may be due to body composition, dietary factors, and endogenous hormones.

It is not clear if smoking is a risk factor for prostate cancer. As mentioned earlier, neither is it clear if having BPH increases the risk of developing prostate cancer.[2,3]

Dietary factors and obesity may be associated with prostate cancer. A diet high in red and processed meat and high-fat dairy products along with a low intake of vegetables and fruits may increase the risk of prostate cancer. The role of dietary carotenoids (e.g., lycopene) and antioxidants (e.g., vitamins D and E and selenium) in the risk for prostate cancer is not clear. A large research study found that men who took vitamin E had an increased incidence of prostate cancer, with selenium supplements showing no benefit.[17]

⚕ Genetic Link

Currently no known single gene causes prostate cancer. Some genes or gene mutations are more common in men with prostate cancer. From a genetics viewpoint, prostate cancer can be classified into three categories.

Most prostate cancers (about 75%) are considered *sporadic,* which means that damage to the genes occurs by chance after a person is born. Prostate cancer that runs in a family, called *familial prostate cancer,* is less common (about 20%). It occurs because of a combination of shared genes and shared environment or lifestyle factors. Familial prostate cancer is when two or more first-degree relatives (father, brother, son) are diagnosed with prostate cancer.

Hereditary (inherited) prostate cancer is rare (5% to 10%) and occurs when gene mutations are passed down in a family from one generation to the next. In hereditary prostate cancer a family has any of the following characteristics: (1) three or more first-degree relatives with prostate cancer, (2) prostate cancer in three generations on the same side of the family, and (3) two or more close relatives (father, brother, son, grandfather, uncle, nephew) on the same side of the family diagnosed with prostate cancer before age 55.

Only genetic testing can determine whether a man has a genetic mutation. However, no genetic tests are available to determine if a man is predisposed to developing prostate cancer.

Having a family history does not mean that a man will develop prostate cancer; it indicates that he has an increased risk. Men with a family history of prostate cancer should talk with their health care provider about their concerns. It is important for the health care provider to obtain a detailed family history, including a family pedigree (see Figs. 13-4 and 13-5). Depending on the findings of the family history, a referral to a genetic counselor may be appropriate.

Hereditary breast and ovarian cancer (HBOC) syndrome is associated with mutations in the *BRCA1* and/or *BRCA2* genes (BRCA stands for BReast CAncer). HBOC is most commonly associated with an increased risk of breast and ovarian cancer in women. However, men with HBOC also have an increased risk of breast cancer and prostate cancer. Mutations in *BRCA1* and *BRCA2* cause only a small percentage of familial prostate cancers. Genetic testing may be appropriate for families with prostate cancer that also have HBOC.

Clinical Manifestations and Complications

Prostate cancer is usually asymptomatic in the early stages. Eventually the patient may have symptoms similar to those of BPH, including dysuria, hesitancy, dribbling, frequency, urgency, hematuria, nocturia, retention, interruption of urinary stream, and inability to urinate. Pain in the lumbosacral area that radiates down to the hips or the legs, when combined with urinary symptoms, may indicate metastasis.

The tumor can spread to pelvic lymph nodes, bones, bladder, lungs, and liver. Once the tumor has spread to distant sites, the major problem becomes the management of pain. As the cancer spreads to the bones (a common site of metastasis), pain can become severe, especially in the back and the legs because of compression of the spinal cord and destruction of bone (Fig. 55-5).

🌐 CULTURAL & ETHNIC HEALTH DISPARITIES

Cancers of the Male Reproductive System

Prostate Cancer
- African American men have the highest rate of prostate cancer in the world (except Jamaican men of African descent).
- African American men tend to be diagnosed with prostate cancer at an earlier age, have more advanced disease at the time of diagnosis, and have a higher mortality rate than do white men.
- Although the mortality rate for prostate cancer among African American men is higher than that among whites, the mortality rate is declining.
- Asian American men have a lower incidence and lower mortality rates from prostate cancer than white men.

Testicular Cancer
- Testicular cancer occurs more frequently among whites than in other ethnic groups.

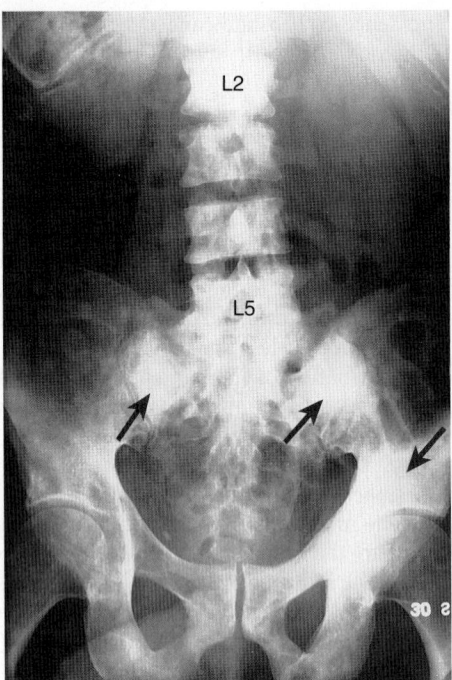

FIG. 55-5 Metastasis of prostate cancer to the pelvis and lumbar spine indicated by arrows.

Diagnostic Studies

Most men in the United States with prostate cancer are diagnosed by PSA screening. Health care providers' recommendations for screening vary. Some encourage yearly screening for men over age 50, and some advise men who are at a higher risk for prostate cancer to begin screening at age 40 or 45. Others caution against routine screening.[18] Although specific recommendations regarding PSA screening vary, there is general agreement that men should be informed about the potential risks (e.g., subsequent evaluation and treatment that may be unnecessary) and benefits (early detection of prostate cancer) of PSA screening before being tested.

At the core of the controversy over routine screening is that many men live and die *with* prostate cancer but not *from* it. As screening has become more widespread, smaller cancers are being found in older men. Slow-growing cancers, in most cases, probably do not need to be treated. However, early detection of aggressive cancers by PSA testing has saved lives.

Patients need to discuss the use of PSA screening in their particular situation with their health care provider. This discussion should start earlier for men ages 40 to 45 who are at high risk of developing prostate cancer (e.g., African American, positive family history). After this discussion, men who want to be screened may have an annual DRE and PSA test. On DRE, an abnormal prostate may feel hard, nodular, and asymmetric.

Elevated levels of PSA (normal level, 0 to 4 ng/mL [0 to 4 mcg/L]), a glycoprotein produced by the prostate, does not necessarily indicate prostate cancer. Mild elevations in PSA may occur with aging, BPH, recent ejaculation, or acute or chronic prostatitis or after long bike rides. In addition, cystoscopy, indwelling urethral catheters, and prostate biopsies may also produce elevated PSA levels. Decreases in the PSA level can occur with drugs such as finasteride and dutasteride.

PSA is used not only to detect prostate cancer, but also to monitor the success of treatment. When treatment has been successful in removing prostate cancer, PSA levels should fall to undetectable levels. The regular measurement of PSA levels after treatment is important to evaluate the effectiveness of treatment and possible recurrence of prostate cancer.

An elevated level of prostatic isoenzyme of serum acid phosphatase (prostatic acid phosphatase [PAP]) is another indicator of prostate cancer, especially if there is extracapsular spread. With advanced prostate cancer, serum alkaline phosphatase is increased as a result of bone metastasis. Investigations to locate a serum biomarker for prostate cancer are ongoing.

Neither PSA nor DRE is a definitive diagnostic test for prostate cancer. If PSA levels are continually elevated or if the DRE is abnormal, a biopsy of the prostate tissue is usually indicated. Biopsy of prostate tissue is necessary to confirm the diagnosis of prostate cancer. The biopsy is typically done by a transrectal resection of the prostate (TRUS) because it allows the physician to visualize the prostate and pinpoint abnormalities. When a suspicious area is located, a biopsy needle is inserted into the prostate to obtain a tissue sample. A pathologic examination of the specimen is done to assess for malignant changes. Other tests used to determine the location and extent of the spread of the cancer may include bone scan, computed tomography (CT), and magnetic resonance imaging (MRI) using an endorectal probe.

Collaborative Care

Chemoprevention of prostate cancer is an active area of research. As discussed earlier in this chapter, finasteride and other drugs used to treat BPH may reduce the chance of getting prostate cancer by up to 25%.[8] Which men may benefit from these drugs is unknown given the increased risk of developing aggressive (high-grade) prostate cancer from these drugs. Men who are concerned about prostate cancer should discuss with their health care provider the potential risks and benefits of taking finasteride.

Early recognition and treatment are important to control tumor growth, prevent metastasis, and preserve quality of life. Most patients (90%) with prostate cancer are initially diagnosed when the cancer is in either a local or a regional stage. The 5-year survival rate with an initial diagnosis at this stage is 100%.

The most common classification system for determining the extent of the prostate cancer is the tumor, node, and metastasis (TNM) system (Table 55-5). The tumor is graded on the basis of tumor histology using the Gleason scale.[19] The scale grades the tumor from 1 to 5 based on the degree of glandular differentiation. Grade 1 represents the most well-differentiated or lowest grade (most like the original cells), and grade 5 represents the most poorly differentiated (unlike the original cells) or highest grade. The two most commonly occurring patterns of cells are graded, and then the two scores are added together to create a Gleason score, which ranges from 2 to 10. The PSA level at diagnosis and the patient's Gleason score are used with the TNM system to determine the stage grouping of the tumor.

The collaborative care of the patient with prostate cancer depends on the stage of the cancer and the patient's overall health. At all stages, there is more than one possible treatment option (Table 55-6). The decision of which treatment course to pursue should be made jointly by patients, their partners, and the health care team.[20]

Active Surveillance. Prostate cancer is relatively slow growing. Therefore a conservative approach to management of

TABLE 55-5 STAGE GROUPING OF PROSTATE CANCER

Stage	Tumor Size	Lymph Node Involvement	Metastasis	PSA Level	Gleason Score
I	Not felt on DRE. Not seen by visual imaging.	No	No	<10	≤6
II	Felt on DRE. Seen by imaging. Tumor confined to prostate.	No	No	10-20	6-7
III	Cancer outside prostate. Possible spread to seminal vesicles.	No	No	Any level	Any score
IV	Any size.	Any nodal involvement.	Yes	Any level	Any score

Adapted from American Cancer Society: How is prostate cancer staged? Retrieved from *www.cancer.org/Cancer/ProstateCancer/DetailedGuide/prostate-cancer-staging;* and National Cancer Institute: Stages of prostate cancer. Retrieved from *www.cancer.gov/cancertopics/pdq/treatment/prostate.*
DRE, Digital rectal examination.

TABLE 55-6 COLLABORATIVE CARE

Prostate Cancer

Diagnostic and Staging Workup
- History and physical examination
- Digital rectal examination (DRE)
- Prostate-specific antigen (PSA)
- Prostatic acid phosphatase (PAP)
- Transrectal ultrasound (TRUS)
- Biopsy of prostate and lymph nodes
- Computed tomography (CT)
- Magnetic resonance imaging (MRI)
- Bone scan (to evaluate for metastatic disease)

Collaborative Therapy
Active Surveillance
- Annual PSA and DRE

Surgery
- Radical prostatectomy
- Cryotherapy
- Orchiectomy (for metastatic disease)

Radiation Therapy
- External beam for primary, adjuvant, and recurrent disease
- Brachytherapy

Drug Therapy
- Androgen deprivation therapy (see Table 55-7)
- Chemotherapy for metastatic disease

EVIDENCE-BASED PRACTICE

Applying the Evidence

You are working as an occupational health nurse at a large manufacturing company. G.N. is a 56-yr-old African American who has come to you for his regular blood pressure check. His father and uncle have a history of prostate cancer. He tells you that he has heard that screening for prostate cancer is "all over the news." He has been getting a blood test for prostate-specific antigen (PSA) yearly and asks you if he needs to continue.

Best Available Evidence	Clinician Expertise	Patient Preferences and Values
PSA screening saves lives when performed appropriately in men at high risk of developing prostate cancer.	You know that G.N. is in a high-risk category for prostate cancer. He is African American, is more than 50 yr old, and has first-degree relatives with prostate cancer. Based on these risk factors, you encourage him to continue to get yearly PSA screening.	G.N. wants the best preventive measures to screen for prostate cancer. He was involved in the care of both his father and uncle when they were sick, and does not want that to happen to him.

Your Decision and Action
You encourage G.N. to discuss his concerns about annual PSA testing with his primary health care provider. You also discuss the potential influence of risk factors and diet on developing prostate cancer and teach him about food to avoid or limit (e.g., red meat, high-fat dietary products) and those to increase (e.g., vegetables, fruits).

Reference for Evidence
National Comprehensive Cancer Network: NCCN stresses importance of PSA testing in high-risk men. Retrieved from *www.nccn.org/about/news/newsinfo.asp?NewsID=218.*

prostate cancer is active surveillance, or "watchful waiting." This strategy is appropriate when the patient has (1) a life expectancy of less than 10 years (low risk of dying of the disease); (2) a low-grade, low-stage tumor; and (3) serious coexisting medical conditions. With active surveillance, patients are typically followed with frequent PSA measurements, along with DRE, to monitor the progress of the disease. Significant changes in the PSA level or the DRE, or the development of symptoms, warrant a reevaluation of treatment options.

Surgical Therapy
Radical Prostatectomy. With radical prostatectomy, the entire prostate gland, seminal vesicles, and part of the bladder neck (ampulla) are removed. The entire prostate is removed because the cancer tends to be in many different locations within the gland. In addition, a retroperitoneal lymph node dissection is usually done as a separate procedure. Surgery is usually not considered an option for advanced stage disease (except to relieve symptoms associated with obstruction) because metastasis has already occurred.

Traditional surgical approaches for a radical prostatectomy include retropubic and perineal resection (Fig. 55-6). With the

retropubic approach, a low midline abdominal incision is made to access the prostate gland, and the pelvic lymph nodes can be dissected. With the *perineal* resection, an incision is made between the scrotum and anus.

A *laparoscopic* approach to prostatectomy is being used in some settings. In this method four small incisions are made into the abdomen. It results in less bleeding, less pain, and a faster recovery compared with other approaches.

A *robotic-assisted* (e.g., da Vinci system) prostatectomy is a type of laparoscopy in which the surgeon sits at a computer console while controlling high-resolution cameras and micro-surgical instruments. Robotics is being used more, since it allows for increased precision, visualization, and dexterity by the surgeon when removing the prostate gland. Compared with traditional approaches, a robotic-assisted radical prostatectomy

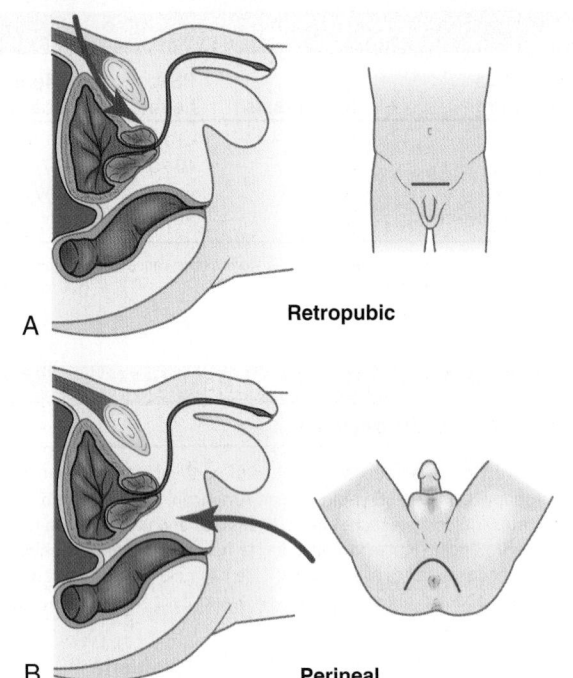

FIG. 55-6 Common approaches used to perform a prostatectomy. **A,** Retropubic approach involves a midline abdominal incision. **B,** Perineal approach involves an incision between the scrotum and the anus.

has resulted in similar surgical outcomes with improved recovery time.[21]

After surgery, the patient has a large indwelling catheter with a 30-mL balloon placed in the bladder via the urethra. A drain is left in the surgical site to aid in the removal of drainage from the area. This drain is typically removed after a couple of days. Because the perineal approach has a higher risk of postoperative infection (because of the location of the incision related to the anus), careful dressing changes and perineal care after each bowel movement are important for comfort and to prevent infection. Depending on the type of surgery, the length of hospital stay postoperatively ranges from 1 to 3 days.

Two major adverse outcomes after a radical prostatectomy are ED and urinary incontinence.[22] The incidence of ED depends on the patient's age, preoperative sexual function, whether nerve-sparing surgery was performed, and the surgeon's expertise. Sexual function after surgery tends to return gradually over at least 24 months or more. Medications such as sildenafil (Viagra) may help improve sexual function.

Problems with urinary control may occur for the first few months after surgery because the bladder must be reattached to the urethra after the prostate is removed. Over time, the bladder adjusts and most men regain control.[23] Kegel exercises strengthen the urinary sphincter and may help improve continence. (Kegel exercises are presented in Table 46-19.) Other complications associated with surgery include hemorrhage, urinary retention, infection, wound dehiscence, deep vein thrombosis, and pulmonary emboli.

Nerve-Sparing Procedure. Near the prostate gland are neurovascular bundles that maintain erectile functioning. The preservation of these bundles during a prostatectomy is possible while still removing all of the cancer. Nerve-sparing prostatectomy is not indicated for patients with cancer outside of the prostate gland. Although the risk of ED is significantly reduced

with this procedure, there is no guarantee that potency will be maintained. However, most men younger than 50 years of age with good preoperative erectile function and low-stage prostate cancer can expect a return of potency after nerve-sparing prostatectomy.

Cryotherapy. *Cryotherapy* (cryoablation) is a surgical technique for prostate cancer that destroys cancer cells by freezing the tissue.[24] It has been used both as an initial treatment and as a second-line treatment after radiation therapy failed. A TRUS probe is inserted to visualize the prostate gland. Probes containing liquid nitrogen are then inserted into the prostate. Liquid nitrogen delivers freezing temperatures, thus destroying the tissue. The treatment takes about 2 hours under general or spinal anesthesia and does not involve an abdominal incision.

Possible complications include damage to the urethra and, in rare cases, a urethrorectal fistula (an opening between the urethra and the rectum) or a urethrocutaneous fistula (an opening between the urethra and the skin). Tissue sloughing, ED, urinary incontinence, prostatitis, and hemorrhage can also occur.

Radiation Therapy. Radiation therapy is another common treatment option for prostate cancer. Radiation therapy may be the only treatment, or it may be used in combination with surgery or with hormone therapy. Salvage radiation therapy given for prostate cancer recurrence after a radical prostatectomy may improve survival in some men.

External Beam Radiation. External beam is the most widely used method of delivering radiation treatments for those with prostate cancer. This therapy can be used to treat patients with prostate cancer confined to the prostate and/or surrounding tissue. Patients are usually treated on an outpatient basis 5 days a week for 4 to 8 weeks. Each treatment lasts only a few minutes.

Side effects from radiation can be acute (occurring during treatment or within 90 days that follow) or delayed (occurring months or years after treatment). The most common side effects involve changes to the skin (dryness, redness, irritation, pain), gastrointestinal tract (diarrhea, abdominal cramping, bleeding), urinary tract (dysuria, frequency, hesitancy, urgency, nocturia), and sexual function (ED).[25] Fatigue may also occur. These problems may lessen 2 to 3 weeks after the completion of radiation therapy. In patients with localized prostate cancer, cure rates with external beam radiation are comparable to those with radical prostatectomy.[15]

Brachytherapy. *Brachytherapy* involves placing radioactive seed implants into the prostate gland, allowing higher radiation doses directly in the tissue while sparing the surrounding tissue (rectum and bladder). The radioactive seeds are placed in the prostate gland with a needle through a grid template guided by TRUS (Fig. 55-7). The grid template and the ultrasound ensure accurate placement of the seeds.

Because brachytherapy is a one-time outpatient procedure, many patients find this more convenient than external beam radiation treatment. Brachytherapy is best suited for patients with early stage disease. The most common side effect is the development of urinary irritative or obstructive problems. Some men may also experience ED. The AUA Symptom Index (see Table 55-1) can be used to measure urinary function for patients undergoing brachytherapy and can be incorporated into postoperative nursing management. For those with more advanced tumors, brachytherapy may be offered in combination with external beam radiation treatment.[26] (Brachytherapy is discussed further in Chapter 16.)

Drug Therapy. The forms of drug therapy available for the treatment of prostate cancer are androgen deprivation (hormone) therapy, chemotherapy, or a combination of both.

Androgen Deprivation Therapy. Prostate cancer growth is largely dependent on the presence of androgens. *Androgen*

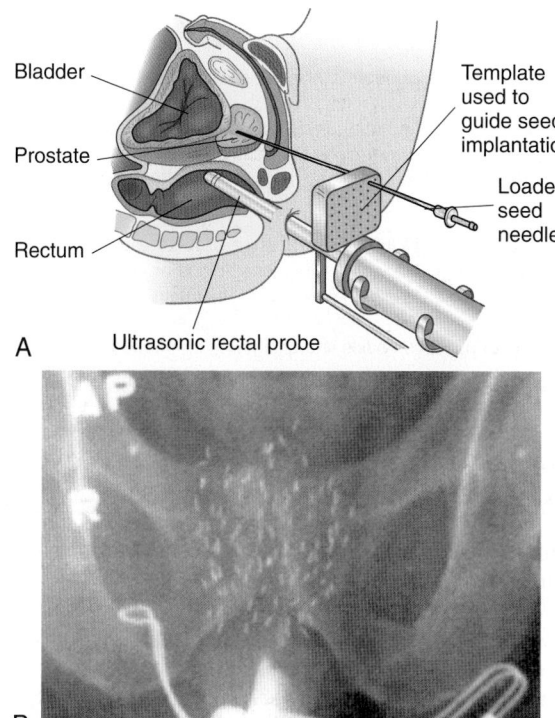

A

FIG. 55-7 A, Prostate brachytherapy. Implantation of radioactive seeds with a needle guided by ultrasound and a template grid. **B,** Radioactive seeds.

deprivation therapy (ADT) reduces the levels of circulating androgens to reduce the tumor growth. Androgen deprivation can be produced by inhibiting androgen production or blocking androgen receptors (Table 55-7).

One of the biggest challenges with ADT is that almost all tumors treated become resistant to this therapy *(hormone refractory)* within a few years. An elevated PSA level is often the first sign that this therapy is no longer effective. Patients taking ADT have an increased risk of cardiovascular side effects, including elevated serum cholesterol and triglyceride levels and coronary artery disease.[27] Research is also examining whether ADT may increase the risk of developing metabolic syndrome.

Osteoporosis and fractures may occur in prostate cancer patients receiving ADT. Drugs recommended to reduce bone mineral loss in these patients include zoledronic acid (Reclast) and raloxifene (Evista).[28] Denosumab (Prolia), a drug that slows the breakdown of bone, may also be used to increase bone mass in men with nonmetastatic prostate cancer.

Androgen Synthesis Inhibitors. The hypothalamus produces luteinizing hormone–releasing hormone (LH-RH), which stimulates the anterior pituitary to produce luteinizing hormone (LH) and follicle-stimulating hormone (FSH). LH stimulates the testicular Leydig cells to produce testosterone. *LH-RH agonists* superstimulate the pituitary. This ultimately results in downregulation of the LH-RH receptors, leading to a refractory condition in which the anterior pituitary is unresponsive to LH-RH. These drugs cause an initial transient increase in LH and testosterone called a *flare*. Symptoms may worsen during this time. However, with continued administration, LH and testosterone levels are decreased.

LH-RH agonists include leuprolide (Lupron, Lupron Depot, Eligard, Viadur,) goserelin (Zoladex), triptorelin (Trelstar), and buserelin (Suprefact) (see Table 55-7). These drugs essentially produce a chemical castration similar to the effects of an orchiectomy. These drugs are given by subcutaneous or intramuscu-

TABLE 55-7 DRUG THERAPY

Androgen Deprivation Therapy for Prostate Cancer

Therapy	Mechanism of Action	Side Effects
Androgen Synthesis Inhibitors		
LH-RH Agonists		
leuprolide (Lupron, Lupron Depot, Eligard, Viadur) goserelin (Zoladex) triptorelin (Trelstar) buserelin (Suprefact)	Reduce secretion of LH and FSH Decrease testosterone production	Hot flashes, gynecomastia, decreased libido, erectile dysfunction Depression and mood changes
LH-RH Antagonist		
degarelix	Blocks LH receptors Immediate testosterone suppression	Pain, redness, and swelling at injection site Elevated liver enzymes
CYP17 Enzyme Inhibitor		
abiraterone (Zytiga)	Inhibits CYP17, an enzyme needed for production of testosterone Inhibits testosterone synthesis from testes, adrenal glands, and prostate cancer cells	Joint swelling, fluid retention, muscle discomfort, hot flashes, diarrhea
Androgen Receptor Blockers		
bicalutamide (Casodex) flutamide (Eulexin) nilutamide (Nilandron) enzalutamide (Xtandi)	Block action of testosterone by competing with receptor sites	Loss of libido, erectile dysfunction, and hot flashes Breast pain and gynecomastia may also occur

FSH, Follicle-stimulating hormone; *LH,* luteinizing hormone; *LH–RH,* luteinizing hormone–releasing hormone.

lar injections on a regular basis. Viadur is an implant that is placed subcutaneously and delivers leuprolide continuously for 1 year.

Degarelix is an *LH-RH antagonist* that lowers testosterone levels. Unlike the LH-RH agonists, degarelix does not cause a testosterone flare because it acts directly to block LH and FSH receptors. It is given as a subcutaneous injection.

Abiraterone (Zytiga) works by inhibiting an enzyme, CYP17, which is needed for the production of testosterone. This drug is given orally.

Androgen Receptor Blockers. Another classification of antiandrogens is drugs that compete with circulating androgens at the receptor sites. Flutamide (Eulexin), nilutamide (Nilandron), bicalutamide (Casodex), and enzalutamide (Xtandi) are androgen receptor blockers. They are taken daily as an oral medication and can be used in combination with an LH-RH agonist (e.g., goserelin, leuprolide). Combining an androgen receptor blocker with an LH-RH agonist is an often-used treatment, which results in combined androgen blockade.

Chemotherapy. The use of chemotherapy has primarily been limited to treatment for those with hormone-refractory prostate cancer (HRPC) in late-stage disease. In HRPC the cancer is progressing despite treatment. This occurs in patients who have taken an antiandrogen for a certain period. The goal of chemotherapy is mainly palliative.

Some commonly used chemotherapy drugs include docetaxel (Taxotere), cabazitaxel (Jevtana), paclitaxel (Abraxane), mitoxantrone (Novantrone), vinblastine (Velban), cyclophosphamide (Cytoxan), and estramustine (Emcyt).

Men with advanced prostate cancer who have HRPC may receive a vaccine (sipuleucel-T [Provenge]). The vaccine stimulates the patient's system against the cancer and may prolong survival.

Radiotherapy. Radium-223 dichloride (Xofigo) can be used in the treatment of patients with castration-resistant prostate cancer, symptomatic bone metastases, and no known visceral metastatic disease. It is an alpha particle–emitting radiotherapy drug that mimics calcium and forms complexes with hydroxyapatite at areas of increased bone turnover, such as bone metastases.

Orchiectomy. Testosterone, produced by the testes, stimulates growth of the prostate cancer. A bilateral orchiectomy is the surgical removal of the testes that may be done alone or in combination with prostatectomy. For advanced stages of prostate cancer, an orchiectomy is one treatment option for cancer control. Another possible benefit of this procedure is the rapid relief of bone pain associated with advanced tumors. Orchiectomy may also shrink the prostate, thus relieving urinary obstruction in the later stages of disease when surgery is not an option.

After an orchiectomy, the weight gain and loss of muscle mass can alter a man's physical appearance. These physical changes can affect self-esteem, leading to grief and depression. Because this procedure is permanent, many men prefer drug therapy over an orchiectomy.

CULTURALLY COMPETENT CARE

PROSTATE CANCER

You need to be aware of ethnic and cultural considerations when providing information about the risk for prostate cancer and screening recommendations. Consider not only the ethnic

---

DELEGATION DECISIONS
Caring for the Patient Receiving Bladder Irrigation

Intermittent or continuous bladder irrigation (CBI) is usually required after invasive prostate surgery to prevent bladder obstruction by clots or mucus.

Role of Registered Nurse (RN)
- Assess for bleeding and clots.
- Assess catheter patency by measuring intake and output and presence of bladder spasms.
- Manually irrigate catheter if bladder spasms or decreased outflow occurs.
- Discontinue CBI and notify physician if obstruction occurs.
- Teach patient Kegel exercises after catheter removal.
- Provide care instructions for patient discharged with indwelling catheter.

Role of Licensed Practical/Vocational Nurse (LPN/LVN)
- Monitor catheter drainage for increased blood or clots.
- Increase flow of irrigating solution to maintain light pink color in outflow.
- Administer antispasmodics and analgesics as needed.

Role of Unlicensed Assistive Personnel (UAP)
- Clean around catheter daily.
- Record intake and output.
- Notify RN if large amount of bright red blood in urine.
- Report complaints of pain or bladder spasms to RN.

---

differences in the incidence of prostate cancer, but also differences in health promotion practices.

African American men have higher mortality rates from prostate cancer than white men. In part this is because their prostate cancer often is more advanced at the time of diagnosis. Despite the availability of early screening measures (PSA and DRE), African American men and those in lower socioeconomic groups frequently do not use them. This is partially related to knowledge levels about prostate cancer. In comparison to white men, African American men with prostate cancer reported more problems with financial access to transportation and health care costs, and they indicated using more religious coping strategies. White men were also perceived as receiving more favorable treatment from their physicians than African Americans.[29]

Although exposure to electronic and print media is successful in informing some men about prostate cancer, the effectiveness differs significantly based on demographic variables such as ethnicity, age, education level, and socioeconomic level. Ideally, all men should be aware of the risks associated with prostate cancer and the screening methods available. Consider the best method to communicate this information to men of all cultures and ethnicities that will result in the greatest degree of understanding and participation in prostate cancer screening.

NURSING MANAGEMENT
PROSTATE CANCER

NURSING ASSESSMENT

Subjective and objective data that should be obtained from a patient with prostate cancer are presented in Table 55-8.

NURSING DIAGNOSES

Nursing diagnoses for the patient with prostate cancer depend on the stage of the cancer. General nursing diagnoses may include, but are not limited to, the following.

TABLE 55-8 **NURSING ASSESSMENT**
Prostate Cancer
Subjective Data **Important Health Information** *Medications:* Testosterone supplements; use of any medications affecting urinary tract such as morphine, anticholinergics, monoamine oxidase inhibitors, and tricyclic antidepressants **Functional Health Patterns** *Health perception–health management:* Positive family history; increasing fatigue and malaise *Nutritional-metabolic:* High-fat diet; anorexia, weight loss (possible indicators of metastasis) *Elimination:* Hesitancy or straining to start stream, urinary urgency, frequency, retention with dribbling, weak stream, hematuria *Sleep:* Nocturia *Cognitive-perceptual:* Dysuria; low back pain radiating to legs or pelvis, bone pain (possible indicators of metastasis) *Self-perception–self-concept:* Anxiety regarding self-concept **Objective Data** **General** Older adult male; pelvic lymphadenopathy (late sign) **Urinary** Distended bladder on palpation; unilaterally hard, enlarged, fixed prostate on rectal examination **Musculoskeletal** Pathologic fractures (metastasis) **Possible Diagnostic Findings** Serum PSA; ↑ serum PAP (metastasis); nodular and irregular prostate on ultrasonography, positive biopsy results; anemia

PAP, Prostatic acid phosphatase; *PSA,* prostate-specific antigen.

- Decisional conflict *related to* numerous alternative treatment options
- Acute pain *related to* surgery, prostatic enlargement, bone metastasis, and bladder spasms
- Urinary retention and impaired urinary elimination *related to* obstruction of the urethra by the prostate and loss of bladder tone
- Sexual dysfunction *related to* effects of treatment
- Anxiety *related to* uncertain outcome of disease process on life and lifestyle and effect of treatment on sexual function

PLANNING

The overall goals are that the patient with prostate cancer will (1) be an active participant in the treatment plan, (2) have satisfactory pain control, (3) follow the therapeutic plan, (4) understand the effect of the therapeutic plan on sexual function, and (5) find a satisfactory way to manage the impact on bladder and bowel function.

NURSING IMPLEMENTATION

HEALTH PROMOTION. One of your most important roles in relation to prostate cancer is to encourage patients, in consultation with their health care providers, to have annual prostate screening (PSA and DRE) starting at age 50 (or younger if risk factors are present). Because of their increased risk of prostate cancer, African American men and other men with a family history of prostate cancer should have an annual PSA and DRE beginning at ages 40 to 45.

ACUTE INTERVENTION. Preoperative and postoperative phases of radical prostatectomy are similar to surgical procedures for BPH (see pp. 1310-1312). Nursing interventions for the patient who undergoes radiation therapy and chemotherapy are discussed in Chapter 16. An additional consideration is the patient's psychologic response to a diagnosis of cancer. Provide sensitive, caring support for the patient and his family to help them cope with the diagnosis. Prostate cancer support groups are available for men and their families to encourage them to be active, informed participants in their own care.

AMBULATORY AND HOME CARE. Teach appropriate catheter care if the patient is discharged with an indwelling catheter in place. Instruct the patient to clean the urethral meatus with soap and water once a day; maintain a high fluid intake; keep the collecting bag lower than the bladder at all times; keep the catheter securely anchored to the inner thigh or abdomen; and report any signs of bladder infection, such as bladder spasms, fever, or hematuria.

If urinary incontinence is a problem, encourage the patient to practice pelvic floor muscle exercises (Kegel exercises) at every urination and throughout the day. Continuous practice during the 4- to 6-week healing process improves the success rate. Products used for incontinence specifically designed for men are available through home care product catalogs and retail stores.

Palliative and end-of-life care is often appropriate and beneficial to the patient with advanced disease and his family (see Chapter 10). Common problems experienced by the patient with advanced prostate cancer include fatigue, bladder outlet obstruction and ureteral obstruction (caused by compression of the urethra and/or ureters from tumor mass or lymph node metastasis), severe bone pain and fractures (caused by bone metastasis), spinal cord compression (from spinal metastasis), and leg edema (caused by lymphedema, deep vein thrombosis, and other medical conditions). Nursing interventions must focus on all of these problems. However, pain management is one of the most important aspects of your care for these patients. Pain control involves ongoing pain assessment, administration of prescribed medications (both opioid and nonopioid agents), and nonpharmacologic methods of pain relief (e.g., relaxation breathing). (Pain management is discussed further in Chapter 9.)

EVALUATION

The outcomes are that the patient with prostate cancer will
- Be an active participant in the treatment plan
- Have satisfactory pain control
- Follow the therapeutic plan
- Understand the effect of the treatment on sexual function
- Find a satisfactory way to manage the impact on bladder or bowel function

PROSTATITIS

Etiology and Pathophysiology

Prostatitis is a broad term that describes a group of inflammatory and noninflammatory conditions affecting the prostate gland. Prostatitis is one of the most common urologic disorders. It is estimated that 12% of all men experience prostatitis in their lifetime.[30] Almost 2 million men are treated for prostatitis every year. The four categories of prostatitis syndromes are (1) acute bacterial prostatitis, (2) chronic bacterial prostatitis, (3) chronic prostatitis/chronic pelvic pain syndrome, and (4) asymptomatic inflammatory prostatitis.

Both acute and chronic bacterial prostatitis generally results from organisms reaching the prostate gland by one of the following routes: ascending from the urethra, descending from the bladder, and invading via the bloodstream or the lymphatic channels. Common causative organisms are *Escherichia coli; Klebsiella, Pseudomonas, Enterobacter,* or *Proteus; Chlamydia trachomatis; Neisseria gonorrhoeae;* and group D streptococci. Chronic bacterial prostatitis differs from acute prostatitis in that it involves recurrent episodes of infection.

Chronic prostatitis/chronic pelvic pain syndrome describes a syndrome of prostate and urinary pain in the absence of an obvious infectious process. The etiology of this syndrome is not known. It may occur after a viral illness, or it may be associated with sexually transmitted infections (STIs), particularly in younger adults. A culture reveals no causative organisms. However, leukocytes may be found in prostatic secretions.

Asymptomatic inflammatory prostatitis is usually diagnosed in individuals who have no symptoms, but are found to have an inflammatory process in the prostate. These patients are usually diagnosed during the evaluation of other genitourinary tract problems. Leukocytes are present in the seminal fluid from the prostate, but the cause of this process is unclear.

Clinical Manifestations and Complications

In acute bacterial prostatitis, common manifestations include fever, chills, back pain, and perineal pain, along with acute urinary symptoms such as dysuria, urinary frequency, urgency, and cloudy urine. The patient may also have acute urinary retention caused by prostatic swelling. With DRE, the prostate is extremely swollen, very tender, and firm. The complications of prostatitis are epididymitis and cystitis. Sexual function may be affected as manifested by postejaculation pain, libido problems, and ED. Prostatic abscess is also a potential, but uncommon, complication.

In chronic bacterial prostatitis and chronic prostatitis/chronic pelvic pain syndrome, manifestations are similar but generally milder than those of acute bacterial prostatitis. These include irritative voiding symptoms (frequency, urgency, dysuria), backache, perineal and pelvic pain, and ejaculatory pain. Obstructive symptoms are uncommon unless there is coexisting BPH. With DRE, the prostate feels enlarged and firm (often described as boggy) and is slightly tender with palpation. Chronic prostatitis can predispose the patient to recurrent UTIs.

The clinical features of prostatitis can mimic those of a UTI. However, it is important to remember that acute cystitis is not common in men.

Diagnostic Studies

Because patients with prostatitis have urinary symptoms, a urinalysis (UA) and urine culture are indicated. Often WBCs and bacteria are present. If the patient has a fever, WBC count and blood cultures are also indicated. The PSA test may be done to rule out prostate cancer. However, PSA levels are often elevated with prostatic inflammation. Thus it is not considered diagnostic in itself.

Microscopic evaluation and culture of expressed prostate secretion are considered useful in the diagnosis of prostatitis.

Expressed prostate secretion is obtained using a premassage and postmassage test.[31] The patient is asked to void into a specimen cup just before and just after a vigorous prostate massage. Prostatic massage (for expressed prostate secretion) should be avoided if acute bacterial prostatitis is suspected, since compression is extremely painful and can increase the risk of bacterial spread. TRUS has not been useful in the diagnosis of prostatitis. However, transabdominal ultrasound or MRI may be done to rule out an abscess on the prostate.

NURSING AND COLLABORATIVE MANAGEMENT PROSTATITIS

Antibiotics commonly used for acute and chronic bacterial prostatitis include trimethoprim/sulfamethoxazole (Bactrim), ciprofloxacin (Cipro), ofloxacin (Floxin), carbachol (Miostat), carbenicillin (Geocillin), cephalexin (Keflex), and doxycycline (Vibramycin) or tetracycline. These antibiotics may be prescribed for those patients with multiple sex partners. Antibiotics are usually given orally for up to 4 weeks for acute bacterial prostatitis. However, if the patient has high fever or other signs of impending sepsis, hospitalization and IV antibiotics are prescribed. Patients with chronic bacterial prostatitis may be given oral antibiotic therapy for 4 to 12 weeks. Antibiotics may be given for a lifetime if the patient is immunocompromised. A short course of oral antibiotics is usually prescribed for those with chronic prostatitis/chronic pelvic pain syndrome. However, antibiotic therapy often is ineffective for patients whose prostatitis is not due to bacteria.

Although patients with acute and chronic bacterial prostatitis tend to experience a great amount of discomfort, the pain resolves as the infection is treated. Pain management for patients with chronic prostatitis/chronic pelvic pain syndrome is more difficult because the pain persists for weeks to months. No single approach has been shown to provide relief for everyone with this condition. Antiinflammatory agents (e.g., ibuprofen, indomethacin) may be used for pain control in prostatitis, but these drugs provide only moderate pain relief. Warm sitz baths may also help. Relaxation of muscle tissue in the prostate using α-adrenergic blockers (e.g., tamsulosin, alfuzosin) has been shown to be effective in reducing discomfort for some men.

Acute urinary retention can develop in acute prostatitis, requiring insertion of a urinary catheter. However, passage of a catheter through an inflamed urethra is contraindicated in acute prostatitis. The placement of a suprapubic catheter may then be indicated. Repetitive prostatic massage may be recommended as adjunct therapy for prostatitis for men.[31] This measure relieves congestion within the prostate by squeezing out excess prostatic secretions, thus providing pain relief. Prostatic massage is performed using the index finger of a gloved hand and pressing down on the prostate, covering the entire gland's surface in longitudinal strokes. Similar to massage, measures to stimulate ejaculation (masturbation and intercourse) may help to drain the prostate and provide some relief.

Because the prostate can serve as a source of bacteria, fluid intake should be kept at a high level for all patients experiencing prostatitis. Encourage the patient to drink plenty of fluids. This is especially important for those with acute bacterial prostatitis because of the increased fluid needs associated with fever and infection. Management of fever is also an important nursing intervention.

PROBLEMS OF THE PENIS

Health problems of the penis are rare if STIs are excluded (see Chapter 53). Problems of the penis may be classified as congenital, problems of the prepuce, problems with the erectile mechanism, and cancer.

CONGENITAL PROBLEMS

Hypospadias is a urologic abnormality in which the urethral meatus is located on the ventral surface of the penis anywhere from the corona to the perineum. Possible causes are hormonal influences in utero, environmental factors, and genetic factors. Surgical repair of hypospadias may be necessary if it is associated with *chordee* (a painful downward curvature of the penis during erection) or if it prevents intercourse or normal urination. Surgery may also be done for cosmetic reasons or emotional well-being.

PROBLEMS OF PREPUCE

Problems of the prepuce in the United States are not common because circumcision has been a routine procedure for many male infants. Circumcision, the surgical removal of the foreskin of the penis, is a procedure done to male infants for religious or cultural reasons.

Phimosis is a tightness or constriction of the foreskin around the head of the penis, making retraction difficult (Fig. 55-8, *A*). It is caused by edema or inflammation of the foreskin, usually associated with poor hygiene techniques that allow bacterial and yeast organisms to become trapped under the foreskin. The goal of treatment is to return the foreskin to its natural position over the glans penis through manual reduction. One strategy involves pushing the glans back through the prepuce by applying constant thumb pressure while the index fingers pull the prepuce over the glans. Ice and/or hand compression on the foreskin, glans, and penis may be done before this technique to reduce edema. Topical corticosteroid cream applied two or three times daily to the exterior and interior of the tip of the foreskin may also be effective.

Paraphimosis is tightness of the foreskin resulting in the inability to pull it forward from a retracted position and preventing normal return over the glans. An ulcer can develop if the foreskin remains contracted (Fig. 55-8, *B*). Paraphimosis can occur when the foreskin is pulled back during bathing, use of urinary catheters, or intercourse and is not placed back in the forward position. Replacement of the foreskin after careful cleaning helps to prevent this condition. Treatment may include antibiotics; warm soaks; and, in some situations, circumcision or dorsal slit of the prepuce.

PROBLEMS OF ERECTILE MECHANISM

Priapism is a painful erection lasting longer than 6 hours that may constitute a medical emergency. Priapism is caused by complex vascular and neurologic factors that result in an obstruction of venous outflow in the penis. Conditions that may be associated with priapism include sickle cell disease, diabetes mellitus, trauma to the spinal cord, degenerative lesions of the spine, and medications (e.g., cocaine, trazodone). Vasoactive medications (e.g., sildenafil) injected into the corpora cavernosa for ED can also cause priapism.

Complications include penile tissue necrosis caused by lack of blood flow or hydronephrosis from bladder distention. With immediate medical treatment, the risk of permanent ED is low.

Treatment varies depending on the cause. In patients with sickle cell disease, a blood exchange transfusion may be done, whereas other patients may be treated with sedatives, an injection of a smooth muscle relaxant directly into the penis, or aspiration and irrigation of the corpora cavernosa with a large-bore needle.

Peyronie's disease, sometimes referred to as curved or crooked penis, is caused by plaque formation in one of the corpora cavernosa of the penis. The palpable, nontender, hard plaque formation is usually found on the posterior surface. It may occur spontaneously or result from trauma to the penile shaft. The plaque prevents adequate blood flow into the spongy tissue, which results in a curvature during erection. The condition is not dangerous but can result in painful erections, ED, or embarrassment. Patients may improve over time, stabilize, or need surgery.

CANCER OF PENIS

Cancer of the penis is rare, with about 1500 cases diagnosed annually. It occurs more commonly in men who have cancers associated with human papillomavirus (HPV) and in men who were not circumcised as infants.[32] The tumor may appear as a superficial ulceration or a pimple-like nodule. The nontender warty lesion may be mistaken for a venereal wart. The majority of malignancies (95%) are well-differentiated squamous cell carcinomas.

Treatment in the early stages is laser removal of the growth. A radical resection of the penis may be done if the cancer has spread. Surgery, radiation, or chemotherapy may be tried depending on the extent of the disease, lymph node involvement, or metastasis.

PROBLEMS OF SCROTUM AND TESTES

INFLAMMATORY AND INFECTIOUS PROBLEMS

Skin Problems

The skin of the scrotum is susceptible to a number of common skin diseases. The most common are fungal infections, dermatitis (neurodermatitis, contact dermatitis, seborrheic dermatitis), and parasitic infections (scabies, lice). These conditions involve discomfort for the patient but are associated with few severe complications (see Chapter 24).

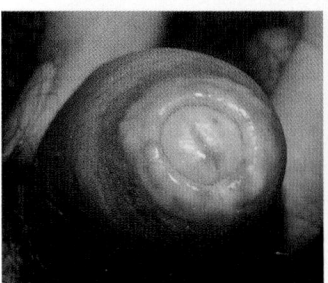 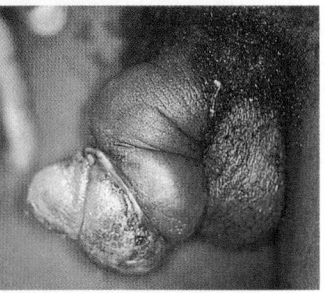

A   B

FIG. 55-8 A, Phimosis: inability to retract the foreskin due to secondary lesions on the prepuce. **B,** Paraphimosis: ulcer with edema from foreskin remaining contracted over the prepuce.

Epididymitis

Epididymitis is an acute, painful inflammatory process of the epididymis (Fig. 55-9), which is often due to an infectious process, trauma, or urinary reflux down the ductus (vas) deferens. It is usually unilateral. Swelling may progress to the point that the epididymis and testis are indistinguishable. In men younger than 40 years of age, the most common cause is gonorrhea or chlamydial infection. UTI and prostatitis are common causes in older men.

The use of antibiotics is important for both partners if the transmission is through sexual contact. Encourage patients to refrain from sexual intercourse during the acute phase. If they do engage in intercourse, a condom should be used. Conservative treatment consists of bed rest with elevation of the scrotum, ice packs, and analgesics. Ambulation places the scrotum in a dependent position and increases pain. Most tenderness subsides within 1 week, although swelling may last for weeks or months.

Orchitis

Orchitis refers to an acute inflammation of the testis. In orchitis, the testis is painful, tender, and swollen. It generally occurs after an episode of bacterial or viral infection such as mumps,

pneumonia, tuberculosis, or syphilis. It can also be a side effect of epididymitis, prostatectomy, trauma, infectious mononucleosis, influenza, catheterization, or complicated UTI. Mumps orchitis is a condition contributing to infertility that could be avoided by childhood vaccination against mumps. Treatment involves the use of antibiotics (if the organism is known), pain medications, or bed rest with the scrotum elevated on an ice pack.

CONGENITAL PROBLEMS

Cryptorchidism (undescended testes) is failure of the testes to descend into the scrotal sac before birth. It is the most common congenital testicular condition. It may occur bilaterally or unilaterally and may be the cause of infertility if corrective surgery is not done by 2 years of age. The incidence of testicular cancer is also higher if the condition is not corrected before puberty. Surgery is performed to locate and suture the testis or testes to the scrotum.

ACQUIRED PROBLEMS

Hydrocele

A *hydrocele* is a nontender, fluid-filled mass that results from interference with lymphatic drainage of the scrotum and swelling of the tunica vaginalis that surrounds the testis (Fig. 55-10; also see Fig. 55-9). Diagnosis is fairly simple because the mass can be seen by shining a flashlight through the scrotum (transillumination). No treatment is indicated unless the swelling becomes large and uncomfortable, in which case aspiration or surgical drainage of the mass is performed.

Spermatocele

A *spermatocele* is a firm, sperm-containing, painless cyst of the epididymis that may be visible with transillumination (see Fig. 55-9). The cause is unknown, and surgical removal is the treatment. It is important for the patient to see his health care provider if he feels any scrotal lumps. He would be unable to distinguish this cyst from cancer when performing self-examination.

Varicocele

A *varicocele* is a dilation of the veins that drain the testes (see Fig. 55-9). The scrotum feels wormlike when palpated. The cause of the problem is unknown. The varicocele is usually located on the left side of the scrotum as a consequence of ret-

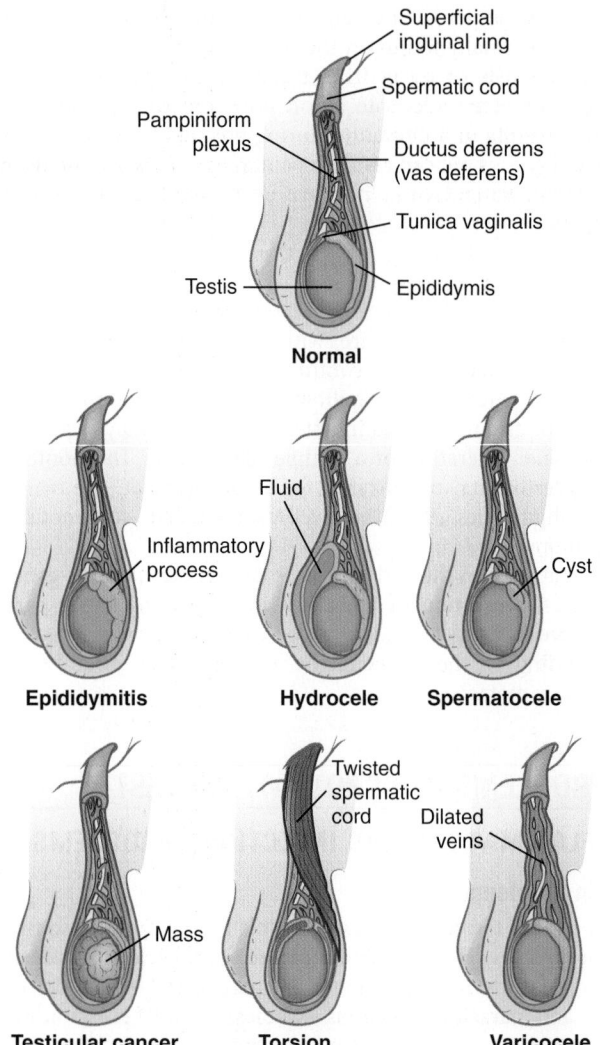

FIG. 55-9 Scrotal masses.

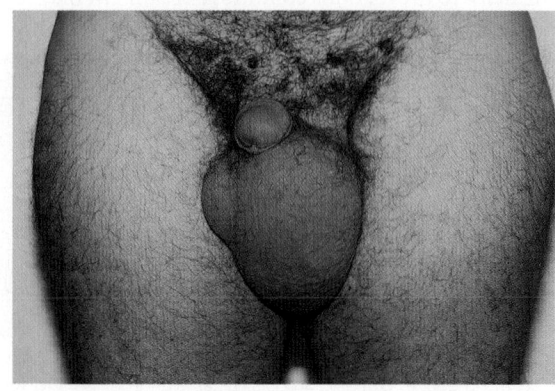

FIG. 55-10 Hydrocele.

rograde blood flow from the left renal vein. Surgery is indicated if the patient is infertile, since persistent varicoceles are associated with 40% to 50% of cases of infertility. Sperm is thought to be damaged by varicoceles. Repair of the varicocele may be through injection of a sclerosing agent or by surgical ligation of the spermatic vein.

Testicular Torsion

Testicular torsion involves a twisting of the spermatic cord that supplies blood to the testes and epididymis (see Fig. 55-9). It is most commonly seen in males younger than age 20. It can occur spontaneously, as a result of trauma, or as a result of an anatomic abnormality. The patient experiences severe scrotal pain, tenderness, swelling, nausea, and vomiting. Urinary symptoms, fever, and WBCs or bacteria in the urine are absent. The pain does not usually subside with rest or elevation of the scrotum.

The *cremasteric reflex* is elicited by lightly stroking (with a reflex hammer or tongue blade) the inner aspect of the thigh in a downward direction. The normal response is a contraction of the cremaster muscle that pulls up the scrotum and testis on the side stroked. In testicular torsion, this reflex is absent on the side of the swelling.

Nuclear scan of the testes or Doppler ultrasound is typically performed to assess blood flow within the testicle. Decreased or absent blood flow confirms the diagnosis. Torsion constitutes a surgical emergency because, if the blood supply to the affected testicle is not restored within 4 to 6 hours, ischemia to the testis will occur, leading to necrosis and the possible need for removal. Unless the torsion resolves spontaneously, surgery to untwist the cord and restore the blood supply must be performed immediately.

TESTICULAR CANCER

Etiology and Pathophysiology

Testicular cancer is rare and accounts for less than 1% of all cancers found in males. However, testicular cancer is the most common type of cancer in young men between 15 and 35 years of age.[33] In the United States about 8600 new cases occur annually with a median age at diagnosis of 33 years old.[16] It is one of the most curable types of cancer. Testicular tumors are more common in males who have had undescended testes (cryptorchidism) or a family history of testicular cancer or anomalies. Other predisposing factors include orchitis, human immunodeficiency virus (HIV) infection, maternal exposure to exogenous estrogen, and testicular cancer in the contralateral testis.

Most testicular cancers develop from two types of embryonic germ cells: seminomas and nonseminomas. Although seminoma germ cell cancers are the most common, they are the least aggressive. Nonseminoma testicular germ cell tumors are rare, but very aggressive. Non–germ cell tumors arise from other testicular tissue and include Leydig cell and Sertoli cell tumors. These account for less than 10% of testicular cancers.

Clinical Manifestations and Complications

Testicular cancer may have a slow or rapid onset depending on the type of tumor (see Fig. 55-9). The patient may notice a painless lump in his scrotum, scrotal swelling, and a feeling of heaviness. The scrotal mass usually is nontender and firm. Some patients complain of a dull ache or heavy sensation in the lower abdomen, the perianal area, or the scrotum. Acute pain is the

initial symptom in about 10% of patients. Manifestations associated with advanced disease are varied and include lower back or chest pain, cough, and dyspnea.

Diagnostic Studies

Palpation of the scrotal contents is the first step in diagnosing testicular cancer. A cancerous mass is firm and does not transilluminate. Ultrasound of the testes is indicated whenever testicular cancer is suspected (e.g., palpable mass) or when persistent or painful testicular swelling is present. If a testicular neoplasm is suspected, blood is obtained to determine the serum levels of α-fetoprotein (AFP), lactate dehydrogenase (LDH), and human chorionic gonadotropin (hCG).[34] (These tumor markers are discussed in Chapter 16.) A chest x-ray and CT scan of the abdomen and the pelvis are done to detect metastasis. Anemia may be present, and liver function levels may be elevated in metastatic disease.

NURSING AND COLLABORATIVE MANAGEMENT TESTICULAR CANCER

TESTICULAR SELF-EXAMINATION

The scrotum is easily examined, and beginning tumors are usually palpable. Instruct and encourage every male starting at puberty to perform a monthly testicular self-examination for the purpose of detecting testicular tumors or other scrotal abnormalities such as varicoceles. Teach male patients, especially those with a history of an undescended testis or a previous testicular tumor, how to perform self-examination.

The procedure for self-examination is not difficult. The man may indicate some reluctance to examine his own genitalia, but with your encouragement he can learn this simple procedure. Guidelines for self-examination of the scrotum are presented in Table 55-9 and Fig. 55-11 on the following page. Encourage him to perform self-examinations frequently until he is comfortable with the procedure. The scrotum should then be examined once a month. Use teaching aids such as videotapes and illustrations on shower hangers, and introduce students to them during high school or college physical education classes.

COLLABORATIVE CARE

Collaborative care of testicular cancer generally involves a radical orchiectomy (surgical removal of the affected testis, spermatic cord, and regional lymph nodes). Some patients with early stage disease do not need further treatment after an orchiectomy. Retroperitoneal lymph node dissection and removal may also be done in early stage disease. These nodes are the primary route for metastasis.

Postorchiectomy treatment may also involve surveillance, radiation therapy, or chemotherapy, depending on the stage of the cancer. Radiation therapy is mainly used for patients with a seminoma, which is very sensitive to radiation. Radiation does not seem to work well for nonseminomas.

Chemotherapy protocols use a combination of agents, including bleomycin (Blenoxane), etoposide (VePesid), ifosfamide (Ifex), and cisplatin (Platinol). (Testicular germ cell tumors are more sensitive to systemic chemotherapy than any other adult solid tumor.) Retroperitoneal lymph node dissection may be done after chemotherapy as adjunct therapy in patients with advanced testicular cancer.[34]

The prognosis for patients with testicular cancer in recent years has greatly improved, and 95% of the patients obtain

TABLE 55-9 PATIENT TEACHING GUIDE

Testicular Self-Examination

Include the following instructions when teaching a patient testicular self-examination.

1. During a shower or bath is the easiest time to examine the testes. Warm temperatures make the testes hang lower in the scrotum (see Fig. 55-11).
2. Use both hands to feel each testis. Roll the testis between the thumb and first three fingers until the entire surface has been covered. Palpate each one separately.
3. Identify the structures. The testis should feel round and smooth, like a hard-boiled egg. Differentiate the testis from the epididymis. The epididymis is not as smooth as the egg-shaped testis. One testis may be larger than the other. Size is not as important as texture. Check for lumps, irregularities, pain in the testes, or a dragging sensation. Locate the spermatic cord, which is usually firm and smooth and goes up toward the groin.
4. Choose a consistent day of the month (one that is easy to remember, such as a birth date) on which to examine the testes. The examination can be performed more frequently if desired.
5. Notify the health care provider at once if any abnormalities are found.

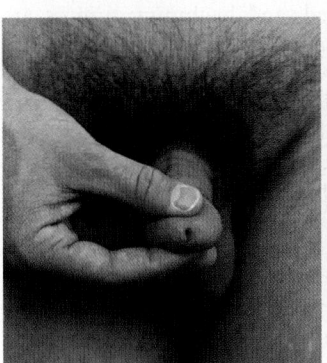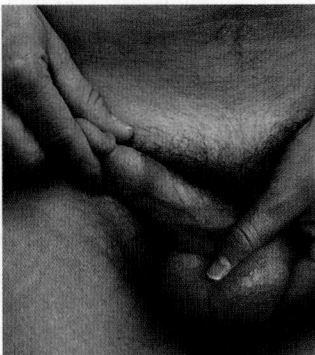

FIG. 55-11 Testicular self-examination.

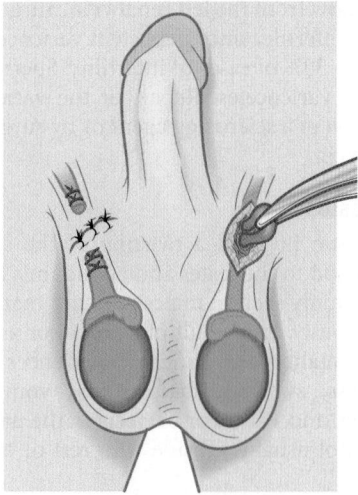

FIG. 55-12 Vasectomy procedure. The ductus deferens is ligated or resected for the purpose of sterilization.

SEXUAL FUNCTION

VASECTOMY

Vasectomy is the bilateral surgical ligation or resection of the ductus deferens performed for the purpose of sterilization (Fig. 55-12). The procedure requires only 15 to 30 minutes and is usually performed with the patient under local anesthesia on an outpatient basis. Although vasectomy is considered a permanent form of sterilization, successful reversals *(vasovasotomy)* have been done.

After vasectomy, the patient should not notice any difference in the look or feel of the ejaculate because its major component is seminal and prostatic fluid. The patient needs to use an alternative form of contraception until semen examination reveals no sperm. This usually requires at least 10 ejaculations or 6 weeks to evacuate sperm distal to the surgical site. Sperm cells continue to be produced by the testes but are absorbed by the body rather than being passed through the ductus deferens. Occasionally postoperative hematoma and swelling of the scrotum occur.

Vasectomy does not affect the production of hormones, ability to ejaculate, or physiologic mechanisms related to erection or orgasm. Psychologic adjustment may be a problem after surgery. It may be difficult for the patient to separate vasectomy from castration at a subconscious level. Some men may develop ED or may feel the need to become more sexually active than they were in the past to prove their masculinity. Careful discussion of the procedure and its outcome before the surgery can help detect patients who may have problems with psychologic adjustment. Surgery should be delayed for these patients.

ERECTILE DYSFUNCTION

Erectile dysfunction (ED) is the inability to attain or maintain an erect penis that allows satisfactory sexual performance. Although sexual function is a topic that many individuals are uncomfortable discussing, health care providers must be able and willing to address ED.[36]

ED is a condition that is significant because of its prevalence, with more than 10 million men in the United States estimated to have ED. It can occur at any age, although the incidence

complete remission if the disease is detected in the early stages. As a result of treatment successes, a majority of men with testicular cancer are long-term survivors.

However, some of the drugs used to treat testicular cancer can cause serious long-term side effects. These include pulmonary toxicity, kidney damage, nerve damage (which can cause numbness and tingling), and hearing loss (from nerve damage). Secondary malignancies can occur as a result of chemotherapy (see Chapter 16).

All patients with testicular cancer, regardless of pathology or stage, require surveillance and regular physical examinations, chest x-rays, CT scans, and assessment of hCG and AFP. The goal is to detect relapse when the tumor burden is minimal.

Prior infertility or impaired fertility is often present at diagnosis. In treatment of testicular cancer, chemotherapy with cisplatin and/or pelvic irradiation often damages the testicular germ cells.[35] However, spermatogenesis can return in some patients. Because of the high risk for infertility, the cryopreservation of sperm in a sperm bank before treatment begins should be sensitively discussed and recommended for the man with testicular cancer. Ejaculatory dysfunction may result from retroperitoneal lymph node dissection. These issues may be hard to discuss with the newly diagnosed patient. Men may think that the disease is a threat to their maleness and self-worth.

ETHICAL/LEGAL DILEMMAS
Sterilization

Situation
C.R., a 43-year-old male patient requesting a vasectomy, informs you that he does not wish to discuss this with his wife. The physician's policy is to have the spouse or partner sign a form acknowledging the patient's desire to be sterilized. C.R. explains that although his wife wants to have more children, the one that they already have is all he wants.

Ethical/Legal Points for Consideration
- Legally, for the competent adult, the only person with the right to consent to or refuse health care treatment including sterilization is that competent adult. It is considered a violation of the right to privacy and the Fourteenth Amendment to limit an adult's right to consent or approve by requiring the consent of another.
- Between consenting and competent adults where there is a legally valid marriage contract, there has been some interest in requiring spousal notification of sterilization and abortion.
- Spousal consent or consent of the husband for sterilization of the wife is certainly a common practice in other countries. However, it has never been successfully required in the United States.
- Prior to sterilization procedures, health care providers can require documentation from the other spouse (not having the procedure) that substantiates the informed consent or refusal, including some document showing that the other spouse has been informed of the procedure and the consequences for childbearing.
- The requesting spouse certainly has the right to select another health care provider for the procedure if that spouse wants to avoid creating that documentation.
- In some religions where the ability to terminate a marriage contract by divorce is very limited, the intentional act by one spouse to permanently limit childbearing by sterilization does provide acceptable grounds to break the marriage contract.

Discussion Questions
1. How would you approach this situation?
2. Are there ever circumstances in which deception of a patient or family would be justified?

EVIDENCE-BASED PRACTICE
Translating Research Into Practice

Do Lifestyle Changes and Cardiovascular Medication Improve Erectile Dysfunction?
Clinical Question
For patients with erectile dysfunction (P), what is the effect of lifestyle modifications and drugs for cardiovascular risk factors (I) on severity of dysfunction (O)?

Best Available Evidence
Systematic review and meta-analysis of randomized controlled trials (RCTs)

Critical Appraisal and Synthesis of Evidence
- Six RCTs (n = 740, mean age of 55 yr old) that examined the effect of lifestyle interventions and drugs targeting cardiovascular (CV) risk factors on erectile dysfunction (ED).
- Interventions lasting at least 6 wk included diet, exercise, maintaining an active lifestyle, and drugs to reduce CV risk factors (i.e., statins to lower cholesterol).
- Changes in lifestyle with improved lipid values were related to a decrease in the severity of ED.

Conclusion
- Sexual function was significantly improved in men with ED through lifestyle modification and drugs for CV risk factors.

Implications for Nursing Practice
- Emphasize the importance of a healthy diet and regular physical activity with men experiencing ED.
- Counsel men that declining sexual health should be brought to the attention of the health care provider for early identification of CV risk factors.

Reference for Evidence
Gupta BP, Murad MH, Clifton MM, et al: The effect of lifestyle modification and cardiovascular risk factor reduction on erectile dysfunction: a systematic review and meta-analysis, *Arch Intern Med* 171:1797, 2011.

P, Patient population of interest; *I*, intervention or area of interest; *O*, outcomes of interest (see p. 12).

increases with age. In fact, it is estimated that about 50% of all men between ages 40 and 70 have at least some degree of ED. ED is increasing in all sexually active males regardless of age. In younger men, the increase is attributed to substance abuse (e.g., recreational drugs, alcohol). Middle-aged men are affected by medical conditions (e.g., diabetes, hypertension) or treatment for these conditions (e.g., antihypertensive drugs) that may cause ED.

Etiology and Pathophysiology
ED can result from a large number of etiologic factors (Table 55-10). Common causes include diabetes, vascular disease, side effects from medications, result of surgery (such as prostatectomy), trauma, chronic illness, stress, difficulty in a relationship, or depression. Although studies suggest a link between cardiovascular disease (CVD) and ED, whether ED is a risk factor for CVD is controversial.[37] A reduction in blood flow is a major factor in ED and CVD, and both of these disorders share many of the same risk factors. Physical inactivity may also be linked to ED (see Evidence-Based Practice box).

Normal physiologic age-related changes are associated with changes in erectile function and may be an underlying cause of ED for some men. Table 51-3 lists age-related changes in sexual function. Explain these age-related changes (if necessary) to reassure an anxious older man regarding normal changes in his sexual abilities. (The male sexual response is discussed in Chapter 51.)

Clinical Manifestations and Complications
The typical symptom of ED is a patient's self-report of problems associated with sexual performance. He usually describes an inability to attain or maintain an erection. The symptoms may occur only occasionally, may be continual with a gradual onset, or may occur with a sudden onset. A gradual onset of symptoms is usually associated with physiologic factors, whereas a sudden or rapid onset of symptoms may be associated with psychologic issues.

A man's inability to perform sexually can cause great distress in his interpersonal relationships and may interfere with his concept of himself as a man. It can also affect the relationship between the man and his partner. Problems with ED can lead to a number of personal issues, including anger, anxiety, and depression.

Diagnostic Studies
The first step in diagnosis and management of ED begins with a thorough sexual, health, and psychosocial history. Self-administered assessment and treatment-related questionnaires

TABLE 55-10 RISK FACTORS FOR ERECTILE DYSFUNCTION

Vascular
- Atherosclerosis
- Hypertension
- Peripheral vascular disease

Drug Induced
- Alcohol
- Antiandrogens
- Antilipidemic agents
- Antihypertensives
- Diuretics (chlorothiazide [Diuril], spironolactone [Aldactone])
- Major tranquilizers (diazepam [Valium], alprazolam [Xanax])
- Marijuana, cocaine
- Nicotine
- Tricyclic antidepressants (e.g., amitriptyline [Elavil])

Endocrine
- Diabetes mellitus
- Obesity
- Testosterone deficiency

Genitourinary
- Radical prostatectomy
- Prostatitis
- Renal failure

Neurologic
- Parkinson's disease
- Cerebrovascular disease
- Trauma to the spinal cord
- Tumors or transection of spinal cord

Psychologic
- Stress
- Depression
- Anxiety
- Fear of failure to perform

Other
- Aging

TABLE 55-11 COLLABORATIVE CARE

Erectile Dysfunction

Diagnostic
- History and physical examination
- Sexual history
- Serum glucose and lipid profile
- Testosterone, prolactin, and thyroid hormone levels
- Nocturnal penile tumescence and rigidity testing
- Vascular studies

Collaborative Therapy
- Modify reversible causes
- Drug therapy
  - sildenafil (Viagra)
  - vardenafil (Levitra, Staxyn)
  - tadalafil (Cialis)
  - avanafil (Stendra)
- Vacuum constriction device (VCD)
- Intraurethral medication pellet
- Intracavernosal self-injection
- Penile implants
- Sexual counseling

have been developed and may prove useful as primary screening tools. For example, the International Index of Erectile Function (IIEF) identifies a man's response to five key areas of male sexual function: erectile function, orgasmic function, sexual desire, intercourse satisfaction, and overall satisfaction.[38]

Second, a physical examination should be performed that focuses on secondary sexual characteristics, including size and appearance of the penis and scrotum. A DRE should be done to assess prostate size, consistency, and presence of nodules. Assessment of blood pressure with palpation and auscultation of the femoral arteries and peripheral pulses should also be included.

Further examination or diagnostic testing is typically based on findings from the history and physical examination. A serum glucose and lipid profile is recommended to rule out diabetes mellitus. Hormonal levels for testosterone, prolactin, LH, and thyroid hormones may help identify endocrine-related problems. Blood chemistries (e.g., PSA level) and a complete blood count may help identify systemic diseases.

Other diagnostic tests may be done to diagnose ED. Nocturnal penile tumescence and rigidity testing is a noninvasive method that involves the continuous measurement of penile circumference and axial rigidity during sleep. Such measurements are used to differentiate between physiologic or psychogenic causes of ED and to evaluate the effectiveness of drug therapy. Vascular studies, including penile arteriography, penile blood flow study, and duplex Doppler ultrasound studies, are used to assess penile blood inflow and outflow. Such studies help assess vascular problems interfering with erection.

Collaborative Care

The goal of ED therapy is for the patient and his partner to achieve a satisfactory sexual relationship. The treatment for ED is based on the underlying cause.

A variety of treatment options are available (Table 55-11). Advise patients that none of the options will restore ejaculation

or tactile sensations if they were absent before treatment. The results of these interventions are usually most satisfactory when both partners are involved in the decision-making process and have realistic expectations of the treatment.

It is important to determine if ED is reversible before treatment is started. For example, if ED appears to be a side effect of prescribed drugs, alternative treatments should be explored. With an established diagnosis of testicular failure (hypogonadism), androgen replacement therapy may sometimes be effective. For individuals who have ED that is psychologic in nature, counseling for the patient (and possibly his partner) is recommended. This counseling should be carried out by a qualified therapist.

Erectogenic Drugs. Sildenafil, tadalafil, vardenafil (Levitra, Staxyn), and avanafil (Stendra) are erectogenic drugs.[39] These drugs are phosphodiesterase type 5 (PDE5) inhibitors that cause smooth muscle relaxation and increased blood flow into the corpus cavernosum, thus promoting penile erection. They are taken orally about 30 to 60 minutes before sexual activity, but not more than once a day. These drugs have been found to be generally safe and effective for the treatment of most types of ED.

Side effects include headaches, dyspepsia, flushing, and nasal congestion. Additional rare side effects are blurred or blue-green visual disturbances, sudden hearing loss, and an erection lasting more than 4 hours that will not go away (priapism). Instruct the patient to seek immediate medical attention if any of these rare reactions occur. Because these drugs may potentiate the hypotensive effect of nitrates, they are contraindicated for individuals taking nitrates (e.g., nitroglycerin).

DRUG ALERT: Sildenafil (Viagra)
- Should not be used with nitrates (nitroglycerin) in any form.
- Can potentiate hypotensive effects of nitrates.

Vacuum Constriction Devices. Vacuum constriction devices (VCDs) are suction devices that can be applied to the flaccid penis to produce an erection by pulling blood up into the corporeal bodies. A penile ring or constrictive band is placed around the base of the penis to retain venous blood, thereby preventing the erection from subsiding. (A VCD is shown in eFig. 55-1, available on the website for this chapter.)

Intraurethral Devices. Intraurethral devices include the use of vasoactive drugs administered as a topical gel, an injection into the penis (intracavernosal self-injection), or a medication pellet inserted into the urethra (intraurethral) using a medicated urethral system for erection (MUSE) device. These vasoactive drugs enhance blood flow into the penile arteries. Current vasoactive drugs include papaverine (topical gel or injection), alprostadil (Caverject) (topical gel, transurethral pellet, or injection), and phentolamine (Vasomax). (These devices are shown in eFig. 55-2, available on the website for this chapter.)

Penile Implants. Surgical implants of semirigid or inflatable penile prostheses are shown in eFig. 55-3, available on the website for this chapter. These surgical procedures are highly invasive and associated with potential complications. Thus they are usually indicated for men with severe ED for which other interventions are ineffective.

The devices are implanted into the corporeal bodies to provide an erection firm enough for penetration. The inflatable implant consists of cylinders in the penis, a small pump in the scrotum, and a reservoir in the lower abdomen. The main problems associated with penile prostheses are mechanical failure, infection, and erosions.

Sexual Counseling. Sexual counseling is often recommended before and after treatment. The ability to please both partners enhances satisfaction levels. Counseling should address psychologic or interpersonal factors that may enhance sexual expression, as well as other factors that are of concern. Counseling can be effective for the individual patient, but it is typically best to include his partner, particularly if he is involved in a long-term relationship.[40] Counseling should begin before the start of medical treatment for ED.

NURSING MANAGEMENT ERECTILE DYSFUNCTION

The man experiencing ED requires a great deal of emotional support for both himself and his partner. Men often do not feel comfortable discussing their problems with others because of society's expectations of a man's sexual abilities. Reassure the patient that confidentiality will be maintained. The majority of men delay seeking medical assistance. They are often highly motivated and expect immediate solutions to their problems. The health care team should provide a support system and accurate information as soon as possible.

Conducting routine health assessments on men seeking any form of medical treatment places you in a unique position. It provides an opportunity to ask the patient questions pertaining to general health, as well as sexual health and function. Given the opportunity, men will be less hesitant to answer these questions when they know that someone cares and can provide them with answers.

ANDROPAUSE

Andropause is a gradual decline in androgen secretion that occurs in most men as they age. The primary male androgen that is reduced is testosterone (Fig. 55-13). Andropause, also called late onset hypogonadism and male menopause, can begin as early as age 40. Factors that determine the rate of decline are not clearly known. Signs and symptoms associated with a lowered level of testosterone include loss of libido, fatigue, ED, depression and mood swings, and sleep disturbances. Symptoms are often attributed to normal aging and frequently are not reported by the patient. The long-term effects, including a loss of muscle mass and strength, may contribute to an increased risk of falls and fractures.[41]

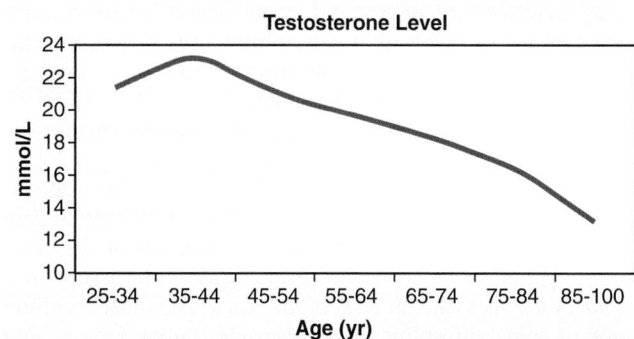

FIG. 55-13 Changes in testosterone plasma level in men as they age.

A diagnosis of andropause is made after a complete physical examination and serum total testosterone levels have been obtained. Normal testosterone levels can range from 280 to 1000 ng/dL. Replacement therapy is generally considered once levels drop below 200 ng/dL.[42] Therapy may be started earlier depending on severity of symptoms. Testosterone replacement therapy (TRT) should not be started until the patient, in consultation with his health care provider, considers the risks and benefits of therapy. Symptoms may improve with TRT, but potential risks include lowered levels of high-density lipoprotein (HDL) cholesterol, increased hematocrit, and worsening sleep apnea. The effect of testosterone on prostatic tissue makes this therapy contraindicated in patients with BPH or prostate cancer. Before treatment is initiated, a DRE and PSA test should be performed. Once TRT begins, patients should be closely monitored by their health care provider.

Replacement therapy is available in different forms. Oral TRT (e.g., methyltestosterone, fluoxymesterone) is not recommended because it is less effective and liver damage can occur with high doses.[43] Intramuscular injections such as cypionate (Depo-Testosterone) and enanthate (Delatestryl) are available in varying doses. These drugs create a cyclic rise and fall in serum testosterone levels with the highest levels 2 or 3 days after the injection. Then the testosterone levels slowly decrease until the next injection. Mood swings can occur with these fluctuations.

Transdermal preparations, including patches and gels (e.g., Androderm, Testim), are more convenient. They are generally applied to the skin daily at various sites, including the back, the arm, and the abdomen. Skin irritation is the most common side effect. Triamcinolone creams (diacetate [Amcort], acetonide [Kenalog]) rubbed into the skin before application of the patch may decrease and prevent irritation. Testosterone may also be given as a buccal tablet (Striant) or as an underarm application (Axiron).

Women of childbearing age and children should avoid direct contact with these products, since they may cause early signs of puberty in young children and changes (virilization) in the external genitalia of a female fetus. Emphasize to the patient the importance of hand washing with soap and water after applying testosterone preparations to the skin. Covering the area with clothing until the preparation has dried is also recommended.

INFERTILITY

Infertility in a couple is defined as the inability to conceive after 1 year of frequent unprotected intercourse. Infertility is a disorder of a couple, not of one individual. For this reason, both partners must be involved in determining the cause of infertility. In about 33% of cases, infertility is primarily caused by factors involving the man. Male infertility can be caused by disorders of the hypothalamic-pituitary system, disorders of the testes, and abnormalities of the ejaculatory system.

The physical causes are generally divided into three categories: pretesticular, testicular, and posttesticular. The *pretesticular* or endocrine causes occur only in about 3% of the cases and can generally be treated with medication or surgery. *Testicular problems* make up 50% of the cases. The most common cause of male infertility is a varicocele. Other factors that influence the testes include infection (e.g., mumps virus, STIs, bacterial infections), congenital anomalies, medications, radiation, substance abuse (alcohol, nicotine, drugs), and environmental hazards. *Posttesticular* causes account for approximately 5% to 7% of the cases, with obstruction, infection, and the result of a surgical procedure being the primary causes. The remaining 40% are classified as *idiopathic,* or of unknown causes.

A careful health history and examination may reveal the cause of a patient's infertility. Thus the history is a starting point for determining cause and treatment. The history should include age; occupation; past injury, surgery, or infections to the genital tract; lifestyle issues such as hot tubs, weight training, or wearing tight undergarments; sexual practices; frequency of intercourse; and emotional factors such as stress levels and the desire for children. Document the use of drugs, such as chemotherapeutic agents, anabolic steroids (testosterone), sulfasalazine (Azulfidine), cimetidine (Tagamet), and recreational drugs, since these drugs can reduce the sperm count. A physical examination can disclose a varicocele, Peyronie's disease, or other physical abnormalities.

The first test in an infertility study is a semen analysis. The test determines the sperm concentration, motility, and morphology. Additional tests that may be helpful in determining the etiology include plasma testosterone and serum LH and FSH measurements. A test for sperm penetration abilities may also be done. The specific cause of infertility is often not determined.

Be concerned and tactful in dealing with the male patient undergoing infertility studies. Many men equate fertility and masculinity.

Treatment options for the man include medications, conservative lifestyle changes (e.g., avoidance of scrotal heat, substance abuse, and high stress), in vitro fertilization techniques, and corrective surgery. Infertility can seriously strain a relationship, and the couple may require counseling and discussion of alternatives if conception is not achieved. (Female infertility is discussed in Chapter 54.)

CASE STUDY

Benign Prostatic Hyperplasia With Acute Urinary Retention

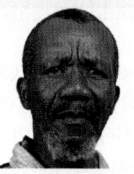

iStockphoto/Thinkstock

Patient Profile

B.G., a 60-yr-old married African American man, comes to the primary health outpatient clinic because of an inability to void for the past 13 hr and pain in the lower abdomen.

Subjective Data
- Complains of the urge to void
- Is restless, anxious, and agitated

Objective Data
- Has prostate enlargement on digital rectal examination
- Has hematuria, bacteria, and WBCs in urine
- Has a tender and palpable bladder above the umbilicus
- PSA test: 8 ng/mL

Collaborative Care
- Indwelling catheter inserted by a urology resident
- Admitted to the hospital

Discussion Questions

1. What risk factors for prostate problems are present in B.G.?
2. Explain the etiology of the objective symptoms B.G. exhibited.
3. Offer possible reasons for B.G.'s elevated PSA level.
4. Discuss the drug and surgical options available to B.G.
5. B.G. asks you about the effect of the various surgical options on his ability to have sex. How would you respond?
6. *Priority Decision:* Based on the assessment data, what are the priority nursing diagnoses? Are there any collaborative problems?
7. *Priority Decision:* What is the priority nursing intervention for B.G.?
8. On further assessment, you note that B.G. has a nursing diagnosis of decisional conflict. How would you help him resolve this conflict related to treatment options?
9. *Evidence-Based Practice:* What information would you offer to B.G. when he asks if he should start taking saw palmetto to prevent future UTIs?

evolve Answers available at *http://evolve.elsevier.com/Lewis/medsurg.*

▌ BRIDGE TO NCLEX EXAMINATION

The number of the question corresponds to the same-numbered outcome at the beginning of the chapter.

1. An older male patient is experiencing difficulty in initiating voiding and a feeling of incomplete bladder emptying. These symptoms of BPH are primarily caused by
   a. obstruction of the urethra.
   b. untreated chronic prostatitis.
   c. decreased bladder compliance.
   d. excessive secretion of testosterone.

2. Postoperatively, a patient who has had a laser prostatectomy has continuous bladder irrigation with a three-way urinary catheter with a 30-mL balloon. When he complains of bladder spasms with the catheter in place, the nurse should
   a. deflate the catheter balloon to 10 mL to decrease bulk in the bladder.
   b. deflate the catheter balloon and then reinflate to ensure that it is patent.
   c. encourage the patient to try to have a bowel movement to relieve colon pressure.
   d. explain that this feeling is normal and that he should not try to urinate around the catheter.

3. Which factors would place a patient at higher risk for prostate cancer *(select all that apply)*?
   a. Older than 65 years
   b. Asian or Native American
   c. Long-term use of an indwelling urethral catheter
   d. Father diagnosed and treated for early stage prostate cancer
   e. Previous history of undescended testicle and testicular cancer

4. A patient scheduled for a prostatectomy for prostate cancer expresses the fear that he will have erectile dysfunction. In responding to this patient, the nurse should keep in mind that
   a. erectile dysfunction can occur even with a nerve-sparing procedure.
   b. retrograde ejaculation affects sexual function more frequently than erectile dysfunction.
   c. the most common complication of this surgery is postoperative bowel incontinence.
   d. preoperative sexual function is the most important factor in determining postoperative erectile dysfunction.

5. The nurse explains to the patient with chronic bacterial prostatitis who is undergoing antibiotic therapy that *(select all that apply)*
   a. all patients require hospitalization.
   b. pain will lessen once treatment has ended.
   c. course of treatment is generally 2 to 4 weeks.
   d. long-term therapy may be indicated in immunocompromised patient.
   e. if the condition is unresolved and untreated, he is at risk for prostate cancer.

6. In assessing a patient for testicular cancer, the nurse understands that the manifestations of this disease often include
   a. acute back spasms and testicular pain.
   b. rapid onset of scrotal swelling and fever.
   c. fertility problems and bilateral scrotal tenderness.
   d. painless mass and heaviness sensation in the scrotal area.

7. The nurse should explain to the patient who has had a vasectomy that
   a. the procedure blocks the production of sperm.
   b. erectile dysfunction is temporary and will return with sexual activity.
   c. the ejaculate will be about half the volume it was before the procedure.
   d. an alternative form of contraception will be necessary for 6 to 8 weeks.

8. To decrease the patient's discomfort over care related to his reproductive organs, the nurse should
   a. relate his sexual concerns to his sexual partner.
   b. arrange to have male nurses care for the patient.
   c. maintain a nonjudgmental attitude toward his sexual practices.
   d. use technical terminology when discussing reproductive function.

1. a, 2. d, 3. a, d, 4. a, 5. b, d, 6. d, 7. d, 8. c

🔁volve

For rationales to these answers and even more NCLEX review questions, visit *http://evolve.elsevier.com/Lewis/medsurg*.

REFERENCES

1. Roehrborn C: Male lower urinary tract symptoms (LUTS) and benign prostatic hyperplasia (BPH), *Med Clin North Am* 95:8, 2011.
*2. Schenk J, Kristal A, Arnold B, et al: Association of symptomatic benign prostatic hyperplasia and prostate cancer: results from the prostate cancer prevention trial, *Am J Epidemiol* 173:1419, 2011.
*3. Ørsted D, Bojesen S, Nielsen S, et al: Association of clinical benign prostate hyperplasia with prostate cancer incidence and mortality revisited: a nationwide cohort study of 3,009,258 men, *Eur Urol* 60:691, 2011.
4. American Urological Association Foundation: Management of benign prostatic hypertrophy. Retrieved from *www.urology health.org/about*.
5. Gerber G, Brendler C: Evaluation of the urologic patient. In Wien A, editor-in-chief: *Campbell-Walsh urology*, ed 10, St Louis, 2011, Saunders.
6. Barry M, Fowler F, O'Leary M, et al: The American Urologic Association symptom index for benign prostatic hyperplasia, *J Urol* 148:1549, 1992. (Classic)
7. Cleveland Clinic: Benign prostatic hypertrophy. Retrieved from *www.clevelandclinic.org/disorders/benign_prostatic_ enlargement_bph*.
8. National Cancer Institute: Prostate cancer prevention trial, National Institutes of Health. Retrieved from *www.cancer.gov*.
9. US Food and Drug Administration: FDA approves Cialis to treat benign prostatic hyperplasia. Retrieved from *www.fda.gov/ NewsEvents/Newsroom/PressAnnouncements/2011*.

10. Barry M, Meleth S, Lee J, et al: Effect of increasing doses of saw palmetto extract on lower urinary tract symptoms: a randomized trial, *JAMA* 306:1344, 2011.
*11. MacDonald R, Tacklind J, Rutks I: *Serenoa repens* monotherapy for benign prostatic hyperplasia (BPH): an updated Cochrane systematic review, *BJU Intern* 109:1756, 2012.
*12. Ahyai S, Gilling P, Kaplan S, et al: Meta-analysis of functional outcomes and complications following transurethral procedures for lower urinary tract symptoms resulting from benign prostatic enlargement, *Eur Urol* 58:384, 2010.
*13. Hermann T, Liatsikos E, Nagele U, et al: EAU guidelines on laser technologies, *Eur Urol* 61:783, 2012.
14. National Kidney and Urologic Diseases Information Clearinghouse: Prostate enlargement: benign prostatic hyperplasia, US Department of Health and Human Services. Retrieved from *www.niddk.nih.gov/kudiseases/pubs/ prostateenlargemen*.
15. American Cancer Society: Cancer facts and figures 2012. Retrieved from *www.cancer.org*.
16. Siegel R, DeSantis C, Virgo K, et al: Cancer treatment and survivorship statistics, 2012, *CA Cancer J Clin* 62:220, 2012.
*17. Klein E, Thompson I, Tangen C, et al: Vitamin E and the risk of prostate cancer: the selenium and vitamin E cancer prevention trial (SELECT), *JAMA* 306:1549, 2011.
*18. Agency for Healthcare Research and Quality: Screening for prostate cancer: summary of recommendations. Retrieved from *www.uspreventiveservicestaskforce.org/uspstf12/prostate/ prostateart.htm*.
19. Cao D: The Gleason score of tumor at the margin in radical prostatectomy is predictive of biochemical recurrence, *Am J Surg Pathol* 34:994, 2010.

*Evidence-based information for clinical practice.

20. National Institutes of Health, National Cancer Institute: Treatment choices for men with early-stage prostate cancer. Retrieved from *www.cancer.gov/cancertopics/treatment/prostate/understanding-prostate-cancer-treatment*.

*21. Quoc-Dien Trinh Q, Sammon J, Sun M, et al: Perioperative outcomes of robot-assisted radical prostatectomy compared with open radical prostatectomy: results from the nationwide inpatient sample, *Eur Urol* 61:679, 2012.

22. Boorjian S, Eastham J, Graefen M, et al: A critical analysis of the long-term impact of radical prostatectomy on cancer control and function outcomes, *Eur Urol* 61:664, 2012.

23. Gandaglia G, Nazareno S, Gallina A, et al: Preoperative erectile function represents a significant predictor of postoperative urinary continence recovery in patients treated with bilateral nerve sparing radical prostatectomy, *J Urol* 187:569, 2012.

24. Dunn M, Kazer M: Prostate cancer overview, *Semin Oncol Nurs* 27:241, 2011.

*25. Cameron S, Springer C, Fox-Wasylyshyn S, et al: A descriptive study of functions, symptoms, and perceived health state after radiotherapy for prostate cancer, *Eur J Oncol Nurs* 16:310, 2012.

*26. Forsythe K, Blacksburg S, Stone N, et al: Intensity-modulated radiotherapy causes fewer side effects than three-dimensional conformal radiotherapy when used in combination with brachytherapy for the treatment of prostate cancer, *Int J Radiat Oncol Biol Phys* 83:630, 2012.

*27. Levine G, D'Amico A, Berger P, et al: Androgen-deprivation therapy in prostate cancer and cardiovascular risk: a science advisory from the American Heart Association, American Cancer Society, and American Urological Association: endorsed by the American Society for Radiation Oncology, *CA Cancer J Clin* 60:194, 2010.

28. VanderWalde A, Hurria A: Aging and osteoporosis, *CA Cancer J Clin* 61:139, 2011.

*29. Dilori C, Steenland K, Goodman M, et al: Differences in treatment-based beliefs and coping between African American and white men with prostate cancer, *J Commun Health* 36:505, 2011.

30. National Institute of Diabetes and Digestive and Kidney Disorders Information Clearinghouse: Prostatitis: disorders of the prostate. Retrieved from *www.niddk.nih.gov/kudiseases/pubs/prostatitis*.

31. Touma N, Nickel J: Prostatitis and chronic pelvic pain syndrome in men, *Med Clin North Am* 95:75, 2011.

32. Lawindy S, Rodriguez A, Horenblas S, et al: Current and future strategies in the diagnosis and management of penile cancer, *Adv Urol* 2011: 593751 (published online 2011 May 30). Retrieved from *www.hindawi.com/journals/au/2011/593751*.

33. National Cancer Institute: Testicular cancer factsheet. Retrieved from *www.nci.nih.gov/cancertopics/factsheet/sites-types/testicular*.

34. Zoltick B: Shedding light on testicular cancer, *Nurse Pract* 36:32, 2011.

35. Bradford B: Chemotherapy-induced infertility in patients with testicular cancer, *Oncol Nurs Forum* 39:27, 2012.

36. Sadovsky R, Brock G, Gerald B, et al: Optimizing treatment outcomes with phosphodiesterase type 5 inhibitors for erectile dysfunction: opening windows to enhanced sexual function and overall health, *J Am Acad Nurse Pract* 23:320, 2011.

*37. Dong J, Zhang Y, Qin L: Erectile dysfunction and risk of cardiovascular disease: meta-analysis of prospective cohort studies, *J Am Coll Cardiol* 58:1378, 2011.

38. Rosen R, Riley A, Wagner G, et al: The International Index of Erectile Function (IIEF): a multidimensional scale for assessment of erectile dysfunction, *Urology* 49:822, 1997. (Classic)

39. Lee M: Focus on phosphodiesterase inhibitors for the treatment of erectile dysfunction in older men, *Clin Therap* 33:1590, 2011.

40. Cleveland Clinic: Erectile dysfunction: sex therapy. Retrieved from *clevelandclinic.org/disorders/erectile_disorder_impotence/hic_sex_therapy.aspx*.

*41. LeBlanc E, Wang P, Lee C, et al: Higher testosterone levels are associated with less loss of lean body mass in older men, *J Clin Endocrinol Metab* 96:3855, 2011.

42. American Association of Clinical Endocrinologists: Medical guidelines for clinical practice for the evaluation and treatment of hypogonadism in adult male patients—2002 update, *Endocrinol Pract* 8:440, 2002. (Classic)

43. Johns Hopkins Medical Letter: Men, should you try testosterone therapy? *HealthAfter50* 22:6, 2011.

RESOURCES

American Cancer Society
www.cancer.org

American Urological Association
www.auanet.org

LiveStrong
www.livestrong.org

National Cancer Institute
www.cancer.gov/cancertopics/types/prostate

National Kidney and Urologic Diseases Information Clearinghouse
www.kidney.niddk.nih.gov

Prostatitis Foundation
www.prostatitis.org

Sexuality Information and Education Council of the United States (SIECUS)
www.siecus.org

Managing Multiple Patients

Introduction

You are working on the medical-surgical unit and have been assigned to care for the following six patients. You have one LPN and one UAP on your team to help you.

Patients

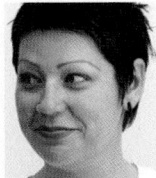

iStockphoto/Thinkstock

L.M. is a 35-yr-old Hispanic woman who went to the clinic 3 days ago complaining of "just not feeling well." She was admitted to the hospital for treatment of hypertension caused by newly diagnosed Cushing syndrome. She has been very depressed and crying because of her physical appearance. Her most recent blood pressure was 150/84 mm Hg.

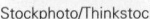

iStockphoto/Thinkstock

N.B. is a 34-yr-old Native American man admitted to the ICU 2 days ago with a diagnosis of diabetic ketoacidosis. He was transferred to the nursing unit yesterday evening. His fasting blood glucose this morning is 296 mg/dL.

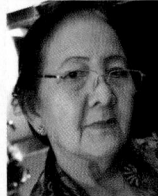

iStockphoto/Thinkstock

A.K. is a 68-yr-old Asian American woman recently diagnosed with adenocarcinoma of her right breast. She had a lumpectomy and axillary node dissection yesterday. She has a Jackson-Pratt drain in her right chest. Her last pain medication was administered 1 hour ago, at which time she rated her pain as a 7 on a scale of 0-10.

B.G. is a 60-yr-old African American man who was admitted to the hospital because of an inability to void for 13 hours and pain in the lower abdomen. He has a urinary tract infection and prostatic enlargement. An indwelling catheter was inserted by a urology resident. B.G. is scheduled to undergo a transurethral resection of his prostate (TURP) this morning.

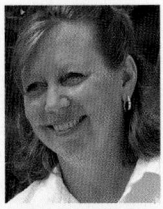

iStockphoto/Thinkstock

R.D. is a 47-yr-old white woman who was diagnosed with Graves' disease 2 months ago. She was treated with antithyroid medication for 2 months and underwent a subtotal thyroidectomy yesterday. She has been complaining of slight numbness and tingling in her fingers.

Jupiterimages/Photos.com/Thinkstock

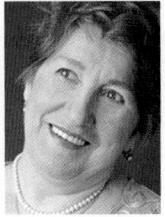

N.B. is a 65-yr-old white woman who underwent a vaginal hysterectomy and anterior/posterior repair 1 day ago. She has vaginal packing and a urinary catheter in place. Her vital signs are stable and she is not complaining of pain.

Jupiterimages/Photos.com/Thinkstock

Management Discussion Questions

1. ***Priority Decision:*** After receiving report, which patient should you see first? Second? Provide a rationale.
2. ***Delegation Decision:*** Which tasks could you delegate to UAP *(select all that apply)?*
   a. Assist N.B. to sit out of bed in a chair.
   b. Teach B.G. what to expect postoperatively.
   c. Take R.D.'s vital signs and report the results to you.
   d. Assess A.K.'s mastectomy incision for manifestations of infection.
   e. Listen to L.M. talk about her feelings while helping her with AM care.
3. ***Priority and Delegation Decision:*** As you are assessing R.D., the LPN informs you that A.K.'s chest dressing is totally saturated with bloody drainage. Which initial action would be most appropriate?
   a. Ask the LPN to call the lab for a stat Hgb and Hct on A.K.
   b. Have the LPN reinforce the dressing with sterile 4 × 4 gauze pads.
   c. Have the LPN stay with R.D. while you assess the patency of A.K.'s Jackson-Pratt drain.
   d. Ask the LPN to stay with A.K. and the UAP to monitor R.D. while you call A.K.'s surgeon.

Case Study Progression

A.K.'s Jackson-Pratt drain was not functioning properly. You get it working and change the chest dressing. The incision is well approximated without signs of infection. When you leave the room, the Jackson-Pratt has a small amount of serosanguineous drainage in it. As you enter R.D.'s room you notice that the patient is having a carpopedal spasm on the same arm that the LPN is taking her blood pressure on. You recognize this as a manifestation of hypocalcemia and notify the health care provider.

4. Which interventions would you expect the health care provider to order for R.D. *(select all that apply)?*
   a. IV calcium gluconate
   b. IV sodium bicarbonate
   c. Have patient hold breath
   d. Rebreathing into paper bag
   e. Parathyroid hormone replacement therapy
5. Which intervention would be most appropriate in caring for L.M.?
   a. Assess her for signs and symptoms of hypoglycemia.
   b. Teach her the need for a high-carbohydrate, low-protein diet.
   c. Administer IV methylprednisolone (Solu-Medrol) over 2 min.
   d. Reassure her that her physical appearance will improve with treatment.
6. B.G. asks you what to expect when he returns from surgery. You explain that he will have a(n)
   a. dressing in his groin as well as a urinary catheter.
   b. 3-way urinary catheter connected to an irrigation system.
   c. patient-controlled analgesia (PCA) pump for pain control.
   d. abdominal and a perineal drain that will be recharged q4h.
7. ***Priority and Management Decision:*** The LPN is assigned to administer medications to N.B., including his sliding scale Novolog insulin with breakfast. The UAP, who is also a senior nursing student, tells you that the LPN administered N.B.'s insulin at least 30 min after the patient ate his breakfast. What is your best initial action?
   a. Report the incident to the charge nurse for follow-up.
   b. Talk to the LPN about the importance of timely medication administration.
   c. Ask the LPN what time the insulin was given and when the patient ate breakfast.
   d. Ask the UAP to first discuss the concern with the LPN so as to follow proper channels of communication.

SECTION 11

Problems Related to Movement and Coordination

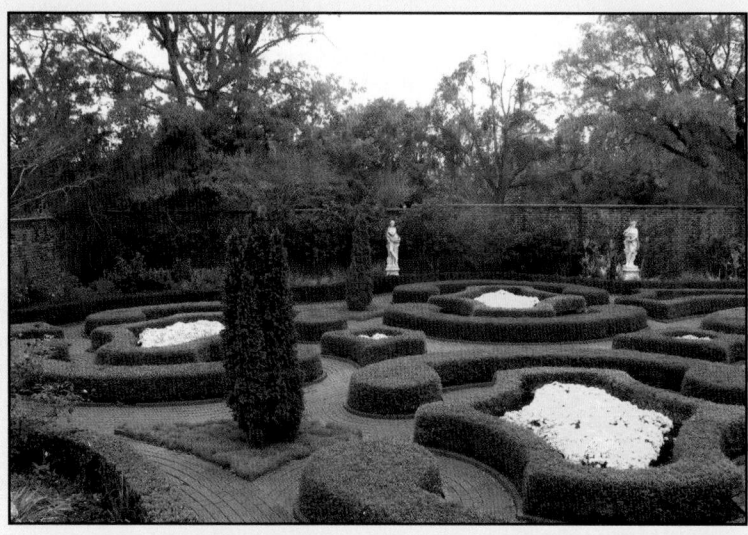

Peter Bonner

If you don't know where you are going, any road will get you there.
Lewis Carroll

The greatest conflicts are not between two people, but between one person and himself.
Garth Brooks

Nursing Assessment
Nervous System

DaiWai Olson

ⓔvolve WEBSITE

http://evolve.elsevier.com/Lewis/medsurg

LEARNING OUTCOMES

1. Differentiate between the functions of neurons and glial cells.
2. Explain the anatomic location and functions of the cerebrum, brainstem, cerebellum, spinal cord, peripheral nerves, and cerebrospinal fluid.
3. Identify the major arteries supplying the brain.
4. Describe the functions of the 12 cranial nerves.
5. Compare the functions of the two divisions of the autonomic nervous system.
6. Link the age-related changes in the neurologic system to the differences in assessment findings.
7. Select significant subjective and objective data related to the nervous system that should be obtained from a patient.
8. Select appropriate techniques to use in the physical assessment of the nervous system.
9. Differentiate normal from abnormal findings of a physical assessment of the nervous system.
10. Describe the purpose, significance of results, and nursing responsibilities related to diagnostic studies of the nervous system.

KEY TERMS

autonomic nervous system (ANS), p. 1340
blood-brain barrier, p. 1342
central nervous system (CNS), p. 1336
cerebrospinal fluid (CSF), p. 1340
cranial nerves (CNs), p. 1340

dermatome, p. 1340
glial cells, p. 1336
lower motor neurons (LMNs), p. 1338
meninges, p. 1342
neurons, p. 1336

neurotransmitters, p. 1337
peripheral nervous system (PNS), p. 1336
reflex, p. 1338
synapse, p. 1337
upper motor neurons (UMNs), p. 1338

Reviewed by Jane A. Madden, RN, MSN, Professor of Nursing, Pikes Peak Community College, Colorado Springs, Colorado.

STRUCTURES AND FUNCTIONS OF NERVOUS SYSTEM

The human nervous system is responsible for the control and integration of the body's many activities. The nervous system can be divided into the central nervous system and the peripheral nervous system. The central nervous system (CNS) consists of the brain, spinal cord, and cranial nerves I and II. The peripheral nervous system (PNS) consists of cranial nerves III to XII, spinal nerves, and the peripheral components of the autonomic nervous system (ANS).

Cells of Nervous System

The nervous system is made up of two types of cells: neurons and glial cells.

Neurons. Neurons are the primary functional unit of the nervous system, Although neurons come in many shapes and sizes, they share three characteristics: (1) *excitability,* or the ability to generate a nerve impulse; (2) *conductivity,* or the ability to transmit an impulse; and (3) *influence,* or the ability to influence other neurons, muscle cells, or glandular cells by transmitting nerve impulses to them.

A typical *neuron* consists of a cell body, multiple dendrites, and an axon (Fig. 56-1). The cell body containing the nucleus and cytoplasm is the metabolic center of the neuron. *Dendrites* are short processes extending from the cell body that receive impulses from the axons of other neurons and conduct impulses toward the cell body. The *axon* projects varying distances from the cell body, ranging from several micrometers to more than a meter. The axon carries nerve impulses to other neurons or to end organs. The end organs are smooth and striated muscles and glands.

Many axons in the CNS and PNS are covered by a *myelin sheath,* a white, lipid substance that acts as an insulator for the conduction of impulses. Axons may be myelinated or unmyelinated. Generally, the smaller fibers are unmyelinated.

Neurons have long been thought to be nonmitotic. That is, after being damaged neurons could not be replaced. The discovery of neuronal stem cells now demonstrates that neurogenesis occurs in adult brains after cerebral injury.[1]

Glial Cells. Glial cells (glia or neuroglia) provide support, nourishment, and protection to neurons. Glial cells constitute almost half of the brain and spinal cord mass and are 5 to 10 times more numerous than neurons.

Glial cells are divided into microglia and macroglia. *Microglia,* specialized macrophages capable of phagocytosis, protect the neurons. These cells are mobile within the brain and multiply when the brain is damaged.

Different types of *macroglial cells* include the astrocytes (most abundant), oligodendrocytes, and ependymal cells.[2] *Astrocytes* are found primarily in gray matter and provide structural support to neurons. Their delicate processes form the blood-brain barrier with the endothelium of the blood vessels. They also play a role in synaptic transmission (conduction of impulses between neurons). When the brain is injured, astrocytes act as phagocytes for neuronal debris. They help restore the neurochemical milieu and provide support for repair. Proliferation of astrocytes contributes to the formation of scar tissue *(gliosis)* in the CNS.

Oligodendrocytes are specialized cells that produce the myelin sheath of nerve fibers in the CNS and are primarily found in the white matter of the CNS. (*Schwann cells* myelinate the nerve fibers in the periphery.) *Ependymal cells* line the brain ventricles and aid in the secretion of cerebrospinal fluid (CSF).

Neuroglia are mitotic and can replicate. In general, when neurons are destroyed, the tissue is replaced by the proliferation of neuroglial cells. Most primary CNS tumors involve glial cells. Primary malignancies involving neurons are rare.

Nerve Regeneration

If the axon of the nerve cell is damaged, the cell attempts to repair itself. Damaged nerve cells attempt to grow back to their original destinations by sprouting many branches from the damaged ends of their axons. Axons in the CNS are generally less successful than peripheral axons in regeneration.[3]

Injured nerve fibers in the PNS can regenerate by growing within the protective myelin sheath of the supporting Schwann cells if the cell body is intact. The final result of nerve regeneration depends on the number of axon sprouts that join with the appropriate Schwann cell columns and reinnervate appropriate end organs.

Nerve Impulse

The purpose of a neuron is to initiate, receive, and process messages about events both within and outside the body. The initiation of a neuronal message *(nerve impulse)* involves the generation of an action potential. Once an action potential is initiated, a series of action potentials travels along the axon. When the impulse reaches the end of the nerve fiber, it is trans-

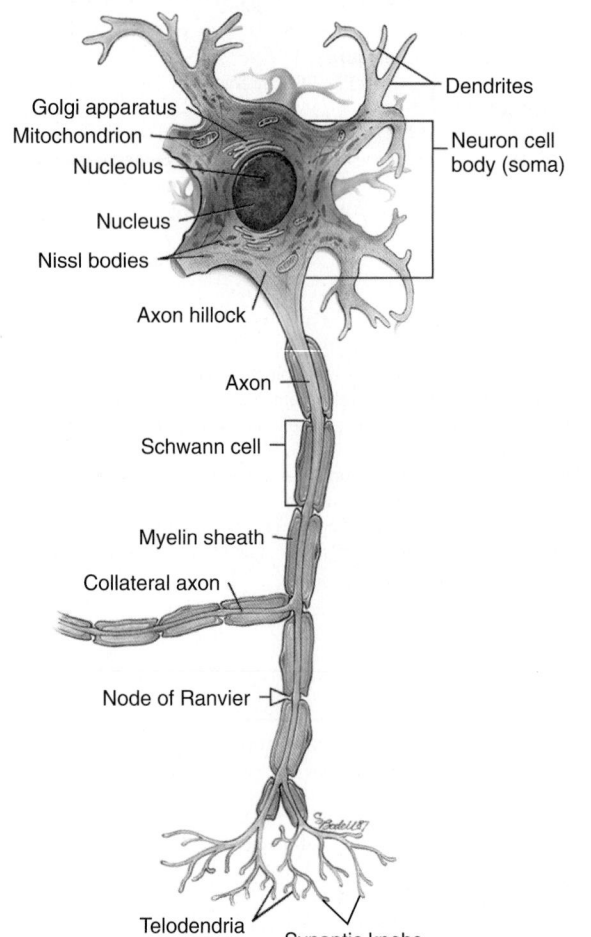

Golgi apparatus
Mitochondrion
Nucleolus
Nucleus
Nissl bodies
Axon hillock
Axon
Schwann cell
Myelin sheath
Collateral axon
Node of Ranvier
Telodendria
Synaptic knobs
Dendrites
Neuron cell body (soma)

FIG. 56-1 Structural features of neurons: dendrites, cell body, and axons.

mitted across the junction between nerve cells *(synapse)* by a chemical interaction involving neurotransmitters. This chemical interaction generates another set of action potentials in the next neuron. These events are repeated until the nerve impulse reaches its destination.

Because of its insulating capacity, myelination of nerve axons facilitates the conduction of an action potential. Many peripheral nerve axons have *nodes of Ranvier* (gaps in the myelin sheath) that allow an action potential to travel much faster by jumping from node to node without traversing the insulated membrane segment. This is called *saltatory* (hopping) conduction. In an unmyelinated fiber, the wave of depolarization travels the entire length of the axon, with each portion of the membrane becoming depolarized in turn.

Synapse. A synapse is the structural and functional junction between two neurons. It is the point at which the nerve impulse is transmitted from one neuron to another. The nerve impulse can also be transmitted from neurons to glands or muscles. The essential structures of synaptic transmission are a presynaptic terminal, a synaptic cleft, and a receptor site on the postsynaptic cell.

Neurotransmitters. Neurotransmitters are chemicals that affect the transmission of impulses across the synaptic cleft. (Examples of neurotransmitters are presented in Table 56-1.) Excitatory neurotransmitters activate postsynaptic receptors that increase the likelihood that an action potential will be generated. Inhibitory neurotransmitters activate postsynaptic receptors that inhibit the likelihood that an action potential will be generated.

Each of the hundreds to thousands of synaptic connections of a single neuron has an influence on that neuron. In general, the net effect (excitatory or inhibitory) depends on the number of presynaptic neurons that are releasing neurotransmitters on the postsynaptic cell. A presynaptic cell that releases an excitatory neurotransmitter does not always cause the postsynaptic cell to depolarize enough to generate an action potential.

Neurotransmitters can be affected by drugs and toxins, which can modify their function or block their attachment to receptor sites on the postsynaptic membrane. When many presynaptic cells release excitatory neurotransmitters on a single neuron, the sum of their input is enough to generate an action potential. Neurotransmitters continue to combine with the receptor sites at the postsynaptic membrane until they are inactivated by enzymes, are taken up by the presynaptic endings, or diffuse away from the synaptic region. With the use of cerebral microdialysis (minimally invasive sampling technique), neurotransmitter levels can now be measured in the cerebral cortex.[4]

Central Nervous System

The components of the CNS include the cerebrum (cerebral hemispheres), brainstem, cerebellum, and spinal cord.

Spinal Cord. The spinal cord is continuous with the brainstem and exits from the cranial cavity through the foramen magnum. A cross section of the spinal cord reveals gray matter that is centrally located in an H shape and is surrounded by white matter. The gray matter contains the cell bodies of voluntary motor neurons, preganglionic autonomic motor neurons, and association neurons (interneurons). The white matter contains the axons of the ascending sensory and the descending (suprasegmental) motor fibers. The myelin surrounding these fibers gives them their white appearance. The spinal pathways or tracts are named for the point of origin and the point of

TABLE 56-1	NEUROTRANSMITTERS*
Neurotransmitter	**Clinical Relevance**
Acetylcholine	A decrease in acetylcholine-secreting neurons is seen in Alzheimer's disease. Myasthenia gravis results from a reduction in acetylcholine receptors.
Amines	
Epinephrine (adrenalin)	Is both a hormone and neurotransmitter. Produced in neurons of CNS and neurosecretory cells of adrenal medulla. Critical component of the fight-or-flight response of SNS.
Norepinephrine	Is both a hormone and neurotransmitter. Has important role as neurotransmitter released from SNS affecting the heart. Along with epinephrine, has important role in fight-or-flight response, increasing heart rate, triggering the release of glucose from energy stores, and increasing blood flow to skeletal muscle.
Serotonin	Primarily found in GI tract, platelets, and CNS. Involved in moods, emotions, and sleep.
Dopamine	Produced in several areas of brain. Involved in emotions and moods and regulating motor control. Parkinson's disease results from destruction of dopamine-secreting neurons.
Amino Acids	
γ-Aminobutyric acid (GABA)	Chief inhibitory neurotransmitter in CNS. Has a role in regulating neuronal excitability throughout the nervous system. Drugs that increase GABA function have been used to treat seizure disorders.
Glutamate and aspartate	Plays key role in learning and memory. Sustained release of glutamate and prolonged excitation is toxic to nerve cells. Glutamate is a destructive factor in amyotrophic lateral sclerosis.
Neuropeptides	
Endorphins and enkephalins	Endogenous opioids that function as neurotransmitters. Produced in pituitary gland and hypothalamus. Produce analgesia and a feeling of well-being. The opioids morphine and heroin bind to endorphin and enkephalin receptors and produce the same effect as the endogenous opioids.
Substance P	Neurotransmitter in pain transmission pathways. Morphine blocks its release.

*These are examples only. Most of the neurotransmitters are also found in other locations and may have additional functions.
CNS, Central nervous system; *SNS,* sympathetic nervous system.

destination (e.g., spinocerebellar tract [ascending], corticospinal tract [descending]).

Ascending Tracts. In general, the ascending tracts carry specific sensory information to higher levels of the CNS. This information comes from special sensory receptors in the skin, muscles and joints, viscera, and blood vessels and enters the spinal cord by way of the dorsal roots of the spinal nerves. The fasciculus gracilis and the fasciculus cuneatus (commonly called the dorsal or posterior columns) carry information and transmit impulses concerned with touch, deep pressure, vibration, position sense, and kinesthesia (appreciation of movement,

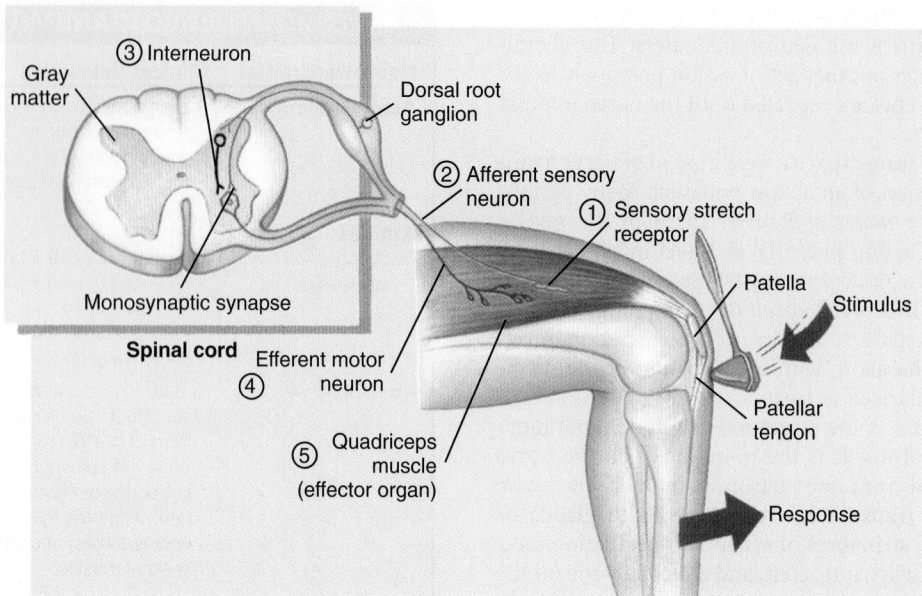

FIG. 56-2 Basic diagram of the patellar "knee jerk" reflex arc, including the *(1)* sensory stretch receptor, *(2)* afferent sensory neuron, *(3)* interneuron, *(4)* efferent motor neuron, and *(5)* quadriceps muscle (effector organ).

weight, and body parts). The *spinocerebellar tracts* carry information about muscle tension and body position to the cerebellum for coordination of movement. The *spinothalamic tracts* carry pain and temperature sensations. Therefore the ascending tracts are organized by sensory modality, as well as by anatomy.

Although the functions of these pathways are generally accepted, other ascending tracts may also carry sensory modalities. The symptoms of various neurologic diseases suggest that additional pathways for touch, position sense, and vibration exist.

Descending Tracts. Descending tracts carry impulses that are responsible for muscle movement. Among the most important descending tracts are the corticobulbar and corticospinal tracts, collectively termed the *pyramidal tract.* These tracts carry volitional (voluntary) impulses from the cerebral cortex to the cranial and peripheral nerves. Another group of descending motor tracts carries impulses from the extrapyramidal system (all motor systems except the pyramidal) concerned with voluntary movement. It includes pathways originating in the brainstem, basal ganglia, and cerebellum. The motor output exits the spinal cord by way of the ventral roots of the spinal nerves.

Lower and Upper Motor Neurons. Lower motor neurons (LMNs) are the final common pathway through which descending motor tracts influence skeletal muscle. The cell bodies of LMNs, which send axons to innervate the skeletal muscles of the arms, trunk, and legs, are located in the anterior horn of the corresponding segments of the spinal cord (e.g., cervical segments contain LMNs for the arms). LMNs for skeletal muscles of the eyes, face, mouth, and throat are located in the corresponding segments of the brainstem. These cell bodies and their axons make up the somatic motor components of the cranial nerves. LMN lesions generally cause weakness or paralysis, denervation atrophy, hyporeflexia or areflexia, and decreased muscle tone (flaccidity).

Upper motor neurons (UMNs) originate in the cerebral cortex and project downward. The corticobulbar tract ends in the brainstem, and the corticospinal tract descends into the spinal cord. These neurons influence skeletal muscle movement.

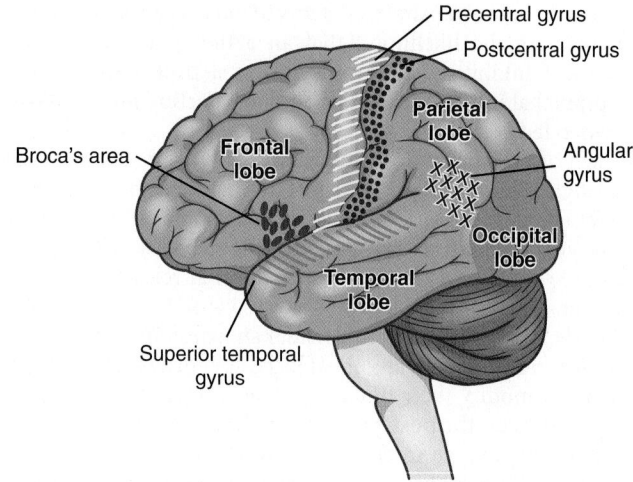

FIG. 56-3 Left hemisphere of cerebrum, lateral surface, showing major lobes and areas of the brain.

UMN lesions generally cause weakness or paralysis, disuse atrophy, hyperreflexia, and increased muscle tone (spasticity).

Reflex Arc. A reflex is an involuntary response to stimuli. In the spinal cord, reflex arcs play an important role in maintaining muscle tone, which is essential for body posture. The components of a monosynaptic reflex arc (Fig. 56-2) are a receptor organ, an afferent neuron, an effector neuron, and an effector organ (e.g., skeletal muscle). The afferent neuron synapses with the efferent neuron in the gray matter of the spinal cord. More complex reflex arcs have other neurons (interneurons) in addition to the afferent neuron influencing the effector neuron.

Brain. The term *brain* usually refers to the three major intracranial components: cerebrum, brainstem, and cerebellum.

Cerebrum. The *cerebrum* is composed of the right and left cerebral hemispheres and divided into four lobes: frontal, temporal, parietal, and occipital (Fig. 56-3). The functions of the cerebrum are multiple and complex (Table 56-2). The *frontal lobe* controls higher cognitive function, memory retention, vol-

TABLE 56-2 FUNCTION OF CEREBRUM

Part	Location	Function
Cortical Areas		
Motor		
Primary	Precentral gyrus	Motor control and movement on opposite side of body
Supplemental	Anterior to precentral gyrus	Facilitates proximal muscle activity, including activity for stance and gait, and spontaneous movement and coordination
Sensory		
Somatic	Postcentral gyrus	Sensory response from opposite side of body
Visual	Occipital lobe	Registers visual images
Auditory	Superior temporal gyrus	Registers auditory input
Association areas	Parietal lobe	Integrates somatic and sensory input
	Posterior temporal lobe	Integrates visual and auditory input for language comprehension
	Anterior temporal lobe	Integrates past experiences
	Anterior frontal lobe	Controls higher-order processes (e.g., judgment, reasoning)
Language		
Comprehension	Wernicke's area	Integrates auditory language (understanding of spoken words)
Expression	Broca's area	Regulates verbal expression
Basal Ganglia	Near lateral ventricles of both cerebral hemispheres	Control and facilitate learned and automatic movements
Thalamus	Below basal ganglia	Relays sensory and motor input to and from the cerebrum
Hypothalamus	Below thalamus	Regulates endocrine and autonomic functions
Limbic System	Lateral to hypothalamus	Influences emotional behavior and basic drives such as feeding and sexual behavior

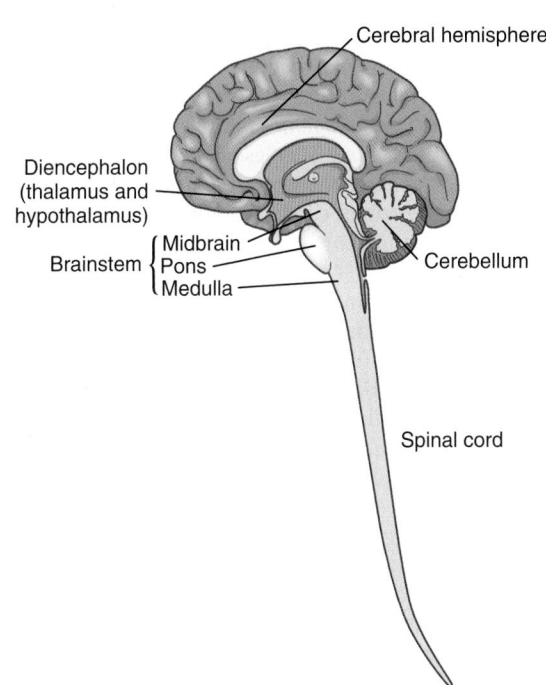

FIG. 56-4 Major divisions of the central nervous system (CNS).

midbrain. Most of them are on both sides of the thalamus. The function of the basal ganglia includes the initiation, execution, and completion of voluntary movements, learning, emotional response, and automatic movements associated with skeletal muscle activity (e.g., swinging the arms while walking, swallowing saliva, and blinking).

The *thalamus* (part of the diencephalon) lies directly above the brainstem (Fig. 56-4) and is the major relay center for afferent inputs to the cerebral cortex. The *hypothalamus* is located just inferior to the thalamus and slightly in front of the midbrain. It regulates the ANS and the endocrine system. The *limbic system* is located near the inner surfaces of the cerebral hemispheres and is concerned with emotion, aggression, feeding behavior, and sexual response.

Brainstem. The *brainstem* includes the midbrain, pons, and medulla (see Fig. 56-4). Ascending and descending fibers to and from the cerebrum and cerebellum pass through the brainstem. The nuclei of cranial nerves III through XII are in the brainstem. The vital centers concerned with respiratory, vasomotor, and cardiac function are located in the medulla.

Also located in the brainstem is the *reticular formation,* a diffusely arranged group of neurons and their axons that extends from the medulla to the thalamus and hypothalamus. The functions of the reticular formation include relaying sensory information, influencing excitatory and inhibitory control of spinal motor neurons, and controlling vasomotor and respiratory activity. The *reticular activating system* (RAS) is a complex system that requires communication among the brainstem, reticular formation, and cerebral cortex. The RAS is responsible for regulating arousal and sleep-wake transitions. The brainstem also contains the centers for sneezing, coughing, hiccupping, vomiting, sucking, and swallowing.

Cerebellum. The *cerebellum* is located in the posterior part of the cranial fossa inferior to the occipital lobe. The cerebellum coordinates voluntary movement and maintains trunk stability and equilibrium. The cerebellum receives information from the

untary eye movements, voluntary motor movement, and speech in Broca's area. The *temporal lobe* integrates somatic, visual, and auditory data and contains Wernicke's speech area. The *parietal lobe* interprets spatial information and contains the sensory cortex. Processing of sight takes place in the *occipital lobe.*

The division of the cerebrum into lobes is useful to delineate portions of the neocortex (gray matter), which makes up the outer layer of the cerebral hemispheres. Neurons in specific parts of the neocortex are essential for various highly complex and sophisticated aspects of mental function, such as language, memory, and appreciation of visual-spatial relationships.

The basal ganglia, thalamus, hypothalamus, and limbic system are also located in the cerebrum. The *basal ganglia* are a group of structures located centrally in the cerebrum and

cerebral cortex, muscles, joints, and inner ear. It influences motor activity through axonal connections to the motor cortex, the brainstem nuclei, and their descending pathways.

Ventricles and Cerebrospinal Fluid. The ventricles are four interconnected fluid-filled cavities. The lower portion of the fourth ventricle becomes the central canal in the lower part of the brainstem. The spinal canal extends centrally through the full length of the spinal cord.

Cerebrospinal fluid (CSF) circulates within the subarachnoid space that surrounds the brain, brainstem, and spinal cord. This fluid provides cushioning for the brain and the spinal cord, allows fluid shifts from the cranial cavity to the spinal cavity, and carries nutrients. The formation of CSF in the choroid plexus in the ventricles involves both passive diffusion and active transport of substances. CSF resembles an ultrafiltrate of blood. Although CSF is produced at an average rate of about 500 mL/day, many factors influence CSF production and absorption. The ventricles and central canal are normally filled with an average of 135 mL of CSF. Changes in the rate of production or absorption will result in a change in the volume of CSF that remains in the ventricles and central canal. Excessive buildup of CSF results in a condition known as *hydrocephalus*.

The CSF circulates throughout the ventricles and seeps into the subarachnoid space surrounding the brain and spinal cord. It is absorbed primarily through the *arachnoid villi* (tiny projections into the subarachnoid space), into the intradural venous sinuses, and eventually into the venous system.

The analysis of CSF composition provides useful diagnostic information related to certain nervous system diseases. CSF pressure is often measured in patients with actual or suspected intracranial injury. Increased intracranial pressure, indicated by increased CSF pressure, can force downward (central) herniation of the brain and brainstem. The signs marking this event are part of the herniation syndrome (see Chapter 57).

Peripheral Nervous System

The PNS includes all the neuronal structures that lie outside the CNS. It consists of the spinal and cranial nerves, their associated ganglia (groupings of cell bodies), and portions of the ANS.

Spinal Nerves. The spinal cord can be seen as a series of spinal segments, one on top of another. In addition to the cell bodies, each segment contains a pair of dorsal (afferent) sensory nerve fibers or roots and ventral (efferent) motor fibers or roots, which innervate a specific region of the body. This combined motor-sensory nerve is called a *spinal nerve* (Fig. 56-5). The cell bodies of the voluntary motor system are located in the anterior horn of the spinal cord gray matter. The cell bodies of the autonomic (involuntary) motor system are located in the anterolateral portion of the spinal cord gray matter. The cell bodies of sensory fibers are located in the dorsal root ganglia just outside the spinal cord. On exiting the spinal column, each spinal nerve divides into ventral and dorsal rami, a collection of motor and sensory fibers that eventually goes to peripheral structures (e.g., skin, muscles, viscera).

A dermatome is the area of skin innervated by the sensory fibers of a single dorsal root of a spinal nerve (Fig. 56-6). The dermatomes give a general picture of somatic sensory innervation by spinal segments. A *myotome* is a muscle group innervated by the primary motor neurons of a single ventral root. The dermatomes and myotomes of a given spinal segment

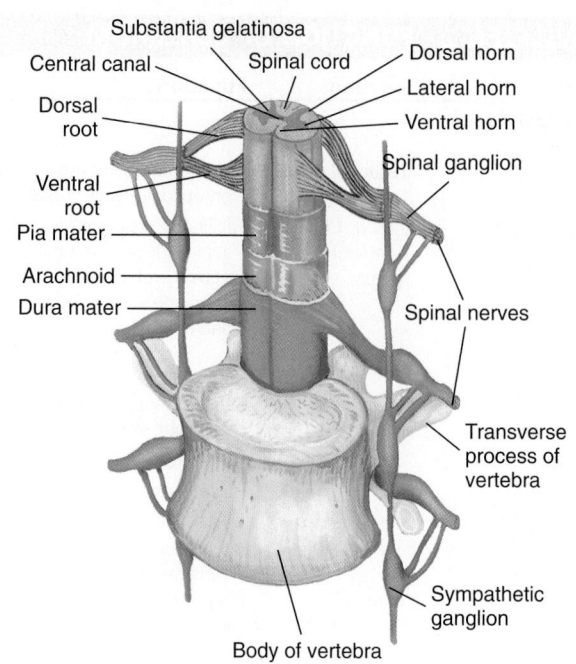

FIG. 56-5 Cross section of spinal cord showing attachments of spinal nerves and coverings of the spinal cord.

overlap with those of adjacent segments because of the development of ascending and descending collateral branches of nerve fibers.

Cranial Nerves. The cranial nerves (CNs) are the 12 paired nerves composed of cell bodies with fibers that exit from the cranial cavity. Unlike the spinal nerves, which always have both afferent sensory and efferent motor fibers, some CNs are only sensory, some only motor, and some both.

Table 56-3 summarizes the motor and sensory components of the CNs. Fig. 56-7 shows the position of the CNs in relation to the brain and spinal cord. Just as the cell bodies of the spinal nerves are located in specific segments of the spinal cord, so are the cell bodies (nuclei) of the CNs located in specific segments of the brain. Exceptions are the nuclei of the olfactory and optic nerves. The primary cell bodies of the olfactory nerve are located in the nasal epithelium, and those of the optic nerve are in the retina.

Autonomic Nervous System. The autonomic nervous system (ANS) is divided into the sympathetic and parasympathetic systems. The ANS governs involuntary functions of cardiac muscle, smooth muscle, and glands through both efferent and afferent pathways. The two systems function together to maintain a relatively balanced internal environment. The preganglionic cell bodies of the *sympathetic nervous system* (SNS) are located in spinal segments T1 through L2. The major neurotransmitter released by the postganglionic fibers of the SNS is norepinephrine, and the neurotransmitter released by the preganglionic fibers is acetylcholine.

The preganglionic cell bodies of the *parasympathetic nervous system* (PSNS) are located in the brainstem and the sacral spinal segments (S2 through S4). Acetylcholine is the neurotransmitter released at both preganglionic and postganglionic nerve endings. (The effects of the SNS and PSNS are compared in eTable 56-1 available on the website for this chapter.)

SNS stimulation activates the mechanisms required for the "fight-or-flight" response that occurs throughout the body. In

TABLE 56-3 CRANIAL NERVES

Nerve	Connection With Brain	Function
I Olfactory	Anterior ventral cerebrum	*Sensory:* from olfactory (smell)
II Optic	Lateral geniculate body of the thalamus	*Sensory:* from retina of eyes (vision)
III Oculomotor	Midbrain	*Motor:* to four eye movement muscles and levator palpebrae muscle *Parasympathetic:* smooth muscle in eyeball
IV Trochlear	Midbrain	*Motor:* to one eye movement muscle, the superior oblique muscle
V Trigeminal		
• Ophthalmic branch	Pons	*Sensory:* from forehead, eye, superior nasal cavity
• Maxillary branch	Pons	*Sensory:* from inferior nasal cavity, face, upper teeth, mucosa of superior mouth
• Mandibular branch	Pons	*Sensory:* from surfaces of jaw, lower teeth, mucosa of lower mouth, and anterior tongue *Motor:* to muscles of mastication
VI Abducens	Pons	*Motor:* to the lateral rectus of the eye
VII Facial	Junction of pons and medulla	*Motor:* to facial muscles of expression and cheek muscle *Sensory:* taste from anterior two thirds of tongue
VIII Vestibulocochlear		
• Vestibular branch	Junction of pons and medulla	*Sensory:* from equilibrium sensory organ, the vestibular apparatus
• Cochlear branch	Junction of pons and medulla	*Sensory:* from auditory sensory organ, the cochlea
IX Glossopharyngeal	Medulla	*Sensory:* from pharynx and posterior tongue, including taste *Motor:* to superior pharyngeal muscles
X Vagus	Medulla	*Sensory:* from much of viscera of thorax and abdomen *Motor:* to larynx and middle and inferior pharyngeal muscles *Parasympathetic:* heart, lungs, most of digestive system
XI Accessory	Medulla and superior spinal segments	*Motor:* to sternocleidomastoid and trapezius muscles
XII Hypoglossal	Medulla	*Motor:* to muscles of tongue

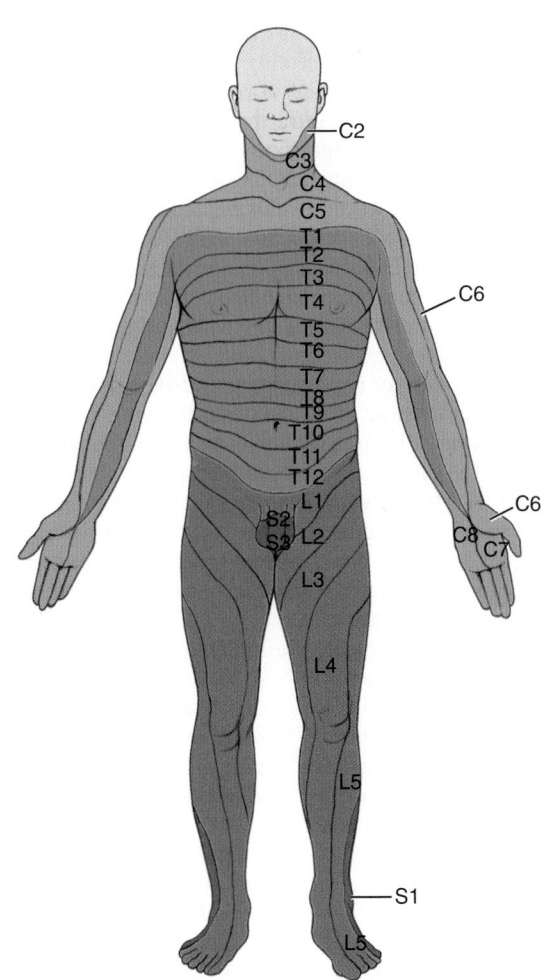

FIG. 56-6 Dermatomes of the body.

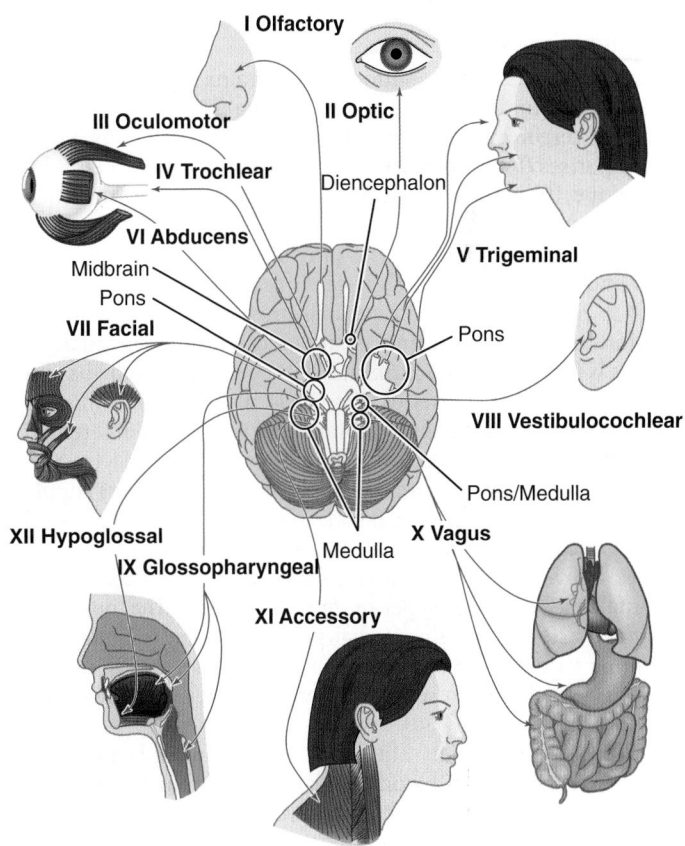

FIG. 56-7 The cranial nerves are numbered according to the order in which they leave the brain.

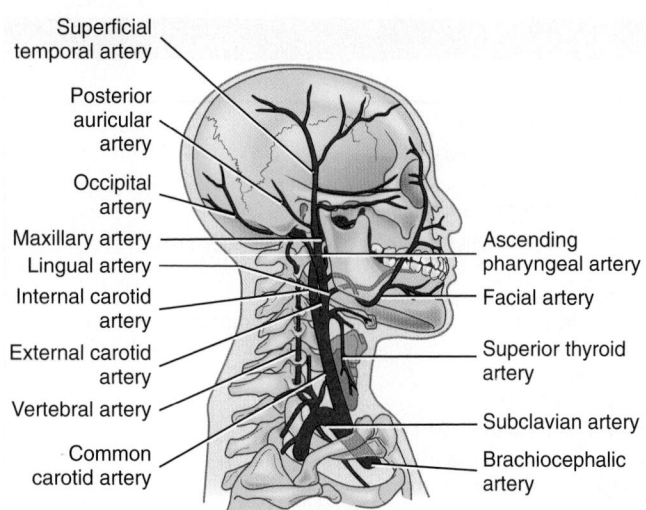

FIG. 56-8 Arteries of the head and neck. Brachiocephalic artery, right common carotid artery, right subclavian artery, and their branches. The major arteries to the head are the common carotid and vertebral arteries.

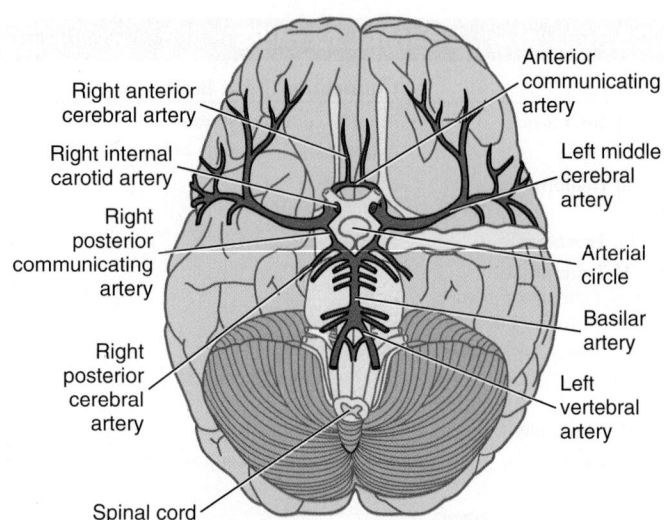

FIG. 56-9 Arteries at the base of the brain. The arteries that compose the circle of Willis are the two anterior cerebral arteries joined to each other by the anterior communicating cerebral artery and to the posterior cerebral arteries by the posterior communicating arteries.

contrast, the PSNS is geared to act in localized and discrete regions. It serves to conserve and restore the body's energy stores. The ANS provides dual and often reciprocal innervation to many structures. For example, the SNS increases the rate and force of heart contraction, and the PSNS decreases the rate and force.

Cerebral Circulation

Knowledge of the distribution of the brain's major arteries is essential for understanding and evaluating the signs and symptoms of cerebrovascular disease and trauma. The brain's blood supply arises from the internal carotid arteries (anterior circulation) and the vertebral arteries (posterior circulation), which are shown in Fig. 56-8.

The internal carotid arteries provide blood flow to the anterior and middle portions of the cerebrum. The vertebral arteries join to form the basilar artery and provide blood flow to the brainstem, cerebellum, and posterior cerebrum. The *circle of Willis* is formed by communicating arteries that join the basilar and internal carotid arteries (Fig. 56-9). The circle of Willis is a safety valve for regulating cerebral blood flow when differential pressures or vascular occlusions are present.

Superior to the circle of Willis, three pairs of arteries supply blood to the left and right hemispheres. The anterior cerebral artery feeds the medial and anterior portions of the frontal lobes. The middle cerebral artery feeds the outer portions of the frontal, parietal, and superior temporal lobes. The posterior cerebral artery feeds the medial portions of the occipital and inferior temporal lobes. Venous blood drains from the brain through the dural sinuses, which form channels that drain into the two jugular veins.

Blood-Brain Barrier. The blood-brain barrier is a physiologic barrier between blood capillaries and brain tissue.[5] This barrier protects the brain from harmful agents, while allowing nutrients and gases to enter. The structure of brain capillaries differs from that of other capillaries, so substances that normally pass into most tissues are prevented from entering brain tissue. Lipid-soluble compounds enter the brain easily, whereas water-soluble and ionized drugs enter the brain and the spinal cord slowly. Thus the blood-brain barrier affects the penetration of drugs. Only certain drugs can enter the CNS from the bloodstream.

Protective Structures

Meninges. The meninges consist of three protective membranes that surround the brain and spinal cord: dura mater, arachnoid, and pia mater (see eFig. 56-1 on the website for this chapter). The thick *dura mater* forms the outermost layer. The *falx cerebri* is a fold of the dura that separates the two cerebral hemispheres and slows expansion of brain tissue in conditions such as a rapidly growing tumor or acute hemorrhage. The *tentorium cerebelli* is a fold of dura that separates the cerebral hemispheres from the posterior fossa (which contains the brainstem and cerebellum). Expansion of mass lesions in the cerebrum forces the brain to herniate through the opening created by the brainstem. This is termed *infratentorial herniation* (see Fig. 57-4).

The *arachnoid* layer is a delicate membrane that lies between the dura mater and the *pia mater* (the delicate innermost layer of the meninges). The area between the arachnoid layer and the pia mater is the *subarachnoid space* and is filled with CSF. Structures such as arteries, veins, and cranial nerves passing to and from the brain and the skull must pass through the subarachnoid space. A larger subarachnoid space in the region of the third and fourth lumbar vertebrae is the area used to obtain CSF during a lumbar puncture.

Skull. The skull protects the brain from external trauma. It is composed of eight cranial bones and 14 facial bones. Although the top and sides of the inside of the skull are relatively smooth, the bottom surface is uneven. It has many ridges, prominences, and foramina (holes through which blood vessels and nerves enter the intracranial vault). The largest hole is the *foramen magnum*, through which the brainstem extends to the spinal cord. This foramen offers the only major space for the expansion of brain contents when increased intracranial pressure occurs.

Vertebral Column. The *vertebral column* protects the spinal cord, supports the head, and provides flexibility. The vertebral column is made up of 33 individual vertebrae: 7 cervical, 12 thoracic, 5 lumbar, 5 sacral (fused into one), and 4 coccygeal

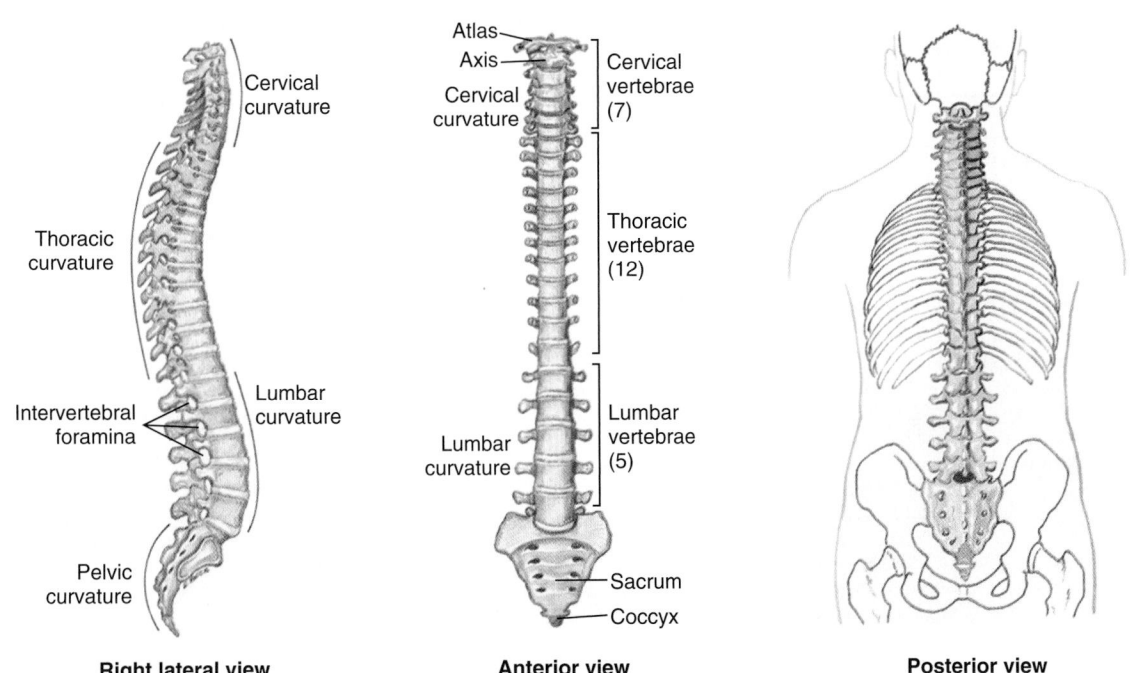

FIG. 56-10 The vertebral column (three views).

(fused into one). Each vertebra has a central opening through which the spinal cord passes. The vertebrae are held together by a series of ligaments. Intervertebral discs occupy the spaces between vertebrae. Fig. 56-10 shows the vertebral column in relation to the trunk.

GERONTOLOGIC CONSIDERATIONS

EFFECTS OF AGING ON NERVOUS SYSTEM

Several parts of the nervous system are affected by aging. In the CNS the gradual loss of neurons in certain areas of the brainstem, cerebellum, and cerebral cortex begins in early adulthood. With loss of neurons, the ventricles widen or enlarge, brain weight decreases,[6] cerebral blood flow decreases, and CSF production declines.

In the PNS, degenerative changes in myelin cause a decrease in nerve conduction. Coordinated neuromuscular activity, such as the maintenance of blood pressure in response to changing from a lying to a standing position, is altered with aging. As a result, older adults are more likely to experience orthostatic hypotension. Similarly, coordination of neuromuscular activity to maintain body temperature is also less efficient with aging. Older adults are less able to adapt to extremes in environmental temperature and are more vulnerable to both hypothermia and hyperthermia.

Additional relevant changes associated with aging include decreases in memory, vision, hearing, taste, smell, vibration and position sense, muscle strength, and reaction time. Sensory changes, including decreases in taste and smell perception, may result in decreased dietary intake in the older adult. Reduced hearing and vision can result in perceptual confusion. Problems with balance and coordination can put the older adult at risk for falls and subsequent fractures.

Changes in assessment findings result from age-related alterations in the various components of the nervous system (Table 56-4).

ASSESSMENT OF NERVOUS SYSTEM

Subjective Data

Important Health Information

Past Health History. Consider three points when taking a history of a patient with neurologic problems. First, avoid suggesting symptoms or asking leading questions. Second, the mode of onset and the course of the illness are especially important aspects of the history. Often the nature of a neurologic disease process can be described by these facts alone. Obtain all pertinent data in the history of the present illness, especially data related to the characteristics and progression of the symptoms. In some cases the history may include birth injury (e.g., cerebral palsy as a consequence of hypoxia). Third, if the patient is not considered a reliable historian, confirm or obtain the history from someone with firsthand knowledge of the patient.

Medications. Obtain a careful medication history, especially the use of sedatives, opioids, tranquilizers, and mood-elevating drugs. Many other drugs can also cause neurologic side effects.

Surgery or Other Treatments. Inquire about any surgery involving any part of the nervous system, such as head, spine, or sensory organs. If a patient had surgery, determine the date, cause, procedure, recovery, and current status.

Growth and developmental history can be important in ascertaining whether nervous system dysfunction was present at an early age. Specifically inquire about major developmental tasks such as walking and talking.

Functional Health Patterns. Key questions to ask a patient with a neurologic problem are presented in Table 56-5.

Health Perception–Health Management Pattern. Ask about the patient's health practices related to the nervous system, such as substance abuse, smoking, adequate nutrition, blood pressure control, safe participation in physical and recreational activities, and use of seat belts or helmets. Also ask about previous hospitalizations for neurologic problems.

TABLE 56-4   GERONTOLOGIC ASSESSMENT DIFFERENCES

Nervous System

Component	Changes	Differences in Assessment Findings
Central Nervous System		
Brain	↓ Cerebral blood flow and metabolism	Alterations in mental functioning.
	↓ Efficiency of temperature-regulating mechanism	Impaired ability to adapt to environmental temperature.
		Conduction of nerve impulses slowed, response time slowed.
	↓ Neurotransmitters, loss of neurons	Changes in gait and ambulation. Diminished kinesthetic sense.
	↓ O₂ supply	Altered balance, vertigo, syncope. ↑ Postural hypotension.
	Cerebral tissue atrophy and ↑ size of ventricles	Proprioception diminished. ↓ Sensory input.
Peripheral Nervous System		
Cranial and spinal nerves	Loss of myelin and ↓ conduction time	↓ Reaction time in specific nerves.
	Cellular degeneration, death of neurons	↓ Speed and intensity of neuronal reflexes.
Functional Divisions		
Motor	↓ Muscle bulk	Diminished strength and agility.
Sensory*	↓ Sensory receptors	Diminished sense of touch, pain, and temperature.
	↓ Electrical activity	Slowing of or alteration in sensory reception.
	Atrophy of taste buds	Signs of malnutrition, weight loss.
	Degeneration and loss of fibers in olfactory bulb	Diminished sense of smell.
	Degenerative changes in nerve cells in inner ear, cerebellum, and proprioceptive pathways	Poor ability to maintain balance, widened gait.
Reflexes	↓ Deep tendon reflexes	Below-average reflex score.
	↓ Sensory conduction velocity	Sluggish reflexes, slowing of reaction time.
Reticular Formation		
Reticular activating system	Modification of hypothalamic function, ↓ stage IV sleep	Disturbances in sleep patterns.
Autonomic Nervous System		
Sympathetic nervous system and parasympathetic nervous system	Morphologic features of ganglia, slowing of autonomic nervous system responses	Orthostatic hypotension, systolic hypertension.

*Specific changes related to the eye are listed in Table 21-1, and specific changes related to the ear are listed in Table 21-7.
ANS, Autonomic nervous system.

CASE STUDY

Patient Introduction

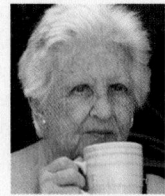

iStockphoto/Thinkstock

A.J. is a 66-yr-old white woman who arrives in the emergency department after falling in the middle of the night when she tried to get up to go to the bathroom. She states that she fell because she could not control her left leg. Her husband brought her to the hospital, but states that he had a really hard time getting her to the car.

Critical Thinking
As you read through this assessment chapter, think about A.J.'s concerns with the following questions in mind:
1. What are the possible causes for her acute leg weakness?
2. What type of assessment would be most appropriate for A.J.: comprehensive, focused, or emergency? What would be your priority assessment?
3. What questions would you ask A.J.?
4. What should be included in the physical assessment? What would you be looking for?
5. What diagnostic studies might you expect to be ordered?

evolve Answers available at *http://evolve.elsevier.com/Lewis/medsurg.*

If the patient has an existing neurologic problem, assess how it affects daily living and the ability to carry out self-care. After a careful review of information, ask someone who knows the patient well whether he or she has noticed any mental or physical changes in the patient. The patient with a neurologic problem may not be aware of it or may be a poor historian.

 GENETIC RISK ALERT
- Huntington's disease is a genetically transmitted, autosomal dominant disorder.
- Major neurologic disorders that may have a genetic basis are multiple sclerosis, headaches, Parkinson's disease, and Alzheimer's disease. The presence of these problems in a family history increases the likelihood of similar problems occurring in the patient.
- A careful family history may determine whether a neurologic problem has a genetic basis.

Nutritional-Metabolic Pattern. Neurologic problems can result in poor nutrition. Problems related to chewing, swallowing, facial nerve paralysis, and muscle coordination could make it difficult for the patient to ingest adequate nutrients.[7] Also, certain vitamins such as thiamine (B₁), niacin, and pyridoxine (B₆) are essential for the maintenance and health of the CNS. Deficiencies in one or more of these vitamins could result in such nonspecific complaints as depression, apathy, neuritis, weakness, mental confusion, and irritability. Cobalamin (vitamin B₁₂) deficiency can occur in older adults, who tend to have problems with vitamin absorption from both supplements and natural food sources such as meat, fish, and poultry. Untreated, cobalamin deficiency can cause mental function decline.

Elimination Pattern. Bowel and bladder problems are often associated with neurologic problems such as stroke, head injury, spinal cord injury, multiple sclerosis, and dementia. It is impor-

TABLE 56-5   HEALTH HISTORY

Nervous System

Health Perception–Health Management
- What are your usual daily activities?
- Do you use alcohol, tobacco, or recreational drugs?*
- What safety practices do you perform in a car? On a motorcycle? On a bicycle?
- Do you have hypertension? If so, is it controlled?
- Have you ever been hospitalized for a neurologic problem?*

Nutritional-Metabolic
- Are you able to feed yourself?
- Do you have any problems getting adequate nutrition because of chewing or swallowing difficulties, facial nerve paralysis, or poor muscle coordination?*
- Give a 24-hr dietary recall.

Elimination
- Do you have incontinence of your bowels or bladder?*
- Do you ever experience problems with hesitancy, urgency, retention?*
- Do you postpone defecation?*
- Do you take any medication to manage neurologic problems? If so, what?

Activity-Exercise
- Describe any problems you experience with usual activities and exercise as a result of a neurologic problem.
- Do you have weakness or lack of coordination?*
- Are you able to perform your personal hygiene needs independently?*

Sleep-Rest
- Describe your sleep pattern.
- When you have trouble sleeping, what do you do?

Cognitive-Perceptual
- Have you noticed any changes in your memory?*
- Do you experience dizziness, heat or cold sensitivity, numbness, or tingling?*
- Do you have chronic pain?*
- Do you have any difficulty with verbal or written communication?*
- Have you noticed any changes in vision or hearing?*

Self-Perception–Self-Concept
- How do you feel about yourself, about who you are?
- Describe your general emotional pattern.

Role-Relationship
- Have you experienced changes in roles such as spouse, parent, or breadwinner?*

Sexuality-Reproductive
- Are you dissatisfied with sexual functioning?*
- Are problems related to sexual functioning causing tension in an important relationship?*
- Do you feel the need for professional counseling related to your sexual functioning?*

Coping–Stress Tolerance
- Describe your usual coping pattern.
- Do you think your present coping pattern is adequate to meet the stressors of your life?*
- What needs are unmet by your current support system?

Value-Belief
- Describe any culturally specific beliefs and attitudes that may influence your care.

*If yes, describe.

---

tant to determine if the bowel or bladder problem was present before or after the neurologic event to plan appropriate interventions. Incontinence of urine and feces and urinary retention are the most common elimination problems associated with a neurologic problem or its treatment.[8] For example, nerve root compression (as occurs in cauda equina conditions) leads to a sudden onset of incontinence. Document key details, such as number of episodes, accompanying sensations or lack of sensations, and measures to control the problem.

Activity-Exercise Pattern. Many neurologic disorders can cause problems in the patient's mobility, strength, and coordination. Neurologic problems can result in changes in the patient's usual activity and exercise patterns. These problems can also result in falls.[9] Assess the person's activities of daily living, since neurologic diseases can affect the ability to perform motor tasks, which increases the possibility of injury.

Sleep-Rest Pattern. Sleep pattern alteration can be both a cause and a response to neurologic problems. Pain and reduced ability to change position because of muscle weakness and paralysis could interfere with sleep quality. Hallucinations resulting from dementia or drugs can also interrupt sleep. Carefully assess and document the patient's sleep pattern and bedtime routines.

Cognitive-Perceptual Pattern. Because the nervous system controls cognition and sensory integration, many neurologic disorders affect these functions. Assess memory, language, calculation ability, problem-solving ability, insight, and judgment.

Ask the patient hypothetical questions such as, "What is a reasonable price for a cup of coffee?" or "What would you do if you saw a car crash outside your house?" Often a structured mental status questionnaire is used to evaluate these functions and provide baseline data.

Delirium is an acute and transient disorder of cognition that can be seen at any time during a patient's illness. As discussed in Chapter 60, delirium is often an early indicator of various illnesses (see Table 60-14). The Confusion Assessment Method tool is used to assess for delirium (see Table 60-16).

Assess a person's ability to use and understand language. Appropriateness of responses is a useful indicator of cognitive and perceptual ability. Determine the patient's understanding and ability to carry out necessary treatments. Neurologic-related cognitive changes can interfere with the patient's understanding of the disease and adherence to related treatment.

Pain is commonly associated with many neurologic problems and is often the reason a patient seeks care. Carefully assess the patient's pain. (Pain and pain assessment are discussed in Chapter 9.)

Self-Perception–Self-Concept Pattern. Neurologic diseases can drastically alter control over one's life and create dependency on others for meeting daily needs. Also, the patient's physical appearance and emotional control can be affected. Sensitively inquire about the patient's evaluation of self-worth, perception of abilities, body image, and general emotional pattern.

Role-Relationship Pattern. Physical impairments such as weakness and paralysis can alter or limit participation in usual roles and activities. Cognitive changes can permanently alter a person's ability to maintain previous roles. These changes can dramatically affect the patient, caregiver, and family. Ask patients if their role (e.g., spouse or breadwinner) has changed as a result of their neurologic problems.

Sexuality-Reproductive Pattern. Assess the person's ability to participate in sexual activity because many neurologic disorders can affect sexual response. Cerebral lesions may inhibit the desire phase or the reflex responses of the excitement phase. The hypothalamus stimulates the pituitary gland to release hormones that influence sexual desire. Brainstem and spinal cord lesions may partially or completely interrupt the desire or ability to have intercourse. Neuropathies and spinal cord lesions may prevent reflex activities of the sexual response or affect sensation and decrease desire. Despite neurologically related changes in sexual function, many persons can achieve satisfying expression of intimacy and affection.

Coping–Stress Tolerance Pattern. The physical sequelae of a neurologic problem can seriously strain a patient's coping patterns. Often the problem is chronic and requires that the patient learn new coping skills. Assess the patient's usual coping pattern to determine if coping skills are adequate to meet the stress of a problem. Also assess the patient's support system.

Value-Belief Pattern. Many neurologic problems have serious, long-term, life-changing effects. Determine what these effects are, since they can strain the patient's belief system. Also determine if any religious or cultural beliefs could interfere with the planned treatment regimen.

Objective Data

Physical Examination. The standard neurologic examination helps determine the presence, location, and nature of disease of the nervous system. The examination assesses six categories of functions: mental status, cranial nerve function, motor function, sensory function, cerebellar function, and reflexes. Develop a consistent pattern of completing the neurologic examination so you remember to include each element every time you examine a patient.

Mental Status. Assessment of mental status (cerebral function) gives a general impression of how the patient is functioning. It involves determining complex and high-level cerebral functions that are governed by many areas of the cerebral cortex. Much of the mental status examination can be assessed as you interact with the patient. For example, assess language and memory when asking the patient for details of the illness and significant past events. Consider the patient's cultural and educational background when evaluating mental status.

The components of the mental status examination include:

- *General appearance and behavior:* This component includes level of consciousness (awake, asleep, comatose), motor activity, body posture, dress and hygiene, facial expression, and speech pattern.
- *Cognition:* Note orientation to time, place, person, and situation, as well as memory, general knowledge, insight, judgment, problem solving, and calculation. Common questions are "Who were the last three presidents?" "Does a rock float on water?" "How much money is a quarter, two dimes, and a nickel?" Consider whether the patient's plans and goals match the physical and mental capabilities. Note the presence of factors affecting intellectual capacity such as cognitive impairment, hallucinations, delusions, and dementia.
- *Mood and affect:* Note any agitation, anger, depression, or euphoria and the appropriateness of these states. Use suitable questions to bring out the patient's feelings.

Cranial Nerves. Testing each CN is an essential part of the neurologic examination (see Table 56-3).

Olfactory Nerve. After determining that both nostrils are patent, test the olfactory nerve (CN I) by asking the patient to close one nostril and identify easily recognized odors (e.g., coffee). Do the same for the other nostril. Chronic rhinitis, sinusitis, and heavy smoking may decrease the sense of smell. Disturbance in ability to smell may be associated with a tumor involving the olfactory bulb, or it may be the result of a basilar skull fracture that has damaged the olfactory fibers as they pass through the delicate cribriform plate of the skull.

Optic Nerve. Assess visual fields and acuity to determine the function of the optic nerve (CN II). Examine each eye independently. Position yourself opposite the patient and ask him or her to look directly at the bridge of your nose and indicate when an object (finger, pencil tip) presented from the periphery of each of the visual fields is seen (Fig. 56-11). Visual field defects may arise from lesions of the optic nerve, optic chiasm, or tracts

---

Subjective Data

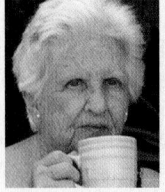

iStockphoto/Thinkstock

A subjective assessment of A.J. revealed the following information:

PMH: Hyperlipidemia, hypertension.

Medications: pravastatin 40 mg/day PO; lisinopril 10 mg/day PO.

Health Perception–Health Management: Smokes one pack of cigarettes per day since she was 28 yr old. Drinks alcohol occasionally. Hypertension controlled when on medication but has not taken her lisinopril for a few weeks because she did not have enough money for the refill and was waiting for her next Social Security check. Has never been hospitalized for a neurologic problem.

Nutritional-Metabolic: A.J. is 5 ft, 3 in tall and weighs 160 lb.

Activity-Exercise: States that up until tonight she was able to walk slowly, but her knees and hips hurt.

Cognitive-Perceptual: States had a brief episode of left-sided weakness and tingling of the face, arm, and hand 3 mo ago. The symptoms totally resolved and she did not seek treatment. Denies dizziness, change in hearing, or memory deficits.

Coping–Stress Tolerance: Is depressed and fearful. Concerned she is having a stroke and she does not know if she has enough money to cover the copay for coming to the emergency department.

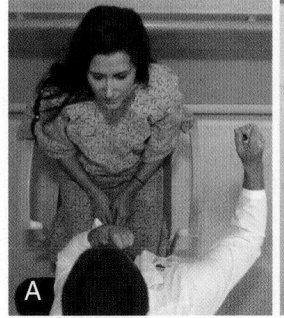
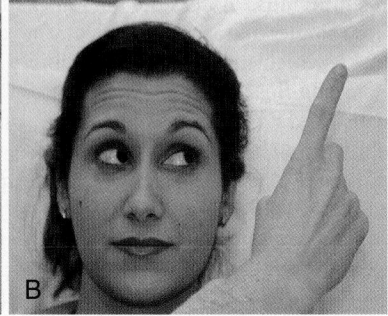

FIG. 56-11 A, Nurse checking visual fields. **B,** Nurse checking extraocular movement (EOM).

that extend through the temporal, parietal, or occipital lobes. Visual field changes resulting from brain lesions are usually either a *hemianopsia* (one half of the visual field is affected), a *quadrantanopsia* (one fourth of the visual field is affected), or monocular.

Test visual acuity by asking the patient to read a Snellen chart. Record the number on the lowest line that the patient can read with 50% accuracy. The patient who wears glasses should wear them during testing, unless they are used only for close reading. If a Snellen chart is not available, ask the patient to read newsprint for a gross assessment of acuity. Record the distance from the patient to the newsprint required for accurate reading. Acuity may not be testable by these means if the patient does not read English or is aphasic.

Oculomotor, Trochlear, and Abducens Nerves. Because the oculomotor (CN III), trochlear (CN IV), and abducens (CN VI) nerves all help move the eye, they are tested together. Ask the person to hold the head steady and to follow the movement of your finger, pen, or penlight only with the eyes. Hold the target back about 12 inches so the person can focus on it comfortably. Move the target to each of the six positions (right and up, right, right and down, left and up, left, left and down), hold it momentarily, and then move back to center. Progress clockwise. A normal response is parallel tracking of the object with both eyes.

With weakness or paralysis of one of the eye muscles, the eyes do not move together, and the patient has a *disconjugate gaze*. The presence and direction of *nystagmus* (fine, rapid jerking movements of the eyes) are observed at this time, even though this condition most often indicates vestibulocerebellar problems.

Test other functions of the oculomotor nerve by checking for pupillary constriction and *accommodation* (pupils constricting with near vision). To test pupillary constriction, shine a light into the pupil of one eye and look for ipsilateral constriction of the same pupil and contralateral (consensual) constriction of the opposite eye. Note the size and shape of the pupils. The optic nerve must be intact for this reflex to occur.

Because the oculomotor nerve exits at the top of the brainstem at the tentorial notch, it can be easily compressed by expanding mass lesions. When this occurs, sympathetic input to the pupil is unopposed and the pupil remains dilated. The lack of pupillary constriction is an early sign of central herniation (see Chapter 57).

Two abbreviations commonly used to record the reaction of the pupils are *PERRL* (*P*upils are *E*qual [in size], *R*ound, and *R*eactive to *L*ight) and *PERRLA* (*P*upils are *E*qual, *R*ound, and *R*eactive to *L*ight and *A*ccommodation). The PERRL abbreviation is appropriate when accommodation cannot be assessed such as in an unconscious patient. Convergence and accommodation are tested by having the patient focus on the examiner's finger as it moves toward the patient's nose.

Newly developed tools such as the pupilometer are being explored for their ability to objectively evaluate the pupillary response (Fig. 56-12). The pupilometer measures the pupil's response to a visual stimulus (e.g., light).

Another function of the oculomotor nerve is to keep the eyelid open. Damage to the nerve can cause *ptosis* (drooping eyelid), pupillary abnormalities, and eye muscle weakness.

Trigeminal Nerve. The sensory component of the trigeminal nerve (CN V) is tested with the patient's eyes closed, by having the patient identify light touch and pinprick in each of the three

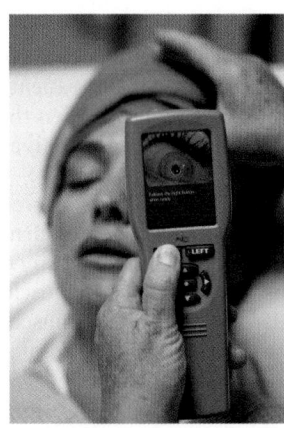

FIG. 56-12 A pupilometer can be used to measure the pupillary response using a light stimulus.

divisions (ophthalmic, maxillary, and mandibular) of the nerve on both sides of the face. Test the motor component by asking the patient to clench the teeth and palpating the masseter muscles just above the mandibular angle. The corneal reflex test evaluates CN V and CN VII simultaneously. Initially, assess blink-to-threat in the unconscious patient. A drop of saline may be applied to the cornea to assess movement of the eyelid as evidence of corneal reflex. The sensory component of this reflex (corneal sensation) is innervated by the ophthalmic division of CN V. The motor component (eye blink) is innervated by the facial nerve (CN VII).

Facial Nerve. The facial nerve (CN VII) innervates the muscles of facial expression. Test its function by asking the patient to raise the eyebrows, close the eyes tightly, purse the lips, draw back the corners of the mouth in an exaggerated smile, and frown. Note any asymmetry in the facial movements because they can indicate damage to the facial nerve. Although taste discrimination of salt and sugar in the anterior two thirds of the tongue is a function of this nerve, it is not routinely tested unless a peripheral nerve lesion is suspected.

Vestibulocochlear (Acoustic) Nerve. The cochlear portion of the vestibulocochlear nerve (CN VIII) is tested by having the patient close the eyes and indicate when he or she hears the rustling of the examiner's fingertips. For more precise assessment of hearing, perform the Weber and Rinne tests or use an audiometer (see Chapter 21).

The vestibular portion of this nerve is not routinely tested unless the patient complains of dizziness, vertigo, or unsteadiness or has auditory dysfunction. In the unconscious patient the oculocephalic reflex (movement of the eyes when the head is briskly turned to the side) may be assessed.

Glossopharyngeal and Vagus Nerves. The glossopharyngeal and vagus nerves (CN IX and X) are tested together because both innervate the pharynx. Test the gag reflex (bilateral contraction of the palatal muscles) by touching the sides of the posterior pharynx or soft palate with a tongue blade. Assess the sensory component of the glossopharyngeal nerve and the major motor component of the vagus nerve. It is important to assess the gag reflex in patients who have a decreased level of consciousness, a brainstem lesion, or a disease involving the throat musculature. If the reflex is weak or absent, the patient is in danger of aspirating food or secretions. The strength and efficiency of swallowing are important to test in these patients for the same reason.

Another test for the awake, cooperative patient is to have the patient phonate by saying "ah," and note the bilateral symmetry of elevation of the soft palate. If the patient is endotracheally intubated, the cough reflex (elicited when the suction catheter contacts the *carina* of the respiratory tree) is a method of assessing the vagus nerve.

Accessory Nerve. Test the accessory nerve (CN XI) by asking the patient to shrug the shoulders and to turn the head to either side against resistance. There should be smooth contraction of the sternocleidomastoid and trapezius muscles. Also note symmetry, atrophy, or fasciculation of the muscle.

Hypoglossal Nerve. Test the hypoglossal nerve (CN XII) by asking the patient to protrude the tongue. It should protrude in the midline. Next ask the patient to move the tongue up and down and side to side. Finally, the patient should also be able to push the tongue to either side against the resistance of a tongue blade. Again, note any asymmetry, atrophy, or fasciculation.

Motor System. The motor system examination includes assessment of strength, tone, coordination, and symmetry of the major muscle groups. Test muscle strength by asking the patient to push and pull against the resistance of your arm as it opposes flexion and extension of the patient's muscle. Ask the patient to offer resistance at the shoulders, elbows, wrists, hips, knees, and ankles. Mild weakness of the arm is demonstrated by downward drifting of the arm or pronation of the palm *(pronator drift)*. Note any weakness or asymmetry of strength between the same muscle groups of the right and left sides.

Test muscle tone by passively moving the limbs through their range of motion. There should be a slight resistance to these movements. Abnormal tone is described as *hypotonia* (flaccidity) or *hypertonia* (spasticity). Note any involuntary movements such as tics, tremor, *myoclonus* (spasm of muscles), *athetosis* (slow, writhing, involuntary movements of extremities), *chorea* (involuntary, purposeless, rapid motions), and *dystonia* (impairment of muscle tone).

Test cerebellar function by assessing balance and coordination. A good screening test for both balance and muscle strength is to observe the patient's stature (posture while standing) and gait. Note the pace and rhythm of the gait and observe for normal symmetric and oppositional arm swing. The patient's ability to ambulate helps to determine the level of nursing care required and the risk of falling.

The finger-to-nose test (having the patient alternately touch the nose, then touch the examiner's finger) and the heel-to-shin test (having the patient stroke the heel of one foot up and down the shin of the opposite leg) test coordination and cerebellar function. Reposition your finger while the patient is touching the nose so that the patient must adjust to a new distance each time your finger is touched. These movements should be performed smoothly and accurately. Other tests include asking the patient to pronate and supinate both hands rapidly and to do a shallow knee bend, first on one leg and then on the other. Note dysarthria or slurred speech because it is a sign of incoordination of the speech muscles.

Sensory System. Several modalities are tested in the somatic sensory examination. Each modality is carried by a specific ascending pathway in the spinal cord before it reaches the sensory cortex. As a rule, perform the examination with the patient's eyes closed and avoid providing the patient with clues. Ask "How does this feel?" rather than "Is this sharp?" In the routine neurologic examination, sensory testing of the anterior torso, posterior torso, and the four extremities is sufficient. However, if a disturbance in sensory function of the skin is identified, the boundaries of that dysfunction should be carefully delineated along the dermatome.

Touch, Pain, and Temperature. Light touch is usually tested first using a cotton wisp or light pin prick. Gently touch each of the four extremities and ask the patient to indicate when he or she feels the stimulus. Test pain by alternately touching the skin with the sharp and dull end of a pin. Tell the patient to respond "sharp" or "dull." Evaluate each limb separately.

Extinction is assessed by simultaneously touching both sides of the body symmetrically. Normally, the simultaneous stimuli are both perceived (sensed). An abnormal response occurs when the patient perceives the stimulus on only one side. The other stimulus is "extinguished."

The sensation of temperature (only to be tested when the response to deep pain is abnormal) can be tested by applying tubes of warm and cold water to the skin and asking the patient to identify the stimuli with the eyes closed. If pain sensation is intact, assessment of temperature sensation may be omitted because both sensations are carried by the same ascending pathways.

Vibration Sense. Assess vibration sense by applying a vibrating tuning fork to the fingernails and the bony prominences of the hands, legs, and feet. Ask the patient if the vibration or "buzz" is felt. Then ask the patient to indicate when the vibration ceases.

Position Sense. Assess position sense *(proprioception)* by placing your thumb and forefinger on either side of the patient's forefinger or great toe and gently moving his or her digit up or down. Ask the patient to indicate the direction in which the digit is moved.

Another test of proprioception is the Romberg test. Ask the patient to stand with feet together and then close his or her eyes. If the patient is able to maintain balance with the eyes open but sways or falls with the eyes closed (i.e., a positive Romberg test), vestibulocochlear dysfunction or disease in the posterior columns of the spinal cord may be indicated. Be aware of patient safety during this test.

Cortical Sensory Functions. Several tests evaluate cortical integration of sensory perceptions (which occurs in the parietal lobes). Assess *two-point discrimination* by placing the two points of a calibrated compass on the tips of the fingers and toes. The minimum recognizable separation is 4 to 5 mm in the fingertips and a greater degree of separation elsewhere. This test is important in diagnosing diseases of the sensory cortex and PNS.

Graphesthesia (ability to feel writing on skin) is tested by having the patient identify numbers traced on the palm of the hands. *Stereognosis* (ability to perceive the form and nature of objects) is tested by having the patient close the eyes and identify the size and shape of easily recognized objects (e.g., coins, keys, safety pin) placed in the hands.

Reflexes. Tendons have receptors that are sensitive to stretch. A reflex contraction of the skeletal muscle occurs when the tendon is stretched. In general, the biceps, triceps, brachioradialis, and patellar and Achilles tendon reflexes are tested. Initiate a simple muscle stretch reflex by briskly tapping the tendon of a stretched muscle, usually with a reflex hammer (Fig. 56-13). The response (muscle contraction of the corresponding muscle) is measured as follows: 0/5 = absent, 1/5 = weak response, 2/5 = normal response, 3/5 = exaggerated response,

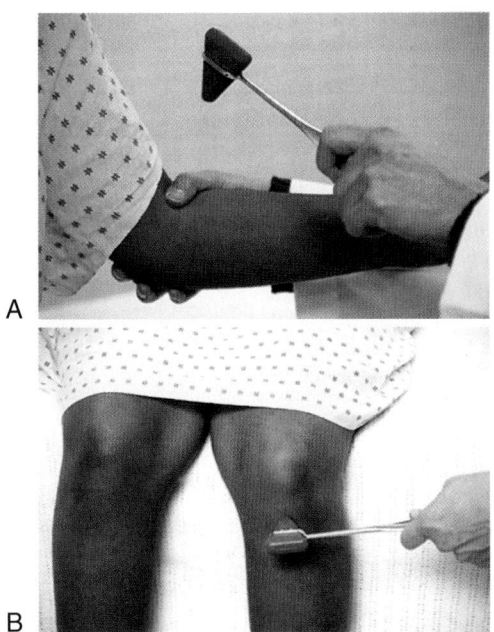

FIG. 56-13 The examiner strikes a swift blow over a stretched tendon to elicit a stretch reflex. **A,** Biceps reflex. **B,** Patellar reflex.

Parameter	Findings
TABLE 56-6	**NORMAL PHYSICAL ASSESSMENT OF NERVOUS SYSTEM***
Mental status	• Alert and oriented, orderly thought processes. • Appropriate mood and affect.
Cranial nerves†	• Smell intact to soap or coffee. • Visual fields full to confrontation. • Intact extraocular movements. • No nystagmus. Pupils equal, round, reactive to light and accommodation. • Intact facial sensation to light touch and pinprick. • Facial movements full. • Intact gag and swallow reflexes. Symmetric smile. Midline protrusion of tongue. • Full strength with head turning and shoulder shrugging.
Motor system	• Normal gait and station. Normal tandem walk. Negative Romberg test. • Normal and symmetric muscle bulk, tone, and strength. • Smooth performance of finger-nose, heel-shin movements.
Sensory system	• Intact sensation to light touch, position sense, pinprick, heat and cold.
Reflexes‡	• Biceps, triceps, brachioradialis, patellar, and Achilles tendon reflexes 2/5 bilaterally. • Downgoing toes with plantar stimulation.

*If some portion of the neurologic examination was not done, this should be indicated (e.g., "Smell not tested").
†May also be recorded as "CN I to XII intact."
‡May also be recorded as drawing of stick figure indicating reflex strength at appropriate sites.

and 4/5 = hyperreflexia with clonus. *Clonus,* an abnormal response, is a continued rhythmic contraction of the muscle with continuous application of the stimulus.

Elicit the *biceps reflex,* with the patient's arm partially flexed and palm up, by placing your thumb over the biceps tendon in the antecubital space and striking the thumb with a hammer. The normal response is flexion of the arm at the elbow or contraction of the biceps muscle that can be felt by your thumb.

Elicit the *triceps reflex* by striking the triceps tendon above the elbow while the patient's arm is flexed. The normal response is extension of the arm or visible contraction of the triceps.

Elicit the *brachioradialis reflex* by striking the radius 3 to 5 cm above the wrist while the patient's arm is relaxed. The normal response is flexion and supination at the elbow or visible contraction of the brachioradialis muscle.

Elicit the *patellar reflex* by striking the patellar tendon just below the patella. The patient can be sitting or lying as long as the leg being tested hangs freely. The normal response is extension of the leg with contraction of the quadriceps.

Elicit the *Achilles tendon reflex* by striking the Achilles tendon while the patient's leg is flexed at the knee and the foot is gently dorsiflexed, by the examiner, at the ankle. The normal response is plantar flexion at the ankle.

A *focused assessment* is used to evaluate the status of previously identified neurologic problems and to monitor for signs of new problems (see Table 3-6). A focused assessment of the neurologic system is presented in the box on p. 1351.

Table 56-6 is an example of a normal neurologic physical assessment. Abnormal assessment findings of the neurologic system are presented in Table 56-7.

DIAGNOSTIC STUDIES OF NERVOUS SYSTEM

Numerous diagnostic studies are available to assess the nervous system. Tables 56-8 and 56-9 present the most common studies, and select studies are described in more detail below.

Objective Data: Physical Examination

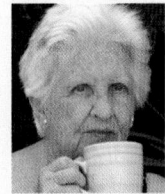

iStockphoto/Thinkstock

A physical assessment of A.J. reveals the following:
• BP 180/110, HR 94, RR 22, T 37°C
• Alert, oriented, and able to answer questions appropriately but mild slowness in responding
• Left-sided arm weakness (3/5) and leg weakness (4/5)
• NIH Stroke score is 3
As you continue to read this chapter, consider diagnostic studies you would anticipate being performed for A.J.

Cerebrospinal Fluid Analysis

CSF analysis provides information about a variety of CNS diseases. Normal CSF fluid is clear, colorless, odorless, and free of red blood cells and contains little protein. Normal CSF values are listed in Table 56-9. CSF may be obtained through lumbar puncture or ventriculostomy.

Lumbar Puncture. Lumbar puncture is the most common method of sampling CSF. A lumbar puncture is contraindicated in the presence of increased intracranial pressure or infection at the site of puncture.

Before the procedure, have the patient void. Most commonly, the patient is side lying. However, a seated position may also be used. Inform the patient that, as a sterile needle is passed between two lumbar vertebrae, he or she may feel temporary pain radiating down the leg.

TABLE 56-7 **ASSESSMENT ABNORMALITIES**

Nervous System

Finding	Description	Possible Etiology and Significance
Mental Status		
Altered consciousness	Stuporous, mute, diminished response to verbal cues or pain	Intracranial lesions, metabolic disorder, psychiatric disorders
Anosognosia	Inability to recognize bodily defect or disease	Lesions in right parietal cortex
Speech		
Aphasia, dysphasia	Loss of or impaired language faculty (comprehension, expression, or both)	Left cerebral cortex lesion
Dysarthria	Lack of coordination in articulating speech	Cerebellar or cranial nerve lesion Antiseizure drugs, sedatives, hypnotic drug toxicity (including alcohol)
Eyes		
Anisocoria	Inequality of pupil size	Optic nerve injury
Diplopia	Double vision	Lesions affecting nerves of extraocular muscles, cerebellar damage
Homonymous hemianopsia	Loss of vision in one side of visual field	Lesions in the contralateral occipital lobe
Cranial Nerves		
Dysphagia	Difficulty in swallowing	Lesions involving motor pathways of CNs IX, X (including lower brainstem)
Ophthalmoplegia	Paralysis of eye muscles	Lesions in brainstem
Papilledema	"Choked disc," swelling of optic nerve head	Increase in intracranial pressure
Motor System		
Apraxia	Inability to perform learned movements despite having desire and physical ability to perform them	Cerebral cortex lesion
Ataxia	Lack of coordination of movement	Lesions of sensory or motor pathways, cerebellum Antiseizure drugs, sedatives, hypnotic drug toxicity (including alcohol)
Dyskinesia	Impairment of voluntary movement, resulting in fragmentary or incomplete movements	Disorders of basal ganglia, idiosyncratic reaction to psychotropic drugs
Hemiplegia	Paralysis on one side	Stroke and other lesions involving motor cortex
Nystagmus	Jerking or bobbing of eyes as they track moving object	Lesions in cerebellum, brainstem, vestibular system Antiseizure drugs, sedatives, hypnotic toxicity (including alcohol)
Sensory System		
Analgesia	Loss of pain sensation	Lesion in spinothalamic tract or thalamus, specific medications
Anesthesia	Absence of sensation	Lesions in spinal cord, thalamus, sensory cortex, or peripheral sensory nerve Specific medications
Paresthesia	Alteration in sensation	Lesions in the posterior column or sensory cortex
Astereognosis	Inability to recognize form of object by touch	Lesions in parietal cortex
Reflexes		
Extensor plantar response	Upgoing toes with plantar stimulation	Suprasegmental or upper motor neuron lesion
Deep tendon reflexes	Diminished or absent motor response	Lower motor neuron lesions
Spinal Cord		
Bladder dysfunction		
• Atonic (autonomous)	Absence of muscle tone and contractility, enlargement of capacity, no sensation of discomfort, overflow with large residual, inability to voluntarily empty	Early stage of spinal cord injury
• Hypotonic	More ability than atonic bladder but less than normal	Interruption of afferent pathways from bladder
• Hypertonic	Increase in muscle tone, diminished capacity, reflex emptying, dribbling, incontinence	Lesions in pyramidal tracts (efferent pathways)
Paraplegia	Paralysis of lower extremities	Spinal cord transection or mass lesion (thoracolumbar region)
Tetraplegia (quadriplegia)	Paralysis of all extremities	Spinal cord transection or mass lesion (cervical region)

FOCUSED ASSESSMENT

Nervous System

Use this checklist to make sure the key assessment steps have been done.

Subjective
Ask the patient about any of the following and note responses.

Blackouts/loss of memory	Y	N
Weakness, numbness, tingling in arms or legs	Y	N
Headaches, especially new onset	Y	N
Loss of balance/coordination	Y	N
Orientation to person, place, and time	Y	N

Objective: Diagnostic
Check the following laboratory results for critical values.

Lumbar puncture	✓
CT or MRI of brain	✓
EEG	✓

Objective: Physical Examination
Inspect/Observe

General level of consciousness/orientation	✓
Oropharynx for gag reflex and soft palate movement	✓
Peripheral sensation of light touch and pinprick (face, hands, feet)	✓
Smell with an alcohol wipe	✓
Eyes for extraocular movements, PERRLA, peripheral vision, nystagmus	✓
Gait for smoothness and coordination	✓

Palpate

Strength of neck, shoulders, arms, and legs full and symmetric	✓

Percuss

Reflexes	✓

CT, Computed tomography; *EEG,* electroencephalogram; *MRI,* magnetic resonance imaging; *PERRLA,* pupils equal, round, and reactive to light and accommodation.

A manometer is attached to the needle to obtain a CSF pressure. CSF is withdrawn in a series of tubes and sent for analysis. Monitor for headache intensity, meningeal irritation *(nuchal rigidity),* or signs and symptoms of local trauma (e.g., hematoma, pain).

Radiologic Studies

Computed Tomography. Computed tomography (CT) scans provide a rapid means of obtaining radiographic images of the brain (see Fig. 56-15, *A*). When viewed in succession, these images provide a three-dimensional representation of the intracranial contents. Denser material appears white, whereas fluid and air appear dark or black. Brain CT can be completed both with and without contrast media in only a few minutes.

Magnetic Resonance Imaging. Magnetic resonance imaging (MRI) provides greater detail than CT and improved resolution (detail) of the intracranial structures (see Fig. 56-15, *B*). However, MRI requires a longer time to complete and may not be appropriate in life-threatening emergencies. Techniques of functional MRI (fMRI) provide time-related (temporal) images that can be used to evaluate how the brain responds to various stimuli.

Cerebral Angiography. Cerebral angiography is indicated when vascular lesions or tumors are suspected. A catheter is inserted into the femoral (sometimes brachial) artery and

Objective Data: Diagnostic Studies

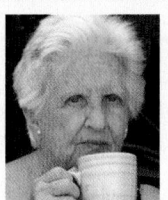

The emergency department physician immediately orders a stat CT scan of the head. The CT scan rules out a hemorrhagic stroke. Stat laboratory test results include a blood glucose of 138 mg/dL, and PT/INR of 12.0/1.1.
Case study continued in Ch. 58 on p. 1410.

iStockphoto/Thinkstock

passed through the aortic arch and into the base of a carotid or a vertebral artery for injection of contrast media. Timed-sequence radiographic images are obtained as contrast flows through arteries, smaller vessels, and veins (see Fig. 56-14). This study can help to identify and localize abscesses, aneurysms, hematomas, arteriovenous malformations, arterial spasm, and certain tumors.

Because this is an invasive procedure, adverse reactions may occur. The patient may have an allergic (anaphylactic) reaction to the contrast medium. This reaction usually occurs immediately after injection of the contrast medium and may require emergency resuscitation measures in the procedure room. Once the patient returns to his or her room after the procedure, observe for bleeding at the catheter puncture site (usually the groin).

Electrographic Studies

Electroencephalography. *Electroencephalography* (EEG) involves recording electrical activity of the surface cortical neurons of the brain by electrodes placed on specific areas of the scalp. Specific tests may be done to evaluate the brain's electrical response to lights and loud noises. This test is done to evaluate not only cerebral disease but also the CNS effects of many metabolic and systemic diseases. Among the cerebral diseases assessed by EEG are seizure disorders, sleep disorders, cerebrovascular lesions, and brain injury. Prolonged EEG monitoring is becoming a common test to diagnose and treat seizure disorders.[10] An EEG is noninvasive. Assure patients that there is no risk of electric shock.

Electromyography and Nerve Conduction Studies. *Electromyography* (EMG) is the recording of electrical activity associated with innervation of skeletal muscle. Needle electrodes are inserted into the muscle to record specific motor units because recording from the skin is not sufficient. Normal muscle at rest shows no electrical activity. Electrical activity occurs only when the muscle contracts. This activity may be altered in diseases of muscle itself (e.g., myopathic conditions) or in disorders of muscle innervation (e.g., segmental or LMN lesions, peripheral neuropathic conditions).

Nerve conduction studies involve applying a brief electrical stimulus to a distal portion of a sensory or mixed nerve and recording the resulting wave of depolarization at some point proximal to the stimulation. For example, a stimulus can be applied to the forefinger and a recording electrode placed over the median nerve at the wrist. The time between the stimulus onset and the initial wave of depolarization at the recording electrode is measured. This is termed *nerve conduction velocity.* Damaged nerves have slower conduction velocities.

TABLE 56-8 **DIAGNOSTIC STUDIES**

Nervous System

Study	Description and Purpose	Nursing Responsibility
Cerebrospinal Fluid Analysis		
Lumbar puncture	CSF is aspirated by needle insertion in L3-4 or L4-5 interspace to assess many CNS diseases (see Table 56-9).	Ensure that patient does not have signs of increased ICP because of the risk of downward herniation from CSF removal. Patient assumes and maintains lateral recumbent position. Use strict aseptic technique. Ensure labeling of CSF specimens in proper sequence. Encourage fluids. Monitor neurologic signs and VS. Administer analgesia as needed.
Radiology		
Skull and spine x-rays	Simple x-ray of skull and spinal column is done to detect fractures, bone erosion, calcifications, abnormal vascularity.	Explain that procedure is noninvasive. Explain positions to be assumed.
Cerebral angiography	Serial x-ray visualization of intracranial and extracranial blood vessels is performed to detect vascular lesions and tumors of brain (Fig. 56-14). Contrast medium is used.	*Preprocedure:* Assess patient for stroke risk before procedure, since thrombi may be dislodged during procedure. Withhold preceding meal. Explain that patient will have hot flush of head and neck when contrast medium is injected. Administer premedication. Explain need to be absolutely still during procedure. *Postprocedure:* Monitor neurologic signs and VS every 15-30 min for first 2 hr, every hour for next 6 hr, then every 2 hr for 24 hr. Maintain bed rest until patient is alert and VS are stable. Report any neurologic status changes.
Computed tomography (CT) scan	Computer-assisted x-ray of multiple cross sections of body parts to detect problems such as hemorrhage, tumor, cyst, edema, infarction, brain atrophy, and other abnormalities (Fig. 56-15, *A*). Contrast media may be used to enhance visualization of brain structures.	Assess for contraindications to contrast media, including allergy to shellfish, iodine, or dye. Explain appearance of scanner. Instruct patient to remain still during procedure.
Magnetic resonance imaging (MRI)	Imaging of brain, spinal cord, and spinal canal by means of magnetic energy (Fig. 56-15, *B*). Used to detect strokes, multiple sclerosis, tumors, trauma, herniation, and seizures. No invasive procedures are required. Contrast media may be used to enhance visualization. Has greater contrast in images of soft tissue structures than CT scan.	Screen patient for metal parts and pacemaker in body. Instruct patient on need to lie very still for up to 1 hr. Sedation may be necessary if patient is claustrophobic.
Magnetic resonance angiography (MRA)	Uses differential signal characteristics of flowing blood to evaluate extracranial and intracranial blood vessels. Provides both anatomic and hemodynamic information. Can be used in conjunction with contrast media.	Similar to MRI (see above).
Positron emission tomography (PET)	Measures metabolic activity of brain to assess cell death or damage. Uses radioactive material that shows up as a bright spot on the image (see Fig. 16-7). Used for patients with stroke, Alzheimer's disease, seizure disorders, Parkinson's disease, and tumors.	Explain procedure to patient. Explain that two IV lines will be inserted. Instruct patient not to take sedatives or tranquilizers. Have patient empty bladder before procedure. Patient may be asked to perform different activities during test.
Single-photon emission computed tomography (SPECT)	A method of scanning similar to PET, but it uses more stable substances and different detectors. Radiolabeled compounds are injected, and their photon emissions can be detected. Images made are accumulation of labeled compound. Used to visualize blood flow or O_2 or glucose metabolism in the brain. Useful in diagnosing strokes, brain tumors, and seizure disorders.	Similar to PET (see above).
Myelogram	X-ray of spinal cord and vertebral column after injection of contrast medium into subarachnoid space. Used to detect spinal lesions (e.g., herniated or ruptured disc, spinal tumor).	*Preprocedure:* Administer sedative as ordered. Instruct patient to empty bladder. Inform patient that test is performed with patient on tilting table that is moved during test. *Postprocedure:* Patient should lie flat for a few hours. Encourage fluids. Monitor neurologic signs and VS. Headache, nausea, and vomiting may occur after procedure.

TABLE 56-8 DIAGNOSTIC STUDIES—cont'd

Nervous System

Study	Description and Purpose	Nursing Responsibility
Electrographic Studies		
Electroencephalography (EEG)	Electrical activity of brain is recorded by scalp electrodes to evaluate seizure disorders, cerebral disease, CNS effects of systemic diseases, brain death.	Inform patient that procedure is noninvasive and without danger of electric shock. Determine whether any medications (e.g., tranquilizers, antiseizure drugs) should be withheld. Resume medications and instruct patient to wash electrode paste out of hair after test.
Magnetoencephalography (MEG)	Uses a biomagnetometer to detect magnetic fields generated by neural activity. It can accurately pinpoint the part of the brain involved in a stroke, seizure, or other disorder or injury. Measures extracranial magnetic fields and scalp electric field (EEG).	MEG, a passive sensor, does not make physical contact with patient. Explain procedure to patient.
Electromyography (EMG) and nerve conduction studies	Electrical activity associated with nerve and skeletal muscle is recorded by insertion of needle electrodes to detect muscle and peripheral nerve disease.	Inform patient that pain and discomfort are associated with insertion of needles.
Evoked potentials	Electrical activity associated with nerve conduction along sensory pathways is recorded by electrodes placed on skin and scalp. Stimulus generates the impulse. Procedure is used to diagnose disease (e.g., multiple sclerosis), locate nerve damage, and monitor function intraoperatively.	Explain procedure to patient.
Ultrasound		
Carotid duplex studies	Combined ultrasound and pulsed Doppler technology. Probe is placed over the carotid artery and slowly moved along the course of the common carotid artery. Frequency of reflected ultrasound signal corresponds to the blood velocity. Increased blood flow velocity can indicate stenosis of a vessel.	Explain procedure to patient. Duplex scanning is a noninvasive study that evaluates the degree of stenosis of the carotid and vertebral arteries.
Transcranial Doppler	Same technology as carotid duplex, but evaluates blood flow velocities of the intracranial blood vessels. Probe is placed on the skin at various "windows" in the skull (areas in the skull that have only a thin bony covering) to register velocities of the blood vessels.	Explain procedure to patient. Noninvasive technique that is useful in assessing vasospasm associated with subarachnoid hemorrhage, altered intracranial blood flow dynamics associated with occlusive vascular disease, presence of emboli, and cerebral autoregulation.

CNS, Central nervous system; *CSF,* cerebrospinal fluid; *ICP,* intracranial pressure.

TABLE 56-9 NORMAL CEREBROSPINAL FLUID VALUES

Parameter	Normal Value
Specific gravity	1.007
pH	7.35
Appearance	Clear, colorless
Red blood cells (RBCs)	None
White blood cells (WBCs)	0-5 cells/μL (0-5 × 10⁶ cells/L)
Protein	
• Lumbar	15-45 mg/dL (0.15-0.45 g/L)
• Cisternal	15-25 mg/dL (0.15-0.25 g/L)
• Ventricular	5-15 mg/dL (0.05-0.15 g/L)
Glucose	40-70 mg/dL (2.2-3.9 mmol/L)
Microorganisms	None
Pressure	60-150 mm H₂O

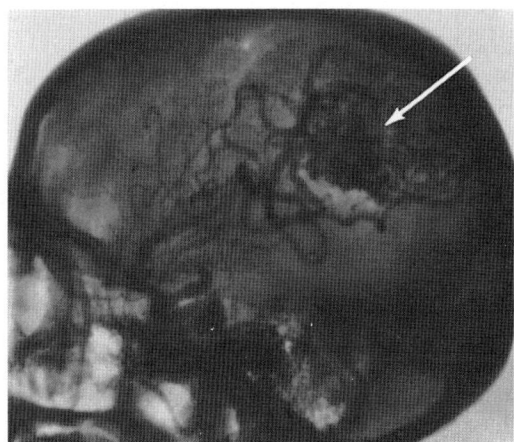

FIG. 56-14 Cerebral angiogram illustrating an arteriovenous malformation *(arrow).*

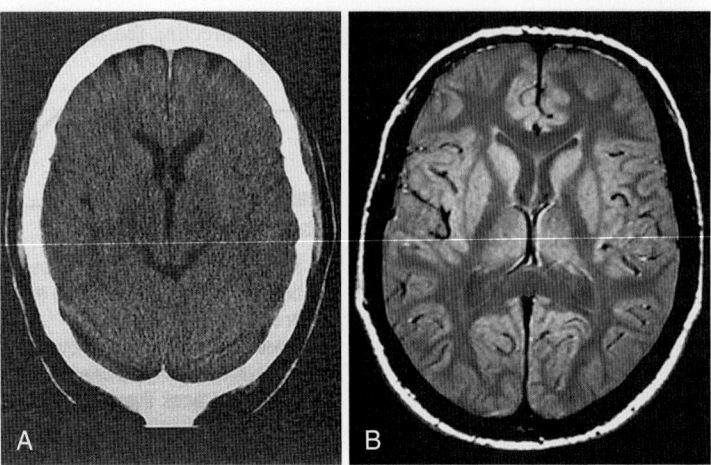

FIG. 56-15 Normal images of the brain. **A,** Computed tomography scan. **B,** Magnetic resonance imaging.

Evoked Potentials. *Evoked potentials* are recordings of electrical activity associated with nerve conduction along sensory pathways. The electrical activity is generated by a specific sensory stimulus related to the type of study (e.g., clicking sounds for auditory evoked potentials, mild electrical pulses for somatosensory evoked potentials).[11] Electrodes placed on specific areas of the skin and the scalp record the electrical activity. Increases in the normal time from stimulus onset to a given peak (latency) indicate slowed nerve conduction or nerve damage.

This technique is useful in diagnosing abnormalities of the visual or auditory systems because it reveals whether a sensory impulse is reaching the appropriate part of the brain. Indications for these tests include evaluation of consciousness, multiple sclerosis (optic neuritis), and acoustic neuroma.

BRIDGE TO NCLEX EXAMINATION

The number of the question corresponds to the same-numbered outcome at the beginning of the chapter.

1. In a patient with a disease that affects the myelin sheath of nerves, such as multiple sclerosis, the glial cells affected are the
   a. microglia.
   b. astrocytes.
   c. ependymal cells.
   d. oligodendrocytes.

2. Drugs or diseases that impair the function of the extrapyramidal system may cause loss of
   a. sensations of pain and temperature.
   b. regulation of the autonomic nervous system.
   c. integration of somatic and special sensory inputs.
   d. automatic movements associated with skeletal muscle activity.

3. An obstruction of the anterior cerebral arteries will affect functions of
   a. visual imaging.
   b. balance and coordination.
   c. judgment, insight, and reasoning.
   d. visual and auditory integration for language comprehension.

4. Paralysis of lateral gaze indicates a lesion of cranial nerve
   a. II.
   b. III.
   c. IV.
   d. VI.

5. A result of stimulation of the parasympathetic nervous system is *(select all that apply)*
   a. constriction of the bronchi.
   b. dilation of skin blood vessels.
   c. increased secretion of insulin.
   d. increased blood glucose levels.
   e. relaxation of the urinary sphincters.

6. Assessment of muscle strength of older adults cannot be compared with that of younger adults because
   a. stroke is more common in older adults.
   b. nutritional status is better in young adults.
   c. most young people exercise more than older people.
   d. aging leads to a decrease in muscle bulk and strength.

7. Data regarding mobility, strength, coordination, and activity tolerance are important for the nurse to obtain because
   a. many neurologic diseases affect one or more of these areas.
   b. patients are less able to identify other neurologic impairments.
   c. these are the first functions to be affected by neurologic diseases.
   d. aspects of movement are the most important function of the nervous system.

8. During neurologic testing, the patient is able to perceive pain elicited by pinprick. Based on this finding, the nurse may omit testing for
   a. position sense.
   b. patellar reflexes.
   c. temperature perception.
   d. heel-to-shin movements.

9. A patient's eyes jerk while the patient looks to the left. You will record this finding as
   a. nystagmus.
   b. CN VI palsy.
   c. oculocephalia.
   d. ophthalmic dyskinesia.

10. The nurse is caring for a patient with peripheral neuropathy who is going to have EMG studies tomorrow morning. The nurse should
    a. ensure the patient has an empty bladder.
    b. instruct the patient that there is no risk of electric shock.
    c. ensure the patient has no metallic jewelry or metal fragments.
    d. instruct the patient that she or he may experience pain during the study.

1. d, 2. d, 3. c, 4. d, 5. a, b, c, 6. c, 7. a, 8. c, 9. a, 10. b

⊝volve

For rationales to these answers and even more NCLEX review questions, visit *http://evolve.elsevier.com/Lewis/medsurg.*

REFERENCES

1. Gopurappilly R, Pal R, Mamidi MK, et al: Stem cells in stroke repair: current success and future prospects, *CNS Neurol Disorders Drug Targets* 10:741, 2011.

2. Zhang H, Wang FW, Yao LL, et al: Microglia—friend or foe, *Front Biosci (Schol Ed)* 3:869, 2011.

3. Otsuka S, Adamson C, Sankar V, et al: Delayed intrathecal delivery of RhoA siRNA to the contused spinal cord inhibits allodynia, preserves white matter, and increases serotonergic fiber growth, *J Neurotrauma* 28:1063, 2011.

4. Timofeev I, Carpenter KL, Nortje J, et al: Cerebral extracellular chemistry and outcome following traumatic brain injury: a microdialysis study of 223 patients, *Brain* 134:484, 2011.

5. Chen JW, Gombart ZJ, Rogers S, et al: Pupillary reactivity as an early indicator of increased intracranial pressure: the introduction of the neurological pupil index, *Surg Neurol Int* 2:82, 2011.

6. Takahashi R, Ishii K, Kakigi T, et al: Gender and age differences in normal adult human brain: voxel-based morphometric study, *Hum Brain Mapp* 32:1050, 2011.

7. Medin J, Windahl J, von Arbin M, et al: Eating difficulties among stroke patients in the acute state: a descriptive, cross-sectional, comparative study, *J Clin Nurs* 20:2563, 2011.

8. Pinder C, Young C: Adverse cognitive effects of phenytoin in severe brain injury: a case report, *Brain Inj* 25:634, 2011.

9. Hunderfund AN, Sweeney CM, Mandrekar JN, et al: Effect of a multidisciplinary fall risk assessment on falls among neurology inpatients, *Mayo Clinic Proc* 86:19, 2011.

10. Swisher CB, Doreswamy M, Gingrich KJ, et al: Phenytoin, levetiracetam, and pregabalin in the acute management of refractory status epilepticus in patients with brain tumors, *Neurocrit Care* 16(1):109, 2012.

11. Guo L, Gelb AW: The use of motor evoked potential monitoring during cerebral aneurysm surgery to predict pure motor deficits due to subcortical ischemia, *Clin Neurophysiol* 122:648, 2011.

RESOURCES

Resources for this chapter are listed after Chapter 57 on p. 1387, Chapter 58 on p. 1412, Chapter 59 on p. 1442, Chapter 60 on p. 1462, and Chapter 61 on p. 1488.

57

*Most people do not listen
with the intent to understand;
they listen with the intent to reply.*
Stephen Covey

Nursing Management
Acute Intracranial Problems

Meg Zomorodi

LEARNING OUTCOMES

1. Explain the physiologic mechanisms that maintain normal intracranial pressure.
2. Describe the common etiologies, clinical manifestations, and collaborative care of the patient with increased intracranial pressure.
3. Describe the collaborative and nursing management of the patient with increased intracranial pressure.
4. Differentiate types of head injury by mechanism of injury and clinical manifestations.
5. Describe the collaborative care and nursing management of the patient with a head injury.
6. Compare the types, clinical manifestations, and collaborative care of patients with brain tumors.
7. Discuss the nursing management of the patient with a brain tumor.
8. Describe the nursing management of the patient undergoing cranial surgery.
9. Differentiate among the primary causes, collaborative care, and nursing management of brain abscess, meningitis, and encephalitis.

KEY TERMS

brain abscess, p. 1381
cerebral edema, p. 1359
coma, p. 1359
concussion, p. 1369
contusion, p. 1370
diffuse axonal injury (DAI), p. 1370

encephalitis, p. 1384
epidural hematoma, p. 1370
Glasgow Coma Scale (GCS), p. 1365
head injury, p. 1368
intracerebral hematoma, p. 1371

intracranial pressure (ICP), p. 1357
meningitis, p. 1381
nuchal rigidity, p. 1382
subdural hematoma, p. 1371
unconsciousness, p. 1359

Acute intracranial problems include diseases and disorders that can increase intracranial pressure (ICP). This chapter discusses the mechanisms that maintain normal ICP and increase ICP. In addition, head injury, brain tumors, and cerebral inflammatory disorders are discussed.

INTRACRANIAL PRESSURE

Understanding the dynamics associated with ICP is important in caring for patients with many different neurologic prob-

lems. The skull is like a closed box with three essential volume components: brain tissue, blood, and cerebrospinal fluid (CSF) (Fig. 57-1). The intracellular and extracellular fluids of brain tissue make up approximately 78% of this volume. Blood in the arterial, venous, and capillary network makes up 12% of the volume, and the remaining 10% is the volume of the CSF.

Primary versus secondary injury is another important concept in understanding ICP. *Primary injury* occurs at the initial time of an injury (e.g., impact of car accident,

---

Reviewed by Sarah Livesay, RN, DNP, ACNP, CNS-A, System Director of Service Line Development, St. Luke's Episcopal Health System, Houston, Texas; Molly M. McNett, RN, PhD, Director, Nursing Research, MetroHealth Medical Center, Cleveland, Ohio; and Susan Yeager, RN, MS, CCRN, ACNP, Neurocritical Care Nurse Practitioner, The Ohio State University Medical Center, Columbus, Ohio.

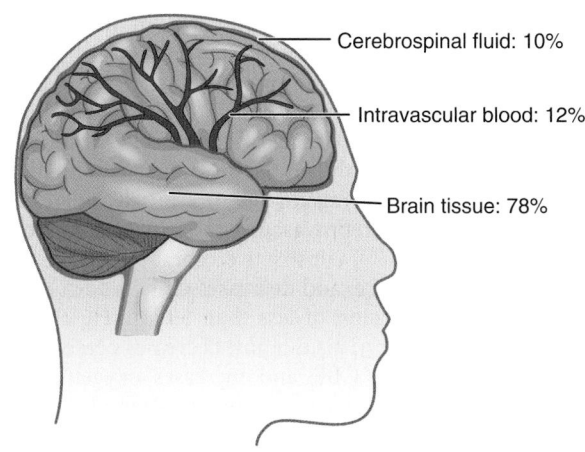

- Cerebrospinal fluid: 10%
- Intravascular blood: 12%
- Brain tissue: 78%

FIG. 57-1 Components of the brain.

TABLE 57-1	**CALCULATION OF CEREBRAL PERFUSION PRESSURE**

CPP = MAP − ICP

$$MAP = DBP + 1/3\,(SBP - DBP) \text{ or } = \frac{SBP + 2\,(DBP)}{3}$$

Example: Systemic blood pressure = 122/84 mm Hg
MAP = 97 mm Hg
ICP = 12 mm Hg
CPP = 85 mm Hg

CPP, Cerebral perfusion pressure; *DBP*, diastolic blood pressure; *ICP*, intracranial pressure; *MAP*, mean arterial pressure; *SBP*, systolic blood pressure.

blunt-force trauma) that results in displacement, bruising, or damage of the three components. *Secondary injury* is the resulting hypoxia, ischemia, hypotension, edema, or increased ICP that follows the primary injury. Secondary injury, which could occur several hours to days after the initial injury, is a primary concern when managing brain injury. Nursing management of the patient with an acute intracranial problem must include management of secondary injury, and thus increased ICP.

Regulation and Maintenance of Intracranial Pressure

Normal Intracranial Pressure. Intracranial pressure (ICP) is the hydrostatic force measured in the brain CSF compartment. Under normal conditions in which intracranial volume remains relatively constant, the balance among the three components (brain tissue, blood, CSF) maintains the ICP. Factors that influence ICP under normal circumstances are changes in (1) arterial pressure; (2) venous pressure; (3) intraabdominal and intrathoracic pressure; (4) posture; (5) temperature; and (6) blood gases, particularly carbon dioxide levels. The degree to which these factors increase or decrease the ICP depends on the brain's ability to adapt to changes.

The Monro-Kellie doctrine states that the three components must remain at a relatively constant volume within the closed skull structure. If the volume of any one of the three components increases within the cranial vault and the volume from another component is displaced, the total intracranial volume will not change.[1] This hypothesis is only applicable in situations in which the skull is closed. The hypothesis is not valid in persons with displaced skull fractures or hemicraniectomy.

ICP can be measured in the ventricles, subarachnoid space, subdural space, epidural space, or brain tissue using a pressure transducer.[2] Normal ICP ranges from 5 to 15 mm Hg. A sustained pressure greater than 20 mm Hg is considered abnormal and must be treated.

Normal Compensatory Adaptations. In applying the Monro-Kellie doctrine, the body can adapt to volume changes within the skull in three different ways to maintain a normal ICP. First, compensatory mechanisms can include changes in the CSF volume. The CSF volume can be changed by altering CSF absorption or production and by displacing CSF into the spinal subarachnoid space. Second, changes in intracranial blood volume can occur through the collapse of cerebral veins and dural sinuses, regional cerebral vasoconstriction or dilation, and changes in venous outflow. Third, brain tissue volume compensates through distention of the dura or compression of brain tissue.

Initially an increase in volume produces no increase in ICP as a result of these compensatory mechanisms. However, the ability to compensate for changes in volume is limited. As the volume increase continues, the ICP rises and decompensation ultimately occurs, resulting in compression and ischemia.

Cerebral Blood Flow

Cerebral blood flow (CBF) is the amount of blood in milliliters passing through 100 g of brain tissue in 1 minute. The global CBF is approximately 50 mL/min/100 g of brain tissue.[3] The maintenance of blood flow to the brain is critical because the brain requires a constant supply of oxygen and glucose. The brain uses 20% of the body's oxygen and 25% of its glucose.[4]

Autoregulation of Cerebral Blood Flow. The brain regulates its own blood flow in response to its metabolic needs despite wide fluctuations in systemic arterial pressure. *Autoregulation* is the automatic adjustment in the diameter of the cerebral blood vessels by the brain to maintain a constant blood flow during changes in arterial blood pressure (BP). The purpose of autoregulation is to ensure a consistent CBF to provide for the metabolic needs of brain tissue and to maintain cerebral perfusion pressure within normal limits.

The lower limit of systemic arterial pressure at which autoregulation is effective in a normotensive person is a mean arterial pressure (MAP) of 70 mm Hg. Below this, CBF decreases, and symptoms of cerebral ischemia, such as syncope and blurred vision, occur. The upper limit of systemic arterial pressure at which autoregulation is effective is a MAP of 150 mm Hg.[3] When this pressure is exceeded, the vessels are maximally constricted, and further vasoconstrictor response is lost.

The *cerebral perfusion pressure* (CPP) is the pressure needed to ensure blood flow to the brain. CPP is equal to the MAP minus the ICP (CPP = MAP − ICP) (see example in Table 57-1). This formula is clinically useful, although it does not consider the effect of cerebrovascular resistance. Cerebrovascular resistance, generated by the arterioles within the cranium, links CPP and blood flow as follows: CPP = Flow × Resistance.

When cerebrovascular resistance is high, blood flow to brain tissue is impaired. Transcranial Doppler is a noninvasive technique used in intensive care units (ICUs) to monitor changes in cerebrovascular resistance.

As the CPP decreases, autoregulation fails and CBF decreases. Normal CPP is 60 to 100 mm Hg. A CPP of less than 50 mm Hg is associated with ischemia and neuronal death. A CPP of less than 30 mm Hg results in ischemia and is incompatible with life.

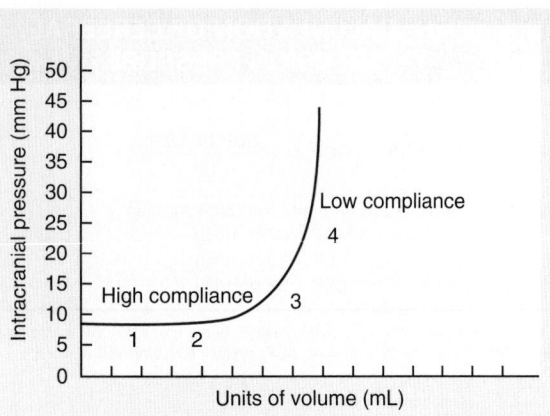

FIG. 57-2 Intracranial pressure-volume curve. (See text for descriptions of *1, 2, 3,* and *4.*)

Normally, autoregulation maintains an adequate CBF and perfusion pressure primarily by adjusting the diameter of cerebral blood vessels and metabolic factors that affect ICP. It is critical to maintain MAP when ICP is elevated.

Remember that CPP may not reflect perfusion pressure in all parts of the brain. There may be local areas of swelling and compression limiting regional perfusion pressure. Thus a higher CPP may be needed for these patients to prevent localized tissue damage. For example, a patient with an acute stroke may require a higher BP, increasing MAP and CPP, in order to increase perfusion to the brain and prevent further tissue damage.

Pressure Changes. The relationship of pressure to volume is depicted in the pressure-volume curve (Fig. 57-2). The curve is affected by the brain's compliance. *Compliance* is the expandability of the brain. It is represented as the volume increase for each unit increase in pressure. With low compliance, small changes in volume result in greater increases in pressure.

$$\text{Compliance} = \text{Volume} / \text{Pressure}$$

The concept of the pressure-volume curve can be used to represent the stages of increased ICP. At stage 1 on the curve, there is high compliance. The brain is in total compensation, with accommodation and autoregulation intact. An increase in volume (in brain tissue, blood, or CSF) does not increase the ICP.

At stage 2, the compliance is beginning to decrease, and an increase in volume places the patient at risk of increased ICP and secondary injury. At stage 3, there is significant reduction in compliance. Any small addition of volume causes a great increase in ICP. Compensatory mechanisms fail, there is a loss of autoregulation, and the patient exhibits manifestations of increased ICP (e.g., headache, changes in level of consciousness or pupil responsiveness).

With a loss of autoregulation, the body attempts to maintain cerebral perfusion by increasing systolic BP. However, decompensation is imminent. The patient's response is characterized by systolic hypertension with a widening pulse pressure, bradycardia with a full and bounding pulse, and altered respirations. This is known as *Cushing's triad* and is a neurologic emergency.

As the patient enters stage 4, the ICP rises to lethal levels with little increase in volume. *Herniation* occurs as the brain tissue is forcibly shifted from the compartment of greater pressure to a compartment of lesser pressure. In this situation, intense pressure is placed on the brainstem, and if herniation continues, brainstem death is imminent.

Factors Affecting Cerebral Blood Flow. Carbon dioxide, oxygen, and hydrogen ion concentration affect cerebral blood vessel tone. An increase in the partial pressure of carbon dioxide in arterial blood ($PaCO_2$) relaxes smooth muscle, dilates cerebral vessels, decreases cerebrovascular resistance, and increases CBF. A decrease in $PaCO_2$ constricts cerebral vessels, increases cerebrovascular resistance, and decreases CBF.

Cerebral oxygen tension of less than 50 mm Hg results in cerebrovascular dilation. This dilation decreases cerebrovascular resistance, increases CBF, and increases oxygen tension. However, if oxygen tension is not increased, anaerobic metabolism begins, resulting in an accumulation of lactic acid. As lactic acid increases and hydrogen ions accumulate, the environment becomes more acidic. Within this acidic environment, further vasodilation occurs in a continued attempt to increase blood flow. The combination of a severely low partial pressure of oxygen in arterial blood (PaO_2) and an elevated hydrogen ion concentration (acidosis), which are both potent cerebral vasodilators, may produce a state where autoregulation is lost and compensatory mechanisms fail to meet tissue metabolic demands.

CBF can be affected by cardiac or respiratory arrest, systemic hemorrhage, and other pathophysiologic states (e.g., diabetic coma, encephalopathies, infections, toxicities). Regional CBF can also be affected by trauma, tumors, cerebral hemorrhage, or stroke. When regional or global autoregulation is lost, CBF is no longer maintained at a constant level but is directly influenced by changes in systemic BP, hypoxia, or catecholamines.

INCREASED INTRACRANIAL PRESSURE

Any patient who becomes unconscious acutely, regardless of the cause, should be suspected of having increased ICP.

Mechanisms of Increased Intracranial Pressure

Increased ICP is a potentially life-threatening situation that results from an increase in any or all of the three components (brain tissue, blood, CSF) within the skull. Elevated ICP is clinically significant because it diminishes CPP, increases risks of brain ischemia and infarction, and is associated with a poor prognosis.[5] Common causes of increased ICP include a mass (e.g., hematoma, contusion, abscess, tumor) and cerebral edema (associated with brain tumors, hydrocephalus, head injury, or brain inflammation).

These cerebral insults, which may result in hypercapnia, cerebral acidosis, impaired autoregulation, and systemic hypertension, increase the formation and spread of cerebral edema. This edema distorts brain tissue, further increasing the ICP, and leads to even more tissue hypoxia and acidosis. Fig. 57-3 illustrates the progression of increased ICP.

It is critical to maintain CBF to preserve tissue and thus minimize secondary injury. Sustained increases in ICP result in brainstem compression and herniation of the brain from one compartment to another.

Displacement and herniation of brain tissue can cause a potentially reversible process to become irreversible. Ischemia and edema are further increased, compounding the preexisting problem. Compression of the brainstem and cranial nerves may be fatal. (Fig. 57-4 illustrates types of herniation.) Herniation

PATHOPHYSIOLOGY MAP

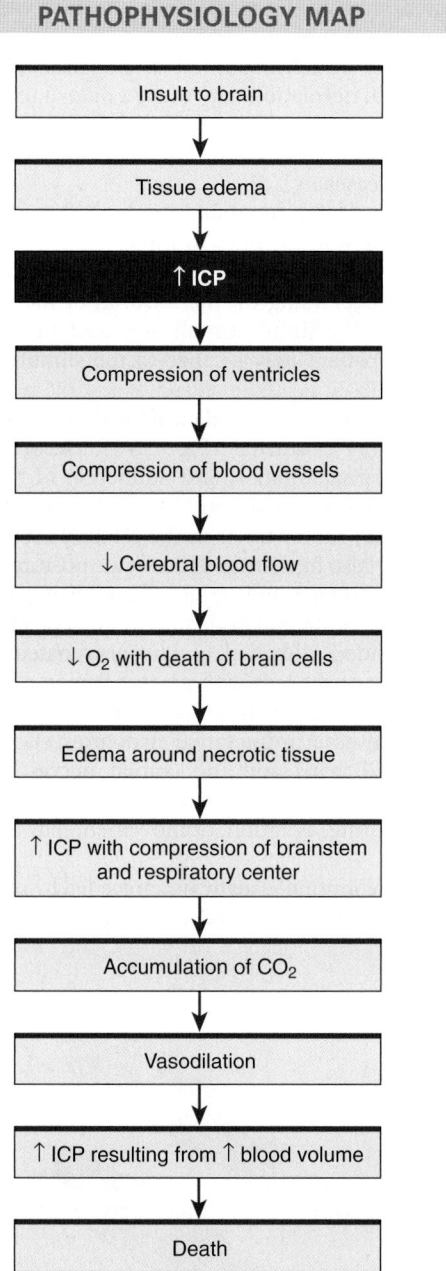

FIG. 57-3 Progression of increased intracranial pressure *(ICP)*.

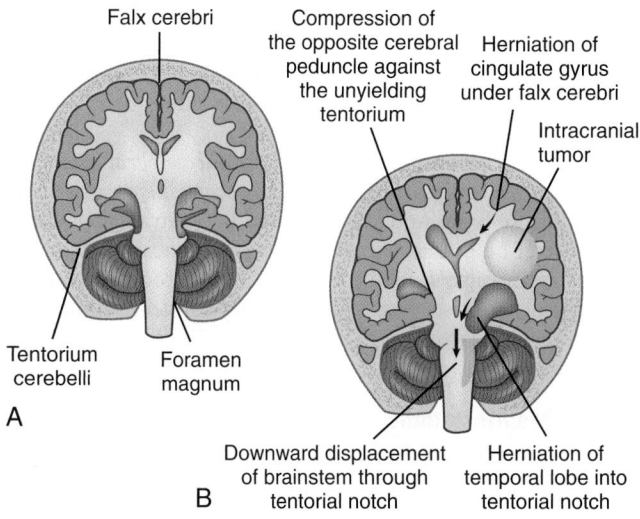

FIG. 57-4 Herniation. **A,** Normal relationship of intracranial structures. **B,** Shift of intracranial structures.

TABLE 57-2	**CAUSES OF CEREBRAL EDEMA**	
Mass Lesions		**Cerebral Infections**

Mass Lesions
- Brain abscess
- Brain tumor (primary or metastatic)
- Hematoma (intracerebral, subdural, epidural)
- Hemorrhage (intracerebral, cerebellar, brainstem)

Head Injuries and Brain Surgery
- Contusion
- Hemorrhage
- Posttraumatic brain swelling

Cerebral Infections
- Meningitis
- Encephalitis

Vascular Insult
- Anoxic and ischemic episodes
- Cerebral infarction (thrombotic or embolic)
- Venous sinus thrombosis

Toxic or Metabolic Encephalopathic Conditions
- Lead or arsenic intoxication
- Hepatic encephalopathy
- Uremia

forces the cerebellum and the brainstem downward through the foramen magnum. If compression of the brainstem is unrelieved, respiratory arrest will occur due to compression of the respiratory control center in the medulla.

Cerebral Edema

As shown in Table 57-2, there are a variety of causes of cerebral edema (increased accumulation of fluid in the extravascular spaces of brain tissue). Regardless of the cause, cerebral edema results in an increase in tissue volume that can increase ICP. The extent and severity of the original insult are factors that determine the degree of cerebral edema.

There are three types of cerebral edema: vasogenic, cytotoxic, and interstitial. The same patient may have more than one type.

Vasogenic Cerebral Edema. *Vasogenic cerebral edema,* the most common type of cerebral edema, occurs mainly in the white matter and is characterized by leakage of macromolecules from the capillaries into the surrounding extracellular space. This results in an osmotic gradient that favors the flow of fluid from the intravascular to the extravascular space. A variety of insults, such as brain tumors, abscesses, and ingested toxins, may cause an increase in the permeability of the blood-brain barrier and produce an increase in the extracellular fluid volume. The speed and extent of the spread of the edema fluid are influenced by the systemic BP, the site of the brain injury, and the extent of the blood-brain barrier defect.

This edema may produce a continuum of symptoms ranging from headache to disturbances in consciousness, including coma (profound state of unconsciousness) and focal neurologic deficits. It is important to recognize that although a headache may seem to be a benign symptom, in cases of cerebral edema it can quickly progress to coma and death. Therefore you must be vigilant in your assessment.

Cytotoxic Cerebral Edema. *Cytotoxic cerebral edema* results from disruption of the integrity of the cell membranes. It develops from destructive lesions or trauma to brain tissue resulting in cerebral hypoxia or anoxia and syndrome of inappropriate antidiuretic hormone (SIADH) secretion. In this type of edema the blood-brain barrier remains intact, with cerebral edema occurring as a result of a fluid and protein shift from the extracellular space directly into the cells, with subsequent swelling and loss of cellular function.

Interstitial Cerebral Edema. *Interstitial cerebral edema* is usually a result of hydrocephalus. *Hydrocephalus* is a build up of fluid in the brain and is manifested by ventricular enlargement. It can be due to excess CSF production, obstruction of flow, or an inability to reabsorb the CSF. Hydrocephalus treatment usually consists of a ventriculostomy or ventriculoperitoneal shunt. (Management of hydrocephalus is discussed later in this chapter.)

Clinical Manifestations

The clinical manifestations of increased ICP can take many forms, depending on the cause, location, and rate of increases in ICP.

Change in Level of Consciousness. The *level of consciousness* (LOC) is the most sensitive and reliable indicator of the patient's neurologic status. Changes in LOC are a result of impaired CBF, which deprives the cells of the cerebral cortex and the reticular activating system (RAS) of oxygen. The RAS is located in the brainstem, with neural connections to many parts of the nervous system. An intact RAS can maintain a state of wakefulness even in the absence of a functioning cerebral cortex. Interruptions of impulses from the RAS or alterations in functioning of the cerebral hemispheres can cause unconsciousness (abnormal state of complete or partial unawareness of self or environment).

The patient's state of consciousness is defined by both the behavior and the pattern of brain activity recorded by an electroencephalogram (EEG). A change in consciousness may be dramatic, as in coma, or subtle, such as a flattening of affect, change in orientation, or decrease in level of attention. In the deepest state of unconsciousness (i.e., coma), the patient does not respond to painful stimuli. Corneal and pupillary reflexes are absent. The patient cannot swallow or cough and is incontinent of urine and feces. The EEG pattern demonstrates suppressed or absent neuronal activity.

Changes in Vital Signs. Changes in vital signs are caused by increasing pressure on the thalamus, hypothalamus, pons, and medulla. Manifestations such as *Cushing's triad* (systolic hypertension with a widening pulse pressure, bradycardia with a full and bounding pulse, and irregular respirations) may be present but often do not appear until ICP has been increased for some time or is suddenly and markedly increased (e.g., head trauma). Always recognize Cushing's triad as a medical emergency, since this is a sign of brainstem compression and impending death. A change in body temperature may also occur because increased ICP affects the hypothalamus.

Ocular Signs. Compression of cranial nerve (CN) III, the oculomotor nerve, results in dilation of the pupil on the same side *(ipsilateral)* as the mass lesion, sluggish or no response to light, inability to move the eye upward, and ptosis of the eyelid. These signs can be the result of the brain shifting from midline, compressing the trunk of CN III, and paralyzing the muscles controlling pupillary size and shape. In this situation, a fixed, unilateral, dilated pupil is considered a neurologic emergency that indicates herniation of the brain.

Other cranial nerves may also be affected, such as the optic (CN II), trochlear (CN IV), and abducens (CN VI) nerves. Signs of dysfunction of these cranial nerves include blurred vision, diplopia, and changes in extraocular eye movements. Central herniation may initially manifest as sluggish but equal pupil response. Uncal herniation may cause a dilated unilateral pupil. *Papilledema* (an edematous optic disc seen on retinal examination) is also noted and is a nonspecific sign associated with persistent increases in ICP.

Decrease in Motor Function. As the ICP continues to rise, the patient manifests changes in motor ability. A *contralateral* (opposite side of the mass lesion) hemiparesis or hemiplegia may develop, depending on the location of the source of the increased ICP. If painful stimuli are used to elicit a motor response, the patient may localize to the stimuli or withdraw from it.

Noxious stimuli may also elicit *decorticate* (flexor) or *decerebrate* (extensor) posturing (Fig. 57-5). Decorticate posture consists of internal rotation and adduction of the arms with flexion of the elbows, wrists, and fingers as a result of interruption of voluntary motor tracts in the cerebral cortex. Extension of the legs may also be seen. A decerebrate posture may indicate more serious damage and results from disruption of motor fibers in the midbrain and brainstem. In this position, the arms are stiffly extended, adducted, and hyperpronated. There is also hyperextension of the legs with plantar flexion of the feet.

Headache. Although the brain itself is insensitive to pain, compression of other intracranial structures, such as the walls of arteries and veins and the cranial nerves, can produce headache. The headache is often continuous but worse in the morning. Straining, agitation, or movement may accentuate the pain.

Vomiting. Vomiting, usually not preceded by nausea, is often a nonspecific sign of increased ICP. This is called unexpected

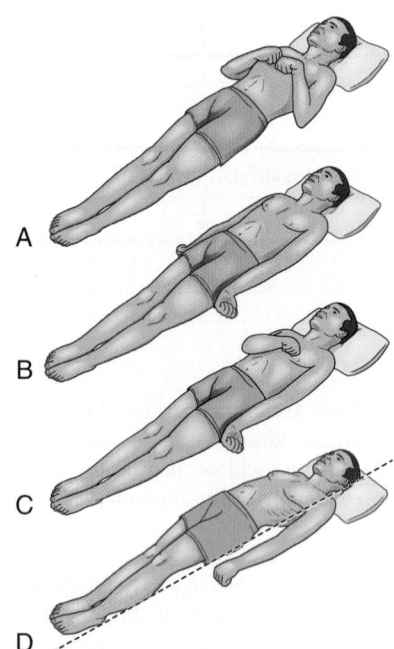

FIG. 57-5 Decorticate and decerebrate posturing. **A,** Decorticate response. Flexion of arms, wrists, and fingers with adduction in upper extremities. Extension, internal rotation, and plantar flexion in lower extremities. **B,** Decerebrate response. All four extremities in rigid extension, with hyperpronation of forearms and plantar flexion of feet. **C,** Decorticate response on right side of body and decerebrate response on left side of body. **D,** Opisthotonic posturing.

vomiting and is related to pressure changes in the cranium. Projectile vomiting may also occur and is related to increased ICP.

Complications

The major complications of uncontrolled increased ICP are inadequate cerebral perfusion and cerebral herniation (see Fig. 57-4). To better understand cerebral herniation, two important structures in the brain must be described. The *falx cerebri* is a thin wall of dura that folds down between the cortex, separating the two cerebral hemispheres. The *tentorium cerebelli* is a rigid fold of dura that separates the cerebral hemispheres from the cerebellum (see Fig. 57-4). It is called the tentorium (meaning tent) because it forms a tentlike cover over the cerebellum.

Tentorial herniation (central herniation) occurs when a mass lesion in the cerebrum forces the brain to herniate downward through the opening created by the brainstem. *Uncal herniation* occurs when there is lateral and downward herniation. *Cingulate herniation* occurs when there is lateral displacement of brain tissue beneath the falx cerebri.

Diagnostic Studies

Diagnostic studies can identify the cause of increased ICP (Table 57-3). Computed tomography (CT) and magnetic

TABLE 57-3 COLLABORATIVE CARE

Increased Intracranial Pressure

Diagnostic
- History and physical examination
- Vital signs, neurologic assessments, ICP measurements
- Skull, chest, and spinal x-ray studies
- CT scan, MRI, cerebral angiography, EEG, PET
- Transcranial Doppler studies
- Infrascanner
- ECG
- Evoked potential studies
- Laboratory studies, including CBC, coagulation profile, electrolytes, serum creatinine, ABGs, ammonia level, drug and toxicology screen, CSF analysis for protein, cells, glucose*

Collaborative Therapy
- Elevation of head of bed to 30 degrees with head in a neutral position
- Intubation and mechanical ventilation
- ICP monitoring
- Cerebral oxygenation monitoring (PbtO₂, SjvO₂)
- Maintenance of PaO₂ ≥100 mm Hg
- Maintenance of fluid balance and assessment of osmolality
- Maintenance of systolic arterial pressure between 100 and 160 mm Hg
- Maintenance of CPP >60 mm Hg
- Reduction of cerebral metabolism (e.g., high-dose barbiturates)
- Drug therapy
  - Osmotic diuretic (mannitol)
  - Hypertonic saline
  - Antiseizure drugs (e.g., phenytoin [Dilantin])
  - Corticosteroids (dexamethasone [Decadron]) for brain tumors, bacterial meningitis
  - Histamine (H₂)-receptor antagonist (e.g., cimetidine [Tagamet]) or proton pump inhibitor (e.g., pantoprazole [Protonix]) to prevent GI ulcers and bleeding

*A lumbar puncture to obtain CSF for analysis should not be done if there is a possibility of herniation.
CPP, Cerebral perfusion pressure; *ICP,* intracranial pressure; *PaO₂,* partial pressure of oxygen in arterial blood; *PbtO₂,* pressure of oxygen in brain tissue; *SjvO₂,* jugular venous oxygen saturation.

resonance imaging (MRI) have revolutionized the diagnosis of increased ICP. These tests are used to differentiate the many conditions that can cause increased ICP and to assess the effect of treatment.

Additional tests include EEG, cerebral angiography, ICP measurement, brain tissue oxygenation measurement via the LICOX catheter (described later), transcranial Doppler studies, and evoked potential studies. Positron emission tomography (PET) is also used to diagnose the cause of increased ICP. In general, a lumbar puncture is not performed when increased ICP is suspected. The reason for this is that cerebral herniation could occur from the sudden release of the pressure in the skull from the area above the lumbar puncture.

In some institutions a hand-held Infrascanner can be used to detect life-threatening intracranial bleeding. The scanner directs a wavelength of light that can penetrate tissue and bone. Blood from intracranial hematomas absorbs the light differently than other areas of the brain.

Monitoring Intracranial Pressure and Cerebral Oxygenation

Indications for Intracranial Pressure Monitoring. ICP monitoring is used to guide clinical care when the patient is at risk for or has elevations in ICP. It may be used in patients with a variety of neurologic insults, including hemorrhage, stroke, tumor, infection, or traumatic brain injury. ICP should be monitored in patients admitted with a Glasgow Coma Scale (GCS) score of 8 or less and an abnormal CT scan or MRI (hematomas, contusion, edema). (The GCS is presented later in Table 57-5.)

Methods of Measuring Intracranial Pressure. Patients with conditions known to elevate ICP, except those with irreversible problems or advanced neurologic disease, usually undergo ICP monitoring in an ICU. Multiple methods and devices are available to monitor ICP in various sites (Fig. 57-6).

The gold standard for monitoring ICP is the *ventriculostomy,* in which a specialized catheter is inserted into the lateral ventricle and coupled to an external transducer (Figs. 57-7 and 57-8). This technique directly measures the pressure within the ventricles, facilitates removal and/or sampling of CSF, and allows for intraventricular drug administration. In this system the transducer is external, and it is important to ensure that the transducer of the ventriculostomy is level with the foramen of Monro (interventricular foramen). The ventriculostomy system must also be at the ideal height (Fig. 57-9, *A*). A reference point

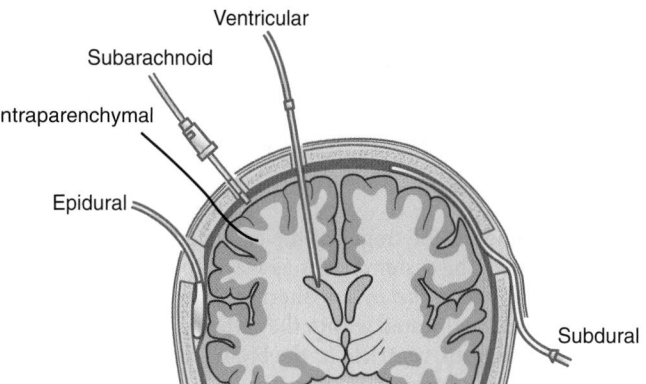

FIG. 57-6 Coronal section of brain showing potential sites for placement of intracranial pressure monitoring devices.

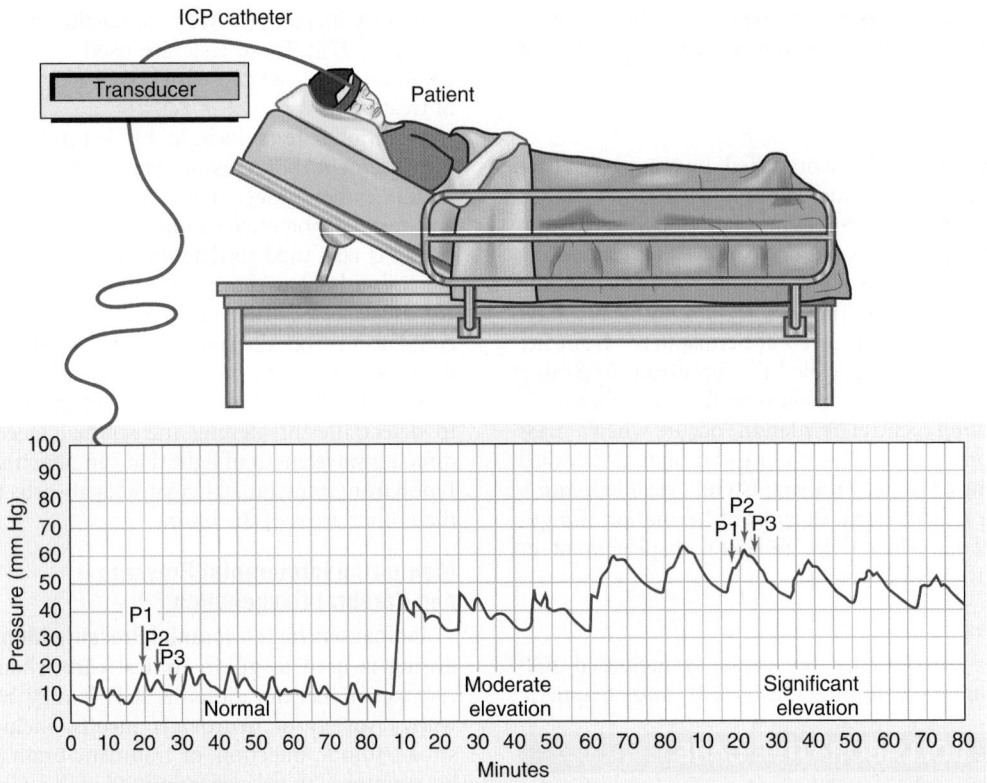

FIG. 57-7 Intracranial pressure *(ICP)* monitoring can be used to continuously measure ICP. The ICP tracing shows normal, elevated, and plateau waves. At high ICP the P2 peak is higher than the P1 peak, and the peaks become less distinct and plateau.

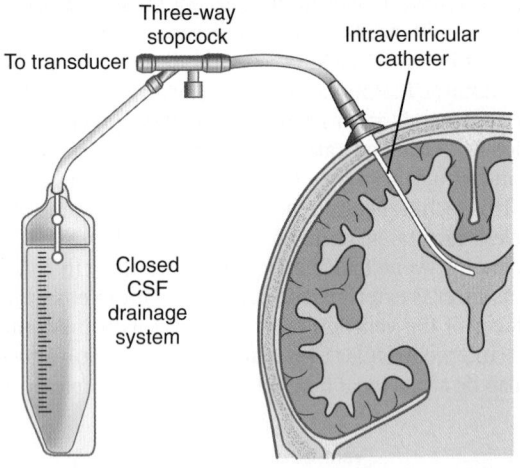

FIG. 57-8 Ventriculostomy in place. Cerebrospinal fluid *(CSF)* can be drained via a ventriculostomy when intracranial pressure (ICP) exceeds the upper pressure parameter set by the physician. Intermittent drainage involves opening the three-way stopcock to allow CSF to flow into the drainage bag for brief periods (30 to 120 seconds) until the pressure is below the upper pressure parameters.

TABLE 57-4	NORMAL INTRACRANIAL PRESSURE WAVEFORMS*	
Waveform		**Meaning**
P1 Percussion wave		Represents arterial pulsations. Normally the highest of the three waveforms.
P2 Rebound wave or tidal wave		Reflects intracranial compliance or relative brain volume. When P2 is higher than P1, intracranial compliance is compromised.
P3 Dicrotic wave		Follows dicrotic notch. Represents venous pulsations. Normally the lowest waveform.

*See Fig. 57-7.

for this foramen is the tragus of the ear. Every time the patient is repositioned, the system needs assessed to ensure it is level.

The *fiberoptic catheter,* an alternative technology, uses a sensor transducer located within the catheter tip. The sensor tip is placed within the ventricle or the brain tissue and provides a direct measurement of brain pressure.

The *subarachnoid bolt* or *screw* is another method of monitoring ICP. It is placed just through the skull between the arach-noid membrane and the cerebral cortex. It does not allow for CSF drainage but is ideal for patients with mild or moderate head injury. It can easily be converted into a ventriculostomy if the patient decompensates.

Infection is a serious complication with ICP monitoring. Factors that contribute to the development of infection include ICP monitoring more than 5 days, use of a ventriculostomy, a CSF leak, and a concurrent systemic infection. Routinely assessing the insertion site, using aseptic technique, and monitoring the CSF for a change in drainage color or clarity are important nursing interventions.

ICP should be measured as a mean pressure. If a CSF drainage device is in place, the drain must be closed for at least 6 minutes to ensure an accurate reading. Record the waveform strip along with other pressure monitoring waveforms. The normal ICP waveform has three phases (see Fig. 57-7 and Table 57-4). It is important to monitor the ICP waveform, as well as

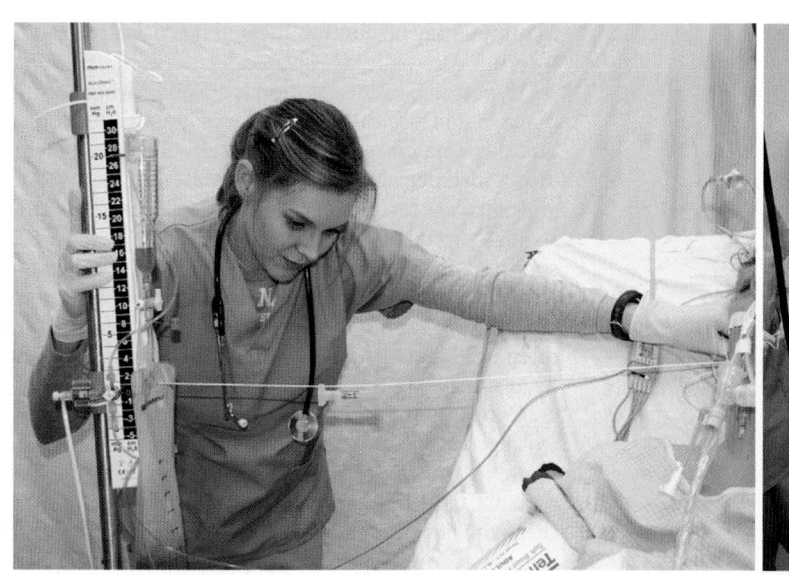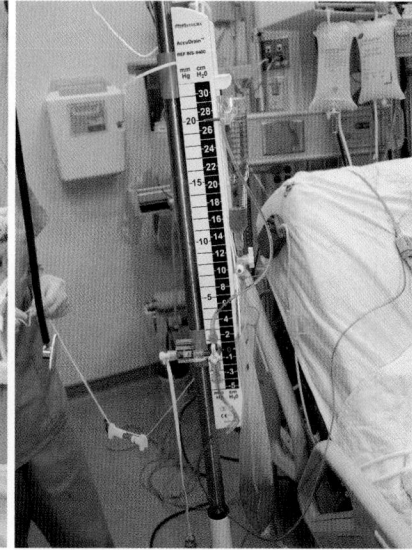

FIG. 57-9 A, Leveling a ventriculostomy. **B,** Cerebrospinal fluid is drained into a drainage system.

the mean CPP. When ICP is normal, P1, P2, and P3 resemble a staircase.[6] As ICP increases, P2 rises above P1, indicating poor ventricular compliance (see Fig. 57-7). Consider the rate at which changes occur and the patient's clinical condition. Neurologic deterioration might not occur until ICP elevation is pronounced and sustained. Immediately report to the health care provider any ICP elevation, either as a mean increase in pressure or as an abnormal waveform configuration.

Inaccurate ICP readings can be caused by CSF leaks around the monitoring device, obstruction of the intraventricular catheter or bolt (from tissue or blood clot), a difference between the height of the bolt and the transducer, kinks in the tubing, and incorrect height of the drainage system relative to the patient's reference point. Bubbles or air in the tubing can also dampen the waveform.

Cerebrospinal Fluid Drainage. With the ventricular catheter, it is possible to control ICP by removing CSF (see Fig. 57-8). The physician typically orders a specific level at which to initiate drainage (e.g., if ICP is greater than 20 mm Hg) and the frequency of drainage (intermittent or continuous). When the ICP is above the indicated level, the ventriculostomy system is opened by turning a stopcock and allowing the drainage of CSF, thus relieving pressure inside the cranial vault (see Fig. 57-9, *B*).

The two options for CSF drainage are intermittent or continuous. If intermittent drainage is ordered, open the ventriculostomy system at the indicated ICP and allow CSF to drain for 2 to 3 minutes. Then close the stopcock to return the ventriculostomy to a closed system. If continuous ICP drainage is ordered, careful monitoring of the volume of CSF drained is essential, keeping in mind that normal CSF production is about 20 to 30 mL/hr, with a total CSF volume of 90 to 150 mL within the ventricles and subarachnoid space. It is also recommended that a sign be posted above the patient's bed to notify anyone before turning, moving, or suctioning the patient to prevent the removal of too much CSF, which can result in other complications.

Strict aseptic technique during dressing changes or sampling of CSF is imperative to prevent infection. The system must remain intact to ensure that the ICP readings are accurate because treatment is initiated based on the pressures.

Complications of this type of drainage system include ventricular collapse, infection, and herniation or subdural hematoma formation from rapid decompression. Although it is generally recognized that CSF removal decreases ICP and improves CPP, guidelines for CSF removal are not universally accepted, but are typically based on institution or physician preference.[7]

Cerebral Oxygenation Monitoring. Technology is available to measure cerebral oxygenation and assess perfusion. Two such devices used in ICU settings are the *LICOX brain tissue oxygenation catheter* and the *jugular venous bulb catheter*. The LICOX catheter, which measures brain oxygenation and temperature, is placed in viable (healthy) white matter of the brain (Fig. 57-10). The LICOX system provides continuous monitoring of the pressure of oxygen in brain tissue ($PbtO_2$). The normal range for $PbtO_2$ is 20 to 40 mm Hg. A lower than normal $PbtO_2$ level is indicative of ischemia. Another advantage of the LICOX catheter is the ability to measure brain temperature. A cooler brain temperature (96.8° F [36° C]) may produce better outcomes.[8]

The jugular venous bulb catheter is placed in the internal jugular vein and positioned so that the catheter tip is located in the jugular bulb. Placement is verified by an x-ray. This catheter provides a measurement of jugular venous oxygen saturation ($SjvO_2$), which indicates total venous brain tissue extraction of oxygen. This is a measure of cerebral oxygen supply and demand. The normal $SjvO_2$ range is 55% to 75%. Values less than 50% demonstrate impaired cerebral oxygenation.

Collaborative Care

The goals of collaborative care (see Table 57-3) are to identify and treat the underlying cause of increased ICP and to support brain function. The earlier the condition is recognized and treated, the better the patient outcome. A careful history is an important diagnostic aid in the search for the underlying cause. The underlying cause of increased ICP is usually an increase in blood (hemorrhage), brain tissue (tumor or edema), or CSF (hydrocephalus) in the brain.

For any patient with increased ICP, it is important to maintain adequate oxygenation to support brain function. An endo-

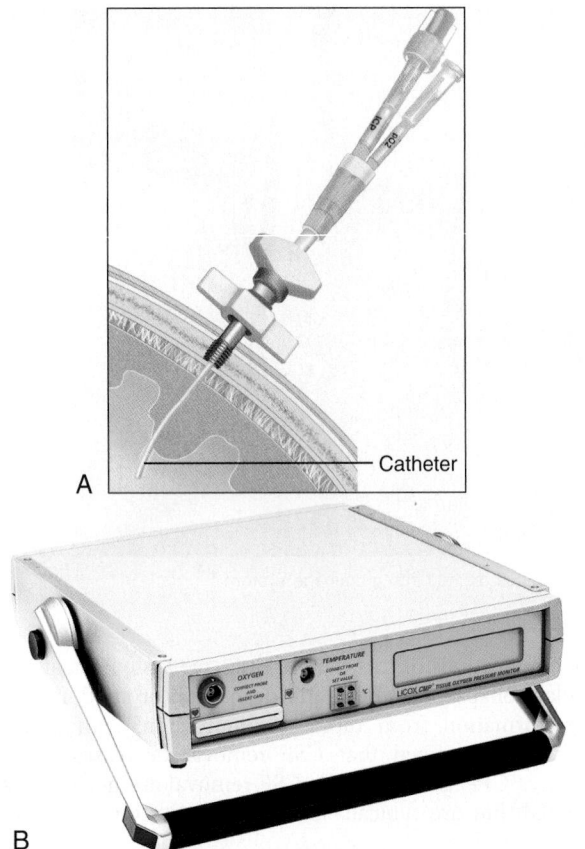

FIG. 57-10 A, The LICOX brain tissue oxygen system involves a catheter inserted through an intracranial bolt. **B,** The system measures oxygen in the brain (PbtO$_2$), brain tissue temperature, and intracranial pressure. (**B,** Permission granted by Integra LifeSciences Corporation, Plainsboro, NJ.)

tracheal tube or tracheostomy may be necessary to maintain adequate ventilation. Arterial blood gas (ABG) analysis guides the oxygen therapy. The goal is to maintain the PaO$_2$ at greater than or equal to 100 mm Hg and to keep PaCO$_2$ in normal range at 35 to 45 mm Hg. The patient may need to be on a mechanical ventilator to ensure adequate oxygenation.

If increased ICP is caused by a mass lesion (e.g., tumor, hematoma), surgical removal of the mass is the best treatment (see the sections on brain tumors and cranial surgery later in this chapter). Nonsurgical intervention for the reduction of tissue volume related to cerebral tissue swelling and cerebral edema includes the use of diuretics and corticosteroids. In aggressive situations, a craniectomy (removal of part of skull) may be performed to reduce ICP and prevent herniation (see head injury section for further details).

Drug Therapy. Drug therapy plays an important part in the management of increased ICP. Mannitol (Osmitrol) (25%) is an osmotic diuretic given IV. Mannitol acts to decrease the ICP in two ways: plasma expansion and osmotic effect. The immediate plasma-expanding effect reduces the hematocrit and blood viscosity, thereby increasing CBF and cerebral oxygen delivery. A vascular osmotic gradient is created by mannitol. Thus fluid moves from the tissues into the blood vessels, reducing the ICP because of the decrease in the total brain fluid content. Monitor fluid and electrolyte status when osmotic diuretics are used.

Mannitol may be contraindicated if renal disease is present and if serum osmolality is elevated.[5]

Hypertonic saline solution is another drug treatment used to manage increased ICP. It produces massive movement of water out of edematous swollen brain cells and into the blood vessels. This movement of water out of the brain can reduce swelling and improve cerebral blood flow. Hypertonic solution infusion requires frequent monitoring of blood pressure and serum sodium levels because intravascular fluid volume excess can occur. Hypertonic saline infusion has been shown to be just as effective as mannitol when treating increased ICP, and both are often used concurrently when caring for a patient with a severe head injury.[9]

Corticosteroids (e.g., dexamethasone [Decadron]) are used to treat vasogenic edema surrounding tumors and abscesses. However, these drugs are not recommended for head-injured patients. Corticosteroids stabilize the cell membrane and inhibit the synthesis of prostaglandins (see Fig. 12-2), thus preventing the formation of proinflammatory mediators. Corticosteroids also improve neuronal function by improving CBF and restoring autoregulation.

Complications associated with the use of corticosteroids include hyperglycemia, increased incidence of infections, and gastrointestinal (GI) bleeding. Regularly monitor fluid intake and sodium levels, and perform blood glucose monitoring at least every 6 hours until hyperglycemia is ruled out. Patients receiving corticosteroids should concurrently be given antacids or histamine (H$_2$)-receptor blockers (e.g., cimetidine [Tagamet], ranitidine [Zantac]) or proton pump inhibitors (e.g., omeprazole [Prilosec], pantoprazole [Protonix, Protonix IV]) to prevent GI ulcers and bleeding.

Metabolic demands such as fever (greater than 100.4° F [38° C]), agitation or shivering, pain, and seizures can also increase ICP. The health care team should plan to reduce these metabolic demands to lower the ICP in the at-risk patient. Monitor patients for seizure activity. They may need to be placed on prophylactic antiseizure medication. Fever should be well controlled to maintain a temperature of 96.8° to 98.6° F (36° to 37° C) by using antipyretics (e.g., acetaminophen), cool baths, cooling blankets, ice packs, or intravascular cooling devices as necessary. However, avoid letting the patient shiver or shake, since this increases the metabolic workload on the brain. If this occurs, sedatives may be needed or a different cooling method selected.

Manage pain while being careful not to oversedate or overmedicate. Finally, the patient should remain in a quiet, calm environment with minimal noise and interruptions. Observe the patient for signs of agitation, irritation, or frustration. Also teach the caregiver and the family about decreasing stimulation, and coordinate with the health care team to minimize procedures that may produce agitation.

Drug therapy for reducing cerebral metabolism may be an effective strategy to control ICP. Reducing the metabolic rate decreases the CBF and therefore the ICP. High doses of barbiturates (e.g., pentobarbital [Nembutal], thiopental [Pentothal]) are used in patients with increased ICP refractory to other treatments. Barbiturates decrease cerebral metabolism, causing a decrease in ICP and a reduction in cerebral edema.[5] When this treatment is used, monitor the patient's ICP, blood flow, and EEG. Barbiturate dosing is typically based on analysis of the bedside EEG tracing and the ICP. The physician orders the barbiturate infusion at a rate that achieves a desired level of brain wave suppression as a means to control ICP. Total *burst suppression*, recognized by the absence of spikes showing brain activity on the EEG monitor, indicates that maximal therapeutic effect has been achieved.[5]

Nutritional Therapy. Patients must have their nutritional needs met, regardless of their state of consciousness. Because malnutrition promotes continued cerebral edema, maintenance of optimal nutrition is imperative. The patient with increased ICP is in a hypermetabolic and hypercatabolic state that increases the need for glucose as fuel for metabolism of the injured brain. If the patient cannot maintain an adequate oral intake, other means of meeting the nutritional requirements, such as enteral feedings or parenteral nutrition, should be initiated.

Early feeding after brain injury may improve patient outcome.[10] Nutritional replacement should begin within 3 days after injury to reach full nutritional replacement within 7 days after the injury is sustained.[10] (Nutritional therapy is discussed in Chapter 40.) Feedings or supplements should be guided by the patient's fluid and electrolyte status and metabolic needs. The patient should remain in a normovolemic fluid state. Continuously evaluate the patient based on clinical factors such as urine output, insensible fluid loss, serum and urine osmolality, and serum electrolytes.

IV 0.9% sodium chloride is the preferred solution for administration of piggyback medications. If 5% dextrose in water or 0.45% sodium chloride is used, serum osmolarity decreases and an increase in cerebral edema may occur.

NURSING MANAGEMENT
INCREASED INTRACRANIAL PRESSURE

NURSING ASSESSMENT

Subjective data about the patient with increased ICP can be obtained from the patient, caregiver, or family who are familiar with the patient. Learn appropriate neurologic assessment techniques. Describe the LOC by noting the specific behaviors observed. When a deviation from the normal state of consciousness occurs, use a more structured method of observation. This type of systematic approach to nursing assessment is illustrated in eFig. 57-1 (available on the website for this chapter). Assess the LOC using the Glasgow Coma Scale (Table 57-5). Also assess body functions, especially circulation and respiration.

GLASGOW COMA SCALE. The Glasgow Coma Scale (GCS) is a quick, practical, and standardized system for assessing the LOC. The three areas assessed in the GCS are the patient's ability to (1) speak, (2) obey commands, and (3) open the eyes when a verbal or painful stimulus is applied. Specific assessments evaluate the patient's response to varying degrees of stimulus. Three indicators of response are evaluated: (1) opening of the eyes, (2) the best verbal response, and (3) the best motor response (see Table 57-5).

Specific behaviors observed as responses to the testing stimulus are given a numeric value. Your responsibility is to elicit the best response on each of the scales: the higher the scores, the higher the level of brain functioning. The subscale scores are particularly important if a patient is untestable in one area. For example, severe periorbital edema may make eye opening impossible.

TABLE 57-5 GLASGOW COMA SCALE

Appropriate Stimulus	Response	Score
Eyes Open		
• Approach to bedside	Spontaneous response.	4
• Verbal command	Opening of eyes to name or command.	3
• Pain	Lack of opening of eyes to previous stimuli but opening to pain.	2
	Lack of opening of eyes to any stimulus.	1
	Untestable.*	U
Best Verbal Response		
• Verbal questioning with maximum arousal	Appropriate orientation, conversant. Correct identification of self, place, yr, and mo.	5
	Confusion. Conversant, but disorientation in one or more spheres.	4
	Inappropriate or disorganized use of words (e.g., cursing), lack of sustained conversation.	3
	Incomprehensible words, sounds (e.g., moaning).	2
	Lack of sound, even with painful stimuli.	1
	Untestable.*	U
Best Motor Response		
• Verbal command (e.g., "raise your arm, hold up two fingers")	Obedience of command.	6
	Localization of pain, lack of obedience but presence of attempts to remove offending stimulus.	5
• Pain (pressure on proximal nail bed)	Flexion withdrawal,* flexion of arm in response to pain without abnormal flexion posture.	4
	Abnormal flexion, flexing of arm at elbow and pronation, making a fist.	3
	Abnormal extension, extension of arm at elbow usually with adduction and internal rotation of arm at shoulder.	2
	Lack of response.	1
	Untestable.*	U

*Added to the original scale by some centers.

The total GCS score is the sum of the numeric values assigned to each of the three areas evaluated. The highest GCS score is 15 for a fully alert person, and the lowest possible score is 3. A GCS score of 8 or less generally indicates coma. Plot the results of the GCS scores on a graph, which can be used to determine whether the patient is stable, improving, or deteriorating.

The GCS offers several advantages in the assessment of the unconscious patient. It allows different health care professionals to arrive at the same conclusion regarding the patient's status and can be used to discriminate between different or changing states.

Although the GCS is the gold standard assessment tool for LOC, other scales are also used in the clinical setting.[11] In cases of stroke or hemorrhage associated with increased ICP, use the NIH Stroke Scale (see Table 58-9). Other components of the neurologic assessment include cranial nerve assessment and motor and sensory testing.

NEUROLOGIC ASSESSMENT. Compare the pupils with one another for size, shape, movement, and reactivity (Fig. 57-11).

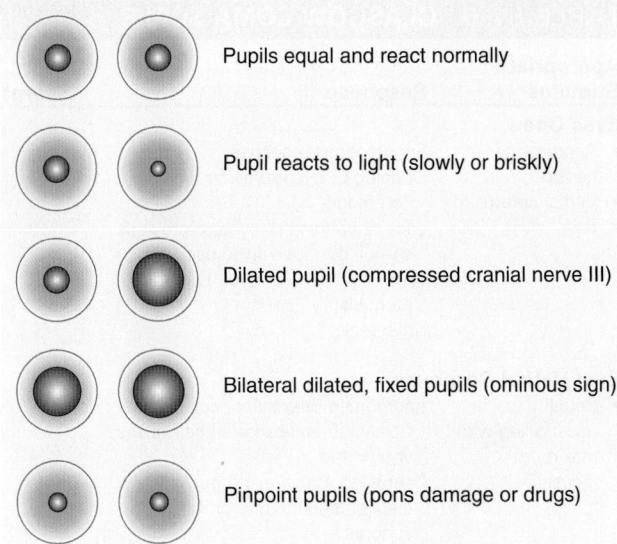

FIG. 57-11 Pupillary check for size and response.

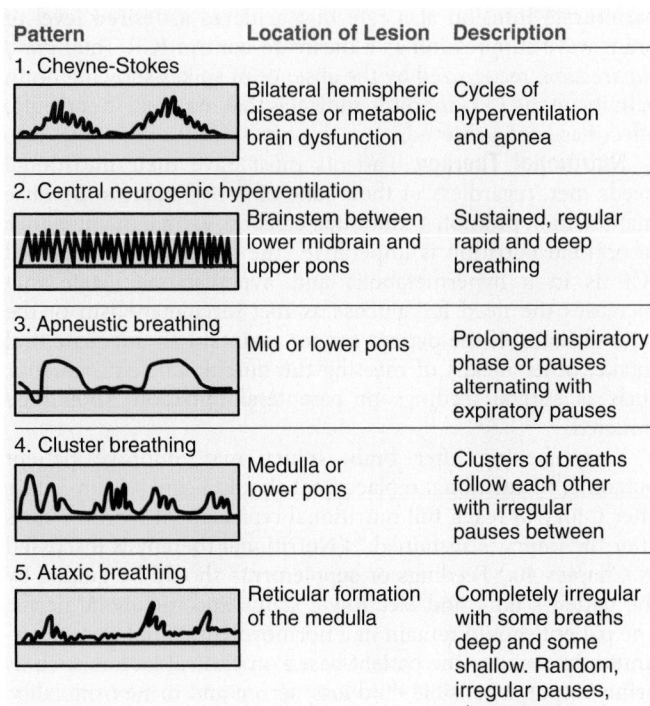

FIG. 57-12 Common abnormal respiratory patterns associated with coma.

If the oculomotor nerve (CN III) is compressed, the pupil on the affected side (ipsilateral) becomes larger until it fully dilates. If ICP continues to increase, both pupils dilate.

Test pupillary reaction with a penlight. The normal reaction is brisk constriction when the light is shone directly into the eye. Also note a consensual response (a slight constriction in the opposite pupil) at the same time. A sluggish reaction can indicate early pressure on CN III. A fixed pupil unresponsive to light stimulus usually indicates increased ICP. However, note that there are other causes of a fixed pupil, including direct injury to CN III, previous eye surgery, administration of atropine, and use of mydriatic eyedrops.

Evaluation of other cranial nerves can be included in the neurologic assessment. Eye movements controlled by CN III, IV, and VI can be examined in the patient who is awake and able to follow commands, and can be used to assess the function of the brainstem. Testing the corneal reflex gives information about the functioning of CN V and VII. If this reflex is absent, initiate routine eye care to prevent corneal abrasion (see Chapters 21 and 22).

Eye movements of the uncooperative or unconscious patient can be elicited by reflex with the use of head movements (oculocephalic) and caloric stimulation (oculovestibular) (see Chapters 21 and 22). To test the oculocephalic reflex (doll's eye reflex), turn the patient's head briskly to the left or right while holding the eyelids open. A normal response is movement of the eyes across the midline in the direction opposite that of the turning. Next, quickly flex and then extend the neck. Eye movement should be opposite to the direction of head movement—up when the neck is flexed and down when it is extended. Abnormal responses can help locate the intracranial lesion. This test should not be attempted if a cervical spine problem is suspected. (The oculovestibular reflex is discussed in Chapter 21.)

Test motor strength by asking the awake and cooperative patient to squeeze your hands to compare strength in the hands. The palmar drift test is an excellent measure of strength in the upper extremities. The patient raises the arms in front of the body with the palms facing upward. If there is any weakness in the upper extremity, the palmar surface turns downward and the arm drifts down. Asking the patient to raise the foot from the bed or to bend the knees up in bed is a good assessment of lower extremity strength. Test all four extremities for strength and for any asymmetry in strength or movement.

Assess the motor response of the unconscious or uncooperative patient by observation of spontaneous movement. If no spontaneous movement is possible, apply a pain stimulus to the patient, and note the response. Resistance to movement during passive range-of-motion exercises is another measure of strength. Do not include hand squeezing as part of the assessment of motor movement in the unconscious or uncooperative patient, since this is a reflex action and can misrepresent the patient's status.

Also record the vital signs, including BP, pulse, respiratory rate, and temperature. Be aware of Cushing's triad, which indicates severely increased ICP. Besides recording respiratory rate, also note the respiratory pattern. Specific respiratory patterns are associated with severely increased ICP (Fig. 57-12).

NURSING DIAGNOSES

Nursing diagnoses for the patient with increased ICP include, but are not limited to, the following:

- Decreased intracranial adaptive capacity *related to* decreased cerebral perfusion or increased ICP
- Risk for ineffective cerebral tissue perfusion *related to* reduction of venous and/or arterial blood flow and cerebral edema
- Risk for disuse syndrome *related to* altered LOC, immobility, and altered nutritional intake

Additional information on nursing diagnoses for patients with increased ICP is presented in eNursing Care Plan 57-1 (available on the website for this chapter).

PLANNING

The overall goals for the patient with increased ICP are to (1) maintain a patent airway; (2) have ICP within normal limits; (3) have normal fluid, electrolyte, and nutritional balance; and (4) prevent complications secondary to immobility and decreased LOC.

NURSING IMPLEMENTATION

ACUTE INTERVENTION

Respiratory Function. Maintaining a patent airway is critical in the patient with increased ICP and is a primary nursing responsibility. As the LOC decreases, the patient is at an increased risk of airway obstruction from the tongue dropping back and occluding the airway or from accumulation of secretions.

SAFETY ALERT
- Be alert to altered breathing patterns.
- Snoring sounds indicate obstruction and require immediate intervention.

Remove accumulated secretions by suctioning as needed. An oral airway facilitates breathing and provides an easier suctioning route in the comatose patient. In general, any patient with a GCS of 8 or less or an altered LOC who is unable to maintain a patent airway or effective ventilation needs intubation and mechanical ventilation.

Prevent hypoxia and hypercapnia to minimize secondary injury. Proper positioning of the head is important. Elevation of the head of the bed to 30 degrees enhances respiratory exchange and aids in decreasing cerebral edema. Suctioning and coughing cause transient decreases in the PaO$_2$ and increases in the ICP. Keep suctioning to a minimum and less than 10 seconds in duration, with administration of 100% oxygen before and after to prevent decreases in the PaO$_2$. To avoid cumulative increases in the ICP with suctioning, limit suctioning to two passes per suction procedure, if possible. Patients with elevated ICP are at risk for lower CPP during suctioning. CPP must be maintained above 60 mm Hg to preserve cerebral perfusion.

Try to prevent abdominal distention, since it can interfere with respiratory function. Insertion of a nasogastric tube to aspirate the stomach contents can prevent distention, vomiting, and possible aspiration. However, in patients with facial and skull fractures, a nasogastric tube is contraindicated unless a basilar skull fracture (at base of skull) has been ruled out, and oral insertion of a gastric tube is preferred.

Pain, anxiety, and fear related to the primary injury, therapeutic procedures, or noxious stimuli can increase ICP and BP, thus complicating the management and recovery of the brain-injured patient. The appropriate choice or combination of sedatives, paralytics, and analgesics for symptom management presents a challenge to the ICU team. Administration of these agents may alter the neurologic state, thus masking true neurologic changes. It may be necessary to temporarily suspend drug therapy to appropriately assess neurologic status. The choice, dose, and combination of agents may vary depending on the patient's history, neurologic state, and overall clinical presentation.

Opioids, such as morphine sulfate and fentanyl (Sublimaze), are rapid-onset analgesics with minimal effect on CBF or oxygen metabolism. The IV anesthetic sedative propofol (Diprivan) has gained popularity in the management of anxiety and agitation in the ICU because of its rapid onset and short half-life. An accurate neurologic assessment can be performed soon after turning off the infusion of propofol.[5] A side effect of this drug is hypotension.

Dexmedetomidine (Precedex), an α$_2$-adrenergic agonist, is used for continuous IV sedation of intubated and mechanically ventilated patients in the ICU setting for up to 24 hours. It is another ideal agent for neurologic patients because of the ease in obtaining a neurologic assessment without altering the dose because of its anxiolytic properties. When using continuous IV sedatives, be aware of the side effects of these drugs, especially hypotension, since this can result in a lower CPP value.

Nondepolarizing neuromuscular blocking agents (e.g., vecuronium [Norcuron], cisatracurium besylate [Nimbex]) are useful for achieving complete ventilatory control in the treatment of refractory intracranial hypertension. Because these agents paralyze muscles without blocking pain or noxious stimuli, they are used in combination with sedatives, analgesics, or benzodiazepines.

Benzodiazepines, although useful for sedation, are usually avoided in the management of the patient with increased ICP because of the hypotensive effect and long half-life, unless they are used as an adjunct to neuromuscular blocking agents.

Frequently monitor and evaluate the ABG values, and take measures to maintain the levels within prescribed or acceptable parameters (see Chapter 26). The appropriate ventilatory support can be ordered on the basis of the PaO$_2$ and PaCO$_2$ values.

Fluid and Electrolyte Balance. Fluid and electrolyte disturbances can have an adverse effect on ICP. Closely monitor IV fluids with the use of an accurate IV infusion control device or pump. Intake and output, with insensible losses and daily weights taken into account, are important parameters in the assessment of fluid balance.

Make electrolyte determinations daily, and discuss any abnormal values with the physician. It is especially important to monitor serum glucose, sodium, potassium, magnesium, and osmolality.

Monitor urine output to detect problems related to diabetes insipidus and SIADH. Diabetes insipidus is caused by a decrease in antidiuretic hormone (ADH). It results in increased urine output and hypernatremia. The usual treatment of diabetes insipidus is fluid replacement, vasopressin (Pitressin), or desmopressin acetate (DDAVP) (see Chapter 50). If it is not treated, severe dehydration will occur.

SIADH is caused by an excess secretion of ADH. SIADH results in decreased urine output and dilutional hyponatremia. It may result in cerebral edema, changes in LOC, seizures, and coma. (Treatment of SIADH is described in Chapter 50.)

Monitoring Intracranial Pressure. ICP monitoring is used in combination with other physiologic parameters to guide the care of the patient and assess the patient's response to treatment. Valsalva maneuver, coughing, sneezing, suctioning, hypoxemia, and arousal from sleep are factors that can increase ICP. Be alert to these factors and attempt to minimize them.

Body Position. Maintain the patient with increased ICP in the head-up position. Take care to prevent extreme neck flexion, which can cause venous obstruction and contribute to elevated ICP. Adjust the body position to decrease the ICP maximally and to improve the CPP. Elevation of the head of the bed promotes drainage from the head and decreases the vascular congestion that can produce cerebral edema. However, raising the head of the bed above 30 degrees may decrease the CPP by lowering systemic BP. Carefully evaluate the effects of elevation of the head of the bed on both the ICP and the CPP. Position the bed so that it lowers the ICP while optimizing the CPP and other indices of cerebral oxygenation.

Take care to turn the patient with slow, gentle movements because rapid changes in position may increase the ICP. Prevent discomfort in turning and positioning the patient because pain or agitation also increases pressure. Increased intrathoracic pressure contributes to increased ICP by impeding the venous return. Thus coughing, straining, and the Valsalva maneuver should be avoided. Avoid extreme hip flexion to decrease the risk of raising the intraabdominal pressure, which increases ICP. Turn the patient at least every 2 hours.

Decorticate or decerebrate posturing is a reflex response in some patients with increased ICP. Turning, skin care, and even passive range of motion can elicit the posturing reflexes. Provide the physical care to minimize complications of immobility, such as atelectasis and contractures.

Protection From Injury. The patient with increased ICP and decreased LOC needs protection from self-injury. Confusion, agitation, and the possibility of seizures increase the risk for injury. Use restraints judiciously in the agitated patient. If restraints are absolutely necessary to keep the patient from removing tubes or falling out of bed, they should be secure enough to be effective, and the skin area under the restraints should be observed regularly for irritation. Agitation may increase with the use of restraints, which indicates the need for other measures to protect the patient from injury. Light sedation with agents such as midazolam (Versed) or lorazepam (Ativan) may be needed. Having a family member stay with the patient may have a calming effect.

For the patient with seizures or the patient at risk for such activity, institute seizure precautions. Seizures are most likely to occur in the first 7 days after traumatic injury, so prophylactic antiseizure therapy is usually used during this time.[12] Additional seizure precautions include padded side rails, an airway at the bedside, suction readily available, accurate and timely administration of antiseizure drugs, and close observation.

The patient can benefit from a quiet, nonstimulating environment. Always use a calm, reassuring approach. Touch and talk to the patient, even one who is in a coma.

Psychologic Considerations. In addition to carefully planned physical care, also be aware of the psychologic well-being of patients and their families. Anxiety over the diagnosis and the prognosis can be distressing to the patient, caregiver and family, and nursing staff. Your competent and assured manner in performing care is reassuring to everyone involved. Short, simple explanations are appropriate and allow the patient and caregiver to acquire the amount of information they desire. There is a need for support, information, and teaching of both patients and families. Assess the family members' desires to assist in providing care for the patient, and allow for their participation as appropriate. Encourage interdisciplinary management (social work, chaplain, etc.) of the patient and family in decision making as much as possible.

EVALUATION

The expected outcomes are that the patient with increased ICP will
- Maintain ICP and cerebral perfusion within normal parameters
- Experience no serious increases in ICP during or after care activities
- Experience no complications of immobility

Additional expected outcomes for the patient with increased ICP are addressed in eNursing Care Plan 57-1 (available on the website for this chapter).

HEAD INJURY

Head injury includes any injury or trauma to the scalp, skull, or brain. A serious form of head injury is *traumatic brain injury* (TBI). Statistics regarding the occurrence of head injuries are incomplete because many victims die at the injury scene or because the condition is considered minor and health care services are not sought. In U.S. hospital emergency departments, an estimated 1.7 million persons are treated and released with TBI. Fifty thousand people die and 275,000 persons are hospitalized with TBI. Of individuals hospitalized, 20% of the patients die.[13] At least 5.3 million Americans (2% of the U.S. population) currently live with disabilities resulting from TBI *(www.braintrauma.org)*.

Motor vehicle collisions and falls are the most common causes of head injury. Other causes of head injury include firearms, assaults, sports-related trauma, recreational injuries, and war-related injuries.[14] Males are twice as likely to sustain a TBI as females.

Head trauma has a high potential for a poor outcome. Deaths from head trauma occur at three points after injury: immediately after the injury, within 2 hours after injury, and approximately 3 weeks after injury.[14] Factors that predict a poor outcome include an intracranial hematoma, older age of the patient, abnormal motor responses, impaired or absent eye movements or pupillary light reflexes, early sustained hypotension, hypoxemia or hypercapnia, and sustained ICP levels greater than 20 mm Hg.[15]

The GCS score on arrival at the hospital is also a strong predictor of survival. A GCS below 8 indicates a 30% to 70% chance of survival, and a score above 8 indicates a greater than 90% survival rate. The majority of deaths after a head injury occur immediately after the injury, either from the direct head trauma or from massive hemorrhage and shock. Deaths occurring within a few hours of the trauma are caused by progressive worsening of the head injury or internal bleeding. Immediate recognition of changes in neurologic status and rapid surgical intervention are critical in the prevention of deaths.[5]

Deaths occurring 3 weeks or more after the injury result from multisystem failure. Expert nursing care in the weeks after the injury is crucial in decreasing the mortality risk and in optimizing patient outcomes.

Types of Head Injuries

Scalp Lacerations. *Scalp lacerations* are an easily recognized type of external head trauma. Because the scalp contains many blood vessels with poor constrictive abilities, most scalp lacerations are associated with profuse bleeding. Even relatively small wounds can bleed significantly. The major complications associated with scalp laceration are blood loss and infection.

Skull Fractures. *Skull fractures* frequently occur with head trauma. Skull fractures can be described in several ways: (1) linear or depressed; (2) simple, comminuted, or compound; and (3) closed or open (Table 57-6). Fractures may be closed or open, depending on the presence of a scalp laceration or extension of the fracture into the air sinuses or dura. The type and severity of a skull fracture depend on the velocity, momentum,

TABLE 57-6 TYPES OF SKULL FRACTURES

Type	Description	Cause
Linear	Break in continuity of bone without alteration of relationship of parts	Low-velocity injuries
Depressed	Inward indentation of skull	Powerful blow
Simple	Linear or depressed skull fracture without fragmentation or communicating lacerations	Low to moderate impact
Comminuted	Multiple linear fractures with fragmentation of bone into many pieces	Direct, high-momentum impact
Compound	Depressed skull fracture and scalp laceration with communicating pathway to intracranial cavity	Severe head injury

TABLE 57-7 MANIFESTATIONS OF SKULL FRACTURES

Location	Manifestations
Frontal fracture	Exposure of brain to contaminants through frontal air sinus, possible association with air in forehead tissue, CSF rhinorrhea, or pneumocranium (air between the cranium and the dura mater)
Orbital fracture	Periorbital ecchymosis (raccoon eyes), optic nerve injury
Temporal fracture	Boggy temporal muscle because of extravasation of blood, oval-shaped bruise behind ear in mastoid region (Battle's sign), CSF otorrhea, middle meningeal artery disruption, epidural hematoma
Parietal fracture	Deafness, CSF or brain otorrhea, bulging of tympanic membrane caused by blood or CSF, facial paralysis, loss of taste, Battle's sign
Posterior fossa fracture	Occipital bruising resulting in cortical blindness, visual field defects, rare appearance of ataxia or other cerebellar signs
Basilar skull fracture	CSF or brain otorrhea, bulging of tympanic membrane caused by blood or CSF, Battle's sign, tinnitus or hearing difficulty, rhinorrhea, facial paralysis, conjugate deviation of gaze, vertigo

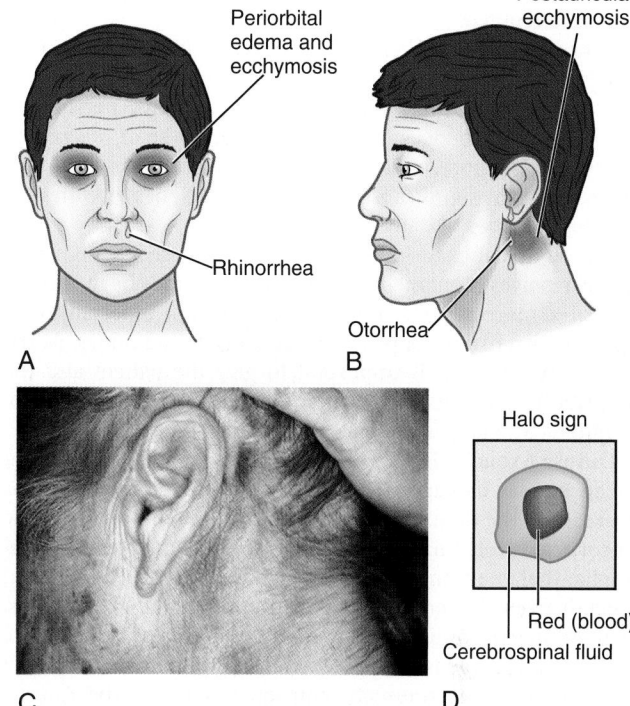

FIG. 57-13 A, Raccoon eyes and rhinorrhea. **B,** Battle's sign (postauricular ecchymosis) with otorrhea. **C,** Battle's sign. **D,** Halo or ring sign (see text).

direction and shape (blunt or sharp) of the injuring agent, and site of impact.

The location of the fracture determines the clinical manifestations (Table 57-7). For example, a basilar skull fracture is a specialized type of linear fracture involving the base of the skull. Manifestations can evolve over the course of several hours; vary with the location and severity of fracture; and may include cranial nerve deficits, Battle's sign (postauricular ecchymosis), and periorbital ecchymosis (raccoon eyes) (Fig. 57-13). This fracture generally is associated with a tear in the dura and subsequent leakage of CSF. *Rhinorrhea* (CSF leakage from the nose) or *otorrhea* (CSF leakage from the ear) generally confirms that the fracture has traversed the dura (see Fig. 57-13). Rhinorrhea may also manifest as postnasal sinus drainage. The significance of rhinorrhea may be overlooked unless the patient is specifically assessed for this finding. The risk of meningitis is high with a CSF leak, and antibiotics should be administered as a preventive measure.

Two methods of testing can be used to determine whether the fluid leaking from the nose or ear is CSF. The first method is to test the leaking fluid with a Dextrostix or Tes-Tape strip to determine whether glucose is present. CSF gives a positive reading for glucose. If blood is present in the fluid, testing for glucose is unreliable because blood also contains glucose. In this event, look for the *halo* or *ring* sign (see Fig. 57-13, *D*). Allow the leaking fluid to drip onto a white gauze pad (4 × 4) or towel, and then observe the drainage. Within a few minutes, the blood coalesces into the center, and a yellowish ring encircles the blood if CSF is present. Note the color, appearance, and amount of leaking fluid because both tests can give false-positive results.

The major potential complications of skull fractures are intracranial infections, hematoma, and meningeal and brain tissue damage. Note that in cases where a basilar skull fracture is suspected, a nasogastric or oral gastric tube should be inserted under fluoroscopy.

Head Trauma. Brain injuries are categorized as diffuse (generalized) or focal (localized). In a *diffuse* injury (e.g., concussion, diffuse axonal injury), damage to the brain cannot be localized to one particular area. In a *focal injury* (e.g., contusion, hematoma), damage can be localized to a specific area of the brain. Brain injury can be classified as *minor* (GCS 13 to 15), *moderate* (GCS 9 to 12), and *severe* (GCS 3 to 8).

Diffuse Injury. Concussion (a sudden transient mechanical head injury with disruption of neural activity and a change in the LOC) is considered a minor diffuse head injury. The patient may or may not lose total consciousness with this injury.

Typical signs of concussion include a brief disruption in LOC, amnesia regarding the event (retrograde amnesia), and headache. The manifestations are generally of short duration. If the patient has not lost consciousness, or if the loss of consciousness lasts less than 5 minutes, the patient is usually discharged from the care facility with instructions to notify the health care provider if symptoms persist or if behavioral changes are noted.

Postconcussion syndrome may develop in some patients, usually anywhere from 2 weeks to 2 months after the injury. Symptoms include persistent headache, lethargy, personality and behavioral changes, shortened attention span, decreased short-term memory, and changes in intellectual ability. This syndrome can significantly affect the patient's abilities to perform activities of daily living.

Although concussion is generally considered benign and usually resolves spontaneously, the symptoms may be the beginning of a more serious, progressive problem, especially in a patient with a history of prior concussion or head injury. At the time of discharge, it is important to give the patient and the caregiver instructions for observation and accurate reporting of symptoms or changes in neurologic status.

Diffuse Axonal Injury. Diffuse axonal injury (DAI) is widespread axonal damage occurring after a mild, moderate, or severe TBI. The damage occurs primarily around axons in the subcortical white matter of the cerebral hemispheres, basal ganglia, thalamus, and brainstem.[16] Initially, DAI was believed to occur from the tensile forces of trauma that sheared axons, resulting in axonal disconnection. There is increasing evidence that axonal damage is not preceded by an immediate tearing of the axon from the traumatic impact, but rather the trauma changes the function of the axon, resulting in axon swelling and disconnection. This process takes approximately 12 to 24 hours to develop and may persist longer.

The clinical signs of DAI are varied, but may include a decreased LOC, increased ICP, decortication or decerebration, and global cerebral edema. Approximately 90% of patients with DAI remain in a persistent vegetative state.[17] Patients with DAI who survive the initial event are rapidly triaged to an ICU, where they will be vigilantly watched for signs of increased ICP and treated accordingly (as previously discussed).

Focal Injury. Focal injury can be minor to severe and can be localized to an area of injury. Focal injury consists of lacerations, contusions, hematomas, and cranial nerve injuries.

Lacerations involve actual tearing of the brain tissue and often occur in association with depressed and open fractures and penetrating injuries. Tissue damage is severe, and surgical repair of the laceration is impossible because of the nature of brain tissue. Medical management consists of antibiotics until meningitis is ruled out, and prevention of secondary injury related to increased ICP. If bleeding is deep into the brain tissue, focal and generalized signs develop.

When major head trauma occurs, many delayed responses are seen, including hemorrhage, hematoma formation, seizures, and cerebral edema. Intracerebral hemorrhage is generally associated with cerebral laceration. This hemorrhage manifests as a space-occupying lesion accompanied by unconsciousness, hemiplegia on the contralateral side, and a dilated pupil on the ipsilateral side. As the hematoma expands, signs of increased ICP become more severe. Prognosis is generally poor for the patient with a large intracerebral hemorrhage. Subarachnoid hemorrhage and intraventricular hemorrhage can also occur secondary to head trauma.

A contusion is bruising of the brain tissue within a focal area. It is usually associated with a closed head injury. A contusion may contain areas of hemorrhage, infarction, necrosis, and edema, and it frequently occurs at a fracture site.

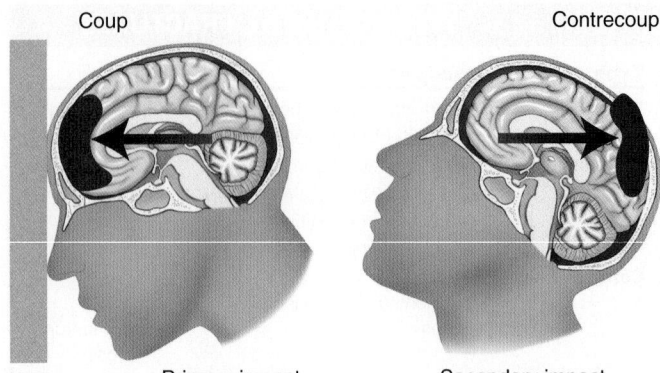

FIG. 57-14 Coup-contrecoup injury. After the head strikes the wall, a coup injury occurs as the brain strikes the skull (primary impact). The contrecoup injury (the secondary impact) occurs when the brain strikes the skull surface opposite the site of the original impact.

With contusion, the phenomenon of *coup-contrecoup injury* is often noted (Fig. 57-14), and injuries can range from minor to severe. Damage from coup-contrecoup injury occurs when the brain moves inside the skull due to high-energy or high-impact injury mechanisms. Contusions or lacerations occur both at the site of the direct impact of the brain on the skull *(coup)* and at a secondary area of damage on the opposite side away from injury *(contrecoup),* leading to multiple contused areas. *Contrecoup* injuries tend to be more severe, and overall patient prognosis depends on the amount of bleeding around the contusion site.

Contusions may continue to bleed or rebleed and appear to "blossom" on subsequent CT scans of the brain, which worsens the neurologic outcome. Neurologic assessment may demonstrate focal and generalized manifestation, depending on the contusion's size and location. Seizures are a common complication of brain contusion, especially in the first 7 days after injury.[12] Anticoagulant use and coagulopathy are associated with increased hemorrhage, more severe head injury, and a higher mortality rate.[18] This is especially important when considering older individuals who are taking warfarin (Coumadin) or aspirin at home. If they fall, their contusion is likely to be more severe due to the use of anticoagulants. Thus risk for falls should be assessed (see Table 63-1).

Complications

Epidural Hematoma. An epidural hematoma results from bleeding between the dura and the inner surface of the skull (Figs. 57-15 and 57-16). An epidural hematoma is a neurologic emergency and is usually associated with a linear fracture crossing a major artery in the dura, causing a tear. It can have a venous or an arterial origin. Venous epidural hematomas are associated with a tear of the dural venous sinus and develop slowly. With arterial hematomas, the middle meningeal artery lying under the temporal bone is often torn. Hemorrhage occurs into the epidural space, which lies between the dura and inner surface of the skull (see Fig. 57-15). Because this is an arterial hemorrhage, the hematoma develops rapidly.

Classic signs of an epidural hematoma include an initial period of unconsciousness at the scene, with a brief lucid interval followed by a decrease in LOC. Other manifestations may be a headache, nausea and vomiting, or focal findings. Rapid surgical intervention to evacuate the hematoma and prevent

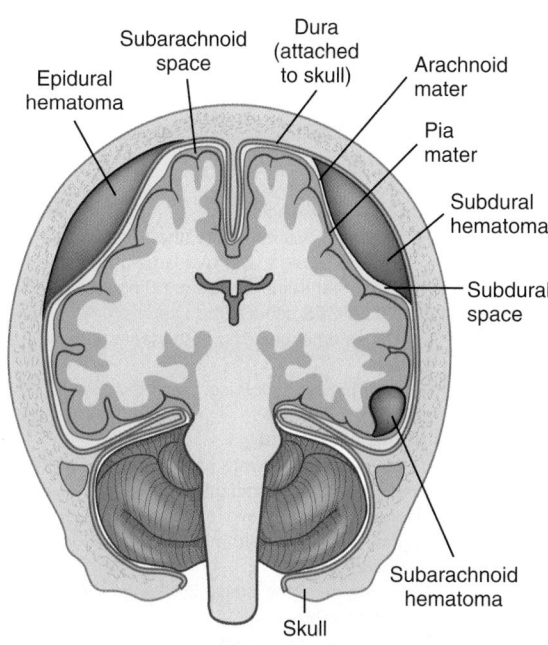

FIG. 57-15 Locations of epidural, subdural, and subarachnoid hematomas.

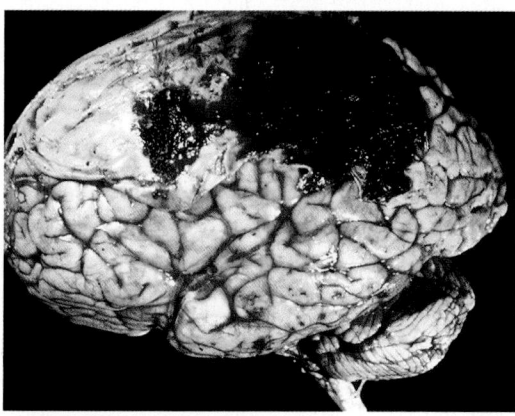

FIG. 57-16 Epidural hematoma covering a portion of the dura. Multiple small contusions are seen in the temporal lobe.

TABLE 57-8	**TYPES OF SUBDURAL HEMATOMAS**	
Occurrence After Injury	**Progression of Symptoms**	**Treatment**
Acute		
24-48 hr after severe trauma.	Immediate deterioration.	Craniotomy, evacuation and decompression.
Subacute		
48 hr–2 wk after severe trauma.	Alteration in mental status as hematoma develops. Progression dependent on size and location of hematoma.	Evacuation and decompression.
Chronic		
Weeks or months, usually >20 days after injury. Often injury seemed trivial or was forgotten by patient.	Nonspecific, nonlocalizing progression. Progressive alteration in LOC.	Evacuation and decompression, membranectomy.

LOC, Level of consciousness.

cerebral herniation, along with medical management for increasing ICP, can dramatically improve outcomes.

Subdural Hematoma. A subdural hematoma occurs from bleeding between the dura mater and the arachnoid layer of the meninges (see Fig. 57-15). A subdural hematoma usually results from injury to the brain tissue and its blood vessels. The veins that drain from the surface of the brain into the sagittal sinus are the source of most subdural hematomas. Because it is usually venous in origin, the subdural hematoma may be slower to develop. However, a subdural hematoma may be caused by an arterial hemorrhage, in which case it develops more rapidly.[19] Subdural hematomas may be acute, subacute, or chronic (Table 57-8).

An *acute subdural hematoma* manifests within 24 to 48 hours of the injury. The signs and symptoms are similar to those associated with brain tissue compression in increased ICP and include decreasing LOC and headache. The size of the hematoma determines the patient's clinical presentation and prognosis. The patient's appearance may range from drowsy and confused to unconscious. The ipsilateral pupil dilates and becomes fixed if ICP is significantly elevated. Blunt force injuries that produce acute subdural hematomas may also cause significant underlying brain injury, resulting in cerebral edema. The resulting increase in ICP from the cerebral edema can cause an increased morbidity and mortality risk despite surgical intervention to evacuate the hematoma.

A *subacute subdural hematoma* usually occurs within 2 to 14 days of the injury. After the initial bleeding, a subdural hematoma may appear to enlarge over time as the breakdown products of the blood draw fluid into the subdural space.

A *chronic subdural hematoma* develops over weeks or months after a seemingly minor head injury. Chronic subdural hematomas are more common in older adults because of a potentially larger subdural space as a result of brain atrophy. With atrophy, the brain remains attached to the supportive structures, but tension is increased, and it is subject to tearing. Because the subdural space is larger, the presenting complaint is focal symptoms, rather than signs of increased ICP.[20] Chronic alcoholics are also prone to cerebral atrophy and subsequent development of subdural hematoma because of an increased incidence of falls.

Diagnosis of a subdural hematoma in the older adult may be delayed because symptoms mimic other health problems in this age-group, such as somnolence, confusion, lethargy, and memory loss. The manifestations of a subdural hematoma are often misinterpreted as vascular disease (stroke, transient ischemic attack [TIA]) and dementia.

Intracerebral Hematoma. Intracerebral hematoma occurs from bleeding within the brain tissue in approximately 16% of head injuries. It usually occurs within the frontal and temporal lobes, possibly from rupture of intracerebral vessels at the time of injury. The size and location of the hematoma are key determinants of the patient's outcome.

Diagnostic Studies and Collaborative Care

CT scan is the best diagnostic test to evaluate for head trauma because it allows rapid diagnosis and intervention in the acute care setting. MRI, PET, and evoked potential studies may also

---

✚ TABLE 57-9   EMERGENCY MANAGEMENT

Head Injury

Etiology	Assessment Findings	Interventions
Blunt • Motor vehicle collision • Pedestrian event • Fall • Assault • Sports injury **Penetrating** • Gunshot wound • Arrow	**Surface Findings** • Scalp lacerations • Fracture or depressions in skull • Bruises or contusions on face, Battle's sign (bruising behind ears) • Raccoon eyes (dependent bruising around eyes) **Respiratory** • Central neurogenic hyperventilation • Cheyne-Stokes respirations • Decreased O_2 saturation • Pulmonary edema **Central Nervous System** • Unequal or dilated pupils • Asymmetric facial movements • Garbled speech, abusive speech • Confusion • Decreased level of consciousness • Combativeness • Involuntary movements • Seizures • Bowel and bladder incontinence • Flaccidity • Depressed or hyperactive reflexes • Decerebrate or decorticate posturing • GCS score <12 • CSF leaking from ears or nose	**Initial** • Ensure patent airway. • Stabilize cervical spine. • Administer O_2 via non-rebreather mask. • Establish IV access with two large-bore catheters to infuse normal saline or lactated Ringer's solution. • Intubate if GCS score <8. • Control external bleeding with sterile pressure dressing. • Remove patient's clothing. **Ongoing Monitoring** • Maintain patient warmth using blankets, warm IV fluids, overhead warming lights, warm humidified O_2. • Monitor vital signs, level of consciousness, O_2 saturation, cardiac rhythm, GCS score, pupil size and reactivity. • Anticipate need for intubation if gag reflex is impaired or absent. • Assume neck injury with head injury. • Assess for rhinorrhea, otorrhea, scalp wounds. • Administer fluids cautiously to prevent fluid overload and increasing ICP.

GCS, Glasgow Coma Scale, *ICP,* intracranial pressure.

---

be used in the diagnosis and differentiation of head injuries. An MRI scan is more sensitive than the CT scan in detecting small lesions. Transcranial Doppler studies allow for the measurement of CBF velocity. A cervical spine x-ray series, CT scan, or MRI of the spine may also be indicated, since cervical spine trauma often occurs at the same time as a head injury. In general, the diagnostic studies are similar to those used for a patient with increased ICP (see Table 57-3).

Emergency management of the patient with a head injury is presented in Table 57-9. In addition to measures to prevent secondary injury by treating cerebral edema and managing increased ICP, the principal treatment of head injuries is timely diagnosis and surgery (if necessary). For the patient with concussion and contusion, observation and management of increased ICP are the primary management strategies.

The treatment of skull fractures is usually conservative. For depressed fractures and fractures with loose fragments, a craniotomy is necessary to elevate the depressed bone and remove the free fragments. If large amounts of bone are destroyed, the bone may be removed (craniectomy), and a cranioplasty will be needed later (see the section on cranial surgery later in this chapter).

In cases of large acute subdural and epidural hematomas, or those associated with significant neurologic impairment, the blood must be removed through surgical evacuation. A craniotomy is generally performed to visualize and allow control of the bleeding vessels. Burr-hole openings may be used in an extreme emergency for a more rapid decompression, followed by a craniotomy. A drain may be placed postoperatively for several days to prevent reaccumulation of blood. In cases where extreme swelling is expected (e.g., DAI, hemorrhage), a craniectomy may be performed, which involves removing a piece of skull to reduce the pressure inside the cranial vault, thus reducing the risk of herniation.

NURSING MANAGEMENT
HEAD INJURY

NURSING ASSESSMENT

A patient with a head injury always has the potential to develop increased ICP. Increased ICP is associated with higher mortality rates and poorer functional outcomes.[6] Objective data are obtained by applying the GCS (see Table 57-5), assessing and monitoring the neurologic status (see eFig. 57-1 on the website for this chapter), and determining whether a CSF leak has occurred. (Nursing assessment related to increased ICP is discussed on pp. 1365-1366.) Nursing assessment of the patient with a head injury is presented in Table 57-10.

NURSING DIAGNOSES

Nursing diagnoses and a potential complication for the patient who has sustained a head injury may include, but are not limited to, the following:

• Risk for ineffective cerebral tissue perfusion *related to* interruption of CBF associated with cerebral hemorrhage, hematoma, and edema
• Hyperthermia *related to* increased metabolism, infection, and hypothalamic injury

TABLE 57-10 NURSING ASSESSMENT

Head Injury

Subjective Data

Important Health Information

Past health history: Mechanism of injury: motor vehicle collision, sports injury, industrial incident, assault, falls
Medications: Anticoagulant medications

Functional Health Patterns

Health perception–health management: Alcohol or recreational drugs; risk-taking behaviors
Cognitive-perceptual: Headache, mood or behavioral change, mentation changes, aphasia, dysphasia, impaired judgment
Coping–stress tolerance: Fear, denial, anger, aggression, depression

Objective Data

General

Altered mental status

Integumentary

Lacerations, contusions, abrasions, hematoma, Battle's sign, periorbital edema and ecchymosis, otorrhea, exposed brain matter

Respiratory

Rhinorrhea, impaired gag reflex, inability to maintain a patent airway; impending herniation: altered/irregular respiratory rate and pattern

Cardiovascular

Impending herniation: Cushing's triad (systolic hypertension with widening pulse pressure, bradycardia with full and bounding pulse, irregular respirations)

Gastrointestinal

Vomiting, projectile vomiting, bowel incontinence

Urinary

Bladder incontinence

Reproductive

Uninhibited sexual expression

Neurologic

Altered level of consciousness, seizure activity, pupil dysfunction, cranial nerve deficit(s)

Musculoskeletal

Motor deficit/impairment, weakness, palmar drift, paralysis, spasticity, decorticate or decerebrate posturing, muscular rigidity or increased tone, flaccidity, ataxia

Possible Diagnostic Findings

Location and type of hematoma, edema, skull fracture, and/or foreign body on CT scan and/or MRI; abnormal EEG; positive toxicology screen or alcohol level, ↓ or ↑ blood glucose level; ↑ ICP

ICP, Intracranial pressure.

- Impaired physical mobility *related to* decreased LOC
- Anxiety *related to* abrupt change in health status, hospital environment, and uncertain future
- Potential complication: increased ICP *related to* cerebral edema and hemorrhage

PLANNING

The overall goals are that the patient with an acute head injury will (1) maintain adequate cerebral oxygenation and perfusion; (2) remain normothermic; (3) achieve control of pain and

---

ETHICAL/LEGAL DILEMMAS

Brain Death

Situation

The emergency nurse receives a radio call from emergency medical service (EMS) personnel about R.G., a young man involved in a motorcycle crash. He was not wearing a helmet and has a large open skull fracture. Transport from the accident scene was delayed by 45 min as a result of a severe thunderstorm and traffic congestion. On the way to the hospital, R.G. exhibits fixed, dilated pupils and experiences cardiac arrest. Estimated arrival at the hospital is still an additional 45 min as a result of the severe weather. EMS personnel request permission to stop resuscitation efforts.

Ethical/Legal Points for Consideration

- Criteria for brain death include coma or unresponsiveness, absence of brainstem reflexes, and apnea (see Chapter 10).
- The definition of death has changed with the advent of new technology, monitoring devices, and interventions.
- These changes and their effect on the legal diagnosis of death will be accepted by the courts through expert witness testimony.
- Another circumstance that influences the manner in which a state of death is determined is the customary practice or best practice for the specific situation.
- In a situation where the professional responsible for determining a state of death is in remote contact with the patient, but the monitoring devices available provide virtual contact with the patient, a remote diagnosis of death may be legally acceptable.
- Brain death criteria do not address patients in a permanent vegetative state, since the brainstem activity in these patients is adequate to maintain heart and lung function.

Discussion Questions

1. What are your feelings about cessation of brain function vs. cessation of heart and lung function as the criteria for death of a patient?
2. What are your state's laws or practices about stopping cardiopulmonary resuscitation (CPR) efforts by EMS personnel in the field?
3. When brain death has occurred, what is your obligation for education of the family or significant other regarding organ donation?

---

discomfort; (4) be free from infection; (5) have adequate nutrition; and (6) attain maximal cognitive, motor, and sensory function.

NURSING IMPLEMENTATION

HEALTH PROMOTION. One of the best ways to prevent head injuries is to prevent car and motorcycle collisions. The use of helmets by cyclists has led to fewer TBIs. The use of car seat belts and child car seats is also associated with reduced TBI mortality rates.

Be active in campaigns that promote driving safety, and speak to driver education classes regarding the dangers of unsafe driving and of driving after drinking alcohol and using drugs. Wearing seat belts in cars and helmets for riding on motorcycles is the most effective measure for increasing survival after crashes. Protective helmets should also be worn by lumberjacks, construction workers, miners, horseback riders, bicycle riders, snowboarders, and skydivers. Additionally, individuals who are at risk for falls (e.g., older adults) should be evaluated for safety in the home, since falls are the second leading cause of head injuries.

ACUTE INTERVENTION. Management at the injury scene can have a significant impact on the outcome of the head injury. Emergency management of head injury is presented in Table 57-9. The general goal of nursing management of the head-injured patient is to maintain cerebral oxygenation and perfusion and prevent secondary cerebral ischemia.

Surveillance or monitoring for changes in neurologic status is critically important because the patient's condition may deteriorate rapidly, necessitating emergency surgery. Appropriate preoperative and postoperative nursing interventions are initiated if surgery is anticipated. Because of the close association between hemodynamic status and cerebral perfusion, be aware of any coexisting injuries or conditions.

Explain the need for frequent neurologic assessments to both the patient and the caregiver. Behavioral manifestations associated with head injury can result in a frightened, disoriented patient who is combative and resists help. Your approach should be calm and gentle. A family member may be available to stay with the patient and thus decrease anxiety and fear. One of the most important needs for the caregiver and family members in the acute injury phase is information about the patient's diagnosis, treatment plan, and rationale for the interventions. Other teaching points are presented in Table 57-11.

Perform neurologic assessments at intervals based on the patient's condition. The GCS is useful in assessing the LOC (see Table 57-5). Indications of a deteriorating neurologic state, no matter how subtle, such as a decreasing LOC or decreasing motor strength, should be reported to the health care provider. Monitor the patient's condition closely.[21]

The major focus of nursing care for the brain-injured patient relates to increased ICP (see eNursing Care Plan 57-1). However, some problems may require specific nursing intervention.

Eye problems may include loss of the corneal reflex, periorbital ecchymosis and edema, and diplopia. Loss of the corneal reflex may necessitate administering lubricating eyedrops or taping the eyes shut to prevent abrasion. Periorbital ecchymosis and edema decrease with time, but cold and, later, warm compresses provide comfort and hasten the process. Diplopia can be relieved by use of an eye patch. Consider a consult with an ophthalmologist.

TABLE 57-11 PATIENT & CAREGIVER TEACHING GUIDE

Head Injury

Include the following instructions when teaching the patient and caregiver about care during the first 2 or 3 days after a head injury.

1. Notify your health care provider immediately if experiencing signs and symptoms that may indicate complications. These include the following:
   - Increased drowsiness (e.g., difficulty arousing, confusion)
   - Nausea or vomiting
   - Worsening headache or stiff neck
   - Seizures
   - Vision difficulties (e.g., blurring)
   - Behavioral changes (e.g., irritability, anger)
   - Motor problems (e.g., clumsiness, difficulty walking, slurred speech, weakness in arms or legs)
   - Sensory disturbances (e.g., numbness)
   - A heart rate <60 beats/min
2. Have someone stay with you.
3. Abstain from alcohol.
4. Check with your health care provider before taking drugs that may increase drowsiness, including muscle relaxants, tranquilizers, and opioid pain medications.
5. Avoid driving, using heavy machinery, playing contact sports, and taking hot baths.

Hyperthermia may occur from injury to or inflammation of the hypothalamus. Elevations in body temperature can result in increased CBF, cerebral blood volume, and ICP. Increased metabolism secondary to hyperthermia increases metabolic waste, which in turn produces further cerebral vasodilation. Avoid hyperthermia with a goal of a temperature of 96.8° to 98.6° F (36° to 37° C) as the standard of care. Use interventions to reduce temperature as previously discussed (see p. 1364) in conjunction with sedation as necessary to prevent shivering.

If CSF rhinorrhea or otorrhea occurs, inform the physician immediately. The head of the bed may be raised to decrease the CSF pressure so that a tear can seal. A loose collection pad may be placed under the nose or over the ear. Do not place a dressing in the nasal or ear cavities. Instruct the patient not to sneeze or blow the nose. Nasogastric tubes should not be used, and nasotracheal suctioning should not be performed on these patients because of the high risk of meningitis.

Nursing measures specific to the care of the immobilized patient, such as those related to bladder and bowel function, skin care, and infection, are also indicated. Nausea and vomiting may be a problem and can be alleviated by antiemetic drugs. Headache can usually be controlled with acetaminophen or small doses of codeine.

If the patient's condition deteriorates, intracranial surgery may be necessary (see the section on cranial surgery later in this chapter). A burr-hole opening or craniotomy may be indicated, depending on the underlying injury that is causing the symptoms. The emergency nature of the surgery may hasten the usual preoperative preparation. Consult with the neurosurgeon to determine specific preoperative nursing measures.

The patient is often unconscious before surgery, making it necessary for a family member to sign the consent form for surgery. This is a difficult and frightening time for the patient's caregiver and family and requires sensitive nursing management. The suddenness of the situation makes it especially difficult for the family to cope.

AMBULATORY AND HOME CARE. Once the condition has stabilized, the patient is usually transferred for acute rehabilitation management. There may be chronic problems related to motor and sensory deficits, communication, memory, and intellectual functioning. Many of the principles of nursing management of the patient with a stroke are appropriate for these patients (see Chapter 58).

Conditions that may require nursing and collaborative management include poor nutritional status, bowel and bladder management, spasticity, dysphagia, deep vein thrombosis, and hydrocephalus. The patient's outward appearance is not a good indicator of how well he or she will ultimately function in the home or work environment. The outward physical appearance does not necessarily reflect what has happened in the brain.

Seizure disorders are seen in approximately 5% of patients with a nonpenetrating head injury. Seizures are most likely to develop during the first week after the head injury,[12] but some patients may not develop a seizure disorder until years later. Antiseizure drugs may be used prophylactically to manage posttraumatic seizure activity.

The mental and emotional sequelae of brain trauma are often the most incapacitating problems. One of the consequences of TBI is that the person may not realize that a brain injury has occurred. Many of the patients with head injuries who have been comatose for more than 6 hours undergo some personality change. They may suffer loss of concentration and memory and defective memory processing. Personal drive may decrease. Apathy may increase. Euphoria and mood swings, along with a seeming lack of awareness of the seriousness of the injury, may occur. The patient's behavior may indicate a loss of social restraint, judgment, tact, and emotional control.

Progressive recovery may continue for 6 months or more before a plateau is reached and a prognosis for recovery can be determined. Specific nursing management in the posttraumatic phase depends on specific residual deficits.

In all cases, the family must be given special consideration. They need to understand what is happening and be taught appropriate interaction patterns. Provide guidance and referrals for financial aid, child care, and other personal needs. Assist the family in involving the patient in family activities whenever possible. Help the patient and the family remain hopeful. The family often has unrealistic expectations of the patient as the coma begins to recede. The family expects full return to pretrauma status. In reality, the patient usually experiences a reduced awareness and ability to interpret environmental stimuli. Prepare the family for the patient's emergence from coma and explain that the process of awakening often takes several weeks. Arrange for social work and chaplain consultations for the family in addition to providing open visitation and frequent status updates.

When it is the time for discharge planning, the patient, caregiver, and family may benefit from specific posthospitalization instructions to avoid family-patient friction. Special "no" policies that may be appropriately suggested by the neurosurgeon, neuropsychologist, and nurse include no drinking of alcoholic beverages, no driving, no use of firearms, no working with hazardous implements and machinery, and no unsupervised smoking. Family members, particularly spouses, go through role transition as the role changes from that of spouse to that of caregiver. (The stresses and needs of family caregivers are discussed in Chapter 4.)

EVALUATION

The expected outcomes are that the patient with a head injury will

- Maintain normal CPP
- Achieve maximal cognitive, motor, and sensory function
- Experience no infection or hyperthermia

BRAIN TUMORS

The annual rate of newly diagnosed brain tumors in the United States is 22,910, with an estimated 13,700 deaths related to brain tumors. The brain is also a frequent site for metastasis from other sites. The 5-year survival rate for primary site brain tumors is approximately 36%.[22] Males have a slightly higher incidence of brain tumors than females. Brain tumors are more commonly seen in middle-aged persons, but they may occur at any age.

Types

Brain tumors can occur in any part of the brain or spinal cord. Tumors of the brain may be *primary*, arising from tissues within the brain, or *secondary*, resulting from a metastasis from a malignant neoplasm elsewhere in the body.[23] Metastatic brain tumors are the most common brain tumor. The cancers that most commonly metastasize to the brain are lung and breast.

Primary brain tumors are generally classified according to the tissue from which they arise (Table 57-12). Meningiomas represent 34% of all primary brain tumors, making them the most common primary brain tumor. Gliomas (e.g., astrocytoma, glioblastoma multiforme) account for 30% of all brain tumors and 80% of all malignant tumors. Glioblastoma multiforme is the most common form of glioma.

⊕ CULTURAL & ETHNIC HEALTH DISPARITIES

Brain Tumors

- Whites have a higher incidence of malignant brain tumors than African Americans.
- White males have the highest incidence of malignant brain tumors.
- African Americans have a higher incidence of benign brain tumors (e.g., meningiomas) than whites.

TABLE 57-12 TYPES OF BRAIN TUMORS

Type	Tissue of Origin	Characteristics
Gliomas		
• Astrocytoma	Supportive tissue, glial cells, and astrocytes	Can range from low-grade to moderate-grade malignancy.
• Glioblastoma multiforme	Primitive stem cell (glioblast)	Highly malignant and invasive. Among the most devastating of primary brain tumors.
• Oligodendroglioma	Oligodendrocytes	Benign (encapsulation and calcification).
• Ependymoma	Ependymal epithelium	Range from benign to highly malignant. Most are benign and encapsulated.
• Medulloblastoma	Primitive neuroectodermal cell	Highly malignant and invasive. Metastatic to spinal cord and remote areas of brain.
Meningioma	Meninges	Can be benign or malignant. Most are benign.
Acoustic neuroma (Schwannoma)	Cells that form myelin sheath around nerves Commonly affects cranial nerve VIII	Many grow on both sides of the brain. Usually benign or low-grade malignancy.
Pituitary adenoma	Pituitary gland	Usually benign.
Hemangioblastoma	Blood vessels of brain	Rare and benign. Surgery is curative.
Primary central nervous system lymphoma	Lymphocytes	Increased incidence in transplant recipients and acquired immunodeficiency syndrome (AIDS) patients.
Metastatic tumors	Lungs, breast	Malignant.

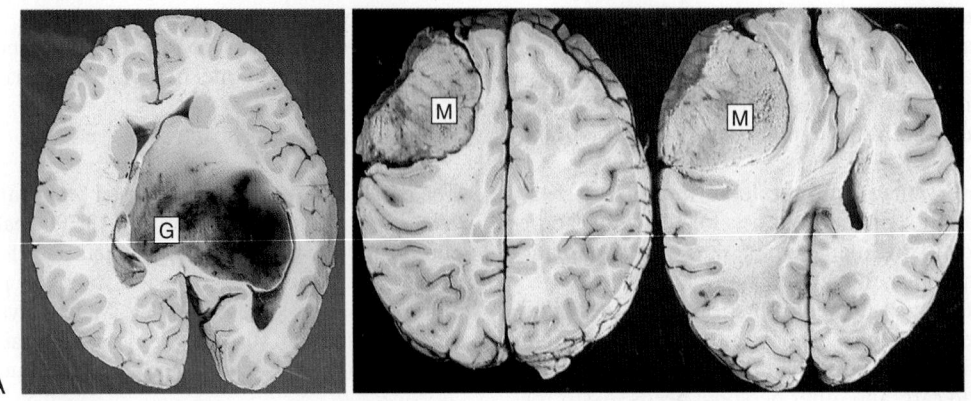

FIG. 57-17 A, A large glioblastoma *(G)* arises from one cerebral hemisphere and has grown to fill the ventricular system. **B,** Meningioma. These two different sections from different levels in the same brain show a meningioma *(M)* compressing the frontal lobe and distorting underlying brain.

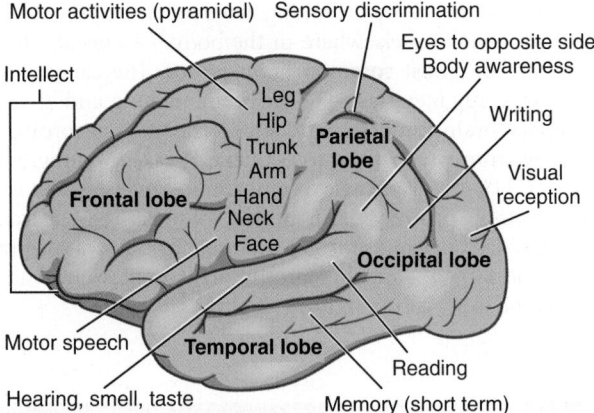

FIG. 57-18 Each area of the brain controls a particular activity.

TABLE 57-13	MANIFESTATIONS OF BRAIN TUMORS
Tumor Location	**Manifestations**
Cerebral hemisphere	
• Frontal lobe (unilateral)	Unilateral hemiplegia, seizures, memory deficit, personality and judgment changes, visual disturbances.
• Frontal lobe (bilateral)	Symptoms associated with unilateral frontal lobe tumors. Ataxic gait.
• Parietal lobe	Speech disturbance (if tumor is in the dominant hemisphere), inability to write, spatial disorders, unilateral neglect.
• Occipital lobe	Vision disturbances and seizures.
• Temporal lobe	Few symptoms. Seizures, dysphagia.
Subcortical	Hemiplegia. Other symptoms may depend on area of infiltration.
Meningeal tumors	Symptoms associated with compression of the brain and depend on tumor location.
Metastatic tumors	Headache, nausea, or vomiting because of ↑ ICP. Other symptoms depend on tumor location.
Thalamus and sellar tumors	Headache, nausea, vision disturbances, papilledema, and nystagmus occur from ↑ ICP. Diabetes insipidus may occur.
Fourth ventricle and cerebellar tumors	Headache, nausea, and papilledema from ↑ ICP. Ataxic gait and changes in coordination.
Cerebellopontine tumors	Tinnitus and vertigo, deafness.
Brainstem tumors	Headache on awakening, drowsiness, vomiting, ataxic gait, facial muscle weakness, hearing loss, dysphagia, dysarthria, "crossed eyes" or other visual changes, hemiparesis.

ICP, Intracranial pressure.

More than half of brain tumors are malignant. They infiltrate the brain tissue and are not amenable to complete surgical removal. Other tumors may be histologically benign but are located such that complete removal is not possible.

Brain tumors rarely metastasize outside the central nervous system (CNS) because they are contained by structural (meninges) and physiologic (blood-brain) barriers. Table 57-12 compares the most common brain tumors. A glioblastoma and meningioma are shown in Fig. 57-17.

Clinical Manifestations and Complications

The clinical manifestations of brain tumors depend mainly on their location and size (Table 57-13). The rate of growth and the appearance of manifestations depend on the location, size, and mitotic rate of the cells of the tissue of origin. Fig. 57-18 illustrates the functional areas of the cerebral cortex and can be used as a guide to correlate the clinical manifestations with the location of the tumor, as indicated by an alteration in the function controlled by the affected area.

Wide ranges of possible clinical manifestations are associated with brain tumors. Headache is a common problem. Tumor-related headaches tend to be worse at night and may awaken the patient. The headaches are usually dull and constant but occasionally throbbing. Seizures are common in gliomas and brain metastases. Brain tumors can cause nausea and vomiting from increased ICP. Cognitive dysfunction, including memory problems and mood or personality changes,

is another common manifestation, especially in patients with brain metastases. Muscle weakness, sensory losses, aphasia, and visual-spatial dysfunction are also manifestations of brain tumors.

If the tumor mass obstructs the ventricles or occludes the outlet, ventricular enlargement (hydrocephalus) can occur. As the brain tumor expands, it may also produce manifestations of increased ICP, cerebral edema, or obstruction of the CSF pathways. Unless treated, all brain tumors eventually cause death from increasing tumor volume leading to increased ICP.

Diagnostic Studies

An extensive history and a comprehensive neurologic examination must be done in the workup of a patient with a suspected brain tumor. A careful history and physical examination may provide data with respect to location. New onset of seizures or adult-onset migraines may be indicative of a brain tumor and should be investigated. Diagnostic studies are similar to those used for a patient with increased ICP (see Table 57-3).

The sensitivity of techniques such as MRI and PET scans allows for detection of small tumors and may provide more reliable diagnostic information than a CT scan. CT and brain scanning are used to identify the lesion's location. Other tests include magnetic resonance spectroscopy, functional MRI, and single-photon emission computed tomography (SPECT). The EEG is useful for ruling out seizures, but is of less importance. A lumbar puncture is seldom diagnostic and carries with it the risk of cerebral herniation. Angiography can be used to determine blood flow to the tumor and further localize the tumor. Other studies are done to rule out a primary lesion elsewhere in the body. Endocrine studies are helpful when a pituitary adenoma is suspected (see Chapter 50).

The correct diagnosis of a brain tumor can be made by obtaining tissue for histologic study. In most patients, tissue is obtained at the time of surgery. Computer-guided stereotactic biopsy is also an option. A smear or frozen section can be performed in the operating room for a preliminary interpretation of the histologic type. With this information, the neurosurgeon can make a better decision about the extent of surgery. In some cases, immunohistochemical stains or electron microscopy may be necessary to ascertain the correct diagnosis. Determination of the MIB-1 index, a measure of mitotic rate, is often helpful in assessing the tumor's mitotic activity.

Collaborative Care

Treatment goals are aimed at (1) identifying the tumor type and location, (2) removing or decreasing tumor mass, and (3) preventing or managing increased ICP.

Surgical Therapy. Surgical removal is the preferred treatment for brain tumors (see the section on cranial surgery later in this chapter). Stereotactic surgical techniques are used with greater frequency to perform a biopsy and remove small brain tumors. The outcome of surgical therapy depends on the tumor's type, size, and location. Meningiomas and oligodendrogliomas can usually be completely removed, whereas the more invasive gliomas and medulloblastomas may only be partially removed. Computer-guided stereotactic biopsy, ultrasound, functional MRI, and cortical mapping can be used to localize brain tumors intraoperatively.

Complete surgical removal of brain tumors is not always possible because the tumor is not always accessible or may involve vital parts of the brain. Surgery can reduce tumor mass, which decreases ICP, provides relief of symptoms, and extends survival time.

Ventricular Shunts. Hydrocephalus can be treated with the placement of a ventricular shunt. A catheter with one-way valves is placed in the lateral ventricle and then tunneled through the skin to drain CSF into the jugular vein, peritoneum, or pelvis. Rapid decompression of ICP can cause total body collapse and weakness, including a headache that may be prevented by gradually introducing the patient to the upright position.

Manifestations of shunt malfunction, which are related to increased ICP, include decreasing LOC, restlessness, headache, blurred vision, or vomiting. This may necessitate shunt revision or replacement. Infection may also occur, as exhibited by high fever, persistent headache, and stiff neck. Antibiotics are used to treat the infection. In some situations the shunt must be replaced.

Radiation Therapy and Stereotactic Radiosurgery. Radiation therapy may be used as a follow-up measure after surgery. Radiation seeds can also be implanted into the brain. Cerebral edema and rapidly increasing ICP may be a complication of radiation therapy, but these problems can be managed with high doses of corticosteroids (dexamethasone, prednisone, or methylprednisolone [Solu-Medrol]). (Radiation therapy is discussed in Chapter 16.)

Stereotactic radiosurgery is a method of delivering a highly concentrated dose of radiation to a precise location within the brain. Stereotactic radiosurgery may be used when conventional surgery has failed or is not an option because of the tumor location. (Radiosurgery is discussed on p. 1379.)

Chemotherapy and Targeted Therapy. The effectiveness of chemotherapy has been limited by difficulty getting drugs across the blood-brain barrier, tumor cell heterogeneity, and tumor cell drug resistance. Chemotherapy drugs called nitrosoureas (e.g., carmustine [BCNU], lomustine [CCNU]) are used to treat brain tumors. Normally the blood-brain barrier prohibits the entry of most drugs into the brain. The most malignant tumors cause a breakdown of the blood-brain barrier in the area of the tumor, thus allowing chemotherapy agents to be used to treat the malignancy. Chemotherapy-laden biodegradable wafers (e.g., Gliadel wafer [polifeprosan with carmustine implant]) implanted at the time of surgery can deliver chemotherapy directly to the tumor site. Other drugs being used include methotrexate and procarbazine (Matulane). One method used to deliver chemotherapy drugs directly to the CNS is intrathecal administration via an Ommaya reservoir.

Temozolomide (Temodar) is the first oral chemotherapy agent found to cross the blood-brain barrier. In contrast with many traditional chemotherapy drugs, which require metabolic activation to exert their effects, temozolomide can convert spontaneously to a reactive agent that directly interferes with tumor growth. It does not interact with other drugs commonly taken by patients with brain tumors, such as antiseizure medications, corticosteroids, and antiemetics.

> **DRUG ALERT: Temozolomide (Temodar)**
> - Causes myelosuppression. Before using, it is recommended that absolute neutrophil count be ≥1500/μL and platelet count be ≥100,000/μL.
> - To reduce nausea and vomiting, take on empty stomach.

Bevacizumab (Avastin) is used to treat patients with glioblastoma multiforme that continues to progress after standard therapy. Bevacizumab is a targeted therapy that inhibits the action of vascular endothelial growth factor, which helps form new blood vessels. These vessels can feed a tumor, helping it to grow, and can also provide a pathway for cancer cells to circulate in the body. (Targeted therapy is discussed in Chapter 16 and Table 16-13.)

Other Therapies. A medical device system, NovoTTF-100A System, is used to treat glioblastoma multiforme that recurs or progresses after receiving chemotherapy and radiation therapy. With this system, electrodes are placed on the surface of the patient's scalp to deliver low-intensity, changing electrical fields called *tumor treatment fields* (TTFs) to the tumor site.

Many techniques to control and treat brain tumors are currently under investigation. Although progress in treatment has increased length and quality of life for patients with brain tumors, outcomes still remain poor for patients with gliomas.[24]

NURSING MANAGEMENT
BRAIN TUMORS

NURSING ASSESSMENT

Structure the initial assessment to provide baseline data of the patient's neurologic status. Use this information to design a realistic, individualized care plan. Assess the patient's LOC, motor abilities, sensory perception, integrated function (including bowel and bladder function), and balance and proprioception, and also assess the coping abilities of the patient, caregiver, and family. Watching a patient perform activities of daily living and listening to the patient's conversation can be part of the neurologic assessment. Having the patient or caregiver explain the problem can be helpful to determine the patient's limitations and obtain information about the patient's insight into the problems. Record all initial data to provide a baseline for comparison to determine whether the patient's condition is improving or deteriorating.

Interview data are as important as the actual physical assessment. Ask questions about the medical history, intellectual abilities and educational level, and history of nervous system infections and trauma. Determine the presence of seizures, syncope, nausea and vomiting, and headaches or other pain to help better plan care for the patient.

NURSING DIAGNOSES

Nursing diagnoses for the patient with a brain tumor may include, but are not limited to, the following:

- Risk for ineffective cerebral tissue perfusion *related to* cerebral edema
- Acute pain (headache) *related to* cerebral edema and increased ICP
- Anxiety *related to* diagnosis and treatment
- Potential complication: seizures *related to* abnormal electrical activity of the brain
- Potential complication: increased ICP *related to* tumor and failure of normal compensatory mechanisms

PLANNING

The overall goals are that the patient with a brain tumor will (1) maintain normal ICP, (2) maximize neurologic functioning, (3) achieve control of pain and discomfort, and (4) be aware of the long-term implications with respect to prognosis and cognitive and physical functioning.

NURSING IMPLEMENTATION

A primary or metastatic tumor of the frontal lobe can cause behavioral and personality changes. Loss of emotional control, confusion, disorientation, memory loss, impulsivity, and depression may be signs of a frontal lobe lesion. These behavioral changes are often not perceived by the patient but can be disturbing and even frightening to the caregiver and family. These changes can also cause a distancing to occur between the family and patient. Assist the caregiver and family in understanding what is happening to the patient, and support the family.

The confused patient with behavioral instability can be a challenge. Protecting the patient from self-harm is an important part of nursing care. Close supervision of activity, use of side rails, judicious use of restraints, appropriate sedative medications, padding of the rails and the area around the bed, and a calm reassuring approach are all essential techniques in the care of these patients.

Perceptual problems associated with frontal and parietal lobe tumors contribute to a patient's disorientation and confusion. Minimize environmental stimuli, create a routine, and use reality orientation for the confused patient.

Seizures, which often occur with brain tumors, are managed with antiseizure drugs. Also use seizure precautions for the patient's protection. Some behavioral changes seen in the patient with a brain tumor are a result of seizure disorders and can improve with adequate seizure control. Patients at risk for seizures may be unable to drive, so be aware of the extra resources needed and collaborate with the social worker and the family. (Seizure disorders are discussed in Chapter 59.)

Motor and sensory dysfunctions interfere with the activities of daily living.[25] Alterations in mobility must be managed. Encourage the patient to provide as much self-care as physically possible. Self-image often depends on the patient's ability to participate in care within the limitations of the physical deficits.

Language deficits can also occur in patients with brain tumors. Motor (expressive) or sensory (receptive) dysphasia may occur. The disturbance in communication can be frustrating for the patient and may interfere with your ability to meet the patient's needs. Make attempts to establish a communication system that can be used by both the patient and the staff.

Nutritional intake may be decreased because of the patient's inability to eat, loss of appetite, or loss of desire to eat. Assess the patient's nutritional status, and ensure adequate nutritional intake. Encourage the patient to eat. Some patients may need enteral or parenteral nutrition (see Chapter 40). The patient with a brain tumor who undergoes cranial surgery requires complex nursing care. This is discussed in the next section.

Although progress is continually being made in helping patients with brain tumors, the prognosis remains grim for those with highly invasive tumors.[24] Provide help and support during the adjustment phase and in long-range planning. Social work and home health nurses may be needed to assist the caregiver with discharge planning and to help the family adjust to role changes and psychosocial and socioeconomic factors. Issues related to palliative and end-of-life care need to be discussed with both the patient and the family (see Chapter 10).

EVALUATION

The expected outcomes are that the patient with a brain tumor will

- Achieve control of pain, vomiting, and other discomforts
- Maintain ICP within normal limits
- Demonstrate maximal neurologic function (cognitive, motor, sensory) given the location and extent of the tumor
- Maintain optimal nutritional status
- Accept the long-term consequences of the tumor and its treatment

TABLE 57-14   INDICATIONS FOR CRANIAL SURGERY

Indication	Cause	Surgical Procedure
Brain abscess	Bacteria that caused intracranial infection	Excision or drainage of abscess
Hydrocephalus	Overproduction of CSF, obstruction to flow, defective reabsorption	Placement of ventriculoatrial or ventriculoperitoneal shunt
Brain tumors	Benign or malignant cell growth	Excision or partial resection of tumor
Intracranial bleeding	Rupture of cerebral vessels because of trauma or stroke	Surgical evacuation through burr holes or craniotomy
Skull fractures	Trauma to skull	Debridement of fragments and necrotic tissue, elevation and realignment of bone fragments
Arteriovenous (AV) malformation	Congenital tangle of arteries and veins (frequently in middle cerebral artery)	Excision of malformation
Aneurysm repair	Dilation of weak area in arterial wall (usually near anterior portion of circle of Willis)	Dissection and clipping or coiling of aneurysm

CSF, Cerebrospinal fluid.

TABLE 57-15   TYPES OF CRANIAL SURGERY

Type	Description
Burr hole	Opening into the cranium with a drill. Used to remove localized fluid and blood beneath the dura.
Craniotomy	Opening into cranium with removal of bone flap and opening the dura to remove a lesion, repair a damaged area, drain blood, or relieve ↑ ICP.
Craniectomy	Excision into the cranium to cut away bone flap.
Cranioplasty	Repair of cranial defect resulting from trauma, malformation, or previous surgical procedure. Artificial material used to replace damaged or lost bone.
Stereotactic procedure	Precise localization of a specific area of the brain using a frame or a frameless system based on three-dimensional coordinates. Procedure is used for biopsy, radiosurgery, or dissection.
Shunt procedures	Alternate pathway to redirect cerebrospinal fluid from one area to another using a tube or implanted device. Examples include ventricular shunt and Ommaya reservoir.

ICP, Intracranial pressure.

CRANIAL SURGERY

The indication for cranial surgery may be related to a brain tumor, CNS infection (e.g., abscess), vascular abnormalities, craniocerebral trauma, seizure disorder, or intractable pain (Table 57-14).

Types

Various types of cranial surgical procedures are presented in Table 57-15.

Craniotomy. Depending on the location of the pathologic condition, a *craniotomy* may be frontal, parietal, occipital, temporal, suboccipital, or a combination of any of these. The surgeon drills a set of burr holes and uses a saw to connect the holes to remove the bone flap. Sometimes operating microscopes are used to magnify the site. After surgery, the bone flap is wired or sutured. Sometimes drains are placed to remove fluid and blood. Patients are usually cared for in an ICU until stable.

Stereotactic Radiosurgery. Stereotactic procedures use precision apparatus (often computer guided) to help the physician precisely target an area of the brain. Stereotactic biopsy can be performed to obtain tissue samples for histologic examination. CT scanning and MRI are used to image the targeted tissue.

With the patient under general or local anesthesia, the surgeon drills a burr hole or creates a bone flap for an entry site and then introduces a probe and biopsy needle. Stereotactic procedures are used for removal of small brain tumors and abscesses, drainage of hematomas, ablative procedures for extrapyramidal diseases (e.g., Parkinson's disease), and repair of arteriovenous malformations. A major advantage of the stereotactic approach is a reduction in damage to surrounding tissue.

Stereotactic radiosurgery is not a form of surgery in the traditional sense. Instead, radiosurgery uses precisely focused radiation to destroy tumor cells and other abnormal growths in the brain. Computers create three-dimensional images of the brain, and these images are used to guide the focused radiation while the patient's head is held still in a stereotactic frame (Fig. 57-19). Radiosurgical techniques can use ionizing radiation generated by a linear accelerator, gamma knife, or CyberKnife. In these procedures, a high dose of cobalt radiation is delivered to precisely targeted tumor tissue. The dose of radiation is delivered in a single treatment lasting a few hours or in multiple sessions. Side effects of stereotactic radiosurgery may include fatigue, headache, and nausea.

In combination with stereotactic procedures to identify and localize tumor sites, surgical lasers can be used to destroy tumors. Three surgical lasers currently used are the carbon dioxide, argon, and neodymium:yttrium-aluminum-garnet (Nd:YAG) lasers. All three work by creating thermal energy, which destroys the tissue on which it is focused. Laser therapy also provides the benefit of reducing damage to surrounding tissue.

NURSING MANAGEMENT
CRANIAL SURGERY

NURSING IMPLEMENTATION

ACUTE INTERVENTION. The general preoperative and postoperative nursing care for the patient undergoing cranial surgery is similar regardless of the cause. Nursing management is similar to that for the patient with increased ICP (presented in eNursing Care Plan 57-1). The patient (if conscious and coherent), caregiver, and family will be concerned about the potential physical and emotional problems that can result from surgery. The uncertainty regarding prognosis and outcome requires compassionate nursing care in the preoperative period.

Preoperative teaching is important in allaying the fears of the patient, caregiver, and family, and also in preparing them for the postoperative period. Provide general information concerning the type of operation that will be performed and what can

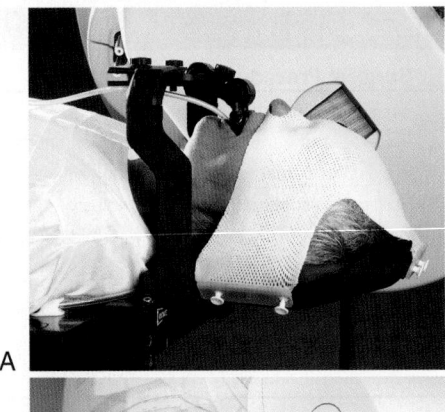

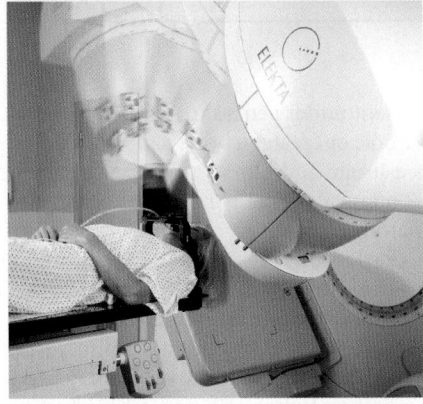

FIG. 57-19 A, Patient in a stereotactic frame. **B,** Elekta's Fraxion head frame helps ensure accuracy and precision in stereotactic radiation therapy (SRT) of cancer targets in the brain and cranium. (Courtesy Elekta.)

ETHICAL/LEGAL DILEMMAS
Withholding Treatment

Situation

C.J., a 26-yr-old patient in a permanent vegetative state, is diagnosed with her fifteenth bladder infection. As her home care nurse, you must determine whether to seek antibiotics for this infection. The family members have expressed a concern that no heroic measures be used to extend the biologic life of their daughter and sister. However, they have been unwilling to withdraw the existing treatment, which is enteral nutrition through a gastrostomy tube. Should antibiotics be withheld?

Ethical/Legal Points for Consideration

- Patients in a persistent vegetative state do not recover.
- The primary legal issue here is who has the legal right to refuse or consent to treatment for this incapacitated patient. You would need to know if a guardian has been appointed by the court or if her parents retain a form of guardianship to make health care decisions for her.
- You also need to know when the vegetative state began; that is, did the patient ever have the right to consent having reached the age of majority as a competent adult, or did the vegetative state begin while she was a minor? If the patient did become a competent adult before the vegetative state, did she ever express any preference for quality-of-life and end-of-life decision making?
- The courts have widespread legal precedents for accepting the decision of the patient's guardian or parents or the patient's clearly expressed preferences for quality-of-life decision making.
- Some courts have made a distinction between medical treatment (antibiotics) and comfort care (enteral feeding tube). The antibiotics may be seen as medical treatment that could be legally refused.

Discussion Questions

1. How would you approach C.J.'s family?
2. What are your feelings about providing nutrition, hydration, and treatments that will prolong life in a patient for whom there is no hope of recovery?
3. What options are available to the family for the care of their daughter once a decision is made about withholding antibiotics?

be expected immediately after the operation. Explain that some hair may be shaved to allow for better exposure and to prevent contamination. The hair is usually removed in the operating room after induction of anesthesia. Also inform the family that the patient will be taken to an ICU or to a special care unit after surgery. The primary goal of care after cranial surgery is prevention of increased ICP. (Nursing management of the patient with increased ICP is presented on pp. 1356-1368.) Frequent assessment of the patient's neurologic status is essential during the first 48 hours. In addition to the neurologic functions, closely monitor fluid and electrolyte levels and serum osmolality to detect changes in sodium regulation, the onset of diabetes insipidus, or severe hypovolemia. Turning and positioning the patient may depend on the site of the operation.

Monitor the patient for pain and nausea. Although the brain itself does not possess pain receptors, patients often report headache caused by edema or pain at the incision site. Control pain with short-acting opioids and monitor neurologic status. Nausea and vomiting are common after surgery and are usually treated with antiemetics. The use of promethazine (Phenergan) is discouraged because it can increase somnolence, thus altering the accuracy of a neurologic assessment.

The surgical dressing is usually in place for a few days. With an incision over the skull in the anterior or middle fossa, the patient will return from the operating room with the head elevated at an angle of 30 to 45 degrees. The head of the bed should remain elevated at least 30 degrees unless the surgical approach is in the posterior fossa or a burr hole has been made. In these cases, the patient is generally kept flat or at a slight elevation (10 to 15 degrees) during the postoperative phase.

If a bone flap has been removed (craniectomy), do not position the patient on the operative side. Observe the dressing for color, odor, and amount of drainage. Notify the surgeon immediately of any excessive bleeding or clear drainage. Checking drains for placement and assessing the area around the dressing are also important. Scalp care should include meticulous care of the incision to prevent wound infection. Cleanse the area and treat it in accordance with hospital protocol or the neurosurgeon's orders. Once the dressing is removed, use an antiseptic soap for washing the scalp. The psychologic impact of hair removal can be alleviated by the use of a wig, turban, scarves, or cap after the incision has completely healed. For the patient who is receiving radiation, instruct the patient to use a sunblock and head covering if any exposure to the sun is anticipated.

AMBULATORY AND HOME CARE. The rehabilitative potential for a patient after cranial surgery depends on the reason for the surgery, the postoperative course, and the patient's general state of health. Base your nursing interventions on a realistic appraisal of these factors. An overall goal is to foster independence for as long as possible and to the highest degree possible.

Specific rehabilitation potential cannot be determined until cerebral edema and increased ICP subside postoperatively. Take care to maintain as much function as possible through measures such as careful positioning, meticulous skin and mouth care, regular range-of-motion exercises, bowel and bladder care, and adequate nutrition.

Referrals may be made to other specialists on the health care team. For example, the speech therapist may be helpful to the patient who has a speech problem, or the physical therapist may

TABLE 57-16	COMPARISON OF CEREBRAL INFLAMMATORY CONDITIONS		
	Meningitis	**Encephalitis**	**Brain Abscess**
Cause	Bacteria (*Streptococcus pneumoniae, Neisseria meningitidis*, group B streptococci, viruses, fungi)	Bacteria, fungi, parasites, herpes simplex virus (HSV), other viruses (e.g., West Nile virus)	Streptococci, staphylococci through bloodstream
CSF (Reference Interval)			
• Pressure (70-150 mm H₂O)	Increased	Normal to slight increase	Increased
• WBC count (0-5 cells/μL)	*Bacterial:* >1000/μL (mainly neutrophils) *Viral:* 25-500/μL (mainly lymphocytes)	500/μL, neutrophils (early), lymphocytes (later)	25-300/μL (neutrophils)
• Protein (15-45 mg/dL [0.15-0.45 g/L])	*Bacterial:* >500 mg/dL *Viral:* 50-500 mg/dL	Slight increase	Normal
• Glucose (40-70 mg/dL [2.2-3.9 mmol/L])	*Bacterial:* Decreased *Viral:* Normal or low	Normal	Low or absent
• Appearance	*Bacterial:* Turbid, cloudy *Viral:* Clear or cloudy	Clear	Clear
Diagnostic Studies	CT scan, Gram stain, smear, culture, PCR*	CT scan, EEG, MRI, PET, PCR, IgM antibodies to virus in serum or CSF	CT scan
Treatment	Antibiotics, dexamethasone, supportive care, prevention of ↑ ICP	Supportive care, prevention of ↑ ICP, acyclovir (Zovirax) for HSV	Antibiotics, incision and drainage Supportive care

*PCR is used to detect viral RNA or DNA.
CSF, Cerebrospinal fluid; *ICP*, intracranial pressure; *PCR*, polymerase chain reaction.

provide an exercise plan to regain functional deficits. Address the needs and problems of each patient individually because many variables affect the plan. The patient's mental and physical deterioration, including seizures, personality disorganization, apathy, and wasting, is difficult for both family and health care professionals to watch. Cognitive and emotional residual deficits are often harder to accept than are motor and sensory losses.

INFLAMMATORY CONDITIONS OF THE BRAIN

Brain abscesses, meningitis, and encephalitis are the most common inflammatory conditions of the brain and spinal cord (Table 57-16). Inflammation can be caused by bacteria, viruses, fungi, and chemicals (e.g., contrast media used in diagnostic tests, blood in the subarachnoid space). CNS infections may occur via the bloodstream, by extension from a primary site, or along cranial and spinal nerves.

The mortality rate for inflammatory conditions of the brain is approximately 2% to 30% in the general population, with higher rates in older patients. Up to 40% of those who recover can have long-term neurologic deficits, including hearing loss.[26]

BRAIN ABSCESS

Brain abscess is an accumulation of pus within the brain tissue that can result from a local or systemic infection. Direct extension from an ear, tooth, mastoid, or sinus infection is the primary cause. Other causes for brain abscess formation include spread from a distant site (e.g., pulmonary infection, bacterial endocarditis), skull fracture, and prior brain trauma or surgery. Streptococci and *Staphylococcus aureus* are the primary infective organisms.

Manifestations of brain abscess, which are similar to those of meningitis and encephalitis, include headache, fever, and nausea and vomiting. Signs of increased ICP may include drowsiness, confusion, and seizures. Focal symptoms may reflect the local area of the abscess. For example, visual field defects or

psychomotor seizures are common with a temporal lobe abscess, whereas an occipital abscess may be accompanied by visual impairment and hallucinations. CT and MRI are used to diagnose a brain abscess.

Antimicrobial therapy is the primary treatment for brain abscess. Other manifestations are treated symptomatically. If drug therapy is not effective, the abscess may need to be drained, or removed if it is encapsulated. In untreated cases the mortality rate approaches 100%.

Nursing measures are similar to those for management of meningitis or increased ICP. If surgical drainage or removal is the treatment of choice, nursing care is similar to that described under cranial surgery.

BACTERIAL MENINGITIS

Meningitis is an acute inflammation of the meningeal tissues surrounding the brain and spinal cord. Meningitis usually occurs in fall, winter, or early spring and is often secondary to viral respiratory disease. Older adults and persons who are debilitated are affected more frequently than the general population. College students living in dormitories and individuals living in institutions (e.g., prisoners) are also at a high risk for contracting meningitis.

Bacterial meningitis is considered a medical emergency. Untreated bacterial meningitis has a mortality rate near 100%.

Etiology and Pathophysiology

Streptococcus pneumoniae and *Neisseria meningitidis* are the leading causes of bacterial meningitis. *Haemophilus influenzae* was once the most common cause of bacterial meningitis. However, the use of *H. influenzae* vaccine has resulted in a significant decrease in meningitis related to this organism.

The organisms usually gain entry to the CNS through the upper respiratory tract or the bloodstream. However, they may enter by direct extension from penetrating wounds of the skull or through fractured sinuses in basilar skull fractures.

The inflammatory response to the infection tends to increase CSF production with a moderate increase in ICP. In bacterial meningitis the purulent secretions produced quickly spread to other areas of the brain through the CSF and cover the cranial nerves and other intracranial structures. If this process extends into the brain parenchyma or if concurrent encephalitis is present, cerebral edema and increased ICP become more of a problem. Closely observe all patients with meningitis for manifestations of increased ICP, which is thought to be a result of swelling around the dura and increased CSF volume.

Clinical Manifestations

Fever, severe headache, nausea, vomiting, and nuchal rigidity (neck stiffness) are key signs of meningitis. Photophobia, a decreased LOC, and signs of increased ICP may also be present. Coma is associated with a poor prognosis and occurs in 5% to 10% of patients with bacterial meningitis. Seizures occur in one third of all cases. The headache becomes progressively worse and may be accompanied by vomiting and irritability. If the infecting organism is a meningococcus, a skin rash is common and petechiae may be seen.

Complications

The most common acute complication of bacterial meningitis is increased ICP. Most patients have increased ICP, and it is the major cause of an altered mental status. Another complication of bacterial meningitis is residual neurologic dysfunction.

Dysfunction often occurs involving many cranial nerves. Cranial nerve irritation can have serious sequelae. The optic nerve (CN II) is compressed by increased ICP. Papilledema is often present, and blindness may occur. When the oculomotor (CN III), trochlear (CN IV), and abducens (CN VI) nerves are irritated, ocular movements are affected. Ptosis, unequal pupils, and diplopia are common. Irritation of the trigeminal nerve (CN V) results in sensory losses and loss of the corneal reflex. Irritation of the facial nerve (CN VII) results in facial paresis. Irritation of the vestibulocochlear nerve (CN VIII) causes tinnitus, vertigo, and deafness. The dysfunction usually disappears within a few weeks. However, hearing loss may be permanent after bacterial meningitis.

Hemiparesis, dysphasia, and hemianopsia may also occur. These signs usually resolve over time. If they do not, a cerebral abscess, subdural empyema, subdural effusion, or persistent meningitis is suspected. Acute cerebral edema may cause seizures, CN III palsy, bradycardia, hypertensive coma, and death.

Headaches may occur for months after the diagnosis of meningitis until the irritation and inflammation have completely resolved. It is important to implement pain management for chronic headaches.

A noncommunicating hydrocephalus may occur if the exudate causes adhesions that prevent the normal flow of CSF from the ventricles. CSF reabsorption by the arachnoid villi may also be obstructed by the exudate. In this situation, surgical implantation of a shunt is the only treatment.

Waterhouse-Friderichsen syndrome is a complication of meningococcal meningitis. The syndrome is manifested by petechiae, disseminated intravascular coagulation (DIC), adrenal hemorrhage, and circulatory collapse. DIC and shock, which are some of the most serious complications of meningitis, are associated with meningococcemia. (DIC is discussed in detail in Chapter 31.)

Diagnostic Studies

When a patient has manifestations suggestive of bacterial meningitis, a blood culture and CT scan should be done. Diagnosis is usually verified by doing a lumbar puncture with analysis of the CSF. A lumbar puncture should be completed only after the CT scan has ruled out an obstruction in the foramen magnum in order to prevent a fluid shift resulting in herniation.

Specimens of the CSF, sputum, and nasopharyngeal secretions are taken for culture before the start of antibiotic therapy to identify the causative organism. A Gram stain is done to detect bacteria.

Variations in the CSF depend on the causative organism. Protein levels in the CSF are usually elevated and are higher in bacterial than in viral meningitis. The CSF glucose concentration is commonly decreased in bacterial meningitis but may be normal in viral meningitis. The CSF is purulent and turbid in bacterial meningitis. It may be the same or clear in viral meningitis. The predominant white blood cell type in the CSF during bacterial meningitis is neutrophils (see Table 57-16).

X-rays of the skull may demonstrate infected sinuses. CT scans and MRI may be normal in uncomplicated meningitis. In other cases, CT scans may reveal evidence of increased ICP or hydrocephalus.

Collaborative Care

Bacterial meningitis is a medical emergency. Rapid diagnosis based on history and physical examination is crucial because the patient is usually in a critical state when health care is sought. When meningitis is suspected, antibiotic therapy is instituted after the collection of specimens for cultures, even before the diagnosis is confirmed (Table 57-17).

Ampicillin, penicillin, vancomycin, cefuroxime (Ceftin), cefotaxime (Claforan), ceftriaxone (Rocephin), ceftizoxime (Cefizox), and ceftazidime (Ceptaz) are some commonly prescribed drugs for treating bacterial meningitis. Dexamethasone (a corticosteroid) may also be prescribed before or with the first

---

TABLE 57-17 COLLABORATIVE CARE

Bacterial Meningitis

Diagnostic
- History and physical examination
- Analysis of CSF for protein, glucose, WBC, Gram stain, and culture
- CBC, coagulation profile, electrolyte levels, glucose, platelet count
- Blood culture
- CT scan, MRI, PET scan
- Skull x-ray studies

Collaborative Therapy
- Rest
- IV fluids
- Hypothermia

Drug Therapy
- IV antibiotics
  - ampicillin, penicillin
  - cephalosporin (e.g., cefotaxime [Claforan], ceftriaxone [Rocephin])
- codeine for headache
- dexamethasone (Decadron)
- acetaminophen or aspirin for temperature >100.4° F (38° C)
- phenytoin (Dilantin) IV
- mannitol (Osmitrol) IV for diuresis

CSF, Cerebrospinal fluid; *PET,* positron emission tomography.

dose of antibiotics. Collaborate with the health care provider to manage the headache, fever, and nuchal rigidity often associated with meningitis.

NURSING MANAGEMENT BACTERIAL MENINGITIS

NURSING ASSESSMENT

Initial assessment should include vital signs, neurologic evaluation, fluid intake and output, and evaluation of the lungs and skin (see eFig. 57-1 available on the website for this chapter).

NURSING DIAGNOSES

Nursing diagnoses for the patient with bacterial meningitis may include, but are not limited to, the following:

- Decreased intracranial adaptive capacity *related to* decreased cerebral perfusion or increased ICP
- Risk for ineffective cerebral tissue perfusion *related to* reduction of blood flow and cerebral edema
- Hyperthermia *related to* infection
- Acute pain *related to* headache and muscle aches

Additional information on nursing diagnoses for the patient with bacterial meningitis is presented in eNursing Care Plan 57-2 (available on the website for this chapter).

PLANNING

The overall goals for the patient with bacterial meningitis are to (1) return to maximal neurologic functioning, (2) resolve the infection, and (3) control pain and discomfort.

NURSING IMPLEMENTATION

HEALTH PROMOTION. Prevention of respiratory tract infections through vaccination programs for pneumococcal pneumonia and influenza is important. Two meningococcal vaccines are available in the United States: meningococcal polysaccharide vaccine (MPSV4) and meningococcal conjugate vaccine (MCV4). MPSV4 has been available since the 1970s. It is the only meningococcal vaccine licensed for people older than 55. MCV4 is the preferred vaccine for people 55 years of age and younger. Two doses of MCV4 are recommended for adolescents 11 through 18 years of age: the first dose at 11 or 12 years of age, with a booster dose at age 16.

Early and vigorous treatment of respiratory tract and ear infections is important. Persons who have close contact with anyone who has bacterial meningitis should be given prophylactic antibiotics.

ACUTE INTERVENTION. The patient with bacterial meningitis is usually acutely ill. The fever is high, and head pain is severe. Irritation of the cerebral cortex may result in seizures. The changes in mental status and LOC depend on the degree of increased ICP. Assess and record vital signs, neurologic status, fluid intake and output, skin, and lung fields at regular intervals based on the patient's condition.

Head and neck pain secondary to movement requires attention. Codeine provides some pain relief without undue sedation for most patients. Assist the patient to a position of comfort, often curled up with the head slightly extended. The head of the bed should be slightly elevated. A darkened room and a cool cloth over the eyes relieve the discomfort of photophobia.

For the delirious patient, additional low lighting may be necessary to decrease hallucinations. All patients suffer some degree of mental distortion and hypersensitivity, and they may be frightened and misinterpret the environment. Make every attempt to minimize environmental stimuli and prevent injury. A familiar person at the bedside may have a calming effect. Be efficient with care but also convey an attitude of caring and of unhurried gentleness. The use of touch and a soothing voice to give simple explanations of activities is helpful. If seizures occur, make appropriate observations and take protective measures. Administer antiseizure drugs such as phenytoin (Dilantin) or levetiracetam (Keppra) as ordered. Problems associated with increased ICP need to be managed (see the section on increased ICP earlier in this chapter).

Fever must be vigorously treated because it increases cerebral edema and the frequency of seizures. In addition, neurologic damage may result from an extremely high temperature over a prolonged time. Acetaminophen or aspirin may be used to reduce fever. However, if the fever is resistant to aspirin or acetaminophen, more vigorous means are necessary, such as a cooling blanket. Take care not to reduce the temperature too rapidly because shivering may result, causing a rebound effect and increasing the temperature. Wrap the extremities in soft towels or a blanket covered with a sheet to reduce shivering (which can raise ICP). If a cooling blanket is not available or desirable, tepid sponge baths with water may be effective in lowering the temperature. Protect the skin from excessive drying and injury and prevent breaks in the skin.

Because high fever greatly increases the metabolic rate and thus insensible fluid loss, assess the patient for dehydration and adequacy of fluid intake. Diaphoresis further increases fluid losses, which should be noted on the output record. Calculate replacement fluids as 800 mL/day for respiratory losses and 100 mL for each degree of temperature above 100.4° F (38° C). Supplemental feeding (e.g., enteral nutrition) to maintain adequate nutritional intake may be necessary. Follow the designated antibiotic schedule to maintain therapeutic blood levels.

Meningitis generally requires respiratory isolation until the cultures are negative. Meningococcal meningitis is highly contagious, whereas other causes of meningitis may pose minimal to no infection risk with patient contact. However, standard precautions are essential to protect the patient and the nurse.

AMBULATORY AND HOME CARE. After the acute period has passed, the patient requires several weeks of convalescence before resuming normal activities. In this period, stress the importance of adequate nutrition, with an emphasis on a high-protein, high-calorie diet in small, frequent feedings.

Muscle rigidity may persist in the neck and the backs of the legs. Progressive range-of-motion exercises and warm baths are useful. Have the patient gradually increase activity as tolerated, but encourage adequate rest and sleep.

Residual effects can result in sequelae such as dementia, seizures, deafness, hemiplegia, and hydrocephalus. Assess vision, hearing, cognitive skills, and motor and sensory abilities after recovery, with appropriate referrals as indicated. Throughout the acute and convalescent periods, be aware of the anxiety and stress experienced by the caregiver and other family members.

EVALUATION

The expected outcomes are that the patient with bacterial meningitis will

- Demonstrate appropriate cognitive function
- Be oriented to person, place, and time
- Maintain body temperature within normal range
- Report satisfaction with pain control

Additional information on expected outcomes for the patient with bacterial meningitis is addressed in eNursing Care Plan 57-2.

VIRAL MENINGITIS

The most common causes of viral meningitis are enteroviruses, arboviruses, human immunodeficiency virus, and herpes simplex virus (HSV). Enteroviruses are most often spread through direct contact with respiratory secretions. Viral meningitis usually manifests as a headache, fever, photophobia, and stiff neck.[26] The fever may be moderate or high.

The Xpert EV test is used to rapidly diagnose viral meningitis. A sample of CSF is used to determine if enterovirus is present, and results are available within hours of symptom onset.[27] An important diagnostic test is examination of the CSF via lumbar puncture. The CSF can be clear or cloudy, and the typical finding is lymphocytosis (see Table 57-16). Organisms are not seen on Gram stain or acid-fast smears. Polymerase chain reaction (PCR) used to detect viral-specific deoxyribonucleic acid (DNA) or ribonucleic acid (RNA) is a highly sensitive method for diagnosing CNS viral infections.

Antibiotics should be administered after the lumbar puncture while awaiting the results of the CSF analysis. Antibiotics are the best defense for bacterial meningitis and can be easily discontinued if the meningitis is found to be viral.[26]

Viral meningitis is managed symptomatically because the disease is self-limiting. Full recovery from viral meningitis is expected. Rare sequelae include persistent headaches, mild mental impairment, and incoordination.

ENCEPHALITIS

Encephalitis, an acute inflammation of the brain, is a serious, and sometimes fatal, disease. In the United States, encephalitis is responsible for about 20,000 cases and 1400 deaths annually.[28]

Encephalitis is usually caused by a virus. Many different viruses have been implicated in encephalitis. Some of the viruses are associated with certain seasons of the year and endemic to certain geographic areas.

Ticks and mosquitoes transmit epidemic encephalitis. Examples include eastern equine encephalitis, La Crosse encephalitis, St. Louis encephalitis, West Nile encephalitis, and western equine encephalitis.[28] Nonepidemic encephalitis may occur as a complication of measles, chickenpox, or mumps. HSV encephalitis is the most common cause of acute nonepidemic viral encephalitis. Cytomegalovirus encephalitis is a common complication in patients with acquired immunodeficiency syndrome (AIDS).

Clinical Manifestations and Diagnostic Studies

The onset of infection is typically nonspecific, with fever, headache, nausea, and vomiting. Encephalitis can be acute or subacute. Signs of encephalitis appear on day 2 or 3 and may vary from minimal alterations in mental status to coma. Virtually any CNS abnormality can occur, including hemiparesis, tremors, seizures, cranial nerve palsies, personality changes, memory impairment, amnesia, and dysphasia.

Early diagnosis and treatment of viral encephalitis are essential for favorable outcomes. Diagnostic findings related to viral encephalitis are shown in Table 57-16. Brain imaging techniques include CT, MRI, and PET. PCR tests allow for early detection of HSV and West Nile encephalitis. West Nile virus should be strongly considered in adults over 50 years old who develop encephalitis or meningitis in summer or early fall. The best diagnostic test for West Nile virus is a blood test that detects viral RNA. This test is also used in screening blood, organs, cells, and tissues that have been donated.

NURSING AND COLLABORATIVE MANAGEMENT ENCEPHALITIS

Prevention of encephalitis requires mosquito control, including cleaning rain gutters, removing old tires, draining bird baths, and removing water where mosquitoes can breed. In addition, insect repellant should be used during mosquito season.

Collaborative and nursing management of encephalitis, including West Nile virus infection, is symptomatic and supportive. In the initial stages of encephalitis, many patients require intensive care.

Acyclovir (Zovirax) and vidarabine (Vira-A) are used to treat encephalitis caused by HSV infection. Acyclovir has fewer side effects than vidarabine and is often the preferred treatment. Use of these antiviral agents has been shown to reduce mortality rates, although neurologic complications may not be reduced. For maximal benefit, antiviral agents should be started before the onset of coma. Treat seizure disorders with antiseizure drugs. Prophylactic treatment with antiseizure drugs may be used in severe cases of encephalitis. Treatment of cytomegalovirus encephalitis in AIDS patients is discussed in Chapter 15.

RABIES

Although 30,000 to 70,000 people die each year from rabies worldwide, only one to three people die annually in the United States. The threat is much greater in developing countries. Rabies vaccine is encouraged for individuals who travel globally, since it remains a serious public health concern.

The etiology of rabies is an RNA virus that causes an acute, progressive viral encephalitis. Although rabies is generally transmitted via saliva from the bite of an infected animal, it can also be spread by scratches, mucous membrane contact with infected secretions, and inhalation of aerosolized virus into the respiratory tract. Any warm-blooded mammal, including livestock, can carry rabies. Throughout the world, rabid dogs are the most common disease vector. However, in developed countries, raccoons, skunks, bats, and foxes are the primary animal carriers.

The rabies virus spreads from the contact site through the CNS via peripheral nerve and possibly muscle fibers. During this time (2 to 14 days after exposure), patients experience flu-like symptoms, pain, paresthesias, or numbness. Then an acute neurologic syndrome occurs 2 to 7 days later and is manifested by agitation, hypersalivation, hydrophobia, dysarthria, vertigo, diplopia, hallucinations, and other neurologic sequelae (e.g., hyperactive reflexes, nuchal rigidity). Coma develops within 7 to 10 days of the neurologic syndrome. Patients experience flaccid paralysis, apnea, hydrophobia, and seizures. Death ensues as a result of respiratory and cardiovascular collapse within a few days after the onset of coma.

Because rabies is nearly always fatal, management efforts are directed at preventing the transmission and onset of the disease. Rabies postexposure prophylaxis is discussed in Chapter 69.

CASE STUDY

Traumatic Brain Injury

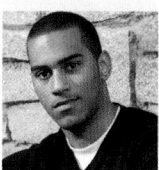

Comstock/Thinkstock

Patient Profile
C.G. is a 24-yr-old African American man who has just returned from a 15-mo Army deployment to Afghanistan. He comes to the outpatient clinic with a report of chronic headaches (pain rating of 8/10) and difficulty sleeping. His wife has noticed some personality changes since his return from deployment and is concerned that he has posttraumatic stress disorder (PTSD).

Subjective Data
- Reports that he has been depressed lately but attributes it to headache and difficulty returning home.
- Headache is worse in the morning or when he lies down.
- Uses tobacco and drinks coffee throughout the day.
- Has difficulty sleeping.
- Reports "incidents" of heavy combat and blasts with a loss of consciousness. Cannot remember how many times. Unable to obtain a more through history as he becomes quite agitated.

Objective Data
- During your assessment, you note that C.G. is looking around the room and jumps when the phone rings next door.
- Loss of short-term memory (remembers one of three items).
- Heart rate ranges from 100 to 130 beats/min.
- ECG strip is shown at right:

- Systolic BP ranges from 120 to 160 mm Hg.
- Right pupil, 3 mm sluggishly reactive; left pupil, 3 mm briskly reactive.

Diagnostic Studies
- CT of the head: negative for skull fracture, hematoma, or hemorrhage. Cerebral edema is noted with cingulate herniation on the right side.
- MRI performed following CT; mild diffuse axonal injury noted.

Discussion Questions
1. What could be the cause of C.G.'s hypertension, tachycardia, and ECG rhythm?
2. In addition to PTSD, what do his clinical manifestations suggest?
3. *Priority Decision:* What are the priority nursing interventions that should be implemented?
4. *Priority Decision:* Based on the assessment data presented, what are the priority nursing diagnoses? Are there any collaborative problems?
5. *Evidence-Based Practice:* What interventions and support can help his wife?

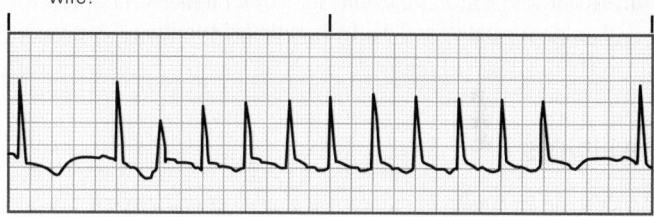

Ⓔvolve Answers available at *http://evolve.elsevier.com/Lewis/medsurg.*

▌ BRIDGE TO NCLEX EXAMINATION

The number of the question corresponds to the same-numbered outcome at the beginning of the chapter.

1. Vasogenic cerebral edema increases intracranial pressure by
   a. shifting fluid in the gray matter.
   b. altering the endothelial lining of cerebral capillaries.
   c. leaking molecules from the intracellular fluid to the capillaries.
   d. altering the osmotic gradient flow into the intravascular component.

2. A patient with intracranial pressure monitoring has a pressure of 12 mm Hg. The nurse understands that this pressure reflects
   a. a severe decrease in cerebral perfusion pressure.
   b. an alteration in the production of cerebrospinal fluid.
   c. the loss of autoregulatory control of intracranial pressure.
   d. a normal balance between brain tissue, blood, and cerebrospinal fluid.

3. A nurse plans care for the patient with increased intracranial pressure with the knowledge that the best way to position the patient is to
   a. keep the head of the bed flat.
   b. elevate the head of the bed to 30 degrees.
   c. maintain patient on the left side with the head supported on a pillow.
   d. use a continuous-rotation bed to continuously change patient position.

4. The nurse is alerted to a possible acute subdural hematoma in the patient who
   a. has a linear skull fracture crossing a major artery.
   b. has focal symptoms of brain damage with no recollection of a head injury.
   c. develops decreased level of consciousness and a headache within 48 hours of a head injury.
   d. has an immediate loss of consciousness with a brief lucid interval followed by decreasing level of consciousness.

5. During admission of a patient with a severe head injury to the emergency department, the nurse places the highest priority on assessment for
   a. patency of airway.
   b. presence of a neck injury.
   c. neurologic status with the Glasgow Coma Scale.
   d. cerebrospinal fluid leakage from the ears or nose.

6. A patient is suspected of having a brain tumor. The signs and symptoms include memory deficits, visual disturbances, weakness of right upper and lower extremities, and personality changes. The nurse recognizes that the tumor is most likely located in the
   a. frontal lobe.
   b. parietal lobe.
   c. occipital lobe.
   d. temporal lobe.

7. Nursing management of a patient with a brain tumor includes *(select all that apply)*

   a. discussing with the patient methods to control inappropriate behavior.

   b. using diversion techniques to keep the patient stimulated and motivated.

   c. assisting and supporting the family in understanding any changes in behavior.

   d. limiting self-care activities until the patient has regained maximum physical functioning.

   e. planning for seizure precautions and teaching the patient and the caregiver about antiseizure drugs.

8. The nurse on the clinical unit is assigned to four patients. Which patient should she assess first?

   a. Patient with a skull fracture whose nose is bleeding

   b. Older patient with a stroke who is confused and whose daughter is present

   c. Patient with meningitis who is suddenly agitated and reporting a headache of 10 on a 0-to-10 scale

   d. Patient who had a craniotomy for a brain tumor who is now 3 days postoperative and has had continued vomiting

9. A nursing measure that is indicated to reduce the potential for seizures and increased intracranial pressure in the patient with bacterial meningitis is

   a. administering codeine for relief of head and neck pain.

   b. controlling fever with prescribed drugs and cooling techniques.

   c. keeping the room dark and quiet to minimize environmental stimulation.

   d. maintaining the patient on strict bed rest with the head of the bed slightly elevated.

1. b, 2. d, 3. b, 4. c, 5. a, 6. a, 7. c, e, 8. c, 9. b

⊜volve

For rationales to these answers and even more NCLEX review questions, visit *http://evolve.elsevier.com/Lewis/medsurg.*

REFERENCES

1. Cushing H: *Studies in intracranial physiology and surgery,* London, 1925, Oxford University Press. (Classic)

*2. Vender J, Waller J, Dhandapani K, et al: An evaluation and comparison of intraventricular, intraparenchymal, and fluid-coupled techniques for intracranial pressure monitoring in patients with severe traumatic brain injury, *J Clin Monit Comput* 25:231, 2011.

3. Seidman R: Cerebrovascular disease, Stonybrook University Medical Center. Retrieved from *www.stonybrookmedicalcenter. org/pathology/neuropathology/chapter2.*

4. Oddo M, Villa F, Citerio G: Brain multimodality monitoring: an update, *Curr Opin Crit Care* 18(2):111, 2012.

*5. Haddad S, Arabi Y: Critical care management of severe traumatic brain injury in adults, *Scand J Trauma Resusc Emerg Med* 20:12, 2012.

6. Fan J, Kirkness C, Vicini P, et al: Intracranial pressure waveform morphology and intracranial adaptive capacity, *Am J Crit Care* 17:545, 2008.

*7. Kim G, Amato A, James M, et al: Continuous and intermittent CSF diversion after subarachnoid hemorrhage: a pilot study, *Neurocrit Care* 14:68, 2011.

*8. Choi H, Badjatia N, Mayer S: Hypothermia for acute brain injury: mechanisms and practical aspects, *Nat Rev Neurol* 28:214, 2012.

9. Scalfani M, Dhar R, Zazulia A, et al: Effect of osmotic agents on regional cerebral blood flow in traumatic brain injury, *J Crit Care* 27(5):526.e7, 2012.

10. Justo Meirelles C, de Aguilar-Nascimento J: Enteral or parenteral nutrition in traumatic brain injury: a prospective randomized trial, *Nutricion Hospitalaria* 26:1120, 2011.

11. Kornbluth J, Bhardwaj A: Evaluation of coma: a critical appraisal of popular scoring systems, *Neurocrit Care* 14:134, 2011.

*12. Pieracci F, Moore E, Beauchamp K, et al: A cost-minimization analysis of phenytoin versus levetiracetam for early seizures pharmacoprophylaxis after traumatic brain injury, *J Trauma* 72: 276, 2012.

13. Centers for Disease Control and Prevention: Injury prevention and control: traumatic brain injury. Retrieved from *www.cdc .gov/traumaticbraininjury/statistics.html.*

14. Sayer N: Traumatic brain injury and its neuropsychiatric sequelae in war, *Ann Rev Med* 63:405, 2012.

15. American Association of Neurological Surgeons: Traumatic brain injury: fact sheets. Retrieved from *www.aans.org/ Patient%20Information/Conditions%20and%20Treatments/ Traumatic%20Brain%20Injury.aspx.*

16. Johnson V, Stewart W, Smith D: Axonal pathology in traumatic brain injury, *Exper Neurol* 136(Pt 1):28–42, 2012.

17. Wasserman J, Koenigsberg RA: Diffuse axonal injury. Retrieved from *http://emedicine.medscape.com/article/339912-overview.*

*18. Wong D, Lurie F, Wong L: The effects of clopidogrel on elderly traumatic brain injured patients, *J Trauma* 65:1303, 2008.

19. Phan N, Hemphill J: Management of acute severe traumatic brain injury. Retrieved from *www.uptodate.com/contents/ management-of-acute-severe-traumatic-brain-injury.*

20. Chronic subdural hematoma. Retrieved from *www.nlm.nih.gov/ medlineplus/ency/article/000781.htm.*

21. Ganz J: Head injury management guidelines for general practitioners, *J Neurosci Rural Pract* 2:198, 2011.

22. National Cancer Institute: Brain tumor, approved by the US National Institutes of Health. Retrieved from *www.cancer.gov/ cancertopics/types/brain.*

23. University of Pittsburgh: Types of brain tumors. Retrieved from *www.neurosurgery.pitt.edu/neuro_oncology/brain/types.html.*

24. Wakabayashi T: Clinical trial updates for malignant brain tumors, *Clin Neurol* 51:853, 2011.

25. Davis M, Stoiber A: Glioblastoma multiforme: enhancing survival and quality of life, *Clin J Oncol Nurs* 15:291, 2011.

26. Centers for Disease Control and Prevention: Meningitis questions and answers. Retrieved from *www.cdc.gov/meningitis/ about/faq.html.*

*Evidence-based information for clinical practice.

27. Nordqvist C: Rapid test approved by FDA. Retrieved from *www.medicalnewstoday.com/articles/65448.php.*

28. Solomon T, Michael BD, Smith PE, et al: National guideline for the management of suspected viral encephalitis in adults, *J Infect* 64(4):347, 2012.

RESOURCES

American Association of Neuroscience Nurses
www.aann.org
American Brain Tumor Association
www.abta.org
Brain Injury Association of America
www.biausa.org

Brain Trauma Foundation
www.braintrauma.org
Brain Tumor Center
http://btc.mgh.harvard.edu
Centers for Disease Control and Prevention: Traumatic Brain Injury
www.cdc.gov/TraumaticBrainInjury
National Brain Tumor Society
www.braintumor.org
TraumaticBrainInjury.com
www.traumaticbraininjury.com
Tug McGraw Foundation
www.tugmcgraw.org

Motivation is like food for the brain.
You cannot get enough in one sitting.
It needs continual and regular top ups.
Peter Davies

Nursing Management

Stroke

Meg Zomorodi

evolve WEBSITE

http://evolve.elsevier.com/Lewis/medsurg

- NCLEX Review Questions
- Key Points
- Pre-Test
- Answer Guidelines for Case Study on p. 1410
- Rationales for Bridge to NCLEX Examination Questions

- Case Studies
  - Patient With Hypertension and Stroke
  - Patient With Stroke
- Nursing Care Plan (Customizable)
  - NCP 58-1: Patient With Stroke

- Concept Map Creator
- Concept Map for Case Study on p. 1410
- Glossary
- Content Updates

LEARNING OUTCOMES

1. Describe the incidence of and risk factors for stroke.
2. Explain mechanisms that affect cerebral blood flow.
3. Compare and contrast the etiology and pathophysiology of ischemic and hemorrhagic strokes.
4. Correlate the clinical manifestations of stroke with the underlying pathophysiology.
5. Identify diagnostic studies performed for patients with strokes.

6. Differentiate among the collaborative care, drug therapy, and surgical therapy for patients with ischemic strokes and hemorrhagic strokes.
7. Describe the acute nursing management of a patient with a stroke.
8. Describe the rehabilitative nursing management of a patient with a stroke.
9. Explain the psychosocial impact of a stroke on the patient, caregiver, and family.

KEY TERMS

aneurysm, p. 1392
aphasia, p. 1394
brain attack, p. 1388
cerebrovascular accident (CVA), p. 1388
dysarthria, p. 1394

dysphasia, p. 1394
embolic stroke, p. 1392
hemorrhagic strokes, p. 1392
intracerebral hemorrhage, p. 1392
ischemic stroke, p. 1391

stroke, p. 1388
subarachnoid hemorrhage (SAH), p. 1392
thrombotic stroke, p. 1391
transient ischemic attack (TIA), p. 1391

Stroke occurs when there is (1) *ischemia* (inadequate blood flow) to a part of the brain or (2) hemorrhage into the brain that results in death of brain cells. Functions such as movement, sensation, or emotions that were controlled by the affected area of the brain are lost or impaired. The severity of the loss of function varies according to the location and extent of the brain damage.

The terms brain attack and cerebrovascular accident (CVA) are also used to describe stroke. The term *brain attack* communicates the urgency of recognizing the clinical manifestations of a stroke and treating this as a medical emergency, as would be done with a heart attack (Table 58-1). After the onset of a stroke, immediate medical attention is crucial to decrease disability and the risk of death.

Stroke is a major public health concern. An estimated 7 million people over the age of 20 in the United States have had a stroke, with 795,000 individuals affected annually.[1] With an aging population, a further increase in the incidence of stroke can be expected. However, stroke can occur at any age. About 28% of strokes occur in people younger than 65 years old.[2]

Stroke is the fourth most common cause of death in the United States, behind cancer, heart disease, and lung disease. More than 275,000 deaths occur annually from stroke. Women are more likely than men to die from a stroke because of the greater number of women over age 65.[1]

Stroke is the leading cause of serious, long-term disability. Of those who survive a stroke, 50% to 70% are functionally independent, and 15% to 30% live with permanent disability.

Reviewed by Carol C. Annesser, RN, MSN, BC, CNE, Assistant Professor, Nursing, Mercy College of Northwest Ohio, Toledo, Ohio; and Molly L. McClelland, RN, PhD, Assistant Professor of Nursing, University of Detroit Mercy, Detroit, Michigan.

TABLE 58-1 PATIENT & CAREGIVER TEACHING GUIDE

Warning Signs of Stroke

Include the following information in the teaching plan for a patient at risk for stroke and the patient's caregiver.

- Call 911 and get medical help immediately if someone has one or more of the following symptoms or signs. Also, check the time so you will know when the first symptoms appeared. It is important to take immediate action.
  - Sudden numbness, weakness, paralysis of the face, arm, or leg, especially on one side of the body
  - Sudden confusion, trouble speaking or understanding
  - Slurred speech
  - Sudden trouble seeing in one or both eyes
  - Sudden trouble walking, dizziness, loss of balance or coordination
  - Sudden, severe headache with no known cause

Source: American Stroke Association: Learn to recognize a stroke, 2009. Retrieved from *www.strokeassociation.org/presenter.jhtml?identifier=1020.*

Twenty-six percent require long-term care after 3 months.[3] Common long-term disabilities include hemiparesis, inability to walk, complete or partial dependence for activities of daily living (ADLs), aphasia, and depression. In addition to the physical, cognitive, and emotional impact of the stroke on the stroke survivor, the stroke affects the lives of the stroke victim's caregiver and family.[4] A stroke is a lifelong change for both the stroke survivor and the family.

PATHOPHYSIOLOGY OF STROKE

Anatomy of Cerebral Circulation

Blood is supplied to the brain by two major pairs of arteries: the internal carotid arteries (anterior circulation) and the vertebral arteries (posterior circulation). The carotid arteries branch to supply most of the frontal, parietal, and temporal lobes; the basal ganglia; and part of the diencephalon (thalamus and hypothalamus). The major branches of the carotid arteries are the middle cerebral and anterior cerebral arteries. The vertebral arteries join to form the basilar artery, which branches to supply the middle and lower parts of the temporal lobes, occipital lobes, cerebellum, brainstem, and part of the diencephalon. The main branch of the basilar artery is the posterior cerebral artery. The anterior and posterior cerebral circulation is connected at the *circle of Willis* by the anterior and posterior communicating arteries (Fig. 58-1). (Fig. 56-9 illustrates the arteries at the base of the brain.) Genetic variations in this area are common, and all connecting vessels may not be present.

Regulation of Cerebral Blood Flow

The brain requires a continuous supply of blood to provide the oxygen and glucose that neurons need to function. Blood flow must be maintained at 750 to 1000 mL/min (55 mL/100 g of brain tissue), or 20% of the cardiac output, for optimal brain functioning. If blood flow to the brain is totally interrupted (e.g., cardiac arrest), neurologic metabolism is altered in 30 seconds, metabolism stops in 2 minutes, and cellular death occurs in 5 minutes.

The brain is normally well protected from changes in mean systemic arterial blood pressure (BP) over a range from 50 to 150 mm Hg by a mechanism known as *cerebral autoregulation.*

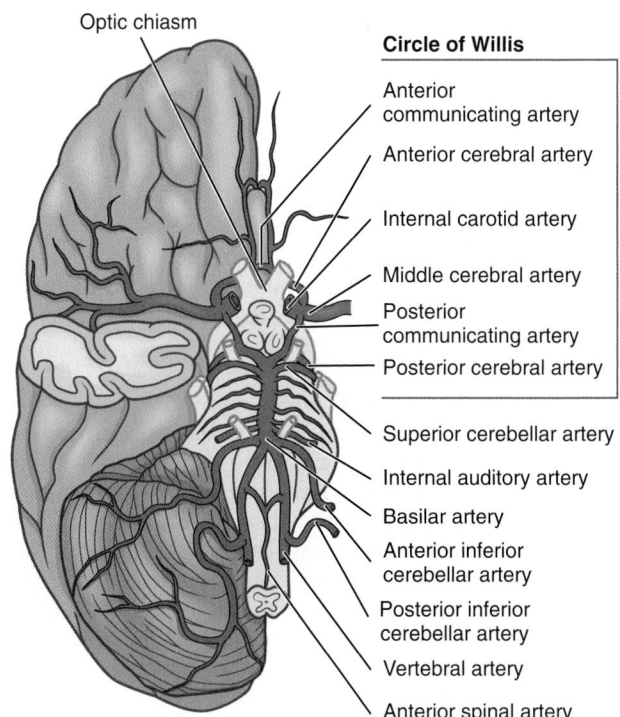

FIG. 58-1 Cerebral arteries and the circle of Willis. The top of the temporal lobe has been removed to show the course of the middle cerebral artery.

This involves changes in the diameter of cerebral blood vessels in response to changes in pressure so that the blood flow to the brain stays constant. When cerebral ischemia occurs, cerebral autoregulation may be impaired, and it is often dependent on changes in BP. Carbon dioxide is a potent cerebral vasodilator, and changes in arterial carbon dioxide levels have a dramatic effect on cerebral blood flow (increased carbon dioxide levels increase cerebral blood flow, and decreased carbon dioxide levels decrease cerebral blood flow). Very low arterial oxygen levels (partial pressure of arterial oxygen less than 50 mm Hg) or increases in hydrogen ion concentration also increase cerebral blood flow.

Factors that affect blood flow to the brain include systemic BP, cardiac output, and blood viscosity. During normal activity, oxygen requirements vary considerably, but changes in cardiac output, vasomotor tone, and distribution of blood flow normally maintain adequate blood flow to the head. Cardiac output has to be reduced by one third before cerebral blood flow is reduced. Changes in blood viscosity affect cerebral blood flow, with decreased viscosity increasing flow.

Collateral circulation may develop over time to compensate for a decrease in cerebral blood flow. An area of the brain can potentially receive blood supply from another blood vessel even if blood supply from the original vessel has been cut off (e.g., because of thrombosis). In other words, the vessels in the brain make an "alternate route" for blood flow to reach damaged areas. Individual differences in collateral circulation partly determine the degree of brain damage and functional loss when a stroke occurs. For example, the bloodstreams of the internal carotid system and the basilar system meet in the posterior communicating arteries. In normal situations the pressure of the arteries is equal and blood will not mix. However, if one of the vessels is blocked, blood will flow from the intact artery to the damaged one, preventing a CVA.

Intracranial pressure (ICP) also influences cerebral blood flow. Increased ICP causes brain compression and reduced cerebral blood flow. One of your major goals when caring for a stroke patient is to reduce secondary injury related to increased ICP (see Chapter 57).

RISK FACTORS FOR STROKE

The most effective way to decrease the burden of stroke is prevention and teaching, especially about risk factors. Risk factors can be divided into nonmodifiable and modifiable. Stroke risk increases with multiple risk factors.

Nonmodifiable Risk Factors

Nonmodifiable risk factors include age, gender, ethnicity or race, and family history or heredity. Stroke risk increases with age, doubling each decade after 55 years of age. Two thirds of all strokes occur in individuals older than 65 years, but stroke can occur at any age. Strokes are more common in men, but more women die from stroke than men. Because women tend to live longer than men, they have more opportunity to suffer a stroke.[1]

African Americans have a higher incidence of stroke and a higher death rate from stroke than whites. This may be related in part to a higher incidence of hypertension, obesity, and diabetes mellitus in African Americans.

Genetic risk factors are important in the development of all vascular diseases, including stroke. A person with a family history of stroke has an increased risk of having a stroke. Genes encoding products involved in lipid metabolism, thrombosis, and inflammation are believed to be potential genetic factors for stroke.

Modifiable Risk Factors

Modifiable risk factors are those that can potentially be altered through lifestyle changes and medical treatment, thus reducing the risk of stroke. Modifiable risk factors include hypertension, heart disease, diabetes mellitus, smoking, excessive alcohol consumption, obesity, sleep apnea, metabolic syndrome, lack of physical exercise, poor diet, and drug abuse.

Hypertension is the single most important modifiable risk factor, but it is still often undetected and inadequately treated. Increases in systolic and diastolic BP independently increase the risk of stroke. Stroke risk can be reduced by up to 50% with appropriate treatment of hypertension.[1-3]

Heart disease, including atrial fibrillation, myocardial infarction, cardiomyopathy, cardiac valve abnormalities, and cardiac congenital defects, is also a risk factor for stroke. Atrial fibrillation is responsible for about 20% of all strokes.[1] The incidence of atrial fibrillation increases with age.

Diabetes mellitus is a significant risk factor for stroke. The risk for stroke in people with diabetes mellitus is five times higher than in the general population.[1]

Increased serum cholesterol and smoking are risk factors for stroke. Smoking nearly doubles the risk of stroke. The risk associated with smoking decreases substantially over time after the smoker quits. After 5 to 10 years of no tobacco use, former smokers have the same risk of stroke as nonsmokers.[5]

The effect of alcohol on stroke risk appears to depend on the amount consumed. Women who drink more than one alcoholic drink per day and men who drink more than two alcoholic drinks per day are at higher risk for hypertension, which increases their chance of stroke. Illicit drug use, especially cocaine use, has been associated with stroke risk.[1]

Abdominal obesity increases ischemic stroke risk in all ethnic groups. In addition, obesity is also associated with hypertension, high blood glucose, and elevated blood lipid levels, all of which increase the risk of stroke.[1] An association of physical inactivity and increased stroke risk is present in both men and women, regardless of ethnicity. Benefits of physical activity can occur with even light to moderate regular activity and may be related to the beneficial impact of exercise on other risk factors. Nutrition teaching is important for the individual at risk for stroke, since a diet high in fat and low in fruits and vegetables may increase stroke risk.

The early forms of birth control pills that contained high levels of progestin and estrogen increased a woman's chance of experiencing a stroke, especially if the woman also smoked heavily. Newer, low-dose oral contraceptives have lower risks for stroke except in those individuals who are hypertensive and smoke.

Other conditions that may increase the risk for strokes include migraine headaches, inflammatory conditions, and hyperhomocysteinemia. Sickle cell disease is another known risk factor for stroke.

GENDER DIFFERENCES

Stroke

Men	Women
• Stroke is more common in men than in women.	• At all ages, more women than men die from strokes.
• In most age-groups, more men than women will have a stroke in a given year.	• Women are more likely to have a hemorrhagic stroke.
• Men are more likely to have a thrombotic stroke.	• Women with atrial fibrillation have an increased risk for stroke.
• Men are more likely to have an embolic stroke.	• Oral contraceptive use and pregnancy contribute to stroke risk.
• Men have a better chance of surviving a stroke than women do.	• tPA is used less frequently to treat women who have strokes.

tPA, Recombinant tissue plasminogen activator.

⊕ CULTURAL & ETHNIC HEALTH DISPARITIES

Stroke

African Americans
- Have a higher incidence of strokes than whites.
- The rate of first strokes is almost twice that of whites.
- Are three times more likely than whites to have an ischemic stroke and four times more likely to have a hemorrhagic stroke.
- High incidence of strokes may be related to their increased rates of hypertension, diabetes mellitus, and sickle cell anemia.
- Have a higher incidence of smoking and obesity than whites, which are two risk factors for stroke.
- Are twice as likely to die from a stroke as whites.

Other Ethnicities
- Hispanics, Native Americans, and Asian Americans have a higher incidence of strokes than whites.
- Diabetes (an important risk factor for strokes) is common among Hispanics.
- Native Americans are more likely than whites to have at least two risk factors for stroke.

Transient Ischemic Attack

Another risk factor associated with stroke is a past history of a transient ischemic attack (TIA). A TIA is a transient episode of neurologic dysfunction caused by focal brain, spinal cord, or retinal ischemia, but without acute infarction of the brain. Clinical symptoms typically last less than 1 hour. In the past, TIAs were operationally defined as any focal cerebral ischemic event with symptoms lasting less than 24 hours. However, it is important to teach the patient to seek treatment for any stroke symptoms, since there is no way to predict if a TIA will resolve or if it is in fact the development of a stroke.[6] In general, one third of individuals who experience a TIA do not experience another event, one third have additional TIAs, and one third progress to stroke.[7]

TIAs may be due to microemboli that temporarily block the blood flow. TIAs are a warning sign of progressive cerebrovascular disease. The signs and symptoms of a TIA depend on the blood vessel that is involved and the area of the brain that is ischemic. If the carotid system is involved, patients may have a temporary loss of vision in one eye *(amaurosis fugax),* transient hemiparesis, numbness or loss of sensation, or a sudden inability to speak. Signs of a TIA involving the vertebrobasilar system may include tinnitus, vertigo, darkened or blurred vision, diplopia, ptosis, dysarthria, dysphagia, ataxia, and unilateral or bilateral numbness or weakness.

TIAs should be treated as medical emergencies. Teach people at risk for TIA to seek medical attention immediately with any stroke-like symptom and to identify the time of symptom onset.[8]

TYPES OF STROKE

Unlike a TIA, where ischemia occurs without infarction, a stroke results in infarction and cell death. Strokes are classified as ischemic or hemorrhagic based on the cause and underlying pathophysiologic findings (Fig. 58-2 and Table 58-2).

Ischemic Stroke

An ischemic stroke results from inadequate blood flow to the brain from partial or complete occlusion of an artery. Nearly 80% of strokes are ischemic.[1] A TIA attack is usually a precursor to ischemic stroke. Ischemic strokes are further divided into thrombotic and embolic strokes.

Thrombotic Stroke. A thrombotic stroke occurs from injury to a blood vessel wall and formation of a blood clot (see Fig. 58-2, *A*). The lumen of the blood vessel becomes narrowed and, if it becomes occluded, infarction occurs. Thrombosis develops readily where atherosclerotic plaques have already narrowed blood vessels. Thrombotic stroke, which is the result of thrombosis or narrowing of the blood vessel, is the most common cause of stroke, accounting for about 60% of strokes.[1] Two thirds of thrombotic strokes are associated with hyperten-

TABLE 58-2   TYPES OF STROKE

Gender and Age	Warning and Onset	Prognosis
Ischemic		
Thrombotic		
Men more than women Oldest median age	*Warning:* TIA (30%-50% of cases) *Onset:* Often during or after sleep	Stepwise progression, signs and symptoms develop slowly, usually some improvement, recurrence in 20%-25% of survivors.
Embolic		
Men more than women	*Warning:* TIA (uncommon) *Onset:* Lack of relationship to activity, sudden onset	Single event, signs and symptoms develop quickly, usually some improvement, recurrence common without aggressive treatment of underlying disease.
Hemorrhagic		
Intracerebral		
Slightly higher in women	*Warning:* Headache (25% of cases) *Onset:* Activity (often)	Progression over 24 hr. Poor prognosis, fatality more likely with presence of coma.
Subarachnoid		
Slightly higher in women Youngest median age	*Warning:* Headache (common) *Onset:* Activity (often), sudden onset, most commonly related to head trauma	Usually single sudden event, fatality more likely with presence of coma.

TIA, Transient ischemic attack.

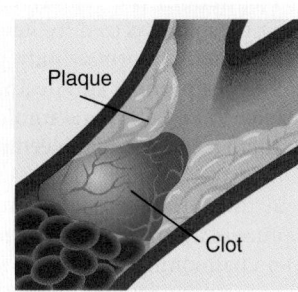

Thrombotic stroke. The process of clot formation (thrombosis) results in a narrowing of the lumen, which blocks the passage of the blood through the artery.

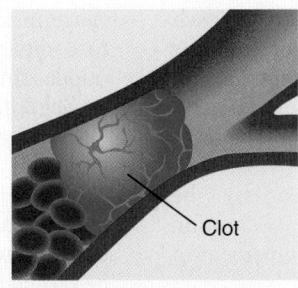

Embolic stroke. An embolus is a blood clot or other debris circulating in the blood. When it reaches an artery in the brain that is too narrow to pass through, it lodges there and blocks the flow of blood.

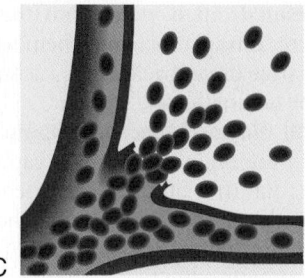

Hemorrhagic stroke. A burst blood vessel may allow blood to seep into and damage brain tissues until clotting shuts off the leak.

FIG. 58-2 Major types of stroke.

sion or diabetes mellitus, both of which accelerate atherosclerosis. In 30% to 50% of individuals, thrombotic strokes are preceded by a TIA.

The extent of the stroke depends on rapidity of onset, the size of the damaged area, and the presence of collateral circulation. Most patients with ischemic stroke do not have a decreased level of consciousness in the first 24 hours, unless it is due to a brainstem stroke or other conditions such as seizures, increased ICP, or hemorrhage. Ischemic stroke symptoms may progress in the first 72 hours as infarction and cerebral edema increase.

Embolic Stroke. Embolic stroke occurs when an embolus lodges in and occludes a cerebral artery, resulting in infarction and edema of the area supplied by the involved vessel (see Fig. 58-2, *B*). Embolism is the second most common cause of stroke, accounting for about 24% of strokes.[1] Most emboli originate in the endocardial (inside) layer of the heart, with plaque breaking off from the endocardium and entering the circulation. The embolus travels upward to the cerebral circulation and lodges where a vessel narrows or bifurcates (splits). Heart conditions associated with emboli include atrial fibrillation, myocardial infarction, infective endocarditis, rheumatic heart disease, valvular prostheses, and atrial septal defects. Less common causes of emboli include air and fat from long bone (e.g., femur) fractures.

The patient with an embolic stroke commonly has severe clinical symptoms that occur suddenly. Embolic strokes can affect any age-group. Rheumatic heart disease is one cause of embolic stroke in young to middle-aged adults. An embolus arising from an atherosclerotic plaque is more common in older adults.

Warning signs are less common with embolic than with thrombotic stroke. The embolic stroke often occurs rapidly, giving little time to accommodate by developing collateral circulation. The patient usually remains conscious, although he or she may have a headache. Prognosis is related to the amount of brain tissue deprived of its blood supply. The effects of the emboli are initially characterized by severe neurologic deficits, which can be temporary if the clot breaks up and allows blood to flow. Smaller emboli then continue to obstruct smaller vessels, which in turn involve smaller portions of the brain with fewer deficits noted. Recurrence of embolic stroke is common unless the underlying cause is aggressively treated.

Hemorrhagic Stroke

Hemorrhagic strokes account for approximately 15% of all strokes and result from bleeding into the brain tissue itself (intracerebral or intraparenchymal hemorrhage) or into the subarachnoid space or ventricles (subarachnoid hemorrhage or intraventricular hemorrhage).[1]

Intracerebral Hemorrhage. Intracerebral hemorrhage is bleeding within the brain caused by a rupture of a vessel and accounts for about 10% of all strokes (see Fig. 58-2, *C*). The prognosis of patients with intracerebral hemorrhage is poor, with the 30-day mortality rate at 40% to 80%. Fifty percent of the deaths occur within the first 48 hours.[1]

Hypertension is the most common cause of intracerebral hemorrhage (Fig. 58-3). Other causes include vascular malformations, coagulation disorders, anticoagulant and thrombolytic drugs, trauma, brain tumors, and ruptured aneurysms. Hemorrhage commonly occurs during periods of activity. Most often there is a sudden onset of symptoms, with progression over minutes to hours because of ongoing bleeding.

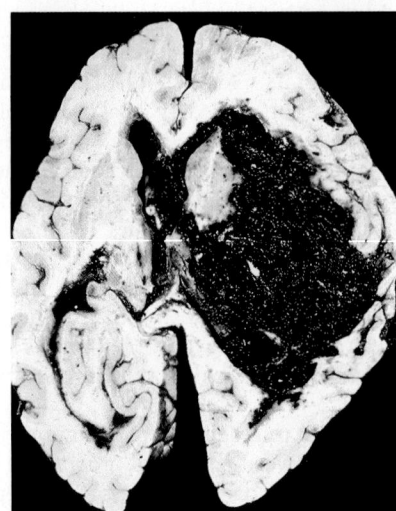

FIG. 58-3 Massive hypertensive hemorrhage rupturing into a lateral ventricle of the brain.

Manifestations include neurologic deficits, headache, nausea, vomiting, decreased level of consciousness (in about 50% of patients), and hypertension. The extent of the symptoms varies depending on the amount, location, and duration of the bleeding. A blood clot within the closed skull can result in a mass that causes pressure on brain tissue, displaces brain tissue, and decreases cerebral blood flow, leading to ischemia and infarction.

Approximately half of intracerebral hemorrhages occur in the putamen and internal capsule, central white matter, thalamus, cerebellar hemispheres, and pons. Initially, patients experience a severe headache with nausea and vomiting. Clinical manifestations of putaminal and internal capsule bleeding include weakness of one side (including the face, arm, and leg), slurred speech, and deviation of the eyes. Progression of symptoms related to a severe hemorrhage includes hemiplegia, fixed and dilated pupils, abnormal body posturing, and coma. Thalamic hemorrhage results in hemiplegia with more sensory than motor loss. Bleeding into the subthalamic areas of the brain leads to problems with vision and eye movement. Cerebellar hemorrhages are characterized by severe headache, vomiting, loss of ability to walk, dysphagia, dysarthria, and eye movement disturbances.

Hemorrhage in the pons is the most serious because basic life functions (e.g., respiration) are rapidly affected. Hemorrhage in the pons can be characterized by hemiplegia leading to complete paralysis, coma, abnormal body posturing, fixed pupils (small in size), hyperthermia, and death.

Subarachnoid Hemorrhage. Subarachnoid hemorrhage (SAH) occurs when there is intracranial bleeding into the cerebrospinal fluid–filled space between the arachnoid and pia mater membranes on the surface of the brain.[9] SAH is commonly caused by rupture of a cerebral aneurysm (congenital or acquired weakness and ballooning of vessels). Aneurysms may be saccular or berry aneurysms, ranging from a few millimeters to 20 to 30 mm in size, or fusiform atherosclerotic aneurysms. The majority of aneurysms are in the circle of Willis. Other causes of SAH include trauma and illicit drug (cocaine) abuse. About 40% of people who have a hemorrhagic stroke due to a ruptured aneurysm die during the first episode. Fifteen percent die from subsequent bleeding.[9] The incidence increases with age and is higher in women than men.

The patient may have warning symptoms if the ballooning artery applies pressure to brain tissue, or minor warning symptoms may result from leaking of an aneurysm before major rupture. In general, cerebral aneurysms are viewed as a "silent killer," since individuals do not have warning signs of an aneurysm until rupture has occurred.

SAFETY ALERT
- Sudden onset of a severe headache that is different from a previous headache and typically the "worst headache of one's life" is a characteristic symptom of a ruptured aneurysm.

Loss of consciousness may or may not occur. The patient's level of consciousness may range from alert to comatose, depending on the severity of the bleed. Other manifestations include focal neurologic deficits (including cranial nerve deficits), nausea, vomiting, seizures, and stiff neck. Despite improvements in surgical techniques and management, many patients with SAH die. Survivors may be left with significant morbidity, including cognitive difficulties.

Complications of aneurysmal SAH include rebleeding before surgery or other therapy is initiated and cerebral vasospasm (narrowing of the blood vessels), which can result in cerebral infarction. Cerebral vasospasm is most likely due to an interaction between the metabolites of blood and the vascular smooth muscle. During the lysis of subarachnoid blood clots, metabolites are released. These metabolites can cause endothelial damage and vasoconstriction. In addition, release of endothelin (a potent vasoconstrictor) may play a major role in the induction of cerebral vasospasm after SAH. Patients with SAH who are at risk for vasospasm are often kept in the intensive care unit for 14 days until the threat of vasospasm is reduced. Peak time for vasospasm occurs 6 to 10 days after the initial bleed.

CLINICAL MANIFESTATIONS OF STROKE

The neurologic manifestations do not significantly differ between ischemic and hemorrhagic stroke. The reason for this is that destruction of neural tissue is the basis for neurologic dysfunction caused by both types of stroke. The clinical manifestations are related to the location of the stroke. Specific manifestations related to the type of stroke are discussed in the previous section. The general clinical manifestations of ischemic and hemorrhagic stroke are discussed together here.

A stroke can affect many body functions, including motor activity, bladder and bowel elimination, intellectual function, spatial-perceptual alterations, personality, affect, sensation, swallowing, and communication. The functions affected are directly related to the artery involved and area of the brain it supplies (Table 58-3). Manifestations related to right- and left-brain damage differ somewhat and are shown in Fig. 58-4.

An additional assessment question that you need to ask is the time of the onset of symptoms. This is important for all types of stroke, especially ischemic strokes, since the time can affect treatment decisions.

Motor Function

Motor deficits are the most obvious effect of stroke. Motor deficits include impairment of (1) mobility, (2) respiratory function, (3) swallowing and speech, (4) gag reflex, and (5) self-care abilities. Symptoms are caused by the destruction of motor neurons in the pyramidal pathway (nerve fibers from the brain that pass through the spinal cord to the motor cells). The characteristic motor deficits include loss of skilled voluntary movement (aki-

TABLE 58-3	STROKE MANIFESTATIONS RELATED TO ARTERY INVOLVEMENT
Artery	**Deficit**
Anterior cerebral	Motor and/or sensory deficit (contralateral), sucking or rooting reflex, rigidity, gait problems, loss of proprioception and fine touch
Middle cerebral	*Dominant side:* Aphasia, motor and sensory deficit, hemianopsia *Nondominant side:* Neglect, motor and sensory deficit, hemianopsia
Posterior cerebral	Hemianopsia, visual hallucination, spontaneous pain, motor deficit
Vertebral	Cranial nerve deficits, diplopia, dizziness, nausea, vomiting, dysarthria, dysphagia, and/or coma

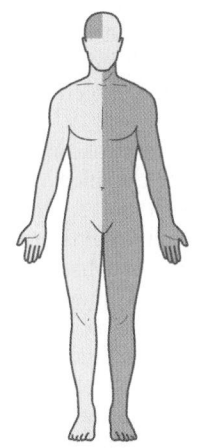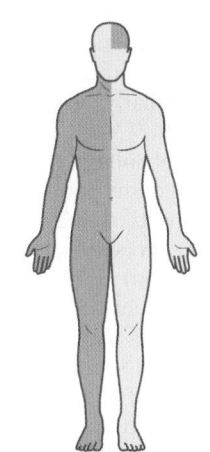

Right-brain damage (stroke on right side of the brain)	**Left-brain damage** (stroke on left side of the brain)
• Paralyzed left side: hemiplegia	• Paralyzed right side: hemiplegia
• Left-sided neglect	• Impaired speech/language aphasias
• Spatial-perceptual deficits	• Impaired right/left discrimination
• Tends to deny or minimize problems	• Slow performance, cautious
• Rapid performance, short attention span	• Aware of deficits: depression, anxiety
• Impulsive, safety problems	• Impaired comprehension related to language, math
• Impaired judgment	
• Impaired time concepts	

FIG. 58-4 Manifestations of right-brain and left-brain stroke.

nesia), impairment of integration of movements, alterations in muscle tone, and alterations in reflexes. The initial *hyporeflexia* (depressed reflexes) progresses to *hyperreflexia* (hyperactive reflexes) for most patients.

Motor deficits after a stroke follow certain specific patterns. Because the pyramidal pathway crosses at the level of the medulla, a lesion on one side of the brain affects motor function on the opposite side of the body (contralateral). The arms and legs of the affected side may be weakened or paralyzed to different degrees depending on which part of and to what extent the cerebral circulation was compromised. A stroke affecting the middle cerebral artery leads to a greater weakness in the upper extremity than the lower extremity. The affected shoulder tends to rotate internally, and the hip rotates externally. The affected foot is plantar flexed and inverted. An initial period of flaccidity may last from days to several weeks and is related to nerve damage. Spasticity of the muscles, which follows the flaccid stage, is related to interruption of upper motor neuron influence.

Communication

The left hemisphere is dominant for language skills in right-handed persons and in most left-handed persons.[10] Language disorders involve expression and comprehension of written and spoken words. The patient may experience aphasia, which may be *receptive aphasia* (loss of comprehension), *expressive aphasia* (inability to produce language), or *global aphasia* (total inability to communicate). Aphasia occurs when a stroke damages the dominant hemisphere of the brain.

Dysphasia refers to impaired ability to communicate. However, in most settings the terms *aphasia* and *dysphasia* are used interchangeably, with aphasia often being the more common term used. (Dysphasia should not be confused with the similarly pronounced *dysphagia*, which is difficulty swallowing.)

Patterns of aphasia may differ, since the stroke affects different portions of the brain. Aphasia may be classified as *nonfluent* (minimal speech activity with slow speech that requires obvious effort) or *fluent* (speech is present but contains little meaningful communication) (Table 58-4). Most types of aphasia are mixed, with impairment in both expression and understanding. A massive stroke may result in global aphasia. Many stroke patients also experience dysarthria, a disturbance in the muscular control of speech. Impairment may involve pronunciation, articulation, and phonation. Dysarthria does not affect the meaning of communication or the comprehension of language, but it does affect the mechanics of speech. Some patients experience a combination of aphasia and dysarthria.

Affect

Patients who have had a stroke may have difficulty controlling their emotions. Emotional responses may be exaggerated or unpredictable. Depression and feelings associated with changes in body image and loss of function can make this worse.[11] Patients may also be frustrated by mobility and communication problems.

An example of unpredictable affect is as follows: a well-respected 63-year-old lawyer has returned home from the hospital after a stroke. During a meal with his family, he becomes frustrated and begins to cry because of the difficulty getting food into his mouth and chewing, something that he was able to do easily before his stroke. His family cannot understand why a previously very competent man is so emotional. As a nurse, it is important for you to help this patient and family understand that frustration and depression are common in the first year after a stroke.

Intellectual Function

Both memory and judgment may be impaired as a result of stroke. These impairments can occur with strokes affecting either side of the brain. A left-brain stroke is more likely to result in memory problems related to language. Patients with a left-brain stroke often are cautious in making judgments. The patient with a right-brain stroke tends to be impulsive and to move quickly.

TABLE 58-4	**TYPES OF APHASIA**
Type	**Characteristics**
Broca's	• A type of nonfluent aphasia. • Damage to frontal lobe of brain. • Frequently speak in short phrases that make sense but are produced with great effort. • Often omit small words such as "is," "and," and "the." • May say, "Walk dog," meaning, "I will take the dog for a walk," or "book book two table," for "There are two books on the table." • Typically understand speech of others fairly well. • Often aware of their difficulties and can become easily frustrated.
Wernicke's	• A type of fluent aphasia. • Damage occurs in left temporal lobe, although it can result from damage to right lobe. • May speak in long sentences that have no meaning, add unnecessary words, and even create made-up words. • May say, "You know that smoodle pinkered and that I want to get him round and take care of him like you want before." • Often difficult to follow what person is trying to say. • Usually have great difficulty understanding speech. • Often unaware of their mistakes.
Global	• A type of nonfluent aphasia. • Results from damage to extensive portions of language areas of brain. • Have severe communication difficulties. • May be extremely limited in ability to speak or comprehend language.
Other	• Results from damage to different language areas in brain. • Some people may have difficulty repeating words and sentences even though they can speak and they understand the meaning of the word or sentence. • Others may have difficulty naming objects even though they know what the object is and what its use is.

An example of behavior in people with right-brain stroke is that they try to rise quickly from a wheelchair without locking the wheels or raising the footrests. On the other hand, people with a left-brain stroke would move slowly and cautiously from the wheelchair. Patients with either type of stroke may have difficulty making generalizations, which interferes with their ability to learn.

Spatial-Perceptual Alterations

Individuals who have had a stroke on the right side of the brain are more likely to have problems with spatial-perceptual orientation. However, this can also occur in people with left-brain stroke.

Spatial-perceptual problems may be divided into four categories. The first is the result of damage of the parietal lobe and causes the patient to have an incorrect perception of self and illness. In this situation, patients may deny their illnesses or their own body parts. The second category occurs when the patient neglects all input from the affected side (erroneous perception of self in space). This may be worsened by *homonymous hemianopsia,* in which blindness occurs in the same half of the visual fields of both eyes. The patient also has difficulty with spatial orientation, such as judging distances. The third spatial-perceptual deficit is *agnosia,* the inability to recognize an object by sight, touch, or hearing. The fourth deficit is *apraxia,* the inability to carry out learned sequential movements on command. Because patients may or may not be aware of their spatial-perceptual alterations, you need to assess for this potential problem, since it will affect rehabilitation and recovery.

Elimination

Most problems with urinary and bowel elimination occur initially and are temporary. When a stroke affects one hemisphere of the brain, the prognosis for normal bladder function is excellent. At least partial sensation for bladder filling remains, and voluntary urination is present. Initially, the patient may experience frequency, urgency, and incontinence. Although motor control of the bowel is usually not a problem, patients are frequently constipated. Constipation is associated with immobility, weak abdominal muscles, dehydration, and diminished response to the defecation reflex. Urinary and bowel elimination problems may also be related to inability to express needs and to manage clothing.

DIAGNOSTIC STUDIES FOR STROKE

When manifestations of a stroke occur, diagnostic studies are done to (1) confirm that it is a stroke and not another brain lesion and (2) identify the likely cause of the stroke (Table 58-5). Tests also guide decisions about therapy.

Important diagnostic tools for patients who have experienced a stroke are a noncontrast computed tomography (CT) scan or magnetic resonance imaging (MRI).[12] These tests can rapidly distinguish between ischemic and hemorrhagic stroke and help determine the size and location of the stroke. Serial CT scans may be used to assess the effectiveness of treatment and to evaluate recovery. Once the individual suspected of TIA or stroke arrives in the emergency department, it is important to rapidly assess and diagnose the patient (usually through a noncontrast head CT or MRI).[12] Rapid access to these diagnostic tools is important, since the results will determine treatment options for the patient.

CT angiography (CTA) provides visualization of cerebral blood vessels. It can be performed after or at the same time as the noncontrast CT scan. CTA can provide an estimate of perfusion and detect filling defects in the cerebral arteries. Magnetic resonance angiography (MRA) can detect vascular lesions and blockages, similar to CTA. CT/MRI perfusion and diffusion imaging may also be done.

Cardiac imaging is also recommended because many strokes are caused by blood clots from the heart. Angiography can identify cervical and cerebrovascular occlusion, atherosclerotic plaques, and malformation of vessels. Cerebral angiography is a definitive study to identify the source of SAH. Risks of angiography include dislodging an embolus, causing vasospasm, inducing further hemorrhage, and provoking an allergic reaction to contrast media.

Intraarterial digital subtraction angiography (DSA) reduces the dose of contrast material, uses smaller catheters, and shortens the length of the procedure compared with conventional angiography. DSA involves the injection of a contrast agent to visualize blood vessels in the neck and the large vessels of the circle of Willis. It is considered safer than cerebral angiography because less vascular manipulation is required.

Transcranial Doppler (TCD) ultrasonography is a noninvasive study that measures the velocity of blood flow in the major cerebral arteries. TCD is effective in detecting microemboli and vasospasm and is ideal for the patient suspected of having an SAH. Carotid duplex scanning is used not only to detect the cause of the stroke, but also to stratify patients for either medical management or carotid intervention if they have carotid stenoses.

A lumbar puncture may be done to look for evidence of red blood cells in the cerebrospinal fluid if an SAH is suspected but the CT does not show hemorrhage. A lumbar puncture is avoided if the patient is suspected of having an obstruction in the foramen magnum or other signs of increased ICP because of the danger of herniation of the brain downward, leading to pressure on cardiac and respiratory centers in the brainstem and potentially death.

If the suspected cause of the stroke includes emboli from the heart, diagnostic cardiac tests should be done. Blood tests are also done to help identify conditions contributing to stroke and to guide treatment (see Table 58-5).

The LICOX system may be used as a diagnostic tool to evaluate the progression of stroke. LICOX measures brain oxygenation and temperature (see discussion in Chapter 57 on p. 1365 and Fig. 57-10). Secondary brain injury adds significantly to mortality risk and poor functional outcome after a stroke.

COLLABORATIVE CARE FOR STROKE

Preventive Therapy

Primary prevention is a priority for decreasing morbidity and mortality risk from stroke (Table 58-6). The goals of stroke prevention include health promotion for a healthy lifestyle and management of modifiable risk factors to prevent a stroke. Health promotion focuses on (1) healthy diet, (2) weight control, (3) regular exercise, (4) no smoking, (5) limitation on alcohol consumption, and (6) routine health assessments. Patients with known risk factors such as diabetes mellitus, hypertension,

---

TABLE 58-5 DIAGNOSTIC STUDIES

Stroke

Diagnosis of Stroke (Including Extent of Involvement)	Cardiac Assessment
• Computed tomography (CT) scan	• Electrocardiogram
• CT angiography (CTA)	• Chest x-ray
• Magnetic resonance imaging (MRI)	• Cardiac markers (troponin, creatine kinase-MB)
• Magnetic resonance angiography (MRA)	• Echocardiography (transthoracic, transesophageal)
• CT/MRI perfusion and diffusion imaging	
	Additional Studies
Cerebral Blood Flow	• Complete blood count, including platelets
• Cerebral angiography	• Coagulation studies: prothrombin time, activated partial thromboplastin time
• Carotid angiography	
• Digital subtraction angiography	• Electrolytes, blood glucose
• Transcranial Doppler ultrasonography	• Renal and hepatic studies
	• Lipid profile
• Carotid duplex scanning	• Cerebrospinal fluid analysis*

*A lumbar puncture to obtain cerebrospinal fluid is avoided if increased intracranial pressure is suspected.

TABLE 58-6   COLLABORATIVE CARE

Stroke

Diagnostic (see Table 58-5)
- History and physical examination

Collaborative Therapy
Prevention
- Control of hypertension
- Control of diabetes mellitus
- Treatment of underlying cardiac problem
- No smoking
- Limiting alcohol intake

Drug Therapy
- Platelet inhibitors (e.g., aspirin)
- Anticoagulation therapy for patients with atrial fibrillation

Surgical Therapy
- Carotid endarterectomy
- Stenting of carotid artery
- Transluminal angioplasty
- Extracranial-intracranial bypass
- Surgical interventions for aneurysms at risk of bleeding

Acute Care
- Maintenance of airway
- Fluid therapy
- Treatment of cerebral edema
- Prevention of secondary injury

Ischemic Stroke
- Tissue plasminogen activator (tPA) IV or intraarterial
- Stent retrievers
- MERCI retriever

Hemorrhagic Stroke
- Surgical decompression if indicated
- Clipping or coiling of aneurysm

Rehabilitation
- Focus on helping patient achieve independence and functional recovery

MERCI, Mechanical embolus removal in cerebral ischemia.

HEALTHY PEOPLE

Prevention of Stroke

- Reduce salt and sodium intake.
- Maintain a normal body weight.
- Maintain a normal blood pressure.
- Increase level of physical exercise.
- Avoid cigarette smoking or tobacco products.
- Limit consumption of alcohol to moderate levels.
- Follow a diet that is low in saturated fat, total fat, and dietary cholesterol and high in fruits and vegetables.

EVIDENCE-BASED PRACTICE

Translating Research Into Practice

Can Mirror Therapy Improve Functioning After Stroke?
Clinical Question
For stroke patients (P), what is the effect of mirror therapy (I) versus control interventions (C) on motor function, activities of daily living (ADLs), and pain (O) at therapy completion and after 6 mo of therapy (T)?

Best Available Evidence
Randomized controlled trials (RCTs) and randomized crossover trials

Critical Appraisal and Synthesis of Evidence
- Fourteen trials (*n* = 567) of patients with stroke comparing mirror therapy to control interventions of no treatment, sham or placebo, or usual care.
- In mirror therapy, which is used to improve motor function after a stroke, a mirror is placed between a person's arms or legs so the image of the unaffected limb gives illusion of normal movement in the affected limb (see Fig. 63-24).
- Mirror therapy has a positive effect on motor function and ADLs in stroke patients, and on relieving pain in patients with complex regional pain syndrome, compared with control interventions.
- The effect of mirror therapy on motor function was stable at a 6-mo follow-up.

Conclusion
- Mirror therapy may improve motor function, ADLs, and pain compared with other interventions with effects lasting after 6 mo.

Implications for Nursing Practice
- Consult with rehabilitation care team if mirror therapy is available as an additional intervention for stroke patients.
- Motivate and encourage patients engaged in mirror therapy to practice as instructed.
- Mirror therapy may be helpful in osteoarthritis and with chronic and phantom limb pain.

Reference for Evidence
Thieme H, Mehrholz J, Pohl M, et al: Mirror therapy for improving motor function after stroke, *Cochrane Database Syst Rev* 3:CD 008449, 2012.

P, Patient population of interest; *I,* intervention or area of interest; *C,* comparison of interest or comparison group; *O,* outcomes of interest; *T,* timing (see p. 12).

obesity, high serum lipids, or cardiac dysfunction require close management.

Preventive Drug Therapy. Measures to prevent the development of a thrombus or an embolus are used in patients with TIAs, since they are at high risk for stroke. Antiplatelet drugs are usually the chosen treatment to prevent stroke in patients who have had a TIA. Aspirin is the most frequently used antiplatelet agent, commonly at a dose of 81 to 325 mg/day. Other drugs include ticlopidine (Ticlid), clopidogrel (Plavix), dipyridamole (Persantine), and combined dipyridamole and aspirin (Aggrenox).[13]

> **DRUG ALERT: Ticlopidine (Ticlid) and Clopidogrel (Plavix)**
> - All health care providers and dentists must be informed that the drug is being taken, especially before scheduling surgery or major dental procedures.
> - Drug may need to be discontinued 10 to 14 days before surgery if antiplatelet effect is not desired.

For patients who have atrial fibrillation, oral anticoagulation can include warfarin (Coumadin), rivaroxaban (Xarelto), and dabigatran etexilate (Pradaxa). The primary advantage of rivaroxaban and dabigatran over warfarin is that these drugs do not need close monitoring or dosage adjustments. Statins (simvastatin [Zocor], lovastatin [Mevacor]) have also been shown to be effective in the prevention of stroke for individuals who have experienced a TIA in the past.[14]

Surgical Therapy for TIA and Stroke Prevention. Surgical interventions for the patient with TIAs due to carotid disease include carotid endarterectomy, transluminal angioplasty, stenting, and extracranial-intracranial (EC-IC) bypass. In a *carotid endarterectomy* (CEA), the atheromatous lesion is removed from the carotid artery to improve blood flow (Fig. 58-5).

Transluminal angioplasty is the insertion of a balloon to open a stenosed artery in the brain and improve blood flow. The balloon is threaded up to the carotid artery via a catheter inserted in the femoral artery.

Stenting involves intravascular placement of a stent in an attempt to maintain patency of the artery (Fig. 58-6). The stent can be inserted during an angioplasty. Once in place, the system can be used with a tiny filter that opens like an umbrella. The filter catches and removes the debris that is stirred up during the stenting procedure before it floats to the brain, where it can trigger a stroke. Stenting is a less invasive strategy for revascularization in patients unable to withstand the CEA because of coexisting medical conditions. Initial research has shown the procedure to be as effective as the CEA.[15]

EC-IC bypass involves anastomosing (surgically connecting) a branch of an extracranial artery to an intracranial artery (most commonly, superficial temporal to middle cerebral artery)

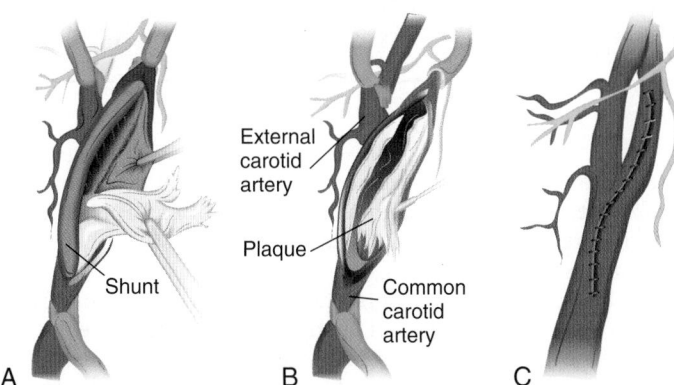

FIG. 58-5 Carotid endarterectomy is performed to prevent impending cerebral infarction. **A,** A tube is inserted above and below the blockage to reroute the blood flow. **B,** Atherosclerotic plaque in the common carotid artery is removed. **C,** Once the artery is stitched closed, the tube can be removed. A surgeon may also perform the technique without rerouting the blood flow.

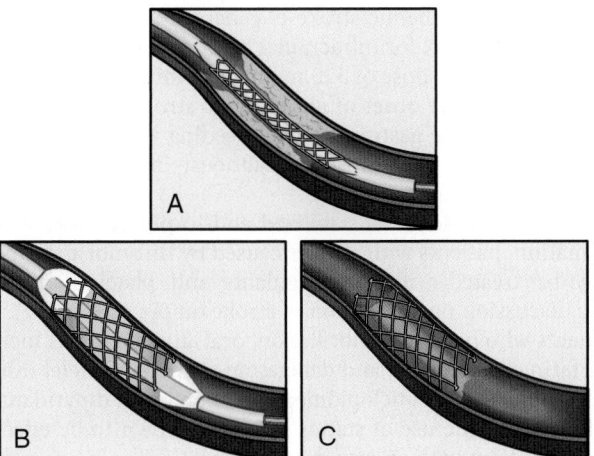

FIG. 58-6 Brain stent used to treat blockages in cerebral blood flow. **A,** A balloon catheter is used to implant the stent into an artery of the brain. **B,** The balloon catheter is moved to the blocked area of the artery and then inflated. The stent expands due to inflation of the balloon. **C,** The balloon is deflated and withdrawn, leaving the stent permanently in place holding the artery open and improving the flow of blood.

beyond an area of obstruction with the goal of increasing cerebral perfusion. This procedure is generally reserved for patients who do not benefit from other forms of therapy. Postoperatively nursing care for these patients consists of neurovascular assessment, BP management, assessment of stent occlusion or retroperitoneal hemorrhage as complications, and minimization of complications at the insertion site by keeping the patient's leg straight for the prescribed time.

Acute Care for Ischemic Stroke

During initial evaluation, the single most important point in the patient's history is the time of onset of symptoms. The goals for collaborative care during the acute phase are preserving life, preventing further brain damage, and reducing disability.

Table 58-7 outlines the emergency management of the patient with a stroke. Acute care begins with managing circulation, airway, and breathing. Patients may have difficulty keeping an open and clear airway because of a decreased level of consciousness or decreased or absent gag and swallowing reflexes. Maintaining adequate oxygenation is important. Oxygen administration, artificial airway insertion, intubation, and mechanical ventilation may be required. Baseline neurologic assessment is carried out, and patients are monitored closely for signs of increasing neurologic deficit. About 25% of patients worsen in the first 24 to 48 hours.

For emergency care, patients should be transported to the closest certified stroke center or, when such an institution is not available, the closest facility offering emergency stroke care. The American Heart Association recommends that acute care facilities have stroke teams in place. The stroke team generally consists of the registered nurse, neurologist, radiologist, and CT technician.[16]

Elevated BP is common immediately after a stroke and may be a protective response to maintain cerebral perfusion. However, it can also be detrimental. Immediately after an ischemic stroke in those patients who do not receive fibrinolytic therapy (discussed below), the use of drugs to lower BP is recommended only if BP is markedly increased (systolic BP greater than 220 mm Hg or diastolic greater than 120 mm Hg). In a patient who is going to have fibrinolytic therapy, the BP needs to be less than 185/110 mm Hg and then maintained at or below 180/105 mm Hg for at least 24 hours after fibrinolytic therapy. In an acute stroke, IV antihypertensives such as labetalol (Normodyne) and nicardipine (Cardene) are preferred. Although low BP immediately after a stroke is uncommon, hypotension and hypovolemia should be corrected if present.

Fluid and electrolyte balance must be controlled carefully. Generally the goal is to keep the patient adequately hydrated to promote perfusion and decrease further brain injury. Overhydration may compromise perfusion by increasing cerebral edema. Adequate fluid intake during acute care via oral, IV, or tube feedings is a priority. Also monitor urine output to make sure the patient does not become dehydrated.

If secretion of antidiuretic hormone (ADH) increases in response to the stroke, urine output decreases and fluid is retained. Low serum sodium (hyponatremia) may occur. IV solutions with glucose and water are avoided because they are hypotonic and may further increase cerebral edema and ICP. In addition, hyperglycemia may be associated with further brain damage and should be treated. In general, decisions regarding individualized fluid and electrolyte replacement therapy are based on the extent of intracranial edema, symptoms of

✚ TABLE 58-7   EMERGENCY MANAGEMENT
Stroke

Etiology	Assessment Findings	Interventions
• Sudden vascular compromise causing disruption of blood flow to brain • Thrombosis • Trauma • Aneurysm • Embolism • Hemorrhage • Arteriovenous malformation	• Altered level of consciousness • Weakness, numbness, or paralysis of portion of body • Speech or visual disturbances • Severe headache • Heart rate ↑ or ↓ • Respiratory distress • Unequal pupils • Hypertension • Facial drooping on affected side • Difficulty swallowing • Seizures • Bladder or bowel incontinence • Nausea and vomiting • Vertigo	**Initial** • Ensure patent airway. • Call stroke code or stroke team. • Remove dentures. • Perform pulse oximetry. • Maintain adequate oxygenation (SaO$_2$ >95%) with supplemental O$_2$, if necessary. • Establish IV access with normal saline. • Maintain BP according to guidelines (e.g., Cardiac Life Support).* • Remove clothing. • Obtain CT scan or MRI immediately. • Perform baseline laboratory tests (including blood glucose) immediately, and treat if hypoglycemic. • Position head in midline. • Elevate head of bed 30 degrees if no symptoms of shock or injury. • Institute seizure precautions. • Anticipate thrombolytic therapy for ischemic stroke. • Keep patient NPO until swallow reflex evaluated. **Ongoing Monitoring** • Monitor vital signs and neurologic status, including level of consciousness (NIH Stroke Scale), motor and sensory function, pupil size and reactivity, SaO$_2$, and cardiac rhythm. • Reassure patient and family.

*See Appendix A.
NIH, National Institutes of Health; *SaO$_2$,* arterial oxygen saturation.

increased ICP, central venous pressure levels, laboratory values for electrolytes, and intake and output.

Increased ICP is more likely to occur with hemorrhagic strokes but can occur with ischemic strokes. Increased ICP from cerebral edema usually peaks in 72 hours and may cause brain herniation. Management of increased ICP includes practices that improve venous drainage, such as elevating the head of the bed, maintaining head and neck in alignment, and avoiding hip flexion. Additional measures for reducing ICP include management of hyperthermia (goal temperature of 96.8° to 98.6° F [36° to 37° C]), drug therapy to prevent seizures, pain management, avoidance of hypervolemia, and management of constipation. Cerebrospinal fluid drainage may be used in some patients to reduce ICP. (The specific management of increased ICP is discussed in Chapter 57.)

Drug Therapy for Ischemic Stroke. Fibrinolytic therapy should not be delayed. Recombinant tissue plasminogen activator (tPA) is used to produce localized fibrinolysis by binding to the fibrin in the thrombi. The fibrinolytic action of tPA occurs as the plasminogen is converted to plasmin, whose enzymatic action then digests fibrin and fibrinogen, and thus lyses the clot. Other fibrinolytic agents cannot be substituted for tPA. (Fibrinolytic [thrombolytic] therapy is discussed in Chapter 34.)

tPA is administered IV to reestablish blood flow through a blocked artery to prevent cell death in patients with the acute onset of ischemic stroke. tPA must be administered within 3 to 4½ hours of the onset of clinical signs of ischemic stroke.[16,17] Patients are screened carefully before tPA can be given. Screening includes a noncontrast CT or MRI scan to rule out hemorrhagic stroke; blood tests for glucose level and coagulation disorders; and screening for recent history of gastrointestinal bleeding, stroke, or head trauma within the past 3 months, or major surgery within 14 days.[16,17] If tPA is expected as a treatment option, insert a urinary catheter, nasogastric tube, and multiple IVs before tPA administration. During infusion of the drug, closely monitor the patient's vital signs and neurologic

status to assess for improvement or for potential deterioration related to intracerebral hemorrhage. Control of BP is critical during treatment and for 24 hours following.

Intraarterial infusion of tPA may also be used for patients with an ischemic stroke. Intraarterial tPA can be administered up to 6 hours after the onset of stroke symptoms. In the intraarterial tPA procedure, the neurovascular specialist inserts a thin, flexible catheter into an artery (usually the femoral artery) and guides the catheter to the area of the clot by angiogram. The tPA is administered through the catheter and immediately targets the clot. Less tPA is needed when it is delivered directly to the clot, which can reduce the possibility of intracranial hemorrhage.[17]

The use of anticoagulants (e.g., heparin) in the emergency phase after an ischemic stroke is generally not recommended because of the risk for intracranial hemorrhage. Acetylsalicylic acid (aspirin) at a dose of 325 mg may be initiated within 24 to 48 hours after the onset of an ischemic stroke. Complications of aspirin include gastrointestinal bleeding with higher doses. Aspirin should be administered cautiously if the patient has a history of peptic ulcer disease.[18]

After the patient has stabilized and to prevent further clot formation, patients with strokes caused by thrombi and emboli may be treated with anticoagulants and platelet inhibitors (see discussion on prevention of stroke on pp. 1396-1397). For patients who have atrial fibrillation, oral anticoagulants include warfarin, rivaroxaban, and dabigatran etexilate. Platelet inhibitors include aspirin, ticlopidine, clopidogrel, and dipyridamole. Additionally, the use of statins has been shown to be effective for the patient with an ischemic stroke.[14]

Surgical Therapy for Ischemic Stroke. Stent retrievers (e.g., Solitaire FR, Trevo) are a way of opening blocked arteries in the brain by using a removable stent system. During the procedure, a catheter is used to guide the small stent from the femoral artery in the groin area to the affected artery in the brain. The stent is guided into the part of the artery where a blood clot has

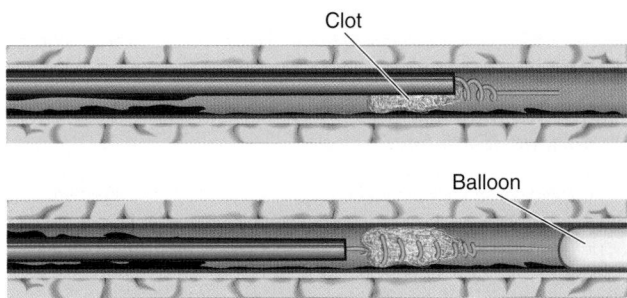

FIG. 58-7 The MERCI retriever removes blood clots in patients who are experiencing ischemic strokes. The retriever is a long, thin wire that is threaded through a catheter into the femoral artery. The wire is pushed through the end of the catheter up to the carotid artery. The wire reshapes itself into tiny loops that latch onto the clot, and the clot can then be pulled out. To prevent the clot from breaking off, a balloon at the end of the catheter inflates to stop blood flow through the artery. *MERCI*, Mechanical embolus removal in cerebral ischemia.

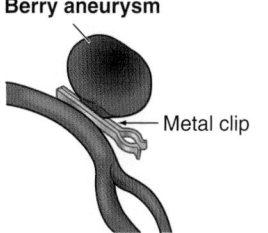

FIG. 58-8 Clipping of aneurysms.

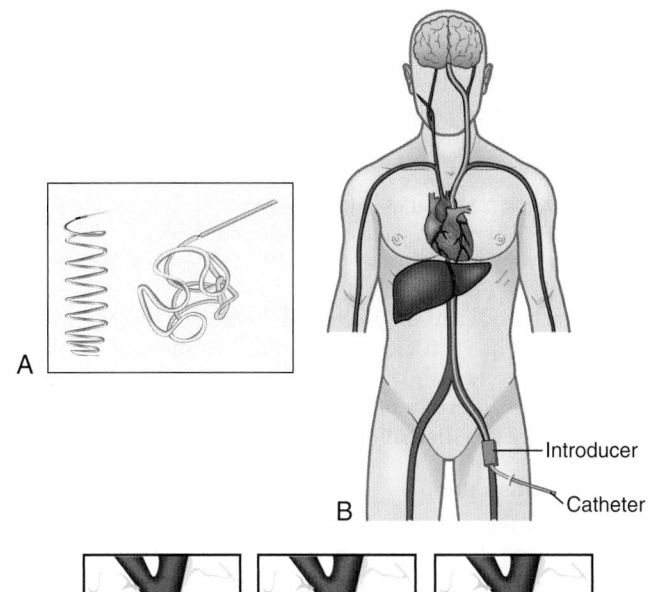

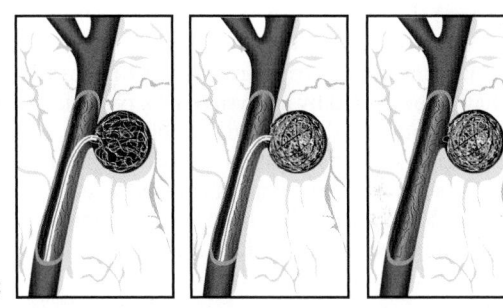

FIG. 58-9 Guglielmi detachable coil (GDC). **A,** A coil is used to occlude an aneurysm. Coils are made of soft, springlike platinum. The softness of the platinum allows the coil to assume the shape of irregularly shaped aneurysms while posing little threat of rupture of the aneurysm. **B,** A catheter is inserted through an introducer (small tube) in an artery in the leg. The catheter is threaded up to the cerebral blood vessels. **C,** Platinum coils attached to a thin wire are inserted into the catheter and then placed in the aneurysm until the aneurysm is filled with coils. Packing the aneurysm with coils prevents the blood from circulating through the aneurysm, reducing the risk of rupture.

formed. The stent expands the interior walls of the artery and allows blood to get to the patient's brain immediately to prevent as much brain damage as possible. The clot seeps into the mesh of the stent. Then, after a few minutes the stent and clot are removed together.

Another surgical approach uses the mechanical embolus removal in cerebral ischemia (MERCI) retriever (Fig. 58-7), which allows the surgeon to go inside the blocked artery of a patient who is experiencing ischemic strokes. The MERCI retriever has a tiny, corkscrew-like device that uses a microcatheter inserted through a femoral artery balloon catheter. Once the corkscrew device reaches the clot in the brain, the device penetrates the clot, allowing it to be removed. A guidewire and the microcatheter are deployed through the balloon catheter and then placed just beyond the clot. The physician then deploys the MERCI retriever device to engage and ensnare the clot. Once the clot is captured, the balloon catheter is inflated to temporarily arrest forward flow while the clot is being withdrawn. The clot is pulled into the balloon catheter and completely out of the body. The balloon is then deflated and blood flow is restored. Research is also being conducted on other mechanical thrombectomy devices for the removal of clots, including acute balloon angioplasty and stenting, snare devices, and ultrasonic aspirators.[19]

Acute Care for Hemorrhagic Stroke

Drug Therapy for Hemorrhagic Stroke. Anticoagulants and platelet inhibitors are contraindicated in patients with hemorrhagic strokes. The main drug therapy for patients with hemorrhagic stroke is the management of hypertension. Oral and IV agents may be used to maintain BP within a normal to high-normal range (systolic BP less than 160 mm Hg). Seizure prophylaxis in the acute period after intracerebral and subarachnoid hemorrhages is situation specific and should be discussed with the collaborative care team.[20]

Surgical Therapy for Hemorrhagic Stroke. Surgical interventions for hemorrhagic stroke include immediate evacuation of aneurysm-induced hematomas or cerebellar hematomas larger than 3 cm. Individuals who have an arteriovenous malformation (AVM) may experience a hemorrhagic stroke if the AVM ruptures. The treatment of AVM is surgical resection and/or radiosurgery (i.e., gamma knife). Both may be preceded by interventional neuroradiology to embolize the blood vessels that supply the AVM.

SAH is usually caused by a ruptured aneurysm. Approximately 20% of patients have multiple aneurysms. Treatment of an aneurysm involves clipping or coiling the aneurysm to prevent rebleeding (Figs. 58-8 and 58-9). In *clipping* the aneurysm, the neurosurgeon places a metallic clip on the neck of the aneurysm to block blood flow and prevent rupture. The clip remains in place for life. In the procedure known as *coiling*, a metal coil is inserted into the lumen of the aneurysm via interventional neuroradiology (see Fig. 58-9). Guglielmi detachable coils (GDCs) provide immediate protection against hemorrhage by reducing the blood pulsations within the aneurysm. Eventually, a thrombus forms within the aneurysm and the aneurysm becomes sealed off from the parent vessel by the formation of an endothelialized layer of connective tissue.

Goals for managing ICP are the same for patients with SAH as they are for patients dealing with acute stroke. After aneurysmal occlusion via clipping or coiling, hyperdynamic therapy (hemodilution-induced hypertension using vasoconstricting agents such as phenylephrine or dopamine [Intropin] and hypervolemia) may be instituted in an effort to increase the mean arterial pressure and increase cerebral perfusion. Volume expansion is achieved via crystalloid or colloid solution.

Interventions to treat cerebral vasospasm either before or after aneurysm clipping or coiling include administration of the calcium channel blocker nimodipine (Nimotop), which is given to patients with SAH to decrease the effects of vasospasm and minimize cerebral damage. Nimodipine restricts the influx of calcium ions into cells by reducing the number of open calcium channels. Although nimodipine is a calcium channel blocker, its exact mechanism of action in reducing vasospasm is not well understood.

DRUG ALERT: Nimodipine (Nimotop)
- Assess BP and apical pulses before administration.
- If pulse is ≤60 beats/min or systolic BP is <90 mm Hg, hold medication and contact physician.

Subarachnoid and intracerebral hemorrhage can involve bleeding into the ventricles of the brain. This situation produces hydrocephalus, which further damages brain tissue from increased ICP. Insertion of a ventriculostomy for cerebrospinal fluid drainage can dramatically improve these situations.[21]

Rehabilitation Care

After the stroke patient has stabilized for 12 to 24 hours, collaborative care shifts from preserving life to lessening disability and attaining optimal function. Many of the interventions discussed in the acute phase are maintained during this phase. The patient may be evaluated by a physiatrist (a physician who specializes in physical medicine and rehabilitation). Remember that some aspects of rehabilitation actually begin in the acute care phase as soon as the patient is stabilized. Specific measures related to rehabilitation are discussed in the section on Ambulatory and Home Care on pp. 1408-1410.

NURSING MANAGEMENT STROKE

NURSING ASSESSMENT

Subjective and objective data that should be obtained from a person who has had a stroke are presented in Table 58-8. Primary assessment focuses on cardiac and respiratory status and neurologic assessment. If the patient is stable, the nursing history is obtained as follows: (1) description of the current illness with attention to initial symptoms, particularly symptom onset and duration, nature (intermittent or continuous), and changes; (2) history of similar symptoms previously experienced; (3) current medications; (4) history of risk factors and other illnesses such as hypertension; and (5) family history of stroke or cardiovascular diseases. This information is gained through an interview of the patient, family members, significant others, and/or caregiver.

Secondary assessment includes a comprehensive neurologic examination of the patient. This includes (1) level of consciousness, including assessment using the National Institutes of Health (NIH) Stroke Scale (Table 58-9); (2) cognition; (3) motor abilities; (4) cranial nerve function; (5) sensation; (6) proprioception; (7) cerebellar function; and (8) deep tendon reflexes.

TABLE 58-8   NURSING ASSESSMENT

Stroke

Subjective Data
Important Health Information
Past health history: Hypertension; previous stroke, TIA, aneurysm, cardiac disease (including recent myocardial infarction), dysrhythmias, heart failure, valvular disease, infective endocarditis; hyperlipidemia, polycythemia, diabetes, gout; previous head injury, family history of hypertension, diabetes, stroke, or coronary artery disease
Medications: Oral contraceptives; use of and compliance with antihypertensive and anticoagulant therapy; illegal substances and drug use (cocaine)

Functional Health Patterns
Health perception–health management: Positive family history of stroke; alcohol abuse, smoking, drug abuse
Nutritional-metabolic: Anorexia, nausea, vomiting; dysphagia, altered sense of taste and smell
Elimination: Change in bowel and bladder patterns
Activity-exercise: Loss of movement and sensation; syncope; weakness on one side; generalized weakness, easy fatigability
Cognitive-perceptual: Numbness, tingling of one side of the body; loss of memory; alteration in speech, language, problem-solving ability; pain; headache, possibly sudden and severe (hemorrhage); visual disturbances; denial of illness

Objective Data
General
Emotional lability, lethargy, apathy or combativeness, fever

Respiratory
Loss of cough reflex, labored or irregular respirations, tachypnea, rhonchi (aspiration), airway occlusion (tongue), apnea, coughing when eating or delayed coughing

Cardiovascular
Hypertension, tachycardia, carotid bruit

Gastrointestinal
Loss of gag reflex, bowel incontinence, decreased or absent bowel sounds, constipation

Urinary
Frequency, urgency, incontinence

Neurologic
Contralateral motor and sensory deficits, including weakness, paresis, paralysis, anesthesia; unequal pupils, hand grasps; akinesia, aphasia (expressive, receptive, global), dysarthria (slurred speech), agnosias, apraxia, visual deficits, perceptual or spatial disturbances, altered level of consciousness (drowsiness to deep coma) and Babinski's sign, ↓ followed by ↑ deep tendon reflexes, flaccidity followed by spasticity, amnesia, ataxia, personality change, nuchal rigidity, seizures

Possible Diagnostic Findings
Positive CT, CTA, MRI, MRA, or other neuroimaging scans showing size, location, and type of lesion; positive Doppler ultrasonography and angiography indicating stenosis

CTA, Computed tomographic angiography; *MRA,* magnetic resonance angiography; *TIA,* transient ischemic attack.

Clear documentation of initial and ongoing neurologic examinations is essential to note changes in the patient's status.

NURSING DIAGNOSES

Nursing diagnoses for the person with a stroke may include, but are not limited to, those presented in Nursing Care Plan 58-1.

TABLE 58-9 NATIONAL INSTITUTES OF HEALTH STROKE SCALE (NIHSS)

Description

The National Institutes of Health Stroke Scale (NIHSS) is a 15-item neurologic examination used to evaluate the effect of an acute stroke.

Procedure for Use

A trained observer rates the patient's ability to answer questions and perform activities. Ratings for each item are scored and there is an allowance for untestable (UN) items. If an item is left untested, a detailed explanation must be clearly written on the form. Training can be completed free at *www.nihstrokescale.org*.

Item	Scale Definition
Level of consciousness	0 = Alert 1 = Not alert, but arousable by minor stimulation 2 = Not alert, requires repeated stimulation to get attention 3 = Responds only with reflex motor or autonomic effects or totally unresponsive, flaccid, areflexic
Level of consciousness questions	0 = Answers both questions correctly 1 = Answers one question correctly 2 = Answers neither question correctly
Level of consciousness commands	0 = Performs both tasks correctly 1 = Performs one task correctly 2 = Performs neither task correctly
Best gaze	0 = Normal 1 = Partial gaze palsy 2 = Forced deviation, or total gaze paresis
Visual	0 = No visual loss 1 = Partial hemianopia 2 = Complete hemianopia 3 = Bilateral hemianopia or blind
Facial palsy	0 = Normal symmetric movement 1 = Minor paralysis 2 = Partial paralysis 3 = Complete paralysis of one or both sides
Motor and drift (for each extremity)	0 = No drift 1 = Drift 2 = Some effort against gravity 3 = No effort against gravity, limb falls 4 = No movement UN = Amputation
Limb ataxia	0 = Absent 1 = Present in one limb 2 = Present in two limbs
Sensory	0 = Normal 1 = Mild to moderate sensory loss 2 = Severe to total sensory loss
Best language	0 = No aphasia, normal 1 = Mild to moderate aphasia 2 = Severe aphasia 3 = Mute, no usable speech or auditory comprehension
Dysarthria	0 = Normal 1 = Mild to moderate 2 = Severe UN = Intubated or other physical barrier
Extinction or inattention	0 = No abnormality 1 = Inattention or extinction to bilateral stimulation 2 = Does not recognize own hand
Distal motor function	0 = Normal (no flexion after 5 sec) 1 = At least some extension but not fully extended 2 = No voluntary extension after 5 sec

Source: American Stroke Association: NIH stroke scale, 2009. Retrieved from *www.ninds.nih.gov/doctors/NIH_Stroke_Scale.pdf*.

PLANNING

Together with the patient, caregiver, and family, establish the goals of nursing care. Typical goals are that the patient will (1) maintain a stable or improved level of consciousness, (2) attain maximum physical functioning, (3) attain maximum self-care abilities and skills, (4) maintain stable body functions (e.g., bladder control), (5) maximize communication abilities, (6) maintain adequate nutrition, (7) avoid complications of stroke, and (8) maintain effective personal and family coping.

NURSING IMPLEMENTATION

HEALTH PROMOTION. You have a major role in the promotion of a healthy lifestyle. Teaching should focus on stroke prevention, particularly for persons with known risk factors. Nursing measures to reduce risk factors for stroke are similar to those for coronary artery disease (see Chapter 34, Table 34-1) and are discussed earlier in this chapter on pp. 1394-1396.

Uncontrolled or undiagnosed hypertension is the primary cause of stroke. Therefore you need to be involved in BP screening and ensuring that patients adhere to the use of their antihypertensive medications. If a person is a diabetic, it is important that the diabetes is well controlled. If an individual has atrial fibrillation, an anticoagulant (see p. 1398) or aspirin may be used to reduce the risk of stroke. Because smoking is a major risk factor for stroke, you need to be actively involved in helping patients to stop smoking (see Chapter 11, Tables 11-4 to 11-6).

Another important aspect of health promotion is teaching patients and families about early symptoms associated with stroke or TIA. Table 58-1 presents information on when to seek health care for these symptoms.

ACUTE INTERVENTION

Respiratory System. During the acute phase after a stroke, management of the respiratory system is a nursing priority.[22] Stroke patients are particularly vulnerable to respiratory problems. Advancing age and immobility increase the risk for atelectasis and pneumonia.

Risk for aspiration pneumonia is high because of impaired consciousness or dysphagia. Dysphagia after stroke is common.[23] Airway obstruction can occur because of problems with chewing and swallowing, food pocketing (food remaining in the buccal cavity of the mouth), and the tongue falling back. Some stroke patients, especially those with brainstem or hemorrhagic stroke, may require endotracheal intubation and mechanical ventilation initially. Enteral tube feedings also place the patient at risk for aspiration pneumonia. All patients should be screened for their ability to swallow and kept on nothing-by-mouth (NPO) status until dysphagia has been ruled out.

Nursing interventions to support adequate respiratory function are individualized to meet the patient's needs. An oropharyngeal airway may be used in comatose patients to prevent the tongue from falling back and obstructing the airway and to provide access for suctioning. Alternatively, a nasopharyngeal airway may be used to provide airway protection and access. When an artificial airway is required for a prolonged time, a tracheostomy may be performed.

Nursing interventions include frequently assessing airway patency and function, providing oxygenation, suctioning, promoting patient mobility, positioning the patient to prevent aspiration, and encouraging deep breathing. In patients who are on mechanical ventilation, oral care at least every 2 hours reduces the occurrence of ventilator-assisted pneumonia.[24]

◎ NURSING CARE PLAN 58-1

Patient With Stroke

NURSING DIAGNOSIS* **Decreased intracranial adaptive capacity** *related to* decreased cerebral perfusion pressure of ≤50-60 mm Hg and sustained increase in ICP secondary to thrombus, embolus, or hemorrhage *as evidenced by* baseline ICP ≥15 mm Hg, elevated systolic blood pressure, bradycardia, widened pulse pressure, and increasing NIH Stroke Scale score

PATIENT GOAL Demonstrates signs of stable or improved cerebral perfusion

Outcomes (NOC)	Interventions (NIC) and *Rationales*
Tissue Perfusion: Cerebral • Intracranial pressure _____ • Systolic blood pressure _____ • Diastolic blood pressure _____ **Measurement Scale** 1 = Severe deviation from normal range 2 = Substantial deviation from normal range 3 = Moderate deviation from normal range 4 = Mild deviation from normal range 5 = No deviation from normal range • Restlessness _____ • Decreased level of consciousness _____ • Impaired cognition _____ • Impaired neurologic reflexes _____ **Measurement Scale** 1 = Severe 2 = Substantial 3 = Moderate 4 = Mild 5 = None	**Cerebral Perfusion Promotion** • Consult with physician to determine hemodynamic parameters, and maintain hemodynamic parameters within this range. • Monitor neurologic status *to detect changes indicative of worsening or improving condition.* • Calculate and monitor cerebral perfusion pressure (CPP) *to detect change in condition.* • Monitor respiratory status (e.g., rate, rhythm, and depth of respirations; PaO_2, $PaCO_2$, pH, and bicarbonate levels) *because high $PaCO_2$ and a high hydrogen ion concentration (acidosis) are potent vasodilators that increase cerebral blood flow.* • Monitor patient's ICP and neurologic responses to care activities, *since changes in positioning and movement can increase ICP.* • Monitor determinants of tissue oxygen delivery (e.g., $PaCO_2$, SaO_2, hemoglobin levels, and cardiac output) *to ensure adequate cerebral oxygenation.* • Administer and titrate vasoactive drugs, as ordered, *to maintain hemodynamic parameters.* • Avoid neck flexion or extreme hip or knee flexion *to avoid obstruction of arterial and venous blood flow.*

NURSING DIAGNOSIS **Risk for aspiration** *related to* decreased level of consciousness and decreased or absent gag and swallowing reflexes

PATIENT GOALS 1. Demonstrates ability to swallow oral foods without aspiration
2. Maintains a clear airway

Outcomes (NOC)	Interventions (NIC) and *Rationales*
Respiratory Status: Airway Patency • Depth of inspiration _____ • Ability to clear secretions _____ **Measurement Scale** 1 = Severe deviation from normal range 2 = Substantial deviation from normal range 3 = Moderate deviation from normal range 4 = Mild deviation from normal range 5 = No deviation from normal range • Adventitious breath sounds _____ • Accumulation of sputum _____ **Measurement Scale** 1 = Severe 2 = Substantial 3 = Moderate 4 = Mild 5 = None	**Aspiration Precautions** • Monitor level of consciousness, cough reflex, gag reflex, and swallowing ability *to determine patient's ability to swallow foods without aspiration.* • Avoid liquids or use thickening agent *to facilitate swallowing.* • Feed in small amounts until patient is no longer at risk for aspiration. • Offer foods or liquids that can be formed into a bolus before swallowing. **Airway Management** • Auscultate breath sounds, noting areas of decreased or absent ventilation and presence of adventitious sounds *to identify airway obstruction and accumulation of secretions.* • Remove secretions by encouraging coughing or by suctioning *to clear airway.* • Encourage slow, deep breathing; turning; and coughing *to increase airway clearance without increasing ICP.* • Assist with incentive spirometer *to open collapsed alveoli, promote deep breathing, and prevent atelectasis.* • Keep patient NPO until swallow evaluation completed *to prevent aspiration.*

NURSING DIAGNOSIS **Impaired physical mobility** *related to* neuromuscular and cognitive impairment and decreased muscle strength and control *as evidenced by* limited ability to perform gross and fine motor skills, limited range of motion, and difficulty turning

PATIENT GOALS 1. Demonstrates increased muscle strength and ability to move
2. Uses adaptive equipment to increase mobility

Outcomes (NOC)	Interventions (NIC) and *Rationales*
Mobility • Balance _____ • Muscle movement _____ • Joint movement _____ • Transfer performance _____ • Walking _____ **Measurement Scale** 1 = Severely compromised 2 = Substantially compromised 3 = Moderately compromised 4 = Mildly compromised 5 = Not compromised	**Exercise Therapy: Muscle Control** • Collaborate with physical, occupational, and recreational therapists in developing and executing exercise program *to determine extent of problem and plan appropriate interventions.* • Determine patient's readiness to engage in activity or exercise protocol *to assess expected level of participation.* • Apply splints to achieve stability of proximal joints involved with fine motor skills *to prevent contractures.* • Encourage patient to practice exercises independently *to promote patient's sense of control.* • Reinforce instructions provided to patient about the proper way to perform exercises *to minimize injury and maximize effectiveness.* • Provide restful environment for patient after periods of exercise *to facilitate recuperation.*

*Nursing diagnoses listed in order of priority.

◎ NURSING CARE PLAN 58-1—cont'd

Patient With Stroke

NURSING DIAGNOSIS **Impaired verbal communication** *related to* aphasia *as evidenced by* refusal or inability to speak, difficulty forming words and sentences to express thoughts, and inappropriate verbalization

PATIENT GOALS
1. Uses effective oral and written communication techniques
2. Demonstrates congruency of verbal and nonverbal communication

Outcomes (NOC)	Interventions (NIC) and *Rationales*
Communication • Use of spoken language _____ • Use of written language _____ • Use of nonverbal language _____ • Exchanges messages accurately with others _____ **Measurement Scale** 1 = Severely compromised 2 = Substantially compromised 3 = Moderately compromised 4 = Mildly compromised 5 = Not compromised	**Communication Enhancement: Speech Deficit** • Listen attentively *to convey the importance of patient's thoughts and to promote a positive environment for learning.* • Provide positive reinforcement and praise *to build self-esteem and confidence.* • Use simple words and short sentences *to avoid overwhelming patient with verbal stimuli.* • Perform prescriptive speech-language therapies during informal interactions with patient *to reinforce prescribed therapies.* • Provide verbal prompts and reminders *to help patient to express self.*

NURSING DIAGNOSIS **Unilateral neglect** *related to* visual field cut and loss on one side of body (hemianopsia) and brain injury from cerebrovascular problems *as evidenced by* consistent inattention to stimuli on affected side

PATIENT GOALS
1. Cares for both sides of the body appropriately
2. Uses strategies to minimize unilateral neglect

Outcomes (NOC)	Interventions (NIC) and *Rationales*
Heedfulness of Affected Side • Acknowledges affected side as being integral to self _____ • Protects affected side when positioning _____ • Protects affected side when ambulating _____ • Performs activities of daily living to affected side _____ • Arranges environment to compensate for physical or sensory deficits _____ • Uses visual scanning as a compensatory strategy _____ **Measurement Scale** 1 = Never demonstrated 2 = Rarely demonstrated 3 = Sometimes demonstrated 4 = Often demonstrated 5 = Consistently demonstrated	**Unilateral Neglect Management** • Monitor for abnormal responses to three types of stimuli: sensory, visual, and auditory *to determine the presence of and degree to which unilateral neglect exists (e.g., inability to see objects on affected side, leaving food on a plate that corresponds to affected side, lack of sensation on affected side).* • Instruct patient to scan from left to right *to visualize the entire environment.* • Position bed in room so that individuals approach and care for patient on unaffected side. • Rearrange the environment to use the right or left visual field; position personal items, television, or reading materials within view on unaffected side *to compensate for visual field deficits.* • Touch unaffected shoulder when initiating conversation *to attract patient's attention.* • Gradually move personal items and activity to affected side as patient demonstrates an ability to compensate for neglect. • Include caregivers in rehabilitation process *to support the patient's efforts and assist with care to promote reintegration with the whole body.*

NURSING DIAGNOSIS **Impaired urinary elimination** *related to* impaired impulse to void or inability to reach toilet or manage tasks of voiding *as evidenced by* loss of urinary control and involuntary loss of urine at unpredictable times

PATIENT GOALS
1. Perceives impulse to void, removes clothing for toileting, and uses toilet
2. Demonstrates ability to urinate when the urge arises or with a timed schedule

Outcomes (NOC)	Interventions (NIC) and *Rationales*
Urinary Continence • Recognizes urge to void _____ • Maintains predictable pattern of voiding _____ • Responds to urge in timely manner _____ • Starts and stops stream _____ **Measurement Scale** 1 = Never demonstrated 2 = Rarely demonstrated 3 = Sometimes demonstrated 4 = Often demonstrated 5 = Consistently demonstrated • Urine leakage between voidings _____ • Wets clothing during the day _____ • Wets clothing or bedding during night _____ **Measurement Scale** 1 = Consistently demonstrated 2 = Often demonstrated 3 = Sometimes demonstrated 4 = Rarely demonstrated 5 = Never demonstrated	**Urinary Habit Training** • Keep a continence specification record for 3 days *to establish voiding pattern and plan appropriate interventions.* • Establish interval of initial toileting schedule (based on voiding pattern and usual routine) *to initiate process of improving bladder functioning and increased muscle tone.* • Assist patient to toilet and prompt to void at prescribed intervals *to assist patient in adapting to new toileting schedule.* • Teach patient to consciously hold urine until the scheduled toileting time *to improve muscle tone.* • Discuss daily record of continence with staff *to provide reinforcement and encourage compliance with toileting schedule.* • Give positive feedback or positive reinforcement to patient when he or she voids at scheduled toileting times, and make no comment when patient is incontinent, *to reinforce desired behavior.*

Continued

◎ **NURSING CARE PLAN 58-1—cont'd**

Patient With Stroke

NURSING DIAGNOSIS **Impaired swallowing** *related to* weakness or paralysis of affected muscles *as evidenced by* drooling, difficulty in swallowing, choking

PATIENT GOAL Demonstrates effective swallowing without choking, coughing, or aspiration

Outcomes (NOC)	Interventions (NIC) and *Rationales*
Swallowing Status	*Swallowing Therapy*
• Maintains food in mouth _____	• Collaborate with other members of health care team (e.g., occupational therapist, speech pathologist, dietitian) *to provide continuity in patient's rehabilitative plan*.
• Handles oral secretions _____	• Assist patient to sit in an erect position (as close to 90 degrees as possible) for feeding/exercise *to provide optimal position for chewing and swallowing without aspirating*.
• Ability to clear oral cavity _____	• Assist patient to position head in forward flexion in preparation for swallowing ("chin tuck").
Measurement Scale	• Assist patient to maintain sitting position for 30 min after completing meal *to prevent regurgitation of food*.
1 = Severely compromised	• Instruct patient or caregiver on emergency measures for choking *to prevent complications in the home setting*.
2 = Substantially compromised	• Check mouth for pocketing of food after eating *to prevent collection and putrefaction of food and/or aspiration*.
3 = Moderately compromised	• Provide mouth care as needed *to promote comfort and oral health*.
4 = Mildly compromised	• Monitor body weight *to determine adequacy of nutritional intake*.
5 = Not compromised	
• Choking _____	
• Coughing _____	
• Gagging _____	
Measurement Scale	
1 = Severe	
2 = Substantial	
3 = Moderate	
4 = Mild	
5 = None	

NURSING DIAGNOSIS **Situational low self-esteem** *related to* actual or perceived loss of function and altered body image *as evidenced by* refusal to participate in self-care and expressions of helplessness and uselessness

PATIENT GOALS
1. Expresses positive feelings of self-worth
2. Participates in self-care of affected body parts

Outcomes (NOC)	Interventions (NIC) and *Rationales*
Self-Esteem	*Self-Esteem Enhancement*
• Verbalizations of self-acceptance _____	• Monitor patient's statements of self-worth *to determine effect of stroke on self-esteem*.
• Maintenance of grooming and hygiene _____	• Encourage patient to identify strengths *to facilitate patient's recognition of intrinsic value*.
• Acceptance of self-limitations _____	• Assist in setting realistic goals *to achieve higher self-esteem*.
• Description of self _____	• Reward or praise patient's progress toward reaching goals.
• Feelings about self-worth _____	• Encourage increased responsibility for self *to promote sense of satisfaction, independence, and control, and to reduce frustrations*.
Measurement Scale	• Monitor levels of self-esteem over time *to determine stressors or situations that trigger low self-esteem and to teach coping mechanisms*.
1 = Never positive	
2 = Rarely positive	
3 = Sometimes positive	
4 = Often positive	
5 = Consistently positive	

ICP, Intracranial pressure; *NIH*, National Institutes of Health; *PaCO₂*, partial pressure of carbon dioxide in arterial blood; *PaO₂*, partial pressure of oxygen in arterial blood; *SaO₂*, arterial oxygen saturation.

Patients who have an unclipped or uncoiled aneurysm may experience rebleeding and the possibility of increasing ICP further with coughing or suctioning, so nursing management is aimed at reducing these interventions while maintaining a proper airway.

Interventions related to maintenance of airway function are described in Nursing Care Plan 58-1.

Neurologic System. The primary clinical assessment tool to evaluate and document neurologic status in acute stroke patients is the NIH Stroke Scale (NIHSS),[25] which measures stroke severity (see Table 58-9). The NIHSS is a predictor of both short- and long-term outcomes of stroke patients. Additionally, it serves as a data collection tool for planning patient care and exchanging information among health care providers.

Additional neurologic assessment includes mental status, pupillary responses, and extremity movement and strength. Also closely monitor vital signs. A decreasing level of consciousness may indicate increasing ICP. Monitor ICP and cere-bral perfusion pressure if the patient is in a critical care environment. Record your nursing assessment on flow sheets to communicate the patient's neurologic status to the stroke team.

Cardiovascular System. Nursing goals for the cardiovascular system are aimed at maintaining homeostasis. Many patients with stroke have decreased cardiac reserves secondary to cardiac disease. Cardiac efficiency may be further compromised by fluid retention, overhydration, dehydration, or BP variations. Central venous pressure, pulmonary artery pressure, or hemodynamic monitoring may be used as indicators of fluid balance or cardiac function in the critical care unit.

Nursing interventions include (1) monitoring vital signs frequently; (2) monitoring cardiac rhythms; (3) calculating intake and output, noting imbalances; (4) regulating IV infusions; (5) adjusting fluid intake to individual patient needs; (6) monitoring lung sounds for crackles and rhonchi indicating pulmonary congestion; and (7) monitoring heart sounds for murmurs or for S_3 or S_4 heart sounds. Bedside monitors or telemetry may record cardiac rhythms.

Hypertension is sometimes seen after a stroke as the body attempts to increase cerebral blood flow. It is important to monitor for orthostatic hypotension before ambulating the patient for the first time. Neurologic changes can occur with a sudden decrease in BP.

After a stroke, the patient is at risk for venous thromboembolism (VTE), especially in the weak or paralyzed lower extremity. VTE is related to immobility, loss of venous tone, and decreased muscle pumping activity in the leg. The most effective prevention is to keep the patient moving. Teach the patient active range-of-motion exercises if the patient has voluntary movement in the affected extremity. For the patient with hemiplegia, perform passive range-of-motion exercises several times a day. Additional measures to prevent VTE include positioning to minimize the effects of dependent edema and using elastic compression gradient stockings or support hose. Sequential compression devices may be ordered for bedridden patients. VTE prophylaxis may include low-molecular-weight heparin (e.g., enoxaparin [Lovenox]). The nursing assessment for VTE includes measuring the calf and thigh daily, observing swelling of the lower extremities, noting unusual warmth of the leg, and asking the patient about pain in the calf.

Musculoskeletal System. The nursing goal for the musculoskeletal system is to maintain optimal function by preventing joint contractures and muscular atrophy. In the acute phase, range-of-motion exercises and positioning are important nursing interventions. Passive range-of-motion exercise is begun on the first day of hospitalization. Muscle atrophy secondary to lack of innervation and activity can develop after stroke, so exercise is an important intervention for rehabilitation and recovery.

The paralyzed or weak side needs special attention when the patient is positioned. Position each joint higher than the joint proximal to it to prevent dependent edema. Specific deformities on the weak or paralyzed side that may be present in patients with stroke include internal rotation of the shoulder; flexion contractures of the hand, wrist, and elbow; external rotation of the hip; and plantar flexion of the foot. Subluxation of the shoulder on the affected side is common. Careful positioning and moving of the affected arm may prevent development of a painful shoulder condition. Immobilization of the affected upper extremity may precipitate a painful shoulder-hand syndrome.

Nursing interventions to optimize musculoskeletal function include (1) trochanter roll at the hip to prevent external rotation; (2) hand cones (not rolled washcloths) to prevent hand contractures; (3) arm supports with slings and lap boards to prevent shoulder displacement; (4) avoidance of pulling the patient by the arm to avoid shoulder displacement; (5) posterior leg splints, footboards, or high-top tennis shoes to prevent footdrop; and (6) hand splints to reduce spasticity.

Use of a footboard for the patient with spasticity is controversial. Rather than preventing plantar flexion (footdrop), the sensory stimulation of a footboard against the bottom of the foot increases plantar flexion. Likewise, experts disagree on whether hand splints facilitate or diminish spasticity. The decision regarding the use of footboards or hand splints is made on an individual patient basis.

Integumentary System. The skin of the patient with stroke is particularly susceptible to breakdown related to loss of sensation, decreased circulation, and immobility. This is compounded by advanced age, poor nutrition, dehydration, edema, and incontinence.

The nursing plan for prevention of skin breakdown includes (1) pressure relief by position changes, special mattresses, or wheelchair cushions; (2) good skin hygiene; (3) emollients applied to dry skin; and (4) early mobility. An example of a position change schedule is side-backside, with a maximum duration of 2 hours for any position. Position the patient on the weak or paralyzed side for only 30 minutes. If an area of redness develops and does not return to normal color within 15 minutes of pressure relief, the epidermis and dermis are damaged.

Do not massage the damaged area because this may cause additional damage. Control of pressure is the single most important factor in both the prevention and treatment of skin breakdown. Pillows can be used under lower extremities to reduce pressure on the heels. Vigilance and good nursing care are required to prevent pressure sores.

Gastrointestinal System. The most common bowel problem for the stroke patient is constipation. Patients may be prophylactically placed on stool softeners and/or fiber (psyllium [Metamucil]). If a patient has liquid stools, check for stool impaction. Fluid and fiber intake goals should be discussed with the stroke team and are based on the patient's nutritional and fluid status.

Physical activity also promotes bowel function. Laxatives, suppositories, or additional stool softeners may be ordered if the patient does not respond to increased fluid and fiber. Enemas are used only if suppositories and digital stimulation are ineffective because they cause vagal stimulation and increase ICP.

Bowel retraining may be needed and continues into the rehabilitation phase. A bowel management program consists of placing the patient on the bedpan or bedside commode or taking the patient to the bathroom at a regular time daily to reestablish bowel regularity. A good time for the bowel program is 30 minutes after breakfast because eating stimulates the gastrocolic reflex and peristalsis, but timing may need to be adjusted, since individual bowel habits may vary.

Urinary System. In the acute stage of stroke the primary urinary problem is poor bladder control, resulting in incontinence. Take steps to promote normal bladder function and avoid the use of indwelling catheters. If an indwelling catheter must be used initially, remove it as soon as the patient is medically and neurologically stable. Long-term use of an indwelling catheter is associated with urinary tract infections and delayed bladder retraining.

An intermittent catheterization program may be used for patients with urinary retention because of the lower incidence of urinary infections. An alternative to intermittent catheterizations is the external catheter for male patients with urinary incontinence. External catheters do not alleviate the problem of urine retention. Avoid bladder overdistention.

Assist the patient with urinary difficulties or incontinence. Often the patient with stroke has functional incontinence, which is associated with communication difficulties, mobility problems, and dressing or undressing difficulties. A bladder retraining program consists of (1) adequate fluid intake with most of it given between 7:00 AM and 7:00 PM; (2) scheduled toileting every 2 hours using bedpan, commode, or bathroom while encouraging the usual position for urinating (standing for men and sitting for women); (3) observation for signs of restlessness, which may indicate the need for urination; and (4) assessment for bladder distention by palpation.

Assessment of postvoid residual volume is often done using bladder ultrasound. The ultrasound measures how much urine is in the bladder after voiding. If urine remains in the bladder, incomplete emptying is a problem and may cause urinary tract infections. A coordinated program by the entire nursing staff is needed to achieve urinary continence.

Nutrition. The patient's nutritional needs require quick assessment and treatment. The patient may initially receive IV infusions to maintain fluid and electrolyte balance and to administer drugs. Patients with severe impairment may require enteral or parenteral nutrition support. Patients should have their nutritional needs addressed in the first 72 hours of admission to the hospital because nutrition is important for recovery and healing.[26]

SAFETY ALERT
- The first oral feeding should be approached carefully because the gag reflex may be impaired due to dysphagia.

Speech therapists (if available) should perform a swallowing evaluation before patients are started on oral intake. The majority of patients experience dysphagia after a stroke.[23] Before initiating feeding, assess the gag reflex by gently stimulating the back of the throat with a tongue blade. If a gag reflex is present, the patient will gag spontaneously. If it is absent, defer the feeding, and begin exercises to stimulate swallowing. The speech therapist or occupational therapist is usually responsible for designing this program. However, you may be called on to develop the program in some clinical settings.

To assess swallowing ability, elevate the head of the bed to an upright position (unless contraindicated) and give the patient a small amount of crushed ice or ice water to swallow. If the gag reflex is present and the patient is able to swallow safely, you may proceed with feeding.

After careful assessment of swallowing, chewing, gag reflex, and pocketing, oral feedings can be initiated. Mouth care before feeding helps stimulate sensory awareness and salivation and can facilitate swallowing. The patient should remain in a high Fowler's position, preferably in a chair with the head flexed forward, for the feeding and for 30 minutes afterward.

The speech therapist may recommend various dietary items. Foods should be easy to swallow and provide enough texture, temperature (warm or cold), and flavor to stimulate a swallow reflex. Crushed ice can be used as a stimulant. Instruct the patient to swallow and then swallow again. Pureed foods are not usually the best choice because they are often bland and too smooth. Thin liquids are often difficult to swallow and may promote coughing. Thin liquids can be thickened with a commercially available thickening agent (e.g., Thick-It). Avoid milk products because they tend to increase the viscosity of mucus and increase salivation.

Place food on the unaffected side of the mouth. Feedings must be followed by scrupulous oral hygiene because food may collect on the affected side of the mouth. During the acute and rehabilitation phase of the stroke, a dietitian can assist in determining the appropriate daily caloric intake based on the patient's size, weight, and activity level. If the patient is unable to take in an adequate oral diet and dysphagia persists, a percutaneous endoscopic gastrostomy (PEG) tube (see Chapter 40, Fig. 40-7) may be used for nutritional support. Most commercially prepared formulas provide about 1 cal/mL. (Enteral feedings are described in Chapter 40.)

The inability to feed oneself can be frustrating and may result in malnutrition and dehydration. Interventions to promote self-feeding include using the unaffected upper extremity to eat; employing assistive devices such as rocker knives, plate guards, and nonslip pads for dishes (Fig. 58-10); removing unnecessary items from the tray or table, which can reduce spills; and providing a calm environment to decrease sensory overload and distraction. The effectiveness of the dietary program is evaluated in terms of maintenance of weight, adequate hydration, and patient satisfaction. Introduce these interventions in the acute care setting so that maximum rehabilitation can occur once the patient is discharged.

Communication. During the acute stage of stroke, your role in meeting the patient's psychologic needs is primarily supportive. Speech, comprehension, and language deficits are the most difficult problems for the patient and caregiver. Assess the patient for both the ability to speak and the ability to understand. The patient's response to simple questions can guide you in structuring explanations and instructions. If the patient cannot understand words, use gestures to support verbal cues. Collaborate with the speech therapist to assess and formulate a plan of care to enhance communication.

Nursing interventions that support communication include (1) communicating frequently and meaningfully; (2) allowing time for the patient to comprehend and answer; (3) using simple, short sentences; (4) using visual cues; (5) structuring conversation so that it permits simple answers by the patient; and (6) praising the patient honestly for improvements with speech.[27]

An alert patient is usually anxious because of lack of understanding about what has happened and because of difficulty with communication or inability to communicate. The stroke patient with aphasia may easily be overwhelmed by verbal stimuli. Give the patient extra time to comprehend and respond to communication. (Guidelines for communicating with a

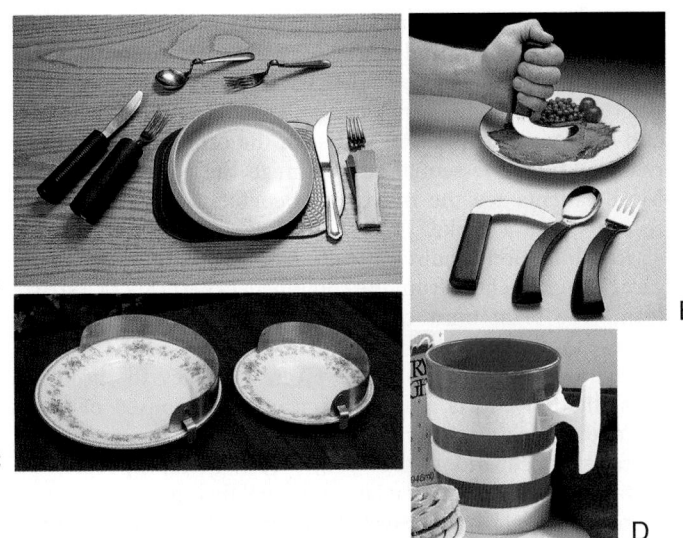

FIG. 58-10 Assistive devices for eating. **A,** The curved fork fits over the hand. The rounded plate helps keep food on the plate. Special grips and swivel handles are helpful for some persons. **B,** Knives with rounded blades are rocked back and forth to cut food. The person does not need a fork in one hand and a knife in the other. **C,** Plate guards help keep food on the plate. **D,** Cup with special handle. (Courtesy Sammons Preston, Bolingbrook, Ill.)

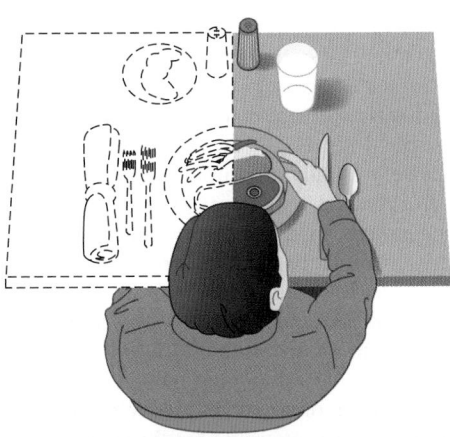

FIG. 58-11 Spatial and perceptual deficits in stroke. Perception of a patient with homonymous hemianopsia shows that food on the left side is not seen and thus is ignored.

TABLE 58-10	**COMMUNICATION WITH A PATIENT WITH APHASIA**

1. Decrease environmental stimuli that may be distracting and disrupting to communication efforts.
2. Treat the patient as an adult.
3. Speak with normal volume and tone.
4. Present one thought or idea at a time.
5. Keep questions simple or ask questions that can be answered with "yes" or "no."
6. Let the person speak. Do not interrupt. Allow time for the individual to complete thoughts.
7. Make use of gestures or demonstration as an acceptable alternative form of communication. Encourage this by saying, "Show me . . ." or "Point to what you want."
8. Do not pretend to understand the person if you do not. Calmly say you do not understand and encourage the use of nonverbal communication, or ask the person to write out what he or she wants.
9. Give the patient time to process information and generate a response before repeating a question or statement.
10. Allow body contact (e.g., the clasp of a hand, touching) as much as possible. Realize that touching may be the only way the patient can express feelings.
11. Organize the patient's day by preparing and following a schedule (the more familiar the routine, the easier it will be).
12. Do not push communication if the person is tired or upset. Aphasia worsens with fatigue and anxiety.

patient who has aphasia are presented in Table 58-10.) A picture board may be helpful for communicating with the stroke patient. Further evaluation and treatment of language and communication deficits are often done by the speech therapist once the patient has stabilized.

Sensory-Perceptual Alterations. Patients who have had a stroke frequently have perceptual deficits. Patients with a stroke on the right side of the brain usually have difficulty judging position, distance, and rate of movement. These patients are often impulsive and impatient and tend to deny problems related to strokes. They may fail to correlate spatial-perceptual problems with the inability to perform activities, such as guiding a wheelchair through the doorway. The patient with a right-brain stroke (left hemiplegia) is at higher risk for injury because of mobility difficulties. Directions for activities are best given verbally for comprehension. Break the task down into simple steps for ease of understanding. Environmental control, such as removing clutter and obstacles and using good lighting, aids in concentration and safer mobility. Provide nonslip socks at all times. One-sided neglect is common for people with right-brain stroke, so you may assist or remind the patient to dress the weak or paralyzed side or shave the forgotten side of the face.

Patients with a left-brain stroke (right hemiplegia) commonly are slower in organization and performance of tasks. They tend to have impaired spatial discrimination. These patients usually admit to deficits and have a fearful, anxious response to a stroke. Their behaviors are slow and cautious. Nonverbal cues and instructions are helpful for comprehension with patients who have had a left-brain stroke.

Homonymous hemianopsia (blindness in the same half of each visual field) is a common problem after a stroke. Persistent disregard of objects in part of the visual field should alert you to this possibility. Initially, help the patient to compensate by arranging the environment within the patient's perceptual field, such as arranging the food tray so that all foods are on the right side or the left side to accommodate for field of vision (Fig. 58-11). Later, the patient learns to compensate for the visual defect by consciously attending or by scanning the neglected side. The weak or paralyzed extremities are carefully checked for adequacy of dressing, for hygiene, and for trauma.

In the clinical situation, it is often difficult to distinguish between a visual field cut and a neglect syndrome. Both problems may occur with strokes affecting either the right or the left side of the brain. A person may be unfortunate enough to have both homonymous hemianopsia and a neglect syndrome, which increases the inattention to the weak or paralyzed side. A neglect syndrome results in decreased safety awareness and places the patient at high risk for injury. Immediately after the stroke, anticipate safety hazards and provide protection from injury. Safety measures can include closely observing the patient, elevating side rails, lowering the height of the bed, and using video monitors. Avoid the use of restraints and soft vests because this may agitate the patient.

Other visual problems may include *diplopia* (double vision), loss of the corneal reflex, and *ptosis* (drooping eyelid), especially if the stroke is in the vertebrobasilar distribution. Diplopia is often treated with an eye patch. If the corneal reflex is absent, the patient is at risk for corneal abrasion and should be observed closely and protected against eye injuries. Corneal abrasion can be prevented with artificial tears or gel to keep the eyes moist and an eye shield (especially at night). Ptosis is generally not treated because it usually does not inhibit vision.

Coping. A stroke is usually a sudden, extremely stressful event for the patient, caregiver, family, and significant others. A stroke is often a family disease, affecting the family emotionally, socially, and financially and changing roles and responsibilities within the family.[28] An older couple may perceive the stroke as a threat to life and to accustomed lifestyle. Reactions to this threat vary considerably but may involve fear, apprehension, denial of the severity of stroke, depression, anger, and sorrow. During the acute phase of caring for the stroke patient and the family, nursing interventions designed to facilitate coping involve providing information and emotional support.

Explanations to the patient about what has happened and about diagnostic and therapeutic procedures should be clear and understandable. Decision making and upholding the patient's wishes during this challenging time are of upmost importance. Advance directives should be honored, and family meetings or updates should be held daily about feeding tube placement or tracheostomy.

Give the caregiver and family a careful, detailed explanation of what has happened to the patient. However, if the family is extremely anxious and upset during the acute phase, explanations may need to be repeated at a later time. Because family members usually have not had time to prepare for the illness, they may need assistance in arranging care for family members or pets and for transportation and finances. A social services referral is often helpful.

It is particularly challenging to keep the aphasic patient adequately informed. Tone, demeanor, and touch may also be used to convey support. When communicating with a patient who has a communication deficit, speak in a normal volume and tone, keep questions simple, and present one thought or idea at a time. To decrease frustration, always let the patient speak without interruption and make use of gestures. Do not forget to use writing and communication boards.[27]

AMBULATORY AND HOME CARE. The patient is usually discharged from the acute care setting to home, an intermediate or long-term care facility, or a rehabilitation facility. Ideally, discharge planning with the patient and the caregiver starts early in the hospitalization and promotes a smooth transition from one care setting to another. The stroke team provides guidance for the appropriate care necessary after discharge. If the patient requires a short- or long-term health care facility, the team can make appropriate referrals that allow time to select and arrange for care. A critical factor in discharge planning is the patient's level of independence in performing ADLs. If the patient is returning home, the team can make referrals for needed equipment and services in preparation for discharge.

You have an excellent opportunity to prepare the patient and caregiver for discharge through teaching, demonstration and return demonstration, practice, and evaluation of self-care skills. Total care is considered in discharge planning: medications, nutrition, mobility, exercises, hygiene, and toileting. Follow-up care is carefully planned to permit continuing nursing care; physical, occupational, and speech therapy; and medical care. Identify community resources to provide recreational activities, group support, spiritual assistance, respite care, adult day care, and home assistance based on the patient's needs.

Rehabilitation. *Rehabilitation* is the process of maximizing the patient's capabilities and resources to promote optimal functioning related to physical, mental, and social well-being. The goals of rehabilitation are to prevent deformity and maintain and improve function. Regardless of the care setting, ongoing rehabilitation is essential to maximize the patient's abilities. Most patients see the maximum benefit in the first year of recovery after a stroke.[29]

Rehabilitation requires a team approach so the patient and caregiver can benefit from the combined, expert care of a stroke team. The team must communicate and coordinate care to achieve the patient's goals. As a nurse, you are in a good position to facilitate this process and are often the key to successful rehabilitation efforts. The stroke team is composed of many members, including nurses, physicians, psychiatrist, physical therapist, occupational therapist, speech therapist, registered dietitian, respiratory therapist, vocational therapist, recreational therapist, social worker, psychologist, pharmacist, and chaplain. Physical therapy focuses on mobility, progressive ambulation, transfer techniques, and equipment needed for mobility. Occupational therapy emphasizes retraining for skills of daily living such as eating, dressing, hygiene, and cooking. Occupational therapists are also skilled in cognitive and perceptual evaluation and training. Speech therapy focuses on speech, communication, cognition, and eating abilities.

Many of the nursing interventions outlined in Nursing Care Plan 58-1 for the patient with a stroke are initiated in the acute phase of care and continue throughout rehabilitation. Some of the interventions are independent nursing actions, whereas others involve the entire rehabilitation team.

The rehabilitation nurse assesses the patient, caregiver, and family with attention to (1) the patient's rehabilitation potential, (2) physical status of all body systems, (3) complications caused by the stroke or other chronic conditions, (4) the patient's cognitive status, (5) family resources and support, and (6) expectations of the patient and caregiver related to the rehabilitation program.

Musculoskeletal Function. Initially emphasize the musculoskeletal functions of eating, toileting, and walking for rehabilitation of the patient. Initial assessment consists of determining the stage of recovery of muscle function. If the muscles are still flaccid several weeks after the stroke, the prognosis for regaining function is poor and care focuses on preventing additional loss (Fig. 58-12).

Most patients begin to show signs of spasticity with exaggerated reflexes within 48 hours after the stroke. Spasticity at this phase of stroke denotes progress toward recovery. As improvement continues, small voluntary movements of the hip or shoulder may be accompanied by involuntary movements in the rest of the extremity *(synergy)*. The final stage of recovery occurs when the patient has voluntary control of isolated muscle groups.

INFORMATICS IN PRACTICE

Video Games for Stroke Recovery

- Patients dealing with the effects of a stroke often have difficulty performing activities of daily living. Playing active video games, like Nintendo Wii or Xbox Kinect, brings some fun into stroke recovery and may get patients to spend more time in therapy.
- Gaming helps patients regain lost strength, improve motor skills, and improve problem solving and short- and long-term memory.
- Patients can play with their families, including children, making gaming a way to involve others in rehabilitation.

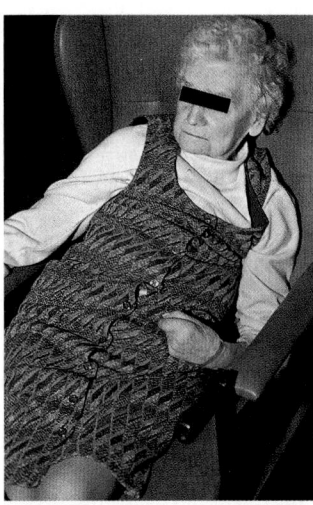

FIG. 58-12 Loss of postural stability is common after stroke. When the nondominant hemisphere is involved, walking apraxia and loss of postural control are usually apparent. The patient is unable to sit upright and tends to fall sideways. Provide appropriate support with pillows or cushions.

Interventions for the musculoskeletal system advance in a manner of progressive activity. Balance training is the initial step and begins with the patient sitting up in bed or dangling the legs over the edge of the bed. Evaluate tolerance by noting dizziness or syncope caused by vasomotor instability.

Also assess whether patients autocorrect their posture when sitting on the edge of the bed. If the patient can straighten his or her posture instead of leaning to the weaker side, the patient may be ready for the next step of transferring from bed to chair. Place the chair beside the bed so that the patient can lead with the stronger arm and leg. The patient sits on the side of the bed, stands, places the strong hand on the far wheelchair arm, and sits down. You may either supervise the transfer or provide minimal assistance by guiding the patient's strong hand to the wheelchair arm, standing in front of the patient while blocking the patient's knees with your knees to prevent knee buckling, and guiding the patient into a sitting position.

In some rehabilitation units the Bobath method is used as an approach to mobility *(http://ibita.org)*. The goal of this approach is to help the patient gain control over patterns of spasticity by inhibiting abnormal reflex patterns. Therapists and nurses use the Bobath approach to encourage normal muscle tone, normal movement, and bilateral function of the body. An example is to have the patient transfer into the wheelchair using the weak or paralyzed side and the stronger side to facilitate more bilateral functioning.

Another approach to stroke rehabilitation is constraint-induced movement therapy (CIMT). CIMT encourages the patient to use the weakened extremity by restricting movement of the normal extremity. Complying with this approach can be challenging for patients and may limit its use. Movement training, skill acquisition, splinting, and exercise are additional therapies offered for rehabilitation of the stroke patient.[29]

Supportive or assistive equipment, such as canes, walkers, and leg braces, may be needed on a short- or long-term basis for mobility. The physical therapist usually selects the most appropriate supportive device(s) to meet individual needs and instructs the patient regarding use. Incorporate physical therapy activities into the patient's daily routine for additional practice and repetition of rehabilitation efforts.

Stroke Survivorship and Coping. Patients who have had strokes often exhibit emotional responses that are not appropriate or typical for the situation. Patients may appear apathetic, depressed, fearful, anxious, weepy, frustrated, and angry. Some patients, especially those with a stroke on the left side of the brain (right hemiplegia), have exaggerated mood swings. The patient may be unable to control emotions and may suddenly burst into tears or laughter. This behavior is out of context and often is unrelated to the patient's underlying emotional state. Nursing interventions for atypical emotional response are to (1) distract the patient who suddenly becomes emotional, (2) explain to the patient and family that emotional outbursts may occur after a stroke, (3) maintain a calm environment, and (4) avoid shaming or scolding the patient during emotional outbursts.

The patient with a stroke may experience many losses, including sensory, intellectual, communicative, functional, role behavior, emotional, social, and vocational losses. The patient, caregiver, and family often go through the process of grief and mourning associated with the losses. Some patients experience long-term depression with symptoms such as anxiety, weight loss, fatigue, poor appetite, and sleep disturbances. In addition, the time and energy required to perform previously simple tasks can result in anger and frustration.

The patient, caregiver, and family need help coping with the losses associated with stroke. Provide assistance by (1) supporting communication between the patient and family; (2) discussing lifestyle changes resulting from stroke deficits; (3) discussing changing roles and responsibilities within the family; (4) being an active listener to allow the expression of fear, frustration, and anxiety; (5) including the family and patient in short- and long-term goal planning and patient care; and (6) supporting family conferences.

Maladjusted dependence with inadequate coping occurs when the patient does not maintain optimal functioning for self-care, family responsibilities, decision making, or socialization. This situation can cause resentment from both the patient and family with a negative cycle of interpersonal dependency and control.[28] Caregivers and family members must cope with three aspects of the patient's behavior: (1) recognition of behavioral changes resulting from neurologic deficits that are not changeable, (2) responses to multiple losses by both the patient and the family, and (3) behaviors that may have been reinforced during the early stages of stroke as continued dependency.

The patient, caregiver, and family may express guilt over not living healthy lifestyles or not seeking professional help sooner. Family therapy is a helpful adjunct to rehabilitation. Open communication, information regarding the total effects of stroke, teaching regarding stroke treatment, and therapy are helpful. Stroke support groups in rehabilitation facilities and in the community are helpful in terms of mutual sharing, education, coping skills, and understanding.

Sexual Function. A patient who has had a stroke may be concerned about the loss of sexual function. Many patients are comfortable talking about their anxieties and fears regarding sexual function if you are comfortable and open to the topic. You may initiate the topic with the patient and spouse or significant other. Common concerns regarding sexual activity are impotence and the occurrence of another stroke during sex. Nursing interventions for sexual activity include teaching about (1) optional positioning of partners, (2) timing for peak energy times, and (3) patient and partner counseling.

Community Integration. Traditionally, successful community integration after stroke has been difficult for the patient because of persistent problems with cognition, coping, physical deficits, and emotional lability that interfere with functioning. Older patients who have had a stroke often have more severe deficits and frequently experience multiple health problems. Failure to continue the rehabilitation regimen at home may result in deterioration and further complications.

Community resources can be an asset to patients and their families. The National Stroke Association provides information, resources, referral services, and quarterly newsletters on stroke. The American Stroke Association, a division of the American Heart Association, has information regarding stroke, hypertension, diet, exercise, and assistive devices. This association sponsors self-help groups in many areas. Easter Seals provides wheelchairs and other assistive devices for stroke patients. Local groups can offer more daily assistance such as meals and transportation. These resources can be identified by nurse case managers, home health nurses, discharge planners, and clinical nurse specialists. (Resources are listed at the end of the chapter.)

GERONTOLOGIC CONSIDERATIONS

STROKE

Stroke is a significant cause of death and disability. The highest incidence of stroke occurs among older adults. Stroke can result in a profound disruption in the life of an older person. The magnitude of disability and changes in total function can leave patients wondering if they can ever return to their "old self," and loss of independence may be a major concern. The ability to perform ADLs may require many adaptive changes because of physical, emotional, perceptual, and cognitive deficits. Home management may be a particular challenge if the patient has an older spouse caregiver who also has health problems. There may be limited family members (including adult children) living in close proximity to provide help.

The rehabilitative phase and helping the older patient deal with the residual deficits of stroke, as well as aging, can provide a challenging nursing experience. Patients may become fearful and depressed because they think they may have another stroke or die. The fear can become immobilizing and interfere with effective rehabilitation.

Changes may occur in the patient-spouse relationship. The dependency resulting from a stroke may threaten the relationship. The spouse may also have chronic medical problems that can affect the ability to take care of the stroke survivor. The patient may not want anyone other than the spouse to provide care, thus putting a significant burden on the spouse.

You have the opportunity to assist the patient and caregiver in the transition through acute hospitalization, rehabilitation, long-term care, and home care. The needs of the patient, the caregiver, and the family require ongoing nursing assessment and adaptation of interventions in response to changing needs to optimize quality of life for all of them.

CASE STUDY

Stroke

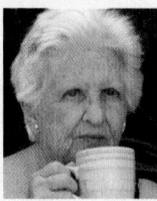

iStockphoto/Thinkstock

Patient Profile

A.J., a 66-yr-old white woman, awoke in the middle of the night and fell when she tried to get up and go to the bathroom (see Chapter 56 case study on p. 1344). She fell because she was not able to control her left leg. Her husband took her to the hospital, where she was diagnosed with an acute ischemic stroke. Because she had awakened with symptoms, the actual time of onset was unknown and she was not a candidate for tPA.

Subjective Data

- Left arm and leg are weak and feel numb
- Feeling depressed and fearful
- Requires help with ADLs
- Concerned about having another stroke
- Says she has not taken her medications for high cholesterol and high blood pressure for several weeks
- History of a brief episode of left-sided weakness and tingling of the face, arm, and hand 3 mo earlier, which totally resolved and for which she did not seek treatment

Objective Data

- BP 180/110 mm Hg
- ECG is as follows:

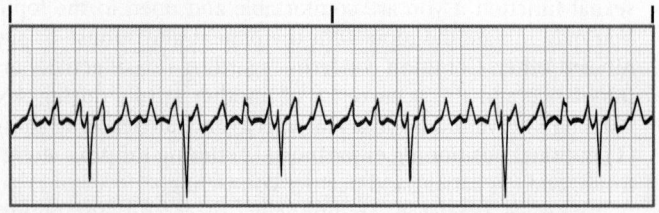

- Left-sided arm weakness (3/5) and leg weakness (4/5)
- Decreased sensation on the left side, particularly the hand
- Left homonymous hemianopsia
- Height 5 ft, 3 in, weight 160 lb
- Alert, oriented, and able to answer questions appropriately but mild slowness in responding

Past Medical History

- Migraines
- Hypertension
- Hyperlipidemia

Discussion Questions

1. How do A.J.'s prior health history and current findings put her at risk for another stroke?
2. How can you address A.J.'s concerns regarding having another stroke?
3. How can A.J. and her family address activity issues such as driving after the stroke?
4. What strategies can you use to help A.J. and her family cope with her depression?
5. ***Priority Decision:*** What are the priority lifestyle changes that A.J. should make to reduce the likelihood of another stroke?
6. How will homonymous hemianopsia affect A.J.'s hygiene, eating, driving, and community activities?
7. What factors should you assess for related to outpatient rehabilitation for A.J.?
8. ***Priority Decision:*** What are the priority nursing interventions for A.J.?
9. ***Priority Decision:*** Based on the assessment data provided, what are the priority nursing diagnoses? Are there any collaborative problems?
10. ***Delegation Decision:*** What nursing interventions for A.J. can the RN delegate to unlicensed assistive personnel (UAP)?
11. ***Evidence-Based Practice:*** A.J.'s family wants to know if her atrial flutter caused her stroke and, if so, what she can do to prevent additional problems with her atrial flutter.

BRIDGE TO NCLEX EXAMINATION

The number of the question corresponds to the same-numbered outcome at the beginning of the chapter.

1. Of the following patients, the nurse recognizes that the one with the highest risk for a stroke is a(n)
   a. obese 45-year-old Native American.
   b. 35-year-old Asian American woman who smokes.
   c. 32-year-old white woman taking oral contraceptives.
   d. 65-year-old African American man with hypertension.

2. The factor related to cerebral blood flow that most often determines the extent of cerebral damage from a stroke is the
   a. amount of cardiac output.
   b. oxygen content of the blood.
   c. degree of collateral circulation.
   d. level of carbon dioxide in the blood.

3. Information provided by the patient that would help differentiate a hemorrhagic stroke from a thrombotic stroke includes
   a. sensory disturbance.
   b. a history of hypertension.
   c. presence of motor weakness.
   d. sudden onset of severe headache.

4. A patient with right-sided hemiplegia and aphasia resulting from a stroke most likely has involvement of the
   a. brainstem.
   b. vertebral artery.
   c. left middle cerebral artery.
   d. right middle cerebral artery.

5. The nurse explains to the patient with a stroke who is scheduled for angiography that this test is used to determine the
   a. presence of increased ICP.
   b. site and size of the infarction.
   c. patency of the cerebral blood vessels.
   d. presence of blood in the cerebrospinal fluid.

6. A patient experiencing TIAs is scheduled for a carotid endarterectomy. The nurse explains that this procedure is done to
   a. decrease cerebral edema.
   b. reduce the brain damage that occurs during a stroke in evolution.
   c. prevent a stroke by removing atherosclerotic plaques blocking cerebral blood flow.
   d. provide a circulatory bypass around thrombotic plaques obstructing cranial circulation.

7. For a patient who is suspected of having a stroke, one of the most important pieces of information that the nurse can obtain is
   a. time of the patient's last meal.
   b. time at which stroke symptoms first appeared.
   c. patient's hypertension history and management.
   d. family history of stroke and other cardiovascular diseases.

8. Bladder training in a male patient who has urinary incontinence after a stroke includes
   a. limiting fluid intake.
   b. keeping a urinal in place at all times.
   c. assisting the patient to stand to void.
   d. catheterizing the patient every 4 hours.

9. Common psychosocial reactions of the stroke patient to the stroke include (select all that apply)
   a. depression.
   b. disassociation.
   c. intellectualization.
   d. sleep disturbances.
   e. denial of severity of stroke.

1. d, 2. c, 3. d, 4. c, 5. c, 6. c, 7. b, 8. c, 9. a, d, e

⟳evolve

For rationales to these answers and even more NCLEX review questions, visit http://evolve.elsevier.com/Lewis/medsurg.

REFERENCES

1. American Heart Association: AHA statistical update, *Circulation* 125:e2, 2012. Retrieved from *http://circ .ahajournals.org/content/125/1/e2.full#sec-81*.
2. University of Medicine and Dentistry of New Jersey: Stroke statistics. Retrieved from *www.theuniversityhospital.com/stroke/ stats.htm*.
3. Centers for Disease Control and Prevention: Faststats: cerebrovascular disease or stroke, 2012. Retrieved from *www.cdc.gov/nchs/fastats/stroke.htm*.
*4. Haley WE, Roth DL, Howard G, et al: Caregiving strain and estimated risk for stroke and coronary heart disease among spouse caregiver: differential effects by race and sex, *Stroke* 41:331, 2010.
5. Centers for Disease Control and Prevention: Health effects of cigarette smoking, 2012. Retrieved from *www.cdc.gov/tobacco/ data_statistics/fact_sheets/health_effects/effects_cig_smoking*.
*6. Jakel A, Plested M, Chapman A, et al: Management of patients with transient ischemic attack: insight from real-life clinical practice in Europe and the United States, *Curr Med Res Opin* 28:429, 2012.

7. American Stroke Association: Transient ischemic attack, 2012. Retrieved from *www.strokeassociation.org/STROKEORG/ AboutStroke/TIA-Transient-Ischemic-Attack_UCM_310942_ Article.jsp*.
8. American Heart Association: The imperative of primary stroke prevention: first things first, 2010. Retrieved from *http:// myamericanheart.org/professional/General/The-Imperative-of- Primary-Stroke-Prevention-First-Things-First_UCM_432544_ Article.jsp*.
9. Dupont S, Wijdicks E, Lanzino G, et al: Aneurysmal subarachnoid hemorrhage: an overview for the practicing neurologist, *Semin Neurol* 30:545, 2010.
10. McCaffrey P: Neuroanatomy of speech, swallowing and language: the blood supply. Retrieved from *www.csuchico.edu/ ~pmccaffrey//syllabi/CMSD%2020/362unit11.html*.
*11. Naess H, Lunde L, Brogger J: The triad of pain, fatigue, and depression in ischemic stroke patients: the Bergen Stroke Study, *Cerebrovasc Dis* 33:461, 2012.
*12. Mazzucco S, Turri G, Mirandola R, et al: What is still missing in acute-phase treatment of stroke: a prospective observational study, *Neurol Sci* 34(4):449, 2013.
*13. Kessler C, Thomas K, Kao J: Antiplatelet therapy for secondary prevention of acute coronary syndrome, transient ischemic attack, and noncardioembolic stroke in an era of cost containment, *J Invest Med* 60(5):792, 2012.

*Evidence-based information for clinical practice.

*14. Fisher M, Moonis M: Neuroprotective effects of statins: evidence from preclinical and clinical studies, *Curr Treatment Options Cardiovasc Medicine* 14(3):252, 2012.

*15. Liu Z, Fu W, Guo Z, et al: Updated systematic review and meta-analysis of randomized clinical trial comparing carotid artery stenting and carotid endarterectomy in the treatment of carotid stenosis, *Ann Vasc Surg* 26(4):576, 2012.

*16. Jauch EC, Saver JL, Adams HP, et al: Guidelines for the early management of patients with acute ischemic stroke: a guideline for healthcare professionals from the American Heart Association/American Stroke Association, *Stroke* 44:870, 2013.

*17. Miller J, Hartwell C, Lewandowski C: Stroke treatment using intravenous and intra-arterial tissue plasminogen activator, *Curr Treat Options Cardiovasc Med* 14(3):273, 2012.

*18. Fujita K, Komatsu Y, Sato N, et al: Pilot study of the safety of starting administration of low-dose aspirin and cilostazol in acute ischemic stroke, *Neurol Med Chir* 51:819, 2011.

19. deCarvalho F, deFigueiredo M, Silva G: Acute stroke: post-procedural care and management of complications, *Tech Vasc Interv Radiol* 15:78, 2012.

20. Alberti A: Seizures, *Front Neurol Neurosci* 30:3, 2012.

21. Lazaridis C, Naval N: Risk factors and medical management of vasospasm after subarachnoid hemorrhage, *Neurosurg Clin North Am* 21:353, 2010.

22. Green T, Kelloway L, Davies-Schinkel C, et al: Nurses' accountability for stroke quality of care, part one: review of the literature on nursing-sensitive outcomes, *Can J Neurosci Nurs* 33:13, 2011.

23. Martino R, Martin R, Black S: Dysphagia after stroke and its management, *Can Med Assoc J* 184(10):1127, 2012.

*24. Heck K: Decreasing ventilator-associated pneumonia in the intensive care unit: a sustainable comprehensive quality improvement program, *Am J Infect Control* 40(9):877, 2012.

25. American Stroke Association: NIH stroke scale international, 2011. Retrieved from *www.nihstrokescale.org*.

26. Rowat A: Malnutrition and dehydration after stroke, *Nurs Stand* 26:42, 2011.

27. Borthwick S: Communication impairment in patients following stroke, *Nurs Stand* 26:35, 2011.

28. Smeets S, van Heugten C, Geboers J: Respite care after acquired brain injury: the well-being of caregivers and patients, *Arch Phys Med Rehabil* 93(5):834, 2012.

29. Flansbjer U, Lexell J, Brogardh C: Long term benefits of progressive resistance training in chronic stroke: a 4-year follow up, *J Rehabil Med* 44:218, 2012.

RESOURCES

American Association of Neuroscience Nurses (AANN)
www.aann.org
American Stroke Association
www.strokeassociation.org
Association of Rehabilitation Nurses (ARN)
www.rehabnurse.org
National Institute of Neurological Disorders and Stroke
www.ninds.nih.gov
National Institutes of Health Stroke Scale (NIHSS)
www.nihstrokescale.org
National Stroke Association
www.stroke.org

If we take care of the moments,
the years will take care of themselves.
Maria Edgeworth

Nursing Management
Chronic Neurologic Problems

Mariann M. Harding

evolve WEBSITE

http://evolve.elsevier.com/Lewis/medsurg

- NCLEX Review Questions
- Key Points
- Pre-Test
- Answer Guidelines for Case Study on p. 1441
- Rationales for Bridge to NCLEX Examination Questions

- Case Studies
  - Patient With Parkinson's Disease and Hip Fracture
  - Patient With Seizures
- Nursing Care Plans (Customizable)
  - eNCP 59-1: Patient With Headache
  - eNCP 59-2: Patient With Seizure Disorder or Epilepsy
  - eNCP 59-3: Patient With Multiple Sclerosis

- eNCP 59-4: Patient With Parkinson's Disease
- Concept Map Creator
- Concept Map for Case Study on p. 1441
- Glossary
- Content Updates

eFigure
- eFig. 59-1: Pathogenesis of amyotrophic lateral sclerosis

LEARNING OUTCOMES

1. Compare and contrast the etiology, clinical manifestations, collaborative care, and nursing management of tension-type, migraine, and cluster headaches.
2. Differentiate the etiology, clinical manifestations, diagnostic studies, collaborative care, and nursing management of seizure disorders, multiple sclerosis, Parkinson's disease, and myasthenia gravis.

3. Describe the clinical manifestations and nursing and collaborative management of restless legs syndrome, amyotrophic lateral sclerosis, and Huntington's disease.
4. Explain the potential impact of chronic neurologic disease on physical and psychologic well-being.
5. Outline the major goals of treatment for the patient with a chronic, progressive neurologic disease.

KEY TERMS

This chapter discusses headaches, chronic neurologic disorders, and degenerative neurologic disorders. Chronic neurologic disorders include seizure disorders and restless legs syndrome. Degenerative neurologic disorders include multiple sclerosis, Parkinson's disease, myasthenia gravis, amyotrophic lateral sclerosis, and Huntington's disease.

HEADACHES

Headache is probably the most common type of pain that humans experience. The majority of people have functional headaches, such as migraine or tension-type headaches. The others have organic headaches caused by intracranial or extracranial disease.

Headache pain can arise from both intracranial and extracranial sources. The pain-sensitive structures in the head include venous sinuses, dura, cranial blood vessels, three divisions of the trigeminal nerve (cranial nerve [CN] V), facial nerve (CN VII), glossopharyngeal nerve (CN IX), vagus nerve (CN X), and the first three cervical nerves.

Headaches are classified as primary or secondary headaches. *Primary headaches* are those not caused by a disease or another medical condition. Primary headache classifications include tension-type, migraine, and cluster headaches. The

Reviewed by Margie Francisco, RN, MSN, EdD, Nursing Professor, Illinois Valley Community College, Oglesby, Illinois; and Linda R. Littlejohns, RN, MSN, CNRN, FAAN, Vice President of Clinical Development, Integra Neurosurgery, San Juan Capistrano, California.

TABLE 59-1	COMPARISON OF TYPES OF HEADACHES		
Pattern	**Tension-Type Headache**	**Migraine Headache**	**Cluster Headache**
Site (see Fig. 59-1)	Bilateral, bandlike pressure at base of skull	Unilateral (in 60%), may switch sides, commonly anterior	Unilateral, radiating up or down from one eye
Quality	Constant, squeezing tightness	Throbbing, synchronous with pulse	Severe, bone-crushing
Frequency	Cycles for many years	Periodic, cycles of several months to years	May have months or years between attacks Attacks occur in clusters over a period of 2-12 wk
Duration	30 min–7 days	4-72 hr	5 min–3 hr
Time and mode of onset	Not related to time	May be preceded by prodrome Onset after awakening Gets better with sleep	Nocturnal, commonly awakens patient from sleep
Associated symptoms	Palpable neck and shoulder muscle tension, stiff neck, tenderness	Nausea, vomiting Irritability, sweating Photophobia Phonophobia Prodrome of sensory, motor, or psychic phenomena Family history (in 65%)	Facial flushing or pallor Unilateral lacrimation, ptosis, and rhinitis

type of primary headache is determined using the International Headache Society (IHS) guidelines based on characteristics of the headache (Table 59-1). *Secondary headaches* are caused by another condition or disorder, such as sinus infection, neck injury, and stroke. A patient may have more than one type of headache. The history and neurologic examination are diagnostic keys to determining the type of headache.

TENSION-TYPE HEADACHE

Tension-type headache, also called stress headache, is the most common type of headache. These headaches are characterized by their bilateral location and pressing or tightening quality. Tension-type headaches are usually of mild or moderate intensity and can last from minutes to days. Tension-type headaches are divided by frequency into episodic and chronic types.[1]

Etiology and Pathophysiology

Although the cause of tension-type headaches is not fully understood, the development of this type of headache is believed to be associated with neurovascular factors similar to those involved in migraine headaches. Many patients gradually progress over years from episodic to chronic headaches, with the

increasing frequency associated with increasing intensity of the headache.[1]

Clinical Manifestations

Patients usually are initially seen with a bilateral frontal-occipital headache described as a constant, dull pressure, or bandlike headache associated with neck pain and increased tone in the cervical and neck muscles. The headache may involve sensitivity to light (*photophobia*) or sound (*phonophobia*), but does not involve nausea or vomiting. There is no *prodrome* (early manifestation of impending disease), and physical activity does not aggravate symptoms. The headaches may occur intermittently for weeks, months, or even years. Many patients can have a combination of migraine and tension-type headaches, with features of both occurring simultaneously. Patients with migraine headaches may experience tension-type headaches between migraine attacks. Fig. 59-1 shows the location of pain for common headache syndromes.

Diagnostic Studies

Careful history taking is probably the most important tool for diagnosing tension-type headache (Table 59-2). If tension-type headache is present during physical examination, increased

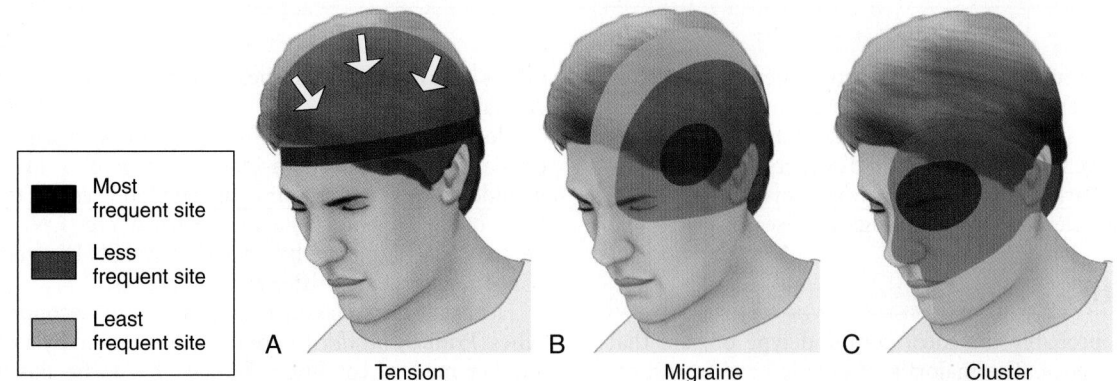

Most frequent site
Less frequent site
Least frequent site

A   Tension   B   Migraine   C   Cluster

FIG. 59-1 Location of pain for common headache syndromes. **A,** Tension headache is often described as feeling of a weight in or on the head or a band squeezing the head. **B,** Migraine headache is described as an intense throbbing or pounding pain that involves one temple. The pain usually is unilateral (on one side of the head), although it can be bilateral. **C,** Cluster headache pain is focused in and around one eye and is often described as sharp, penetrating, or burning.

TABLE 59-2 DIAGNOSTIC STUDIES

Headaches

History and physical examination
- Neurologic examination (often negative)
- Inspection for local infections
- Palpation for tenderness, bony swellings
- Auscultation for bruits over major arteries

Routine laboratory studies
- Complete blood count (CBC)
- Electrolytes
- Urinalysis

Computed tomography (CT) scan of sinuses

Special studies (e.g., CT scan, angiography, EMG, EEG, MRI, MRA, lumbar puncture)

EEG, Electroencephalography; *EMG*, electromyography; *MRA*, magnetic resonance angiography.

GENDER DIFFERENCES

Headaches

Men	Women
• Cluster headaches are more common than in women (6:1). • Exercise-induced headaches are more common than in women.	• Migraine headaches are more common than in men (3:1). • Tension headaches are more common than in men.

resistance to passive movement of the head and tenderness of the head and neck may be present. Electromyography (EMG) may reveal sustained contraction of the neck, scalp, or facial muscles. However, many patients may not show increased muscle tension with this test, even when the test is done during the actual headache.

MIGRAINE HEADACHE

Migraine headache is a recurring headache characterized by unilateral (sometimes bilateral) throbbing pain, a triggering event or factor, and manifestations associated with neurologic and autonomic nervous system dysfunction. The most common age for onset of migraine is between 20 and 30 years. Migraine affects as many as 17% of females and 6% of males in the United States. Migraines are more common in women than men (see Gender Differences box). Risk factors for migraine include family history, low level of education, low socioeconomic status, high workload, and frequent tension-type headaches.[2]

The IHS subdivides migraines into categories. *Migraine without aura* (formerly called common migraine) is the most common type of migraine headache. *Migraine with aura* (formerly called classic migraine) occurs in only 10% of migraine headache episodes.

Etiology and Pathophysiology

Although many theories have addressed the cause of migraine headaches, the exact etiology is not known. The current theory is that a complex series of neurovascular events initiates a migraine headache.[3] People who have migraines have a state of neuronal hyperexcitability in the cerebral cortex, especially in the occipital cortex.

Approximately 70% of those with migraine have a first-degree relative who also had migraine headaches. Migraine is associated with seizure disorders, ischemic stroke, asthma, depression, anxiety, myocardial infarction, Raynaud's syndrome, and irritable bowel syndrome.[3]

In many cases, migraine headaches have no known precipitating events. However, for some patients, specific factors trigger or precipitate a headache. These include foods, menstruation, head trauma, physical exertion, fatigue, stress, missed meals, weather, and drugs. Food triggers include chocolate, cheese, oranges, tomatoes, onions, monosodium glutamate, aspartame, and alcohol (particularly red wine).

Clinical Manifestations

A prodrome and an aura may precede the headache phase by several hours or several days. The *prodrome* may include neurologic (e.g., photophobia), psychologic (e.g., hyperactivity, irritability), and other (e.g., food craving) manifestations. An aura is a complex of neurologic symptoms characterized by visual (e.g., bright lights, scotomas [patchy blindness], visual distortions, zigzag lines), sensory (voices or sounds that do not exist, strange smells), and/or motor (e.g., weakness, paralysis, feeling that limbs are moving) phenomena. The aura immediately precedes the headache and may last 10 to 30 minutes before the headache starts.

A migraine headache may last 4 to 72 hours. The headache is described as a steady, throbbing pain that is synchronous with the pulse. Although the headache is usually unilateral, it may switch to the opposite side in another episode. During the headache phase, some patients with migraine may tend to "hibernate." They seek shelter from noise, light, odors, people, and problems.

The presentation of migraine varies in severity. Not all migraine headaches are disabling, and many patients who have migraine headaches do not seek health care treatment for them. In some patients the symptoms of the migraine headaches may become worse over time.

Diagnostic Studies

The diagnosis of migraine headache is usually based on the patient history. The neurologic and other diagnostic examinations are often normal (see Table 59-2).

There is no specific laboratory or radiologic test for migraine headache. Neuroimaging techniques (e.g., head computed tomography [CT], with or without contrast, and magnetic resonance imaging [MRI]) are not recommended for routine evaluation of headache unless the neurologic examination reveals abnormal findings. If atypical features are present, then additional testing is done to rule out a secondary headache.

CLUSTER HEADACHE

Cluster headaches are a rare form of headache, affecting less than 0.1% of the population.[1] Cluster headaches involve repeated headaches that can occur for weeks to months at a time, followed by periods of remission.

Etiology and Pathophysiology

Neither the cause nor the pathophysiologic mechanism of cluster headache is fully known. The trigeminal nerve has a role in the production of pain, but cluster headaches also involve dysfunction of intracranial blood vessels, the sympathetic nervous system, and pain modulation systems. Imaging studies show hypothalamic activation at the onset of cluster headache.[3]

Alcohol is the only dietary trigger. Strong odors, weather changes, and napping are other triggers.[4]

Clinical Manifestations

The cluster headache is one of the most severe forms of headache, with intense pain lasting from a few minutes to 3 hours. The pain of cluster headache is sharp and stabbing, which is in contrast to the pulsing pain of the migraine headache. The pain is generally located around the eye, radiating to the temple, forehead, cheek, nose, or gums. Other manifestations may include swelling around the eye, lacrimation (tearing), facial flushing or pallor, nasal congestion, and constriction of the pupil. During the headache, the patient is often agitated and restless, unable to sit still or relax.

Cluster headaches can occur every other day and as often as eight times a day. The attacks occur in clusters. The clusters occur with regularity, usually at the same time each day, during the same seasons of the year. A cluster typically lasts 2 weeks to 3 months, and then the patient goes into remission for months to years.

Diagnostic Studies

The diagnosis of cluster headache is based on the patient history. Asking patients to keep a headache diary can be useful. CT scan, MRI, or magnetic resonance angiography (MRA) may rule out an aneurysm, a tumor, or an infection. A lumbar puncture may rule out other disorders that may cause similar symptoms.

OTHER TYPES OF HEADACHES

Although tension, migraine, and cluster headaches are by far the most common types of headaches, other types can occur. These headaches may be the first symptom of a more serious illness. Headache can accompany subarachnoid hemorrhage; brain tumors; other intracranial masses; vascular abnormalities; trigeminal neuralgia (tic douloureux); diseases of the eyes, nose, and teeth; and systemic illness (e.g., bacteremia, carbon monoxide poisoning, mountain sickness, polycythemia vera). The symptoms vary greatly. Because of the variety of causes of headache, clinical evaluation must be thorough. It should include an evaluation of personality, life adjustment, environment, and family situation, as well as a comprehensive evaluation of neurologic and physical status.

COLLABORATIVE CARE FOR HEADACHES

If no systemic underlying disease is the cause, the type of headache guides therapy. Table 59-2 outlines the general workup for a patient with headache to rule out any intracranial or extracranial disease. Table 59-3 summarizes the current therapies for prophylaxis and symptom relief of common headaches. These therapies include drugs, meditation, yoga, biofeedback, cognitive-behavioral therapy, and relaxation training.

Cognitive-behavioral therapy and relaxation therapy used alone or in conjunction with drug therapy may be beneficial to some patients. Biofeedback involves the use of physiologic monitoring equipment to give the patient information regarding muscle tension and peripheral blood flow (e.g., skin temperature of the fingers). The patient is trained to relax the muscles and raise the finger temperature, and is given reinforcement (operant conditioning) in accomplishing these changes.

Acupuncture, acupressure, and hypnosis also work well in some patients with headaches. See Chapters 6 and 7 for further description of these therapies.

Drug Therapy

Tension-Type Headache. Drug treatment for tension-type headache usually involves aspirin, acetaminophen (Tylenol), or nonsteroidal antiinflammatory drugs (NSAIDs) used alone or in combination with a sedative, muscle relaxant, or tranquilizer. However, many of these drugs have serious side effects. Caution the patient about the long-term use of aspirin and aspirin-containing drugs because they can cause upper gastrointestinal (GI) bleeding and coagulation abnormalities in susceptible patients. Drugs containing acetaminophen can cause kidney damage with chronic use and liver damage when taking large doses or when combined with alcohol. To decrease the recurrence of tension-type headache, the patient may receive preventive therapy with a tricyclic antidepressant (e.g., amitriptyline [Elavil], nortriptyline) or topiramate (Topamax), divalproex (Depakote), or mirtazapine (Remeron).

Migraine Headache. The aim of drug treatment of an acute migraine attack is terminating or decreasing the symptoms. Many people with mild or moderate migraine can obtain relief with NSAIDs, aspirin, or caffeine-containing combination analgesics. For moderate to severe headaches, the triptans have become the first line of therapy. Triptans (e.g., sumatriptan [Imitrex]) affect selected serotonin receptors, thus reducing neurogenic inflammation of the cerebral blood vessels and producing vasoconstriction (see Table 59-3). They are most effective when taken at the onset of migraine headache or during the aura. Sumatriptan is available in various forms: oral, subcutaneous, nasal spray.

Some patients respond better to one triptan than to others, so health care providers need to be knowledgeable about all of them. Because these drugs cause vasoconstriction, patients with heart disease or stroke should avoid their use. The combination drug sumatriptan/naproxen (Treximet) combines a triptan with an antiinflammatory drug. Risk of serious cardiovascular events such as myocardial infarction, thromboembolic events, and stroke may increase over time with Treximet. When triptans are contraindicated, other drugs can be used (see Table 59-3).

> **DRUG ALERT: Sumatriptan (Imitrex)**
> - Should not be given to patients with the following:
>   - History or manifestations of ischemic cardiac, cerebrovascular, or peripheral vascular problems
>   - Uncontrolled hypertension, since it may increase blood pressure
> - Excess dosage may produce tremor and decrease respirations.

Preventive treatment is important in the management of migraine headaches. The decision to initiate prophylactic treatment is individually determined based on frequency, severity, and any disability related to headaches. Several different classes of medications are used.

Topiramate, an antiseizure drug, taken daily is an effective therapy for migraine prevention. Common side effects include hypoglycemia, paresthesia, weight loss, and cognitive changes. Usually these side effects are mild to moderate and transient. Topiramate must be used for 2 to 3 months to determine its effectiveness. Not all patients will become pain free on this medication. Health care providers must provide adequate teaching regarding topiramate to promote patient adherence.

TABLE 59-3   COLLABORATIVE CARE

Headaches

Tension-Type Headache	Migraine Headache	Cluster Headache
Diagnostic		
History*	History*	History
Collaborative Therapy		
Abortive/Symptomatic Drugs		
Nonopioid analgesics: aspirin, acetaminophen, NSAIDs	Nonopioid analgesics: aspirin, NSAIDs	α-Adrenergic blocker
Analgesic combinations	Serotonin receptor agonists	• ergotamine tartrate
• butalbital/aspirin/caffeine (Fiorinal)	• almotriptan (Axert)	O₂ 100%
• butalbital/acetaminophen/caffeine (Fioricet)	• eletriptan (Relpax)	Serotonin receptor agonists
• dichloralphenazone/acetaminophen/isometheptene (Midrin)	• frovatriptan (Frova)	• almotriptan
Muscle relaxants	• naratriptan (Amerge)	• eletriptan
	• rizatriptan (Maxalt)	• frovatriptan
	• sumatriptan (Imitrex)	• naratriptan
	• zolmitriptan (Zomig)	• rizatriptan
	Combination	• sumatriptan
	• sumatriptan/naproxen (Treximet)	• zolmitriptan
	α-Adrenergic blockers	
	• ergotamine tartrate (Ergomar)	
	• dihydroergotamine (DHE)	
	Analgesic combinations	
	• acetaminophen/caffeine/aspirin	
	• acetaminophen/isometheptene/dichloralphenazone	
	Corticosteroids	
	• dexamethasone (Decadron)	
Preventive/Prophylactic Drugs		
Tricyclic antidepressants	β-Adrenergic blocker	α-Adrenergic blocker
• amitriptyline (Elavil)	• propranolol	• ergotamine tartrate
• nortriptyline (Pamelor)	Antidepressants	Serotonin antagonist
• doxepin (Sinequan)	• amitriptyline	• methysergide
Selective serotonin reuptake inhibitors	• imipramine (Tofranil)	Corticosteroid
• fluoxetine (Prozac)	Antiseizure	• prednisone
• paroxetine (Paxil)	• valproic acid (Depakene)	Calcium channel blocker
β-Adrenergic blocker:	• divalproex	• verapamil
• propranolol (Inderal)	• topiramate (Topamax)	Lithium
Other drugs	• gabapentin (Neurontin)	Biofeedback
• topiramate (Topamax)	Calcium channel blockers	
• divalproex (Depakote)	• verapamil (Calan)	
• mirtazapine (Remeron)	• flunarizine (Sibelium)	
Biofeedback	Serotonin antagonist†	
Psychotherapy	• methysergide (Sansert)	
Muscle relaxation training	Botulinum toxin A (Botox)	
	Biofeedback	
	Relaxation therapy	
	Cognitive-behavioral therapy	

*Diagnostic imaging should be considered in nonacute headache patients with unexplained abnormal neurologic examination, atypical headache, headache features, or an additional risk factor such as immunodeficiency.

†Only for patients suffering from one or more severe headaches per week.

DRUG ALERT: Topiramate (Topamax)
- Instruct patient to do the following:
  - Not abruptly discontinue, since this may cause seizures.
  - Avoid tasks that require alertness until response to drug is established.
  - Take adequate fluids to decrease risk of renal stone development.

Botulinum toxin A (Botox) may be an effective prophylactic treatment for patients who have chronic migraines lasting for 4 hours or more at least 15 days each month, or migraines that do not respond to other medications. Botox is given by multiple injections around the head and neck. Its effects last 2 to 4 months; the injections are repeated every 3 months. The most common adverse reactions are neck pain and headache. There is a slight risk of the toxin migrating from the injection site to other areas of the face and neck, causing swallowing and breath-

ing difficulties. Teach the patient to seek immediate medical attention if this occurs.[5]

Additional antiseizure drugs used in migraine prevention are divalproex and gabapentin (Neurontin). Antidepressants used in migraine prophylaxis include tricyclic antidepressants (e.g., amitriptyline) and selective serotonin reuptake inhibitors (e.g., fluoxetine [Prozac]). Other drugs used for migraine headache prevention are listed in Table 59-3.

Cluster Headache. Because cluster headaches occur suddenly, often at night, and do not last long, drug therapy is not as useful as it is for other types of headaches. Acute treatment of cluster headache is inhalation of 100% oxygen delivered at a rate of 6 to 8 L/min for 10 minutes, which may relieve headache by causing vasoconstriction and increasing synthesis of sero-

EVIDENCE-BASED PRACTICE

Translating Research Into Practice

Can Botulinum Toxin A Prevent Headaches?

Clinical Question

For adults with chronic headaches (P), does prophylactic botulinum toxin A (I) vs. placebo vs. medication (C) decrease headache frequency or severity (O)?

Best Available Evidence

Meta-analysis of randomized controlled trials (RCTs) and comparative effectiveness trials

Critical Appraisal and Synthesis of Evidence

- Twenty-seven RCTs (*n* = 5313) comparing botulinum toxin A (Botox) with placebo, and four trials comparing Botox with medication (amitriptyline [Elavil], topiramate [Topamax], valproic acid [Depakote]).
- Headaches assessed were migraine or tension, episodic (<15 headaches per month) or chronic (>15 headaches per month), and a chronic daily headache.
- Botox resulted in decreased frequency of chronic daily and chronic migraine headaches. It had no effect on episodic migraine or chronic tension-type headaches.
- Botox was not related to fewer migraine headaches when compared with valproic acid, topiramate, or amitriptyline.

Conclusion

- Botox is beneficial for chronic daily headaches and chronic migraine headaches.

Implications for Nursing Practice

- Inform patients that Botox can prevent some types of headaches.
- Advise patients of Botox side effects, including blepharoptosis, paresthesia, neck stiffness and pain, and muscle weakness.

Reference for Evidence

Jackson JL, Kuriyama A, Hayashino Y: Botulinum toxin A for prophylactic treatment of migraine and tension headaches in adults: a meta-analysis, *JAMA* 307:1736, 2012.

P, Patient population of interest; *I,* intervention or area of interest; *C,* comparison of interest or comparison group; *O,* outcomes of interest (see p. 12).

tonin in the central nervous system. This can be repeated after a 5-minute rest. However, a drawback to this treatment is that the patient must have continuous access to the oxygen supply. The triptans (e.g., sumatriptan) are also effective in treating acute cluster headache. Intranasal administration of lidocaine is useful as an adjunctive therapy.[6]

Prophylactic drugs may include verapamil, lithium, ergotamine, divalproex, melatonin, or antiseizure medications. If the cluster headache recurs at a known time, prophylactic methysergide may be used. Options for patients with refractory cluster headaches include invasive nerve blocks, deep brain stimulation, and ablative neurosurgical procedures (e.g., percutaneous radiofrequency).

Other Headaches. Patients with frequent headaches may overuse analgesic drugs. *Medication overuse headache* (MOH) is the term used to describe an analgesic rebound headache. Drugs known to cause this problem are acetaminophen, aspirin, NSAIDs (e.g., ibuprofen), butalbital, sumatriptan, and opioids. Patients with daily headaches may complain of early awakening with decreased appetite, nausea, restlessness, decreased memory, and irritability. Treatment involves abrupt withdrawal of the offending drug (except for opioids, which need to be tapered) and initiation of alternative drugs such as amitriptyline.

TABLE 59-4 NURSING ASSESSMENT

Headaches

Subjective Data
Important Health Information

Past health history: Seizures, cancer, recent fall or trauma, cranial infection, stroke; asthma or allergies; mental illness; relationship of headache to overwork, stress, menstruation, exercise, food, sexual activity, travel, bright lights, or noxious environmental stimuli

Medications: Hydralazine (Apresoline), bromides, nitroglycerin, ergotamine (withdrawal), nonsteroidal antiinflammatory drugs (in high daily doses), estrogen preparations, oral contraceptives, over-the-counter or prescription remedies

Surgery or other treatments: Craniotomy, sinus surgery, facial surgery

Functional Health Patterns

Health perception–health management: Positive family history; malaise

Nutritional-metabolic: Ingestion of alcohol, caffeine, cheese, chocolate, monosodium glutamate, aspartame, lunch meats (nitrites in cured meats), sausage, hot dogs, onions, avocados; anorexia, nausea, vomiting (migraine prodrome); unilateral lacrimation (cluster)

Activity-exercise: Vertigo, fatigue, weakness, paralysis, fainting

Sleep-rest: Insomnia

Cognitive-perceptual

- *Migraine:* Aura; unilateral, severe, throbbing (possible switching of side) headache; visual disturbances; photophobia; phonophobia; dizziness; tingling or burning sensations
- *Cluster:* Unilateral and severe, nocturnal headache; nasal stuffiness
- *Tension-type:* Bilateral, bandlike, dull and persistent, base-of-skull headache, neck tenderness

Self-perception–self-concept: Depression

Coping–stress tolerance: Stress, anxiety, irritability, withdrawal

Objective Data
General

Anxiety, apprehension

Integumentary

Cluster: Forehead diaphoresis, pallor, unilateral facial flushing with cheek edema, conjunctivitis

Migraine: Generalized edema (prodrome), pallor, diaphoresis

Neurologic

Horner's syndrome, restlessness (cluster), hemiparesis (migraine)

Musculoskeletal

Resistance of head and neck movement, nuchal rigidity (meningeal, tension-type), palpable neck and shoulder muscle tension (tension-type)

Possible Diagnostic Findings

Evidence of disease, deformity, or infection on brain imaging (CT, MRI, MRA), cerebral angiogram, lumbar puncture, EEG, EMG; nonspecific brain imaging or laboratory tests

EMG, Electromyography; *MRA,* magnetic resonance angiography.

NURSING MANAGEMENT
HEADACHES

NURSING ASSESSMENT

Table 59-4 outlines subjective and objective data you should obtain from a patient with headache. Because the history provides the key to assessment of headache, it should include specific details of the headache itself, such as the location and type of pain, onset, frequency, duration, relation to events (emotional, psychologic, physical), and time of day of the occurrence. Obtain information about previous illnesses, surgery, trauma, allergies, family history, and response to medication.

Suggest that the patient keep a diary of headache episodes with specific details. This type of record can be of great help in determining the type of headache and the precipitating events. If the patient has a history of migraine, tension-type, or cluster headaches, it is important to determine if the character, intensity, or location of the headache has changed. This may be an important clue as to the cause of the headache.

NURSING DIAGNOSES

Nursing diagnoses for the patient with headache may include, but are not limited to, the following:

- Acute pain *related to* headache
- Ineffective self-health management *related to* drug therapy and lifestyle adjustments

Additional information on nursing diagnoses is presented in eNursing Care Plan 59-1 for the patient with headache (available on the website for this chapter).

PLANNING

The overall goals are that the patient with a headache will (1) have reduced or no pain, (2) demonstrate understanding of triggering events and treatment strategies, (3) use positive coping strategies to deal with pain, and (4) experience increased quality of life and decreased disability.

NURSING IMPLEMENTATION

Patients with chronic headache present a great challenge to health care providers. Since an inability to cope with daily stresses can cause headaches, an effective therapy may be to help patients examine their lifestyle, recognize stressful situations, and learn to cope with them more appropriately. Help the patient identify precipitating factors and develop ways to avoid them. Encourage daily exercise, relaxation periods, and socialization because each can help decrease the recurrence of headache. Suggest alternative ways of handling headache pain through techniques such as relaxation, meditation, and yoga.

In addition to using analgesics and analgesic combinations for symptomatic relief of headache, encourage the migraine sufferer to seek a quiet, dimly lit environment. Massage and moist hot packs to the neck and head can help a patient with tension-type headaches. The patient should learn about the drugs prescribed for preventive/prophylactic and abortive/symptomatic treatment of headache and should be able to describe the purpose, action, dosage, and side effects of the drugs. To prevent accidental overdose, the patient should make a written note of each dose of drug or headache remedy.

For the patient with headaches triggered by food, provide dietary counseling. Encourage the patient to eliminate foods that may provoke headaches, such as chocolate, cheese, oranges, tomatoes, onions, monosodium glutamate, aspartame, alcohol (particularly red wine), excessive caffeine, and fermented or marinated foods. Active challenge and provocative testing with specific foods may be necessary to determine the specific causative agents. However, food triggers may change over time.

Teach patients to avoid smoking and exposure to triggers such as strong perfumes, volatile solvents, and gasoline fumes. Cluster headache attacks may occur at high altitudes with low oxygen levels during air travel. Ergotamine, taken before the plane takes off, may decrease the likelihood of these attacks. See Table 59-5 for a teaching guide for the patient with a headache.

TABLE 59-5 PATIENT & CAREGIVER TEACHING GUIDE

Headaches

Include the following instructions when teaching the patient with a headache and the patient's caregiver.

1. Keep a diary or calendar of headaches and possible precipitating events.
2. Avoid factors that can trigger a headache:
   - Foods containing amines (cheese, chocolate), nitrites (meats such as hot dogs), vinegar, onions, monosodium glutamate
   - Fermented or marinated foods
   - Caffeine
   - Oranges
   - Tomatoes
   - Aspartame
   - Nicotine
   - Ice cream
   - Alcohol (particularly red wine)
   - Emotional stress
   - Fatigue
   - Drugs such as ergot-containing preparations (ergotamine tartrate [Ergomar]) and monoamine oxidase inhibitors (e.g., rasagiline [Azilect])
3. Learn the purpose, action, dosage, and side effects of drugs taken.
4. Self-administer sumatriptan (Imitrex) subcutaneously if prescribed.
5. Use stress management techniques such as relaxation.
6. Participate in regular exercise.
7. Contact health care provider if any of the following occurs:
   - Symptoms become more severe, last longer than usual, or are resistant to medication.
   - Nausea and vomiting (if severe or not typical), change in vision, or fever occurs with the headache.
   - Problems occur with any drugs.

EVALUATION

Expected outcomes are that the patient with headache will

- Report satisfaction with pain relief
- Use drug and nondrug measures appropriately to manage pain

Additional information on expected outcomes for the patient with headache is presented in eNursing Care Plan 59-1 (available on the website for this chapter).

CHRONIC NEUROLOGIC DISORDERS

SEIZURE DISORDERS AND EPILEPSY

Seizure is a paroxysmal, uncontrolled electrical discharge of neurons in the brain that interrupts normal function. Seizures may accompany a variety of disorders, or they may occur spontaneously without any apparent cause. Seizures resulting from systemic and metabolic disturbances are not considered epilepsy if the seizures cease when the underlying problem is corrected. Metabolic disturbances that cause seizures include acidosis, electrolyte imbalances, hypoglycemia, hypoxia, alcohol and barbiturate withdrawal, dehydration, and water intoxication. Extracranial disorders that can cause seizures are heart, lung, liver, or kidney diseases; systemic lupus erythematosus; diabetes mellitus; hypertension; and septicemia.

Epilepsy is a condition in which a person has spontaneous recurring seizures caused by a chronic underlying condition. In the United States, it is estimated that more than 3 million people have active epilepsy, with 200,000 new cases diagnosed each year. National trends show that the incidence of epilepsy is increasing in older adults. New cases of epilepsy are more common in African Americans and in socially disadvantaged populations. Males are slightly more likely to develop epilepsy than females. People at high risk for developing epilepsy include those with Alzheimer's disease or those who have had a stroke. The risk is also increased in the child of a person who has epilepsy.[7]

Etiology and Pathophysiology

Seizure disorders have many possible causes, with the most common causes varying by age. The most common causes of seizure disorder during the first 6 months of life are severe birth injury, congenital defects involving the central nervous system (CNS), infections, and inborn errors of metabolism. In people between 2 and 20 years of age, the primary causes are birth injury, infection, trauma, and genetic factors. In individuals between 20 and 30 years of age, seizure disorder usually occurs as the result of structural lesions, such as trauma, brain tumors, or vascular disease. After 50 years of age, the primary causes of seizure disorders are stroke and metastatic brain tumors. However, nearly 30% of all epilepsy cases are idiopathic, called *idiopathic generalized epilepsy (IGE)*, meaning they are not attributable to a specific cause.

The etiology of recurring seizures (epilepsy) has long been attributed to a group of abnormal neurons *(seizure focus)* that seem to undergo spontaneous firing. This firing spreads by physiologic pathways to involve adjacent or distant areas of the brain. If this activity spreads to involve the whole brain, a generalized seizure occurs. The factor that causes this abnormal firing is not clear. Any stimulus that causes the cell membrane of the neuron to depolarize induces a tendency for spontaneous firing.

Scar tissue (gliosis) is often found in the area of the brain from which the epileptic activity arises. Scarring is believed to interfere with the normal chemical and structural environment of the brain neurons, making them more likely to fire abnormally.

In addition to neuronal alterations, changes in the function of astrocytes may play several key roles in recurring seizures. Activation of astrocytes by hyperactive neurons is one of the crucial factors that predispose neurons nearby to the generation of an epileptic discharge.

🧬 Genetic Link

Genetic abnormalities may be the most important factor contributing to IGE. Some types of epilepsy tend to run in families, suggesting a genetic influence. Other types of IGE are related to abnormalities in specific genes that control the flow of ions in and out of cells and regulate neuron signaling or are involved with protein and carbohydrate metabolism. Some researchers estimate that more than 500 genes could play a role in IGE.[8]

The role of genetics in the etiology of seizure disorders has been difficult to determine because of the problem of separating genetic from environmental or acquired influences. In some forms of epilepsy, families carry a predisposition to seizure disorders in the form of an inherently low threshold to seizure-producing stimuli, such as trauma, disease, and high fever.

Abnormal genes may influence the disorder in subtle ways. For example, a person with epilepsy may have an abnormally active version of a gene that increases resistance to drugs. This may help explain why antiseizure drugs do not work for some people.

TABLE 59-6	**CLASSIFICATION OF SEIZURE DISORDERS**
Generalized Seizures (Nonfocal Origin)	**Focal Seizures (Focal Origin)**

• Tonic-clonic seizures
• Absence seizures
  • Typical
  • Atypical
  • Absence with special features
• Myoclonic seizures
• Tonic seizures
• Atonic seizures (drop attacks)
• Clonic seizures
	• Simple focal seizures (no impairment of consciousness)
	• Complex focal seizures (impairment of consciousness)
	• Focal seizures evolving to secondary generalized seizures
	Unknown

Adapted from Berg AT, Berkovic SF, Brodie MJ, et al: Revised terminology and concepts for organization of seizures and epilepsies: report of the ILAE Commission on Classification and Terminology, 2005-2009, International League Against Epilepsy, *Epilepsia* 5:676, 2010.

Clinical Manifestations

The specific clinical manifestations of a seizure are determined by the site of the electrical disturbance.[9] The preferred method of classifying seizures is presented in Table 59-6. This system, which is based on the clinical and electroencephalographic manifestations of seizures, divides seizures into two major classes: *generalized* and *focal* (Fig. 59-2). Depending on the type, a seizure may progress through several phases: (1) the *prodromal phase,* with signs or activity that precede a seizure; (2) the *aural phase,* with a sensory warning; (3) the *ictal phase,* with full seizure; and (4) the *postictal phase,* the period of recovery after the seizure.

Generalized Seizures. Generalized seizures involve both sides of the brain and are characterized by bilateral synchronous epileptic discharges in the brain from the onset of the seizure. In most cases the patient loses consciousness for a few seconds to several minutes.

Tonic-Clonic Seizures. The most common generalized seizure is the generalized tonic-clonic (formerly known as *grand mal*) seizure. Tonic-clonic seizure is characterized by losing consciousness and falling to the ground if the patient is upright, followed by stiffening of the body (tonic phase) for 10 to 20 seconds and subsequent jerking of the extremities (clonic phase) for another 30 to 40 seconds. Cyanosis, excessive salivation, tongue or cheek biting, and incontinence may accompany the seizure.

In the postictal phase the patient usually has muscle soreness, is tired, and may sleep for several hours. Some patients may not feel normal for several hours or days after a seizure. The patient has no memory of the seizure.

Typical Absence Seizures. The absence seizure (formerly called petit mal) usually occurs only in children and rarely continues beyond adolescence. This type of seizure may cease altogether as the child matures, or it may evolve into another type of seizure. The typical clinical manifestation is a brief staring spell resembling "daydreaming" that lasts only a few seconds, so it often goes unnoticed. When untreated, the seizures may occur up to 100 times a day. The electroencephalogram (EEG) demonstrates a 3-Hz (cycles per second) spike-and-wave pattern that is unique to this type of seizure. Hyperventilation and flashing lights can precipitate absence seizures.

Atypical Absence Seizures. Another type of generalized seizure is *atypical absence seizure,* which is characterized by a

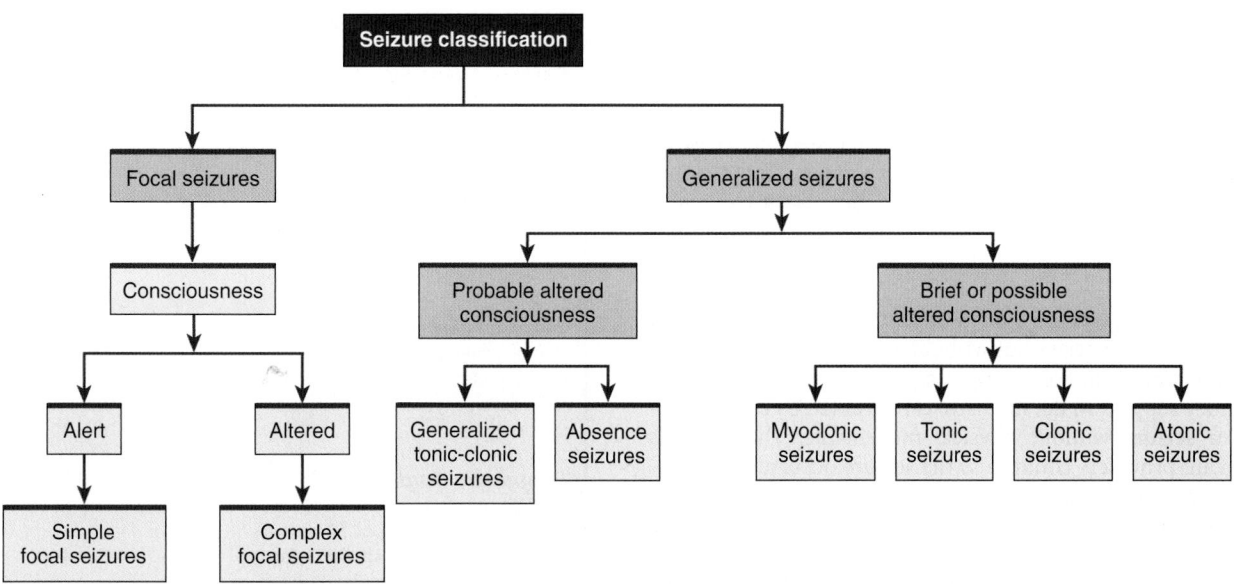

FIG. 59-2 Algorithm for classification of seizures.

staring spell accompanied by other signs and symptoms, including brief warnings, peculiar behavior during the seizure, or confusion after the seizure. It is longer lasting than a typical absence seizure and may be associated with loss of postural tone. The EEG demonstrates atypical spike-and-wave patterns, usually greater or less than 3 Hz.

Other Types of Generalized Seizures. Other generalized seizures are myoclonic, atonic, tonic, and clonic seizures. A *myoclonic seizure* is characterized by a sudden, excessive jerk of the body or extremities. The jerk may be forceful enough to hurl the person to the ground. These seizures are brief and may occur in clusters.

An *atonic* ("drop attack") seizure involves either a tonic episode or a paroxysmal loss of muscle tone and begins suddenly with the person falling to the ground. Consciousness usually returns by the time the person hits the ground, and normal activity can be resumed immediately. Patients with this type of seizure are at a great risk of head injury and often have to wear protective helmets.

A *tonic* seizure involves a sudden onset of maintained increased tone in the extensor muscles. These patients often fall.

Clonic seizures begin with loss of consciousness and sudden loss of muscle tone, followed by limb jerking that may or may not be symmetric.

Focal Seizures. Focal seizures, also called partial or partial focal seizures, are the other major class of seizures (see Table 59-6). Focal seizures begin in one hemisphere of the brain in a specific region of the cortex, as indicated by the EEG. They produce signs and symptoms related to the function of the area of the brain involved. For example, if the discharging focus is located in the medial aspect of the postcentral gyrus, the patient may experience paresthesias and tingling or numbness in the leg on the side opposite the focus. If the discharging focus is located in the part of the brain that governs a particular function, sensory, motor, cognitive, or emotional manifestations may occur.

Focal seizures are divided according to their clinical expression into (1) simple focal seizures (the person remains conscious) and (2) complex focal seizures (the person has a change or loss of consciousness).[8] In a *simple focal seizure*, patients

remain conscious but experience unusual feelings or sensations that can take many forms. They may experience sudden and unexplainable feelings of joy, anger, sadness, or nausea. They also may hear, smell, taste, see, or feel things that are not real.

In a *complex focal seizure*, patients have a loss of consciousness or an alteration in their consciousness, producing a dreamlike experience. They display strange behavior such as lip smacking and *automatisms* (repetitive movements that may not be appropriate). Patients may continue an activity started before the seizure, such as counting out change or picking items from a grocery shelf, but after the seizure they do not remember the activity performed during the seizure. Other automatisms are less organized, such as picking at clothing, fumbling with objects (real or imaginary), or simply walking away. These seizures usually last just a few seconds.

Focal seizures may be confined to one side of the brain and remain focal (partial) in nature, or they may spread to involve the entire brain, culminating in a generalized tonic-clonic seizure. Any tonic-clonic seizure that is preceded by an aura or warning is a focal seizure that generalizes secondarily. Many tonic-clonic seizures that appear to be generalized from the outset may actually be secondary generalized seizures, but the preceding partial component may be so brief that it is undetected by the patient, by the observer, or even on the EEG. Unlike the primary generalized tonic-clonic seizure, the secondary generalized seizure may result in a transient residual neurologic deficit postictally. This is called *Todd's paralysis* (focal weakness), which resolves after varying lengths of time.

Psychogenic Seizures. Psychogenic seizures, also called pseudoseizures, are seizures that are psychiatric in origin. Since they closely resemble epileptic seizures, psychogenic seizures may be misdiagnosed as epilepsy. Proper diagnosis usually requires video-EEG monitoring to capture a typical episode. Patients with psychogenic seizures frequently have a history of emotional abuse, physical neglect, or a specific traumatic episode.[10]

Complications

Physical. Status epilepticus is a state of continuous seizure activity or a condition in which seizures recur in rapid succession without return to consciousness between seizures. It is the most serious complication of epilepsy and is a neurologic emergency. Status epilepticus can occur with any type of seizure. During repeated seizures the brain uses more energy than can be supplied. Neurons become exhausted and cease to function. Permanent brain damage may result. Tonic-clonic status epilepticus is the most dangerous because it can cause ventilatory insufficiency, hypoxemia, cardiac dysrhythmias, hyperthermia, and systemic acidosis, all of which can be fatal.

Subclinical seizures are a form of status epilepticus in which the sedated patient seizes but without external signs because of sedating medication. For example, a patient under sedation for ventilatory support in the intensive care unit (ICU) could experience a seizure without physical movements. The patient's health care providers could miss the seizure occurrence.

Another complication of seizures is severe injury and even death from trauma suffered during a seizure. Patients who lose consciousness during a seizure are at greatest risk.

Persons with epilepsy have a mortality rate that is two or three times the rate of the general population. Forty percent of these deaths are related to epilepsy because of accidents occurring during seizures, suicide, treatment-related death, death from an underlying disease, and sudden unexplained or unexpected death in epilepsy (SUDEP). SUDEP is higher in males, those on multiple antiseizure medications, and patients with long-standing epilepsy. The direct cause of SUDEP is unknown, but is thought to be related to respiratory dysfunction, cardiac dysrhythmias, or cerebral depression.[11]

Psychosocial. Perhaps the most common complication of seizure disorders is the effect it has on a patient's lifestyle. The patient may develop ineffective coping methods because of the psychosocial problems related to having a seizure disorder. Although attitudes have improved in recent years, epilepsy still carries a social stigma. The patient with epilepsy may experience discrimination in employment and educational opportunities. Transportation may be difficult because of legal sanctions against driving.

Diagnostic Studies

A diagnosis of epilepsy or seizure disorder has many socioeconomic, physical, and psychologic consequences for the patient. Therefore an accurate diagnosis is crucial. The most useful diagnostic tools are an accurate and comprehensive description of the seizures and the patient's health history (Table 59-7). The EEG is a useful diagnostic adjuvant to the history, but only if it shows abnormalities. Abnormal findings help determine the type of seizure and help pinpoint the seizure focus. Ideally, an EEG should be done within 24 hours of a suspected seizure. Unfortunately, only a small percentage of patients with seizure disorders have abnormal findings on the EEG the first time the test is done. Either repeated EEGs or continuous EEG monitoring may be needed to detect abnormalities. An EEG is not a definitive test because some patients who do not have seizure disorders have abnormal patterns on their EEGs, whereas many patients with seizure disorders have normal EEGs between seizures. If abnormal discharges do not occur during the 30 to 40 minutes of sampling during EEG, the test may not indicate an abnormality. Magnetoencephalography may be done in conjunction with the EEG. This test has greater sensitivity in detecting small magnetic fields generated by neuronal activity.

TABLE 59-7 COLLABORATIVE CARE

Seizure Disorders and Epilepsy

Diagnostic
History and Physical Examination
- Birth and developmental history
- Significant illnesses and injuries
- Family history
- Febrile seizures
- Comprehensive neurologic assessment

Seizure History
- Precipitating factors
- Antecedent events
- Seizure description (including onset, duration, frequency, postictal state)

Diagnostic Studies
- CBC, urinalysis, electrolytes, creatinine, fasting blood glucose
- Lumbar puncture for CSF analysis
- CT, MRI, MRA, MRS, PET scan
- Electroencephalography (EEG)

Collaborative Therapy
- Antiseizure drugs (see Table 59-9)
- Surgery (see Table 59-10)
- Vagal nerve stimulation
- Psychosocial counseling

MRA, Magnetic resonance angiography; *MRS,* magnetic resonance spectroscopy; *PET,* positron emission tomography.

A complete blood count, serum chemistries, studies of liver and kidney function, and a urinalysis should be done to rule out metabolic disorders. A CT scan or MRI should be done in any new-onset seizure to rule out a structural lesion. Cerebral angiography, single-photon emission computed tomography (SPECT), magnetic resonance spectroscopy (MRS), MRA, and positron emission tomography (PET) may be used in selected clinical situations.

If a patient is diagnosed with a seizure disorder, it is important to classify the seizure type correctly (see Fig. 59-2 and Table 59-6). The choice of treatment depends on the type of seizure.

Collaborative Care

Most seizures do not require professional emergency medical care because they are self-limiting and rarely cause bodily injury. However, if status epilepticus occurs, if significant bodily harm occurs, or if the event is a first-time seizure, medical care should be sought immediately. Table 59-8 summarizes emergency care of the patient with a generalized tonic-clonic seizure, the seizure most likely to warrant professional emergency medical care. Table 59-7 outlines the diagnostic studies and collaborative care of seizure disorders.

Drug Therapy. The primary treatment for seizure disorders is antiseizure drugs (Table 59-9). Because a cure is not possible, the goal of therapy is to prevent seizures with a minimum of toxic side effects from drug therapy. Medications control seizures in about 70% of the patients. Drugs generally act by stabilizing nerve cell membranes and preventing spread of the epileptic discharge. The principle of drug therapy is to begin with a single drug based on the patient's age and weight; type, frequency, and cause of seizure; and then increase the dosage until seizures are controlled or toxic side effects occur.

✚ TABLE 59-8 EMERGENCY MANAGEMENT

Tonic-Clonic Seizures

Etiology	Assessment Findings	Interventions
Head Trauma • Epidural hematoma • Subdural hematoma • Intracranial hematoma • Cerebral contusion • Traumatic birth injury **Drug-Related Processes** • Overdose • Withdrawal of alcohol, opioids, antiseizure drugs • Ingestion, inhalation **Infectious Processes** • Meningitis • Septicemia • Encephalitis **Intracranial Events** • Brain tumor • Subarachnoid hemorrhage • Stroke • Hypertensive crisis • Increased ICP secondary to clogged shunt **Metabolic Imbalances** • Fluid and electrolyte imbalance • Hypoglycemia **Medical Disorders** • Heart, liver, lung, or kidney disease • Systemic lupus erythematosus **Other** • Cardiac arrest • Idiopathic • Psychiatric disorders • High fever	• Aura (peculiar sensations that precede seizure) • Loss of consciousness • Bowel and bladder incontinence • Tachycardia • Diaphoresis • Warm skin • Pallor, flushing, or cyanosis • *Tonic phase:* Continuous muscle contractions • *Hypertonic phase:* Extreme muscular rigidity lasting 5–15 sec • *Clonic phase:* Rigidity and relaxation alternating in rapid succession • *Postictal phase:* Lethargy, altered level of consciousness • Confusion and headache • Repeated tonic-clonic seizures for several min	**Initial** • Ensure patent airway. • Protect patient from injury during seizure. *Do not restrain.* Pad side rails. • Remove or loosen tight clothing. • Establish IV access. • Stay with patient until seizure has passed. • Anticipate administration of phenobarbital, phenytoin (Dilantin), or benzodiazepines (e.g., diazepam [Valium], midazolam [Versed], lorazepam [Ativan]) to control seizures. • Suction as needed. • Assist ventilations if patient does not breathe spontaneously after seizure. Anticipate need for intubation if gag reflex absent. **Ongoing Monitoring** • Monitor vital signs, level of consciousness, O₂ saturation, Glasgow Coma Scale results, pupil size and reactivity. • Reassure and orient the patient after seizure. • Never force an airway between a patient's clenched teeth. • Give IV dextrose for hypoglycemia.

ICP, Intracranial pressure.

If seizure control is not achieved with a single drug, the drug dosage or timing of administration may be changed or a second drug may be added. About one third of patients require a combination regimen for adequate control.

The therapeutic range for each drug indicates the serum level above which most patients experience toxic side effects and below which most continue to have seizures. Therapeutic drug ranges are only guides for therapy. If the patient's seizures are well controlled with a subtherapeutic level, the drug dosage need not be increased. Likewise, if a drug level is above the therapeutic range and the patient has good seizure control without toxic side effects, the drug dosage does not need to be decreased. Serum drug levels are monitored if seizures continue to occur, if seizure frequency increases, or if drug adherence is questioned. Many of the newer drugs do not require drug-level monitoring because the therapeutic range is very large.

The primary drugs to treat generalized tonic-clonic and focal seizures are phenytoin (Dilantin), carbamazepine (Tegretol), phenobarbital, divalproex, and primidone (Mysoline). The drugs used to treat absence and myoclonic seizures include ethosuximide (Zarontin), divalproex, and clonazepam (Klonopin).

TABLE 59-9 DRUG THERAPY

Seizure Disorders and Epilepsy

Generalized Tonic-Clonic and Focal Seizures	Absence and Myoclonic Seizures
• carbamazepine (Tegretol) • divalproex (Depakote) • ezogabine (Potiga) • felbamate (Felbatol) • gabapentin (Neurontin) • lacosamide (Vimpat) • lamotrigine (Lamictal) • levetiracetam (Keppra) • oxcarbazepine (Trileptal) • perampanel (Fycompa) • phenobarbital (Luminal) • phenytoin (Dilantin) • pregabalin (Lyrica) • primidone (Mysoline) • tiagabine (Gabitril) • topiramate (Topamax) • valproic acid (Depakene) • vigabatrin (Sabril) • zonisamide (Zonegran)	• clonazepam (Klonopin) • divalproex (Depakote) • ethosuximide (Zarontin) • zonisamide (Zonegran)

DRUG ALERT: Carbamazepine (Tegretol)
- Do not take with grapefruit juice.
- Instruct patient to report visual abnormalities.
- Abrupt withdrawal after long-term use may precipitate seizures.

Other antiseizure drugs include gabapentin, topiramate, lamotrigine (Lamictal), tiagabine (Gabitril), levetiracetam (Keppra), and zonisamide (Zonegran). Some of these drugs are broad spectrum and appear to be effective for multiple seizure types. Pregabalin (Lyrica) is used as an "add-on" for control of focal seizures that are not successfully managed with a single medication.

Treatment of status epilepticus requires initiation of a rapid-acting IV antiseizure drug. The drugs most commonly used are lorazepam (Ativan) and diazepam (Valium). Because these are short-acting drugs, their administration is followed with long-acting drugs such as phenytoin or phenobarbital.

Because many of the antiseizure drugs (e.g., phenytoin, phenobarbital, ethosuximide, lamotrigine, topiramate) have a long half-life, they can be given in once- or twice-daily doses. This increases the patient's adherence to the drug regimen by simplifying it and avoiding the need to take the drug at work or school.

DRUG ALERT: Antiseizure Drugs
- Abrupt withdrawal after long-term use may precipitate seizures.
- If weaning is to occur, the patient must be seizure free for a prolonged period (e.g., 2 to 5 yr) and have a normal neurologic examination and EEG.

Side effects of antiseizure drugs involve the CNS and include diplopia, drowsiness, ataxia, and mental slowness. Neurologic assessment for dose-related toxicity involves testing the eyes for nystagmus, hand and gait coordination, cognitive functioning, and general alertness.

As a nurse, you need to be knowledgeable about these side effects so that patients can be informed and institute proper treatment. A common side effect of phenytoin is gingival hyperplasia (excessive growth of gingival tissue) and hirsutism, especially in young adults. Good dental hygiene, including regular tooth brushing and flossing, can limit gingival hyperplasia. If gingival hyperplasia is extensive, the hyperplastic tissue may have to be surgically removed (gingivectomy), and phenytoin replaced with another antiseizure drug.

Medication nonadherence can be a problem in persons with a seizure disorder. Take measures to increase patient adherence to the prescribed drug regimens. If made aware of the issue, health care providers can work with the patient to find an acceptable drug regimen. For example, using pregabalin in some cases as an adjunct medication will allow a decreased dose of the primary antiseizure drug, thus decreasing undesirable side effects.

GERONTOLOGIC CONSIDERATIONS

DRUG THERAPY FOR SEIZURE DISORDERS

The incidence of new-onset seizure disorders is high among older adults. Closely consider the relationship between the action of antiseizure drugs and the normal changes that occur with aging. For example, phenytoin is widely used to treat seizure disorders. However, because the liver metabolizes phenytoin, its use can be a problem for older patients with compromised liver function. Age-related changes in liver enzymes decrease the liver's ability to metabolize drugs. Phenobarbital, carbamazepine, and primidone have potential effects on cogni-

TABLE 59-10	SURGERY FOR SEIZURE DISORDERS
Type of Seizure	**Surgical Procedure**
Complex focal seizure of temporal lobe origin	Resectioning of epileptogenic tissue
Focal seizures of frontal lobe origin	Resectioning of epileptogenic tissue (if in resectable area)
Generalized seizures (Lennox-Gastaut syndrome or drop attacks)	Sectioning of corpus callosum
Intractable unilateral multifocal epilepsy associated with infantile hemiplegia	Hemispherectomy or callosotomy

tive function, so their use may be less desirable for the older adult. Carbamazepine, phenytoin, and phenobarbital have many significant drug interactions.[12]

Several of the newer antiseizure medications offer greater treatment benefit to older adults. Compared with older drugs, gabapentin, lamotrigine, oxcarbazepine, and levetiracetam may be safer, have fewer effects on cognitive function, and have fewer interactions with other drugs.[12]

Surgical Therapy. A significant number of patients whose epilepsy is not controlled with drug therapy are candidates for surgical intervention to remove the epileptic focus or prevent spread of epileptic activity in the brain (Table 59-10). The most common surgical intervention is an anterior temporal lobe resection. Approximately 70% of patients are essentially seizure free after this procedure.[8]

The benefits of surgery include cessation or reduction in frequency of the seizures. However, not all types of epilepsy benefit from surgery. An extensive preoperative evaluation is important, including continuous EEG monitoring and other specific tests to ensure precise localization of the focal point. Surgical candidates must meet three requirements: (1) a confirmed diagnosis of epilepsy, (2) an adequate trial with drug therapy without satisfactory results, and (3) a defined electroclinical syndrome (type of seizure disorder).

Other Therapies. Vagal nerve stimulation is used as an adjunct to medications when surgery is not feasible. The exact mechanism of action is unknown, but it is thought to interrupt the synchronization of epileptic brain wave activity and stop excessive discharge of neurons. A surgically implanted electrode in the neck is programmed to deliver the electrical impulse to the vagus nerve. The patient can activate it with a magnet when he or she senses a seizure is imminent. Vagal nerve stimulation can cause adverse effects such as coughing, hoarseness, dyspnea, and tingling in the neck. Battery replacement is required via surgery about every 5 years.

The ketogenic diet is a special high-fat, low-carbohydrate diet that has been used to control seizures in some people with epilepsy. When a person is on this diet, ketones are produced and pass into the brain and replace glucose as an energy source. The diet may be effective for some patients with drug-resistant epilepsy, but the long-term effects of the diet are not clear. Patients on this diet who use anticoagulants need close monitoring for bleeding.[13]

Biofeedback to control seizures is aimed at teaching the patient to maintain a certain brain wave frequency that is refractory to seizure activity. Further trials are needed to assess the effectiveness of biofeedback for seizure control.

NURSING MANAGEMENT
SEIZURE DISORDERS AND EPILEPSY

NURSING ASSESSMENT

Subjective and objective data to obtain from a patient with a seizure disorder are presented in Table 59-11. Obtain data related to a specific seizure episode from a witness.

NURSING DIAGNOSES

Nursing diagnoses for the patient with seizure disorders and epilepsy may include, but are not limited to, the following:

- Ineffective breathing pattern *related to* neuromuscular impairment
- Ineffective self-health management *related to* drug therapy and lifestyle adjustments
- Risk for injury *related to* loss of consciousness during seizure activity and postictal physical weakness

Additional information on nursing diagnoses for the patient with a seizure disorder is presented in eNursing Care Plan 59-2 (available on the website for this chapter).

PLANNING

The overall goals are that the patient with seizures will (1) be free from injury during a seizure, (2) have optimal mental and physical functioning while taking antiseizure drugs, and (3) have satisfactory psychosocial functioning.

NURSING IMPLEMENTATION

HEALTH PROMOTION. Some cases of seizure disorders can be prevented by promoting general safety measures, such as wearing helmets in situations involving risk of head injury. Improved perinatal, labor, and delivery care have reduced fetal trauma and hypoxia and thereby have reduced brain damage leading to seizure disorders.

The patient with a seizure disorder should practice good general health habits (e.g., maintaining a proper diet, getting adequate rest, exercising). Help the patient identify events or situations that precipitate the seizures and provide suggestions for avoiding them or handling them better. Teach the patient to avoid excessive alcohol intake, fatigue, and loss of sleep. Help the patient handle stress constructively.

ACUTE INTERVENTION. Nursing care for a hospitalized patient with a seizure disorder or a patient who has had seizures from metabolic factors involves several responsibilities, including observation and treatment of the seizure, education, and psychosocial intervention.

When a seizure occurs, carefully observe and record details of the event because the diagnosis and subsequent treatment often rest solely on the seizure description. Note all aspects of the seizure. What events preceded the seizure? When did the seizure occur? How long did each phase (aural [if any], ictal, postictal) last? What occurred during each phase?

Both subjective data (usually the only type of data in the aural phase) and objective data are important. Note the exact onset of the seizure (which body part was affected first and how); the course and nature of the seizure activity (loss of consciousness, tongue biting, automatisms, stiffening, jerking, total lack of muscle tone); the body parts involved and their sequence of involvement; and autonomic signs, such as dilated pupils, excessive salivation, altered breathing, cyanosis, flushing, diaphoresis, or incontinence. Assessment of the postictal period should include a detailed description of the level of conscious-

---

TABLE 59-11   NURSING ASSESSMENT
Seizure Disorders and Epilepsy

Subjective Data
Important Health Information
Past health history: Previous seizures, birth defects or injuries, anoxic episodes; CNS trauma, tumors, or infections; stroke; metabolic disorders, alcoholism; exposure to metals and carbon monoxide; hepatic or renal failure; fever; pregnancy, systemic lupus erythematosus
Medications: Adherence to antiseizure medication regimen; barbiturate or alcohol withdrawal; use and overdose of cocaine, amphetamines, lidocaine, theophylline, penicillin, lithium, phenothiazines, tricyclic antidepressants, benzodiazepines

Functional Health Patterns
Health perception–health management: Positive family history
Cognitive-perceptual: Headaches, aura, mood or behavioral changes before seizure; mentation changes; abdominal pain, muscle pain (postictal)
Self-perception–self-concept: Anxiety, depression; loss of self-esteem, social isolation
Sexuality-reproductive: Decreased sexual drive, erectile dysfunction; increased sexual drive (postictal)

Objective Data
General
Precipitating factors, including severe metabolic acidosis or alkalosis, hyperkalemia, hypoglycemia, dehydration, or water intoxication

Integumentary
Bitten tongue, soft tissue damage, cyanosis, diaphoresis (postictal)

Respiratory
Abnormal respiratory rate, rhythm, or depth; apnea (ictal); absent or abnormal breath sounds, possible airway occlusion

Cardiovascular
Hypertension, tachycardia or bradycardia (ictal)

Gastrointestinal
Bowel incontinence; excessive salivation

Urinary
Incontinence

Neurologic
Generalized
Tonic-clonic: Loss of consciousness, muscle tightening, then jerking; dilated pupils; hyperventilation, then apnea; postictal somnolence
Absence: Altered consciousness (5–30 sec), minor facial motor activity

Focal
Simple: Aura; consciousness; focal sensory, motor, cognitive, or emotional phenomena (focal motor); unilateral "marching" motor seizure (jacksonian)
Complex: Altered consciousness with inappropriate behaviors, automatisms, amnesia of event

Musculoskeletal
Weakness, paralysis, ataxia (postictal)

Possible Diagnostic Findings
Positive toxicology screen or alcohol level; altered serum electrolytes, acidosis or alkalosis, very low blood glucose level, ↑ blood urea nitrogen or serum creatinine, abnormal liver function tests, ammonia; abnormal CT scan or MRI of head, abnormal findings from lumbar puncture; abnormal discharges on EEG

DELEGATION DECISIONS

Caring for the Patient With a Seizure Disorder

Since any nursing staff member may be present when a patient experiences a seizure, all staff members are responsible for maintaining patient safety.

Role of Registered Nurse (RN)

- Teach patient about factors that increase risk for seizures, such as alcohol use, fatigue, inadequate sleep, and stress.
- Teach patient about prescribed antiseizure medications, including drug regimen, side effects, and required monitoring of drug levels.
- Assess and document details of seizure events, including events preceding the seizure; length of each phase of the seizure; course and nature of the seizure activity; and the level of consciousness, vital signs, and activity during the postictal period.
- Assess airway patency and position patient to maintain airway after any seizures.
- Administer IV antiseizure medications to the patient experiencing status epilepticus.
- Make appropriate referrals to the Epilepsy Foundation and community agencies to assist patient with financial problems, work training, employment, and living arrangements.
- Teach family members and caregivers about management of seizures and status epilepticus.
- In the ambulatory and home care setting, evaluate patient self-management of medications and lifestyle.

Role of Licensed Practical/Vocational Nurse (LPN/LVN)

- Administer oral antiseizure medications as scheduled.
- In the ambulatory and home setting, monitor patient adherence with medications and lifestyle changes and report problems to the RN.

Role of Unlicensed Assistive Personnel (UAP)

- Place suction equipment, Ambu bag, and O2 at the patient bedside.
- Remove potentially harmful objects from the bedside and pad side rails.
- Immediately report any seizure activity to the RN.
- Observe and report events of the seizure to the RN.
- Obtain vital signs during the postictal period.
- Provide oropharyngeal suctioning after a seizure (after being trained and evaluated in this procedure).

TABLE 59-12   PATIENT & CAREGIVER TEACHING GUIDE

Seizure Disorders and Epilepsy

Include the following information in the teaching plan for the patient with a seizure disorder.

1. Take drugs as prescribed. Report any and all side effects of drugs to the health care provider. When necessary, blood is drawn to ensure that therapeutic levels are maintained.
2. Use nondrug techniques, such as relaxation therapy and biofeedback training, to potentially reduce the number of seizures.
3. Be aware of availability of resources in the community.
4. Wear a medical alert bracelet or necklace, and carry an identification card.
5. Avoid excessive alcohol intake, fatigue, and loss of sleep.
6. Eat regular meals and snacks in between if feeling shaky, faint, or hungry.

Caregivers should receive the following information.

1. For first aid treatment of tonic-clonic seizure, it is not necessary to call an ambulance or send the patient to the hospital after a single seizure unless the seizure is prolonged, another seizure immediately follows, or extensive injury has occurred.
2. During an acute seizure, it is important to protect the patient from injury. This may involve supporting and protecting the head, turning the patient to the side, loosening constrictive clothing, and easing the patient to the floor, if seated.

---

ness, vital signs, pupil size and position of the eyes, memory loss, muscle soreness, speech disorders (aphasia, dysarthria), weakness or paralysis, sleep period, and the duration of each sign or symptom.

> **SAFETY ALERT**
> During a seizure, you should do the following:
> - Maintain a patent airway for the patient.
> - Protect the patient's head, turn the patient to the side, loosen constrictive clothing, ease patient to the floor (if seated).
> - Do not restrain the patient.
> - Do not place any objects in the patient's mouth.

After the seizure the patient may require repositioning to open and maintain the airway, suctioning, and oxygen. A seizure can be frightening for the patient and for others who witnessed it. Assess the level of their understanding and provide information about how and why the event occurred. This is an excellent opportunity for you to dispel many common misconceptions about seizures.

AMBULATORY AND HOME CARE. Prevention of recurring seizures is the major goal in the treatment of epilepsy. For treatment to be effective, drugs must be taken regularly and continuously, often for a lifetime. Ensure that the patient knows this, the specifics of the drug regimen, and what to do if a dose

is missed. Usually the dose is made up if the omission is remembered within 24 hours. Caution the patient not to adjust drug dosages without professional guidance because this can increase seizure frequency and even cause status epilepticus. Encourage the patient to report any medication side effects and to keep regular appointments with the health care provider.

You have an important role in teaching the patient and caregiver. Review the guidelines for teaching shown in Table 59-12. Teach the caregiver, family members, and significant others the emergency management of tonic-clonic seizures (see Table 59-8). Remind them that it is not necessary to call an ambulance or send a person to the hospital after a single seizure unless the seizure is prolonged, another seizure immediately follows, or extensive injury has occurred.

Patients with a seizure disorder may experience concerns or fears related to recurrent seizures, incontinence, or loss of self-control. Support the patient through teaching and by helping him or her use effective coping mechanisms.

Perhaps the greatest challenge for a patient with a seizure disorder is adjusting to the personal and societal limitations imposed by the illness. Discrimination in employment is the most serious problem facing the person with a seizure disorder. For issues relating to job discrimination, refer patients to the state department of vocational rehabilitation or the U.S. Equal Employment Opportunity Commission (EEOC).

Assist the patient who has a specific problem in finding appropriate resources. If you believe that associating with others who have a seizure disorder would be beneficial, refer the patient to the local chapter of the Epilepsy Foundation (EF), a volunteer agency that offers a variety of services to patients with epilepsy. Refer the patient who is an eligible veteran to a Department of Veterans Affairs medical center that provides comprehensive care. If intensive psychologic counseling is needed, refer the patient to a community mental health center.

Social workers and welfare agencies can help with financial problems and living arrangements. State agencies specializing in vocational rehabilitation services can provide vocational assessment, counseling, funding for training, and assistance with job placement for patients whose seizures are not well controlled. They can also offer financial assistance for transportation and medical costs related to vocational rehabilitation or job maintenance.

Driving laws for patients who have had a seizure vary from state to state. For example, some states require a 3-month seizure-free period before issuing or reissuing a driver's license, whereas others require up to 1 year. The EF provides current information on driving laws for each state.

Inform the patient that medical alert bracelets, necklaces, and identification cards are available through the EF, local pharmacies, or companies specializing in identification devices (e.g., Medic Alert). However, the use of these medical identification tags is optional. Some patients have found them beneficial, but others prefer not to be identified as having a seizure disorder.

Encourage the patient to learn more about epilepsy through self-education materials. The EF provides several information pamphlets and may facilitate support groups. Many agencies that offer services to epileptic patients, as well as local chapters of EF, have these available as teaching aids.

▋ EVALUATION

Expected outcomes are that the patient with seizures will
- Experience breathing pattern adequate to meet oxygen needs
- Experience no seizure-related injury
- Express acceptance of seizure disorder by admitting presence of epilepsy and maintaining adherent behavior

Additional expected outcomes are presented in eNursing Care Plan 59-2 available on the website.

RESTLESS LEGS SYNDROME

Etiology and Pathophysiology

Restless legs syndrome (RLS), also called Willis-Ekbom disease, is a relatively common condition characterized by unpleasant sensory (paresthesias) and motor abnormalities of one or both legs. Prevalence rates vary from 5% to 15%. However, the numbers may be higher because the condition is underdiagnosed. RLS is more common in older adults. It is also more common in women than men, and women may have an earlier age of onset.[14]

There are two distinct types of RLS: primary (idiopathic) and secondary. The majority of cases are primary, and many patients with this type of RLS report a positive family history. Secondary RLS can occur with metabolic abnormalities associated with iron deficiency, renal failure, hypertension, diabetes mellitus, or rheumatoid arthritis. Conditions such as anemia, pregnancy, and certain medications can cause or worsen symptoms.

Although the exact pathophysiology of primary RLS is unknown, it is believed that RLS is related to a dysfunction in the brain's basal ganglia circuits that use the neurotransmitter dopamine, which controls movements. In RLS this dysfunction causes the urge to move the legs. Abnormal iron metabolism or brain iron deficiencies may result in abnormalities of the dopamine system, thus leading to RLS.[15]

Clinical Manifestations

The severity of RLS sensory symptoms ranges from infrequent minor discomfort (paresthesias, including numbness, tingling, and "pins and needles" sensation) to severe pain. Sensory symptoms often appear first. Patients describe annoying and uncomfortable (but usually not painful) sensations in the legs. Some describe the sensations like bugs creeping or crawling on the legs. The leg pain is localized within the calf muscles. Patients can also experience pain in the upper extremities and the trunk. The discomfort occurs when the patient is sedentary and is most common in the evening or at night.

The pain at night can disrupt sleep. Physical activity, such as walking, stretching, rocking, or kicking, often relieves the pain. In the most severe cases, patients sleep only a few hours at night, resulting in daytime fatigue and disruption of the daily routine. The motor abnormalities associated with RLS consist of voluntary restlessness and stereotyped, periodic, involuntary movements. The involuntary movements usually occur during sleep. Fatigue further aggravates symptoms. Over time, RLS advances to more frequent and severe episodes.

Diagnostic Studies

RLS is a clinical diagnosis, based in large part on the patient's history or the report of the bed partner related to nighttime activities. The diagnosis of RLS is based on four specific criteria: (1) desire to move the extremities, often associated with paresthesias; (2) motor restlessness; (3) worsening of symptoms at rest with at least temporary relief from activity; and (4) worsening of symptoms in the evening or night.[15]

The patient may undergo polysomnography studies during sleep to distinguish RLS from other clinical conditions that can disturb sleep (e.g., sleep apnea). However, periodic leg movements in sleep are a common feature in RLS patients. Blood tests, such as a complete blood count, serum ferritin levels, and renal function tests (e.g., serum creatinine), may help exclude secondary causes of RLS. A patient's history of diabetes mellitus and its management may provide information to determine whether paresthesias are caused by peripheral neuropathy related to diabetes or RLS.

▋ NURSING AND COLLABORATIVE MANAGEMENT RESTLESS LEGS SYNDROME

The goal of collaborative management is to reduce patient discomfort and distress and to improve sleep quality. When RLS is secondary to renal failure or iron deficiency, treatment of these conditions will decrease symptoms. Nondrug approaches to RLS management include establishing regular sleep habits; exercising; avoiding activities that cause symptoms; and eliminating aggravating factors such as alcohol, caffeine, and certain drugs (neuroleptics, lithium, antihistamines, antidepressants).

If nondrug measures fail to provide symptom relief, drug therapy is an option. No single medication effectively manages RLS for all patients. The main drugs used in RLS include dopamine precursors (e.g., carbidopa/levodopa [Sinemet]) and dopamine agonists (e.g., ropinirole [Requip], pramipexole [Mirapex]) to increase the amount of dopamine in the brain. The antiseizure drug gabapentin enacarbil (Horizant) is used to decrease the sensory sensations. If the patient has iron deficiency or low serum ferritin levels, iron supplementation is considered.

Other drugs may relieve some symptoms of RLS. These include opioids and benzodiazepines. Low doses of opioids (e.g., oxycodone) are usually reserved for patients with severe symptoms who fail to respond to other drug therapies. The main side effect of opioids is constipation, so the patient may need to take a stool softener or laxative. Clonidine (Catapres) and propranolol (Inderal) are also effective in some patients.

DEGENERATIVE NEUROLOGIC DISORDERS

Degenerative nerve diseases lead to nerve damage that worsens as the disease progresses. These diseases affect many activities, including balance, movement, speech, and respiratory and heart function. There are more than 200 degenerative neurologic disorders. These include the disorders discussed in the remainder of this chapter, as well as disorders such as cerebellar degeneration, Friedreich's ataxia, Creutzfeldt-Jakob disease, and neurofibromatosis. Some have no known cause. However, many of these diseases have a genetic basis. Most degenerative nerve diseases have no cure. Treatment aims to reduce symptoms and help the patient maintain an optimal level of function.

Patients with these diseases have similar concerns and problems. They must deal with not only their disease, but also the impact that the disease has on their quality of life. Many patients have concerns regarding safety, mobility, self-care, and coping. The patient and family often require psychosocial support, especially as the disease progresses and the patient's disability gets worse.

MULTIPLE SCLEROSIS

Multiple sclerosis (MS) is a chronic, progressive, degenerative disorder of the CNS characterized by disseminated demyelination of nerve fibers of the brain and spinal cord. The onset of MS is usually between 20 and 50 years of age, although it can occur in young teens and much older adults. Women are affected two to three times more often than men.

MS is five times more prevalent in temperate climates (between 45 and 65 degrees of latitude), such as those found in the northern United States, Canada, and Europe, as compared with tropical regions. Migration from one geographic area to another may alter a person's risk of developing MS. Immigrants and their descendants tend to take on the risk level (either higher or lower) of the area to which they move. However, the change in risk may not appear immediately. For example, African Americans (in the United States) have a prevalence rate that is 40% that of European Americans, whereas Africans (in Africa) are thought to have a prevalence rate that is approximately 1% that of European Americans. The variations in incidence of MS suggest that geography, ethnicity, and other factors interact in a complex way to cause MS.[16]

Etiology and Pathophysiology

The cause of MS is unknown, although research suggests that it is unlikely MS is related to a single cause. Researchers believe the disease develops in a genetically susceptible person as a result of environmental exposure, like an infection. Multiple genes are believed to be involved in the inherited susceptibility to MS, and first-, second-, and third-degree relatives of patients with MS are at an increased risk.[16]

Possible precipitating factors include infection, smoking, physical injury, emotional stress, excessive fatigue, pregnancy, and a poor state of health. The role of precipitating factors such as exposure to pathogenic agents is controversial. It is possible that their association with MS is random and that there is no cause-and-effect relationship.

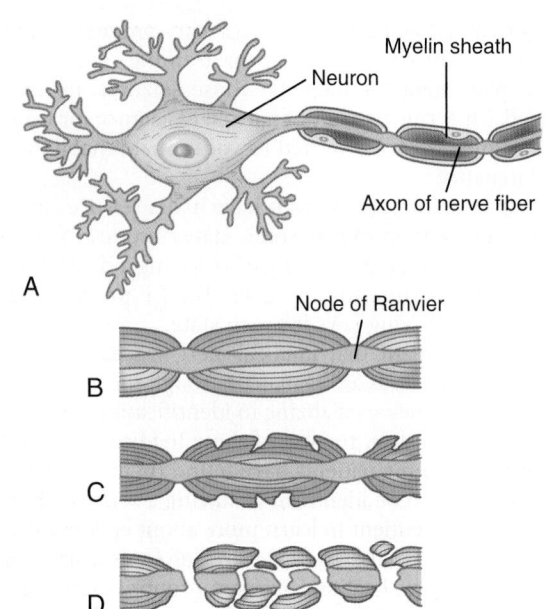

FIG. 59-3 Pathogenesis of multiple sclerosis. **A,** Normal nerve cell with myelin sheath. **B,** Normal axon. **C,** Myelin breakdown. **D,** Myelin totally disrupted; axon not functioning.

Three pathologic processes characterize MS: chronic inflammation, demyelination, and gliosis (scarring) in the CNS. The primary neuropathologic condition is an autoimmune process orchestrated by activated T cells (lymphocytes). An environmental factor or virus in genetically susceptible individuals may initially trigger this process. The activated T cells in the systemic circulation migrate to the CNS, disrupting the blood-brain barrier. This is likely the initial event in the development of MS. Subsequent antigen-antibody reaction within the CNS activates the inflammatory response and leads to the demyelination of axons.

Initially, attacks on the myelin sheaths of the neurons in the brain and spinal cord result in damage to the myelin sheath (Fig. 59-3, *A* to *C*). However, the nerve fiber is not affected. Transmission of nerve impulses still occurs, though transmission is slowed. The patient may complain of a noticeable impairment of function (e.g., weakness). However, the myelin can regenerate, and when it does, symptoms disappear. At that point, the patient experiences a remission.

As ongoing inflammation occurs, the nearby oligodendrocytes are affected, and the myelin loses the ability to regenerate. Eventually damage occurs to the underlying axon. Nerve impulse transmission is disrupted, resulting in the permanent loss of nerve function (Fig. 59-3, *D*). As inflammation subsides, glial scar tissue replaces the damaged tissue, leading to the formation of hard, sclerotic plaques (Fig. 59-4). These plaques are found throughout the white matter of the CNS.

Clinical Manifestations

The onset of MS is often insidious and gradual, with vague symptoms occurring intermittently over months or years that often dissuade the patient from seeking medical attention. Thus the disease may not be diagnosed until long after the onset of the first symptom. The disease is characterized by chronic, progressive deterioration in some patients, and remissions and exacerbations in others. With repeated exacerbations, the overall trend is progressive deterioration in neurologic function.

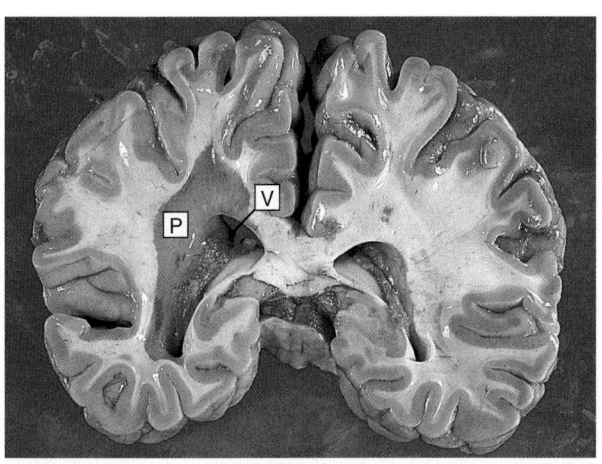

FIG. 59-4 Chronic multiple sclerosis. Demyelination plaque *(P)* at gray-white junction and adjacent partially remyelinated shadow plaque *(V)*.

TABLE 59-13 PATTERNS OF MULTIPLE SCLEROSIS

Category	Characteristics
Relapsing-remitting	• Clearly defined relapses with full recovery or sequelae and residual deficit on recovery. • Approximately 85% of people are initially diagnosed with this type of multiple sclerosis (MS).
Primary-progressive	• Slowly worsening neurologic function from the beginning with no distinct relapses or remissions. • About 10% of people are diagnosed with this type of MS.
Secondary-progressive	• A relapsing-remitting initial course, followed by progression with or without occasional relapses, minor remissions, and plateaus. • New treatments may slow progression. • About 50% of people with relapsing-remitting MS develop this type within 10 yr.
Progressive-relapsing	• Progressive disease from onset, with clear acute relapses, with or without full recovery. Periods between relapses are characterized by continuing progression. • Only 5% of people experience this type of MS.

Since the disease process has a spotty distribution in the CNS, the clinical manifestations vary with each patient according to the areas of the CNS involved. Some patients have severe, long-lasting symptoms early in the course of the disease. Others may experience only occasional and mild symptoms for several years after onset. A classification scheme, with four primary patterns of MS, has been developed based on the clinical course[16,17] (Table 59-13).

Common manifestations of MS include motor, sensory, cerebellar, and emotional problems. Motor symptoms include weakness or paralysis of the limbs, the trunk, or the head; diplopia; scanning speech; and spasticity of the muscles that are chronically affected. Patients with MS experience a variety of sensory abnormalities, including numbness and tingling and other paresthesias, patchy blindness *(scotomas)*, blurred vision, vertigo, tinnitus, decreased hearing, and chronic neuropathic pain. Radicular (nerve root) pains may be present, particularly in the low thoracic and abdominal regions. *Lhermitte's sign* is a transient sensory symptom described as an electric shock radiating down the spine or into the limbs with flexion of the neck. Cerebellar signs include nystagmus, ataxia, dysarthria, and dys-

phagia. Many patients have severe fatigue, sometimes with significant disability. The fatigue is aggravated by heat, humidity, deconditioning, and medication side effects.[16]

Bowel and bladder function can be affected if the sclerotic plaque is located in areas of the CNS that control elimination. Problems with defecation usually involve constipation rather than fecal incontinence. Urinary problems are variable. A common problem in MS patients is a *spastic* (uninhibited) bladder. As a result, the bladder has a small capacity for urine, and its contractions are unchecked. This is accompanied by urinary urgency and frequency and results in dribbling or incontinence.

A *flaccid* (hypotonic) bladder indicates a lesion in the reflex arc controlling bladder function. A flaccid bladder has a large capacity for urine because there is no sensation or desire to void, no pressure, and no pain. Generally, the patient has urinary retention, but urgency and frequency may also occur with this type of lesion. Another urinary problem is a combination of the previous two. Urinary problems cannot be adequately diagnosed and treated without urodynamic studies.

Sexual dysfunction occurs in many persons with MS. Physiologic erectile dysfunction may result from spinal cord involvement in men. Women may experience decreased libido, difficulty with orgasmic response, painful intercourse, and decreased vaginal lubrication. Diminished sensation can prevent a normal sexual response in both sexes. The emotional effects of chronic illness and the loss of self-esteem also contribute to loss of sexual response.

Some women with MS who become pregnant experience remission or an improvement in their symptoms during the gestation period. The hormonal changes associated with pregnancy appear to affect the immune system. However, during the postpartum period, women are at greater risk for exacerbation of the disease.

About half of people with MS experience some problems with cognitive function. For most, the problems are difficulties with short-term memory, attention, information processing, planning, visual perception, and word finding. General intellect remains unchanged and intact, including long-term memory, conversational skills, and reading comprehension. In only about 5% to 10% of MS patients, the cognitive changes are so severe that they significantly impair the person's ability to carry out activities of daily living. Most of the time, cognitive difficulties occur later in the course of the disease. However, they can occur much earlier in the disease process, and occasionally they are present at the onset of MS.

Persons with MS may also experience emotional changes such as anger, depression, or euphoria. Physical and emotional trauma, fatigue, and infection may aggravate or trigger signs and symptoms.

The average life expectancy after the onset of symptoms is more than 25 years. Death usually occurs due to infectious complications (e.g., pneumonia) of immobility or because of an unrelated disease.

Diagnostic Studies

Because there is no definitive diagnostic test for MS, factors considered are the history, clinical manifestations, and results of certain diagnostic tests (Table 59-14). An MRI of the brain and spinal cord may show plaques, inflammation, atrophy, and tissue breakdown and destruction. Cerebrospinal fluid (CSF) analysis may show an increase in immunoglobulin G and the

TABLE 59-14 COLLABORATIVE CARE

Multiple Sclerosis

Diagnostic
- History and physical examination
- CSF analysis
- CT scan
- MRI, MRS
- Evoked potential testing
  - Somatosensory evoked potential (SSEP)
  - Auditory evoked potential (AEP)
  - Visual evoked potential (VEP)

Collaborative Therapy
- Drug therapy (see Table 59-15)
- Surgical therapy
  - Thalamotomy (unmanageable tremor)
  - Neurectomy, rhizotomy, cordotomy (unmanageable spasticity)

MRS, Magnetic resonance spectroscopy.

presence of oligoclonal banding.[17] Evoked potential responses are often delayed in persons with MS because of decreased nerve conduction from the eye and the ear to the brain.

To be diagnosed with MS, the patient must have (1) evidence of at least two inflammatory demyelinating lesions in at least two different locations within the CNS, (2) damage or an attack occurring at different times (usually 1 month or more apart), and (3) all other possible diagnoses ruled out.

Collaborative Care

Drug Therapy. Because currently there is no cure for MS, collaborative care is aimed at treating the disease process and providing symptomatic relief (see Table 59-14). Since no two cases of MS are alike, therapy is tailored specifically to the disease pattern and manifestations that the patient is experiencing (Table 59-15).

The initial treatment of MS is the use of immunomodulator drugs to modify the disease progression and prevent relapses. These drugs include interferon β-1b (Betaseron) and glatiramer acetate (Copaxone), which are given subcutaneously every other day, and interferon β-1a (Avonex), which is given intramuscularly (IM). Another formulation of interferon β-1a is Rebif, which is administered subcutaneously three times weekly.

DRUG ALERT: β-Interferon (Avonex, Betaseron, Rebif)
- Rotate injection sites with each dose.
- Assess for depression, suicidal ideation.
- Wear sunscreen and protective clothing while exposed to sun.
- Know that flu-like symptoms are common after initiation of therapy.

Fingolimod (Gilenya) reduces MS disease activity by preventing lymphocytes from reaching the CNS and causing damage. Teriflunomide (Aubagio) is an immunomodulatory agent with antiinflammatory properties. The exact mechanism of action is unknown but may involve a reduction in the number of activated lymphocytes in the CNS. Teriflunomide is specifically indicated for treatment of relapsing forms of MS.

For more active and aggressive forms of MS, IV natalizumab (Tysabri) and mitoxantrone (Novantrone) may be used. Natalizumab, a monoclonal antibody, is given monthly when patients have had an inadequate response to other drugs. Natalizumab increases the risk of progressive multifocal leukoencephalopathy, a potentially fatal viral infection of the brain. Mitoxantrone, an antineoplastic medication, has serious effects, including cardiotoxicity, leukemia, and infertility.[17]

TABLE 59-15 DRUG THERAPY

Multiple Sclerosis

Drug	Patient Teaching
Disease-Modifying Drugs	
Immunomodulators	
β-Interferon (Betaseron, Extavia, Avonex, Rebif) glatiramer acetate (Copaxone) teriflunomide (Aubagio)	• Perform self-injection techniques. • Report side effects. • Treat flu-like symptoms with an NSAID or acetaminophen. • Because it may cause serious liver disease, monitor liver tests. • Avoid pregnancy.
Immunosuppressant	
mitoxantrone (Novantrone) dimethyl fumarate (Tecfidera)	• Report side effects. • Avoid pregnancy. • Avoid contact with large crowds and people who have an infection.
Sphingosine 1-Phosphate Receptor Modulator	
fingolimod (Gilenya)	• Report side effects. • Monitor blood pressure regularly. • Avoid pregnancy.
Monoclonal Antibody	
natalizumab (Tysabri)	• Report side effects. • Avoid pregnancy.
Drugs for Managing Exacerbations	
Corticosteroids	
ACTH prednisone methylprednisolone	• Restrict salt intake. • Do not abruptly stop therapy. • Know drug interactions.
Drugs for Symptom Management	
Cholinergics	
bethanechol (Urecholine) neostigmine (Prostigmin)	• Consult with health care provider before using other drugs, including over-the-counter drugs.
Anticholinergics	
propantheline (Pro-Banthine) oxybutynin (Ditropan)	• Consult health care provider before using other drugs, especially sleeping aids, antihistamines (possibly leading to potentiated effect).
Muscle Relaxants	
diazepam (Valium) baclofen (Lioresal) dantrolene (Dantrium) tizanidine (Zanaflex)	• Avoid driving and similar activities because of sedative effects. • Do not abruptly stop therapy. • Avoid use with tranquilizers and alcohol.
Nerve Conduction Enhancer	
dalfampridine (Ampyra)	• Be aware that it may cause seizures, especially at higher doses. • Take the tablet whole. Do not take more than 2 in 24 hr.

ACTH, Adrenocorticotropic hormone.

Dimethyl fumarate (Tecfidera) provides a new approach to treating MS by activating the Nrf2 pathway. This pathway provides a way for cells in the body to defend themselves against the inflammation and oxidative stress caused by MS. Dimethyl fumarate is used to treat relapsing-remitting MS.

Corticosteroids (e.g., methylprednisolone, prednisone) are most helpful to treat acute exacerbations of MS. They work by reducing edema and acute inflammation at the site of demyelin-

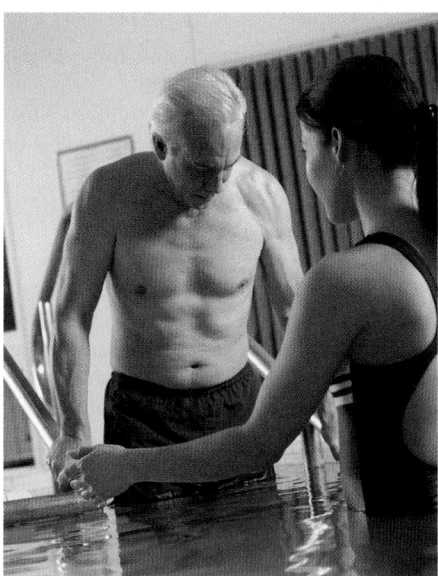

FIG. 59-5 Water therapy provides exercise and recreation for the patient with a chronic neurologic disease. (Photos.com/AbleStock.com/Thinkstock.)

ation. However, these drugs do not affect the ultimate outcome or the degree of residual neurologic impairment from the exacerbation.

Many other drugs are used to treat the various symptoms of MS, which may include fatigue, spasticity, tremor, vertigo or dizziness, depression, pain, bowel problems, bladder problems, sexual dysfunction, and cognitive changes. For example, muscle relaxants are used for spasticity. Amantadine (Symmetrel) and CNS stimulants (pemoline [Cylert], methylphenidate [Ritalin], and modafinil [Provigil]) are used to treat fatigue. Anticholinergics are used to treat bladder symptoms. Tricyclic antidepressants and antiseizure drugs are used for chronic pain syndromes. Dalfampridine (Ampyra) is used to improve walking speed in MS patients. It is a selective potassium channel blocker and improves nerve conduction in damaged nerve segments. It should not be used in patients with a history of seizure disorders or in those with moderate to severe kidney disease.

Other Therapies. Spasticity is primarily treated with muscle relaxants. However, surgery (e.g., neurectomy, rhizotomy, cordotomy), dorsal-column electrical stimulation, or intrathecal baclofen (Lioresal) delivered by pump may be required. Tremors that become unmanageable with drugs are sometimes treated by thalamotomy or deep brain stimulation.

Neurologic dysfunction sometimes improves with physical and speech therapies. Exercise improves the daily functioning for patients with MS not experiencing an exacerbation. Exercise decreases spasticity, increases coordination, and retrains unaffected muscles to substitute for impaired ones. An especially beneficial type of physical therapy is water exercise (Fig. 59-5). Water gives buoyancy to the body and allows the patient to perform activities that would normally be impossible because the patient has more control over the body.

NURSING MANAGEMENT
MULTIPLE SCLEROSIS

NURSING ASSESSMENT

Subjective and objective data that should be obtained from a patient with MS are presented in Table 59-16.

TABLE 59-16 NURSING ASSESSMENT

Multiple Sclerosis

Subjective Data
Important Health Information
Past health history: Recent or past viral infections or vaccinations, other recent infections, residence in cold or temperate climates, recent physical or emotional stress, pregnancy, exposure to extremes of heat and cold
Medications: Adherence to regimen of corticosteroids, immunomodulators, immunosuppressants, cholinergics, anticholinergics, antispasmodics

Functional Health Patterns
Health perception–health management: Positive family history; malaise
Nutritional-metabolic: Weight loss; difficulty in chewing, dysphagia
Elimination: Urinary frequency, urgency, dribbling or incontinence, retention; constipation
Activity-exercise: Generalized muscle weakness, muscle fatigue; tingling and numbness, ataxia (clumsiness)
Cognitive-perceptual: Eye, back, leg, joint pain; painful muscle spasms; vertigo; blurred or lost vision; diplopia; tinnitus
Sexuality-reproductive: Impotence, decreased libido
Coping–stress tolerance: Anger, depression, euphoria, social isolation

Objective Data
General
Apathy, inattentiveness

Integumentary
Pressure ulcers

Neurologic
Scanning speech, nystagmus, ataxia, tremor, spasticity, hyperreflexia, decreased hearing

Musculoskeletal
Muscle weakness, paresis, paralysis, spasms, foot dragging, dysarthria

Possible Diagnostic Findings
↓ T suppressor cells, demyelinating lesions on MRI or MRS scans, ↑ IgG or oligoclonal banding in cerebrospinal fluid, delayed evoked potential responses

IgG, Immunoglobulin G; *MRS,* magnetic resonance spectroscopy.

NURSING DIAGNOSES

Nursing diagnoses for the patient with MS may include, but are not limited to, the following:

- Impaired physical mobility *related to* muscle weakness or paralysis and muscle spasticity
- Impaired urinary elimination *related to* sensorimotor deficits
- Ineffective self-health management *related to* knowledge deficit regarding management of MS

Additional information on nursing diagnoses for the patient with MS is presented in the eNursing Care Plan 59-3 (available on the website for this chapter).

PLANNING

The overall goals are that the patient with MS will (1) maximize neuromuscular function, (2) maintain independence in activities of daily living for as long as possible, (3) manage disabling fatigue, (4) optimize psychosocial well-being, (5) adjust to the illness, and (6) reduce factors that precipitate exacerbations.

NURSING IMPLEMENTATION

The patient with MS should be aware of triggers that may cause exacerbations or worsening of the disease. Exacerbations of MS are triggered by infection (especially upper respiratory and urinary tract infections), trauma, immunization, childbirth, stress, and change in climate. Each person responds differently to these triggers. Assist the patient in identifying particular triggers and develop ways to avoid them or minimize their effects.

During the diagnostic phase the patient needs reassurance that, even though there is a tentative diagnosis of MS, certain diagnostic studies must be done to rule out other neurologic disorders. Assist the patient in dealing with the anxiety caused by a diagnosis of a disabling illness. The patient with recently diagnosed MS may need assistance with the grieving process.

During an acute exacerbation, the patient may be immobile and confined to bed. The focus of nursing interventions at this phase is to prevent major complications of immobility, such as respiratory and urinary tract infections and pressure ulcers.

Focus patient teaching on building general resistance to illness, including avoiding fatigue, extremes of heat and cold, and exposure to infection. Encourage vigorous and early treatment of infection when it does occur. Teach the patient to achieve a good balance of exercise and rest; minimize caffeine intake; and eat nutritious, well-balanced meals. A diet high in roughage may help relieve the problem of constipation. Patients should know their treatment regimens, drug side effects, how to watch for and manage side effects, and drug interactions with over-the-counter medications. The patient should consult a health care provider before taking nonprescription drugs.

Bladder control is a major problem for many patients with MS. Although anticholinergics may be beneficial for some patients to decrease spasticity, you may need to teach others self-catheterization (discussed in Chapter 46 on pp. 1092-1094). Bowel problems, particularly constipation, frequently occur in patients with MS. Increasing the dietary fiber intake may help some patients achieve regularity in bowel habits.

The patient with MS and the caregiver need to make many emotional adjustments because of the unpredictability of the disease, the need to change lifestyles, and the challenge of avoiding or decreasing precipitating factors. The National Multiple Sclerosis Society and its local chapters can offer a variety of services to meet the needs of patients with MS.

EVALUATION

The expected outcomes are that the patient with MS will
- Maintain or improve muscle strength and mobility
- Use assistive devices appropriately for ambulation and mobility
- Maintain urinary continence
- Make decisions about health and lifestyle modifications necessary for management of MS

Additional information on expected outcomes for the patient with MS are presented in eNursing Care Plan 59-3 (available on the website for this chapter).

PARKINSON'S DISEASE

Parkinson's disease (PD) is a chronic, progressive neurodegenerative disorder characterized by slowness in the initiation and execution of movement *(bradykinesia),* increased muscle tone *(rigidity),* tremor at rest, and gait disturbance. It is the most common form of *parkinsonism* (a syndrome characterized by similar symptoms).

The prevalence of PD is about 160 per 100,000. The diagnosis of PD increases with age, with the condition affecting about 2% of people over 60 years old. However, as many as 15% of those diagnosed with PD are less than 50 years old. PD is more common in men by a ratio of 3:2.[18]

Etiology and Pathophysiology

Although the exact cause of PD is unknown, a complex interplay of environmental and genetic factors is involved. Between 10% and 15% of PD patients have a family history of the disease, indicating a strong genetic basis. In other persons, exposure to toxins or certain viruses may trigger PD.[18]

There are many forms of parkinsonism other than PD. Parkinsonism-like symptoms have occurred after intoxication with a variety of chemicals, including carbon monoxide and manganese (among copper miners) and the product of meperidine analog synthesis, MPTP. Drug-induced parkinsonism can follow therapy with metoclopramide (Reglan), reserpine (Serpasil), methyldopa (Aldomet), lithium, haloperidol (Haldol), and chlorpromazine (Thorazine). Parkinsonism can also be seen after the use of illicit drugs, including amphetamine and methamphetamine. Other causes of parkinsonism include hydrocephalus, MS, encephalitis, infections, stroke, tumor, Huntington's disease, and trauma.[19]

Many changes found in the brains of people with PD may play a role in development of the disease, including a lack of dopamine (DA). The pathologic process of PD involves degeneration of the DA-producing neurons in the substantia nigra of the midbrain (Figs. 59-6 to 59-8), which in turn disrupts the normal balance between DA and acetylcholine (ACh) in the basal ganglia. DA is a neurotransmitter essential for normal functioning of the extrapyramidal motor system, including control of posture, support, and voluntary motion. Manifestations of PD do not occur until 80% of neurons in the substantia nigra are lost.

Lewy bodies, unusual clumps of protein, are found in the brains of patients with PD. It is not known what causes these bodies to form, but their presence indicates abnormal functioning of the brain. Lewy body dementia is discussed in Chapter 60.

Genetic Link

Approximately 20% of PD patients have a family history of PD. Many autosomal dominant and recessive genes have been linked to familial PD. The most common genetic contributor to PD is the *LRRK2* gene. Mutations in this gene also appear to have a role in sporadic, or noninherited, cases of PD. *LRRK2* and mutations in another gene, α-synuclein *(SNCA)*, have manifestations similar to those of the common, age-related PD. Other genes involved in familial PD are parkin *(PARK2)*, *DJ-1*, and *PINK1*. Mutations in these genes are often associated with a younger age of onset and have additional manifestations than those typically seen with age-related PD. *PINK1* mutations are related to a rare, early-onset form of PD.[18,20,21]

Clinical Manifestations

The onset of PD is gradual and insidious, with an ongoing progression. It may involve only one side of the body initially. The classic manifestations of PD are a triad of tremor, rigidity, and bradykinesia. In the beginning stages, only a mild tremor, a slight limp, or a decreased arm swing may be evident. Later in the disease the patient may have a shuffling, propulsive gait with arms flexed and loss of postural reflexes. Some patients have a slight change in speech patterns. None of these manifestations alone is sufficient evidence for a diagnosis of the disease.

Tremor. *Tremor*, often the first sign, may be minimal initially, so the patient is the only one who notices it. This tremor can affect handwriting, causing it to trail off, particularly toward the ends of words. Parkinsonian tremor is more prominent at

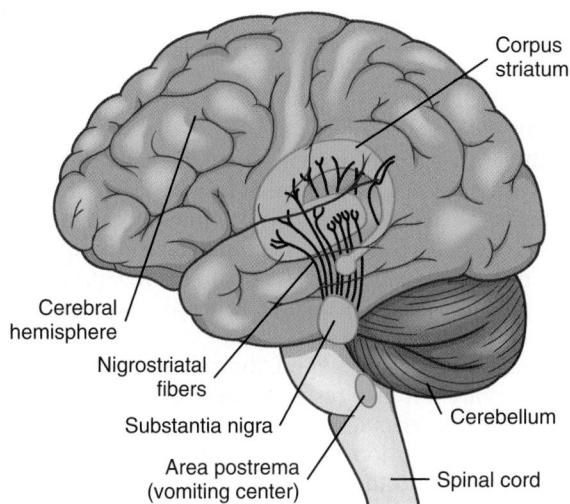

FIG. 59-6 Nigrostriatal disorders produce parkinsonism. Left-sided view of the human brain showing the substantia nigra and the corpus striatum *(shaded area)* lying deep within the cerebral hemisphere. Nerve fibers extend upward from the substantia nigra, divide into many branches, and carry dopamine to all regions of the corpus striatum.

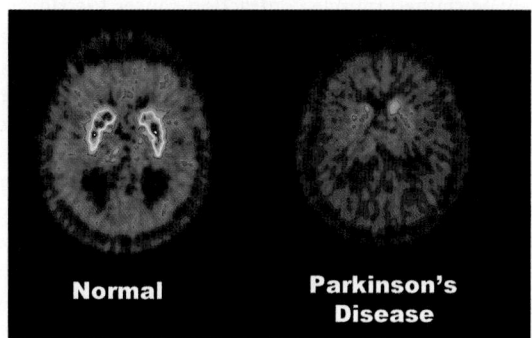

FIG. 59-8 In Parkinson's disease, positron emission tomography (PET) scan showing reduced fluorodopa uptake in the basal ganglia *(right)* compared with a normal control *(left)*.

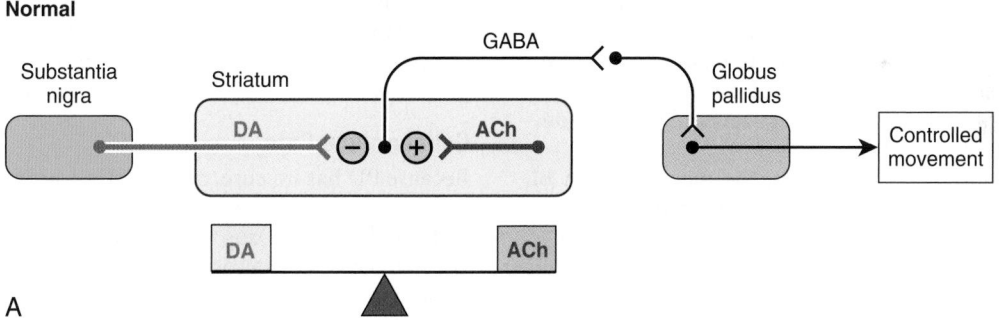

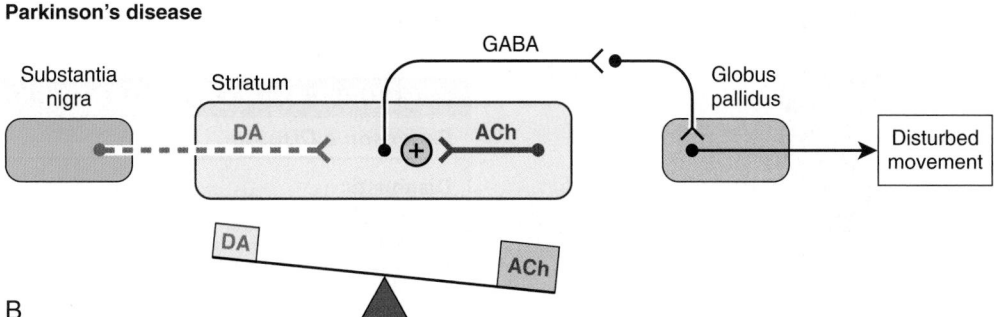

FIG. 59-7 In Parkinson's disease there is a deficit in dopamine. These deficits create an imbalance between dopamine and the excitatory neurotransmitter acetylcholine. **A,** In a healthy person, dopamine *(DA)* released from neurons originating in the substantia nigra inhibits the firing of neurons in the striatum that release γ-aminobutyric acid *(GABA)*. Conversely, neurons located within the striatum, which release acetylcholine *(ACh)*, excite the GABAergic neurons. Under normal conditions, the inhibitory actions of DA are balanced by the excitatory actions of ACh, and controlled movement results. **B,** In Parkinson's disease, the neurons in the substantia nigra that supply DA to the striatum degenerate. When there is a deficit of DA, the excitatory effects of ACh go unopposed, resulting in disturbed movements (tremor, rigidity).

rest and is aggravated by emotional stress or increased concentration. The hand tremor is described as "pill rolling" because the thumb and forefinger appear to move in a rotary fashion as if rolling a pill, coin, or other small object. Tremor can also involve the diaphragm, tongue, lips, and jaw but rarely causes shaking of the head.

Unfortunately, in many people a benign essential tremor is mistakenly diagnosed as PD. Essential tremor occurs during voluntary movement, has a more rapid frequency than parkinsonian tremor, and is often familial.

Rigidity. *Rigidity,* the second sign of the triad, is the increased resistance to passive motion when the limbs are moved through their range of motion. Parkinsonian rigidity is typified by cogwheel rigidity, or a jerky quality, as if there were intermittent catches in the movement of a cogwheel, when the joint is moved passively. Sustained muscle contraction causes the rigidity and consequently elicits complaints of muscle soreness; feeling tired and achy; or pain in the head, the upper body, the spine, or the legs. Another consequence of rigidity is slowness of movement because it inhibits the alternating of contraction and relaxation in opposing muscle groups (e.g., biceps and triceps).

Bradykinesia. *Bradykinesia* is particularly evident in the loss of automatic movements, which is secondary to the physical and chemical alteration of the basal ganglia and related structures in the extrapyramidal portion of the CNS. In the unaffected patient, automatic movements are involuntary and occur subconsciously. They include blinking of the eyelids, swinging of the arms while walking, swallowing of saliva, self-expression with facial and hand movements, and minor movement of postural adjustment.

The patient with PD does not execute these movements and lacks spontaneous activity. This accounts for the stooped posture, masked face (deadpan expression), drooling of saliva, and shuffling gait *(festination)* that are characteristic of a person with this disease. The posture is that of a slowed "old man" image, with the head and trunk bent forward and the legs constantly flexed (Fig. 59-9).

Postural instability is common. Patients may complain of being unable to stop themselves from going forward (propulsion) or backward (retropulsion). Assessment of postural instability includes the "pull test," in which the examiner stands behind the patient and gives a tug backward on the shoulder, causing the patient to lose his or her balance and fall backward.

In addition to the motor signs of PD, many nonmotor symptoms are common. They include depression, anxiety, apathy, fatigue, pain, constipation, impotence, and short-term memory impairment. Sleep problems are common in patients with PD and include difficulty staying asleep at night, restless sleep, nightmares, and drowsiness or sudden sleep onset during the day.[18]

Complications

As the disease progresses, complications increase. These include motor symptoms (e.g., dyskinesias [spontaneous, involuntary movements], weakness, *akinesia* [total immobility]), neurologic problems (e.g., dementia), and neuropsychiatric problems (e.g., depression, hallucinations, psychosis). As PD progresses, it often results in a severe dementia, which is associated with an increase in mortality.

As swallowing becomes more difficult (dysphagia), malnutrition or aspiration may result. General debilitation may lead to pneumonia, urinary tract infections, and skin breakdown. Orthostatic hypotension may occur in some patients and, along with loss of postural reflexes, may result in falls or other injury.[22]

Diagnostic Studies

Because there is no specific diagnostic test for PD, the diagnosis is based on the history and the clinical features. A firm diagnosis can be made only when at least two of the three signs of the classic triad are present: tremor, rigidity, and bradykinesia. The ultimate confirmation of PD is a positive response to antiparkinsonian drugs. Research is ongoing regarding the role of genetic testing and MRI in diagnosing patients with PD.[23]

Collaborative Care

Because PD has no cure, collaborative care focuses on relieving the symptoms (Table 59-17).

Drug Therapy. Drug therapy for PD is aimed at correcting the imbalance of neurotransmitters within the CNS. Antiparkinsonian drugs either enhance the release or the supply of DA (dopaminergic) or antagonize or block the effects of the overactive cholinergic neurons in the striatum (anticholinergic) (see Fig. 59-7). Levodopa with carbidopa (Sinemet) is often the first drug used. Levodopa is a chemical precursor of DA and can

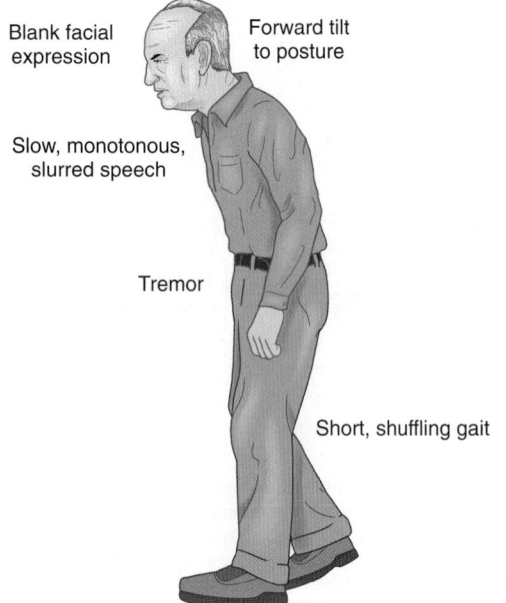

Blank facial expression

Forward tilt to posture

Slow, monotonous, slurred speech

Tremor

Short, shuffling gait

FIG. 59-9 Characteristic appearance of a patient with Parkinson's disease.

TABLE 59-17 **COLLABORATIVE CARE**
Parkinson's Disease
Diagnostic
• History and physical examination
• Tremor, rigidity, and bradykinesia
• Positive response to antiparkinsonian drugs
• MRI
• Rule out side effects of phenothiazines, reserpine, benzodiazepines, haloperidol
Collaborative Therapy
• Antiparkinsonian drugs (see Table 59-18)
• Deep brain stimulation
• Ablation surgery

cross the blood-brain barrier. It is converted to DA in the basal ganglia. Sinemet is the preferred drug because it also contains carbidopa, an agent that inhibits the enzyme dopa-decarboxylase in the peripheral tissues. Dopa-decarboxylase breaks down levodopa before it reaches the brain. The net result of the combination of levodopa and carbidopa is that more levodopa reaches the brain, and therefore less drug is needed. Levodopa has many side effects and drug interactions. Prolonged use can often result in dyskinesias and "off/on" periods when the medication will unpredictably start or stop working.

DRUG ALERT: Carbidopa/Levodopa (Sinemet)
- Monitor for signs of dyskinesia.
- Effects may be delayed for several weeks to months.
- Instruct patient or caregiver to report any uncontrolled movement of face, eyelids, mouth, tongue, arms, hands, or legs; mental changes; palpitations; severe nausea and vomiting; and difficulty urinating.

Many patients are given Sinemet early in the disease course. It is effective for the management of akinetic symptoms. Tremor and rigidity may also respond to this drug.[21] However, some health care providers believe that, after a few years of therapy, the effectiveness of Sinemet wears off. Therefore they prefer to initiate therapy with a DA receptor agonist. These drugs include bromocriptine (Parlodel), pergolide (Permax), ropinirole (Requip), pramipexole (Mirapex), and rotigotine (Neupro). These drugs directly stimulate DA receptors. Sinemet is then added to the drug regimen when more moderate to severe symptoms are present.

DRUG ALERT: Bromocriptine (Parlodel)
- Patient may become dizzy or faint due to orthostatic hypotension, especially after the first dose.
- Notify physician immediately if a severe headache develops that does not let up or continues to get worse.

Selegiline (Eldepryl) and rasagiline (Azilect), monoamine oxidase type B (MAO-B) inhibitors, are sometimes used in combination with Sinemet. By inhibiting MAO-B, the degradative enzyme for DA, these agents increase the levels of DA and prolong the half-life of levodopa. Rasagiline can also be used alone as therapy in early PD.

Entacapone (Comtan) and tolcapone (Tasmar) block the enzyme catechol O-methyltransferase (COMT), which breaks down levodopa in the peripheral circulation, thus prolonging the effect of Sinemet. These drugs are used only as adjuncts to levodopa.[18]

Anticholinergic drugs such as trihexyphenidyl (Artane) and benztropine (Cogentin) are also used to manage PD. These drugs decrease the activity of ACh, thus providing balance between cholinergic and dopaminergic actions. Antihistamines (e.g., diphenhydramine [Benadryl]) with anticholinergic properties may be used to manage tremors.

The antiviral agent amantadine is also an effective antiparkinsonian drug. Although its exact mechanism of action is not known, amantadine promotes the effect of DA.[18] Rivastigmine (Exelon) or donepezil (Aricept) is used to treat mild to moderate Parkinson's dementia. Amitriptyline may be used to treat depression.

Table 59-18 summarizes the drugs commonly used in PD. The use of only one drug is preferred because fewer side effects occur and the drug dosage is easier to adjust than when several drugs are used. However, as the disease progresses, combination therapy is often required. Excessive amounts of dopaminergic drugs can lead to *paradoxic intoxication* (aggravation rather than relief of symptoms).

TABLE 59-18 DRUG THERAPY

Parkinson's Disease

Drug	Mechanism of Action
Dopaminergics	
Dopamine Precursors	
levodopa (L-dopa)	Converted to dopamine in basal
levodopa/carbidopa (Sinemet, Parcopa [orally dissolving tablet])	ganglia
Dopamine Receptor Agonists	
bromocriptine (Parlodel)	Stimulate dopamine receptors
pergolide (Permax)	
pramipexole (Mirapex)	
ropinirole (Requip, Requip XL)	
rotigotine (Neupro [skin patch])	
Dopamine Agonists	
amantadine (Symmetrel)	Blocks reuptake of dopamine into presynaptic neurons
apomorphine (Apokyn)	Stimulates postsynaptic dopamine receptors
Anticholinergics	
trihexyphenidyl (Artane)	Block cholinergic receptors, thus
benztropine (Cogentin)	helping to balance cholinergic
biperiden (Akineton)	and dopaminergic activity
Antihistamine	
diphenhydramine (Benadryl)	Has anticholinergic effect
Monoamine Oxidase Inhibitors	
selegiline (Eldepryl, Carbex)	Block breakdown of dopamine
rasagiline (Azilect)	
Catechol O-Methyltransferase (COMT) Inhibitors	
entacapone (Comtan)	Block COMT and slow the
tolcapone (Tasmar)	breakdown of levodopa, thus prolonging the action of levodopa

Within 3 to 5 years of standard Parkinson's drug treatments, many patients experience episodes of hypomobility (e.g., inability to rise from chair, to speak, or to walk). The episodes can occur toward the end of a dosing interval with standard medications (so-called end-of-dose wearing off) or at unpredictable times (spontaneous "on/off").

A combination of carbidopa, levodopa, and entacapone (Stalevo) is available for patients with end-of-dose wearing off. Apomorphine (Apokyn) can also be used to treat Parkinson's patients during these episodes of "hypomobility," or "off periods," in which the patient becomes immobile or unable to perform activities of daily living. Apomorphine, which is given by a subcutaneous injection, needs to be taken with an antiemetic drug (e.g., trimethobenzamide [Tigan]) because, when taken alone, it causes severe nausea and vomiting. It must not be taken with the antiemetics in the serotonin (5-HT3) receptor antagonist class (e.g., ondansetron [Zofran]) because the combination of apomorphine and these drugs can lead to very low blood pressure and loss of consciousness.

Surgical Therapy. Surgical procedures are aimed at relieving symptoms of PD and are usually used in patients who are unresponsive to drug therapy or who have developed severe motor complications. Surgical procedures fall into three categories: deep brain stimulation (DBS), ablation (destruction), and transplantation. Today, the most common surgical treatment is

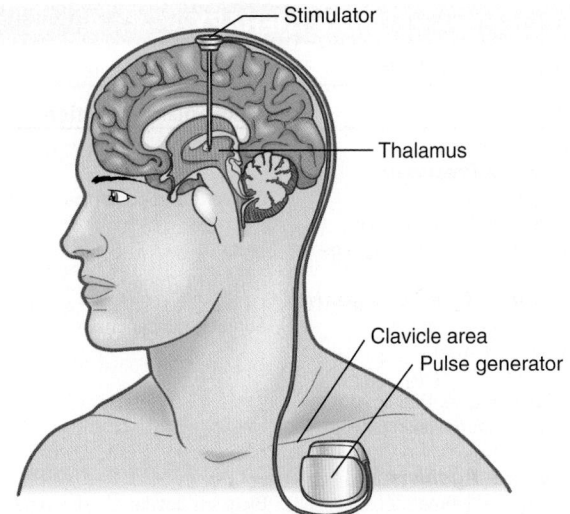

FIG. 59-10 A deep brain stimulator can be used to treat the tremors and uncontrolled movements in Parkinson's disease. Electrodes are surgically placed in the brain and connected to a neurostimulator (pacemaker device) in the chest.

DBS. DBS involves placing an electrode in either the thalamus, globus pallidus, or subthalamic nucleus and connecting it to a generator placed in the upper chest (like a pacemaker) (Fig. 59-10). The device is programmed to deliver a specific current to the targeted brain location. Unlike ablation procedures, DBS can be adjusted to control symptoms better and is reversible (the device can be removed). These ablative and DBS procedures work by reducing the increased neuronal activity produced by DA depletion. DBS has been shown to improve motor function and reduce dyskinesia and medication usage.[18]

Ablation surgery involves stereotactic ablation of areas in the thalamus (*thalamotomy*), globus pallidus (*pallidotomy*), and subthalamic nucleus (*subthalamic nucleotomy*). *Transplantation* of fetal neural tissue into the basal ganglia is designed to provide DA-producing cells in the brains of patients with PD. This form of therapy is still in the experimental stages.

Nutritional Therapy. Diet is of major importance to the patient with PD because malnutrition and constipation can be serious consequences of inadequate nutrition. Patients who have dysphagia and bradykinesia need appetizing foods that are easily chewed and swallowed. The diet should contain adequate roughage and fruit to avoid constipation. Cut food into bite-sized pieces before it is served, and serve it on a warmed plate to preserve its appeal.

Eating six small meals a day may be less exhausting than eating three large meals a day. Plan ample time for eating to avoid frustration. The absorption of levodopa can be impaired by protein ingestion and vitamin B_6. Therefore some patients are advised to limit their protein intake to the evening meal to decrease this problem. They also need to consult with their health care provider regarding the possible supplementation of vitamin B_6 in their multivitamins and fortified cereals.

NURSING MANAGEMENT PARKINSON'S DISEASE

NURSING ASSESSMENT

Subjective and objective data that should be obtained from a patient with PD are presented in Table 59-19.

TABLE 59-19   NURSING ASSESSMENT

Parkinson's Disease

Subjective Data
Important Health Information
Past health history: Central nervous system trauma, cerebrovascular disorders, exposure to metals and carbon monoxide, encephalitis
Medications: Major tranquilizers, especially haloperidol (Haldol), and phenothiazines, reserpine, methyldopa, amphetamines

Functional Health Patterns
Health perception–health management: Fatigue
Nutritional-metabolic: Excessive salivation, dysphagia; weight loss
Elimination: Constipation, incontinence; excessive sweating
Activity-exercise: Difficulty in initiating movements; frequent falls; loss of dexterity; micrographia (handwriting deterioration)
Sleep-rest: Insomnia, nightmares, daytime sleepiness
Cognitive-perceptual: Diffuse pain in head, shoulders, neck, back, legs, and hips; muscle soreness and cramping
Self-perception–self-concept: Depression; mood swings, hallucinations

Objective Data
General
Blank (masked) faces, slow and monotonous speech, infrequent blinking

Integumentary
Seborrhea, dandruff; ankle edema

Cardiovascular
Postural hypotension

Gastrointestinal
Drooling

Neurologic
Tremor at rest, first in hands (pill rolling), later in legs, arms, face, and tongue; aggravation of tremor with anxiety, absence in sleep; poor coordination; subtle dementia; impaired postural reflexes

Musculoskeletal
Cogwheel rigidity, dysarthria, bradykinesia, contractures, stooped posture, shuffling gait

Possible Diagnostic Findings
No specific tests; diagnosis on basis of history and physical findings and ruling out of other diseases

---

NURSING DIAGNOSES

Nursing diagnoses for the patient with PD may include, but are not limited to, the following:

- Impaired physical mobility *related to* rigidity, bradykinesia, and akinesia
- Imbalanced nutrition: less than body requirements *related to* inability to ingest food
- Impaired swallowing *related to* neuromuscular impairment (e.g., decreased or absent gag reflex)
- Impaired verbal communication *related to* dysarthria, tremor, and bradykinesia

Additional information on nursing diagnoses for the patient with PD is presented in eNursing Care Plan 59-4 (available on the website for this chapter).

PLANNING

The overall goals are that the patient with PD will (1) maximize neurologic function, (2) maintain independence in activities of daily living for as long as possible, and (3) optimize psychosocial well-being.

NURSING IMPLEMENTATION

Because PD is a chronic degenerative disorder with no acute exacerbations, teaching and nursing care are directed toward maintenance of good health, encouragement of independence, and avoidance of complications such as contractures and falls. Problems secondary to bradykinesia can be alleviated by relatively simple measures.

Promotion of physical exercise and a well-balanced diet are major concerns for nursing care. Exercise can limit the consequences of decreased mobility, such as muscle atrophy, contractures, and constipation. The American Parkinson Disease Association (see Resources at the end of this chapter) publishes a series of booklets and videotapes with helpful exercises that can be used by family members and health care professionals.

A physical therapist may be consulted to design a personal exercise program aimed at strengthening and stretching specific muscles. Overall muscle tone and specific exercises to strengthen the muscles involved with speaking and swallowing should be included. Although exercise will not halt the progress of the disease, it will enhance the patient's functional ability. An occupational therapist can also assist the patient with strategies to increase self-care measures, including eating and dressing.

SAFETY ALERT
- Have patients who are at risk for falling and tend to "freeze" while walking do the following:
  - Consciously think about stepping over imaginary or real lines on the floor.
  - Drop rice kernels and step over them.
  - Rock from side to side.
  - Lift the toes when stepping.
  - Take one step backward and two steps forward.

Work closely with the patient's caregiver and family in exploring creative adaptations that allow maximum independence and self-care. The patient can facilitate getting out of a chair by using an upright chair with arms and placing the back legs of the chair on small (2-in) blocks. Encourage environmental alterations, such as removing rugs and excess furniture to avoid stumbling, using an elevated toilet seat to facilitate getting on and off the toilet, and elevating the legs on an ottoman to decrease dependent ankle edema. Clothing can be simplified by the use of slip-on shoes and Velcro hook-and-loop fasteners or zippers on clothing, instead of buttons and hooks.

Effective management of sleep problems can greatly improve the quality of life for patients with PD. Some PD patients find the use of satin nightwear or satin sheets beneficial. Information on teaching regarding sleep hygiene practices is presented in Chapter 8.

In the early stages of PD, many patients experience depression and anxiety. Patients need to adjust their lifestyle, including work and home responsibilities. As the disease progresses, the impact on the patient's psychologic well-being also increases. Assist the patient by listening, providing teaching, challenging distorted thoughts, and encouraging social interactions. Psychologic therapy and counseling can be helpful.

In the early stage of the disease, the patient has subtle changes in cognitive function, which can progress to dementia. This results in increased caregiver burden and the potential for long-term care placement. Information on care of the patient with dementia is provided in Chapter 60.

Family caregivers (e.g., spouse, children) care for the majority of patients with PD. As the disease progresses, the caregiver burden increases, often while the caregiver's physical and mental health decline. Strategies to reduce caregiver burden are described in Chapter 4. Other interventions for the patient with PD are presented in eNursing Care Plan 59-4 (available on the website for this chapter).

EVALUATION

The expected outcomes are that the patient with PD will
- Perform physical exercise to deter muscle atrophy and joint contractures
- Use assistive devices appropriately for ambulation and mobility
- Maintain nutritional intake adequate for metabolic needs
- Experience safe passage of fluids and/or solids from the mouth to the stomach
- Use methods of communication that meet needs for interaction with others

Additional information on expected outcomes for the patient with PD are presented in eNursing Care Plan 59-4 (available on the website).

MYASTHENIA GRAVIS

Myasthenia gravis (MG) is an autoimmune disease of the neuromuscular junction characterized by the fluctuating weakness of certain skeletal muscle groups. MG occurs in either gender and in persons of any ethnicity. The prevalence rate is 20 per 100,000; currently about 60,000 people have MG in the United States.[24] The peak age at onset in women is during the childbearing years; in men the peak onset of MG is between the ages of 50 and 70 years. However, it does occur in men and women outside of these age ranges.

Etiology and Pathophysiology

MG is caused by an autoimmune process in which antibodies attack acetylcholine (ACh) receptors, resulting in a decreased number of ACh receptor (AChR) sites at the neuromuscular junction. This prevents ACh molecules from attaching and stimulating muscle contraction. Anti-AChR antibodies are detectable in the serum of 90% of patients with generalized MG. In the 10% of patients who lack autoantibodies to AChR, their muscular weakness may be related to autoantibodies to muscle-specific receptor tyrosine kinase, although other autoantibodies may be involved.[25] Thymic tumors are found in about 15% of patients, and abnormal thymus tissue is found in most others.

Clinical Manifestations and Complications

The primary feature of MG is fluctuating weakness of skeletal muscle. The muscles most often involved are those used for moving the eyes and eyelids, chewing, swallowing, speaking, and breathing. These muscles are generally the strongest in the morning and become exhausted with continued activity. A period of rest usually restores strength. Consequently, by the end of the day, muscle weakness is prominent.

In 90% of cases the eyelid muscles or extraocular muscles are involved (Fig. 59-11). Facial mobility and expression can be impaired. The patient may have difficulty chewing and swallowing food. Speech is affected, and the voice often fades after a long conversation. The muscles of the trunk and limbs are less often affected. Of these, the proximal muscles of the neck,

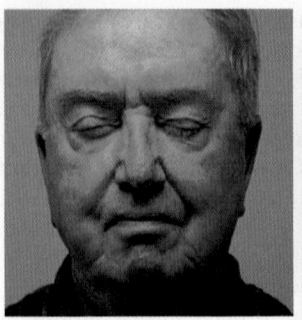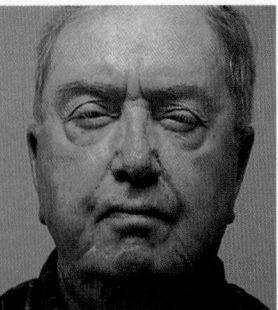

FIG. 59-11 "Peek" sign in myasthenia gravis. During sustained forced eyelid closure he is unable to bury his eyelashes *(left)* and, after 30 sec, he is unable to keep the lids fully closed *(right)*.

TABLE 59-20   **COLLABORATIVE CARE**
Myasthenia Gravis

Diagnostic	**Collaborative Therapy**
• History and physical examination	• Drugs
	• Anticholinesterase agents
• Fatigability with prolonged upward gaze (2-3 min)	• Corticosteroids
• Muscle weakness	• Immunosuppressive agents
• EMG	• Surgery (thymectomy)
• Tensilon test	• Plasmapheresis
• Acetylcholine receptor antibodies	• IV immunoglobulin G
• Chest x-ray	

EMG, Electromyography.

shoulder, and hip are more often affected than the distal muscles. No other signs of neural disorder accompany MG. There is no sensory loss, reflexes are normal, and muscle atrophy is rare.

The course of this disease is highly variable. Some patients may have short-term remissions, others may stabilize, and others may have severe, progressive involvement.[24] Exacerbations of MG can be precipitated by emotional stress, pregnancy, menses, another illness, trauma, temperature extremes, and hypokalemia. Ingestion of drugs, including aminoglycoside antibiotics, β-adrenergic blockers, procainamide, quinidine, and phenytoin, can aggravate MG. Psychotropic drugs (e.g., lithium carbonate, phenothiazines, benzodiazepines, tricyclic antidepressants) have also been associated with worsening of myasthenia, as have neuromuscular blocking agents (tubocurarine chloride, pancuronium, succinylcholine [Anectine]).

Myasthenic crisis is an acute exacerbation of muscle weakness triggered by infection, surgery, emotional distress, drug overdose, or inadequate drugs. The major complications of MG result from muscle weakness in areas that affect swallowing and breathing. This results in aspiration, respiratory insufficiency, and respiratory tract infection.

Diagnostic Studies

The diagnosis of MG can be made based on history and physical examination. However, other tests may be used if the diagnosis is still in doubt. EMG may show a decreased response to repeated stimulation of the hand muscles, indicative of muscle fatigue. Single-fiber EMG is sensitive in confirming the diagnosis of MG. Use of drugs may also aid in the diagnosis.

The Tensilon test in a patient with MG reveals improved muscle contractility after IV injection of the anticholinesterase agent edrophonium chloride (Tensilon). (Anticholinesterase blocks the enzyme acetylcholinesterase.) This test also aids in the diagnosis of cholinergic crisis (secondary to overdose of anticholinesterase drug), which occurs when there is too much cholinesterase inhibition. Clinical features include muscle fasciculation, sweating, excessive salivation, and constricted pupils. In this condition, Tensilon does not improve muscle weakness but may actually increase it. Atropine, a cholinergic antagonist, should be readily available to counteract the effects of Tensilon when it is used diagnostically. In patients with a confirmed diagnosis of MG, a chest CT scan may be done to evaluate the thymus.

Collaborative Care

Drug Therapy. Drug therapy for MG includes anticholinesterase drugs, alternate-day corticosteroids, and immunosup-

pressants (Table 59-20). Anticholinesterase drugs are aimed at enhancing function of the neuromuscular junction. Acetylcholinesterase is the enzyme that breaks down ACh. Thus inhibition of this enzyme by an anticholinesterase inhibitor will prolong the action of ACh and facilitate transmission of impulses at the neuromuscular junction. Pyridostigmine (Mestinon) is the most successful drug of this group in long-term treatment of MG.

Tailoring the dose to avoid a myasthenic or cholinergic crisis often presents a clinical challenge. Corticosteroids (specifically prednisone) are used to suppress the immune response. Drugs such as azathioprine (Imuran), mycophenolate (CellCept), and cyclosporine (Sandimmune) may also be used for immunosuppression.

Many drugs are contraindicated or must be used with caution in patients with MG. Classes of drugs that should be cautiously evaluated before use include anesthetics, antidysrhythmics, antibiotics, quinine, antipsychotics, barbiturates and sedative-hypnotics, cathartics, diuretics, opioids, muscle relaxants, thyroid preparations, and tranquilizers.

Surgical Therapy. Because the presence of the thymus gland in the patient with MG appears to enhance the production of AChR antibodies, removal of the thymus gland results in improvement in a majority of patients. Thymectomy is indicated for almost all patients with thymoma, for patients with generalized MG between the ages of puberty and about 65 years, and for patients with purely ocular MG.

Other Therapies. Plasmapheresis and IV immunoglobulin G can yield a short-term improvement in symptoms and are indicated for patients in myasthenic crisis or in preparation for surgery when corticosteroids must be avoided. Plasmapheresis directly removes circulating AChR antibodies, leading to a decrease in symptoms. (Plasmapheresis is discussed in Chapter 14.) It is not certain how IV immunoglobulin works, but it is probably related to a decrease in antibody production.[24]

NURSING MANAGEMENT
MYASTHENIA GRAVIS

NURSING ASSESSMENT

Assess the severity of MG by asking the patient about fatigability, what body parts are affected, and how severely they are affected. Assess the patient's coping abilities and strategies and understanding of the disorder. Some patients become so fatigued that they are no longer able to work or even walk.

Objective data should include respiratory rate and depth, oxygen saturation, arterial blood gas analyses, pulmonary function tests, and evidence of respiratory distress in patients with acute myasthenic crisis. Assess muscle strength of all face and limb muscles, swallowing, speech (volume and clarity), and cough and gag reflexes.

NURSING DIAGNOSES

Nursing diagnoses for the patient with MG may include, but are not limited to, the following.

- Ineffective airway clearance *related to* intercostal muscle weakness and impaired cough and gag reflex
- Impaired verbal communication *related to* weakness of the larynx, lips, mouth, pharynx, and jaw
- Activity intolerance *related to* muscle weakness and fatigability
- Disturbed body image *related to* inability to maintain usual lifestyle and role responsibilities

PLANNING

The overall goals are that the patient with MG will (1) have a return of normal muscle endurance, (2) manage fatigue, (3) avoid complications, and (4) maintain a quality of life appropriate to the disease course.

NURSING IMPLEMENTATION

The patient with MG who is admitted to the hospital usually has a respiratory tract infection or is in an acute myasthenic crisis. Nursing care is aimed at maintaining adequate ventilation, continuing drug therapy, and watching for side effects of therapy. Be able to distinguish cholinergic from myasthenic crisis (Table 59-21) because the causes and treatment of the two conditions differ greatly.

As with other chronic illnesses, focus care on the neurologic deficits and their impact on daily living. Teach the patient about a balanced diet that can easily be chewed and swallowed. Semisolid foods may be easier to eat than solids or liquids. Schedul-

ing doses of drugs so that peak action is reached at mealtime may make eating less difficult. Arrange diversional activities that require little physical effort and match the patient's interests. Help the patient plan activities of daily living to avoid fatigue. Teaching should focus on the importance of following the medical regimen, complications of the disease, potential adverse reactions to specific drugs, and complications of therapy (crisis conditions) and what to do about them. Explore community resources such as the Myasthenia Gravis Foundation of America and MG support groups.

EVALUATION

The expected outcomes are that the patient with MG will
- Maintain optimal muscle function
- Be free from side effects of drugs
- Not experience complications (myasthenic or cholinergic crises) from the disease
- Maintain a quality of life appropriate to the disease course

AMYOTROPHIC LATERAL SCLEROSIS

Amyotrophic lateral sclerosis (ALS) is a rare progressive neurologic disorder characterized by loss of motor neurons. ALS usually leads to death 2 to 6 years after diagnosis, but a few patients may survive for more than 10 years.[26] This disease became known as Lou Gehrig's disease after the famous baseball player was stricken with it in 1939. The onset is usually between 40 and 70 years of age. ALS is more common in men than women by a ratio of 2:1. Approximately 5000 people in the United States are diagnosed with ALS every year.[26]

For unknown reasons, in ALS motor neurons in the brainstem and the spinal cord gradually degenerate (see eFig. 59-1 available on the website for this chapter). Dead motor neurons cannot produce or transport signals to muscles. Consequently, electrical and chemical messages originating in the brain do not reach the muscles to activate them.

The typical symptoms of ALS are limb weakness, dysarthria, and dysphagia. Muscle wasting and fasciculations result from the denervation of the muscles and lack of stimulation and use. Other symptoms include pain, sleep disorders, spasticity, drooling, emotional lability, depression, constipation, and esophageal reflux.[26] Death usually results from respiratory tract infection secondary to compromised respiratory function.

Unfortunately, there is no cure for ALS. Riluzole (Rilutek) slows the progression of ALS. This drug works to decrease the amount of glutamate (an excitatory neurotransmitter) in the brain.

The illness trajectory for ALS is devastating because the patient remains cognitively intact while wasting away. Guide the patient in the use of moderate-intensity, endurance-type exercises for the trunk and limbs, since this may help reduce ALS spasticity. Nursing interventions include (1) facilitating communication, (2) reducing risk of aspiration, (3) facilitating early identification of respiratory insufficiency, (4) decreasing pain secondary to muscle weakness, (5) decreasing risk of injury related to falls, and (6) providing diversional activities such as reading and companionship,

Support the patient's cognitive and emotional functions. Help the patient and family manage the disease process, including grieving related to the loss of motor function and ultimately death. Discuss with the patient and caregiver issues such as artificial methods of ventilation and advance directives.

TABLE 59-21 COMPARISON OF MYASTHENIC AND CHOLINERGIC CRISES	
Myasthenic Crisis	**Cholinergic Crisis**
Causes	
Exacerbation of myasthenia following precipitating factors or failure to take drug as prescribed or drug dose too low	Overdose of anticholinesterase drugs resulting in increased ACh at the receptor sites, remission (spontaneous or after thymectomy)
Differential Diagnosis	
Improved strength after IV administration of anticholinesterase drugs	Weakness within 1 hr after ingestion of anticholinesterase
Increased weakness of skeletal muscles manifesting as ptosis, bulbar signs (e.g., difficulty swallowing, difficulty articulating words), or dyspnea	Increased weakness of skeletal muscles manifesting as ptosis, bulbar signs, dyspnea
	Effects on smooth muscle include pupillary miosis, salivation, diarrhea, nausea or vomiting, abdominal cramps, increased bronchial secretions, sweating, or lacrimation

ACh, Acetylcholine.

⚕ GENETICS IN CLINICAL PRACTICE

Huntington's Disease (HD)

Genetic Basis
- Autosomal dominant disorder.
- Caused by mutation in *HTT* gene located on chromosome 4.

Incidence
- 1 in 10,000.
- Higher incidence in people of European ancestry.
- With each pregnancy a heterozygous affected parent has a 5% chance of having a child with HD.

Genetic Testing
- DNA testing is available.
- DNA testing can be done on fetal cells obtained by amniocentesis or chorionic villus sampling.
- Preimplantation genetic diagnosis can be done on embryos before implantation and pregnancy.
- One copy of altered gene is sufficient to cause HD.
- No test is available to predict when symptoms will develop.

Clinical Implications
- HD is a progressive, degenerative brain disorder.
- Onset of disease usually occurs at 30–50 yr of age. No cure is available.
- Drugs are available to control movements and behavioral problems.
- Genetic counseling may be considered if there is a family history of HD.
- Because HD is an autosomal dominant disorder, individuals who are at risk have a strong motivation to seek genetic testing.
- A positive result is not considered a diagnosis, since it may be obtained decades before the symptoms begin.
- A negative test means that the individual does not carry the mutated gene and will not develop HD.

INFORMATICS IN PRACTICE

Social Networking in Huntington's Disease

- Many patients with Huntington's disease experience social isolation and depression.
- Encourage the patient to participate in an online community where people who have Huntington's disease discuss their condition.
- Social contact and a social network with others who have Huntington's disease will help patients deal better with their illness and improve their quality of life.

HUNTINGTON'S DISEASE

Huntington's disease (HD) is a genetically transmitted, autosomal dominant disorder that affects both men and women of all races. The offspring of a person with this disease have a 50% risk of inheriting it (see Genetics in Clinical Practice box above). The onset of HD is usually between 30 and 50 years of age. Often the diagnosis is made after the affected individual has had children. About 15,000 Americans are symptomatic, and 150,000 are at risk for HD.[27]

The diagnostic process begins with a review of the family history and clinical symptoms. Genetic testing confirms the disease in a person with symptoms. People who are asymptomatic but who have a positive family history of HD face the dilemma of whether to be genetically tested. If the test is positive, the person will develop HD, but when and to what extent the disease develops cannot be determined.

Like PD, the pathologic process of HD involves the basal ganglia and the extrapyramidal motor system. However, instead of a deficiency of DA, HD involves a deficiency of the neurotransmitters ACh and γ-aminobutyric acid (GABA). The net effect is an excess of DA, which leads to symptoms that are the opposite of those of parkinsonism.

The clinical manifestations are a movement disorder and cognitive and psychiatric disorders. The movement disorder is characterized by abnormal and excessive involuntary movements *(chorea)*. These are writhing, twisting movements of the face, the limbs, and the body. The movements get worse as the disease progresses. Facial movements involving speech, chewing, and swallowing are affected and may cause aspiration and malnutrition. The gait deteriorates, and ambulation eventually becomes impossible.

Psychiatric symptoms are frequently present in the early stage of the disease, often before the onset of motor symptoms. Depression is common. Other psychiatric symptoms include anxiety, agitation, impulsivity, apathy, social withdrawal, and obsessiveness. Cognitive deterioration is more variable and involves perception, memory, attention, and learning. Eventually all psychomotor processes, including the ability to eat and talk, are impaired.

Death usually occurs 10 to 20 years after the onset of symptoms. The most common cause of death is pneumonia, followed by suicide. Other causes of death include injuries related to a fall and other complications.[27]

Because HD has no cure, collaborative care is palliative. Tetrabenazine (Xenazine) is used to treat the chorea and works to decrease the amount of DA available at synapses in the brain and thus decreases the involuntary movements of chorea.

Other medications used for the movement disorder include neuroleptics such as haloperidol and risperidone (Risperdal), benzodiazepines such as diazepam and clonazepam, and DA-depleting agents such as reserpine and tetrabenazine. Cognitive disorders are treated as needed with nondrug therapies (e.g., counseling, memory books). The psychiatric disorders can be treated with selective serotonin reuptake inhibitors such as sertraline (Zoloft) and paroxetine (Paxil). Antipsychotic medication, such as haloperidol or risperidone, may also be needed.

HD presents a great challenge to health care professionals. The goal of nursing management is to provide the most comfortable environment possible for the patient and caregiver by maintaining physical safety, treating the physical symptoms, and providing emotional and psychologic support.

Because of the choreic movements, caloric requirements are high. Patients may require as many as 4000 to 5000 cal/day to maintain body weight. As the disease progresses, meeting caloric needs becomes a greater challenge when the patient has difficulty swallowing and holding the head still. Depression and mental deterioration can also compromise nutritional intake. Alternative sources of nutrition may be indicated as the disease progresses.

End-of-life issues need to be discussed with the patient and caregiver. These include care in the home or long-term care facility, artificial methods of feeding, advance directives and cardiopulmonary resuscitation (CPR), use of antibiotics to treat infections, and guardianship. These topics should be addressed throughout the course of the disease as the patient and caregiver adapt to increasing disability.

CASE STUDY

Epilepsy With Headache

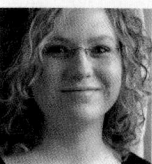

Purestock/Thinkstock

Patient Profile

J.P. is a 24-yr-old woman who was diagnosed with epilepsy at age 15. At that time, she had a tonic-clonic seizure and was given a prescription for phenytoin (Dilantin). She had a second witnessed seizure 4 mo later, but has since been seizure free. J.P. now has complaints of headaches and says she is afraid that her seizures are going to return. She is single, lives alone, and describes her job as stressful.

Subjective Data

- Describes headache pain on the left side of her forehead as throbbing
- Has vomited with headache
- Describes changes in vision, including flashing lights
- Headache occurs nearly every month on a regular cycle

Objective Data

- Alert and oriented to person
- Neurologic examination negative

- Phenytoin level within normal limits
- EEG normal
- CT of head normal

Discussion Questions

1. What is epilepsy?
2. What is the pathophysiology of epilepsy?
3. What is the significance of the laboratory and diagnostic findings?
4. Is the headache related to seizure activity?
5. *Priority Decision:* What is a priority nursing intervention for J.P.?
6. What should be included in the teaching plan for J.P. regarding the course of the disease?
7. *Priority Decision:* Based on the assessment data, what are the priority nursing diagnoses?
8. *Evidence-Based Practice:* Based on current treatment guidelines, what medication may be effective in managing both J.P.'s epilepsy and her migraine headaches?

ⓔvolve Answers available at *http://evolve.elsevier.com/Lewis/medsurg.*

▌ BRIDGE TO NCLEX EXAMINATION

The number of the question corresponds to the same-numbered outcome at the beginning of the chapter.

1. A 50-year-old man complains of recurring headaches. He describes these as sharp, stabbing, and located around his left eye. He also reports that his left eye seems to swell and get teary when these headaches occur. Based on this history, you suspect that he has
   a. cluster headaches.
   b. tension headaches.
   c. migraine headaches.
   d. medication overuse headaches.

2. A 65-year-old woman was just diagnosed with Parkinson's disease. The priority nursing intervention is
   a. searching the Internet for educational videos.
   b. evaluating the home for environmental safety.
   c. promoting physical exercise and a well-balanced diet.
   d. designing an exercise program to strengthen and stretch specific muscles.

3. The nurse finds that an 87-year-old woman with Alzheimer's disease is continually rubbing, flexing, and kicking out her legs throughout the day. The night shift reports that this same behavior escalates at night, preventing her from obtaining her required sleep. The next step the nurse should take is to
   a. ask the physician for a daytime sedative for the patient.
   b. request soft restraints to prevent her from falling out of her bed.
   c. ask the physician for a nighttime sleep medication for the patient.
   d. assess the patient more closely, suspecting a disorder such as restless legs syndrome.

4. Social effects of a chronic neurologic disease include *(select all that apply)*
   a. divorce.
   b. job loss.
   c. depression.
   d. role changes.
   e. loss of self-esteem.

5. The nurse is reinforcing teaching with a newly diagnosed patient with amyotrophic lateral sclerosis. Which statement would be appropriate to include in the teaching?
   a. "ALS results from an excess chemical in the brain, and the symptoms can be controlled with medication."
   b. "Even though the symptoms you are experiencing are severe, most people recover with treatment."
   c. "You need to consider advance directives now, since you will lose cognitive function as the disease progresses."
   d. "This is a progressing disease that eventually results in permanent paralysis, though you will not lose any cognitive function."

1, a, 2, c, 3, d, 4, a, b, c, d, e, 5, d

ⓔvolve

For rationales to these answers and even more NCLEX review questions, visit *http://evolve.elsevier.com/Lewis/medsurg.*

REFERENCES

*1. Mathew PG, Garza I: Headache, *Semin Neurol* 31:5, 2011.
*2. Lipton RB: Chronic migraine, classification, differential diagnosis, and epidemiology, *Headache* 51:77, 2011.

3. Goldman L, Schafer AI: *Goldman's Cecil medicine,* ed 24, St Louis, 2012, Mosby.
*4. Rozen TD, Fishman RS: Cluster headache in the United States of America, *Headache* 52:99, 2012.
*5. Rothrock JF: Onabotulinumtoxin A for the treatment of chronic migraine, *Headache* 51:659, 2011.
*6. Halker R, Vargas B, Dodick DW: Cluster headache: diagnosis and treatment, *Semin Neurol* 30:175, 2010.

*Evidence-based information for clinical practice.

7. Epilepsy Foundation: Epilepsy and seizure statistics. Retrieved from *www.epilepsyfoundation.org/about/statistics.cfm*.

8. National Institute of Neurologic Disorders and Stroke: Seizures and epilepsy. Retrieved from *www.ninds.nih.gov/disorders/ epilepsy/detail_epilepsy.htm*.

9. Berg AT, Berkovic SF, Brodie MJ, et al: Revised terminology and concepts for organization of seizures and epilepsies: report of the ILAE Commission on Classification and Terminology, 2005-2009, International League Against Epilepsy, *Epilepsia* 5:676, 2010.

*10. Kranick S, Ekanayake V, Martinez V, et al: Psychopathology and psychogenic movement disorders, *Mov Disord* 26:1844, 2011.

*11. Shorvon S, Tomson T: Sudden unexpected death in epilepsy, *Lancet* 378:2028, 2011.

*12. Stefan H: Epilepsy in the elderly, *Acta Neurol Scand* 124:223, 2011.

*13. Payne NE, Cross JH, Sander JW, et al: The ketogenic and related diets in adolescents and adults, *Epilepsia* 52:1941, 2011.

*14. Cuellar NG: Advances in the science of genomics in restless legs syndrome, *Biol Res Nurs* 12:178, 2010.

15. National Institute of Neurologic Disorders and Stroke: Restless legs syndrome. Retrieved from *www.ninds.nih.gov/disorders/ restless_legs/detail_restless_legs.htm*.

16. National Multiple Sclerosis Society: About MS. Retrieved from *www.nationalmssociety.org/about-multiple-sclerosis/index.aspx*.

17. Brodkey MB, Ben-Zacharia AB, Reardon JD: Living well with multiple sclerosis, *Am J Nurs* 111:40, 2011.

18. National Institute of Neurologic Disorders and Stroke: Parkinson's disease. Retrieved from *www.ninds.nih.gov/ disorders/parkinsons_disease/detail_parkinsons_disease.htm*.

*19. Vilensky JA, Gilman S, McCall S: A historical analysis of the relationship between encephalitis lethargica and postencephalitic parkinsonism, *Mov Disord* 25:1116, 2010.

*20. Falcone DC, Wood EM, Xie SX, et al: Genetic testing and Parkinson disease: assessment of patient knowledge, attitudes, and interest, *J Genet Counsel* 20:384, 2011.

*21. Bonifati V: Autosomal recessive parkinsonism, *Parkinsonism Relat Disord* 18:S4, 2012.

*22. Gershanik OS: Clinical problems in late-stage Parkinson's disease, *J Neurol* 257:S288, 2010.

*23. Chahine LM, Stern MB: Diagnostic markers for Parkinson's disease, *Curr Opin Neurol* 24:309, 2011.

24. Myasthenia Gravis Foundation of America: What is myasthenia gravis? Retrieved from *www.myasthenia.org/WhatisMG.aspx*.

*25. Vrolix K, Fraussen J, Molenaar PC, et al: The auto-antigen repertoire in myasthenia gravis, *Autoimmunity* 43:380, 2010.

*26. Gordon PH: Amyotrophic lateral sclerosis, *CNS Drugs* 25:1, 2011.

27. National Institute of Neurologic Disorders and Stroke: Huntington's disease. Retrieved from *www.ninds.nih.gov/ disorders/huntington/detail_huntington.htm*.

RESOURCES

ALS Association
www.alsa.org

American Association of Neuroscience Nurses (AANN)
www.aann.org

American Headache Society
www.americanheadachesociety.org

American Parkinson Disease Association
www.apdaparkinson.org

Epilepsy Foundation
www.epilepsyfoundation.org

Huntington's Disease Society of America
www.hdsa.org

International Headache Society
www.ihs-headache.org

Myasthenia Gravis Foundation of America
www.myasthenia.org

National Headache Foundation
www.headaches.org

National Institute of Neurological Disorders and Stroke
www.ninds.nih.gov

National Multiple Sclerosis Society
www.nationalmssociety.org

National Parkinson Foundation
www.parkinson.org

Willis-Ekbom Disease Foundation
www.rls.org

The more you use your brain, the more brain you have to lose.
George Dorsey

Nursing Management
Alzheimer's Disease, Dementia, and Delirium

Sharon L. Lewis

evolve WEBSITE

http://evolve.elsevier.com/Lewis/medsurg

- NCLEX Review Questions
- Key Points
- Pre-Test
- Answer Guidelines for Case Study on p. 1461
- Rationales for Bridge to NCLEX Examination Questions

- Case Study
  - Patient With Alzheimer's Disease
- Nursing Care Plans (Customizable)
  - eNCP 60-1: Patient With Alzheimer's Disease
  - eNCP 60-2: Family Caregivers
- Concept Map Creator

- Glossary
- Content Updates

eTable
- eTable 60-1: Mini-Mental State Examination (MMSE)

LEARNING OUTCOMES

1. Define dementia and describe its impact on society.
2. Compare and contrast different etiologies of dementia.
3. Describe the clinical manifestations, diagnostic studies, and collaborative management of dementia.
4. Describe the clinical manifestations of mild cognitive impairment.
5. Describe the clinical manifestations, diagnostic studies, and collaborative management of Alzheimer's disease.
6. Describe the nursing management of the patient with Alzheimer's disease.
7. Differentiate among other neurodegenerative disorders associated with dementia, including dementia with Lewy bodies, frontotemporal lobar degeneration, Creutzfeldt-Jakob disease, and normal pressure hydrocephalus.
8. Describe the etiology, pathophysiology, clinical manifestations, diagnostic studies, and collaborative management of delirium.

KEY TERMS

Alzheimer's disease (AD), p. 1445
Creutzfeldt-Jakob disease (CJD), p. 1458
delirium, p. 1458
dementia, p. 1443
dementia with Lewy bodies (DLB), p. 1457

familial Alzheimer's disease (FAD), p. 1446
frontotemporal lobar degeneration (FTLD), p. 1458
mild cognitive impairment (MCI), p. 1450
mixed dementia, p. 1458

neurofibrillary tangles, p. 1446
normal pressure hydrocephalus, p. 1458
retrogenesis, p. 1448
sundowning, p. 1454
vascular dementia, p. 1444

This chapter discusses the cognitive disorders of dementia and delirium, with a focus on the nursing management of patients with Alzheimer's disease. The etiology and pathophysiology of dementia and delirium are differentiated, and the collaborative and nursing management of patients with these cognitive disorders are described.

The three most common cognitive problems in adults are dementia, delirium (acute confusion), and depression (Table 60-1). Although this chapter focuses on dementia and delirium, depression is often associated with these conditions.

▌DEMENTIA

Dementia is a syndrome characterized by dysfunction or loss of memory, orientation, attention, language, judgment,

and reasoning. Personality changes and behavioral problems such as agitation, delusions, and hallucinations may occur. Ultimately these problems result in alterations in the individual's ability to work, fulfill social and family responsibilities, and perform activities of daily living. Dementia is often diagnosed when two or more brain functions, such as memory loss or language skills, are significantly impaired.

Fifteen percent of older Americans have dementia. As the average life span increases, the number of those affected with dementia is growing. There are about 100 causes of dementia, with about 60% to 80% of the patients with dementia having a diagnosis of Alzheimer's disease (AD) (Fig. 60-1). In the United States, about half of all patients in long-term care facilities have AD or a related dementia.[1]

Reviewed by Anna M. Bruch, RN, MSN, Professor of Nursing, Illinois Valley Community College, Oglesby, Illinois.

TABLE 60-1   COMPARISON OF DEMENTIA, DELIRIUM, AND DEPRESSION

Feature	Dementia	Delirium	Depression
Onset	Usually insidious.	Rapid, often at night.	Often coincides with life changes. Often abrupt.
Progression	Slow.	Abrupt.	Variable, rapid to slow but may be uneven.
Duration	Years (usually 8-20).	Hours to days to weeks.	Can be several months to years, especially if not treated.
Thinking	Difficulty with abstract thinking, impaired judgment, words difficult to find.	Disorganized, distorted. Slow or accelerated incoherent speech.	Intact but with apathy, fatigue. May be indecisive. Feels sense of hopelessness. May not want to live.
Perception	Misperceptions often present. Delusions and hallucinations.	Distorted. Delusions and hallucinations.	May deny or be unaware of depression. May have feelings of guilt.
Psychomotor behavior	May pace or be hyperactive. As disease progresses, may not be able to perform tasks or movements when asked.	Variable. Can be hyperactive or hypoactive, or mixed.	Often withdrawn and hypoactive.
Sleep-wake cycle	Sleeps during day. Frequent awakenings at night. Fragmented sleep.	Disturbed sleep. Reversed sleep-wake cycle.	Disturbed, often with early morning awakening.

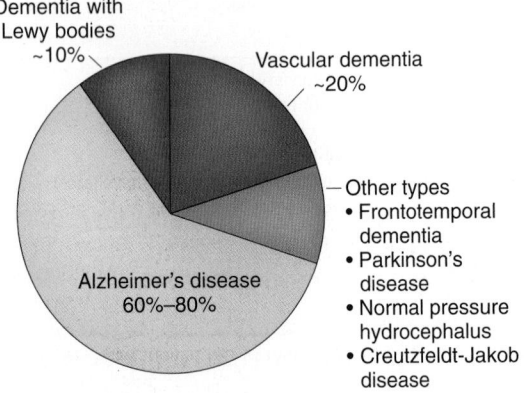

FIG. 60-1 Causes of dementia.

TABLE 60-2   CAUSES OF DEMENTIA

Type of Dementia	Cause
Neurodegenerative disorders	• Alzheimer's disease • Dementia with Lewy bodies (DLB) • Frontotemporal lobar degeneration (FTLD) • Down syndrome • Amyotrophic lateral sclerosis (ALS) • Parkinson's disease • Huntington's disease
Vascular diseases	• Vascular (multiinfarct) dementia • Subarachnoid hemorrhage* • Chronic subdural hematoma*
Toxic, metabolic, or nutritional diseases	• Alcoholism • Thiamine (vitamin B_1) deficiency* • Cobalamin (vitamin B_{12}) deficiency* • Folate deficiency* • Hyperthyroidism* • Hypothyroidism*
Immunologic diseases or infections	• Multiple sclerosis • Chronic fatigue syndrome • Infections (e.g., Creutzfeldt-Jakob disease) • Acquired immunodeficiency syndrome (AIDS) • Meningitis* • Encephalitis* • Neurosyphilis* • Systemic lupus erythematosus*
Systemic diseases	• Uremic encephalopathy* • Dialysis dementia* • Hepatic encephalopathy* • Wilson's disease
Trauma	• Head injury*
Tumors	• Brain tumors (primary)* • Metastatic tumors*
Ventricular disorders	• Hydrocephalus*
Drugs†	• Anticholinergics • phenytoin (Dilantin) • Opioids • Hypnotics • Tranquilizers • Antiparkinsonian drugs • Cardiac drugs: digoxin, methyldopa (Aldomet) • Cocaine • Heroin

*Potentially reversible.
†These are examples of drugs that may cause cognitive impairment that is potentially reversible.

Etiology and Pathophysiology

Dementia is due to both treatable and nontreatable conditions (Table 60-2). The two most common causes of dementia are neurodegenerative conditions (e.g., AD) and vascular disorders. Dementia is sometimes caused by conditions that may initially be reversible (see Table 60-2). However, with prolonged exposure or disease, irreversible changes may occur.

Vascular conditions are the second most common cause of dementia.[1] **Vascular dementia,** also called *multiinfarct dementia,* is loss of cognitive function resulting from ischemic or hemorrhagic brain lesions caused by cardiovascular disease. This type of dementia is the result of decreased blood supply from narrowing and blocking of arteries that supply the brain. Vascular dementia may be caused by a single stroke (infarct) or by multiple strokes.

Risk Factors. The greatest risk factor for dementia is aging, although it is not a normal part of aging. Family history is also an important risk factor, since those with a first-degree relative with dementia are more likely to develop the disease. Those who have more than one first-degree relative with dementia are even at higher risk of developing the disease.[1]

Other risk factors for dementia are diabetes mellitus, obesity, smoking, cardiac dysrhythmias (e.g., atrial fibrillation), hypertension, hypercholesterolemia, and coronary artery disease. Genetic factors (discussed on pp. 1446-1447) also contribute to the risk of dementia.

Diabetes dramatically increases a person's risk of developing AD or other types of dementia. Diabetes can contribute to dementia in several ways. Insulin resistance, which causes high blood glucose and in some cases leads to type 2 diabetes, may interfere with the body's ability to break down amyloid, a protein that forms brain plaques in AD. High blood glucose also produces oxygen-containing molecules that can damage cells, in a process known as oxidative stress. In addition, high blood glucose along with high cholesterol has a role in atherosclerosis, which contributes to vascular dementia.[2]

Diabetes may contribute to poor memory and diminished mental function in various other ways. The disease causes microangiopathy, which damages small blood vessels throughout the body. Ongoing damage to blood vessels in the brain may be one reason why people with diabetes are at a higher risk of cognitive problems as they grow older. [2]

Head trauma is also a risk factor for dementia. Professional football players and military veterans who had traumatic brain injury or posttraumatic stress disorder have an increased risk for AD and other types of dementia.[3,4]

Clinical Manifestations

Depending on the cause of the dementia, the onset of manifestations may be insidious and gradual or more abrupt. Often dementia associated with neurologic degeneration is gradual and progressive over time. Causes of vascular dementia often result in symptoms that appear suddenly or progress in a stepwise pattern. However, it is difficult to distinguish the etiology of dementia (vascular versus neurodegenerative) based on symptom progression alone. An acute (days to weeks) or subacute (weeks to months) pattern of change may be indicative of an infectious or metabolic cause, including encephalitis, meningitis, hypothyroidism, or drug-related dementia. The manifestations of different types of dementia overlap and can be further complicated by coexisting medical conditions.

Depression is often mistaken for dementia in older adults, and, conversely, dementia for depression. Manifestations of depression (especially in the older adult) include sadness, difficulty thinking and concentrating, fatigue, apathy, feelings of despair, and inactivity. When the depression is severe, poor concentration and attention may result, causing memory and functional impairment. When dementia and depression occur together (as happens in many patients with dementia), the intellectual deterioration can be extreme. Depression, alone or in combination with dementia, is treatable. The challenge is to make an accurate and early assessment and diagnosis (see Table 60-1).

Other clinical manifestations of dementia are discussed in the section on clinical manifestations of AD on pp. 1447-1448.

Diagnostic Studies

The diagnosis of dementia is focused on determining the cause (e.g., reversible versus irreversible factors). An important first step is a thorough medical, neurologic, and psychologic history. A thorough physical examination is performed to rule out other potential medical conditions. Screening for cobalamin (vitamin B_{12}) deficiency and hypothyroidism is often performed. Based on patient history, testing for neurosyphilis (see Chapter 59) may be performed.

Diagnosis of dementia related to vascular causes is based on cognitive loss, vascular brain lesions demonstrated by neuroimaging techniques (computed tomography [CT] or magnetic resonance imaging [MRI]), and the exclusion of other causes of dementia (e.g., AD).

NURSING AND COLLABORATIVE MANAGEMENT DEMENTIA

In many ways, management of the patient with dementia is similar to management of the patient with AD (described later in this chapter). One form of dementia, vascular dementia, can often be prevented. Preventive measures include treatment of risk factors such as hypertension, diabetes, smoking, hypercholesterolemia, and cardiac dysrhythmias. (Stroke is discussed in Chapter 58.) Drugs that are used for patients with AD are also useful in patients with vascular dementia. Drug therapy is discussed on p. 1452 later in this chapter.

ALZHEIMER'S DISEASE

Alzheimer's disease (AD) is a chronic, progressive, degenerative disease of the brain. It is the most common form of dementia, accounting for 60% to 80% of all cases of dementia.[1] AD is named after Alois Alzheimer, a German physician who in 1906 described changes in the brain tissue of a 55-year-old woman who had died of an unusual mental illness.

Approximately 5.2 million Americans suffer from AD. It is estimated that 11% of people age 65 and older, and nearly one third of those over age 85, have AD. Ultimately the disease is fatal, with death typically occurring 4 to 8 years after diagnosis, although some patients live for 20 years. AD is the sixth leading cause of death in the United States.[1] It is the only cause of death among the top 10 in United States that cannot be prevented or cured, or its progression even slowed. The burden of care for the patient with AD on the family, caregivers, and society is staggering. AD has often been referred to as the "long good-bye" or "death in slow motion."

The incidence of AD is slightly higher in African Americans and Hispanic Americans than in whites. AD has been associated with lower socioeconomic status and education level and poor access to health care. Women are more likely than men to develop AD, primarily because they live longer (see the Gender Differences box).

Etiology and Pathophysiology

The exact etiology of AD is unknown, but is likely a combination of genetic and environmental factors. AD is not a normal part of aging, but as with other forms of dementia, age is the most important risk factor for developing AD. Only a small percentage of people younger than 60 years old develop AD. When AD develops in someone younger than 60 years old, it is referred to as *early-onset AD*. AD that becomes evident in individuals more than 60 years old is called *late-onset AD* (see the Genetics in Clinical Practice box).

GENDER DIFFERENCES

Alzheimer's Disease and Dementia

Men	Women
• Men have a higher incidence of vascular dementia than women.	• Nearly two thirds of people with Alzheimer's disease are women. • Women are more likely to develop Alzheimer's disease than men, probably because they live longer. • About twice as many women as men die each year from Alzheimer's disease.

⚕ GENETICS IN CLINICAL PRACTICE

Alzheimer's Disease (AD)

Genetic Basis

Early Onset (Familial) (<60 Yr Old at Onset)
- Autosomal dominant disorder.
- Various mutations in the following genes:
  - Amyloid precursor protein *(APP)* gene on chromosome 21
  - Presenilin-1 *(PSEN1)* gene on chromosome 14
  - Presenilin-2 *(PSEN2)* gene on chromosome 1

Late Onset (Sporadic) (>60 Yr Old at Onset)
- Genetically more complex than early-onset form.
- Apolipoprotein E-4 *(ApoE-4)* allele on chromosome 19 increases the likelihood of developing AD.
- Presence of *ApoE-2* allele is associated with a lower risk of AD.

Incidence

Early Onset
- Rare form of AD, accounting for <5% of cases.
- Fifty percent risk of disease for children of affected parents.
- May occur in people as young as 30 yr old.

Late Onset
- *ApoE-4* is present in about 40% of people with late-onset AD. (It is present in 25%–30% of normal population.)
- Many *ApoE-4*-positive people do not develop AD, and many *ApoE-4*-negative people do.

Genetic Testing

Early Onset
- Genetic screening is available for mutations on chromosomes 1, 14, and 21.

Late Onset
- Blood test can identify which *ApoE* allele a person has but cannot predict who will develop disease.*
- *ApoE* testing is mainly used in research to identify people who may have an increased risk of developing AD.

Clinical Implications
- AD is the most common cause of dementia.
- Genetic testing and counseling for family members of patients with early-onset AD may be appropriate.
- If person tests positive for *ApoE-4*, it does not mean that the person will develop AD.

**ApoE testing is useful for studying AD risk in large groups of people, but not for determining an individual's specific risk.*

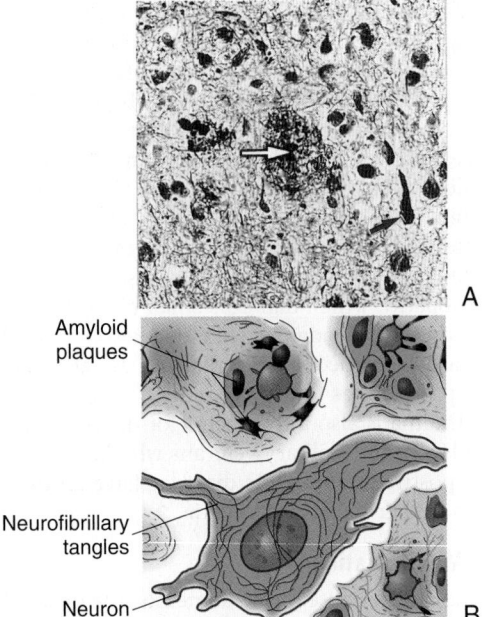

FIG. 60-2 Pathologic changes in Alzheimer's disease **A,** Plaque with central amyloid core *(white arrow)* next to a neurofibrillary tangle *(red arrow)* on the histologic specimen from a brain autopsy. **B,** Schematic representation of amyloid plaque and neurofibrillary tangle.

Individuals with a clear pattern of inheritance within a family have familial Alzheimer's disease (FAD). Other cases where no familial connection can be made are termed *sporadic.* FAD is associated with an early onset (before 60 years of age) and a more rapid disease course. In both FAD and sporadic AD, the pathogenesis of AD is similar.

Characteristic findings of AD relate to changes in the brain's structure and function: (1) amyloid plaques, (2) neurofibrillary tangles, (3) loss of connections between neurons, and (4) neuron death. Fig. 60-2 shows the pathologic changes in AD.

As part of aging, people develop some plaques in their brain tissue, but in AD more plaques appear in certain parts of the brain. These plaques consist of clusters of insoluble deposits of a protein called *β-amyloid,* other proteins, remnants of neurons, non-nerve cells such as microglia (cells that surround and digest damaged cells or foreign substances), and other cells such as astrocytes.

β-Amyloid is cleaved from amyloid precursor protein (APP), which is associated with the cell membrane (Fig. 60-3). The normal function of APP is unknown. In AD, plaques develop first in areas of the brain used for memory and cognitive function, including the hippocampus (a structure that is important in forming and storing short-term memories). Eventually AD attacks the cerebral cortex, especially the areas responsible for language and reasoning.

Neurofibrillary tangles are abnormal collections of twisted protein threads inside nerve cells. The main component of these structures is a protein called *tau.* Tau proteins in the central nervous system (CNS) are involved in providing support for intracellular structure through their support of microtubules. Tau proteins hold the microtubules together like railroad ties hold railroad tracks together. In AD the tau protein is altered, and as a result, the microtubules twist together in a helical fashion (see Fig. 60-3). This ultimately forms the neurofibrillary tangles found in the neurons of persons with AD.

Plaques and neurofibrillary tangles are not unique to patients with AD or dementia. They are also found in the brains of individuals without evidence of cognitive impairment. However, they are more abundant in the brains of individuals with AD.

The other feature of AD is the loss of connections between neurons and neuron death. These processes result in structural damage. Affected parts of the brain begin to shrink in a process called brain atrophy. By the final stage of AD, brain tissue has shrunk significantly (Fig. 60-4).

⚕ Genetic Link

Genetic factors may play a critical role in how the brain processes the β-amyloid protein. Overproduction of β-amyloid appears to be an important risk factor for AD. Abnormally high levels of β-amyloid cause cell damage either directly or by eliciting an inflammatory response and ultimately neuron death. Understanding why neurons produce β-amyloid led

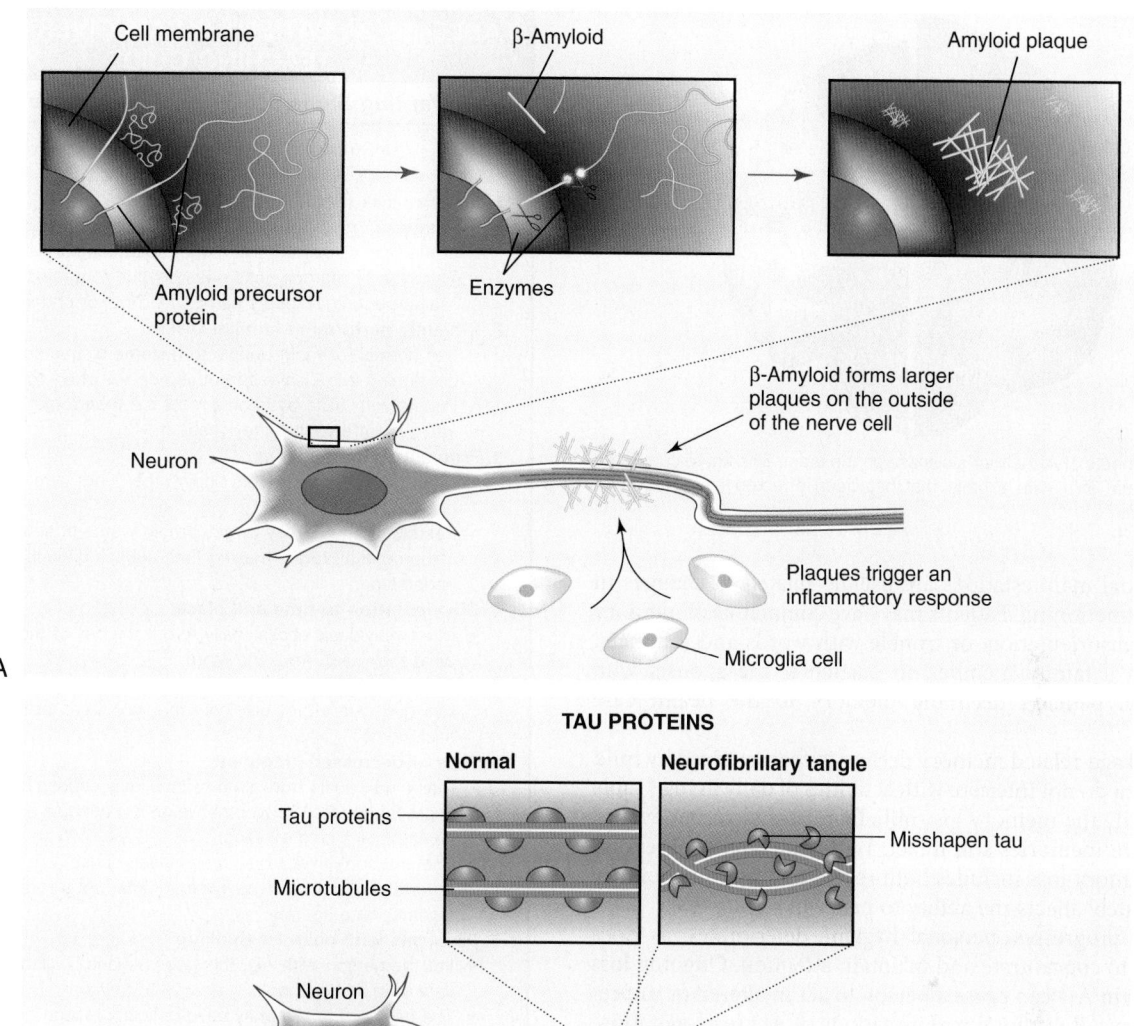

FIG. 60-3 Current etiologic theories for the development of Alzheimer's disease. **A,** Abnormal amounts of β-amyloid are cleaved from the amyloid precursor protein *(APP)* and released into the circulation. The β-amyloid fragments come together in clumps to form plaques that attach to the neuron. Microglia react to the plaque, and an inflammatory response results. **B,** Tau proteins provide structural support for the neuron microtubules. Chemical changes in the neuron produce structural changes in tau proteins. This results in twisting and tangling (neurofibrillary tangles).

researchers to examine the enzymes (and their genes) that are responsible for both the synthesis and processing of APP.

In patients with early-onset AD, three genes have been identified as important in the etiology (see the Genetics in Clinical Practice box on p. 1446). When the *presenilin-1, presenilin-2,* and *APP* genes are mutated, they cause brain cells to overproduce β-amyloid.[5]

The first gene associated with AD was the *epsilon (E)-4* allele of the *apolipoprotein E (ApoE)* gene on chromosome 19. *ApoE* comes in several different alleles or forms, but three alleles occur most commonly. People inherit one allele (i.e., *ApoE-2, ApoE-3, or ApoE-4*) from each parent. *ApoE* contains the instructions to make a protein that helps to carry cholesterol and other types of fat in the bloodstream. *ApoE* may have a role in clearing amyloid plaques. Mutations in this gene result in greater amyloid deposition. The presence of *ApoE-4*, which is a risk-factor gene, increases the risk of a person developing late-

onset AD.[5] However, the presence of the gene alone is not adequate to account for AD, since many people with *ApoE-4* do not develop AD.

Environmental Factors. As previously mentioned in the section on risk factors for dementia (pp. 1444-1445), diabetes mellitus, hypertension, current smoking, hypercholesterolemia, obesity, and trauma are associated with an increased risk of dementia, including AD.

Clinical Manifestations

Pathologic changes often precede clinical manifestations of dementia by anywhere from 5 to 20 years.[6] The Alzheimer's Association has developed a list of warning signs that include common manifestations of AD (Table 60-3). The stages of AD can be categorized as mild, moderate, and severe (Table 60-4). The rate of progression from mild to severe is highly variable and ranges from 3 to 20 years.

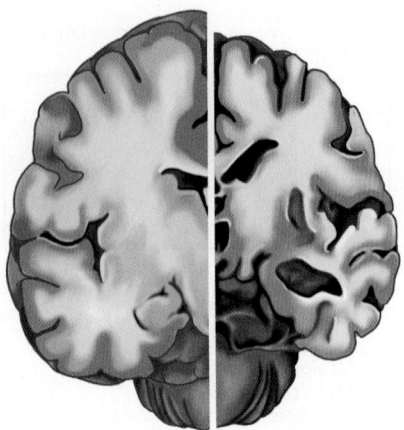

FIG. 60-4 Effects of Alzheimer's disease on the brain. This figure compares a normal brain *(left)* with a brain that has been affected by Alzheimer's disease *(right)*.

The initial manifestations are usually related to changes in cognitive functioning. Patients may have complaints of memory loss, mild disorientation, or trouble with words and numbers. Often it is a family member, in particular the spouse, who reports the patient's declining memory to the health care provider.

Normal age-related memory decline is characterized by mild changes that do not interfere with activities of daily living (Table 60-5). In AD the memory loss initially relates to recent events, with remote memories still intact. With time and progression of AD, memory loss includes both recent and remote memory and ultimately affects the ability to perform self-care.

As AD progresses, personal hygiene deteriorates, as does the ability to concentrate and maintain attention. Ongoing loss of neurons in AD can cause a person to act in altered or unpredictable ways. Behavioral manifestations of AD (e.g., agitation, aggression) result from changes that take place within the brain. They are neither intentional nor controllable by the individual with the disease. Some patients develop delusions and hallucinations.

With progression of AD, additional cognitive impairments are noted. These include *dysphasia* (difficulty comprehending language and oral communication), *apraxia* (inability to manipulate objects or perform purposeful acts), *visual agnosia* (inability to recognize objects by sight), and *dysgraphia* (difficulty communicating via writing). Eventually long-term memories cannot be recalled, and patients lose the ability to recognize family members and friends. Other problems include aggression and a tendency to wander.

Later in the disease, the ability to communicate and to perform activities of daily living is lost. In the late stages of AD, the patient is unresponsive and incontinent and requires total care.

Retrogenesis. Retrogenesis is the process in AD patients in which degenerative changes occur in the reverse order in which they were acquired.[7] This theory compares the developmental stages in children with the deterioration in AD patients. As seen in Table 60-6, a relationship exists between the developmental stage and deterioration of function. For example, it is appropriate for a person with AD in the moderate stage to feel good about putting together puzzles that belong to his 3-year-old grandson. In fact, they may play well together on the same task or project.

TABLE 60-3   PATIENT & CAREGIVER TEACHING GUIDE

Early Warning Signs of Alzheimer's Disease

Include the following information in the teaching plan for the patient with Alzheimer's disease.

1. **Memory loss that affects job skills**
   - Frequent forgetfulness or unexplainable confusion at home or in the workplace may signal that something is wrong.
   - This type of memory loss goes beyond forgetting an assignment, colleague's name, deadline, or phone number.
2. **Difficulty performing familiar tasks**
   - It is normal for most people to become distracted and to forget something (e.g., leave something on the stove too long).
   - People with AD may cook a meal but then forget not only to serve it but also that they made it.
3. **Problems with language**
   - Most people have trouble finding the "right" word from time to time.
   - Persons with AD may forget simple words or substitute inappropriate words, making their speech difficult to understand.
4. **Disorientation to time and place**
   - Most individuals occasionally forget the day of the week or what they need from the store.
   - People with AD can become lost on their own street, not knowing where they are, how they got there, or how to get back home.
5. **Poor or decreased judgment**
   - Many individuals from time to time may choose not to dress appropriately for the weather (e.g., not bringing a coat or sweater on a cold evening).
   - The person with AD may dress inappropriately in more noticeable ways, such as wearing a bathrobe to the store or a sweater on a hot day.
6. **Problems with abstract thinking**
   - For the person with AD, this goes beyond challenges such as balancing a checkbook.
   - The person with AD may have difficulty recognizing numbers or doing even basic calculations.
7. **Misplacing things**
   - For many individuals, temporarily misplacing keys, purses, or wallets is a normal albeit frustrating event.
   - The person with AD may put items in inappropriate places (e.g., eating utensils in clothing drawers) but have no memory of how they got there.
8. **Changes in mood or behavior**
   - Most individuals experience mood changes.
   - The person with AD tends to exhibit more rapid mood swings for no apparent reason.
9. **Changes in personality**
   - As most individuals age, they may demonstrate some change in personality (e.g., become less tolerant).
   - The person with AD can change dramatically, either suddenly or over time. For example, someone who is generally easygoing may become angry, suspicious, or fearful.
10. **Loss of initiative**
    - The person with AD may become and remain uninterested and uninvolved in many or all of his or her usual pursuits.

Adapted from Alzheimer's Association: *Early warning signs,* Chicago, The Association.

Diagnostic Criteria for Alzheimer's Disease

The original 1984 clinical criteria for AD defined it as having a single stage, dementia, and based the diagnosis solely on clinical symptoms. It assumed that people free of dementia symptoms were disease-free. Since then, research has determined that AD may cause changes in the brain many years before symptoms

TABLE 60-4 STAGES OF ALZHEIMER'S DISEASE

Mild	Moderate	Severe
• Forgetfulness beyond what is seen in a normal person • Short-term memory impairment, especially for new learning • Loss of initiative and interests • May forget recent events or the names of people or things • Small personality changes • May no longer be able to solve simple math problems • Slowly loses the ability to plan and organize	• Memory loss and confusion become more obvious • Has more trouble organizing, planning, and following directions • May need help getting dressed • May start having incontinence • Trouble recognizing family members and friends • Agitation, restlessness • May lack judgment and begin to wander, gets lost • May have trouble sleeping • Delusions, hallucinations, paranoia • Behavioral problems	• Severe impairment of all cognitive functions • Little memory, unable to process new information • Unable to perform self-care activities • Often needs help with daily needs • May not be able to talk • Cannot understand words • May have difficulty eating, swallowing • May not be able to walk or sit up without help • Immobility • Incontinence

TABLE 60-5 COMPARISON OF NORMAL FORGETFULNESS AND MEMORY LOSS

Normal Forgetfulness	Memory Loss in Mild Cognitive Impairment	Memory Loss in Alzheimer's Disease
• Sometimes misplaces keys, eyeglasses, or other items • Momentarily forgets an acquaintance's name • Occasionally has to search for a word • Occasionally forgets to run an errand • May forget an event from the distant past • When driving, may momentarily forget where to turn, but quickly orients self • Jokes about memory loss	• Frequently misplaces items • Frequently forgets people's names and is slow to recall them • Has increasing difficulty finding desired words • Begins to forget important events and appointments • May forget recent events or newly learned information • Becomes temporarily lost more often, may have trouble understanding and following a map • Worries about memory loss, family and friends notice lapses	• Forgets what an item is used for or puts it in an inappropriate place • May not remember knowing a person • Begins to lose language skills and may withdraw from social interaction • Loses sense of time, does not know what day it is • Has seriously impaired recent memory and difficulty learning and remembering new information • Becomes easily disoriented or lost in familiar places, sometimes for hours • May have little or no awareness of cognitive problems

Adapted from Rabins P: Memory. In *The Johns Hopkins white papers,* Baltimore, 2007, Johns Hopkins University.

TABLE 60-6 RETROGENESIS IN ALZHEIMER'S DISEASE

Stage	Alzheimer's Disease	Reisberg Stage*	Developmental Age	Diversion/Distraction Activities
Mild	No difficulty at all.	1	Adult	—
	Some memory trouble begins to affect job and home. Forgets familiar names.	2	—	—
	Much difficulty maintaining job performance. Withdrawal from difficult situations.	3	12+ yr	Can function with understanding. Enjoy things they have always enjoyed—watch TV, play and listen to music, play games.
	Can no longer hold a job, plan and prepare meals, handle personal finances, etc. Driving becomes difficult, although can drive to familiar places.	4	8-12 yr	Can still enjoy simple games, watch TV and videos. Enjoys family photos and memories.
Moderate	Can no longer select proper clothing for occasion or season. Needs help to remain safe in home. Forgets to bathe.	5	5-7 yr	Needs age-appropriate toys and games.
	Requires help with dressing.	6a	5 yr	Needs activities appropriate for preschoolers. Enjoys many of the same activities as preschoolers.
	Requires help with bathing.	6b	4 yr	
	Requires help with toileting.	6c	4 yr	
	Urinary incontinence.	6d	3-4 yr	
	Fecal incontinence.	6e	2-3 yr	
Severe	Speech limited to 5-6 intelligent words/day.	7a	15 mo	Enjoys infant toys, mobiles, dangling ribbons.
	Speech limited to one word/day.	7b	1 yr	
	Can no longer walk without assistance.	7c	1 yr	
	Can no longer sit up without assistance.	7d	6-10 mo	
	Can no longer smile.	7e	2-4 mo	
	Can no longer hold up head.	7f	1-3 mo	

*These stages are based on Functional Assessment Staging. Reisberg B: Functional assessment staging (FAST), *Psychopharmacol Bull* 24:653, 1988.

TABLE 60-7   DIAGNOSTIC CRITERIA FOR ALZHEIMER'S DISEASE*

Stage and Description		Recommendations for Biomarkers
Preclinical Alzheimer's Disease (AD)	• Brain changes, including amyloid buildup and other early neuron changes, may already be in process. • At this point, significant clinical symptoms are not yet evident. • In some people, amyloid buildup can be detected with positron emission tomography (PET) scans and cerebrospinal fluid (CSF) analysis.	• Use of imaging and biomarker tests at this stage are recommended only for research. • Biomarkers are still being developed and standardized and are not used by clinicians in general practice.
Mild Cognitive Impairment (MCI) due to Alzheimer's Disease	• The MCI stage is marked by symptoms of memory problems, enough to be noticed and measured, but not compromising a person's independence. • People with MCI may or may not progress to Alzheimer's dementia.	• Used primarily by researchers. • May be used in specialized clinical settings to supplement standard clinical tests to help determine possible causes of MCI. • May help confirm that the person's impairment is related to AD.
Dementia due to Alzheimer's Disease	• Characterized by memory, thinking, and behavioral symptoms that impair a person's ability to function in daily life. • Dementia marks the terminal stage of AD. • Encompasses all stages presented in Table 60-4.	• May be used in some cases to increase the level of certainty about a diagnosis of AD. • Also may be used to distinguish AD from other dementias.

Source: Jack CR, Albert MS, Knopman DS, et al: Introduction to the recommendations from the National Institute on Aging–Alzheimer's Association workgroups on diagnostic guidelines for Alzheimer's disease, *Alzheimers Dement* 7:257, 2011.
*Note that these are recommended criteria and guidelines. More research is needed, especially biomarker research, before the new criteria and guidelines can be used in clinical settings.

appear and that symptoms do not always directly relate to abnormal changes in the brain caused by AD.

In 2011 updated criteria and guidelines classified AD as a spectrum, where dementia marks the terminal stage of the disease (Table 60-7). The stages in the new classification spectrum are preclinical AD, mild cognitive impairment, and dementia due to AD.[8] The guidelines address the use of imaging and biomarkers (discussed in section on diagnostic studies below) that may help determine whether changes are due to AD.[9]

Preclinical Stage. A long lag exists between pathologic changes in the brain and manifestations of AD. The future goal would be to modify the disease process of AD before it becomes symptomatic. Once plaques and tangles have formed in sufficient quantity, it may be too late to intervene to prevent the disease or its progression. Although currently all attempts at modifying the disease process have failed, research is ongoing. The model for early intervention is seen in other diseases, such as removing polyps to prevent colon cancer, controlling blood glucose in diabetes before the disease progresses to heart and kidney disease, and treating cardiac risk factors before a person has a myocardial infarction.

Mild Cognitive Impairment. Mild cognitive impairment (MCI), the second stage in the AD spectrum, is a state of cognitive function in which individuals have problems with memory, language, or another essential cognitive function that are severe enough to be noticeable to others and show up on tests, but not severe enough to interfere with activities of daily living. Because the problems do not interfere with daily activities, the person does not meet the criteria for being diagnosed with dementia.[10] To the casual observer, an individual with MCI may seem fairly normal. However, the person with MCI is often aware of a significant change in memory, and family members may observe changes in the individual's abilities (see Table 60-5).

Between 10% and 20% of people 65 years old and older have MCI and are at high risk of developing AD. Some individuals with MCI show no progression and do not go on to develop AD, but an estimated 15% of people with MCI eventually do. Although not in clinical use, biomarkers can be a useful tool to predict who will develop dementia.[10]

No drugs have been approved for the treatment of MCI. Research is being conducted to determine whether patients with MCI would benefit from the medications used in AD (e.g., cholinesterase inhibitors). There is little evidence that cholinesterase inhibitors affect progression to dementia or cognitive test scores in people with MCI.[11]

Currently the primary treatment of MCI consists of ongoing monitoring. Recognize the importance of monitoring the patient with MCI for changes in memory and thinking skills that would indicate a worsening of symptoms or a progression to dementia. It is critical that you understand the 10 early warning signs of AD (see Table 60-3).

Diagnostic Studies

No definitive diagnostic test exists for AD. The diagnosis of AD is primarily a diagnosis of exclusion. In patients with cognitive impairment, there is increased emphasis on early and careful evaluation. As indicated earlier in this chapter, many conditions can cause manifestations of dementia, some of which are treatable or reversible (see Table 60-2).

When all other possible conditions that can cause cognitive impairment have been ruled out, a clinical diagnosis of AD can be made. A comprehensive patient evaluation includes a complete health history, physical examination, neurologic and mental status assessments, and laboratory tests (Table 60-8). Brain imaging tests (e.g., CT or MRI) may show brain atrophy in the later stages of the disease, although this finding occurs in other diseases and can also be seen in persons without cognitive impairment. Positron emission tomography (PET) scanning can be used to differentiate AD from other forms of dementia (Fig. 60-5). Neuroimaging techniques allow for detection of changes early in the disease and monitoring of treatment response. A definitive diagnosis of AD usually requires examination of brain tissue at autopsy and findings of neurofibrillary tangles and neuritic plaques.

The new criteria and guidelines identify two biomarker categories: (1) biomarkers showing the level of β-amyloid accumulation in the brain and (2) biomarkers showing that nerve cells in the brain are injured or actually degenerating. Biomarkers include (1) cerebrospinal fluid (CSF) neurochemical markers:

TABLE 60-8 COLLABORATIVE CARE

Alzheimer's Disease

Diagnostic

- History and physical examination, including psychologic evaluation
- Neuropsychologic testing, including Mini-Cog (Table 60-9), Mini-Mental State Examination (eTable 60-1)
- Brain imaging tests: CT, MRI, MRS, PET
- Complete blood count
- Electrocardiogram
- Serum glucose, creatinine, BUN
- Serum levels of vitamins B_1, B_6, B_{12}
- Thyroid function tests
- Liver function tests
- Screening for depression

Collaborative Therapy

- Drug therapy for cognitive problems (see Table 60-10)
- Behavioral modification
- Moderate exercise
- Assistance with functional independence
- Assistance and support for caregiver

MRS, Magnetic resonance spectroscopy; *PET,* positron emission tomography

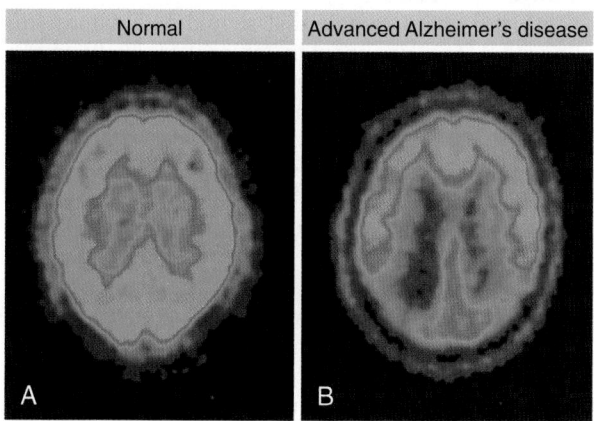

Normal	Advanced Alzheimer's disease
A	B

FIG. 60-5 Positron emission tomography (PET) scan can be used to assist in the diagnosis of Alzheimer's disease (AD). Radioactive fluorine is applied to glucose (fluorodeoxyglucose), and the yellow areas indicate metabolically active cells. **A,** A normal brain. **B,** Advanced AD is recognized by hypometabolism in many areas of the brain.

TABLE 60-9 THE MINI-COG

Introduction

The Mini-Cog is used as a brief assessment tool for cognitive impairment. It can be quickly administered and can guide the need for further evaluation.

Administration

1. Instruct the patient to listen carefully to and remember three unrelated words and then to repeat the words. *Example:* apple, table, penny. (This initial step is not scored.)
   The same three words may be repeated to the patient up to three tries to register all three words.
2. Instruct the patient to draw the face of a clock, either on a blank sheet of paper or on a sheet with the clock circle already drawn on the page. After the patient puts the numbers on the clock face, ask him or her to draw the hands of the clock to read a specific time (11:10). The test is considered normal if all numbers are present in the correct sequence and position, and the hands readably display the requested time.
3. Ask the patient to repeat the three previously stated words.
   Scoring (out of total of 5 points)
   Give 1 point for each recalled word after the clock drawing test.
   - Patients recalling none of the three words are classified as cognitively impaired (score = 0).
   - Patients recalling all three words are classified as not cognitively impaired (score = 3).
   - Patients with intermediate word recall of one or two words are classified on the clock drawing test:
     The clock drawing test is scored 2 if normal and 0 if abnormal.
     Interpretation of results
     0-2: Positive screen for dementia
     3-5: Negative screen for dementia

Source: Borson S, Scanlan J, Brush M, et al: The Mini-Cog: a cognitive "vital signs" measure for dementia screening in multi-lingual elderly, *Intern J Geriatr Psychiatry* 15(11):1021, 2000.

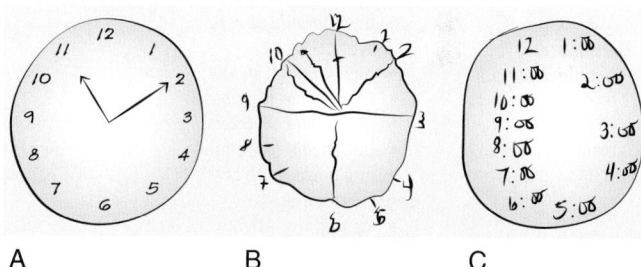

A B C

FIG. 60-6 Clock drawing is a simple test that can be used as an assessment technique in dementia. The person undergoing testing is asked to draw a clock, put in all of the numbers, and set the hands at 10 past 11. **A,** Shows a clock drawn by a person with no dementia. **B** and **C** show clocks drawn by people with dementia.

β-amyloid and tau proteins and (2) imaging biomarkers: volumetric MRI and PET. The level of tau in the CSF is an indication of neurodegeneration. (Plasma levels of tau or β-amyloid are not of any value in diagnosing AD.) In AD multiple brain structures atrophy and the volume of the brain correlates with neurodegeneration. PET determines brain metabolism using glucose tracers (see Fig. 60-5). PET can also be used to detect amyloid.

Some imaging biomarkers are used in specialized clinical settings. CSF biomarkers are mainly used for research. Biomarkers may be used in some cases to increase the level of certainty about a diagnosis of Alzheimer's dementia and to distinguish Alzheimer's dementia from other dementias. However, more research is needed with biomarkers before they are used routinely in clinical practice.

Neuropsychologic testing with tools such as the Mini-Cog (Table 60-9) and the Mini-Mental State Examination (see eTable 60-1, available on the website for this chapter) can help document the degree of cognitive impairment. The clock drawing test can be used as part of the Mini-Cog or by itself to assess cognitive function (Fig. 60-6). Neuropsychologic testing is important not only for diagnostic purposes but also to establish a baseline for evaluating changes over time.

Collaborative Care

At this time there is no cure for AD. No treatment is available to stop the deterioration of brain cells in AD. Nothing stops or really slows the progression of the disease.

The collaborative management of AD is aimed at (1) controlling the undesirable behavioral manifestations that the patient may exhibit and (2) providing support for the family caregiver.

Drug Therapy. Although drug therapy for AD is available (Table 60-10), these drugs do not cure or reverse the progression of the disease. Drugs help many people, but not for very long and not very well. The use of drugs may lead to a modest decrease in the rate of decline of cognitive function. However, the drugs have no effect on overall disease progression.[12,13]

Cholinesterase inhibitors block cholinesterase, the enzyme responsible for the breakdown of acetylcholine in the synaptic cleft (Fig. 60-7). Cholinesterase inhibitors include donepezil (Aricept), rivastigmine (Exelon), and galantamine (Razadyne). Rivastigmine is available as a patch.

Memantine (Namenda) protects the brain's nerve cells against excess amounts of glutamate, which is released in large amounts by cells damaged by AD. The attachment of glutamate to N-methyl-D-aspartate (NMDA) receptors permits calcium to flow freely into the cell, which in turn may lead to cell degenera-tion. Memantine may prevent this destructive sequence by blocking the action of glutamate.

Treating the depression that is often associated with AD may improve cognitive ability. Depression is often treated with selec-tive serotonin reuptake inhibitors, including fluoxetine (Prozac), sertraline (Zoloft), fluvoxamine (Luvox), and citalopram (Celexa). The antidepressant trazodone (Desyrel) may help with problems related to sleep.

Although antipsychotic drugs are approved for treating psy-chotic conditions (e.g., schizophrenia), they have been used for the management of behavioral problems (e.g., agitation, aggres-sive behavior) that occur in patients with AD. However, these drugs have been shown to increase the risk of death in older dementia patients.[14] The U.S. Food and Drug Administration (FDA) has warned that antipsychotics are not indicated for the treatment of dementia-related psychosis. However, the warning does not mean that the drugs cannot be used for these patients with dementia.

TABLE 60-10 DRUG THERAPY

Alzheimer's Disease

Problem	Drugs
Decreased memory and cognition	Cholinesterase inhibitors • donepezil (Aricept) • rivastigmine (Exelon) • galantamine (Razadyne) N-methyl-D-aspartate (NMDA) receptor antagonist • memantine (Namenda)
Depression	Selective serotonin reuptake inhibitors (SSRIs) • sertraline (Zoloft) • fluvoxamine (Luvox) • citalopram (Celexa) • fluoxetine (Prozac) Atypical antidepressants • mirtazapine (Remeron) • trazodone (Desyrel)
Behavioral problems (e.g., agitation, physical aggression, disinhibition)	Antipsychotics* • haloperidol (Haldol) • risperidone (Risperdal) • olanzapine (Zyprexa) • quetiapine (Seroquel) • aripiprazole (Abilify) Benzodiazepines • lorazepam (Ativan) • clonazepam (Klonopin)
Sleep disturbances	zolpidem (Ambien)

*The use of these drugs in older patients with dementia is associated with an increased risk of death.

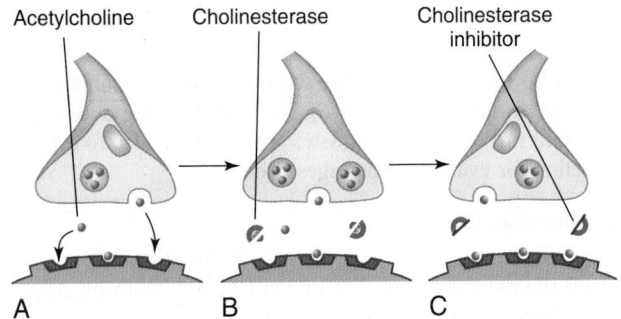

FIG. 60-7 Mechanism of action of cholinesterase inhibitors. **A,** Acetylcho-line is released from the nerve synapses and carries a message across the synapse. **B,** Cholinesterase breaks down acetylcholine. **C,** Cholinesterase inhibitors block cholinesterase, thus giving acetylcholine more time to trans-mit the message.

NURSING MANAGEMENT ALZHEIMER'S DISEASE

NURSING ASSESSMENT

Subjective and objective data that should be obtained from a person with AD are presented in Table 60-11. Useful questions for the patient and caregiver are, "When did you first notice the memory loss?" and "How has the memory loss progressed since then?"

NURSING DIAGNOSES

Nursing diagnoses for AD may include, but are not limited to, the following:
- Impaired memory *related to* the effects of dementia
- Self-neglect *related to* memory deficit, cognitive impairment, and neuromuscular impairment
- Risk for injury *related to* impaired judgment, gait instability, muscle weakness, and sensory/perceptual alteration
- Wandering *related to* cognitive impairment

Additional information on nursing diagnoses for the patient with AD is presented in eNursing Care Plan 60-1 (available on the website for this chapter).

PLANNING

The overall goals are that the patient with AD will (1) maintain functional ability for as long as possible, (2) be maintained in a safe environment with a minimum of injuries, (3) have personal care needs met, and (4) have dignity maintained. The overall goals for the caregiver of a patient with AD are to (1) reduce caregiver stress; (2) maintain personal, emotional, and physical health; and (3) cope with the long-term effects of caregiving.

NURSING IMPLEMENTATION

HEALTH PROMOTION. Can AD be prevented? Although there is no known definitive way to prevent AD, several steps can help keep your brain healthy:
- *Avoid harmful substances.* Excessive drinking and drug abuse can damage brain cells.
- *Challenge yourself.* Read frequently, do crossword puzzles. Keep mentally active. Learn new skills. This strengthens the brain connections and promotes new ones.
- *Exercise regularly.* Even low to moderate level activity such as walking or gardening three to five times per

TABLE 60-11 NURSING ASSESSMENT

Alzheimer's Disease

Subjective Data
Important Health Information
Past health history: Repeated head trauma, stroke, previous CNS infection, family history of dementia
Medications: Use of any drug to decrease symptoms (e.g., tranquilizers, hypnotics, antidepressants, antipsychotics)

Functional Health Patterns
Health perception–health management: Positive family history; emotional lability
Nutritional-metabolic: Anorexia, malnutrition, weight loss
Elimination: Incontinence
Activity-exercise: Poor personal hygiene; gait instability, weakness; inability to perform activities of daily living
Sleep-rest: Frequent nighttime awakening, daytime napping
Cognitive-perceptual: Forgetfulness, inability to cope with complex situations, difficulty with problem solving (early signs); depression, withdrawal, suicidal ideation (early)

Objective Data
General
Disheveled appearance, agitation

Neurologic
Mild: Loss of recent memory; disorientation to date and time; flat affect; lack of spontaneity; impaired abstraction, cognition, and judgment
Moderate: Agitation; impaired ability to recognize close family and friends; loss of remote memory; confusion, apraxia, agnosia, alexia (inability to understand written language); aphasia; inability to do simple tasks
Severe: Inability to do self-care; incontinence; immobility; limb rigidity; flexor posturing

Possible Diagnostic Findings
Diagnosis by exclusion, cerebral cortical atrophy on CT scan, poor scores on mental status tests, hippocampal atrophy on MRI scan, abnormal changes on PET

---

week can make you feel better. Daily physical activity, even in older adults, can decrease the risk for cognitive decline.[15]

- *Stay socially active.* Family, friends, church, and a sense of community may all contribute to better brain health.
- *Avoid trauma to the brain.* Because traumatic brain injury may be a risk factor for developing AD, promote safety in physical activities and driving.
- *Treat depression.* Recognize and treat depression early. Depression may cause or worsen memory loss and other cognitive impairment.

Early recognition and treatment of AD are important. You have a responsibility to inform patients and their families regarding the early signs of AD (see Table 60-3).

ACUTE INTERVENTION. The diagnosis of AD is traumatic for both the patient and the family. It is not unusual for the patient to respond with depression, denial, anxiety, fear, withdrawal, and feelings of loss. In the early stages of AD, patients are often aware that their memory is faulty and do things to cover up or mask the problem. See the Resources at the end of this chapter for a link to *What Happens Next?*, a booklet specifically for people dealing with the beginning stages of dementia.

You are in an important position to assess for depression. Antidepressant drugs and counseling may be indicated. Family

caregivers may also be in denial and may not seek medical attention early in the disease. Along with patient assessment, assess family caregivers and their ability to accept and cope with the diagnosis.

Although no current treatment is available for reversing AD, there is a need for ongoing monitoring of both the patient with AD and the patient's caregiver. An important nursing responsibility is to work collaboratively with the caregiver to manage clinical manifestations effectively as they change over time. You are often responsible for teaching the caregiver to perform the many tasks that are required to manage the patient's care. Consider both the patient with AD and the caregiver as patients with overlapping but unique problems.[16]

Patients with AD may be hospitalized for other health problems. Patients with AD are subject to acute and other chronic illnesses and may require surgical interventions. Their inability to communicate symptoms of health problems places the responsibility for assessment and diagnosis on caregivers and health care professionals. Hospitalization of the patient with AD can be a traumatic event for both the patient and caregiver and can precipitate a worsening of the disease or delirium. Patients with AD in the acute care setting need to be observed more closely because of concerns for safety, frequently oriented to place and time, and given reassurance. Anxiety or disruptive behavior may be reduced through the use of consistent nursing staff.

AMBULATORY AND HOME CARE. Currently, family members and friends care for most individuals with AD in their homes. Others with AD reside in various facilities, including long-term care and assisted living facilities. A facility that is good for one person may not be suitable for another. Also, what is helpful for a person at one point in the disease process may be completely different from what is best when the disease progresses.

Patients with AD move through the stages at variable rates. The nursing care required by the patient with AD changes as the disease progresses, emphasizing the need for regular assessment and support. Regardless of the setting, the severity of the problems and the amount of nursing care required intensify over time. The specific manifestations of the disease depend on the area of the brain involved. Nursing care focuses on decreasing clinical manifestations, preventing harm, and supporting the patient and caregiver throughout the disease process.

In the early stages of AD, memory aids (e.g., calendars) may be beneficial. Patients often develop depression during this phase. Depression may be related to the diagnosis of an incurable disorder and the impact of the disease on activities of daily living (e.g., driving, socializing with friends, participating in hobbies or recreational activities).

After the initial diagnosis, patients need to be aware that the progression of the disease is variable. Effective management of the disease may slow the progress of the disease and decrease the burden on the patient, caregiver, and family. However, decisions related to care should be made with the patient, family members, and health care team early in the disease. You have a role in advising the patient and caregiver to initiate health care decisions, including advance directives, while the patient has the capacity to do so. This can ease the burden for the caregiver as the disease progresses.

Adult day care is one of the options available to the person with AD. Although programs vary in size, structure, physical environment, and staff experience, the common goals of all day care programs are to provide respite for the family and a protective environment for the patient. During the early and moderate stages of AD, the person can still benefit from stimulating activities that encourage independence and decision making in a protective environment.[17] The patient returns home tired, content, less frustrated, and ready to be with the family. The respite from the demands of care allows the caregiver to be more responsive to the patient's needs.

As the disease progresses, the demands on the caregiver eventually exceed the resources, and the person with AD may need to be placed in a long-term care facility. Special units to care for persons with AD are becoming increasingly common in long-term care settings. The Alzheimer's unit is designed with an emphasis on safety. For example, many facilities have designated areas that allow the patient to walk freely within the unit, while the unit is secured so that the patient cannot wander outside of it.

As the patient with AD progresses to the late stages (severe impairment) of AD, he or she has increased difficulty with the most basic functions, including walking and talking. Total care is required.

Specific problems relate to the care of the patient with AD in all phases of the disease. These problems are described below.

Behavioral Problems. Behavioral problems occur in about 90% of patients with AD. These problems include repetitiveness (asking the same question repeatedly), delusions (false beliefs), hallucinations, agitation, aggression, altered sleeping patterns, wandering, and resisting care. Many times these behaviors are unpredictable and may challenge caregivers. Caregivers need to be aware that these behaviors are not intentional and are often difficult to control. Behavioral symptoms often lead to the placement of patients in institutional care settings.

These behaviors are often the patient's way of responding to a precipitating factor (e.g., pain, frustration, temperature extremes, anxiety). When these behaviors become problematic, you must plan interventions carefully. Initially assess the patient's physical status. Check the patient for changes in vital signs, urinary and bowel patterns, and pain that could account for behavioral problems. Then assess the environment to identify factors that may trigger behavior disruptions. Extremes in temperature or excessive noise may lead to behavior changes. When the patient is agitated by the environment, either move the patient or remove the stimulus.

When a patient resists or pulls tubes or dressings, cover these items with stretch tube gauze or remove them from the visual field. Reassure the patient that you are present to keep him or her safe. Do not ask the confused or agitated patient challenging "why" questions. If the patient cannot verbalize distress, validate his or her mood. Rephrase the patient's statement to validate its meaning. Closely observe the patient's emotional state.

Nursing strategies that address difficult behavior include redirection, distraction, and reassurance. For the patient who is restless or agitated, redirecting involves changing the patient's focus (e.g., having the patient perform activities such as sweeping, raking, or dusting). Ways to distract the agitated patient may include providing snacks, taking a car ride, sitting on a porch swing or rocker, listening to favorite music, watching videotapes, looking at family photographs, or walking. Reassurance involves communicating to the patient that he or she will be protected from danger, harm, or embarrassment. Use of repetitive activities, songs, poems, music, massage, aromas, or a favorite object can be soothing to patients.[18]

When dealing with the difficult patient, do not threaten to restrain the patient or call the physician. A calming family member can be asked to stay with the patient until the patient becomes calmer. Monitor the patient frequently, and document all interventions. As verbal skills decline, you and the caregiver must rely more on the patient's body language to communicate care needs. The use of positive nurse actions can reduce the use of chemical (drug therapy) restraints.

Disruptive behaviors have been treated with antipsychotic drugs (see Table 60-10). However, as discussed on p. 1452, these drugs have adverse side effects. Before these drugs are used, all other measures of treating behavioral issues should be exhausted.

A specific type of agitation, termed sundowning, is when the patient becomes more confused and agitated in the late afternoon or evening. Behaviors commonly exhibited include agitation, aggressiveness, wandering, resistance to redirection, and increased verbal activity such as yelling. The cause of sundowning is unclear, but several theories propose that it is due to a disruption of circadian rhythms. Other possible causes include fatigue, unfamiliar environment and noise (especially in an acute care setting), medications, reduced lighting, and sleep fragmentation. When a patient experiences sundowning, remain calm and avoid confrontation. Assess the situation for possible causes of the agitation. Nursing interventions that may be helpful include (1) creating a quiet, calm environment; (2) maximizing exposure to daylight (open blinds and turn on lights during the day); (3) evaluating medications to determine if any could cause sleep disturbance; (4) limiting naps and caffeine; and (5) consulting with the health care provider regarding drug therapy. Management of sundowning can be challenging for you, the patient, and the family.

Safety. The person with AD is at risk for problems related to personal safety. Potential hazards include falling, ingesting dangerous substances, wandering, injuring others and self with sharp objects, being burned, and being unable to respond to crisis situations. These concerns require careful attention to the home environment to minimize risk. Supervision is also required. As the patient's cognitive function declines over time, the patient may have difficulty navigating physical spaces and interpreting environmental cues. Assist the caregiver in assessing the home environment for safety risks.

SAFETY ALERT
Teach the caregiver to take the following steps:
- Have stairwells well lit.
- Handrails should be graspable.
- Tack down carpet edges.
- Remove throw rugs and extension cords.
- Use nonskid mats in tub or shower.
- Install handrails in the bath and by the commode.

Wandering is a major concern for caregivers. Wandering may be related to loss of memory or to side effects of drugs, or it may be an expression of a physical or emotional need, restlessness, curiosity, or stimuli that trigger memories of earlier routines. As with other behaviors, observe for factors or events that may precipitate wandering. For example, the patient may be sensitive to stress and tension in the environment. In such cases, wandering may reflect an attempt to leave.[19]

When someone with AD is discovered missing, every second counts. To assist caregivers with locating them, the Alzheimer's Association and the MedicAlert Foundation have created an alliance called MedicAlert + Alzheimer's Association Safe Return.[20] This program includes identification products (e.g.,

DELEGATION DECISIONS
Caring for the Patient With Alzheimer's Disease

All staff members who care for a patient with Alzheimer's disease (AD) are responsible for ensuring the patient's physiologic and psychosocial safety. The registered nurse (RN) is responsible for ongoing assessments of the patient's level of function and for development of the plan of care. Since most patients with AD are cared for at home or in long-term care settings, many routine nursing activities are delegated to licensed practical/vocational nurses (LPN/LVNs), unlicensed assistive personnel (UAP), or family caregivers.

Role of Registered Nurse (RN)
- Assess patient memory and level of function.
- Teach patient and caregivers memory enhancement aids (e.g., calendars, notes).
- Monitor for physiologic problems associated with AD, such as pain, swallowing difficulties, urinary tract infection, pneumonia, skin breakdown, and constipation.
- Assess patient's nutritional and fluid intake and develop a plan to ensure adequate intake.
- Evaluate patient's safety risk factors.
- Determine possible precipitating factors for behavioral changes and develop strategies to address difficult behavior.
- Assess the family caregiver's stress level and coping strategies.
- Make referrals for community services such as adult day care and respite care.

Role of Licensed Practical/Vocational Nurse (LPN/LVN)
- Monitor for behavioral changes that may indicate physiologic problems.
- Check patient environment for potential safety hazards.
- Administer enteral feedings to patients who are unable to swallow (if ordered).
- Administer ordered drug therapy.

Role of Unlicensed Assistive Personnel (UAP)
- Assist patient to use the toilet, commode, or bedpan at frequent intervals.
- Provide personal hygiene, skin care, oral care.
- Help patients with eating.
- Assist patients with daily activities.
- Use bed alarms and surveillance to decrease risk for falls.

bracelet, necklace, wallet cards), a national photo and information database, a 24-hour toll-free emergency crisis line, local chapter support, and wandering behavior education and training for caregivers and families.

Pain Management. Because of difficulties with oral and written language, AD patients may have difficulty expressing physical complaints, including pain. You need to rely on other clues such as the patient's behavior. Pain can result in alterations in the patient's behavior, such as increased vocalization, agitation, withdrawal, and changes in function. Pain should be recognized and treated promptly and the patient's response monitored.

Eating and Swallowing Difficulties. Undernutrition is a problem in the moderate and severe stages of AD, with patients in long-term facilities having the highest incidence of undernutrition. Loss of interest in food and decreased ability to self-feed (*feeding apraxia),* as well as co-morbid conditions, can result in significant nutritional deficiencies in the patient with AD. In long-term care facilities, inadequate assistance with feeding may add to the problem.

Use pureed foods, thickened liquids, and nutritional supplements when chewing and swallowing become problematic for the patient. Patients may need reminders to chew their food

and to swallow. Patients need a quiet and unhurried environment for eating. Avoid distractions at mealtimes, including the television. Low lighting, music, and simulated nature sounds may improve eating behaviors. Easy-grip eating utensils and finger foods may allow the patient to self-feed. Offer liquids frequently.

When oral feeding is not possible, explore alternative routes. Nasogastric (NG) feeding may be used for short periods. However, for the long term the NG tube is uncomfortable and may add to the patient's agitation. A percutaneous endoscopic gastrostomy (PEG) tube provides another option (see Fig. 40-7). However, PEG tubes can be problematic, since patients with AD are particularly vulnerable to aspiration of feeding formula and tube dislodgment. The potential positive outcomes to be gained from nutritional therapies are considered in light of overall outcome goals and potential adverse effects of the specific therapy. Nutritional support therapies are described in Chapter 40.

Oral Care. In the late stages of AD the patient is unable to perform oral self-care. With decreased tooth brushing and flossing, dental problems are likely to occur. Because of swallowing difficulties, patients may retain food in the mouth, adding to the potential for tooth decay. Dental caries and tooth abscess can add to patient discomfort or pain and subsequently may increase agitation. Inspect the mouth regularly and provide mouth care to those patients unable to do self-care.

Infection Prevention. Urinary tract infection and pneumonia are the most common infections in patients with AD. Such infections are ultimately the cause of death in many patients with AD. Because of feeding and swallowing problems, the patient is at risk for aspiration pneumonia. Immobility can also predispose the patient to pneumonia. Reduced fluid intake, prostate hyperplasia in men, poor hygiene, and urinary drainage devices (e.g., catheters) can predispose patients to bladder infection. Any manifestations of infection, such as a change in behavior, fever, cough (pneumonia), or pain on urination (bladder), need prompt evaluation and treatment.

Skin Care. It is important to monitor the patient's skin over time. Note and treat rashes, areas of redness, and skin breakdown. In the late stages, incontinence along with immobility and undernutrition can place the patient at risk for skin breakdown. Keep the skin dry and clean, and change the patient's position regularly to avoid areas of pressure over bony prominences.

Elimination Problems. During the moderate and severe stages of AD, urinary and fecal incontinence lead to increased need for nursing care. When possible, habit or behavioral retraining of bladder and bowel function (e.g., scheduled toileting) may help decrease episodes of incontinence.

Another common elimination problem is constipation. Causes may relate to immobility, dietary intake (e.g., reduced fiber intake), and decreased fluid intake. Increased dietary fiber, fiber supplements, and stool softeners are the first lines of management. The combination of aging, other health problems, and swallowing difficulties may increase the risk of complications associated with the use of mineral oil, stimulants, osmotic agents, and enemas. Management of constipation is discussed in Chapter 43.

Caregiver Support. An estimated 15 million Americans provide unpaid care for people with AD or other dementia.[1] The majority of these are family members providing care in the home (Fig. 60-8). AD is a disease that disrupts all aspects of personal and family life. Caregivers for persons with AD describe it as very

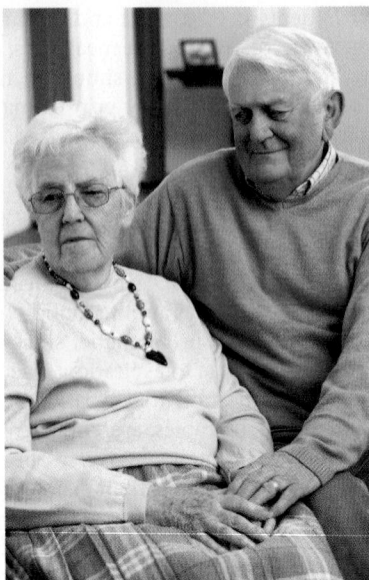

FIG. 60-8 Caregivers of patients with dementia face an incredible challenge that often causes deterioration in their own physical and emotional health. (iStockphoto/Thinkstock.)

TABLE 60-12	**FAMILY & CAREGIVER TEACHING GUIDE**

Alzheimer's Disease

Include the following instructions when teaching families and caregivers the management of the patient with Alzheimer's disease.

Mild Stage
- Many treatable (and potentially reversible) conditions can mimic dementia (see Table 60-2). Try to get a definitive diagnosis.
- Get the person to stop driving. Confusion and poor judgment can impair driving skills and potentially put others at risk.
- Encourage activities such as visiting with friends and family, listening to music, participating in hobbies, and exercising.
- Provide cues in the home, establish a routine, and determine a specific location where essential items (e.g., glasses) need to be kept.
- Do not correct misstatements or faulty memory.
- Register with MedicAlert + Alzheimer's Association Safe Return, a program established by the MedicAlert Foundation and the Alzheimer's Association to locate individuals who wander from their homes.
- Make plans for the future in terms of advance directives, care options, financial concerns, and personal preference for care.

Moderate Stage
- Install door locks for patient safety.
- Provide protective wear for urinary and fecal incontinence.
- Ensure that the home has good lighting, install handrails in stairways and bathroom, and remove area rugs.
- Label drawers and faucets (hot and cold) to ensure safety.
- Develop strategies such as distraction and diversion to cope with behavioral problems. Identify and reduce potential triggers (e.g., reduce stress, extremes in temperature) for disruptive behavior.
- Provide memory triggers, such as pictures of family and friends.

Severe Stage
- Provide a regular schedule for toileting to reduce incontinence.
- Provide care to meet needs, including oral care and skin care.
- Monitor diet and fluid intake to ensure their adequacy.
- Continue communication through talking and touching.
- Consider placement in a long-term care facility when providing total care becomes too difficult.

stressful (see Table 4-5). These caregivers also exhibit adverse consequences relating to their own emotional and physical health.

The chronic and often severe stress associated with dementia caregiving increases the risk for the development of dementia in spouse caregivers. One mechanism proposed is that the detrimental effects of the chronic stress of caregiving can affect the hippocampus, a region of the brain responsible for memory.[21]

As the disease progresses, the relationship of the caregiver to the patient changes. Family roles may be altered or reversed (e.g., son caring for father). Decisions must be made, including when to tell the patient about the diagnosis, when to have the patient stop driving or doing activities that might be dangerous, when to ask for assistance, and when to place the patient in adult day care or a long-term care facility. With early-onset AD, the patient is affected during his or her most productive years in terms of career and family. The consequences can be devastating for the patient and the family.[22]

Sexual relations for couples are also seriously affected by AD. As the disease progresses, sexual interest may decline for both the patient and partner. A number of reasons account for this, including fatigue, memory impairment, and episodes of incontinence. The patient may also become sexually driven as the disease progresses and the patient becomes more uninhibited.

Work with the caregiver to assess stressors (see Table 4-4) and to identify coping strategies to reduce the burden of caregiving.[23] For example, ask which behaviors are most disruptive to family life at a given time, while remembering that this is likely to change as the disease progresses. Determining what the caregiver views as most disruptive or distressful can help to establish priorities for care. Risk to the safety of the patient and caregiver is given high priority. It is also important to assess what the caregiver's expectations are regarding the patient's behavior. Are the expectations reasonable given the progression of the disease? A family and caregiver teaching guide based on the disease stages is provided in Table 60-12. Other tips for caregivers are listed in Table 60-13. A nursing care plan for the family caregiver (eNursing Care Plan 60-2) is available on the website for this chapter.

Support groups for caregivers and family members (Fig. 60-9) can provide an atmosphere of understanding and give current information about the disease itself and related topics such as safety, legal, ethical, and financial issues. The needs of family caregivers are discussed in Chapter 4 on pp. 51-52. Strategies related to stress management are discussed in Chapter 7.

The Alzheimer's Association has many educational and support systems available to help family caregivers. The link to a booklet for caregivers, *Caring for a Person With Alzheimer's Disease*, is provided in the Resources section at the end of this chapter.

EVALUATION

Expected outcomes are that the patient with AD will
- Function at the highest level of cognitive ability
- Perform basic personal care activities of daily living, including bathing, dressing, feeding, and toileting by self or with assistance as needed

TABLE 60-13 GUIDELINES FOR DEALING WITH DEMENTIA PATIENTS

Do

- Treat them like adults, with respect and dignity, even when their behavior is childlike.
- Use gentle touch and direct eye contact.
- Remain patient, flexible, calm, and understanding.
- Anticipate challenging behaviors, since the patient's ability to think logically has been affected.
- Give directions using gestures or pictures.
- Simplify tasks. Focus on one thing at a time.
- Avoid questions or topics that require extensive thought, memory, or words.
- Be flexible. If one approach does not work, try another.
- Use distraction, changing the subject, redirecting to another activity.
- Provide reassurance. Praise sincerely for success.

Do Not

- Criticize, correct, or argue.
- Rush or hurry the patient.
- Force participation in activities or events.
- Talk about the patient as if he or she is not there.
- Blame the person with AD. Instead blame the disease.
- Take challenging behaviors personally. These behaviors are due to the patient's disease.
- Use condescending terms, such as "honey" or "sweetie."
- Use threatening gestures.
- Overreact to the person with AD.
- Try to explain "why" or rationalize.

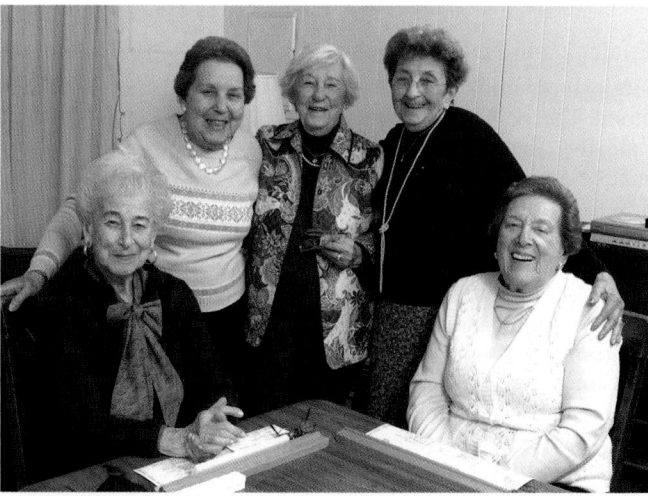

FIG. 60-9 Support groups are an effective way to help caregivers cope. (iStockphoto/Thinkstock.)

- Experience no injury
- Remain in restricted area during ambulation and activity

Additional information on the expected outcomes for the patient with AD is addressed in eNursing Care Plan 60-1 (available on the website for this chapter).

OTHER NEURODEGENERATIVE DISEASES

Parkinson's disease and Huntington's disease are both neurodegenerative diseases (see Chapter 59). Both diseases are chronic, progressive, and incurable. Despite differences in the

EVIDENCE-BASED PRACTICE

Translating Research Into Practice

Does Cognitive Reframing Help Caregivers of Patients With Dementia?

Clinical Question
What are the effects of cognitive reframing interventions (I) on psychologic morbidity and stress (O) in family caregivers (P) of patients with dementia?

Best Available Evidence
Systematic review of randomized controlled trials (RCTs)

Critical Appraisal and Synthesis of Evidence
- Eleven RCTs (n = 1139) on family caregivers of community-dwelling people with dementia.
- Cognitive reframing is changing distressing cognitions and thoughts into ones that support adaptive behavior.
- Interventions focused on (1) family caregivers' beliefs about their own responsibilities and interpretation of problem behaviors of their relatives with dementia and/or (2) beliefs about their own need for support and assistance.
- Outcomes were psychologic morbidity (depression, anxiety); caregiver stress; and caregiver appraisals of burden, coping, and problem behaviors in their relative with dementia.
- Cognitive reframing reduced caregivers' anxiety, depression, and stress but did not affect their appraisals of coping or burden or reactions to their relatives' behaviors.

Conclusion
- Cognitive reframing for family caregivers reduces psychologic morbidity and stress.

Implications for Nursing Practice
- Assess the intensity and complexity of family caregivers' responsibilities and demands.
- Help caregivers access stress management resources (e.g., support groups) in their communities.
- Support and encourage caregivers to identify and implement strategies to reduce their stress, depression, and anxiety.

Reference for Evidence
Vernooij-Dassen M, Draskovic I, McCleery J, et al: Cognitive reframing for carers of people with dementia, *Cochrane Database Syst Rev* 11: CD005318, 2011.

P, Patient population of interest; *I*, intervention or area of interest; *O*, outcomes of interest (see p. 12).

etiology and pathophysiology of these diseases, both are associated with the development of dementia in the later stages of disease.

Dementia with Lewy bodies (DLB) is a condition characterized by the presence of Lewy bodies (abnormal deposits of the protein α-synuclein) in the brainstem and cortex. Patients typically have symptoms of parkinsonism, hallucinations, short-term memory loss, unpredictable cognitive shifts, and sleep disturbances. A possible diagnosis of DLB is indicated by dementia plus two of the following symptoms: (1) extrapyramidal signs such as bradykinesia, rigidity, and postural instability, but not always a tremor; (2) fluctuating cognitive ability; and (3) hallucinations. This disease has features of both AD and Parkinson's disease, and it is imperative that a correct diagnosis be reached.

Medications for DLB are determined on an individual basis. Medications may include levodopa/carbidopa and acetylcholinesterase inhibitors. Nursing care for these patients relates to management of the dementia and of problems related to dysphagia and immobility. Swallowing problems can lead to impaired nutrition. These patients are at risk for falls from impaired mobility and balance. Pneumonia is a common complication. The diagnostic criteria for LBD are based on clinical signs and symptoms and confirmed at autopsy by histologic examination of brain tissue.

Frontotemporal lobar degeneration (FTLD) is a clinical syndrome associated with shrinking of the frontal and temporal anterior lobes of the brain. In Pick's disease, one type of FTLD, the brain has abnormal microscopic deposits called Pick bodies (though these are not always present). In FTLD, portions of the frontal and temporal lobes atrophy. FTLD is often misdiagnosed as a psychiatric problem or as AD. However, FTLD tends to occur at a younger age than does AD, typically between ages 40 and 70. The major distinguishing characteristic between these disorders and AD is marked symmetric lobar atrophy of the temporal and/or frontal lobes.

FTLD is characterized by disturbances in behavior, sleep, personality, and eventually memory. The disease progresses relentlessly and may ultimately include language impairment, erratic behavior, and dementia. Because of the strange behavior associated with FTLD, psychiatrists often see these patients first. There is no specific treatment. The diagnosis can be confirmed at autopsy.

Normal pressure hydrocephalus is an uncommon disorder characterized by an obstruction in the flow of CSF, causing a buildup of CSF in the brain. Symptoms of the condition include dementia, urinary incontinence, and difficulty walking. Meningitis, encephalitis, or head injury may cause the condition. If diagnosed early, normal pressure hydrocephalus is treatable by surgery in which a shunt is inserted to divert the fluid away from the brain.

Creutzfeldt-Jakob disease (CJD) is a rare and fatal brain disorder caused by a prion protein. A *prion* is a small infectious pathogen containing protein but lacking nucleic acids. The source of infection of a variant form of CJD (vCJD) is beef obtained from animals contaminated with bovine spongiform encephalopathy, which is also called *mad cow disease*. The risk of contracting vCJD is extremely low.

The earliest symptom of the disease may be memory impairment and behavior changes. The disease progresses rapidly with mental deterioration, involuntary movements (muscle jerks), weakness in the limbs, blindness, and eventually coma. There is no diagnostic test for CJD. Only autopsy and examination of brain tissue can confirm the diagnosis. There is no treatment for CJD.

Mixed dementia occurs when two or more types of dementia are present at the same time. It is characterized by the hallmark abnormalities of Alzheimer's and another type of dementia. Usually the other type of dementia is vascular dementia, but it can be other types, such as DLB.

DELIRIUM

Delirium, a state of temporary but acute mental confusion, is a common, life-threatening, and possibly preventable syndrome. Delirium is the most frequent complication of hospitalization in older patients. In the hospital setting, 15% to 53% of older adults experience delirium postoperatively, and as many as 80% of patients in an intensive care unit (ICU) experience delirium.[24]

TABLE 60-14	**FACTORS THAT PRECIPITATE DELIRIUM**
Demographic Characteristics	**Decreased Oral Intake**
• Age 65 yr or older	• Dehydration
• Male gender	• Malnutrition
Cognitive Status	**Drugs**
• Dementia	• Sedative-hypnotics
• Cognitive impairment	• Opioids
• History of delirium	• Anticholinergic drugs
• Depression	• Aminoglycosides
	• Treatment with multiple drugs
Environmental	• Alcohol or drug abuse or withdrawal
• Admission to an intensive care unit	
• Use of physical restraints	**Coexisting Medical Conditions**
• Pain (especially untreated)	• Severe acute illness
• Emotional stress	• Electrolyte imbalances
• Sleep deprivation	• Chronic renal or hepatic disease
	• History of stroke
Functional Status	• Neurologic disease
• Functional dependence	• Acute infection, sepsis, fever
• Immobility	• Fracture or trauma
• History of falls	• Terminal illness
	Surgery
Sensory	• Orthopedic surgery
• Sensory deprivation	• Cardiac surgery
• Sensory overload	• Prolonged cardiopulmonary bypass
• Visual or hearing impairment	• Noncardiac surgery

Etiology and Pathophysiology

The pathophysiologic mechanism of delirium is poorly understood. The main hypothesis is reversible impairment of cerebral oxidative metabolism and multiple neurotransmitter abnormalities. Cholinergic deficiency, excess release of dopamine, and both increased and decreased serotonergic activity may contribute to delirium. Proinflammatory cytokines, including interleukin-1, interleukin-2, interleukin-6, tumor necrosis factor-α (TNF-α), and interferon, appear to play a role. Stress and sleep deprivation have also been linked to the onset of delirium.[25]

Clinically, delirium is rarely caused by a single factor. It is often the result of the interaction of the patient's underlying condition with a precipitating event. Delirium can occur after a relatively minor insult in a vulnerable patient. For example, a patient with underlying health problems such as heart failure, cancer, cognitive impairment, or sensory limitations may develop delirium in response to a relatively minor change (e.g., use of a sleeping medication). In other nonvulnerable patients, it may take a combination of factors (e.g., anesthesia, major surgery, infection, prolonged sleep deprivation) to precipitate delirium. Delirium can also be a symptom of a serious medical illness such as bacterial meningitis.

Understanding factors that can lead to delirium can help in determining effective interventions. Several factors that can precipitate or cause delirium are listed in Tables 60-14 and 60-15. Many of these factors are more common in older patients.[26] In addition, older patients have limited compensatory mechanisms to deal with physiologic insults such as hypoxia, hypoglycemia, and dehydration. Older adults are more susceptible to drug-induced delirium, in part because of their

TABLE 60-15	MNEMONIC FOR CAUSES OF DELIRIUM

Dementia, dehydration
Electrolyte imbalances, emotional stress
Lung, liver, heart, kidney, brain
Infection, intensive care unit
Rx Drugs
Injury, immobility
Untreated pain, unfamiliar environment
Metabolic disorders

TABLE 60-16	CONFUSION ASSESSMENT METHOD (CAM)

Delirium is diagnosed with the presence of features 1 and 2, and either 3 or 4.

Feature 1 **Acute Onset** **and Fluctuating** **Course**	Data usually obtained from a family member or nurse. Shown by positive responses to following questions: • Is there evidence of an acute change in mental status from the patient's baseline? • Did the (abnormal) behavior fluctuate during the day (i.e., tend to come and go, or increase and decrease in severity)?
Feature 2 **Inattention**	Shown by positive response to following question: • Did the patient have difficulty focusing attention (e.g., being easily distractible, or having difficulty keeping track of what was being said)?
Feature 3 **Disorganized** **Thinking**	Shown by a positive response to following question: • Was the patient's thinking disorganized or incoherent, such as rambling or irrelevant conversation, unclear or illogical flow of ideas, or unpredictable switching from subject to subject?
Feature 4 **Altered Level of** **Consciousness**	Shown by any answer other than "alert" to the following question: • Overall, how would you rate this patient's level of consciousness (alert [normal], vigilant [hyperalert], lethargic [drowsy, easily aroused], stupor [difficult to arouse], or coma [unarousable])?

Adapted from Inouye S, van Dyck C, Alessi C, et al: Clarifying confusion: the Confusion Assessment Method, *Ann Intern Med* 113(12):941, 1990.

increased use of multiple drugs. Many medications, including sedative-hypnotics, opioids (especially meperidine [Demerol]), benzodiazepines, and drugs with anticholinergic properties, can cause or contribute to delirium, especially in older or vulnerable patients. An important risk factor for delirium is preexisting dementia.[27]

Clinical Manifestations

Patients with delirium can have a variety of manifestations ranging from hypoactivity and lethargy to hyperactivity, agitation, and hallucinations. Patients can also have mixed delirium, manifesting both hypoactive and hyperactive symptoms. Delirium can develop over the course of hours to days. In most patients, delirium usually develops over a 2- to 3-day period. The early manifestations often include inability to concentrate, irritability, insomnia, loss of appetite, restlessness, and confusion. Later manifestations may include agitation, misperception, misinterpretation, and hallucinations.

Acute delirium occurs frequently in hospitalized older adults. This transient condition is characterized by disorganized thinking, difficulty concentrating, and sensory misperceptions that last from 1 to 7 days. However, some delirium manifestations may persist up to and after discharge. Delirium is one of the most frequent consequences of unscheduled surgery on the older adult, especially when the patient has not been stabilized physically or prepared emotionally. Often this patient experiences a decline in ability to perform activities of daily living and an increased risk for falls.

Manifestations of delirium are sometimes confused with those of dementia. A key distinction between delirium and dementia is that the person who exhibits sudden cognitive impairment, disorientation, or clouded sensorium is more likely to have delirium rather than dementia. (A comparison of delirium and dementia is presented in Table 60-1.)

Diagnostic Studies

Diagnosing delirium is complicated because many critically ill patients cannot communicate their needs. A careful medical and psychologic history and physical examination are the first steps in diagnosing delirium. This includes careful attention to medications, both prescription and over-the-counter drugs. The Confusion Assessment Method (CAM) has been extensively studied and is a reliable tool for assessing delirium (Table 60-16). It is important to distinguish whether the delirium is part of an underlying problem of dementia.

Once delirium has been diagnosed, explore potential causes. Carefully review the patient's health history and medication record. Laboratory tests include complete blood count, serum electrolytes, blood urea nitrogen, and creatinine levels; electrocardiogram; urinalysis; liver and thyroid function tests;

and oxygen saturation level. Drug and alcohol levels may be obtained. If unexplained fever or nuchal rigidity is present and meningitis or encephalitis is suspected, a lumbar puncture may be performed. CSF is examined for glucose, protein, and bacteria. If the patient's history includes head injury, appropriate x-rays or scans may be ordered. In general, brain imaging studies such as CT and MRI are used only in situations in which head injury is known or suspected.

NURSING AND COLLABORATIVE MANAGEMENT
DELIRIUM

In caring for the patient with delirium, your roles include prevention, early recognition, and treatment. Prevention of delirium involves recognition of high-risk patients.[28] Patient groups at risk include those with neurologic disorders (e.g., stroke, dementia, CNS infection, Parkinson's disease), sensory impairment, and advanced age. Other risk factors, including hospitalization in an ICU and untreated pain, are listed in Table 60-14.

Care of the patient with delirium focuses on eliminating precipitating factors.[29] If it is drug induced, medications are discontinued. Keep in mind that delirium can also accompany drug and alcohol withdrawal. Depending on patient history, drug screening may be performed. Fluid and electrolyte imbalances and nutritional deficiencies (e.g., thiamine) are corrected

ETHICAL/LEGAL DILEMMAS
Board of Nursing Disciplinary Action

Situation

The State Board of Nursing has received multiple complaints about J.R., a registered nurse (RN) who works in a long-term care facility. J.R. has signed off on three controlled substances count sheets that have been determined to be inaccurate. During an investigation it was discovered that several members of the nursing staff knew about J.R.'s reported behavior, but they did not report their observations to the unit administrator. After the investigation, the board of nursing subpoenas J.R. to a meeting to discuss charges in preparation for a disciplinary hearing.

Ethical/Legal Points for Consideration

- Regulation of professional nursing practice is the right of each of the 50 states, most of which have separate regulatory agencies charged with writing regulations and rules to implement the State Nurse Practice Act. The regulations approved by these agencies carry the weight of law. Failure to behave accordingly places a nurse at risk for disciplinary action.
- The RN who is charged with unprofessional behavior has been charged with an offense and is entitled to the same legal rights as any other individual, including a fair and timely hearing, opportunity to confront the accusers, right to be represented by an attorney, and right to prepare a defense.
- Possible disciplinary actions include temporary suspension of the nursing license, revocation of the nursing license, mandatory rehabilitation for substance abuse, and mandated supervision and evaluation of practice. Sometimes the disciplinary action includes fines and requires re-education. In addition, the State Board of Nursing may report the action to the state attorney general if evidence suggests that a crime has been committed. The RN who has been found guilty of unprofessional practice must report this action on all future applications for nursing positions.
- All RNs should be familiar with their state's nurse practice act and regulations, as well as the composition and actions of the State Board of Nursing. Nurses should pay particular attention to the regulation that lists examples of actionable behavior and disciplinary actions sanctioned by the state.
- RNs have a legal and ethical obligation to report suspected illegal behavior to their administrators and to continue reporting until the situation is resolved. By failing to report, the RN may be charged as an accessory to the act or aiding and abetting the behavior. This RN may be charged with unprofessional behavior and risks losing his or her nursing license. Shifting the obligation to someone else to report or failure to continue reporting each incident does not satisfy this duty.

Discussion Questions

1. How would you handle a situation where retaliation for reporting unprofessional behavior is likely?
2. What would you do if the nurse suspected of illegal behavior is related to someone in the administrative hierarchy?

---

if appropriate. If the problem is related to environmental conditions (e.g., an overstimulating or understimulating environment), changes should be made. If delirium is secondary to infection, appropriate antibiotic therapy is started. Similarly, if delirium is secondary to chronic illness such as chronic kidney disease or heart failure, treatment focuses on these conditions.[30]

Care of the patient experiencing delirium includes protecting the patient from harm. Give priority to creating a calm and safe environment. This may include encouraging family members to stay at the bedside, providing familiar objects, transferring the patient to a private room or one closer to the nurses' station, and planning for consistent nursing staff if possible. Use reorientation and behavioral interventions in patients with delirium. Provide the patient with reassurance and reorienting information as to place, time, and procedures. Clocks, calendars, and lists of the patient's scheduled activities are also useful in reducing confusion. Reduce environmental stimuli, including noise and light levels.

Personal contact through touch and verbal communication can be an important reorienting strategy. If the patient uses eyeglasses or a hearing aid, they should be readily available because sensory deprivation can precipitate delirium. Avoid the use of restraints. Other interventions, including relaxation techniques, music therapy, and massage, may also be appropriate for some patients with delirium.

Comprehensive, multicomponent interventions to prevent delirium are the most effective and should be implemented through institution-based programs that are interdisciplinary. These interdisciplinary teams may also address issues related to polypharmacy, pain, nutritional status, and potential for incontinence. The patient experiencing delirium is also at risk for the adverse consequences of immobility, including skin breakdown. Give attention to increasing physical activity or providing range-of-motion exercises, when appropriate, and maintaining skin integrity.

Also focus on supporting the family and caregivers during episodes of delirium. Family members need to understand factors that may have precipitated the delirium, as well as the potential outcomes. *Delirium in the ICU: A Guide for Patients and Families* is available in eTable 66-1 (available on the website for Chapter 66).

▌DRUG THERAPY

Drug therapy is reserved for patients with severe agitation, especially when it interferes with needed medical therapy (e.g., fluid replacement, intubation, dialysis). Agitation can put the patient at risk for falls and injury. Drug therapy is used cautiously because many of the drugs used to manage agitation have psychoactive properties. Drugs should be used only when nonpharmacologic interventions have failed.

Dexmedetomidine (Precedex), an α-adrenergic receptor agonist, has been used in ICU settings for sedation. In addition, low-dose antipsychotics (neuroleptics) may be used such as haloperidol (Haldol), risperidone (Risperdal), olanzapine (Zyprexa), and quetiapine (Seroquel). Haloperidol can be administered IV, intramuscularly, or orally and will produce sedation. In addition to sedation, other side effects of antipsychotics include hypotension; extrapyramidal side effects, including *tardive dyskinesia* (involuntary muscle movements of face, trunk, and arms) and *athetosis* (involuntary writhing movements of the limbs); muscle tone changes; and anticholinergic effects. Carefully monitor older patients receiving antipsychotic agents.

Short-acting benzodiazepines (e.g., lorazepam [Ativan]) can be used to treat delirium associated with sedative and alcohol withdrawal or in conjunction with antipsychotics to reduce extrapyramidal side effects. However, these drugs may worsen delirium caused by other factors and must be used cautiously.

CASE STUDY

Alzheimer's Disease

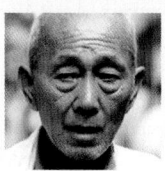

iStockphoto/Thinkstock

Patient Profile

M.Y., an 80-yr-old Asian American man, was diagnosed with Alzheimer's disease (AD) 3 yr ago. Today his 78-yr-old wife brings him to the emergency department because he wandered from his home, fell, and injured his left hip.

Subjective Data

- Can state his name
- Confused as to place and time
- Denies memory of wandering or falling
- Agitated, trying to get up
- Denies pain

Objective Data

Physical Examination

- Left leg shorter than right leg
- Tense and anxious

Diagnostic Studies

- X-ray of left hip indicates a fracture
- Mini-Cog testing indicates cognitive impairment

Discussion Questions

1. What is the pathogenesis of AD?
2. What precipitating factors may have resulted in M.Y.'s fall?
3. What precautions need to be taken regarding the inpatient care of M.Y.?
4. *Priority Decision:* What is the priority nursing intervention for M.Y.?
5. What teaching plan should you develop for M.Y. and his wife?
6. Surgery is planned to repair his fractured hip. Why is he at risk for delirium?
7. *Priority Decision:* Based on the assessment data, what are the priority nursing diagnoses? Are there any collaborative problems?
8. *Delegation Decision:* What nursing activities can the RN delegate to unlicensed assistive personnel (UAP)?
9. *Evidence-Based Practice:* M.Y.'s wife asks you if she should give her husband ginkgo to help his memory. How would you respond?

ⓔvolve Answers available at *http://evolve.elsevier.com/Lewis/medsurg.*

BRIDGE TO NCLEX EXAMINATION

The number of the question corresponds to the same-numbered outcome at the beginning of the chapter.

1. Dementia is defined as a
   a. syndrome that results only in memory loss.
   b. disease associated with abrupt changes in behavior.
   c. disease that is always due to reduced blood flow to the brain.
   d. syndrome characterized by cognitive dysfunction and loss of memory.

2. Vascular dementia is associated with
   a. transient ischemic attacks.
   b. bacterial or viral infection of neuronal tissue.
   c. cognitive changes secondary to cerebral ischemia.
   d. abrupt changes in cognitive function that are irreversible.

3. The clinical diagnosis of dementia is based on
   a. CT or MRS.
   b. brain biopsy.
   c. electroencephalogram.
   d. patient history and cognitive assessment.

4. Which statement(s) accurately describe(s) mild cognitive impairment *(select all that apply)*?
   a. Always progresses to AD
   b. Caused by variety of factors and may progress to AD
   c. Should be aggressively treated with acetylcholinesterase drugs
   d. Caused by vascular infarcts that, if treated, will delay progression to AD
   e. Patient is usually not aware that there is a problem with his or her memory

5. The early stage of AD is characterized by
   a. no noticeable change in behavior.
   b. memory problems and mild confusion.
   c. increased time spent sleeping or in bed.
   d. incontinence, agitation, and wandering behavior.

6. A major goal of treatment for the patient with AD is to
   a. maintain patient safety.
   b. maintain or increase body weight.
   c. return to a higher level of self-care.
   d. enhance functional ability over time.

7. Creutzfeldt-Jakob disease is characterized by
   a. remissions and exacerbations over many years.
   b. memory impairment, muscle jerks, and blindness.
   c. parkinsonian symptoms, including muscle rigidity and tremors at rest.
   d. increased intracranial pressure secondary to decreased CSF drainage.

8. Which patient is most at risk for developing delirium?
   a. A 50-year-old woman with cholecystitis
   b. A 19-year-old man with a fractured femur
   c. A 42-year-old woman having an elective hysterectomy
   d. A 78-year-old man admitted to the medical unit with complications related to heart failure

1. d, 2. c, 3. d, 4. b, 5. b, 6. a, 7. b, 8. d

ⓔvolve

For rationales to these answers and even more NCLEX review questions, visit *http://evolve.elsevier.com/Lewis/medsurg.*

REFERENCES

1. Alzheimer's Association: 2013 Alzheimer's Association facts and figures report. Retrieved from *www.alz.org/downloads/facts_figures_2013.pdf.*
2. Ohara T, Doi Y, Ninomiya T, et al: Glucose tolerance status and risk of dementia in the community: the Hisayama study, *Neurology* 77:1126, 2011.
3. Lehman EJ, Hein MJ, Baron SL, et al: Neurodegenerative causes of death among retired National Football League players, *Neurology* 79(19):1970, 2012.
4. Yaffe K, Vittinghoff E, Lindquist K, et al: Post-traumatic stress disorder and risk of dementia among U.S. veterans, *Arch Gen Psychiatry* 67(6):608, 2010.
5. Alzheimer's Disease Education and Referral Center: Alzheimer's disease genetics: facts sheet. Retrieved from

www.nia.nih.gov/sites/default/files/alzheimers_disease_genetics_fact_sheet.pdf.

6. Reiman EM, Quiroz YT, Fleisher AS, et al: Brain imaging and fluid biomarker analysis in young adults at genetic risk for autosomal dominant Alzheimer's disease in the presenilin 1 E280A kindred: a case-control study, *Lancet Neurol* 11(12):1048, 2012.

7. Reisberg B, Franssen EH, Souren LE, et al: Evidence and mechanisms of retrogenesis in Alzheimer's and other dementias: management and treatment import, *Am J Alzheimers Dis Other Demen* 17(4):202, 2002. (Classic)

8. Jack CR, Albert MS, Knopmana DS, et al: Introduction to the recommendations from the National Institute on Aging–Alzheimer's Association workgroups on diagnostic guidelines for Alzheimer's disease, *Alzheimers Dement* 7:257, 2011.

9. McKhann GM, Knopman DS, Chertkow H, et al: The diagnosis of dementia due to Alzheimer's disease: recommendations from the National Institute on Aging and the Alzheimer's Association workgroup, *Alzheimers Dement* 7:263, 2011.

*10. Albert MS, DeKoskyb ST, Dickson D, et al: The diagnosis of mild cognitive impairment due to Alzheimer's disease: recommendations from the National Institute on Aging and Alzheimer's Association workgroup, *Alzheimers Dement* 7:270, 2011.

*11. Russ TC, Morling JR: Cholinesterase inhibitors for mild cognitive impairment, *Cochrane Database Syst Rev* 9:CD009132, 2012.

*12. Howard R, McShane R, Lindesay J, et al: Donepezil and memantine for moderate-to-severe Alzheimer's disease, *N Engl J Med* 366(10):893, 2012.

13. Dwolatzky T, Clarfield AM: Cholinesterase inhibitors and memantine in more advanced Alzheimer's disease: the debate continues, *Aging Health* 8(3):233, 2012.

14. Huybrechts KF, Gerhard T, Crystal S, et al: Differential risk of death in older residents in nursing homes prescribed specific antipsychotic drugs: population based cohort study, *BMJ* 344:e977, 2011.

15. Buchman AS, Boyle PA, Yu L, et al: Total daily physical activity and the risk of AD and cognitive decline in older adults, *Neurology* 78:1323, 2012.

16. Levine C: The hospital nurse's assessment of family caregiver needs, *Am J Nurs* 111:47, 2011.

*17. Woods B, Aguirre E, Spector AE, et al: Cognitive stimulation to improve cognitive functioning in people with dementia, *Cochrane Database Syst Rev* 2:CD005562, 2012.

18. Budson AE, Solomon PR: *Memory loss: a practical guide for clinicians*, St Louis, 2011, Saunders.

19. Rowe MA, Greenblum CA, D'Aoust RF: Missing incidents in community-dwelling people with dementia, *Am J Nurs* 112:30, 2012.

20. Alzheimer's Association: MedicAlert + Alzheimer's Association Safe Return. Retrieved from *www.alz.org/care/dementia-medic-alert-safe-return.asp.*

21. Norton MC, Smith KR, Østbye T: Greater risk for dementia when spouse has dementia? The Cache County study, *J Am Geriatr Society* 58:895, 2010.

22. Lewis SL, Arevalo-Flechas LC, Miner-Williams D: Caregiving. In Giddens J, editor: *Concept-based nursing*, St Louis, 2012, Mosby.

23. Walton MK: Communicating with family caregivers, *Am J Nurs* 111:47, 2011.

24. American Association of Critical-Care Nurses: Delirium assessment and management. Retrieved from *www.aacn.org/WD/practice/content/practicealerts/delirium-practice-alert.content.*

25. Delirium in the intensive care unit: an under-recognized syndrome of organ dysfunction. Retrieved from *www.medscape.com/viewarticle/410883_4.*

26. Brooks PB: Postoperative delirium in elderly patients, *Am J Nurs* 112:38, 2012.

27. Fong TG, Jones RN, Marcantonio ER: Adverse outcomes after hospitalization and delirium in persons with Alzheimer's disease, *Ann Intern Med* 156:848, 2012.

*28. Rathier MO, Baker WL: A review of recent clinical trials and guidelines on the prevention and management of delirium in hospitalized older patients, *Hosp Pract* 39(4):96, 2011.

29. Balas MC, Rice M, Chaperon C, et al: Management of delirium in critically ill older adults, *Crit Care Nurse* 32(4):15, 2012.

*30. Neto AS, Nassar AP, Cardoso SO, et al: Delirium screening in critically ill patients: a systematic review and meta-analysis, *Crit Care Med* 40(6):1946, 2012.

RESOURCES

Alzheimer's Association
www.alz.org
Alzheimer's Disease Education and Referral Center
www.alzheimers.org
Caregiver Action Network
http://caregiveraction.org
Lewy Body Dementia Association
www.lewybodydementia.org
National Alliance for Caregiving
www.caregiving.org
National Council on Aging (NCOA)
www.ncoa.org
National Institute of Neurological Disorders and Strokes
www.ninds.nih.gov
National Institute on Aging
www.nia.nih.gov
   Caring for a Person With Alzheimer's Disease
      www.nia.nih.gov/sites/default/files/caring_for_a_person_with_alzheimers_disease_0.pdf
   What Happens Next?
      www.nia.nih.gov/sites/default/files/84206ADEARWhatHappensNextEarlyStageBookletab09OCT01_0.pdf
Stress-Busting Program for Family Caregivers (developed by Sharon Lewis)
www.caregiverstressbusters.org

*Evidence-based information for clinical practice.

So many of our dreams at first seem impossible, then they seem improbable, and then when we summon the will, they soon become inevitable.
Christopher Reeve

Nursing Management
Peripheral Nerve and Spinal Cord Problems

Teresa E. Hills

⊝volve WEBSITE

http://evolve.elsevier.com/Lewis/medsurg

- NCLEX Review Questions
- Key Points
- Pre-Test
- Answer Guidelines for Case Study on p. 1485
- Rationales for Bridge to NCLEX Examination Questions

- Case Study
  - Patient With Spinal Cord Injury
- Nursing Care Plan (Customizable)
  - eNCP 61-1: Patient With a Spinal Cord Injury
- Concept Map Creator
- Glossary
- Content Updates

eFigures
- eFig. 61-1: Syndromes associated with incomplete cord injuries
- eFig. 61-2: Standard neurologic classification of spinal cord injury

eTable
- eTable 61-1: Comparison of Multiple Sclerosis and Guillain-Barré Syndrome

LEARNING OUTCOMES

1. Explain the etiology, clinical manifestations, collaborative care, and nursing management of trigeminal neuralgia and Bell's palsy.
2. Explain the etiology, clinical manifestations, collaborative care, and nursing management of Guillain-Barré syndrome, botulism, tetanus, and neurosyphilis.
3. Describe the classification of spinal cord injuries and associated clinical manifestations.
4. Describe the clinical manifestations, collaborative care, and nursing management of neurogenic and spinal shock.

5. Relate the clinical manifestations of spinal cord injury to the level of disruption and rehabilitation potential.
6. Describe the nursing management of the major physical and psychologic problems of the patient with a spinal cord injury.
7. Describe the effects of spinal cord injury on the older adult.
8. Explain the types, clinical manifestations, collaborative care, and nursing management of spinal cord tumors.

KEY TERMS

anterior cord syndrome, Table 61-3, p. 1472
autonomic dysreflexia, p. 1479
Bell's palsy, p. 1466
botulism, p. 1468
Brown-Séquard syndrome, Table 61-3, p. 1472
central cord syndrome, Table 61-3, p. 1472
Guillain-Barré syndrome, p. 1467
neurogenic bladder, p. 1480
neurogenic bowel, p. 1481

neurogenic shock, p. 1470
neurosyphilis, p. 1468
paraplegia, p. 1470
posterior cord syndrome, Table 61-3, p. 1472
spinal shock, p. 1470
tetanus, p. 1468
tetraplegia, p. 1470
trigeminal neuralgia, p. 1464

Reviewed by Jean Burt, RN, MSN, Instructor, Wilbur Wright College, Chicago, Illinois; and Fernande E. Deno, RN, MSN, CNE, Instructor, Anoka Ramsey Community College, Coon Rapids, Minnesota.

This chapter discusses peripheral nerve and spinal cord problems, including cranial nerve disorders, polyneuropathies, spinal cord injuries, and spinal cord tumors. A focus of this chapter is the nursing management of the many problems encountered by the patient with a spinal cord injury.

CRANIAL NERVE DISORDERS

Cranial nerve disorders are commonly classified as peripheral neuropathies. The 12 pairs of cranial nerves are considered the peripheral nerves of the brain. The disorders usually involve the motor or sensory (or both) branches of a single nerve (*mononeuropathies*). Causes of cranial nerve problems include tumors, trauma, infections, inflammatory processes, and idiopathic (unknown) causes. Two cranial nerve disorders discussed in this chapter are trigeminal neuralgia and Bell's palsy.

TRIGEMINAL NEURALGIA

Trigeminal neuralgia *(tic douloureux)* is sudden, usually unilateral, severe, brief, stabbing, recurrent episodes of pain in the distribution of the trigeminal nerve. It is diagnosed in approximately 150,000 Americans each year and is the most commonly diagnosed neuralgic condition. It is seen approximately twice as often in women as in men. The majority of cases (more than 90%) are diagnosed in individuals over age 40.[1]

Etiology and Pathophysiology

The trigeminal nerve is the fifth cranial nerve (CN V) and has both motor and sensory branches. In trigeminal neuralgia the sensory or afferent branches, primarily the maxillary and mandibular branches, are involved (Fig. 61-1).

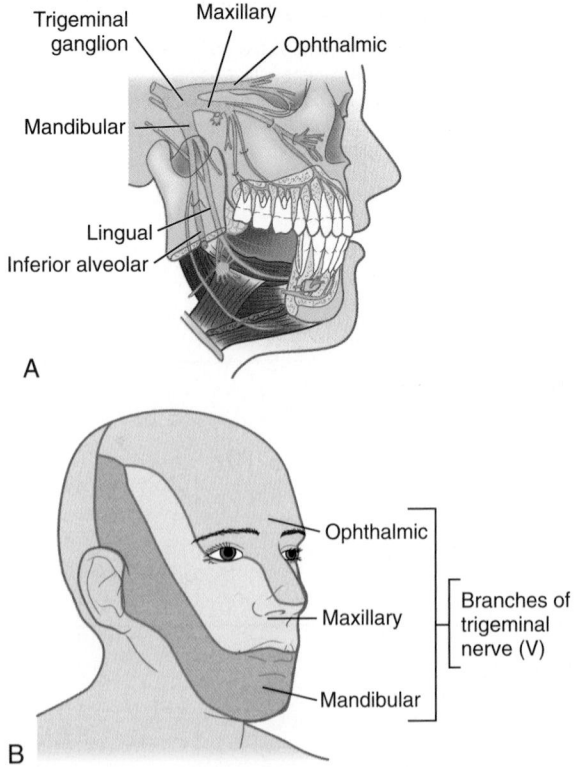

A

B

FIG. 61-1 A, Trigeminal (fifth cranial) nerve and its three main divisions: ophthalmic, maxillary, and mandibular nerves. **B,** Cutaneous innervation of the head.

The etiology and pathophysiology of trigeminal neuralgia is not fully understood.[2] One theory is that blood vessels, especially the superior cerebellar artery, become compressed, resulting in chronic irritation of the trigeminal nerve at the root entry zone. This irritation leads to increased firing of the afferent or sensory fibers. Risk factors are multiple sclerosis and hypertension. Other factors that may cause neuralgia include herpesvirus infection, infection of the teeth and jaw, and a brainstem infarct.

Clinical Manifestations

The classic feature of trigeminal neuralgia is an abrupt onset of paroxysms of excruciating pain described as a burning, knife-like, or lightning-like shock in the lips, upper or lower gums, cheek, forehead, or side of the nose. Intense pain, twitching, grimacing, and frequent blinking and tearing of the eye occur during the acute attack (giving rise to the term *tic*). Some patients may also experience facial sensory loss. The attacks are usually brief, lasting only seconds to 2 or 3 minutes, and are generally unilateral.

Recurrences, which are unpredictable, may occur several times a day, or weeks or months apart. After the refractory (pain-free) period, a phenomenon known as clustering can occur. *Clustering* is characterized by a cycle of pain and refractoriness that continues for hours.

The painful episodes are usually initiated by a triggering mechanism of light touch at a specific point *(trigger zone)* along the distribution of the nerve branches. Precipitating stimuli include chewing, tooth brushing, feeling a hot or cold blast of air on the face, washing the face, yawning, or even talking. As a result, the patient may eat improperly, neglect hygienic practices, wear a cloth over the face, and withdraw from interaction with other individuals. The patient may sleep excessively as a means of coping with the pain.

Although this condition is considered benign, the severity of the pain and the disruption of lifestyle can result in almost total physical and psychologic dysfunction or even suicide.

Diagnostic Studies

A computed tomography (CT) scan or magnetic resonance imaging (MRI) of the brain is performed to rule out any lesions (including multiple sclerosis), tumors, or vascular abnormalities. A complete neurologic assessment is done, including audiologic evaluation. The results are usually normal.

Collaborative Care

Once the diagnosis is made, the goal of treatment is relief of pain either medically or surgically (Tables 61-1 and 61-2).

Drug Therapy. Antiseizure drug therapy may reduce pain by stabilizing the neuronal membrane and blocking nerve

TABLE 61-1 **COLLABORATIVE CARE**	
Trigeminal Neuralgia	
Diagnostic	**Collaborative Therapy**

• History and physical examination (including neurologic examination)
 • CT scan
 • MRI
	• Drug therapy
	   • Antiseizure drugs (e.g., carbamazepine [Tegretol], oxcarbazepine [Trileptal])
	   • gabapentin (Neurontin)
	   • Tricyclic antidepressants (e.g., amitriptyline [Elavil])
	 • Local nerve block
	 • Surgical therapy (see Table 61-2)

TABLE 61-2	SURGICAL THERAPY FOR TRIGEMINAL NEURALGIA	
Procedure	**Description**	**Effect**
Peripheral		
Glycerol rhizotomy (injection into one or more branches of the trigeminal nerve)	Chemical ablation	Total pain relief with sparing of touch and corneal reflex.
Intracranial		
Percutaneous radiofrequency rhizotomy	Destruction of sensory fibers by low-voltage current	Total pain relief, sparing of touch and corneal reflex (increased risk for sensory changes).
Microvascular decompression	Lifting of artery pressing on nerve root in posterior fossa with wedge of sponge, leading to removal of pressure at nerve-root entry zone, or removing the involved vessel	Pain relief without loss of sensation.
Gamma knife radiosurgery	Technique that uses high doses of radiation focused on the trigeminal nerve root using stereotactic localization	Pain relief 1 day– 4 mo posttreatment. Noninvasive with no loss of sensation.

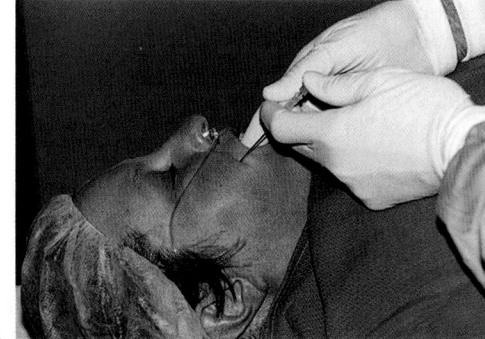

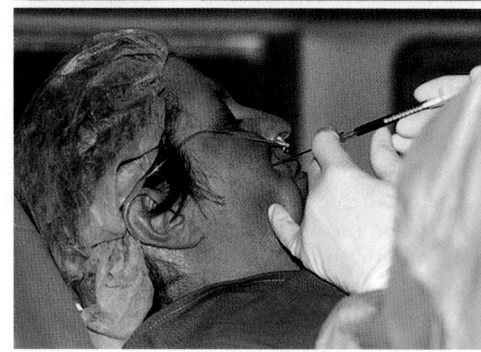

FIG. 61-2 A, Patient with trigeminal neuralgia having needle placed. **B,** Physician injecting glycerol.

firing.[2] These first-line drugs include carbamazepine (Tegretol), oxcarbazepine (Trileptal), topiramate (Topamax), clonazepam (Klonopin), phenytoin (Dilantin), lamotrigine (Lamictal), and divalproex (Depakote). Gabapentin (Neurontin) or baclofen (Lioresal) can be used in combination with any of the antiseizure drugs if a single agent is not effective. Tricyclic antidepressants such as amitriptyline (Elavil) or nortriptyline (Pamelor, Aventyl) can be used to treat constant burning, or aching pain.[2] Analgesics or opioids are usually not effective in controlling pain.

Conservative Therapy. Nerve blocking with local anesthetics is another treatment option. Relief of pain is temporary, lasting from 6 to 18 months. This treatment is usually tolerated well by older adults.

Some patients use complementary and alternative therapies, usually in combination with drug treatment. These techniques include acupuncture, biofeedback, vitamin therapy, nutritional therapy, and electrical stimulation of the nerves.

Surgical Therapy. If a conservative approach including drug therapy is not effective, surgical therapy is available (see Table 61-2). *Glycerol rhizotomy* is a percutaneous procedure that consists of an injection of glycerol through the foramen ovale into the trigeminal cistern (Fig. 61-2).

Percutaneous radiofrequency rhizotomy is an outpatient procedure consisting of placing a needle into the trigeminal rootlets that are adjacent to the pons and destroying the area by means of a radiofrequency current. This can result in facial numbness (although some degree of sensation may be retained), corneal anesthesia, and trigeminal motor weakness.[3]

Microvascular decompression of the trigeminal nerve is another commonly used procedure for neuralgia. It is done by first performing a small craniotomy behind the ear (suboccipi-

tal craniotomy). The next step involves displacing and repositioning the blood vessels that appear to be compressing the nerve at the root entry zone where it exits the pons. This procedure relieves pain without residual sensory loss.[3]

Gamma knife radiosurgery is another surgical treatment that is used to treat trigeminal neuralgia. Radiosurgery (see Chapter 57) using a gamma knife provides precise radiation of the proximal trigeminal nerve identified on high-resolution imaging.

NURSING MANAGEMENT TRIGEMINAL NEURALGIA

Patients with trigeminal neuralgia are primarily treated on an outpatient basis. Assessment of the attacks, including the triggering factors, characteristics, frequency, and pain management techniques, helps you plan for patient care. The nursing assessment should include the patient's nutritional status, hygiene (especially oral), and behavior (including withdrawal). Evaluate the degree of pain and its effects on the patient's lifestyle, drug use, emotional state, and suicidal tendencies.

Monitor the patient's response to drug therapy and note any side effects. Alternative pain relief measures, such as acupuncture and biofeedback, should be explored for the patient who is not a surgical candidate and whose pain is not controlled by other measures. Environmental management is essential during an acute period to decrease triggering stimuli. The room should be kept at an even, moderate temperature and free of drafts. Many patients prefer to carry out their own care, fearing that someone else will inadvertently injure them.

Teach the patient about the importance of nutrition, hygiene, and oral care and convey understanding if previous oral neglect is apparent. A small, soft-bristled toothbrush or a warm mouthwash assists in promoting oral care. Hygiene activities are best carried out when analgesia is at its peak.

Food should be high in protein and calories and easy to chew. It should be served lukewarm and offered frequently. When oral intake is sharply reduced and the patient's nutritional status is compromised, a nasogastric tube can be inserted on the unaffected side for enteral feedings.

Appropriate teaching related to surgical procedures depends on the type of procedure planned (e.g., percutaneous). Patients need to know that they will be awake during local procedures so that they can cooperate when corneal and ciliary reflexes and facial sensations are checked. After the procedure the patient's pain is compared with the preoperative level. The corneal reflex, extraocular muscles, hearing, sensation, and facial nerve function are evaluated frequently (see Chapter 56). If the corneal reflex is impaired, take special care to protect the eyes. This includes the use of artificial tears or eye shields.

If intracranial surgery is performed, general postoperative nursing care after a craniotomy is appropriate. (Nursing care related to craniotomy is discussed in Chapter 57 on p. 1379.)

After a percutaneous radiofrequency procedure, apply an ice pack to the jaw on the operative side for 3 to 5 hours. To avoid injuring the mouth, the patient should not chew on the operative side until sensation has returned.

Plan for regular follow-up care, and instruct the patient on the dosage and side effects of medications. Although relief of pain may be complete, encourage the patient to keep environmental stimuli to a moderate level and to use stress management techniques. Long-term management after surgical intervention depends on the residual effects of the procedure. If anesthesia is present or the corneal reflex is altered, teach the patient to (1) chew on the unaffected side; (2) avoid hot foods or beverages, which can burn the mucous membranes; (3) check the oral cavity after meals to remove food particles; (4) practice meticulous oral hygiene and continue with semiannual dental visits; (5) protect the face against extremes of temperature; (6) use an electric razor; (7) wear a protective eye shield or avoid rubbing eyes; and (8) examine eye regularly for symptoms of infection or irritation.

BELL'S PALSY

Bell's palsy (peripheral facial paralysis, acute benign cranial polyneuritis) is a disorder characterized by inflammation of the facial nerve (CN VII) on one side of the face in the absence of any other disease such as a stroke. Bell's palsy is an acute, peripheral facial paresis of unknown cause. Each year approximately 40,000 Americans are diagnosed with Bell's palsy. It can affect any age-group. Despite its good prognosis, Bell's palsy leaves more than 8000 people a year in the United States with permanent, potentially disfiguring facial weakness.[4]

Etiology and Pathophysiology

Although the exact etiology is not known, it is believed that a viral infection such as viral meningitis or activation of herpes simplex virus 1 (HSV1) may trigger Bell's palsy. The viral infection causes inflammation, edema, ischemia, and eventual demyelination of the nerve, creating pain and alterations in motor and sensory function. Bell's palsy has also been associated with influenza or a flu-like illness, headaches, chronic middle ear infection, hypertension, diabetes, sarcoidosis, tumors, Lyme disease, and trauma such as skull fracture or facial injury.[4]

Bell's palsy is considered benign, with full recovery in 3 to 6 months, especially if treatment is begun immediately. A small group of patients have long-term facial paralysis.[4]

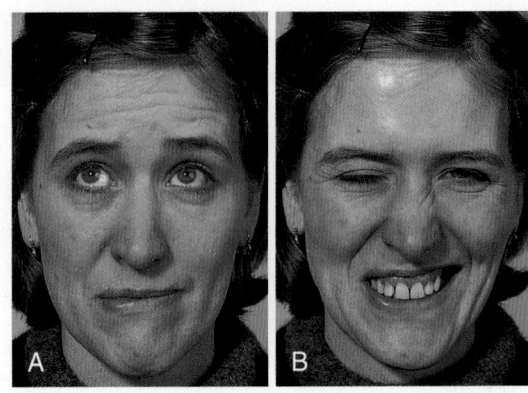

FIG. 61-3 Facial characteristics of Bell's palsy. **A,** At rest the face may look almost normal, but the patient is not able to wrinkle her forehead on the affected side and the right corner of the mouth droops. **B,** When she is asked to close her eyes and show her teeth, the differences between the affected and unaffected sides become more obvious.

Clinical Manifestations and Diagnostic Studies

The onset of Bell's palsy is often accompanied by an outbreak of herpes vesicles in or around the ear. Patients may complain of pain around and behind the ear. Additional manifestations may include fever, tinnitus, and hearing deficit. Paralysis of the motor branches of the facial nerve typically results in flaccidity of the affected side of the face, with drooping of the mouth accompanied by drooling (Fig. 61-3).

An inability to close the eyelid, with an upward movement of the eyeball when closure is attempted, is also evident. Other manifestations include a widened *palpebral fissure* (the opening between the eyelids); flattening of the nasolabial fold; and inability to smile, frown, or whistle. Unilateral loss of taste is common. Decreased muscle movement may alter chewing ability. Although some patients experience a loss of tearing, many patients complain of excessive tearing. The muscle weakness causes the lower lid to turn out, allowing overflow of normal tear production. Pain may be present behind the ear on the affected side, especially before the onset of paralysis.

Complications include psychologic withdrawal because of changes in appearance, malnutrition, dehydration, mucous membrane trauma, corneal abrasions, muscle stretching, and facial spasms and contractures.

The diagnosis of Bell's palsy is one of exclusion. There is no definitive test. The diagnosis and prognosis are indicated by observing the typical pattern of onset and signs and testing percutaneous nerve excitability by electromyography (EMG).

Collaborative Care

Methods of treatment for Bell's palsy include moist heat, gentle massage, and electrical stimulation of the nerve and prescribed exercises. Stimulation may maintain muscle tone and prevent atrophy. Care is primarily focused on relief of symptoms, prevention of complications, and protection of the eye on the affected side.

Corticosteroids (prednisone) are started immediately, with best results if corticosteroids are initiated before paralysis is complete. When the patient improves to the point that the corticosteroids are no longer necessary, the drug should be tapered over a 2-week period. Because HSV is implicated in approximately 70% of cases of Bell's palsy, treatment with acyclovir (Zovirax), alone or in conjunction with prednisone, may be used. Additional antiviral agents, including valacyclovir

(Valtrex) and famciclovir (Famvir), have also been used in the management of Bell's palsy.

NURSING MANAGEMENT
BELL'S PALSY

The patient with Bell's palsy is treated on an outpatient basis. Mild analgesics can relieve pain. Hot wet packs can reduce the discomfort of herpetic lesions, aid circulation, and relieve pain. Tell the patient to protect the face from cold and drafts because trigeminal *hyperesthesia* (extreme sensitivity to pain or touch) may occur. Maintenance of good nutrition is important. Teach the patient to chew on the unaffected side of the mouth to avoid trapping food and to enjoy the taste of food. Thorough oral hygiene must be carried out after each meal to prevent parotitis, caries, and periodontal disease from accumulated residual food.

The patient may wear dark glasses for protective and cosmetic reasons. Artificial tears (methylcellulose) should be instilled frequently during the day to prevent drying of the cornea. Ointment and an impermeable eye shield can be used at night to retain moisture. In some patients, taping the lids closed at night may be necessary to provide protection. Instruct the patient to report ocular pain, drainage, or discharge.

A facial sling may be helpful to support affected muscles, improve lip alignment, and facilitate eating. The facial sling is usually made and fitted by a physical or occupational therapist. When function begins to return, active facial muscle exercises are performed several times a day.

The change in physical appearance as a result of Bell's palsy can be devastating. Reassure the patient that a stroke did not occur and that chances for a full recovery are good. Enlisting support from family and friends is important. Tell the patient that most patients recover within about 6 weeks of the onset of symptoms.

POLYNEUROPATHIES

GUILLAIN-BARRÉ SYNDROME

Guillain-Barré syndrome (Landry-Guillain-Barré-Strohl syndrome, postinfectious polyneuropathy, ascending polyneuropathic paralysis) is an acute, rapidly progressing, and potentially fatal form of polyneuritis. It is characterized by ascending, symmetric paralysis that usually affects cranial nerves and the peripheral nervous system. The syndrome is rare, affecting an estimated 3000 to 6000 Americans each year. It affects males and females equally.[5,6]

Etiology and Pathophysiology

The etiology of this disorder is unknown. Both cellular and humoral immune mechanisms play a role in the immune reaction directed at the nerves. The result is a loss of myelin (a segmental demyelination) and edema and inflammation of the affected nerves. As demyelination occurs, the transmission of nerve impulses is stopped or slowed down. The muscles innervated by the damaged peripheral nerves undergo denervation and atrophy. In the recovery phase, remyelination occurs slowly, and neurologic function returns in a proximal-to-distal pattern.[6] Guillain-Barré syndrome is similar in presentation to multiple sclerosis (MS), and therefore a full diagnostic workup should be performed to rule out MS (see Chapter 59).

The syndrome is often preceded by immune system stimulation from a viral infection, trauma, surgery, or viral immuniza-

tions. *Campylobacter jejuni* gastroenteritis is thought to precede Guillain-Barré syndrome in approximately 30% of cases.[5-7]

Clinical Manifestations and Complications

Guillain-Barré syndrome is a heterogeneous condition with manifestations ranging from mild to severe. Weakness of the lower extremities (evolving more or less symmetrically) occurs over hours to days to weeks, usually peaking about the fourteenth day. *Paresthesia* (numbness and tingling) is common, with paralysis usually following in the extremities. *Hypotonia* (reduced muscle tone) and *areflexia* (lack of reflexes) are common manifestations.[5-7]

In Guillain-Barré syndrome, autonomic nervous system dysfunction results, with manifestations of orthostatic hypotension, hypertension, and abnormal vagal responses (bradycardia, heart block, asystole). Other autonomic dysfunctions include bowel and bladder dysfunction, facial flushing, and diaphoresis. Patients may also have syndrome of inappropriate antidiuretic hormone (SIADH) secretion.[8] (SIADH is discussed in Chapter 50.) Cranial nerve involvement is manifested as facial weakness, extraocular eye movement difficulties, dysphagia, and paresthesia of the face.

Pain is a common symptom in the patient with Guillain-Barré syndrome. The pain can be paresthesias, muscular aches and cramps, and hyperesthesias. Pain appears to be worse at night. Opioids may be indicated for those experiencing severe pain. Pain may lead to a decrease in appetite and may interfere with sleep.

The most serious complication is respiratory failure, which occurs as the paralysis progresses to the nerves that innervate the thoracic area. Constant monitoring of the respiratory system by checking respiratory rate and depth provides information about the need for immediate intervention, including intubation and mechanical ventilation. Respiratory or urinary tract infections (UTIs) may occur. Immobility from the paralysis can cause problems such as paralytic ileus, muscle atrophy, deep vein thrombosis, pulmonary emboli, skin breakdown, orthostatic hypotension, and nutritional deficiencies.

Diagnostic Studies

Diagnosis is based primarily on the patient's history and clinical signs. Cerebrospinal fluid (CSF) is normal or has a low protein content initially, but after 7 to 10 days it shows an elevated protein level (normal protein is 15 to 45 mg/dL [0.15 to 0.45 g/L]) with a normal cell count. Results of EMG and nerve conduction studies are markedly abnormal (reduced nerve conduction velocity) in the affected extremities. A brain MRI can be done to rule out MS.

NURSING AND COLLABORATIVE MANAGEMENT
GUILLAIN-BARRÉ SYNDROME

Management of Guillain-Barré syndrome is aimed at supportive care, particularly ventilatory support, during the acute phase. Plasmapheresis is used in the first 2 weeks. (Plasmapheresis is discussed in Chapter 14.) IV administration of high-dose immunoglobulin (Sandoglobulin) has been as effective as plasma exchange and is more readily available.

Beyond 3 weeks after disease onset, plasmapheresis and immunoglobulin therapies have little value. Corticosteroids appear to have little effect on the prognosis or duration of the disease.

Assessment of the patient is the most important aspect of nursing care during the acute phase. During the routine assessment, monitor the ascending paralysis; assess respiratory function; monitor arterial blood gases (ABGs); and assess the gag, corneal, and swallowing reflexes. Reflexes are usually decreased or absent.

Monitor blood pressure (BP) and cardiac rate and rhythm during the acute phase because dysrhythmias may occur. Autonomic dysfunction is common and usually takes the form of bradycardia and dysrhythmias. Orthostatic hypotension secondary to muscle atony may occur in severe cases. Vasopressor agents and volume expanders may be needed to treat the low BP. However, the presence of SIADH may require fluid restriction.

The objective of therapy is to support body systems until the patient recovers. Respiratory failure and infection are serious threats. Monitoring the vital capacity and ABGs is essential. If the vital capacity drops to less than 800 mL or the ABGs deteriorate, endotracheal intubation or tracheostomy may be done so that the patient can be mechanically ventilated (see Chapter 68). If fever develops, obtain sputum cultures to identify the pathogen. Appropriate antibiotic therapy is then initiated.

Nutritional needs must be met in spite of possible problems associated with delayed gastric emptying, paralytic ileus, and potential for aspiration if the gag reflex is lost. In addition to testing for the gag reflex, note drooling and other difficulties with secretions that may indicate an inadequate gag reflex. Initially, enteral or parenteral nutrition may be used to ensure adequate caloric intake. Because of delayed gastric emptying, assess residual volumes of the feedings at regular intervals or before feedings (see Chapter 40).

Throughout the course of the illness, provide support and encouragement to the patient, caregiver, and family. Although 85% to 95% of patients almost completely recover, it is generally a slow process that takes months or years. About 30% of those with Guillain-Barré have some residual weakness.[5-7]

BOTULISM

Botulism is rare but the most serious type of food poisoning. It is caused by gastrointestinal (GI) absorption of the neurotoxin produced by *Clostridium botulinum*. This organism is found in the soil, and the spores are difficult to destroy. It can grow in any food contaminated with the spores. Improper home canning of foods is often the cause.[9] It is thought that the neurotoxin destroys or inhibits the neurotransmission of acetylcholine at the myoneural junction, resulting in disturbed muscle innervation.

Neurologic manifestations can develop rapidly or evolve over several days. They include a descending paralysis with muscle incoordination and weakness, difficulty swallowing, seizures, and respiratory muscle weakness that can rapidly deteriorate to respiratory and/or cardiac arrest.

The clinical manifestations, prevention, and treatment are presented in Table 42-24. Patient and caregiving teaching related to food poisoning are presented in Table 42-25. Nursing care during the acute illness is similar to that for Guillain-Barré syndrome. Supportive nursing interventions include rest, activities to maintain respiratory function, adequate nutrition, and prevention of loss of muscle mass.

TETANUS

Tetanus (lockjaw) is a severe infection of the nervous system affecting spinal and cranial nerves. It results from the effects of a potent neurotoxin released by the anaerobic bacillus *Clostridium tetani*. The spores of the bacillus are present in soil, garden mold, and manure. *C. tetani* enters the body through a wound that provides an appropriate low-oxygen environment for the organisms to mature and produce toxin. Examples of possible wounds include IV drug use injection sites, human and animal bites, burns, frostbite, open fractures, and gunshot wounds.[10,11]

Initial manifestations of tetanus include stiffness in the jaw *(trismus)* and neck and signs of infection (e.g., fever). As the disease progresses, the neck muscles, back, abdomen, and extremities become progressively rigid. In severe forms, continuous tonic seizures may occur with *opisthotonos* (extreme arching of the back and retraction of the head). Laryngeal and respiratory spasms cause apnea and anoxia. The slightest noise, jarring motion, or bright light can set off a seizure. These seizures are agonizingly painful. Mortality rate is almost 100% in the severe form.[11]

Tetanus prevention and immunizations, which are the most important factors influencing the incidence of this disease, are summarized in Table 69-6. Adults should receive a tetanus and diphtheria toxoid booster every 10 years. Teach the patient that immediate, thorough cleansing of all wounds with soap and water is important to prevent tetanus. If an open wound occurs and the patient has not been immunized within 5 years, the health care provider should be contacted so that a tetanus booster can be given.

The management of tetanus includes administration of a tetanus toxoid, diphtheria toxoid, and pertussis (Tdap) booster and tetanus immune globulin (TIG) in different sites before the onset of symptoms to neutralize circulating toxins (see Table 69-6). A much larger dose of TIG is administered to patients with clinical manifestations of tetanus.[10-12]

Control of spasms is essential and is managed by sedation and skeletal muscle relaxation, usually with diazepam (Valium), barbiturates, and, in severe cases, neuromuscular blocking agents such as vecuronium (Norcuron) that act to paralyze skeletal muscles. Opioid analgesics such as morphine or fentanyl are also indicated for pain management. A 10- to 14-day course of penicillin, metronidazole, tetracycline, or doxycycline is recommended to inhibit further growth of *C. tetani*.[11]

Because of laryngospasm and the potential need for neuromuscular blocking drugs, a tracheostomy is usually performed early and the patient is maintained on mechanical ventilation. Sedative agents and opioid analgesics are given concomitantly to all patients who are pharmacologically paralyzed. Any recognized wound should be debrided or an abscess drained. Antibiotics may be given to prevent secondary infections.

NEUROSYPHILIS

Neurosyphilis is caused by *Treponema pallidum,* the bacteria that cause syphilis. It usually occurs about 10 to 20 years after a person is first infected with syphilis. Not everyone who has syphilis will develop this complication. It is the result of untreated or inadequately treated syphilis (see Chapter 53). The organism can invade the central nervous system within a few months of the original infection. Untreated neurosyphilis, although not contagious, can be fatal.

Late neurosyphilis results from degenerative changes in the spinal cord (tabes dorsalis) and brainstem (general paresis). *Tabes dorsalis* (progressive locomotor ataxia) is characterized by vague, sharp pains in the legs; ataxia; "slapping" gait; loss of proprioception and deep tendon reflexes; and zones of hyperesthesia. *Charcot's joints,* which are characterized by enlargement, bone destruction, and hypermobility, also occur as a result of joint effusion and edema. Other manifestations of neurosyphilis include seizures, vision and hearing problems, and cognitive impairment.[13]

Management includes treatment with penicillin, symptomatic care, and protection from physical injury.[13] The prognosis after treatment depends on how severe the neurosyphilis is before treatment. The neurologic deficits may remain or progress after treatment.

SPINAL CORD PROBLEMS

SPINAL CORD INJURY

Spinal cord injury (SCI) is caused by trauma or damage to the spinal cord. It can result in either a temporary or permanent alteration in the function of the spinal cord. About 12,000 Americans suffer SCIs each year. About 260,000 persons in the United States are living with SCI.[14,15] With improved treatment strategies, even the very young patient with an SCI can anticipate a long life. The potential for disruption of individual growth and development, altered family dynamics, economic loss in terms of employment, and the high cost of rehabilitation and long-term health care make SCI a major problem.

Young adult men between ages 16 and 30 years have the greatest risk for SCI. Eighty-one percent of people with SCI are male. There has also been an increase in the number of older adults with SCIs. This trend toward older age at time of injury is reflected in the overall increase in mean age of people with SCI from 28 years in the 1970s to 40 years at this time.[15]

Although many people with SCIs can care for themselves independently, those with the highest level of injury may require round-the-clock care at home or in a long-term care facility. Almost 90% of patients with SCI are discharged from the hospital to home or another noninstitutional residence. The remaining 10% are discharged to nursing homes, chronic care facilities, or group homes.

Etiology and Pathophysiology

SCIs are usually a result of trauma. The most common causes are motor vehicle collisions (42%), falls (27%), violence (15%), sports injuries (7%), and other miscellaneous causes (8%).[15]

Types of Injury. The extent of the neurologic damage caused by an SCI results from *primary injury* (actual physical disruption of axons) and *secondary injury* (ischemia, hypoxia, hemorrhage, and edema).

Primary Injury. The spinal cord is wrapped in tough layers of dura and is rarely torn or transected by direct trauma. SCI can be due to cord compression by bone displacement, interruption of blood supply to the cord, or traction resulting from pulling on the cord. Penetrating trauma, such as gunshot and stab wounds, can result in tearing and transection. The initial mechanical disruption of axons as a result of stretch or laceration is referred to as the *primary injury.*

Secondary Injury. *Secondary injury* refers to the ongoing, progressive damage that occurs after the primary injury.[16] Several theories exist on what causes this ongoing damage, including free radical formation, uncontrolled calcium influx, ischemia, and lipid peroxidation. *Apoptosis* (cell death) occurs

and sometimes may continue for weeks or months after the initial injury. Thus the complete cord damage (previously thought to be transection) in severe trauma is related to autodestruction of the cord. Hemorrhagic areas in the center of the spinal cord appear within 1 hour, and by 4 hours there may be infarction in the gray matter.[16] This ongoing destructive process makes it critical that the initial care and management of the patient with an SCI be initiated as soon as possible to limit further destruction of the spinal cord.

Fig. 61-4 illustrates the cascade of events causing secondary injury after traumatic SCI. The resulting hypoxia reduces the oxygen levels below the metabolic needs of the spinal cord. Lactate metabolites and an increase in vasoactive substances, including norepinephrine, serotonin, and dopamine, are noted. At high levels, these vasoactive substances cause vasospasms and hypoxia, leading to subsequent necrosis. Unfortunately, the spinal cord has minimal ability to adapt to vasospasm.

By 24 hours or less, permanent damage may occur because of the development of edema. The edema secondary to the inflammatory response is particularly harmful because of lack

PATHOPHYSIOLOGY MAP

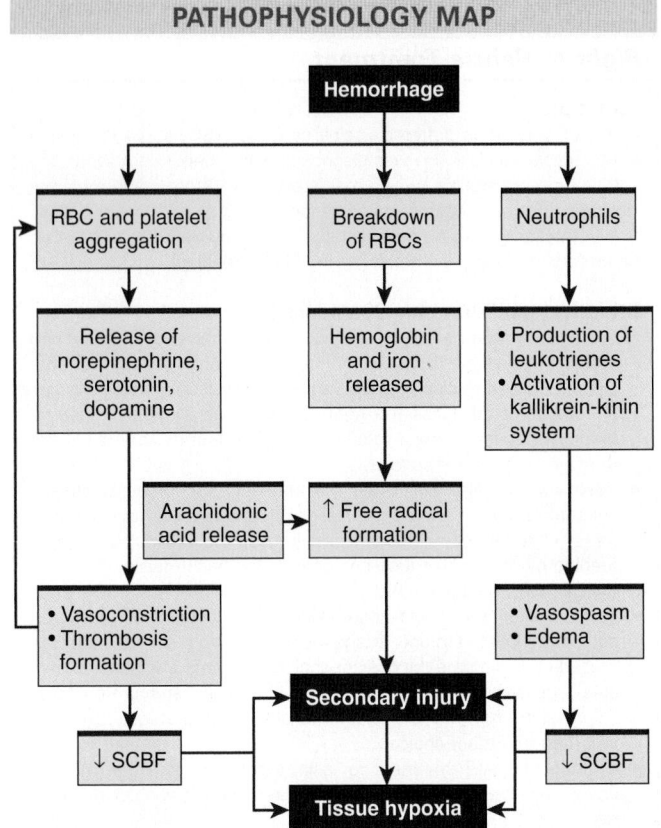

FIG. 61-4 Cascade of metabolic and cellular events that leads to spinal cord ischemia and hypoxia of secondary injury. *RBCs,* Red blood cells; *SCBF,* spinal cord blood flow.

of space for tissue expansion. Therefore compression of the spinal cord occurs. Edema extends above and below the injury, thus increasing the ischemic damage. Because secondary injury progresses over time, the extent of the injury and prognosis for recovery are most accurately determined at least 72 hours or more after injury.

Spinal and Neurogenic Shock. About 50% of people with acute SCI experience a temporary neurologic syndrome known as spinal shock. This type of shock is characterized by decreased reflexes, loss of sensation, and flaccid paralysis below the level of injury.[16] This syndrome lasts days to months and may mask postinjury neurologic function.

Neurogenic shock, in contrast to spinal shock, is due to the loss of vasomotor tone caused by injury and is characterized by hypotension and bradycardia. Loss of sympathetic nervous system innervation causes peripheral vasodilation, venous pooling, and a decreased cardiac output. These effects are generally associated with a cervical or high thoracic injury (T6 or higher).

Classification of Spinal Cord Injury. SCIs are classified by the (1) mechanism of injury, (2) level of injury, and (3) degree of injury.

Mechanisms of Injury. The major mechanisms of injury are flexion, hyperextension, flexion-rotation, extension-rotation, and compression[17] (Fig. 61-5). The flexion-rotation injury is the most unstable of all because the ligamentous structures that stabilize the spine are torn. This injury is most often implicated in severe neurologic deficits.

Level of Injury. *Skeletal level* of injury is the vertebral level where there is the most damage to vertebral bones and ligaments. *Neurologic level* is the lowest segment of the spinal cord

with normal sensory and motor function on both sides of the body. The level of injury may be cervical, thoracic, lumbar, or sacral. Cervical and lumbar injuries are most common because these levels are associated with the greatest flexibility and movement. If the cervical cord is involved, paralysis of all four extremities occurs, resulting in tetraplegia (formerly termed *quadriplegia*). However, when the damage is low in the cervical cord, the arms are rarely completely paralyzed.

If the thoracic, lumbar, or sacral spinal cord is damaged, the result is paraplegia (paralysis and loss of sensation in the legs). Fig. 61-6 shows affected structures and functions at different levels of cord injury.

Degree of Injury. The degree of spinal cord involvement may be either complete or incomplete (partial). *Complete cord involvement* results in total loss of sensory and motor function below the level of injury. *Incomplete cord involvement* results in a mixed loss of voluntary motor activity and sensation and leaves some tracts intact. The degree of sensory and motor loss varies depending on the level of injury and reflects the specific nerve tracts damaged.[16]

Six syndromes are associated with incomplete injuries: central cord syndrome, anterior cord syndrome, Brown-Séquard syndrome, posterior cord syndrome, cauda equina syndrome, and conus medullaris syndrome[16] (Table 61-3).

Clinical Manifestations

The manifestations of SCI are generally the direct result of trauma that causes cord compression, ischemia, edema, and possible cord transection. Manifestations of SCI are related to the level and degree of injury. The patient with an incomplete injury may demonstrate a mixture of manifestations. The higher the injury, the more serious the sequelae because of the proximity of the cervical cord to the medulla and brainstem.[16,17]

American Spinal Injury Association (ASIA) Impairment Scale. The American Spinal Injury Association (ASIA) Impairment Scale is commonly used for classifying the severity of impairment resulting from SCI. It combines assessments of motor and sensory function to determine neurologic level and completeness of injury (Fig. 61-7, and eFig. 61-2, available on the website for this chapter).

The sensory regions are called *dermatomes,* with each segment of the spinal cord innervating a particular area of skin. Each dermatome has a specific point recommended for testing, as shown in eFig. 61-2. A dermatome map is also shown in Fig. 56-6.

The ASIA Impairment Scale is useful for recording changes in neurologic status and identifying appropriate goals for rehabilitation. Movement and rehabilitation potential related to specific locations of the SCI are described in Table 61-4. In general, sensory function closely parallels motor function at all levels.

Respiratory System. Respiratory complications closely correspond to the level of injury. Cervical injuries above the level of C4 present special problems because of the total loss of respiratory muscle function. Mechanical ventilation is required to keep the patient alive. At one time the majority of these patients died at the scene of the injury, but with improved emergency medical services, more of these patients are surviving the initial events of their SCI.

Injury or fracture below the level of C4 results in diaphragmatic breathing if the phrenic nerve is functioning. Even if the injury is below C4, spinal cord edema and hemorrhage can affect the function of the phrenic nerve and cause respiratory insufficiency. Hypoventilation almost always occurs with dia-

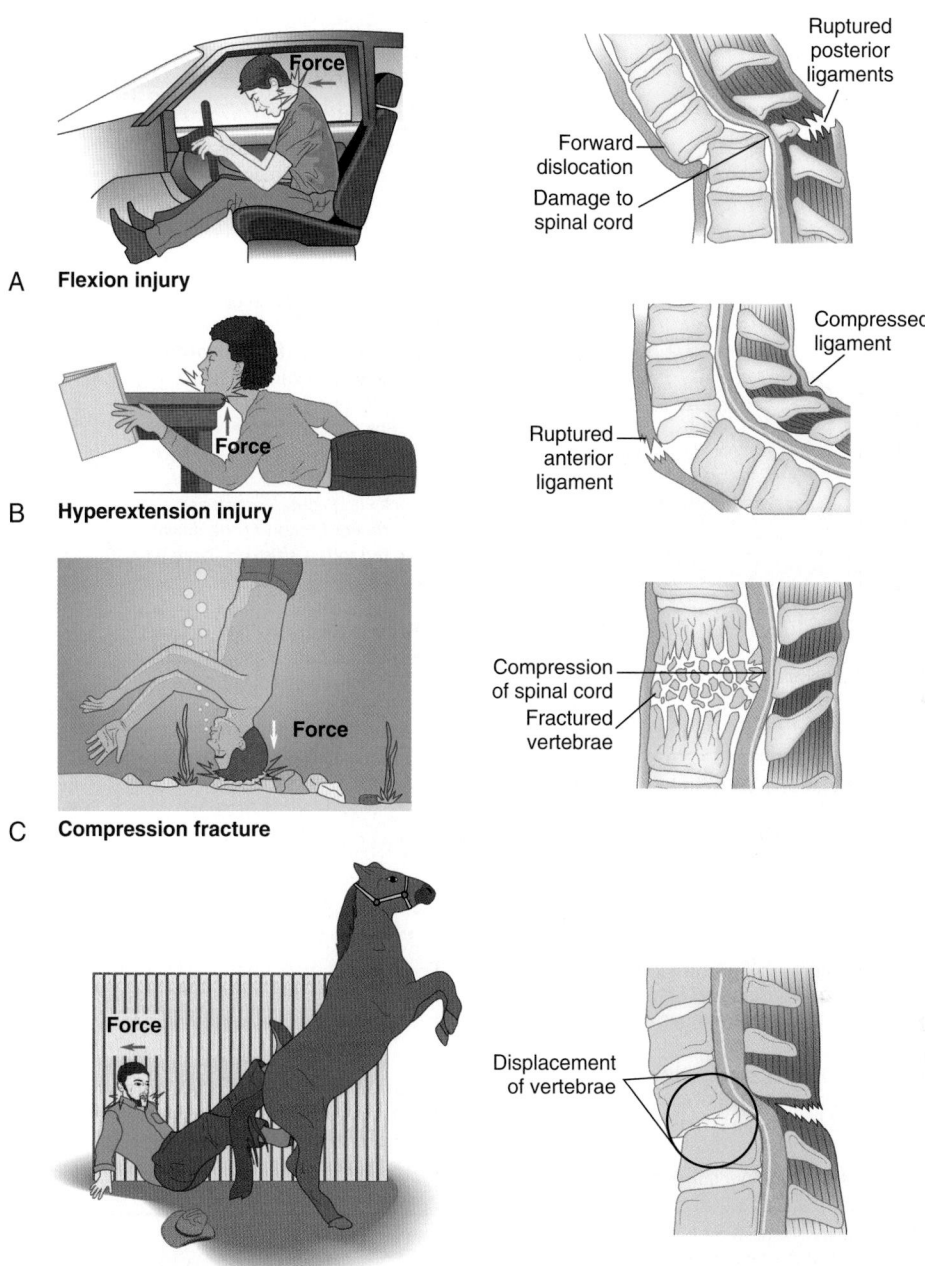

A **Flexion injury**

B **Hyperextension injury**

C **Compression fracture**

D **Flexion-rotation injury**

FIG. 61-5 Mechanisms of spinal cord injury. Many situations may produce these injuries. This only shows some examples. **A,** Flexion injury of the cervical spine ruptures the posterior ligaments. **B,** Hyperextension injury of the cervical spine ruptures the anterior ligaments. **C,** Compression fractures crush the vertebrae and force bony fragments into the spinal canal. **D,** Flexion-rotation injury of the cervical spine often results in tearing of ligamentous structures that normally stabilize the spine.

phragmatic respirations because of the decrease in vital capacity and tidal volume, a result of impairment of the intercostal muscles.

Cervical and thoracic injuries cause paralysis of abdominal muscles and often the intercostal muscles. Therefore the patient cannot cough effectively enough to remove secretions, leading to atelectasis and pneumonia. An artificial airway provides direct access for pathogens, making bronchial hygiene and chest physiotherapy extremely important measures to reduce infection. Neurogenic pulmonary edema may occur secondary to a dramatic increase in sympathetic nervous system activity at the time of injury, which shunts blood to the lungs. In addition, pulmonary edema may occur in response to fluid overload.

Cardiovascular System. Any cord injury above the level of T6 greatly decreases the affect of the sympathetic nervous system. Bradycardia occurs. Peripheral vasodilation results in hypotension. A relative hypovolemia exists because of the increase in the capacity of the dilated veins. Cardiac monitoring is necessary. In marked bradycardia (heart rate less than 40 beats/minute), appropriate drugs (e.g., atropine) to increase the heart rate and prevent hypoxemia are necessary. The peripheral vasodilation reduces the venous return of blood to the

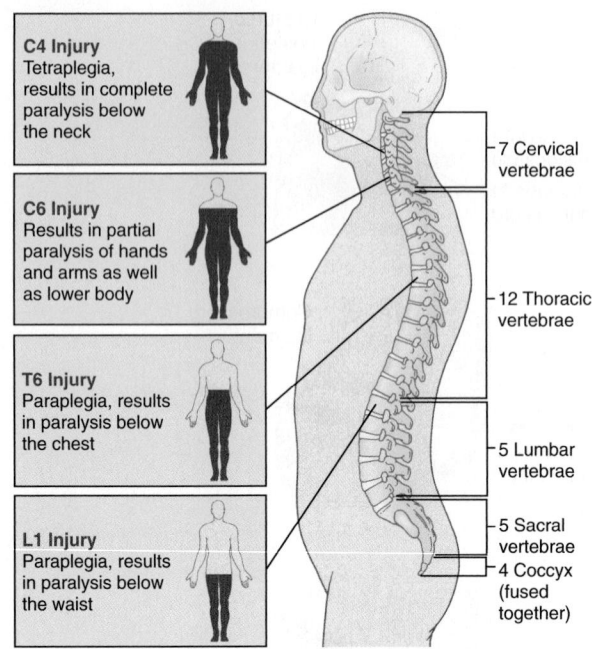

FIG. 61-6 Symptoms, degree of paralysis, and potential for rehabilitation depend on the level of the injury.

American Spinal Injury Association (ASIA) Impairment Scale

☐ **A = Complete:** No motor or sensory function is preserved in the sacral segments S4-5.

☐ **B = Incomplete:** Sensory but not motor function is preserved below the neurologic level and includes the sacral segments S4-5.

☐ **C = Incomplete:** Motor function is preserved below the neurologic level, and more than half of key muscles below the neurologic level have a muscle grade less than 3.

☐ **D = Incomplete:** Motor function is preserved below the neurologic level, and at least half of key muscles below the neurologic level have a muscle grade of 3 or more.

☐ **E = Normal:** Motor and sensory function are normal.

FIG. 61-7 The American Spinal Injury Association Impairment Scale. See eFig. 61-2 on the website for this chapter for standard neurologic classification of spinal cord injury.

TABLE 61-3	**INCOMPLETE SPINAL CORD INJURY SYNDROMES**
Description	**Manifestations**
Central Cord Syndrome	
• Caused by damage to the central spinal cord (see eFig. 61-1). • Occurs most commonly in the cervical cord region. • More common in older adults.	• Motor weakness and sensory loss are present in both upper and lower extremities. • Upper extremities are affected more than the lower ones.
Anterior Cord Syndrome	
• Caused by damage to the anterior spinal artery. • Results in compromised blood flow to the anterior spinal cord. • Typically results from injury causing acute compression of anterior portion of the spinal cord, often a flexion injury (see eFig. 61-1).	• Motor paralysis and loss of pain and temperature sensation below the level of injury. • Because posterior cord tracts are not injured, sensations of touch, position, vibration, and motion remain intact.
Brown-Séquard Syndrome	
• Results from damage to one half of the spinal cord (see eFig. 61-1). • Typically results from penetrating injury to spinal cord.	• *Ipsilateral* (same side as injury): Loss of motor function and position and vibratory sense, vasomotor paralysis. • *Contralateral* (opposite side of injury): Loss of pain and temperature sensation below the level of injury.
Posterior Cord Syndrome	
• Results from compression or damage to the posterior spinal artery. • Very rare condition.	• Generally the dorsal columns are damaged, resulting in loss of proprioception. • Pain, temperature sensation, and motor function below the level of injury remain intact.
Conus Medullaris Syndrome and Cauda Equina Syndrome	
• Result from damage to conus (lowest portion of the spinal cord) and cauda equina (lumbar and sacral nerve roots).	• Flaccid paralysis of the lower limbs and areflexic (flaccid) bladder and bowel.

---

heart and subsequently decreases cardiac output, resulting in hypotension. IV fluids or vasopressor drugs may be required to support the BP.

Urinary System. Urinary retention is a common development in acute SCI and spinal shock. While the patient is in spinal shock, the bladder is atonic and becomes overdistended. An indwelling catheter is inserted to drain the bladder. In the postacute phase the bladder may become hyperirritable, with a loss of inhibition from the brain resulting in reflex emptying. Chronic indwelling catheterization increases the risk of infection.

Gastrointestinal System. If the SCI has occurred above the level of T5, the primary GI problems are related to hypomotility. Decreased GI motor activity contributes to the development of paralytic ileus and gastric distention. A nasogastric tube for intermittent suctioning may relieve the gastric distention. Metoclopramide (Reglan) may be used to treat delayed gastric emptying. The development of stress ulcers is common because of excessive release of hydrochloric (HCl) acid in the stomach.

Intraabdominal bleeding may occur and is difficult to diagnose because the person with an SCI may experience no pain or tenderness. Continued hypotension in spite of vigorous treatment and decreased hemoglobin and hematocrit may be indications of bleeding. Expanding girth of the abdomen may also be noted.

Loss of voluntary neurologic control over the bowel results in a *neurogenic bowel*. In the early period after injury when spinal shock is present and for patients with an injury level of T12 or below, the bowel is *areflexic* and sphincter tone is decreased. As reflexes return, the bowel becomes *reflexic*, sphincter tone is enhanced, and reflex emptying occurs. Both areflexic and reflexic neurogenic bowel can be managed successfully with a regular bowel program coordinated with the gastrocolic reflex to minimize fecal incontinence.

Integumentary System. A major consequence of lack of movement is the potential for skin breakdown over bony prom-

TABLE 61-4 LEVEL OF SPINAL CORD INJURY AND REHABILITATION POTENTIAL

Movement Remaining	Rehabilitation Potential	Movement Remaining	Rehabilitation Potential
Tetraplegia		**C7-8**	
C1-3		All triceps to elbow extension, finger extensors and flexors, good grasp with some decreased strength, decreased respiratory reserve.	Ability to transfer self to wheelchair. Roll over and sit up in bed. Push self on most surfaces. Perform most self-care. Independent use of wheelchair. Ability to drive car with powered hand controls (in some patients). Attendant care 0-6 hr/day.
Often fatal injury. Movement in neck and above, loss of innervation to diaphragm, absence of independent respiratory function.	Ability to drive electric wheelchair equipped with portable ventilator by using chin control or mouth stick, headrest to stabilize head. Computer use with mouth stick, head wand, or noise control. Attendant care 24 hr/day, able to instruct others.		
		Paraplegia	
		T1-6	
C4		Full innervation of upper extremities. Back, essential intrinsic muscles of hand; full strength and dexterity of grasp. Decreased trunk stability, decreased respiratory reserve.	Full independence in self-care and in wheelchair. Ability to drive car with hand controls (in most patients). Independent standing in standing frame.
Sensation and movement in neck and above. May be able to breathe without a ventilator.	Same as C1-3.		
C5		**T6-12**	
Full neck, partial shoulder, back, biceps. Gross elbow, inability to roll over or use hands. Decreased respiratory reserve.	Ability to drive electric wheelchair with mobile hand supports. Indoor mobility in manual wheelchair. Able to feed self with setup and adaptive equipment. Attendant care 10 hr/day.	Full, stable thoracic muscles and upper back. Functional intercostals, resulting in increased respiratory reserve.	Full independent use of wheelchair. Ability to stand erect with full leg brace, ambulate on crutches with swing (although gait difficult). Inability to climb stairs.
		L1-2	
C6		Varying control of legs and pelvis, instability of lower back.	Good sitting balance. Full use of wheelchair. Ambulation with long leg braces.
Shoulder and upper back abduction and rotation at shoulder, full biceps to elbow flexion, wrist extension, weak grasp of thumb, decreased respiratory reserve.	Ability to assist with transfer and perform some self-care. Feed self with hand devices. Push wheelchair on smooth, flat surface. Drive adapted van from wheelchair. Independent computer use with adaptive equipment. Attendant care 6 hr/day.	**L3-4**	
		Quadriceps and hip flexors, absence of hamstring function, flail ankles.	Completely independent ambulation with short leg braces and canes. Inability to stand for long periods.

inences in areas of decreased or absent sensation. Pressure ulcers can occur quickly and can lead to major infection and sepsis.

Thermoregulation. *Poikilothermism* is the adjustment of the body temperature to the room temperature. This occurs in SCIs because the interruption of the sympathetic nervous system prevents peripheral temperature sensations from reaching the hypothalamus. With spinal cord disruption there is also decreased ability to sweat or shiver below the level of injury, which also affects the ability to regulate body temperature. The degree of poikilothermism depends on the level of injury. Patients with high cervical injuries have a greater loss of ability to regulate temperature than do those with thoracic or lumbar injuries.

Metabolic Needs. Nasogastric suctioning may lead to metabolic alkalosis, and decreased tissue perfusion may lead to acidosis. Electrolyte levels, including sodium and potassium, can be altered by gastric suctioning. Monitor these electrolytes until suctioning is discontinued and a normal diet is resumed. Loss of weight (greater than 10%) is common. The person with an SCI has greater nutritional needs than other patients who are immobilized. A high-protein diet helps prevent skin breakdown and infections and decreases the rate of muscle atrophy.

Peripheral Vascular Problems. Venous thromboembolism (VTE) is a common problem accompanying SCI during the first 3 months.[18] It is more difficult to detect a deep venous thrombosis (DVT) in a person with an SCI because the usual signs and symptoms, such as pain and tenderness, are not present. Pulmonary embolism is one of the leading causes of death in patients with SCI.

Diagnostic Studies

CT scan is the preferred imaging study to diagnose the location and degree of injury and degree of spinal canal compromise. Cervical x-rays are obtained when CT scan is not readily available. However, it is often difficult to visualize C7 and T1 on a cervical x-ray, compromising the ability to fully evaluate cervical spine injury. MRI is used to assess for soft tissue and neurologic changes and for unexplained neurologic deficits or worsening of neurologic status. A comprehensive neurologic examination is performed along with assessment of the head, chest, and abdomen for additional injuries or trauma. Patients with cervical injuries who demonstrate altered mental status may also need a CT angiogram to rule out vertebral artery damage.

Duplex Doppler ultrasound, impedance plethysmography, venous occlusion plethysmography, venography, and the clinical examination are recommended for use as diagnostic tests for DVT.

Collaborative Care

Immediate postinjury goals include maintaining a patent airway, adequate ventilation, and adequate circulating blood volume and preventing extension of cord damage (secondary

➕ TABLE 61-5 EMERGENCY MANAGEMENT

Spinal Cord Injury

Etiology	Assessment Findings	Interventions
Blunt Trauma • Compression, flexion, extension, or rotational injuries to spinal column • Motor vehicle collisions • Pedestrian incidents • Falls • Diving **Penetrating Trauma** • Stretched, torn, crushed, or lacerated spinal cord • Gunshot wounds • Stab wounds	• Pain, tenderness, deformities, or muscle spasms adjacent to vertebral column • Numbness, paresthesias • Alterations in sensation: temperature, light touch, deep pressure, proprioception • Weakness or heaviness in limbs • Weakness, paralysis, or flaccidity of muscles • Spinal shock • Cuts; bruises; open wounds over head, face, neck, or back • Neurogenic shock: hypotension, bradycardia, dry, flushed skin • Bowel and bladder incontinence • Urinary retention • Difficulty breathing • Priapism • Diminished rectal sphincter tone	**Initial** • Ensure patent airway. • Immobilize and stabilize cervical spine.* • Administer O_2 via nasal cannula or non-rebreather mask. • Establish IV access with two large-bore catheters to infuse normal saline or lactated Ringer's solution as appropriate. • Assess for other injuries. • Control external bleeding. • Obtain CT scan or cervical spine x-rays. **Ongoing Monitoring** • Monitor vital signs, level of consciousness, O_2 saturation, cardiac rhythm, urine output. • Keep warm. • Monitor for urinary retention, hypertension. • Anticipate need for intubation if gag reflex absent.

*Spinal immobilization is not recommended in patients who have penetrating trauma.

TABLE 61-6 COLLABORATIVE CARE

Cervical Cord Injury

Diagnostic
- History and physical examination, including complete neurologic examination
- Arterial blood gases
- Serial bedside PFTs
- Electrolytes, glucose level, coagulation profile, hemoglobin and hematocrit levels
- Urinalysis
- CT scan, MRI
- X-rays of spine
- Anteroposterior, lateral, and odontoid spinal x-ray studies
- EMG to measure evoked potentials
- Duplex Doppler ultrasound, impedance plethysmography

Collaborative Therapy
Acute Care
- Immobilization of vertebral column
- Maintenance of heart rate (e.g., atropine) and blood pressure (e.g., dopamine [Intropin])
- Insertion of nasogastric tube and attachment to suction
- Intubation (if indicated by ABGs and PFTs)
- O_2 by high-humidity mask
- Indwelling urinary catheter
- Administration of IV fluids
- Stress ulcer prophylaxis
- Deep vein thrombosis prophylaxis
- Bowel and bladder training

Rehabilitation and Home Care
- Physical therapy
  - Range-of-motion exercises
  - Mobility training
  - Muscle strengthening
- Occupational therapy (splints, activities of daily living training)
- Bowel and bladder training
- Autonomic dysreflexia prevention
- Pressure ulcer prevention
- Recreational therapy
- Patient and caregiver teaching

injury). Table 61-5 outlines the emergency management of the patient with an SCI. Recommended immobilization includes a combination of a rigid cervical collar and supportive blocks on a backboard with straps. Spinal immobilization with sandbags and tape is insufficient and is not recommended. Spinal immobilization in patients with penetrating trauma is not recommended because of increased mortality. The concern during the initial management of patients with potential cervical spinal injuries is that neurologic function may be impaired as a result of movement of the injured vertebrae. [19,20]

Systemic and neurogenic shock must be treated to maintain BP. For injury at the cervical level, all body systems must be maintained until the full extent of the damage can be evaluated.

Collaborative care during the acute phase for a patient with a cervical injury is described in Table 61-6. Compared to cervical injury, patients with SCIs of the thoracic and lumbar vertebrae require less intense support. Respiratory compromise is not as severe, and bradycardia is usually not a problem. Specific problems are treated symptomatically.

After stabilization at the injury scene, the person is transferred to a medical facility. A thorough assessment is done to specifically evaluate the degree of deficit and to establish the level and degree of injury. A history is obtained, with emphasis on how the incident occurred and the extent of injury as perceived by the patient immediately after the event. Assessment involves testing muscle groups rather than individual muscles. Test muscle groups with and against gravity, alone and against resistance, and on both sides of the body. Note spontaneous movement. Ask the patient to move legs and then hands, spread fingers, extend wrists, and shrug shoulders. After assessing motor status, carry out a sensory examination, including touch and pain as tested by pinprick, starting at the toes and working upward toward the head. If time and conditions permit, also assess position sense and vibration.

The types of injury mechanisms that cause spinal cord trauma, especially those involving the cervical cord, may also result in brain injury. Therefore assess for a history of unconsciousness, signs of concussion, and increased intracranial pressure (see Chapter 57). In addition, perform a careful assessment for musculoskeletal injuries and trauma to internal organs.

Because the patient has no muscle, bone, or visceral sensations, the only clue to internal trauma with hemorrhage may be a rapidly increasing BP and pulse. Examine the urine for hematuria, which is also indicative of internal injuries.

Move the patient in alignment as a unit *(logroll)* during transfers and when repositioning to prevent further injury. Monitor respiratory, cardiac, urinary, and GI functions. The patient may go directly to surgery after initial immobilization and stabilization or to the intensive care unit (ICU) for monitoring and management.

Nonoperative Stabilization. Nonoperative treatments involve stabilization of the injured spinal segment and decompression, either through traction or realignment. Stabilization methods eliminate damaging motion at the injury site. These methods are intended to prevent secondary spinal cord damage caused by repeated contusion or compression.

Surgical Therapy. The decision to perform surgery on a patient with an SCI often depends on the particular physician's preference. When cord compression is certain or the neurologic disorder progresses, immediate surgery may be beneficial. Surgery decompresses and stabilizes the spinal column. Early cord decompression may reduce secondary injury to the spinal cord and therefore improve the outcome. Other criteria used in the decision for early surgery include (1) evidence of cord compression, (2) progressive neurologic deficit, (3) compound fracture of the vertebrae, (4) bony fragments (may dislodge and penetrate the cord), and (5) penetrating wounds of the spinal cord or surrounding structures.

Surgery to stabilize the spine can be performed from the back of the spine *(posterior approach)* or from the front of the spine *(anterior approach)*. In some cases, both approaches may be needed. A fusion procedure involves attaching metal screws, plates, or other devices to the bones of the spine to help keep them properly aligned. This is usually done when two or more vertebrae have been injured. Small pieces of bone may also be attached to the injured bones to help them fuse into one solid piece. The bone used for this procedure is usually taken from another bone in the body, most often from the hip. (Specific surgical and nursing interventions for these techniques are discussed in Chapter 64 on pp. 1548-1550.)

Drug Therapy. Methylprednisolone (MP), which was used for many years to treat acute SCI, is no longer recommended. It is not approved by the Food and Drug Administration (FDA) for this use and there is no evidence of clinical benefit of MP to treat acute SCI. High-dose MP is associated with harmful side effects including immunosuppression, increased frequency of upper GI bleeding, increased risk of infection, sepsis, longer stays in the ICU, and sometimes death.[21]

Low-molecular-weight heparin (e.g., enoxaparin [Lovenox]) is used to prevent VTE unless contraindicated. Contraindications include internal bleeding and recent surgery. Oral anticoagulation alone is not recommended as a prophylactic treatment strategy.[22]

Vasopressor agents such as dopamine (Intropin) are used in the acute phase as adjuvants to treatment. These agents are used to maintain the mean arterial pressure at a level greater than 90 mm Hg so that perfusion to the spinal cord is improved.

Drug metabolism is altered in patients with an SCI. Therefore drug interactions may occur. The differences in drug metabolism correlate with level and completeness of injury, with greater change apparent in people with cervical cord injury than in those with injury at lower spinal levels.

NURSING MANAGEMENT SPINAL CORD INJURY

NURSING ASSESSMENT

Subjective and objective data that should be obtained from a patient with a recent SCI are presented in Table 61-7.

NURSING DIAGNOSES

Nursing diagnoses for the patient with an SCI depend on the severity of the injury and the level of dysfunction. The nursing diagnoses for a patient with an SCI may include, but are not limited to, the following:

- Ineffective breathing pattern *related to* respiratory muscle fatigue, neuromuscular paralysis, and/or retained secretions
- Impaired skin integrity *related to* immobility and/or poor tissue perfusion
- Impaired urinary elimination *related to* spinal injury and/or limited fluid intake
- Constipation *related to* neurogenic bowel, inadequate fluid intake, and/or immobility
- Risk for autonomic dysreflexia *related to* reflex stimulation of sympathetic nervous system

Additional information on nursing diagnoses for the patient with an SCI is presented in eNursing Care Plan 61-1 (available on the website for this chapter). The care plan is for a patient with a complete cervical cord injury.

PLANNING

The overall goals are that the patient with an SCI will (1) maintain an optimal level of neurologic functioning; (2) have minimal or no complications of immobility; (3) learn new skills, gain new knowledge, and acquire new behaviors to be able to care for self or successfully direct others to do so; and (4) return to home and the community at an optimal level of functioning.

NURSING IMPLEMENTATION

HEALTH PROMOTION. Nursing interventions for the prevention of an SCI include identification of high-risk populations, counseling, and teaching. Support of legislation related to seat belt use in cars, helmets for motorcyclists and bicyclists, child safety seats, and tougher penalties for drunk-driving offenses is a professional responsibility.

Emphasize the importance of other health promotion and health screening in addition to SCI care. After injury, health-promoting behaviors can have a significant impact on the general health and well-being of the individual with an SCI. Nursing interventions include teaching and counseling; referral to programs such as smoking cessation classes, recreation and exercise programs, and alcohol treatment programs; and performing routine physical examinations for non-neurologic problems. Outpatient health care requires that the facilities for the screening and prevention programs must be accessible to and accommodate people with SCI. Nurses in these clinical settings should advocate for wheelchair-accessible examination rooms, adjustable-height examination tables, and scheduling that allows extra time if needed.

ACUTE INTERVENTION. High cervical cord injury caused by flexion-rotation is the most complex SCI and is discussed in this section. Interventions for this type of injury can be modified for patients with less severe injuries.

TABLE 61-7 **NURSING ASSESSMENT**
Spinal Cord Injury

Subjective Data
Important Health Information
Health history: Motor vehicle collision, sports injury, industrial incident, gunshot or stabbing injury, falls

Functional Health Patterns
Health perception–health management: Use of alcohol or recreational drugs; risk-taking behaviors
Activity-exercise: Loss of strength, movement, and sensation below level of injury; dyspnea, inability to breathe adequately ("air hunger")
Cognitive-perceptual: Tenderness, pain at or above level of injury; numbness, tingling, burning, twitching of extremities
Coping–stress tolerance: Fear, denial, anger, depression

Objective Data
General
Poikilothermism (unable to regulate body heat)

Integumentary
Warm, dry skin below level of injury (neurogenic shock)

Respiratory
Injury at C1-3: Apnea, inability to cough
Injury at C4: Poor cough, diaphragmatic breathing, hypoventilation
Injury at C5-T6: Decreased respiratory reserve

Cardiovascular
Injury above T5: Bradycardia, hypotension, postural hypotension, absence of vasomotor tone

Gastrointestinal
Decreased or absent bowel sounds (paralytic ileus in injuries above T5), abdominal distention, constipation, fecal incontinence, fecal impaction

Urinary
Retention (for injuries at T1-L2); flaccid bladder (acute stages); spasticity with reflex bladder emptying (later stages)

Reproductive
Priapism, loss of sexual function

Neurologic
Complete: Flaccid paralysis and anesthesia below level of injury resulting in tetraplegia (for injuries above C8) or paraplegia (for injuries below C8), hyperactive deep tendon reflexes, bilaterally positive Babinski test (after resolution of spinal shock)
Incomplete: Mixed loss of voluntary motor activity and sensation

Musculoskeletal
Muscle atony (in flaccid state), contractures (in spastic state)

Possible Diagnostic Findings
Location of level and type of bony involvement on spinal x-ray: injury, edema, compression on CT scan and MRI; positive finding on myelogram

Immobilization. Proper immobilization of the neck involves the maintenance of a neutral position.

SAFETY ALERT
- Use a hard cervical collar, and a backboard to stabilize the neck to prevent lateral rotation of the cervical spine.
- The body should always be correctly aligned.
- Perform turning so that the patient is moved as a unit (i.e., logrolling) to prevent movement of the spine.

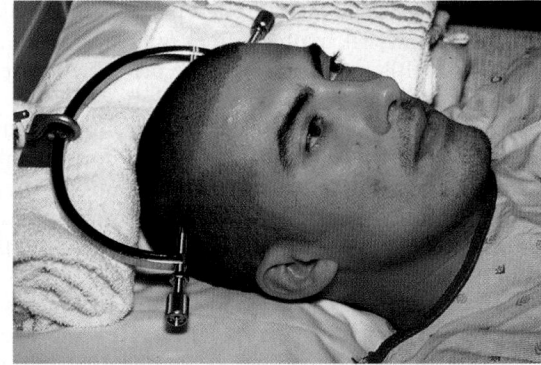
FIG. 61-8 Cervical traction is attached to tongs inserted in the skull.

For cervical injuries, skeletal traction is used less frequently since the development of better surgical stabilization. When skeletal traction is used, the goal is realignment or reduction of the injury. Crutchfield (Fig. 61-8), Vinke, or Gardner-Wells tongs or other types of devices can provide this type of traction, using a rope that extends from the center of the tongs over a pulley and has weights attached at the end. Traction must be maintained at all times. Depending on the type of injury and the goal of treatment, the tongs and traction may be removed 1 to 4 weeks after the injury. One disadvantage of skull tongs is that the skull pins can be displaced. If this occurs, hold the head in a neutral position and get help. Stabilize the head while the physician reinserts the tongs.

Infection at the sites of tong insertion is another potential problem. Preventive care includes cleansing the sites twice a day with normal saline solution and applying an antibiotic ointment, which acts as a mechanical barrier to the entrance of bacteria. The procedures for preventive care of insertion sites may vary depending on individual hospital standards of care.

Special beds are often used in the management of the patient with SCI (Fig. 61-9). Kinetic therapy is the continuous side-to-side rotation of a patient to 40 degrees or more to help prevent pulmonary complications. This lateral rotation also redistributes pressure, helping prevent pressure ulcers.

After cervical fusion or other stabilization surgery, a hard cervical collar or sternal-occipital-mandibular immobilizer brace can be worn (Fig. 61-10). In a stable injury for which surgery is not done, a halo fixation apparatus may be applied. The halo is the most frequently used method of stabilizing cervical injuries. The halo apparatus can be used to apply cervical traction by means of a jacket-like arrangement (Fig. 61-11). Hanging weights, such as those used with tongs, can be incorporated with the halo. In addition, the apparatus can be attached to a body vest, stabilizing the injured area and allowing ambulation if the patient is neurologically intact. Another alternative is to use the halo after the patient has had traction removed. It allows the patient to be more mobile and to begin active rehabilitation.

Patients with thoracic or lumbar spine injuries are immobilized with a custom thoracolumbar orthosis ("body jacket"), which inhibits spinal flexion, extension, and rotation, or with a Jewett brace, which restricts forward flexion.

Immobilization of the neck of the patient with an SCI prevents further injury, but the effects of immobility are profound. Meticulous skin care is critical because decreased sensation and circulation make the patient particularly susceptible to skin breakdown. Remove the patient's backboard as soon as possible

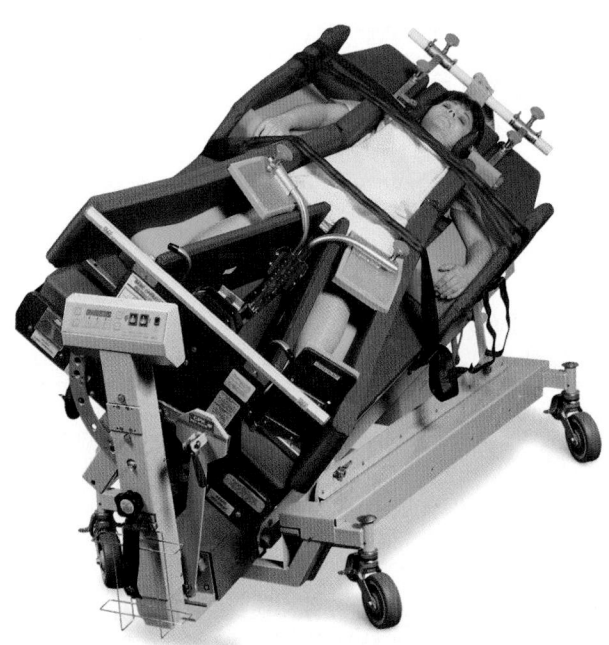

FIG. 61-9 The RotoRest Therapy System helps prevent and treat pulmonary complications for immobile patients, including those with unstable cervical, thoracic, and lumbar fractures. Kinetic therapy, the continual side-to-side bilateral rotation of the patient, redistributes pulmonary blood flow and mobilizes secretions to improve ventilation and perfusion matching. The therapy system also helps to prevent pressure ulcers. (Courtesy Arjo Huntleigh, Addison, Ill.)

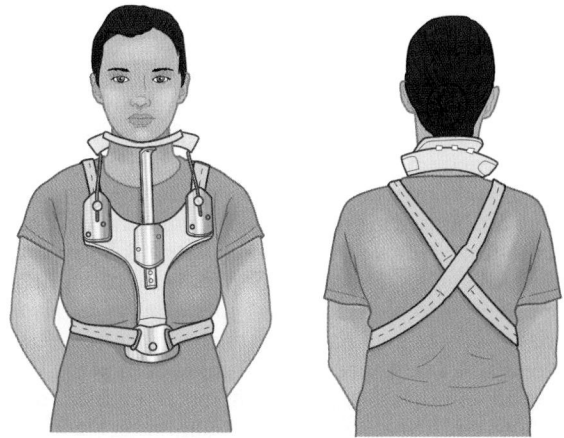

FIG. 61-10 Sternal-occipital-mandibular immobilizer brace.

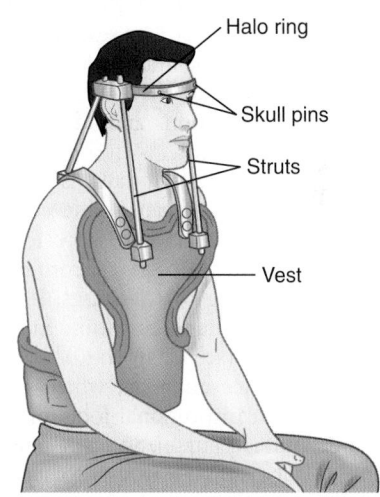

FIG. 61-11 Halo vest. The halo traction brace immobilizes the cervical spine, which allows the patient to ambulate and participate in self-care.

and replace it with other forms of immobilization to prevent coccygeal and occipital area skin breakdown. Properly fit cervical collars. Inspect the areas under the halo vest or jacket or under braces or orthoses to assess the skin condition.

Respiratory Dysfunction. During the first 48 hours after injury, spinal cord edema may increase the level of dysfunction, and respiratory distress may occur. If the injury is at or above C3, or if the patient is exhausted from labored breathing or ABGs deteriorate (indicating inadequate oxygenation or ventilation), initiate endotracheal intubation or tracheostomy and mechanical ventilation. The possibility of respiratory arrest requires careful monitoring and prompt action should it occur. Pneumonia and atelectasis are potential problems because of reduced vital capacity and the loss of intercostal and abdominal muscle function, resulting in diaphragmatic breathing, pooled secretions, and an ineffective cough.

The older adult has a more difficult time responding to hypoxia and hypercapnia. Therefore aggressive chest physiotherapy, adequate oxygenation, and proper pain management are essential to maximize respiratory function and gas exchange. Other respiratory problems include nasal stuffiness and bronchospasm.

Regularly assess (1) breath sounds, (2) ABGs, (3) tidal volume, (4) vital capacity, (5) skin color, (6) breathing patterns (especially the use of accessory muscles), (7) subjective comments about the ability to breathe, and (8) the amount and color of sputum. A PaO$_2$ (partial pressure of oxygen in arterial blood) greater than 60 mm Hg and a PaCO$_2$ (partial pressure of carbon dioxide in arterial blood) less than 45 mm Hg are acceptable values in a patient with uncomplicated tetraplegia. A patient who is unable to count to 10 aloud without taking a breath needs immediate attention.

In addition to monitoring, you can intervene to maintain ventilation. Administer oxygen until ABGs stabilize. Chest physiotherapy and assisted coughing help to clear secretions. Assisted (augmented) coughing simulates the action of the ineffective abdominal muscles during the expiratory phase of a cough. Place the heels of both hands just below the xiphoid process and exert firm upward pressure to the area timed with the patient's efforts to cough (see Fig. 68-7). Perform tracheal suctioning if crackles or rhonchi are present. Incentive spirometry is an additional technique that can be used to improve the patient's respiratory status.

Cardiovascular Instability. Because of unopposed vagal response, the heart rate is slowed, often to less than 60 beats/minute. Any increase in vagal stimulation, such as turning or suctioning, can result in cardiac arrest. Loss of sympathetic nervous system tone in peripheral vessels results in chronic low BP with potential postural hypotension. Lack of muscle tone to aid venous return can result in sluggish blood flow and predispose the patient to DVT.

Frequently assess vital signs. If bradycardia is symptomatic, administer an anticholinergic drug such as atropine. A temporary or permanent pacemaker may be inserted in some patients. Hypotension is managed with a vasopressor agent, such as dopamine or norepinephrine, and fluid replacement.

In the older adult, consider the effects of aging on the cardiovascular system. The older patient is less able to handle the stress of traumatic injury because heart contractions weaken and cardiac output is reduced. Maximum heart rate is also reduced. In addition to the effects of aging, the older person may also have cardiovascular disease.

Sequential compression devices or compression gradient stockings can be used to prevent thromboemboli and to promote venous return. Remove the stockings every 8 hours for skin care. Venous duplex studies may be performed before applying compression devices. Also regularly perform range-of-motion exercises and stretching. Assess the thighs and calves every shift for signs of DVT (e.g., deep reddish color, edema).

If blood loss has occurred from other injuries, monitor hemoglobin and hematocrit levels and administer blood according to protocol. Also monitor the patient for indications of hypovolemic shock secondary to hemorrhage.

Fluid and Nutritional Maintenance. During the first 48 to 72 hours after the injury, the GI tract may stop functioning (paralytic ileus) and a nasogastric tube must be inserted. Because the patient cannot have oral intake, carefully monitor fluid and electrolyte status. Specific solutions and additives are ordered based on individual requirements.

Once bowel sounds are present or flatus is passed, gradually introduce oral food and fluids. Because of severe catabolism, a high-protein, high-calorie diet is necessary for energy and tissue repair. In patients with high cervical cord injuries, evaluate swallowing before starting oral feedings. If the patient is unable to resume eating, enteral nutrition may be used to provide nutritional support (see Chapter 40).

Some patients experience anorexia, which can be due to depression, boredom with institutional food, or discomfort at being fed (often by a hurried nurse). Some patients have a normally small appetite. Occasionally, refusal to eat is a means of maintaining control over the environment because of diminished or absent body control. If the patient is not eating adequately, thoroughly assess the cause.

On the basis of this assessment, make a contract with the patient using mutual goal setting regarding the diet. This gives the patient increased control of the situation and often results in improved nutritional intake. General measures such as providing a pleasant eating environment, allowing adequate time to eat (including any self-feeding the patient can achieve), encouraging the family to bring in special foods, and planning social rewards for eating may be useful. Keep a calorie count, and record the patient's daily weight to evaluate progress. If feasible, the patient should participate in recording calorie intake. Dietary supplements may be necessary to meet nutritional needs. Increased dietary fiber should be included to promote bowel function. Avoid allowing the patient's nutritional intake to become a basis for a power struggle.

Bladder and Bowel Management. Immediately after the injury, urine is retained because of the loss of autonomic and reflex control of the bladder and sphincter. Because there is no sensation of fullness, overdistention of the bladder can result in reflux into the kidney with eventual renal failure. Bladder overdistention may even result in rupture of the bladder. Consequently, an indwelling catheter is usually inserted as soon as possible after injury. Ensure the patency of the catheter by frequent inspection and irrigation if necessary. In some institutions a physician's order is required for this procedure. Strict aseptic technique for catheter care is essential to avoid introducing

infection. During the period of indwelling catheterization, a large fluid intake is required. Check the catheter to prevent kinking and ensure free flow of urine.

UTIs are a common problem. The best method for preventing UTIs is regular and complete bladder drainage. After the patient is stabilized, assess the best means of managing long-term urinary function. Usually the patient is started on an intermittent catheterization program. (Intermittent catheterization is discussed on p. 1481 later in this chapter and in Chapter 46.)

Intermittent catheterization should be done every 3 to 4 hours to prevent bacterial overgrowth from urinary stasis. If the appearance or odor of the urine is suspicious or if the patient develops symptoms of a UTI (e.g., chills, fever, malaise), send a specimen for culture.

Consider age-related changes in renal function. The older adult is more likely to develop renal calculi. Older men may have benign prostatic hyperplasia, which may interfere with urinary flow and complicate management of urinary problems.

Constipation is generally a problem during spinal shock because no voluntary or involuntary (reflex) evacuation of the bowels occurs. A bowel program should be started during acute care. This consists of choosing a rectal stimulant (suppository or small-volume enema) to be inserted daily at a regular time, followed by gentle digital stimulation or manual evacuation until evacuation is complete.[23] Initially the program may be done in bed with the patient in the side-lying position, but as soon as the patient has resumed sitting, it should be done in the upright position on a padded bedside commode chair.

Temperature Control. Because there is no vasoconstriction, piloerection, or heat loss through perspiration below the level of injury, temperature control is largely external to the patient. Monitor the environment closely to maintain an appropriate temperature. Also regularly monitor body temperature. Do not overload patients with covers or unduly expose them (such as during bathing). If an infection with high fever develops, more extensive means of temperature control, such as a cooling blanket, may be necessary.

Stress Ulcers. Stress ulcers are a problem for the patient with an SCI because of the physiologic response to severe trauma and psychologic stress. Peak incidence of stress ulcers is 6 to 14 days after injury. Test stool and gastric contents daily for blood, and monitor the hematocrit for a slow drop. Histamine (H₂)-receptor blockers (e.g., ranitidine [Zantac], famotidine [Pepcid]) or proton pump inhibitors (e.g., pantoprazole [Protonix], omeprazole [Prilosec]) may be given prophylactically to decrease the secretion of HCl acid and prevent ulcers during the initial phase.

Sensory Deprivation. You need to compensate for the patient's absent sensations to prevent sensory deprivation. Do this by stimulating the patient above the level of injury. Conversation, music, and interesting foods can be a part of the nursing care plan. Provide prism glasses so that the patient can read and watch television. Make every effort to prevent the patient from withdrawing from the environment.

Patients with SCI often report altered sensorium and vivid dreams during the acute phase of their treatment. Whether this is due to drugs used to manage pain and anxiety is not known. Patients may also experience disrupted sleep patterns as a result of the hospital environment or posttraumatic stress disorder.[24]

Reflexes. Once spinal cord shock is resolved, the return of reflexes may complicate rehabilitation. Lacking control from the higher brain centers, reflexes are often hyperactive and produce exaggerated responses. Penile erections can occur from a variety of stimuli, causing embarrassment and discomfort. Spasms ranging from mild twitches to convulsive movements below the level of injury may also occur. The patient or caregiver may interpret this reflex activity as a return of function. Tactfully explain the reason for the activity. Inform the patient of the positive use of these reflexes in sexual, bowel, and bladder retraining. Spasms may be controlled with the use of antispasmodic drugs such as baclofen, dantrolene (Dantrium), and tizanidine (Zanaflex). Botulism toxin injections may also be given to treat severe spasticity.

Autonomic Dysreflexia. The return of reflexes after the resolution of spinal shock means that patients with an injury level at T6 or higher may develop autonomic dysreflexia. Autonomic dysreflexia (also known as *autonomic hyperreflexia*) is a massive uncompensated cardiovascular reaction mediated by the sympathetic nervous system.[25] It involves stimulation of sensory receptors below the level of the SCI. The intact sympathetic nervous system below the level of injury responds to the stimulation with a reflex arteriolar vasoconstriction that increases BP, but the parasympathetic nervous system is unable to directly counteract these responses via the injured spinal cord. Baroreceptors in the carotid sinus and the aorta sense the hypertension and stimulate the parasympathetic system. This results in a decrease in heart rate, but the visceral and peripheral vessels do not dilate because efferent impulses cannot pass through the injured spinal cord.

The most common precipitating cause of autonomic dysreflexia is a distended bladder or rectum. However, autonomic dysreflexia can be caused by any sensory stimulation, including contraction of the bladder or rectum, stimulation of the skin, or stimulation of pain receptors.

Manifestations include hypertension (up to 300 mm Hg systolic), throbbing headache, marked diaphoresis above the level of injury, bradycardia (30 to 40 beats/minute), *piloerection* (erection of body hair) as a result of pilomotor spasm, flushing of the skin above the level of injury, blurred vision or spots in the visual fields, nasal congestion, anxiety, and nausea. It is important to measure BP when a patient with an SCI complains of a headache.

This is a life-threatening condition that requires immediate resolution. If uncorrected, autonomic dysreflexia can lead to status epilepticus, stroke, myocardial infarction, and even death.

Nursing interventions in this serious emergency are elevating the head of the bed 45 degrees or sitting the patient upright, notifying the physician, and determining the cause. The most common cause is bladder irritation. Immediate catheterization to relieve bladder distention may be necessary. Instill lidocaine jelly in the urethra before catheterization. If a catheter is already in place, check it for kinks or folds. If it is plugged, perform small-volume irrigation slowly and gently to open a plugged catheter, or insert a new catheter.

Stool impaction can also result in autonomic dysreflexia. Perform a digital rectal examination only after application of an anesthetic ointment to decrease rectal stimulation and to avoid increasing symptoms. Remove all skin stimuli, such as constrictive clothing and tight shoes. Monitor BP frequently during the episode. If symptoms persist after the source has been relieved, administer an α-adrenergic blocker or an arteriolar vasodilator (e.g., nifedipine [Procardia]). Continue careful monitoring until vital signs stabilize.

Teach the patient and caregiver to recognize the causes and symptoms of autonomic dysreflexia (Table 61-8). They must understand the life-threatening nature of this dysfunction and know how to relieve the cause.

REHABILITATION AND HOME CARE. Rehabilitation of the person with an SCI is complex. With physical and psychologic care and intensive and specialized rehabilitation, the patient with an SCI can learn to function at the highest level of wellness. It is recommended that all patients with a new SCI receive comprehensive inpatient rehabilitation in a rehabilitation unit or center that specializes in spinal cord rehabilitation.

Many of the problems identified in the acute period become chronic and continue throughout life. Rehabilitation focuses on retraining of physiologic processes and extensive patient, caregiver, and family teaching about how to manage the physiologic and life changes resulting from the injury (Fig. 61-12).

Rehabilitation is an interdisciplinary endeavor carried out through a team approach. Team members include rehabilitation nurses, physicians, physical therapists, occupational therapists, speech therapists, vocational counselors, psychologists, therapeutic recreation specialists, prosthetists, orthotists, and dietitians.

Rehabilitation care is organized around the individual patient's goals and needs. Patients are expected to be involved in therapies and learn self-care for several hours each day. Such intensive work at a time when the patient is dealing with the sudden change in health and functional status can be stressful. Progress may be slow. The rehabilitation nurse has a pivotal role in providing encouragement, specialized nursing care, and patient and caregiver teaching, and in helping to coordinate the efforts of the rehabilitation team.

Respiratory Rehabilitation. The patient with a high cervical SCI may have greatly increased mobility with phrenic nerve stimulators or electronic diaphragmatic pacemakers. These devices are not appropriate for all ventilator-dependent patients but may be helpful for those with an intact phrenic nerve. Ventilators are also reasonably portable, and ventilator-dependent tetraplegic patients can be mobile and somewhat independent. Patients and caregivers should be taught all aspects of home ventilator care, with referrals made to appropriate community agencies. Teach patients with cervical-level injuries who are not ventilator dependent assisted coughing, regular use of incentive spirometry, or deep breathing exercises.

Neurogenic Bladder. A neurogenic bladder is any type of bladder dysfunction related to abnormal or absent bladder innervation. After spinal cord shock resolves, depending on the completeness of the SCI, patients usually have some degree of neurogenic bladder. Normal voiding requires nervous system coordination of urethral and pelvic floor relaxation with simultaneous contraction of the detrusor muscle. Depending on the injury, a neurogenic bladder may have no reflex detrusor contractions (areflexic, flaccid), may have hyperactive reflex detrusor contractions (hyperreflexic, spastic), or may lack coordination between detrusor contraction and urethral relaxation (*dyssynergia*). Common problems with a neurogenic bladder include urgency, frequency, incontinence, inability to void, and high bladder pressures resulting in reflux of urine into the kidneys.[26]

Types of neurogenic bladder are presented in Table 61-9. Diagnostic and collaborative care of neurogenic bladder is described in Table 61-10. The patient with an SCI and a neurogenic bladder requires a comprehensive program to manage bladder function.

After the patient's overall condition is stable and there is evidence of neurologic reflexes, urodynamic testing (see Table 45-8) and a urine culture are done. Many factors are considered when selecting a bladder management strategy. These include patient preference, upper extremity function, and availability of a caregiver. The type of bladder dysfunction (see Table 61-9) also determines management options.

TABLE 61-8   PATIENT & CAREGIVER TEACHING GUIDE

Autonomic Dysreflexia

For a patient at risk for autonomic dysreflexia, include the following information in the teaching plan for the patient and caregiver.

1. Signs and symptoms
   - Sudden onset of acute headache
   - Elevation in blood pressure and/or reduction in pulse rate
   - Flushed face and upper chest (above the level of injury) and pale extremities (below the level of injury)
   - Sweating above the level of injury
   - Nasal congestion
   - Feeling of apprehension
2. Immediate interventions
   - Raise the person to a sitting position.
   - Remove the noxious stimulus (fecal impaction, kinked urinary catheter, tight clothing).
   - Call the health care provider if above actions do not relieve the signs and symptoms.
3. Measures to decrease the incidence of autonomic dysreflexia
   - Maintain regular bowel function.
   - If manual rectal stimulation is used to promote bowel function, local anesthetics may prevent autonomic dysreflexia.
   - Monitor urine output.
   - Wear a Medic Alert bracelet indicating a history of risk for autonomic dysreflexia.

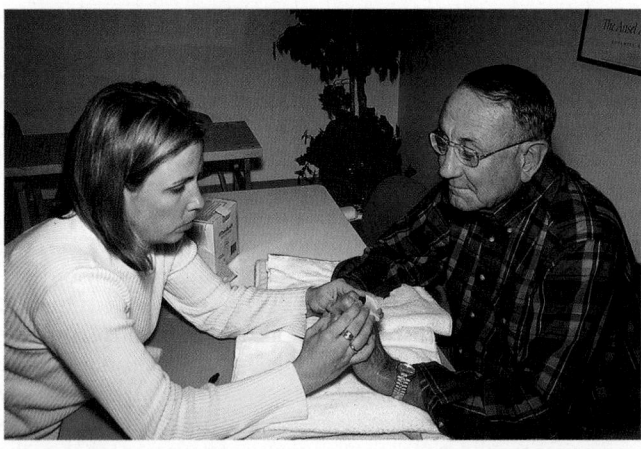

FIG. 61-12 Patient participating in occupational therapy.

TABLE 61-9   TYPES OF NEUROGENIC BLADDER

	Characteristics	Causes	Manifestations
Reflexic (spastic, uninhibited)	No inhibitions influence time and place of voiding. Bladder empties in response to stretching of bladder wall.	Results from upper motor neuron injury, corticospinal tract injury. Observed in spinal cord injury, stroke, multiple sclerosis, brain tumor, brain trauma.	Incontinence, frequency, urgency. Voiding is unpredictable and incomplete.
Areflexic (autonomous, flaccid)	Bladder acts as if there were paralysis of all motor functions, fills without emptying.	Results from lower motor neuron injury caused by trauma involving S2-4. Lesions of cauda equina, pelvic nerves.	If sensory function intact, patient feels bladder distention and hesitancy. No control of micturition, resulting in overdistention of bladder and overflow incontinence.
Sensory (lack of sensation of need to urinate)	Damage to sensory limb of bladder spinal reflex arc.	Seen in multiple sclerosis, diabetes mellitus.	Poor bladder sensation, infrequent voiding of large residual volume.

TABLE 61-10 COLLABORATIVE CARE

Neurogenic Bladder

Diagnostic
- History and physical examination, including neurologic examination
- Urodynamic testing
- CT urogram
- Intravenous pyelogram
- Urine culture

Collaborative Therapy
- Drug therapy
  - Anticholinergics
  - α-Adrenergic blockers
  - Antispasmodics
- Fluid intake of 1800-2000 mL/day
- Urine drainage
  - Voluntary or reflex voiding
  - Intermittent catheterization
  - Indwelling catheter
- Surgical therapy
  - Sphincterotomy
  - Electrical stimulation
  - Urinary diversion

TABLE 61-11 PATIENT & CAREGIVER TEACHING GUIDE

Bowel Management After Spinal Cord Injury

For the patient with a spinal cord injury include the following information about bowel management in the teaching plan for the patient and caregiver.

1. Optimal nutritional intake includes the following:
   - Three well-balanced meals each day
   - Two servings from the milk group
   - Two or more servings from the meat group, including beef, pork, poultry, eggs, fish
   - Four or more servings from the vegetable and fruit groups
   - Four or more servings from the bread and cereal group
2. Fiber intake should be approximately 20-30 g/day. The amount of fiber eaten should be increased gradually over 1-2 wk.
3. Two to three quarts of fluid per day should be consumed unless contraindicated. Water or fruit juices should be used (fluid softens hard stools). Caffeinated beverages such as coffee, tea, and cola should be limited (caffeine stimulates fluid loss through urination).
4. Avoid foods that produce gas (e.g., beans) or upper GI upset (spicy foods).
5. *Timing:* Establish a regular schedule for bowel evacuation. A good time is 30 min after the first meal of the day.
6. *Position:* If possible, an upright position with feet flat on the floor or on a stepstool enhances bowel evacuation. Staying on the toilet, commode, or bedpan for longer than 20-30 min may cause skin breakdown. Based on stability, someone may need to stay with the patient.
7. *Activity:* Exercise is important for bowel function. In addition to improving muscle tone, it also increases GI transit time and increases appetite. Muscles should be exercised. This includes stretching, range-of-motion, position changing, and functional movement.
8. *Drug treatment:* Suppositories may be necessary to stimulate a bowel movement. Manual stimulation of the rectum may also be helpful in initiating defecation. Use stool softeners as needed to regulate stool consistency. Use oral laxatives only if necessary.

Various drugs can be used to treat neurogenic bladders. Anticholinergic drugs (oxybutynin [Ditropan], tolterodine [Detrol]) may be used to suppress bladder contraction. α-Adrenergic blockers (e.g., terazosin [Hytrin], doxazosin [Cardura]) may be used to relax the urethral sphincter, and antispasmodic drugs (e.g., baclofen) may be used to decrease spasticity of pelvic floor muscles.

Numerous drainage methods are possible, including bladder reflex retraining if partial voiding control remains, indwelling catheter, intermittent catheterization, and external catheter (condom catheter). Evaluate the long-term use of an indwelling catheter because of the associated high incidence of UTI, fistula formation, and diverticula. However, for some patients this may be the best option. Patients with indwelling catheters need to have an adequate fluid intake (at least 3 to 4 L/day). Regularly check the patency of the indwelling catheter. The frequency of routine catheter changes ranges widely depending on the type of catheter used and agency policy.

Intermittent catheterization is the most commonly recommended method of bladder management (see Chapter 46). Nursing assessment is important in selecting the time interval between catheterizations. Initially, catheterization is done every 4 hours. Bladder volume can be assessed before catheterization using the portable bladder ultrasound machine. If less than 200 mL of urine is measured, the time interval may be extended. If more than 500 mL of urine is measured, the time interval is shortened. Usually five or six intermittent catheterizations are done per day.

Urinary diversion surgery may be necessary if the patient has repeated UTIs with renal involvement or repeated stones or if therapeutic interventions have been unsuccessful. Surgical treatment of neurogenic bladder includes bladder neck revision (sphincterotomy), bladder augmentation (augmentation cystoplasty), penile prosthesis, artificial sphincter, perineal ureterostomy, cystotomy, vesicotomy, and anterior urethral transplantation. (Urinary diversion procedures are discussed in Chapter 46.)

No matter which bladder management strategy is selected, teach the patient, caregiver, and family how to accomplish successful self-management. Inform them about management techniques, how to obtain necessary supplies, care of supplies and equipment, and when to seek health care. Arrange for resources and referrals for supplies and ongoing care.

Neurogenic Bowel. Careful management of bowel evacuation is necessary in the patient with an SCI because voluntary control of this function may be lost. This condition is called **neurogenic bowel**. The usual measures for preventing constipation include a high-fiber diet and adequate fluid intake (see Table 43-6). Patient and caregiver teaching guidelines related to bowel management are presented in Table 61-11. However, these measures by themselves may not be adequate to stimulate evacuation. In addition, suppositories (bisacodyl [Dulcolax] or glycerin) or small-volume enemas and digital stimulation (performed 20 to 30 minutes after suppository insertion) by the nurse or patient may be necessary. In the patient with an upper motor neuron injury, digital stimulation is necessary to relax the external sphincter to promote defecation. A stool softener such as docusate sodium (Colace) can be used to regulate stool consistency. Oral stimulant laxatives should be used only if absolutely necessary for a day or two and not on a regular basis.

Valsalva maneuver and manual stimulation are useful in patients with lower motor neuron injuries. The Valsalva maneuver requires intact abdominal muscles, so it is used in those patients with injuries below T12. In general, a bowel movement every other day is considered adequate. However, preinjury patterns should be considered. Fecal incontinence can result from too much stool softener or a fecal impaction.

Carefully record bowel movements, including amount, time, and consistency. Timing of defecation may also be an important factor. Planning bowel evacuation for 30 to 60 minutes after the first meal of the day may enhance success by taking advantage of the gastrocolic reflex induced by eating. This reflex may also be stimulated by drinking a warm beverage immediately after the meal. Remember that patient, caregiver, and family teaching is required to promote successful independent bowel management.

Neurogenic Skin. Prevention of pressure ulcers and other types of injury to insensitive skin is essential for every patient with SCI.[27] Nurses in rehabilitation are responsible for teaching these skills and providing information about daily skin care. A comprehensive visual and tactile examination of the skin should be done at least once daily, with special attention given to areas over bony prominences. The areas most vulnerable to breakdown include ischia, trochanters, heels, and sacrum. Initially carefully position and reposition every 2 hours, with gradual increases in the times between turns if no redness over bony prominences is seen at the time of turning. Pressure-relieving cushions must be used in wheelchairs, and special mattresses may also be needed. Movement during turns and transfers should be done carefully to avoid stretching and folding of soft tissues (shear), friction, or abrasion.

Assess nutritional status regularly. Both body weight loss and weight gain can contribute to skin breakdown. Adequate intake of protein is essential for skin health. Measurement of prealbumin, total protein, and albumin can help identify inadequate protein intake. Stress the importance of nutrition to skin health to the patient and caregiver.

Protection of the skin also requires avoidance of thermal injury. Burns can be caused by hot food or liquids, bath or shower water that is too warm, radiators, heating pads, and uninsulated plumbing. Thermal injury also can result from extreme cold (frostbite). Injuries may not be noticed until severe damage is done. Anticipatory guidance about potential risks is essential. Patient and caregiver teaching related to skin care is provided in Tables 61-12 and 61-13.

Sexuality. Sexuality is an important issue regardless of the patient's age or gender. To provide accurate and sensitive counseling and teaching about sexuality, you need to be aware of your own sexuality and understand the human sexual responses. When discussing sexual potential, use scientific terminology rather than slang whenever possible. Knowledge of the level and completeness of injury is needed to understand the male patient's potential for orgasm, erection, and fertility and the patient's capacity for sexual satisfaction.[28]

Men normally have two types of erections: psychogenic and reflex. The process of *psychogenic erections* begins in the brain with sexual thoughts. Signals from the brain are then sent through the nerves of the spinal cord down to the T10-L2 levels. The signals are then relayed to the penis and trigger an erection. A *reflex erection* occurs with direct physical contact to the penis or other erotic areas. A reflex erection is involuntary and can occur without sexually stimulating thoughts. These reflex erections are often short lived and uncontrolled and cannot be maintained or summoned at the time of coitus. The nerves that control a man's ability to have a reflex erection are located in the sacral nerves (S2-4) of the spinal cord.[29]

For men with SCI, the ability to have a psychogenic erection depends on the level and extent of injury. Generally, men with low-level incomplete injuries are more likely to have psychogenic erections than men with higher-level incomplete injuries. Men with complete injuries are less likely to experience psychogenic erections. However, most men with SCI are able to have a reflex erection with physical stimulation regardless of the extent of the injury if the S2-4 nerve pathways are not damaged.

TABLE 61-12 PATIENT & CAREGIVER TEACHING GUIDE

Skin Care After Spinal Cord Injury

To prevent skin breakdown in a patient with a spinal cord injury, include the following instructions when teaching the patient and caregiver.

Change Position Frequently
- If in a wheelchair, lift self up and shift weight every 15-30 min.
- If in bed, change positions with a regular turning schedule (at least every 2 hr) that includes sides, back, and abdomen.
- Use special mattresses and wheelchair cushions to reduce pressure.
- Use pillows to protect bony prominences when in bed.

Monitor Skin Condition
- Inspect skin frequently for areas of redness, swelling, and breakdown.
- Keep fingernails trimmed to avoid scratches and abrasions.
- If a wound develops, follow standard wound care management procedures.

TABLE 61-13 PATIENT & CAREGIVER TEACHING GUIDE

Halo Vest Care

Include the following instructions when teaching the patient and caregiver management of a halo vest.

1. Inspect the pins on the halo traction ring. Report to health care provider if pins are loose or if there are signs of infection, including redness, tenderness, swelling, or drainage at the insertion sites.
2. Clean around pin sites carefully with hydrogen peroxide, water, or alcohol on a cotton swab as directed.
3. Apply antibiotic ointment as prescribed.
4. To provide skin care, the patient should lie down on a bed with his or her head resting on a pillow to reduce pressure on the brace. Loosen one side of the vest. Gently wash the skin under the vest with soap and water, rinse it, and then dry it thoroughly. At the same time, check the skin for pressure points, redness, swelling, bruising, or chafing. Close the open side and repeat the procedure on the opposite side.
5. If the vest becomes wet or damp, carefully dry it with a blow dryer.
6. An assistive device (e.g., cane, walker) may be used to provide greater balance. Flat shoes should be worn.
7. Turn the entire body, not just the head and neck, when trying to view sideways.
8. In case of an emergency, keep a set of wrenches close to the halo vest at all times.
9. Mark the vest strap to maintain consistent buckling and fit.
10. Avoid grabbing bars or vest to assist the patient.
11. Keep sheepskin pad under vest. Change and wash at least weekly.
12. If perspiration or itching is a problem, a cotton T-shirt can be worn under the sheepskin. The T-shirt can be modified with a Velcro seam closure on one side.

Because each SCI is different, the impact of injury on sexual function can also differ.[29]

Treatment for erectile dysfunction includes drugs, vacuum devices, and surgical procedures. Sildenafil (Viagra) has become the treatment of choice in men with SCI. Penile injection of vasoactive substances (papaverine, prostaglandin E) is another medical treatment. Risks include *priapism* (prolonged penile erection) and scarring, so these substances are often considered only after failure of sildenafil. Vacuum suction devices use negative pressure to encourage blood flow into the penis. Erection is maintained by a constriction band placed at the base of the penis. The main surgical option is implantation of a penile prosthesis. (Erectile dysfunction is discussed in Chapter 55.)

Male fertility is affected by SCI, causing poor sperm quality and ejaculatory dysfunction. Recent advances in methods of retrieving sperm (penile vibratory stimulation and electroejaculation) combined with ovulation induction and intrauterine insemination of the female partner have changed the prognosis for men with SCI to father children from unlikely to a reasonable possibility of successful outcomes.

The effect of SCI on female sexual response is less clear. Lubrication is similar to erections in males, with reflex and psychogenic components. Women with upper motor neuron injuries may retain the capacity for reflex lubrication, whereas psychogenic lubrication depends on the completeness of injury. Orgasm is reported by about 50% of women with SCI.[28]

The woman of childbearing age with an SCI usually remains fertile. The injury does not affect the ability to become pregnant or to deliver normally through the birth canal. Menses may cease for as long as 6 months after injury. If sexual activity is resumed, protection against an unplanned pregnancy is necessary. A normal pregnancy may be complicated by UTIs, anemia, and autonomic dysreflexia. Because uterine contractions are not felt, a precipitous delivery is always a danger.

Open discussion with the patient regarding sexual rehabilitation is essential. This important aspect of rehabilitation should be handled by someone specially trained in sexual counseling. A nurse or other rehabilitation professional with such expertise works with the patient and the partner to provide support, with an emphasis on open communication. As a nurse, you should respect every couple's religious and cultural beliefs. Alternative methods of obtaining sexual satisfaction, such as oral-genital sex (cunnilingus and fellatio), may be suggested. Explicit films may also be used, such as a film demonstrating the sexual activities of a patient with paraplegia and a nondisabled partner. Use graphics cautiously because they may be too limiting or focus too much on the mechanics of sex rather than on the relationship.

Care should be taken not to dislodge an indwelling catheter during sexual activity. If an external catheter is used, it should be removed before sexual activity and the patient should refrain from fluids. The bowel program should include evacuation the morning of sexual activity. The partner should be informed that incontinence is always possible. The woman may need a water-soluble lubricant to supplement diminished vaginal secretions and facilitate vaginal penetration.

Grief and Depression. Patients with SCIs may feel an overwhelming sense of loss. They may temporarily lose control over everyday activities and must depend on others for activities of daily living and for life-sustaining measures. Patients may believe that they are useless and burdens to their families. At a stage when independence is often of great importance, they may be totally dependent on others.

The patient's response and recovery differ in some important aspects from those of patients experiencing loss from amputation or terminal illness. First, regression can and does occur at different stages. Working through grief is a difficult, lifelong process with which the patient needs support and encouragement. With recent advances in rehabilitation, patients are often independent physically and discharged from the rehabilitation center before completion of the grief process.

The goal of recovery is related more to adjustment than to acceptance. Adjustment implies the ability to go on with living with certain limitations. Although the patient who is cooperative and accepting is easier to treat, expect a wide fluctuation of emotions from a patient with an SCI. Your role in grief work is to allow mourning as a component of the rehabilitation process. Table 61-14 summarizes the grief response to an SCI and appropriate nursing interventions. Maintaining hope is an important strategy during the grieving process and should not be interpreted as denial. During the shock and denial stage, reassure the patient. During the anger stage, assist the patient in achieving control over the environment, particularly by allowing the patient's input into the plan of care. Do not respond to anger or manipulation or become involved in a power struggle with the patient. As self-care abilities increase, the patient's independence increases.

TABLE 61-14	GRIEF RESPONSE IN SPINAL CORD INJURY	
Patient Behavior	**Nursing Intervention**
Shock and Denial	
Struggle for survival, complete dependence, excessive sleep, withdrawal, fantasies, unrealistic expectations	• Provide honest information. • Use simple diagrams to explain injury. • Encourage patient to begin road to recovery. • Establish agreement to use and improve all current abilities while not denying the possibility of future improvement.
Anger	
Refusal to discuss paralysis, decreased self-esteem, manipulation, hostile and abusive language	• Coordinate care with patient and encourage self-care. • Support family members. • Use humor appropriately. • Allow patient outbursts. • Do not allow fixation on injury.
Depression	
Sadness, pessimism, anorexia, nightmares, insomnia, agitation, "blues," suicidal preoccupation, refusal to participate in any self-care activities	• Encourage family involvement and the use of community resources. • Plan graded steps in rehabilitation to give success with minimal opportunity for frustration. • Give cheerful and willing assistance with activities of daily living. • Avoid sympathy. • Use firm kindness.
Adjustment and Acceptance	
Planning for future, active participation in therapy, finding personal meaning in experience and continuation of growth, return to premorbid personality.	• Remember that patients have individual personalities. • Balance support systems to encourage independence. • Set goals with patient input. • Emphasize potential.

The patient's caregiver and family also require counseling to avoid promoting dependency in the patient through guilt or misplaced sympathy. The family is also experiencing an intense grieving process. A support group of family members and friends of patients with SCI can help family members increase their participation and knowledge of the grieving process, physical difficulties, rehabilitation plan, and meaning of the disability in society.

During the stage of depression, be patient. Sympathy is not helpful. Treat the patient as an adult and encourage participation in care planning. A primary nurse relationship is helpful. Staff planning and sessions in which staff members can express their feelings help provide consistency of care. To achieve the stage of adjustment, the patient needs continual support throughout the rehabilitation process in the forms of acceptance, affection, and caring. Be attentive when the patient needs to talk and sensitive to needs at the various stages of the grief process.

Although the stage of depression during the grief process usually lasts days to weeks, some individuals may become clinically depressed and require treatment for depression. Evaluation by a psychiatric nurse or psychiatrist is recommended. Treatment may include drugs and therapy.

EVALUATION

Expected outcomes are that the patient with an SCI will

- Maintain adequate ventilation and have no signs of respiratory distress
- Maintain intact skin over bony prominences
- Establish a bowel management program based on neurologic function and personal preference
- Establish a bladder management program based on neurologic function, caregiver status, and lifestyle choices
- Experience no episodes of autonomic dysreflexia

Additional information on expected outcomes for the patient with an SCI is addressed in eNursing Care Plan 61-1 on the website for this chapter.

GERONTOLOGIC CONSIDERATIONS

SPINAL CORD INJURY

Because of increased work and recreational activities of older adults, more older adults are experiencing SCI. Falls are the leading cause of SCI for people 65 and older. Besides having greater mortality rates, older adults with traumatic injuries experience more complications than younger ones, and they are hospitalized longer.

The demographics of patients living with SCI are changing. Given the longer life spans of persons with SCI, an increasing number of older adults are now living with an SCI. Aging is also associated with more chronic illnesses, which can have a serious impact on these older adults. As patients with SCI age, both individual aging changes and length of time since injury can affect functional ability. For example, bowel and bladder dysfunction can increase with the duration and severity of SCI.

Health promotion and screening are important for the older patient with an SCI. Daily skin inspections, UTI prevention measures, and monthly breast examinations for women and regular prostate cancer screening for men are recommended. Cardiovascular disease is the most common cause of morbidity and mortality among older adults with an SCI. The lack of sensation, including chest pain, in those with high-level injuries may mask acute myocardial ischemia. Altered autonomic nervous system function and decreases in physical activity can place the patient at risk for cardiovascular problems, including hypertension.

Health promotion to decrease the risk of injuries includes fall prevention strategies (e.g., using a stepstool or a grab bar to reach high shelves, handrails on stairs). Rehabilitation for the older person who has had an SCI may take longer because of preexisting conditions and poorer health status at the time of the initial injury. An interdisciplinary team approach to rehabilitation is essential in preventing secondary complications associated with SCI, especially in older adults.

SPINAL CORD TUMORS

Spinal cord tumors account for 0.5% to 1% of all neoplasms. These tumors are classified as *primary* (arising from some component of cord, dura, nerves, or vessels) or *secondary* (from primary growths in other places in the body that have metastasized to the spinal cord).

Etiology and Pathophysiology

Spinal cord tumors are further classified as *extradural* (outside the spinal cord), *intradural extramedullary* (within the dura but outside the actual spinal cord), and *intradural intramedullary* (within the spinal cord itself) (Fig. 61-13, Table 61-15).

Extradural tumors are usually metastatic and most often arise in the vertebral bodies.[30] These metastatic lesions can invade intradurally and compress the spinal cord. Tumors that commonly metastasize to the spinal epidural space are those that spread to bone, such as prostate, breast, lung, and kidney cancer.

Because many spinal cord tumors are slow growing, their symptoms are due to the mechanical effects of slow compression and irritation of nerve roots, displacement of the cord, or gradual obstruction of the vascular supply. The slowness of growth does not cause autodestruction (secondary injury) as in traumatic SCIs. Therefore complete functional restoration may be possible when the tumor is removed.

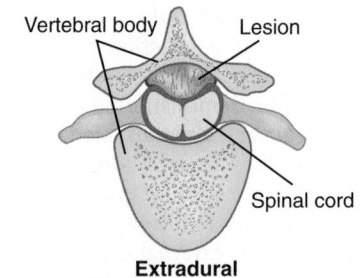

Extradural

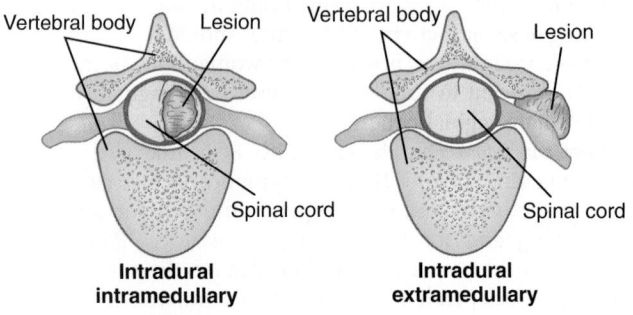

Intradural intramedullary   **Intradural extramedullary**

FIG. 61-13 Types of spinal cord tumors.

TABLE 61-15	**CLASSIFICATION OF SPINAL CORD TUMORS**		
Type	**Incidence**	**Treatment**	**Prognosis**
Extradural			
Outside the spinal cord in extradural space	Ninety percent of all spinal cord tumors. Mostly malignant metastatic lesions.	Relief of cord pressure by surgical laminectomy, radiation, chemotherapy, or combination approach.	Poor. Treatment is usually palliative.
Intradural			
Intradural Extramedullary			
Within dura mater but outside cord	Most frequent of intradural tumors. Mostly benign. Meningiomas, neurofibromas, and schwannomas.	Complete surgical removal of tumor (if possible). Partial removal followed by radiation.	Usually very good if lack of damage to cord from compression.
Intradural Intramedullary			
Within the spinal cord	Least frequent of intradural tumors. Mostly benign. Astrocytomas, ependymomas.	Complete surgical removal of tumor (if possible). Partial removal followed by radiation.	Usually very good if lack of damage to cord from compression. Complete surgical resection of astrocytomas difficult.

Clinical Manifestations

Both sensory and motor problems may result, with the location and extent of the tumor determining the severity and extent of the problem. The most common early symptom of a spinal cord tumor is back pain. The location of the pain depends on the level of compression. The pain worsens with activity, coughing, straining, and lying down. Sensory disruption is later manifested by coldness, numbness, and tingling in an extremity or in several extremities.

Motor weakness accompanies the sensory disturbances and consists of slowly increasing clumsiness, weakness, and spasticity. Paralysis can develop. The sensory and motor disturbances are ipsilateral (on the same side) to the injury. Bladder disturbances are marked by urgency with difficulty in starting the flow and progressing to retention with overflow incontinence.

NURSING AND COLLABORATIVE MANAGEMENT SPINAL CORD TUMORS

Extradural tumors are seen early on routine spinal x-rays, whereas intradural and intramedullary tumors require MRI or CT scans for detection. CSF analysis may reveal tumor cells.

Compression of the spinal cord is an emergency. Relief of the ischemia related to the compression is the goal of therapy. Corticosteroids are generally prescribed immediately to relieve tumor-related edema. Dexamethasone (Decadron) (often in large doses) is also usually used to treat edema.

Indications for surgery vary depending on the type of tumor. Primary spinal tumors may be removed with the goal of cure. In patients with metastatic tumors, treatment is primarily palliative, with the goal of restoring or preserving neurologic function, stabilizing the spine, and alleviating pain.[30]

Radiation therapy after surgery is fairly effective. Chemotherapy has also been used in conjunction with radiation therapy.

Relief of pain and return of function are the ultimate goals of treatment. Be aware of the patient's neurologic status before and after treatment. Ensuring that the patient receives pain medication as needed is an important nursing responsibility. Depending on the amount of neurologic dysfunction exhibited, the care of the patient may be similar to that of a patient recovering from an SCI. Rehabilitation of patients with spinal cord tumors is similar to rehabilitation for the patient with an SCI.

CASE STUDY

Spinal Cord Injury

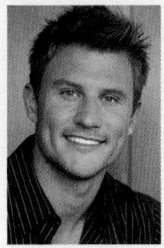

iStockphoto/Thinkstock

Patient Profile
Acute Phase
B.V., a 24-yr-old white man, is admitted to the emergency department with the diagnosis of a cervical spinal cord injury (SCI). B.V. was swimming at a neighbor's backyard pool. He dove into the shallow end, striking his head on the bottom of the pool. His friends noticed that he did not resurface. They rescued him and brought him to the side of the pool. They maintained neck immobilization until the rescue crews arrived.

Subjective Data
- Is awake and alert
- Is complaining of neck pain
- Is anxious and asking why he cannot move his legs
- Is asking to see his family

Objective Data
Physical Examination
- Weak biceps movement bilaterally
- No triceps movement bilaterally
- Gross elbow movement present bilaterally
- No movement in bilateral lower extremities
- Decreased sensation from the shoulders down
- No bladder or bowel control
- BP 85/50 mm Hg; pulse 56 beats/min; respirations 32 breaths/min and labored

Diagnostic Studies
- CT C-spine shows C5 subluxation and compression fracture
- MRI C-spine shows a severe spinal cord compression at C5-6

Collaborative Care
- Intubated in the emergency department
- Started on mechanical ventilation
- Placed in tongs and traction on arrival to the ICU

Discussion Questions (Acute Phase)
1. **Priority Decision:** What nursing activities would be a priority on B.V.'s arrival in the ICU?
2. What physiologic problems are causing B.V. to have hypotension and bradycardia?

3. What would be the first line of treatment for B.V.'s hypotension and bradycardia?
4. What signs and symptoms would indicate respiratory distress, and what physiologic problem would cause respiratory distress in B.V.'s injury state?
5. What can you do to decrease B.V.'s anxiety?
6. **Priority Decision:** Based on the assessment data provided, what are the priority nursing diagnoses? Are there any collaborative problems?
7. **Delegation Decision:** Identify activities that can be delegated to unlicensed assistive personnel (UAP).

Patient Profile
Rehabilitation Phase
B.V. is now 1 mo postinjury and is currently at a local inpatient SCI rehabilitation facility. He has since been extubated and uses a wheelchair to mobilize. He eats three meals a day with assistance and is on a strict bowel and bladder program.

Subjective Data
- Awake and alert but anxious
- Complaining of severe headache, blurred vision, and nausea

Objective Data
Physical Examination
- Flushed and diaphoretic above the level of injury
- No bowel movement for 2 days
- BP 235/106 mm Hg, pulse 32 beats/min, respirations 30 breaths/min and labored

Discussion Questions (Rehabilitation Phase)
1. **Priority Decision:** What initial priority nursing interventions would be appropriate?
2. What physiologic problem is causing B.V.'s hypertension and bradycardia?
3. Once the physician has been notified, what other interventions would be appropriate?
4. **Priority Decision:** Based on the assessment data provided, what are the priority nursing diagnoses?
5. Patient and family involvement in the rehabilitation process is vital. What teaching will you provide about bowel management?
6. **Evidence-Based Practice:** B.V. and his family are concerned about the potential risk of autonomic dysreflexia. What information would you provide the patient and family?

evolve Answers available at *http://evolve.elsevier.com/Lewis/medsurg.*

■ BRIDGE TO NCLEX EXAMINATION

The number of the question corresponds to the same-numbered outcome at the beginning of the chapter.

1. During assessment of the patient with trigeminal neuralgia, the nurse should *(select all that apply)*
   a. inspect all aspects of the mouth and teeth.
   b. assess the gag reflex and respiratory rate and depth.
   c. lightly palpate the affected side of the face for edema.
   d. test for temperature and sensation perception on the face.
   e. ask the patient to describe factors that initiate an episode.

2. During routine assessment of a patient with Guillain-Barré syndrome, the nurse finds the patient is short of breath. The patient's respiratory distress is caused by
   a. elevated protein levels in the CSF.
   b. immobility resulting from ascending paralysis.
   c. degeneration of motor neurons in the brainstem and spinal cord.
   d. paralysis ascending to the nerves that stimulate the thoracic area.

3. A patient is admitted to the ICU with a C7 spinal cord injury and diagnosed with Brown-Séquard syndrome. On physical examination, the nurse would most likely find
   a. upper extremity weakness only.
   b. complete motor and sensory loss below C7.
   c. loss of position sense and vibration in both lower extremities.
   d. ipsilateral motor loss and contralateral sensory loss below C7.

4. A patient is admitted to the hospital with a C4 spinal cord injury after a motorcycle collision. The patient's BP is 84/50 mm Hg, his pulse is 38 beats/minute, and he remains orally intubated. The nurse determines that this pathophysiologic response is caused by
   a. increased vasomotor tone after injury.
   b. a temporary loss of sensation and flaccid paralysis below the level of injury.
   c. loss of parasympathetic nervous system innervation resulting in vasoconstriction.
   d. loss of sympathetic nervous system innervation resulting in peripheral vasodilation.

5. Goals of rehabilitation for the patient with an injury at the C6 level include (select all that apply)
   a. stand erect with leg brace.
   b. feed self with hand devices.
   c. assist with transfer activities.
   d. drive adapted van from wheelchair.
   e. push a wheelchair on a flat surface.

6. A patient with a C7 spinal cord injury undergoing rehabilitation tells the nurse he must have the flu because he has a bad headache and nausea. The nurse's first priority is to
   a. call the physician.
   b. check the patient's temperature.
   c. take the patient's blood pressure.
   d. elevate the head of the bed to 90 degrees.

7. For a 65-year-old woman who has lived with a T1 spinal cord injury for 20 years, which health teaching instructions should the nurse emphasize?
   a. A mammogram is needed every year.
   b. Bladder function tends to improve with age.
   c. Heart disease is not common in persons with spinal cord injury.
   d. As a person ages, the need to change body position is less important.

8. The most common early symptom of a spinal cord tumor is
   a. urinary incontinence.
   b. back pain that worsens with activity.
   c. paralysis below the level of involvement.
   d. impaired sensation of pain, temperature, and light touch.

1. a, d, e, 2. d, 3. d, 4. d, 5. b, c, e, 6. c, 7. a, 8. b

ⓔvolve

For rationales to these answers and even more NCLEX review questions, visit *http://evolve.elsevier.com/Lewis/medsurg*.

REFERENCES

1. National Institute of Neurological Disorders and Stroke: Trigeminal neuralgia fact sheet.. Retrieved from *www.ninds.nih.gov/disorders/trigeminal_neuralgia/detail_trigeminal_neuralgia.htm*.
2. Brisman R: Trigeminal neuralgia: diagnosis and treatment, *World Neurosurg* 76(6):533, 2011.
*3. Zakrzewska JM, Akram H: Neurosurgical interventions for the treatment of classical trigeminal neuralgia, *Cochrane Database Syst Rev* 9:CD007312, 2011. DOI:10.1002/14651858.CD007312.pub2.
4. National Institute of Neurological Disorders and Stroke: Bell's palsy fact sheet. Retrieved from *www.ninds.nih.gov/disorders/bells/detail_bells.htm*.
5. National Institute of Neurological Disorders and Stroke: Guillain-Barré syndrome fact sheet. Retrieved from *www.ninds.nih.gov/disorders/gbs/detail_gbs.htm*.
6. Bowyer HR, Glover M: Guillain-Barré syndrome: management and treatment options for patients with moderate to severe progression, *J Neurosci Nurs* 42(5):288, 2010.
7. Lugg J: Recognizing and managing Guillain-Barré syndrome, *Emerg Nurse* 18(3):27, 2010.
8. Saifudheen K, Jose J, Gafoor VA, et al: Guillain-Barré and SIADH, *Neurology* 76(8):1, 2011.
9. Centers for Disease Control and Prevention: Botulism. Retrieved from *http://emergency.cdc.gov/agent/Botulism/clinicians/epidemiology.asp*.
10. Centers for Disease Control and Prevention: Tetanus. Retrieved from *www.cdc.gov/vaccines/pubs/pinkbook/downloads/tetanus.pdf*.
11. Ataro P, Mushatt D, Shagufta A: Tetanus: a review, *South Med J* 104(8):613, 2011.
12. Centers for Disease Control and Prevention. Updated recommendations for use of tetanus toxoid, reduced diphtheria toxoid and acellular pertussis (Tdap) vaccine from the Advisory Committee on Immunization Practices, 2010, *MMWR* 60:13, 2011.
13. National Institute of Neurological Disorders and Stroke: Neurosyphilis information page. Retrieved from *www.ninds.nih.gov/disorders/neurosyphilis/neurosyphilis.htm*.
14. Centers for Disease Control and Prevention, National Center for Injury Prevention and Control: Spinal cord injury (SCI): fact sheet. Retrieved from *www.cdc.gov/ncipc/factsheets/scifacts.htm*.
15. Dawodu ST, Campagnolo DI: Spinal cord injury: definition, epidemiology, pathophysiology. Retrieved from *http://emedicine.medscape.com/article/322480-overview*.
16. Nayduch DA: Back to the basics: identifying and managing acute spinal cord injury, *Nursing* 40(9):24, 2010.
17. Looby S, Flanders A: Spine trauma, *Radiol Clin North Am* 49(1):1, 2011.
*18. Chung SB, Lee SH, Kim ES, et al: Incidence of deep vein thrombosis after spinal cord injury: a prospective study in 37 consecutive patients with traumatic or nontraumatic spinal cord injury treated with mechanical prophylaxis, *J Trauma* 71(4):867, 2011.
*19. Hadley MN, Walters BC: Introduction to the guidelines for the management of acute cervical spine and spinal cord injuries, *Neurosurgery* 72(suppl):1, 2013.
*20. Nicholas T, Hadley MN, Aarabi B, et al: Prehospital cervical spinal immobilization after trauma, *Neurosurgery* 72(suppl):22, 2013.

*Evidence-based information for clinical practice.

*21. Hurlbert RJ, Hadley MN, Walters B, et al: Pharmacological therapy for acute spinal cord injury, *Neurosurgery* 72(suppl):93, 2013.

*22. Dhall SS, Hadley MN, Aarabi B, et al: Deep venous thrombosis and thromboembolism in patients with cervical spinal cord injuries, *Neurosurgery* 72(suppl):244, 2013.

23. Wyndaele JJ: Neurogenic bowel management after spinal cord injury, *Spinal Cord* 48(10):710, 2010.

24. National Spinal Cord Injury Association. Retrieved from *www.spinalcord.org.*

25. Ho CP, Krassioukov AV: Autonomic dysreflexia and myocardial ischemia, *Spinal Cord* 48(9):714, 2010.

26. McGuire EJ: Urodynamics of the neurogenic bladder, *Urol Clin North Am* 37:507, 2010.

*27. Saunders LL, Krause JS, Peters BA, et al: The relationship of pressure ulcers, race, and socioeconomic conditions after spinal cord injury, *J Spinal Cord Med* 33(4):387, 2010.

*28. Consortium for Spinal Cord Medicine: Sexuality and reproductive health in adults with spinal cord injury: a clinical practice guideline for health-care professionals, *J Spinal Cord Med* 33(3):281, 2010.

29. Sexual function for men with SCI. Retrieved from *http://images.main.uab.edu/spinalcord/SCI%20Infosheets%20in%20PDF/Sexual%20Function%20for%20Men%20with%20SCI.pdf.*

30. Spinal Cord Tumor Association. Retrieved from *www.spinalcordtumor.org.*

RESOURCES

American Spinal Injury Association (ASIA)
www.asia-spinalinjury.org
Christopher and Dana Reeve Foundation
www.christopherreeve.org
GBS-CIDP Foundation International
www.gbs-cidp.org
National Institute of Neurological Disorders and Stroke (NINDS)
www.ninds.nih.gov
National Rehabilitation Information Center (NARIC)
www.naric.com
National Spinal Cord Injury Association
www.spinalcord.org
Paralyzed Veterans of America
www.pva.org
Spinal Cord Society
www.scsus.org
Spinal Cord Tumor Association, Inc,
www.spinalcordtumor.org

We must be the change we want to see.
Mahatma Gandhi

Nursing Assessment
Musculoskeletal System

Dottie Roberts

LEARNING OUTCOMES

1. Describe the gross anatomic and microscopic composition of bone.
2. Explain the classification system for joints and movements at synovial joints.
3. Compare and contrast the types and structure of muscle tissue.
4. Describe the functions of cartilage, muscles, ligaments, tendons, fascia, and bursae.
5. Link age-related changes in the musculoskeletal system to the differences in assessment findings.

6. Select significant subjective and objective data related to the musculoskeletal system that should be obtained from a patient.
7. Select appropriate techniques to use in the physical assessment of the musculoskeletal system.
8. Differentiate normal from abnormal findings of a physical assessment of the musculoskeletal system.
9. Describe the purpose, significance of results, and nursing responsibilities related to diagnostic studies of the musculoskeletal system.

KEY TERMS

This chapter provides a review of the structures and functions of the musculoskeletal system to facilitate nursing assessment and evaluation of the assessment findings of this system. The musculoskeletal system is composed of voluntary muscle and five types of connective tissue: bones, cartilage, ligaments, tendons, and fascia. The purpose of the musculoskeletal system is to protect body organs, provide support and stability for the body, and allow for coordinated movement.

STRUCTURES AND FUNCTIONS OF MUSCULOSKELETAL SYSTEM

Bone

Function. The main functions of bone are support, protection of internal organs, voluntary movement, blood cell production, and mineral storage.[1] Bones provide the supporting framework that keeps the body from collapsing and also

Reviewed by Damien Zsiros, RN, MSN, CNE, CRNP, Nursing Instructor, The Pennsylvania State University School of Nursing, Fayette/The Eberly Campus, Uniontown, Pennsylvania; Jan Foecke, RN, MS, ONC, Director of Programs, National Association of Orthopaedic Nurses, Kansas City, Missouri; and Clemma K. Snider, RN, MSN, Assistant Professor, Associate Degree Nursing, Eastern Kentucky University, Richmond, Kentucky.

allows the body to bear weight. Bones also protect underlying vital organs and tissues. For example, the skull encloses the brain, the vertebrae surround the spinal cord, and the rib cage contains the lungs and heart. Bones serve as a point of attachment for muscles, which are connected to bones by tendons. Bones act as a lever for muscles, and movement occurs as a result of muscle contractions applied to these levers. Bones contain hematopoietic tissue for the production of red and white blood cells. Bones also serve as a site for storage of inorganic minerals such as calcium and phosphorus.

Bone is a dynamic tissue that continuously changes form and composition. It contains both organic material (collagen) and inorganic material (calcium, phosphate). The internal and external growth and remodeling of bone are ongoing processes.

Microscopic Structure. Bone is classified according to structure as *cortical* (compact and dense) or *cancellous* (spongy). In *cortical bone,* cylindric structural units called **osteons** *(Haversian systems)* fit closely together, creating a dense bone structure (Fig. 62-1, *A*). Within the systems, the Haversian canals run parallel to the bone's long axis and contain the blood vessels that travel to the bone's interior from the periosteum. Surrounding each osteon are concentric rings known as *lamellae,* which characterize mature bone. Smaller canals *(canaliculi)* extend from the Haversian canals to the *lacunae,* where mature bone cells are embedded.

Cancellous bone lacks the organized structure of cortical bone. The lamellae are not arranged in concentric rings but rather along the lines of maximum stress placed on the bone. Cancellous bone tissue is filled with red or yellow marrow, and blood reaches the bone cells by passing through spaces in the marrow.

The three types of bone cells are osteoblasts, osteocytes, and osteoclasts.[2] *Osteoblasts* synthesize organic bone matrix (collagen) and are the basic bone-forming cells. *Osteocytes* are the mature bone cells. *Osteoclasts* participate in bone remodeling by assisting in the breakdown of bone tissue. *Bone remodeling* is the removal of old bone by osteoclasts *(resorption)* and the deposition of new bone by osteoblasts *(ossification).* The inner layer of bone is composed primarily of osteoblasts with a few osteoclasts.

Gross Structure. The anatomic structure of bone is best represented by a typical long bone such as the tibia (see Fig. 62-1, *B*). Each long bone consists of the epiphysis, diaphysis, and metaphysis. The *epiphysis,* the widened area found at each end of a long bone, is composed primarily of cancellous bone. The wide epiphysis allows for greater weight distribution and provides stability for the joint. The epiphysis is also the location of muscle attachment. Articular cartilage covers the ends of the epiphysis to provide a smooth surface for joint movement. The *diaphysis* is the main shaft of the bone. It provides structural support and is composed of compact bone. The tubular structure of the diaphysis allows it to more easily withstand bending and twisting forces. The *metaphysis* is the flared area between the epiphysis and the diaphysis. Like the epiphysis, it is composed of cancellous bone.

The *epiphyseal plate,* or growth zone, is the cartilaginous area between the epiphysis and metaphysis. It actively produces bone to allow longitudinal growth in children. Injury to the epiphyseal plate in a growing child can lead to a shorter extremity that can cause significant functional problems. In the adult, the metaphysis and the epiphysis become joined as this plate hardens to mature bone.

The *periosteum* is composed of fibrous connective tissue that covers the bone. Tiny blood vessels penetrate the periosteum to provide nutrition to underlying bone. Musculotendinous fibers anchor to the outer layer of the periosteum. The inner layer of the periosteum is attached to the bone by bundles of collagen. No periosteum exists on the articular surfaces of long bones. These bone ends are covered by articular cartilage.

The medullary (marrow) cavity is in the center of the diaphysis and contains either red or yellow bone marrow.[3] In the growing child, red bone marrow is actively involved in blood cell production (hematopoiesis). In the adult, the medullary

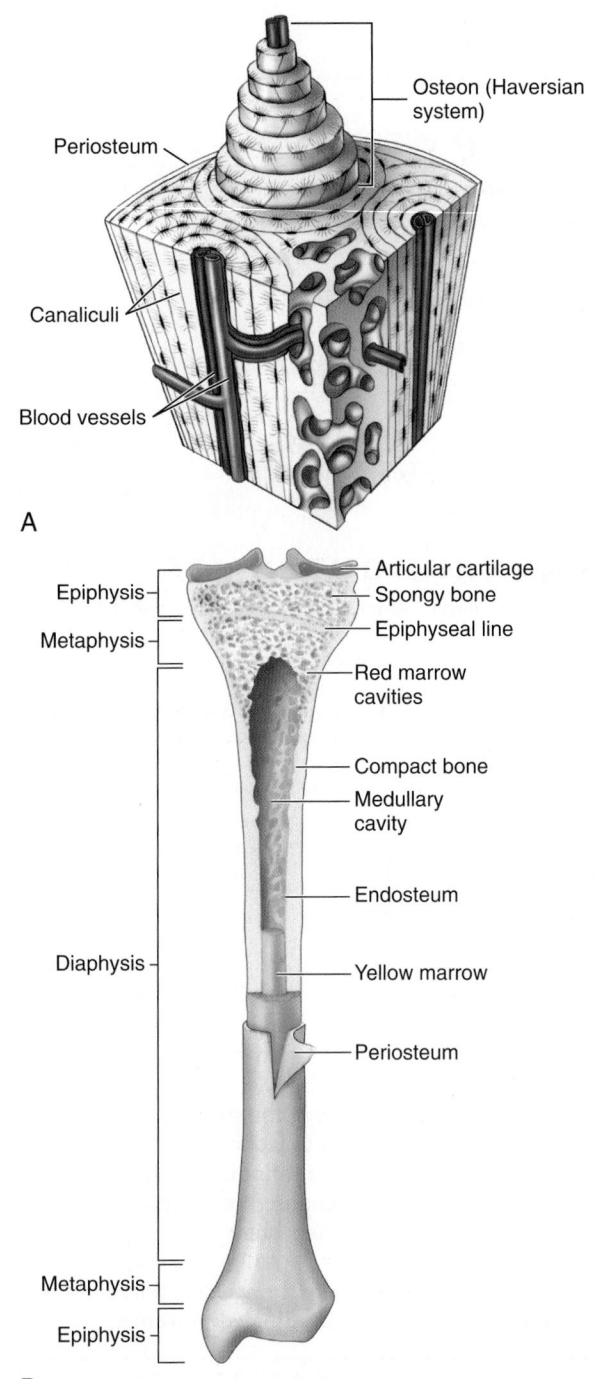

FIG. 62-1 Bone structure. **A,** Cortical (compact) bone showing numerous structural units called osteons. **B,** Anatomy of a long bone (tibia) showing cancellous and compact bone.

cavity of long bones contains yellow bone marrow, which is mainly adipose tissue. Yellow marrow is involved in hematopoiesis only in times of great blood cell need. In adults, red marrow is found mainly in the *flat bones,* such as the pelvis, skull, sternum, cranium, ribs, vertebrae, and scapulae, and in the *cancellous* ("spongy") material at the epiphyseal ends of long bones such as the femur and the humerus.

Types. The skeleton consists of 206 bones, which are classified according to shape as long, short, flat, or irregular.

Long bones are characterized by a central shaft (diaphysis) and two widened ends (epiphyses) (see Fig. 62-1, *B*). Examples include the femur, humerus, and tibia. *Short bones* are composed of cancellous bone covered by a thin layer of compact bone. Examples include the carpals in the hand and the tarsals in the foot.

Flat bones have two layers of compact bone separated by a layer of cancellous bone. Examples include the ribs, skull, scapula, and sternum. The spaces in the cancellous bone contain bone marrow. *Irregular bones* appear in a variety of shapes and sizes. Examples include the sacrum, mandible, and ear ossicles.

Joints

A *joint* (articulation) is a place where the ends of two bones are in proximity and move in relation to each other. Joints are classified by the degree of movement that they allow (Fig. 62-2).

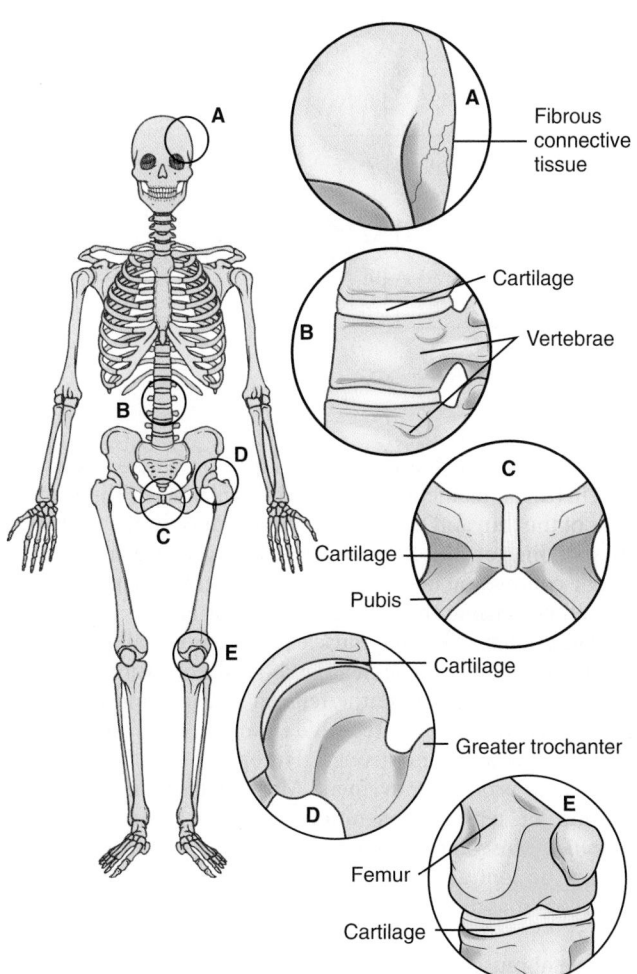

FIG. 62-2 Classification of joints. **A** to **C,** Synarthrotic (immovable) and amphiarthrotic (slightly movable) joints. **D** and **E,** Diarthrodial (freely movable) joints.

The most common joint is the freely movable *diarthrodial* (synovial) type. Each joint is enclosed in a capsule of fibrous connective tissue, which joins the two bones together to form a cavity (Fig. 62-3). The capsule is lined by a synovial membrane, which secretes a thick synovial fluid to lubricate the joint, reduce friction, and allow opposing surfaces to slide smoothly over each other. The end of each bone is covered with articular (hyaline) cartilage. Supporting structures (e.g., ligaments, tendons) reinforce the joint capsule and provide limits and stability to joint movement. Types of diarthrodial joints are shown in Fig. 62-4.

Cartilage

The three types of *cartilage* tissue are hyaline, elastic, and fibrous. *Hyaline cartilage,* the most common, contains a moderate amount of collagen fibers. It is found in the trachea, bronchi, nose, epiphyseal plate, and articular surfaces of bones. *Elastic cartilage,* which contains both collagen and elastic fibers, is more flexible than hyaline cartilage. It is found in the ear, epiglottis, and larynx. *Fibrous cartilage* (fibrocartilage) consists mostly of collagen fibers and is a tough tissue that often functions as a shock absorber. It is found between the vertebral discs and also forms a protective cushion between the bones of the pelvic girdle, knee, and shoulder.

Cartilage in synovial joints serves as a support for soft tissue and provides the articular surface for joint movement. It protects underlying tissues. The cartilage in the epiphyseal plate is also involved in the growth of long bones before physical maturity is reached. Because articular cartilage is considered to be avascular, it must receive nourishment by the diffusion of material from the synovial fluid. The lack of a direct blood supply contributes to the slow metabolism of cartilage cells and explains why healing and repair of cartilage tissue occur slowly.

Muscle

Types. The three types of muscle tissue are cardiac (striated, involuntary), smooth (nonstriated, involuntary), and skeletal (striated, voluntary) muscle. *Cardiac muscle* is found in the

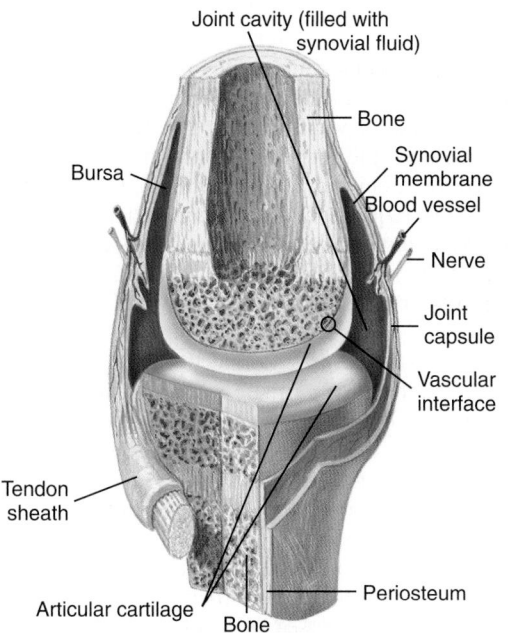

FIG. 62-3 Structure of diarthrodial (synovial) joint.

Joint	Movement	Examples	Illustration
Hinge joint	Flexion, extension	Elbow joint (shown), interphalangeal joints, knee joint	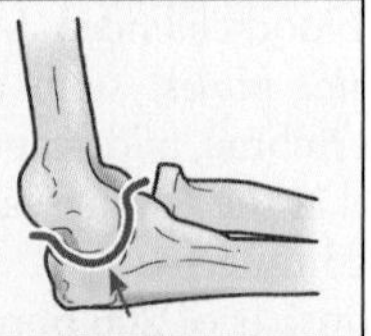
Ball and socket (spheroidal)	Flexion, extension; adduction, abduction; circumduction	Shoulder (shown), hip	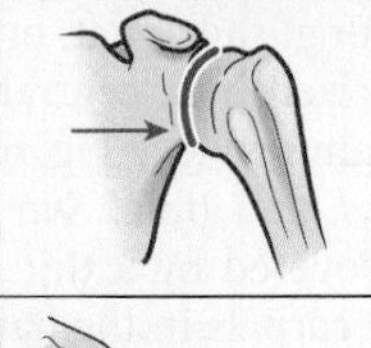
Pivot (rotary)	Rotation	Atlas-axis, proximal radioulnar joint (shown)	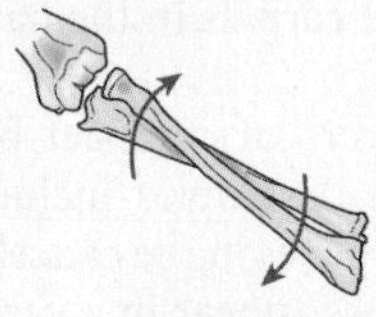
Condyloid	Flexion, extension; abduction, adduction; circumduction	Wrist joint (between radial and carpals) (shown)	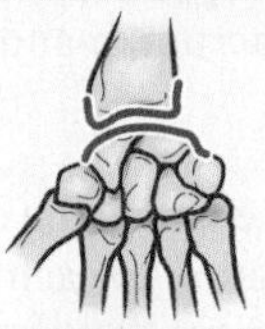
Saddle	Flexion, extension; abduction, adduction; circumduction, thumb-finger opposition	Carpometacarpal joint of thumb (shown)	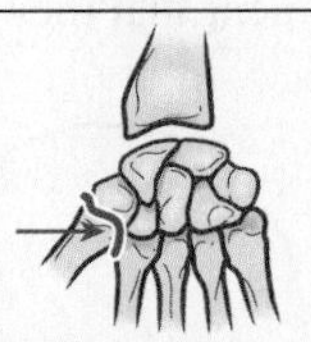
Gliding	One surface moves over another surface	Between tarsal bones, sacroiliac joint, between articular processes of vertebrae, between carpal bones (shown)	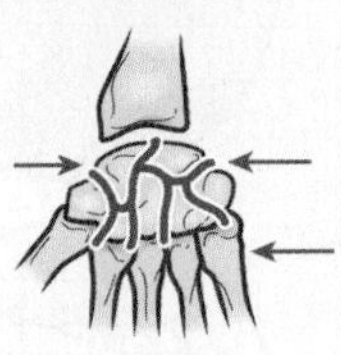

FIG. 62-4 Types of diarthrodial (synovial) joints.

heart. Its spontaneous contractions propel blood through the circulatory system. *Smooth muscle* occurs in the walls of hollow structures such as airways, arteries, gastrointestinal (GI) tract, urinary bladder, and uterus. Smooth muscle contraction is modulated by neuronal and hormonal influences. *Skeletal muscle,* which requires neuronal stimulation for contraction, accounts for about half of a human being's body weight. It is the focus of the following discussion.

Structure. The skeletal muscle is enclosed by the *epimysium,* a continuous layer of deep fascia. The epimysium helps muscles slide over nearby structures. Connective tissue surrounding and extending into the muscle can be subdivided into fiber bundles, or *fasciculi.* These bundles are covered by *perimysium* and an innermost connective tissue layer called the *endomysium* that surrounds each fiber (Fig. 62-5).

The structural unit of skeletal muscle is the muscle cell or muscle fiber, which is highly specialized for contraction. Skeletal muscle fibers are long, multinucleated cylinders that contain many mitochondria to support their high metabolic activity. Muscle fibers are composed of myofibrils, which in turn are made up of contractile filaments (protein). The *sarcomere* is the contractile unit of the myofibrils. Each sarcomere consists of myosin (thick) filaments and actin (thin) filaments. The arrangement of the thin and thick filaments accounts for the characteristic banding of muscle when it is seen under a microscope. Muscle contraction occurs as thick and thin filaments slide past each other, causing the sarcomeres to shorten.

Contractions. Skeletal muscle contractions allow posture maintenance, body movement, and facial expressions. Isometric contractions increase the tension within a muscle but do not produce movement. Repeated isometric contractions make muscles grow larger and stronger. Isotonic contractions shorten a muscle to produce movement. Most contractions are a combination of tension generation (*isometric*) and shortening (*isotonic*). Muscular *atrophy* (decrease in size) occurs with the absence of contraction that results from immobility, whereas increased muscular activity leads to *hypertrophy* (increase in size).

Skeletal muscle fibers are divided into two groups based on the type of activity they demonstrate. *Slow-twitch muscle fibers* support prolonged muscle activity such as marathon running. Because they also support the body against gravity, they assist

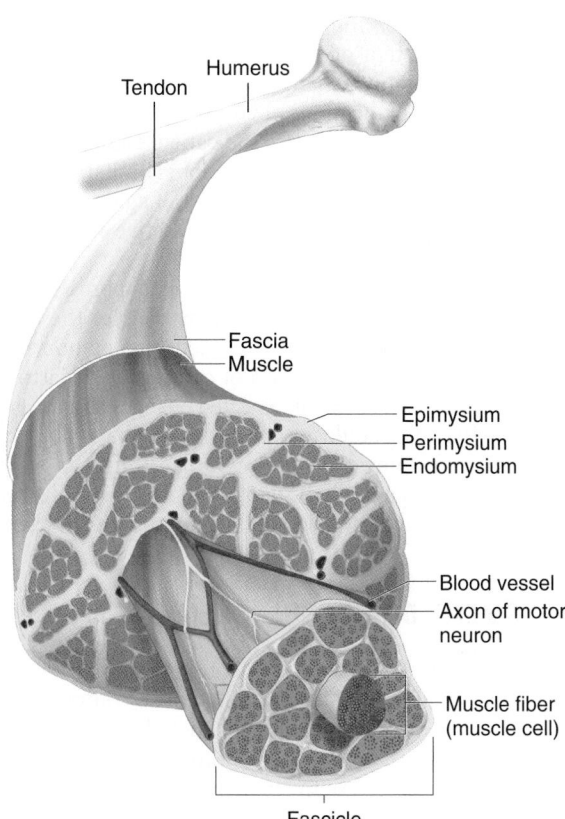

FIG. 62-5 Structure of a muscle.

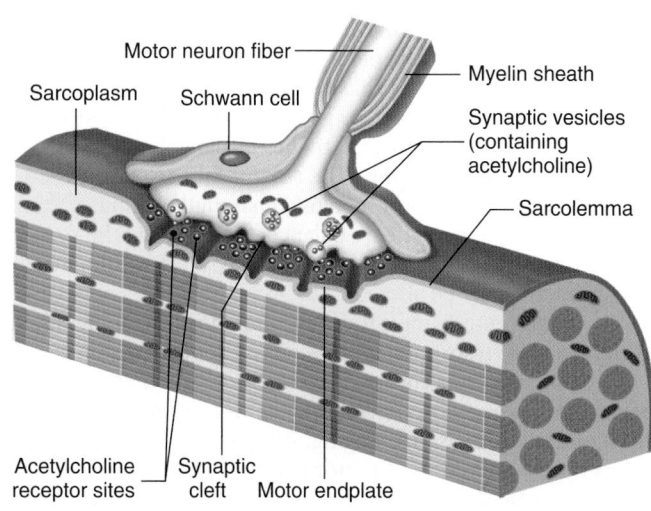

FIG. 62-6 Neuromuscular junction.

in posture maintenance. *Fast-twitch muscle fibers* are used for rapid muscle contraction required for activities such as blinking the eye, jumping, or sprinting. Fast-twitch fibers tend to tire more quickly than slow-twitch fibers.

Neuromuscular Junction. Skeletal muscle fibers require a nerve impulse to contract. A nerve fiber and the skeletal muscle fibers it stimulates are called a *motor endplate*. The junction between the axon of the nerve cell and the adjacent muscle cell is called the *myoneural* or *neuromuscular junction* (Fig. 62-6).

Acetylcholine is released from the presynaptic neuron and diffuses across the neuromuscular junction to bind with receptors on the motor endplate of the muscle. In response to this stimulation, the sarcoplasmic reticulum releases calcium ions into the cytoplasm. The presence of calcium triggers the contraction in the myofibrils. When calcium is low, *tetany* (involuntary contractions of skeletal muscle) can occur.

Energy Source. The direct energy source for muscle fiber contractions is adenosine triphosphate (ATP). ATP is synthesized by cellular oxidative metabolism in numerous mitochondria located close to the myofibrils. It is rapidly depleted through conversion to adenosine diphosphate (ADP) and must be rephosphorylated. Phosphocreatine provides a rapid source for the resynthesis of ATP, but it is in turn converted to creatine and must be recharged. Glycolysis can serve as a source of ATP when the oxygen supply is inadequate for the metabolic needs of the muscle tissue. Glucose is broken down to pyruvic acid, which can be further converted to lactic acid to make more oxygen available. An accumulation of lactic acid in tissues leads to fatigue and pain.

Ligaments and Tendons

Ligaments and tendons are both composed of dense, fibrous connective tissue that contains bundles of closely packed collagen fibers arranged in the same plane for additional strength. *Tendons* attach muscles to bones as an extension of the muscle sheath that adheres to the periosteum. *Ligaments* connect bones to bones (e.g., tibia to femur at knee joint). They have a higher elastic content than tendons.[4] Ligaments provide stability while permitting controlled movement at the joint.

Ligaments and tendons have a relatively poor blood supply, usually making tissue repair a slow process after injury. For example, the stretching or tearing of ligaments that occurs with a sprain may require a long time to mend.

Fascia

Fascia refers to layers of connective tissue with intermeshed fibers that can withstand limited stretching. Superficial fascia lies immediately under the skin. Deep fascia is a dense, fibrous tissue that surrounds muscle bundles, nerves, and blood vessels. It also encloses individual muscles, allowing them to act independently and to glide over each other during contraction. In addition, fascia provides strength to muscle tissues.

Bursae

Bursae are small sacs of connective tissue lined with synovial membrane and containing viscous synovial fluid. They are typically located at bony prominences or joints to relieve pressure and decrease friction between moving parts.[5] For example, bursae are found between the patella and the skin (prepatellar bursae), between the olecranon process of the elbow and the skin (olecranon bursae), between the head of the humerus and the acromion process of the scapula (subacromial bursae), and between the greater trochanter of the proximal femur and the skin (trochanteric bursae). *Bursitis* is an inflammation of a bursa sac. The inflammation may be acute or chronic.

GERONTOLOGIC CONSIDERATIONS

EFFECTS OF AGING ON MUSCULOSKELETAL SYSTEM

Many of the functional problems experienced by the aging adult are related to changes of the musculoskeletal system. Although some changes begin in early adulthood, obvious signs of musculoskeletal impairment may not appear until later adult years. Alterations may affect the older adult's ability to complete self-care tasks and pursue other customary activities. Effects of musculoskeletal changes may range from mild discomfort and decreased ability to perform activities of daily living to severe, chronic pain and immobility. The risk for falls also increases in the older adult due in part to a loss of strength. Aging can also bring changes in the patient's balance, thus making the person unsteady, and *proprioception* (awareness of self in relation to the environment) may be altered.

The bone remodeling process is altered in the aging adult. Increased bone resorption and decreased bone formation cause a loss of bone density, contributing to the development of osteopenia and osteoporosis (see Chapter 64). Muscle mass and strength also decrease with aging. Almost 30% of muscle mass is lost by age 70. A loss of motor neurons can cause additional problems with skeletal muscle movement. Tendons and ligaments become less flexible, and movement becomes more rigid. Joints in the aging adult are also more likely to be affected by osteoarthritis[6] (see Chapter 65).

Perform a musculoskeletal assessment with a particular emphasis on exercise practices. Obtain information on the type of exercise performed, including frequency and warm-up activ-

ities. Determine the impact of age-related changes of the musculoskeletal system on the older adult's functional status. Specifically inquire about changes in self-care habits and ability to be self-sufficient in the home environment. Identify any musculoskeletal changes that increase the patient's risk for falls, and discuss fall prevention strategies. Functional limitations that are accepted by older adults as a normal part of aging can often be halted or reversed with appropriate preventive strategies (see Table 63-1).

Diseases such as osteoarthritis and osteoporosis are not a normal part of growing older for many people. These metabolic bone diseases involve the deterioration of bone tissue (osteoporosis) and the destruction of cartilage (osteoarthritis). Carefully differentiate between expected changes and the effects of disease in the aging adult. Symptoms of disease can be treated in many cases, helping the older adult to return to a higher functional level. Age-related changes in the musculoskeletal system and differences in assessment findings are presented in Table 62-1.

ASSESSMENT OF MUSCULOSKELETAL SYSTEM

Subjective Data

Important Health Information. The most common symptoms of musculoskeletal impairment include pain, weakness, deformity, limitation of movement, stiffness, and joint crepitation (crackling sound). Ask the patient about changes in sensation or in the size of a muscle.

Past Health History. Because certain illnesses are known to affect the musculoskeletal system either directly or indirectly, question the patient about past medical problems, including tuberculosis, poliomyelitis, diabetes mellitus, parathyroid problems, hemophilia, rickets, soft tissue infection, and neuromuscular disabilities. In addition, past or developing musculoskeletal problems can affect the patient's overall health. Trauma to the musculoskeletal system is a common reason for seeking medical evaluation. Questions should also focus on symptoms of arthritic and connective tissue diseases (e.g., gout, psoriatic arthritis, systemic lupus erythematosus), osteomalacia, osteo-

TABLE 62-1 GERONTOLOGIC ASSESSMENT DIFFERENCES

Musculoskeletal System

Changes	Differences in Assessment Findings
Muscle	
• Decreased number and diameter of muscle cells. Replacement of muscle cells by fibrous connective tissue. • Loss of elasticity in ligaments, tendons, and cartilage. • Reduced ability to store glycogen. Decreased ability to release glycogen as quick energy during stress. • Decreased basal metabolic rate.	• Decreased muscle strength and mass. Abdominal protrusion. Flabby muscles. • Increased rigidity in neck, shoulders, back, hips, and knees. • Decreased fine motor dexterity, decreased agility. • Slowed reaction times and reflexes as a result of slowing of impulse conduction along motor units. Earlier fatigue with activity.
Joints	
• Increased risk for cartilage erosion that contributes to direct contact between bone ends and overgrowth of bone around joint margins. • Loss of water from discs between vertebrae, decreased height of intervertebral spaces.	• Joint stiffness, decreased mobility, limited ROM, possible crepitation on movement. Pain with motion and/or weight bearing. • Loss of height and shortening of trunk from disc compression. Posture change.
Bone	
• Decreased bone density and strength, brittleness. • Slowed remodeling process.	• Loss of height and deformity such as dowager's hump (kyphosis) from vertebral compression and degeneration. • Back pain, stiffness. • Bony prominences more pronounced. • Increased risk of osteopenia and osteoporosis.

Patient Introduction

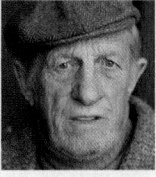

T.K. is a 78-yr-old white man brought to the emergency department by ambulance after falling on a patch of ice outside his home. He lay outside in the cold for 2 hr before neighbors found him. He is pale, diaphoretic, and complaining of excruciating pain in his left hip. The paramedics applied O_2 at 2 L via nasal cannula.

iStockphoto/Thinkstock

Critical Thinking
As you read through this assessment chapter, think about T.K.'s symptoms with the following questions in mind:
1. What is the most likely cause for T.K.'s acute hip pain?
2. What type of assessment would be most appropriate for T.K.: comprehensive, focused, or emergency? What would be your priority assessment(s)?
3. What questions would you ask T.K.?
4. What should be included in the physical assessment? What would you be looking for?
5. What diagnostic studies might you expect to be ordered?

myelitis, and fungal infection of bones or joints. Ask the patient about possible sources of a secondary bacterial infection, such as ears, tonsils, teeth, sinuses, lungs, or genitourinary tract. These infections can enter the bones, resulting in osteomyelitis or joint destruction. Obtain a detailed account of the course and treatment of any of these problems.

Medications. Question the patient regarding prescription and over-the-counter drugs and herbal products and nutritional supplements (see the Complementary & Alternative Therapies box in Chapter 3 on p. 39). Obtain detailed information about each treatment, including its name, the dose and frequency, length of time it was taken, its effects, and any possible side effects. Inquire about the use of skeletal muscle relaxants, opioids, nonsteroidal antiinflammatory drugs, and systemic and topical corticosteroids. Question the patient who has taken antiinflammatory drugs about GI distress or signs of bleeding.

In addition to drugs taken for treatment of a musculoskeletal problem, ask the patient about drugs that can have detrimental effects on this system. Some of these drugs and their potential side effects include antiseizure drugs (osteomalacia), phenothiazines (gait disturbances), corticosteroids (avascular necrosis, decreased bone and muscle mass), and potassium-depleting diuretics (muscle cramps and weakness). Question women about their menstrual history. Episodes of premenopausal amenorrhea can contribute to the development of osteoporosis.[7] Ask postmenopausal women about their use of hormone therapy. Inquire about calcium and vitamin D supplements for both women and men.

Surgery or Other Treatments. Obtain information about past hospitalizations related to a musculoskeletal problem. Document the reason for hospitalization; the date and the duration; and the treatment, including ongoing rehabilitation. Also record details of emergency treatment for musculoskeletal injuries. Obtain specific information regarding any surgical procedure, postoperative course, and complications. If the patient experienced a period of prolonged immobilization, consider the possible development of osteoporosis and muscle atrophy.

Functional Health Patterns. The use of functional health patterns assists in organizing the assessment data. Table 62-2 summarizes specific questions to ask in relation to functional health patterns.

Health Perception–Health Management Pattern. Ask about the patient's health practices related to the musculoskeletal system, such as maintenance of a normal body weight, avoidance of excessive stress on muscles and joints, and use of proper body mechanics when lifting objects. Question the patient

TABLE 62-2 HEALTH HISTORY

Musculoskeletal System

Health Perception–Health Management Pattern
- Describe your usual daily activities.
- Do you experience any difficulties performing these activities?* Describe what you do if you experience difficulty in dressing, preparing meals and feeding yourself, performing basic hygiene, writing or using the phone, or maintaining your home.
- Do you have to lift heavy objects? Do your work or exercise habits require repetitive motion or joint stress? Describe any specialized equipment you use or wear when you work or exercise that helps protect you from injury.
- Do you take any drugs or herbal products to manage your musculoskeletal problem? If so, what are their names and what are the expected effects?

Nutritional-Metabolic Pattern
- What is your usual daily intake of food and snacks?
- Do you have difficulties preparing your food?
- What dietary supplements do you take? (Ask specifically about calcium, vitamin D supplements, and herbal products.)
- What is your weight? Describe any recent weight loss or gain.

Elimination Pattern
- Does your musculoskeletal problem make it difficult for you to reach the toilet in time?*
- Do you need any assistive devices or equipment to achieve satisfactory toileting?*
- Do you experience constipation related to decreased mobility or to drugs taken for your musculoskeletal problem?*

Activity-Exercise Pattern
- Do you require assistance in completing your usual daily activities because of a musculoskeletal problem?*
- Describe your usual exercise pattern. Do you experience musculoskeletal symptoms before, during, or after exercising?*
- Are you able to move all your joints comfortably through full range of motion?
- Do you use any prosthetic or orthotic devices?*

Sleep-Rest Pattern
- Do you experience any difficulty sleeping because of a musculoskeletal problem?* Do you require frequent position changes at night?*
- Do you wake up at night because of musculoskeletal pain?*
- Do you use complementary and alternative therapies to help you sleep at night?*

Cognitive-Perceptual Pattern
- Describe any musculoskeletal pain you experience. How do you manage your pain? (Ask specifically about adjunctive therapies such as heat and cold or complementary and alternative therapies such as acupuncture.)

Self-Perception–Self-Concept Pattern
- Describe how changes in your musculoskeletal system (posture, walking, muscle strength) and decreased ability to do certain things may affect how you feel about yourself. Have these changes affected your lifestyle?*

Role-Relationship Pattern
- Do you live alone?
- Describe how family, friends, or others assist you with your musculoskeletal problem.
- Describe the effect of your musculoskeletal problem on your work and on your social relationships.

Sexuality-Reproductive Pattern
- Describe any sexual concerns related to your musculoskeletal problem.

Coping–Stress Tolerance Pattern
- Describe how you deal with problems such as pain, weakness, or immobility that have resulted from your musculoskeletal problem.

Value-Belief Pattern
- Describe any cultural practices or religious beliefs that may influence the treatment of your musculoskeletal problem.

*If yes, describe.

specifically about tetanus and polio immunizations. Obtain the most current date and reaction to a tuberculin skin test.

Patients who are good historians can recount numerous minor and major injuries of their musculoskeletal system. Record information chronologically and include the following:

- Mechanism and circumstances of the injury (e.g., twist, crush, stretch)
- Methods and duration of treatment
- Current status related to the injury
- Need for assistive devices
- Interference with activities of daily living

Safety practices can affect the patient's predisposition for certain injuries and illnesses. Therefore ask the patient about safety practices as they relate to the work environment, home life, recreation, and exercise. For example, if the patient is a computer programmer, ask about ergonomic adaptations in the office that decrease the risk of carpal tunnel syndrome or low back pain. Identification of problems in this area will direct your plan for patient teaching.

⚕ GENETIC RISK ALERT

Autoimmune Diseases
- Many autoimmune diseases of the musculoskeletal system have a genetic basis involving human leukocyte antigens (HLAs).
- These diseases include ankylosing spondylitis, rheumatoid arthritis, and systemic lupus erythematosus.

Osteoporosis
- Genetic factors contribute to osteoporosis by influencing not only bone mineral density but also bone size, bone quality, and bone turnover.

Osteoarthritis, Gout, and Scoliosis
- A genetic predisposition is a contributing risk factor in all these diseases.

Muscular Dystrophy
- The most common types of muscular dystrophy are X-linked recessive disorders.

Obtain a family history related to rheumatoid arthritis, systemic lupus erythematosus, ankylosing spondylitis, osteoarthritis, gout, osteoporosis, and scoliosis because a patient may have a genetic predisposition to these or other musculoskeletal disorders.

Nutritional-Metabolic Pattern. The patient's description of a typical day's diet provides clues to areas of nutritional concern that can affect the musculoskeletal system. An adequate intake of vitamins C and D, calcium, and protein is essential for a healthy, intact musculoskeletal system. Abnormal nutritional patterns can predispose individuals to problems such as osteomalacia and osteoporosis. In addition, maintenance of normal weight is an important nutritional goal. Obesity places additional stress on weight-bearing joints such as the knees, hips, and spine, and it predisposes individuals to instability of the ligaments.

Elimination Pattern. Questions about the patient's mobility may reveal difficulty with ambulating to the toilet. Ask the patient if an assistive device such as an elevated toilet seat or a grab bar is necessary to accomplish toileting. Decreased mobility secondary to a musculoskeletal problem can lead to constipation. In addition, musculoskeletal problems can contribute to bowel or bladder incontinence when ambulation is a problem.

Activity-Exercise Pattern. Obtain a detailed account of the type, duration, and frequency of exercise and recreational activities. Compare daily, weekend, and seasonal patterns because occasional or sporadic exercise can be more problematic than regular exercise. Many musculoskeletal problems can affect the patient's activity-exercise pattern. Question the patient about clumsiness or limitations in movement, pain, weakness, crepitus, or any change in the bones or joints that interferes with daily activities.

Extremes of activity related to occupation can also affect the musculoskeletal system. A sedentary occupation can negatively affect muscle flexibility and strength. Jobs that require extreme effort through heavy lifting or pushing can lead to damage of joints and supporting structures. Specifically question the patient about work-related injuries to the musculoskeletal system, including treatment and time lost from work.

Sleep-Rest Pattern. The discomfort caused by musculoskeletal disorders can interfere with the patient's normal sleep pattern. Ask the patient about possible alterations in sleep patterns. If the patient describes sleep interference related to a musculoskeletal problem, inquire further about the type of bedding and pillows used, bedtime routine, sleeping partner, and sleeping positions.

Cognitive-Perceptual Pattern. Fully explore and document any pain experienced by the patient as a result of a musculoskeletal problem. To provide a baseline for later reassessment, ask the patient to describe the intensity of the pain on a numeric scale from 0 to 10 (0 = no pain, 10 = most severe pain imaginable).[8] Reassessments over time assist in determining the effectiveness of any treatment plan. Question the patient about measures used at home for managing pain. Ask about related problems such as joint swelling or muscle weakness and any accommodations that help with the problem. (Pain is discussed in Chapter 9.)

Self-Perception–Self-Concept Pattern. Many chronic musculoskeletal problems lead to deformities and a reduction in activities that can have a serious negative impact on the patient's body image and sense of personal worth. Assess the patient's feelings about these changes and the effect they may have on interactions with family and friends.

Role-Relationship Pattern. Impaired mobility and chronic pain from musculoskeletal problems can negatively affect the patient's ability to perform in roles of spouse, parent, or employee. The ability to pursue and maintain meaningful social and personal relationships can also be affected by musculoskeletal problems. Carefully question the patient about role performance and relationships.

If the patient lives alone, the current musculoskeletal problem and rehabilitation may make it difficult or impossible to continue this arrangement. Determine the degree of assistance available from family, friends, and other caregivers. Find out if additional resources are needed such as physical therapy and home health care.

Sexuality-Reproductive Pattern. The pain of musculoskeletal problems can impede the patient's ability to obtain sexual satisfaction. Explore this area with a sensitive and nonjudgmental attitude. Help the patient feel comfortable discussing any sexual problems related to pain, movement, and positioning. Additional information in obtaining patient data in this area is presented in Chapter 51.

Coping–Stress Tolerance Pattern. Mobility limitations and pain, whether acute or chronic, are serious potential stressors that challenge the patient's coping resources. Recognize the potential for ineffective coping in the patient and family or significant other. Additional questioning will help to determine if a musculoskeletal problem is causing difficulties in coping and adjusting.

CASE STUDY—cont'd

Subjective Data

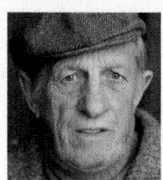

iStockphoto/Thinkstock

A focused subjective assessment of T.K. revealed the following information:

PMH: Type 2 diabetes for 11 yr. COPD for 15 yr. 40 pack-year smoking history.

Medications: Metformin (Glucophage) 500 mg PO bid; glyburide (DiaBeta) 5 mg/day PO; fluticasone and salmeterol combination (Advair) 250/50 mcg 1 inhalation bid; albuterol 2 puffs q4hr PRN as rescue inhaler.

Health Perception–Health Management: Currently smokes 2 to 3 packs of cigarettes per day. Is trying to quit but finding it difficult. Drinks alcohol at night.

Nutritional-Metabolic: T.K. is 6 ft, 2 in tall and weighs 195 lb. Does not take any nutritional supplements and tends to shy away from milk and other dairy products, since they make him "gassy."

Activity-Exercise: Leads a fairly sedentary lifestyle because of dyspnea on exertion. Until this current fall, has been able to perform ADLs without assistance. Denies any history of musculoskeletal problems.

Cognitive-Perceptual: Rates left hip pain at a 9 on a scale of 0-10. Describes pain as sharp spasms that increase in intensity with any movement.

Coping–Stress Tolerance: Is asking for pain medicine "as strong as you can give me."

Value-Belief Pattern. Ask the patient about cultural or religious beliefs that might influence the patient's acceptance of treatment for the musculoskeletal problem. These may include recommendations for diet, exercise, medication, and lifestyle modifications.

Objective Data

Physical Examination. Examination involves observation, palpation, motion, and muscular assessment. Conduct a general overview, while obtaining data in a careful health history to provide guidance in choosing areas to concentrate on during the local examination. Take specific measurements as indicated by the local examination.

Inspection. A systematic inspection is performed starting at the head and neck and proceeding to the upper extremities, lower extremities, and trunk. The regular use of a systematic approach is important to avoid missing important aspects of the examination. Inspect the skin for general color, scars, or other overt signs of previous injury or surgery. Certain cutaneous lesions require additional investigation because they can indicate underlying disorders. For example, butterfly rash over the cheeks and nose is a characteristic marker of systemic lupus erythematosus.

Note the patient's general body build, muscle configuration, and symmetry of joints. Observe for any swelling, deformity, nodules or masses, and discrepancies in limb length or muscle size. Use the patient's opposite body part for comparison when an abnormality is suspected.

Palpation. Carefully palpate any area that has aroused concern because of a subjective complaint or that appears abnormal on inspection. As with inspection, palpation usually proceeds cephalopedally (head to toe) to examine the neck, shoulders, elbows, wrists, hands, back, hips, knees, ankles, and feet. Both superficial and deep palpation are usually performed consecutively.

Warm your hands to prevent muscle spasm, which can interfere with identification of essential landmarks or soft tissue

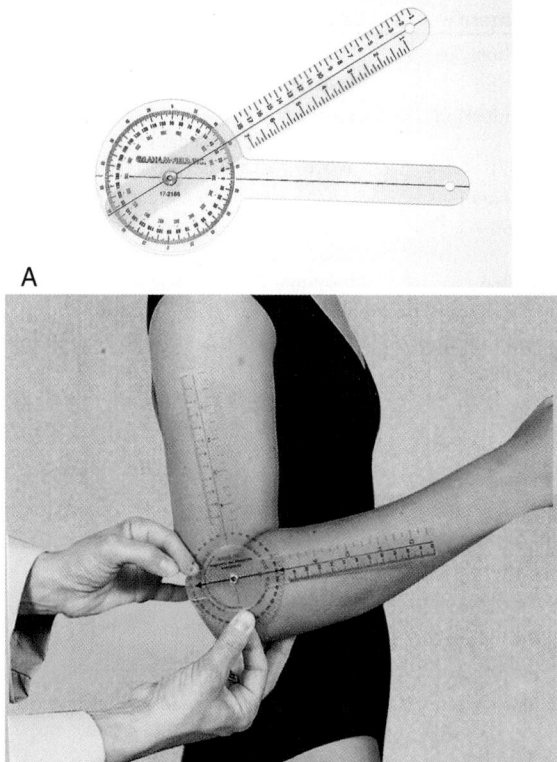

FIG. 62-7 A, Goniometer. **B,** Measurement of joint range of motion using a goniometer.

structures. Palpate both muscles and joints to allow for evaluation of skin temperature, local tenderness, swelling, and crepitation. Establish the relationship of adjacent structures, and evaluate the general contour, abnormal prominences, and local landmarks.

Motion. When assessing the patient's joint mobility, carefully evaluate both active and passive range of motion (full movement potential of a joint). Measurements should be similar for both active and passive maneuvers. *Active range of motion* means the patient takes his or her own joints through all movements without assistance. *Passive range of motion* occurs when someone else moves the patient's joints without his or her assistance through the full range of motion. Be careful in performing passive range of motion because of the risk of injury to underlying structures. If pain or resistance is encountered, stop manipulation immediately.

If you note deficits in active or passive range of motion, also assess functional range of motion to determine if performance of activities of daily living has been affected by joint changes. This is done by asking the patient if activities such as eating and bathing need to be performed with assistance or cannot be done at all.

Range of motion is most accurately assessed with a goniometer, which measures the angle of the joint (Fig. 62-7). Specific degrees of range of motion of all joints are usually not measured unless a musculoskeletal problem has been identified. A less exact but valuable assessment method is to compare the range of motion of one extremity with that on the opposite side. Common movements that occur at the synovial joints, includ-

TABLE 62-3   SYNOVIAL JOINT MOVEMENTS

Movement	Description
Abduction	Movement of part away from midline of body
Adduction	Movement of part toward midline of body
Circumduction	Combination of flexion, extension, abduction, and adduction resulting in circular motion of a body part
Dorsiflexion	Flexion of the ankle and toes toward the shin
Eversion	Turning of sole outward away from midline of body
Extension	Straightening of joint that increases angle between two bones
External rotation	Movement along longitudinal axis away from midline of body
Flexion	Bending of joint as a result of muscle contraction that results in decreased angle between two bones
Hyperextension	Extension in which angle exceeds 180 degrees
Internal rotation	Movement along longitudinal axis toward midline of body
Inversion	Turning of sole inward toward midline of body
Opposition	Moving the first and fifth metacarpals anteriorly from a flattened palm ("cupping position"); makes it possible to hold objects between the thumb and fingers
Plantar flexion	Flexion of the ankle and toes toward the plantar surface of the foot ("toes pointed")
Pronation	Turning of palm downward
Supination	Turning of palm upward

ing *abduction, adduction, flexion,* and *extension,* are described in Table 62-3.

Muscle-Strength Testing. Grade the strength of individual muscles or groups of muscles during contraction (Table 62-4). Grade normal muscle strength as a 5 bilaterally, with full resistance to opposition. Have the patient apply resistance to the force the examiner is exerting. For example, try to pull the bent arm down while the patient attempts to raise it. Compare muscle strength with the strength of the opposite extremity. Note any subtle variations in muscle strength when comparing the patient's dominant and nondominant sides. Variations in strength also exist when comparing individuals.

Measurement. When length discrepancies or subjective problems are noted, obtain limb length and circumferential muscle mass measurements. For example, measure leg length when gait disorders are observed. Measure the affected limb between the anterosuperior iliac crest and the bottom of the medial malleolus. Then compare it with the similar measure-

TABLE 62-4   MUSCLE STRENGTH SCALE

0	No detection of muscular contraction
1	A barely detectable flicker or trace of contraction with observation or palpation
2	Active movement of body part with elimination of gravity
3	Active movement against gravity only and not against resistance
4	Active movement against gravity and some resistance
5	Active movement against full resistance without evident fatigue (normal muscle strength)

ment of the opposite extremity. Measure muscle mass circumferentially at the largest area of the muscle. When recording measurements, document the exact location at which the measurements were obtained (e.g., the quadriceps muscle is measured 15 cm above the patella). This informs the next examiner of the exact area to measure and ensures consistency during reassessment.

Other. Note the patient's use of an assistive device such as a walker or cane. Assess the patient for a proper fit while reviewing the safe and correct technique for using these devices. Regularly review with the patient the use of the assistive device to ensure it remains appropriate and safe.[9] If the patient is able to move independently, assess posture and gait by watching the patient walk, stand, and sit. Musculoskeletal and neurologic problems can result in abnormal gait patterns.

Scoliosis is a lateral S-shaped curvature of the thoracic and lumbar spine. Unequal shoulder and scapula height is usually noted when the patient is observed from the back (Fig. 62-8). Also ask the patient to place the fingertips together as if diving into a swimming pool and slowly bend forward, allowing for assessment of thoracic rib prominence or paravertebral muscle prominence in the lumbar spine. If the deformity is greater than 45 degrees, lung and cardiac function is usually impaired.

The *straight-leg-raising test* is performed on the supine patient with sciatica or leg pain. Passively raise the patient's leg 60 degrees or less. The test is positive if the patient complains of pain along the distribution of the sciatic nerve. A positive test indicates nerve root irritation from intervertebral disc prolapse and herniation, particularly at the level of L4-5 or L5-S1.

Assessment of reflexes is discussed in Chapter 56. Neurovascular assessment is discussed in Chapter 63. Table 62-5 is an example of how to record a normal physical assessment of the musculoskeletal system. Abnormal assessment findings of the musculoskeletal system are presented in Table 62-6.

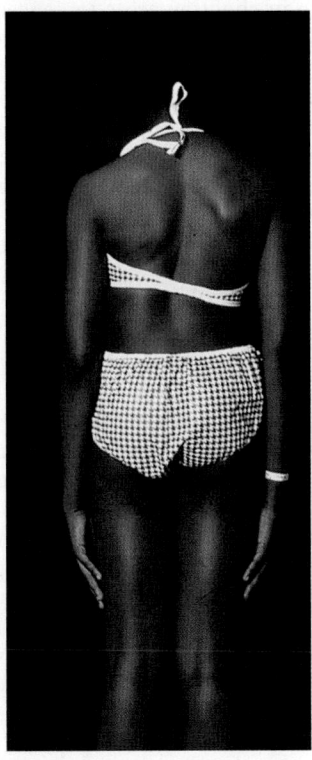

FIG. 62-8 Scoliosis in a standing erect posture.

TABLE 62-5 NORMAL PHYSICAL ASSESSMENT OF THE MUSCULOSKELETAL SYSTEM

- Normal spinal curvatures
- No muscle atrophy or asymmetry
- No joint swelling, deformity, or crepitation
- No tenderness on palpation of spine, joints, or muscles
- Full range of motion of all joints without pain or laxity
- Muscle strength of 5

FOCUSED ASSESSMENT
Musculoskeletal System

Use this checklist to make sure the key assessment steps have been done.

Subjective
Ask the patient about any of the following and note responses.

Joint pain or stiffness	Y	N
Muscle weakness	Y	N
Bone pain	Y	N

Objective: Diagnostic
Check the results of the following diagnostic studies.

X-ray results	✓
Bone scans	✓
Erythrocyte sedimentation rate	✓

Objective: Physical Examination
Inspect and Palpate

Skeleton and extremities (and compare sides) for alignment, contour, symmetry, size, and gross deformities	✓
Joints for range of motion, tenderness or pain, heat, crepitus, and swelling	✓
Muscles (and compare sides) for size, symmetry, tone, and tenderness or pain	✓
Bones for tenderness or pain	✓

A *focused assessment* is used to evaluate the status of previously identified musculoskeletal problems and to monitor for signs of new problems (see Table 3-6). A focused assessment of the musculoskeletal system is presented in the box above.

DIAGNOSTIC STUDIES OF MUSCULOSKELETAL SYSTEM

Numerous diagnostic studies are available to assess the musculoskeletal system. Table 62-7 presents the most common studies, and select studies are described in more detail below.

The use of studies such as x-rays, magnetic resonance imaging (MRI), and bone scans has greatly improved orthopedic care. The x-ray, or roentgenogram, is the most common diagnostic study used to assess musculoskeletal problems and to monitor the effectiveness of treatment. Because bones are denser than other tissues, x-rays do not penetrate them. Dense areas show as white on the standard x-ray. X-rays provide information about bone deformity, joint congruity, bone density, and calcification in soft tissue. Fracture diagnosis and management are the primary indications for x-rays, but they are also useful in the evaluation of genetic, developmental, infectious, inflammatory, neoplastic, metabolic, and degenerative disorders.

A small fiberoptic tube called an arthroscope is used to directly examine the interior of a joint cavity in a procedure

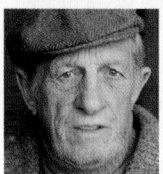
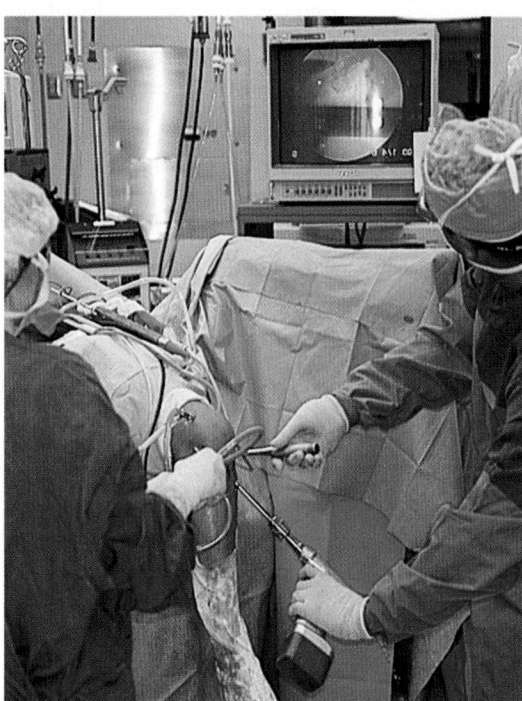

FIG. 62-9 Knee arthroscopy in progress. Notice the monitor in the background.

known as **arthroscopy.** After anesthesia has been administered, a large-bore needle is inserted into the joint, and the joint is distended with fluid or air (Fig. 62-9). When the arthroscope is inserted, the surgeon is able to perform extensive, accurate visualization of the joint cavity. Photographs or videotapes can be made through the scope, and a biopsy of the synovium or cartilage can be obtained. Torn tissue can be repaired through arthroscopic surgery, eliminating the need for a larger incision and greatly decreasing the recovery time.

An **arthrocentesis** (joint aspiration) is usually performed for synovial fluid analysis. It may also be done to remove fluid from joints to relieve pain. First, the skin is cleansed and a local anesthetic is given. After an 18-gauge or larger needle is inserted into the joint, the fluid is withdrawn. The appropriate sterile container should be readily available to receive the aspirated fluid, which must be transported immediately to the laboratory. Patients with inflammatory joint conditions (e.g., rheumatoid arthritis, septic arthritis, osteoarthritis) may be treated with an

Text continued on p. 1503

TABLE 62-6 ASSESSMENT ABNORMALITIES

Musculoskeletal System

Finding	Description	Possible Etiology and Significance
Achilles tendonitis	Pain in posterior leg, initially when running or walking. Can progress to pain at rest.	Cumulative stress on Achilles tendon resulting in inflammation.
Ankylosis	Stiffness and fixation of a joint.	Chronic joint inflammation and destruction (e.g., rheumatoid arthritis).
Antalgic gait	Shortened stride with as little weight bearing as possible on the affected side.	Pain or discomfort in the lower extremity on weight bearing. Can be related to trauma or other disorders.
Ataxic gait	Staggering, uncoordinated gait often with sway.	Neurogenic disorders (e.g., spinal cord lesion).
Atrophy	Flabby appearance of muscle leading to decreased function and tone.	Muscle denervation, contracture, prolonged disuse as a result of immobilization.
Boutonnière deformity	Finger abnormality, flexion of proximal interphalangeal (PIP) joint and hyperextension of the distal interphalangeal (DIP) joint of the fingers (see Fig. 65-4, B).	Typical deformity of rheumatoid and psoriatic arthritis caused by rupture of extensor tendons over the fingers.
Contracture	Resistance of movement of muscle or joint as a result of fibrosis of supporting soft tissues.	Shortening of muscle or ligaments, tightness of soft tissue, incorrect positioning of immobilized extremity.
Crepitation (crepitus)	Frequent, audible crackling sound with palpable grating that accompanies movement.	Fracture, dislocation, temporomandibular joint dysfunction, osteoarthritis.
Dislocation	Separation of two bones from their normal position within a joint.	Trauma, disorders of surrounding soft tissues.
Festinating gait	While walking, neck, trunk, and knees flex while the body is rigid. Delayed start with short, quick, shuffling steps. Speed may increase as if patient is unable to stop (festination).	Neurogenic disorders (e.g., Parkinson's disease).
Ganglion cyst	Small fluid-filled bump or mass over a tendon sheath or joint, usually on dorsal surface of wrist or foot.	Inflammation of tissues around a joint, which can increase in size or disappear.
Kyphosis (dowager's hump)	Exaggerated thoracic curvature.	Poor posture, tuberculosis, arthritis, osteoporosis, growth disturbance of vertebral epiphyses.
Lateral epicondylitis (tennis elbow)	Dull ache along outer aspect of elbow, worsens with twisting and grasping motions.	Partial tearing of tendon at its insertion on epicondyle.
Limited range of motion (ROM)	Joint does not achieve the expected degrees of motion.	Injury, inflammation, contracture.
Lordosis (swayback)	Asymmetric scapulae and shoulders, exaggerated lumbar curvature.	Secondary to other spinal deformities, muscular dystrophy, obesity, flexion contracture of hip, congenital dislocation of hip.
Muscle spasticity	Increased muscle tone (rigidity) with sustained muscle contractions (spasms); stiffness or tightness may interfere with gait, movement, speech.	Neuromuscular disorders such as multiple sclerosis (MS) or cerebral palsy.
Myalgia	General muscle tenderness and pain.	Chronic rheumatic syndromes (e.g., fibromyalgia). Overuse, injury, or strain.
Paresthesia	Numbness and tingling, often described as a "pins and needles" sensation.	Compromised sensory nerves, often due to edema in a closed space such as a cast or bulky dressing. May also result from spinal stenosis.
Pes planus (flatfoot)	Abnormal flatness of the sole and arch of the foot.	Hereditary, muscle paralysis, mild cerebral palsy, early muscular dystrophy, injury to posterior tibial tendon.
Plantar fasciitis	Burning, sharp pain on sole of foot; worse in the morning.	Chronic degenerative/reparative cycle resulting in inflammation.
Scoliosis	Asymmetric elevation of shoulders, scapulae, and iliac crests with lateral spine curvature (see Fig. 62-8).	Idiopathic or congenital condition, fracture or dislocation, osteomalacia.
Short-leg gait	A limp, unless corrective footwear used.	Leg length discrepancy of ≥1 in, generally of structural origin (arthritis, fracture).
Spastic gait	Short steps with dragging of foot. Jerky, uncoordinated, cross-knee (scissor) movement.	Neurogenic (e.g., cerebral palsy, hemiplegia).
Steppage gait	Increased hip and knee flexion to clear the foot from the floor. Footdrop is evident, foot slaps down and along walking surface.	Neurogenic disorders (e.g., peroneal nerve injury, paralyzed dorsiflexor muscles).
Subluxation	Partial dislocation of joint.	Instability of joint capsule and supporting ligaments (e.g., trauma, arthritis).
Swan neck deformity	Hyperextension of the PIP joint with flexion of the metacarpophalangeal (MCP) and DIP joints of the fingers (see Fig. 65-4, D).	Typical deformity of rheumatoid and psoriatic arthritis caused by contracture of muscles and tendons.
Swelling	Enlargement, often of a joint due to fluid collection. Generally leads to pain, stiffness.	Trauma or inflammation.
Tenosynovitis	Superficial swelling, pain, and tenderness along a tendon sheath.	Inflammation that often occurs with infection, injury, or overuse.
Torticollis (wryneck)	Neck is twisted in unusual position to one side.	Prolonged contraction of neck muscles, congenital or acquired.
Ulnar deviation (ulnar drift)	Fingers drift to ulnar side of forearm (see Fig. 65-4, A).	Typical deformity of rheumatoid arthritis due to tendon contracture.
Valgum deformity (knock-knees)	When knees are together and there is >1 in (2.5 cm) between the medial malleoli.	Poliomyelitis, congenital deformity, arthritis.
Varum deformity (bowlegs)	When knees are apart and the medial malleoli are together, a space of >1 in (2.5 cm) exists.	Arthritis, congenital deformity.

TABLE 62-7 DIAGNOSTIC STUDIES

Musculoskeletal System

Study	Description and Purpose	Nursing Responsibility
Radiologic Studies		
Standard x-ray	Determines density of bone. Evaluates structural or functional changes of bones and joints. In anteroposterior view, x-ray beam passes from front to back, allowing one-dimensional view. Lateral position provides two-dimensional view.	Avoid excessive exposure of patient and self. Before procedure, remove any radiopaque objects that can interfere with results. Explain procedure to patient.
Diskogram	X-ray of cervical or lumbar intervertebral disc is done after injection of contrast media into nucleus pulposus. Permits visualization of intervertebral disc abnormalities.	Assess patient for possible allergy to contrast medium. Explain procedure.
Computed tomography (CT) scan	X-ray beam is used with a computer to provide a three-dimensional picture. Used to identify soft tissue abnormalities, bony abnormalities, and various types of musculoskeletal trauma.	Inform patient that procedure is painless. Inform patient of importance of remaining still during procedure. If contrast medium is being used, verify that patient does not have shellfish allergy.
Myelogram with or without CT	Involves injecting a radiographic contrast medium into sac around nerve roots. CT scan may follow to show how the bone is affecting the nerve roots. Sensitive test for nerve impingement and can detect subtle lesions and injuries.	Main risk is the potential for spinal headache. Inform patient that headache should resolve in 1–2 days with rest and fluids, but should be reported to health care provider.
Magnetic resonance imaging (MRI)	Radio waves and magnetic field are used to view soft tissue. Especially useful in the diagnosis of avascular necrosis, disc disease, tumors, osteomyelitis, ligament tears, and cartilage tears. Patient is placed inside scanning chamber. Gadolinium may be injected IV to enhance visualization of structures. Open MRI does not require patient to be placed inside a chamber. Contraindicated in patient with aneurysm clips, metallic implants, pacemakers, electronic devices, hearing aids, and shrapnel.	Inform patient that procedure is painless. Explain that the machine will make loud tapping noises intermittently and there is no cause for alarm. Ear plugs can be requested or music to listen to. Ensure that patient has no metal on clothing (e.g., snaps, zippers, jewelry, credit cards). Inform patient to remain still throughout procedure. Inform patients who are claustrophobic that they may experience symptoms during examination. Administer antianxiety agent if indicated and ordered. Open MRI may be indicated for obese patient or patient with large chest and abdominal girth or severe claustrophobia.
Bone Mineral Density (BMD) Measurements		
Dual energy x-ray absorptiometry (DXA)	Measures bone mass of spine, femur, forearm, and total body. Allows assessment of bone density with minimal radiation exposure. Used to diagnose metabolic bone disease and to monitor changes in bone density with treatment.	Inform patient that procedure is painless.
Quantitative ultrasound (QUS)	Evaluates density, elasticity, and strength of bone using ultrasound rather than radiation. Common area assessed is calcaneus (heel).	Same as above.
Radioisotope Studies		
Bone scan	Involves injection of radioisotope (usually technetium [Tc]-99m) that is taken up by bone. A uniform uptake of the isotope is normal. Increased uptake is seen in osteomyelitis, osteoporosis, primary and metastatic malignant lesions of bone, and certain fractures. Decreased uptake is seen in areas of avascular necrosis.	Explain that radioisotope is given 2 hr before procedure. Ensure that bladder is emptied before scan. Inform patient that procedure requires 1 hr while patient lies supine and that no pain or harm will result from isotopes. Increase fluids after the examination.
Endoscopy		
Arthroscopy	Involves insertion of arthroscope into joint (usually knee) for visualization of structure and contents. Can be used for exploratory surgery (removal of loose bodies and biopsy); repair of joint structures; and diagnosis of abnormalities of meniscus, articular cartilage, ligaments, or joint capsule. Other structures that can be visualized through an arthroscope include shoulder, elbow, wrist, jaw, hip, and ankle.	Inform patient that procedure can be performed in outpatient setting and that local or general anesthesia may be used. After procedure, cover wound with sterile dressing. Explain any postprocedure activity restrictions.
Mineral Metabolism		
Alkaline phosphatase	This enzyme, produced by osteoblasts of bone, is needed for mineralization of organic bone matrix. Elevated levels are found in healing fractures, bone cancers, osteoporosis, osteomalacia, and Paget's disease. *Reference interval:* 38-126 U/L (0.65-2.14 µkat/L)	Obtain blood samples by venipuncture. Observe venipuncture site for bleeding or hematoma formation. Inform patient that procedure does not require fasting.
Calcium	Bone is primary organ for calcium storage. Calcium provides bone with rigid structure. Decreased serum level is found in osteomalacia, renal disease, and hypoparathyroidism. Increased level is found in hyperparathyroidism and some bone tumors. *Reference interval:* 8.6-10.2 mg/dL (2.20-2.55 mmol/L)	Same as above.

Continued

TABLE 62-7 DIAGNOSTIC STUDIES—cont'd

Musculoskeletal System

Study	Description and Purpose	Nursing Responsibility
Phosphorus	Amount present is indirectly related to calcium metabolism. Decreased level is found in osteomalacia. Increased level is found in chronic kidney disease, healing fractures, and osteolytic metastatic tumor. *Reference interval:* 2.4-4.4 mg/dL (0.78-1.42 mmol/L)	Same as above.
Serologic Studies		
Rheumatoid factor (RF)	Assesses presence of autoantibody (rheumatoid factor) in serum. Factor is not specific for rheumatoid arthritis and is seen in other connective tissue diseases and in a small percentage of normal population. *Reference interval:* Negative or titer <1:17	Same as above.
Erythrocyte sedimentation rate (ESR)	Nonspecific index of inflammation. Measures rapidity with which red blood cells settle from unclotted blood in 1 hr. Results influenced by physiologic factors and diseases. Elevated levels are seen with any inflammatory process (especially rheumatoid arthritis, rheumatic fever, osteomyelitis, and respiratory tract infections). *Reference interval:* <30 mm/hr (some gender variation)	Same as above.
Antinuclear antibody (ANA)	Assesses presence of antibodies capable of destroying nucleus of body's tissue cells. Finding is positive in 95% of patients with systemic lupus erythematosus and may also be positive in individuals with scleroderma or rheumatoid arthritis and in a small percentage of normal population. *Reference interval:* Negative at 1:40 dilution	Same as above.
Anti-DNA antibody	Detects serum antibodies that react with DNA. Most specific test for systemic lupus erythematosus. *Reference interval:* <70 IU/mL	Same as above.
Complement, total hemolytic (CH_{50})	Complement, a normal body protein, is essential to both immune and inflammatory reactions. Complement components used in these reactions are depleted. Complement depletions may be found in patients with rheumatoid arthritis or systemic lupus erythematosus. *Reference interval:* 75-160 U/mL (75-160 kU/L)	Same as above.
Uric acid	End product of purine metabolism is normally excreted in urine. Although not specific, levels are usually elevated in gout. *Male:* 4.4-7.6 mg/dL (262-452 µmol/L) *Female:* 2.3-6.6 mg/dL (137-393 µmol/L)	Same as above.
C-reactive protein (CRP)	Used to diagnose inflammatory diseases, infections, and active widespread malignancy. Synthesized by the liver and is present in large amounts in serum 18-24 hr after onset of tissue damage. *Reference interval:* 6.8-820 mcg/dL (68-8200 mcg/L)	Same as above.
Human leukocyte antigen (HLA)–B27	Antigen often present in autoimmune disorders such as ankylosing spondylitis and rheumatoid arthritis.	Same as above.
Markers of Muscle Injury		
Creatine kinase (CK)	Highest concentration found in skeletal muscle. Increased levels found in progressive muscular dystrophy, polymyositis, and traumatic injuries. *Male:* 20-200 U/L *Female:* 20-180 U/L	Same as above.
Potassium	Increased in muscle trauma as cell destruction releases this electrolyte into serum. Cardiac dysrhythmias can be caused by hyperkalemia or hypokalemia. *Reference interval:* 3.5-5.0 mEq/L (3.5-5.0 mmol/L)	Same as above.
Aldolase	Useful in monitoring muscular dystrophy and dermatomyositis. *Reference interval:* 1.5-8.1 U/L	Same as above.
Invasive Procedures		
Arthrocentesis	Incision or puncture of joint capsule to obtain samples of synovial fluid from within joint cavity or to remove excess fluid. Local anesthesia and aseptic preparation are used before needle is inserted into joint and fluid aspirated. Useful in diagnosis of joint inflammation, infection, meniscal tears, and subtle fractures.	Inform patient that procedure is usually done at bedside or in examination room. Send samples of synovial fluid to laboratory for examination (if indicated). After procedure apply compression dressing. Observe for leakage of blood or fluid on dressing.

TABLE 62-7 DIAGNOSTIC STUDIES—cont'd

Musculoskeletal System

Study	Description and Purpose	Nursing Responsibility
Electromyogram (EMG)	Evaluates electrical potential associated with skeletal muscle contraction. Small-gauge needles are inserted into certain muscles. Needle probes are attached to leads that feed information to EMG machine. Recordings of electrical activity of muscle are traced on audio transmitter and on oscilloscope and recording paper. Useful in providing information related to lower motor neuron dysfunction and primary muscle disease.	Inform patient that procedure is usually done in EMG laboratory while patient lies supine on special table. Keep patient awake to cooperate with voluntary movement. Inform patient that procedure involves some discomfort from needle insertion. Avoid stimulants, including caffeine, and sedatives 24 hr before procedure.
Miscellaneous		
Duplex venous Doppler	Ultrasound of the veins, usually of the lower extremities, to detect blood flow abnormalities that could indicate deep vein thrombosis.	Inform patient that procedure is painless and noninvasive.
Thermography	Uses infrared detector that measures degree of heat radiating from skin surface. Useful in investigating cause of inflamed joint and in determining patient response to antiinflammatory drug therapy.	Same as above.
Plethysmography	Records variations in volume and pressure of blood passing through tissues. Test is nonspecific.	Same as above.
Somatosensory evoked potential (SSEP)	Evaluates evoked potential of muscle contractions. Electrodes are placed on skin and provide recordings of electrical activity of muscle. Useful in identifying subtle dysfunction of lower motor neuron and primary muscle disease. Measures nerve conduction along pathways not accessible by EMG. Transcutaneous or percutaneous electrodes are applied to the skin and help identify neuropathy and myopathy. Often used during spinal surgery for scoliosis to detect neurologic compromise when patient is under anesthesia.	Inform patient that procedure is similar to EMG but does not involve needles. Electrodes are applied to the skin.

intraarticular injection of corticosteroids after the joint fluid has been aspirated.[10]

The fluid is examined grossly for volume, color, clarity, viscosity, and mucin clot formation. Normal synovial fluid is transparent and colorless or straw colored. It should be scant in amount and of low viscosity. Fluid from an infected joint may be purulent and thick or gray and thin. In gout, the fluid may be whitish yellow. Blood may be aspirated if there is hemarthrosis due to injury or a bleeding disorder. The mucin clot test indicates the character of the protein portion of the synovial fluid. Normally a white, ropelike mucin clot is formed. In the presence of inflammation, the clot fragments easily. The fluid is examined grossly for floating fat globules, which indicate bone injury. In septic arthritis, protein content is elevated and glucose is considerably decreased. Presence of uric acid crystals suggests a diagnosis of gout. A Gram stain and culture may also be done.

Diagnostic Studies

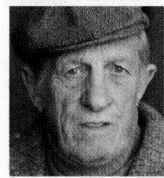

iStockphoto/Thinkstock

The emergency department physician immediately orders the following diagnostic studies:

- X-ray of left hip
- Chest x-ray
- CBC, electrolytes, aPTT, PT/INR
- Arterial blood gases (ABGs)

The x-ray of the left hip reveals an extracapsular fracture. The chest x-ray findings are consistent with COPD without any evidence of pneumonia at present. Hematocrit is 43%, hemoglobin 15 g/dL, and WBC is 15,100/μL (15.1 × 10⁹/L). The remainder of CBC, electrolytes, aPTT, and PT/INR are WNL. The ABGs demonstrate compensated respiratory acidosis. This case is continued in Chapter 63 on p. 1536.

BRIDGE TO NCLEX EXAMINATION

The number of the question corresponds to the same-numbered outcome at the beginning of the chapter.

1. The bone cells that function in the resorption of bone tissue are called
   a. osteoids.
   b. osteocytes.
   c. osteoclasts.
   d. osteoblasts.

2. While performing passive range of motion for a patient, the nurse puts the ankle joint through the movements of (select all that apply)
   a. flexion and extension.
   b. inversion and eversion.
   c. pronation and supination
   d. flexion, extension, abduction, and adduction.
   e. pronation, supination, rotation, and circumduction.

3. To prevent muscle atrophy, the nurse teaches the patient with a leg immobilized in traction to perform *(select all that apply)*
   a. flexion contractions.
   b. tetanic contractions.
   c. isotonic contractions.
   d. isometric contractions.
   e. extension contractions.

4. A patient with tendonitis asks what the tendon does. The nurse's response is based on the knowledge that tendons
   a. connect bone to muscle.
   b. provide strength to muscle.
   c. lubricate joints with synovial fluid.
   d. relieve friction between moving parts.

5. The increased risk for falls in the older adult is most likely due to
   a. changes in balance.
   b. decrease in bone mass.
   c. loss of ligament elasticity.
   d. erosion of articular cartilage.

6. While obtaining subjective assessment data related to the musculoskeletal system, it is particularly important to ask a patient about other medical problems such as
   a. hypertension.
   b. thyroid problems.
   c. diabetes mellitus.
   d. chronic bronchitis.

7. When grading muscle strength, the nurse records a score of 3, which indicates
   a. no detection of muscular contraction.
   b. a barely detectable flicker of contraction.
   c. active movement against full resistance without fatigue.
   d. active movement against gravity but not against resistance.

8. A normal assessment finding of the musculoskeletal system is
   a. no deformity or crepitation.
   b. muscle and bone strength of 4.
   c. ulnar deviation and subluxation.
   d. angulation of bone toward midline.

9. A patient is scheduled for an electromyogram (EMG). The nurse explains that this diagnostic test involves
   a. incision or puncture of the joint capsule.
   b. insertion of small needles into certain muscles.
   c. administration of a radioisotope before the procedure.
   d. placement of skin electrodes to record muscle activity.

1. c, 2. a, b, 3. d, 4. a, 5. a, 6. c, 7. d, 8. a, 9. b

evolve

For rationales to these answers and even more NCLEX review questions, visit *http://evolve.elsevier.com/Lewis/medsurg*.

REFERENCES

1. Cleveland Clinic: Normal structure and function of the musculoskeletal system. Retrieved from *my.clevelandclinic.org/anatomy/musculoskeletal_system*.

2. Huether S, McCance K: *Understanding pathophysiology*, ed 5, St Louis, 2012, Mosby.

3. Thibodeau GA, Patton KT: *Structure and function of the human body*, ed 14, St Louis, 2012, Mosby.

4. Brinker M, O'Connor D, Almekinders L, et al: Basic science and injury of muscle, tendon, and ligament. In DeLee J, Drez DD, Miller M, editors: *DeLee and Drez's orthopaedic sports medicine*, ed 3, Philadelphia, 2010, Saunders.

5. Jarvis C: *Physical examination and health assessment*, ed 6, St Louis, 2012, Saunders.

6. National Institute of Arthritis and Musculoskeletal and Skin Diseases: Handout on health: osteoarthritis, National Institutes of Health. Retrieved from *www.niams.nih.gov/Health_Info/Osteoarthritis*.

7. Mehler P, Cleary B, Gaudiani J: Osteoporosis in anorexia nervosa, *Eat Disord* 19:194, 2011.

*8. Nworah U: From documentation to the problem: controlling postoperative pain, *Nurs Forum* 47:91, 2012.

9. Thomas S, Halbert J, Mackintosh S, et al: Walking aid use after discharge following hip fracture is rarely reviewed and often inappropriate: an observational study, *J Physiother* 56:267, 2010.

10. Bettencourt RB, Linder M: Arthrocentesis and therapeutic joint injection: an overview for the primary care physician, *Prim Care* 37:691, 2010.

RESOURCES

Resources for this chapter are listed after Chapter 63 on p. 1538, Chapter 64 on p. 1560, and Chapter 65 on p. 1595.

---

*Evidence-based information for clinical practice.

Dreams are the touchstones of our character.
Henry David Thoreau

Nursing Management
Musculoskeletal Trauma and Orthopedic Surgery

Damien Zsiros and Mary Wollan

evolve WEBSITE

LEARNING OUTCOMES

1. Differentiate among the etiology, pathophysiology, clinical manifestations, and collaborative care of soft tissue injuries, including strains, sprains, dislocations, subluxations, bursitis, repetitive strain injury, carpal tunnel syndrome, and injuries to the rotator cuff, meniscus, and anterior cruciate ligament.
2. Relate the sequential events involved in fracture healing.
3. Compare closed reduction, cast immobilization, open reduction, and traction in terms of purpose, complications, and nursing management.
4. Evaluate the neurovascular assessment of an injured extremity.

5. Explain common complications associated with a fracture and fracture healing.
6. Describe the collaborative care and nursing management of patients with various kinds of fractures.
7. Describe the indications for and the collaborative care and nursing management of the patient with an amputation.
8. Describe the types of joint replacement surgery for arthritis and connective tissue disorders.
9. Prioritize the preoperative and postoperative management of the patient having joint replacement surgery.

KEY TERMS

arthrodesis, p. 1535
arthroplasty, p. 1534
bursitis, p. 1511
carpal tunnel syndrome (CTS), p. 1509
compartment syndrome, p. 1522
dislocation, p. 1508

fat embolism syndrome (FES), p. 1523
fracture, p. 1511
osteotomy, p. 1534
phantom limb sensation, p. 1531
repetitive strain injury (RSI), p. 1508

sprain, p. 1506
strain, p. 1506
subluxation, p. 1508
synovectomy, p. 1534
traction, p. 1514

Musculoskeletal problems resulting from trauma, along with common orthopedic surgical procedures, are discussed in this chapter. The nurse's role in prevention of complications and promotion of function in patients with fractures and orthopedic surgery is emphasized.

The most common cause of musculoskeletal injuries is a traumatic event resulting in fracture, dislocation, and/or soft tissue injuries. Although most of these injuries are not fatal, the cost in terms of pain, disability, medical expense, and lost wages is enormous. For all age-groups, accidents are exceeded

only by heart disease, cancer, chronic lower respiratory tract diseases, and strokes as a cause of death.[1] Accidental injuries (e.g., motor vehicle collisions, drowning, burns) are the leading cause of death in young adults in the United States.

It is important to teach the public about the basic principles of safety and accident prevention. The morbidity associated with accidents can be significantly reduced if people are aware of environmental hazards, use appropriate safety equipment, and apply safety and traffic rules. In the occupational and industrial setting, teach employees and employers about the

Reviewed by Julie Darby, RN, MSN, Assistant Professor, Baptist College of Health Sciences, Memphis, Tennessee.

use of proper safety equipment and avoidance of hazardous working situations.

SAFETY ALERT
- Falls account for many musculoskeletal injuries in the home environment.
- Provide preventive teaching to high-risk individuals (e.g., people with gait instability or visual or cognitive impairment).
- Stress the importance of wearing shoes with functional and stable soles and heels, avoiding wet or slippery surfaces, and removing throw rugs in the home.

TABLE 63-1   PATIENT & CAREGIVER TEACHING GUIDE

Prevention of Musculoskeletal Problems in Older Adults

To prevent musculoskeletal problems, include the following instructions when teaching older adults and their caregivers.
1. Use ramps in buildings and at street corners instead of steps to prevent falls.
2. Eliminate scatter rugs in the home.
3. Treat pain and discomfort from osteoarthritis.
   - Rest in positions that decrease discomfort.
   - Discuss use of medication for pain.
4. Use a walker or cane to help prevent falls.
5. Eat the amount and kind of foods to prevent excess weight gain because obesity adds stress to joints, which may predispose to osteoarthritis.
6. Get regular and frequent exercise.
   - Activities of daily living provide range-of-motion exercises. Tai Chi may also be helpful.
   - Hobbies (e.g., jigsaw puzzles, needlework, model building) exercise finger joints and prevent stiffness.
   - Performing weight-bearing exercise (e.g., walking) is essential and should be done on a daily basis.
7. Use shoes with good support to provide for safety and promote comfort.
8. Gradually initiate activities to promote optimal coordination. Rise slowly to a standing position to prevent dizziness, falls, and fractures.
9. Avoid walking on uneven surfaces and wet floors.

Ways to prevent common musculoskeletal problems in the older adult are listed in Table 63-1.

SOFT TISSUE INJURIES

Soft tissue injuries, which include sprains, strains, dislocations, and subluxations, are usually caused by trauma. The increasing number of people involved in a fitness program or participating in sports has contributed to the increased incidence of soft tissue injuries. Common sports-related injuries are summarized in Table 63-2. The most common sports injuries that result in a visit to the emergency department for younger patients are bruises, sprains and strains, tendinitis, and fractures.[2]

SPRAINS AND STRAINS

Sprains and strains are common injuries from abnormal stretching or twisting forces that may occur during vigorous activities. These injuries tend to occur around joints and in the spinal musculature.

A **sprain** is an injury to the ligamentous structures surrounding a joint, usually caused by a wrenching or twisting motion. Most sprains occur in the ankle, wrist, and knee joints.[3] A sprain is classified according to the degree of ligament damage. A *first-degree (mild) sprain* involves tears in only a few fibers, resulting in mild tenderness and minimal swelling. A *second-degree (moderate) sprain* is partial disruption of the involved tissue with more swelling and tenderness. A *third-degree (severe) sprain* is complete tearing of the ligament in association with moderate to severe swelling. A gap in the muscle may be apparent or palpated through the skin if the muscle is torn. Because areas around joints are rich in nerve endings, the injury can be extremely painful.

A **strain** is an excessive stretching of a muscle, its fascial sheath, or a tendon. Most strains occur in the large muscle groups, including the lower back, calf, and hamstrings. Strains may also be classified as first degree (mild or slightly pulled muscle), second degree (moderate or moderately

---

TABLE 63-2   SPORTS-RELATED INJURIES

Injury	Description	Treatment
Impingement syndrome	Entrapment of soft tissue structures under coracoacromial arch of shoulder.	NSAIDs. Rest until symptoms decrease and then gradual ROM and strengthening exercises.
Rotator cuff tear	Tear within muscle or tendinoligamentous structures around shoulder.	*If minor tear:* Rest, NSAIDs, and gradual mobilization with ROM and strengthening exercises. *If major tear:* Surgical repair.
Shin splints	Inflammation along anterior aspect of calf from periostitis caused by improper shoes, overuse, or running on hard pavement.	Rest, ice, NSAIDs, proper shoes. Gradual increase in activity. If pain persists, x-ray to rule out stress fracture of tibia.
Tendinitis	Inflammation of tendon as a result of overuse or incorrect use.	Rest, ice, NSAIDs. Gradual return to sport activity. Protective brace (orthosis) may be necessary if symptoms recur.
Ligament injury	Tearing or stretching of ligament. Usually occurs as a result of inversion, eversion, shearing, or torque applied to a joint. Characterized by sudden pain, swelling, and instability.	Rest, ice, elevation of extremity if possible, NSAIDs. Protection of affected extremity by use of brace. If symptoms persist, surgical repair may be necessary.
Meniscus injury	Injury to fibrocartilage of knee characterized by popping, clicking, tearing sensation, effusion, and/or swelling.	Rest, ice, elevation of extremity if possible, NSAIDs. Gradual return to regular activities. If symptoms persist, MRI to diagnose meniscus injury and possible arthroscopic surgery.
Anterior cruciate ligament tear	Traumatic tearing of ligament by deceleration forces together with pivoting or odd positions of the knee or leg.	Physical therapy with rehabilitation, knee brace. If knee instability or continued injuries, reconstructive surgery may be done.

torn muscle), and third degree (severely torn or ruptured muscle).

The clinical manifestations of sprains and strains are similar and include pain, edema, decreased function, and contusion. Pain aggravated by continued use is common. Edema develops in the injured area because of the local inflammatory response.

Mild sprains and strains are usually self-limiting, with full function returning within 3 to 6 weeks. X-rays of the affected part may be taken to rule out a fracture. A severe sprain can result in a concomitant *avulsion fracture,* in which the ligament pulls loose a fragment of bone. Alternatively, the joint structure may become unstable and result in subluxation or dislocation. At the time of injury, *hemarthrosis* (bleeding into a joint space or cavity) or disruption of the synovial lining may occur. Severe strains may require surgical repair of the muscle, tendon, or surrounding fascia.

NURSING MANAGEMENT
SPRAINS AND STRAINS

NURSING IMPLEMENTATION

HEALTH PROMOTION. Warming up muscles before exercising and vigorous activity, followed by stretching, may significantly reduce the risk of sprains and strains. Strength, balance, and endurance exercises are also important. Strengthening exercises that involve working against resistance build up muscle strength and bone density. Balance exercises, which may overlap with some strengthening exercises, help to prevent falling. Endurance exercises should start at a low level of effort and progress gradually to a moderate level.[4] Exercise instructions for these types of physical activity are available at *www.weboflife.ksc. nasa.gov/exerciseandaging.*

ACUTE INTERVENTION. If an injury occurs, the immediate care focuses on (1) stopping the activity and limiting movement, (2) applying ice compresses to the injured area, (3) compressing the involved extremity, (4) elevating the extremity, and (5) providing analgesia as necessary (Table 63-3).

RICE (*R*est, *I*ce, *C*ompression, *E*levation) may decrease local inflammation and pain for most musculoskeletal injuries. Movement should be restricted and the extremity rested as soon as pain is felt. Unless the injury is severe, prolonged rest is usually not indicated.

Cold *(cryotherapy)* in several forms can be used to produce hypothermia in the involved part. The cold induces physiologic changes in soft tissue, including vasoconstriction and a reduction in the transmission and perception of nerve pain impulses. In addition to pain relief, these changes reduce muscle spasms, inflammation, and edema. Cold is most useful when applied immediately after the injury has occurred. Ice applications should not exceed 20 to 30 minutes per application, and ice should not be applied directly to the skin.

An elastic compression bandage can be wrapped around the injured part. To prevent edema and encourage fluid return, wrap the bandage starting distally (at the point farthest from the midline of the body) and progress proximally (toward the midline of the body). The bandage is too tight if numbness is felt below the area of compression or there is additional pain or swelling beyond the edge of the bandage. The bandage can be left in place for 30 minutes and then removed for 15 minutes. However, some elastic wraps are left on during training, athletic, and occupational activities.

The injured part should be elevated above the heart level to help mobilize excess fluid from the area and prevent further

HEALTHY PEOPLE

Health Impact of Regular Physical Activity

- Assists in weight control.
- Helps maintain bone mass.
- Helps prevent high blood pressure.
- Increases lean muscle and decreases body fat.
- Increases muscle strength, flexibility, and endurance.
- Appears to reduce symptoms of depression and anxiety.
- Reduces the risk of heart disease, diabetes, and colon cancer.
- Enhances psychologic well-being and may reduce risk of depression.

✚ TABLE 63-3   EMERGENCY MANAGEMENT

Acute Soft Tissue Injury

Etiology	Assessment Findings	Interventions
• Falls • Direct blows • Crush injury • Motor vehicle collisions • Sports injuries	• Edema • Ecchymosis, contusion • Pain, tenderness • Decreased sensation with severe edema • Decreased pulse, coolness, and capillary refill >2 sec • Decreased movement • Pallor • Shortening or rotation of extremity • Inability to bear weight when lower extremity involved • Limited or decreased function with upper extremity involvement • Muscle spasms	**Initial** • Ensure airway, breathing, and circulation. • Assess neurovascular status of involved limb. • Elevate involved limb. • Apply compression bandage unless dislocation present. • Apply ice packs to affected area. • Immobilize affected extremity in the position found. Do *not* attempt to realign or reinsert protruding bones. • Anticipate x-rays of injured extremity. • Give analgesia as necessary. • Administer tetanus and diphtheria prophylaxis if there is a break in skin integrity or open fracture. • Administer antibiotic prophylaxis for open fracture, large tissue defects, or mangled extremity injury. **Ongoing Monitoring** • Monitor for changes in neurovascular status. • Eliminate weight bearing when lower extremity involved. • Anticipate compartment pressure monitoring if neurovascular status changes and compartment syndrome suspected.

edema. The injured part should be elevated even during sleep. Mild analgesics and nonsteroidal antiinflammatory drugs (NSAIDs) may be necessary to manage patient discomfort.

After the acute phase (usually 24 to 48 hours), warm, moist heat may be applied to the affected part to reduce swelling and provide comfort. Heat applications should not exceed 20 to 30 minutes, allowing a "cool-down" time between applications. Encourage the patient to use the limb, provided that the joint is protected by means of casting, bracing, taping, or splinting. Movement of the joint maintains nutrition to the cartilage, and muscle contraction improves circulation and resolution of the contusion and swelling.

AMBULATORY AND HOME CARE. Most sprains and strains are treated in the outpatient setting. Instruct the patient to use ice and elevate for 24 to 48 hours after the injury to reduce edema. Encourage the use of mild analgesics to promote comfort. Use of an elastic wrap may provide additional support during activity. Emphasize to the patient the importance of strengthening and conditioning exercises to prevent reinjury.

The physical therapist may help provide pain relief by modalities such as ultrasound. The therapist may also teach the patient exercises to perform for flexibility and strength.

DISLOCATION AND SUBLUXATION

A **dislocation** is a severe injury of the ligamentous structures that surround a joint. Dislocation results in the complete displacement or separation of the articular surfaces of the joint. A **subluxation** is a partial or incomplete displacement of the joint surface. The clinical manifestations of a subluxation are similar to those of a dislocation but are less severe.

Dislocations characteristically result from forces transmitted to the joint that disrupt the soft tissue support structures surrounding it. The joints most frequently dislocated in the upper extremity include the thumb, elbow, and shoulder. In the lower extremity, the hip is vulnerable to dislocation as a result of severe trauma, often associated with motor vehicle collisions (Fig. 63-1). The patella may dislocate because of a sharp blow to the kneecap or after a sudden twisting inward motion while the planted foot is pointed outward.[5]

The most obvious clinical manifestation of a dislocation is deformity. For example, if a hip is dislocated in a posterior (or backward) direction, the limb can be shorter and is often internally rotated on the affected side. Additional manifestations include local pain, tenderness, loss of function of the injured part, and swelling of the soft tissues in the joint region. The major complications of a dislocated joint are open joint injuries, intraarticular fractures, *avascular necrosis* (bone cell death as a result of inadequate blood supply), and damage to adjacent neurovascular tissue.

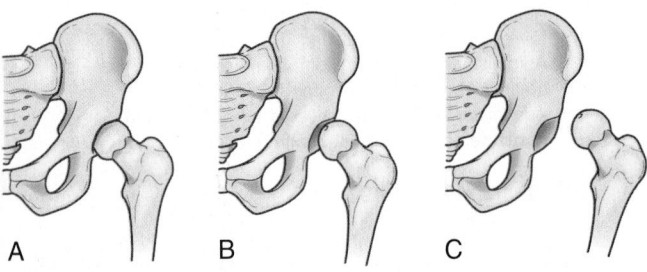

FIG. 63-1 Soft tissue injury of the hip. **A,** Normal. **B,** Subluxation (partial dislocation). **C,** Dislocation.

X-ray studies are performed to determine the extent of displacement of the involved structures. The joint may also be aspirated to assess for hemarthrosis or fat cells. Fat cells in the aspirate indicate a probable intraarticular (within the joint) fracture.

NURSING AND COLLABORATIVE MANAGEMENT DISLOCATION

A dislocation requires prompt attention and is often considered an orthopedic emergency. It may be associated with significant vascular injury. The longer the joint remains unreduced, the greater the possibility of avascular necrosis. The hip joint is particularly susceptible to avascular necrosis. Compartment syndrome (discussed on p. 1522) may also occur after a dislocation. Neurovascular assessment is critical (see pp. 1517–1518).

The first goal of management is to realign the dislocated portion of the joint in its original anatomic position. This can be accomplished by a closed reduction, which may be performed under local or general anesthesia or IV conscious sedation. Anesthesia is often necessary to relax the muscle so that the bones can be manipulated. In some situations, surgical open reduction may be necessary. After reduction, the extremity is usually immobilized by bracing, splinting, taping, or using a sling to allow the torn ligaments and capsular tissue time to heal.

Nursing management of subluxation or dislocation is directed toward relief of pain and support and protection of the injured joint. After the joint has been reduced and immobilized, motion is usually restricted. A carefully monitored rehabilitation program can prevent fracture instability and joint dysfunction. Gentle range-of-motion (ROM) exercises may be recommended if the joint is stable and well supported. An exercise program slowly restores the joint to its original ROM without causing another dislocation. The patient should gradually return to normal activities.

A patient who has dislocated a joint may be at greater risk for repeated dislocations because of loose ligaments. Activity restrictions may be imposed on the affected joint to decrease the risk of repeated dislocations.

REPETITIVE STRAIN INJURY

Repetitive strain injury (RSI) and *cumulative trauma disorder* are terms used to describe injuries resulting from prolonged force or repetitive movements and awkward postures. RSI is also referred to as repetitive trauma disorder, nontraumatic musculoskeletal injury, overuse syndrome (sports medicine), regional musculoskeletal disorder, and work-related musculoskeletal disorder. Repeated movements strain the tendons, ligaments, and muscles, causing tiny tears that become inflamed. The exact cause of these disorders is unknown. There are no specific diagnostic tests, and diagnosis is often difficult.

Persons at risk for RSI include musicians, dancers, butchers, grocery clerks, vibratory tool workers, and those who frequently use a computer mouse and keyboard. Competitive athletes and poorly trained athletes may also develop RSI. Swimming, overhead throwing (e.g., baseball), weight lifting, gymnastics, tennis, skiing, and kicking sports (e.g., soccer) require repetitive motion, and overtraining compounds the effects of RSI.

In addition to repetitive movements, other factors related to RSI include poor posture and positioning, poor workspace ergonomics, badly designed workplace equipment (e.g., computer keyboard), and repetitive lifting of heavy objects without sufficient muscle rest. The result may be inflammation, swelling, and pain in the muscles, tendons, and nerves of the neck, spine, shoulder, forearm, and hand. Symptoms of RSI include pain, weakness, numbness, or impairment of motor function. RSI can be prevented through education and *ergonomics* (the science that promotes efficiency and safety in the interaction of humans and their work environment). Ergonomic considerations for persons who work at a desk and use a computer include keeping the hips and knees flexed to 90 degrees with the feet flat, keeping the wrist straight to type, having the top of the computer monitor even with the forehead, and taking at least hourly stretch breaks. Once RSI is diagnosed, treatment consists of identification of the precipitating activity; modification of equipment or activity; pain management, including heat or cold application and NSAIDs; rest; physical therapy for strengthening and conditioning exercises; and lifestyle changes.

CARPAL TUNNEL SYNDROME

Carpal tunnel syndrome (CTS) is a condition caused by compression of the median nerve, which enters the hand through the narrow confines of the carpal tunnel (Fig. 63-2). The carpal tunnel is formed by ligaments and bones. CTS is the most common compression neuropathy in the upper extremity. This syndrome is associated with hobbies or occupations that require continuous wrist movement (e.g., musicians, carpenters, computer operators).

This condition is often caused by pressure from trauma or edema caused by inflammation of a tendon (tenosynovitis), neoplasm, rheumatoid arthritis, or soft tissue masses such as ganglia. Hormones may be involved, since initial manifestations of CTS often occur during the premenstrual period, pregnancy, and menopause. Persons with diabetes mellitus, peripheral vascular disease, and rheumatoid arthritis have a higher incidence of CTS because of swelling that changes blood flow to the nerve and narrows the carpal tunnel.[6] Women are more likely than men to develop CTS, possibly because of a smaller carpal tunnel.

The clinical manifestations of CTS are weakness, pain, numbness, or impaired sensation in the distribution of the median nerve (see Fig. 63-2). Numbness and tingling may awaken the patient at night. Shaking the hands often relieves these symptoms. Clumsiness in performing fine hand movements is also common.

Manifestations of CTS include a positive Tinel's sign and Phalen's sign. *Tinel's sign* can be elicited by tapping over the median nerve as it passes through the carpal tunnel in the wrist. A positive response is a sensation of tingling in the distribution of the median nerve over the hand. *Phalen's sign* can be elicited by allowing the wrists to fall freely into maximum flexion and maintain the position for longer than 60 seconds. A positive response is a sensation of tingling in the distribution of the median nerve over the hand. In late stages there is atrophy of the thenar muscles around the base of the thumb, resulting in recurrent pain and eventual dysfunction of the hand.

NURSING AND COLLABORATIVE MANAGEMENT
CARPAL TUNNEL SYNDROME

To prevent CTS, teach employees and employers to identify risk factors. Adaptive devices such as wrist splints may be worn to hold the wrist in a slight extension and relieve pressure on the median nerve. Special keyboard pads and mouses that help prevent repetitive pressure on the median nerve are available for computer users. Other ergonomic changes include workstation modifications, change in body positions, and frequent breaks from work-related activities.

Collaborative care of the patient with CTS is directed toward relieving the underlying cause of the nerve compression. The early symptoms associated with CTS can usually be relieved by stopping the aggravating movement and by resting the hand and wrist by immobilizing them in a hand splint. Splints worn at night help keep the wrist in a neutral position and may reduce night pain and numbness. Physical therapy with hand and wrist exercises may lessen symptom severity. Injection of a corticosteroid drug directly into the carpal tunnel may provide short-term relief. The patient may need to consider a change in occupation because of discomfort and sensory changes.

Carpal tunnel release is generally recommended if symptoms last for more than 6 months. Surgery involves severing the band of tissue around the wrist to reduce pressure on the median nerve (see Fig. 63-2). Surgery is done in the outpatient setting using local anesthesia. The types of carpal tunnel release surgery include open release and endoscopic surgery.[6] In *open release surgery* an incision is made in the wrist and then the carpal ligament is cut to enlarge the carpal tunnel. *Endoscopic carpal tunnel release* is performed through one or more small puncture incisions in the wrist and palm. A camera is attached to a tube, and the carpal ligament is cut. The endoscopic approach may allow for a faster recovery and less postoperative discomfort than traditional open release surgery.

Although symptoms may be relieved immediately after surgery, full recovery may take months. After surgery, assess the hand's neurovascular status. Instruct the patient about wound care and the appropriate assessments to perform at home.

ROTATOR CUFF INJURY

The rotator cuff is a complex of four muscles in the shoulder: the supraspinatus, infraspinatus, teres minor, and subscapularis muscles. These muscles act to stabilize the humeral head in the glenoid fossa while assisting with the ROM of the shoulder joint and rotation of the humerus.

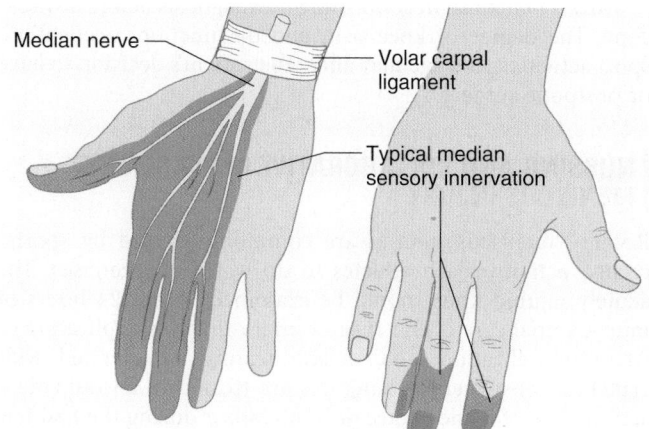

FIG. 63-2 Wrist structures involved in carpal tunnel syndrome. Median nerve distribution. Shaded areas depict the locations of pain in carpal tunnel syndrome.

Median nerve

Volar carpal ligament

Typical median sensory innervation

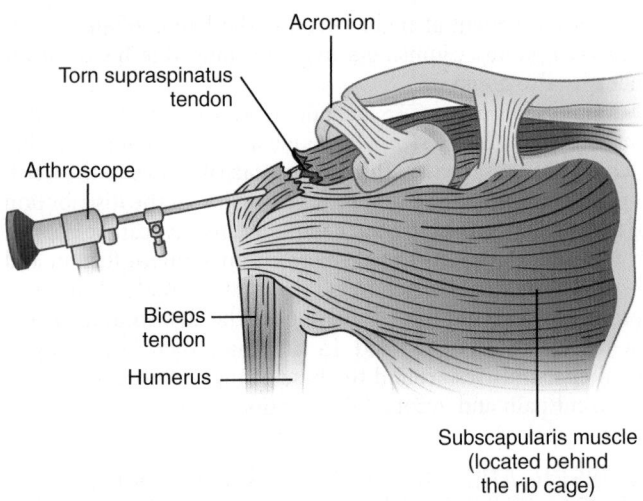

FIG. 63-3 A torn rotator cuff is repaired using arthroscopic surgery.

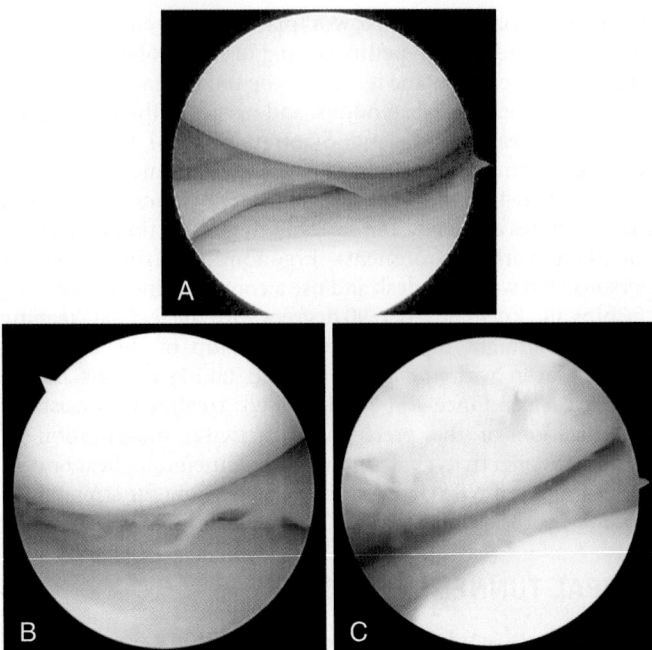

FIG. 63-4 Arthroscopic views of the meniscus. **A,** Normal meniscus. **B,** Torn meniscus. **C,** Surgically repaired meniscus.

A tear in the rotator cuff may occur as a gradual, degenerative process resulting from aging, repetitive stress (especially overhead arm motions), or injury to the shoulder while falling. The rotator cuff can tear as a result of sudden adduction forces applied to the cuff while the arm is held in abduction. In sports, repetitive overhead motions, such as in swimming, weight lifting, and swinging a racquet (tennis, racquetball) often cause injury. Other causes include (1) falling onto an outstretched arm and hand, (2) a blow to the upper arm, (3) heavy lifting, or (4) repetitive work motions.

Manifestations of a rotator cuff injury include shoulder weakness and pain and decreased ROM. The patient usually experiences severe pain when the arm is abducted between 60 and 120 degrees (the painful arc). The *drop arm test,* in which the arm falls suddenly after the patient is asked to slowly lower the arm to the side after it has been abducted 90 degrees, is another sign of rotator cuff injury. An x-ray alone is usually not beneficial in the diagnosis. A tear can usually be confirmed by magnetic resonance imaging (MRI).

The patient with a partial tear or cuff inflammation may be treated conservatively with rest, ice and heat, NSAIDs, corticosteroid injections into the joint, ultrasound, and physical therapy.[7] If the patient does not respond to conservative treatment or if a complete tear is present, surgical repair may be necessary. Most surgical repairs are performed as outpatient procedures through an arthroscope (Fig. 63-3). If the tear is extensive, an *acromioplasty* (surgical removal of part of the acromion to relieve compression of the rotator cuff during movement) may be done. A sling or, more commonly, a shoulder immobilizer may be used immediately after surgery to limit shoulder movement. However, the shoulder should not be immobilized for too long because "frozen" shoulder or arthrofibrosis may occur. Pendulum exercises and physical therapy begin the first postoperative day. Restrictions for lifting weights are usually given, with full recovery taking up to 6 months.

MENISCUS INJURY

The menisci are crescent-shaped pieces of fibrocartilage in the knee. Menisci are also found in other joints. Meniscus injuries are closely associated with ligament sprains common among athletes in sports such as basketball, football, soccer, and hockey.

These activities produce rotational stress when the knee is in varying degrees of flexion and the foot is planted or fixed. A blow to the knee can cause the meniscus to be sheared between the femoral condyles and the tibial plateau, resulting in a torn meniscus. (The knee joint is shown in eFig. 63-1 on the website for this chapter.) People who work in occupations that require squatting or kneeling and older patients may be at risk for degenerative tears.

Meniscus injuries alone do not usually cause significant edema because most of the cartilage is avascular. However, an acutely torn meniscus may be suspected when localized tenderness, pain, and effusion are noted (Fig. 63-4). Pain is elicited by flexion, internal rotation, and then extension of the knee (called *McMurray's test*). The patient may feel that the knee is unstable and often reports that the knee "clicks," "pops," "locks," or "gives way." Quadriceps atrophy is usually evident if the injury has been present for some time. Traumatic arthritis may occur from repeated meniscus injury and chronic inflammation.

MRI is beneficial in confirming the diagnosis before arthroscopy. The degree of knee pain and dysfunction, occupation, sport activities, and age may affect the patient's decision to have or postpone surgery.

NURSING AND COLLABORATIVE MANAGEMENT MENISCUS INJURY

Because meniscus injuries are commonly caused by sports-related activity, teach athletes to do warm-up exercises. The acutely injured knee should be examined within 24 hours of injury. Initial care of this type of injury involves application of ice, immobilization, and weight bearing as tolerated with crutches. Most meniscus injuries are treated in an outpatient setting. Use of a knee brace or immobilizer during the first few days after the injury protects the knee and offers some pain relief. After acute pain has decreased, physical therapy can help the patient regain knee flexion and muscle strength to assist in returning to full function. In older adults with degenerative meniscus tears, progressive exercise therapy may improve neuromuscular function and muscle strength.[8]

Surgical repair or excision of part of the meniscus (meniscectomy) may be necessary (see Fig. 63-4). Meniscal surgery is performed by arthroscopy. Pain relief may include NSAIDs or other analgesics. Rehabilitation starts soon after surgery, including quadriceps and hamstring strengthening exercises and ROM. When the patient's strength is back to its preinjury level, normal activities may be resumed.

ANTERIOR CRUCIATE LIGAMENT INJURY

Knee injuries account for more than 50% of all sport injuries. The most commonly injured knee ligament is the anterior cruciate ligament (ACL). ACL injuries are usually noncontact injuries that occur when the athlete pivots, lands from a jump, or slows down when running. Patients often report coming down on the knee, twisting, and hearing a pop, followed by acute knee pain and swelling. Athletes usually cannot continue playing, and the knee may feel unstable. An injury to the ACL can result in a partial tear, a complete tear, or an *avulsion* (tearing away) from the bone attachments that form the knee (Fig. 63-5).

Examination of the knee with an ACL tear may produce a positive *Lachman's test*.[9] This test is performed by flexing the knee 15 to 30 degrees and pulling the tibia forward while the femur is stabilized. The test is considered positive for an ACL tear if there is forward motion of the tibia with the feeling of a soft or indistinct endpoint. MRI is often used to diagnose coexisting conditions, including a fracture, meniscus tearing, and collateral ligament injuries.

NURSING AND COLLABORATIVE MANAGEMENT ANTERIOR CRUCIATE LIGAMENT INJURY

Prevention programs have been shown to significantly reduce ACL injuries in athletes.[10] Conservative treatment for an intact ACL injury includes rest, ice, NSAIDs, elevation, and ambulation as tolerated with crutches. If there is a tight, painful effu-

sion, it may be aspirated. A knee immobilizer or hinged knee brace may be helpful in supporting the knee. Physical therapy often assists the patient in maintaining knee joint motion and muscle tone.

Reconstructive surgery is usually recommended in physically active patients who have sustained severe injury to the ligament and the meniscus. In reconstruction the torn ACL tissue is removed and replaced with autologous or allograft tissue. ROM is encouraged soon after surgery, and the knee is placed in a brace or immobilizer. Rehabilitation with physical therapy is critical with progressive weight bearing determined by the degree of surgical repair. A safe return to the patient's prior level of physical functioning may take 6 to 8 months.

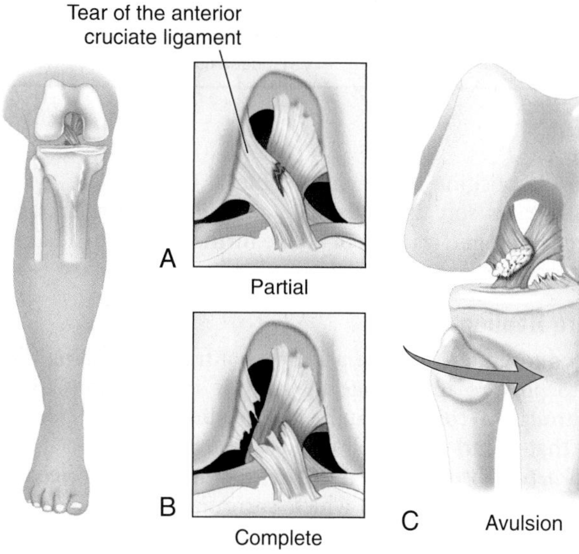

BURSITIS

Bursae are closed sacs that are lined with synovial membrane and contain a small amount of synovial fluid. They are located at sites of friction, such as between tendons and bones and near the joints. Bursitis (inflammation of the bursa) results from repeated or excessive trauma or friction, gout, rheumatoid arthritis, or infection.

The primary clinical manifestations of bursitis are warmth, pain, swelling, and limited ROM in the affected part. Sites at which bursitis commonly occurs include hands, knees, greater trochanters of the hip, shoulders, and elbows. Improper body mechanics, repetitive kneeling (carpet layers, coal miners, and gardeners), jogging in worn-out shoes, and prolonged sitting with crossed legs are common precipitating activities.

Attempts are made to determine and correct the cause of the bursitis. Rest is often the only treatment needed. The affected part may be immobilized in a compression dressing or splint. Ice and NSAIDs may be used to reduce pain and inflammation.[11] Aspiration of the bursal fluid and intraarticular injection of a corticosteroid may be necessary. If the bursal wall has become thickened and continues to interfere with normal joint function, surgical excision (bursectomy) is often done. Septic bursae usually require surgical incision and drainage.

FRACTURES

Classification

A fracture is a disruption or break in the continuity of the structure of bone. Although traumatic injuries account for the majority of fractures, some fractures are secondary to a disease process (pathologic fractures from cancer or osteoporosis).

Fractures can be classified as *open* (formerly called compound) or *closed* (formerly called simple) depending on communication or noncommunication with the external environment (Fig. 63-6). In an *open fracture* the skin is broken, exposing bone and causing soft tissue injury. In a *closed fracture* the skin has not been ruptured and remains intact.

Fractures can also be classified as complete or incomplete. Fractures are termed *complete* if the break is completely through the bone and *incomplete* if the fracture occurs partly across a bone shaft but the bone is still in one piece. An incomplete fracture is often the result of bending or crushing forces applied to a bone.

Fractures are also described and classified according to the direction of the fracture line. Types include linear, oblique, transverse, longitudinal, and spiral fractures (Fig. 63-7).

FIG. 63-5 Anterior cruciate ligament (ACL) injury. **A,** Partial tear. **B,** Complete tear. **C,** Avulsion.

Tear of the anterior cruciate ligament

A Partial

B Complete

C Avulsion

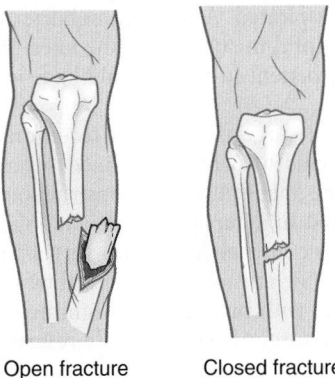

Open fracture   Closed fracture

FIG. 63-6 Fracture classification according to communication with the external environment.

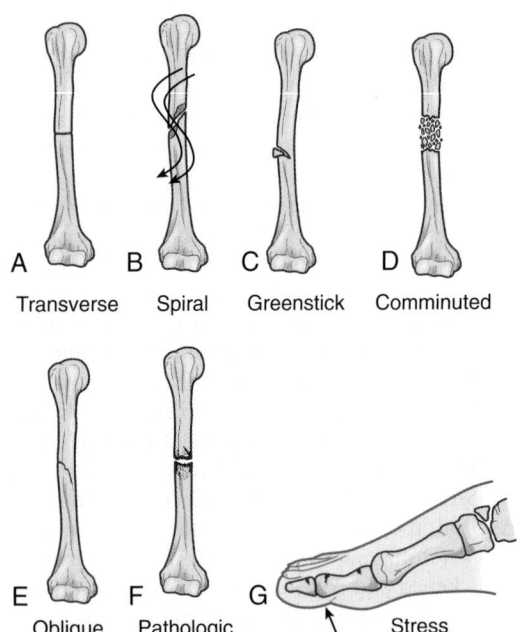

FIG. 63-7 Types of fractures. **A,** Transverse fracture: the line of the fracture extends across the bone shaft at a right angle to the longitudinal axis. **B,** Spiral fracture: the line of the fracture extends in a spiral direction along the bone shaft. **C,** Greenstick fracture: an incomplete fracture with one side splintered and the other side bent. **D,** Comminuted fracture: a fracture with more than two fragments. The smaller fragments appear to be floating. **E,** Oblique fracture: the line of the fracture extends in an oblique direction. **F,** Pathologic fracture: a spontaneous fracture at the site of a bone disease. **G,** Stress fracture: occurs in normal or abnormal bone that is subject to repeated stress, such as from jogging or running.

TABLE 63-4	**MANIFESTATIONS OF FRACTURE**
Manifestation	**Significance**
Edema and Swelling Disruption and penetration of bone through skin or soft tissues, or bleeding into surrounding tissues.	Unchecked bleeding, swelling, and edema in closed space can occlude circulation and damage nerves (e.g., risk of compartment syndrome).
Pain and Tenderness Muscle spasm as a result of involuntary reflex action of muscle, direct tissue trauma, increased pressure on nerves, movement of fracture parts.	Pain and tenderness encourage splinting of muscle around fracture with reduction in motion of injured area.
Muscle Spasm Irritation of tissues and protective response to injury and fracture.	Muscle spasms may displace nondisplaced fracture or prevent it from reducing spontaneously.
Deformity Abnormal position of extremity or part as result of original forces of injury and action of muscles pulling fragment into abnormal position. Seen as a loss of normal bony contours.	Deformity is cardinal sign of fracture. If uncorrected, it may result in problems with bony union and restoration of function of injured part.
Ecchymosis, Contusion Discoloration of skin as a result of extravasation of blood in subcutaneous tissues.	Ecchymosis may appear immediately after injury and may appear distal to injury. Reassure patient that process is normal and discoloration will eventually resolve.
Loss of Function Disruption of bone or joint, preventing functional use of limb or part.	Fracture must be managed properly to ensure restoration of function to limb or part.
Crepitation Grating or crunching together of bony fragments, producing palpable or audible crunching or popping sensation.	Crepitation may increase chance for nonunion if bone ends are allowed to move excessively. Micromovement of bone-end fragments (postfracture) assists in osteogenesis (new bone growth).

Fractures can also be classified as displaced or nondisplaced. In a *displaced* fracture the two ends of the broken bone are separated from one another and out of their normal positions. Displaced fractures are usually *comminuted* (more than two fragments) or *oblique* (see Fig. 63-7). In a *nondisplaced* fracture the periosteum is intact across the fracture and the bone is still in alignment. Nondisplaced fractures are usually transverse, spiral, or greenstick (see Fig. 63-7).

Clinical Manifestations

The clinical manifestations include immediate localized pain, decreased function, and inability to bear weight on or use the affected part (Table 63-4). The patient guards and protects the extremity against movement. Obvious bone deformity may not be present. If a fracture is suspected, the extremity is immobi-

lized in the position in which it is found. Unnecessary movement increases soft tissue damage and may convert a closed fracture to an open fracture or create further injury to adjacent neurovascular structures.

Fracture Healing

You need to understand the principles of fracture healing (Fig. 63-8) to provide appropriate therapeutic interventions. Bone goes through a complex multistage healing process (termed *union*) that occurs in the following stages:[12]

1. *Fracture hematoma:* When a fracture occurs, bleeding creates a hematoma, which surrounds the ends of the fragments. The hematoma is extravasated blood that changes from a liquid to a semisolid clot. This occurs in the initial 72 hours after injury.

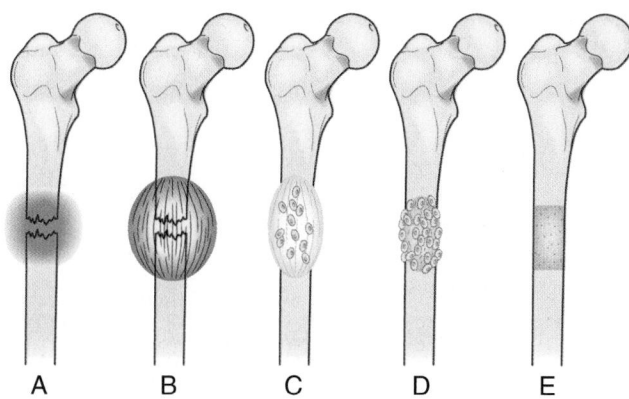

FIG. 63-8 Bone healing (schematic representation). **A,** Bleeding at fractured ends of the bone with subsequent hematoma formation. **B,** Organization of hematoma into fibrous network. **C,** Invasion of osteoblasts, lengthening of collagen strands, and deposition of calcium. **D,** Callus formation: new bone is built up as osteoclasts destroy dead bone. **E,** Remodeling is accomplished as excess callus is resorbed and trabecular bone is laid down.

TABLE 63-5 COMPLICATIONS OF FRACTURE HEALING

Complication	Description
Delayed union	Fracture healing progresses more slowly than expected. Healing eventually occurs.
Nonunion	Fracture fails to heal despite treatment. No x-ray evidence of callus formation.
Malunion	Fracture heals in expected time but in unsatisfactory position, possibly resulting in deformity or dysfunction.
Angulation	Fracture heals in abnormal position in relation to midline of structure (type of malunion).
Pseudoarthrosis	Type of nonunion occurring at fracture site in which a false joint is formed with abnormal movement at site.
Refracture	New fracture occurs at original fracture site.
Myositis ossificans	Deposition of calcium in muscle tissue at site of significant blunt muscle trauma or repeated muscle injury.

TABLE 63-6 COLLABORATIVE CARE

Fractures

Diagnostic
- History and physical examination
- X-ray
- CT scan, MRI

Collaborative Therapy
Fracture Reduction
- Manipulation
- Closed reduction
- Skin traction
- Skeletal traction
- Open reduction

Fracture Immobilization
- Casting or splinting
- Traction
- External fixation
- Internal fixation

Open Fractures
- Surgical debridement and irrigation
- Tetanus and diphtheria immunization
- Prophylactic antibiotic therapy
- Immobilization

2. *Granulation tissue:* During this stage, active phagocytosis absorbs the products of local necrosis. The hematoma converts to granulation tissue. Granulation tissue (consisting of new blood vessels, fibroblasts, and osteoblasts) produces the basis for new bone substance called *osteoid* during days 3 to 14 postinjury.
3. *Callus formation:* As minerals (calcium, phosphorus, and magnesium) and new bone matrix are deposited in the osteoid, an unorganized network of bone is formed that is woven about the fracture parts. *Callus* is primarily composed of cartilage, osteoblasts, calcium, and phosphorus. It usually appears by the end of the second week after injury. Evidence of callus formation can be verified by x-ray.
4. *Ossification:* Ossification of the callus occurs from 3 weeks to 6 months after the fracture and continues until the fracture has healed. Callus ossification is sufficient to prevent movement at the fracture site when the bones are gently stressed. However, the fracture is still evident on x-ray. During this stage of *clinical union,* the patient may be allowed limited mobility or the cast may be removed.
5. *Consolidation:* As callus continues to develop, the distance between bone fragments diminishes and eventually closes. During this stage ossification continues. It can be equated with *radiologic union,* which occurs when there is x-ray evidence of complete bony union. This phase can occur up to 1 year after injury.
6. *Remodeling:* Excess bone tissue is resorbed in the final stage of bone healing, and union is complete. Gradual return of the injured bone to its preinjury structural strength and shape occurs. Bone remodels in response to physical loading stress or Wolf's law. Initially, stress is provided through exercise. Weight bearing is gradually introduced. New bone is deposited in sites subjected to stress and resorbed at areas where there is little stress.

Many factors influence the time required for complete fracture healing, including displacement and site of the fracture, blood supply to the area, immobilization, and internal fixation devices (e.g., screws, pins). The ossification process may be arrested by inadequate reduction and immobilization, excessive movement of the fracture fragments, infection, poor nutrition, and systemic disease. Healing time for fractures increases with age. For example, an uncomplicated midshaft fracture of the femur heals in 3 weeks in a newborn and in 20 weeks in an adult. Smoking also increases fracture healing time. Fracture healing may not occur in the expected time (*delayed union*) or may not occur at all (*nonunion*). Table 63-5 summarizes complications of fracture healing.

Collaborative Care

The overall goals of fracture treatment are (1) anatomic realignment of bone fragments (reduction), (2) immobilization to maintain realignment, and (3) restoration of normal or near-normal function of the injured part. Table 63-6 summarizes the collaborative care of fractures.

Fracture Reduction

Closed Reduction. *Closed reduction* is a nonsurgical, manual realignment of bone fragments to their previous anatomic position. Traction and countertraction are manually applied to the bone fragments to restore position, length, and alignment. Closed reduction is usually performed while the patient is under local or general anesthesia. After reduction, traction, casting, external fixation, splints, or orthoses (braces) immobilize the injured part to maintain alignment until healing occurs.

Open Reduction. *Open reduction* is the correction of bone alignment through a surgical incision. It usually includes internal fixation of the fracture with wires, screws, pins, plates, intramedullary rods, or nails. The type and location of the fracture, patient age, and concurrent disease may influence the decision to use open reduction. The main disadvantages of this form of fracture management are the possibility of infection, complications associated with anesthesia, and effect of preexisting medical conditions (e.g., diabetes).

If open reduction with internal fixation (ORIF) is used for intraarticular fractures, early initiation of ROM of the joint is indicated. Machines that provide continuous passive motion (CPM) to various joints (e.g., knee, shoulder) are used to prevent extraarticular and intraarticular adhesions. The use of CPM results in faster reconstruction of the subchondral (beneath cartilage) bone plate, more rapid healing of the articular cartilage, and decreased incidence of posttraumatic arthritis. ORIF facilitates early ambulation, thus decreasing the risk of complications related to prolonged immobility.

Traction. Traction is the application of a pulling force to an injured or diseased part of the body or an extremity. *Countertraction* pulls in the opposite direction. Traction is used to (1) prevent or reduce pain and muscle spasm associated with low back pain or cervical sprain (e.g., whiplash), (2) immobilize a joint or part of the body, (3) reduce a fracture or dislocation, and (4) treat a pathologic joint condition (e.g., tumor, infection). Traction is also indicated to (1) provide immobilization to prevent soft tissue damage, (2) promote active and passive exercise, (3) expand a joint space during arthroscopic procedures, and (4) expand a joint space before major joint reconstruction.

Traction devices apply a pulling force on a fractured extremity to attain realignment while countertraction pulls in the opposite direction. The two most common types of traction are skin traction and skeletal traction. *Skin traction* is generally used for short-term treatment (48 to 72 hours) until skeletal traction or surgery is possible. Tape, boots, or splints are applied directly to the skin to maintain alignment, assist in reduction, and help diminish muscle spasms in the injured extremity. The traction weights are usually limited to 5 to 10 lb (2.3 to 4.5 kg). A *Buck's traction* boot is a type of skin traction used to immobilize a fracture, prevent hip flexion contractures, and reduce muscle spasms (Fig. 63-9). Pelvic or cervical skin traction may require heavier weights applied intermittently. In skin traction, assessment of the skin is a priority, since pressure points and skin breakdown may develop quickly. Assess key pressure points every 2 to 4 hours.

Skeletal traction, generally in place for longer periods than skin traction, is used to align injured bones and joints or to treat joint contractures and congenital hip dysplasia. It provides a long-term pull that keeps the injured bones and joints aligned. To apply skeletal traction, the physician inserts a pin or wire into the bone, either partially or completely, to align and immobilize the injured body part.[13] Weight for skeletal traction ranges

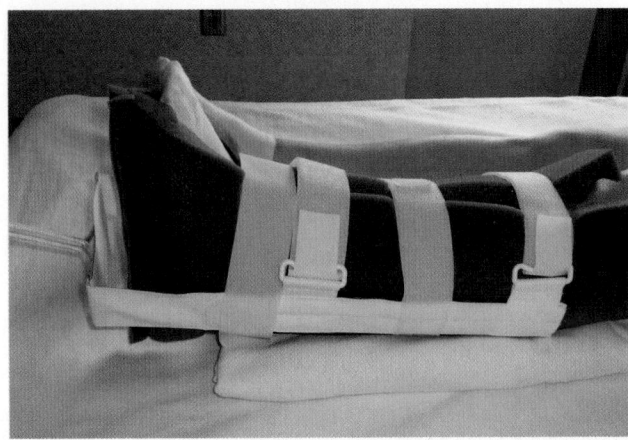

FIG. 63-9 Buck's traction is most commonly used for fractures of the hip and femur.

from 5 to 45 lb (2.3 to 20.4 kg). The use of too much weight can result in delayed union or nonunion. The major complications of skeletal traction are infection in the area of the bone where the skeletal pin is inserted and the consequences of prolonged immobility.

When traction is used to treat fractures, the forces are usually exerted on the distal fragment to align it with the proximal fragment. Several types of traction are used for this purpose. One of the more common types of skeletal traction is balanced suspension traction (Fig. 63-10). Fracture alignment depends on

---

DELEGATION DECISIONS

Caring for the Patient With a Cast or Traction

Role of Registered Nurse (RN)
- Perform neurovascular assessments on the affected extremity.
- Assess for clinical manifestations of compartment syndrome.
- Monitor cast during drying for denting or flattening.
- Teach patient and caregiver about cast care and complications of casting.
- Determine correct body alignment to enhance traction.
- Instruct patient and caregiver about traction and correct body positioning.
- Teach patient and caregiver range-of-motion (ROM) exercises.
- Assess for complications associated with immobility or fracture (e.g., wound infection, constipation, deep vein thrombosis, renal calculi, atelectasis).
- Develop plan to minimize complications associated with immobility or fracture.

Role of Licensed Practical/Vocational Nurse (LPN/LVN)
- Check color, temperature, capillary refill, and pulses distal to the cast.
- Mark circumference of any drainage on the cast.
- Monitor skin integrity around cast and at traction connections.
- Pad cast edges and traction connections to prevent skin irritation.
- Monitor pain level and administer prescribed analgesics.
- Notify RN of changes in pain or if pain persists after prescribed analgesics are administered.

Role of Unlicensed Assistive Personnel (UAP)
- Position casted extremity above heart level.
- Apply ice to cast as directed by RN.
- Maintain body position and integrity of traction (after being trained and evaluated in this procedure).
- Assist patient with passive and active ROM exercises.
- Notify RN about patient complaints of pain, tingling, or decreased sensation in the affected extremity.

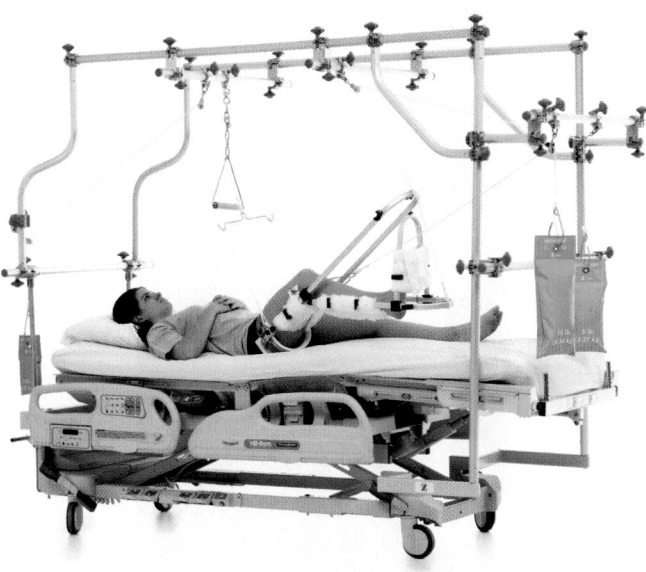

FIG. 63-10 Balanced suspension skeletal traction. Most commonly used for fractures of the femur, hip, and lower leg. Courtesy Zimmer, Inc.

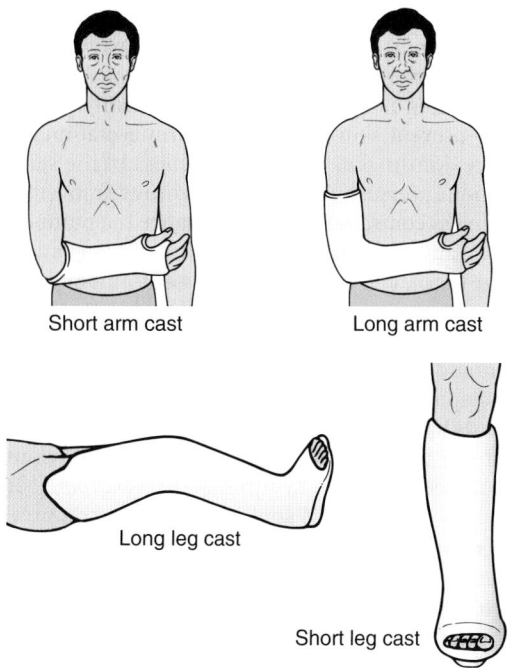

Short arm cast   Long arm cast

Long leg cast

Short leg cast

FIG. 63-11 Common types of casts.

the correct positioning and alignment of the patient while the traction forces remain constant. For extremity traction to be effective, forces must be pulling in the opposite direction (countertraction). Countertraction is commonly supplied by the patient's body weight or by weights pulling in the opposite direction, and it may be augmented by elevating the end of the bed. It is imperative to maintain traction continuously and to keep the weights off the floor and moving freely through the pulleys.

Fracture Immobilization. Fracture immobilization can be done using casts, braces, splints, immobilizers, and external and internal fixation devices.

Casts. A *cast* is a temporary circumferential immobilization device. Casting is a common treatment following closed reduction. It allows the patient to perform many normal activities of daily living while providing sufficient immobilization to ensure stability. Cast materials are natural (plaster of paris), synthetic acrylic, fiberglass-free, latex-free polymer, or a hybrid of materials. A cast generally incorporates the joints above and below a fracture. Immobilization above and below a joint restricts tendon and ligament movement, thereby assisting with joint stabilization while the fracture heals.

To apply a cast on an extremity, first cover the affected part with a stockinette that is cut longer than the extremity.[14] Then place padding over the stockinette with the bony prominences given extra padding. If plaster of paris casting material is used, it is usually immersed in warm water, then wrapped and molded around the affected part. The number of layers of plaster bandage and the technique of application determine the strength of the cast. The plaster sets within 15 minutes, so the patient may move around without difficulty. However, it is not strong enough for weight bearing until about 24 to 72 hours after application. (The decision about weight bearing is determined by the physician.)

A fresh plaster cast should never be covered because air cannot circulate, heat builds up in the cast that may cause a burn, and drying is delayed. Avoid direct pressure on the cast during the drying period. Handle the cast gently with an open palm to avoid denting the cast. Once the cast is thoroughly dry, the edges may need to be *petaled* to avoid skin irritation from

rough edges and to prevent plaster of paris debris from falling into the cast and causing irritation or pressure necrosis. The health care provider places several strips (petals) of tape over the rough areas to ensure a smooth cast edge.

Casts made of synthetic materials are being used more than plaster because they are lightweight, stronger, and relatively waterproof and provide for early weight bearing. The synthetic casting materials (thermolabile plastic, thermoplastic resins, polyurethane, and fiberglass) are activated by submersion in cool or tepid water. Then they are molded to fit the torso or extremity.

Upper Extremity Injuries. Immobilization of an acute fracture or soft tissue injury of the upper extremity is often accomplished by use of a (1) sugar-tong splint, (2) posterior splint, (3) short arm cast, or (4) long arm cast (Fig. 63-11). The *sugar-tong splint* is typically used for acute wrist injuries or injuries that may result in significant swelling. Plaster splints are applied over a well-padded forearm, beginning at the phalangeal joints of the hand, extending up the dorsal aspect of the forearm around the distal humerus, and then extending down the volar aspect of the forearm to the distal palmar crease. The splinting material is wrapped with either elastic bandage or bias stockinette. The sugar-tong posterior splint accommodates postinjury swelling in the fractured extremity.

The *short arm cast* is often used for the treatment of stable wrist or metacarpal fractures. An aluminum finger splint can be incorporated into the short arm cast for concurrent treatment of phalangeal injuries. The short arm cast is a circular cast extending from the distal palmar crease to the proximal forearm. This cast provides wrist immobilization and permits unrestricted elbow motion.

The *long arm cast* is commonly used for stable forearm or elbow fractures and unstable wrist fractures. It is similar to the short arm cast but extends to the proximal humerus, restricting motion at the wrist and elbow. Direct your care in supporting the extremity and reducing the effects of edema by elevating the extremity with a sling. However, when a hanging arm cast is used for a proximal humerus fracture, elevation or a supportive sling is contraindicated because hanging provides traction and maintains fracture alignment.

When a sling is used, ensure that the axillary area is well padded to prevent skin excoriation and maceration associated with direct skin-to-skin contact. Placement of the sling should not put undue pressure on the neck. Encourage movement of the fingers (unless contraindicated) to enhance the pumping action of vascular and soft tissue structures to decrease edema. Also encourage the patient to actively move nonimmobilized joints of the upper extremity to prevent stiffness and contractures.

Vertebral Injuries. The *body jacket brace* is used for immobilization and support for stable spine injuries of the thoracic or lumbar spine. The brace goes around the chest and abdomen and extends from above the nipple line to the pubis. After application of the brace, assess the patient for the development of superior mesenteric artery syndrome *(cast syndrome)*. This condition occurs if the brace is applied too tightly, compressing the superior mesenteric artery against the duodenum. The patient generally complains of abdominal pain, abdominal pressure, nausea, and vomiting. Assess the abdomen for decreased bowel sounds (a window in the brace may be left over the umbilicus). Treatment includes gastric decompression with a nasogastric (NG) tube and suction. Assessment also includes monitoring respiratory status, bowel and bladder function, and areas of pressure over the bony prominences, especially the iliac crest. The brace may need to be adjusted or removed if any complications occur.

Lower Extremity Injuries. Injuries to the lower extremity are often immobilized by a long leg cast, a short leg cast, a cylinder cast, a Robert Jones dressing, or a prefabricated splint or immobilizer. The usual indications for applying a long leg cast are an unstable ankle fracture, soft tissue injuries, a fractured tibia, and knee injuries. The cast usually extends from the base of the toes to the groin and gluteal crease. The short leg cast can be used for a variety of conditions, but primarily for stable ankle and foot injuries. A cylinder cast, which is used for knee injuries or fractures, extends from the groin to the malleoli of the ankle. A Robert Jones dressing is composed of bulky padding materials (absorption dressing and cotton sheet wadding), splints, and an elastic wrap or bias-cut stockinette.

After application of a lower extremity cast or dressing, the extremity should be elevated on pillows above the heart level for the first 24 hours. After the initial phase, a casted extremity should not be placed in a dependent position because of the possibility of excessive edema. After cast application, observe for signs of compartment syndrome (discussed on p. 1522 later in this chapter) and increased pressure, especially in the heel, anterior tibia, head of the fibula, and malleoli. This increased pressure is manifested by pain or a burning feeling in these areas.

Prefabricated knee and ankle splints and immobilizers are used in many settings. This type of immobilization is easy to apply and remove, which permits close observation of the affected joint for swelling and skin breakdown (Fig. 63-12). Depending on the injury, removal of the splint or immobilizer facilitates ROM of the affected joint and a faster return to function.

The *hip spica cast* is now mainly used for femur fractures in children. The purpose of the hip spica cast is to immobilize the affected extremity and the trunk. The hip spica cast extends from above the nipple line to the base of the foot (single spica) and may include the opposite extremity up to an area above the

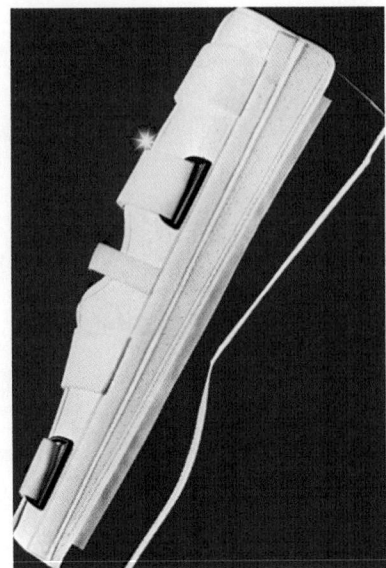

FIG. 63-12 Knee immobilizer.

knee (spica and a half) or both extremities (double spica). Assess the patient with a hip spica cast for the same problems that are associated with the body jacket brace.

External Fixation. An external fixator is a metallic device composed of metal pins that are inserted into the bone and attached to external rods to stabilize the fracture while it heals. It can be used to apply traction or to compress fracture fragments and to immobilize reduced fragments when the use of a cast or other traction is not appropriate. The external device holds fracture fragments in place similar to a surgically implanted internal device. The external fixator is attached directly to the bones by percutaneous transfixing pins or wires (Fig. 63-13). External fixation is indicated in simple fractures, complex fractures with extensive soft tissue damage, correction of bony defects (congenital), nonunion or malunion, and limb lengthening.

External fixation is often used in an attempt to salvage extremities that otherwise might require amputation. Because the use of an external device is a long-term process, ongoing assessment for pin loosening and infection is critical. Infection signaled by exudate, erythema, tenderness, and pain may require removal of the device. Instruct the patient and caregiver about meticulous pin care. Although each physician has a protocol for pin care cleaning, half-strength hydrogen peroxide with normal saline is often used.

Internal Fixation. Internal fixation devices (pins, plates, intramedullary rods, and metal and bioabsorbable screws) are surgically inserted to realign and maintain bony fragments (Fig. 63-14 and eFig. 63-2 on the website for this chapter). These metal devices are biologically inert and made from stainless steel, vitallium, or titanium. Proper alignment is evaluated by x-ray studies at regular intervals.

Electrical Bone Growth Stimulation. Electrical bone growth stimulation is used to facilitate the healing process for certain types of fractures, especially those with nonunion or delayed healing. The mechanism of action of electrical bone growth stimulation may include (1) increasing the calcium uptake of bone, (2) activating intracellular calcium stores, and (3) increasing the production of bone growth factors (e.g., bone morphogenic protein).

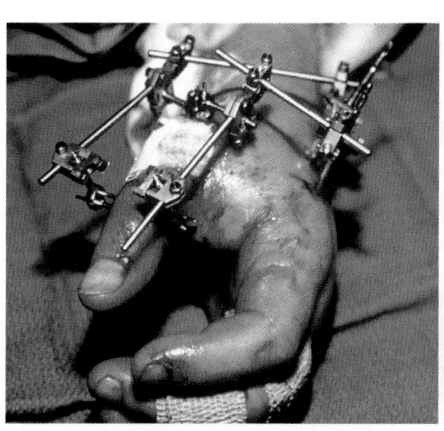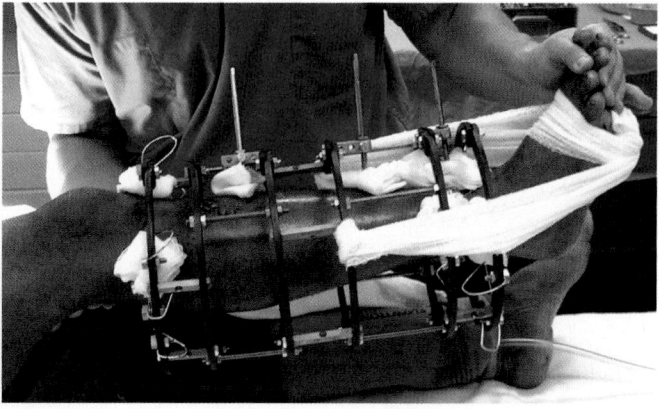

A   B

FIG. 63-13 External fixators. **A,** Stabilization of hand injury. **B,** Stabilization of a tibial fracture.

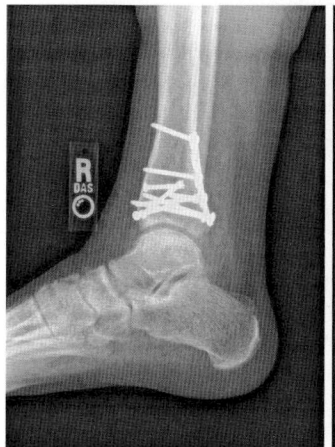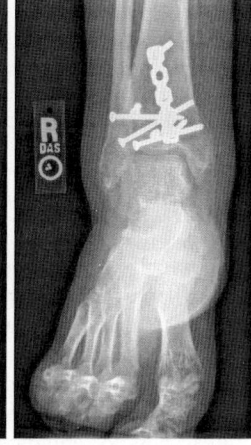

FIG. 63-14 Views of internal fixation devices to stabilize a fractured tibia and fibula.

Noninvasive, semi-invasive, and invasive methods of electrical bone growth stimulation are used. Noninvasive stimulators use direct current or pulsed electromagnetic fields (PEMFs) to generate a weak electrical current. Electrodes are placed over the patient's skin or cast and are used 10 to 12 hours each day, usually while the patient is sleeping. Semi-invasive or percutaneous bone growth stimulators use an external power supply and electrodes that are inserted through the skin and into the bone. Invasive stimulators require surgical implantation of a current generator in an intramuscular or subcutaneous space. An electrode is implanted in the bone fragments.

Drug Therapy. Patients with fractures experience varying degrees of pain associated with muscle spasms. Central and peripheral muscle relaxants, such as carisoprodol (Soma), cyclobenzaprine (Flexeril), or methocarbamol (Robaxin), may be prescribed for relief of pain associated with muscle spasms.[15]

Acute pain management for the patient with a fracture is presented in eNursing Care Plan 63-1 (on the website for this chapter).

In an open fracture the threat of tetanus can be reduced with tetanus and diphtheria toxoid or tetanus immunoglobulin for the patient who has not been previously immunized (see Table 69-6). Bone-penetrating antibiotics, such as a cephalosporin (e.g., cefazolin [Kefzol, Ancef]), are used prophylactically before surgery.

Nutritional Therapy. Proper nutrition is an essential component of the healing process in injured tissue. An adequate energy source is needed to promote muscle strength and tone, build endurance, and provide energy for ambulation and gait-training skills. The patient's dietary requirements must include adequate protein (e.g., 1 g/kg of body weight), vitamins (especially B, C, and D), calcium, phosphorus, and magnesium to ensure optimal soft tissue and bone healing. Low serum protein levels and vitamin C deficiencies interfere with tissue healing. Immobility and bone healing increase calcium needs.

Three well-balanced meals a day usually provide the necessary nutrients. The well-balanced meals should be supplemented by a fluid intake of 2000 to 3000 mL/day to promote optimal bladder and bowel function. Adequate fluid and a high-fiber diet with fruits and vegetables prevent constipation. If immobilized in bed with skeletal traction or in a body jacket brace, the patient should eat six small meals to avoid overeating and thus abdominal pressure and cramping.

NURSING MANAGEMENT
FRACTURES

NURSING ASSESSMENT

A brief history of the traumatic episode, the mechanism of injury, and the position in which the victim was found can be obtained from the patient or witnesses. As soon as possible, the patient should be transported to an emergency department where a thorough assessment and treatment can be initiated (Table 63-7). Subjective and objective data that should be obtained from an individual with a fracture are presented in Table 63-8 on p. 1519.

Place special emphasis on the region distal to the site of injury. Document clinical findings before fracture treatment to avoid doubts about whether a problem discovered later was missed during the original examination or was caused by the treatment.

NEUROVASCULAR ASSESSMENT. Musculoskeletal injuries may cause changes in the neurovascular status of an injured extremity. Application of a cast or constrictive dressing, poor positioning, and the physiologic responses to the traumatic injury can cause nerve or vascular damage, usually distal to the injury. The neurovascular assessment should consist of a *peripheral vascular assessment* (color, temperature, capillary refill, peripheral pulses, and edema) and a *peripheral neurologic assessment* (sensation, motor function, and pain). Throughout the neurovascular assessment, compare both extremities to obtain an accurate assessment.

✚ TABLE 63-7 EMERGENCY MANAGEMENT
Fractured Extremity

Etiology	Assessment Findings	Interventions
Blunt Trauma • Motor vehicle collision • Pedestrian event • Falls • Direct blows • Forced flexion or hyperextension • Twisting forces **Penetrating Trauma** • Gunshot • Blast **Other** • Pathologic conditions • Violent muscle contractions (seizures) • Crush injury	• Deformity (loss of normal bony contours) or unnatural position of affected limb • Edema and ecchymosis • Muscle spasm • Tenderness and pain • Warmth at site • Loss of function • Numbness, tingling, loss of distal pulses • Grating (crepitus) • Open wound over injured site, exposure of bone	**Initial** • Treat life-threatening injuries first. • Ensure airway, breathing, and circulation. • Control external bleeding with direct pressure or sterile pressure dressing and elevation of the extremity. • Check neurovascular status distal to injury before and after splinting. • Elevate injured limb if possible. • Do *not* attempt to straighten fractured or dislocated joints. • Do *not* manipulate protruding bone ends. • Apply ice packs to affected area. • Obtain x-rays of affected limb. • Administer tetanus and diphtheria prophylaxis if there is a break in skin integrity. • Mark location of pulses to facilitate repeat assessment. • Splint fracture site, including joints above and below fracture site. **Ongoing Monitoring** • Monitor vital signs, level of consciousness, O₂ saturation, neurovascular status, and pain. • Monitor for compartment syndrome characterized by excessive pain, pain with passive stretch of the affected extremity muscles, pallor, paresthesia, and late signs of paralysis and pulselessness. • Monitor for fat embolism (dyspnea, chest pain, temperature elevation).

Assess an extremity's color (pink, pale, cyanotic) and temperature (hot, warm, cool, cold) in the area of the injury. Pallor or a cool to cold extremity below the injury could indicate arterial insufficiency. A warm, cyanotic extremity could indicate poor venous return. Next assess capillary refill (blanching of the nail bed). The standard for a compressed nail bed to return to its original color is within 3 seconds.

Compare pulses on both the unaffected and injured extremity to identify differences in rate or quality. Pulses are described as strong, diminished, audible by Doppler, or absent. A diminished or absent pulse distal to the injury can indicate vascular dysfunction and insufficiency. Also assess peripheral edema. Pitting edema may be present with severe injury.

Evaluate the ulnar, median, and radial nerves by assessing sensation and motor innervation in the upper extremity. Assess neurovascular status by abduction and adduction of the fingers, opposition of the fingers, and supination and pronation of the hand. In the lower extremity, dorsiflexion and plantar flexion indicate motor function of the peroneal and tibial nerves. Sensory innervation is evaluated for the peroneal nerve on the dorsal part of the foot between the web space of the great and second toes. Tibial nerve assessment is performed by stroking the plantar surface (sole) of the foot. Contralateral evaluation is critical.

Paresthesia (abnormal sensation [e.g., numbness, tingling]) and hypersensation or hyperesthesia may be reported by the patient. Partial or full loss of sensation (paresis or paralysis) may be a late sign of neurovascular damage. Instruct patients to report any changes in their neurovascular status.

NURSING DIAGNOSES
Nursing diagnoses for the patient with a fracture may include, but are not limited to, the following:
- Impaired physical mobility *related to* loss of integrity of bone structures, movement of bone fragments, and prescribed movement restrictions

- Risk for peripheral neurovascular dysfunction *related to* vascular insufficiency and nerve compression secondary to edema and/or mechanical compression by traction, splints, or casts
- Acute pain *related to* edema, movement of bone fragments, and muscle spasms
- Readiness for enhanced self–health management

Additional information on nursing diagnoses for the patient with a fracture is presented in eNursing Care Plan 63-1 (on the website for this chapter).

PLANNING
The overall goals are that the patient with a fracture will (1) have healing with no associated complications, (2) obtain satisfactory pain relief, and (3) achieve maximal rehabilitation potential.

NURSING IMPLEMENTATION
HEALTH PROMOTION. Teach people in the community to take appropriate safety precautions to prevent injuries while at home, at work, when driving, or when participating in sports. Be an advocate for personal actions known to reduce injuries, such as regularly using seat belts; driving within posted speed limits; avoiding distracted driving; warming up muscles before exercise; using protective athletic equipment (helmets and knee, wrist, and elbow pads); using safety equipment at work; and not combining driving and drinking or the use of illicit drugs.

Encourage individuals (especially older adults) to participate in moderate exercise to help maintain muscle strength and balance. To reduce falls, they should wear adequate footwear and assess their living environment for safety (e.g., remove scatter rugs, maintain good lighting, clear paths to the bathroom for nighttime use) (see Table 63-1). Also stress the importance of adequate calcium and vitamin D intake.

ACUTE INTERVENTION. Patients with fractures may be treated in an emergency department or a physician's office and released to home care, or they may require hospitalization for varying

TABLE 63-8 NURSING ASSESSMENT

Fracture

Subjective Data
Important Health Information
Past health history: Traumatic injury; long-term repetitive forces (stress fracture); bone or systemic diseases, prolonged immobility, osteopenia, osteoporosis
Medications: Corticosteroids (osteoporotic fractures); analgesics
Surgery or other treatments: First aid treatment of fracture, previous musculoskeletal surgeries

Functional Health Patterns
Health perception–health management: Estrogen replacement therapy, calcium supplementation
Activity-exercise: Loss of motion or weakness of affected part; muscle spasms
Cognitive-perceptual: Sudden and severe pain in affected area; numbness, tingling, loss of sensation distal to injury; chronic pain that increases with activity (stress fracture)

Objective Data
General
Apprehension, guarding of injured site

Integumentary
Skin lacerations, pallor and cool skin or bluish and warm skin distal to injury; ecchymosis, hematoma, edema at site of fracture

Cardiovascular
Reduced or absent pulse distal to injury, ↓ skin temperature, delayed capillary refill

Neurovascular
Paresthesias, absent or ↓ sensation, hypersensation

Musculoskeletal
Restricted or lost function of affected part; local bony deformities, abnormal angulation; shortening, rotation, or crepitation of affected part; muscle weakness

Possible Diagnostic Findings
Identification and extent of fracture on x-ray, bone scan, CT scan, or MRI

EVIDENCE-BASED PRACTICE

Translating Research Into Practice

Do Vitamin D Supplements Improve Strength in Older Adults?

Clinical Question
In older adults (P) does vitamin D supplementation (I) improve strength, balance, and gait (O)?

Best Available Evidence
Systematic review of randomized controlled trials (RCTs)

Critical Appraisal and Synthesis of Evidence
- Thirteen RCTs (*n* = 2268) of older adults (mainly women) were done to determine the effect of supplemental vitamin D without an exercise intervention on muscle strength, gait, and balance.
- Supplemental vitamin D with daily doses of 800 to 1000 IU consistently demonstrated beneficial effects on strength and balance. An effect on gait was not demonstrated, although further evaluation is recommended.
- Increasing serum vitamin D levels to normal levels resulted in better muscle strength.

Conclusion
- Supplemental vitamin D has beneficial effects on strength and balance in older adults.

Implications for Nursing Practice
- Assess for vitamin D deficiencies and offer strategies to improve nutritional uptake, brief sunlight exposure, and supplementation.
- Discuss the importance of vitamin D in reducing the risk of falls.

Reference for Evidence
Muir SW, Montero-Odasso M: Effect of vitamin D supplementation on muscle strength, gait and balance in older adults: a systematic review and meta-analysis, *J Am Geriatr Soc* 59:2291, 2011.

P, Patient population of interest; *I,* intervention or area of interest; *O,* outcomes of interest (see p. 12).

---

amounts of time. Specific nursing measures depend on the setting and the type of treatment used.

Preoperative Management. If surgical intervention is required to treat a fracture, patients need preoperative preparation. In addition to the usual preoperative nursing measures (see Chapter 18), inform patients of the type of immobilization and assistive devices that will be used and the expected activity limitations after surgery. Assure patients that their needs will be met by the nursing staff until they can resume self-care. Knowing that pain medication will be available if needed is often beneficial.

Postoperative Management. In general, postoperative nursing care and management are directed toward monitoring vital signs and applying the general principles of postoperative nursing care (see Chapter 20). Frequent neurovascular assessments of the affected extremity are necessary to detect early and subtle neurovascular changes. Closely monitor any limitations of movement or activity related to turning, positioning, and extremity support. Pain and discomfort can be minimized through proper alignment and positioning. Carefully observe dressings or casts for any signs of bleeding or drainage. Report

a significant increase in size of the drainage area. If a wound drainage system is in place, regularly measure the volume of drainage and assess the patency of the system, using aseptic technique to avoid contamination.

Additional nursing responsibilities depend on the type of immobilization used. A blood salvage and reinfusion system that allows for recovery and reinfusion of the patient's own blood may be used. The blood is retrieved from a joint space or cavity, and the patient receives this blood in the form of an autotransfusion. (Autotransfusion is discussed in Chapter 31.) Additional nursing measures for the patient who has had orthopedic surgery are discussed in eNursing Care Plan 63-2 (on the website for this chapter).

Other Measures. Patients often have reduced mobility as a result of the fracture. Plan care to prevent the many complications associated with immobility. Prevent constipation by increased patient activity and maintenance of a high fluid intake (more than 2500 mL/day unless contraindicated by the patient's health status) and a diet high in bulk and roughage (fresh fruits and vegetables). If these measures are not effective in maintaining the patient's normal bowel pattern, warm fluids, stool softeners, laxatives, or suppositories may be necessary. Maintain a regular time for elimination to promote bowel regularity.

Renal calculi can develop as a result of bone demineralization. The hypercalcemia from demineralization causes a rise in urine pH and stone formation from the precipitation of calcium. Unless contraindicated, a fluid intake of 2500 mL/day is recommended. (Renal calculi are discussed in Chapter 46.)

Rapid deconditioning of the cardiopulmonary system can occur as a result of prolonged bed rest, resulting in orthostatic hypotension and decreased lung capacity. Unless contraindicated, these effects can be diminished by having the patient sit on the side of the bed, allowing the patient's lower limbs to dangle over the bedside, and having the patient perform standing transfers. When the patient is allowed to increase activity, assess for orthostatic hypotension. Also assess patients for deep vein thrombosis (DVT) and pulmonary emboli. (DVT is discussed in Chapter 38.)

Traction. When slings are used with traction, inspect exposed skin areas regularly. Pressure over a bony prominence created by the wrinkling of sheets or bedclothes may cause pressure necrosis. Persistent skin pressure may impair blood flow and cause injury to the peripheral neurovascular structures. Observe skeletal traction pin sites for signs of infection. Pin site care varies but usually includes regularly removing exudate with half-strength hydrogen peroxide, rinsing pin sites with sterile saline, and drying the area with sterile gauze.

External rotation of the hip can occur when skin traction is used on the lower extremity. Correct this position by placing a pillow or rolled-up towels along the greater trochanter of the femur. Generally, the patient should be in the center of the bed in a supine position. Incorrect alignment can result in increased pain and nonunion or malunion.

To offset some of the problems associated with prolonged immobility, discuss specific patient activity with the health care provider. If exercise is permitted, encourage patient participation in a simple exercise regimen based on activity restrictions. Activities that the patient should participate in include frequent position changes, ROM exercises of unaffected joints, deep-breathing exercises, isometric exercises, and use of the trapeze bar (if permitted) to raise the body off the bed for linen changes and use of the bedpan. These activities should be performed several times each day. Encourage and help the hospitalized patient to stay connected with friends and family through social media resources (see Informatics in Practice box).

AMBULATORY AND HOME CARE

Cast Care. Because many fractures are treated in an outpatient setting, the patient often requires only a short hospitalization or none at all. Regardless of the type of cast material, a cast can interfere with circulation and nerve function if it is applied too tightly or excessive edema occurs after application. Frequent neurovascular assessments of the immobilized extremity are critical. Teach the patient the signs of cast complications so that they can be reported promptly. Elevation of the extremity above the level of the heart to promote venous return and applications

of ice to control or prevent edema are measures frequently used during the initial phase. (If compartment syndrome is suspected, do not elevate the extremity above the heart.) Instruct the patient to exercise joints above and below the cast. Discourage pulling out cast padding and scratching or placing foreign objects inside the cast because it predisposes the patient to skin breakdown and infection. For itching, instruct the patient that a hair dryer set on a cool setting can be directed under the cast.

Patient and caregiver teaching is important to prevent complications. In addition to specific instructions for cast care and recognition of complications, encourage the patient to contact the health care provider should questions arise. Table 63-9 summarizes patient and caregiver instructions for cast care. Validate the patient's and caregiver's understanding of these instructions before discharge. A follow-up phone call is appropriate, and home care nursing visits are warranted, especially for the patient with a body jacket brace.

The cast is removed in the outpatient setting. Patients often fear being cut by the oscillating blade of the cast saw. Reassure the patient that damage to the skin is unlikely. Teach the patient about possible alterations in the appearance of the extremity (e.g., dry, wrinkled skin, atrophied muscle) that has been beneath the cast. The patient may also have anxiety related to using the injured extremity after the cast is removed.

Psychosocial Problems. Short-term rehabilitative goals are directed toward the transition from dependence to independence in performing simple activities of daily living and preserving or increasing strength and endurance. Long-term rehabilitative goals are aimed at preventing problems associated with musculoskeletal injury (Table 63-10). An important part

---

INFORMATICS IN PRACTICE

Staying Connected While Immobilized

- A patient in traction or other immobilization devices for a long period may feel lonely or isolated.
- There are a number of ways to use a computer or smart phone to ease separation anxiety and help the patient reconnect with family and friends.
- Set up video chat. Encourage personal contact through instant messaging and e-mail. Have the patient catch up on the latest news and blog on social networking sites.

TABLE 63-9 PATIENT & CAREGIVER TEACHING GUIDE

Cast Care

After a cast is applied, include the following instructions when teaching the patient and the caregiver.

Do
1. Apply ice directly over fracture site for first 24 hr (avoid getting cast wet by keeping ice in plastic bag and protecting cast with cloth).
2. Check with health care provider before getting fiberglass cast wet.
3. Dry cast thoroughly after exposure to water.
   - Blot dry with towel.
   - Use hair dryer on low setting until cast is thoroughly dry.
4. Elevate extremity above level of heart for first 48 hr.
5. Move joints above and below cast regularly.
6. Use hair dryer on cool setting for itching.
7. Report signs of possible problems to health care provider.
   - Increasing pain despite elevation, ice, and analgesia.
   - Swelling associated with pain and discoloration of toes or fingers.
   - Pain during movement.
   - Burning or tingling under the cast.
   - Sores or foul odor under the cast.
8. Keep appointment to have fracture and cast checked.

Do Not
1. Get cast wet.
2. Remove any padding.
3. Insert any objects inside cast.
4. Bear weight on new cast for 48 hr (not all casts are made for weight bearing; check with health care provider when unsure).
5. Cover cast with plastic for prolonged periods.

TABLE 63-10	PROBLEMS ASSOCIATED WITH MUSCULOSKELETAL INJURIES	
Problem	**Description**	**Nursing Considerations**
Muscle atrophy	• Decreased muscle mass normally occurs as a result of disuse after prolonged immobilization. • Loss of nerve innervation can precipitate muscle atrophy.	• Isometric muscle-strengthening exercise regimen within confines of immobilization device assists in reducing amount of atrophy. • Muscle atrophy interferes with and prolongs rehabilitation process.
Contracture	• Abnormal condition of joint characterized by flexion and fixation. • Caused by atrophy and shortening of muscle fibers or by loss of normal elasticity of skin over joint.	• Can be prevented by frequent position change, correct body alignment, and active-passive range-of-motion exercises several times a day. • Intervention requires gradual and progressive stretching of muscles or ligaments in region of joint.
Footdrop	• Plantar-flexed position of the foot (footdrop) occurs when Achilles tendon in ankle shortens because it has been allowed to assume an unsupported position. • Peroneal nerve palsy (a compression neuropathy) can cause footdrop and spinal nerve compression.	• Management of patient with long-term injuries must include preventive measures by supporting foot in neutral position. • Once footdrop has developed, ambulation and gait training may be significantly hindered. • May require splint to keep foot (feet) in neutral position. • High-top athletic shoes may also help.
Pain	• Frequently associated with fractures, edema, and muscle spasm. • Pain varies in intensity from mild to severe and is described as aching, dull, burning, throbbing, sharp, or deep.	• Causes of pain include incorrect positioning and alignment of extremity, incorrect support of extremity, sudden movement of extremity, immobilization device that is applied too tightly or in an incorrect position, constrictive dressings, and motion occurring at fracture site. • Determine causes of pain so that corrective action can be taken.
Muscle spasms	• Caused by involuntary muscle contraction after fracture, muscle strain, or nerve injury and may last several weeks. • Pain associated with muscle spasms is often intense and can last from several seconds to several minutes.	• Measures to reduce the intensity of the muscle spasms are similar to corrective actions for pain control. • Do not massage muscle spasms because it may stimulate muscle tissue contraction that increases spasm and pain. • Thermotherapy, especially heat, may reduce muscle spasm.

of care during the rehabilitative phase is helping the patient adjust to any problems caused by the injury (e.g., separation from family, financial impact of medical care, loss of income from inability to work, potential for lifetime disability). Offer support and encouragement while actively listening to the patient's and the caregiver's concerns.

Ambulation. Know the overall goals of physical therapy in relation to the patient's abilities, needs, and tolerance. Mobility training and instruction in the use of assistive aids (cane, crutches, walker) are major areas of responsibility of the physical therapist. Reinforce these instructions to the patient. The patient with lower extremity dysfunction usually starts mobility training when able to sit in bed and dangle the feet over the side. Collaborate with the physical therapist to coordinate pain management before a physical therapy session.

When the patient begins to ambulate, know the patient's weight-bearing status and the correct technique if the patient is using an assistive device. Weight-bearing ambulation occurs in different degrees: (1) non–weight-bearing (no weight borne) ambulation, (2) touch-down/toe-touch weight-bearing ambulation (contact with floor but no weight borne), (3) partial–weight-bearing ambulation (25% to 50% of patient's weight borne), (4) weight bearing as tolerated (dictated by patient's pain and tolerance), and (5) full–weight-bearing ambulation (no limitations).

Assistive Devices. Devices for ambulation range from a cane (can relieve up to 40% of the weight normally borne by a lower limb) to a walker or crutches (may allow for complete non–weight-bearing ambulation). The health care provider decides which device is appropriate,, balancing the need for maximum stability and safety versus maneuverability (this is required in small spaces such as bathrooms). Discuss with the patient his or her lifestyle requirements and select a device with which each patient feels most secure and independent. The technique for using assistive ambulation devices varies. The involved limb is usually advanced at the same time or immediately after advance of the device. The uninvolved limb is advanced last. In almost all cases, canes are held in the hand opposite the involved extremity.

Place a transfer belt around the patient's waist to provide stability while he or she is learning to use an assistive device. Discourage the patient from reaching for furniture or relying on another person for support. When there is inadequate upper limb strength or poorly fitted crutches, the patient bears weight at the axilla rather than at the hands, endangering the neurovascular bundle that passes across the axilla. If verbal coaching does not correct the problem, instruct the patient in another form of ambulation (e.g., crutches, walker) until strength is adequate.

Patients who must ambulate without weight bearing require sufficient upper limb strength to lift their own weight at each step. Because the muscles of the shoulder girdle are not accustomed to this work, they require vigorous and diligent training in preparation for this task. Push-ups, pull-ups using the overhead trapeze bar, and weight lifting develop the triceps and biceps. Straight-leg raises and quadriceps-setting exercises strengthen the quadriceps.

Counseling and Referrals. During the rehabilitative process, the patient's caregiver assumes an important role in the provision and follow-through of long-term care plans. Instruct the caregiver in the techniques of strength and endurance exercises, assistance with mobility training, and promotion of activities that enhance the quality of daily living. Also evaluate patients for posttraumatic stress disorder. This is especially important if significant injury to others or fatalities were associated with the patient's injuries.

EVALUATION

The expected outcomes are that the patient with a fracture will
- Report satisfactory relief of pain
- Demonstrate appropriate care of cast or immobilizer
- Experience no peripheral neurovascular dysfunction
- Experience uncomplicated bone healing

COMPLICATIONS OF FRACTURES

The majority of fractures heal without complications. If death occurs after a fracture, it is usually the result of damage to underlying organs and vascular structures or from complications of the fracture or immobility. Complications of fractures may be either direct or indirect. *Direct complications* include problems with bone infection, bone union, and avascular necrosis. *Indirect complications* are associated with blood vessel and nerve damage resulting in conditions such as compartment syndrome, venous thromboembolism, fat embolism, rhabdomyolysis (breakdown of skeletal muscle), and hypovolemic shock. Although most musculoskeletal injuries are not life threatening, open fractures, fractures accompanied by severe blood loss, and fractures that damage vital organs (e.g., lung, heart) are medical emergencies requiring immediate attention.

Infection

Open fractures and soft tissue injuries have a high incidence of infection. An open fracture usually results from the impact of severe external forces. Massive or blunt soft tissue injury often has more serious consequences than the fracture. Devitalized and contaminated tissue is an ideal medium for many common pathogens, including gas-forming (anaerobic) bacilli such as *Clostridium tetani*. Treatment of infection is costly in terms of extended nursing and medical care, time for treatment, and loss of patient income. Osteomyelitis can become chronic[16] (see Chapter 64).

Open fractures require aggressive surgical debridement. The wound is initially cleansed by pulsating saline lavage in the operating room. Gross contaminants are irrigated and mechanically removed. Contused, contaminated, and devitalized tissue such as muscle, subcutaneous fat, skin, and fragments of bone are surgically excised *(debridement)*. The extent of the soft tissue damage determines whether the wound is closed at the time of surgery and whether it requires repeat debridement, closed suction drainage, and skin grafting. Depending on the location and extent of the fracture, reduction may be maintained by external fixation or traction. During surgery the open wound may be irrigated with antibiotic solution. Antibiotic-impregnated beads may also be placed in the surgical site. During the postoperative phase the patient may have antibiotics administered IV for 3 to 7 days. Antibiotics, in conjunction with aggressive surgical management, have greatly reduced the occurrence of infection.

Compartment Syndrome

Compartment syndrome is a condition in which swelling and increased pressure within a limited space (a compartment) press on and compromise the function of blood vessels, nerves, and/or tendons that run through that compartment. Compartment syndrome causes capillary perfusion to be reduced below a level necessary for tissue viability. Compartment syndrome usually involves the leg, but can also occur in the arm, shoulder, and buttock.

Thirty-eight compartments are located in the upper and lower extremities. Two basic causes of compartment syndrome are (1) decreased compartment size resulting from restrictive dressings, splints, casts, excessive traction, or premature closure of fascia; and (2) increased compartment contents related to bleeding, inflammation, edema, or IV infiltration.

Edema can create sufficient pressure to obstruct circulation and cause venous occlusion, which further increases edema. Eventually arterial flow is compromised, resulting in ischemia to the extremity. As ischemia continues, muscle and nerve cells are destroyed over time, and fibrotic tissue replaces healthy tissue. Contracture, disability, and loss of function can occur. Delays in diagnosis and treatment cause irreversible muscle and nerve ischemia, resulting in a functionally useless or severely impaired extremity.

Compartment syndrome is usually associated with trauma, fractures (especially the long bones), extensive soft tissue damage, and crush injury. Fractures of the distal humerus and proximal tibia are the most common fractures associated with compartment syndrome. Compartment injury can also occur after knee or leg surgery. Prolonged pressure on a muscle compartment may result when someone is trapped under a heavy object or a person's limb is trapped beneath the body because of an obtunded state such as drug or alcohol overdose.

Clinical Manifestations. Compartment syndrome may occur initially from the body's physiologic response to the injury, or it may be delayed for several days after the original insult or injury. Ischemia can occur within 4 to 8 hours after the onset of compartment syndrome.

One or more of the following six *P*s are characteristic of compartment syndrome: (1) *pain* distal to the injury that is not relieved by opioid analgesics and *pain* on passive stretch of muscle traveling through the compartment; (2) increasing *pressure* in the compartment; (3) *paresthesia* (numbness and tingling); (4) *pallor,* coolness, and loss of normal color of the extremity; (5) *paralysis* or loss of function; and (6) *pulselessness,* or diminished or absent peripheral pulses.

Collaborative Care. Prompt, accurate diagnosis of compartment syndrome is critical.[17] Perform and document regular neurovascular assessments on all patients with fractures, especially those with an injury of the distal humerus or proximal tibia or soft tissue injuries in these areas. Early recognition and effective treatment of compartment syndrome are essential to avoid permanent damage to muscles and nerves.

Carefully assess the location, quality, and intensity of the pain (see Chapter 9). Evaluate the patient's level of pain on a scale of 0 to 10. Pain unrelieved by drugs and out of proportion to the level of injury is one of the *first* indications of impending compartment syndrome. Pulselessness and paralysis (in particular) are later signs of compartment syndrome. Notify the health care provider immediately of a patient's changing condition.

Because of the possibility of muscle damage, assess urine output. Myoglobin released from damaged muscle cells precipitates and causes obstruction in renal tubules. This condition results in acute tubular necrosis and acute kidney injury. Common signs are dark reddish brown urine and clinical manifestations associated with acute kidney injury (see Chapter 47).

Elevation of the extremity may lower venous pressure and slow arterial perfusion. Therefore the extremity should not be elevated above heart level. Similarly, the application of cold compresses may result in vasoconstriction and exacerbate compartment syndrome. It may also be necessary to remove or loosen the bandage and split the cast in half (bivalving). A reduction in traction weight may also decrease external circumferential pressures.

Surgical decompression (e.g., fasciotomy) of the involved compartment may be necessary (Fig. 63-15). The fasciotomy site is left open for several days to ensure adequate soft tissue

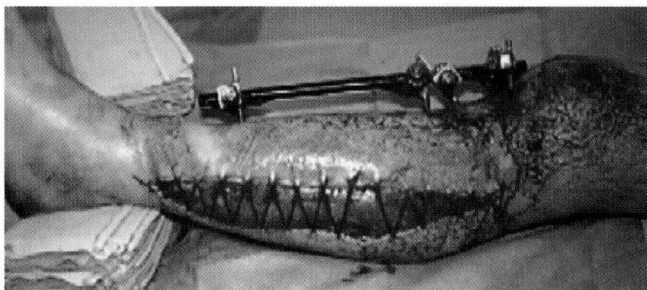

FIG. 63-15 Fasciotomy associated with compartment syndrome. Stabilization of fracture with external fixator.

decompression. Infection resulting from delayed wound closure is a potential problem after a fasciotomy. In severe cases of compartment syndrome, an amputation may be required.

Venous Thromboembolism

The veins of the lower extremities and the pelvis are highly susceptible to thrombus formation after a fracture, especially a hip fracture. Venous thromboembolism (VTE) may also occur after total hip or total knee replacement surgery.[18] In patients with limited mobility, venous stasis is aggravated by inactivity of the muscles that normally assist in the pumping action of venous blood returning to the extremities.

Because of the high risk of VTE in the orthopedic surgical patient, prophylactic anticoagulant drugs such as warfarin (Coumadin), low-molecular-weight heparin (LMWH) such as enoxaparin (Lovenox), fondaparinux (Arixtra), or rivaroxaban (Xarelto) may be ordered. In addition to wearing compression gradient stockings (antiembolism hose) and using sequential compression devices, the patient should move (dorsiflex and plantar flex) the fingers or toes of the affected extremity against resistance and perform ROM exercises on the unaffected lower extremities. (Assessment and management of VTE are discussed in Chapter 38.)

Fat Embolism Syndrome

Fat embolism syndrome (FES) is characterized by systemic fat globules from fractures that are distributed into tissues and organs after a traumatic skeletal injury. FES is a contributory factor in mortality associated with fractures. The fractures that most often cause FES are those of the long bones, ribs, tibia, and pelvis. FES has also been known to occur after total joint replacement, spinal fusion, liposuction, crush injuries, and bone marrow transplantation.

Two theories about fat embolism exist. First, the mechanical theory is that fat emboli may originate from the fat that is released from the marrow of injured bone. The fat then enters the systemic circulation where it embolizes to other organs such as the brain.[19] Microvascular lodging of droplets produces local ischemia and inflammation. Second, the biochemical theory is that hormonal changes caused by trauma or sepsis stimulate the systemic release of free fatty acids such as chylomicrons, which form the fat emboli.

Clinical Manifestations. Early recognition of FES is crucial to prevent a potentially lethal course. Most patients manifest symptoms within 24 to 48 hours after injury. Severe forms have occurred within hours of injury. The fat emboli in the lungs cause a hemorrhagic interstitial pneumonitis that produces signs and symptoms of acute respiratory distress syndrome (ARDS), such as chest pain, tachypnea, cyanosis, dyspnea,

apprehension, tachycardia, and decreased partial pressure of arterial oxygen (PaO_2). All of these symptoms are caused by poor oxygen exchange. Because they are frequently the presenting manifestations, changes in mental status (a result of hypoxemia) are important to recognize. Memory loss, restlessness, confusion, elevated temperature, and headache should prompt further investigation so that central nervous system involvement is not mistaken for alcohol withdrawal or acute head injury. The continued change in level of consciousness and petechiae located around the neck, anterior chest wall, axilla, buccal membrane, and conjunctiva of the eye help distinguish fat emboli from other problems. Petechiae may appear due to intravascular thromboses caused by decreased oxygenation.

The clinical course of a fat embolus may be rapid and acute. Frequently the patient expresses a feeling of impending disaster. In a short time, skin color changes from pallor to cyanosis, and the patient may become comatose. No specific laboratory examinations are available to aid in the diagnosis.[19] However, certain diagnostic abnormalities may be present. These include fat cells in blood, urine, or sputum; a decrease of the PaO_2 to less than 60 mm Hg; ST segment changes on ECG; a decrease in the platelet count and hematocrit levels; and a prolonged prothrombin time. A chest x-ray may reveal areas of pulmonary infiltrate or multiple areas of consolidation. This is sometimes referred to as the "white-out effect."

Collaborative Care. Treatment of fat embolism is directed at prevention. Careful immobilization of a long bone fracture is probably the most important factor in prevention of fat embolism. Management of FES is mostly supportive and related to management of symptoms. Treatment includes fluid resuscitation to prevent hypovolemic shock, correction of acidosis, and replacement of blood loss. Encourage coughing and deep breathing. Reposition the patient as little as possible before fracture immobilization or stabilization because of the danger of dislodging more fat droplets into the general circulation.

Use of corticosteroids to prevent or treat fat embolism is controversial. Oxygen is administered to treat hypoxia. Intubation or intermittent positive pressure ventilation may be considered if a satisfactory PaO_2 cannot be obtained with supplemental oxygen alone. Some patients may develop pulmonary edema, ARDS, or both, leading to an increased mortality rate. Most persons survive FES with few sequelae.

TYPES OF FRACTURES

COLLES' FRACTURE

A *Colles' fracture* is a fracture of the distal radius and is one of the most common fractures in adults (Fig. 63-16). The styloid process of the ulna may be involved as well. The injury usually occurs when the patient attempts to break a fall with an outstretched arm and hand. This type of fracture most often occurs in patients over 50 years old whose bones are osteoporotic. A younger person with a Colles' fracture caused by a low-energy force should be referred for an osteoporosis evaluation.

The clinical manifestations of Colles' fracture are pain in the immediate area of injury, pronounced swelling, and dorsal displacement of the distal fragment (silver-fork deformity). This displacement appears as an obvious deformity of the wrist. The major complication associated with a Colles' fracture is vascular insufficiency secondary to edema. Carpal tunnel syndrome can be a later complication.

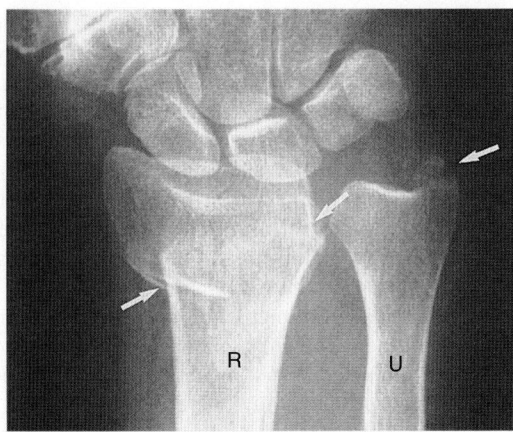

FIG. 63-16 Colles' fracture. Fracture of the distal radius *(R)* and ulnar *(U)* styloid from patient falling on the outstretched hand.

A Colles' fracture is usually managed by closed manipulation of the fracture and immobilization by either a splint or a cast or, if displaced, by internal or external fixation. Nursing management includes measures to prevent or reduce edema and frequent neurovascular assessments. Provide support and protection of the extremity, and encourage active movement of the thumb and fingers to reduce edema and increase venous return. Instruct the patient to perform active movements of the shoulder to prevent stiffness or contracture.

FRACTURE OF HUMERUS

Fractures involving the shaft of the humerus are common among young and middle-aged adults (see eFig. 63-3 on the website for this chapter). The most common clinical manifestations are an obvious displacement of the humerus shaft, shortened extremity, abnormal mobility, and pain. The major complications associated with fracture of the humerus are radial nerve injury and vascular injury to the brachial artery as a result of laceration, transection, or muscle spasm.

The treatment for a fracture of the humerus depends on the location and displacement of the fracture. Nonoperative treatment may include a hanging arm cast; shoulder immobilizer; or sling and swathe, which is a type of immobilizer that prevents glenohumeral movement. The swathe encircles the trunk and humerus as an additional binder. It is often used after surgical repairs and shoulder dislocation.

When these devices are used, elevate the head of the bed to assist gravity in reducing the fracture. Allow the arm to hang freely when the patient is sitting or standing. Include measures to protect the axilla and prevent skin breakdown. Carefully place absorbable composite dressing pads (i.e., ABD pads) in the axilla and change them twice daily or as needed. Skin or skeletal traction may be used for reduction and immobilization.

During the rehabilitative phase, an exercise program to improve strength and motion of the injured extremity is extremely important. Exercises should include assisted motion of the hand and fingers. The shoulder can also be exercised if the fracture is stable. This helps prevent stiffness secondary to frozen shoulder or fibrosis of the shoulder capsule.

FRACTURE OF PELVIS

Pelvic fractures range from benign to life threatening, depending on the mechanism of injury and associated vascular insult. Although only a small percentage of all fractures are pelvic

---

ETHICAL/LEGAL DILEMMAS
Entitlement to Treatment

Situation

H.Z., a 35-yr-old German tourist, had a hang gliding accident while touring the United States. He was taken to the regional trauma center for treatment of internal injuries, loss blood, and severe pelvic fractures. He has become septic, is now in renal failure, and has acute respiratory distress syndrome. He has no health insurance. Despite a poor chance of survival, his wife and parents want all possible measures to be taken.

Ethical/Legal Points for Consideration

• Federal law requires hospitals receiving federal funds through Medicare and Medicaid, under the Emergency Medical Treatment and Active Labor Act (EMTALA), to provide emergency evaluation and treatment to stabilize patients. They are under no obligation to continue treatment and may transfer the patient to another facility.
• In addition, the Hill-Burton Act requires states to have sufficient hospitals to provide necessary services for those unable to pay.
• Discussions with the family need to take place to clarify the goals of treatment (i.e., recovery, survival, continued biologic existence, nonabandonment of the patient), and what they mean by wanting "everything done." There is no legal or ethical obligation to continue medical treatment when the treatment goals cannot be met.
• Contact with the German consulate may result in collaboration to stabilize the patient and transport him to Germany.
• Neither health care providers nor hospitals are required to provide medically futile care (care that provides no benefit to the patient).
• H.Z. intentionally participated in a potentially dangerous activity, although he had no health insurance coverage.

Discussion Questions

1. How can the nurse facilitate discussions with the family regarding their goals for H.Z.?
2. If a person engages in risky behavior, is withholding treatment an option because of the behavior?

---

fractures, this type of injury is associated with a high mortality rate. Preoccupation with more obvious injuries at the time of a traumatic event may result in an oversight of pelvic injuries.

Pelvic fractures may cause serious intraabdominal injury such as paralytic ileus; hemorrhage; and laceration of the urethra, bladder, or colon. Pelvic fractures can cause acute pelvic compartment syndrome.[20] Patients may survive the initial pelvic injury, only to die from sepsis, FES, or thromboembolism.

Physical examination of the abdomen demonstrates local swelling, tenderness, deformity, unusual pelvic movement, and ecchymosis. Assess the neurovascular status of the lower extremities and manifestations of associated injuries. Pelvic fractures are diagnosed by x-ray and computed tomography (CT) scan.

Treatment of a pelvic fracture depends on the severity of the injury. Stable, nondisplaced fractures require limited intervention, and early mobilization is encouraged. Bed rest for stable pelvic fractures is maintained from a few days to 6 weeks. More complex fractures may be treated with pelvic sling traction, skeletal traction, external fixation, open reduction, or a combination of these methods. ORIF of a pelvic fracture may be necessary if the fracture is displaced. Use extreme care in handling or moving the patient to prevent serious injury from a displaced fracture fragment. Turn the patient only when ordered by the health care provider. Because a pelvic fracture can damage other organs, assess bowel and urinary elimination and distal neurovascular status. Provide back care while the patient is raised from the bed either by independent use of the trapeze or with adequate assistance.

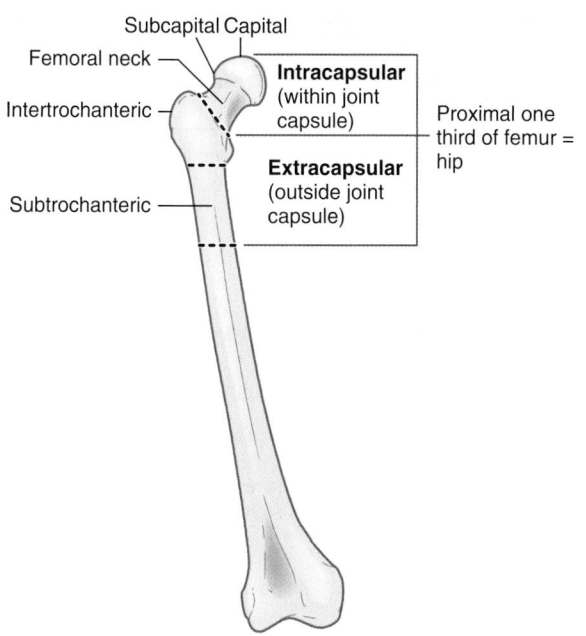

FIG. 63-17 Femur with location of various types of fracture.

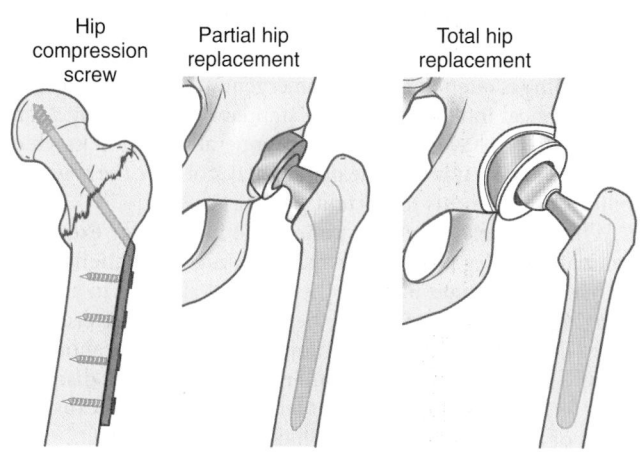

FIG. 63-18 Types of surgical repair for a hip fracture.

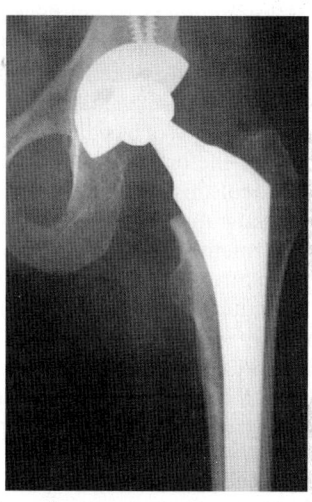

FIG. 63-19 Total hip replacement (arthroplasty) with a cementless femoral prosthesis of metal alloy with a plastic acetabular socket.

FRACTURE OF HIP

Hip fractures are common in older adults, with 90% of these fractures resulting from a fall.[21] More than 320,000 patients are admitted to hospitals annually because of a hip fracture. By age 90, approximately 33% of all women and 17% of all men will have sustained a hip fracture. In adults more than 65 years old, hip fracture occurs more frequently in women than in men because of osteoporosis.[22] By age 80, one in five women will have a hip fracture. Many older adults with a hip fracture develop disabilities that require long-term care.

A fracture of the hip (Fig. 63-17) refers to a fracture of the proximal (upper) third of the femur, which extends to 5 cm below the lesser trochanter. Fractures that occur within the hip joint capsule are called *intracapsular fractures.* Intracapsular fractures (femoral neck) are further identified by their specific locations: (1) capital (fracture of the head of the femur), (2) subcapital (fracture just below the head of the femur), and (3) transcervical (fracture of the neck of the femur). These fractures are often associated with osteoporosis and minor trauma. *Extracapsular fractures* occur outside the joint capsule. They are termed (1) *intertrochanteric* (in a region between the greater and lesser trochanter) or (2) *subtrochanteric* (below the lesser trochanter). Extracapsular fractures are usually caused by severe direct trauma or a fall.

Clinical Manifestations

The clinical manifestations of hip fractures are external rotation, muscle spasm, shortening of the affected extremity, and severe pain and tenderness around the fracture site. Displaced femoral neck fractures cause serious disruption of blood supply to the femoral head, which can result in avascular necrosis of the femoral head.

Collaborative Care

Initially the affected extremity may be temporarily immobilized by Buck's traction (see Fig. 63-9) until the patient's physical condition is stabilized and surgery can be performed. Buck's traction relieves painful muscle spasms and is used for up to 24 to 48 hours.

Surgical treatment of hip fractures permits early mobilization and decreases the risk of major complications. The type of surgery depends on the location and severity of the fracture and the person's age. Surgical options include (1) repair with internal fixation devices (e.g., hip compression screw, intramedullary devices) (Fig. 63-18), (2) replacement of part of the femur with a prosthesis (partial hip replacement) (see Fig. 63-18), and (3) total hip replacement (involves both the femur and acetabulum) (see Figs. 63-18 and 63-19).

NURSING MANAGEMENT HIP FRACTURE

NURSING IMPLEMENTATION

PREOPERATIVE MANAGEMENT. The majority of people who have hip fractures are older adults. When planning treatment of the hip fracture, consider the patient's chronic health problems (e.g., diabetes mellitus, cardiac and pulmonary disease). Surgery may be delayed for a brief time until the patient's general health is stabilized.[23]

Before surgery, severe muscle spasms can increase pain. Appropriate analgesics or muscle relaxants, comfortable positioning (unless contraindicated), and properly adjusted traction (if used) can help to manage the spasms.

Teaching is often done in the emergency department because quick surgical intervention is the standard of care today. Many patients do not have an overnight preoperative period in which to receive instructions, or the patient may not have the cognitive abilities to retain this important patient teaching.

When possible, teach the patient the method for exercising the unaffected leg and both arms. Encourage the patient to use the overhead trapeze bar and the opposite side rail to assist in changing positions. A physical therapist can begin to teach out-of-bed and chair transfers. Inform the caregiver about the patient's weight-bearing status after surgery. Plans for discharge begin as soon as the patient enters the hospital because the length of stay postoperatively will only be a few days.

POSTOPERATIVE MANAGEMENT. Similar principles of patient care apply to any of the surgical procedures for hip fractures. The content described in this section is also appropriate for the patient who has a total hip replacement for joint disease.

In the initial postoperative period assess vital signs, intake, and output; monitor respiratory function and deep breathing and coughing; administer pain medication; and observe the dressing and incision for signs of bleeding and infection. eNursing Care Plan 63-2 for the orthopedic surgical patient is presented on the website for this chapter.

In the early postoperative period there is a potential for neurovascular impairment. Assess the patient's extremity for (1) color, (2) temperature, (3) capillary refill, (4) distal pulses, (5) edema, (6) sensation, (7) motor function, and (8) pain. Edema is alleviated by elevating the leg whenever the patient is in a chair. The pain resulting from poor alignment of the affected extremity can be reduced by keeping pillows (or an abductor pillow) between the knees when the patient is turning to either side.

If the hip fracture has been treated by insertion of a prosthesis with a *posterior approach* (accessing the hip joint from the back), measures to prevent dislocation must be used (Table 63-11). Inform the patient and caregiver about positions and activities that predispose the patient to dislocation (more than 90 degrees of flexion, adduction across the midline [crossing of legs and ankles], internal rotation). Many daily activities may reproduce these positions, including putting on shoes and socks; crossing the legs or feet while seated; assuming the side-lying position incorrectly; standing up or sitting down while the body is flexed more than 90 degrees relative to the chair; and sitting on low seats, especially low toilet seats. Until the soft tissue capsule surrounding the hip has healed sufficiently to stabilize the prosthesis, teach the patient to avoid these activities (usually for at least 6 weeks).

Elevated toilet seats and chair alterations (e.g., raising the seat with pillows, maintaining a straight back) are necessary. Towel rolls (i.e., a trochanter roll) or pillows placed on the lateral side of the leg are also used to prevent external rotation. If a foam abduction pillow is used, it should be placed between the legs to prevent dislocation of the new joint (Fig. 63-20). Ensure that the top straps are above the knee to avoid placing pressure on the peroneal nerve at the lateral tibial tubercle.

In addition to teaching the patient and caregiver how to prevent prosthesis dislocation, you should also (1) place an abductor pillow or several pillows between the patient's legs when turning and (2) avoid turning the patient on the affected side until approved by the surgeon. In addition, some health

TABLE 63-11	**PATIENT & CAREGIVER TEACHING GUIDE**

Hip Replacement*

After a hip replacement, include the following instructions when teaching a patient and caregiver.

Do
- Use an elevated toilet seat.
- Place chair inside shower or tub and remain seated while washing.
- Use pillow between legs for first 6 wk after surgery when lying on nonoperative side or when supine.
- Keep hip in neutral, straight position when sitting, walking, or lying.
- Notify surgeon if severe pain, deformity, or loss of function occurs.
- Inform dentist of presence of prosthesis before dental work so that prophylactic antibiotics can be given if indicated.

Do Not
- Force hip into greater than 90 degrees of flexion (e.g., sitting in low chairs or toilet seats).
- Force hip into adduction.
- Force hip into internal rotation.
- Cross legs at knees or ankles.
- Put on own shoes or stockings without adaptive device (e.g., long-handled shoehorn or stocking-helper) until 4-6 wk after surgery.
- Sit on chairs without arms. They are needed to aid rising to a standing position.

*For patients having surgery by a posterior approach.

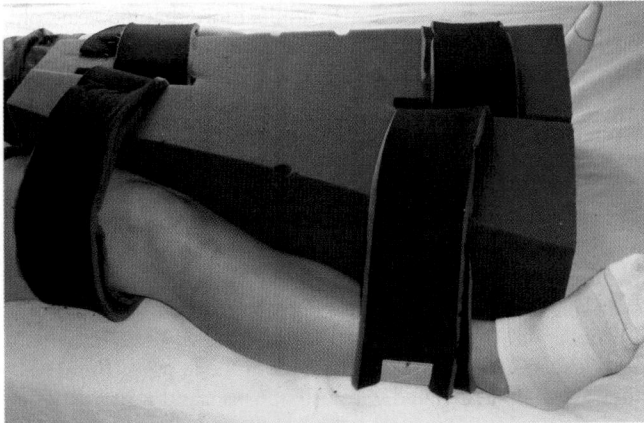

FIG. 63-20 Maintaining postoperative abduction following total hip replacement.

care providers prefer that the patient keep the leg abductor pillow on except when bathing.

Taking a tub bath and driving a car are not allowed for 4 to 6 weeks. An occupational therapist may teach the patient to use assistive devices, such as reachers or grabbers to avoid bending over to pick something off the floor, long-handled shoehorns, or sock assists. The knees must be kept apart. Instruct the patient to never cross the legs or twist to reach behind.

If the hip fracture has been treated by insertion of a prosthesis with an *anterior approach* (joint reached from front of body), the hip muscles are left intact. This approach generally results in a more stable hip in the postoperative period with a lower rate of complications. Patient precautions related to motion and weight bearing are few and may include instructions to avoid hyperextension.

The physical therapist usually supervises exercises for the affected extremity and ambulation when the surgeon permits it. The patient is usually out of bed on the first postoperative day. In collaboration with the physical therapist, monitor the patient's ambulation status for proper use of crutches or a walker. For the patient to be discharged home, have the patient demonstrate the proper use of crutches or a walker, the ability to transfer into and from a chair and bed, and the ability to ascend and descend stairs.

Weight bearing on the involved extremity varies. Weight bearing of especially fragile fractures may be restricted until x-ray examination indicates adequate healing, usually 6 to 12 weeks.

Complications associated with femoral neck fracture include nonunion, avascular necrosis, dislocation, and degenerative arthritis. As a result of an intertrochanteric fracture, the affected leg may be shortened. A cane or built-up shoe may be required for safe ambulation.

Sudden severe pain, a lump in the buttock, limb shortening, and external rotation indicate prosthesis dislocation. This requires a closed reduction with conscious sedation or open reduction to realign the femoral head in the acetabulum. If this occurs (regardless of the setting), keep the patient on nothing-by-mouth (NPO) status in anticipation of a possible surgical intervention.

Assist both the patient and caregiver in adjusting to the restrictions and dependence imposed by the hip fracture. Anxiety and depression can easily occur, but creative nursing care and awareness of potential problems can help to prevent them. Inform the patient and caregiver about community referral services that can assist in the postdischarge rehabilitation phase.

AMBULATORY AND HOME CARE. Hospitalization averages 3 or 4 days. Patients frequently require care in a subacute unit, at a skilled nursing facility, or in a rehabilitation facility for a few weeks before returning home. Arrange regular follow-up care after discharge, including home health nursing.

Home care considerations include ongoing assessment of pain management, monitoring for infection, and prevention of DVT. The incision may be closed with metal staples, which are removed at the surgeon's office. If warfarin is used to decrease the high risk for thromboembolism, determine prothrombin times weekly and adjust anticoagulation accordingly. Alternatives to warfarin include enoxaparin, fondaparinux, and rivaroxaban. These newer anticoagulants require less monitoring than warfarin. Teach the patient who is receiving an anticoagulant to immediately report signs of bleeding to the health care provider (see Chapter 38).

Exercises designed to restore strength and muscle tone in the quadriceps and muscles about the hip are essential to improve function and ROM. These include quadriceps setting (e.g., tightening the kneecap), gluteal muscle setting (e.g., tightening the buttocks), leg raises in supine and prone positions, and abduction exercises from the supine and standing positions (e.g., swinging the leg out but never crossing midline). The patient continues these exercises for many months after discharge. It is important to teach the exercise program to the caregiver who will be encouraging the patient at home.

A physical therapist assesses ROM, ambulation, and compliance with the exercise regimen. The patient gradually increases the number of repetitions of exercises, adds weights to ankles,

and swims, and may eventually use a stationary bicycle to tone quadriceps and improve cardiovascular fitness. High-impact exercises and sports, such as jogging and tennis, may loosen the implant and should be avoided.

▌EVALUATION

The expected outcomes are that the patient with a fracture of the hip will

- Report satisfactory pain relief
- Participate in exercise therapy
- Understand prescribed treatment plan

▌GERONTOLOGIC CONSIDERATIONS

HIP FRACTURE

Factors that increase the risk of a hip fracture in older adults include a tendency to fall, inability to correct a postural imbalance, inadequacy of local tissue shock absorbers (e.g., fat, muscle bulk), and reduced skeletal strength. Factors that increase the older adult's risk of falling include gait and balance problems, decreased vision and hearing, slowed reflexes, orthostatic hypotension, and medication use. Leading hazards of falls are loose rugs and slippery or uneven surfaces.[24]

Many falls are associated with getting in or out of a chair or bed. Falls to the side, the most common type seen in frail older adults, are more likely to result in a hip fracture than a forward fall.[24] External hip protectors may help prevent hip fractures in the frail older patient.[25] Older women often have osteoporosis and accompanying low bone density, which increases their risk of hip and other types of fractures.

Calcium and vitamin D supplementation, estrogen replacement, and bisphosphonate drug therapy decrease bone loss or increase bone density and thus reduce the likelihood of fracture, especially in patients with osteoporosis. (Osteoporosis is discussed in Chapter 64.)

FEMORAL SHAFT FRACTURE

Femoral shaft fracture occurs with a severe direct force because the femur can bend slightly before an actual fracture occurs. Young adults have a higher incidence of this type of fracture. The force exerted to cause the fracture such as from a motor vehicle collision or gunshot wound frequently damages the adjacent soft tissue structures. These injuries may be more serious than the bone injury.

Displacement of the fracture fragments often results in open fracture and increased soft tissue damage. This can lead to considerable blood loss (1 to 1.5 L). The most common types of femoral shaft fracture include transverse, spiral, comminuted, oblique, and open (see Figs. 63-6 and 63-7).

The clinical manifestations of a fracture of the femoral shaft are usually obvious. They include marked deformity and angulation, shortening of the extremity, inability to move either the hip or the knee, and pain. The common complications associated with fracture of the femoral shaft include fat embolism; nerve and vascular injury; and problems associated with bone union, open fracture, and soft tissue damage.

Initial management of a femoral shaft fracture is directed toward stabilization of the patient and immobilization of the fracture. Traction may be used as a temporary measure before surgical treatment or in patients unable to undergo surgery. The method of treatment most often used for a femoral shaft fracture is *intermedullary nailing.*[26] A metal rod is placed into the marrow canal of the femur. The rod passes across the fracture to keep it in position. Internal fixation is preferred because it reduces the hospital stay and the complications associated with prolonged bed rest.

In the postoperative period teach the patient to carefully follow the health care provider's instructions for weight bearing. Promotion and maintenance of strength in the affected extremity usually include gluteal and quadriceps isometric exercises. Ensure that the patient performs ROM and strengthening exercises for all uninvolved extremities in preparation for ambulation. The patient may be allowed to begin non–weight-bearing activities with an ambulatory assistive device (e.g., walker, crutches). Full weight bearing is usually restricted until there is x-ray evidence of union of the fracture fragments.

FRACTURE OF TIBIA

Although the tibia is vulnerable to injury because it lacks a covering of anterior muscle, strong force is required to produce a fractured tibia. As a result, soft tissue damage, devascularization, and open fracture are frequent. The tibia is one of the more common sites of a stress fracture. Complications associated with tibial fractures are compartment syndrome, fat embolism, problems associated with bony union, and possible infection associated with open fracture.

The recommended management for closed tibial fracture is closed reduction followed by immobilization in a long leg cast. ORIF with intramedullary rods, plate fixation, or external fixation is indicated for complex tibial fractures and those with extensive soft tissue damage. Locking plates (screw and plate system) are another type of surgical device. In both types of reduction, the emphasis is on maintaining the strength of the quadriceps.

Assess the neurovascular status of the affected extremity at least every 2 hours during the first 48 hours. Instruct patients to perform active ROM exercises with the uninvolved leg and the upper extremities to build the strength required for crutch walking. When the health care provider has determined that the patient is ready for gait training, instruct the patient in the principles of crutch walking. The patient may be non–weight bearing for 6 to 12 weeks, depending on healing. Home nursing visits can be initiated to augment outpatient appointments and monitor the patient's progress.

STABLE VERTEBRAL FRACTURE

Stable fractures of the vertebral column are usually caused by motor vehicle collisions, falls, diving, or athletic injuries. More than 700,000 vertebral compression fractures occur annually (many of these are stable) in patients with osteoporosis.[27] A stable fracture is one in which the fracture or the fragment is not likely to move or cause spinal cord damage. This type of injury is frequently confined to the anterior element (vertebral body) of the spinal column in the lumbar region, and less frequently involves the cervical and thoracic regions. The vertebral bodies are usually protected from displacement by the intact spinal ligaments.

Most patients with stable spinal fractures experience only brief periods of disability. However, if the ligamentous structures are significantly disrupted, dislocation of the vertebral structures may occur, resulting in instability and injury to the spinal cord (unstable fracture). These injuries generally require

surgery. The most serious complication of vertebral fractures is fracture displacement, which can cause damage to the spinal cord (see Chapter 61). Although stable vertebral fractures are not associated with abnormal spinal cord pathologic conditions, all spinal injuries should be considered unstable and potentially serious until diagnostic tests are performed and the fracture is determined to be stable.

The patient usually complains of pain and tenderness in the affected region of the spine. Sudden loss of function below the level of fracture indicates spinal cord impingement and paraplegia. Stable compression fractures are associated with a kyphotic deformity (flexion angulation of several vertebrae). This deformity may be noted during the physical examination. In patients with a stable vertebral fracture secondary to osteoporosis, several vertebral levels may be involved as evidenced by a *dowager's hump* (abnormal curvature of thoracic spine) (see Fig. 64-9) or *lordosis* (extreme inward curve of lumbar spine). The cervical spine may also be involved. Bowel and bladder dysfunction may indicate an interruption of the autonomic nervous system nerves or injury to the spinal cord.

The overall goal in management of stable vertebral fractures is to keep the spine in good alignment until union has been accomplished. Many nursing interventions are aimed at assessing for the possibility of spinal cord trauma. Regularly evaluate vital signs and bowel and bladder function. Also monitor the motor and sensory status of the peripheral nerves distal to the injured region. Promptly report any deterioration in the patient's neurovascular status.

Treatment includes pain medication followed by early mobilization and bracing. If hospitalized, the patient is usually placed in a standard hospital bed with firm support from the mattress. The aim is to support the spinal column, relax muscles, decrease edema, and prevent potential compression on nerve roots. Teach the patient to keep the spine straight when turning by turning the shoulders and pelvis together. Nursing assistance is necessary for the patient to learn the technique of logrolling. Several days after the initial injury, the health care provider may apply a specially constructed orthotic device (e.g., Milwaukee, Jewett, or Taylor brace), a jacket cast, or a removable corset if there is no evidence of neurologic deficit.

Vertebral compression fractures (which are often due to osteoporosis) may be treated with two outpatient procedures: vertebroplasty or kyphoplasty. *Vertebroplasty* uses radioimaging to guide the injection of bone cement into a fractured vertebral body. The cement (when hardened) serves to stabilize and prevent further vertebral compression. *Kyphoplasty* initially involves inserting a balloon into the vertebral body and then inflating it. This creates a cavity that is filled with bone cement under low pressure. Kyphoplasty results in less leakage of bone cement compared with vertebroplasty and helps restore the height of the vertebral body. Vertebroplasty and kyphoplasty result in improved healing, better pain relief, and decreased complications compared to conservative treatment.[28]

If the fracture is in the cervical spine, the patient may wear a hard cervical collar. Some cervical fractures are immobilized by use of a halo vest (see Fig. 61-11). This consists of a plastic jacket or cast fitted about the chest and attached to a halo that is held in place by skeletal pins inserted into the cranium. These devices immobilize the spine in the fracture area but allow the patient to ambulate.

The patient with a stable vertebral fracture is discharged after (1) regaining ambulation skills, (2) learning care of the cast or orthotic device, and (3) learning how to cope with the safety and security issues imposed by the injury and the treatment. Unstable vertebral fractures and spinal cord injuries are discussed in Chapter 61.

FACIAL FRACTURE

Any bone of the face can be fractured as a result of trauma, such as a motor vehicle collision, assault, or falls.[29] The primary concern after facial injury is to establish and maintain a patent airway and to provide adequate ventilation. Foreign material and blood need to be removed. Suctioning may be necessary. An alternative airway (tracheostomy) may be needed if a patent airway cannot be maintained.

Concurrent facial fractures and cervical spine injuries are common. All patients with facial injuries should be treated as if they have a cervical injury until proven otherwise by examination and imaging studies (e.g., CT scan, x-ray). Table 63-12 describes the clinical manifestations of common facial fractures.

Associated soft tissue injury often makes assessment of a facial injury difficult. Perform oral and facial examinations after the patient has been stabilized and any life-threatening situations have been treated. Careful assessment is made of the ocular muscles and cranial nerve involvement (cranial nerves III, IV, and VI).[30] X-rays are used to determine the extent of the injury. CT scanning helps differentiate between bone and soft tissue.

Suspect injury to the eye when a facial injury occurs, particularly if the injury is near the orbit. If an eye-globe rupture is suspected, stop the examination and place a protective shield over the eye. Signs of globe rupture include the extrusion of vitreous humor, or brown tissue (iris or ciliary body), on the surface of the globe or penetrating through a laceration with an eccentric or teardrop-shaped pupil.

Specific treatment depends on the site and extent of the facial fracture and the associated soft tissue injury. Immobilization or surgical stabilization may be necessary. Maintain a patent airway and adequate nutrition throughout the recovery period.

You need to be sensitive about the alterations in appearance that may occur after a facial fracture. The changes in appearance may be drastic. Edema and discoloration subside with time, but concurrent soft tissue injuries may result in permanent scarring.

Mandibular Fracture

A fracture of the mandible may result from trauma to the face or the jaws. Maxillary fractures may also occur, but they are less common than mandibular fractures. The mandibular fracture may be simple, with no bone displacement, or it may involve loss of tissue and bone. The fracture may require immediate and sometimes long-term treatment to ensure survival and restore satisfactory appearance and function.

Mandibular fracture may also be therapeutically performed to correct an underlying malocclusion problem that cannot be corrected by orthodontic procedures alone. The mandible is resected during surgery and manipulated forward or backward depending on the occlusion problem.

Surgery consists of immobilization, usually by wiring the jaws (*intermaxillary fixation*). Internal fixation may be done with screws and plates. In a simple fracture with no loss of teeth, the lower jaw is wired to the upper jaw. Wires are placed around the teeth, and then cross-wires or rubber bands are used to hold the lower jaw tight against the upper jaw (Fig. 63-21). Arch bars may be placed on the maxillary and mandibular arches of the teeth. Vertical wires are placed between the arch bars, holding the jaws together. If teeth are missing or bone is displaced, other forms of fixation such as metal arch bars in the mouth or insertion of a pin in the bone may be needed. Bone grafting may also be required. Immobilization is usually necessary for only 4 to 6 weeks because the fractures often heal rapidly.

NURSING MANAGEMENT
MANDIBULAR FRACTURE

Inform the patient preoperatively about the surgical procedure, including what it involves, how the face will look afterward, and alterations caused by the surgery. Reassure the patient about the ability to breathe normally, speak, and swallow liquids. Hospitalization for respiratory monitoring is brief unless there are other injuries or problems.

Postoperative care focuses on a patent airway, oral hygiene, communication, pain management, and adequate nutrition. Two potential problems in the immediate postoperative period are airway obstruction and aspiration of vomitus. Because the patient cannot open the jaws, it is essential that an airway is maintained. Observe for signs of respiratory distress (e.g., dyspnea; alterations in rate, quality, and depth of respirations). Place the patient on the side with the head slightly elevated immediately after surgery.

Tape a wire cutter or scissors (for rubber bands) to the head of the bed and send it with the patient on all appointments and examinations away from the bedside. The wire cutter or scissors may be used to cut the wires or elastic bands in case of an emergency (e.g., cardiac arrest or respiratory distress) requiring

TABLE 63-12	MANIFESTATIONS OF FACIAL FRACTURES
Fracture	**Manifestation**
Frontal bone	Rapid edema that may mask underlying fractures
Periorbital bone	Possible frontal sinus involvement, entrapment of ocular muscles
Nasal bone	Displacement of nasal bones, epistaxis
Zygomatic arch	Depression of zygomatic arch and entrapment of ocular muscles
Maxilla	Segmental motion of maxilla and alveolar fracture of teeth
Mandible	Tooth fractures, bleeding, limited motion of mandible

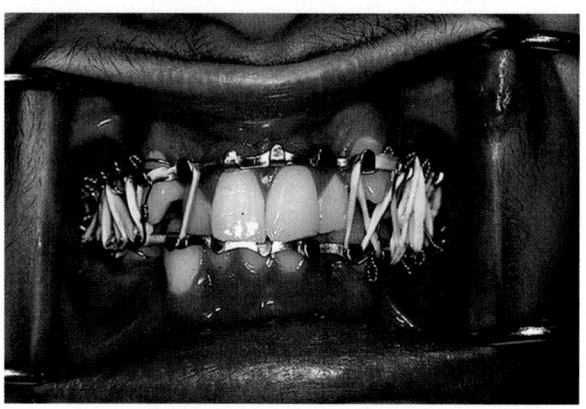

FIG. 63-21 Intermaxillary fixation.

access to the pharynx or lungs. Information including a picture on the appropriate wires to cut should be included in the care plan. In some cases, cutting the wires may cause the entire facial and upper jaw structure to shift or collapse and worsen the problem. A tracheostomy or endotracheal tray should always be available.

If the patient begins to vomit or choke, try to clear the mouth and airway. Suctioning may be necessary and may be done by the nasopharyngeal or oral route, depending on the extent of injury and the type of repair. An NG tube may be used for decompression to remove fluids and gas from the stomach to help prevent aspiration. An NG tube also helps prevent vomiting. Antiemetics may also be used. The NG tube can later be used as a feeding tube. Teach the patient to clear secretions and vomitus.

Oral hygiene is an extremely important part of nursing care. The mouth should be rinsed frequently, particularly after meals and snacks, to remove food debris. Warm normal saline solution, water, or alkaline mouthwashes may be used. A syringe and soft irrigation catheter or a Water Pik is effective for a thorough oral cleansing. Inspect the mouth several times a day to see that it is clean. Use a tongue depressor to retract the cheeks. Keep the lips, corners of the mouth, and buccal mucosa moist. Dental wax may be used to cover any sharp edges of the wires to prevent irritation of the buccal mucosa.

Communication may be a problem, particularly in the early postoperative period. Establish an effective way of communicating preoperatively (e.g., use of dry erase board, pad and pencil). Usually the patient can speak well enough to be understood, especially after the first few postoperative days.

Ingestion of sufficient nutrients poses a challenge because the diet must be liquid. The patient easily tires of sucking through a straw or laboriously using a spoon. Work with the dietitian and the patient to plan a diet that includes adequate calories, protein, and fluids. Liquid protein supplements may be helpful for improving the nutritional status. The low-bulk, high-carbohydrate diet and the intake of air through the straw create a problem with constipation and flatus. Ambulation, prune juice, and bulk-forming laxatives may help relieve these problems.

The patient is usually discharged with the wires in place. Encourage the patient to verbalize feelings about the altered appearance. Discharge teaching should include oral care, techniques for handling secretions, diet, how and when to use wire cutters or scissors, and when to notify the health care provider about concerns and problems.

AMPUTATION

An *amputation* is the removal of a body extremity by trauma or surgery. An estimated 2 million people in the United States are living with limb loss.[31] The middle and older age-groups have the highest incidence of amputation because of the effects of peripheral vascular disease (PVD), atherosclerosis, and vascular changes related to diabetes mellitus. Amputation in young people is usually secondary to trauma (e.g., motor vehicle crashes, land mines, farm-related injury). In the past decade more than 1600 American military personnel have undergone a service-related amputation.[32]

Clinical Indications

Most amputations are performed due to PVD, especially in older patients with diabetes mellitus. These patients often expe-

TABLE 63-13   **COLLABORATIVE CARE**

Amputation

Diagnostic
- History and physical examination
- Physical appearance of soft tissues
- Skin temperature
- Sensory function
- Presence of peripheral pulses
- Arteriography
- Venography
- Plethysmography
- Transcutaneous ultrasonic Doppler recordings

Collaborative Therapy
Medical
- Appropriate management of underlying disease
- Stabilization of trauma victim

Surgical
- Residual limb management
- Immediate or delayed prosthetic fitting

Rehabilitation
- Coordination of prosthesis-fitting and gait-training activities
- Coordination of muscle-strengthening and physical therapy regimens

rience peripheral neuropathy that progresses to trophic ulcers and subsequent gangrene. Other common reasons for amputation are trauma and thermal injuries, tumors, osteomyelitis, and congenital limb disorders. Although pain is often present, it is not usually the primary reason for an amputation.

Diagnostic Studies

The types of diagnostic studies performed depend on the underlying problem that makes the amputation necessary (Table 63-13). An elevated white blood cell (WBC) count with abnormal differential may indicate infection. Vascular tests such as arteriography, Doppler studies, and venography provide information about the circulatory status of the extremity.

Collaborative Care

If amputation is considered "elective," carefully assess the patient's general health. Chronic illnesses and infection are important considerations before performing an amputation. Help the patient and caregiver understand the need for the amputation and assure them that rehabilitation can result in an active, useful life. If the amputation is performed on an emergency basis as a result of trauma, management of the patient is physically and emotionally more complicated.

The goal of amputation surgery is to preserve extremity length and function while removing all infected, pathologic, or ischemic tissue. (Levels of amputation of upper and lower extremities are illustrated in Fig. 63-22.) The type of amputation depends on the reason for the surgery. A closed amputation is performed to create a weight-bearing *residual limb* (or stump). An anterior skin flap with dissected soft tissue padding covers the bony part of the residual limb. The skin flap is sutured posteriorly so that the suture line will not be positioned in a weight-bearing area. Special care is necessary to prevent accumulation of drainage, which can produce pressure and harbor bacteria that may cause infection.

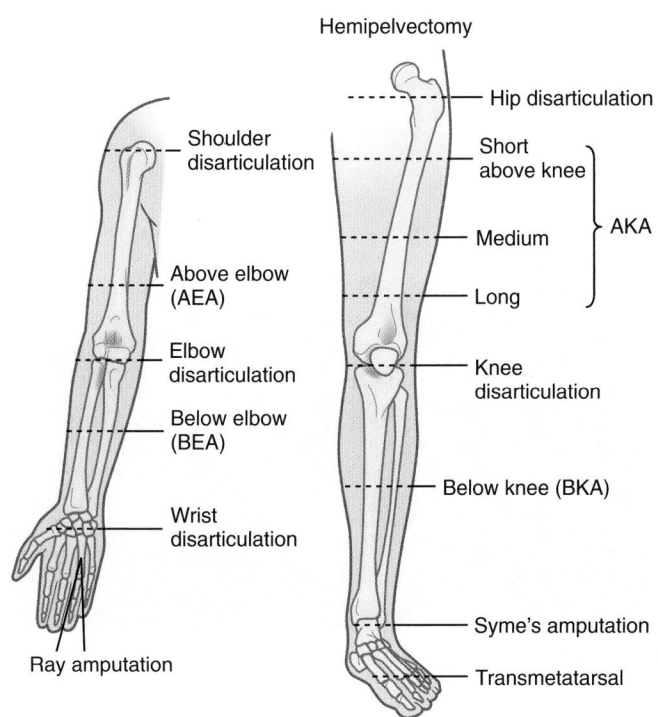

FIG. 63-22 Location and description of amputation sites of the upper and lower extremities. *AKA,* Above-the-knee amputation.

Disarticulation is an amputation performed through a joint. A *Syme's amputation* is a form of disarticulation at the ankle. An open amputation leaves a surface on the residual limb that is not covered with skin. This type of surgery is generally indicated for control of actual or potential infection. The wound is usually closed later by a second surgical procedure or closed by skin traction surrounding the residual limb. This is often called a *guillotine amputation.*

NURSING MANAGEMENT AMPUTATION

NURSING ASSESSMENT
Assess any preexisting illnesses because most amputations are performed as a result of vascular problems. Assessment of vascular and neurologic status is an important part of the assessment process (see Chapters 32 and 56).

NURSING DIAGNOSES
Nursing diagnoses for the patient with an amputation may include, but are not limited to, the following:
- Disturbed body image *related to* loss of body part and impaired mobility
- Impaired skin integrity *related to* immobility and improperly fitted prosthesis
- Chronic pain *related to* phantom limb sensation or residual limb pain
- Impaired physical mobility *related to* amputation of lower limb

PLANNING
The overall goals are that the patient with an amputation will (1) have adequate relief from the underlying health problem, (2) have satisfactory pain control, (3) reach maximum rehabili-

tation potential with the use of a prosthesis (if indicated), (4) cope with the body image changes, and (5) make satisfying lifestyle adjustments.

NURSING IMPLEMENTATION
HEALTH PROMOTION. Control of causative illnesses such as PVD, diabetes mellitus, chronic osteomyelitis, and pressure ulcers can eliminate or delay the need for amputation. Teach patients with these problems to carefully examine their lower extremities daily for signs of potential problems. If the patient cannot assume this responsibility, the caregiver should help. Instruct patients and their caregivers to report changes in the feet or toes to the health care provider, including changes in skin color or temperature, decrease or absence of sensation, tingling, burning pain, or lesions.

Instruct people in proper safety precautions for recreational activities and potentially hazardous work. This responsibility is especially critical for the occupational health nurse.

ACUTE INTERVENTION. The reasons for an amputation and the rehabilitation potential depend on a person's age, diagnosis, occupation, personality, resources, and support system. It is important for you to recognize the tremendous psychologic and social implications of an amputation. The disruption in body image caused by an amputation often results in a patient going through the grieving process (see Chapter 10). Use therapeutic communication to assist the patient and caregiver through this process to arrive at a realistic attitude about the future.

Preoperative Management. Before surgery, reinforce information that the patient and caregiver have received about the reasons for the amputation, proposed prosthesis, and mobility-training program. To meet the patient's educational needs, know the level of amputation, type of postsurgical dressings to be applied, and type of prosthesis to be used. Instruct the patient in the performance of upper extremity exercises such as push-ups in bed or the wheelchair to promote arm strength. This instruction is essential for crutch walking and gait training. Discuss general postoperative nursing care, including positioning, support, and residual limb care. If a compression bandage is to be used after surgery, instruct the patient about its purpose and how it will be applied. If an immediate prosthesis is planned, discuss general ambulation expectations.

Tell the patient that the amputated limb may feel like it is still present after surgery. This phenomenon, termed phantom limb sensation, occurs in many amputees. (Nursing management of phantom limb sensation is discussed in the next section.)

Postoperative Management. General postoperative care for the patient who has had an amputation depends largely on the patient's general state of health, reason for the amputation, and patient's age. Monitor individuals who undergo amputation as a result of a traumatic injury for posttraumatic stress disorder because they have had no time to prepare or perhaps even to participate in the decision to have a limb amputated.

Prevention and detection of complications are important during the postoperative period. Carefully monitor the patient's vital signs and dressings for hemorrhage in the operative area. Careful attention to sterile technique during dressing changes reduces the potential for wound infection.

If an *immediate* postoperative prosthesis has been applied, careful surveillance of the surgical site is required. A surgical tourniquet must always be available for emergency use. If excessive bleeding occurs, notify the surgeon immediately.

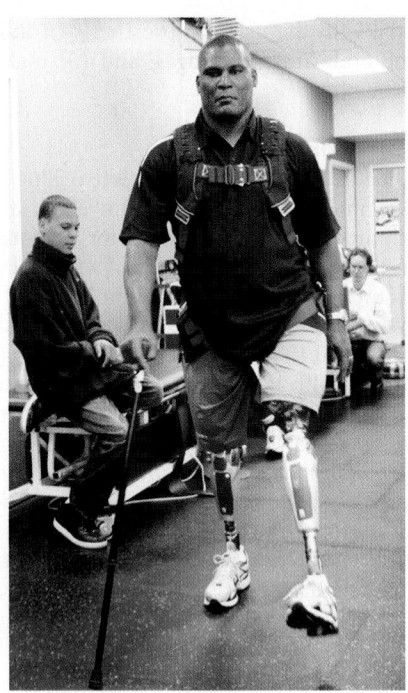

FIG. 63-23 A double amputee fitted with prostheses. (Photo courtesy United States Army.)

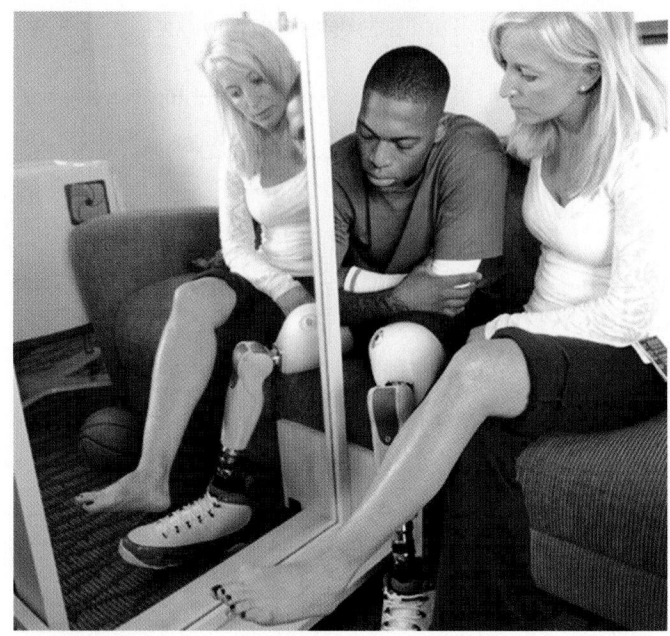

FIG. 63-24 Mirror therapy, a type of treatment that may reduce phantom limb sensation and pain. (U.S. Navy photo courtesy Mass Communication Specialist Seaman Joseph A. Boomhower.)

The *delayed* prosthetic fitting may be the best choice for patients who have had amputations above the knee or below the elbow, older adults, debilitated individuals, and those with infection (Fig. 63-23). The appropriate timing for use of a prosthesis depends on satisfactory healing of the residual limb and on the patient's general condition. A temporary prosthesis may be used for partial weight bearing once the sutures are removed. Barring any problems, patients can bear full weight on permanent prostheses approximately 3 months after amputation.

Not all patients are candidates for prostheses. The seriously ill or debilitated patient may not have the upper body strength and energy required to use a lower extremity prosthesis. Mobility with a wheelchair may be the most realistic goal for these patients.

Often patients may be extremely anxious about phantom limb sensation because they still perceive pain in the missing portion of the limb. As recovery and ambulation progress, phantom limb sensation and pain usually subside, although the pain may become chronic. The patient may also complain of shooting, burning, or crushing pain and feelings of coldness, heaviness, and cramping,

Mirror therapy reduces phantom limb sensation and pain in some patients[33] (Fig. 63-24). The mirror is thought to provide visual information to the brain, replacing the sensory feedback expected from the missing limb. However, it is unknown why looking in the mirror at the remaining limb would decrease phantom limb sensation and pain. Mirror therapy may also improve patient functioning after a stroke (see Evidence-Based Practice box on p. 1396 in Chapter 58).

Success of the rehabilitation program depends on the patient's physical and emotional health. Chronic illness and deconditioning can complicate rehabilitation efforts. Both physical and occupational therapy must be an integral component of the patient's overall plan of care.

Flexion contractures may delay the rehabilitation process. The most common and debilitating contracture is hip flexion. Hip adduction contracture is rare. To prevent flexion contractures, have patients avoid sitting in a chair for more than 1 hour with hips flexed or having pillows under the surgical extremity. Unless specifically contraindicated, patients should lie on their abdomen for 30 minutes three or four times each day and position the hip in extension while prone.

Proper residual limb bandaging fosters shaping and molding for eventual prosthesis fitting (Fig. 63-25). The physician usually orders a compression bandage to be applied immediately after surgery to support the soft tissues, reduce edema, hasten healing, minimize pain, and promote residual limb shrinkage and maturation. This bandage may be an elastic roll applied to the residual limb or a residual limb shrinker, which is an elastic stocking that fits tightly over the residual limb and lower trunk area.

The compression bandage is initially worn at all times except during physical therapy and bathing. The bandage is taken off and reapplied several times daily, and care is taken to apply it snugly but not so tight as to interfere with circulation. Shrinker bandages should be washed and changed daily. After it is healed, the residual limb is bandaged only when the patient is not wearing the prosthesis. Instruct the patient to avoid dangling the residual limb over the bedside to minimize edema.

As the patient's overall condition improves, an exercise regimen is normally started under the supervision of the health care provider and the physical therapist. Active ROM exercises of all joints should be started as soon after surgery as the patient's pain level and medical status permit. In preparation for mobility, the patient should increase triceps and shoulder strength and lower limb support and learn balance of the altered body. The loss of the weight of an amputated limb requires adaptation of the patient's proprioceptive and coordination mechanisms to prevent falls and injury.

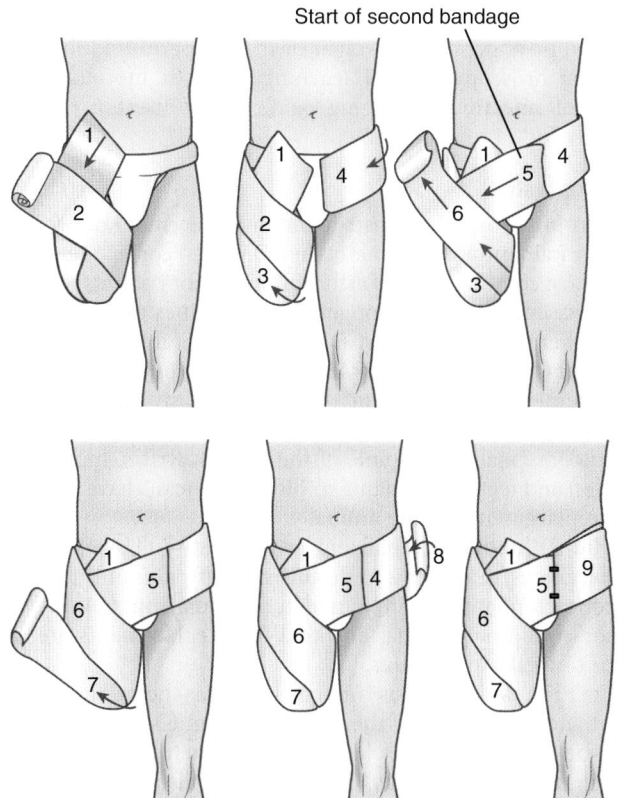

Start of second bandage

FIG. 63-25 Bandaging for the above-the-knee amputation residual limb. Figure-eight style covers progressive areas of the residual limb. Two elastic wraps are required.

Crutch walking is started as soon as the patient is physically able. After an immediate postsurgical fitting, orders related to weight bearing must be carefully followed to avoid injury to the skin flap and delay of tissue healing. Before discharge, instruct the patient and caregiver in residual limb care, ambulation, prevention of contractures, recognition of complications, exercise, and follow-up care (Table 63-14).

AMBULATORY AND HOME CARE. When healing has occurred satisfactorily and the residual limb is well molded, the patient is ready for fitting of the prosthesis. A prosthetist initially makes a mold of the residual limb and measures landmarks for fabrication of the prosthesis. The molded limb socket allows the residual limb to fit snugly into the prosthesis. The limb is covered with a residual limb stocking to ensure good fit and prevent skin breakdown. The residual limb may continue to shrink, causing a loose fit, in which case a new socket has to be fabricated. The patient may need to have the prosthesis adjusted to prevent rubbing and friction between the residual limb and socket. Excessive movement of a loose prosthesis can cause severe skin irritation, breakdown, and gait disturbances.

Artificial limbs become an integral part of the patient's changed body image. Instruct the patient to clean the prosthesis socket daily with a mild soap and rinse thoroughly to remove irritants. Leather and metal parts of the prosthesis should not get wet. Encourage the patient to have regular maintenance of the prosthesis. Consideration of the condition of the shoe is also necessary. A badly worn shoe alters the gait and may damage the prosthesis.

SPECIAL CONSIDERATIONS IN UPPER LIMB AMPUTATION. The emotional implications of an upper limb amputation are often

TABLE 63-14 **PATIENT & CAREGIVER TEACHING GUIDE**

Following an Amputation

After an amputation, include the following instructions when teaching the patient and caregiver.
1. Inspect the residual limb daily for signs of skin irritation, especially erythema, excoriation, and odor. Pay particular attention to areas prone to pressure.
2. Discontinue use of the prosthesis if irritation develops. Have the area checked before resuming use of the prosthesis.
3. Wash the residual limb thoroughly each night with warm water and a bacteriostatic soap. Rinse thoroughly and dry gently. Expose the residual limb to air for 20 min.
4. Do not use any substance such as lotions, alcohol, powders, or oil on residual limb unless prescribed by the health care provider.
5. Wear only a residual limb sock that is in good condition and supplied by the prosthetist.
6. Change residual limb sock daily. Launder in a mild soap, squeeze, and lay flat to dry.
7. Use prescribed pain management techniques.
8. Perform ROM to all joints daily. Perform general strengthening exercises, including the upper extremities, daily.
9. Do not elevate the residual limb on a pillow.
10. Lay prone with hip in extension for 30 min three or four times daily.

more devastating than those for lower limb amputation. The enforced dependency brought about by one-handedness may be depressing and frustrating to the patient. Because most upper extremity amputations result from trauma, the patient has had little time to adjust psychologically to an amputation or to participate in the decision-making process.

Both immediate and delayed prosthetic fittings are possible for the below-the-elbow amputee. Prosthetic fitting is delayed for the above-the-elbow amputee. The usual functional prosthesis is the arm and hook. A cosmetic hand is available but has limited functional value. As with the lower limb prosthesis, patient motivation and perseverance are major factors contributing to a satisfactory outcome. Technologic advances to improve the functionality of upper limb prostheses are an active area of research.[34]

EVALUATION

The expected outcomes are that the patient with an amputation will

- Accept changed body image and integrate changes into lifestyle
- Have no evidence of skin breakdown
- Have reduction or absence of pain
- Become mobile within limitations imposed by amputation

GERONTOLOGIC CONSIDERATIONS

AMPUTATION

If a lower limb amputation has been performed on an older adult, the patient's previous ability to ambulate may affect the extent of recovery. Use of a prosthesis requires significant strength and energy for ambulation. For example, walking with a below-the-knee prosthesis requires 40% additional energy, and an above-the-knee prosthesis requires 60% more energy than walking on two legs. Older adults whose general health is altered and weakened by disorders such as cardiac or pulmonary dysfunction may not be candidates for prosthesis use. The patient's ability to ambulate may be limited. If possible, discuss these issues with the patient and caregiver before surgery so that realistic expectations can be set.

COMMON JOINT SURGICAL PROCEDURES

Surgery plays an important role in the treatment and rehabilitation of patients with various types of joint disease. Surgery is aimed at relieving chronic pain, improving joint motion, correcting deformity and malalignment, and removing intraarticular erosion. If decreased functional ability of the joint is not corrected, contraction with permanent limitation of motion often occurs. Limitation of motion at the joint can be demonstrated on physical examination and by joint-space narrowing on x-ray examination.

TYPES OF JOINT SURGERIES

Synovectomy

Synovectomy (removal of synovial membrane) is used as a prophylactic measure and as a palliative treatment of rheumatoid arthritis (RA). Removal of the synovial membrane, thought to be the location of the basic pathologic changes in joint destruction, helps prevent further progression of joint damage. A synovectomy is best performed early in the disease process to prevent serious destruction of joint surfaces. Removal of the thickened synovium prevents extension of the inflammatory process into adjacent cartilage, ligaments, and tendons.

It is impossible to surgically remove all the synovium in a joint. The underlying disease process is still present and will again affect the regenerating synovium. However, the disease appears to be milder after synovectomy, and definite improvements in pain, weight bearing, and ROM can be expected. Common sites for this surgery include the elbow, wrist, and fingers. Synovectomy in the knee is done less frequently because knee joint replacement is usually performed.

Osteotomy

An osteotomy involves removing a wedge or slice of bone to change alignment (joint and vertebral) and to shift weight bearing, thereby correcting deformity and relieving pain. Cervical osteotomy may be used to correct deformity in some patients with ankylosing spondylitis. Halo vests and body jacket braces are worn until fusion occurs (3 to 4 months). Subtrochanteric or femoral osteotomy may provide some relief of pain and improve motion in selected patients with hip osteoarthritis (OA). Osteotomy has proven ineffective in patients with inflammatory joint disease. Osteotomy of the knee (tibia) provides relief of pain in selected patients, but advanced joint destruction is usually corrected by joint replacement surgery.

The postoperative care of the patient with an osteotomy is similar to the treatment of an internal fixation of a fracture at a comparable site (see p. 1519). Internal wires, screws and plates, bone grafts, or an external fixator usually fixes the bone in place.

Debridement

Debridement is the removal of degenerative debris such as loose bodies, osteophytes, joint debris, and degenerated menisci from a joint. This procedure is usually performed on the knee or shoulder using a fiberoptic arthroscope. The procedure is usually done on an outpatient basis. A compression dressing is applied postoperatively. Weight bearing is permitted following knee arthroscopy. Patient teaching includes monitoring for signs of infection, managing pain, and restricting excessive activity for 24 to 48 hours.

Arthroplasty

Arthroplasty is the reconstruction or replacement of a joint to relieve pain, improve or maintain ROM, and correct deformity. The most common uses of arthroplasty are for patients with OA, RA, avascular necrosis, congenital deformities or dislocations, and other systemic problems. There are several types of arthroplasty, including surgical reshaping of the bones of the joints, replacement of part of a joint (hemiarthroplasty), and total joint replacement. Replacement arthroplasty is available for elbows, shoulders, phalangeal joints of the fingers, wrists, hips, knees, ankles, and feet. More than 1 million Americans have knee and hip replacement surgery annually.[35]

Hip Arthroplasty. Total hip arthroplasty (THA) (total hip replacement) provides significant relief of pain and improved function for patients with joint deterioration from OA, RA, and other conditions. Partial and total hip replacements are also used to treat hip fractures.

In THA the prosthesis (implant) replaces the ball and socket joint and upper shaft of the femur (see Fig. 63-19). The socket can be "cemented" in place with polymethyl methacrylate, which bonds to the bone. The socket may also be inserted and not cemented ("cementless"). Cementless THAs may provide longer-term prosthesis stability by facilitating biologic ingrowth of new bone tissue into the porous surface coating of the prosthesis. Although some surgeons use cementless devices for all patients, they are most often recommended for younger, more active patients and patients with good bone quality where bone ingrowth into the components can be readily achieved.

The nursing care for a patient who has a THA is discussed in the section on nursing management of a patient with a hip fracture on pp. 1526–1527.

Hip Resurfacing. An alternative to hip replacement is hip resurfacing, which allows the femoral head to be preserved and reshaped rather than replaced. (In contrast, in a THA the prosthesis replaces the femoral head.) The resurfaced femoral head (ball) is then capped by a metal prosthesis. The metal appears to have a lower rate of wear, and thus the prosthesis may have a longer lifetime. Hip resurfacing is a more favorable option for younger, active patients. After surgery there is generally a 6-month waiting period before strenuous activity until strong muscles are built around the joint. Patients receiving a smaller femoral head (including many women) have a higher failure rate with a resurfaced implant when compared with patients receiving a THA.[36]

Knee Arthroplasty. Unremitting pain and instability as a result of severe destructive deterioration of the knee joint are the main indications for total knee arthroplasty (TKA).[37] Osteoporosis may necessitate bone grafting to augment defects and to correct bone deficiencies. Either part of or the entire knee joint may be replaced with a metal and plastic prosthetic device. A compression dressing may be used to immobilize the knee in extension immediately after the operation. This dressing is removed before discharge and may be replaced with a knee immobilizer or posterior plastic shell, which maintains extension during ambulation and at rest for about 4 weeks. Dislocation is not typical with TKA.

After surgery an emphasis is placed on physical therapy. Isometric quadriceps setting usually begins the first postoperative day. The patient progresses to straight-leg raises and gentle ROM to increase muscle strength and obtain 90-degree knee flexion. Active flexion exercises or passive flexion exercises with a continuous passive motion (CPM) machine may promote joint mobility. Full weight bearing is begun before discharge. An active home exercise program involves progressive ROM with muscle strengthening and flexibility exercises. After TKA, many older patients with advanced OA have shown significant improvement in mobility, motor function tests, and ability to complete daily tasks.

Finger Joint Arthroplasty. A silicone rubber arthroplastic device is used to help restore function in the fingers of the patient with RA. Ulnar deviation is often present, which results in severe functional limitations of the hand. The goal of hand surgery is primarily to restore function related to grasp, pinch, stability, and strength rather than to correct cosmetic deformity. Before surgery the patient is instructed in hand exercises, including flexion, extension, abduction, and adduction of the fingers.

Postoperatively the hand is kept elevated with a bulky dressing in place. After surgery, conduct a neurovascular assessment and look for signs of infection. The success of the surgery depends largely on the postoperative treatment plan, which is usually implemented by an occupational therapist. After the dressing is removed, a guided splinting program is initiated. The patient is discharged with splints to use while sleeping and hand exercises to perform at least three or four times a day for 10 to 12 weeks. Also instruct the patient to avoid lifting heavy objects.

Elbow and Shoulder Arthroplasty. Although available, total replacement of elbow and shoulder joints is not as common as other forms of arthroplasty. Shoulder replacements are performed in patients with severe pain because of RA, OA, avascular necrosis, or previous trauma. The shoulder replacement is usually considered if the patient has adequate surrounding muscle strength and bone stock. If joint replacement is necessary for both elbow and shoulder, the elbow is usually done first because a severely painful elbow interferes with the shoulder rehabilitation program.

Significant pain relief has been achieved after elbow and shoulder arthroplasty, with most patients having no pain at rest or minimal pain with activity. Functional improvements have also resulted in better hygiene and increased ability to perform activities of daily living. However, rehabilitation is longer and more difficult than with other joint surgeries.

Ankle Arthroplasty. Total ankle arthroplasty (TAA) is indicated for RA, OA, trauma, and avascular necrosis. Although the use of TAA is not widespread, it is becoming a viable alternative to fusion for the treatment of severe ankle arthritis in selected patients. Devices available include several fixed-bearing devices and a mobile-bearing cementless prosthesis. This device more closely imitates natural ankle function.

Ankle fusion is often selected over arthroplasty because the result is more durable. However, the patient is left with a stiff foot and the inability to change heel height. TAA is advantageous because it achieves a more normal gait pattern. Postoperatively, the patient may not bear weight for 6 weeks and must elevate the extremity to reduce and prevent edema, be extremely careful to prevent postoperative infection, and maintain immobilization as directed by the physician.

Arthrodesis

Arthrodesis is the surgical fusion of a joint. This procedure is indicated only if articular surfaces are too severely damaged or infected to allow joint replacement or if reconstructive surgery fails. Arthrodesis relieves pain and provides a stable but immobile joint. The fusion is usually accomplished by removal of the articular hyaline cartilage and the addition of bone grafts across the joint surface. The affected joint must be immobilized until bone healing has occurred. Common areas of fusion are wrist, ankle, cervical spine, lumbar spine, and metatarsophalangeal (MTP) joint of the great toe.

Complications of Joint Surgery

Infection is a serious complication of joint surgery, particularly joint replacement surgery.[37] The most common causative organisms are gram-positive aerobic streptococci and staphylococci. Infection may lead to pain and loosening of the prosthesis, generally requiring extensive surgery. Efforts to reduce the incidence of infection include the use of specially designed self-contained operating suites, operating rooms with laminar airflow, and prophylactic antibiotic administration.

Thromboembolism is another potentially serious complication after joint surgeries, particularly those involving the lower extremities. Prophylactic measures such as warfarin, LMWH, and sequential compression devices of the legs are usually instituted. Patients may be followed postoperatively with venous Doppler ultrasound to detect DVT, the source of most pulmonary emboli.

Collaborative Care

Preoperative Management. The primary goal of preoperative assessment is to identify risk factors associated with postoperative complications so that nursing strategies can be implemented to promote optimal positive outcomes. A careful history includes previous medical diagnoses and complications such as diabetes and thromboembolism, pain tolerance and management preferences, current functional status and expectations following surgery, and level of social support and home care needs after discharge. The patient should be free from infection and acute joint inflammation.

If lower extremity surgery is planned, assess upper extremity muscle strength and joint function to determine the type of assistive devices needed postoperatively for ambulation and activities of daily living. Preoperative teaching is important for the patient and caregiver related to the expected hospital course and postoperative management at home. In addition, it prepares them to maximize the usefulness and longevity of the prosthesis. Patients also need to realize that recovery is "not going to happen overnight." Talking with other people who have had a total joint arthroplasty may help the patient better understand the reality of rehabilitation.

Postoperative Management. Postoperatively, perform neurovascular assessment to assess nerve function and circulatory status. Anticoagulation therapy, analgesia, and parenteral antibiotics are administered. In general, the affected joint is exercised and ambulation is encouraged as early as possible to prevent complications of immobility. Specific protocols vary according to the patient, type of prosthesis, and surgeon preference. Pain management techniques may include epidural or intrathecal analgesia, femoral nerve block, patient-controlled IV analgesia, and oral opioids or NSAIDs. Assess patient comfort frequently during the postoperative period.

The hospital stay after arthroplasty is 3 to 5 days depending on the patient's course and need for physical therapy. Physical therapy and ambulation enhance mobility, build muscle strength, and reduce the risk of thromboembolism. If the patient is taking warfarin, therapy starts on the day of surgery, and prothrombin time is measured on a regular basis. For those taking LMWH (e.g., enoxaparin), therapy starts soon after surgery and continues for 2 weeks postoperatively. Daily monitoring of the patient's coagulation status is not necessary when the patient is taking LMWH.

NURSING MANAGEMENT
JOINT SURGERY

The nursing management of the patient undergoing joint surgery begins with preoperative teaching and realistic goal setting. It is important that the patient understands and accepts the limitations of the proposed surgery and realizes that in some cases surgery will not remove or treat the underlying disease. Explain postoperative procedures such as turning, deep breathing, use of bedpan and bedside commode, and use of abductor pillows. Provide opportunities for practice. Reassure the patient that pain relief will be available. Patient-controlled analgesia can be helpful. A preoperative visit from a physical therapist allows practice of postoperative exercises and measurement for crutches or other assistive devices.

Discharge planning begins immediately. Discuss the duration of the hospital stay and the expected postoperative events because the patient and caregiver must prepare. The home environment must be assessed for safety (e.g., scatter rugs, electric cords) and accessibility. Are the bathroom and bedroom on the first floor? Are door frames wide enough to accommodate a walker? Assess the patient's social support. Is a friend or family member available to assist the patient in the home? Will the patient require homemaker or meal services? The older patient may need the rehabilitation services of a subacute or extended care facility for a few weeks postoperatively to progressively develop independent living skills. Nursing interventions for the patient having orthopedic surgery are presented in eNursing Care Plan 63-2 (on the website for this chapter).

Instruct the patient on reporting complications, including infection (e.g., fever, increased pain, drainage) and dislocation of the prosthesis (e.g., pain, loss of function, shortening or malalignment of an extremity). Your role in the home care setting is to act as the liaison between the patient and surgeon, while monitoring for postoperative complications. Also assess the patient's comfort level and ROM at regular intervals to facilitate the goal of improved functional performance.

CASE STUDY

Hip Fracture Surgery

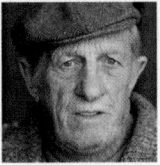

iStockphoto/Thinkstock

Patient Profile

T.K. is a 78-yr-old white man admitted to the hospital through the emergency department. It appears that he may have sustained a fracture to his left hip (see Chapter 62 case study on p. 1494). He is scheduled for a surgical hip repair in the morning.

Subjective Data

See the case study in Chapter 62 on p. 1497.

Collaborative Care
Preoperative
• Pain not relieved by morphine.
• Accompanying T.K. is his wife of 40 yr who is crying and anxious. Her anxiety is also causing T.K. to become anxious.

Operative Procedure
• Left hip repair using hip compression plate and bone screws

Postoperative
• Cefazolin (Ancef) 1 g IV q8hr
• Intake and output for 48 hr
• Morphine via patient-controlled analgesia pump

Discussion Questions
1. How do T.K.'s preexisting medical conditions predispose him to postoperative complications?

2. What actions can you take to help decrease the wife's anxiety?
3. **Priority Decision:** As you plan care for T.K., what are the preoperative and postoperative priority nursing interventions?
4. What are the most likely postoperative complications that T.K. could develop?
5. **Priority Decision:** On assessment of T.K. on the second postoperative day, you note an irregular pulse, which is a new finding. The pulse rate is 66 and the ECG tracing is shown below. You identify this as which dysrhythmia? What is the priority action at this time?

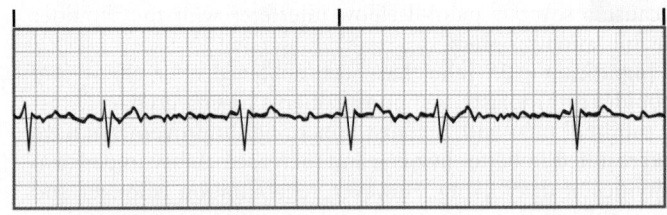

6. **Priority Decision:** What are the priority teaching interventions that should be done before discharge?
7. **Evidence-Based Practice:** Why is satisfactory pain relief an important nursing goal in the postoperative period for T.K?

BRIDGE TO NCLEX EXAMINATION

The number of the question corresponds to the same-numbered outcome at the beginning of the chapter.

1. The nurse suspects an ankle sprain when a patient at the urgent care center relates
   a. being hit by another soccer player during a game.
   b. having ankle pain after sprinting around the track.
   c. dropping a 10-lb weight on his lower leg at the health club.
   d. twisting his ankle while running bases during a baseball game.

2. The nurse explains to a patient with a fracture of the distal shaft of the humerus who is returning for a 4-week checkup that healing is indicated by
   a. formation of callus.
   b. complete bony union.
   c. hematoma at fracture site.
   d. presence of granulation tissue.

3. A patient with a comminuted fracture of the tibia is to have an open reduction with internal fixation (ORIF) of the fracture. The nurse explains that ORIF is indicated when
   a. the patient is unable to tolerate prolonged immobilization.
   b. the patient cannot tolerate the surgery of a closed reduction.
   c. a temporary cast would be too unstable to provide normal mobility.
   d. adequate alignment cannot be obtained by other nonsurgical methods.

4. An indication of a neurovascular problem noted during assessment of the patient with a fracture is
   a. exaggeration of strength with movement.
   b. increased redness and heat below the injury.
   c. decreased sensation distal to the fracture site.
   d. purulent drainage at the site of an open fracture.

5. A patient with a stable, closed fracture of the humerus caused by trauma to the arm has a temporary splint with bulky padding applied with an elastic bandage. The nurse suspects compartment syndrome and notifies the physician when the patient experiences
   a. increasing edema of the limb.
   b. muscle spasms of the lower arm.
   c. rebounding pulse at the fracture site.
   d. pain when passively extending the fingers.

6. A patient with a fracture of the pelvis should be monitored for
   a. changes in urine output.
   b. petechiae on the abdomen.
   c. a palpable lump in the buttock.
   d. sudden increase in blood pressure.

7. During the postoperative period, the nurse instructs the patient with an above-the-knee amputation that the residual limb should not be routinely elevated because this position promotes
   a. hip flexion contractures.
   b. skin irritation and breakdown.
   c. clot formation at the incision site.
   d. increased risk of wound dehiscence.

8. A patient with osteoarthritis is scheduled for a total hip arthroplasty. The nurse explains that the purpose of this procedure is to (select all that apply)
   a. fuse the joint.
   b. replace the joint.
   c. prevent further damage.
   d. improve or maintain ROM.
   e. decrease the amount of destruction in the joint.

9. In teaching a patient scheduled for a total ankle replacement, it is important to tell the patient that after surgery he should avoid
   a. lifting heavy objects.
   b. sleeping on the back.
   c. abduction exercises of the affected ankle.
   d. bearing weight on the affected leg for 6 weeks.

1. d, 2, a, 3, d, 4, c, 5, d, 6, a, 7, a, 8, b, d, 9, d

ⓔvolve

For rationales to these answers and even more NCLEX review questions, visit *http://evolve.elsevier.com/Lewis/medsurg*.

REFERENCES

1. Centers for Disease Control and Prevention: Ten leading causes of death and injury, causes of death by age group. Retrieved from *www.cdc.gov/nchs/fastats/lcod.htm*.

2. National Institute of Arthritis and Musculoskeletal and Skin Diseases: Childhood sports injuries and their prevention: a guide for parents with ideas for kids. Retrieved from *www.niams.nih.gov/health_info/Sports_Injuries/child_sports_injuries.asp*.

3. American Academy of Orthopaedic Surgeons: Sprains, strains, and other soft-tissue injuries. Retrieved from *www.orthoinfo.aaos.org/topic*.

4. National Institute on Aging and the National Aeronautics and Space Administration: Exercise: guide from the National Institute on Aging. Retrieved from *www.weboflife.ksc.nasa.gov/exerciseandaging*.

5. Buttaravoli P, Leffler S: Patellar dislocation. In Buttaravoli P, editor: *Minor emergencies*, ed 3, St Louis, 2012, Saunders.

6. Cleveland Clinic: Get a grip on carpal tunnel syndrome, *Arthritis Advisor* 11:4, 2012.

*7. Agency for Healthcare Research and Quality: Treatment options for rotator cuff tears: a guide for adults and comparative effectiveness of interventions for rotator cuff tears in adults: a guide for clinicians. Retrieved from *http://effectivehealthcare.ahrq.gov/index.cfm/search-for-guides-reviews-and-reports/?productid=544&pageaction=displayproduct*.

*8. Stensrud S, Roos E, Risberg M: A 12-week exercise therapy program in middle-aged patients with degenerative meniscus tears: a case series with 1-year follow-up, *J Orthop Sports Phys Ther* 42:919, 2012.

*9. Meuffels D, Poldervaart M, Diercks R, et al: Guideline on anterior cruciate ligament injury, *Acta Orthop* 83:379, 2012.

*10. Sadoghi P, von Keudell P: Effectiveness of anterior cruciate ligament injury prevention training programs, *J Bone Joint Surg* 94:769, 2012.

11. Aaron D, Patel A, Kayiaros S, et al: Four common types of bursitis: diagnosis and management, *J Am Acad Orthop Surg* 19:359, 2011.

*Evidence-based information for clinical practice.

12. Fazzalari N: Bone fracture and bone fracture repair, *Osteoporosis Int* 22:2003, 2011.

13. Marshall S, Browner B: Emergency care of musculoskeletal injuries. In Townsend C, Beauchamp R, Evers B, et al, editors: *Townsend: Sabiston textbook of surgery*, ed 19, St Louis, 2012, Saunders.

14. Satryb S, Wilson T, Patterson MM: Casting: all wrapped up, *Orthop Nurs* 30:37, 2011.

15. *Saunders nursing drug handbook*, St Louis, 2014, Saunders.

16. Patrice M, Hatch R: General principles of fracture care. In Patrice M, Hatch R, editors: *Eiff: fracture management for primary care*, ed 3, St Louis, 2011, Mosby.

17. Azar F: Traumatic disorders. In Canale S, Beaty J, editors: *Canale and Beaty: Campbell's operative orthopaedics*, ed 12, St Louis, 2012, Mosby.

18. Welle M: Understanding the new emerging oral anticoagulants for venous thromboembolism prophylaxis, *Orthop Nurs* 31:265, 2012.

19. Tzioupis C, Giannoudis P: Fat embolism syndrome: what have we learned over the years? *Trauma* 13:259, 2011.

*20. Ojike N: Pelvic compartment syndrome: a systematic review, *ACTA Orthop Belg* 78:6, 2012.

21. Centers for Disease Control and Prevention: Hip fractures among older adults. Retrieved from *www.cdc.gov/ HomeandRecreationalSafety/Falls/adulthipfx.html*.

22. Cummings-Vaughn L: Falls, osteoporosis, and hip fractures, *Med Clin North Am* 95:495, 2011.

*23. Hung W, Egol K, Zuckerman J, et al: Hip fracture management: tailoring care for the older patient, *JAMA* 307:2185, 2012.

24. World Health Organization: WHO global report on falls prevention in older age. Retrieved from *www.who.int/ageing/ publications/Falls_prevention7March.pdf*.

*25. Juby A: The challenges of interpreting efficacy of hip protector pads in fracture prevention in high-risk seniors, *Clin Rheumatol* 28:723, 2009. (Classic)

*26. Faucett S, Collinge C, Koval KJ: Is reconstruction nailing of all femoral shaft fractures cost effective? A decision analysis, *J Orthop Trauma* 26:624, 2012.

27. American Academy of Orthopaedic Surgeons: Osteoporosis and spinal fractures. Retrieved from *http://orthoinfo.aaos.org/ topic.cfm?topic=A00538*.

28. Asenjo J, Rossel F: Vertebroplasty and kyphoplasty: new evidence adds heat to the debate, *Curr Opin Anesthesiol* 25:577, 2012.

*29. Smith H, Peek-Asa C, Nesheim D, et al: Etiology, diagnosis, and characteristics of facial fracture at a Midwestern level I trauma center, *J Trauma Nurs* 19:57, 2012.

30. Patrice M, Hatch R: Facial and skull fractures. In Patrice M, Hatch R, editors: *Eiff: fracture management for primary care*, ed 3, St Louis, 2011, Mosby.

31. National Limb Loss Information Center: Fact sheet. Retrieved from *www.amputee-coalition.org/fact_sheets/amp_stats_cause*.

32. Fischer H: U.S. Military casualty statistics: Operation New Dawn, Operation Iraqi Freedom, and Operation Enduring Freedom, *Congressional Research Service 5-5700*, September 28, 2010.

*33. Rothgangel A, Brau S, Beurskens A, et al: The clinical aspects of mirror therapy in rehabilitation: a systematic review of the literature, *Int J Rehab Res*, 34:1, 2011.

34. Velez D, Dellefield M: Provide a helping hand to patients with upper extremity prostheses, *Nursing* 41:49, 2011.

35. National Institute of Arthritis and Musculoskeletal and Skin Diseases: Joint replacement surgery: information for multicultural communities. Retrieved from *www.niams.nih.gov/ health_info/joint_replacement/default.asp*.

*36. Smith A, Dieppe P, Howard P, et al: Failure rates of metal-on-metal hip resurfacings: analysis of data from the National Joint Registry for England and Wales, *Lancet* 380:1759, 2012.

37. Bartlett D: What you need to know about total knee arthroplasty, *OR Nurse* 6:16, 2012.

RESOURCES

American Academy of Orthopedic Surgeons (AAOS)
www.aaos.org
American Association for Hand Surgery
www.handsurgery.org
American College of Sports Medicine (ACSM)
www.acsm.org
Amputee Coalition
www.amputee-coalition.org
Easter Seals Disability Services
www.easterseals.com
National Amputation Foundation
www.nationalamputation.org
National Association of Orthopaedic Nurses (NAON)
www.orthonurse.org
National Institute of Arthritis and Musculoskeletal and Skin Diseases
www.niams.nih.gov

⊝volve

For additional Internet resources, see the website for this book at *http:// evolve.elsevier.com/Lewis/medsurg*.

Courage is like a muscle.
We strengthen it with use.
Ruth Gordon

Nursing Management
Musculoskeletal Problems

Jerry Harvey

⊖volve WEBSITE

http://evolve.elsevier.com/Lewis/medsurg

- NCLEX Review Questions
- Key Points
- Pre-Test
- Answer Guidelines for Case Study on p. 1558
- Rationales for Bridge to NCLEX Examination Questions

- Case Study
  - Patient With Osteoporosis
- Nursing Care Plans (Customizable)
  - eNCP 64-1: Patient With Osteomyelitis
  - eNCP 64-2: Patient With Low Back Pain

- Concept Map Creator
- Glossary
- Content Updates

LEARNING OUTCOMES

1. Describe the pathophysiology, clinical manifestations, collaborative care, and nursing management of osteomyelitis.
2. Differentiate among the types, pathophysiology, clinical manifestations, and collaborative care of bone cancer.
3. Differentiate between the causes and characteristics of acute and chronic low back pain.
4. Explain the conservative and surgical therapy of intervertebral disc damage.
5. Describe the postoperative nursing management of a patient who has undergone vertebral disc surgery.
6. Specify the etiology and nursing management of common foot disorders.
7. Describe the etiology, pathophysiology, clinical manifestations, and collaborative and nursing management of osteomalacia, osteoporosis, and Paget's disease.

KEY TERMS

Acute and chronic musculoskeletal problems are a common source of pain and disability. A variety of problems unrelated to trauma that affect the musculoskeletal system are presented in this chapter, including osteomyelitis, bone cancer, muscular dystrophy, foot disorders, and metabolic bone diseases. Management of the patient with both acute and chronic low back pain is addressed, and spinal surgery is discussed as an intervention for a herniated disc. Throughout the discussion of all of these problems, the nurse's role in prevention of injury and maintenance of mobility is emphasized.

OSTEOMYELITIS

Etiology and Pathophysiology

Osteomyelitis is a severe infection of the bone, bone marrow, and surrounding soft tissue. Although *Staphylococcus aureus* is a common cause of infection, a variety of microorganisms may cause osteomyelitis[1] (Table 64-1).

The infecting microorganisms can invade by indirect or direct entry. The *indirect entry* (hematogenous) of microorganisms most frequently affects growing bone in boys younger than 12 years old, and is associated with their higher incidence of blunt trauma. Adults with vascular insufficiency disorders (e.g., diabetes mellitus) and genitourinary and respiratory tract infections are at higher risk for a primary infection to spread via the blood to the bone. The pelvis, tibia, and vertebrae, which are vascular-rich sites of bone, are the most common sites of infection.

Direct entry osteomyelitis can occur at any age when there is an open wound (e.g., penetrating wounds, fractures) and microorganisms gain entry to the body. Osteomyelitis may also occur in the presence of a foreign body such as an implant

Reviewed by Tammy C. Roman, RN, EdD, CNE, Assistant Professor of Nursing, St. John Fisher College, Wegmans School of Nursing, Rochester, New York; and Dianne Travers Gustafson, RN, PhD, Associate Professor, Creighton University School of Nursing, Omaha, Nebraska.

TABLE 64-1	**ORGANISMS CAUSING OSTEOMYELITIS**
Organism	**Predisposing Problem**
Staphylococcus aureus	Pressure ulcer, penetrating wound, open fracture, orthopedic surgery, vascular insufficiency disorders (e.g., diabetes, atherosclerosis)
Staphylococcus epidermidis	Indwelling prosthetic devices (e.g., joint replacements, fracture fixation devices)
Streptococcus viridans	Abscessed tooth, gingival disease
Escherichia coli	Urinary tract infection
Mycobacterium tuberculosis	Tuberculosis
Neisseria gonorrhoeae	Gonorrhea
Pseudomonas	Puncture wounds, IV drug use
Salmonella	Sickle cell disease
Fungi, mycobacteria	Immunocompromised host

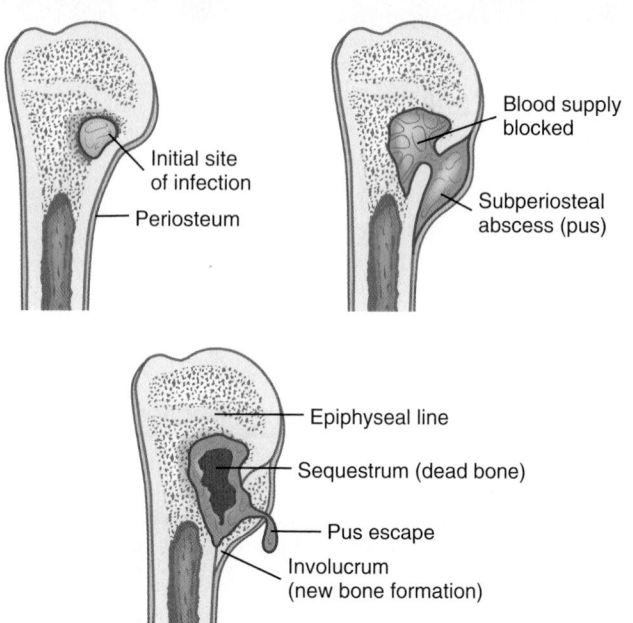

FIG. 64-1 Development of osteomyelitis infection with involucrum and sequestrum.

or an orthopedic prosthetic device (e.g., plate, total joint prosthesis).

After gaining entry into the blood, the microorganisms grow, resulting in an increase in pressure because of the nonexpanding nature of most bone. This increasing pressure eventually leads to ischemia and vascular compromise of the periosteum. The infection spreads through the bone cortex and marrow cavity, ultimately resulting in cortical devascularization and necrosis.

Once ischemia occurs, the bone dies. The area of devitalized bone eventually separates from the surrounding living bone, forming *sequestra*. The part of the periosteum that continues to have a blood supply forms new bone called *involucrum* (Fig. 64-1). It is difficult for blood-borne antibiotics or white blood cells (WBCs) to reach the sequestrum. A sequestrum may become a reservoir for microorganisms that spread to other sites, including the lungs and brain. If the sequestrum does not resolve on its own or is debrided surgically, a sinus tract may develop, resulting in chronic, purulent cutaneous drainage.

Clinical Manifestations and Complications

Acute osteomyelitis refers to the initial infection or an infection of less than 1 month in duration. The clinical manifestations of acute osteomyelitis are both local and systemic. Local manifestations include constant bone pain unrelieved by rest that worsens with activity; swelling, tenderness, and warmth at the infection site; and restricted movement of the affected part. Systemic manifestations include fever, night sweats, chills, restlessness, nausea, and malaise. Later signs include drainage from cutaneous sinus tracts or the fracture site.

Chronic osteomyelitis refers to a bone infection that persists for longer than 1 month or an infection that has failed to respond to the initial course of antibiotic therapy. Chronic osteomyelitis is either a continuous, persistent problem (a result of inadequate acute treatment) or a process of exacerbations and remissions (Fig. 64-2). Systemic signs may be diminished, with local signs of infection more common, including constant bone pain and swelling and warmth at the infection site. Over time, granulation tissue turns to scar tissue. This avascular scar tissue provides an ideal site for continued microorganism growth that cannot be penetrated by antibiotics.

Long-term and mostly rare complications of osteomyelitis include septicemia, septic arthritis, pathologic fractures, and amyloidosis.

Diagnostic Studies

A bone or soft tissue biopsy is the definitive way to determine the causative microorganism. The patient's blood and wound cultures are frequently positive for microorganisms.[2] An elevated WBC count and erythrocyte sedimentation rate (ESR) may also be found. X-ray signs suggestive of osteomyelitis usually do not appear until 10 days to weeks after the initial clinical symptoms, by which time the disease will have progressed. Radionuclide bone scans (gallium and indium) are helpful in diagnosis and are usually positive in the area of infection. Magnetic resonance imaging (MRI) and computed tomography (CT) scans may be used to help identify the extent of the infection.[3]

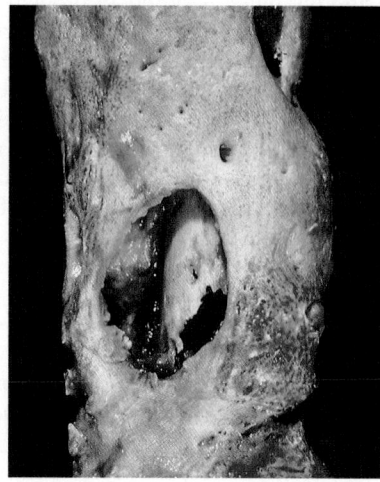

FIG. 64-2 Resection of femur due to osteomyelitis.

Collaborative Care

Vigorous and prolonged IV antibiotic therapy is the treatment of choice for acute osteomyelitis, as long as bone ischemia has not yet occurred. Cultures or a bone biopsy should be done if possible before initiating drug therapy. If antibiotic therapy is delayed, surgical debridement and decompression are often necessary.

Patients are often discharged to home care or a skilled nursing facility with IV antibiotics delivered via a central venous catheter or peripherally inserted central catheter. IV antibiotic therapy may be started in the hospital and continued at home for 4 to 6 weeks or as long as 3 to 6 months. A variety of antibiotics may be prescribed depending on the microorganism. These drugs include penicillin, nafcillin (Nafcil), neomycin, vancomycin, cephalexin (Keflex), cefazolin (Ancef), cefoxitin (Mefoxin), gentamicin (Garamycin), and tobramycin (Nebcin).

DRUG ALERT: Gentamicin (Garamycin)

- Assess patient for dehydration before starting therapy.
- Ensure renal function testing is done before starting therapy, especially in older patients.
- Monitor peak and trough levels for therapeutic effect and to minimize renal and inner ear toxicity.[4]
- Instruct patient to notify health care provider if any visual, hearing, or urinary problems develop.

In adults with chronic osteomyelitis, oral therapy with a fluoroquinolone (ciprofloxacin [Cipro]) for 6 to 8 weeks may be prescribed instead of IV antibiotics. Oral antibiotic therapy may also be given after acute IV therapy is completed to ensure resolution of the infection. The patient's response to drug therapy is monitored through bone scans and ESR tests.

Treatment of chronic osteomyelitis includes surgical removal of the poorly vascularized tissue and dead bone and the extended use of antibiotics.[5] Antibiotic-impregnated polymethyl methacrylate bead chains may also be implanted at this time to help combat the infection. After debridement of the devitalized and infected tissue, the wound may be closed and a suction irrigation system inserted. Intermittent or constant irrigation of the affected bone with antibiotics may also be initiated. Protection of the limb or the surgical site with casts or braces is often done. Negative-pressure wound therapy (vacuum-assisted wound closure) may be used (see pp. 181-182 in Chapter 12).

Hyperbaric oxygen with 100% oxygen may be given as an adjunct therapy in refractory cases of chronic osteomyelitis. This therapy is thought to stimulate circulation and healing in the infected tissue (see pp. 182-183 in Chapter 12). Orthopedic prosthetic devices, if a source of chronic infection, must be removed. Muscle flaps or skin grafting provides wound coverage over the dead space (cavity) in the bone. Bone grafts may help to restore blood flow. Amputation of the extremity may be indicated when bone destruction is extensive and to save the patient's life or to improve quality of life.

NURSING MANAGEMENT OSTEOMYELITIS

NURSING ASSESSMENT

Subjective and objective data that should be obtained from an individual with osteomyelitis are presented in Table 64-2.

NURSING DIAGNOSES

Nursing diagnoses for the patient with osteomyelitis may include, but are not limited to, the following.

- Acute pain *related to* inflammatory process secondary to infection

TABLE 64-2	NURSING ASSESSMENT

Osteomyelitis

Subjective Data
Important Health Information
Past health history: Bone trauma, open fracture, open or puncture wounds, other infections (e.g., streptococcal sore throat, bacterial pneumonia, sinusitis, skin or tooth infection, chronic urinary tract infection)
Medications: Analgesics or antibiotics
Surgery or other treatments: Bone surgery

Functional Health Patterns
Health perception–health management: IV drug and alcohol abuse; malaise
Nutritional-metabolic: Anorexia, weight loss; chills
Activity-exercise: Weakness, paralysis, muscle spasms around affected bone
Cognitive-perceptual: Local tenderness over affected area, increase in pain with movement of affected bone
Coping–stress tolerance: Irritability, withdrawal, dependency, anger

Objective Data
General
Restlessness; high, spiking temperature; night sweats

Integumentary
Diaphoresis; erythema, warmth, edema at infected bone

Musculoskeletal
Restricted movement; wound drainage; spontaneous fractures

Possible Diagnostic Findings
Leukocytosis, positive blood and/or wound cultures, ↑ erythrocyte sedimentation rate; presence of sequestrum and involucrum on x-rays, radionuclide bone scans, CT, and MRI

- Ineffective self–health management *related to* lack of knowledge regarding long-term management of osteomyelitis
- Impaired physical mobility *related to* pain, immobilization devices, and weight-bearing limitations

Additional information on nursing diagnoses for the patient with osteomyelitis is available in eNursing Care Plan 64-1 (on the website for this chapter).

PLANNING

The overall goals are that the patient with osteomyelitis will (1) have satisfactory pain and fever control, (2) not experience any complications associated with osteomyelitis, (3) cooperate with the treatment plan, and (4) maintain a positive outlook on the outcome of the disease.

NURSING IMPLEMENTATION

HEALTH PROMOTION. The control of infections already in the body (e.g., urinary, respiratory tract, deep pressure ulcers) is important in preventing osteomyelitis. Individuals who are especially at risk for osteomyelitis are those who are immunocompromised, have orthopedic prosthetic devices, or have vascular insufficiencies. Instruct these patients regarding the local and systemic manifestations of osteomyelitis. Also make family members aware of their role in monitoring the patient's health. Instruct patients to immediately report symptoms of bone pain, fever, swelling, and restricted limb movement to the health care provider so treatment can be started.

ACUTE INTERVENTION. Some immobilization of the affected limb (e.g., splint, traction) is usually indicated to decrease pain. Carefully handle the involved limb and avoid excessive manipulation, which increases pain and may cause a pathologic fracture. Assess the patient's pain. Minor to severe pain may be experienced with muscle spasms. Nonsteroidal antiinflammatory drugs (NSAIDs), opioid analgesics, and muscle relaxants may be prescribed to provide patient comfort. Encourage nondrug approaches to pain management (e.g., guided imagery, relaxation breathing) (see Chapters 7 and 9).

Dressings are used to absorb the exudate from draining wounds and to debride devitalized tissue from the wound site. Types of dressings include dry, sterile dressings; dressings saturated in saline or antibiotic solution; and wet-to-dry dressings. Handle soiled dressings carefully to prevent cross-contamination of the wound or spread of the infection to other patients. Sterile technique is essential when changing the dressing.

The patient is frequently on bed rest in the early stages of the acute infection. Good body alignment and frequent position changes prevent complications associated with immobility and promote comfort. Flexion contracture of the lower extremity is a common complication of osteomyelitis because the patient frequently positions the affected extremity in a flexed position to promote comfort. Footdrop can develop quickly if the foot is not correctly supported in a neutral position by a splint or if a splint applies excessive pressure, which can injure the peroneal nerve.

Teach the patient the potential adverse and toxic reactions associated with prolonged and high-dose antibiotic therapy (e.g., tobramycin, neomycin). These reactions include hearing deficit, nephrotoxicity, and neurotoxicity. With cephalosporins (e.g., cefazolin) these reactions include hives, severe or watery diarrhea, blood in stools, and throat or mouth sores.

Tendon rupture (especially the Achilles tendon) can occur with use of the fluoroquinolones (e.g., ciprofloxacin, levofloxacin [Levaquin]). Peak and trough blood levels of most antibiotics should be monitored to avoid adverse effects. Lengthy antibiotic therapy can also result in an overgrowth of *Candida albicans* and *Clostridium difficile* in the genitourinary and gastrointestinal (GI) tract, especially in immunosuppressed and older patients. Instruct the patient to report any changes in the oral cavity such as whitish yellow, curdlike lesions or changes in the genitourinary cavity such as any perianal itching or diarrhea.

The patient, caregiver, and family may be anxious and discouraged because of the serious nature of osteomyelitis, the uncertainty of the outcome, and the cost and lengthy course of treatment. Continued psychologic and emotional support is an integral part of nursing management. A nursing care plan for the patient with osteomyelitis (eNursing Care Plan 64-1) is available on the website for this chapter.

AMBULATORY AND HOME CARE. IV antibiotics can be administered to the patient in a skilled nursing facility or home setting. If at home, instruct the patient and caregiver on the proper care and management of the venous access device. Also teach them how to administer the antibiotic when scheduled and the need for follow-up laboratory testing. Stress the importance of continuing to take antibiotics after the symptoms have subsided. If there is an open wound, dressing changes are often necessary. The patient and caregiver may require supplies and instruction in the technique. If the osteomyelitis becomes chronic, patients need continued physical and psychologic support.

EVALUATION

The expected outcomes are that the patient with osteomyelitis will

- Have satisfactory pain relief
- Follow the recommended treatment regimen
- Verbalize confidence in ability to implement treatment regimen at home
- Demonstrate a consistent increase in mobility and range of motion

BONE TUMORS

Primary bone tumors, both benign and malignant, are relatively rare in adults. They account for only about 3% of all tumors. Metastatic bone cancer in which the cancer has spread from another site is a more common problem.

BENIGN BONE TUMORS

Benign bone tumors are more common than primary malignant tumors. The main types of benign bone tumors are osteochondroma, osteoclastoma, and endochroma (Table 64-3). These types of tumors are often removed by surgery.

Osteochondroma

Osteochondroma is the most common primary benign bone tumor. It is characterized by an overgrowth of cartilage and bone near the end of the bone at the growth plate. It is more commonly found in the long bones of the leg, pelvis, or scapula.

Clinical manifestations include a painless, hard, immobile mass; lower-than-normal height for age; soreness of muscles in close proximity to the tumor; one leg or arm longer than the other; and pressure or irritation with exercise. Patients may also be asymptomatic. Diagnosis is confirmed using x-ray, CT scan, and MRI.

No treatment is necessary for asymptomatic osteochondroma. If the tumor is causing pain or neurologic symptoms because of compression, surgical resection is usually done. Patients should have regular screening examinations for early detection of malignant transformation.

MALIGNANT BONE TUMORS

A sarcoma is a malignant tumor that can develop in bone, muscle, fat, nerve, or cartilage. The most common types of malignant bone tumors are osteosarcoma, chondrosarcoma, and Ewing's sarcoma (see Table 64-3). Annually about 2900 new cases of bone (and joint) cancer occur in the United States, with an estimated 1400 deaths.[6] Primary malignant tumors occur most often during childhood and young adulthood. They are characterized by their rapid metastasis and bone destruction.

Osteosarcoma

Osteosarcoma is a primary malignant bone tumor that is extremely aggressive and rapidly metastasizes to distant sites. It usually occurs in the metaphyseal region of the long bones of extremities, particularly in the regions of the distal femur, proximal tibia, and proximal humerus, as well as the pelvis (Fig. 64-3, *A*). Osteosarcoma is the most common malignant bone tumor affecting children and young adults. It can also occur, but not as commonly, in older adults. It is most often associated with Paget's disease and prior radiation.

TABLE 64-3	TYPES OF PRIMARY BONE TUMORS
Types	**Description**
Benign	
Osteochondroma	• Most common benign bone tumor • Frequently located in metaphyseal portion of long bones, particularly leg, pelvis, or scapula • Occurs most often in persons ages 10-25 • Malignant transformation may occur (chondrosarcoma)
Osteoclastoma (giant cell tumor)	• Arises in cancellous ends of arm and leg bones • About 10% are locally aggressive and may spread to lungs • High rate of local recurrence after surgery and chemotherapy
Endochroma	• Intramedullary cartilage tumor usually found in cavity of a single hand or foot bone • Rare malignant transformation can occur • If tumor becomes painful, a surgical resection is done • Peak incidence in persons ages 10-20
Malignant	
Osteosarcoma	• Most common primary bone cancer • Occurs mostly in young males between ages 10 and 25 • Most often in bones of arms, legs, or pelvis (see Fig. 64-3, *A*)
Chondrosarcoma	• Occurs in cartilage most commonly in arm, leg, and pelvic bones of older adults ages 50-70 • Can also arise from benign bone tumors (osteochondromas) • Wide surgical resection is mostly done, since tumor rarely responds to radiation and chemotherapy • Survival rate depends on stage, size, and grade of tumor (see Fig. 64-3, *B*)
Ewing's sarcoma	• Develops in medullary cavity of long bones, especially femur, humerus, pelvis, and tibia • Usually occurs in children and teenagers • Use of wide surgical resection, radiation, and chemotherapy has greatly improved the 5-yr survival rate to 60%

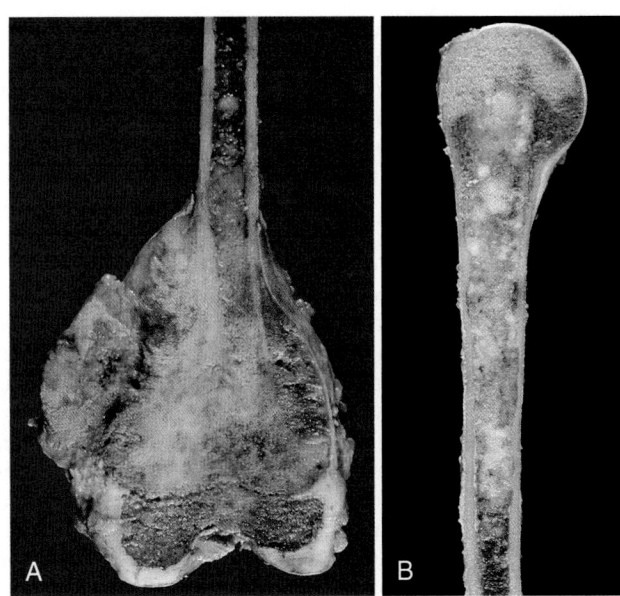

FIG. 64-3 A, Osteosarcoma. **B,** Chondrosarcoma.

The use of adjunct chemotherapy after amputation or limb salvage has increased the 5-year survival rate to 70% in people without metastasis. Chemotherapy includes methotrexate, doxorubicin (Adriamycin), cisplatin (Platinol), cyclophosphamide (Cytoxan), etoposide (VePesid), bleomycin (Blenoxane), dactinomycin (Cosmegen), and ifosfamide (Ifex).[7]

Metastatic Bone Cancer

The most common type of malignant bone tumor occurs as a result of metastasis from a primary tumor located at another site. Common sites for the primary tumor include breast, prostate, lungs, kidney, and thyroid. Metastatic cancer cells travel from the primary tumor to the bone via the lymph and blood supply. The metastatic bone lesions are commonly found in vertebrae, pelvis, femur, humerus, or ribs.[8] Pathologic fractures at the site of metastasis are common because of a weakening of the involved bone. High serum calcium levels result as calcium is released from damaged bones.

Once a primary lesion has been identified, radionuclide bone scans are often done to detect the metastatic lesions before they are visible on x-ray. Metastatic bone lesions may occur at any time (even years later) following diagnosis and treatment of the primary tumor. Metastasis to the bone should be suspected in any patient who has local bone pain and a past history of cancer. Treatment may be palliative and consists of radiation and pain management (see Chapter 9). Surgical stabilization of the bone may be indicated if there is a fracture or the patient is at high risk for a fracture. Prognosis depends on the primary type of cancer and any other sites of metastasis.

NURSING MANAGEMENT
BONE CANCER

Assess the patient with bone cancer for the location and severity of pain. Also note weakness caused by anemia and decreased mobility. Monitor the site of the tumor for swelling; changes in circulation; and decreased movement, sensation, or joint function.

Clinical manifestations of osteosarcoma are usually associated with the gradual onset of pain and swelling, especially around the knee. A minor injury does not cause the neoplasm but may bring the preexisting condition to medical attention. Metastasis is present in 10% to 20% of individuals when they are diagnosed with osteosarcoma.

Diagnosis is confirmed from tissue biopsy, elevation of serum alkaline phosphatase and calcium levels, x-ray, computed tomography (CT) or positron emission tomography (PET) scans, and magnetic resonance imaging (MRI).

Preoperative (neoadjuvant) chemotherapy may be used in the treatment of osteosarcoma to decrease tumor size before surgery. Limb salvage procedures are usually considered when there is a clear (no cancer present) 6- to 7-cm margin surrounding the lesion. Limb salvage is usually contraindicated if there is major neurovascular involvement, pathologic fracture, infection, or extensive muscle involvement.

Nursing care of the patient with a malignant bone tumor does not differ significantly from the care provided to the patient with a malignant disease of any other body system (see Chapter 16). However, special attention is required to prevent pathologic fractures or to reduce the complications associated with them. It is important to prevent fractures by careful handling and support of the affected extremity and logrolling for those on bed rest.

Treatment for hypercalcemia may need to be initiated if bone decalcification occurs (see Chapter 16, p. 278). The patient is often reluctant to participate in exercise or therapeutic activities because of weakness from the disease and the treatment, fear of falling and fracturing a bone, and fear of pain. Provide regular rest periods between activities.

The pain associated with bone cancer can be severe. The pain is often caused by the tumor pressing against nerves and other organs near the bone. Carefully monitor the patient's pain and ensure that he or she has adequate pain medication. Sometimes radiation therapy is used as a palliative therapy to shrink the tumor and decrease the pain.

Assist the patient and caregiver in accepting the poor prognosis associated with bone malignancies. General principles related to cancer nursing are applicable (see Chapter 16). Special attention is necessary for the problems of pain and disability, side effects of chemotherapy, and postoperative care after surgery such as spinal cord decompression or amputation. As with all types of cancer, stress the importance of follow-up examinations.

MUSCULAR DYSTROPHY

Muscular dystrophy (MD) is a group of genetic diseases characterized by progressive symmetric wasting of skeletal muscles without evidence of neurologic involvement. In all forms of MD an insidious loss of strength occurs with increasing disability and deformity. The types of MD differ in the groups of muscles affected, age of onset, rate of progression, and mode of genetic inheritance (Table 64-4). The most common type of MD is Duchenne.

Genetic Link

Both Duchenne and Becker MD are X-linked recessive disorders usually seen only in males. (X-linked recessive disorders are discussed in Chapter 13.) In Duchenne and Becker MD there is a mutation of the dystrophin gene. Dystrophin in normal muscle cells helps skeletal muscle fibers attach to the basement membrane. Abnormal dystrophin can lead to defects in the plasma membrane of muscle fiber with subsequent muscle fiber degeneration.

A family history can be used to obtain a family pedigree. Family pedigrees for X-linked recessive disorders are shown in Figs. 13-4 and 13-5.

Diagnostic studies for MD include muscle serum enzymes (especially creatine kinase), electromyogram (EMG) testing, muscle fiber biopsy, and electrocardiogram abnormalities reflective of cardiomyopathy. Muscle biopsy confirms the diagnosis with classic findings of fat and connective tissue deposits, degeneration and necrosis of muscle fibers, and a deficiency of the muscle protein dystrophin.

Currently no definitive therapy is available to stop the progressive wasting of MD. The primary goals of treatment are to preserve mobility and independence through exercise, physical

TABLE 64-4		TYPES OF MUSCULAR DYSTROPHY
Type	**Genetic Basis**	**Manifestations**
Duchenne (pseudohypertrophic)	X-linked Mutation of dystrophin gene	• Onset before age 5 yr • Progressive weakness of pelvic and shoulder muscles • Unable to walk after age 12 yr • Cardiomyopathy • Respiratory failure in teens or 20s • Mental impairment
Becker (benign pseudohypertrophic)	X-linked Mutation of dystrophin gene	• Onset between 5 and 15 yr • Slower course of pelvic and shoulder muscle wasting than Duchenne • Cardiomyopathy • Respiratory failure • May survive into 30s or 40s
Landouzy-Déjérine (facioscapulohumeral)	Autosomal dominant Deletion of chromosome 4q35	• Onset before age 20 • Slowly progressive weakness of face, shoulder muscles, and foot dorsiflexion • Deafness
Erb (limb-girdle)	Autosomal recessive or autosomal dominant	• Onset ranges from early childhood to early adulthood • Slow progressive weakness of shoulder and hip muscles

therapy, and orthopedic appliances. Progressive weakening of muscles around the trunk can lead to spinal collapse. To prevent injuries, the patient may be fitted early with an orthotic jacket to provide stability and prevent further deformity.

Cardiomyopathy often occurs and results in heart failure. Dysrhythmias are a frequent cause of death.[9] Gradual decreases in respiratory function often lead to the use of continuous positive airway pressure (CPAP). Eventually a tracheostomy and mechanical ventilation are necessary to sustain respiratory function. Corticosteroid therapy may significantly halt the disease progression for up to 2 years.[10]

Encourage communication among family members (and parents) to cope with the emotional and physical strains of MD. Teach the patient and caregiver range-of-motion exercises, nutritional therapy, and signs of progression. Genetic testing and counseling may be recommended for individuals with a family history of MD.

Focus your care on keeping the patient active as long as possible. Prolonged bed rest should be avoided because immobility can lead to further muscle wasting. As the disease progresses, the focus shifts to teaching the patient to limit sedentary periods to prevent skin breakdown and respiratory complications. Ongoing medical and nursing care is required throughout the individual's lifetime. The Muscular Dystrophy Association (*www.mda.org*) is an important resource for health care and support services for MD patients and their caregivers and family.

LOW BACK PAIN

Low back pain is most often due to a musculoskeletal problem. It may be experienced as localized or diffuse. In *localized pain* patients feel soreness or discomfort when they or someone else

GENETICS IN CLINICAL PRACTICE
Duchenne and Becker Muscular Dystrophy (MD)

Genetic Basis
- Caused by different mutations in the same *DMD* gene.
- Gene provides instructions for making dystrophin (protein that keeps muscles intact).
- X-linked recessive disorder.

Incidence
- Between 400 and 600 boys are born with MD each year.
- Together these disorders affect 1 in 3500–5000 newborn males.

Genetic Testing
- DNA testing for mutation in dystrophin gene is available.

Clinical Implications
- Muscular dystrophies are a group of genetic conditions characterized by progressive muscle weakness and atrophy.
- These two conditions differ in their severity, age of onset, and rate of progression (see Table 64-4).
- Few individuals with the disease live to adulthood.
- Genetic testing and counseling should be considered in individuals with a family history of MD.
- Because there are many types of MD with different genetic bases, establishing the type of MD is important to determine treatment and possible genetic counseling recommendations.

palpates or presses on a specific area of the lower back. *Diffuse pain* is spread over a larger area and comes from deep tissue layers.

Low back pain may be radicular or referred. *Radicular pain* is caused by irritation of a nerve root. Sciatica is an example of radicular pain. *Referred pain* is "felt" or perceived in the lower back, but the source of the pain is another location (e.g., kidneys, lower abdomen).

Low back pain is common and has affected about 80% of adults in the United States at least once during their lifetime. Backache is second only to headache as the most common pain complaint. In persons under age 45, low back pain is responsible for more lost working hours than any other medical condition.[11]

Low back pain is a common problem because the lumbar region (1) bears most of the weight of the body, (2) is the most flexible region of the spinal column, (3) contains nerve roots that are vulnerable to injury or disease, and (4) has an inherently poor biomechanical structure. Several risk factors associated with low back pain include lack of muscle tone and excess body weight, stress, poor posture, cigarette smoking, pregnancy, prior compression fractures of the spine, spinal problems since birth, and a family history of back pain. Jobs that require repetitive heavy lifting, vibration (such as a jackhammer operator), and prolonged periods of sitting are also associated with low back pain.

The causes of low back pain of musculoskeletal origin include (1) acute lumbosacral strain, (2) instability of the lumbosacral bony mechanism, (3) osteoarthritis of the lumbosacral vertebrae, (4) degenerative disc disease, and (5) herniation of an intervertebral disc.

Health care personnel who engage in patient care–related tasks are at high risk for the development of low back pain.[12] Lifting and moving patients, excessive time stooping over or leaning forward, and frequent twisting can result in low back pain that contributes to lost time and productivity and disability.

ACUTE LOW BACK PAIN

Acute low back pain is low back pain that lasts 4 weeks or less. Most acute low back pain is caused by trauma or some type of activity that causes undue stress (often hyperflexion) of the lower back. Examples of trauma or activity that could cause acute back pain are heavy lifting, overuse of the back muscles while working in the yard, a sports injury, or a sudden jolt such as a car accident.

Often symptoms do not appear at the time of injury but develop later (usually within 24 hours) because of a gradual increase in pressure on the nerve by an intervertebral disc. Symptoms may range from muscle ache to shooting or stabbing pain, limited flexibility or range of motion, or an inability to stand straight.

Few definitive diagnostic abnormalities are present with nerve irritation and muscle strain. One test is the straight-leg raise (see Chapter 62, p. 1498). MRI and CT scans are generally not done unless trauma or systemic disease (e.g., cancer, spinal infection) is suspected.

NURSING AND COLLABORATIVE MANAGEMENT
ACUTE LOW BACK PAIN

NURSING ASSESSMENT

Subjective and objective data that should be obtained from the patient with low back pain are summarized in Table 64-5.

NURSING IMPLEMENTATION

HEALTH PROMOTION. As a role model, you need to use proper body mechanics at all times. This includes increasing the patient's bed height, bending at the knees, asking for help in lifting and moving patients, and using lifting devices.

Assess the patient's use of body mechanics and offer advice when the person does activities that could produce back strain (Table 64-6). Some health care providers refer patients with back pain to a program called "Back School." It is a formal program usually taught by health professionals such as physicians, nurses, and physical therapists. It is designed to teach the patient how to minimize back pain and avoid repeat episodes of low back pain. Tips for prevention of back injury are listed in Table 64-6.

Advise patients to maintain appropriate body weight. Excess body weight places additional stress on the lower back and weakens the abdominal muscles that support the lower back. Flat shoes or shoes with low heels and shock-absorbing shoe inserts are recommended for women.

The position assumed while sleeping is also important in preventing low back pain. Tell patients to avoid sleeping in a prone position because it produces excessive lumbar lordosis, placing excessive stress on the lower back. The patient should sleep in either a supine or side-lying position with knees and hips flexed to prevent unnecessary pressure on support muscles, ligaments, and lumbosacral joints. A firm mattress is recommended.

Teach patients the importance of stopping smoking, since it has been associated with low back pain. One reason for this is that nicotine decreases circulation to the intervertebral discs.

TABLE 64-5   NURSING ASSESSMENT

Low Back Pain

Subjective Data
Important Health Information
Past health history: Acute or chronic lumbosacral strain/trauma, osteoarthritis, degenerative disc disease, obesity
Medications: Opioid and nonopioid analgesics, muscle relaxants, nonsteroidal antiinflammatory drugs, corticosteroids; over-the-counter remedies, including herbal products and nutritional supplements
Surgery or other treatments: Previous back surgery, epidural corticosteroid injections

Functional Health Patterns
Health perception–health management: Smoking, lack of exercise
Nutritional-metabolic: Obesity
Activity-exercise: Poor posture, muscle spasms, activity intolerance
Elimination: Constipation
Sleep-rest: Interrupted sleep
Cognitive-perceptual: Pain in back, buttocks, or leg associated with walking, turning, straining, coughing, leg raising; numbness or tingling of legs, feet, toes
Role-relationship: In occupations requiring heavy lifting, vibrations, or extended driving; change in role within family structure due to inability to work and provide income

Objective Data
General
Guarded movement

Neurologic
Depressed or absent Achilles tendon reflex or patellar tendon reflex; positive straight-leg-raising test, positive crossover straight-leg-raising test, positive Trendelenburg test

Musculoskeletal
Tense, tight paravertebral muscles on palpation, ↓ range of motion of spine

Possible Diagnostic Findings
Localization of site of lesion or disorder on myelogram, CT scan, or MRI; determination of nerve root impingement on electromyography

HEALTHY PEOPLE

Prevention of Low Back Pain

- Maintain healthy weight.
- Do not sleep in a prone position.
- Sleep on side with knees flexed and a pillow between the knees.
- Avoid cigarette smoking and tobacco products.
- Obtain regular physical activity, including strength and endurance training.
- Use proper body mechanics to avoid low back strain (e.g., when lifting heavy objects, bend at the knees, not at the waist, and stand up slowly while holding object close to your body).

ACUTE INTERVENTION. If the acute muscle spasms and accompanying pain are not severe and debilitating, the patient may be treated on an outpatient basis with NSAIDs (e.g., acetaminophen) and muscle relaxants (e.g., cyclobenzaprine [Flexeril]). Massage and back manipulation, acupuncture, and the application of cold and hot compresses may help some patients.[13] Severe pain may require a brief course of opioid analgesics.

TABLE 64-6   PATIENT & CAREGIVER TEACHING GUIDE

Low Back Problems

Include the following instructions when teaching the patient and caregiver how to manage low back problems.

Do
- Avoid straining the lower back by placing a foot on a step or stool during prolonged standing.
- Sleep in a side-lying position with knees and hips bent.
- Sleep on back with a lift under knees and legs or on back with 10-in-high pillow under knees to flex hips and knees.
- Regularly exercise 15 min in the morning and evening; begin exercises with 2- or 3-min warm-up period by moving arms and legs, alternately relaxing and tightening muscles; exercise slowly with smooth movements.
- Carry light items close to body.
- Maintain appropriate body weight.
- Use local heat and cold application.
- Use a lumbar roll or pillow for sitting.

Do Not
- Lean forward without bending knees.
- Lift anything above level of elbows.
- Stand in one position for prolonged time.
- Sleep on abdomen or on back or side with legs out straight.
- Exercise without consulting health care provider if having severe pain.
- Exceed prescribed amount and type of exercises without consulting health care provider.

A brief period (1 to 2 days) of rest at home may be necessary for some people, but most patients do better with a continuation of their regular activities. Prolonged bed rest should be avoided.[14] Patients should refrain from activities that aggravate the pain, including lifting, bending, twisting, and prolonged sitting. Most cases of acute low back pain show improvement within 2 weeks and often resolve without treatment.

Teach patients about their health problem and ways to prevent recurrent episodes. Muscle stretching and strengthening exercises may be part of the management plan. (See the Resource section at the end of this chapter for a link to exercises to strengthen the back.) Although the actual exercises are often taught by the physical therapist, it is your responsibility to ensure that the patient understands the type and frequency of exercise prescribed and the rationale for the program.

Other nursing interventions for the patient with low back pain are summarized in eNursing Care Plan 64-2 (on the website for this chapter).

AMBULATORY AND HOME CARE. The goal of management is to make an episode of acute low back pain an isolated incident. If the lumbosacral mechanism is unstable, repeated episodes can be anticipated. The lumbosacral spine may be unable to meet the demands placed on it without strain because of factors such as obesity, poor posture, poor muscle support, older age, or trauma. Intervention is aimed at strengthening the supporting muscles by exercise (see above).

Persistent use of poor body mechanics may also result in repeated episodes of low back pain. If the strain is work related, occupational counseling may be necessary. The frustration, pain, and disability imposed on the patient with low back pain require your emotional support and understanding care.

CHRONIC LOW BACK PAIN

Chronic low back pain is low back pain that lasts more than 3 months or is a repeated incapacitating episode. It is often progressive, and the cause can be difficult to determine. Causes include (1) degenerative conditions such as arthritis or disc disease; (2) osteoporosis or other metabolic bone diseases; (3) prior injury (scar tissue weakens the back); (4) chronic strain on the lower back muscles from obesity, pregnancy, or job-related stooping, bending, or other stressful postures; and (5) congenital abnormalities in the spine.

Spinal Stenosis

Spinal stenosis is a narrowing of the spinal canal (hollow vertical hole that contains the spinal cord). Stenosis in the lumbar area of the spine is a common cause of chronic low back pain. Spinal stenosis can be caused by either acquired or inherited conditions. A common acquired cause is osteoarthritis in the spine. Arthritic changes (bone spurs, calcification of spinal ligaments, degeneration of discs) narrow the space around the spinal canal and nerve roots, eventually leading to compression. Inflammation caused by the compression results in pain, weakness, and numbness.

Other acquired conditions that may lead to spinal stenosis include rheumatoid arthritis, spinal tumors, Paget's disease, and traumatic damage to the vertebral column. Inherited conditions that lead to spinal stenosis include congenital spinal stenosis and scoliosis.

The pain associated with lumbar spinal stenosis often starts in the lower back and then radiates to the buttock and leg. It worsens with walking and, in particular, standing without walking. Numbness, tingling, weakness, and heaviness in the legs and buttocks may also be present. A history of the pain lessening when the patient bends forward or sits down is often a sign of spinal stenosis. In most cases the stenosis slowly progresses and does not cause paralysis.

NURSING AND COLLABORATIVE MANAGEMENT CHRONIC LOW BACK PAIN

Nursing management and treatment of chronic low back pain are similar to those recommended for acute low back pain. Relief of pain and stiffness with mild analgesics, such as NSAIDs, is necessary for the patient's daily comfort. Antidepressants (e.g., duloxetine [Cymbalta]) may help with pain relief and sleep problems. The antiseizure drug gabapentin (Neurontin) may improve walking and relieve leg symptoms.

Weight reduction, sufficient rest periods, local heat or cold application, physical therapy, and exercise and activity throughout the day assist in keeping the muscles and joints mobilized. Cold, damp weather aggravates the back pain, which can be relieved with rest and local heat application. Complementary and alternative therapies such as biofeedback, acupuncture, and yoga may help reduce the pain (see the Evidence-Based Practice box). "Back School" (discussed on p. 1545) can significantly reduce pain and improve body posture for both patients and nurses.[15]

Minimally invasive treatments, such as epidural corticosteroid injections and implanted devices that deliver pain medication, may be used for patients with chronic low back pain that is refractory to the usual therapeutic options. Surgical intervention may be indicated in patients with severe chronic low back pain who do not respond to conservative care and/or have continued neurologic deficits. (Surgery for low back pain is discussed on pp. 1548-1550.)

EVIDENCE-BASED PRACTICE

Translating Research Into Practice

Can Yoga Improve Chronic Low Back Pain?

Clinical Question
Among adults with chronic low back pain (P), do interventions of yoga (I) vs. stretching exercises vs. a self-care book (C) improve function and pain (O)?

Best Available Evidence
Randomized controlled trials (RCTs)

Critical Appraisal and Synthesis of Evidence
- One RCT (*n* = 228) of adults with chronic low back pain comparing 12 weekly classes of yoga (*n* = 92) or stretching exercises (*n* = 91) or a self-care book on chronic low back pain (*n* = 45).
- Outcomes of back-related functional status and pain were assessed at 6, 12, and 26 wk.
- At 12 wk patients doing yoga had better functioning and less pain than patients in the self-care group.
- At 26 wk, functioning for the yoga group remained superior to the self-care group.
- Yoga was not better than stretching exercises at any time point.

Conclusion
- Yoga was more effective than a self-care book in improving function and reducing pain for at least several months. Yoga was no better than stretching classes.

Implications for Nursing Practice
- Assist patients in identifying resources and community classes that focus on stretching exercises and yoga.
- Assess and monitor back pain. Encourage regular participation in complementary and alternative therapies that patients find effective for chronic low back pain.

Reference for Evidence
Sherman KJ, Cherkin DC, Wellman RD, et al: A randomized trial comparing yoga, stretching, and a self-care book for chronic low back pain, *Arch Intern Med* 171:2019, 2011.

P, Patient population of interest; *I*, intervention or area of interest; *C*, comparison of interest or comparison group; *O*, outcomes of interest (see p. 12).

INTERVERTEBRAL DISC DISEASE

Intervertebral discs separate the vertebrae of the spinal column and provide shock absorption for the spine. *Intervertebral disc disease* is a condition that involves the deterioration, herniation, or other dysfunction of the intervertebral discs. Disc disorders can involve the cervical, thoracic, and lumbar spine.

Etiology and Pathophysiology

Structural degeneration of discs is often caused by degenerative disc disease (DDD). This progressive degeneration is a normal process of aging and results in the intervertebral discs losing their elasticity, flexibility, and shock-absorbing capabilities.[16] Thinning of the discs occurs as the *nucleus pulposus* (gelatinous center of the disc) starts to dry out and shrink. These changes limit the ability of the discs to distribute pressure loads between the vertebrae. Then these loads are transferred to the *annulus fibrosus* (strong outside portion of the intervertebral disc), causing progressive structural deterioration. With structural damage to the disc, the nucleus pulposus may seep through a torn or stretched annulus. This is called a **herniated disc** *(slipped disc),* a condition in which a spinal disc herniates and bulges outward between the vertebrae (Fig. 64-4).

A herniated disc can be the result of natural degeneration with age or repeated stress and trauma to the spine. The nucleus pulposus may first bulge and then it can herniate, placing pressure on nearby nerves. The most common sites of herniation are the lumbosacral discs, specifically L4-5 and L5-S1. Disc herniation may also occur at C5-6 and C6-7. Disc herniation may be the result of spinal stenosis, in which narrowing of the spinal canal forces the intervertebral disc to bulge.

The spinal nerves emerge from the spinal column through an opening *(intervertebral foramen)* between adjacent vertebrae. Herniated discs can press against these nerves ("pinched nerve") causing *radiculopathy* (radiating pain, numbness, tingling, and diminished strength and/or range of motion).

Osteoarthritis of the spine is associated with DDD and the stresses placed on the vertebrae. The joints, which are not adequately lubricated, rub against each other, leading to damage of the protective cartilage and the formation of painful bone spurs, which are one of the changes found in osteoarthritis.

Clinical Manifestations

In *lumbar disc disease* the most common manifestation is low back pain. Radicular pain that radiates down the buttock and below the knee, along the distribution of the sciatic nerve, generally indicates disc herniation. (Specific manifestations of lumbar disc herniation are summarized in Table 64-7.) The straight-leg-raising test may be positive, indicating nerve root irritation. Back or leg pain may be reproduced by raising the leg and flexing the foot at 90 degrees. Low back pain from other causes may not be accompanied by leg pain. Reflexes may be depressed or absent, depending on the spinal nerve root involved. Paresthesia or muscle weakness in the legs, feet, or toes may occur.

Multiple nerve root *(cauda equina)* compressions from a herniated disc, a tumor, or an epidural abscess may be manifested as bowel and bladder incontinence.[17] This condition is a medical emergency.

In *cervical disc disease* pain radiates into the arms and the hands, following the pattern of the nerve involved. Similar to lumbar disc disease, reflexes may or may not be present, and the handgrip is often weak.

Diagnostic Studies

X-rays are done to detect any structural defects. A myelogram, MRI, or CT scan is helpful in localizing the damaged site. An epidural venogram or diskogram may be necessary if other methods of diagnosis are unsuccessful. An EMG of the extremities can be performed to determine the severity of nerve irritation or to rule out other pathologic conditions such as peripheral neuropathy.

Collaborative Care

The patient with suspected disc damage is usually first managed with conservative therapy (Table 64-8). This includes limitation of extremes of spinal movement (brace, corset, or belt), local heat or ice, ultrasound and massage, traction, and transcutaneous electrical nerve stimulation (TENS). Drug therapy to relieve pain includes NSAIDs, short-term use of opioids, analgesics, muscle relaxants, antiseizure drugs, and antidepressants.[18] Epidural corticosteroid injections may be effective in reducing inflammation and relieving acute pain. If the underlying cause remains, the pain tends to recur.

Once the symptoms subside, back strengthening exercises are begun twice a day and are encouraged for a lifetime. Teach the patient the principles of good body mechanics. Discourage extremes of flexion and torsion. Most patients heal with a conservative treatment plan after 6 months.

Surgical Therapy. If conservative treatment is unsuccessful, radiculopathy becomes progressively worse, or loss of bowel or bladder control (cauda equina) occurs, surgery may then be indicated. Surgery for a damaged disc is generally performed when diagnostic tests indicate that the problem is not responding to conservative treatment and the patient is in constant pain and/or has a persistent neurologic deficit.

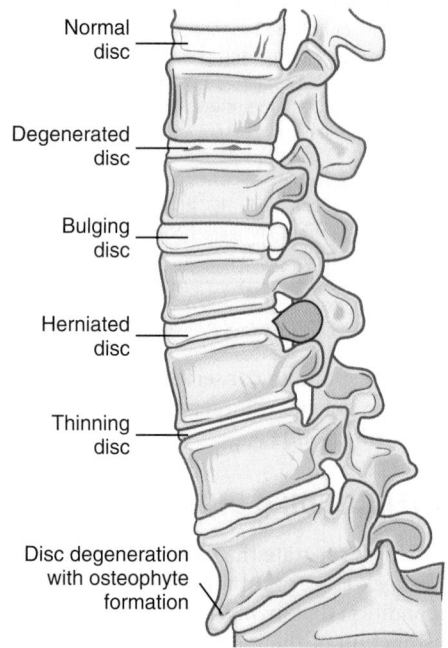

Normal disc

Degenerated disc

Bulging disc

Herniated disc

Thinning disc

Disc degeneration with osteophyte formation

FIG. 64-4 Common causes of degenerative disc damage.

TABLE 64-7	**MANIFESTATIONS OF LUMBAR DISC HERNIATION***			
Intervertebral Level	Pain	Affected Reflex	Motor Function	Sensation
L3-4	Back to buttocks to posterior thigh to inner calf	Patellar	Quadriceps, anterior tibialis	Inner aspect of lower leg, anterior part of thigh
L4-5	Back to buttocks to dorsum of foot and big toe	None	Anterior tibialis, extensor hallucis longus, gluteus medius	Dorsum of foot and big toe
L5-S1	Back to buttocks to sole of foot and heel	Achilles	Gastrocnemius, hamstring, gluteus maximus	Heel and lateral foot

*A disc herniation can involve pressure on more than one nerve root.

An *intradiscal electrothermoplasty* (IDET) is a minimally invasive outpatient procedure that may help treat back and sciatica pain. The procedure involves inserting a needle into the affected disc with the guidance of an x-ray. A wire is then threaded down through the needle and into the disc. The wire is heated, which denervates the small nerve fibers that have grown into the cracks and have invaded the degenerating disc. The heat also partially melts the annulus fibrosus, which triggers the body to generate new reinforcing proteins in the fibers of the annulus.

Another outpatient technique is *radiofrequency discal nucleoplasty* (coblation nucleoplasty). A needle is inserted into the disc similar to IDET. Instead of a heating wire, a special radiofrequency probe is used. The probe generates energy that breaks up the molecular bonds of the gel in the nucleus pulposus. The result is that up to 20% of the nucleus is removed, which decompresses the disc and reduces the pressure on both the disc and the surrounding nerve roots. Relief from pain varies among patients.

A third procedure is the use of an *interspinous process decompression system* (X-Stop). This device is made of titanium and fits onto a mount that is placed on vertebrae in the lower back. The X-Stop is used in patients with pain due to lumbar spinal stenosis. The device works by lifting the vertebrae off the pinched nerve.

A common and traditional surgical procedure for lumbar disc disease is a *laminectomy*. It involves the surgical excision of part of the vertebra (referred to as the lamina) to gain access to the protruding disc to remove it. A minimal hospital stay is usually required after the procedure.

A *diskectomy* is another common surgical procedure to decompress the nerve root.[11] Microsurgical diskectomy is a version of the standard diskectomy in which the surgeon uses a microscope to allow better visualization of the disc and disc space during surgery to aid in the removal of the damaged portion. This helps maintain the bony stability of the spine.

A *percutaneous diskectomy* is an outpatient surgical procedure using a tube that is passed through the retroperitoneal soft tissues to the disc with the aid of fluoroscopy. A laser is then used on the damaged portion of the disc. Small stab wounds are used, and minimal blood loss occurs during the procedure. The procedure is effective and safe and decreases rehabilitation time.

The goals of artificial disc replacement surgery are to restore movement and eliminate pain. The *Charité disc* is used in patients with lumbar disc damage associated with DDD. This artificial disc is made up of a high-density core sandwiched between two cobalt-chromium endplates (Fig. 64-5). This device is surgically placed in the spine (usually through a small incision below the umbilicus) after the damaged disc is removed. The disc allows for movement at the level of the implant.

The *ProDisc-L* is another type of artificial lumbar disc that can be used to treat DDD.[19] The *Prestige cervical disc system* may be used in the treatment of DDD of the cervical spine.

A *spinal fusion* may be performed if the spine is unstable. The spine is stabilized by creating an ankylosis (fusion) of contiguous vertebrae with a bone graft from the patient's fibula or iliac crest or from a donated cadaver bone. Metal fixation with rods, plates, or screws may be implanted at the time of spinal surgery to provide more stability and decrease vertebral motion. A posterior lumbar fusion may be performed in patients to provide extra support for bone grafting or a prosthetic device.

Bone morphogenetic protein (BMP), a genetically engineered protein, may be used to stimulate bone growth of the graft in spinal fusions.[20] A dissolvable sponge soaked with BMP is implanted into the spine. The protein on the sponge stimulates the body's own cells to become active and produce bone. BMP begins the process of fusion, which continues even after the protein and sponge dissolve, leaving living bone behind.

TABLE 64-8	**COLLABORATIVE CARE**

Intervertebral Disc Disease

Diagnostic
- History and physical examination
- X-ray
- CT scan
- MRI
- Myelogram
- Diskogram
- Electromyogram (EMG)

Collaborative Therapy
Conservative
- Restricted activity for several days, limit total bed rest
- Local ice or heat
- Physical therapy
- Drug therapy
  - Analgesics (e.g., tramadol [Ultram, Ryzolt])
  - Nonsteroidal antiinflammatory drugs
  - Muscle relaxants (e.g., cyclobenzaprine [Flexeril])
  - Antiseizure drugs (e.g., gabapentin [Neurontin])
  - Antidepressants (e.g., pregabalin [Lyrica])
  - Epidural corticosteroid injections

Surgical
- Intradiscal electrothermoplasty (IDET)
- Radiofrequency discal nucleoplasty
- Interspinous process decompression system (X-Stop)
- Laminectomy with or without spinal fusion
- Diskectomy
- Percutaneous laser diskectomy
- Artificial disc replacement (e.g., Charité disc)
- Spinal fusion with instrumentation (e.g., plates, screws) or without

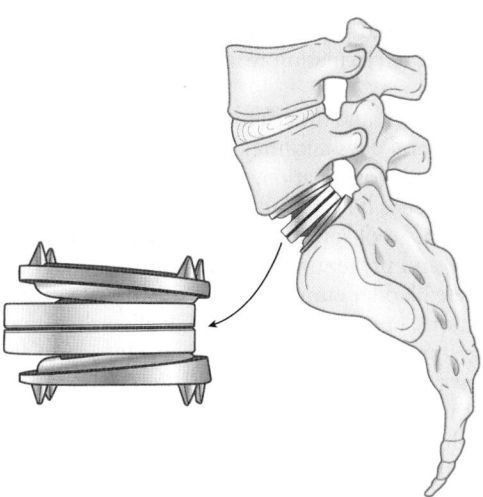

FIG. 64-5 The Charité artificial disc, used in degenerative disc disease to replace a damaged intervertebral disc. The Charité artificial disc consists of two cobalt-chromium alloy endplates sandwiched around a movable high-density plastic core. The disc's design helps align the spine and preserve its natural ability to move.

NURSING MANAGEMENT
VERTEBRAL DISC SURGERY

After vertebral disc surgery, postoperative nursing interventions mainly focus on maintaining proper alignment of the spine until it has healed. Depending on the type and extent of surgery and the surgeon's preference, the patient may be able to dangle the legs at the side of the bed, stand, or even ambulate the same day of surgery.

When a patient has had a lumbar fusion, place pillows under the thighs of each leg when supine and between the legs when in the side-lying position to provide comfort and ensure alignment. The patient often fears turning or any movement that increases pain by straining the surgical area. Reassure the patient that the proper technique is being used to maintain body alignment. Sufficient staff should be available to move the patient without undue pain or strain on staff members or the patient.

Postoperatively, most patients require opioids such as morphine IV for 24 to 48 hours. Patient-controlled analgesia (PCA) allows for optimal analgesic levels and is the preferred method of continued pain management during this time. Once fluids are being taken, the patient may be switched to oral drugs such as acetaminophen with codeine, hydrocodone (Vicodin), or oxycodone (Percocet). Diazepam (Valium) may be prescribed for muscle relaxation. Monitor and document pain management and its effectiveness.

Because the spinal canal may be entered during surgery, there is potential for cerebrospinal fluid (CSF) leakage. Immediately report a severe headache or leakage of CSF on the dressing. CSF appears as clear or slightly yellow drainage on the dressing. It has a high glucose concentration and is positive for glucose when tested with a dipstick. Note the amount, color, and characteristics of drainage.

Frequently monitor the patient's peripheral neurologic signs after spinal surgery. Movement of the arms and the legs and assessment of sensation should be unchanged when compared with the preoperative status. These assessments are usually repeated every 2 to 4 hours during the first 48 hours after surgery and compared with the preoperative assessment. Paresthesias, such as numbness and tingling, may not be relieved immediately after surgery. Document any new muscle weakness or paresthesias and report them to the surgeon immediately. Assess extremity circulation using temperature, capillary refill, and pulses.

Paralytic ileus and interference with bowel function may occur for several days and may manifest as nausea, abdominal distention, and constipation. Assess whether the patient is passing flatus; has bowel sounds in all quadrants; and has a flat, soft abdomen. Stool softeners (e.g., docusate [Colace]) may aid in relieving and preventing constipation.

Adequate bladder emptying may be altered because of activity restrictions, opioids, or anesthesia. If allowed by the surgeon, encourage men to dangle the legs over the side of the bed or stand to urinate. Patients should use the commode or ambulate to the bathroom when allowed to promote adequate emptying of the bladder. Ensure that privacy is maintained. Intermittent catheterization or an indwelling catheter may be necessary for patients who have difficulty urinating.

Loss of sphincter tone or bladder tone may indicate nerve damage. Monitor for incontinence or difficulty evacuating the bowel or bladder, and report significant findings to the surgeon immediately.

In addition to the nursing care appropriate for a patient who has had a laminectomy, there are other nursing responsibilities if the patient has also had a spinal fusion. Because a bone graft is usually involved, the postoperative healing time is prolonged compared with that of a laminectomy. Limitations on activity may be necessary over an extended time. A rigid orthosis (thoracic-lumbar-sacral orthosis [TLSO] or chairback brace) is often used during this period. Some surgeons require that the patient be taught to put it on and take it off by logrolling in bed, whereas others allow their patients to apply the brace in a sitting or standing position. Verify the preferred method before initiating this activity.

If surgery is done on the cervical spine, be alert for manifestations of spinal cord edema such as respiratory distress and a worsening neurologic status of the upper extremities. After surgery, the patient's neck may be immobilized in either a soft or hard cervical collar.

In addition to the primary surgical site, regularly assess the donor site for the bone graft. The posterior iliac crest is the most commonly used donor site, although the fibula may also be used. The donor site usually causes greater pain than the spinal fusion area. The donor site is bandaged with a pressure dressing to prevent excessive bleeding. If the donor site is the fibula, neurovascular assessments of the extremity are a postoperative nursing responsibility.

After a spinal fusion the patient may experience some immobility of the spine at the fusion site. Instruct the patient in proper body mechanics and to avoid sitting or standing for prolonged periods. Encourage activities that include walking, lying down, and shifting weight from one foot to the other when standing. Lifting is usually restricted in the postoperative period after spinal surgery. The patient should learn to mentally think through an activity before starting any potentially injurious task such as bending or stooping. Any twisting movement of the spine is contraindicated. Patients should use the thighs and knees, rather than the back, to absorb the shock of activity and movement. A firm mattress or bed board is essential.

NECK PAIN

Neck pain occurs almost as frequently as low back pain, affecting up to 50% of adults at some point in their life. Neck pain may be the result of many conditions, both benign (e.g., poor posture) and serious (e.g., herniated cervical disc)[21] (Table 64-9).

Cervical neck sprains and strains occur from hyperflexion and hyperextension injury. Patients have symptoms of stiffness and neck pain and possible pain radiating into the arm and hand. Pain may also radiate into the head, anterior chest, thoracic spine region, and shoulders. Cervical nerve root compression from stenosis, DDD, or herniation may be indicated by weakness or paresthesia of the arm and hand.

The cause of neck pain is diagnosed by history, physical examination, x-ray, MRI, CT scan, and myelogram. An

TABLE 64-9	CAUSES OF NECK PAIN
• Poor posture	• Spondylosis
• Strain or sprain	• Rheumatoid arthritis
• Degenerative disc disease, including herniation	• Tumor
• Trauma (e.g., fractures, subluxation)	• Osteoporosis
	• Osteomyelitis
	• Meningitis

Musculoskeletal System

TABLE 64-10	PATIENT & CAREGIVER TEACHING GUIDE

Neck Exercises

When teaching the patient exercises for neck pain, include the following instructions for the patient and caregiver.

- Bend your head backward until you are looking up at the ceiling. Repeat slowly five times. Stop if experiencing dizziness.
- Bring your head forward so that your chin touches your chest and your face is looking down at the floor. Repeat slowly five times.
- Keep your head facing forward, and bend your ear down toward one shoulder. Alternate this movement with your other ear. Repeat slowly five times on each side.
- Turn your head slowly around to one side as far as it will go. Repeat toward the other side. Repeat exercise five times on each side.

EMG of the upper extremities is done to diagnose cervical radiculopathy.

Conservative treatment for neck pain in patients without an underlying disorder includes head support using a soft cervical collar, heat and ice applications, massage, rest until symptoms subside, ultrasound, and NSAIDs. Therapeutic neck exercises[22] and acupuncture may also be used for pain relief. Most neck pain resolves without surgical intervention.

Preventing neck pain that occurs with everyday activities such as prolonged sitting at a computer or television, sleeping in nonaligned spinal positions, or making jarring movements during exercise is important. Preventive strategies can begin by practicing good posture and maintaining neck flexibility (Table 64-10).

FOOT DISORDERS

The foot is the platform that supports the weight of the body and absorbs considerable shock when the person is ambulating. The foot is a complicated structure composed of bony structures, muscles, tendons, and ligaments. It can be affected by (1) congenital conditions, (2) structural weakness, (3) traumatic and stress injuries, and (4) systemic conditions such as diabetes mellitus and rheumatoid arthritis. Much of the pain, deformity, and disability associated with foot disorders can be directly attributed to or accentuated by improperly fitting shoes, which cause crowding and angulation of the toes and inhibit the normal movement of foot muscles.

The purposes of footwear are to (1) provide support, foot stability, protection, shock absorption, and a foundation for orthoses; (2) increase friction with the walking surface; and (3) treat foot abnormalities. (Table 64-11 summarizes common foot disorders.)

NURSING MANAGEMENT
FOOT DISORDERS

NURSING IMPLEMENTATION

HEALTH PROMOTION. Well-constructed and properly fitted shoes are essential for healthy, pain-free feet. The selection of footwear for women is often influenced by fashion styles instead of comfort and support. Stress the importance of having a shoe that conforms to the foot rather than to current fashion trends. The shoe must be long enough and wide enough to avoid crowding the toes and forcing the great toe into a position of

hallux valgus (Fig. 64-6). At the metatarsal head, the shoe should be wide enough to allow foot muscles to move freely and toes to bend. The shank (narrow part of sole under the instep) of the shoe should be rigid enough to give optimal support. The height of the heel should be realistic in relation to the purpose for which the shoe is worn. Ideally, the heel of the shoe should not rise more than 1 in higher than the forefoot support. Wearing higher heeled shoes with a narrow toe box will cause hammertoes and corns over time.[23]

ACUTE INTERVENTION. Many foot problems require a referral to a podiatrist. Depending on the problem, conservative therapies are usually tried first (see Table 64-11). These therapies include NSAIDs, shock-wave therapy, icing, physical therapy, alterations in footwear, stretching, warm soaks, orthotics, ultrasound, and corticosteroid injections. If these methods do not provide relief, then surgery may be recommended.

Depending on the type of surgery performed, pins or wires may extend through the toes, or a protective splint that extends over the end of the foot may be in place. Postoperatively, the foot is usually immobilized by a bulky dressing (Fig. 64-7), short leg cast, slipper (plaster) cast, or a platform "shoe" that fits over the dressing and has a rigid sole (known as a bunion boot).

The foot should be elevated with the heel off the bed to help reduce discomfort and prevent edema. Assess neurovascular status frequently during the immediate postoperative period. The devices inserted may interfere with or preclude assessment for movement. Also be aware that sensation may be hard to evaluate because the patient may have difficulty differentiating pain from surgery and that caused by nerve pressure or circulatory impairment.

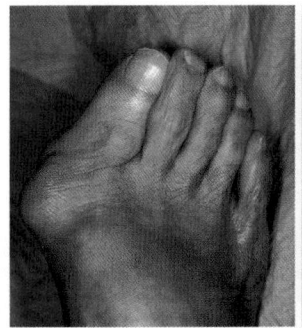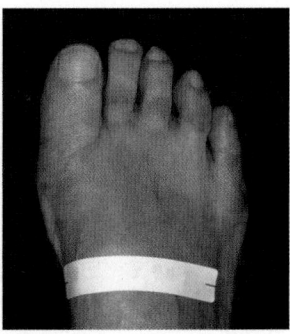

A   B

FIG. 64-6 A, Severe hallux valgus with bursa formation. **B,** Postoperative correction.

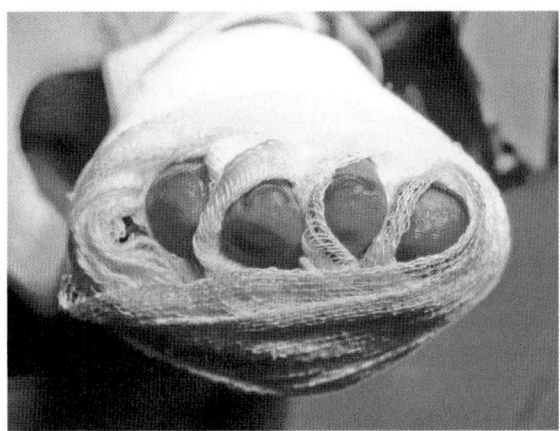

FIG. 64-7 Postoperative supportive dressing for a moderate forefoot deformity. Dressing must be conforming and binding enough to hold toe in exact position.

TABLE 64-11	COMMON FOOT DISORDERS	
Disorder	**Description**	**Treatment**
Forefoot		
Hallux valgus (bunion)	Painful deformity of great toe consisting of lateral angulation of great toe toward second toe, bony enlargement of medial side of first metatarsal head, swelling of bursa and formation of callus over bony enlargement (see Fig. 64-6).	Conservative treatment includes wearing shoes with wide forefoot or "bunion pocket" and use of bunion pads to relieve pressure on bursal sac. Surgical treatment is removal of bursal sac and bony enlargement and correction of lateral angulation of great toe. May include temporary or permanent internal fixation.
Hallux rigidus	Painful stiffness of first MTP joint caused by osteoarthritis or local trauma.	Conservative treatment includes intraarticular corticosteroids and passive manual stretching of first MTP joint. A shoe with a stiff sole decreases pain in the joint during walking. Surgical treatment is joint fusion or arthroplasty with silicone rubber implant.
Hammer toe	Deformity of the 2nd to 5th toes, including flexion deformity of PIP and DIP joints, hyperextension of MTP joint, flexion deformity of DIP joint alone (mallet toe). Callus formation and flexion of PIP and DIP joint hyperextension (claw toe). Complaints related to hammer toe include burning on bottom of foot and pain and difficulty walking when wearing shoes.	Conservative treatment consists of passive manual stretching of PIP joint and use of metatarsal arch support. Surgical correction consists of resection of base of middle phalanx and head of proximal phalanx and bringing raw bone ends together. Kirschner wire maintains straight position.
Morton's neuroma (Morton's toe or plantar neuroma)	Neuroma in web space between third and fourth metatarsal heads, causing sharp, sudden attacks of pain and burning sensations.	Surgical excision is the usual treatment.
Midfoot		
Pes planus (flatfoot)	Loss of metatarsal arch causing pain in foot or leg.	Symptoms are relieved by use of resilient longitudinal arch supports. Surgical treatment consists of triple arthrodesis or fusion of subtalar joint.
Pes cavus	Elevation of longitudinal arch of foot resulting from contracture of plantar fascia or bony deformity of arch.	Surgical correction is necessary if it interferes with ambulation.
Hindfoot		
Painful heels	Complaint of heel pain with weight bearing. Common causes are plantar bursitis, plantar fasciitis, or bone spur.	Corticosteroids are injected locally into inflamed bursa, and sponge-rubber heel cup is used. Surgical excision of bursa or spur is performed. For plantar fasciitis stretching exercises, ice, shoe heel cup, shock-wave therapy, NSAIDs, and corticosteroids are used.
Calcaneus stress fracture	Complaint of heel pain after moderate walking. Common causes are overtraining, running on hard surfaces, or osteoporosis.	Rest, ice, shoe heel pad, and NSAIDs are used. See health care provider to assess for osteoporosis.
Other Problems		
Corn	Localized thickening of skin caused by continual pressure over bony prominences, especially metatarsal head, frequently causing localized pain.	Corn is softened with warm water or preparations containing salicylic acid and trimmed with razor blade or scalpel. Pressure on bony prominences caused by shoes is relieved.
Soft corn	Painful lesion caused by bony prominence of one toe pressing against adjacent toe. Usual location is web space between toes. Softness caused by secretions keeping web space relatively moist.	Pain is relieved by placing cotton or spacers between toes to separate them. Surgical treatment is excision of projecting bone spur (if present).
Callus	Similar formation to corn but covering wider area and usually located on weight-bearing part of foot.	Same as for corn.
Plantar wart	Painful papillomatous growth caused by virus that may occur on any part of skin on sole of foot. Tend to cluster on pressure points.	Remedies containing salicylic acid (e.g., Compound W), excision with electrocoagulation, or surgical removal. Laser treatments may also be used. May disappear without treatment.

DIP, Distal interphalangeal; *MTP*, metatarsophalangeal; *PIP*, proximal interphalangeal.

The type and extent of surgery determine the degree of ambulation allowed. Crutches, a walker, or a cane may be necessary. The patient may experience pain or a throbbing sensation when starting ambulation. Reinforce instructions given by the physical therapist and the importance of walking with an erect posture and with proper weight distribution. Report dysfunction of gait or continued pain to the physician. Instruct the patient on the importance of frequent rest periods with the foot elevated.

AMBULATORY AND HOME CARE. Foot care should include performing daily hygienic care and wearing clean stockings. Stockings should be long enough to avoid wrinkling and causing pressure areas. Trimming toenails straight across helps prevent ingrown toenails and reduces the possibility of infection. Provide detailed instruction to persons with impaired circulation or diabetes mellitus to prevent serious complications associated with blisters, pressure areas, and infections. (See Table 49-21 for guidelines on foot care.)

GERONTOLOGIC CONSIDERATIONS

FOOT PROBLEMS

The older adult is prone to developing foot problems because of poor circulation, atherosclerosis, and decreased sensation in the lower extremities. This is especially a problem for older patients with diabetes mellitus.[24] A patient may develop an open wound but not feel it because of altered sensation. This may be the result of peripheral vascular disease or diabetic neuropathy. Instruct older adults to inspect their feet daily and report any open wounds or breaks in the skin to their health care provider.[25] If left untreated, wounds may become infected, lead to osteomyelitis, and require surgical debridement. If the infection becomes widespread, lower limb amputation may be necessary. Teach the caregiver of the older adult who needs assistance with hygiene practices the importance of carefully assessing the feet at regular intervals.

METABOLIC BONE DISEASES

Normal bone metabolism is affected by hormones, nutrition, and genetic factors. When dysfunction occurs in any of these factors, a generalized reduction in bone mass and strength may result. Metabolic bone diseases include osteomalacia, osteoporosis, and Paget's disease.

OSTEOMALACIA

Osteomalacia is caused by a vitamin D deficiency, resulting in decalcification and softening of bones. In the United States it is an uncommon disease. This disease is the same as rickets in children except that the epiphyseal growth plates are closed in the adult. Vitamin D is required for the absorption of calcium from the intestine. Insufficient vitamin D intake can interfere with the normal mineralization of bone; with little or no calcification, bone softening results.

Causes of osteomalacia include lack of exposure to ultraviolet rays (which is needed for vitamin D synthesis), GI malabsorption, extensive burns, chronic diarrhea, pregnancy, kidney disease, and drugs such as phenytoin (Dilantin). Morbidly obese persons are at higher risk for developing osteomalacia because of inadequate calcium intake, decreased physical activity, vitamin D deficiency, coexisting chronic diseases (e.g., hyperlipidemia), and the use of medications associated with these diseases (e.g., cholestyramine [Questran]).[26]

Common manifestations of osteomalacia are bone pain, difficulty rising from a chair, and difficulty walking.[27] Other manifestations include muscular weakness, especially in the pelvic girdle; weight loss; and progressive deformities of the spine (kyphosis) or extremities. Fractures are common and indicate delayed bone healing.

Laboratory findings commonly include decreased serum calcium or phosphorus levels, decreased serum 25-hydroxyvitamin D, and elevated serum alkaline phosphatase. X-rays may demonstrate the effects of generalized bone demineralization, especially loss of calcium in the bones of the pelvis and associated bone deformity. Looser's transformation zones (ribbons of decalcification in bone found on x-ray) are diagnostic of osteomalacia. However, significant osteomalacia may exist without changes noted on x-ray.

Collaborative care of osteomalacia is directed toward correction of the vitamin D deficiency. When vitamin D$_3$ (cholecalciferol) and vitamin D$_2$ (ergocalciferol) are used as supplements, the patient often shows a dramatic response. Calcium salts or phosphorus supplements may also be prescribed. Encourage dietary ingestion of eggs, meat, oily fish, and milk and breakfast cereals fortified with calcium and vitamin D. Exposure to sunlight (and ultraviolet rays) is also valuable, along with weight-bearing exercise.

Patients who have bariatric surgery to treat obesity should be assessed for osteomalacia. Any vitamin D deficiencies should be corrected before surgery.[26]

OSTEOPOROSIS

Osteoporosis, or porous bone (fragile bone disease), is a chronic, progressive metabolic bone disease characterized by low bone mass and structural deterioration of bone tissue, leading to increased bone fragility (Fig. 64-8). More than 44 million persons in the United States have decreased bone density or osteoporosis.[28] One in two women and one in four men over age 50 will sustain an osteoporosis-related fracture during their lifetime. Osteoporosis is known as the "silent thief" because it slowly and insidiously over many years robs the skeleton of its banked resources. Bones can eventually become so fragile that they cannot withstand normal mechanical stress.

Osteoporosis is more common in women than in men for several reasons: (1) women tend to have lower calcium intake than men throughout their lives (men between 15 and 50 years of age consume twice as much calcium as women); (2) women have less bone mass because of their generally smaller frames; (3) bone resorption begins at an earlier age in women and is accelerated at menopause; (4) pregnancy and breastfeeding deplete a woman's skeletal reserve unless calcium intake is adequate; and (5) longevity increases the likelihood of osteoporosis.

Current guidelines recommend an initial bone scan in women before the age of 65. If the results are normal and the person is at low risk for osteoporosis, another scan is not needed for 15 years.[29] Testing should start earlier and be done more frequently if a person is at high risk for fractures (e.g., low body weight, smoker, prior fractures). Men should be screened before the age of 70 years old and by age 50 if at high risk for fractures (e.g., low body weight, hypogonadism).[30]

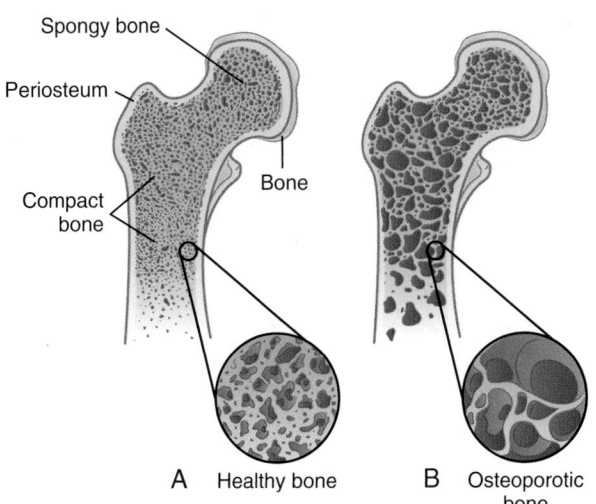

FIG. 64-8 **A,** Normal bone. **B,** Osteoporotic bone.

Etiology and Pathophysiology

Risk factors for osteoporosis are listed in Table 64-12. Decreased risk is associated with regular weight-bearing exercise and fluoride, calcium, and vitamin D ingestion. Low testosterone levels are a major risk factor in men.

Peak bone mass (maximum bone tissue) is primarily achieved before age 20. It is determined by a combination of four major factors: heredity, nutrition, exercise, and hormone function. Heredity may be responsible for up to 70% of a person's peak bone mass. Bone loss from midlife (ages 35 to 40 years) onward is inevitable, but the rate of loss varies. At menopause, women experience rapid bone loss when the decline in estrogen production is the sharpest. This rate of loss then slows, and eventually matches the rate of bone lost by men 65 to 70 years old.

🌐 CULTURAL & ETHNIC HEALTH DISPARITIES

Osteoporosis

- White and Asian American women have a higher incidence of osteoporosis than Native American, Hispanic, and African American women.
- African American women begin menopause with more bone mass and have a lower rate of bone loss after menopause than non–African American women.
- Risk of fracture in white women is higher than in non-white women of the same age.

TABLE 64-12   RISK FACTORS FOR OSTEOPOROSIS

- Advancing age (>65 yr)
- Female gender
- Low body weight
- White or Asian ethnicity
- Current cigarette smoking
- Nontraumatic fracture
- Sedentary lifestyle
- Postmenopausal (estrogen deficiency)
- Family history of osteoporosis
- Diet low in calcium or vitamin D deficiency
- Excessive use of alcohol (>2 drinks/day)
- Low testosterone level in men
- Long-term use of corticosteroids, thyroid replacements, heparin, long-acting sedatives, or antiseizure medications

---

Genetic factors contribute to osteoporosis by influencing not only bone mineral density but also bone size, bone quality, and bone turnover.

Bone is continuously being deposited by osteoblasts and resorbed by osteoclasts, a process called *remodeling.* Normally the rates of bone deposition and resorption are equal to one another so that the total bone mass remains constant.[31] In osteoporosis, bone resorption exceeds bone deposition.

Specific diseases associated with osteoporosis include inflammatory bowel disease, intestinal malabsorption, kidney disease, rheumatoid arthritis, hyperthyroidism, chronic alcoholism, cirrhosis of the liver, hypogonadism, and diabetes mellitus. Many drugs can interfere with bone metabolism, including corticosteroids, antiseizure drugs (e.g., divalproex sodium [Depakote], phenytoin), aluminum-containing antacids, heparin, certain cancer treatments, and excessive thyroid hormones. At the time one of these drugs is prescribed, inform the patient of this possible side effect. Long-term corticosteroid use is a major contributor to osteoporosis.

Clinical Manifestations

Osteoporosis occurs most commonly in the bones of the spine, hips, and wrists. The usual first manifestations are back pain or spontaneous fractures. The loss of bone substance causes the bone to become mechanically weakened and prone to either spontaneous fractures or fractures from minimal trauma. A person who has one spinal vertebral fracture due to osteoporosis has an increased risk of having a second vertebral fracture within 1 year. Over time, wedging and fractures of the vertebrae produce gradual loss of height and a humped back known as *kyphosis,* or "dowager's hump" (Fig. 64-9).

GENDER DIFFERENCES

Osteoporosis

Men	Women
• Men are underdiagnosed and undertreated for osteoporosis as compared to women.	• Osteoporosis is eight times more common in women than in men.
• One in four men over age 50 will have an osteoporosis-related fracture in his lifetime.	• One in two women over age 50 will have an osteoporosis-related fracture in her lifetime.

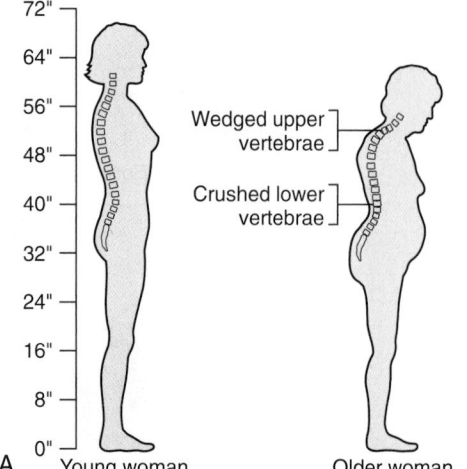

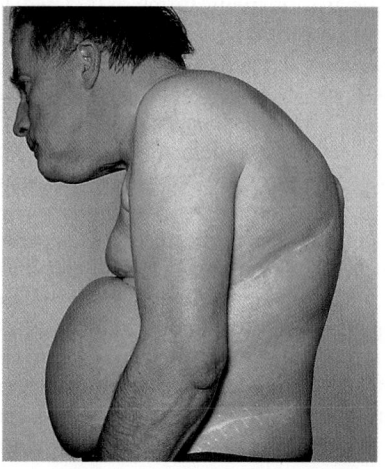

FIG. 64-9 The effects of osteoporosis. **A,** Comparison of young woman with an older woman. **B,** Severe fixed kyphosis producing a question-mark appearance.

Diagnostic Studies

Osteoporosis often goes unnoticed because it cannot be detected by conventional x-ray until more than 25% to 40% of calcium in the bone is lost. Serum calcium, phosphorus, and alkaline phosphatase levels usually are normal, although alkaline phosphatase may be elevated after a fracture.

Bone mineral density (BMD) measurements are typically expressed as the grams of mineral per unit volume.[32] BMD is determined by peak bone mass and amount of bone loss. (BMD measurements are presented in Table 62-7.) Types of BMD measurement include quantitative ultrasound (QUS) and dual-energy x-ray absorptiometry (DXA). QUS measures bone density with sound waves in the heel, kneecap, or shin. DXA (one of the most common BMD studies) measures bone density in the spine, hips, and forearm (the most common sites of fractures resulting from osteoporosis). DXA studies are also useful to evaluate changes in bone density over time and to assess the effectiveness of treatment.

DXA results are reported as T-scores. The T-score is the number of standard deviations below average for normal bone density. A T-score of −1 or higher indicates normal bone density. Osteoporosis is defined as a BMD of −2.5 or lower (at least 2.5 standard deviations) below the mean BMD of young adults. Osteopenia is defined as bone loss that is more than normal (a T-score between −1 and −2.5), but not yet at the level for a diagnosis of osteoporosis.

Sometimes the health care provider asks for a Z-score instead of a T-score. In this case, a person is compared with someone his or her own age and/or ethnic group instead of an individual in the best of health at 30 years of age. A Z-score that is less than −2.0 indicates a bone density problem.

NURSING AND COLLABORATIVE MANAGEMENT OSTEOPOROSIS

Collaborative care for osteoporosis focuses on proper nutrition, calcium supplementation, exercise, prevention of falls and fractures, and drugs (Table 64-13). The National Osteoporosis Foundation (www.nof.org) recommends treatment for osteoporosis for postmenopausal women who have (1) a T-score of less than −2.5, (2) a T-score between −1 and −2.5 with additional risk factors (see Table 64-12), or (3) prior history of a hip or vertebral fracture.

A patient's risk of fracture from osteoporosis can also be calculated with the Fracture Risk Assessment (FRAX) tool (www.shef.ac.uk/FRAX). The FRAX takes into account BMD and additional clinical factors when assessing fracture risk.[33]

Prevention and treatment of osteoporosis focuses on adequate calcium intake (1000 mg/day in premenopausal women and postmenopausal women taking estrogen, and 1500 mg/day in postmenopausal women who are not receiving supplemental estrogen). Foods that are high in calcium content include whole and skim milk, yogurt, turnip greens, cottage cheese, ice cream, sardines, and spinach (Table 64-14). If dietary intake of calcium is inadequate, supplemental calcium may be recommended. Calcium is difficult to absorb in single doses greater than 500 mg.[34] Teach the patient the importance of taking supplemental calcium in divided doses with food. The amount of elemental calcium varies in different calcium preparations (Table 64-15).

Vitamin D is important in calcium absorption and function and may also have a role in bone formation. Most people get enough vitamin D from their diet or naturally through synthesis in the skin from exposure to sunlight. Being in the sun for 20 minutes a day is generally enough. However, supplemental vitamin D (800 to 1000 IU) is recommended for postmenopausal women, older men, those who are homebound, and those who get minimal sun exposure.

Regular physical activity is important to build up and maintain bone mass.[35] Exercise also increases muscle strength, coordination, and balance. The best exercises are weight-bearing exercises that force an individual to work against gravity. These

---

TABLE 64-13 COLLABORATIVE CARE

Osteoporosis

Diagnostic
- History and physical examination
- Serum calcium, phosphorus, alkaline phosphatase, and vitamin D levels
- Bone mineral densitometry
  - Dual-energy x-ray absorptiometry (DXA)
  - Quantitative ultrasound (QUS)

Collaborative Therapy
- Diet high in calcium (see Table 64-14)
- Calcium supplements (see Table 64-15)
- Vitamin D supplements
- Exercise program
- Drug therapy
  - Bisphosphonates
    - alendronate (Fosamax, Binosto)
    - clodronate (Bonefos)
    - etidronate (Didronel)
    - ibandronate (Boniva)
    - pamidronate (Aredia)
    - risedronate (Actonel)
    - tiludronate (Skelid)
    - zoledronic acid (Reclast)
  - salmon calcitonin (Calcimar)
  - Selective estrogen receptor modulator (e.g., raloxifene [Evista])
  - Recombinant form of parathyroid hormone (e.g., teriparatide [Forteo])
  - denosumab (Prolia)
- Minimally invasive procedures
  - Vertebroplasty
  - Kyphoplasty

TABLE 64-14 NUTRITIONAL THERAPY

Sources of Calcium

Food	Calcium (mg)	Food	Calcium (mg)
Good Sources		**Good Sources—cont'd**	
1 cup milk		1 med stalk cooked broccoli	158
• Whole	291		
• Skim	302	1 cup cooked spinach	200
1 oz cheese		1 cup almonds	304
• American	174		
• Cheddar	130	**Poor Sources**	
• Cottage	130	Egg	28
8 oz yogurt	415	3 oz beef, pork, poultry	10
1 cup ice cream	176	Apple, banana	10
• Soft serve	272	1 med potato	14
3 oz seafood		1 med carrot	14
• Salmon	167	¼ head lettuce	27
• Oysters	113		

TABLE 64-15	ELEMENTAL CALCIUM CONTENT OF CALCIUM PREPARATIONS

Calcium Preparation	Elemental Calcium Content
Calcium carbonate (Tums 500)	500 mg/tablet
Calcium carbonate + 5 mcg vitamin D_2 (Os-Cal 250)	250 mg/tablet
Calcium gluconate	40 mg/500 mg
Calcium carbonate	400 mg/g
Calcium lactate	80 mg/600 mg
Calcium citrate	40 mg/300 mg

exercises include walking, hiking, weight training, stair climbing, tennis, and dancing. Walking is preferred to high-impact aerobics or running, both of which may put too much stress on the bones, resulting in stress fractures. Walking 30 minutes, three times a week is recommended. Instruct patients to quit smoking and cut down on alcohol intake to decrease the likelihood of losing bone mass.

Although loss of bone cannot be significantly reversed, further loss can be prevented if the patient follows a regimen of calcium and vitamin D supplementation, exercise, and drugs (see Table 64-13) if indicated. Make an effort to keep patients with osteoporosis ambulatory to prevent further loss of bone substance as a result of immobility.

Treatment may also involve the use of a gait aid as needed and to protect areas of potential pathologic fractures. For example, a thoracic-lumbar-sacral orthosis (TLSO) brace may be used to maintain the spine in proper alignment after a fracture or treatment of a vertebral fracture. (Fractures are discussed in Chapter 63.)

Vertebroplasty and *kyphoplasty* are minimally invasive procedures used to treat osteoporotic vertebral fractures[36] (see Chapter 63). In vertebroplasty, bone cement is injected into the collapsed vertebra to stabilize it, but it does not correct the deformity. In kyphoplasty, an air bladder is inserted into the collapsed vertebra and inflated to regain vertebral body height, and then bone cement is injected.

DRUG THERAPY

Estrogen therapy after menopause is no longer given as a primary treatment to prevent osteoporosis because it is associated with an increased risk of heart disease and breast and uterine cancer. If estrogen therapy is being used to treat menopausal symptoms, it also protects the woman against bone loss and fractures of the hip and vertebrae.[37] It is believed that estrogen inhibits osteoclast activity, leading to decreased bone resorption and preventing both cortical and trabecular bone loss.

Bisphosphonates inhibit osteoclast-mediated bone resorption, thereby increasing total bone mass and BMD. These drugs, which are widely used in the treatment of osteoporosis,[38] are listed in Table 64-13. Common side effects are anorexia, weight loss, and gastritis. Instruct patients on the proper administration of a bisphosphonate to aid in its absorption (see Drug Alert). These precautions have been shown to decrease GI side effects (especially esophageal irritation) and increase absorption. A rare and serious side effect of bisphosphonates is jaw osteonecrosis (bone death). The etiology of this side effect is unknown.

EVIDENCE-BASED PRACTICE

Applying the Evidence

R.F. is a 76-yr-old white woman who fell in her home and sustained a hip fracture. Her recent laboratory work shows a vitamin D deficiency. You discuss her options for improving this deficiency. She tells you that she is moving to Arizona to be with her daughter and is planning to spend "many hours in the sun" every day.

Best Available Evidence	Clinician Expertise	Patient Preferences and Values
Postmenopausal women should receive 1500 mg of calcium and 800–1000 IU of vitamin D daily. Dietary sources and supplements should be used to meet these requirements.	You have worked with many patients recovering from fractures related to osteoporosis. You review R.F.'s usual diet and determine that it is deficient in calcium and vitamin D.	Patient prefers sun exposure over changing her diet (she is a vegetarian) or taking supplements.

Your Action and Decision

You discuss the risks associated with daily sun exposure and that sun exposure will not correct a calcium deficiency. R.F. tells you she understands but wants to try before taking "any more pills." You explain the importance of adding foods high in calcium to her diet. You provide her with a list of some choices that meet her vegetarian diet restrictions.

Reference for Evidence

National Institutes of Health: Dietary supplement fact sheet: vitamin D. Retrieved from *www.ods.od.nih.gov/factsheets/VitaminD-Quick Facts*.

DRUG ALERT: Bisphosphonates
- Instruct patient to
  - Take with full glass of water.
  - Take 30 min before food or other medications.
  - Remain upright for at least 30 min after taking.

Alendronate (Fosamax) is available as a once-per-week oral tablet. Ibandronate (Boniva) and risedronate (Actonel) are available as once-per-month oral tablets. Zoledronic acid (Reclast) is approved for a once-yearly IV infusion and can prevent osteoporosis for 2 years after a single infusion. Flu-like symptoms may occur for the first few days after administration of the drug.

Calcitonin is secreted by the thyroid gland and inhibits osteoclastic bone resorption by directly interacting with active osteoclasts. Salmon calcitonin (Calcimar) is available in intramuscular (IM), subcutaneous, and intranasal forms. Administration of the IM or subcutaneous form of the drug at night has been shown to decrease the side effects of nausea and facial flushing associated with this drug. Nausea does not occur with the nasal spray. If patients are using the nasal form, teach them to alternate nostrils daily. Nasal dryness and irritation are the most frequent side effects. When calcitonin is used, calcium supplementation is necessary to prevent secondary hyperparathyroidism.

Another type of drug used in treating osteoporosis is raloxifene (Evista), which is a selective estrogen receptor modulator (SERM). This drug mimics the effect of estrogen on bone by reducing bone resorption without stimulating the tissues of the breast or uterus. Raloxifene in postmenopausal women significantly increases BMD. Side effects included leg cramps, hot flashes, and blood clots. Raloxifene may decrease breast cancer risk. Similar to tamoxifen, it blocks the estrogen receptor sites of cancer cells.

Teriparatide (Forteo), which is a recombinant form of human parathyroid hormone (PTH), increases the action of osteoblasts. This drug is used to treat osteoporosis in men and postmenopausal women at high risk for fractures. Teriparatide is the first drug approved for the treatment of osteoporosis that stimulates new bone formation (most drugs prevent further bone loss). Teriparatide is administered by subcutaneous injection once a day. Side effects include leg cramps and dizziness.

Denosumab (Prolia) may be used for postmenopausal women with osteoporosis who are at high risk for fractures. It is a monoclonal antibody that binds to a protein (RANKL) involved in the formation and function of osteoclasts. Denosumab is given as a subcutaneous injection every 6 months.

Medical management of patients receiving corticosteroids includes prescribing the lowest effective dose and ensuring an adequate intake of calcium and vitamin D, including supplementation when osteoporosis drugs are prescribed. If osteopenia is evident on bone densitometry in people who are taking corticosteroids, treatment with bisphosphonates may be considered.

PAGET'S DISEASE

Paget's disease *(osteitis deformans)* is a chronic skeletal bone disorder in which excessive bone resorption is followed by replacement of normal marrow by vascular, fibrous connective tissue. The new bone is larger, disorganized, and structurally weaker. The regions of the skeleton commonly affected are pelvis, long bones, spine, ribs, sternum, and cranium. Up to 5% of adults in the United States are affected by Paget's disease.[39] The etiology is unknown, although a viral cause has been proposed. Up to 40% of all patients with Paget's disease have at least one relative with the disorder. Compared with women, men are affected 2:1.

In milder forms of Paget's disease, patients may remain free of symptoms, and the disease may be discovered incidentally on x-ray or serum chemistry findings of a high alkaline phosphatase level.[40] The initial clinical manifestations are usually insidious development of bone pain (which may progress to severe intractable pain), fatigue, and progressive development of a waddling gait. Patients may complain that they are becoming shorter or that their heads are becoming larger. Headaches, dementia, visual deficits, and loss of hearing can result with an enlarged, thickened skull. Increased bone volume in the spine can cause spinal cord or nerve root compression.

Pathologic fracture is the most common complication of Paget's disease and may be the first indication of the disease. Other complications include osteosarcoma, fibrosarcoma, and osteoclastoma (giant cell) tumors.

Serum alkaline phosphatase levels are markedly elevated (indicating high bone turnover) in advanced forms of the disease.[41] X-rays may demonstrate that the normal contour of the affected bone is curved and the bone cortex is thickened and irregular, especially the weight-bearing bones and the cranium. Bone scans using a radiolabeled bisphosphonate demonstrate increased uptake in the affected skeletal areas.

Collaborative care of Paget's disease is usually limited to symptomatic and supportive care and correction of secondary deformities by either surgical intervention or braces. Bisphosphonate drugs (see Table 64-13) are used to retard bone resorption. Zoledronic acid may also be given as a bone-building drug. Calcium and vitamin D are often given to decrease hypocalcemia, a common side effect with these drugs. Drug effectiveness may be monitored by serum alkaline phosphatase levels.

Calcitonin therapy is recommended for patients who cannot tolerate bisphosphonate drugs. Human calcitonin (Cibacalcin) inhibits osteoclastic activity, prevents bone resorption, relieves acute symptoms, and lowers the serum alkaline phosphatase levels. This drug is available as a subcutaneous injection. Salmon calcitonin can also be used as a subcutaneous or IM injection for treating Paget's disease. Salmon calcitonin has a longer half-life and greater milligram potency than human calcitonin. Response to calcitonin therapy is not permanent and often stops when therapy is discontinued.

Pain is usually managed by NSAIDs. Orthopedic surgery for fractures, hip and knee replacements, and knee realignment may be necessary.

A firm mattress should be used to provide back support and relieve pain. The patient may be required to wear a corset or light brace to relieve back pain and provide support when in the upright position. The patient should be proficient in the correct application of such devices and know how to regularly examine areas of the skin for friction damage. Discourage activities such as lifting and twisting. Physical therapy may increase muscle strength. Good body mechanics are essential. A properly balanced nutrition program is important in the management of metabolic disorders of bone, especially pertaining to vitamin D, calcium, and protein, which are necessary to ensure the availability of the components for bone formation. Initiate prevention measures such as patient teaching, use of an assistive device, and environmental changes to prevent falls and subsequent fractures.

SAFETY ALERT
To reduce the risk of patient harm resulting from falls:
- Evaluate patients for fall risk.
- Identify high-risk factors for falls, including medications and uncorrected vision.
- Take action to address any identified risks.

GERONTOLOGIC CONSIDERATIONS

METABOLIC BONE DISEASES
Osteoporosis and Paget's disease are common in older adults. Instruct patients in proper nutritional management to prevent further bone loss. Keep the patient as active as possible to slow demineralization of bone resulting from disuse or extended immobilization.

Because metabolic bone disorders increase the possibility of pathologic fractures, use extreme caution when the patient is turned or moved. Hip fractures in particular can adversely affect quality of life and may lead to admission to a long-term care facility. A supervised exercise program is an essential part of an osteoporosis treatment program. If the patient's condition permits, encourage ambulation without causing fatigue.

CASE STUDY

Osteoporosis

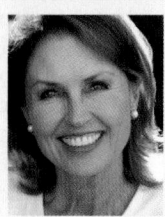

Jupiterimages/
Comstock/Thinkstock

Patient Profile

M.L. is a 58-yr-old white retired nurse who had a total hysterectomy and salpingo-oophorectomy for removal of a benign ovarian cyst 7 yr ago. She also has a history of a seizure disorder since childhood and Addison's disease.

Subjective Data

- Acute, severe lumbar pain and tenderness that radiate to her right hip and lateral thigh after falling and landing on her buttocks last week
- Walking and bending increases pain
- Stress fracture in wrist 5 mo ago
- Reports no noticeable loss of height
- Maternal history of osteoporosis
- Taking corticosteroids and mineralocorticoids for past 6 yr for Addison's disease
- Taking phenytoin (Dilantin) every evening
- Drinks two alcoholic beverages every evening
- Dislikes dairy products

Objective Data

- 5 ft, 7 in tall, 110 lb

Diagnostic Studies

- Tests show decreased bone mineral density at spine and hip
- Lumbar spine radiographs reveal a slightly displaced L4 compression fracture
- Normal serum calcium, phosphorus, and alkaline phosphatase levels

Collaborative Care

- L4 vertebroplasty
- Thoracic-lumbar-sacral orthosis (TLSO) brace postoperatively
- Ibandronate (Boniva) 150 mg/mo PO
- Calcium supplements 1500 mg/day PO
- High-calcium diet
- Reduce alcohol intake
- Regular low-impact weight-bearing exercise program

Discussion Questions

1. What factors increase M.L.'s risk for osteoporosis?
2. Why does walking and bending increase M.L.'s pain?
3. What is the purpose of the TLSO brace prescribed for M.L.?
4. **Priority Decision:** What are the priority teaching needs for M.L.?
5. **Delegation Decision:** Which of the following nursing personnel should be responsible for teaching M.L. related to her osteoporosis and new medication: RN, LPN/LVN, UAP?
6. How might you assist M.L. in increasing her intake of calcium?
7. Why would regular exercise be important for M.L.?
8. **Priority Decision:** Based on the assessment data presented, what are the priority nursing diagnoses? Are there any collaborative problems?
9. **Evidence-Based Practice:** M.L. asks you why taking corticosteroids increases her risk for developing osteoporosis. How would you respond to her?

ⓔvolve Answers available at *http://evolve.elsevier.com/Lewis/medsurg.*

BRIDGE TO NCLEX EXAMINATION

The number of the question corresponds to the same-numbered outcome at the beginning of the chapter.

1. A patient with osteomyelitis is treated with surgical debridement with implantation of antibiotic beads. When the patient asks why the beads are used, the nurse answers *(select all that apply)*
   a. "The beads are used to directly deliver antibiotics to the site of the infection."
   b. "There are no effective oral or IV antibiotics to treat most cases of bone infection."
   c. "This is the safest method of delivering long-term antibiotic therapy for a bone infection."
   d. "The beads are an adjunct to debridement and oral and IV antibiotics for deep infections."
   e. "The ischemia and bone death that occur with osteomyelitis are impenetrable to IV antibiotics."

2. A patient has been diagnosed with osteosarcoma of the humerus. He shows an understanding of his treatment options when he states
   a. "I accept that I have to lose my arm with surgery."
   b. "The chemotherapy before surgery will shrink the tumor."
   c. "This tumor is related to the melanoma I had 3 years ago."
   d. "I'm glad they can take out the cancer with such a small scar."

3. Which individuals would be at high risk for low back pain *(select all that apply)*?
   a. A 63-year-old man who is a long-distance truck driver
   b. A 36-year-old 6 ft, 2 in construction worker who weighs 260 lb
   c. A 28-year-old female yoga instructor who is 5 ft, 6 in and weighs 130 lb
   d. A 30-year-old male nurse who works on an orthopedic unit and smokes
   e. A 44-year-old female chef with prior compression fracture of the spine

4. The nurse's responsibility for a patient with a suspected disc herniation who is experiencing acute pain and muscle spasms is
   a. encouraging total bed rest for several days.
   b. teaching the principles of back strengthening exercises.
   c. stressing the importance of straight-leg raises to decrease pain.
   d. promoting the use of cold and hot compresses and pain medication.

5. In caring for a patient after a spinal fusion, the nurse would immediately report to the physician which patient symptom?
   a. The patient experiences a single episode of emesis.
   b. The patient is unable to move the lower extremities.
   c. The patient is nauseated and has not voided in 4 hours.
   d. The patient complains of pain at the bone graft donor site.
6. Before discharge from the same-day surgery unit, instruct the patient who has had a surgical correction of bilateral hallux valgus to
   a. rest frequently with the feet elevated.
   b. soak the feet in warm water several times a day.
   c. expect the feet to be numb for the next few days.
   d. expect continued pain in the feet, since this is not uncommon.

7. You are teaching a patient with osteopenia. What is important to include in the teaching plan?
   a. Lose weight.
   b. Stop smoking.
   c. Eat a high-protein diet.
   d. Start swimming for exercise.

1. a, d, 2. b, 3. a, b, d, e, 4. d, 5. b, 6. a, 7. b

ⓔvolve

For rationales to these answers and even more NCLEX review questions, visit *http://evolve.elsevier.com/Lewis/medsurg.*

REFERENCES

1. Matteson E, Osmon D: Infections of the bursae, joints, and bones. In Goldman L, Schafer A, editors: *Goldman: Goldman's Cecil medicine*, ed 24, Philadelphia, 2011, Saunders.
2. US National Library of Medicine–PubHealth: Osteomyelitis. Retrieved from *www.ncbi.nlm.nih.gov/pubmedhealth/PMH0001473.*
3. Merck Manual Home Health Handbook: Osteomyelitis. Retrieved from *www.merckmanuals.com/home/bone_joint_and_muscle_disorders/bone_and_joint_infections/osteomyelitis.*
4. Lehne R: *Pharmacology for nursing care*, ed 7, Philadelphia, 2012, Saunders.
5. Rao N: Treating osteomyelitis: antibiotics and surgery, *Plast Reconst Surg* 127:117S, 2011.
6. Siegel R, Naishadham D, Jemal A, et al: Cancer statistics 2012, *CA Cancer J Clin* 62:10, 2012.
*7. Anninga J, Gelderblom H, Fiocco M, et al: Chemotherapeutic adjuvant treatment for osteosarcoma: where do we stand? *Eur J Cancer* 47:2431, 2011.
8. American Cancer Society: What is bone metastasis? Retrieved from *www.cancer.org/treatment/understandingyourdiagnosis/bonemetastasis.*
9. Judge D, Kass D, Thompson W, et al: Pathophysiology and therapy of cardiac dysfunction in Duchenne muscular dystrophy, *Am J Cardiovasc Drugs* 11:287, 2011.
10. Abdel-Hamid H, Clemens P: Pharmacological therapies for muscular dystrophies, *Curr Opin Neurol* 25:604, 2012.
11. National Institute of Neurological Disorders and Stroke: Low back pain, National Institutes of Health. Retrieved from *www.ninds.nih.gov/disorders/backpain.*
*12. Graham P, Dougherty J: Oh, their aching backs! Occupational injuries in nursing assistants, *Orthop Nurs* 31:218, 2012.
13. Cleveland Clinic: Alternative approaches may help ease back pain, *Arthritis Advisor* 11:4, 2012.
14. Casazza B: Diagnosis and treatment of acute low back pain, *Am Fam Physician* 85:343, 2012.
*15. Jaromi M, Nemeth A, Kranicz J, et al: Treatment and ergonomics training of work-related lower back pain and body posture problems for nurses, *J Clin Nurs* 21(11/12):1776, 2012.

16. Johns Hopkins Medicine, Neurology and Neurosurgery: Degenerative disc disease. Retrieved from *www.hopkinsmedicine.org/neurology_neurosurgery/specialty_areas/spine/conditions/degenerative_disc_disease.html.*
17. Dixit R: Low back pain. In Firestein G, Budd R, Gabriel S, et al, editors: *Kelley's textbook of rheumatology*, ed 9, Philadelphia, 2012, Saunders.
18. Mayo Clinic: Herniated disk. Retrieved from *www.mayoclinic.com/health/herniated-disk.*
*19. Cepoiu-Martin M, Faris P, Lorenzetti D, et al: Artificial cervical disc arthroplasty: a systematic review, *Spine* 36:E1623, 2011.
*20. Deyo R, Ching A, Matsen L, et al: Use of bone morphogenetic proteins in spinal fusion surgery for older adults with lumbar stenosis, *Spine* 37:222, 2012.
21. Cleveland Clinic: Don't let the pain in your neck get you down, *Arthritis Advisor* 10:6, 2011.
*22. Kay T, Gross A, Goldsmith CH, et al: Exercises for mechanical neck disorders, *Cochrane Database Syst Rev* 8:CD004250, 2012.
23. American Academy of Orthopedic Surgeons: Shoes: finding the right fit. Retrieved from *www.orthoinfo.aaos.org.*
24. Turns M: The diabetic foot: an overview for community nurses, *Br J Commun Nurs* 17:422, 2012.
*25. Stolt M, Suhonen R, Puukka P, et al: Foot health and self-care activities of older people in home care, *J Clin Nurs* 21:3082, 2012.
26. Williams S: Metabolic bone disease in the bariatric surgery patient, *J Obesity* 2011:634614, 2011. Retrieved from *www.hindawi.com/journals/jobes/2011/634614.*
27. Bhan A, Rao AD, Rao DS: Osteomalacia as a result of vitamin D deficiency, *Rheum Dis Clin North Am* 38:81, 2012.
28. National Osteoporosis Foundation: Debunking the myths. Retrieved from *www.nof.org/articles.*
*29. Gourlay M, Fine J, Preisser J, et al: Bone-density testing interval and transition to osteoporosis in older women, *N Engl J Med* 366:225, 2012.
*30. Watts N, Adler R, Bilezekian J, et al: Osteoporosis in men: an Endocrine Society clinical practice guideline, *J Clin Endocrinol Metab* 97:1802, 2012.
31. Armas L, Recker R: Pathophysiology of osteoporosis, *Endocrinol Metab Clin North Am* 41:475, 2012.
32. Link T: Osteoporosis imaging: state of the art and advanced imaging, *Radiology* 263:3, 2012.
33. Shuler F, Conjeski J, Kendall D, et al: Understanding the burden of osteoporosis and use of the World Health Organization FRAX, *Orthopedics* 35:798, 2012.

*Evidence-based information for clinical practice.

34. Agency for Healthcare Research and Quality: Diagnosis and treatment of osteoporosis. Retrieved from *www .guideline.gov/content.aspx?id=34270&search=treatment+ of+osteoporosis.*

35. Sutcliffe A: Management and prevention of osteoporosis, *Pract Nurse* 42:32, 2012.

36. Asenjo J, Rossel F: Vertebroplasty and kyphoplasty: new evidence adds heat to the debate, *Curr Opin Anesthesiol* 25:577, 2012.

*37. Schmidt P: The 2012 hormone therapy position statement of the North American Menopause Society, *Menopause* 19:257, 2012.

38. Schuiling K, Robinia K, Nye R: Osteoporosis update, *J Midwifery Womens Health* 56:615, 2011.

39. Chung P, Van Hul W: Paget's disease of bone: evidence for complex pathogenetic interactions, *Semin Arthritis Rheum* 41:619, 2012.

40. Cortis K, Micallef K, Mizzi A: Imaging Paget's disease of bone—from head to toe, *Clin Radiol* 66:662, 2011.

41. Klemm K, Klein M, McPherson R: Biochemical markers of bone metabolism. In Dalton H, Pincus M, editors: *McPherson: Henry's clinical diagnosis and management of laboratory methods,* ed 22, St Louis, 2011, Saunders.

RESORCES

American Academy of Orthopedic Surgeons (AAOS)
www.aaos.org
Exercises to strengthen the back
http://orthoinfo.aaos.org/topic.cfm?topic=a00302
American College of Foot and Ankle Surgeons (ACFAS)
www.acfas.org
American Podiatric Medical Association
www.apma.org
International Osteoporosis Foundation
www.osteofound.org
Muscular Dystrophy Association (MDA)
www.mda.org
National Association of Orthopaedic Nurses (NAON)
www.orthonurse.org
National Institutes of Health (NIH) Osteoporosis and Related Bone Diseases National Resource Center
www.niams.nih.gov/Health_Info/bone
National Osteoporosis Foundation
www.nof.org
Paget Foundation
www.paget.org

Most folks are as happy as they make up their minds to be.
Abraham Lincoln

Nursing Management
Arthritis and Connective Tissue Diseases

Dottie Roberts

⊘volve WEBSITE

http://evolve.elsevier.com/Lewis/medsurg

- NCLEX Review Questions
- Key Points
- Pre-Test
- Answer Guidelines for Case Study on p. 1593
- Rationales for Bridge to NCLEX Examination Questions

- Case Studies
  - Patient With Obesity and Osteoarthritis
  - Patient With Rheumatoid Arthritis
  - Patient With Systemic Lupus Erythematosus
- Nursing Care Plans (Customizable)
  - eNCP 65-1: Patient With Rheumatoid Arthritis
  - eNCP 65-2: Patient With Systemic Lupus Erythematosus

- Concept Map Creator
- Concept Map for Case Study on p. 1593
- Glossary
- Content Updates

eFigure
- eFig. 65-1: Comparison of hands in osteoarthritis and rheumatoid arthritis

LEARNING OUTCOMES

1. Compare and contrast the sequence of events leading to joint destruction in osteoarthritis and rheumatoid arthritis.
2. Detail the clinical manifestations, collaborative care, and nursing management of osteoarthritis and rheumatoid arthritis.
3. Describe the pathophysiology, clinical manifestations, and collaborative care of gout, Lyme disease, and septic arthritis.
4. Summarize the pathophysiology, clinical manifestations, collaborative care, and nursing management of ankylosing spondylitis, psoriatic arthritis, and reactive arthritis.
5. Differentiate the pathophysiology, clinical manifestations, collaborative care, and nursing management of systemic lupus erythematosus, scleroderma, polymyositis, dermatomyositis, and Sjögren's syndrome.
6. Explain the drug therapy and related nursing management associated with arthritis and connective tissue diseases.
7. Compare and contrast the possible etiologies, clinical manifestations, and collaborative and nursing management of fibromyalgia and chronic fatigue syndrome.

KEY TERMS

Reviewed by Cheryl A. Waklatsi, RN, MSN, Assistant Professor Nursing Education, The Christ College of Nursing and Health Sciences, Cincinnati, Ohio; Jerry Harvey, RN, MS, BC, Assistant Professor of Nursing, Liberty University, Lynchburg, Virginia; and Geri B. Neuberger, EdD, APRN-CNS, Professor of Nursing, University of Kansas School of Nursing, Kansas City, Kansas.

This chapter discusses *rheumatic diseases,* which primarily affect body joints, tendons, ligaments, muscles, and bones. These diseases are often characterized by inflammation. Rheumatic diseases result from the loss of function in one or more of the connective or bone structures of the body. There are more than 100 kinds of rheumatic diseases. An estimated 46 million people in the United States have rheumatic conditions.[1]

ARTHRITIS

Arthritis, a type of rheumatic disease, involves inflammation of a joint or joints. Most forms of arthritis affect women more frequently than men.[2] The most common types of arthritis are osteoarthritis, rheumatoid arthritis, and gout.

OSTEOARTHRITIS

Osteoarthritis (OA), the most common form of joint (articular) disease in North America, is a slowly progressive noninflammatory disorder of the diarthrodial (synovial) joints. Currently 27 million Americans are affected by OA, with the numbers expected to greatly increase as the population ages.[1]

Etiology and Pathophysiology

OA involves the formation of new joint tissue in response to cartilage destruction.[3] OA is not considered a normal part of the aging process, but aging is one risk factor for disease development.[4] Cartilage destruction may actually begin between ages 20 and 30, and the majority of adults are affected by age 40. Few patients experience symptoms until after age 50 or 60, but more than half of those over 65 years of age have x-ray evidence of OA in at least one joint. After 55 years of age, women are affected by OA more often than men.[5]

OA is usually caused by a known event or condition that directly damages cartilage or causes joint instability (Table 65-1). The increased incidence of OA in aging women is believed to be due to estrogen reduction at menopause. Modifiable risk factors for OA have been identified, including obesity, which contributes to hip and knee OA. Regular moderate exercise, which also helps with weight control, has been shown to decrease the likelihood of disease development and progression. Anterior cruciate ligament injury, which is associated with quick stops and pivoting as in football and soccer, has been linked to an increased risk of knee OA.[6] Occupations that require frequent kneeling and stooping are also linked to a higher risk of knee OA.

The pathogenesis of OA is complex, with genetic, metabolic, and local factors that interact and cause a process of cartilage deterioration. OA results from cartilage damage at the level of the chondrocytes (Fig. 65-1). Progression of OA causes the normally smooth, white, translucent articular cartilage to become dull, yellow, and granular. Affected cartilage gradually becomes softer, less elastic, and less able to resist wear with heavy use.

The body's attempts at cartilage repair cannot keep up with the destruction that is occurring. Continued changes in the collagen structure of the cartilage lead to fissuring and erosion of the articular surfaces. As the central cartilage becomes thinner, cartilage and bony growth *(osteophytes)* increase at the joint margins. The resulting incongruity in joint surfaces creates an uneven distribution of stress across the joint and contributes to a reduction in motion.

Although inflammation is not characteristic of OA, a secondary synovitis may result when phagocytic cells try to rid the joint of small pieces of cartilage torn from the joint surface. These inflammatory changes contribute to the early pain and stiffness of OA. The pain of later disease results from contact between exposed bony joint surfaces after the articular cartilage has deteriorated completely.

Clinical Manifestations

Systemic. Systemic manifestations, such as fatigue, fever, and organ involvement, are not present in OA. This is an important distinction between OA and inflammatory joint disorders such as rheumatoid arthritis.

Joints. Manifestations of OA range from mild discomfort to significant disability. Joint pain is the predominant symptom and the typical reason that the patient seeks medical attention. Pain generally worsens with joint use. In the early stages of OA, joint pain is relieved by rest. However, in advanced disease the patient may complain of pain at rest or experience sleep disruptions caused by increasing joint discomfort. Pain may also become worse as the barometric pressure falls before inclement weather. As OA progresses, increasing pain can contribute significantly to disability and loss of function. The pain of OA may

TABLE 65-1 CAUSES OF OSTEOARTHRITIS

Cause	Effects on Joint Cartilage
Trauma	Dislocations or fractures may lead to avascular necrosis or uneven stress on cartilage.
Mechanical stress	Repetitive physical activities (e.g., sports) cause cartilage deterioration.
Inflammation	Release of enzymes in response to local inflammation can affect cartilage integrity.
Joint instability	Damage to supporting structures causes instability, placing uneven stress on articular cartilage.
Neurologic disorders	Pain and loss of reflexes from neurologic disorders, such as diabetic neuropathy and Charcot's joint, cause abnormal movements that contribute to cartilage deterioration.
Skeletal deformities	Congenital or acquired conditions such as Legg-Calvé-Perthes disease or dislocated hip contribute to cartilage deterioration.
Hematologic or endocrine disorders	Chronic hemarthrosis (e.g., hemophilia) contributes to cartilage deterioration.
Drugs	Drugs such as indomethacin (Indocin), colchicine, and corticosteroids can stimulate collagen-digesting enzymes in joint synovium.

GENDER DIFFERENCES

Osteoarthritis (OA)

Men	Women
• Before age 50, men are affected more often than women.	• After age 50, women are affected twice as often as men.
• After age 55, hip OA is more common in men than in women.	• After age 55, OA in interphalangeal joints and thumb base is more common in women than in men.
• Before age 45, knee OA is more common in men than in women.	• After age 45, knee OA is more common in women than in men.

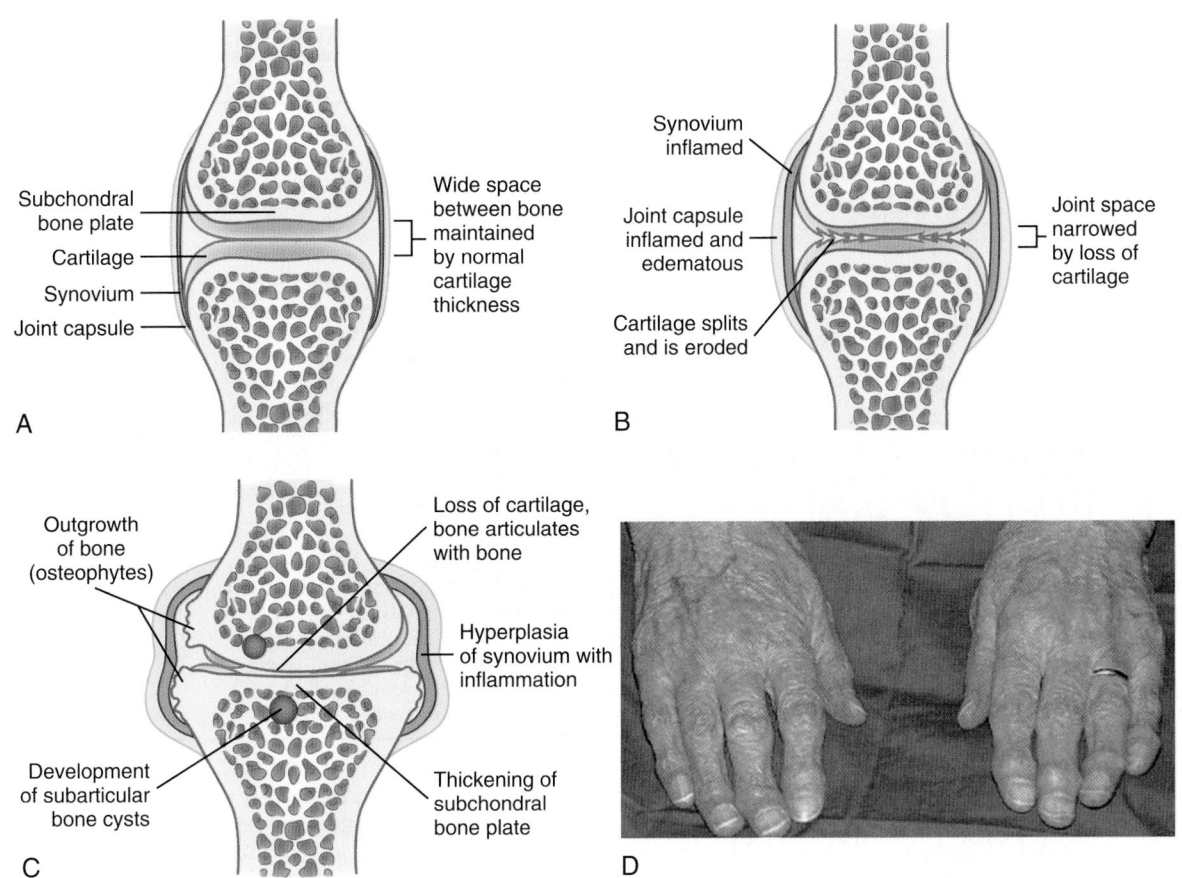

FIG. 65-1 Pathologic changes in osteoarthritis. **A,** Normal synovial joint. **B,** Early change in osteoarthritis is destruction of articular cartilage and narrowing of the joint space. There is inflammation and thickening of the joint capsule and synovium. **C,** With time, thickening of subarticular bone occurs, caused by constant friction of the two bone surfaces. Osteophytes form around the periphery of the joint by irregular overgrowths of bone. **D,** In osteoarthritis of the hands, osteophytes on the distal interphalangeal joints of the fingers, termed *Heberden's nodes,* appear as small nodules.

be referred to the groin, buttock, or medial side of the thigh or knee. Sitting down becomes difficult, as does rising from a chair when the hips are lower than the knees. As OA develops in the intervertebral (apophyseal) joints of the spine, localized pain and stiffness are common.

Unlike pain, which is typically provoked by activity, joint stiffness occurs after periods of rest or static position. Early morning stiffness is common but generally resolves within 30 minutes, a factor distinguishing OA from inflammatory arthritic disorders such as rheumatoid arthritis. Overactivity can cause a mild joint effusion that temporarily increases stiffness. *Crepitation,* a grating sensation caused by loose particles of cartilage in the joint cavity, can also contribute to stiffness. Crepitation is a common sign in patients with knee OA.

OA usually affect joints asymmetrically. The most commonly involved joints are the distal interphalangeal (DIP) and proximal interphalangeal (PIP) joints of the fingers, the metacarpophalangeal (MCP) joint of the thumb, weight-bearing joints (hips, knees), the metatarsophalangeal (MTP) joint of the foot, and the cervical and lower lumbar vertebrae (Fig. 65-2).

Deformity. Deformity or instability associated with OA is specific to the involved joint. For example, *Heberden's nodes* occur on the DIP joints as an indication of osteophyte formation and loss of joint space (see Fig. 65-1, *D*). They can appear as early as age 40 and tend to be seen in family members. *Bouchard's nodes* on the PIP joints indicate similar disease

involvement. Heberden's and Bouchard's nodes are often red, swollen, and tender. Although these bony enlargements usually do not cause significant loss of function, the patient may be distressed by the visible disfigurement.

Knee OA often leads to joint malalignment as a result of cartilage loss in the medial compartment. The patient has a characteristic bowlegged appearance and may develop an altered gait in response to the obvious deformity. In advanced hip OA, one of the patient's legs may become shorter from a loss of joint space.

Diagnostic Studies

A bone scan, computed tomography (CT) scan, or magnetic resonance imaging (MRI) may be useful to diagnose OA because of the sensitivity of these tests in detecting early joint changes. X-rays are helpful in confirming disease and staging the progression of joint damage. As OA progresses, x-rays typically show joint space narrowing, bony sclerosis, and osteophyte formation. However, these changes do not always correlate with the degree of pain that the patient experiences. Despite significant x-ray indications of disease, the patient may be relatively free of symptoms. Conversely, another patient may have severe pain with only minimal x-ray changes.

No laboratory abnormalities or biomarkers have been identified that are specific diagnostic indicators of OA. The erythrocyte sedimentation rate (ESR) is normal except in instances of

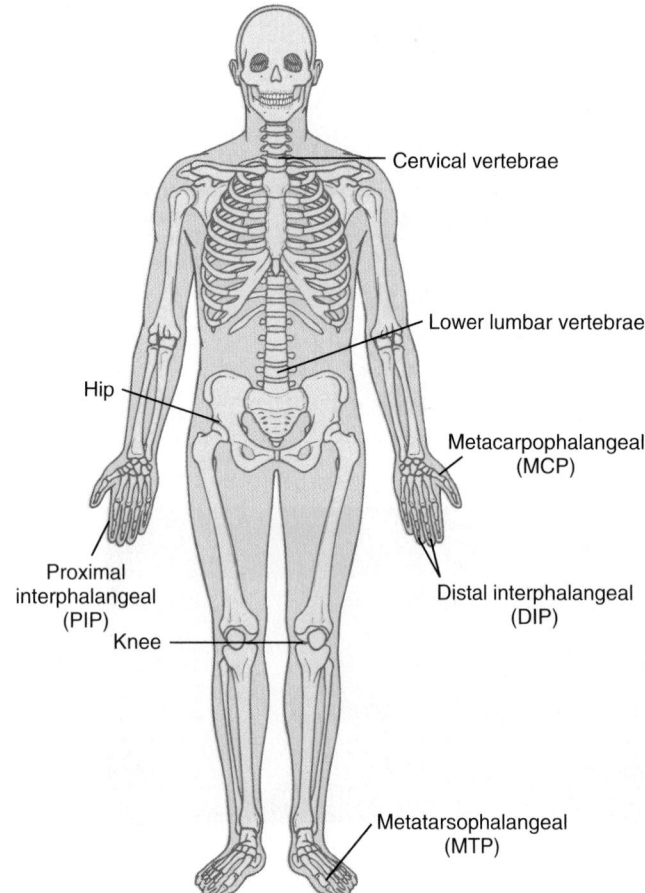

FIG. 65-2 Joints most frequently involved in osteoarthritis.

Labels on figure: Cervical vertebrae; Lower lumbar vertebrae; Hip; Metacarpophalangeal (MCP); Proximal interphalangeal (PIP); Knee; Distal interphalangeal (DIP); Metatarsophalangeal (MTP)

TABLE 65-2   **COLLABORATIVE CARE**
Osteoarthritis

Diagnostic
- History and physical examination
- Radiologic studies of involved joints (e.g., x-ray, CT scan, MRI, bone scan)
- Synovial fluid analysis

Collaborative Therapy
- Nutritional and weight management counseling
- Rest and joint protection, use of assistive devices
- Therapeutic exercise
- Heat and cold applications
- Complementary and alternative therapies
  - Herbs and nutritional supplements (e.g., glucosamine)
  - Movement therapies (e.g., yoga, Tai Chi)
  - Transcutaneous electrical nerve stimulation (TENS)
  - Acupuncture
- Drug therapy*
  - acetaminophen
  - Nonsteroidal antiinflammatory drugs
  - Antibiotics
  - Intraarticular hyaluronic acid
  - Intraarticular corticosteroids
  - Opioid analgesics
- Reconstructive joint surgery

*See Table 65-3.

acute synovitis, when minimal elevations may be noted. Other routine blood tests (e.g., complete blood count [CBC], renal and liver function tests) are useful only in screening for related conditions or for establishing baseline values before the initiation of therapy. Synovial fluid analysis allows differentiation between OA and other forms of inflammatory arthritis. In OA the fluid remains clear yellow with little or no sign of inflammation.

Collaborative Care

Because OA has no cure, collaborative care focuses on managing pain and inflammation, preventing disability, and maintaining and improving joint function (Table 65-2). Nondrug interventions are the foundation for OA management and should be maintained throughout the patient's treatment period. Drug therapy serves as an adjunct to nondrug treatments.

Rest and Joint Protection. The OA patient must understand the importance of a balance of rest and activity. The affected joint should be rested during any periods of acute inflammation and maintained in a functional position with splints or braces if necessary. However, immobilization should not exceed 1 week because of the risk of joint stiffness with inactivity. The patient may need to modify his or her usual activities to decrease stress on affected joints. Teach the patient with knee OA to avoid prolonged periods of standing, kneeling, or squatting. Using an assistive device such as a cane, walker, or crutches can also help decrease stress on arthritic joints.

Heat and Cold Applications. Applications of heat and cold may help reduce complaints of pain and stiffness. Although ice is not used as often as heat in the treatment of OA, it can be appropriate if the patient experiences acute inflammation. Heat therapy, including hot packs, whirlpool baths, ultrasound, and paraffin wax baths, is especially helpful for stiffness.

Nutritional Therapy and Exercise. If the patient is overweight, a weight-reduction program is a critical part of the total treatment plan. Help the patient evaluate the current diet to make appropriate changes. (Chapter 41 discusses ways to assist the patient in attaining and maintaining a healthy body weight.) Because the load on the joints and the degree of joint mobilization are essential to the preservation of articular cartilage integrity, exercise is a fundamental part of OA management.[7] Aerobic conditioning, range-of-motion exercises, and specific programs for strengthening the quadriceps have been beneficial for many patients with knee OA.

Complementary and Alternative Therapies. Complementary and alternative therapies for symptom management of arthritis are popular with patients who have failed to find relief through traditional medical care. Acupuncture is effective in decreasing chronic arthritic pain.[8] Other therapies include yoga, massage, guided imagery, and therapeutic touch (see Chapters 6 and 7). Nutritional supplements such as glucosamine and chondroitin may help relieve arthritic pain and improve joint mobility in some patients[9] (see the Complementary & Alternative Therapies boxes on p. 1565).

Drug Therapy. Drug therapy is based on the severity of the patient's symptoms (Table 65-3). The patient with mild to moderate joint pain may get relief from acetaminophen (Tylenol). The patient may receive up to 1000 mg every 6 hours, with the daily dose not to exceed 4 g. A topical agent such as capsaicin cream (Zostrix) may also be beneficial, either alone or in conjunction with acetaminophen. It blocks pain by locally interfering with substance P, which is responsible for the transmission of pain impulses. A concentrated product is available by prescription, but creams of 0.025% to 0.075% capsaicin are available over the counter (OTC). Other OTC products that contain

COMPLEMENTARY & ALTERNATIVE THERAPIES

Acupuncture

Acupuncture is a traditional Chinese medical practice of inserting very fine needles into the skin to stimulate specific anatomic points in the body (called acupoints) for therapeutic purposes.

Scientific Evidence*
Moderately strong for reducing chronic pain from osteoarthritis; chronic headache; and back, neck, and shoulder pain.

Nursing Implications
- Acupuncture is an effective treatment to suggest to patients with chronic pain.
- Refer interested patients to a practitioner who is appropriately trained and licensed (see Chapter 6).

*Source: Vickers A, Cronin A, Maschino A, et al: Acupuncture for chronic pain: individual patient data meta-analysis, *Arch Int Med* 172(19):1444, 2012.

COMPLEMENTARY & ALTERNATIVE THERAPIES

Glucosamine and Chondroitin

Scientific Evidence*
- Both glucosamine and chondroitin provide some relief for moderate to severe arthritic pain but not for mild arthritic pain.
- Pain outcomes over 2 yr were similar to those of patients taking celecoxib (Celebrex) or placebo.

Nursing Implications
- Can be suggested to patients who are unable to take celecoxib or other NSAIDs.
- Discontinue if no effects after consistent use over 90-120 days.
- May decrease effectiveness of insulin or other drugs used to control blood glucose.
- May increase the risk of bleeding.

*Source: National Center for Complementary and Alternative Medicine: Glucosamine/Chondroitin Arthritis Intervention Trial (GAIT): primary and ancillary study results. Retrieved from *www.nccam.nih.gov/research/results/gait*.

TABLE 65-3 DRUG THERAPY

Arthritis and Connective Tissue Disorders*

Drug	Mechanism of Action	Nursing Considerations
Salicylates aspirin, salicylate (salsalate [Disalcid]) choline salicylate (Arthropan) choline magnesium trisalicylate (Trilisate)	Antiinflammatory Analgesic Antipyretic Act by inhibiting synthesis of prostaglandins	Administer drug with food, milk, antacids as prescribed, or full glass of water. May use enteric-coated aspirin. Report signs of bleeding (e.g., tarry stools, bruising, petechiae, nosebleeds).
Nonsteroidal Antiinflammatory Drugs (NSAIDs) ibuprofen (Motrin, Advil, Novo-Profen) naproxen (Naprosyn, Anaprox, Aleve) ketoprofen (Orudis, Actron) piroxicam (Feldene, Novo-Pirocam) indomethacin (Indocin, Indocid) sulindac (Clinoril, Apo-Sulin, NovoSundac) tolmetin (Tolectin) diclofenac (Voltaren) meclofenamate (Meclomen) nabumetone (Relafen) oxaprozin (Daypro) meloxicam (Mobic) celecoxib (Celebrex)	Antiinflammatory Analgesic Antipyretic Act by inhibiting synthesis of prostaglandins	Administer drug with food, milk, or antacids as prescribed. Report signs of bleeding (e.g., tarry stools, bruising, petechiae, nosebleeds), edema, skin rashes, persistent headaches, visual disturbances. Monitor BP for elevations related to fluid retention. Needs to be used regularly for maximal effect.
Antibiotics doxycycline (Vibramycin) minocycline (Minocin)	Decreases action of enzymes on cartilage degradation Antirheumatic effect possibly related to immunomodulatory/antiinflammatory properties	Possible treatment alternative with mild disease.
Topical Analgesics capsaicin cream (Zostrix, Capzasin-P) diclofenac sodium (Voltaren Gel)	Depletes substance P from nerve endings, interrupting pain signals to the brain Antiinflammatory Analgesic	Must be used regularly over time for maximal effect. Aloe vera cream may moderate burning sensation. Advise patient not to use cream with external heat source (heating pad) because of risk of burns. Available in OTC and prescriptive strengths. Advise patient to avoid sun and ultraviolet (UV) light exposure. Should not be used in combination with other oral NSAIDs or aspirin due to potential for increased side effects.

*eTable 65-1 presents an enhanced version of this table.
TNF-α, Tumor necrosis factor–alpha.

Continued

TABLE 65-3   **DRUG THERAPY**—cont'd

Arthritis and Connective Tissue Disorders*

Drug	Mechanism of Action	Nursing Considerations
Corticosteroids *Intraarticular Injections* methylprednisolone acetate (Depo-Medrol) triamcinolone (Aristospan)	Antiinflammatory Analgesic Act by inhibiting synthesis and/or release of inflammatory mediators	Use strict aseptic technique for joint fluid aspiration or corticosteroid injection. Inform patient that joint may feel worse immediately after injection. Inform patient that improvement lasts weeks to months after injection. Advise patient to avoid overusing affected joint immediately after injection.
Systemic hydrocortisone (Solu-Cortef) methylprednisolone (Solu-Medrol) dexamethasone (Decadron) prednisone triamcinolone (Aristocort)	Antiinflammatory Analgesic Act by inhibiting synthesis and/or release of inflammatory mediators	Use only in life-threatening exacerbation or when symptoms persist after treatment with less potent antiinflammatory drugs. Administer for limited time only, tapering dose slowly. Be aware that exacerbation of symptoms occurs with abrupt withdrawal of drug. Monitor BP, weight, CBC, and potassium level. Limit sodium intake. Report signs of infection.
Disease-Modifying Antirheumatic Drugs (DMARDs) methotrexate (Rheumatrex, Trexall)	Antimetabolite Inhibits DNA, RNA, protein synthesis	Monitor CBC and hepatic and renal function. Advise patient to report signs of anemia (fatigue, weakness). Keep patient well hydrated. Teratogenic effects. Inform female patient that contraception should be used during and 3 mo after treatment.
sulfasalazine (Azulfidine, Salazopyrin)	Sulfonamide Antiinflammatory Blocks prostaglandin synthesis	Advise patient that drug may cause orange-yellow discoloration of urine or skin. Space doses evenly around the clock, taking drug after food with 8 oz water. Treatment may be continued even after symptoms are relieved. Monitor CBC.
leflunomide (Arava)	Antiinflammatory Immunomodulatory agent that inhibits proliferation of lymphocytes	Monitor hepatic function. Evaluate for relief of pain, swelling, stiffness, and increase in joint mobility. Advise women of childbearing age to avoid pregnancy.
penicillamine (Cuprimine, Depen)	Antiinflammatory Exact mechanism unknown but may suppress cell-mediated immune response	Monitor WBC count, platelets, urinalysis. Advise patient to take medication 1 hr before or 2 hr after meals or at least 1 hr away from any other drug, food, or milk.
Gold Compounds *Parenteral:* gold sodium thiomalate (Myochrysine), aurothioglucose (Solganal) *Oral:* auranofin (Ridaura)	Alter immune responses, suppressing synovitis of active RA	Rule out pregnancy before beginning treatment. Monitor CBC, urinalysis, and hepatic and renal function. Advise patient that therapeutic response may not occur for 3-6 mo. Advise patient to immediately report pruritus, rash, sore mouth, indigestion, or metallic taste.
Antimalarials hydroxychloroquine (Plaquenil)	Exact mechanism unknown but may suppress formation of antigens	Monitor CBC and hepatic function. Advise patient that therapeutic response may not occur for up to 6 mo. Advise patient to immediately report visual difficulties, muscular weakness, and decreased hearing or tinnitus.
Immunosuppressants azathioprine (Imuran) cyclophosphamide (Cytoxan)	Inhibit DNA, RNA, protein synthesis	Evaluate for relief of pain, swelling, stiffness, and increase in joint mobility. Advise patient to immediately report unusual bleeding or bruising. Advise patient that therapeutic response may take up to 12 wk. Advise women of childbearing age to avoid pregnancy. Encourage increased fluid intake to decrease risk of hemorrhagic cystitis.
mycophenolate mofetil (CellCept)	Inhibits DNA synthesis	Monitor blood count and liver function tests every 2–4 wk for first 3 mo of treatment, thereafter every 1–3 mo. Inform patient of increased infection risk. Instruct patients not to take antacids at same time, since they may interfere with absorption of immunosuppressant.
JAK (Janus Kinase) Inhibitors tofacitinib (Xeljanz)	Inhibits the action of the JAK enzymes, which are signaling pathways inside the cell and have an important role in the inflammation involved in RA	Patients are at increased risk of serious infections, including opportunistic infections. Monitor patient for any sign or symptom of infection so it can be treated early.

TABLE 65-3	**DRUG THERAPY—cont'd**

Arthritis and Connective Tissue Disorders*

Drug	Mechanism of Action	Nursing Considerations
Biologic and Targeted Therapies		
Tumor Necrosis Factor (TNF) Inhibitors		
etanercept (Enbrel) infliximab (Remicade) adalimumab (Humira) certolizumab (Cimzia) golimumab (Simponi)	Bind to TNF, thus blocking its interaction with TNF cell surface receptors. Decrease inflammatory and immune responses	Evaluate for relief of pain, swelling, stiffness, and increase in joint mobility. Advise patient of increased risk for tuberculosis. Instruct patient to have yearly PPD. Monitor for infection, bleeding, and emergence of malignancies. Advise patient psoriasis may worsen. Advise patient that injection site reaction generally occurs in first month of treatment and decreases with continued therapy. Advise patient to not receive live virus vaccines during treatment.
Interleukin-1 Receptor Antagonist		
anakinra (Kineret)	Blocks the action of interleukin-1, thus decreasing inflammatory response	Evaluate for relief of pain, swelling, stiffness, and increase in joint mobility. Advise patient that injection site reaction generally occurs in first month of treatment and decreases with continued therapy. Evaluate renal function. Monitor for infection. Do not take drug with TNF inhibitors.
Interleukin-6 Receptor Antagonist		
tocilizumab (Actemra)	Blocks action of interleukin-6, thus decreasing inflammatory response	Given to patients with RA who have failed other therapies. Monitor BP and for infection. Advise patient of GI effects (e.g., perforation). Monitor liver enzyme and low-density lipoprotein (LDL) levels.
T Cell Activation Inhibitor		
abatacept (Orencia)	Inhibits T cell activation, thus suppressing immune response	Not recommended for concomitant use with TNF inhibitors. Evaluate for relief of pain, swelling, stiffness, and increase in joint mobility.
B Cell Depleting Agent		
rituximab (Rituxan)	Monoclonal antibody that binds to CD20, an antigen on B cells, destroying B cells and suppressing immune response	Monitor for infection and bleeding. Advise patient to not receive live virus vaccines with treatment. Monitor for low BP if also taking BP medication. Advise patient that fatigue is common with this medication.

camphor, eucalyptus oil, and menthol (e.g., BenGay, Arthricare) may also provide temporary pain relief. Topical salicylates (e.g., Aspercreme) that can be absorbed into the blood are an alternative for patients who are able to take aspirin-containing medication. Because effects of topical agents are not sustained, several applications may be needed daily.

For the patient who fails to obtain adequate pain management with acetaminophen or for a patient with moderate to severe OA pain or signs of joint inflammation, a nonsteroidal antiinflammatory drug (NSAID) may be more effective for pain treatment. NSAID therapy typically is initiated in low-dose OTC strengths (ibuprofen [Motrin, Advil] 200 mg up to four times daily), with the dose increased as symptoms indicate. If the patient is at risk for or experiences gastrointestinal (GI) side effects with a conventional NSAID, supplemental treatment with a protective agent such as misoprostol (Cytotec) may be indicated. Arthrotec, a combination of misoprostol and the NSAID diclofenac, is also available. Diclofenac gel may be applied to the affected joint.

Because traditional NSAIDs block the production of prostaglandins from arachidonic acid by inhibiting the production of cyclooxygenase-1 (COX-1) and cyclooxygenase-2 (COX-2) (see Fig. 12-2), the risk for GI erosion and bleeding is increased. Traditional NSAIDs affect platelet aggregation, leading to a prolonged bleeding time. Patients taking both warfarin (Coumadin) and an NSAID are at high risk for bleeding. Concerns have also been raised regarding the possible negative effects of long-term NSAID treatment on cartilage metabolism, particularly in older patients who may already have diminished cartilage integrity. As an alternative to traditional NSAIDs, treatment with the COX-2 inhibitor celecoxib (Celebrex) may be considered in selected patients.

When given in equivalent antiinflammatory dosages, all NSAIDs are considered comparable in efficacy but vary widely in cost. Individual responses to the NSAIDs are also variable. Some patients still prefer aspirin, but it is no longer a common treatment and should not be used in combination with NSAIDs because both inhibit platelet function and prolong bleeding time. Intraarticular injections of corticosteroids may be appropriate for the patient with local inflammation and effusion. Four or more injections without relief suggest the need for additional intervention. Systemic use of corticosteroids is not indicated and may actually accelerate the disease process.

Another treatment for mild to moderate knee OA is hyaluronic acid (HA), a type of viscosupplementation. HA is found in normal joint fluid and articular cartilage. It contributes to both the viscosity and elasticity of synovial fluid, and its degradation can result in joint damage. Synthetic and naturally occurring HA derivatives (Orthovisc, Synvisc, Supartz, Nuflexxa, Hyalgan) are administered in three weekly injections directly into the joint space. Synvisc-1, a newer single-injection HA drug, may offer pain relief for up to 6 months. HA may also be added to oral supplements of glucosamine, chondroitin, and methylsulfonylmethane (MSM). Few side effects have been reported with HA.

Medications thought to slow the progression of OA or support joint healing are known as disease-modifying osteoarthritis drugs (DMOADs). To date, no drugs have been approved to modify OA progression despite numerous clinical trials. A variety of molecular targets are under investigation, including the use of anticatabolic agents to stimulate new cartilage growth and slow OA progression.[10]

Surgical Therapy. Symptoms of disease are often managed conservatively for many years, but the patient's loss of joint function, unrelieved pain, and diminished ability to independently perform self-care may prompt a recommendation for surgery. In patients less than 55 years of age, arthroscopic surgery for knee OA may delay the need for more serious surgery, such as a knee replacement. The main indication for arthroscopic surgery for OA is to remove debris (e.g., bits of cartilage known as loose bodies) that may be causing problems with joint motion. Reconstructive surgical procedures (e.g., hip and knee replacements) are discussed in Chapter 63.

NURSING MANAGEMENT
OSTEOARTHRITIS

▌NURSING ASSESSMENT

Carefully assess and document the type, location, severity, frequency, and duration of the patient's joint pain and stiffness. Also question the patient about the extent to which these symptoms affect the ability to perform activities of daily living. Note pain management practices and question the patient about the duration and success of each treatment. Physical examination of the affected joint or joints includes assessment of tenderness, swelling, limitation of movement, and crepitation. Compare an involved joint with the contralateral joint if it is not affected.

▌NURSING DIAGNOSES

Nursing diagnoses for the patient with OA may include, but are not limited to, the following:

- Acute and chronic pain *related to* physical activity and lack of knowledge of pain self-management techniques
- Impaired physical mobility *related to* weakness, stiffness, or pain on ambulation
- Imbalanced nutrition: more than body requirements *related to* intake in excess of energy output
- Depression *related to* chronic pain, changing physical appearance, and impaired social and work roles

▌PLANNING

The overall goals are that the patient with OA will (1) maintain or improve joint function through a balance of rest and activity, (2) use joint protection measures (Table 65-4) to improve activity tolerance, (3) achieve independence in self-care and maintain optimal role function, and (4) use drug and nondrug strategies to manage pain satisfactorily.

▌NURSING IMPLEMENTATION

HEALTH PROMOTION. Prevention of OA is possible in many cases. Community education should focus on altering modifiable risk factors by losing weight and reducing occupational and

---

TABLE 65-4	**PATIENT & CAREGIVER TEACHING GUIDE**

Joint Protection and Energy Conservation

Include the following instructions when teaching patients with arthritis to protect joints and conserve energy.

- Maintain appropriate weight.
- Use assistive devices, if indicated.
- Avoid forceful repetitive movements.
- Avoid positions of joint deviation and stress.
- Use good posture and proper body mechanics.
- Seek assistance with necessary tasks that may cause pain.
- Develop organizing and pacing techniques for routine tasks.
- Modify home and work environment to create less stressful ways to perform tasks.

HEALTHY PEOPLE

Prevention of Osteoarthritis

- Avoid trauma to joints.
- Avoid cigarette smoking.
- Maintain healthy weight.
- Use safety measures to protect and decrease risk of injury to joints.
- Exercise regularly, including strength and endurance training.

---

recreational hazards. Athletic instruction and physical fitness programs should include safety measures that protect and reduce trauma to the joints. Traumatic joint injuries should be treated promptly to prevent the development of OA.

ACUTE INTERVENTION. The person with OA most often complains of pain, stiffness, limitation of function, and the frustration of coping with these physical difficulties on a daily basis. The older adult may believe that OA is an inevitable part of aging and that nothing can be done to ease the discomfort and related disability.

The patient with OA is usually treated on an outpatient basis, often by an interdisciplinary team of health care providers that may include an internal medicine physician or family health care provider, a rheumatologist, a nurse, an occupational therapist, and a physical therapist. Health assessment questionnaires are often used to pinpoint areas of decreased function. Complete questionnaires at regular intervals to document disease and treatment progression. Treatment goals can be developed based on data from the questionnaires and the physical examination, with specific interventions to target identified problems. The patient is usually hospitalized only if joint surgery is planned (see Chapter 63).

Drugs are administered for the treatment of pain and inflammation. Nondrug strategies to decrease pain and disability may include gentle exercise, the application of heat (thermal packs) or cold (ice packs), relaxation, and yoga.[11] Splints may be prescribed to rest and stabilize painful or inflamed joints.

Once an acute flare has subsided, a physical therapist can provide valuable assistance in planning an exercise program. Therapists may recommend Tai Chi as a low-impact form of exercise. Tai Chi can be performed by patients of all ages and may be done in a wheelchair. Emphasize the importance of warming up before any exercise to prevent stretch injuries.

Patient and caregiver teaching related to OA is an important nursing responsibility. Provide information about the nature and treatment of the disease, pain management, body mechanics, correct use of assistive devices (e.g., cane, walker), principles of joint protection and energy conservation (see Table 65-4), nutritional choices, weight and stress management, and an exercise program.

Assure the patient that OA is a localized disease and that severe deforming arthritis is not the usual course. The patient can also gain support and understanding of the disease process through community resources such as the Arthritis Foundation's Self-Help Course *(www.arthritis.org)*.

AMBULATORY AND HOME CARE. Individualize home management goals to meet the patient's needs. Include the caregiver, family members, and significant others in goal setting and teaching. Home and work environment modification is essential for patient safety, accessibility, and self-care. Measures include removing scatter rugs, providing rails at the stairs and bathtub, using night-lights, and wearing well-fitting supportive shoes. Assistive devices such as canes, walkers, elevated toilet seats, and grab bars also reduce the load on an affected joint and promote safety. Urge the patient to continue all prescribed therapies at home and also be open to new approaches to symptom management.

Sexual counseling may help the patient and significant other to enjoy physical closeness by introducing the idea of alternate positions and timing for sexual activity. Discussion also increases awareness of each partner's needs. Encourage the patient to take analgesics or a warm bath to decrease joint stiffness before sexual activity.

EVALUATION

The expected outcomes are that the patient with OA will
- Experience adequate rest and activity
- Achieve satisfactory pain management
- Maintain joint flexibility and muscle strength through joint protection and therapeutic exercise
- Verbalize acceptance of OA as a chronic disease, collaborating with health care providers in disease management

RHEUMATOID ARTHRITIS

Rheumatoid arthritis (RA) is a chronic, systemic autoimmune disease characterized by inflammation of connective tissue in the diarthrodial (synovial) joints. RA is typically characterized by periods of remission and exacerbation. RA is frequently accompanied by extraarticular manifestations.

RA occurs globally, affecting all ethnic groups. It can occur at any time of life, but the incidence increases with age, peaking between 30 and 50 years old. An estimated 1.3 million adult Americans are affected by RA. Women are more likely than men to have the disease.[12]

Etiology and Pathophysiology

Although the exact cause of RA is unknown, it probably results from a combination of genetics and environmental triggers. An autoimmune etiology, which is currently the most widely accepted theory, suggests that changes associated with RA begin when a genetically susceptible person has an initial immune response to an antigen. Although a bacterium or virus has been proposed as a possible antigen, to date no infection or organism has been identified as the cause.

The antigen, which is probably not the same in all patients, triggers the formation of an abnormal immunoglobulin G (IgG). RA is characterized by autoantibodies against this abnormal

IgG. The autoantibodies are known as rheumatoid factor (RF), and they combine with IgG to form immune complexes that initially deposit on synovial membranes or superficial articular cartilage in the joints. Immune complex formation leads to the activation of complement, and an inflammatory response results. (Complement activation is discussed in Chapter 12, and immune complex formation is discussed in Chapter 14.)

Neutrophils are attracted to the site of inflammation, where they release proteolytic enzymes that can damage articular cartilage and cause the synovial lining to thicken (Fig. 65-3). Other inflammatory cells include T helper (CD4) cells, which are the primary orchestrators of cell-mediated immune responses. Activated CD4 cells stimulate monocytes, macrophages, and synovial fibroblasts to secrete the proinflammatory cytokines interleukin-1 (IL-1), interleukin-6 (IL-6), and tumor necrosis factor (TNF). These cytokines are the primary factors that drive the inflammatory response in RA. If unarrested, the disease progresses through four stages, which are identified in Table 65-5.

TABLE 65-5 ANATOMIC STAGES OF RHEUMATOID ARTHRITIS

Stage	Characteristics
I: Early	No destructive changes on x-ray, possible x-ray evidence of osteoporosis.
II: Moderate	X-ray evidence of osteoporosis, with or without slight bone or cartilage destruction. No joint deformities (although possibly limited joint mobility). Adjacent muscle atrophy. Possible presence of extraarticular soft tissue lesions (e.g., nodules, tenosynovitis).
III: Severe	X-ray evidence of cartilage and bone destruction in addition to osteoporosis. Joint deformity, such as subluxation, ulnar deviation, or hyperextension, without fibrous or bony ankylosis. Extensive muscle atrophy. Possible presence of extraarticular soft tissue lesions (e.g., nodules, tenosynovitis).
IV: Terminal	Fibrous or bony ankylosis with stage III criteria.

Data from American College of Rheumatology: Classification criteria for determining progression of rheumatoid arthritis. Retrieved from *www.hopkins-arthritis.org/physician-corner/education/acr/acr.html#class_rheum*.
NOTE: These findings describe spontaneous remission or drug-induced disease suppression.

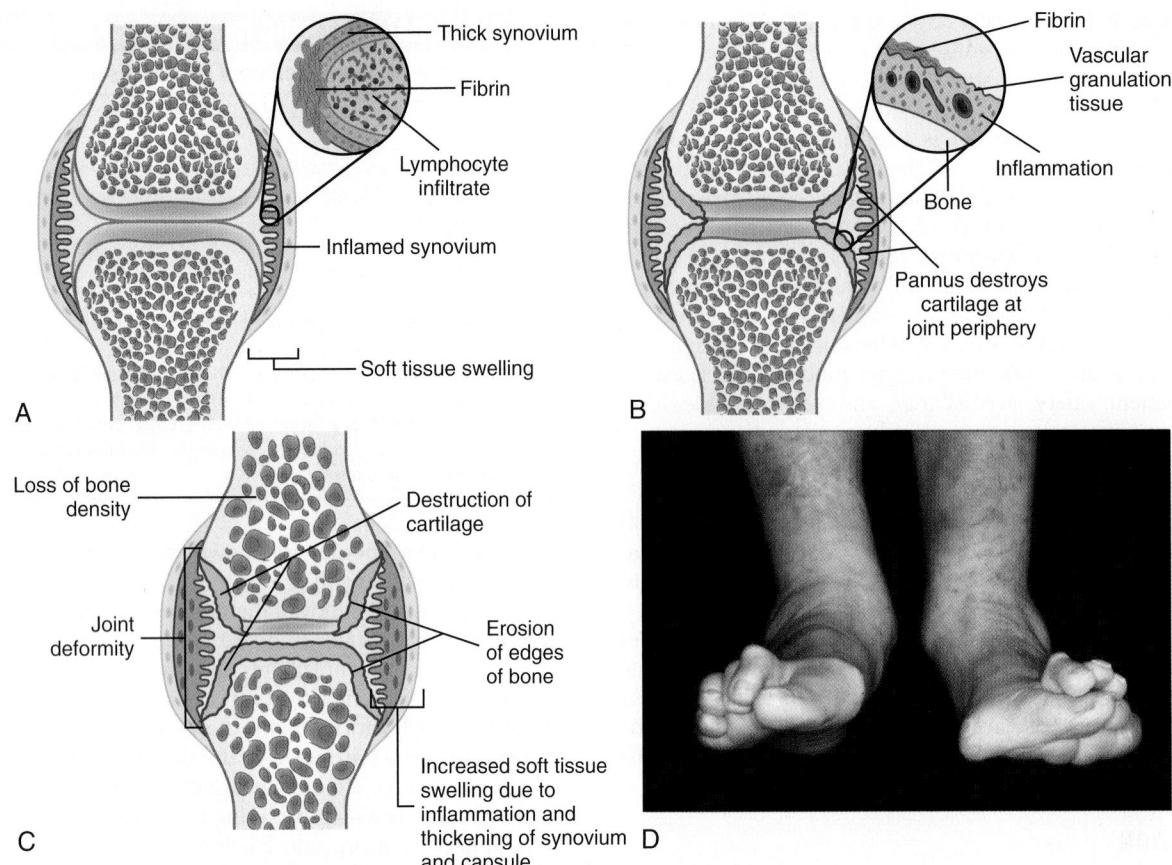

FIG. 65-3 Rheumatoid arthritis. **A,** Early pathologic change in rheumatoid arthritis is rheumatoid synovitis. The synovium is inflamed. Lymphocytes and plasma cells increase greatly. **B,** With time, articular cartilage destruction occurs, vascular granulation tissue grows across the surface of the cartilage (pannus) from the edges of the joint, and the articular surface shows loss of cartilage beneath the extending pannus, most marked at joint margins. **C,** Inflammatory pannus causes focal destruction of bone. At edges of the joint there is osteolytic destruction of bone, responsible for erosions seen on x-rays. This phase is associated with joint deformity. **D,** Multiple deformities of the foot associated with rheumatoid arthritis.

🧬 Genetic Link

Genetic predisposition is important in the development of RA. For example, a higher concurrence of RA has been noted in identical twins compared with fraternal twins.[13] The strongest evidence for a genetic influence is the role of human leukocyte antigens (HLA), especially the HLA-DR4 and HLA-DR1 antigens. (HLA is discussed in Chapter 14.)

Smoking increases the risk of RA for persons who are genetically predisposed to the disease, and makes successful treatment more difficult.

Clinical Manifestations

Joints. The onset of RA is typically insidious. Nonspecific manifestations such as fatigue, anorexia, weight loss, and generalized stiffness may precede the onset of arthritic complaints. The stiffness becomes more localized in the following weeks to months. Some patients report a history of a precipitating stressful event such as infection, work stress, physical exertion, childbirth, surgery, or emotional upset. However, research has been unable to directly correlate such events with the onset of RA.

Specific articular involvement is manifested by pain, stiffness, limitation of motion, and signs of inflammation (e.g., heat, swelling, tenderness). Joint symptoms occur symmetrically and frequently affect the small joints of the hands (PIP and MCP)

and feet (MTP). Larger peripheral joints such as wrists, elbows, shoulders, knees, hips, ankles, and jaw may also be involved. The cervical spine may be affected, but the axial skeleton (the spine and bones connected to it) is generally spared. Table 65-6 compares RA and OA.

The patient characteristically experiences joint stiffness after periods of inactivity. Morning stiffness may last from 60 minutes to several hours or more, depending on disease activity. MCP and PIP joints are typically swollen. In early disease the fingers may become spindle shaped from synovial hypertrophy and thickening of the joint capsule. Joints become tender, painful, and warm to the touch. Joint pain increases with motion, varies in intensity, and may not be proportional to the degree of inflammation. Tenosynovitis frequently affects the extensor and flexor tendons around the wrists, producing manifestations of carpal tunnel syndrome and making it difficult for the patient to grasp objects.

As disease activity progresses, inflammation and fibrosis of the joint capsule and supporting structures may lead to deformity and disability. Atrophy of muscles and destruction of tendons around the joint cause one articular surface to slip past the other *(subluxation).* Metatarsal head dislocation and subluxation in the feet may cause pain and walking disability (Fig. 65-3, *D*). Typical distortions of the hand include ulnar drift

TABLE 65-6	COMPARISON OF RHEUMATOID ARTHRITIS AND OSTEOARTHRITIS	
Parameter	**Rheumatoid Arthritis**	**Osteoarthritis**
Age at onset	Young to middle age.	Usually >40 yr.
Gender	Female/male ratio is 2:1 or 3:1. Less marked sex difference after age 60.	Before age 50, more men than women. After age 50, more women than men.
Weight	Lost or maintained weight.	Often overweight.
Disease	Systemic disease with exacerbations and remissions.	Localized disease with variable, progressive course.
Affected joints	Small joints typically first (PIPs, MCPs, MTPs), wrists, elbows, shoulders, knees. Usually bilateral, symmetric joint involvement.	Weight-bearing joints of knees and hips, small joints (MCPs, DIPs, PIPs), cervical and lumbar spine. Often asymmetric.
Pain characteristics	Stiffness lasts 1 hr to all day and may decrease with use. Pain is variable, may disrupt sleep.	Stiffness occurs on arising but usually subsides after 30 min. Pain gradually worsens with joint use and disease progression, relieved with rest.
Effusions	Common.	Uncommon.
Nodules	Present, especially on extensor surfaces.	Heberden's (DIPs) and Bouchard's (PIPs) nodes.
Synovial fluid	WBC count >20,000/µL with mostly neutrophils.	WBC count <2000/µL (mild leukocytosis).
X-rays	Joint space narrowing and erosion with bony overgrowths, subluxation with advanced disease. Osteoporosis related to corticosteroid use.	Joint space narrowing, osteophytes, subchondral cysts, sclerosis.
Laboratory findings	RF positive in 80% of patients.	RF negative.
	Elevated ESR, CRP indicative of active inflammation.	Transient elevation in ESR related to synovitis.

CRP, C-reactive protein; *DIPs,* distal interphalangeal; *ESR,* erythrocyte sedimentation rate; *MCPs,* metacarpophalangeals; *MTPs,* metatarsophalangeals; *PIPs,* proximal interphalangeal; *RF,* rheumatoid factor.

("zig-zag deformity"), swan neck, and boutonnière deformities (Fig. 65-4).

Extraarticular Manifestations. RA can affect nearly every system in the body (Fig. 65-5). Extraarticular manifestations are more likely to occur in the person with high levels of biomarkers such as RF.

Rheumatoid nodules develop in 20% to 30% of all patients with RA.[14] Rheumatoid nodules appear subcutaneously as firm, nontender, granuloma-type masses and are usually located over the extensor surfaces of joints such as fingers and elbows. Nodules at the base of the spine and back of the head are common in older adults. On the skin, these nodules can ulcerate, similar to pressure ulcers. In later disease, cardiopulmonary effects may occur. These may include pleurisy, pleural effusion, pericarditis, pericardial effusion, and cardiomyopathy.

Sjögren's syndrome is seen in 10% to 15% of patients with RA.[14] Sjögren's syndrome can occur by itself or in conjunction with other arthritic disorders such as RA and systemic lupus erythematosus (SLE). Affected patients have diminished lacrimal and salivary gland secretion, leading to a dry mouth; burning, itchy eyes with decreased tearing; and photosensitivity. (Sjögren's syndrome is discussed later in this chapter on p. 1590.)

Felty syndrome occurs most commonly in patients with severe, nodule-forming RA. It is characterized by splenomegaly and leukopenia.

Flexion contractures and hand deformities cause diminished grasp strength and affect the patient's ability to perform self-care tasks. Nodular myositis and muscle fiber degeneration can lead to pain similar to that of vascular insufficiency. Cataract development and loss of vision can result from scleral nodules. Depression may occur, which is often related to the chronic pain associated with RA.[15]

Diagnostic Studies

An accurate diagnosis is essential to the initiation of appropriate treatment and the prevention of unnecessary disability. A diagnosis is often made based on history and physical findings, but some laboratory tests are useful for confirmation and to monitor disease progression (see Tables 65-7 and 65-8). Positive RF

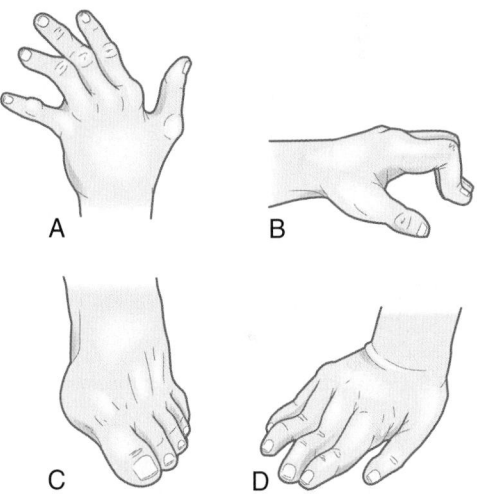

FIG. 65-4 Typical deformities of rheumatoid arthritis. **A,** Ulnar drift. **B,** Boutonnière deformity. **C,** Hallux valgus. **D,** Swan neck deformity.

occurs in approximately 80% of adult RA patients, and titers rise during active disease. ESR and C-reactive protein (CRP) are general indicators of active inflammation. An increase in antinuclear antibody (ANA) titers is also seen in some RA patients. Testing for the anti-citrullinated protein antibody (ACPA) is another important diagnostic test for RA. Levels of ACPA are more specific than those of RF for RA and in some cases may allow for an earlier and more accurate diagnosis.[16]

Synovial fluid analysis in early disease often shows a straw-colored fluid with many fibrin flecks. The enzyme MMP-3 is increased in the synovial fluid of the patient with RA, and it may be a marker of progressive joint damage. The white blood cell (WBC) count of synovial fluid is elevated (up to 25,000/µL). Inflammatory changes in the synovium can be confirmed by tissue biopsy.

X-rays are not specifically diagnostic of RA. They may be inconclusive during early stages of the disease, revealing only soft tissue swelling and possible bone demineralization. In later disease, narrowing of the joint space, destruction of articular

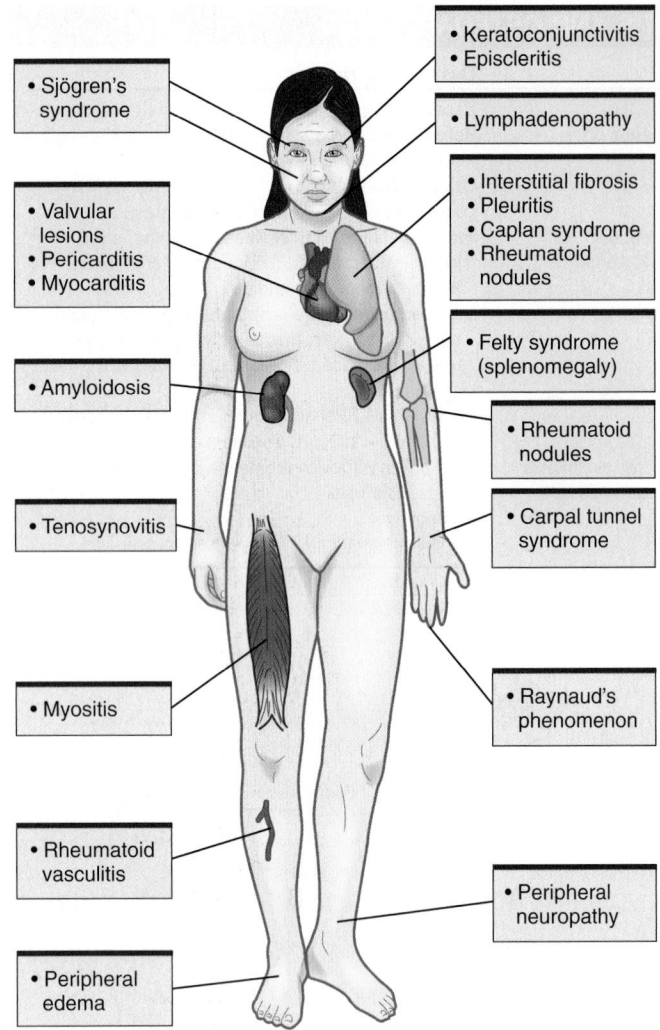

- Keratoconjunctivitis
- Episcleritis
- Sjögren's syndrome
- Lymphadenopathy
- Interstitial fibrosis
- Pleuritis
- Caplan syndrome
- Rheumatoid nodules
- Valvular lesions
- Pericarditis
- Myocarditis
- Felty syndrome (splenomegaly)
- Amyloidosis
- Rheumatoid nodules
- Carpal tunnel syndrome
- Tenosynovitis
- Myositis
- Raynaud's phenomenon
- Rheumatoid vasculitis
- Peripheral neuropathy
- Peripheral edema

FIG. 65-5 Extraarticular manifestations of rheumatoid arthritis.

cartilage, erosion, subluxation, and deformity are seen. Malalignment and ankylosis are often evident in advanced disease. Baseline films may be useful in monitoring disease progression and treatment effectiveness. Bone scans are more useful in detecting early joint changes and confirming a diagnosis so that RA treatment can be initiated.

Criteria for the diagnosis of RA in a newly presenting patient are described in Table 65-7.

Collaborative Care

Care of the patient with RA begins with a comprehensive program of education and drug therapy. Teaching regarding drug therapy includes correct administration, reporting of side effects, and frequent medical and laboratory follow-up visits. Teach the patient and the caregiver about the disease process and home management strategies. NSAIDs are prescribed to promote physical comfort. Physical therapy helps the patient maintain joint motion and muscle strength. Occupational therapy develops upper extremity function and encourages joint protection through the use of splints or other assistive devices and strategies for activity pacing.

An individualized treatment plan considers the nature of the disease activity, joint function, age, gender, family and social roles, and response to previous treatment (see Table 65-8). A

TABLE 65-7	DIAGNOSTIC CRITERIA FOR RHEUMATOID ARTHRITIS*

Patients should be tested for RA who initially are seen with:
- At least 1 joint with definite clinical synovitis
- Synovitis not better explained by another disease

A. Joint Involvement	**Score**
• 1 large joint	0
• 2-10 large joints	1
• 1-3 small joints (with or without large joint involvement)	2
• 4-10 small joints (with or without large joint involvement)	3
• >10 joints (at least 1 small joint)	5
B. Serology (at least 1 test result needed for classification)	
• Negative RF *and* negative ACPA	0
• Low-positive RF *or* low-positive ACPA	2
• High-positive RF *or* high-positive ACPA	3
C. Acute Phase Reactants (at least 1 test needed)	
• Normal CRP *and* normal ESR	0
• Abnormal CRP *or* abnormal ESR	1
D. Duration of Symptoms	
• <6 wk	0
• ≥6 wk	1

From Aletaha D, Neogi T, Silman AJ, et al: 2010 Rheumatoid arthritis classification criteria: an American College of Rheumatology/European League Against Rheumatism Collaborative Initiative, *Arthritis Rheum* 62:2569, 2010. Retrieved from *www .rheumatology.org/practice/clinical/classification/ra/2010_revised_criteria _classification_ra.*
Scoring: Add score of categories A-D. Possible scores range from 0-10. A score of ≥6 indicates the definitive presence of RA.
*Used for newly diagnosed patients.
ACPA, Anti-citrullinated protein antibody; *CRP*, C-reactive protein; *ESR*, erythrocyte sedimentation rate; *RF*, rheumatoid factor.

TABLE 65-8	**COLLABORATIVE CARE**

Rheumatoid Arthritis

Diagnostic
- History and physical examination
- Laboratory studies
  - Complete blood cell (CBC) count
  - Erythrocyte sedimentation rate (ESR)
  - Rheumatoid factor (RF)
  - Anti-citrullinated protein antibody (ACPA)
  - Antinuclear antibody (ANA)
  - C-reactive protein (CRP)
- X-ray studies of involved joints
- Synovial fluid analysis

Collaborative Therapy
- Nutritional and weight management counseling
- Therapeutic exercise
- Psychologic support
- Rest and joint protection, use of assistive devices
- Heat and cold applications
- Complementary and alternative therapies
  - Herbal products
  - Acupuncture
- Drug therapy (See Table 65-3)
  - Disease-modifying antirheumatic drugs (DMARDs)
  - Intraarticular or systemic corticosteroids
  - Nonsteroidal antiinflammatory drugs (NSAIDs)
  - Biologic and targeted therapy
- Reconstructive surgery (e.g., arthroplasty)

caring, long-term relationship with an arthritis health care team can promote the patient's self-esteem and positive coping.

Drug Therapy

Disease-Modifying Antirheumatic Drugs. Drugs remain the cornerstone of RA treatment (see Table 65-3). Because irreversible joint changes can occur as early as the first year of RA, health care providers aggressively prescribe disease-modifying antirheumatic drugs (DMARDs). These drugs have the potential to lessen the permanent effects of RA, such as joint erosion and deformity. The choice of drug is based on disease activity; the patient's level of function; and lifestyle considerations, such as the desire to bear children.

Treatment of early RA often involves DMARD therapy with methotrexate (Rheumatrex).[17] The rapid antiinflammatory effect of methotrexate reduces clinical symptoms in days to weeks. It has a lower toxicity than other drugs. Side effects include bone marrow suppression and hepatotoxicity. Methotrexate therapy requires frequent laboratory monitoring, including CBC and chemistry panel.

Sulfasalazine (Azulfidine) and the antimalarial drug hydroxychloroquine (Plaquenil) may be effective DMARDs for mild to moderate disease. They are rapidly absorbed, relatively safe, and well-tolerated medications. The synthetic DMARD leflunomide (Arava) blocks immune cell overproduction. Its efficacy and side effects are similar to those of methotrexate and sulfasalazine. Because the drug is teratogenic, the possibility of pregnancy in women of childbearing age must be excluded before therapy is initiated.

Tofacitinib (Xeljanz) is a new drug used to treat moderate to severe active RA. This drug is from a new class of medications called JAK (Janus kinase) inhibitors. The drug interferes with the JAK enzymes that contribute to the joint inflammation in RA.

Biologic and Targeted Therapies. Biologic and targeted therapies are also used to slow disease progression in RA. These drugs can be categorized based on their mechanism of action (see Table 65-3). They can be used to treat patients with moderate to severe disease who have not responded to DMARDs, or in combination therapy with an established DMARD such as methotrexate.

Tumor necrosis factor inhibitors include etanercept (Enbrel), infliximab (Remicade), adalimumab (Humira), certolizumab (Cimzia), and golimumab (Simponi). Etanercept is a biologically engineered copy (using recombinant deoxyribonucleic acid [DNA] technology) of the TNF cell receptor. This soluble TNF receptor binds to TNF in circulation before TNF can bind to the cell surface receptor. By inhibiting binding of TNF, etanercept inhibits the inflammatory response. This drug is given as a subcutaneous injection.

> **DRUG ALERT: Etanercept (Enbrel)**
> - Increased risk of serious infection and heart failure is a concern.
> - Report persistent fever, bruising, bleeding, or other signs of infection.

Infliximab and adalimumab are monoclonal antibodies that bind to TNF, thus preventing the TNF from binding to TNF receptors on cells. Infliximab is given IV, in combination with methotrexate. Adalimumab is given subcutaneously.

Certolizumab and golimumab are TNF inhibitors that improve symptoms in patients with moderate to severe RA. Both drugs are given in combination with methotrexate. When compared to other biologic and targeted therapy, certolizumab stays in the system longer and may also show a more rapid (1 to 2 weeks) and significant reduction in RA symptoms. Certolizumab is also used in treating Crohn's disease.

> **DRUG ALERT: Tumor Necrosis Factor Inhibitors**
> - Administer tuberculin test and chest x-ray before initiation of therapy.
> - Monitor for signs of infection and stop drug if acute infection develops.
> - Instruct patients to avoid live vaccination while taking drug.

Anakinra (Kineret) is a recombinant version of IL-1 receptor antagonist (IL-1Ra). It blocks the biologic activity of IL-1 by competitively inhibiting IL-1 binding to the IL-1 receptor. It is given as a subcutaneous injection. Anakinra is used to reduce the pain and swelling associated with moderate to severe RA. It can be used in combination with DMARDs but not with TNF inhibitors. Concurrent use of these agents can cause serious infection and neutropenia.

Tocilizumab (Actemra) blocks the action of IL-6, a proinflammatory cytokine. It is used to treat patients with moderate to severe RA who have not adequately responded to or cannot tolerate other drugs for RA.

Abatacept (Orencia) blocks T cell activation. It is recommended for patients who have an inadequate response to DMARDs or TNF inhibitors. It is given IV. Like anakinra, it should not be used concomitantly with TNF inhibitors.

Rituximab (Rituxan) is a monoclonal antibody that targets B cells (see Fig. 16-16). It may be used in combination with methotrexate for patients with moderate to severe RA not responding to TNF inhibitors (e.g., etanercept, infliximab). It is given IV.

Other Drug Therapy. Additional medications used infrequently for treating RA include antibiotics (minocycline [Minocin]), immunosuppressants (azathioprine [Imuran]), penicillamine (Cuprimine), and gold preparations (auranofin [Ridaura], gold sodium thiomalate [Myochrysine]).

Corticosteroid therapy can be used for symptom control. Intraarticular injections may temporarily reduce the pain and inflammation associated with disease flare-ups. Long-term use of oral corticosteroids should not be a mainstay of RA treatment because of the risk of complications, including osteoporosis and avascular necrosis. However, low-dose prednisone may be used for a limited time in select patients to decrease disease activity until DMARD therapy is effective.

Various NSAIDs and salicylates continue to be included in the drug regimen to treat arthritic pain and inflammation. Enteric-coated aspirin may be used in high dosages of 3.2 to 5.4 g/day (10 to 18 tablets).[18] NSAIDs have antiinflammatory, analgesic, and antipyretic properties. Some relief may be noted within days of the start of treatment with NSAIDs, but full effectiveness may take 2 to 3 weeks. NSAIDs may be used when the patient cannot tolerate high doses of aspirin. Antiinflammatory drugs that are taken only once or twice a day may improve the patient's ability to follow the treatment regimen (see Table 65-3). The newer-generation NSAIDs, the COX-2 inhibitors, are effective in RA as well as OA. Celecoxib is currently the only available COX-2 inhibitor.

Nutritional Therapy. Although there is no special diet for RA, balanced nutrition is important. Fatigue, pain, depression, limited endurance, and mobility deficits often accompany RA and may cause a loss of appetite or interfere with the patient's ability to shop for and prepare food. Weight loss may result. The occupational therapist may help the patient modify the home environment and use assistive devices to make food preparation easier.

Corticosteroid therapy or immobility secondary to pain may result in unwanted weight gain. A sensible weight loss program consisting of balanced nutrition and exercise reduces stress on affected joints. Corticosteroids also increase the appetite, resulting in a higher caloric intake. In addition, the patient may become distressed as signs and symptoms of Cushing syndrome, including moon face and the redistribution of fatty tissue to the trunk, change the physical appearance. Encourage the patient to continue to eat a balanced diet and not to alter the corticosteroid dose or stop therapy abruptly. Weight slowly adjusts to normal several months after cessation of therapy.

Surgical Therapy. Occasionally, surgery is needed to relieve severe pain and improve the function of severely deformed joints. Removal of the joint lining (synovectomy) is one type of surgical therapy. Total joint replacement (arthroplasty) can be done for many different joints in the body. Joint surgery is discussed in Chapter 63.

NURSING MANAGEMENT
RHEUMATOID ARTHRITIS

NURSING ASSESSMENT

Subjective and objective data that should be obtained from the patient with RA are presented in Table 65-9.

NURSING DIAGNOSES

Nursing diagnoses for the patient with RA may include, but are not limited to, the following:

- Impaired physical mobility *related to* joint pain, stiffness, and deformity
- Chronic pain *related to* joint inflammation, misuse of joints, and ineffective pain and/or comfort measures
- Disturbed body image *related to* chronic disease activity, long-term treatment, deformities, stiffness, and inability to perform usual activities

Additional information on nursing diagnoses for the patient with RA is provided in eNursing Care Plan 65-1 (on the website for this chapter).

PLANNING

The overall goals are that the patient with RA will (1) have satisfactory pain management, (2) have minimal loss of functional ability of the affected joints, (3) participate in planning and carrying out the therapeutic regimen, (4) maintain a positive self-image, and (5) perform self-care to the maximum amount possible.

NURSING IMPLEMENTATION

HEALTH PROMOTION. Prevention of RA is not possible based on the current state of knowledge. However, early treatment can help prevent further joint damage. Community education programs should focus on symptom recognition to promote early diagnosis and treatment of RA. The Arthritis Foundation offers many publications, classes, and support activities to assist affected persons (see Resources at the end of this chapter).

ACUTE INTERVENTION. The primary goals in the management of RA are the reduction of inflammation, management of pain, maintenance of joint function, and prevention or minimization of joint deformity. Goals may be met through a comprehensive program of drug therapy, balance of rest and activity with joint protection, heat and cold applications, exercise, and patient and caregiver teaching. Work closely with the health care provider,

TABLE 65-9 **NURSING ASSESSMENT**
Rheumatoid Arthritis

Subjective Data
Important Health Information
Past health history: Recent infections; precipitating factors such as emotional upset, infections, overwork, childbirth, surgery; pattern of remissions and exacerbations
Medications: Aspirin, NSAIDs, corticosteroids, DMARDs
Surgery or other treatments: Any joint surgery

Functional Health Patterns
Health perception–health management: Positive family history for rheumatoid arthritis or other autoimmune disorders; malaise, ability to participate in therapeutic regimen; impact of disease on functional ability
Nutritional-metabolic: Anorexia, weight loss; dry mucous membranes of mouth and pharynx
Activity-exercise: Stiffness and joint swelling, muscle weakness, difficulty walking, fatigue
Cognitive-perceptual: Paresthesias of hands and feet, loss of sensation; symmetric joint pain and aching that increases with motion or stress on joint

Objective Data
General
Lymphadenopathy, fever

Integumentary
Keratoconjunctivitis; subcutaneous rheumatoid nodules on forearms, elbows; skin ulcers; shiny, taut skin over involved joints; peripheral edema

Cardiovascular
Symmetric pallor and cyanosis of fingers (Raynaud's phenomenon); distant heart sounds, murmurs, dysrhythmias

Respiratory
Chronic bronchitis, tuberculosis, histoplasmosis, fibrosing alveolitis

Gastrointestinal
Splenomegaly (Felty syndrome)

Musculoskeletal
Symmetric joint involvement with swelling, erythema, heat, tenderness, and deformities; enlargement of proximal phalangeal and metacarpophalangeal joints; limitation of joint movement; muscle contractures, muscle atrophy

Possible Diagnostic Findings
Positive rheumatoid factor, ↑ ESR, anemia; ↑ WBCs in synovial fluid; evidence of joint space narrowing, and bony erosion and deformity on x-ray (osteoporosis with advanced disease)

DMARDs, Disease-modifying antirheumatic drugs; *ESR,* erythrocyte sedimentation rate; *NSAIDs,* nonsteroidal antiinflammatory drugs.

physical and occupational therapists, and social worker to help the patient restore function and make appropriate lifestyle adjustments to chronic illness.

The newly diagnosed RA patient is usually treated on an outpatient basis. Hospitalization may be necessary for patients with extraarticular complications or advancing disease requiring reconstructive surgery for disabling deformities.

Intervention begins with a careful physical assessment (e.g., joint pain, swelling, range of motion [ROM], and general health status). Also evaluate psychosocial needs (e.g., family support, sexual satisfaction, emotional stress, financial constraints, vocational and career limitations) and environmental concerns (e.g., transportation, home or work modifications). After identifying the patient's problems, coordinate a carefully planned program for rehabilitation and education with the interdisciplinary health care team.

Suppression of inflammation may be effectively achieved through the administration of NSAIDs, DMARDs, and biologic and targeted therapies. Careful attention to timing of drug administration is critical to sustain a therapeutic drug level and reduce early morning stiffness. Discuss the action and side effects of each prescribed drug and the importance of laboratory monitoring. Because many patients with RA take several different drugs, make the drug regimen as understandable as possible. Encourage patients to develop a method for remembering to take their medications (e.g., pill containers).

Nondrug management may include the use of therapeutic heat and cold, rest, relaxation techniques, joint protection (see Tables 65-4 and 65-10), biofeedback (see Chapter 6), transcutaneous electrical nerve stimulation (see Chapter 9), and hypnosis. Allow the patient and the caregiver to choose therapies that promote optimal comfort within the parameters of their lifestyle.

Lightweight splints may be prescribed to rest an inflamed joint and prevent deformity from muscle spasms and contractures. Remove the splints at regular intervals to give skin care and perform ROM exercises. After assessment has been completed and supportive care has been given, reapply the splints as prescribed. The occupational therapist may help identify additional self-help devices for activities of daily living.

Plan your care and procedures around the patient's morning stiffness. Sitting or standing in a warm shower, sitting in a tub with warm towels around the shoulders, or simply soaking the hands in a basin of warm water may help relieve joint stiffness and allow the patient to perform activities of daily living more comfortably.

AMBULATORY AND HOME CARE

Rest. Alternating scheduled rest periods with activity throughout the day helps relieve fatigue and pain. The amount of rest needed varies according to the severity of the disease and the patient's limitations. The patient should rest before becoming exhausted. Total bed rest rarely is necessary and should be avoided to prevent stiffness and other effects of immobility. However, even a patient with mild disease may require daytime rest in addition to 8 to 10 hours of sleep at night. Help the patient identify ways to modify daily activities to avoid overexertion that can lead to fatigue and exacerbate disease activity. For example, the patient may tolerate meal preparation more easily while sitting on a high stool in front of the sink.

Good body alignment while resting can be maintained through use of a firm mattress or bed board. Encourage positions of extension, and teach the patient to avoid positions of flexion. To decrease the risk of joint contracture, never place pillows under the knees. A small, flat pillow may be used under the head and shoulders.

Joint Protection. Protecting joints from stress is important. Help the patient identify ways to modify tasks to put less stress on joints during routine activities (Table 65-10). Energy conservation requires careful planning. The emphasis is on work simplification techniques. Work should be done in short periods with scheduled rest breaks to avoid fatigue (pacing). Activities should be organized to avoid going up and down stairs repeatedly. Carts should be used to carry supplies, or materials that

TABLE 65-10	**PATIENT & CAREGIVER TEACHING GUIDE**

Protection of Small Joints

Include the following instructions when teaching the patient with arthritis how to protect small joints.
1. Maintain joint in neutral position to minimize deformity.
   - Press water from a sponge instead of wringing.
2. Use strongest joint available for any task.
   - When rising from chair, push with palms rather than fingers.
   - Carry laundry basket in both arms rather than with fingers.
3. Distribute weight over many joints instead of stressing a few.
   - Slide objects instead of lifting them.
   - Hold packages close to body for support.
4. Change positions frequently.
   - Do not hold book or grip steering wheel for long periods without resting.
   - Avoid grasping pencil or cutting vegetables with knife for extended periods.
5. Avoid repetitious movements.
   - Do not knit for long periods.
   - Rest between rooms when vacuuming.
   - Modify home environment to include faucets and doorknobs that are pushed rather than turned.
6. Modify chores to avoid stress on joints.
   - Avoid heavy lifting.
   - Sit on stool instead of standing during meal preparation.

are used often can be stored in a convenient, easily reached area. Timesaving joint protective devices (e.g., electric can opener) should be used whenever possible. Tasks can also be delegated to other family members.

Patient independence may be increased by occupational therapy training with assistive devices that simplify tasks, such as built-up utensils, buttonhooks, modified drawer handles, lightweight plastic dishes, and raised toilet seats. Wearing shoes with Velcro fasteners and clothing with buttons or a zipper down the front instead of the back makes dressing easier. A cane or a walker offers support and relief of pain when walking.

Heat and Cold Therapy and Exercise. Heat and cold applications can help relieve stiffness, pain, and muscle spasm. Application of ice is especially beneficial during periods of disease exacerbation, whereas moist heat appears to offer better relief of chronic stiffness. Superficial heat sources such as heating pads, moist hot packs, paraffin baths, and warm baths or showers can relieve stiffness to allow participation in therapeutic exercises. Plastic bags of small frozen vegetables (peas or kernel corn), which can easily mold around the shoulder, wrists, or knees, are an effective home treatment. The patient can also use ice cubes or small paper cups of frozen water to massage areas proximal or distal to a painful joint. Heat and cold can be used as often as desired. However, the heat application should not exceed 20 minutes at one time, and the cold application should not exceed 10 to 15 minutes at one time. Alert the patient to the possibility of a burn and the need to avoid the use of a heat-producing cream (e.g., capsaicin) with another external heat device.

Individualized exercise is an integral part of the treatment plan. A physical therapist usually develops a therapeutic exercise program to improve the flexibility and strength of the affected joints and the patient's overall endurance. Reinforce program participation and ensure correct performance of the exercises. Inadequate joint movement can result in progressive joint immobility and muscle weakness, and overaggressive exercise can result in increased pain, inflammation, and joint damage. Emphasize that participating in a recreational exercise program (e.g., walking, swimming) or performing usual daily activities does not eliminate the patient's need for therapeutic exercise to maintain adequate joint motion.

Gentle ROM exercises are usually done daily to keep the joints functional. The patient should have the opportunity to practice the exercises with supervision. Aquatic exercises in warm water (78° to 86° F [25° to 30° C]) allow easier joint movement because of the buoyancy and warmth of the water. At the same time, although movement seems easier, water provides two-way resistance that makes muscles work harder than they would on land. During acute inflammation, exercise should be limited to one or two repetitions.

Psychologic Support. Self-management and adherence to an individualized home treatment program can be accomplished only if the patient has a thorough understanding of RA, the nature and course of the disease, and the goals of therapy. In addition, consider the patient's value system and perception of the disease.

The patient is challenged constantly by problems of limited function and fatigue, loss of self-esteem, altered body image, and fear of disability and deformity. Discuss alterations in sexuality. Chronic pain or loss of function may make the patient vulnerable to believing the claims of false advertising and attempting unproven or even dangerous remedies. Help the patient recognize fears and concerns that are faced by all people who live with chronic illness.

Evaluation of the family support system is important. Financial planning may be necessary. Community resources such as a home care nurse, homemaker services, and vocational rehabilitation may be considered. Self-help groups are beneficial for some patients.

The presence of chronic pain may lead to depression. Strategies that may help to decrease depressive symptoms include listening to music, reading, exercising, and counseling. Hypnosis and biofeedback may also be of value.

▌GERONTOLOGIC CONSIDERATIONS

ARTHRITIS

The prevalence of arthritis in older adults is high, and the disease is accompanied by problems unique to this age-group. The most problematic areas in older adults include the following:

- The high incidence of OA in older adults often keeps the health care provider from considering other types of arthritis.
- Age alone causes changes in serologic profiles, making interpretation of laboratory values such as RF and ESR more difficult. Drugs taken for co-morbid conditions can also affect laboratory values.
- Polypharmacy in the older adult can result in iatrogenic arthritis.
- Nonorganic musculoskeletal pain syndromes and weakness may be related to depression and physical inactivity.
- Diseases such as SLE, which commonly occurs in younger adults, can develop in a milder form in older adults.

Aging brings many physical and metabolic changes that may increase the older patient's sensitivity to both the therapeutic and toxic effects of some drugs. The older adult who takes NSAIDs has an increased risk for side effects, particularly GI bleeding and renal toxicity. The use of NSAIDs with a shorter half-life may require more frequent dosing but may also produce fewer side effects in the older patient with altered drug metabolism.

The common occurrence of polypharmacy in the older adult makes the use of additional drugs in RA treatment particularly problematic because of the increased likelihood of untoward drug interactions. The drug regimen should be simplified as much as possible to increase adherence (e.g., limited number of drugs with decreased frequency of administration), particularly for the patient without regular assistance.

A major concern in the older patient relates to the use of corticosteroid therapy. Corticosteroid-induced osteopenia can add to the problem of decreased bone density related to age and inactivity. It also increases the risk of pathologic fractures, especially compression fractures of vertebrae. Corticosteroid-induced myopathy can be minimized or prevented by an age-appropriate exercise program. Although important for all age-groups, an adequate support system for the older adult is a critical factor in the ability to follow a treatment regimen that includes nutritional planning, exercise, general health maintenance, and appropriate therapy.

GOUT

Gout is a type of recurring acute arthritis characterized by the accumulation of uric acid crystals in one or more joints. Characteristic deposits of sodium urate crystals occur in articular, periarticular, and subcutaneous tissues. More than 3 million Americans are affected by gout. The incidence among African American men is nearly twice that of white men.[19]

Gout may be classified as primary or secondary. In *primary gout* a hereditary error of purine metabolism leads to the overproduction or retention of uric acid. Primary gout, which accounts for 90% of cases, occurs predominantly in middle-aged men.

Secondary gout may be related to another acquired disorder (Table 65-11) or may be the result of drugs known to inhibit uric acid excretion. Secondary gout may also be caused by drugs that increase the rate of cell death, such as the chemotherapy agents used in treating leukemia. Hyperuricemia may also develop in patients taking thiazide diuretics, postmenopausal women, and organ transplant recipients who are receiving immunosuppressive agents.

Obesity in men increases the risk of gout. Hypertension, diuretic use, and excessive alcohol consumption are additional risk factors. A diet high in purine-rich foods (e.g., shellfish such as crab and shrimp; vegetables such as lentils, asparagus, and spinach; meats such as beef, chicken, and pork) will not cause gout, but can trigger an acute attack if a person is susceptible to gout.

TABLE 65-11	CAUSES OF HYPERURICEMIA
• Acidosis or ketosis • Alcohol use • Atherosclerosis • Chemotherapy drugs • Diabetes mellitus • Drug-induced renal impairment • Hyperlipidemia • Hypertension	• Malignant disease • Myeloproliferative disorders • Obesity or starvation • Renal insufficiency • Sickle cell anemia • Exposure to lead • Use of certain common drugs (low-dose aspirin, thiazide, diuretics, niacin)

Etiology and Pathophysiology

Uric acid is the major end product of purine catabolism and is primarily excreted by the kidneys. Gout is caused by (1) an increase in uric acid production; (2) underexcretion of uric acid by the kidneys; or (3) increased intake of foods containing purines, which are metabolized to uric acid by the body. Underexcretion of uric acid is believed to be the major cause of hyperuricemia in 80% to 90% of affected persons. High dietary intake of purine alone has relatively little effect on uric acid levels. Hyperuricemia may result from prolonged fasting or excessive alcohol drinking because of the increased production of keto acids, which then inhibit uric acid excretion.

Clinical Manifestations and Complications

In the acute phase, gouty arthritis may occur in one or more joints but usually less than four. Affected joints may appear dusky or cyanotic and are extremely tender. Inflammation of the great toe *(podagra)* is the most common initial problem. Other affected joints may include wrists, knees, ankles, and midtarsal area of the foot. Olecranon bursae may also be involved. Acute gouty arthritis is usually precipitated by trigger events such as trauma, surgery, alcohol ingestion, or systemic infection. The onset of symptoms typically occurs at night with sudden swelling and excruciating pain peaking within several hours, often accompanied by low-grade fever. Individual attacks usually subside, treated or untreated, in 2 to 10 days. The affected joint returns to normal and patients are often free of symptoms between attacks.

Chronic gout is characterized by multiple joint involvement and visible deposits of sodium urate crystals *(tophi)*. These are typically noted in the synovium, subchondral bone, olecranon bursae, and vertebrae; along tendons; and in the skin and cartilage (Fig. 65-6). Tophi are rarely present at the initial attack and are generally noted only many years after the onset of disease.

The severity of gouty arthritis varies. The clinical course may consist of infrequent mild attacks or multiple severe episodes (up to 12 per year) associated with a slowly progressive disability. In general, the higher the serum uric acid level, the earlier the appearance of tophi and the greater the tendency toward more frequent, severe episodes of acute gout. Chronic inflammation may result in joint deformity, and cartilage destruction may predispose the joint to secondary OA. Large and unsightly tophaceous deposits may perforate overlying skin, producing draining sinuses that often become infected.

Excessive uric acid excretion may lead to kidney or urinary tract stone formation. Pyelonephritis associated with intrarenal sodium urate deposits and obstruction may contribute to kidney disease.

Diagnostic Studies

In gout, serum uric acid levels are usually elevated above 6 mg/dL. However, hyperuricemia is not specifically diagnostic of gout because increased levels may be related to a variety of drugs or may exist as an asymptomatic abnormality in the general population. Specimens for 24-hour urine uric acid values may be obtained to determine if the disease is caused by decreased renal excretion or overproduction of uric acid.

Synovial fluid aspiration is a controversial part of patient evaluation because an accurate diagnosis of gout is possible in 80% of patients based on clinical symptoms alone. However, aspiration may have therapeutic value by decompressing a swollen joint capsule. Joint aspiration is also the only reliable method of distinguishing gout from septic arthritis and *pseudogout* (calcium phosphate crystals are formed). Affected fluid characteristically contains needle-like monosodium urate crystals.[20] X-rays appear normal in the early stages of gout. In chronic disease, tophi may appear as eroded areas in the bone.

Collaborative Care

Goals for the care of the patient with gout (Table 65-12) include termination of an acute attack using an antiinflammatory agent such as colchicine. Drug therapy is the primary therapy used in treating acute and chronic gout. In addition, weight reduction

GENDER DIFFERENCES

Gout

Men
- Occurs more commonly in men than in women.
- Occurs predominantly in middle-aged men.

Women
- Low occurrence in premenopausal women.

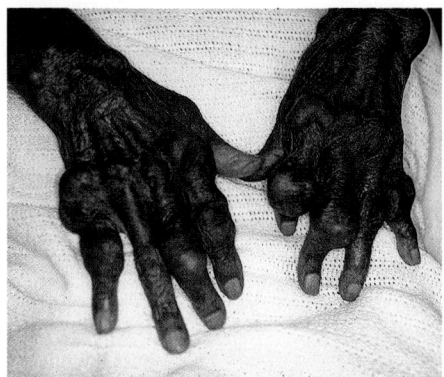

FIG. 65-6 Tophi associated with chronic gout. Nodules are painless and filled with uric acid crystals.

TABLE 65-12 COLLABORATIVE CARE

Gout

Diagnostic
- History and physical examination
- Family history of gout
- Sodium urate crystals in synovial fluid
- Elevated serum uric acid levels
- Elevated 24-hr urine for uric acid levels
- X-ray of affected joints

Collaborative Therapy
- Joint immobilization
- Local application of heat or cold
- Joint aspiration and intraarticular corticosteroids
- Dietary avoidance of food and fluids with high purine content (e.g., anchovies, liver, wine, beer)
- Drug therapy
  - colchicine
  - Nonsteroidal antiinflammatory drugs (e.g., naproxen [Naprosyn])
  - allopurinol (Zyloprim)
  - probenecid (Benemid)
  - febuxostat (Uloric)
  - Corticosteroids (prednisone)
  - Intraarticular corticosteroids (methylprednisolone)
  - Adrenocorticotropic hormone (ACTH)

(as needed) and possible avoidance of alcohol and foods high in purine (red and organ meats) are recommended.

Drug Therapy. Acute gout is treated with colchicine and NSAIDs. Because colchicine has antiinflammatory effects but no analgesic properties, an NSAID is added to the treatment regimen for pain management. Oral administration of colchicine generally produces dramatic pain relief when given within 12 to 24 hours of an attack.[20] Colchicine also has diagnostic merit in that a good response to this drug offers further evidence for the diagnosis of gout.

Future attacks of gout are prevented in part by a maintenance dose of urate-lowering drugs such as a xanthine oxidase inhibitor (allopurinol [Zyloprim, Aloprim]) or a uricosuric drug (probenecid [Benemid, Probalan]). Febuxostat (Uloric), a selective inhibitor of xanthine oxidase, is given for long-term management of hyperuricemia in people with chronic gout.

Patients who cannot take or do not respond to drugs that lower uric acid in the blood may be given pegloticase (Krystexxa). This drug is an enzyme that metabolizes uric acid into a harmless chemical that is excreted in the urine. The drug is given IV. Corticosteroids given either orally or by intraarticular injection can be helpful in treating acute attacks of gout. Systemic corticosteroids may be used only if routine therapies are contraindicated or ineffective. Adrenocorticotropic hormone (ACTH) may also be used for treating acute gout.

For many years, the standard therapy for hyperuricemia caused by urate underexcretion has been uricosuric drugs such as probenecid, which inhibit renal tubular reabsorption of urates. However, these drugs are ineffective when creatinine clearance is reduced, as can occur in patients over 60 years old and those with renal impairment. Aspirin inactivates the effect of uricosuric drugs, resulting in urate retention, and should be avoided while taking uricosuric drugs. Acetaminophen can be used safely if analgesia is required.

Adequate urine volume with normal renal function (2 to 3 L/day) must be maintained to prevent precipitation of uric acid in the renal tubules. Allopurinol, which blocks the production of uric acid, is particularly useful in patients with uric acid stones or renal impairment, in whom uricosuric drugs may be ineffective or dangerous. For patients who cannot tolerate allopurinol because of side effects, oxypurinol can be prescribed. Oxypurinol is the active metabolite of allopurinol. The angiotensin II receptor antagonist losartan (Cozaar) may be especially useful for treatment of older patients with both gout and hypertension. Losartan promotes urate diuresis and may normalize serum urate levels. Combination therapy with losartan and allopurinol may also be given. Regardless of which drugs are prescribed, serum uric acid levels must be checked regularly to monitor treatment effectiveness.

Nutritional Therapy. Dietary restrictions that limit alcohol and foods high in purine help minimize uric acid production (see Table 46-12). Instruct obese patients in a carefully planned weight-reduction program.

NURSING MANAGEMENT
GOUT

Nursing interventions for the patient with an acute episode of gout include supportive care of the inflamed joints. Avoid causing pain by careless handling of an inflamed joint. Bed rest may be appropriate with affected joints properly immobilized. Involvement of a lower extremity may require use of a cradle or

footboard to protect the painful area from the weight of bedclothes. Assess the limitation of motion and degree of pain and document treatment effectiveness.

Help the patient and family understand that hyperuricemia and gout are chronic problems that can be controlled with careful adherence to a treatment program.[21] Explain the importance of drug therapy and the need for periodic determination of serum uric acid levels. Teach the patient about precipitating factors that may cause an attack, including excessive caloric intake or overindulgence in purine-containing foods and alcohol, starvation (fasting), drug use (e.g., niacin, aspirin, diuretics), and major medical events (e.g., surgery, myocardial infarction).

LYME DISEASE

Lyme disease is a spirochetal infection caused by *Borrelia burgdorferi* and transmitted by the bite of an infected deer tick. It was first identified in 1975 in Lyme, Connecticut, after an unusual clustering of arthritis in children. It is now the most common vector-borne disease in the United States. The tick typically feeds on mice, dogs, cats, cows, horses, deer, and humans. Wild animals do not exhibit the illness, but clinical Lyme disease does occur in domestic animals. Person-to-person transmission does not occur.

The peak season for human infection is during the summer months. Most U.S. cases occur in three endemic areas: along the northeastern coast from Maryland to Massachusetts, in the Midwestern states of Wisconsin and Minnesota, and along the northwestern coast of California and Oregon. More than 20,000 cases are reported annually in the United States. Reinfection is not uncommon.

Lyme disease symptoms can mimic those of other diseases such as multiple sclerosis, mononucleosis, and meningitis. The most characteristic clinical symptom of early localized disease is *erythema migrans* (EM), a skin lesion ("bull's eye rash") that occurs in 70% to 80% of infected persons at the site of the tick bite within 3 to 30 days after exposure (Fig. 65-7). The lesion begins as a red macule or papule that slowly expands to form a large round lesion of up to 12 in with a bright red border and central clearing. The EM lesion is often accompanied by acute flu-like symptoms, such as low-grade fever, chills, headache, stiff neck, fatigue, swollen lymph nodes, and migratory joint and muscle pain. Of note, loss of tone in facial muscles can manifest as Bell's palsy. Symptoms usually occur in a week, but may be delayed for up to 30 days. The flu-like symptoms generally resolve over a period of weeks or months, even if untreated.

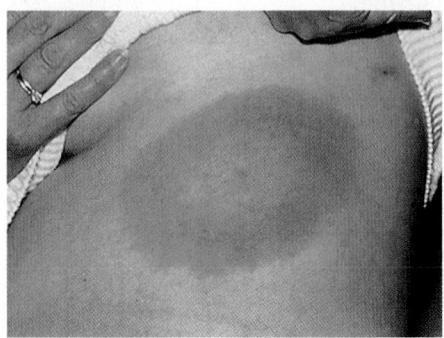

FIG. 65-7 Erythema migrans. Characteristic skin lesion of Lyme disease that occurs at the site of tick bite.

TABLE 65-13 PATIENT & CAREGIVER TEACHING GUIDE

Prevention and Early Treatment of Lyme Disease

Include the following instructions when teaching patients how to prevent Lyme disease.

- Avoid walking through tall grasses and low brush, and sitting on logs.
- Mow grass. Remove brush around paths, buildings, and campsites to create "tick-safe zones."
- Move woodpiles and bird feeders away from house. Discourage deer (main source of food for adult ticks) from being in the area.
- Wear long pants or nylon tights of tightly woven, light-colored fabric so ticks can be easily seen.
- Tuck pants into boots or long socks, wear long-sleeved shirts tucked into pants, and wear closed shoes when hiking.
- Check often for ticks crawling from pant legs to open skin.
- Thoroughly inspect and wash clothes. Placing clothing in dryer on high heat effectively kills ticks.
- Spray insect repellent containing DEET sparingly on skin or apply permethrin to boots, clothes (especially on lower extremities), and camping gear.
- Have pets wear tick collars, inspect them often, and do not allow pets on furniture or beds.

Include the following instructions when teaching patients and caregivers living in endemic areas.

- Remove attached ticks with tweezers (not fingers). Grasp tick's mouth parts as close to skin as possible and gently pull straight out. Do not twist or jerk. Avoid folk solutions such as painting the tick with nail polish or petroleum jelly.
- Save the tick in a bottle of alcohol (if you need it later for identification).
- Wash bitten area with soap and water and apply antiseptic. Wash hands.
- See a health care provider immediately if flu-like symptoms or a bull's-eye rash appears within 2-30 days after removal of tick.

Adapted from Centers for Disease Control and Prevention: It's spring: time to prevent Lyme disease. Retrieved from *www.cdc.gov/features/lymedisease;* and Centers for Disease Control and Prevention: Tick removal. Retrieved from *www.cdc.gov/lyme/removal/index.html.*
DEET, N,N-diethyl-m-toluamide.

If not treated, the spirochete can disseminate within several weeks or months to the heart, joints, and central nervous system (CNS). Carditis may occur.[22] About 60% of persons with untreated infection develop chronic arthritic pain and swelling in the large joints. Nervous system problems may include severe headaches or poor motor coordination. The accompanying neurologic condition known as tertiary neuroborreliosis results in confusion and forgetfulness.

A diagnosis of Lyme disease is often based on clinical manifestations, in particular the EM lesion, and a history of exposure in an endemic area. CBC and ESR are usually normal. A two-step laboratory testing process is recommended by the Centers for Disease Control and Prevention to confirm the diagnosis.[23] The first step is the enzyme immunoassay (EIA), which will have positive results for most people with Lyme disease. If the EIA is positive or inconclusive, a Western blot test is done to confirm the infection. In individuals with neurologic involvement, cerebrospinal fluid should also be examined.

Active lesions can be treated with oral antibiotics. Doxycycline (Vibramycin), cefuroxime (Ceftin), and amoxicillin are often effective in treating early-stage infection and preventing later stages of the disease. Doxycycline prevents Lyme disease when given within 3 days after the bite of a deer tick. Short-term

therapy of 2 to 3 weeks is usually effective for solitary EM, but patients with neurologic or cardiac complications may require IV therapy with ceftriaxone (Rocephin) or penicillin. In most cases, persons with Lyme disease are treated successfully with antibiotics. Approximately 10% to 20% of persons treated with antibiotics for Lyme disease may experience lingering fatigue or joint and muscle pain. This condition, known as post–Lyme disease syndrome, may result from residual damage to tissues and the immune system.[22]

Reducing exposure to ticks is the best way to prevent Lyme disease. Patient and caregiver teaching for people living in endemic areas is outlined in Table 65-13. No vaccine is available for Lyme disease.

SEPTIC ARTHRITIS

Septic arthritis (infectious or bacterial arthritis) is caused by microorganisms invading the joint cavity. Bacteria can travel through the bloodstream from another site of active infection, resulting in hematogenous seeding of the joint. Organisms can also be introduced directly through trauma or surgical incision.

Any bacteria can cause the infection—even nonpathogenic bacteria in the immunocompromised patient. *Staphylococcus aureus* and *Streptococcus hemolyticus* are the most common causative organisms.[24] *Neisseria gonorrhoeae* is the most common cause in sexually active young adults. Factors that increase the risk of infection include (1) diseases in which there is decreased host resistance (e.g., leukemia, diabetes mellitus), (2) treatment with corticosteroids or immunosuppressive drugs, and (3) debilitating chronic illness.

In septic arthritis, large joints such as the knee and hip are most frequently involved. Inflammation of the joint cavity causes severe pain, erythema, and swelling. Because infection has often spread from a primary site elsewhere in the body, fever or shaking chills often accompany articular manifestations. A diagnosis may be made by aspiration of the joint (arthrocentesis) and culture of the synovial fluid. However, WBC counts may be low early in the infectious process, and diagnosis is not possible solely based on WBC counts. Blood cultures for aerobic and anaerobic organisms should also be obtained.

Septic arthritis requires prompt treatment to prevent joint destruction and bone loss.[25] Broad-spectrum antibiotics against gram-negative organisms, pneumococci, and staphylococci are often started before the causative organism is identified. Once the organism is identified, specific treatment can be determined. Infections may respond to treatment within 2 weeks or may take as long as 4 to 8 weeks, depending on the causative organism. Local aspiration and surgical drainage may be required. If diagnosis and treatment are delayed, destruction of articular cartilage can occur, followed by loss of joint function. Chronic infection can also develop. Septic arthritis of the hip can contribute to development of avascular necrosis.

Assess and monitor joint inflammation, pain, and fever. To control pain, use resting splints or traction to immobilize affected joints. Local hot compresses can also help relieve pain. Initiate gentle ROM exercises as soon as tolerated to prevent muscle atrophy and joint contractures. Explain the need for antibiotics and the importance of their continued use until the infection is resolved. Offer support to the patient who requires arthrocentesis or operative drainage. Use strict aseptic technique when assisting with joint aspiration procedures.

SPONDYLOARTHROPATHIES

The spondyloarthropathies are a group of interrelated multi-system inflammatory disorders that affect the spine, peripheral joints, and periarticular structures. These disorders are all negative for rheumatoid factor (RF) and thus are often referred to as seronegative arthropathies.

Inheritance of HLA-B27 is strongly associated with these diseases. Both genetic and environmental factors play a role in the development of this group of diseases, which includes ankylosing spondylitis, psoriatic arthritis, and reactive arthritis. (HLAs and their relationship to autoimmune diseases are discussed in Chapter 14.)

The spondyloarthropathies share clinical and laboratory characteristics that may make it difficult to distinguish among them in early disease. These characteristics include absence of antibodies in the serum, inflammatory arthritis of the spine, peripheral joint involvement predominantly of the lower extremities, sacroiliitis, uveitis, enteric mucosal lesions, and skin lesions.[26]

ANKYLOSING SPONDYLITIS

Ankylosing spondylitis (AS) is a chronic inflammatory disease that primarily affects the axial skeleton, including the sacroiliac joints, intervertebral disc spaces, and costovertebral articulations. HLA-B27 antigen is found in approximately 90% of people with AS. Individuals with the antigen have a significantly greater risk of developing a spondyloarthropathy than those who do not.[19] The usual age of onset of AS is before 40 years old. Men are three to five times more likely to develop AS than women. The disease may go undetected in women because of a milder course.

Etiology and Pathophysiology

Genetic predisposition appears to play an important role in the pathogenesis of AS, but the precise mechanisms of the disease are unknown. Aseptic synovial inflammation in the joints and adjacent tissue causes the formation of granulation tissue *(pannus)* and dense fibrous scars that lead to fusion of articular tissues. Extraarticular inflammation can affect the eyes, lungs, heart, kidneys, and peripheral nervous system.

Clinical Manifestations and Complications

AS is characterized by symmetric sacroiliitis and progressive inflammatory arthritis of the axial skeleton. Symptoms of inflammatory spine pain are the first clues to a diagnosis of AS. The patient typically complains of low back pain, stiffness, and limitation of motion that is worse during the night and in the morning but improves with mild activity. In women, early symptoms of disease may manifest as pain and stiffness in the neck rather than the lower back. General symptoms such as fever, fatigue, anorexia, and weight loss are rarely present. *Uveitis* (intraocular inflammation) is the most common nonskeletal symptom. It can appear as an initial presentation of the disease years before arthritic symptoms develop. AS patients may also experience chest pain and sternal/costal cartilage tenderness that can be distressing.

Severe postural abnormalities and deformity can lead to significant disability for the patient with AS (Fig. 65-8). Impaired spinal ROM and fixed kyphosis contribute to altered visual function, raising concerns about safe ambulation. Aortic insuf-

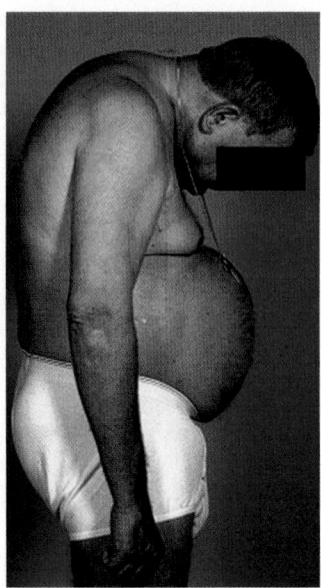

FIG. 65-8 Advanced ankylosing spondylitis. Kyphotic posture causes many patients to have a protuberant abdomen secondary to pulmonary restriction.

GENETICS IN CLINICAL PRACTICE

Ankylosing Spondylitis

Genetic Basis
- Inheritance of human leukocyte antigen (HLA) B27 increases susceptibility to development of ankylosing spondylitis (AS).

Incidence
- About 80%-90% of white people with AS have HLA-B27 antigen.
- Inheriting HLA-B27 does not mean that a person will develop the disease. Of children who inherit HLA-B27 from a parent with AS, 80% do not develop the disease.
- AS is three to five times more common in men than in women.
- It occurs more often in whites than in other ethnic groups.
- It affects 7 in 100,000 people.

Genetic Testing
- Testing for HLA-B27 antigen available.

Clinical Implications
- Diagnosis of AS usually occurs between ages 18 and 40.
- Multiple genetic and environmental factors play a role in pathogenesis of disease.
- It is not known how HLA-B27 increases the risk of AS.
- AS is present in about 3%-10% of patients with inflammatory bowel disease (IBD).
- About 50%-70% of patients with both AS and IBD are HLA-B27 positive.

ficiency and pulmonary fibrosis are frequent complications. Cauda equina syndrome (compression of the nerves at the end of the spinal cord) can also result, contributing to lower extremity weakness and bladder dysfunction. In addition, the patient is at risk for spinal fracture because of associated osteoporosis.

Diagnostic Studies

X-rays are the most important radiographic technique for the diagnosis and follow-up of AS. However, x-rays are limited in detecting early sacroiliitis or subtle changes in posterior vertebrae. MRI can be useful in assessing early cartilage abnormalities, while CT scan is appropriate in specific situations (e.g., cases with subtle x-ray changes). Changes on later spinal films include the appearance of "bamboo spine," which is the result of calcifications (syndesmophytes) that bridge from one vertebra to another.

Laboratory testing is not specific, but an elevated ESR and mild anemia may be seen. When the suspicion of AS is high, the presence of the HLA-B27 antigen improves the likelihood of this diagnosis.

Collaborative Care

Prevention of AS is not possible. However, families with other diagnosed HLA-B27-positive rheumatic diseases (e.g., acute anterior uveitis, juvenile spondyloarthritis) should be alert to signs of low back pain for early identification and treatment of AS.

Care of the AS patient is aimed at maintaining maximal skeletal mobility while decreasing pain and inflammation. Heat applications can help relieve local symptoms. NSAIDs and salicylates are commonly prescribed. DMARDs such as sulfasalazine or methotrexate have little effect on spinal disease but may help with peripheral joint disease. Local corticosteroid injections may be beneficial in relieving symptoms.

TNF, which promotes inflammation, is found in elevated levels in the blood and certain tissues of patients with AS. Etanercept, a biologic and targeted therapy drug, binds TNF and inhibits its action. Etanercept reduces active inflammation and improves spinal mobility. Additional anti-TNF inhibitors (infliximab, adalimumab, golimumab) may also be effective.

Once pain and stiffness are managed, exercise is essential. Postural control is important to minimize spinal deformity. The exercise regimen should include back, neck, and chest stretches. Hydrotherapy has also been shown to decrease pain and facilitate spinal extension. Surgery may be indicated for severe deformity and mobility impairment. Spinal osteotomy and total joint replacement are the most commonly performed procedures (see Chapter 63).

▌ NURSING MANAGEMENT
▌ ANKYLOSING SPONDYLITIS

A key nursing responsibility is to teach the patient with AS about the disease and principles of therapy. The home management program should include regular exercise and attention to posture, local moist heat applications, and knowledgeable use of drugs.

Baseline ROM assessment includes chest expansion (using breathing exercises). Encourage smoking cessation to decrease the risk for lung complications in those with reduced chest expansion. Ongoing physical therapy includes gentle, graded stretching and strengthening exercises to preserve ROM and improve thoracolumbar flexion and extension.

Discourage excessive physical exertion during periods of active flare-up of the disease. Proper positioning at rest is essential. The mattress should be firm, and the patient should sleep on the back with a flat pillow, avoiding positions that encourage flexion deformity. Postural training emphasizes avoiding spinal flexion (e.g., leaning over a desk); heavy lifting; and prolonged walking, standing, or sitting. Encourage sports that facilitate natural stretching, such as swimming and racquet games. Family counseling and vocational rehabilitation are important.

PSORIATIC ARTHRITIS

Psoriatic arthritis (PsA) is a progressive inflammatory disease that affects about 10% of the 3 million people with psoriasis.[27] Psoriasis is a common, benign, inflammatory skin disorder characterized by red, irritated, and scaly patches. Both PsA and psoriasis appear to have a genetic link with the HLA antigens in many patients. Although the exact cause of PsA is unknown, a combination of immune, genetic, and environmental factors is suspected.

PsA can occur in different forms. These include (1) arthritis involving primarily the small joints of the hands and feet (DIP), (2) asymmetric arthritis involving joints of the extremities, (3) symmetric polyarthritis resembling RA, and (4) arthritis of the sacroiliac joints and spine (psoriatic spondylitis).[28]

On x-ray, the cartilage loss and erosion resemble those of RA. Advanced cases of PsA often reveal widened joint spaces. A "pencil in cup" deformity is common in the DIP joints as a result of osteolysis. In this deformity the narrowed end(s) of the metacarpals or phalanges insert into the expanded end of the other (adjacent) bone sharing the joint. Elevated ESR, mild anemia, and elevated blood uric acid levels can be seen in some patients. Therefore the diagnosis of gout must be excluded.

Treatment includes splinting, joint protection, and physical therapy. NSAIDs given early in the course of the disease may help with inflammation. Drug therapy also includes the DMARDs such as methotrexate, which is effective for both articular and cutaneous manifestations. Sulfasalazine and cyclosporine may be used for treating PsA. In addition, biologic and targeted therapy, such as etanercept, golimumab, adalimumab, and infliximab, may also be used.

REACTIVE ARTHRITIS

Reactive arthritis (Reiter's syndrome) occurs more commonly in young men than in young women. It is associated with a symptom complex that includes urethritis, conjunctivitis, and mucocutaneous lesions. Although the exact etiology is unknown, reactive arthritis appears to be a reaction triggered in the body after exposure to specific genitourinary or GI tract infections. Chlamydia trachomatis is most often implicated in sexually transmitted reactive arthritis.[19] Reactive arthritis is also associated with GI infections with Shigella, Salmonella, Campylobacter, or Yersinia species and other microorganisms.

Individuals who are positive for HLA-B27 are at increased risk of developing reactive arthritis after sexual contact or exposure to certain enteric pathogens. This finding supports the likelihood of a genetic predisposition.

Urethritis develops within 1 to 2 weeks after sexual contact or GI infection. In women, symptoms include cervicitis. Low-grade fever, conjunctivitis, and arthritis may occur over the next several weeks. This type of arthritis tends to be asymmetric, frequently involving the large joints of the lower extremities and the toes. Lower back pain may occur with severe disease. Mucocutaneous lesions commonly occur as small, painless, superficial ulcerations on the tongue, oral mucosa, and glans penis. Soft tissue manifestations commonly include Achilles tendinitis or plantar fasciitis. Few laboratory abnormalities occur, although the ESR may be elevated.

Prognosis is favorable, with most patients recovering after 2 to 16 weeks. Because reactive arthritis is often associated with

C. trachomatis infection, treatment of patients and their sexual partners with doxycycline is widely recommended. Conjunctivitis and lesions require no treatment, but topical ophthalmic corticosteroids are typically prescribed for treatment of uveitis. Drug therapy may also include NSAIDs, methotrexate, and sulfasalazine. Physical therapy may be helpful during disease recovery.

Most patients have complete remission with restoration of full joint function. Up to 30% may develop chronic or recurring disease, which can result in major disability.[29] X-ray changes in chronic reactive arthritis closely resemble those of AS. Treatment of chronic reactive arthritis is symptomatic.

SYSTEMIC LUPUS ERYTHEMATOSUS

Systemic lupus erythematosus (SLE) is a multisystem inflammatory autoimmune disease. It is a complex disorder of multifactorial origin resulting from interactions among genetic, hormonal, environmental, and immunologic factors. SLE typically affects the skin, joints, and serous membranes (pleura, pericardium), along with the renal, hematologic, and neurologic systems. SLE is characterized by a chronic unpredictable course marked by alternating periods of exacerbation and remission.

The overall incidence of SLE in the United States is approximately 2 to 8 per 100,000.[30] Most cases of SLE occur in women in their childbearing years. Women are 10 times more likely than men to develop SLE. African Americans (especially), Asian Americans, Hispanics, and Native Americans are more likely than whites to develop the disease.

Etiology and Pathophysiology

The etiology of the abnormal immune response in SLE is unknown.[31] Based on the high prevalence of SLE among family members, a genetic influence is suspected. Multiple susceptibility genes from the HLA complex, including *HLA-DR3*, show associations with SLE.

Hormones are also known to play a role in the etiology of SLE. Onset or exacerbation of disease symptoms sometimes occurs after the onset of menarche, with the use of oral contraceptives, and during and after pregnancy. The disease tends to worsen in the immediate postpartum period.

Environmental factors are believed to contribute to the occurrence of SLE, with sun exposure and sunburns as the most common environmental triggers. Infectious agents may serve as a stimulus for immune hyperactivity. SLE may also be precipitated or aggravated by certain drugs such as procainamide (Pronestyl), hydralazine (Apresoline), and a number of antiseizure drugs.

SLE is characterized by the production of a large variety of autoantibodies against nucleic acids (e.g., single- and double-stranded DNA), erythrocytes, coagulation proteins, lymphocytes, platelets, and many other self-proteins. Autoimmune reactions characteristically are directed against constituents of the cell nucleus (antinuclear antibodies [ANAs]), particularly DNA.

Circulating immune complexes containing antibody against DNA are deposited in the basement membranes of capillaries in the kidneys, heart, skin, brain, and joints. Complement is activated, and inflammation occurs.[32] The overaggressive autoimmune response is also related to activation of B and T cells. The specific manifestations of SLE depend on which cell types or organs are involved. (SLE is a type III hypersensitivity response [see Chapter 14].)

Clinical Manifestations and Complications

SLE is extremely variable in its severity, ranging from a relatively mild disorder to a rapidly progressive one affecting many body systems (Fig. 65-9). No characteristic pattern occurs in the progressive involvement of SLE. Any organ can be affected by an accumulation of circulating immune complexes. The most commonly affected tissues are the skin and muscle, the lining of the lungs, the heart, nervous tissue, and the kidneys. Generalized complaints such as fever, weight loss, arthralgia, and excessive fatigue may precede an exacerbation of disease activity.

Dermatologic Problems. Cutaneous vascular lesions can appear in any location but are most likely to develop in sun-exposed areas. Severe skin reactions can occur in people who are photosensitive. The classic butterfly rash over the cheeks and bridge of the nose occurs in 50% of patients with SLE (Fig. 65-10). About 20% of patients have *discoid* (round, coin-shaped) lesions. A small number of patients have persistent lesions, photosensitivity, and mild systemic disease in a syndrome referred to as *subacute cutaneous lupus.*

Ulcers of the oral or nasopharyngeal membranes occur in up to one third of patients with SLE. Alopecia is also common, with or without underlying scalp lesions. The hair may grow back during remission, but hair loss may be permanent over lesions. The scalp becomes dry, scaly, and atrophied.

Musculoskeletal Problems. Arthritis occurs in more than 90% of patients with SLE. Polyarthralgia with morning stiffness is often the patient's first complaint and may precede the onset of multisystem disease by many years. Diffuse swelling is accompanied by joint and muscle pain and some stiffness. Lupus-related arthritis is generally nonerosive, but it may cause deformities such as swan neck deformity of the fingers (see Fig. 65-4, *D*), ulnar deviation, and subluxation with hyperlaxity of the joints. Patients with SLE have an increased risk of bone loss and fracture.

Cardiopulmonary Problems. Tachypnea and cough in patients with SLE are suggestive of lung disease. Pleurisy is also possible. Cardiac involvement may include dysrhythmias resulting from fibrosis of the sinoatrial and atrioventricular nodes. This is an ominous sign of advanced disease, contributing significantly to the morbidity and mortality seen in SLE. Pericarditis can also occur. Clinical factors such as hypertension and hypercholesterolemia require aggressive therapy and careful monitoring. In addition, people with SLE are at risk for secondary *antiphospholipid syndrome,* a disorder of coagulation that leads to clots in the arteries and veins with associated risk of stroke, gangrene, and heart attack.

Renal Problems. Lupus nephritis (LN) occurs in approximately 40% of patients with SLE. Renal involvement is usually evident within 5 years after symptoms of SLE appear. Manifestations of renal involvement vary from mild proteinuria to rapidly progressive glomerulonephritis. Scarring and permanent damage can lead to end-stage kidney disease.

The primary goal in treating LN is to slow the progression of nephropathy and preserve renal function by managing the underlying disease. The importance of obtaining a renal biopsy is controversial, but findings can help guide treatment. Although LN may be one of the more serious complications of SLE, effective treatments are available. These typically include corticosteroids, cytotoxic agents (cyclophosphamide [Cytoxan]),

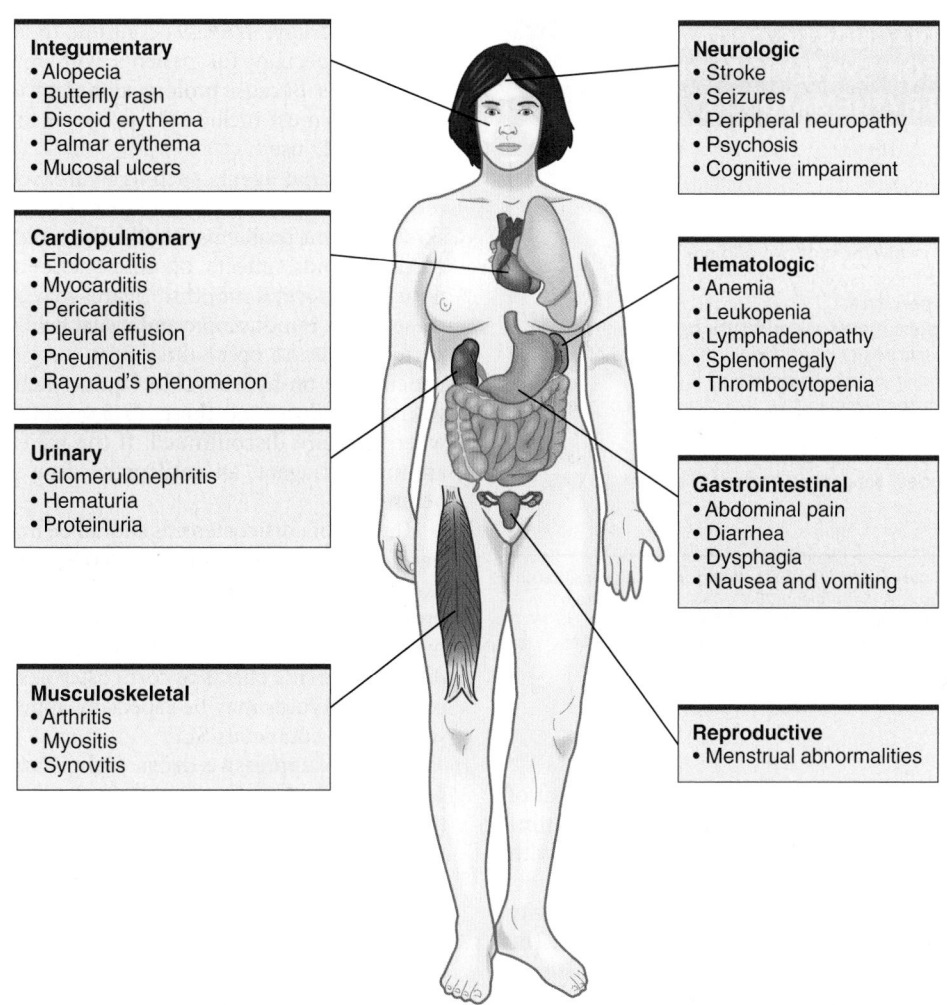

FIG. 65-9 Multisystem involvement in systemic lupus erythematosus.

Integumentary
• Alopecia
• Butterfly rash
• Discoid erythema
• Palmar erythema
• Mucosal ulcers

Cardiopulmonary
• Endocarditis
• Myocarditis
• Pericarditis
• Pleural effusion
• Pneumonitis
• Raynaud's phenomenon

Urinary
• Glomerulonephritis
• Hematuria
• Proteinuria

Musculoskeletal
• Arthritis
• Myositis
• Synovitis

Neurologic
• Stroke
• Seizures
• Peripheral neuropathy
• Psychosis
• Cognitive impairment

Hematologic
• Anemia
• Leukopenia
• Lymphadenopathy
• Splenomegaly
• Thrombocytopenia

Gastrointestinal
• Abdominal pain
• Diarrhea
• Dysphagia
• Nausea and vomiting

Reproductive
• Menstrual abnormalities

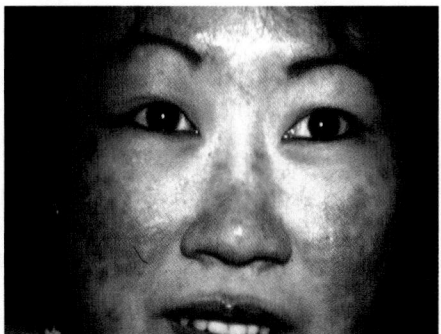

FIG. 65-10 Butterfly rash of systemic lupus erythematosus.

and immunosuppressive agents (azathioprine, cyclosporine, mycophenolate mofetil [CellCept]). Rituximab and eculizumab (Soliris) are being studied as possible treatments. Oral prednisone or pulsed IV methylprednisolone may also be used as an intervention for LN, especially in the initial treatment period when cytotoxic agents have not had time to take effect.

Nervous System Problems. Along with renal involvement, neuropsychiatric manifestations are prevalent in SLE. Generalized or focal seizures are the most common manifestation involving the CNS and occur in as many as 15% of patients with

SLE by the time of diagnosis. Seizures are generally controlled by corticosteroids or antiseizure drugs. Peripheral neuropathy can also occur, leading to sensory and motor deficits.

Cognitive dysfunction, recognized as a CNS manifestation of SLE, may result from the deposition of immune complexes within the brain tissue. It is characterized by disordered thought processes, disorientation, memory deficits, and psychiatric symptoms such as severe depression and psychosis. Various psychiatric disorders are reported in SLE, including mood disorders, anxiety, and psychosis, although they may be related to the stress of having a major illness or to associated drug therapies. Occasionally a stroke or aseptic meningitis may be attributable to SLE. Headaches are also common and can become severe during a flare (exacerbation of disease).

Hematologic Problems. The formation of antibodies against blood cells, such as erythrocytes, leukocytes, thrombocytes, and coagulation factors, is also a common feature of SLE.[32] Anemia, mild leukopenia, and thrombocytopenia are often present. Some patients develop a tendency toward coagulopathy involving either excessive bleeding or blood clot development. A manifestation of antiphospholipid antibody syndrome is a common cause of hypercoagulability in SLE patients, many of whom benefit from high-intensity treatment with warfarin.

Infection. Patients with SLE appear to have increased susceptibility to infections, possibly because of defects in the ability

TABLE 65-14	DIAGNOSTIC CRITERIA FOR SYSTEMIC LUPUS ERYTHEMATOSUS*

- Malar rash
- Discoid rash
- Photosensitivity
- Oral ulcers
- Arthritis: nonerosive, involvement of two or more joints characterized by tenderness, swelling, and effusion
- Serositis: pleuritis or pericarditis
- Renal disorder: persistent proteinuria or cellular casts in urine
- Neurologic disorder: seizures or psychosis (in the absence of causative drugs or known metabolic disorders)
- Hematologic disorder: hemolytic anemia, leukopenia, lymphopenia, or thrombocytopenia
- Immunologic disorder: positive LE preparation, anti-DNA antibody or antibody to Sm nuclear antigen, or false-positive serologic tests for syphilis
- Antinuclear antibody

Source: Tan EM, Cohen AS, Fries JF, et al: The 1982 revised criteria for classification of systemic lupus erythematosus, *Arthritis Rheum* 25:11, 1982. Retrieved from *www.rheumatology.org/practice/clinical/classification/SLE/sle.asp*.
*A person is classified as having SLE if four or more of the criteria are present, serially or simultaneously, during any interval of observation.
LE, Lupus erythematosus; *Sm*, Smith.

to phagocytize invading bacteria, deficiencies in production of antibodies, and the immunosuppressive effect of many antiinflammatory drugs. Infection is a major cause of death, with pneumonia being the most common infection. Fever may indicate an underlying infectious process rather than lupus activity alone. Vaccinations are generally safe for patients with SLE. The exception is the need to avoid live virus vaccines in patients being treated with corticosteroids or cytotoxic agents.

Diagnostic Studies

The diagnosis of SLE is based on distinct criteria revealed through patient history, physical examination, and laboratory findings (Table 65-14). No specific test is diagnostic for SLE, but a variety of abnormalities may be present in the blood. SLE is marked by the presence of ANA in 97% of persons with the disease.

Other antibodies include anti-DNA, antineuronal, anticoagulant, anti-WBC, anti–red blood cell (RBC), antiplatelet, antiphospholipid, and anti–basement membrane. Anti–double-stranded DNA antibodies are found in half the persons with SLE. The anti-Smith (Sm) antibodies are found in 30% to 40% of persons with lupus and are almost always considered diagnostic. The lupus erythematosus (LE) cell prep test is a nonspecific test for SLE and is positive in other rheumatic diseases. ESR and CRP levels are not diagnostic of SLE, but may be used to monitor disease activity and effectiveness of therapy.

Collaborative Care

A major challenge in the treatment of SLE is managing the active phase of the disease while preventing complications of treatments. Survival is influenced by several factors, including age, race, gender, socioeconomic status, accompanying morbid conditions, and severity of disease. The prognosis of SLE can be improved with early diagnosis, prompt recognition of serious organ involvement, and effective therapeutic regimens.

Drug Therapy. NSAIDs continue to be an important intervention, especially for patients with mild polyarthralgias or polyarthritis. Because prolonged therapy is likely, careful patient monitoring must include the potential for GI and renal effects from NSAID use.

Antimalarial agents such as hydroxychloroquine and chloroquine (Aralen) are often used to treat fatigue and moderate skin and joint problems. Unlike the rapid response noted with corticosteroids, effects of antimalarial therapy may not be noticed for several months.[33] Flares may also be prevented with these drugs. Funduscopic and visual field examinations must be performed by an ophthalmologist every 6 to 12 months when patients are on hydroxychloroquine. Retinopathy can develop with high doses of these drugs, but it generally reverses when they are discontinued. If the patient cannot tolerate an antimalarial agent, an antileprosy drug such as dapsone may be used.

The use of corticosteroids should be limited. However, tapering doses of IV methylprednisolone may help control severe exacerbations of polyarthritis. Steroid-sparing immunosuppressants such as methotrexate can serve as an alternative treatment and are prescribed in combination with folic acid to decrease the side effects of corticosteroids. However, high doses of corticosteroids may be especially appropriate for the patient with severe cutaneous SLE.

Immunosuppressive drugs such as azathioprine and cyclophosphamide may be prescribed to reduce the need for long-term corticosteroid therapy. Azathioprine or cyclophosphamide is also appropriate for treatment of severe organ-system disease, especially LN. Close monitoring is necessary to minimize drug toxicity and side effects. Because blood clots can be a life-threatening complication of SLE, anticoagulants such as warfarin or heparin may be prescribed.[33]

Topical immunomodulators are an alternative to corticosteroids for treating serious skin conditions. Tacrolimus (Protopic, Prograf) and pimecrolimus (Elidel) suppress immune activity in the skin, including the butterfly rash and possibly discoid lesions.

Clinical trials are currently investigating the effect of various medications on SLE management. These include biologic and targeted therapy agents that interfere with the immune response such as abatacept, and hormones (prasterone [Prestara]) to combat lupus-induced osteoporosis. Thalidomide as a second-line therapy has been shown to improve cutaneous lupus even in persons who have not responded to other therapies.

When teaching patients about their prescribed drugs, include their indications for use, proper administration, and possible side effects. Help the patient understand that abrupt cessation may exacerbate disease activity.

Disease management is most appropriately monitored by serial anti-DNA titers and serum complement levels (Table 65-15). Simpler and less costly tests such as ESR or CRP may also help in monitoring treatment effectiveness.

NURSING MANAGEMENT
SYSTEMIC LUPUS ERYTHEMATOSUS

NURSING ASSESSMENT

Subjective and objective data that should be obtained from the patient with SLE are presented in Table 65-16. In particular, evaluate the extent to which pain and fatigue influence activities of daily living.

TABLE 65-15 **COLLABORATIVE CARE**

Systemic Lupus Erythematosus

Diagnostic
- History and physical examination
- Antibodies (e.g., anti-DNA, anti-Sm, ANA)
- Complete blood cell count
- LE cell prep
- Serum complement levels
- Urinalysis
- X-ray of affected joints
- Chest x-ray
- ECG to determine extraarticular involvement

Collaborative Therapy
- NSAIDs for mild disease
- Steroid-sparing drugs (e.g., methotrexate)
- Antimalarials (e.g., hydroxychloroquine [Plaquenil])
- Corticosteroids for exacerbations and severe disease
- Immunosuppressive drugs (e.g., cyclophosphamide [Cytoxan], mycophenolate mofetil [CellCept])

ANA, Antinuclear antibody; *LE,* lupus erythematosus; *Sm,* Smith.

NURSING DIAGNOSES

Nursing diagnoses for the patient with SLE may include, but are not limited to, the following:
- Fatigue *related to* chronic inflammation and altered immunity
- Impaired skin integrity *related to* photosensitivity, skin rash, and alopecia
- Impaired comfort *related to* illness-related symptoms, treatment-related side effects, and the potential for variable and unpredictable progression of the disease

Additional information on nursing diagnoses for the patient with SLE is presented in eNursing Care Plan 65-2 (on the website for this chapter).

PLANNING

The overall goals are that the patient with SLE will (1) have satisfactory pain management, (2) adhere to the therapeutic regimen to achieve maximum symptom management, (3) demonstrate awareness of and avoid activities that exacerbate the disease, and (4) maintain optimal role function and a positive self-image.

NURSING IMPLEMENTATION

HEALTH PROMOTION. Prevention of SLE is not possible at this time. However, education of health professionals and the community should promote a clear understanding of the disease and the need for early diagnosis and treatment.

ACUTE INTERVENTION. As in the majority of rheumatic diseases, the unpredictable nature of SLE presents many challenges to the patient and caregiver. The physical, psychologic, and sociocultural problems associated with the long-term management of SLE require the varied approaches and skills of the multidisciplinary health care team.

During an exacerbation of SLE, the patient may become abruptly and dramatically ill. Nursing interventions include accurately recording the severity of symptoms and documenting the response to therapy. Specifically assess fever pattern, joint inflammation, limitation of motion, location and degree of discomfort, and fatigue. Monitor the patient's weight and fluid intake and output if corticosteroids are prescribed because

TABLE 65-16 **NURSING ASSESSMENT**

Systemic Lupus Erythematosus

Subjective Data
Important Health Information
Past health history: Exposure to ultraviolet radiation, drugs, chemicals, viral infections; physical or psychologic stress; states of increased estrogen activity, including early onset of menarche, pregnancy, and postpartum period; pattern of remissions and exacerbations
Medications: Oral contraceptives, procainamide (Pronestyl), hydralazine (Apresoline), isoniazid (INH), antiseizure drugs, antibiotics (possibly precipitating symptoms of SLE); corticosteroids, NSAIDs

Functional Health Patterns
Health perception–health management: Family history of autoimmune disorders; frequent infections; malaise; impact of disease on functional ability
Nutritional-metabolic: Weight loss, oral and nasal ulcers; nausea and vomiting; xerostomia (salivary gland dryness), dysphagia; photosensitivity with rash; frequent infections
Elimination: Decreased urine output; diarrhea or constipation
Activity-exercise: Morning stiffness; joint swelling and deformity; shortness of breath, dyspnea; excessive fatigue
Sleep-rest: Insomnia
Cognitive-perceptual: Visual disturbances; vertigo; headache; polyarthralgia; chest pain (pericardial, pleuritic); abdominal pain; joint pain; painful, throbbing, cold fingers with numbness and tingling
Sexuality-reproductive: Amenorrhea, irregular menstrual periods
Coping–stress tolerance: Depression, withdrawal

Objective Data
General
Fever, lymphadenopathy, periorbital edema

Integumentary
Alopecia; dry, scaly scalp; keratoconjunctivitis, malar "butterfly" rash, palmar or discoid erythema, urticaria, periungual erythema, purpura, or petechiae; leg ulcers

Respiratory
Pleural friction rub, decreased breath sounds

Cardiovascular
Vasculitis; pericardial friction rub; hypertension, edema, dysrhythmias, murmurs; bilateral, symmetric pallor and cyanosis of fingers (Raynaud's phenomenon)

Gastrointestinal
Oral and pharyngeal ulcers; splenomegaly

Neurologic
Facial weakness, peripheral neuropathies, papilledema, dysarthria, confusion, hallucination, disorientation, psychosis, seizures, aphasia, hemiparesis

Musculoskeletal
Myopathy, myositis, arthritis

Urinary
Proteinuria

Possible Diagnostic Findings
Presence of anti-DNA, anti-Sm, and antinuclear antibodies; anemia, leukopenia, thrombocytopenia; ↑ erythrocyte sedimentation rate (ESR); positive LE cell prep; ↑ serum creatinine; microscopic hematuria, cellular casts in urine; pericarditis or pleural effusion evident on chest x-ray

Sm, Smith.

of their fluid-retention effect and the possibility of renal failure. Collection of 24-hour urine samples for protein and creatinine clearance may be ordered. Observe for signs of bleeding that result from drug therapy, such as pallor, skin bruising, petechiae, or tarry stools.

Carefully assess the neurologic status. Observe for visual disturbances, headaches, personality changes, seizures, and forgetfulness. Psychosis may indicate CNS disease or may be an effect of corticosteroid therapy. Irritation of the nerves of the extremities (peripheral neuropathy) may produce numbness, tingling, and weakness of the hands and feet.

Explain the nature of the disease, modes of therapy, and all diagnostic procedures. Emotional support for the patient and family is also essential, especially during an exacerbation.

AMBULATORY AND HOME CARE. Emphasize the importance of patient cooperation for successful home management. Help the patient understand that even strong adherence to the treatment plan is no guarantee against exacerbations because the course of the disease is unpredictable. A variety of factors may increase disease activity, such as fatigue, sun exposure, emotional stress, infection, drugs, and surgery. Help the patient and caregiver eliminate or minimize exposure to precipitating factors (Table 65-17).

Lupus and Pregnancy. Because SLE is most common in women of childbearing age, treatment during pregnancy must be considered. The woman's primary health care provider (or rheumatologist) and obstetrician should thoroughly discuss with the woman her desire to become pregnant. Infertility may have resulted from renal involvement and the previous use of high-dose corticosteroid and chemotherapy drugs. The SLE patient should understand that spontaneous abortion, stillbirth, and intrauterine growth retardation are common problems with pregnancy. They occur because of deposits of immune complexes in the placenta and because of inflammatory responses in the placental blood vessels.

Renal, cardiovascular, pulmonary, and central nervous systems (in particular) may be affected during pregnancy. Women who already demonstrate serious SLE involvement in these systems should be counseled against pregnancy. For the best outcome, pregnancy should be planned at a point when the disease activity is minimal. Exacerbation is common during the postpartum period. Therapeutic abortion offers the same risk of postdelivery exacerbation as carrying the fetus to term.

Psychosocial Issues. The patient with SLE confronts many psychosocial issues. Disease onset and symptoms may be vague, and SLE may be undiagnosed for a long time. Supportive therapies may become as important as medical treatment in helping the patient cope with the disease. Counsel the patient and caregiver that SLE has a good prognosis for the majority of people.

Families worry about hereditary aspects and want to know whether their children will also have SLE. Many couples require pregnancy and sexual counseling. Individuals making decisions about marriage and careers worry about how SLE will interfere with their plans. You may have to educate teachers, employers, and co-workers.

The obvious physical effects of skin lesions and alopecia may cause social isolation for the patient with SLE, affecting his or her self-esteem and body image.[34] Consultation with a dermatologist may be recommended for appropriate treatment and cosmetic products to conceal the rash.

Pain and fatigue may interfere with quality of life. Pacing techniques and relaxation therapy can help the patient remain involved in day-to-day activities. Stress the importance of planning both recreational and occupational activities. Young adults may find sun restrictions and physical limitations particularly difficult to follow. Help the patient develop and accomplish reasonable goals for improving or maintaining mobility, energy levels, and self-esteem.

▍EVALUATION

The expected outcomes are that the patient with SLE will
- Use energy conservation techniques
- Adapt lifestyle to energy level
- Maintain skin integrity with the use of topical treatments
- Prevent exacerbations with the use of sunscreens and limited sun exposure

Additional information on expected outcomes for the patient with SLE is presented in eNursing Care Plan 65-2 (on the website for this chapter).

SCLERODERMA

Scleroderma *(systemic sclerosis)* is a disorder of connective tissue characterized by fibrotic, degenerative, and occasionally inflammatory changes in the skin, blood vessels, synovium, skeletal muscle, and internal organs.

Scleroderma occurs in all ethnic groups but is more common in African Americans than whites. Hispanics and Native Americans may also be at higher risk than whites. Although symptoms may begin at any time, the usual age at onset is between 30 and 50 years. Scleroderma is relatively rare, with approximately 75,000 to 100,000 people in the United States affected. Seventy-five percent of cases are women.[35]

Two types of disease exist: *limited cutaneous scleroderma,* which is the more common (80%), and *diffuse scleroderma.* Both forms are systemic with distinct degrees and types of organ involvement and disease progression. The prognosis of patients with limited disease is generally better than for those with diffuse disease.

Etiology and Pathophysiology

The exact cause of scleroderma is unknown. Immunologic dysfunction and vascular abnormalities are believed to play a role

TABLE 65-17	PATIENT & CAREGIVER TEACHING GUIDE

Systemic Lupus Erythematosus

Include the following information in the teaching plan for a patient with systemic lupus erythematosus and the caregiver.
- Disease process
- Names of drugs, actions, side effects, dosage, administration
- Pain management strategies
- Energy conservation and pacing techniques
- Therapeutic exercise, use of heat therapy (for arthralgia)
- Avoidance of physical and emotional stress
- Avoidance of exposure to individuals with infection
- Avoidance of drying soaps, powders, household chemicals
- Use of sunscreen protection (at least SPF 15) and protective clothing, with minimal sun exposure from 11:00 AM to 3:00 PM
- Regular medical and laboratory follow-up
- Marital and pregnancy counseling as needed
- Community resources and health care agencies

SPF, Sun protection factor.

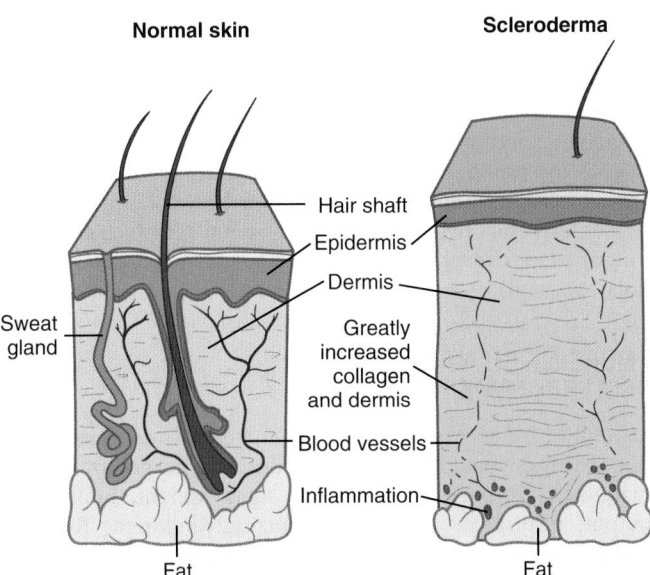

Normal skin   **Scleroderma**

Hair shaft
Epidermis
Dermis
Greatly
increased
collagen
and dermis
Blood vessels
Inflammation

Sweat
gland

Fat   Fat

FIG. 65-11 Skin changes in scleroderma.

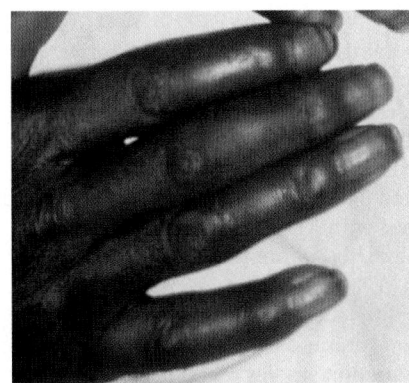

FIG. 65-12 Hand of a patient with scleroderma showing sclerodactyly.

in the development of widespread systemic disease. Other risk factors associated with skin thickening include environmental or occupational exposure to coal, plastics, and silica dust.

In scleroderma, collagen (protein that gives normal skin its strength and elasticity) is overproduced (Fig. 65-11). Excessive production of collagen leads to progressive tissue fibrosis and occlusion of blood vessels. Proliferation of collagen disrupts the normal functioning of internal organs, such as lungs, kidney, heart, and GI tract.

The vascular alterations, which primarily involve the small arteries and arterioles, are almost always present in scleroderma. These changes are some of the earliest alterations in scleroderma.

Clinical Manifestations

Manifestations of scleroderma range from a diffuse cutaneous thickening with rapidly progressive and widespread organ involvement to the more benign limited cutaneous form. The signs of limited disease appear on the face and hands, whereas diffuse disease initially involves the trunk and extremities. Clinical manifestations of scleroderma can be described by the acronym CREST:

Calcinosis: painful deposits of calcium in the skin
Raynaud's phenomenon: abnormal blood flow in response to cold or stress
Esophageal dysfunction: difficulty with swallowing caused by internal scarring
Sclerodactyly: tightening of the skin on the fingers and the toes
Telangiectasia: red spots on hands, forearms, palms, face, and lips

Raynaud's Phenomenon. Raynaud's phenomenon (paroxysmal vasospasm of the digits) is the most common initial complaint in limited scleroderma. Patients have diminished blood flow to the fingers and toes on exposure to cold (blanching or white phase), followed by cyanosis as hemoglobin releases oxygen to the tissues (blue phase), and then erythema during rewarming (red phase). The color changes are often accompanied by numbness and tingling. Raynaud's phenomenon may precede the onset of systemic disease by months, years, or even

decades. (Raynaud's phenomenon is described in more detail in Chapter 38.)

Skin and Joint Changes. Symmetric painless swelling or thickening of the skin of the fingers and hands may progress to diffuse scleroderma of the trunk. In limited disease, skin thickening generally does not extend above the elbow or above the knee, although the face may be affected. In more diffuse disease, the skin loses elasticity and becomes taut and shiny, producing the typical expressionless facies with tightly pursed lips. Skin changes in the face may also contribute to reduced ROM in the temporomandibular joint. The hands may be affected by *sclerodactyly* in which the fingers are in a semiflexed position, with tightened skin to the wrist (Fig. 65-12). Reduced peripheral joint function may occur as an early symptom of polyarthritis.

Internal Organ Involvement. About 20% of people with scleroderma develop secondary Sjögren's syndrome, a condition associated with dry eyes and dry mouth. Dysphagia, gum disease, and dental caries can result. Frequent reflux of gastric acid can also occur as a result of esophageal fibrosis. If swallowing becomes difficult, the patient is likely to decrease food intake and loses weight. Additional GI effects include constipation resulting from colonic hypomotility and diarrhea caused by malabsorption from bacterial overgrowth.

Lung involvement includes pleural thickening, pulmonary fibrosis, and pulmonary function abnormalities. The patient develops a cough and dyspnea. Pulmonary arterial hypertension and interstitial lung disease may occur. Pulmonary arterial hypertension is treated with medications such as extended-release nifedipine (Afeditab CR), bosentan (Tracleer), and ambrisentan (Letairis). (Pulmonary artery hypertension is discussed in Chapter 28.) Lung disease is the main cause of death in scleroderma.

Primary heart disease consists of pericarditis, pericardial effusion, and cardiac dysrhythmias. Myocardial fibrosis resulting in heart failure occurs most frequently in patients with diffuse disease.

Renal disease was previously a major cause of death in diffuse scleroderma. Because malignant hypertension associated with rapidly progressive and irreversible renal insufficiency can occur, early recognition of renal involvement and initiation of therapy are critical. Recent improvements in dialysis, bilateral nephrectomy in patients with uncontrollable hypertension, and kidney transplantation have offered some hope to patients with renal failure. In particular, use of angiotensin-converting enzyme (ACE) inhibitors (e.g., lisinopril [Prinivil]) has had a marked impact on the ability to treat renal disease.

Diagnostic Studies

Laboratory findings in scleroderma are relatively normal. Blood studies may reveal a mild hemolytic anemia as a result of RBC damage in diseased small vessels. ANAs are found in most patients.[36] The scleroderma antibody SCL-70 is found in about 30% of patients with diffuse disease, and serum RF is found in 30% of affected patients. An anticentromere antibody is seen in many patients with CREST. If renal involvement is present, urinalysis may show proteinuria, microscopic hematuria, and casts. Serum levels of creatinine may be elevated. X-ray evidence of subcutaneous calcification, distal esophageal hypomotility, or bilateral pulmonary fibrosis is diagnostic of scleroderma. Pulmonary function studies reveal decreased vital capacity and lung compliance.

Collaborative Care

The collaborative care of scleroderma (Table 65-18) offers no specific treatment. Supportive care is directed toward preventing or treating secondary complications of involved organs. Physical therapy helps to maintain joint mobility and preserve muscle strength. Occupational therapy assists the patient in maintaining functional abilities.

Drug Therapy. No specific drug or combination of drugs has been proven effective for the treatment of scleroderma. Vasoactive agents are often prescribed in early disease, and calcium channel blockers (nifedipine [Adalat, Procardia], diltiazem [Cardizem]) are now a common treatment choice for Raynaud's phenomenon. Reserpine (Serpasil), an α-adrenergic blocking agent, increases blood flow to the fingers. Bosentan, an endothelin-receptor antagonist, and epoprostenol (Flolan), a vasodilator, may help prevent and treat digital ulcers while improving exercise capacity and heart and lung dynamics. Losartan, an angiotensin II blocker, may be used to treat Raynaud's phenomenon.

Corticosteroids may have little effect on scleroderma. Topical agents may provide some relief from joint pain. Capsaicin cream may be useful, not only as a local analgesic, but also as a vasodilator. Other therapies prescribed to treat specific systemic problems include tetracycline for diarrhea caused by bacterial overgrowth, histamine (H_2)-receptor blockers (e.g., cimetidine [Tagamet]) and proton pump inhibitors (e.g., omeprazole [Prilosec]) for esophageal symptoms, an antihypertensive agent (e.g., captopril [Capoten], propranolol [Inderal], methyldopa [Aldomet]) for hypertension with renal involvement, and immunosuppressive drugs (e.g., cyclophosphamide, mycophenolate mofetil).

NURSING MANAGEMENT
SCLERODERMA

Prevention of scleroderma is not possible. Nursing interventions for these patients often begin during a hospitalization for diagnostic purposes. Assess vital signs, weight, intake and output, respiratory and bowel function, and joint ROM at regular intervals as indicated by specific symptoms to plan appropriate care. Emotional stress and cold ambient temperatures may aggravate Raynaud's phenomenon. Instruct patients with scleroderma not to have finger-stick blood testing done because of compromised circulation and poor healing of the fingers.

Teaching is an important nursing intervention as the patient and family begin to live with this disease. Obvious changes in the face and hands often lead to poor self-image and the loss of mobility and function. The patient must actively complete therapeutic exercises at home to prevent skin retraction and promote vascularization. Mouth excursion (yawning with an open mouth) is a good exercise to help with temporomandibular joint function. Isometric exercises are most appropriate if the patient has arthropathy because no joint movement occurs. Encourage the use of moist heat applications or paraffin baths to promote skin flexibility in the hands and feet. Teach the patient to use assistive devices as appropriate and organize activities to preserve strength and reduce disability.

Teach the patient to protect the hands and feet from cold exposure and possible burns or cuts that might heal slowly. Smoking should be avoided because of its vasoconstricting effect. Signs of infection should be reported promptly. Lotions may help alleviate skin dryness and cracking, but they must be rubbed in for an unusually long time because of the thick skin.

Dysphagia may be reduced by eating small, frequent meals; chewing carefully and slowly; and drinking fluids. Heartburn may be minimized by using antacids 45 to 60 minutes after each meal and by sitting upright for at least 2 hours after eating. Using additional pillows or raising the head of the bed on blocks may help reduce nocturnal gastroesophageal reflux.

Job modifications are often necessary because of problems with climbing stairs, using a computer, writing, and being exposed to cold. The patient may become socially withdrawn as skin tightening alters the appearance of the face and hands. Dining out may become socially embarrassing because of the patient's small mouth, difficulty swallowing, and reflux. Some individuals with scleroderma wear gloves to protect fingertip ulcers and to provide extra warmth. Emphasize daily oral hygiene because neglect may lead to increased tooth and gingival problems. The patient needs a dentist who is familiar with scleroderma and can deal with a small mouth.

Psychologic support, biofeedback training, and relaxation can reduce stress and improve sleeping habits. Sexual dys-

---

TABLE 65-18 COLLABORATIVE CARE

Scleroderma

Diagnostic
- History and physical examination
- Antinuclear antibody titers
- Anticentromere antibody
- Nail bed capillary microscopy
- X-ray of chest
- Skin or visceral biopsy
- Urinalysis (proteinuria, hematuria, casts)
- Pulmonary function tests
- ECG

Collaborative Therapy
- Physical therapy
- Occupational therapy
- Drug therapy
  - *Vasoactive agents:* reserpine (Serpasil), bosentan (Tracleer), epoprostenol (Flolan)
  - *Calcium channel blockers:* diltiazem (Cardizem), nifedipine (Adalat, Procardia)
  - *Angiotensin-converting enzyme inhibitors:* lisinopril (Prinivil)
  - *Immunosuppressive drugs:* cyclophosphamide (Cytoxan), mycophenolate mofetil (CellCept)

function resulting from body changes, pain, muscular weakness, limited mobility, decreased self-esteem, erectile dysfunction, and decreased vaginal secretions may require sensitive counseling.

POLYMYOSITIS AND DERMATOMYOSITIS

Polymyositis (PM) is diffuse, idiopathic, inflammatory myopathy of striated muscle that produces bilateral weakness, usually most severe in the proximal or limb girdle muscles. When muscle changes associated with PM are accompanied by characteristic skin changes, the disorder is called dermatomyositis (DM).[37]

Although these relatively rare disorders can be similar in signs, symptoms, and treatment, they are two distinct diseases. They typically affect adults ages 45 to 65 years. Both PM and DM occur twice as often in women as in men. Patients with PM generally have more severe disease than those with DM.

Etiology and Pathophysiology

The exact cause of PM and DM is unknown. Theories include an infectious agent, neoplasms, drugs or vaccinations, and stress. Because T cytotoxic cells and macrophages have been found near the damaged muscle fibers of PM, this disease is believed to be caused by cell-mediated injury. In contrast, DM has been associated with B cells (humoral immunity) and destruction of the muscle microvasculature. An autoimmune response to nuclear and cytoplasm self-antigens has also been noted in many persons with these disorders.[38]

Clinical Manifestations and Complications

Muscular. Patients with PM and DM experience weight loss and increasing fatigue, with a gradually developing weakness of the muscles that leads to difficulty performing routine activities. The most commonly affected muscles are those of the shoulders, legs, arms, and pelvic girdle. The patient may have difficulty rising from a chair or bathtub, climbing stairs, combing hair, or reaching into a high cupboard. Neck muscles may become so weak that the patient is unable to raise the head from the pillow. Muscle discomfort or tenderness is uncommon. Muscle examination reveals an inability to move against resistance or even gravity. Weak pharyngeal muscles may produce dysphagia and dysphonia (nasal or hoarse voice).

Dermal. Skin changes of DM include a classic violet-colored, cyanotic, or erythematous symmetric rash *(heliotrope)* with edema around the eyelids. Violet or erythematous papules and small plaques can develop over the DIP or MCP areas, and at elbow or knee joints in about 70% of patients with DM (Gottron's papules) (Fig. 65-13). These early skin changes usually prompt earlier recognition of DM compared with PM, in which a rash does not appear. Reddened, smooth, or scaly patches appear with the same symmetric distribution but sparing the interphalangeal spaces (Gottron's sign). They can be confused with psoriasis or seborrheic dermatitis. An erythematous scaling rash (poikiloderma) may develop as a late finding on the back, buttocks, and a V-shaped area of the anterior neck and chest. Hyperemia and telangiectasias are often present at the nail beds. Calcium nodules (calcinosis cutis), which can develop throughout the skin, are especially common in long-standing DM.

Other Manifestations. Joint redness, pain, and inflammation often occur and contribute to limitations in joint ROM in

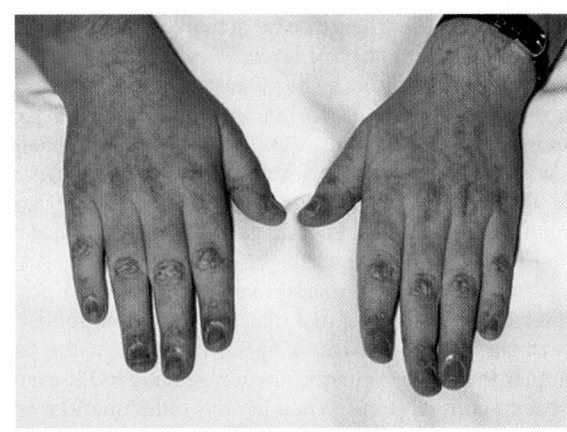

FIG. 65-13 Dermatomyositis skin changes. Gottron's papules.

PM and DM. Contractures and muscle atrophy may occur with advanced disease. Weakened pharyngeal muscles can lead to a poor cough effort, difficulty swallowing, and increased risk for aspiration pneumonia in both disorders. Interstitial lung disease occurs in up to 65% of all patients. People with DM also have an increased risk of cancer, which may be present at the time of diagnosis. Both PM and DM may be associated with other connective tissue disorders (e.g., scleroderma).

Diagnostic Studies

A diagnosis of PM or DM is confirmed by MRI, electromyogram (EMG), muscle biopsy, and serum muscle enzyme levels. An EMG suggestive of PM shows bizarre high-frequency discharges and spontaneous fibrillation, with positive spikes at rest. Muscle biopsy reveals necrosis, degeneration, regeneration, and fibrosis with pathologic findings distinct for DM or PM. Markers such as creatinine kinase and myoglobin are elevated. Elevation of the ESR or CRP is also expected with active disease. In addition, more than 50% of persons with PM have positive RF. The typical skin rash seen with DM is not commonly found with other disorders.

NURSING AND COLLABORATIVE MANAGEMENT POLYMYOSITIS AND DERMATOMYOSITIS

PM and DM are treated initially with high-dose corticosteroids. Improvement generally occurs if corticosteroid therapy is instituted promptly. Dosage can be reduced as the patient improves. Long-term corticosteroid therapy may be required because relapses are common when the drug is withdrawn. If corticosteroids are ineffective after 4 weeks of treatment and/or organ involvement is occurring, immunosuppressive drugs (methotrexate, azathioprine, tacrolimus, cyclophosphamide) may also be administered.

DM has been shown to improve with high doses of IV immunoglobulin. Topical corticosteroids and hydroxychloroquine may be prescribed to treat the skin rash.

The role of newer medications such as TNF inhibitors remains unclear, although their use in refractory cases has shown some success. Ongoing clinical trials continue to explore the use of the monoclonal antibody rituximab and interferon α-2a in the treatment of PM and DM.

Physical therapy can be helpful and should be tailored to disease activity. Massage and passive movement are appropriate during active disease. More aggressive exercises should be reserved for periods when disease activity is minimal, as evidenced by low serum enzyme levels.

Teach the patient about the disease, prescribed therapies, diagnostic tests, and the importance of regular medical care. It is important for the patient to understand that the benefits of therapy are often delayed. For example, weakness may increase during the first few weeks of corticosteroid therapy. Pay special attention to patient safety. Encourage the use of assistive devices as a fall prevention strategy. To prevent aspiration, encourage the patient to rest before meals, maintain an upright position when eating, and choose a diet of easily swallowed foods.

Assist the patient in organizing activities and using pacing techniques to conserve energy. Encourage daily ROM exercises to prevent contractures. When active inflammation is not evident, start muscle-strengthening (repetitive) exercises. Home care and bed rest may become necessary during the acute phase of PM because profound muscle weakness results in the patient's inability to complete activities of daily living.

MIXED (OVERLAPPING) CONNECTIVE TISSUE DISEASE

Patients having a combination of clinical features of several rheumatic diseases are described as having *mixed* or *overlapping connective tissue disease.*[38] The term is used to describe a disorder with features of SLE, Sjögren's syndrome, and PM. About 80% of people with this disease are women.

SJÖGREN'S SYNDROME

Sjögren's syndrome is a relatively common autoimmune disease that targets the moisture-producing exocrine glands, which leads to *xerostomia* (dry mouth) and *keratoconjunctivitis sicca* (dry eyes).[39] The nose, throat, airways, and skin can also become dry. The disease may affect other glands as well, including those in the stomach, pancreas, and intestines (extraglandular involvement). The disease is usually diagnosed in people over age 40, with 90% of them women.

In primary Sjögren's syndrome, symptoms can be traced to problems with lacrimal and salivary glands. The patient with primary disease is likely to have antibodies against the cytoplasmic antigens SSA (or Ro) and SSB (or La), as well as ANA. The patient with secondary Sjögren's syndrome typically had another autoimmune disease (e.g., RA, SLE) before Sjögren's developed.

Sjögren's syndrome appears to be caused by genetic and environmental factors. Several genes seem to be involved. One gene predisposes whites to the disease, whereas other genes are linked to the disease in people of Japanese, Chinese, and African American heritage. The trigger may be a viral or bacterial infection that adversely stimulates the immune system. In Sjögren's syndrome, lymphocytes attack and damage the lacrimal and salivary glands.

Dry eyes cause decreased tearing, which leads to a "gritty" sensation in the eyes, burning, blurred vision, and photosensitivity. Dry mouth produces buccal membrane fissures, altered sense of taste, dysphagia, and increased frequency of mouth infections or dental caries. Dry skin and rashes, joint and muscle pain, and thyroid problems may also be present. Other exocrine glands can be affected. For example, vaginal dryness may lead to dyspareunia (painful intercourse).

Autoimmune thyroid disorders, including Graves' disease and Hashimoto's thyroiditis, are common with Sjögren's syn-

drome. Histologic study reveals lymphocyte infiltration of salivary and lacrimal glands. The disease may become more generalized and involve the lymph nodes, bone marrow, and visceral organs (pseudolymphoma). Persons with severe Sjögren's syndrome have a 5% risk of developing non-Hodgkin's lymphoma.[40]

Ophthalmologic examination (Schirmer's test for tear production), measures of salivary gland function, and lower lip biopsy of minor salivary glands aid in diagnosis. The treatment of Sjögren's syndrome is symptomatic, including (1) instillation of preservative-free artificial tears or ophthalmic antiinflammatory drops (e.g., cyclosporine [Restasis]) as necessary to maintain adequate hydration and lubrication, (2) surgical punctual occlusion, and (3) increased fluids with meals. Dental hygiene is important.

Pilocarpine (Salagen) and cevimeline (Evoxac) can be used to treat symptoms of dry mouth. Increased humidity at home may reduce respiratory tract infections. Vaginal lubrication with a water-soluble product such as K-Y jelly may increase comfort during intercourse.

MYOFASCIAL PAIN SYNDROME

Myofascial pain syndrome is a chronic form of muscle pain. It is characterized as musculoskeletal pain and tenderness, typically in the chest, neck, shoulders, hips, and lower back. Referred pain from these muscle groups can also travel to the buttock, hand, and head, causing severe headaches.

Temporomandibular joint pain may also originate in myofascial pain. Regions of pain are often within the taut bands and fascia of skeletal muscles. When activated by pressure, trigger points are thought to activate a characteristic pattern of pain that can worsen with activity or stress.

Myofascial pain syndrome occurs more often in middle-aged adults, and in women rather than men. Patients complain of the pain as deep and aching and accompanied by a sensation of burning, stinging, and stiffness. Examples of this syndrome include fibromyalgia, myalgia, and myositis.[41]

Physical therapy is one treatment used for myofascial pain syndrome. A typical treatment is the "spray and stretch" method, in which the painful area is iced or sprayed with a coolant such as ethyl chloride and then stretched. Positive results have been seen with topical patches and injection of the trigger points with a local anesthetic (e.g., 1% lidocaine). Massage, acupuncture, biofeedback, and ultrasound therapy have also benefitted some patients.

FIBROMYALGIA

Fibromyalgia is a chronic disorder characterized by widespread, nonarticular musculoskeletal pain and fatigue with multiple tender points. People with fibromyalgia may also experience nonrestorative sleep, morning stiffness, irritable bowel syndrome, and anxiety. Fibromyalgia is a commonly diagnosed musculoskeletal disorder and a major cause of disability. It affects an estimated 5 million Americans, with 75% to 90% of these persons being women.[42] Fibromyalgia and chronic fatigue syndrome share many commonalities (Table 65-19).

Etiology and Pathophysiology

Identifying the underlying causes and pathophysiologic mechanisms of fibromyalgia is an active area of research. There is general agreement that fibromyalgia is a disorder involving neuroendocrine/neurotransmitter dysregulation. The pain amplification experienced by the affected patient is due to abnormal sensory processing in the CNS.

Multiple physiologic abnormalities have been found. They include increased levels of substance P in the spinal fluid, low levels of blood flow to the thalamus, dysfunction of the hypothalamic-pituitary-adrenal (HPA) axis, low levels of serotonin and tryptophan, and abnormalities in cytokine function. Serotonin and substance P play a role in mood regulation, sleep,

and pain perception. Changes in the HPA axis can also negatively affect a person's physical and mental health, leading to an increased incidence of depression and a decreased response to stress. Genetic factors also contribute to the etiology of fibromyalgia, as a familial tendency exists. A recent illness or trauma may serve as a trigger in susceptible people.

Clinical Manifestations and Complications

The patient complains of a widespread burning pain that worsens and improves through the course of a day. It is often difficult for the patient to discriminate whether pain occurs in the muscles, joints, or soft tissues. Head or facial pain often results from stiff or painful neck and shoulder muscles. The pain can accompany temporomandibular joint dysfunction, which affects an estimated one third of patients with fibromyalgia.

Physical examination characteristically reveals point tenderness at 11 or more of 18 identified sites (Fig. 65-14). Patients with fibromyalgia are sensitive to painful stimuli throughout the body, not merely at the identified tender sites. In addition, point tenderness can vary from day to day. On some occasions, the patient may respond to fewer than 11 tender points. At other times, palpation of all sites may elicit pain.

Cognitive effects range from difficulty concentrating to memory lapses and a feeling of being overwhelmed when dealing with multiple tasks. Many individuals report migraine headaches. Depression and anxiety often occur and may require drug therapy. Stiffness, nonrefreshing sleep, fatigue, and numbness or tingling in the hands or feet (paresthesia) often accompany fibromyalgia. Restless legs syndrome is also typical, with the patient describing an irresistible urge to move the legs when at rest or lying down.[43]

Irritable bowel syndrome with manifestations of constipation and/or diarrhea, abdominal pain, and bloating is common. Fibromyalgia patients may also experience difficulty swallowing, perhaps because of abnormalities in esophageal smooth

TABLE 65-19	COMMONALITIES BETWEEN FIBROMYALGIA AND CHRONIC FATIGUE SYNDROME
Commonality	**Description**
Occurrence	Previously healthy, young, and middle-aged women.
Etiology (theories)	Infectious trigger, dysfunction in HPA axis, alteration in CNS.
Clinical manifestations	Generalized musculoskeletal pain, malaise and fatigue, cognitive dysfunction, headaches, sleep disturbances, depression, anxiety, fever.
Course of disease	Variable intensity of symptoms, fluctuates over time.
Diagnosis	No definitive laboratory tests or joint and muscle examinations, mainly a diagnosis of exclusion.
Collaborative therapy	Treatment is symptomatic and may include antidepressant drugs such as amitriptyline (Elavil) and fluoxetine (Prozac). Other measures are heat, massage, regular stretching, biofeedback, stress management, and relaxation training. Patient and caregiver teaching is essential.

HPA, Hypothalamic-pituitary-adrenal.

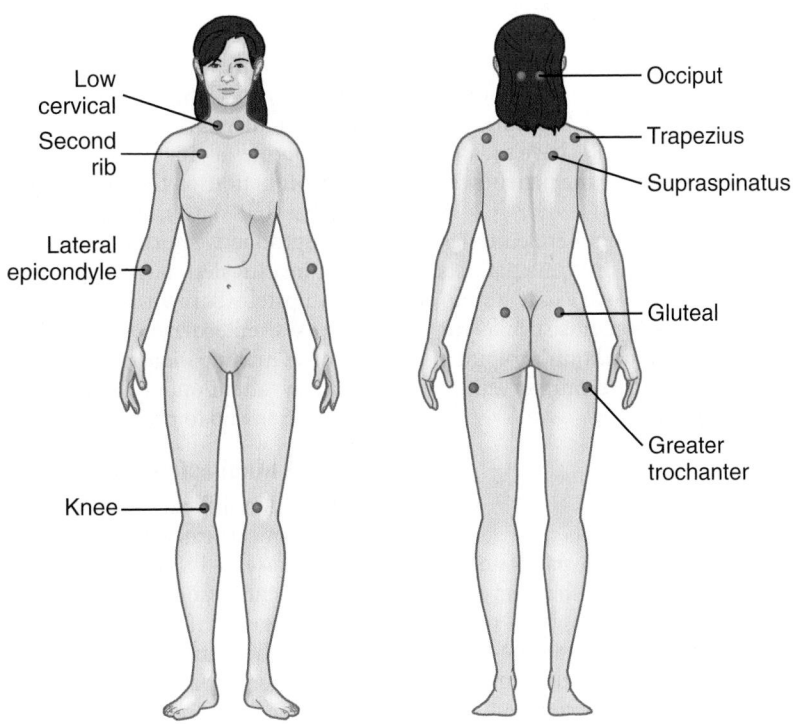

FIG. 65-14 Tender points in fibromyalgia.

muscle function. Increased frequency of urination and urinary urgency, in the absence of a bladder infection, are typical complaints. Women with fibromyalgia may experience more difficult menstruation, with a worsening of disease symptoms during this time.

Diagnostic Studies

A definitive diagnosis of fibromyalgia is often difficult to establish. Lack of knowledge about the disease and its manifestations among health care providers may also cause delays in diagnosis and treatment.

Laboratory results in most cases serve to rule out other suspected disorders. Occasionally a low ANA titer is seen, but it is not considered diagnostic. Muscle biopsy may reveal a nonspecific moth-eaten appearance or fiber atrophy. The American College of Rheumatology classifies an individual as having fibromyalgia if two criteria are met: (1) pain is experienced in 11 of the 18 tender points on palpation (see Fig. 65-14) and (2) a history of widespread pain is noted for at least 3 months.[44] Widespread pain is defined as pain that occurs on both sides of the body and above and below the waist. In addition, fatigue, cognitive symptoms, and extensive somatic symptoms are considered in establishing a diagnosis.

Collaborative Care

The treatment of fibromyalgia is symptomatic and requires a high level of patient motivation. You have a key role in teaching the patient to be an active participant in the therapeutic regimen. Rest can help the pain, aching, and tenderness.

Drug therapy for the chronic widespread pain associated with fibromyalgia includes pregabalin (Lyrica), duloxetine (Cymbalta), and milnacipran (Savella). Low-dose tricyclic antidepressants, selective serotonin reuptake inhibitors (SSRIs), or benzodiazepines (e.g., diazepam [Valium]) may also be prescribed. If the tricyclic antidepressant amitriptyline (Elavil) is not well tolerated, similar drugs can be substituted (e.g., doxepin [Sinequan], imipramine [Tofranil], trazodone [Desyrel]). SSRI antidepressants (e.g., sertraline [Zoloft] or paroxetine [Paxil]) tend to be reserved for fibromyalgia patients who also have depression. SSRIs may need to be prescribed at higher doses than when used to treat depression. Both antidepressants and muscle relaxants (e.g., cyclobenzaprine [Flexeril]) have sedative effects that can help improve nighttime rest for the patient with fibromyalgia.

Long-acting opioids generally are not recommended unless fibromyalgia is refractory to other therapies. In some patients, pain may be managed with OTC analgesics such as acetaminophen, ibuprofen, or naproxen (Aleve). Nonopioids such as tramadol (Ultram) may also be used. In addition, zolpidem (Ambien) is sometimes prescribed for short-term intervention in the patient with severe sleep problems.

NURSING MANAGEMENT
FIBROMYALGIA

Because of the chronic nature of fibromyalgia, the patient needs consistent support from you and other health care team members. Massage is often combined with ultrasound or the application of alternating heat and cold packs to soothe tense, sore muscles and increase blood circulation. Gentle stretching to relieve muscle tension and spasm can be performed by a physical therapist or practiced by the fibromyalgia patient at

home. Yoga and Tai Chi are often appropriate choices. Low-impact aerobic exercise, such as walking, can help prevent muscle atrophy.

Dietitians often urge fibromyalgia patients to limit their consumption of sugar, caffeine, and alcohol because these substances have been shown to be muscle irritants. Vitamin and mineral supplements may help combat stress, correct deficiencies, and support the immune system. However, unproven "miracle diets" or supplements should be carefully investigated by the patient and discussed with the health care provider before using them. Inform the patient that some foods and supplements can cause serious or even dangerous side effects when mixed with certain drugs.

Pain and the related symptoms of fibromyalgia can cause significant stress. Patients with fibromyalgia may not deal effectively with stress. Effective relaxation strategies include biofeedback, mindfulness meditation, and cognitive behavioral therapy. Patients need to receive initial training for these interventions, but they can then continue to practice in their own homes. (Stress management is discussed in Chapter 7.) Psychologic counseling (individual or group) may also be beneficial for the patient with fibromyalgia.

CHRONIC FATIGUE SYNDROME

Chronic fatigue syndrome (CFS), also called *chronic fatigue and immune dysfunction syndrome* or *myalgic encephalomyelitis,* is a disorder characterized by debilitating fatigue and a variety of associated complaints. CFS is a poorly understood condition that can have a devastating impact on the lives of patients and their families.

An estimated 1 million people in the United States have CFS, but less than 20% of them have been diagnosed. Women are affected more often than men. CFS occurs in all ethnic and socioeconomic groups. The prevalence of CFS is difficult to establish because of the lack of validated diagnostic tests.

Etiology and Pathophysiology

Despite numerous attempts to determine the etiology and pathology of CFS, the precise mechanisms remain unknown. However, there are many theories about the cause of CFS. Neuroendocrine abnormalities have been implicated involving a hypofunction of the HPA axis and hypothalamic-pituitary-gonadal (HPG) axis, which together regulate the stress response and reproductive hormone levels. Several microorganisms have been investigated as etiologic agents, including herpesviruses (e.g., Epstein-Barr virus [EBV], cytomegalovirus [CMV]), retroviruses, enteroviruses, *Candida albicans*, and mycoplasma. Because many patients have cognitive deficits (e.g., decreased memory, attention, concentration), it has also been proposed that CFS is due to changes in the CNS.

Clinical Manifestations

CFS is often difficult to distinguish from fibromyalgia because many clinical features are similar (see Table 65-19). In about half the cases, CFS develops insidiously, or the patient may have intermittent episodes that gradually become chronic. Incapacitating fatigue is the most common symptom of CFS and is the problem that causes the patient to seek health care.

In other situations, CFS arises suddenly in a previously active, healthy individual. An unremarkable flu-like illness or other acute stress is often identified as a triggering event.

Associated symptoms (Table 65-20) may fluctuate in intensity over time.

The patient may become angry and frustrated with the inability of health care providers to diagnose a problem. The disorder may have a major impact on work and family responsibilities. Some individuals may even need help with activities of daily living.

Diagnostic Studies

Physical examination and diagnostic studies can be used to rule out other possible causes of the patient's symptoms. No laboratory test can diagnose CFS or measure its severity. The Centers for Disease Control and Prevention has developed a diagnostic algorithm based on the patient's symptoms[45] (see Table 65-20). In general, CFS remains a diagnosis of exclusion.

TABLE 65-20	DIAGNOSTIC CRITERIA FOR CHRONIC FATIGUE SYNDROME*

Major Criterion
- Unexplained, persistent, or relapsing chronic fatigue of new and definite onset (not lifelong). Not due to ongoing exertion. Not substantially alleviated by rest. Results in substantial reduction in occupational, educational, social, or personal activities.

Minor Criteria
- Impaired memory or concentration
- Frequent or recurring sore throat
- Tender cervical or axillary lymph nodes
- Muscle pain
- Multijoint pain without joint swelling or redness
- Headaches of a new type, pattern, or severity
- Unrefreshing sleep
- Postexertional malaise

Adapted from Centers for Disease Control and Prevention: Chronic fatigue syndrome: revised case definition. Retrieved from *www.cdc.gov/cfs/cfsdefinitionHCP.htm.*
*For a diagnosis to be made, the patient must demonstrate the major criterion, plus four or more of the minor criteria for ≥6 mo. These criteria were prepared by the Centers for Disease Control and Prevention, National Institutes of Health, and International Chronic Fatigue Syndrome Study Group.

NURSING AND COLLABORATIVE MANAGEMENT CHRONIC FATIGUE SYNDROME

Because no definitive treatment exists for CFS, supportive management is essential. Tell the patient what is known about the disease. All complaints should be taken seriously.

NSAIDs can be used to treat headaches, muscle and joint aches, and fever. Because many patients with CFS also have allergies and sinusitis, antihistamines and decongestants can be used to treat allergic symptoms. Tricyclic antidepressants (e.g., doxepin, amitriptyline) and SSRIs (e.g., fluoxetine [Prozac], paroxetine) can improve mood and sleep problems. Clonazepam (Klonopin) can also be used to treat sleep disturbances and panic disorders. The use of low-dose hydrocortisone to decrease fatigue and disability is being studied.

Total rest is not advised because it can potentiate the self-image of being an invalid, while strenuous exertion can exacerbate the exhaustion. Therefore it is important to plan a carefully graduated exercise program. A well-balanced diet, including fiber and fresh dark-colored fruits and vegetables for antioxidant action, is essential in treatment. Behavioral therapy may be used to promote a positive outlook and improve overall disability, fatigue, and other symptoms.

One of the major problems facing many CFS patients is financial instability.[46] When the illness strikes, they cannot work or must decrease the amount of time working. Loss of a job often leads to loss of medical insurance. Obtaining disability benefits can be frustrating because of the difficulty of establishing a definitive diagnosis of CFS. Patients with CFS may experience substantial occupational and psychosocial impairments and loss, including the social pressure and isolation from being characterized as lazy or "crazy."

CFS does not appear to progress. Although most patients recover or at least gradually improve over time, some do not show substantial improvement. Recovery is more common in individuals with a sudden onset of CFS.

CASE STUDY

Rheumatoid Arthritis

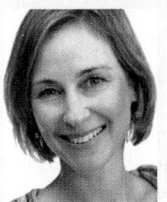
iStockphoto/Thinkstock

Patient Profile
K.R., a 42-yr-old married white woman, is seen at the rheumatology clinic with complaints of tenderness and pain in the small joints of her hands.

Subjective Data
- Complains of tenderness, joint pain, and stiffness in her hands for the last 3 mo
- Experiencing fatigue, anorexia, and morning stiffness
- Mother diagnosed with ankylosing spondylitis 8 yr ago
- Expresses doubt about her ability to manage disease

Objective Data
Physical Examination
- Swelling, warmth, and tenderness of third and fourth metacarpophalangeal joints of both hands
- Mild pain with neck motion
- Tenosynovitis

Diagnostic Studies
- Positive ESR, RF, and ACPA
- Moderate bone demineralization evident bilaterally in hand x-rays

Collaborative Care
- Diagnosed with RA
- Started on methotrexate (Rheumatrex) 7.5 mg PO once per week, etanercept (Enbrel) 50 mg subcutaneously once per week, prednisone 10 mg/day

Discussion Questions
1. How will you explain the pathophysiology of RA to K.R.?
2. K.R. asks you if genetic factors are related to a diagnosis of RA. How will you respond?
3. What are some home and work modifications that you can suggest to K.R. to reduce her symptoms?
4. What suggestions can you make to K.R. about coping with fatigue?
5. *Priority Decision:* Based on the assessment data presented, what are the priority nursing diagnoses? Are there any collaborative problems?
6. *Evidence-Based Practice:* Why is an exercise program important in the treatment plan for K.R.?

Ⓔvolve Answers and a corresponding concept map available at *http://evolve.elsevier.com/Lewis/medsurg.*

BRIDGE TO NCLEX EXAMINATION

The number of the question corresponds to the same-numbered outcome at the beginning of the chapter.

1. In assessing the joints of a patient with osteoarthritis, the nurse understands that Heberden's nodes
   a. are often red, swollen, and tender.
   b. indicate osteophyte formation at the DIP joints.
   c. are the result of pannus formation at the PIP joints.
   d. occur from deterioration of cartilage by proteolytic enzymes.

2. A patient with rheumatoid arthritis is experiencing articular involvement of the joints. The nurse recognizes that these characteristic changes include (select all that apply)
   a. bamboo-shaped fingers.
   b. metatarsal head dislocation in feet.
   c. noninflammatory pain in large joints.
   d. asymmetric involvement of small joints.
   e. morning stiffness lasting 60 minutes or more.

3. When administering medications to the patient with gout, the nurse would recognize that which drug is used as a treatment for this disease?
   a. Colchicine
   b. Febuxostat
   c. Sulfasalazine
   d. Cyclosporine

4. The nurse should teach the patient with ankylosing spondylitis the importance of
   a. regularly exercising and maintaining proper posture.
   b. avoiding extremes in environmental temperatures.
   c. maintaining usual physical activity during flare-ups.
   d. applying hot and cool compresses for relief of local symptoms.

5. In teaching a patient with SLE about the disorder, the nurse knows that the pathophysiology of SLE includes
   a. circulating immune complexes formed from IgG autoantibodies reacting with IgG.
   b. an autoimmune T-cell reaction that results in destruction of the deep dermal skin layer.
   c. immunologic dysfunction leading to chronic inflammation in the cartilage and muscles.
   d. the production of a variety of autoantibodies directed against components of the cell nucleus.

6. In teaching a patient with Sjögren's syndrome about drug therapy for this disorder, the nurse includes instruction on use of which drug?
   a. Pregabalin (Lyrica)
   b. Etanercept (Enbrel)
   c. Cyclosporine (Restasis)
   d. Cyclobenzaprine (Flexeril)

7. Teach the patient with fibromyalgia the importance of limiting intake of which foods (select all that apply)?
   a. Sugar
   b. Alcohol
   c. Caffeine
   d. Red meat
   e. Root vegetables

1. b, 2. b, e, 3. b, 4. a, 5. d, 6. c, 7. a, b, c

ⓔvolve

For rationales to these answers and even more NCLEX review questions, visit *http://evolve.elsevier.com/Lewis/medsurg*.

REFERENCES

1. National Institute of Arthritis and Musculoskeletal and Skin Disease: Questions and answers about arthritis and rheumatic diseases. Retrieved from *www.niams.nih.gov/health_info/arthritis/arthritis_rheumatic_qa.asp*.

2. Centers for Disease Control and Prevention: Arthritis: meeting the challenge. Retrieved from *www.cdc.gov/nccdphp/publications/aag/arthritis.htm*.

3. Roberts D: Arthritis and connective tissue disorders. In National Association of Orthopaedic Nurses: *NAON core curriculum for orthopaedic nursing*, ed 7, Boston, 2012, Pearson Custom Publishing.

4. Centers for Disease Control and Prevention: Arthritis risk factors. Retrieved from *www.cdc.gov/arthritis/basics/risk_factors.htm*.

5. Arthritis Foundation: Who gets osteoarthritis? Retrieved from *www.arthritis.org/who-gets-osteoarthritis.php*.

6. Antonelli M, Starz T: Assessing for risk and progression of osteoarthritis: the nurse's role, *Am J Nurs* 112:S26, 2012.

7. American College of Rheumatology Subcommittee on Osteoarthritis Guidelines: Recommendations for the medical management of osteoarthritis of the hip and knee. Retrieved from *www.rheumatology.org/practice/clinical/guidelines/oa-mgmt.asp*.

*8. Vickers A, Cronin A, Maschino A, et al: Acupuncture for chronic pain: individual patient data meta-analysis, *Arch Inter Med* 172(19):1444, 2012.

*9. National Center for Complementary and Alternative Medicine: Glucosamine/Chondroitin Arthritis Intervention Trial (GAIT): primary and ancillary study results. Retrieved from *http://nccam.nih.gov/research/results/gait*.

10. LeGraverand-Gastineau MP: Disease-modifying osteoarthritis drugs: facing development challenges and choosing molecular targets, *Curr Drug Targets* 11:528, 2010.

11. Robbins L, Kulsea M: The state of the science in the prevention and management of osteoarthritis, *Am J Nurs* 112:S3, 2012.

12. Centers for Disease Control and Prevention: Rheumatoid arthritis. Retrieved from *www.cdc.gov/arthritis/basics/rheumatoid.htm#6*.

13. Firestein G: Etiology and pathogenesis of rheumatoid arthritis. In G Firestein, R Budd, S Gabriel, et al, editors: *Kelley's textbook of rheumatology*, ed 9, Philadelphia, 2012, Saunders.

14. Johns Hopkins Arthritis Center: Rheumatoid arthritis clinical presentation. Retrieved from *www.hopkins-arthritis.org/arthritis-info/rheumatoid-arthritis/rheum_clin_pres*.

15. Cleveland Clinic: RA doldrums: how to cope with joint pain and depression, *Arthritis Advisor* 11:3, 2012.

16. Besada E, Nikolaissen C, Nossent H: Should rheumatoid factor in rheumatoid arthritis be sent to Davy Jones's locker? *Scand J Rheumatol* 41:85, 2012.

17. Simmons S: Recognizing and managing rheumatoid arthritis, *Nursing* 41:34, 2011.

18. Arthritis Foundation: Arthritis drug chart: NSAIDs. Retrieved from *www.arthritistoday.org/DrugGuide/drug-chart.php?drug_type=NSAIDs*.

*Evidence-based information for clinical practice.

19. *Arthritis Keeping Your Joints Healthy,* Boston, 2011, Harvard Health Publications.

20. Hardy E: Gout diagnosis and management: what NPs need to know, *Nurse Pract* 36:15, 2011.

21. Doghramji PP: Managing your patient with gout: a review of treatment options, *Postgrad Med* 123:56, 2011.

22. Bockenstedt L: Lyme disease. In G Firestein, R Budd, S Gabriel, et al, editors: *Kelley's textbook of rheumatology,* ed 9, Philadelphia, 2012, Saunders.

23. Centers for Disease Control and Prevention: Lyme disease. Retrieved from *www.cdc.gov/lyme/.*

24. Xu B, Katz B: Atypical presentation of *Staphylococcus aureus* septic arthritis in an elderly woman, *Clin Geriatr* 20:43, 2012.

25. Horowitz DL, Katzap E, Horowitz S, et al: Approach to septic arthritis, *Am Fam Physician* 84:653, 2011.

26. Akgul O, Ozgocmen S: Classification criteria for spondyloarthropathies, *World J Orthop* 2:107, 2011.

27. Cleveland Clinic: Psoriatic arthritis: when you feel pain above and below your skin, *Arthritis Advisor* 11:1, 2012.

28. National Psoriasis Foundation: The five types of psoriatic arthritis. Retrieved from *www.psoriasis.org/netcommunity/learn_psatypes.*

29. Hill Gaston JS: Reactive arthritis and undifferentiated spondyloarthritis. In G Firestein, R Budd, S Gabriel, et al, editors: *Kelley's textbook of rheumatology,* ed 9, Philadelphia, 2012, Saunders.

30. Bernknop A, Rowley K, Bailey T: A review of systemic lupus erythematosus and current treatment options, *Formulary* 46:178, 2011.

31. Ferenekh-Koroma A: Systemic lupus erythematosus: nurse and patient education, *Nurs Stand* 26:49, 2012.

32. Tsokos GC: Systemic lupus erythematosus, *New Engl J Med* 365:2110, 2011.

33. Lupus Foundation of America: Medications to treat lupus symptoms. Retrieved from *www.lupus.org/webmodules/webarticlesnet/templates/new_learntreating.aspx?articleid=2246&zoneid=525.*

34. Jolly M, Pickard, A, Mikolaitis R, et al: Body image in patients with systemic lupus erythematosus, *Int J Behav Med* 19:157, 2012.

35. American College of Rheumatology: Scleroderma. Retrieved from *www.rheumatology.org/practice/clinical/patients/diseases_and_conditions/scleroderma.pdf.*

36. Varga J: Systemic sclerosis (scleroderma). In L Goldman, A Schafer, editors: *Goldman: Goldman's Cecil medicine,* ed 24, Philadelphia, 2011, Saunders.

37. Cedars-Sinai Health System: Polymyositis and dermatomyositis. Retrieved from *www.cedars-sinai.edu/Patients/Health-Conditions/Polymyositis-and-Dermatomyositis.aspx.*

38. von Mühlen C, Nakamura R: Clinical and laboratory evaluation of systemic rheumatic diseases. In R McPherson, M Pincus, editors: *McPherson: Henry's clinical diagnosis and management by laboratory methods,* ed 22, Philadelphia, 2011, Saunders.

39. Jonsson R, Vogelsang P, Volchenkov R, et al: The complexity of Sjögren's syndrome: novel aspects on pathogenesis, *Immunol Lett* 141:1, 2011.

*40. Covelli ME, Lanciano P, Tartaglia M, et al: Rituximab treatment for Sjögren syndrome–associated non-Hodgkin's lymphoma: case series, *Rheum Int* 32:3281, 2012.

41. Belden J, DeFriez C, Huether S: Pain, temperature, sleep, and sensory function. In S Huether, K McCance, editors: *Understanding pathophysiology,* ed 5, St Louis, 2012, Mosby.

42. Cleveland Clinic: Chronic pain: is it fibromyalgia—or something else? *Arthritis Advisor* 10:4, 2011.

*43. Shillam C, Jones K, Miller L: Fibromyalgia symptoms, physical function, and comorbidity in middle-aged and older adults, *Nurs Res* 60:309, 2011.

44. Wolfe F, Clauw DJ, Fitzcharles M, et al: The American College of Rheumatology preliminary diagnostic criteria for fibromyalgia and measurement of symptom severity, *Arthritis Care Res* 62:600, 2010.

45. Centers for Disease Control and Prevention: Chronic fatigue syndrome: revised case definition. Retrieved from *www.cdc.gov/cfs/cfsdefinitionHCP.htm.*

46. Burns D, Bennett C, McGough A: Chronic fatigue syndrome or myalgic encephalomyelitis, *Nurs Stand* 26:48, 2012.

RESOURCES

American College of Rheumatology
www.rheumatology.org
Arthritis Foundation
www.arthritis.org
International Association for CFS/ME
www.iacfsme.org
Lupus Foundation of America
www.lupus.org
National Fibromyalgia Association
www.fmaware.org
National Institute of Arthritis and Musculoskeletal and Skin Diseases Information Clearinghouse, National Institutes of Health
www.niams.nih.gov
National Psoriasis Foundation
www.psoriasis.org
Scleroderma Foundation
www.scleroderma.org
Sjögren's Syndrome Foundation
www.sjogrens.org
Spondylitis Association of America
www.spondylitis.org

Managing Multiple Patients

You are working on the medical-surgical unit and have been assigned to care for the following five patients. You have one LPN and one UAP on your team to help you.

Patients

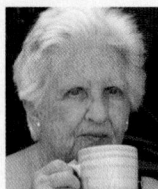

iStockphoto/Thinkstock

A.J. is a 66-yr-old white woman who had an ischemic stroke 2 days ago. She has a history of migraines, hypertension, and atrial fibrillation. She is alert, oriented, and able to answer questions appropriately but has mild slowness in responding. She has left-sided arm weakness (3/5) and left leg weakness (4/5). Her vital signs are BP 160/84, HR 88, RR 20, T 37° C. She is receiving ASA 325 mg po daily, Lovenox 80 mg subcutaneously q12hr, lisinopril 10 mg po daily, Cardizem CD 180 mg po daily, and Coumadin 5 mg po daily. Her most recent INR was 1.7. She is scheduled to receive physical therapy today.

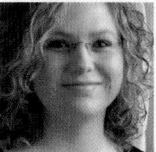

Purestock/Thinkstock

J.P. is a 24-yr-old woman who fell and hit her head after experiencing a tonic-clonic seizure. Her boyfriend found her lying semiconscious on the floor in her apartment. She had an emergency evacuation of a subdural hematoma and was initially admitted to the ICU. She was transferred to the medical-surgical unit yesterday and is scheduled for rehabilitation evaluation. She is oriented to person only and is somewhat restless. A safety sitter is with her at all times.

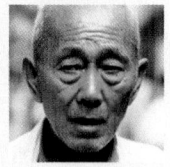

iStockphoto/Thinkstock

M.Y., an 80-yr-old Asian American man, had an ORIF 2 days ago for a fractured left hip. He has a 3-yr history of Alzheimer's disease and is confused to place and time. Although he has a history of agitation, he has been pleasant and cooperative. He has a personal alarm and bed alarm on for safety. His hip dressing is dry and intact and the drainage in the hemovac is minimal.

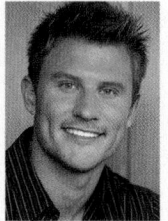

iStockphoto/Thinkstock

B.V., a 24-yr-old white man, was admitted to the ICU 3 weeks ago after suffering a C5-6 cervical spinal cord injury. B.V. dove into the shallow end of a neighbor's backyard pool and struck his head on the bottom. He was initially placed in cervical traction, intubated, and mechanically ventilated. He has since undergone surgical stabilization and the traction was removed. He was weaned from the ventilator 2 days ago. He was transferred to the medical-surgical unit yesterday. He is currently requesting medication for a "severe headache."

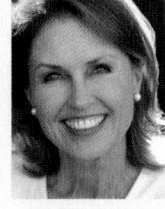

Jupiterimages/Comstock/
Thinkstock

M.L. is a 58-yr-old white retired nurse who suffered an L4 compression fracture after falling 1 week ago. She underwent vertebroplasty yesterday and was kept in the hospital overnight for observation after experiencing some postoperative hypotension. She has a 6-yr history of Addison's disease. She is planning to be discharged home today.

Management Discussion Questions

1. **Priority Decision:** After receiving report, which patient should you see first? Provide a rationale.
2. **Delegation Decision:** Which tasks could you delegate to UAP (select all that apply)?
   a. Explain discharge instructions to M.L.
   b. Change the dressing on M.Y.'s left hip.
   c. Obtain vital signs on M.L. before discharge.
   d. Sit with J.P. while the safety sitter takes a break.
   e. Assess A.J.'s ability to swallow before feeding her breakfast.
3. **Priority and Delegation Decision:** When you enter the room to assess B.V., you find him diaphoretic with a flushed face and pale extremities. His BP is 200/102 mm Hg. Which two initial actions would be most appropriate?
   a. Ask the UAP to obtain a stat bladder scan.
   b. Have the LPN administer his oral antihypertensive meds stat.
   c. Elevate the head of the bed while assessing for any noxious stimuli.
   d. Ask the LPN to stay with B.V. while you call B.V.'s health care provider.
   e. Insert rectal suppository after applying lidocaine to the area around the rectum.

Case Study Progression

B.V.'s bladder scan revealed 700 mL of urine. After you have the LPN catheterize him using a local anesthetic gel, his symptoms subside. You take this time to further teach B.V. about the clinical manifestations of autonomic dysreflexia and the need to report any symptom as soon as it appears. You also take the time to discuss bladder training strategies and how to avoid bladder distention in the future. B.V. is grateful for the information and your caring attitude. Just as you are finishing, the UAP informs you that M.Y. has pulled out his hemovac drain.

4. What should be your initial intervention for M.Y.?
   a. Reinsert the hemovac drain.
   b. Assess the incision site for a hematoma.
   c. Notify M.Y.'s surgeon that the drain was removed.
   d. Apply pressure to the incisional site where the drain had been placed.
5. Which intervention would be most appropriate in caring for A.J.?
   a. Place her left arm in a sling for support.
   b. Arrange the food tray so that all foods are on the right side.
   c. Call the health care provider to decrease her Coumadin dosage.
   d. Position her left leg so that the ankle is lower than the knee to prevent contractures.
6. When teaching J.P.'s boyfriend about what to expect during recovery from a head injury, which statement is most accurate?
   a. "You can tell by how great she looks physically that she will ultimately function well at the home."
   b. "One good thing that will come out of this injury is that her seizures should occur less frequently."
   c. "Most patients are usually transferred for acute rehabilitation management to prepare them for going home."
   d. "She can expect a full recovery without any chronic problems, but it may take a few months to achieve that goal."
7. **Priority and Management Decision:** As you enter M.L.'s room to discuss her discharge plans, you find her all packed up and walking out the door. She tells you the UAP already told her what she needed to do. What is your best initial action?
   a. Ask M.L. if she has any further questions.
   b. Call the UAP to M.L.'s room to find out what she told her.
   c. Review discharge instructions with M.L. to ascertain correct understanding.
   d. Give M.L. a telephone number to call in case she has any concerns when she gets home.

Nursing Care in Critical Care Settings

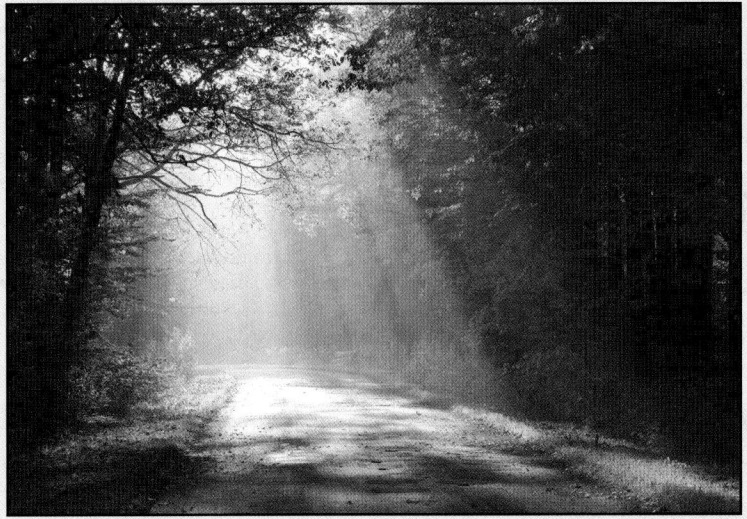

iStockphoto/Thinkstock

If you don't like the road you're walking, start paving another one.
Dolly Parton

CHAPTER

66

You must have long-range goals to keep you
from being frustrated by short-range failures.
Charles C. Noble

Nursing Management
Critical Care

Linda Bucher and Maureen A. Seckel

LEARNING OUTCOMES

1. Differentiate the various certification opportunities for critical care nurses.
2. Select appropriate nursing interventions to manage common problems and needs of critically ill patients.
3. Develop strategies to manage issues related to caregivers of critically ill patients.
4. Apply the principles of hemodynamic monitoring to the collaborative care and nursing management of patients receiving this intervention.
5. Differentiate the purpose of, indications for, and function of circulatory assist devices and related collaborative care and nursing management.
6. Differentiate the indications for and modes of mechanical ventilation.
7. Select appropriate nursing interventions related to the care of an intubated patient.
8. Relate the principles of mechanical ventilation to the collaborative care and nursing management of patients receiving this intervention.

KEY TERMS

arterial pressure–based cardiac output (APCO), p. 1606
assist-control ventilation (ACV), p. 1619
circulatory assist devices (CADs), p. 1610
continuous positive airway pressure (CPAP), p. 1621
endotracheal (ET) intubation, p. 1613

hemodynamic monitoring, p. 1602
high-frequency oscillatory ventilation (HFOV), p. 1622
intraaortic balloon pump (IABP), p. 1610
mechanical ventilation, p. 1618
negative pressure ventilation, p. 1618

positive end-expiratory pressure (PEEP), p. 1621
positive pressure ventilation (PPV), p. 1618
pressure support ventilation (PSV), p. 1621
ventricular assist device (VAD), p. 1612
volume ventilation, p. 1618
weaning, p. 1625

This chapter focuses on the role of the critical care nurse in the management of the critically ill patient in an intensive care setting. The chapter reviews the concepts related to cardiovascular and respiratory dynamics. It emphasizes nursing management of patients requiring aspects of critical care not addressed in other chapters, such as invasive hemodynamic monitoring, circulatory assist devices, artificial airways, and mechanical ventilation.

CRITICAL CARE NURSING

The American Association of Critical-Care Nurses (AACN) defines *critical care nursing* as that specialty dealing with human responses to life-threatening problems.[1] Critical care nurses care for patients with acute and unstable physiologic problems, and their caregivers. This involves assessing life-threatening conditions, initiating appropriate interventions,

Reviewed by Steven J. Palazzo, RN, PhD, Sauvage Fellow, The Hope Heart Institute, and Nurse Faculty Leadership Academy Fellow, STTI, Seattle University, College of Nursing, Seattle, Washington; and Trevah A. Panek, RN, MSN, CCRN, Assistant Professor of Nursing, Saint Francis University, Loretto, Pennsylvania.

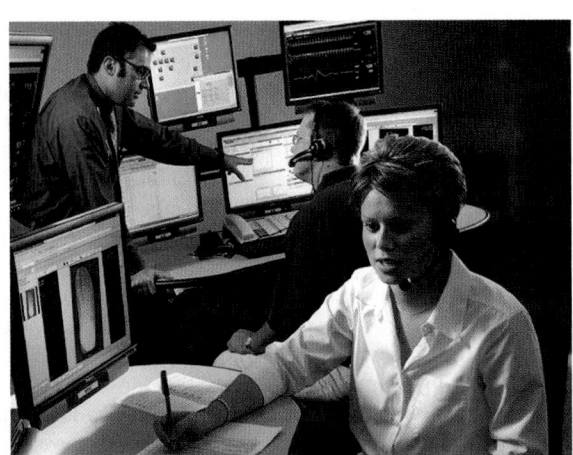

FIG. 66-1 Tele-intensive care unit control room. (From Avera Health, Sioux Falls, S Dak.)

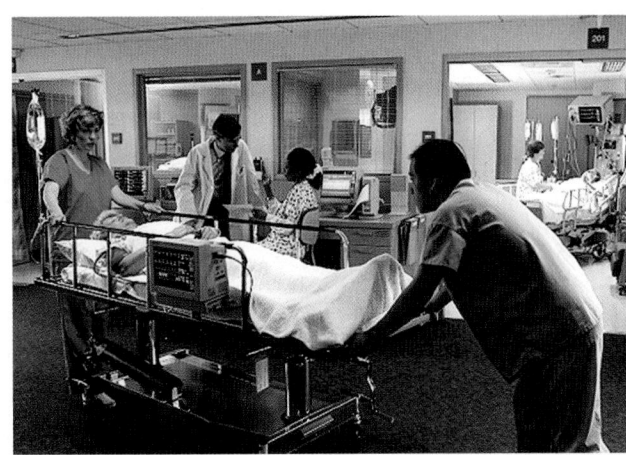

FIG. 66-2 Typical intensive care unit. (Courtesy Spacelabs Medical, Redmond, Wash.)

evaluating the outcomes of the interventions, and providing education and emotional support to caregivers.

Critical Care Units

Critical care units (CCUs) or *intensive care units* (ICUs) are designed to meet the special needs of acutely and critically ill patients. In many hospitals the concept of ICU care has expanded from delivering care in a standard unit to bringing ICU care to patients wherever they might be. For example, the *electronic* or *teleICU* assists the bedside ICU team by monitoring the patient from a remote location (Fig. 66-1).

Similarly, the development of *rapid response teams* (RRTs) provides for the delivery of advanced care by specialized teams usually composed of a critical care nurse, a respiratory therapist, and a critical care physician or an advanced practice registered nurse (APRN). The team brings rapid and immediate care to unstable patients in noncritical care units. Patients often exhibit early and subtle signs of deterioration (e.g., mild confusion, tachypnea) 6 to 8 hours before cardiac or respiratory arrest. Early critical care intervention has made significant contributions to reducing mortality rates in these patients.[2]

The technology available in the ICU is extensive and always evolving. It is possible to continuously monitor the electrocardiogram (ECG), blood pressure (BP), oxygen (O_2) saturation, cardiac output (CO), intracranial pressure, and temperature. More advanced monitoring devices measure cardiac index (CI), stroke volume (SV), stroke volume variation (SVV), ejection fraction (EF), end-tidal carbon dioxide (CO_2), and tissue O_2 consumption. Patients may receive ongoing support from mechanical ventilators, intraaortic balloon pumps (IABPs), circulatory assist devices (CADs), or dialysis machines. Fig. 66-2 shows a typical ICU.

Progressive care units (PCUs), also called intermediate care or step-down units, provide a transition between the ICU and the general care unit or discharge. Generally, PCU patients are at risk for serious complications, but their risk is lower than that of ICU patients. Examples of patients found in PCUs include those scheduled for interventional cardiac procedures (e.g., stent placement), awaiting heart transplant, receiving stable doses of vasoactive IV drugs (e.g., diltiazem [Cardizem]), or being weaned from prolonged mechanical ventilation. Monitoring capabilities in these units include continuous ECG, arterial BP, O_2 saturation, and end-tidal CO_2. The use of PCUs provides

critical care nursing for an at-risk patient population in a more cost-effective environment.

Critical Care Nurse

A critical care nurse has in-depth knowledge of anatomy, physiology, pathophysiology, pharmacology, and advanced assessment skills, as well as the ability to use advanced technology. As a critical care nurse, you perform frequent assessments to monitor trends (patterns) in the patient's physiologic parameters (e.g., BP, ECG). This allows you to rapidly recognize and manage complications while aiding healing and recovery. You must also provide psychologic support to the patient and caregiver. To be effective, you must be able to communicate and collaborate with all members of the interdisciplinary health team (e.g., physician, dietitian, social worker, respiratory therapist, occupational therapist).

As a critical care nurse, you will face ethical dilemmas related to the care of your patients. Moral distress over perceived issues of delivering futile or nonbeneficial care can lead to emotional exhaustion or burnout. Consequently, it is important that all members of the health care team coexist in a healthy work environment.

Specialization in critical care nursing requires formal education combined with a preceptored clinical orientation, often over several months. The AACN Certification Corporation offers critical care certification (CCRN) in adult, pediatric, and neonatal critical care nursing; progressive care certification (PCCN); and teleICU certification (CCRN-E). Subspecialty certifications are available in cardiac medicine (CMC) and cardiac surgery (CSC). The designation requires registered nurse (RN) licensure, practice experience in the related specialty area, and successful completion of a written test. Certification validates basic knowledge of critical or progressive care nursing. It is not the same as advanced practice.

Advanced practice critical care nurses currently have a graduate (master's or doctorate) degree with a proposed transition to a doctor of nursing practice (DNP) by 2015.[3] These nurses function in a variety of roles: patient and staff educators, consultants, administrators, researchers, or expert practitioners. The advanced practice critical care nurse who is a clinical nurse specialist (CNS) typically functions in one or more of these roles. Certification for the CNS in acute and critical care is available through the AACN. Another advanced practice role is the acute care nurse practitioner (ACNP). This APRN provides comprehensive care to select critically ill patients and their caregivers. The ACNP conducts comprehensive assessments, orders and interprets diagnostic tests, manages health problems and disease-related symptoms, prescribes treatments, and coordinates care during transitions in settings. Certification as an ACNP is available through the AACN. Prescriptive authority and licensure regulations for APRNs vary by state.

Critical Care Patient

AACN defines a *critically ill patient* as one who is at high risk for actual or potential life-threatening health problems and who requires intense and vigilant nursing care.[1] A patient is generally admitted to the ICU for one of three reasons. First, the patient may be physiologically unstable, requiring advanced clinical judgments by you and a physician. Second, the patient may be at risk for serious complications and require frequent assessments and often invasive interventions. Third, the patient may require intensive and complicated nursing support related to the use of IV polypharmacy (e.g., sedation, thrombolytics, drugs requiring titration [e.g., vasopressors]) and advanced technology (e.g., mechanical ventilation, intracranial pressure monitoring, continuous renal replacement therapy, hemodynamic monitoring).

ICU patients can be clustered by disease condition (e.g., neurology, pulmonary) or age-group (e.g., neonatal, pediatrics). ICU patients are sometimes clustered by acuity (e.g., acute and unstable versus technology dependent but stable). Patients commonly treated in the ICU include those with respiratory distress, myocardial infarction, or acute neurologic impairment or those receiving care after cardiac surgery or other major surgical procedures (e.g., organ transplantation). Trauma and burn ICUs care for critically injured patients. Patients with medical emergencies (e.g., sepsis, diabetic ketoacidosis, drug overdoses, thyroid crisis) are treated in a medical ICU. The patient who is not expected to recover from an illness is usually not admitted to an ICU. For example, the ICU is not used to manage the patient in a persistent coma or to prolong the natural process of death.

Despite the emphasis on caring for patients who are expected to survive, the incidence of death is higher in ICU patients than in non-ICU patients. In general, nonsurvivors are older, have co-morbidities (e.g., liver disease, obesity), and experience longer ICU stays.[4] Consequently, it is important that you are skilled in palliative and end-of-life care (see Chapter 10).

Common Problems of Critical Care Patients. The patient admitted to the ICU is at risk for numerous complications and special problems. Critically ill patients are usually immobile and at high risk for skin problems (see Chapter 24) and venous thromboembolism (see Chapter 38). The use of multiple, invasive devices predisposes the patient to health care–associated infections (HAIs). Sepsis and multiple organ dysfunction syndrome (MODS) may follow (see Chapter 67). Adequate nutrition for the critically ill patient is essential. Other special problems relate to anxiety, pain, impaired communication, sensory-perceptual problems, and sleep disorders.

Nutrition. Patients often arrive at ICUs with conditions that result in either hypermetabolic states (e.g., burns, sepsis) or catabolic states (e.g., acute kidney injury). Other times, patients are in severely malnourished states (e.g., chronic heart, pulmonary, or liver disease). In general, inadequate nutrition is linked to increased mortality and morbidity rates. One contributing factor to underfeeding patients is the frequent interruptions in enteral feedings because of medication administration and multiple tests and procedures. Determining who to feed, what to feed, when to feed, and how to feed (e.g., route of administration) is crucial when caring for critically ill patients.[5] Collaborate with the physician and the dietitian to determine how best to meet the nutritional needs of ICU patients.

The primary goal of nutritional support is to prevent or correct nutritional deficiencies. This is usually done by the early provision of enteral nutrition (i.e., delivery of calories via the gastrointestinal [GI] tract) or parenteral nutrition (i.e., IV delivery of calories).[5] Enteral nutrition preserves the structure and function of the gut mucosa and stops the movement of gut bacteria across the intestinal wall and into the bloodstream. In addition, early enteral nutrition is associated with fewer complications and shorter hospital stays and is less expensive than parenteral nutrition.[5] (Enteral and parenteral nutrition are discussed in Chapter 40.)

Parenteral nutrition is used when the enteral route cannot provide adequate nutrition or is contraindicated. Examples of these conditions are paralytic ileus, diffuse peritonitis, intestinal obstruction, pancreatitis, GI ischemia, abdominal trauma or surgery, and severe diarrhea.

Anxiety. Anxiety is a common problem for ICU patients. The primary sources of anxiety include the perceived or anticipated threat to health or life, loss of control of body functions, and an environment that is foreign. Many patients and caregivers feel uncomfortable in the ICU with its complex equipment, high noise and light levels, and intense pace of activity. Pain, impaired communication, sleeplessness, immobilization, and loss of control all enhance anxiety.

To help reduce anxiety, encourage patients and caregivers to express concerns, ask questions, and state their needs. Include the patient and caregiver in all conversations and explain the purpose of equipment and procedures. Be sure to structure the patient's environment in a way that decreases anxiety. For example, encourage caregivers to bring in photographs and personal items. Appropriate use of antianxiety drugs (e.g., lorazepam [Ativan]) and relaxation techniques (e.g., music therapy) may reduce the stress response that can be triggered by anxiety.[6]

Pain. The control of pain in the ICU patient is vital. As many as 70% of ICU patients have moderate to severe unrelieved pain. Inadequate pain control is often linked with agitation and anxiety and is known to add to the stress response. ICU patients at high risk for pain include those who (1) have medical conditions that include ischemic, infectious, or inflammatory processes; (2) are immobilized; (3) have invasive monitoring

---

INFORMATICS IN PRACTICE

Smart Infusion Pumps

- Smart infusion pumps, with preprogrammed drug libraries and wireless technology, calculate medication dose and delivery rates to help prevent IV medication errors and reduce the risk of patient harm.
- Smart pumps provide information used in driving safe practices, such as the total number of infusions programmed using the drug library, how many times pumps were manually overridden, or how often an alert resulted in reprogramming an infusion.
- Remember, if you make a mistake and enter incorrect data, you will get incorrect results. Some drugs (e.g., heparin [Hep-Lock]) require that a second nurse confirm the pump settings. Always use your best nursing judgment when using smart infusion pumps or any other technology and follow agency policy.

devices, including endotracheal tubes; and (4) require invasive or noninvasive procedures.[7]

For some critically ill patients (e.g., those needing mechanical ventilation), continuous IV sedation (e.g., propofol [Diprivan]) and an analgesic agent (e.g., fentanyl [Sublimaze]) are effective strategies for sedation and pain control. However, patients getting deep sedation are unresponsive. This prevents you and other health care providers from fully assessing the patient's neurologic status. To address this problem, guidelines should include a daily, scheduled interruption of sedation, or "sedation holiday." These daily interruptions allow you to awaken the patient to conduct a neurologic examination.[8] (Pain management is discussed in Chapter 9.)

Impaired Communication. Inability to communicate is distressing for patients who cannot speak because of the use of sedative and paralyzing drugs or an endotracheal tube. As part of every procedure, explain what will happen or is happening to the patient. When the patient cannot speak, explore alternative methods of communication, such as picture boards, notepads, magic slates, or computer keyboards. When speaking with the patient, look directly at the patient and use hand gestures when appropriate. For patients and caregivers who do not speak English, an approved translator or translator phone service must be provided (see Chapter 4).

Nonverbal communication is important. High levels of procedure-related touch and lower levels of comfort-related touch often characterize the ICU environment. Patients have different levels of tolerance for being touched, usually related to culture and personal history. If appropriate, use comforting touch with ongoing evaluation of the patient's response. Similarly, encourage caregivers to touch and talk with the patient even if the patient is unresponsive.

Sensory-Perceptual Problems. Acute and reversible sensory-perceptual changes are common in ICU patients. The combination of alterations in mentation (e.g., delusions, short attention span, loss of recent memory), psychomotor behavior (e.g., restlessness, lethargy), and sleep-wake cycle (e.g., daytime sleepiness, nighttime agitation) has been inappropriately called *ICU psychosis.* The patient experiencing these changes is not psychotic but is suffering from *delirium.* It is estimated that the prevalence of delirium in ICU patients is as high as 80%.[9] Significant risk factors for delirium include preexisting dementia, history of baseline hypertension or alcohol abuse, and severe illness on admission. Environmental factors that can contribute to delirium include sleep deprivation, anxiety, sensory overload, and immobilization. Physical conditions such as hemodynamic instability, hypoxemia, hypercarbia, electrolyte disturbances, and severe infections can lead to delirium. Last, certain drugs (e.g., sedatives [benzodiazepines], analgesics [opioids], and antimicrobials [aminoglycosides]) have been linked with the development of delirium.[9] (Chapter 60 discusses delirium.)

Monitor all ICU patients for delirium. Assessment tools include the Confusion Assessment Method for the ICU and the Intensive Care Delirium Screening Checklist[9] (both available at *www.icudelirium.org*). It is critical to address physiologic factors (e.g., correction of oxygenation, perfusion, and electrolyte problems). The use of clocks and calendars can help orient the patient. If the patient demonstrates hyperactivity, insomnia, or delusions, management with sedative drugs with anxiolytic effects (e.g., dexmedetomidine [Precedex]) can be considered.[9] In addition, the presence of a caregiver may help orient the patient and reduce agitation. (See eTable 66-1 on the website for this chapter.)

Sensory overload can also result in patient distress and anxiety. Environmental noise levels are particularly high in the ICU.[10] You can limit noise and assist the patient in understanding noises that cannot be prevented. Conversation is a particularly stressful noise, especially when the discussion concerns the patient and is held in the presence of, but without participation from, the patient.[10] Reduce this source of stress by finding suitable places for patient-related discussions. Whenever possible, include the patient or the caregiver in the discussion.

You can also limit noise levels by muting phones, setting alarms based on the patient's condition, and reducing unnecessary alarms. For example, silence the BP alarm when handling invasive lines and then reset the alarm when done. Similarly, silence ventilator alarms when suctioning. Last, limit overhead paging and all unnecessary noise in patient care areas.

Sleep Problems. Nearly all ICU patients have sleep disturbances. Patients may have difficulty falling asleep or have disrupted sleep because of noise, anxiety, pain, frequent monitoring, or treatment procedures. Sleep disturbance has been associated with delirium and delayed recovery.[8,10] Arrange the environment to promote the patient's sleep-wake cycle. Strategies include scheduling rest periods, dimming lights at nighttime, opening curtains during the daytime, getting physiologic measurements without disturbing the patient, limiting noise, and providing comfort measures (e.g., massage).[11] If necessary, use benzodiazepines (e.g., temazepam [Restoril]) and benzodiazepine-like drugs (e.g., zolpidem [Ambien]) to induce and maintain sleep. (Sleep and sleep disorders are discussed in Chapter 8.)

Issues Related to Caregivers

When someone becomes critically ill, care extends beyond the patient to the patient's caregivers. Caregivers play a valuable role in the patient's recovery and are members of the health care team. They contribute to the patient's well-being by

- Providing a link to the patient's personal life (e.g., news of family, job)
- Advising the patient in health care decisions or functioning as the decision maker when the patient cannot
- Helping with activities of daily living (e.g., bathing, oral suctioning)
- Providing positive, loving, and caring support

To be effective in caring for their loved one, caregivers need your guidance and support. The experience of having a friend or relative in the ICU is physically and emotionally difficult, often to the point of exhaustion. Anxiety and concerns regarding the patient's condition, prognosis, and pain are some of the issues caregivers confront. In addition, caregivers commonly experience anxiety over the financial issues related to the provision of care during a critical illness. Consulting with the case manager or social worker is helpful in these instances.

Caregivers often disrupt their daily routines to support the patient. They may be far from their own home, friends, and relatives. Ultimately, caregivers of the critically ill are in crisis, and family-centered care is essential.[12] To provide family-centered care effectively, you must be skilled in crisis intervention. Conduct a family assessment and intervene as necessary. Strategies include active listening, reduction of anxiety, and support of those who become upset or angry. Acknowledge the caregivers' feelings and accept and support their decisions. Consult other health care team members (e.g., chaplains, psychologists, patient representatives) as necessary to help caregivers cope. The extent to which family-centered care is provided can affect the patient's clinical course in the ICU.

The major needs of caregivers of critically ill patients include information, reassurance, and convenience.[13] Lack of information is a major source of anxiety for the caregivers. Assess the caregiver's understanding of the patient's status, treatment plan, and prognosis and provide information as appropriate. Identify a spokesperson for the family to help coordinate information exchange between the health care team and family.

The caregiver needs reassurance regarding the way in which the patient's care is managed and decisions are made. Invite the caregiver to meet the health care team members. Evaluate the appropriateness of including caregivers in interdisciplinary rounds and patient care conferences. It helps caregivers accept and cope with problems when they see that the health care team is caring and competent, decisions are deliberate, and their input is valued. If the patient has an advance directive, the caregiver needs to see that the patient's wishes are followed. If the patient has designated a durable power of attorney for health care, this person must be involved in the patient's plan of care.

Caregivers of critically ill patients need access to the patient. Limiting visitation does not protect the patient from adverse physiologic consequences.[14] AACN strongly recommends less restrictive, individualized visiting policies. This is accomplished by assessing the patient's and caregiver's needs and preferences and incorporating these into the plan of care.[14]

ETHICAL/LEGAL DILEMMAS
Family Presence and Visitation in the Adult ICU

Situation

B.W., a new nurse, is undergoing orientation in the surgical intensive care unit (ICU). He asks his preceptor why the patients' families are permitted on the unit throughout the day and even the night. B.W. states that, in his last position, visiting hours in the ICU were 10 AM to noon and 4 to 6 PM. He adds that families make him nervous when they watch what he is doing and ask him multiple questions. B.W. states that he intends to tell the visitors to leave the patient's room when he is providing care.

Ethical/Legal Points for Consideration

- The majority of nurses in adult ICUs prefer unrestricted visiting policies, but research indicates that most ICU policies limit visitation.
- Family visitation was thought to cause the patient physiologic stress and interfere with care. Additionally, it was believed that family visitation was mentally exhausting to patients and families, and even contributed to increased infection rates. Evidence does not support any of these beliefs.
- Evidence suggests several positive patient benefits to flexible family visitation: decreases in anxiety, confusion, and agitation; reductions in cardiovascular complications; decreases in length of ICU stay; and reports that patients feel more secure and satisfied with care.
- Similar evidence exists for the benefits of flexible visitation for family members: increases in satisfaction, decreases in anxiety, promotion of better communication, and increases in opportunities for patient and family teaching as the family becomes more involved in care.
- Some conditions may require restricting visitation: a legal reason is documented in the chart; visitor behavior presents a risk to the patient, family, staff, or others; visitor behavior disrupts the functioning of the unit; visitor has a contagious illness or has been exposed to a contagious disease that could endanger the patient's health; or the patient requests fewer or no visitors.

Discussion Questions

1. How should the preceptor respond to B.W.'s statement of his intentions?
2. Does B.W. have an ethical or legal obligation to permit family visitation regardless of his personal concerns? Defend your position.

The first time that caregivers visit it is important for you to prepare them for the experience. Briefly describe the patient's appearance and the physical environment (e.g., equipment, noise).[15] Join caregivers as they enter the room, and observe the responses of both the patient and caregivers. Invite the caregivers to participate in the patient's care if they desire. In some ICUs, visitation includes animal-assisted therapy or pet visitation. The positive benefits of these interventions (e.g., decreases in BP and anxiety) far outweigh the risks (e.g., transmission of infection from animal to patient). They should be a part of the visitation policy.

In addition to traditional visiting, caregivers of patients undergoing invasive procedures (e.g., central line insertion) and cardiopulmonary resuscitation (CPR) want the option of being present at the bedside during these events. Even when the outcomes are not favorable, being present helps caregivers overcome doubts about the patient's condition, reduces their anxiety and fear, meets their need to be together and to support their loved one, and aids the grief process if death occurs. AACN encourages critical care nurses to develop policies and procedures that provide for the option of family presence during invasive procedures and CPR.[16]

CULTURALLY COMPETENT CARE

CRITICAL CARE PATIENTS

Providing culturally competent care to critically ill patients and caregivers is challenging. Often, meeting the patient's physiologic needs is a priority and overshadows the influence of the patient's culture on the illness experience. It remains important to consider the cultural aspects of the meaning of sickness and health, pain, dying and death, and grief when caring for critically ill patients and their caregivers (see Chapter 2).

Cultural perspectives on dying and death are complex. Telling some patients that they are dying as a way of letting them prepare for death may infringe on the family's role. Others view a discussion about advance directives as a legal device to deny care.

Customs surrounding dying and death vary widely. Caregiver requests may range from asking you to leave a window open so the spirit of the dead person can leave, to providing the final bath for the deceased. Ask the caregivers about the family's cultural traditions when caring for the dying patient. Several variables influence the expressions of grief that follow the loss of a loved one. These include the relationship between the grieving person and the deceased, whether the loss is sudden or anticipated, the support systems available to the grieving person, past experiences with loss, and the person's religious and cultural beliefs. Proceed cautiously when approaching patients facing death and their caregivers. Asking patients, "What do you want to know?" and "Who do you want with you when discussing options?" are good starting points.[17] (Chapter 10 provides additional information about end-of-life care.)

HEMODYNAMIC MONITORING

Hemodynamic monitoring is the measurement of pressure, flow, and oxygenation within the cardiovascular system. The purpose of hemodynamic monitoring is to assess heart function, fluid balance, and the effects of fluids and drugs on CO. Both invasive (internally placed devices) and noninvasive (external devices) hemodynamic parameters (values) are obtained. These include systemic and pulmonary arterial pressures, central venous pressure (CVP), pulmonary artery wedge pressure (PAWP) (also known as pulmonary artery occlusive pressure [PAOP]), CO/CI, SV/SV index [SVI], SVV, O$_2$ saturation of the hemoglobin of arterial blood (SaO$_2$), and mixed venous oxygen saturation (SvO$_2$). From these measurements you can calculate several values, including the resistance of the systemic and pulmonary arterial vasculature and O$_2$ content, delivery, and consumption. When you integrate these data, you get a picture of the patient's hemodynamic status and the effect of therapy over time (trends). Make all measurements with attention to technical accuracy. Inaccurate data can result in unnecessary or inappropriate treatment.

Hemodynamic Terminology

Cardiac Output and Cardiac Index. *Cardiac output* (CO) is the volume of blood in liters pumped by the heart in 1 minute.

Cardiac index (CI) is the measurement of the CO adjusted for body surface area (BSA). It is a more precise measurement of the efficiency of the heart's pumping action. Although minor beat-to-beat variations may occur, generally the left and right ventricles pump the same volume. The volume ejected with each heartbeat is the *stroke volume* (SV). Like CI, *stroke volume index* (SVI) is the measurement of SV adjusted for BSA. CO and the forces opposing blood flow determine BP. *Systemic vascular resistance* (SVR) (opposition encountered by the left ventricle) or *pulmonary vascular resistance* (PVR) (opposition encountered by the right ventricle) is the resistance to blood flow by the vessels. Preload, afterload, and contractility (see Chapter 32) determine SV (and thus CO and BP). It is essential that you understand these concepts and relationships. In addition, you must understand the effects of manipulating each of these variables. Table 66-1 presents the formulas and values for common hemodynamic parameters.

TABLE 66-1 RESTING HEMODYNAMIC PARAMETERS

Indicators	Normal Range
Preload	
Right atrial pressure (RAP) or central venous pressure (CVP)	2-8 mm Hg
Pulmonary artery wedge pressure (PAWP) or left atrial pressure (LAP)	6-12 mm Hg
Pulmonary artery diastolic pressure (PADP)	4-12 mm Hg
Right ventricular end-diastolic volume (RVEDV) $= \dfrac{\text{Stroke volume (SV)}}{\text{Right ventricular ejection fraction (RVEF)}}$	100-160 mL
Afterload	
Pulmonary vascular resistance (PVR) $= \dfrac{(\text{Pulmonary artery mean pressure [PAMP]} - \text{PAWP}) \times 80}{\text{Cardiac output (CO)}}$	<250 dynes/sec/cm^{-5}
Pulmonary vascular resistance index (PVRI) $= \dfrac{(\text{PAMP} - \text{PAWP}) \times 80}{\text{Cardiac index (CI)}}$	160-380 dynes/sec/cm^{-5}/m^2
Systemic vascular resistance (SVR) $= \dfrac{(\text{Mean arterial pressure [MAP]} - \text{CVP}) \times 80}{\text{CO}}$	800-1200 dynes/sec/cm^{-5}
Systemic vascular resistance index (SVRI) $= \dfrac{(\text{MAP} - \text{CVP}) \times 80}{\text{CI}}$	1970-2390 dynes/sec/cm^{-5}/m^2
MAP $= \dfrac{\text{Systolic blood pressure} + 2(\text{Diastolic blood pressure})}{3^*}$	70-105 mm Hg
PAMP $= \dfrac{\text{Pulmonary artery systolic pressure (PASP)} + 2\,\text{PADP}}{3^*}$	10-20 mm Hg
Other	
Stroke volume $= \dfrac{\text{CO}}{\text{Heart rate}}$	60-150 mL/beat
Stroke volume index (SVI) $= \dfrac{\text{CI}}{\text{Heart rate}}$	30-65 mL/beat/m^2
Stroke volume variation (SVV) $= \dfrac{\text{SV}_{max} - \text{SV}_{min}}{\text{SV}_{mean}}$	<13%
Heart rate (HR)	60-100 beats/min
CO $=$ SV $\times$ HR	4-8 L/min
CI $= \dfrac{\text{CO}}{\text{Body surface area (BSA)}}$	2.2-4 L/min/m^2
RVEF $= \dfrac{\text{SV}}{\text{RVEDV} \times 100}$	40%-60%
Arterial hemoglobin O$_2$ saturation	95%-100%
Mixed venous hemoglobin O$_2$ saturation	60%-80%
Venous hemoglobin O$_2$ saturation	70%

*This formula is an approximation because it does not take into consideration the heart rate. The monitor looks at the area under the pressure curve, as well as the heart rate, to calculate MAP and PAMP.

Preload. *Preload* is the volume within the ventricle at the end of diastole. Unfortunately, chamber volume measurements are difficult to obtain. Instead, various pressures are used to estimate the volume. Left ventricular preload is called *left ventricular end-diastolic pressure.* PAWP, a measurement of pulmonary capillary pressure, reflects left ventricular end-diastolic pressure under normal conditions (i.e., when there is no mitral valve dysfunction, intracardiac defect, or dysrhythmia). CVP, measured in the right atrium or in the vena cava close to the heart, is the right ventricular preload or right ventricular end-diastolic pressure when there is no tricuspid valve dysfunction, intracardiac defect, or dysrhythmia.

Frank-Starling's law explains the effects of preload and states that the more a myocardial fiber is stretched during filling, the more it shortens during systole and the greater the force of the contraction. As preload increases, force generated in the subsequent contraction increases, and thus SV and CO increase. The greater the preload, the greater the myocardial stretch and the greater the O_2 requirement of the myocardium. Hence, increases in CO via increased preload require increased delivery of O_2 to the myocardium. Remember that the change in SV with preload comes about because of stretching and recoil of the heart muscle. However, the clinical measurement made is not a direct measurement of the muscle length. The measurement is of the pressure at the time of the peak stretch (end diastole) (see Table 66-1). This pressure indirectly indicates the amount of stretch and the volume. This pressure is also important because it indicates pressure in the blood vessels of the lung or in the blood returning to the heart. Diuresis and vasodilation decrease preload, and fluid administration increases preload.

Afterload. *Afterload* refers to the forces opposing ventricular ejection. These forces include systemic arterial pressure, the resistance offered by the aortic valve, and the mass and density of the blood to be moved. Clinically, although the measures fail to include all the components of afterload, SVR and arterial pressure are indices of left ventricular afterload. Similarly, PVR and pulmonary arterial pressure are indices of right ventricular afterload. Increased afterload often results in a decreased CO. CO can be restored and myocardial O_2 needs reduced by decreasing afterload (i.e., decreasing forces opposing contraction). Vasodilator drug therapy (e.g., milrinone [Primacor]) can reduce afterload.

Vascular Resistance. *Systemic vascular resistance* (SVR) is the resistance of the systemic vascular bed. *Pulmonary vascular resistance* (PVR) is the resistance of the pulmonary vascular bed. Both these measures reflect afterload as described earlier and can be adjusted for body size (see Table 66-1).

Contractility. *Contractility* describes the strength of contraction. Contractility is said to increase when preload is unchanged yet the heart contracts more forcefully. Epinephrine, norepinephrine (Levophed), isoproterenol (Isuprel), dopamine (Intropin), dobutamine (Dobutrex), digitalis-like drugs, calcium, and milrinone increase or improve contractility. These drugs are termed *positive inotropes.* Contractility is reduced by *negative inotropes.* Examples include certain drugs (e.g., alcohol, calcium channel blockers, β-adrenergic blockers) and clinical conditions (e.g., acidosis). Increased contractility results in increased SV and increased myocardial O_2 requirements. There are no direct clinical measures of cardiac contractility. Measuring the patient's preload (PAWP) and CO and graphing the results indirectly indicates contractility. If preload, heart rate, and afterload remain constant yet CO changes, con-

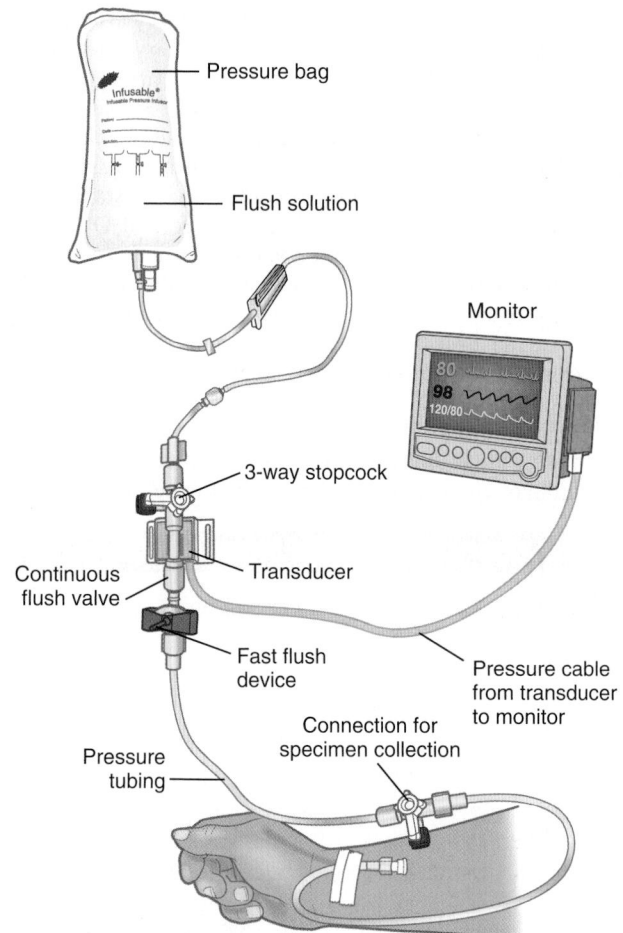

FIG. 66-3 Components of a pressure monitoring system. The cannula, shown entering the radial artery, is connected via pressure (nondistensible) tubing to the transducer. The transducer converts the pressure wave into an electronic signal. The transducer is wired to the electronic monitoring system, which amplifies, conditions, displays, and records the signal. Stopcocks are inserted into the line for specimen withdrawal and for referencing and zero-balancing procedures. A flush system, consisting of a pressurized bag of IV fluid, tubing, and a flush device, is connected to the system. The flush system provides continuous slow (approximately 3 mL/hr) flushing and provides a mechanism for fast flushing of lines.

tractility is changed. Contractility is reduced in the failing heart.

Principles of Invasive Pressure Monitoring

Invasive lines are used in the ICU to measure systemic and pulmonary BPs. Fig. 66-3 shows the components of a typical invasive arterial BP monitoring system. The catheter, pressure tubing, flush system, and transducer are disposable.

Pressure monitoring equipment is referenced and zero balanced to the environment and dynamic response characteristics optimized for accuracy. *Referencing* means positioning the transducer so that the zero reference point is at the level of the atria of the heart. The stopcock nearest the transducer is usually the zero reference for the transducer. To place this level with the atria, use an external landmark, the phlebostatic axis. To identify the *phlebostatic axis,* draw two imaginary lines with the patient supine (Fig. 66-4, *A*). Draw a horizontal line down from the axilla, midway between the anterior and posterior chest walls. Draw a vertical line laterally through the fourth intercos-

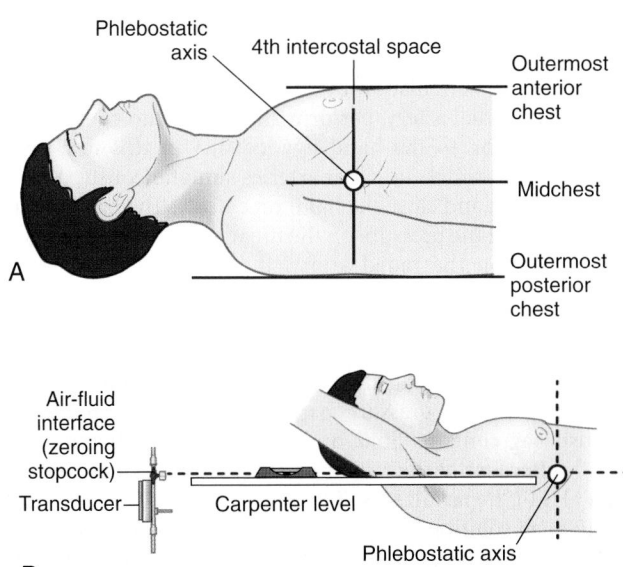

FIG. 66-4 Identification of the phlebostatic axis. **A,** Phlebostatic axis is an external landmark used to identify the level of the atria in the supine patient. It is defined as the intersection of two imaginary lines: one drawn horizontally from the axilla, midway between the anterior and posterior chest walls, and the other drawn vertically through the fourth intercostal space along the lateral chest wall. **B,** Air-fluid interface (zeroing the stopcock) is level with the phlebostatic axis using a carpenter's or laser level.

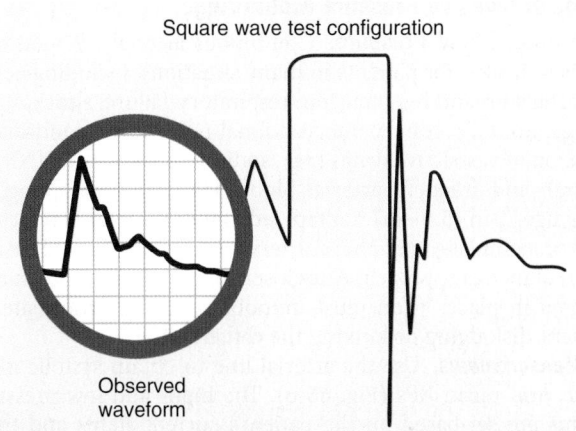

When the fast flush of the continuous flush system is activated and quickly released, a sharp upstroke terminates in a flat line at the maximal indicator on the monitor and hard copy. This is then followed by an immediate rapid downstroke extending below baseline with just 1 or 2 oscillations within 0.12 second (minimal ringing) and a quick return to a baseline. The patient's pressure waveform is also clearly defined with all components of the waveform, such as the dicrotic notch on an arterial waveform, clearly visible.

FIG. 66-5 Optimally damped system. Dynamic response test (square wave test) using the fast flush system: normal response. No adjustment in the monitoring system is required.

tal space along the chest wall. The phlebostatic axis is the intersection of the two imaginary lines. Mark this location on the patient's chest with a permanent marker. Position the port of the stopcock nearest the transducer level with the phlebostatic axis. Tape the transducer to the patient's chest at the phlebostatic axis or mount it on a bedside pole (Fig. 66-4, *B*).

Zeroing confirms that when pressure within the system is zero, the monitor reads zero. To do this, open the reference stopcock to room air (off to the patient) and observe the monitor for a reading of zero. This allows the monitor to use the atmospheric pressure as a reference for zero. Zero the transducer during the initial setup, immediately after insertion of the arterial line, when the transducer has been disconnected from the pressure cable or the pressure cable has been disconnected from the monitor, and when the accuracy of the measurements is questioned. Always follow the manufacturer's guidelines.

Optimizing dynamic response characteristics involves checking that the equipment reproduces, without distortion, a signal that changes rapidly. Perform a *dynamic response test (square wave test)* every 8 to 12 hours and when the system is opened to air or the accuracy of the measurements is questioned. It involves activating the fast flush and checking that the equipment reproduces a distortion-free signal (Fig. 66-5).

Table 66-2 outlines the steps in obtaining BP measurements with an invasive line. Obtain measurements from both digital and printed analog outputs. Readings from a printed pressure tracing at the end of expiration (to limit the effect of the respiratory cycle on arterial BP) are most accurate.[18] Position the patient supine for initial readings. Unless the patient's BP is extremely sensitive to orthostatic changes, values with head-of-bed (HOB) elevation (up to 45 degrees) are generally equal to measurements with the patient supine. Additionally, readings in the prone position are generally accurate. However, there is little support for the accuracy of readings in the lateral posi-

TABLE 66-2	INVASIVE ARTERIAL BLOOD PRESSURE MEASUREMENT

1. Explain the procedure to the patient.
2. Position the patient supine and flat or, if appropriate, with the head of the bed at less than 45 degrees or prone.
3. Confirm that the zero reference (port of the stopcock nearest the transducer) is placed at the level of the phlebostatic axis (see Fig. 66-4). If the reference stopcock is not taped to the patient's chest, use a leveling device to position the stopcock on a bedside pole at the point level with the phlebostatic axis.
4. Observe the monitor tracing and assess the quality of the tracing. Perform a dynamic response test (see Fig. 66-5).
5. Obtain an analog printout, if available, and measure the systolic and diastolic pressures at end expiration (see Fig. 66-6). If no printout is available, freeze the tracing on the oscilloscope screen and use the cursor to measure the pressures at end expiration.
6. Record the pressure measurements promptly, including (if available) the printout marked to identify the points read.

tions.[18] It is not necessary to reposition the patient for each pressure reading. However, it is important to keep the zero reference stopcock level with the phlebostatic axis.

SAFETY ALERT: Positioning the Zero Reference Stopcock
- Mark the location of the phlebostatic axis on the patient's chest with a permanent marker.
- Recheck the leveling of the zero reference stopcock to the phlebostatic axis with any change in the patient's position before obtaining a reading.
- Transducers placed higher than the phlebostatic axis will produce falsely low readings. Transducers placed lower than the phlebostatic axis will produce falsely high readings.

Types of Invasive Pressure Monitoring

Arterial Blood Pressure. Continuous arterial BP monitoring is indicated for patients in many situations, including acute hypertension and hypotension, respiratory failure, shock, neurologic injury, coronary interventional procedures, continuous infusion of vasoactive drugs (e.g., sodium nitroprusside [Nitropress]), and frequent arterial blood gas (ABG) sampling. A 20-gauge, 2-in (5.1-cm) nontapered Teflon catheter is typically used to cannulate a peripheral artery (e.g., radial, femoral) using a percutaneous approach. After insertion, the catheter is usually sutured in place.[18] You must immobilize the insertion site to prevent dislodging or kinking the catheter line.

Measurements. Use the arterial line to obtain systolic, diastolic, and mean BPs (Fig. 66-6). The high- and low-pressure alarms are set based on the patient's current status and then activated. Various patient conditions will change the pressure tracings. In heart failure, the systolic upstroke may be slower. In volume depletion, systolic pressure varies greatly with mechanical ventilation, decreasing during inspiration. Observe simultaneous ECG and pressure tracings with dysrhythmias. Dysrhythmias that significantly diminish arterial BP are more urgent than those that cause only a slight decrease in systolic amplitude.

Complications. Arterial lines carry the risk of hemorrhage, infection, thrombus formation, neurovascular impairment, and loss of limb. Hemorrhage is most likely to occur when the catheter dislodges or the line disconnects. To avoid this serious complication, use Luer-Lok connections, always check the arterial waveform, and activate alarms. If the pressure in the line falls (e.g., when the line is disconnected), the low-pressure alarm sounds immediately, allowing you to promptly correct the problem.

Infection is a risk with any invasive line. To limit the risk of catheter-related infection, inspect the insertion site for local signs of inflammation and monitor the patient for signs of systemic infection. Change the pressure tubing, flush bag, and transducer every 96 hours or according to agency policy. If infection is suspected, remove the catheter and replace the equipment.

Circulatory impairment can result from formation of a thrombus around the catheter, release of an embolus, spasm, or occlusion of the circulation by the catheter. Before inserting a line into the radial artery, perform an *Allen test* to confirm that ulnar circulation to the hand is adequate. In this test, apply pressure to the radial and ulnar arteries simultaneously. Ask the patient to open and close the hand repeatedly. The hand should blanch. Release the pressure on the ulnar artery while maintaining pressure on the radial artery. If pinkness fails to return within 6 seconds, the ulnar artery is inadequate and you should not use the radial artery for line insertion.

To maintain line patency and limit thrombus formation, assess the continuous flush system every 1 to 4 hours to determine that the (1) pressure bag is inflated to 300 mm Hg, (2) flush bag contains fluid, and (3) system is delivering 3 to 6 mL/hr. Because of the risk of heparin-induced thrombocytopenia (HIT), heparinized saline should not be routinely used for the flush solution.[18] (HIT is discussed in Chapter 31.)

Once the catheter is inserted, evaluate the neurovascular status distal to the arterial insertion site hourly. The limb with compromised arterial flow will be cool and pale, with capillary refill time longer than 3 seconds. The patient may have symptoms of neurologic impairment (e.g., paresthesia, pain, paralysis). Neurovascular impairment, which can result in the loss of a limb, is an emergency.

Arterial Pressure–Based Cardiac Output. Arterial pressure–based cardiac output (APCO) monitoring is a minimally invasive technique to determine *continuous CO (CCO)/continuous CI (CCI)*. In addition to measuring CCO, APCO is used to assess a patient's ability to respond to fluids by increasing SV (*preload responsiveness*). This is determined by using *stroke volume variation* (SVV) or by measuring the percent increase in SV after a fluid bolus[19] (see Table 66-1). This technology uses a specialized sensor that attaches to a standard arterial pressure line and a monitor (Fig. 66-7).

SVV is the variation of the arterial pulsation caused by the heart-lung interaction. It is a sensitive indicator of preload responsiveness when used on select patients. SVV is used only for patients on controlled mechanical ventilation with a fixed

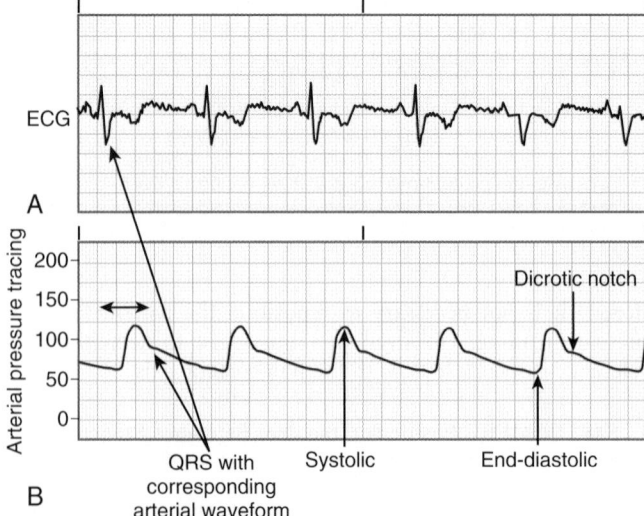

FIG. 66-6 A, Simultaneously recorded electrocardiogram (ECG) tracing and **B,** systemic arterial pressure tracing. Systolic pressure is the peak pressure. The *dicrotic notch* indicates aortic valve closure. Diastolic pressure is the lowest value before contraction. Mean pressure is the average pressure over time calculated by the monitoring equipment.

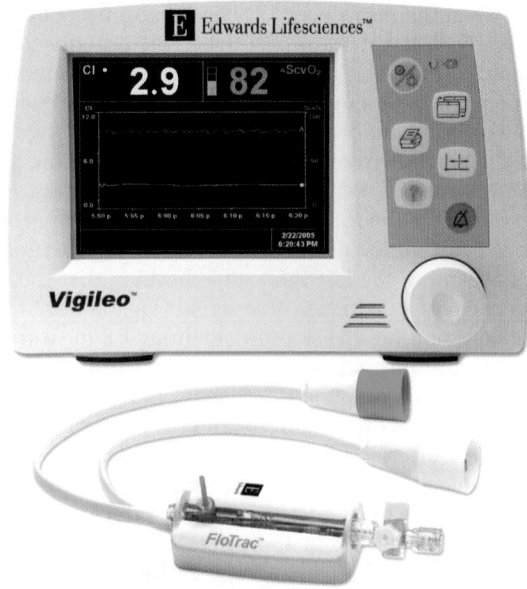

FIG. 66-7 FloTrac sensor and Vigileo monitor. (Courtesy Edwards Lifesciences, Irvine, Calif.)

respiratory rate and a fixed tidal volume of 8 mL/kg. Also, the APCO monitor may not be able to filter certain dysrhythmias—specifically atrial fibrillation—limiting the use of SVV in these patients. These limitations only apply to SVV, not to the use of APCO for CO monitoring.

Measurements. Arterial pressure is the force generated by the ejection of blood from the left ventricle into the arterial circulation. Pulsatile pressure waves are produced by the heart's contractions (systole). The specialized sensor measures the arterial pulse pressure, which is proportional to SV. APCO monitoring uses the arterial waveform characteristics along with patient demographic data (i.e., gender, age, height, and weight) to calculate SV and pulse rate (PR) to calculate CCO/CCI and SV/SVI every 20 seconds. CO is calculated by multiplying the PR and calculated SV and is displayed on a continuous basis.[20] APCO monitoring is frequently used in conjunction with a central venous oximetry catheter. Together, these allow for continuous monitoring of central venous oxygen saturation ($ScvO_2$) and SVR that is derived from the CVP.

APCO is only indicated in adult patients and cannot be used in patients who are on IABP therapy.[20]

Pulmonary Artery Flow-Directed Catheter. Pulmonary artery (PA) pressure monitoring guides the acute-phase management of patients with select complicated heart and lung problems (Table 66-3). PA diastolic (PAD) pressure and PAWP are sensitive indicators of cardiac function and fluid volume status. PAD pressure and PAWP increase in heart failure and fluid volume overload. They decrease with volume depletion. Fluid therapy based on PA pressures can restore fluid balance while avoiding overcorrection or undercorrection of the problem. Monitoring PA pressures permits precise therapeutic manipulation of preload. This allows CO to be maintained without placing the patient at risk for pulmonary edema.

A PA flow-directed catheter (e.g., Swan-Ganz) is used to measure PA pressures, including PAWP. The standard PA catheter is number 7.5F, 43 in (110 cm) long, with multiple lumens (Fig. 66-8). When properly positioned, the distal lumen port (catheter tip) is within the PA. This port is used to monitor PA pressures and sample mixed venous blood (e.g., to evaluate O_2 saturation).

A balloon connected to an external valve surrounds the distal lumen port. Balloon inflation has two purposes: (1) to allow moving blood to float the catheter forward and (2) to allow PAWP measurement. The catheter has one or two proximal lumens, with exit ports in the right atrium or right atrium and right ventricle (if two). The right atrium port is used for

TABLE 66-3	**INDICATIONS AND CONTRAINDICATIONS FOR PULMONARY ARTERY CATHETERIZATION***

Indications
- Assessment of response to therapy in patients with precapillary and mixed types of pulmonary hypertension
- Cardiogenic shock
- Differential diagnosis of pulmonary hypertension
- Myocardial infarction with complications (e.g., heart failure, cardiogenic shock)
- Potentially reversible systolic heart failure (e.g., fulminant myocarditis)
- Severe chronic heart failure requiring inotropic, vasopressor, and vasodilator therapy
- Transplantation work-up

Contraindications
- Coagulopathy
- Endocardial pacemaker
- Endocarditis
- Mechanical tricuspid or pulmonic valve

*List is not all-inclusive.

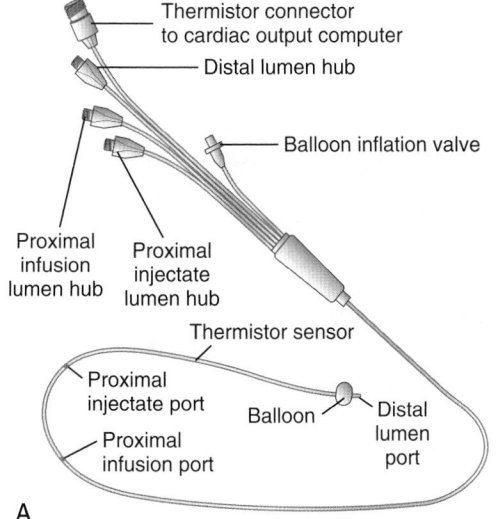

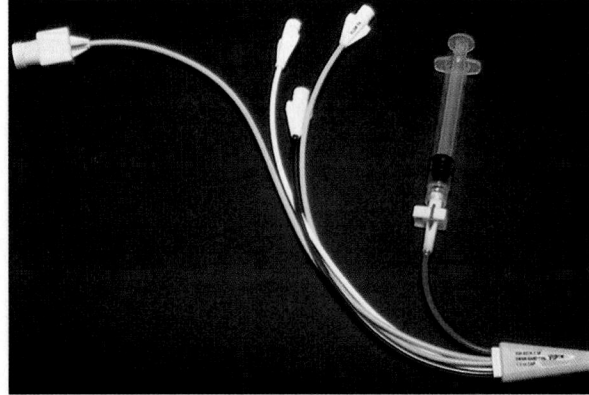

FIG. 66-8 Pulmonary artery (PA) catheter. **A,** Illustrated catheter has five lumens. When properly positioned, the distal lumen exit port is in the PA and the proximal lumen ports are in the right atrium and right ventricle. The distal and one of the proximal ports are used to measure PA and central venous pressures, respectively. A balloon surrounds the catheter near the distal end. The balloon inflation valve is used to inflate the balloon with air to allow reading of the pulmonary artery wedge pressure. A thermistor located near the distal tip senses PA temperature and is used to measure thermodilution cardiac output when solution cooler than body temperature is injected into a proximal port. **B,** Photo of an actual catheter. (**B,** Courtesy Edwards Critical Care Division, Baxter Healthcare Corporation, Santa Ana, Calif.)

measurement of CVP, injection of fluid for CO determination, and withdrawal of blood specimens. The second proximal port (if available) is used for infusion of fluids and drugs or blood sampling. A thermistor (temperature sensor) is located near the distal tip and is wired to an external connector. This is used to monitor blood or core temperature and for the thermodilution method of measuring CO.[21]

In addition to providing most of the same functions as the standard PA catheter, the advanced technology PA catheter can continuously monitor the patient's SvO_2. This provides a global indicator of the balance between oxygen delivery and oxygen consumption. CCO and right ventricular EF (RVEF) also can be measured using advanced thermodilution technology. RVEF provides information regarding RV function and helps to assess right heart contractility. RV end-diastolic volume is continuously measured by dividing SV by RVEF (see Table 66-1). This serves as a key indicator of preload.

The PA catheter sheath (introducer) usually has a side port that serves as a large-bore IV line. Most catheters have a plastic "sleeve" connected to the sheath. This allows the catheter to be advanced or pulled back while maintaining sterility. The physician or other qualified health care provider (e.g., ACNP) usually manipulates the PA catheter, but this practice varies by agency.

Pulmonary Artery Catheter Insertion. Before PA catheter insertion, note the patient's electrolyte, acid-base, oxygenation, and coagulation status. Imbalances such as hypokalemia, hypomagnesemia, hypoxemia, or acidosis can make the heart more irritable and increase the risk of ventricular dysrhythmia during catheter insertion. Coagulopathy increases the risk of hemorrhage. Preparation for the procedure includes arranging the monitor, cables, and infusion and pressurized flush solutions. The system is zero referenced to the phlebostatic axis. The physician or other health care provider explains the procedure to the patient and obtains informed consent. The patient is positioned supine and flat. The PA catheter is inserted through a sheath percutaneously into the internal jugular, subclavian, antecubital, or femoral vein using surgical asepsis. Venous cutdown is rarely required. The catheter is advanced through the venous system to the right side of the heart.

Continuously observe the characteristic waveforms on the monitor as the catheter is moved through the heart to the PA (Fig. 66-9). When the tip reaches the right atrium, the balloon is inflated. Inflation of the balloon should not exceed the balloon's capacity (1.5 mL of air). The catheter is then "floated" through the tricuspid valve into the right ventricle and then through the pulmonic valve to the PA. Monitor the ECG continuously during insertion because of the risk for dysrhythmias, particularly when the catheter reaches the right ventricle. Once a typical PAWP tracing is observed, the balloon is deflated, and the PA waveform should return on the monitor. After insertion and before using the PA catheter, a chest x-ray must confirm the catheter's position. To maintain the catheter in its proper position, secure it at the point of entry into the skin. Note and record the measurement at the exit point. Finally, apply an occlusive dressing, and then change it according to agency policy.

Recently, the use of PA pressure monitoring has decreased dramatically. This is due, in part, to risks associated with the technology (e.g., infection) and the development of less invasive techniques (e.g., APCO monitoring). More detailed information about PA pressure monitoring is available as an eSupplement on the website for this chapter.

Central Venous or Right Atrial Pressure Measurement. CVP is a measurement of right ventricular preload and reflects fluid volume problems. It is most often measured with a central venous catheter placed in the internal jugular or subclavian vein. It can be measured with a PA catheter using the proximal lumen located in the right atrium. CVP waveforms (Fig. 66-10) are similar to PAWP waveforms. CVP is measured as a mean pressure at the end of expiration. An elevated CVP indicates

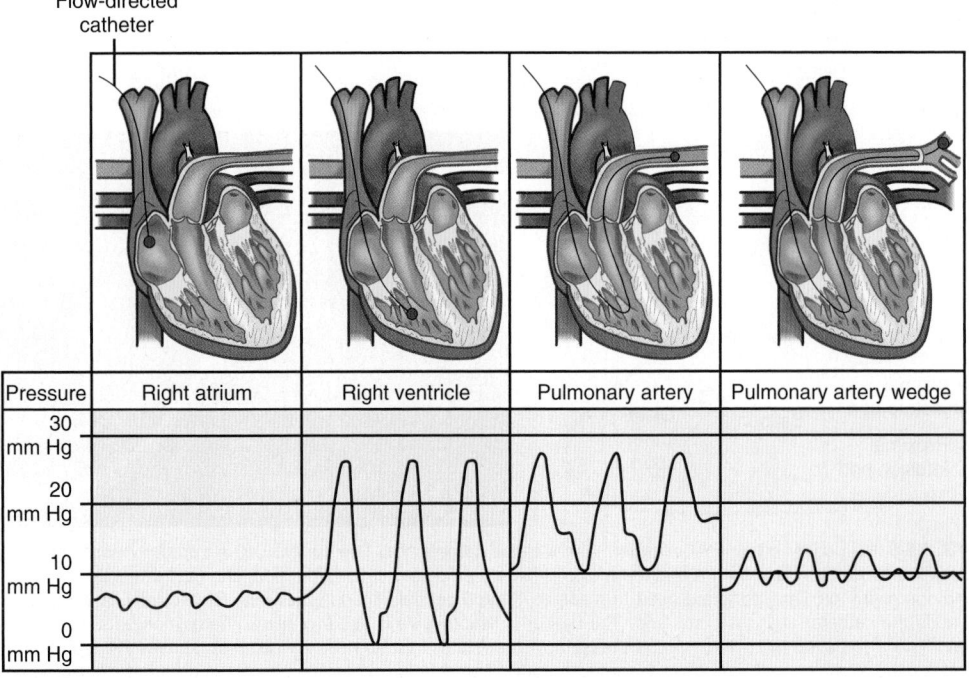

Flow-directed catheter

FIG. 66-9 Position of the pulmonary artery flow-directed catheter during progressive stages of insertion with corresponding pressure waveforms.

right ventricular failure or volume overload. A low CVP indicates hypovolemia.

Venous Oxygen Saturation Monitoring. Both CVP and PA catheters can include sensors to measure O_2 saturation of hemoglobin in venous blood. The O_2 saturation of venous blood from the CVP catheter is termed *central venous oxygen saturation* ($ScvO_2$). Similarly, the O_2 saturation of blood from the PA catheter is termed *mixed venous oxygen saturation* (SvO_2). Either measurement is useful in determining the adequacy of tissue oxygenation. $ScvO_2/SvO_2$ reflects the balance between oxygenation of the arterial blood, tissue perfusion, and tissue O_2 consumption. $ScvO_2/SvO_2$ is useful in assessing hemodynamic status and response to treatments or activities when considered in conjunction with arterial O_2 saturation (Table 66-4). Normal $ScvO_2/SvO_2$ at rest is 60% to 80%.

Carefully review sustained decreases and increases in $ScvO_2/SvO_2$. Decreased $ScvO_2/SvO_2$ may indicate decreased arterial oxygenation, low CO, low hemoglobin level, or increased O_2 consumption or extraction. If the $ScvO_2/SvO_2$ falls below 60%, determine which of these factors has changed. Observe for changes in arterial oxygenation (e.g., monitor pulse oximetry or ABGs) and indirectly assess CO and tissue perfusion. This is done by noting any changes in mental status, strength and quality of peripheral pulses, capillary refill, urine output, and skin color and temperature. If arterial oxygenation, CO, and hemoglobin level are unchanged, a fall in $ScvO_2/SvO_2$ indicates increased O_2 consumption or extraction. This could represent an increased metabolic rate, pain, movement, or fever. If O_2 consumption increases without a comparable increase in O_2 delivery, more O_2 is extracted from the blood, and $ScvO_2/SvO_2$ will continue to fall.[22]

Increased $ScvO_2/SvO_2$ is also clinically significant and may indicate a clinical improvement (e.g., increased arterial O_2 saturation, improved perfusion, decreased metabolic rate) or problem (e.g., sepsis). In sepsis, O_2 is not extracted properly at the tissue level, resulting in increased $ScvO_2/SvO_2$.

Your interventions are guided by changes in $ScvO_2/SvO_2$. For example, you might note that the patient's heart rate increased moderately during repositioning but that the $ScvO_2/SvO_2$ remained stable. In this case, you would conclude that the patient tolerated the position change. If the $ScvO_2/SvO_2$ had dropped, this would be an indication to stop the activity until the $ScvO_2/SvO_2$ returns to baseline.

In many cases, as activity or metabolism increases, heart rate and CO increase, and $ScvO_2/SvO_2$ remains constant or varies slightly. However, critically ill patients often have conditions (e.g., heart failure, shock) that prevent substantial increases in CO. In these cases, $ScvO_2/SvO_2$ can be a useful indicator of the balance between O_2 delivery and consumption.

Noninvasive Arterial Oxygenation Monitoring

Pulse oximetry is a noninvasive and continuous method of determining the oxygen saturation of hemoglobin (SpO_2). Monitoring SpO_2 may reduce the frequency of ABG sampling (see Chapter 26). SpO_2 is normally 95% to 100%. Accurate SpO_2 measurements may be difficult to obtain on patients who are hypothermic, receiving IV vasopressor therapy (e.g., norepinephrine), or experiencing hypoperfusion and vasoconstriction (e.g., shock). Consider alternative locations for placement of the pulse oximetry probe (e.g., forehead, earlobe).

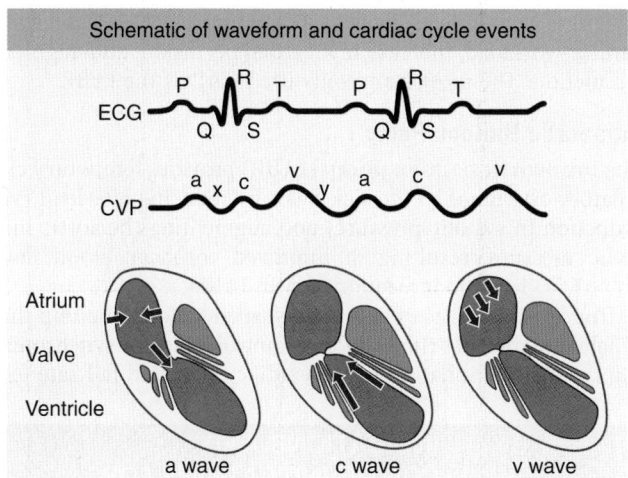

FIG. 66-10 Cardiac events that produce the central venous pressure (CVP) waveform with *a*, *c*, and *v* waves. The *a* wave represents atrial contraction. The *x* descent represents atrial relaxation. The *c* wave represents the bulging of the closed tricuspid valve into the right atrium during ventricular systole. The *v* wave represents atrial filling. The *y* descent represents opening of the tricuspid valve and filling of the ventricle.

TABLE 66-4	**INTERPRETATION OF $ScvO_2/SvO_2$* MEASUREMENTS**	
$ScvO_2/SvO_2$ Measurement	**Physiologic Basis for Change in $ScvO_2/SvO_2$**	**Clinical Diagnosis and Rationale**
High $ScvO_2/SvO_2$ (80%-95%)	Increased O_2 supply Decreased O_2 demand	• Patient receiving more O_2 than required by clinical condition • Anesthesia, which causes sedation and decreased muscle movement • Hypothermia, which lowers metabolic demand (e.g., with cardiopulmonary bypass) • Sepsis caused by decreased ability of tissues to use O_2 at the cellular level • False high positive because pulmonary artery catheter is wedged in a pulmonary capillary (SvO_2 only)
Normal $ScvO_2/SvO_2$ (60%-80%)	Normal O_2 supply and metabolic demand	• Balanced O_2 supply and demand
Low $ScvO_2/SvO_2$ (<60%)	Decreased O_2 supply caused by • Low hemoglobin • Low arterial saturation (SaO_2) • Low cardiac output • Increased O_2 demand	• Anemia or bleeding with compromised cardiopulmonary system • Hypoxemia resulting from decreased O_2 supply or lung disease • Cardiogenic shock caused by left ventricular pump failure • Metabolic demand exceeds O_2 supply in conditions that increase muscle movement and metabolic rate, including physiologic states such as shivering, seizures, and hyperthermia and nursing interventions such as being weighed on a bedside scale and turning

Source: Urden LD, Lough ME, Stacy KM: *Critical care nursing: diagnosis and management*, ed 6, St Louis, 2010, Mosby.
*$ScvO_2$ values are generally slightly higher than SvO_2 values.

A common use for pulse oximetry is to evaluate the effectiveness of O_2 therapy. Decreased SpO_2 indicates inadequate oxygenation of the blood in the pulmonary capillaries. You can correct this by increasing the fraction of inspired oxygen (FIO_2) and evaluating the patient's response. Similarly, use SpO_2 to monitor how the patient tolerates decreases in FIO_2 and responds to interventions. For example, if SpO_2 falls when you position the patient in a left lateral recumbent position, plan position changes that pose less risk for the patient.

Noninvasive Hemodynamic Monitoring: Impedance Cardiography

Impedance cardiography (ICG) is a continuous or intermittent, noninvasive method of obtaining CO and assessing thoracic fluid status. Based on the concepts of *impedance* (the resistance to the flow of electric current [Ω]), ICG uses four sets of external electrodes to deliver a high-frequency, low-amplitude current that is similar to that used in apnea monitors. Blood is an excellent conductor of electricity (lower impedance), and pulsatile blood flow generates electrical impedance changes. ICG measures the change in impedance ($d\Omega$) in the ascending aorta and left ventricle over time (dt) and is represented as $d\Omega/dt$. Ωo is the measurement of the average impedance of the fluid in the thorax. Impedance-based hemodynamic parameters (CO, SV, and SVR) are calculated from Ωo, $d\Omega/dt$, mean arterial pressure (MAP), CVP, and the ECG.

Major indications for ICG include early signs and symptoms of pulmonary or cardiac dysfunction, differentiation of cardiac or pulmonary cause of shortness of breath, evaluation of etiology and management of hypotension, monitoring after discontinuing a PA catheter or justification for insertion of a PA catheter, evaluation of drug therapy, and diagnosis of rejection after cardiac transplantation. ICG is not recommended in patients who have generalized edema or third spacing because the excess volume interferes with accurate signals.

NURSING MANAGEMENT HEMODYNAMIC MONITORING

Assessment of hemodynamic status requires integrating data from many sources and trending these data over time. Thorough, basic nursing observations provide important clues about the patient's hemodynamic status. Begin by obtaining baseline data regarding the patient's general appearance, level of consciousness, skin color and temperature, vital signs, peripheral pulses, capillary refill, and urine output. Does the patient appear tired, weak, exhausted? There may be too little cardiac reserve to sustain even minimum activity. Pallor, cool skin, and diminished pulses may indicate decreased CO. Changes in mental status may reflect problems with cerebral perfusion or oxygenation. Monitor urine output to determine the adequacy of perfusion to the kidneys. The patient with diminished perfusion to the GI tract may develop hypoactive or absent bowel sounds. If the patient is bleeding and developing shock, BP might initially be relatively stable, yet the patient may become increasingly pale and cool from peripheral vasoconstriction. Conversely, the patient experiencing septic shock may remain warm and pink yet develop tachycardia and BP instability. Elevated heart rates are common in stressed, compromised, critically ill patients. However, sustained tachycardia increases myocardial O_2 demand and can result in decreased CO.

Always correlate observational data with data obtained from biotechnology (e.g., ECG, arterial and PA pressures, $ScvO_2$/SvO_2). Single hemodynamic values are rarely helpful. You must monitor trends in these values and evaluate the whole clinical picture with the goals of recognizing early clues and intervening before problems escalate.

CIRCULATORY ASSIST DEVICES

Mechanical **circulatory assist devices (CADs)**, such as the intraaortic balloon pump (IABP) and left or right ventricular assist device (VAD), are used to decrease cardiac work and improve organ perfusion in patients with heart failure when conventional drug therapy is no longer adequate. The type of device used depends on the extent and nature of the heart problem. CADs provide interim support in three types of situations: (1) the left, right, or both ventricles require support while recovering from acute injury (e.g., postcardiotomy); (2) the patient must be stabilized before surgical repair of the heart (e.g., a ruptured septum); and (3) the heart has failed, and the patient is awaiting cardiac transplantation. All CADs decrease cardiac workload, increase myocardial perfusion, and augment circulation. The most commonly used CAD is the IABP.

Intraaortic Balloon Pump

The **intraaortic balloon pump (IABP)** provides temporary circulatory assistance to the sick heart by reducing afterload (via reduction in systolic pressure) and augmenting the aortic diastolic pressure, resulting in improved coronary blood flow. Table 66-5 lists the indications for an IABP.

The IABP consists of a sausage-shaped balloon, a pump that inflates and deflates the balloon, a control panel for synchronizing the balloon inflation to the cardiac cycle, and fail-safe fea-

TABLE 66-5	INDICATIONS AND CONTRAINDICATIONS FOR IABP THERAPY*

Indications
- Refractory unstable angina (when drugs have failed)
- Short-term bridge to heart transplantation
- Acute myocardial infarction with any of the following:†
  - Ventricular aneurysm accompanied by ventricular dysrhythmias
  - Acute ventricular septal defect
  - Acute mitral valve dysfunction
  - Cardiogenic shock
  - Refractory chest pain with or without ventricular dysrhythmias
- Preoperative, intraoperative, and postoperative cardiac surgery (e.g., prophylaxis before surgery, failure to wean from cardiopulmonary bypass, left ventricular failure after cardiopulmonary bypass)
- High-risk interventional cardiology procedures

Contraindications
- Irreversible brain damage
- Major coagulopathy (e.g., disseminated intravascular coagulation [DIC])
- Terminal or untreatable diseases of any major organ system
- Abdominal aortic and thoracic aneurysms
- Moderate to severe aortic insufficiency
- Generalized peripheral vascular disease (e.g., aortoiliac disease)‡

*List is not all-inclusive.
†Allows time for emergent angiography and corrective cardiac surgery to be performed.
‡May inhibit placement of balloon and is considered a relative contraindication; sheathless insertion may be used.

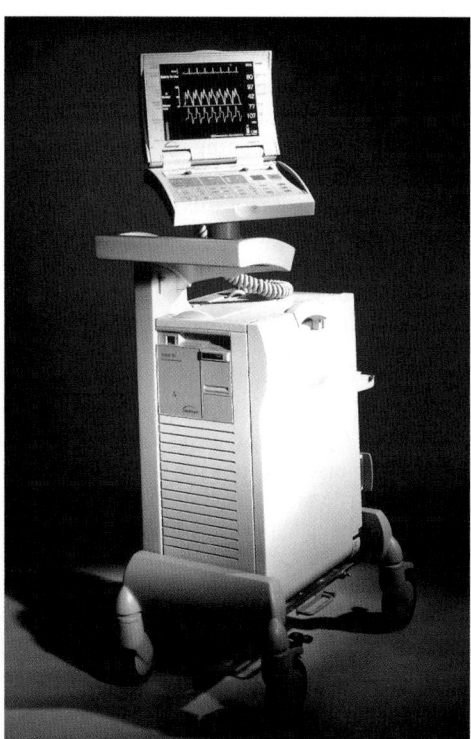

FIG. 66-11 Intraaortic balloon pump machine. (Courtesy Datascope Corp, Fairfield, NJ.)

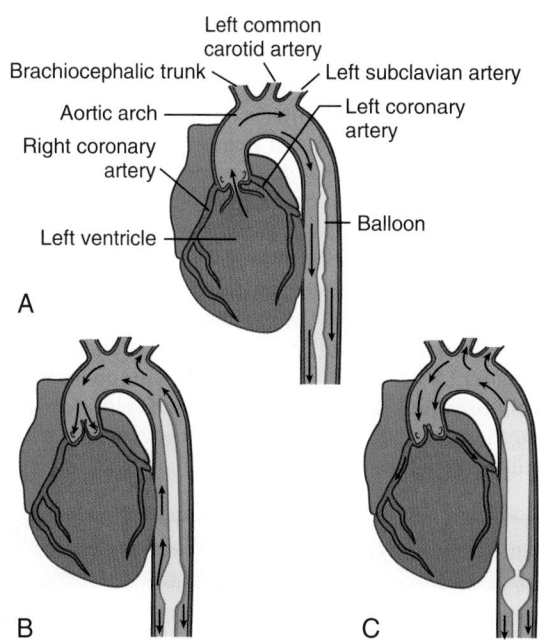

FIG. 66-12 Intraaortic balloon pump. **A,** During systole the balloon is deflated, which facilitates ejection of blood into the periphery. **B,** In early diastole, the balloon begins to inflate. **C,** In late diastole, the balloon is totally inflated, which augments aortic pressure and increases the coronary perfusion pressure with the end result of increased coronary and cerebral blood flow.

tures (Fig. 66-11). The balloon is inserted percutaneously or surgically into the femoral artery. It is moved toward the heart and placed in the descending thoracic aorta just below the left subclavian artery and above the renal arteries (Fig. 66-12). After placement, an x-ray confirms the position. A pneumatic device fills the balloon with helium at the start of diastole (immediately after aortic valve closure) and deflates it just before the next systole. The ECG is the trigger used to start the deflation on the upstroke of the R wave (of the QRS) and inflation on the T wave. The dicrotic notch of the arterial pressure tracing is used to refine timing (see eFig. 66-4 on the website for this chapter). IABP therapy is known as *counterpulsation* because the timing of balloon inflation is opposite to ventricular contraction. The IABP assist ratio is 1:1 in the acute phase of treatment, meaning that one IABP cycle of inflation and deflation occurs for every heartbeat.

Effects of Counterpulsation. In late diastole when the balloon is totally inflated, blood is forcibly displaced distal to the extremities and proximal to the coronary arteries and main branches of the aortic arch. Diastolic arterial pressure rises (diastolic augmentation), increasing coronary artery perfusion pressure and perfusion of vital organs. The rise in coronary artery perfusion pressure causes an increase in blood flow to the myocardium. The balloon is rapidly deflated just before systole. This creates a vacuum that causes aortic pressure to drop. When aortic resistance to left ventricular ejection is reduced (reduced afterload), the left ventricle empties more easily and completely. As with other types of afterload reduction, the SV increases, yet the myocardial O_2 consumption decreases. Table 66-6 summarizes the hemodynamic effects of IABP therapy.

Complications With IABP Therapy. Vascular injuries such as dislodgment of plaque, aortic dissection, and compromised distal circulation are common with IABP therapy. Thrombus

TABLE 66-6 HEMODYNAMIC EFFECTS OF COUNTERPULSATION

Effects of Inflation During Diastole
- Increased diastolic pressure (may exceed systolic pressure)
- Increased pressure in the aortic root during diastole
- Increased coronary artery perfusion pressure
- Improved O_2 delivery to the myocardium
  - Decreased angina
  - Decreased electrocardiographic evidence of ischemia
  - Decreased ventricular ectopy

Effects of Deflation During Systole
- Decreased afterload
- Decreased peak systolic pressure
- Decreased myocardial O_2 consumption
- Increased stroke volume, possibly associated with
  - Improved mentation
  - Warm skin
  - Increased urine output
  - Decreased heart rate
- Increased forward flow of blood, decreasing preload
  - Decreased PA pressures, including PAWP
  - Decreased crackles

PA, Pulmonary artery; *PAWP,* PA wedge pressure.

and embolus formation add to the risk of circulatory compromise to the extremity. The action of the IABP can also destroy platelets and cause thrombocytopenia. Peripheral nerve damage can occur, particularly when a cutdown is performed for insertion. Movement of the balloon can block the left subclavian, renal, or mesenteric arteries. This can result in a weak or absent radial pulse, decreased urine output, and reduced or absent bowel sounds. Patients receiving IABP therapy are prone to infection. Local or systemic signs of infection require catheter removal.[23] To reduce these complications, perform cardiovascular, neurovascular, and hemodynamic assessments every 15 to 60 minutes, depending on the patient's status (Table 66-7).

Mechanical complications from IABP are rare but can occur. Improper timing of balloon inflation may cause increased afterload, decreased CO, myocardial ischemia, and increased myocardial O_2 demand. These complications must be recognized immediately. If the balloon develops a leak, the pump will automatically stop. The catheter is promptly removed to avoid an embolus. Signs of a leak include less effective augmentation, repeated alarms for gas loss, and blood backing up into the catheter. A malfunction of the balloon or console triggers failsafe alarms and automatically shuts down the unit.

The patient with an IABP is relatively immobile, limited to side-lying or supine positions with the HOB elevated less than 45 degrees. The patient may be receiving ventilatory support and will likely have multiple invasive lines that increase the

challenge of comfortable positioning. The patient may experience sleeplessness and anxiety. Adequate sedation, pain relief, skin care, and comfort measures are essential.

As the patient improves, circulatory support provided by the IABP is gradually reduced. Weaning involves reducing the IABP assist ratio from 1:1 to 1:2 and assessing the patient's response (see eFig. 66-4 on the website for this chapter). If hemodynamic parameters remain stable, the ratio can be changed from 1:2 to 1:3 until the IABP catheter is removed. Pumping is continued until the line is removed even if the patient is stable. This reduces the risk of thrombus formation around the catheter.

Ventricular Assist Devices

The **ventricular assist device (VAD)** provides short- and long-term support for the failing heart and allows more mobility than the IABP. VADs are inserted into the path of flowing blood to augment or replace the action of the ventricle. Some VADs are implanted internally (e.g., peritoneum), and others are positioned externally. A typical VAD shunts blood from the left atrium or ventricle to the device and then to the aorta. Some VADs provide right or biventricular support (Fig. 66-13).

Failure to wean from cardiopulmonary bypass (CPB) after surgery is a primary indicator for VAD support. VADs are also used to support patients with ventricular failure caused by myocardial infarction and patients awaiting heart transplantation. A VAD is a temporary device that can partially or totally support circulation until the heart recovers or a donor heart is obtained. Cannula sites depend on the type of device used. For support of the right side of the heart, the right atrium and PA are cannulated. The left ventricular apex can be cannulated for left VADs. Direct cannulation of the atria and great vessels occurs in the operating room through a sternotomy.

Appropriate patient selection for VAD therapy is critical. Indications include (1) failure to wean from CPB or postcardiotomy cardiogenic shock, (2) a bridge to recovery or heart transplantation, and (3) patients with New York Heart Association Class IV heart disease (see Table 35-5) who have failed

TABLE 66-7	**MANAGING COMPLICATIONS OF IABP THERAPY**
Potential Complications	**Nursing Interventions**
Site infection from invasive lines	• Use strict aseptic technique for insertion and dressing changes for all lines. • Cover all insertion sites with occlusive dressings. • Administer prescribed prophylactic antibiotic for entire course of therapy.
Pneumonia associated with immobilization	• Reposition patient q2hr, being careful not to displace balloon. • If patient requires chest physiotherapy, avoid introducing ECG artifact.
Arterial trauma caused by insertion or displacement of balloon	• Evaluate and mark peripheral pulses before insertion of balloon to use as baseline for assessing pulses after insertion. • After insertion of balloon, evaluate perfusion to both upper and lower extremities at least every hour. • Measure urine output at least every hour (occlusion of renal arteries causes severe decrease in urine output). • Observe arterial waveforms for sudden changes. • Keep head of bed no higher than 45 degrees. • Do not flex cannulated leg at the hip. • Immobilize cannulated leg to prevent flexion using a draw sheet tucked under the mattress, soft ankle restraint, or knee immobilizer.
Thromboembolism caused by trauma, balloon obstruction of blood flow distal to catheter	• Administer prophylactic heparin if ordered. • Evaluate pulses, urine output, and level of consciousness at least every hour. • Check circulation, sensation, and movement in both legs at least every hour.
Hematologic complications caused by platelet aggregation along the balloon (e.g., thrombocytopenia)	• Monitor coagulation profiles, hematocrit, and platelet count.
Hemorrhage from insertion site	• Check site for bleeding at least every hour. • Monitor vital signs for signs of hypovolemia with each check.
Balloon leak or rupture	• Prepare for emergent removal and possible reinsertion.

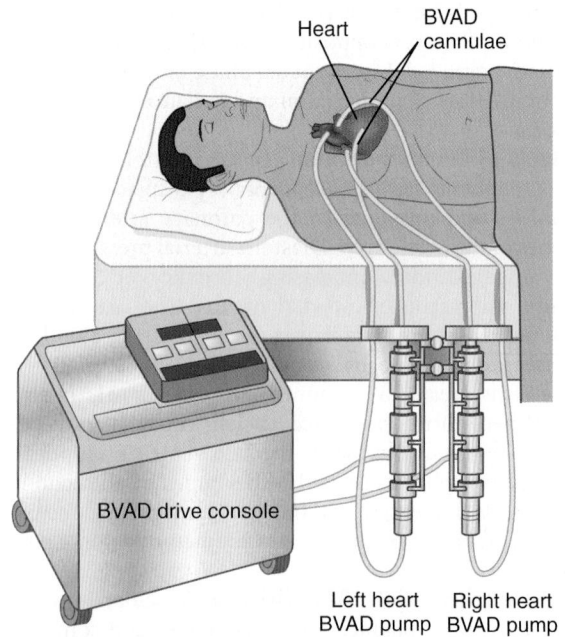

FIG. 66-13 Schematic diagram of a biventricular assist device (BVAD).

Heart

BVAD cannulae

BVAD drive console

Left heart BVAD pump   Right heart BVAD pump

medical therapy. Relative contraindications for VAD therapy include (1) BSA less than manufacturer's limit (e.g., 1.3 m²), (2) renal or liver failure unrelated to a cardiac event, and (3) co-morbidities that would limit life expectancy to less than 3 years.[24]

Implantable Artificial Heart

Every year about 2200 patients receive cardiac transplants, yet the demand for heart transplants far exceeds the supply. Research on mechanical CADs has led to the development of a fully implantable artificial heart that can sustain the body's circulatory system. This device is used to replace the hearts of patients who are not eligible for a transplant and have no other treatment alternative. One major advantage of the artificial heart compared with heart transplantation is decreased costs for implantation and drug therapies. Patients do not require immunosuppression therapy and thus do not experience its inevitable, long-term effects. However, patients do require lifelong anticoagulation.[25]

NURSING MANAGEMENT CIRCULATORY ASSIST DEVICES

The patient with an IABP requires highly skilled nursing care. Perform frequent and thorough cardiovascular assessments. These include measurement of hemodynamic parameters (e.g., arterial BP, CO/CI, SVR), auscultation of the heart and lungs, and evaluation of the ECG (e.g., rate, rhythm). Assess for adequate tissue perfusion (e.g., skin color and temperature, mental status, capillary refill, peripheral pulses, urine output, bowel sounds) at regular intervals. It is expected that IABP therapy will improve these findings.

Nursing care of the patient with a VAD is similar to that of the patient with an IABP. Observe the patient for bleeding, cardiac tamponade, ventricular failure, infection, dysrhythmias, renal failure, hemolysis, and thromboembolism. Unlike the patient with an IABP, who must remain in bed with limited position change, the patient with VAD may be mobile and require an activity plan. In some cases, patients with VADs may go home. Preparation for discharge is complex and requires in-depth teaching about the device and support equipment

(e.g., battery chargers). A competent caregiver must be present at all times.

Ideally, patients with CADs will recover through ventricular improvement, heart transplantation, or artificial heart implantation. However, many patients die, or the decision to terminate the device is made and death follows. Both the patient and caregiver require emotional support. Consult other members of the health care team, such as social workers or clergy, as appropriate.

ARTIFICIAL AIRWAYS

Patients in the ICU often need mechanical assistance to maintain airway patency. Inserting a tube into the trachea, bypassing upper airway and laryngeal structures, creates an artificial airway. The tube is placed into the trachea via the mouth or nose past the larynx (endotracheal [ET] intubation) or through a stoma in the neck (tracheostomy). ET intubation is more common in ICU patients than a tracheostomy. It is performed quickly and safely at the bedside. Indications for ET intubation include (1) upper airway obstruction (e.g., secondary to burns, tumor, bleeding), (2) apnea, (3) high risk of aspiration, (4) ineffective clearance of secretions, and (5) respiratory distress. Fig. 66-14 shows the parts of an ET tube.

A *tracheotomy* is a surgical procedure that is performed when the need for an artificial airway is expected to be long term. There is ongoing debate regarding the timing of a tracheotomy in the patient requiring an ET tube. Research suggests that early tracheotomy (2 to 10 days) may have advantages over delayed tracheotomy, particularly when mechanical ventilation is predicted to be needed for longer than 10 to 14 days.[26] The situation varies with the patient, physician, and institution. Chapter 27 discusses tracheostomy tubes and related nursing management.

Endotracheal Tubes

In *oral intubation* the ET tube is passed through the mouth and vocal cords and into the trachea with the aid of a laryngoscope or a bronchoscope. In *nasal ET intubation* the ET is placed blindly (i.e., without seeing the larynx) through the nose, nasopharynx, and vocal cords. Oral ET intubation is preferred for

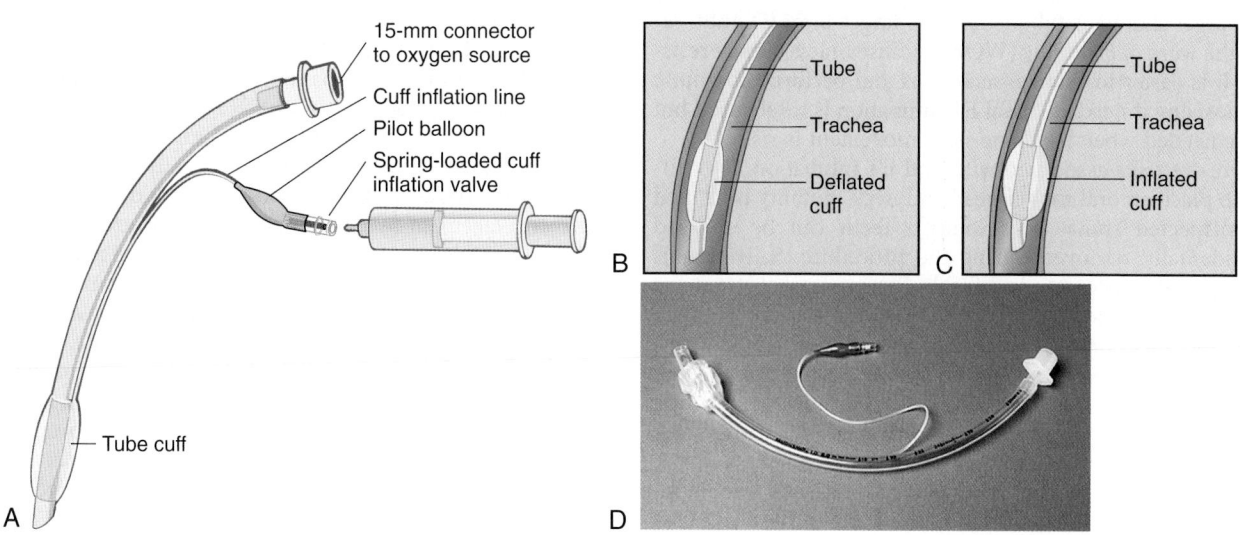

FIG. 66-14 Endotracheal tube. **A,** Parts of an endotracheal tube. **B,** Tube in place with cuff deflated. **C,** Tube in place with the cuff inflated. **D,** Photo of tube before placement.

Translating Research Into Practice

Does Timing of Tracheotomy Affect Critically Ill Patient Outcomes?

Clinical Question
In critically ill patients (P) what is the effect of an early tracheotomy (I) vs. late tracheotomy (C) on short-term mortality and incidence of ventilator-assisted pneumonia (O)?

Best Available Evidence
Systematic review of randomized controlled trials (RCTs)

Critical Appraisal and Synthesis of Evidence
- Seven RCTs (n = 1044) of critically ill adult patients requiring prolonged mechanical ventilation. Early tracheotomy was compared with either late tracheotomy or prolonged endotracheal intubation.
- Primary outcomes were short-term mortality and ventilator-assisted pneumonia (VAP).
- Secondary outcomes were long-term mortality, duration of ventilation and sedation, length of ICU and hospital stay, and complications.
- Early tracheotomy did not significantly reduce short–term or long-term mortality or rate of VAP. Tracheotomy timing was not related to reductions in duration of mechanical ventilation or sedation, shorter stays in ICU or hospital, or more complications.

Conclusion
- Clinically significant outcomes are not affected by timing of a tracheotomy.

Implications for Nursing Practice
- The optimal tracheotomy timing (early vs. late) for patients on prolonged mechanical ventilation is not really known.
- Continue to consider benefits of tracheotomy (e.g., increased patient comfort, improved oral hygiene) compared to the risks and complications (e.g., bleeding, wound infection, tracheal stenosis). The risk/benefit of tracheotomy needs to be weighed against the risk/benefit of prolonged endotracheal intubation.

Reference for Evidence
Wang F, Wu Y, Bo L, et al: The timing of tracheotomy in critically ill patients undergoing mechanical ventilation: a systematic review and meta-analysis of randomized controlled trials, *Chest* 140:1456, 2011.

P, Patient population of interest; *I*, intervention or area of interest; *C*, comparison of interest or comparison group; *O*, outcomes of interest (see p. 12).

most emergencies because the airway can be secured rapidly and a larger-diameter tube is used. A larger-bore ET tube reduces the *work of breathing* (WOB) because of less airway resistance. It is easier to remove secretions and perform fiberoptic bronchoscopy if needed. Nasal ET intubation is rarely used but may be needed when head and neck movement is risky.

There are risks associated with oral ET intubation. It is difficult to place an oral tube if head and neck mobility is limited (e.g., suspected spinal cord injury). Teeth can be chipped or accidentally removed during the procedure. Salivation is increased and swallowing is difficult. Patients can obstruct the ET tube by biting down on it. Sedation along with a bite block or oropharyngeal airway may be used to avoid this. The ET tube and bite block (if used) should be secured (separately) to the face. Mouth care is a challenge because of limited space in the oral cavity. Manage this by using smaller or pediatric-sized oral products for tooth brushing, cleaning, and suctioning.

Nasal intubation is contraindicated in patients with facial fractures or suspected fractures at the base of the skull and postoperatively after cranial surgeries. The WOB is greater because the longer, narrower tube offers more airflow resistance

and may kink. Suctioning and secretion removal are more difficult. Finally, nasal tubes have been linked to an increased incidence of sinus infection and ventilator-associated pneumonia (VAP).[27]

Endotracheal Intubation Procedure

Unless ET intubation is emergent, consent for the procedure is obtained. Tell the patient and caregiver the reason for ET intubation, the steps in the procedure, and the patient's role in the procedure (if indicated). Also explain that, while intubated, the patient will not be able to speak, but that you will provide other means of communication. Tell them that the patient's hands may be briefly restrained for safety purposes.

Have a self-inflating *bag-valve-mask* (BVM) (e.g., *Ambu bag*) available and attached to O_2, suctioning equipment ready at the bedside, and IV access. The BVM contains a reservoir that is filled with O_2 so that concentrations of 90% to 95% are delivered. The slower the bag is deflated and inflated, the higher the O_2 concentration that is delivered. Assemble and check the equipment to be used, remove the patient's dentures or partial plates (for oral intubation), and administer medications as ordered. Premedication varies depending on the patient's level of consciousness (e.g., awake, obtunded) and the nature of the procedure (e.g., emergent, nonemergent).

Rapid-sequence intubation (RSI) is the rapid, concurrent administration of both a sedative and a paralytic agent during emergency airway management to decrease the risks of aspiration and injury to the patient. RSI is not indicated in patients who are in cardiac arrest or have a known difficult airway.[28] A sedative-hypnotic-amnesic (e.g., midazolam [Versed], etomidate [Amidate]) is used to induce unconsciousness, along with a rapid-onset opioid (e.g., fentanyl) to blunt the pain of the procedure. A paralytic drug (e.g., succinylcholine [Anectine]) is then given to produce skeletal muscle paralysis. Monitor the patient's oxygenation status during the procedure with pulse oximetry.

For oral intubation, place the patient supine with the head extended and the neck flexed ("sniffing position"). This position permits visualization of the vocal cords. For nasal intubation, the nasal passages may be sprayed with a local anesthetic and vasoconstrictor (e.g., lidocaine [Xylocaine] with epinephrine) to reduce trauma and bleeding. Before intubation is started, preoxygenate the patient using the BVM and 100% O_2 for 3 to 5 minutes. Each intubation attempt is limited to less than 30 seconds. Ventilate the patient between successive attempts using the BVM and 100% O_2.

After intubation, inflate the cuff and confirm the placement of the ET tube while the patient is manually ventilated using the BVM with 100% O_2. Use an end-tidal CO_2 detector to confirm proper placement by noting the presence of exhaled CO_2 from the lungs. Place the detector between the BVM and the ET tube and either observe for a color change (indicating the presence of CO_2) or a number. If no CO_2 is detected, the tube is in the esophagus and needs to be reinserted.[29] Auscultate the lungs for bilateral breath sounds and the epigastrium for the absence of air sounds. Observe the chest for symmetric chest wall movement. In addition, SpO_2 should be stable or improved.

If the findings support proper ET tube placement, connect the tube to an O_2 source and secure per agency policy (Fig. 66-15). Suction the ET tube and pharynx, and insert a bite block as needed. Obtain a chest x-ray immediately to confirm tube location (2 to 6 cm above the carina in the adult). This position

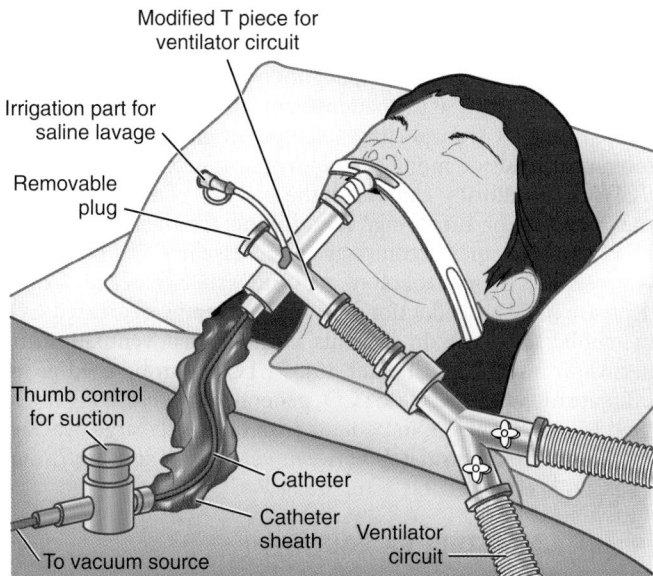

Modified T piece for
ventilator circuit

Irrigation part for
saline lavage

Removable
plug

Thumb control
for suction

Catheter

Catheter
sheath   Ventilator
circuit

To vacuum source

FIG. 66-15 Closed tracheal suction system.

allows the patient to move the neck without moving the tube or causing it to enter the right mainstem bronchus. Once proper positioning is confirmed with x-ray, record and mark the position of the tube at the lip or teeth (usually 21 cm for women and 23 cm for men) or nose. Cut excess tubing to reduce dead air space.

The ET tube is connected to either humidified air, O_2, or a mechanical ventilator. Obtain ABGs immediately after intubation to determine baseline oxygenation and ventilation status. ABG values are reviewed and used to guide oxygenation and ventilation changes. Continuous pulse oximetry and end-tidal CO_2 monitoring provide valuable data related to arterial oxygenation and ventilation.

NURSING MANAGEMENT
ARTIFICIAL AIRWAY

Management of a patient with an artificial airway is often a shared responsibility between you and the respiratory therapist, with specific management tasks determined by agency policy. Nursing responsibilities for the patient with an artificial airway may include some or all of the following: (1) maintaining correct tube placement, (2) maintaining proper cuff inflation, (3) monitoring oxygenation and ventilation, (4) maintaining tube patency, (5) assessing for complications, (6) providing oral care and maintaining skin integrity, and (7) fostering comfort and communication. eNursing Care Plan 66-1 for the patient on a mechanical ventilator is available on the website for this chapter.

MAINTAINING CORRECT TUBE PLACEMENT

Continuously monitor the patient with an ET tube for proper placement. If the tube is dislodged, it could end up in the pharynx or enter the esophagus or the right mainstem bronchus (thus ventilating only the right lung).

SAFETY ALERT: Endotracheal Tube Placement
- Maintain proper ET tube position by placing an "exit mark" on the tube.
- Confirm that the mark remains constant while at rest and during patient care, repositioning, and transport.

Observe for symmetric chest wall movement and auscultate to confirm bilateral breath sounds. If the ET tube is not positioned properly, it is an emergency. Stay with the patient, maintain the airway, support ventilation, and call for the appropriate help to immediately reposition the tube. It may be necessary to ventilate the patient with a BVM and 100% O_2. If a dislodged tube is not repositioned, minimal or no O_2 is delivered to the lungs or the entire tidal volume is delivered to one lung. This places the patient at risk for pneumothorax.

MAINTAINING PROPER CUFF INFLATION

The cuff is an inflatable, pliable sleeve encircling the outer wall of the ET tube (see Fig. 66-14). The high-volume, low-pressure cuff stabilizes and "seals" the ET tube within the trachea and prevents escape of ventilating gases. However, excess volume in the cuff can damage the tracheal mucosa. To avoid this, inflate the cuff with air, and measure and monitor the cuff pressure. To ensure adequate tracheal perfusion, maintain cuff pressure at 20 to 25 cm H_2O.[30] Measure and record cuff pressure after intubation and on a routine basis (e.g., every 8 hours) using the *minimal occluding volume* (MOV) *technique* or *the minimal leak technique* (MLT).

The steps in the MOV technique for cuff inflation are as follows: (1) for the mechanically ventilated patient, place a stethoscope over the trachea and inflate the cuff to MOV by adding air until no air leak is heard at peak inspiratory pressure (end of ventilator inspiration); (2) for the spontaneously breathing patient, inflate until no sound is heard after a deep breath or after inhalation with a BVM; (3) use a manometer to verify that cuff pressure is between 20 and 25 cm H_2O; and (4) record cuff pressure in the chart. If adequate cuff pressure cannot be maintained or larger volumes of air are needed to keep the cuff inflated, there could be a leak in the cuff or tracheal dilation at the cuff site. In these situations, notify the physician to reposition or change the ET tube.

The procedure for MLT is similar with one exception. Remove a small amount of air from the cuff until a slight air leak is auscultated at peak inflation. Both techniques aim to prevent the risks of tracheal damage from high cuff pressures. The use of continuous cuff measurement is being studied.[31]

MONITORING OXYGENATION AND VENTILATION

Vigilantly monitor the patient with an ET tube for adequate oxygenation by assessing clinical findings, ABGs, SpO_2, and, if available, $ScvO_2/SvO_2$. Assess for signs of hypoxemia such as a change in mental status (e.g., confusion), anxiety, dusky skin, and dysrhythmias. Periodic ABGs (specifically PaO_2) and continuous SpO_2 provide objective data regarding oxygenation. Lower values are expected in patients with some disease states, such as chronic obstructive pulmonary disease (COPD). CVP or PA catheters with $ScvO_2$ or SvO_2 capability provide an indirect indication of the patient's tissue oxygenation status (see Table 66-4).

Indicators of ventilation include clinical findings, $PaCO_2$, and continuous partial pressure of end-tidal CO_2 ($PETCO_2$). Assess the patient's respirations for rate, rhythm, and use of accessory muscles. The patient who is hyperventilating will be breathing rapidly and deeply and may experience circumoral and peripheral numbness and tingling. The patient who is hypoventilating will be breathing shallowly or slowly and may appear dusky. $PaCO_2$ is the best indicator of alveolar hyperventilation (e.g., decreased $PaCO_2$, increased pH indicate respira-

TABLE 66-8 SUCTIONING PROCEDURES FOR PATIENT ON MECHANICAL VENTILATOR

General Measures for Open and Closed Suction Techniques

1. Gather all equipment.
2. Wash hands and don personal protective equipment.
3. Explain procedure and patient's role in assisting with secretion removal by coughing.
4. Monitor patient's cardiopulmonary status (e.g., vital signs, SpO_2, $SvO_2/ScvO_2$, ECG, level of consciousness) before, during, and after the procedure.
5. Turn on suction and set vacuum to 100-120 mm Hg.
6. Pause ventilator alarms.

Open-Suction Technique

7. Open sterile catheter package using the inside of the package as a sterile field. NOTE: Suction catheter should be no wider than half the diameter of the ET tube (e.g., for a 7-mm ET tube, select a 10F suction catheter).
8. Fill the sterile solution container with sterile normal saline or water.
9. Don sterile gloves.
10. Pick up sterile suction catheter with dominant hand. Using nondominant hand, secure the connecting tube (to suction) to the suction catheter.
11. Check equipment for proper functioning by suctioning a small volume of sterile saline solution from the container. **(Go to step 13.)**

Closed-Suction Technique

12. Connect the suction tubing to the closed suction port.
13. Hyperoxygenate the patient for 30 sec using one of the following methods:
    - Activate the suction hyperoxygenation setting on the ventilator using nondominant hand.
    - Increase FIO_2 to 100%. NOTE: Remember to return FIO_2 to baseline level at the completion of the procedure if not done automatically after preset time by ventilator.
    - Disconnect the ventilator tubing from the ET tube and manually ventilate the patient with 100% O_2 using a BVM device.* Administer five or six breaths over 30 sec. NOTE: Use of a second person to deliver the manual breaths significantly increases the tidal volume delivered.
14. With suction off, gently and quickly insert the catheter using the dominant hand. When you meet resistance, pull back ½ in.
15. Apply continuous or intermittent suction using the nondominant thumb. Withdraw the catheter over 10 sec or less.
16. Hyperoxygenate for 30 sec as described in step 13.
17. If secretions remain and the patient has tolerated the procedure, perform two or three suction passes as described in steps 14 and 15. NOTE: Rinse the suction catheter with sterile saline solution between suctioning passes as needed.
18. Reconnect patient to ventilator (open-suction technique).
19. At the completion of ET tube suctioning, rinse the catheter and connecting tubing with the sterile saline solution.
20. Suction oral pharynx. NOTE: Use a separate catheter for this step when using the closed-suction technique.
21. Discard the suction catheter and rinse the connecting tubing with the sterile saline solution (open-suction technique).
22. Reset FIO_2 (if necessary) and ventilator alarms.
23. Reassess patient for signs of effective suctioning.

Adapted from Chulay M, Seckel M: Suctioning: endotracheal or tracheostomy tube. In Wiegand DL-M, editor: *AACN procedure manual for critical care*, ed 6, St Louis, 2011, Saunders.
*Attach a PEEP valve to the BVM for patients on >5 cm H_2O PEEP.
BVM, Bag-valve-mask; *ECG*, electrocardiogram; *ET*, endotracheal; *FIO_2*, fraction of inspired oxygen; *PEEP*, positive end-expiratory pressure.

tory alkalosis) or hypoventilation (e.g., increased $PaCO_2$, decreased pH indicate respiratory acidosis).

$PETCO_2$ monitoring (*capnography*) is done by analyzing exhaled gas directly at the patient-ventilator circuit (*mainstream sampling*) or by transporting a sample of gas via a small-bore tubing to a bedside monitor (*sidestream sampling*). Continuous $PETCO_2$ monitoring can assess the patency of the airway and the presence of breathing. In addition, gradual changes in $PETCO_2$ values may accompany an increase in CO_2 production (e.g., sepsis, hypoventilation, neuromuscular blockade) or a decrease in CO_2 production (e.g., hypothermia, decreased CO, metabolic acidosis). In patients with normal ventilation-to-perfusion ratios (see Chapter 68), $PETCO_2$ can be used as an estimate of $PaCO_2$, with $PETCO_2$ generally 1 to 5 mm Hg lower than $PaCO_2$. However, in patients with unusually large dead air space or serious mismatch between ventilation and perfusion, $PETCO_2$ is not a reliable estimate of $PaCO_2$.[29]

MAINTAINING TUBE PATENCY

Do not routinely suction a patient. Regularly assess the patient to determine if suctioning is needed. Indications for suctioning include (1) visible secretions in the ET tube, (2) sudden onset of respiratory distress, (3) suspected aspiration of secretions, (4) increase in peak airway pressures, (5) auscultation of adventitious breath sounds over the trachea or bronchi, (6) increase in respiratory rate or sustained coughing, and (7) sudden or gradual decrease in PaO_2 or SpO_2.

Table 66-8 describes two recommended suctioning methods, the *closed-suction technique* (CST) and the *open-suction technique* (OST). The CST uses a suction catheter that is enclosed in a plastic sleeve connected directly to the patient-ventilator circuit (see Fig. 66-15). With the CST, oxygenation and ventilation are maintained during suctioning, and exposure to the patient's secretions is reduced. The CST should be used for patients who (1) require high levels of positive end-expiratory pressure (PEEP) (greater than 10 cm H_2O), (2) have high levels of FIO_2, (3) have bloody or infected pulmonary secretions, (4) require frequent suctioning, and (5) experience clinical instability with the OST.[32]

Potential complications associated with suctioning include hypoxemia, bronchospasm, increased intracranial pressure, dysrhythmias, hypertension, hypotension, mucosal damage, pulmonary bleeding, pain, and infection.[32] Closely assess the patient before, during, and after the suctioning procedure. If the patient does not tolerate suctioning (e.g., decreased SpO_2, increased or decreased BP, sustained coughing, development of dysrhythmias), stop the procedure and hyperoxygenate until equilibration occurs and before attempting another suction pass. Prevent hypoxemia by hyperoxygenating the patient before and after each suctioning pass and limiting each pass to 10 seconds or less (see Table 66-8). Assess both the ECG and SpO_2 before, during, and after the suctioning procedure.

Causes of dysrhythmias during suctioning include (1) hypoxemia resulting in myocardial ischemia; (2) vagal stimulation caused by tracheal irritation; and (3) sympathetic nervous system stimulation caused by anxiety, discomfort, or pain. Dysrhythmias include tachydysrhythmias and bradydysrhythmias, premature beats, and asystole. Stop suctioning if any new dysrhythmias develop. Avoid excessive suctioning in patients with severe hypoxemia or bradycardia.

Tracheal mucosal damage may occur because of excessive suction pressures (greater than 120 mm Hg), overly vigorous catheter insertion, and the characteristics of the suction catheter itself. Blood streaks or tissue shreds in aspirated secretions may indicate that mucosal damage has occurred. Mucosal damage increases the risk of infection and bleeding, particularly if the patient is receiving anticoagulants.[32] Trauma to the mucosa can be prevented by following the steps described in Table 66-8.

Secretions may be thick and difficult to suction because of inadequate hydration, inadequate humidification, infection, or inaccessibility of the left mainstem bronchus or lower airways. Adequately hydrating the patient (e.g., oral or IV fluids) and providing supplemental humidification of inspired gases may assist in thinning secretions. Instillation of normal saline into the ET tube is discouraged and may be harmful. If infection is the cause of thick secretions, give the patient appropriate antibiotics. Mobilization, postural drainage, percussion, and turning the patient every 2 hours may help move secretions into larger airways.

PROVIDING ORAL CARE AND MAINTAINING SKIN INTEGRITY

When an oral ET tube is in place, the patient's mouth is always open. Moisten the lips, tongue, and gums with saline or water swabs to prevent mucosal drying. Proper oral care provides comfort and prevents injury to the gums and plaque formation (Table 66-9). Meticulous care is required to prevent skin breakdown on the face, lips, tongue, and nares because of pressure from the ET tube or bite block or the method used to secure the ET tube to the patient's face. Reposition and retape the ET tube every 24 hours and as needed. This practice may be shared between nursing and respiratory therapy or limited to respiratory therapy.

For the nasally intubated patient, remove the old tape or ties and clean the skin around the ET tube with saline-soaked gauze or cotton swabs. For the orally intubated patient, remove the bite block (if present) and the old tape or ties. Provide oral hygiene and then reposition the ET tube to the opposite side of the mouth. Replace the bite block (if appropriate) and reconfirm

TABLE 66-9	ORAL CARE PROCEDURES FOR PATIENT ON MECHANICAL VENTILATOR

General Measures
1. Gather all equipment.
2. Wash hands and don personal protective equipment.
3. Explain procedure to the patient and caregiver, if present.
4. Perform oral care using pediatric or adult soft toothbrushes at least twice a day by gently brushing to clean and remove plaque.
5. Use oral swabs with a 1.5% hydrogen peroxide solution every 2-4 hr.
6. Use 0.12% chlorhexidine oral rinse twice daily.
7. Apply a mouth moisturizer to oral mucosa and lips with each cleaning.
8. Suction oral cavity and pharynx frequently. See Fig. 66-16 for example of an endotracheal tube that can provide continuous or intermittent subglottic suctioning.

NOTE:
- Change all oral suction equipment and suction tubing every 24 hr.
- Rinse nondisposable oral suction apparatus with sterile normal saline after each use and place on a dry paper towel.

Adapted from Vollman KM, Sole ML: Endotracheal tube and oral care. In Wiegand DL-M, editor: *AACN procedure manual for critical care*, ed 6, St Louis, 2011, Saunders; and Institute for Healthcare Improvement: How-to guide: prevent ventilator-associated pneumonia. Retrieved from *http://www.ihi.org*.

proper cuff inflation and tube placement. Secure the ET tube again per agency policy (see eFig. 66-5 on the website for this chapter). If a manufactured tube holder is used, loosen the straps, massage the area under the straps, and then reapply the straps. Two staff members should perform the repositioning procedure to prevent accidental dislodgment. Monitor the patient for any signs of respiratory distress throughout the procedure.

FOSTERING COMFORT AND COMMUNICATION

Intubation is a major stressor for the patient.[33,34] The intubated patient may experience anxiety from not being able to talk or knowing what to expect. Communicating with the intubated patient can be frustrating for the patient, caregiver, and you. To communicate more effectively, use a variety of methods[35] (see Common Problems of Critical Care Patients earlier in this chapter on p. 1600).

The physical discomfort associated with ET intubation and mechanical ventilation often requires sedating the patient and giving an analgesic until the ET tube is no longer required. The patient may need morphine, lorazepam, propofol, or other sedatives to blunt the anxiety and discomfort related to intubation. Evaluate the drugs' effectiveness in achieving an acceptable level of patient comfort. In addition, consider using relaxation techniques (e.g., music therapy) to complement drug therapy.

COMPLICATIONS OF ENDOTRACHEAL INTUBATION

Two major complications of ET intubation are unplanned extubation and aspiration. Unplanned *extubation* (i.e., removal of the ET tube from the trachea) can be a catastrophic event and usually complicates the patient's recovery. Unplanned extubations can be due to patient removal of the ET tube or accidental removal during movement or a procedure. Usually the unplanned extubation is obvious (the patient is holding the ET tube). Other times, the tip of the ET tube is in the hypopharynx or esophagus and the extubation is not so obvious.

SAFETY ALERT: Unplanned Extubation
Observe for signs of unplanned extubation, which can be a life-threatening event:
- Patient talking
- Activation of the low-pressure ventilator alarm
- Diminished or absent breath sounds
- Respiratory distress
- Gastric distention

You are responsible for preventing unplanned extubation by ensuring that the ET tube is secured and observing and supporting the ET tube during repositioning, procedures, and patient transfers. Additionally, giving adequate sedation and analgesia and using standardized weaning protocols decrease the incidence of self-extubation.[36] The use of soft wrist restraints or mitts to immobilize the patient's hands has not shown to be an absolute deterrent to self-extubation.[37] Be sure to explain to the patient and caregiver when you use restraints for patient safety. Reassess for the continued need of restraints per agency policy.

Should an unplanned extubation occur, stay with the patient and call for help. Interventions are aimed at maintaining the patient's airway, supporting ventilation (e.g., manually ventilating the patient with a BVM and 100% O_2), securing the appropriate assistance to immediately reintubate the patient (if necessary), and providing psychologic support to the patient.

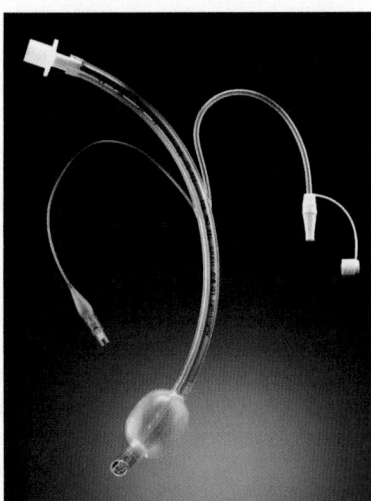

FIG. 66-16 Continuous subglottal suctioning can be provided by the Hi Lo Evac Tube. A dorsal lumen above the cuff allows for suctioning of secretions from the subglottic area. (Reprinted by permission of Nellcor Puritan Bennett Inc, Pleasanton, Calif.)

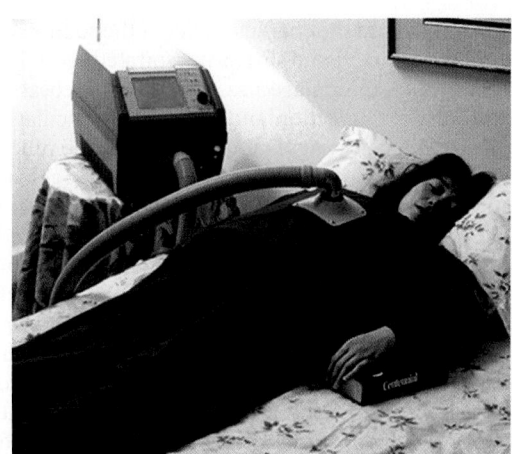

FIG. 66-17 Negative pressure ventilator. (Courtesy Lifecare, Westminster, Colo.)

Aspiration is another potential hazard for the patient with an ET tube. The ET tube passes through the epiglottis, splinting it in an open position. Thus the intubated patient cannot protect the airway from aspiration. The high-volume, low-pressure ET or tracheal cuff cannot totally prevent the trickle of oral or gastric secretions into the trachea. Further, secretions collect above the cuff. When the cuff is deflated, those secretions can move into the lungs. Some ET tubes provide continuous suctioning of secretions above the cuff (Fig. 66-16).

Oral intubation increases salivation, yet swallowing is difficult, so suction the patient's mouth frequently. Use a Yankauer (tonsil-tip) suction catheter or a sterile single-use catheter. Other factors contributing to aspiration include improper cuff inflation, patient positioning, and tracheoesophageal fistula. The patient with an ET tube is at risk for aspiration of gastric contents. Even when the cuff is properly inflated, take precautions to prevent vomiting, which can lead to aspiration.[38] Often, a nasogastric (NG) or an orogastric (OG) tube is inserted and connected to low, intermittent suction when a patient is first intubated. An OG tube is preferred over an NG tube to reduce the risk of sinusitis. All patients who are intubated or receiving enteral feedings must have the HOB elevated a minimum of 30 to 45 degrees unless medically contraindicated.

MECHANICAL VENTILATION

Mechanical ventilation is the process by which the FIO_2 (21% [room air] or more) is moved in and out of the lungs by a mechanical ventilator. Mechanical ventilation is not curative. It is a means of supporting patients until they recover the ability to breathe independently. It can also serve as a bridge to long-term mechanical ventilation, or until a decision is made to withdraw ventilatory support.

Indications for mechanical ventilation include (1) apnea or impending inability to breathe or protect the airway, (2) acute respiratory failure (see Chapter 68), (3) severe hypoxia, and (4) respiratory muscle fatigue.[39] Patients with chronic pulmonary disease and their caregivers should be given the opportunity to discuss mechanical ventilation before end-stage respiratory disease develops. Encourage all patients, particu-

larly those with chronic illnesses, to discuss the subject with their families and health care providers. They should record and place the results of these discussions in an advance directive. The decision to use, withhold, or withdraw mechanical ventilation must be made carefully, respecting the wishes of the patient and caregiver. When the health care team, patient, and/or caregiver disagree over the plan of care, you need to consult the agency's ethics committee for assistance.

Types of Mechanical Ventilation
The two major types of mechanical ventilation are negative pressure and positive pressure ventilation.

Negative Pressure Ventilation. Negative pressure ventilation involves the use of chambers that encase the chest or body and surround it with intermittent subatmospheric (or negative) pressure. The "iron lung" was the first form of negative pressure ventilation, developed during the polio epidemic. Intermittent negative pressure around the chest wall causes the chest to be pulled outward, reducing intrathoracic pressure. Air rushes in via the upper airway, which is outside the sealed chamber. Expiration is passive. The machine cycles off, allowing chest retraction. This type of ventilation is similar to normal ventilation in that decreased intrathoracic pressures produce inspiration, and expiration is passive. Negative pressure ventilation is delivered by noninvasive ventilation and does not require an artificial airway.

Several portable negative pressure ventilators are available for home use for patients with neuromuscular diseases, central nervous system disorders, diseases and injuries of the spinal cord, and severe COPD (Fig. 66-17). Negative pressure ventilators are not routinely used for acutely ill patients.

Positive Pressure Ventilation. Positive pressure ventilation (PPV) is the primary method used with acutely ill patients (Fig. 66-18). During inspiration the ventilator pushes air into the lungs under positive pressure. Unlike spontaneous ventilation, intrathoracic pressure is raised during lung inflation rather than lowered. Expiration occurs passively as in normal expiration. Modes of PPV are categorized into two groups: volume and pressure ventilation.[39]

Volume Ventilation. With volume ventilation a predetermined tidal volume (V_T) is delivered with each inspiration, and the amount of pressure needed to deliver the breath varies based on compliance and resistance factors of the patient-ventilator

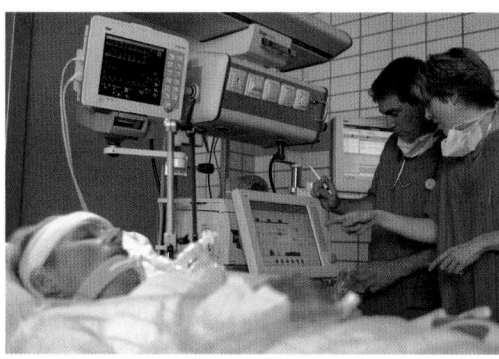

FIG. 66-18 Patient receiving mechanical ventilation. (Courtesy Draeger Medical.)

system. Consequently, the V_T is consistent from breath to breath, but airway pressures vary.

Pressure Ventilation. With *pressure ventilation* the peak inspiratory pressure is predetermined, and the V_T delivered to the patient varies based on the selected pressure and compliance and resistance factors of the patient-ventilator system. With this understanding, careful attention must be given to the V_T to prevent unplanned hyperventilation or hypoventilation. For example, when the patient breathes out of synchrony with the ventilator, the pressure limit may be reached quickly, and the volume of gas delivered may be small. Initially, pressure ventilation was used only in stable patients being weaned from the ventilator. Today, pressure ventilation is frequently used to treat critically ill patients.

Settings of Mechanical Ventilators

Mechanical ventilator settings regulate rate, depth, and other characteristics of ventilation (Table 66-10). Settings are based on the patient's status (e.g., ABGs, ideal body weight, level of consciousness, muscle strength). The ventilator is tuned as finely as possible to match the patient's ventilatory pattern. Settings are evaluated and adjusted frequently until the patient achieves optimal ventilation. Some settings serve as a fail-safe mechanism, alerting staff to problems with ventilation. It is important that you check that all ventilator alarms are always on. Alarms alert the staff to potentially dangerous situations such as mechanical malfunction, apnea, unplanned extubation, or patient asynchrony with the ventilator (Table 66-11). On many ventilators the alarms can be temporarily suspended or silenced for up to 2 minutes for suctioning or testing while a staff member is in the room. After that time, the alarm system automatically becomes functional again.

Modes of Volume Ventilation

The variable methods by which the patient and ventilator interact to deliver effective ventilation are called *ventilator modes.* The selected ventilator mode is based on how much WOB the patient should or can perform. WOB refers to inspiratory effort needed to overcome the elasticity and viscosity of the lungs along with the airway resistance. The mode is determined by the patient's ventilatory status, respiratory drive, and ABGs. Generally, ventilator modes are controlled or assisted.

With controlled ventilatory support, the ventilator does all of the WOB. With assisted ventilatory support, the ventilator and patient share the WOB. Historically, volume modes such as controlled mandatory ventilation (CMV), assist-control ventilation (ACV), and synchronized intermittent mandatory venti-

TABLE 66-10	**SETTINGS OF MECHANICAL VENTILATION**
Parameter	**Description**
Respiratory rate (f)	Number of breaths the ventilator delivers per minute. *Usual setting:* 6-20 breaths/min
Tidal volume (V_T)	Volume of gas delivered to patient during each ventilator breath. *Usual volume:* 6-10 mL/kg
O_2 concentration (FIO$_2$)	Fraction of inspired O_2 (FIO$_2$) delivered to patient. May be set between 21% (essentially room air) and 100%. *Usually adjusted* to maintain PaO$_2$ level >60 mm Hg or SpO$_2$ level >90%
Positive end-expiratory pressure (PEEP)	Positive pressure applied at the end of expiration of ventilator breaths. *Usual setting:* 5 cm H_2O
Pressure support	Positive pressure used to augment patient's inspiratory pressure. *Usual setting:* 6-18 cm H_2O
I:E ratio	Duration of inspiration (I) to duration of expiration (E). *Usual setting:* 1:2 to 1:1.5 unless IRV is desired
Inspiratory flow rate and time	Speed with which the V_T is delivered. *Usual setting:* 40-80 L/min and time is 0.8-1.2 sec
Sensitivity	Determines the amount of effort the patient must generate to initiate a ventilator breath. It may be set for pressure triggering or flow triggering. *Usual setting:* A pressure trigger is set 0.5-1.5 cm H_2O below baseline pressure and a flow trigger is set 1-3 L/min below baseline flow
High-pressure limit	Regulates the maximal pressure the ventilator can generate to deliver the V_T. When the pressure limit is reached, the ventilator terminates the breath and spills the undelivered volume into the atmosphere. *Usual setting:* 10-20 cm H_2O above peak inspiratory pressure

Adapted from Urden LD, Lough ME, Stacy KM: *Critical care nursing: diagnosis and management,* ed 6, St Louis, 2010, Mosby.
IRV, Inverse ratio ventilation.

lation (SIMV) have been used to treat critically ill patients. More recently, pressure modes such as pressure support ventilation (PSV) and pressure-control inverse ratio ventilation (PC-IRV) have become more widespread.[39] Table 66-12 describes these ventilator modes.

Assist-Control Mechanical Ventilation. With assist-control ventilation (ACV), the ventilator delivers a preset V_T at a preset frequency. When the patient initiates a spontaneous breath, the ventilator senses a decrease in intrathoracic pressure and then delivers the preset V_T. The patient can breathe faster than the preset rate but not slower. This mode has the advantage of allowing the patient some control over ventilation while providing some assistance. ACV is used in patients with a variety of conditions, including neuromuscular disorders (e.g., Guillain-Barré syndrome), pulmonary edema, and acute respiratory failure.

In the ACV mode, the patient has the potential for hypoventilation and hyperventilation. The spontaneously breathing

TABLE 66-11 **INTERPRETING MECHANICAL VENTILATION ALARMS**

Alarm	Possible Causes
High-pressure limit	• Secretions, coughing, or gagging • Patient fighting ventilator (ventilator asynchrony) • Condensate (water) in tubing • Kinked or compressed tubing (e.g., patient biting on endotracheal tube [ET] tube) • Increased resistance (e.g., bronchospasm) • Decreased compliance (e.g., pulmonary edema, pneumothorax)
Low-pressure limit	• Total or partial ventilator disconnect • Loss of airway (e.g., total or partial extubation) • ET tube or tracheotomy cuff leak (e.g., patient speaking, grunting)
Apnea	• Respiratory arrest • Oversedation • Change in patient condition • Loss of airway (e.g., total or partial extubation)
High tidal volume, minute ventilation, or respiratory rate	• Pain, anxiety • Change in patient condition • Excess condensate in tubing (i.e., false reading)
Low tidal volume or minute ventilation	• Change in patient's breathing efforts (e.g., rate and volume) • Patient disconnection, loose connection, or leak in circuit • ET tube or tracheotomy cuff leak (e.g., patient speaking, grunting) • Insufficient gas flow
Ventilator inoperative or low battery	• Machine malfunction • Unplugged, power failure, or internal battery not charged

Adapted from Pierce LN: *Management of the mechanically ventilated patient*, ed 2, St Louis, 2007, Saunders.
ET, Endotracheal.

patient can easily be overventilated, resulting in hyperventilation. If the volume or minimum rate is set low and the patient is apneic or weak, the patient will be hypoventilated. Thus these patients require vigilant assessment and monitoring of ventilatory status, including respiratory rate, ABGs, SpO_2, and $ScvO_2$/SvO_2. It is also important that the sensitivity or amount of negative pressure required to initiate a breath is appropriate to the patient's condition. For example, if it is too difficult for the patient to initiate a breath, the WOB is increased and the patient may tire or develop ventilator asynchrony (i.e., the patient "fights" the ventilator).

Synchronized Intermittent Mandatory Ventilation. With *synchronized intermittent mandatory ventilation* (SIMV), the ventilator delivers a preset V_T at a preset frequency in synchrony with the patient's spontaneous breathing. Between ventilator-delivered breaths, the patient is able to breathe spontaneously through the ventilator circuit. Thus the patient receives the preset FIO_2 during the spontaneous breaths but self-regulates the rate and volume of those breaths. This mode of ventilation differs from ACV, in which all breaths are of the same preset volume. It is used during continuous ventilation and during weaning from the ventilator. SIMV may also be combined with PSV (described below). Potential benefits of SIMV include improved patient-ventilator synchrony, lower mean airway pressure, and prevention of muscle atrophy as the patient takes on more of the WOB.

TABLE 66-12 **MODES OF MECHANICAL VENTILATION**

Volume Modes
Assist-Control (AC) or Assisted Mandatory Ventilation (AMV)
• Requires that rate, V_T, inspiratory time, and PEEP be set for the patient.
• The ventilator sensitivity is also set, and when the patient initiates a spontaneous breath, a full-volume breath is delivered.

Intermittent Mandatory Ventilation (IMV) and Synchronized Intermittent Mandatory Ventilation (SIMV)
• Requires that rate, V_T, inspiratory time, sensitivity, and PEEP are set for the patient.
• In between "mandatory breaths," patients spontaneously breathe at their own rates and V_T. With SIMV, the ventilator synchronizes the mandatory breaths with the patient's own inspirations.

Pressure Modes
Pressure Support Ventilation (PSV)
• Provides an augmented inspiration to a spontaneously breathing patient.
• The clinician selects an inspiratory pressure level, PEEP, and sensitivity.
• When the patient initiates a breath, a high flow of gas is delivered to the preselected pressure level, and pressure is maintained throughout inspiration.
• The patient determines the parameters of V_T, rate, and inspiratory time.

Pressure-Control Inverse Ratio Ventilation (PC-IRV)
• Combines pressure-limited ventilation with an inverse ratio of inspiration to expiration.
• The clinician selects the pressure level, rate, inspiratory time (1:1, 2:1, 3:1, 4:1), and the PEEP level.
• With the prolonged inspiratory times, auto-PEEP may result.
• The auto-PEEP may be a desirable outcome of the inverse ratios.
• Some clinicians use PC without IRV.
• Conventional inspiratory times are used and rate, pressure level, and PEEP are selected.

Airway Pressure Release Ventilation (APRV)
• Provides two levels of continuous positive airway pressure (CPAP) with timed releases, and permits spontaneous breathing throughout the respiratory cycle.
• The clinician selects both pressure high and pressure low along with time high and time low. Tidal volume is not a set variable and depends on the CPAP level, the patient's compliance and resistance, and spontaneous breathing effort.

Positive End-Expiratory Pressure (PEEP) and Continuous Positive Airway Pressure (CPAP)
PEEP
• Creates positive pressure at end exhalation and restores functional residual capacity (FRC).
• The term *PEEP* is used when end-expiratory pressure is provided during ventilator positive pressure breaths.

CPAP
• Similar to PEEP, CPAP restores FRC.
• This pressure is continuous during spontaneous breathing; no positive pressure breaths are present.

Modified from Burns SM: Invasive mechanical ventilation (through an artificial airway) volume and pressure modes. In Wiegand DL-M, editor: *AACN procedure manual for critical care*, ed 6, St Louis, 2011, Saunders.

SIMV also has disadvantages. If spontaneous breathing decreases when the preset rate is low, ventilation might not be adequately supported. Only patients with regular, spontaneous breathing should use low-rate SIMV. Weaning with SIMV demands close monitoring and may take longer because the rate of breathing is gradually reduced. Patients being weaned with SIMV may also have increased muscle fatigue associated with spontaneous breathing efforts.

Modes of Pressure Ventilation

Pressure Support Ventilation. With pressure support ventilation (PSV), positive pressure is applied to the airway only during inspiration and is used in conjunction with the patient's spontaneous respirations. The patient must be able to initiate a breath in this modality. The level of positive airway pressure is preset so that the gas flow rate is greater than the patient's inspiratory flow rate. As the patient initiates a breath, the machine senses the spontaneous effort and supplies a rapid flow of gas at the initiation of the breath and variable flow throughout the breath. With PSV the patient determines inspiratory length, V_T, and respiratory rate. V_T depends on the pressure level and airway compliance.

PSV is used with continuous ventilation and during weaning. PSV may also be used with SIMV during weaning. PSV is not used as a sole ventilatory support during acute respiratory failure because of the risk of hypoventilation. Advantages of PSV include increased patient comfort, decreased WOB (because inspiratory efforts are augmented), decreased O_2 consumption (because inspiratory work is reduced), and increased endurance conditioning (because the patient is exercising respiratory muscles).

Pressure-Control Inverse Ratio Ventilation. *Pressure-control inverse ratio ventilation* (PC-IRV) combines pressure-limited ventilation with an inverse ratio of inspiration (I) to expiration (E). Some clinicians use PC without IRV. The I/E ratio is the ratio of duration of inspiration to the duration of expiration. This value is normally a ratio of 1:2. With IRV, the I/E ratio begins at 1:1 and may progress to 4:1. Prolonged positive pressure is applied, increasing inspiratory time. IRV progressively expands collapsed alveoli. The short expiratory time has a PEEP-like effect, preventing alveolar collapse. Because IRV imposes a nonphysiologic breathing pattern, the patient requires sedation with or without paralysis. PC-IRV is indicated for patients with acute respiratory distress syndrome (ARDS) who continue to have refractory hypoxemia despite high levels of PEEP. Not all patients with poor oxygenation respond to PC-IRV.

Airway Pressure Release Ventilation. *Airway pressure release ventilation* (APRV) permits spontaneous breathing at any point during the respiratory cycle with a preset continuous positive airway pressure (CPAP) with short timed pressure releases. The CPAP level (pressure high, pressure low) is adjusted to maintain oxygenation goals while the timed releases (time high, time low) are increased or decreased to meet ventilation goals. V_T is not a set variable and depends on the CPAP level, the patient's compliance and resistance, and spontaneous breathing effort. The mode is designed for patients with ARDS who need high pressure levels for alveolar recruitment (open collapsed alveoli). One advantage of this mode is the ability to permit spontaneous respirations. This may reduce the need for deep sedation or paralytics.

Other Modes. Increases in ventilator technology have led to the development of additional pressure modes. However, because of the nonstandardization of these options, the names and features are manufacturer specific. The superiority of these modes has not been established. Some examples include *volume-assured pressure ventilation* and *adaptive support ventilation.*

Other Ventilatory Maneuvers

Positive End-Expiratory Pressure. Positive end-expiratory pressure (PEEP) is a ventilatory maneuver in which positive pressure is applied to the airway during exhalation. Normally during exhalation, airway pressure drops to zero, and exhalation occurs passively. With PEEP, exhalation remains passive, but pressure falls to a preset level, often 3 to 20 cm H_2O. Lung volume during expiration and between breaths is greater than normal with PEEP. This increases functional residual capacity (FRC) and often improves oxygenation with restoration of lung volume that normally remains at the end of passive exhalation. The mechanisms by which PEEP increases FRC and oxygenation include increased aeration of patent alveoli, aeration of previously collapsed alveoli, and prevention of alveolar collapse throughout the respiratory cycle.

PEEP is titrated to the point that oxygenation improves without compromising hemodynamics. This is termed *best* or *optimal PEEP*. Often 5 cm H_2O PEEP (referred to as *physiologic PEEP*) is used prophylactically to replace the glottic mechanism, help maintain a normal FRC, and prevent alveolar collapse. PEEP of 5 cm H_2O is also used for patients with a history of alveolar collapse during weaning. PEEP improves gas exchange, vital capacity, and inspiratory force when used during weaning.

In contrast, *auto-PEEP* is not purposely set on the ventilator but is a result of inadequate exhalation time. Auto-PEEP is additional PEEP over what is set by the health care provider. This additional PEEP may result in increased WOB, barotrauma, and hemodynamic instability. However, during some ventilator modes (PC-IRV), auto-PEEP may be desirable. Interventions to limit auto-PEEP include sedation and analgesia, large-diameter ET tube, bronchodilators, short inspiratory times, and decreased respiratory rates. Reducing water accumulation in the ventilator circuit by frequent emptying or use of heated circuits also limits auto-PEEP. In patients with short exhalation times and early airway closure (e.g., asthma), setting PEEP can offset auto-PEEP by splinting the airway open during exhalation and preventing "air trapping."

In general, the major purpose of PEEP is to maintain or improve oxygenation while limiting risk of O_2 toxicity. FIO_2 can often be reduced when PEEP is used. PEEP is indicated in lungs with diffuse disease, severe hypoxemia unresponsive to FIO_2 greater than 50%, and loss of compliance or stiffness. It is used in pulmonary edema to provide a counterpressure opposing fluid extravasation. The classic indication for PEEP therapy is ARDS (see Chapter 68). PEEP is contraindicated or used with extreme caution in patients with highly compliant lungs (e.g., COPD), unilateral or nonuniform disease, hypovolemia, and low CO. In these cases the adverse effects of PEEP may outweigh any benefits.

Continuous Positive Airway Pressure. Continuous positive airway pressure (CPAP) restores FRC and is similar to PEEP. However, the pressure in CPAP is delivered continuously during spontaneous breathing, thus preventing the patient's airway pressure from falling to zero. For example, if CPAP is 5 cm H_2O, airway pressure during expiration is 5 cm H_2O. During inspiration, 1 to 2 cm H_2O of negative pressure is generated, thus reducing airway pressure to 3 or 4 cm H_2O. The patient receiving SIMV with PEEP receives CPAP when breathing spontaneously. CPAP is commonly used in the treatment of obstructive sleep apnea.[40] CPAP can be administered noninvasively by a tight-fitting mask or an ET or tracheal tube. CPAP increases WOB because the patient must forcibly exhale against the CPAP. Therefore it must be used with caution in patients with myocardial compromise.

Automatic Tube Compensation. *Automatic tube compensation* (ATC) is an adjunct designed to overcome WOB through an artificial airway. It is currently available on many ventilators. ATC is increased during inspiration and decreased during expiration. It is set by entering the internal diameter of the patient's airway along with the desired percentage of compensation. ATC may increase auto-PEEP in patients with obstructive disease and should be used cautiously in this population.[41]

Bilevel Positive Airway Pressure. In addition to O_2, *bilevel positive airway pressure* (BiPAP) provides two levels of positive pressure support: higher inspiratory positive airway pressure and lower expiratory positive airway pressure. It is a noninvasive modality and is delivered through a tight-fitting face mask, nasal mask, or nasal pillows. As with PSV delivered through an artificial airway, the patient must be able to spontaneously breathe and cooperate with this treatment.[40] BiPAP is used for COPD patients with heart failure and acute respiratory failure and for patients with sleep apnea. BiPAP may also be used after extubation to prevent reintubation. Patients with shock, altered mental status, or increased airway secretions are not candidates for BiPAP because of the risk of aspiration and the inability to remove the mask.

High-Frequency Oscillatory Ventilation. High-frequency oscillatory ventilation (HFOV) involves delivery of a small V_T (usually 1 to 5 mL/kg of body weight) at rapid respiratory rates (100 to 300 breaths/minute) in an effort to recruit and maintain lung volume and reduce intrapulmonary shunting. One benefit of HFOV is the ability to support gas exchange at a fixed mean airway pressure while limiting the risk of ventilator-induced lung injury. HFOV has been widely accepted in neonatal and pediatric ICUs. It is used in adults for the treatment of refractory hypoxemia and ARDS.[42] Patients receiving HFOV must be sedated and may be paralyzed to suppress spontaneous respiration. All patients must receive concurrent sedation and analgesia if using a paralytic drug (see Chapter 68).

Nitric Oxide. *Nitric oxide* (NO) is a gaseous molecule that is made intravascularly and participates in the regulation of pulmonary vascular tone. Inhibition of NO production results in pulmonary vasoconstriction, and administration of continuous inhaled NO results in pulmonary vasodilation. NO may be administered via an ET tube, a tracheostomy, or a face mask. Currently, NO is used in ARDS, as a diagnostic screening tool for pulmonary hypertension during a cardiac catheterization, and during or after cardiac surgery.

Prone Positioning. *Prone positioning* is the repositioning of a patient from a supine or lateral position to a prone (on the stomach, face down) position. This repositioning improves lung recruitment (reexpansion) through various mechanisms. Gravity reverses the effects of fluid in the dependent parts of the lungs as the patient is moved from supine to prone. The heart rests on the sternum, away from the lungs, contributing to an overall uniformity of pleural pressures. The prone position is a relatively safe (although nurse-intensive), supportive therapy used in critically ill patients with acute lung injury or ARDS to improve oxygenation.[43]

Extracorporeal Membrane Oxygenation. *Extracorporeal membrane oxygenation* (ECMO) is an alternative form of pulmonary support for the patient with severe respiratory failure. It is used more frequently in the pediatric and neonatal populations but is increasingly being used in adults. ECMO is a modification of cardiac bypass and involves partially removing blood from a patient with large-bore catheters, infusing O_2, removing CO_2, and returning the blood to the patient. This intensive therapy requires systemic anticoagulation and is a time-limited intervention. A skilled team of specialists, including a perfusionist, is required continuously at the bedside.[44]

Complications of Positive Pressure Ventilation

Although PPV may be essential to maintain ventilation and oxygenation, it can cause adverse effects. It is often difficult to distinguish complications of mechanical ventilation from the underlying disease.

Cardiovascular System. PPV can affect circulation because of the transmission of increased mean airway pressure to the thoracic cavity. With increased intrathoracic pressure, thoracic vessels are compressed. This results in decreased venous return to the heart, decreased left ventricular end-diastolic volume (preload), decreased CO, and hypotension. Mean airway pressure is further increased if titrating PEEP (greater than 5 cm H_2O) to improve oxygenation.

If the lungs are noncompliant (e.g., ARDS), airway pressures are not as easily transmitted to the heart and blood vessels. Thus effects of PPV on CO are reduced. Conversely, with compliant lungs (e.g., emphysema), there is increased danger of transmission of high airway pressures and negative effects on hemodynamics.

Compromised venous return by PPV is worsened by hypovolemia (e.g., hemorrhage) and decreased venous tone (e.g., sepsis, spinal shock). Restoration and maintenance of the circulating blood volume are important in minimizing cardiovascular complications.

Pulmonary System

Barotrauma. As lung inflation pressures increase, risk of *barotrauma* increases. Patients with compliant lungs (e.g., COPD) are at greater risk for barotrauma. This results when the increased airway pressure distends the lungs and possibly ruptures fragile alveoli or emphysematous blebs. Patients with stiff lungs (e.g., ARDS) who are given high inspiratory pressures and high levels of PEEP (greater than 5 cm H_2O) and patients with lung abscesses resulting from necrotizing organisms (e.g., staphylococci) are also susceptible to barotrauma.

Air can escape into the pleural space from alveoli or interstitium and become trapped. Pleural pressure increases and collapses the lung, causing pneumothorax. (Chapter 28 discusses the clinical manifestations of pneumothorax.) The lungs receive air during inspiration but cannot expel it during expiration. Respiratory bronchioles are larger on inspiration than expiration. They may close on expiration, and air becomes trapped. With PPV, a simple pneumothorax can become a life-threatening tension pneumothorax. The mediastinum and contralateral lung are compressed, reducing CO. Immediate treatment of the pneumothorax is required. For some patients, chest tubes are placed prophylactically.

Pneumomediastinum usually begins with rupture of alveoli into the lung interstitium. Progressive air movement occurs into the mediastinum and subcutaneous neck tissue, and a pneumothorax often follows. New, unexplained subcutaneous emphysema is an indication for immediate chest x-ray. Pneumomediastinum and subcutaneous emphysema may be too small to detect on x-ray or clinically before the development of a pneumothorax.

Volutrauma. The concept of *volutrauma* in PPV relates to the lung injury that occurs when a large V_T is used to ventilate noncompliant lungs. Volutrauma results in alveolar fractures and movement of fluids and proteins into the alveolar spaces. Low-volume ventilation rather than pressure ventilation should be used in ARDS patients to protect the lungs.

Alveolar Hypoventilation. *Alveolar hypoventilation* can be caused by inappropriate ventilator settings, leakage of air from the ventilator tubing or around the ET tube or tracheostomy cuff, lung secretions or obstruction, and low ventilation/perfusion ratio. A low V_T or respiratory rate decreases minute ventilation. This results in hypoventilation and leads to respiratory acidosis. A leaking cuff or tubing that is not secured may cause air leakage, lowering the delivered V_T. Excess lung secretions can cause hypoventilation. Mobilizing the patient, turning the patient every 1 to 2 hours, providing chest physiotherapy to lung areas with increased secretions, encouraging deep breathing and coughing, and suctioning (as needed) may limit this. Atelectasis may develop. Increasing the V_T, adding small increments of PEEP, and adding a preset number of sighs to the ventilator settings reduce the risk of atelectasis.

Alveolar Hyperventilation. Respiratory alkalosis can occur if the respiratory rate or V_T is set too high *(mechanical overventilation)* or if the patient receiving assisted ventilation is *hyperventilating.* It is easy to overventilate a patient on PPV. Particularly at risk are patients with chronic alveolar hypoventilation and CO_2 retention. For example, the patient with COPD may have a chronic $PaCO_2$ elevation (acidosis) and compensatory bicarbonate retention by the kidneys. When the patient is ventilated, the patient's "normal baseline" rather than the standard normal values is the therapeutic goal. If the COPD patient is returned to a standard normal $PaCO_2$, the patient will develop alkalosis because of the retained bicarbonate. Such a patient could move from compensated respiratory acidosis to serious metabolic alkalosis. The presence of alkalosis makes weaning from the ventilator difficult. Alkalosis, especially if the onset is abrupt, can have additional serious consequences, including hypokalemia, hypocalcemia, and dysrhythmias. Neuromuscular irritability, seizures, coma, and death can occur. Usually the patient with COPD who is supported on the ventilator does better with a short inspiratory and longer expiratory time.

If hyperventilation is spontaneous, it is important to determine the cause and treat it. Possible causes include hypoxemia, pain, fear, anxiety, or compensation for metabolic acidosis. Patients who fight the ventilator or breathe out of synchrony may be anxious or in pain. If the patient is anxious and fearful, sitting with the patient and verbally coaching the patient to breathe with the ventilator may help. If these measures fail, manually ventilating the patient slowly with a BVM and 100% O_2 may slow breathing enough to bring it in synchrony with the ventilator.

Ventilator-Associated Pneumonia. The risk for hospital-acquired pneumonia is highest in patients requiring mechanical ventilation because the ET or tracheostomy tube bypasses normal upper airway defenses. In addition, a poor nutritional state, immobility, and the underlying disease process (e.g., immunosuppression, organ failure) make the patient more prone to infection. *Ventilator-associated pneumonia* (VAP) is pneumonia that occurs 48 hours or more after ET intubation.[45] It occurs in 9% to 27% of all intubated patients, with half of the cases developing within the first 4 days of mechanical ventilation. In addition, patients who develop VAP have significantly longer hospital stays and higher mortality rates than those who do not.

In patients with early VAP (within 96 hours of mechanical ventilation), sputum cultures often grow gram-negative bacteria (e.g., *Escherichia coli, Klebsiella, Streptococcus pneumoniae, Haemophilus influenzae*). Organisms associated with late VAP include antibiotic-resistant organisms such as *Pseudomonas aeruginosa* and oxacillin-resistant *Staphylococcus aureus.* These organisms are abundant in the hospital environment and the patient's GI tract. They can spread in a number of ways, including contaminated respiratory equipment, inadequate hand washing, adverse environmental factors such as poor room ventilation and high traffic flow, and decreased patient ability to cough and clear secretions. Colonization of the oropharynx tract by gram-negative organisms predisposes the patient to gram-negative pneumonia.

Clinical evidence suggesting VAP includes fever, elevated white blood cell count, purulent or odorous sputum, crackles or rhonchi on auscultation, and pulmonary infiltrates noted on chest x-ray. The patient is treated with antibiotics after appropriate cultures are taken by tracheal suctioning or bronchoscopy and when infection is evident.

Guidelines on VAP prevention include (1) HOB elevation at a minimum of 30 to 45 degrees unless medically contraindicated, (2) no routine changes of the patient's ventilator circuit tubing, and (3) the use of an ET tube with a dorsal lumen above the cuff to allow continuous suctioning of secretions in the subglottic area[46] (see Fig. 66-16). Prevention also includes strict hand washing before and after suctioning, whenever ventilator equipment is touched, and after contact with any respiratory secretions (see Nursing Management: Artificial Airway earlier in this chapter). Always wear gloves when in contact with the patient and change gloves between activities (e.g., emptying urinary catheter drainage, hanging an IV drug). Finally, always drain the water that collects in the ventilator tubing away from the patient as it collects.

Sodium and Water Imbalance. Progressive fluid retention often occurs after 48 to 72 hours of PPV, especially PPV with PEEP. Fluid retention is associated with decreased urine output and increased sodium retention. Fluid balance changes may be due to decreased CO, which in turn results in diminished renal perfusion. Consequently, renin release is stimulated with subsequent production of angiotensin and aldosterone (see Chapter 45, Fig. 45-4). This results in sodium and water retention. It is also possible that pressure changes within the thorax are associated with decreased release of atrial natriuretic peptide, which also causes sodium retention. Mild water retention is also associated with PPV. Less insensible water loss occurs via the airway because ventilated delivered gases are humidified with body-temperature water. In addition, as a part of the stress response, release of antidiuretic hormone and cortisol contributes to sodium and water retention.

Neurologic System. In patients with head injury, PPV (especially with PEEP) can impair cerebral blood flow. The increased intrathoracic positive pressure impedes venous drainage from the head, resulting in jugular venous distention. The patient may exhibit increases in intracranial pressure because of the impaired venous return and increase in cerebral volume. Elevating the

HOB and keeping the patient's head in alignment may decrease the harmful effects of PPV on intracranial pressure.

Gastrointestinal System. Patients receiving PPV are stressed because of the serious illness, immobility, or discomforts associated with the ventilator. This places the ventilated patient at risk for developing stress ulcers and GI bleeding. Patients with a preexisting ulcer or those receiving corticosteroids are at an increased risk. Any kind of circulatory compromise, including reduction of CO caused by PPV, may contribute to ischemia of the gastric and intestinal mucosa and possibly increase the risk of translocation of GI bacteria.

To decrease the risk of VAP, guidelines support the use of routine peptic ulcer prophylaxis in mechanically ventilated patients.[46] Peptic ulcer prophylaxis includes the administration of histamine (H_2)-receptor blockers (e.g., ranitidine [Zantac]), proton pump inhibitors (PPIs) (e.g., esomeprazole [Nexium]), and enteral nutrition to decrease gastric acidity and diminish the risk of stress ulcer and hemorrhage. Some evidence suggests that the use of PPIs may be linked to an increase in the development of *Clostridium difficile*–associated diarrhea.[47] (This is discussed in Chapter 42 on p. 933.)

Gastric and bowel dilation may occur because of gas accumulation in the GI tract from swallowed air. The irritation of an artificial airway may cause excessive air swallowing and subsequent gastric dilation. Gastric or bowel dilation may put pressure on the vena cava, decrease CO, and prohibit adequate diaphragmatic excursion during spontaneous breathing. Elevation of the diaphragm as a result of paralytic ileus or bowel dilation leads to compression of the lower lobes of the lungs. This may cause atelectasis and compromise respiratory function. Decompression of the stomach is done by inserting an OG or NG tube.[48]

Immobility, sedation, circulatory impairment, decreased oral intake, use of opioid pain medications, and stress contribute to decreased peristalsis. The patient's inability to exhale against a closed glottis may make defecation difficult. As a result, the ventilated patient is at risk for constipation, and a bowel regimen should be initiated.

Musculoskeletal System. Maintenance of muscle strength and prevention of the problems associated with immobility are important. Adequate analgesia and nutrition can enhance exercise tolerance. Plan for early and progressive mobility of appropriate patients receiving PPV.[49] (See eFig. 66-6 on the website for this chapter.) In collaboration with physical and occupational therapy, perform passive and active exercises to maintain muscle tone in the upper and lower extremities. Simple maneuvers such as leg lifts, knee bends, quadriceps setting, or arm circles are appropriate. Prevent contractures, pressure ulcers, footdrop, and external rotation of the hip and legs by proper positioning and the use of specialized mattresses or beds. Use a portable ventilator or manually ventilate the patient with a BVM and 100% O_2 while ambulating.

Psychosocial Needs. The patient receiving mechanical ventilation often experiences physical and emotional stress. In addition to the problems related to critical care patients discussed at the beginning of this chapter, the patient supported by a mechanical ventilator is unable to speak, eat, move, or breathe normally. Tubes and machines cause pain, fear, and anxiety. Usual activities of daily living such as eating, elimination, and coughing are extremely complicated.

Feeling safe is an overpowering need of patients on mechanical ventilation. In addition, four related needs include the need

to know (information), the need to regain control, the need to hope, and the need to trust. When patients' needs are met, they feel safe. Work to strengthen the various factors that affect feeling safe. Encourage hope, as appropriate, and build trusting relationships with both the patient and caregiver. Involve patients and caregivers in decision making as much as possible.[14,16]

Patients receiving PPV usually require sedation (e.g., propofol) and/or analgesia (e.g., fentanyl) to facilitate optimal ventilation. Before initiating sedation or analgesia in the mechanically ventilated patient who is agitated or anxious, identify the cause of distress. Common problems that can result in patient agitation or anxiety include PPV, nutritional deficits, pain, hypoxemia, hypercapnia, drugs, and environmental stressors (e.g., sleep deprivation). Delirium is an acute change in mental status. It is a marker of cerebral insufficiency and associated with longer hospital stays and higher mortality rates. ICU patients are particularly vulnerable to delirium, and you must make every effort to assess and treat it.[8]

At times, the decision is made to paralyze the patient with a neuromuscular blocking agent (e.g., cisatracurium [Nimbex]) to provide more effective synchrony with the ventilator and improve oxygenation. Remember that the paralyzed patient can hear, see, think, and feel. It is important to administer IV sedation and analgesia concurrently when the patient is paralyzed. Monitoring patients receiving these medications is challenging. Assessment of the patient should include train-of-four (TOF) peripheral nerve stimulation, physiologic signs of pain or anxiety (changes in heart rate and BP), and ventilator synchrony. The TOF assessment involves using a peripheral nerve stimulator to deliver four successive stimulating currents to elicit muscle twitches (Fig. 66-19). The number of twitches varies with the percentage of neuromuscular blockade. The usual goal is one or two twitches out of four. Noninvasive electroencephalogram-based technology can also help guide sedative and analgesic therapy in these patients. Excessive administration of neuromuscular blocking agents may predispose the patient to prolonged paralysis and muscle weakness even after these agents are stopped.

Many patients have few memories of their time in the ICU, whereas others remember vivid details. Although appearing to be asleep, sedated, or paralyzed, patients may be aware of their surroundings, and you should always address them as if they were awake and alert.[50]

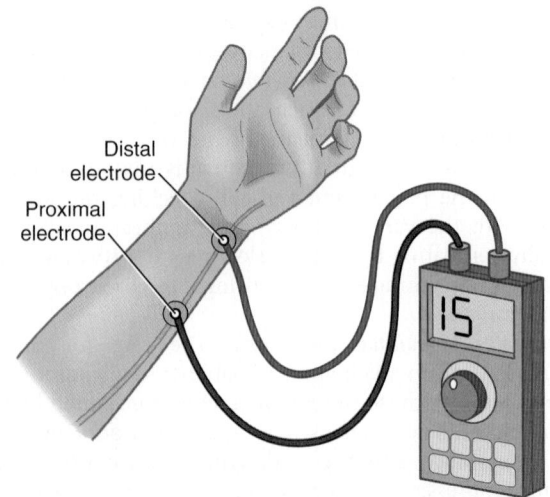

FIG. 66-19 Placement of electrodes along ulnar nerve.

Machine Disconnection or Malfunction. Mechanical ventilators may become disconnected or malfunction. When turned on and operative, alarms alert you to problems (see Table 66-11). Most deaths from accidental ventilator disconnection occur while the alarm is off, and most accidental disconnections in critical care settings are discovered by low-pressure alarms. The most frequent site for disconnection is between the tracheal tube and the adapter. Push connections together and then twist to secure more tightly. Be certain that alarms are set at all times, and chart that this is the case. You can pause alarms (not inactivate) during suctioning or removal from the ventilator, but you must reactivate them before leaving the patient's bedside.

Ventilator malfunction may also occur due to several factors. Although most institutions have emergency generators in the event of a power failure and newer ventilators may have battery backup, power failure is always a possibility. Have a plan for manually ventilating all patients who depend on a ventilator. If, at any time, you determine that the ventilator is malfunctioning (e.g., failure of O_2 supply), disconnect the patient from the machine and manually ventilate with a BVM and 100% O_2 until the ventilator is fixed or replaced.

Nutritional Therapy: Patient Receiving Positive Pressure Ventilation

PPV and the hypermetabolism associated with critical illness can contribute to inadequate nutrition. The presence of an ET tube eliminates the normal route for eating. Patients with a tracheostomy may be able to eat normally once the stoma heals. Swallowing studies and a consultation with a speech therapist are done to assess the patient's readiness. When eating with a tracheostomy tube in place, the patient should tilt the head slightly forward to facilitate swallowing and to prevent aspiration. Diet may be restricted to soft foods (e.g., puddings, ice cream) and thickened liquids.

Patients unlikely to be able to eat for 3 to 5 days should have a nutritional assessment and enteral feeding started within 24 to 48 hours of admission.[5] Inadequate nutrition makes the patient receiving prolonged mechanical ventilation prone to poor O_2 transport secondary to anemia and to poor tolerance of minimal exercise. Critically ill patients have frequent interruptions of enteral feedings because of problems with residuals, transportation to and during procedures, and routine nursing care. Poor nutrition and the disuse of respiratory muscles contribute to decreased respiratory muscle strength. In addition, critical illness, trauma, and surgery are associated with hypermetabolism, anxiety, pain, and increased WOB, which greatly increase caloric expenditure. Serum protein levels (e.g., albumin, prealbumin, transferrin, total protein) are usually decreased. Inadequate nutrition can delay weaning, decrease resistance to infection, and slow down recovery. Enteral gastric or small bowel feeding is the preferred method to meet caloric needs of ventilated patients (see Chapter 40 for discussion of enteral feeding).

Verification of feeding tube placement includes (1) x-ray confirmation before initial use, (2) marking and ongoing assessment of the tube's exit site, and (3) ongoing review of routine x-rays and aspirate.[48] The auscultatory method of assessment (i.e., listening for air after injection) is not a reliable method for verifying the placement of feeding tubes.

A concern regarding the nutritional support of patients receiving PPV is the carbohydrate content of the diet. Metabolism of carbohydrates may increase the serum CO_2 levels. This

DELEGATION DECISIONS

Caring for the Patient Requiring Mechanical Ventilation

In the critically ill patient who requires mechanical ventilation the registered nurse (RN) provides most of the care. Some patients who require chronic mechanical ventilation may be in long-term care settings or at home. In these settings, the RN assesses the patient and plans and evaluates care, but implementation of some activities may be delegated.

Role of Registered Nurse (RN)
- Auscultate breath sounds and respiratory effort, assessing for decreased ventilation or adventitious sounds.
- Monitor ventilator settings and alarms.
- Maintain appropriate cuff inflation on endotracheal (ET) tube.
- Develop plan for communication with the patient who has a tracheostomy or an ET tube.
- Administer sedatives, analgesics, and paralytic medications as needed.
- Determine need for ET tube suctioning. Implement suctioning for unstable patients.
- Reposition and secure ET tube (may delegate to respiratory therapist, depending on agency policy).
- Teach patient and caregiver about mechanical ventilation and weaning procedures.
- Monitor oxygenation level and signs of respiratory fatigue during weaning procedure.

Role of Licensed Practical/Vocational Nurse (LPN/LVN)
- Suction tracheostomy or ET tube for stable patients as directed by RN (after being educated and evaluated in this procedure).
- Administer routinely scheduled medications (consider state Nurse Practice Act and agency policy for IV medications).
- Assist RN or respiratory therapist with repositioning and securing ET tube.
- Administer enteral nutrition to stable patients as directed by RN.

Role of Unlicensed Assistive Personnel (UAP)
- Obtain vital signs and report these to RN.
- Perform bedside glucose testing, if needed.
- Provide personal hygiene and skin care and oral care (after being taught and evaluated in this procedure).
- Assist with frequent position changes, including ambulation, as directed by the RN.
- Perform passive or assisted range-of-motion exercises.
- Measure urine output and report information to RN.

can result in a higher required minute ventilation and increased WOB. Limiting carbohydrate content in the diet may lower CO_2 production. Consult the dietitian to determine the caloric and nutrient needs of these patients.

Weaning From Positive Pressure Ventilation and Extubation

Weaning is the process of reducing ventilator support and resuming spontaneous ventilation. The weaning process differs for patients requiring short-term ventilation (up to 3 days) versus long-term ventilation (longer than 3 days). Patients requiring short-term ventilation (e.g., after cardiac surgery) experience a linear weaning process. Patients likely to require prolonged PPV (e.g., patients with COPD who develop respiratory failure) often experience a weaning process that consists of peaks and valleys. Preparation for weaning begins when PPV is initiated and involves a team approach (e.g., nurse, physician, patient, caregiver, dietitian, respiratory therapist, physical therapist).

Weaning generally consists of three phases: the *preweaning phase*, the *weaning process*, and the *outcome phase*. The preweaning or assessment phase determines the patient's ability to breathe spontaneously. Assessment in this phase depends on a combination of respiratory (Table 66-13) and nonrespiratory factors. Weaning assessment parameters should include criteria to assess muscle strength (negative inspiratory force) and endurance (spontaneous V_T, vital capacity, minute ventilation, and rapid shallow breathing index). In addition, the patient's lungs should be reasonably clear on auscultation and chest x-ray. Nonrespiratory factors include the patient's neurologic status; hemodynamics; fluid, electrolytes, and acid-base balance; nutrition; and hemoglobin. It is important to have an alert, well-rested, and well-informed patient relatively free from pain and anxiety who can cooperate with the weaning plan. This does not mean complete withdrawal from sedatives or analgesics. Instead, drugs should be titrated to achieve comfort without causing excessive drowsiness.

A *spontaneous breathing trial* (SBT) is recommended in patients who demonstrate weaning readiness.[51] An SBT should be at least 30 minutes but no more than 120 minutes. It may be done with low levels of CPAP, low levels of PSV, or a T piece. Tolerance of the trial may lead to extubation. Failure to tolerate an SBT should prompt a search for reversible or complicating factors and a return to a nonfatiguing ventilator modality for the patient. The SBT should be reattempted the next day.

The use of a weaning protocol decreases ventilator days (see eFig. 66-7, available on the website for this chapter). The parts of a protocol are not as important as the use of a protocol to prevent delays in weaning. The patient receiving SIMV can have the ventilator breaths gradually reduced as his or her ventilatory status permits. CPAP or PSV can be added to SIMV. PSV is thought to

---

TABLE 66-13 INDICATORS FOR WEANING

Weaning Readiness

Patients receiving mechanical ventilation for respiratory failure should undergo a formal assessment of weaning potential if the following are satisfied:*

1. Reversal of the underlying cause of respiratory failure
2. Adequate oxygenation
   - PaO_2/FIO_2 >150-200
   - SpO_2 ≥90%
   - PEEP ≤5-8 cm H_2O
   - FIO_2 ≤40%-50%
   - pH ≥7.25

3. Hemodynamic stability
   - Absence of myocardial ischemia
   - Absence of clinically significant hypotension (no vasopressor therapy or low dose)
4. Patient ability to initiate an inspiratory effort
5. Optional criteria
   - Hemoglobin ≥7-10 mg/dL
   - Core temperature ≤38° (100.4° F) to 38.5° C (101.3° F)
   - Mental status awake and alert or easily arousable

Weaning Assessment

Measurement	Significance	Normal Values	Indices for Weaning
Spontaneous respiratory rate (f)	Respiratory rate/frequency over 1 min.	12-20 min	<35 min
Spontaneous tidal volume (V_T)	Amount of air exchanged during normal breathing at rest. Measure of muscle endurance.	7-9 mL/kg	≥5 mL/kg
Minute ventilation (V_E)	Tidal volume multiplied by respiratory rate over 1 min. *For example:* 0.350 (V_T) × 28 (f) = 9.8 L/min	5-10 L/min	≤10 L/min
Negative inspiratory force or pressure (NIF, NIP)	Amount of negative pressure that a patient is able to generate to initiate spontaneous respirations. Measured by clinician: After complete occlusion of inspiratory valve, a pressure manometer is attached to airway or mouth for 10-20 sec while negative inspiratory efforts are noted.	–75 to –100 cm H_2O	>–20 cm H_2O The more negative the number, the better indication for weaning.
Positive expiratory pressure (PEP)	Measure of expiratory muscle strength and ability to cough. Measured by clinician: After complete occlusion of expiratory valve, a pressure manometer is attached to the airway or mouth for 10-20 sec while positive expiratory efforts are noted.	60-85 cm H_2O	≥30 cm H_2O
Compliance, rate, oxygenation, and pressure (CROP) index	Combined index that is complex to calculate. $C_{Dyn} \times NIF \times (PaO_2/PAO_2)/f$ C_{Dyn} = Compliance PaO_2/PAO_2 = Oxygenation ratio of arterial O_2/alveolar O_2	Not applicable	>13
Rapid shallow breathing index (f/V_T)	Spontaneous respiratory rate over 1 min divided by tidal volume (in liters). *For example:* 30 (f)/0.400 (V_T) = 75/L	60-105/L	<105/L
Vital capacity (VC)	Maximum inspiration and then measurement of air during maximal forced expiration. Measure of respiratory muscle endurance or reserve or both. Requires patient cooperation.	65-75 mL/kg	≥10-15 mL/kg
Spontaneous breathing trial (SBT)	If patient passes daily weaning screen, assess patient during spontaneous breathing with little or no ventilator assistance. Trial should be at least 30 min to a maximum of 120 min.		Successful completion of trial is based on an integrated patient assessment.

Adapted from A Collective Task Force Facilitated by the American College of Chest Physicians, the American Association for Respiratory Care, and the American College of Critical Care Medicine. Evidence-based guidelines for weaning and discontinuing ventilatory support. Respiratory Care 47:69, 2002; and Burns SM: Weaning process. In Wiegand DL-M, editor: *AACN procedure manual for critical care*, ed 6, St Louis 2011, Saunders.
*The decision to use these criteria must be individualized to the patient.

provide gentle, slow respiratory muscle conditioning. It may be especially beneficial for patients who are deconditioned or have heart problems. Some patients may be weaned by simply providing humidified oxygen (T-piece or flow-by method).

Weaning may be tried at any time of day, although it is usually done during the day, with the patient ventilated at night in a rest mode. The rest mode should be a stable, nonfatiguing, and comfortable form of support for the patient. Regardless of the weaning mode selected, all health care team members should be familiar with the weaning plan. Additionally, it is important to permit the patient's respiratory muscles to rest between weaning trials. Once the respiratory muscles become fatigued, they may require 12 to 24 hours to recover.

The patient being weaned and the caregiver need ongoing emotional support. Explain the weaning process to them and keep them informed of progress. Place the patient in a comfortable sitting or semirecumbent position. Obtain baseline vital signs and respiratory parameters. During the weaning trial, closely monitor the patient for signs and symptoms that may signal intolerance and a need to end the trial (e.g., tachypnea, dyspnea, tachycardia, dysrhythmias, sustained desaturation [SpO_2 less than 91%], hypertension or hypotension, agitation, diaphoresis, anxiety, sustained V_T less than 5 mL/kg, changes in mentation). Document the patient's tolerance throughout the weaning process and include statements regarding the patient's and the caregiver's perceptions.

The weaning outcome phase is the period when the patient is extubated or weaning is stopped because no further progress is being made. The patient who is ready for extubation should receive hyperoxygenation and suctioning (e.g., oropharynx, ET tube). Instruct the patient to take a deep breath, and at the peak of inspiration, deflate the cuff and remove the tube in one motion. After removal, encourage the patient to deep breathe and cough, and suction the oropharynx as needed. Administer supplemental O_2 and provide naso-oral care. Carefully monitor the patient's vital signs, respiratory status, and oxygenation immediately after extubation, within 1 hour, and per institution policy. If the patient does not tolerate extubation, immediate reintubation or a trial of noninvasive ventilation may be necessary.

Chronic Mechanical Ventilation

Mechanical ventilators are no longer limited to the ICU but are now a part of long-term and home care. In some instances, terminally ill, ventilated patients may be discharged to hospice. The emphasis on controlling hospital costs has increased the early discharge of patients and the need to provide highly technical care such as mechanical ventilation in home settings.[52] The success of home mechanical ventilation depends, in part, on careful predischarge assessment and planning for both the patient and caregivers.

Both negative pressure and positive pressure ventilators are used in the home. Negative pressure ventilators do not require an artificial airway and are less complicated to use. Several types of small, portable (battery-powered) positive pressure ventilators are available and can be attached to a wheelchair or placed on a bedside table. Settings and alarms on these ventilators are simpler to use than on the standard ICU ventilators.

Home mechanical ventilation has advantages and disadvantages. Having the patient in the home eliminates the strain that the hospital setting imposes on family dynamics. Caregivers' feelings of helplessness when they first hear about the necessity for long-term mechanical ventilation is frequently balanced by the opportunity to participate in the patient's care in the home

setting. At home the patient may be able to take part in more activities of daily living around an individualized schedule and, because of the smaller size of the home ventilator, be more mobile. Another advantage of home mechanical ventilation is the reduced risk of HAIs.

Disadvantages of home mechanical ventilation include problems related to equipment, reimbursement, caregiver stress and fatigue, and the patient's complex needs. Ventilated patients are usually dependent, requiring extensive nursing care, at least initially. Disposable products may not be reimbursable. Financial resources must be carefully assessed when arranging home mechanical ventilation. Schedule a meeting with the discharge team before initiating a teaching plan for discharge.

Another disadvantage of home mechanical ventilation is its potential impact on the family. Caregivers may seem enthusiastic about caring for their loved one in the home but may be motivated by numerous, complex factors. They may not understand the sacrifices they may have to make financially and in personal time and commitment. Encourage caregivers to consider respite care to periodically relieve their stress and fatigue.

NURSING MANAGEMENT
MECHANICAL VENTILATION

eNursing Care Plan 66-1 for the patient receiving mechanical ventilation is available on the website for this chapter.

OTHER CRITICAL CARE CONTENT

Table 66-14 lists additional critical care content presented in other chapters of this book.

TABLE 66-14	CROSS-REFERENCES TO CRITICAL CARE CONTENT	
Topic		**Discussed in Chapter**
Acute coronary syndrome		34
Acute heart failure		35
Acute respiratory distress syndrome (ARDS)		68
Acute respiratory failure		68
Basic life support and CPR		Appendix A
Burns		25
Cardiac dysrhythmias		36
Cardiac pacemakers		36
Cardiac surgery		34
Central venous access device (CVAD)		17
Continuous renal replacement therapy (CRRT)		47
Delirium		60
Emergencies		69
End-of-life (EOL) care		10
Enteral nutrition (EN)		40
Head injury, including ICP monitoring		57
Multiple organ dysfunction syndrome (MODS)		67
Myocardial infarction (MI)		34
Oxygen delivery		29
Pain management		9
Parenteral nutrition (PN)		40
Pulmonary edema		35
Renal dialysis		47
Shock		67
Stroke		58
Systemic inflammatory response syndrome (SIRS)		67
Tracheostomy		27
Trauma		69

CPR, Cardiopulmonary resuscitation; *ICP,* intracranial pressure.

CASE STUDY

Critical Care and Mechanical Ventilation

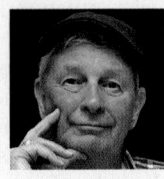

iStockphoto/Thinkstock

Patient Profile

R.K. is a 72-yr-old white man who collapsed on the street. He was unresponsive on admission and remains unresponsive. He has an oral ET tube in place and is receiving mechanical ventilation. He weighs 198 lb (90 kg). A subclavian central line was placed to monitor CVP and administer fluids.

Subjective Data

None. Patient is unresponsive to painful stimuli.

Objective Data

Physical Examination

- Noninvasive BP 100/75 mm Hg; heart rate 128 (atrial fibrillation with a rapid ventricular response); temperature 102° F (38.8° C); SpO$_2$ is 98%
- Purulent secretions from ET tube
- Breath sounds: rhonchi bilaterally, decreased breath sounds on the right

Diagnostic Studies

- Chest x-ray reveals right lower lung consolidation
- ABGs: pH 7.48; PaO$_2$ 94 mm Hg; PaCO$_2$ 30 mm Hg; HCO$_3$ 34 mEq/L
- CT scan is positive for massive hemorrhagic stroke

Collaborative Care

- Positive pressure ventilation settings: assist-control mode
- Settings: FIO$_2$ 70%, V$_T$ 700 mL, respiratory rate 16 breaths/min, PEEP 5 cm H$_2$O
- Enteral feeding at 25 mL/hr via small-bore nasogastric feeding tube
- External condom catheter for urinary drainage
- HOB elevated at 40 degrees

- Reposition every 2 hr
- Azithromycin (Zithromax) 500 mg IV q24hr
- Cefotaxime (Claforan) 2 g IV q6hr
- D$_5$NS with KCl 20 mEq/L at 100 mL/hr

Discussion Questions

1. Identify two reasons for intubating and providing mechanical ventilation for R.K.
2. What do R.K.'s ABGs indicate, and which ventilator setting(s) should be changed?
3. What is his PaO$_2$/FIO$_2$ ratio, and what does it indicate?
4. R.K.'s BP drops to 80 mm Hg. Despite increasing doses of vasopressors and fluid challenges, his BP remains low. A central venous catheter and an arterial line are inserted. APCO monitoring is started. What would be the purpose of hemodynamic monitoring in this patient?
5. *Priority Decision:* What are two priority nursing considerations for a patient with invasive monitoring?
6. R.K.'s pulmonary condition deteriorates. PaO$_2$ drops to 70 mm Hg, and SpO$_2$ is 89%. PEEP is increased to 7.5 cm H$_2$O. What implications does this have for R.K. given his hemodynamic status?
7. *Priority Decision:* Based on the data presented, what are the priority nursing diagnoses? Are there any collaborative problems?
8. *Delegation Decision:* What patient care activities can you delegate to unlicensed assistive personnel?
9. *Evidence-Based Practice:* R.K.'s family wants to know why he is getting tube feedings. What would you tell the family? What is the evidence to support the use of tube feedings?
10. After 4 days, R.K. remains unresponsive and has developed renal failure. The physician believes the patient will not recover from his neurologic injury and wishes to discuss goals of care with the patient's caregiver. What would be your role in this meeting?

⊕volve Answers available at *http://evolve.elsevier.com/Lewis/medsurg.*

▌ BRIDGE TO NCLEX EXAMINATION

The number of the question corresponds to the same-numbered outcome at the beginning of the chapter.

1. Certification in critical care nursing (CCRN) by the American Association of Critical-Care Nurses indicates that the nurse
   a. is an advanced practice nurse who cares for acutely and critically ill patients.
   b. may practice independently to provide symptom management for the critically ill.
   c. has earned a master's degree in the field of advanced acute and critical care nursing.
   d. has practiced in critical care and successfully completed a test of critical care knowledge.

2. What are the appropriate nursing interventions for the patient with delirium in the ICU *(select all that apply)?*
   a. Use clocks and calendars to maintain orientation.
   b. Encourage round-the-clock presence of caregivers at the bedside.
   c. Sedate the patient with appropriate drugs to protect the patient from harmful behaviors.
   d. Silence all alarms, reduce overhead paging, and avoid conversations around the patient.
   e. Identify physiologic factors that may be contributing to the patient's confusion and irritability.

3. The critical care nurse recognizes that an ideal plan for caregiver involvement includes
   a. a caregiver at the bedside at all times.
   b. allowing caregivers at the bedside at preset, brief intervals.
   c. an individually devised plan to involve caregivers with care and comfort measures.
   d. restriction of visiting in the ICU because the environment is overwhelming to caregivers.

4. To establish hemodynamic monitoring for a patient, the nurse zeros the
   a. cardiac output monitoring system to the level of the left ventricle.
   b. pressure monitoring system to the level of the catheter tip located in the patient.
   c. pressure monitoring system to the level of the atrium, identified as the phlebostatic axis.
   d. pressure monitoring system to the level of the atrium, identified as the midclavicular line.

5. The hemodynamic changes the nurse expects to find after successful initiation of intraaortic balloon pump therapy in a patient with cardiogenic shock include *(select all that apply)*
   a. decreased SV.
   b. decreased SVR.
   c. decreased PAWP.
   d. increased diastolic BP.
   e. decreased myocardial oxygen consumption.

6. The purpose of adding PEEP to positive pressure ventilation is to
   a. increase functional residual capacity and improve oxygenation.
   b. increase FIO_2 in an attempt to wean the patient and avoid O_2 toxicity.
   c. determine if the patient is in synchrony with the ventilator or needs to be paralyzed.
   d. determine if the patient is able to be weaned and avoid the risk of pneumomediastinum.

7. The nursing management of a patient with an artificial airway includes
   a. maintaining ET tube cuff pressure at 30 cm H_2O.
   b. routine suctioning of the tube at least every 2 hours.
   c. observing for cardiac dysrhythmias during suctioning.
   d. preventing tube dislodgment by limiting mouth care to lubrication of the lips.

8. The nurse monitors the patient with positive pressure mechanical ventilation for
   a. paralytic ileus because pressure on the abdominal contents affects bowel motility.
   b. diuresis and sodium depletion because of increased release of atrial natriuretic peptide.
   c. signs of cardiovascular insufficiency because pressure in the chest impedes venous return.
   d. respiratory acidosis in a patient with COPD because of alveolar hyperventilation and increased PaO_2 levels.

1. d, 2. a, c, e, 3. c, 4. a, 5. b, c, d, e, 6. a, 7. c, 8. c

ⓔvolve

For rationales to these answers and even more NCLEX review questions, visit *http://evolve.elsevier.com/Lewis/medsurg*.

REFERENCES

1. American Association of Critical-Care Nurses: About critical care nursing. Retrieved from *www.aacn.org/WD/publishing/content/pressroom/aboutcriticalcarenursing.content*.

2. Jones DA, DeVita MA, Bellomo R: Rapid-response teams, *N Engl J Med* 365:139, 2011.

3. American Association of Critical-Care Nurses: Frequently asked questions about APRN Consensus Model implementation for NP programs. Retrieved from *www.aacn.org/WD/Certifications/Content/APRN-NP-FAQs.content*.

4. Wiegand DL-M, Williams LD: End-of-life care. In KK Carlson, editor: *Advanced critical care nursing*, St Louis, 2009, Saunders.

*5. McClave SA, Martindale RG, Vanek VW, et al: Guidelines for the provision and assessment of nutrition support therapy in the adult critically ill patient: Society of Critical Care Medicine and American Society for Parenteral and Enteral Nutrition, *J Parenter Enteral Nutr* 33:277, 2009.

*6. Woods S: Spiritual and complementary therapies to promote healing and reduce stress. In NC Molter, editor: *Protocols for practice: creating healing environments*, ed 2, Sudbury, Mass, 2007, Jones & Bartlett. (Classic)

*7. Arbour RB: Pain management. In NC Molter, editor: *Protocols for practice: creating healing environments*, ed 2, Sudbury, Mass, 2007, Jones & Bartlett. (Classic)

*8. Barr J, Fraser GL, Puntillo K, et al: Clinical practice guidelines for the management of pain, agitation, and delirium in adult patients in the intensive care unit, *Crit Care Med* 41:263, 2013.

*9. American Association of Critical-Care Nurses: Delirium assessment and management. Retrieved from *www.aacn.org/WD/practice/content/practicealerts/delirium-practice-alert.content*.

*10. Lawson N, Thompson K, Saunders G, et al: Sound intensity and noise evaluation in a critical care unit, *Am J Crit Care* 19:e88, 2010.

*11. Hellstrom A, Willman A: Promoting sleep by nursing interventions in health care settings: a systematic review, *Worldviews Evid Based Nurs* 8:128, 2011.

12. Institute for Patient and Family Centered Care: Advancing the practice of patient and family centered care in hospitals: how to get started. Retrieved from *www.ipfcc.org/pdf/getting_started.pdf*.

*13. Leske JS, Pasquale MA: Family needs, interventions and presence. In NC Molter, editor: *Protocols for practice: creating healing environments*, ed 2, Sudbury, Mass, 2007, Jones & Bartlett. (Classic)

*14. American Association of Critical-Care Nurses: AACN practice alert: family presence: visitation in the adult ICU. Retrieved from *www.aacn.org/WD/practice/docs/practicealerts/family-visitation-adult-icu-practicealert.pdf*.

15. Society of Critical Care Medicine: Patient and family resources: ICU issues and answers brochures. Retrieved from *www.myicucare.org/Support_Brochures/Pages/default.aspx*.

*16. American Association of Critical-Care Nurses: AACN practice alert: family presence during CPR and invasive procedures. Retrieved from *www.aacn.org/WD/Practice/Docs/PracticeAlerts/Family%20Presence%2004-2010%20final.pdf*.

*17. Medina J, Puntillo K, editors: *AACN protocols for practice: palliative care and end-of-life issues in critical care*, Sudbury, Mass, 2006, Jones & Bartlett. (Classic)

*18. Shaffer RB: Arterial catheter insertion (assist). In Wiegand DL-M, editor: *AACN procedure manual for critical care*, ed 6, St Louis, 2011, Saunders.

*19. Edwards Lifesciences: Understanding stroke volume variation and its clinical application. Retrieved from *http://ht.edwards.com/presentationvideos/powerpointslides/strokevolumevar/strokevolumevariation.pdf*.

*20. Kern ME: Arterial pressure-based cardiac output monitoring. In DL-M Wiegand, editor: *AACN procedure manual for critical care*, ed 6, St Louis, 2011, Saunders.

*21. Klein DG: Cardiac output measurement techniques (invasive). In DL-M Wiegand, editor: *AACN procedure manual for critical care*, ed 6, St Louis, 2011, Saunders.

*Evidence-based information for clinical practice.

*22. Headley JM, Giuliano KK: Continuous venous oxygenation monitoring. In DL-M Wiegand, editor: *AACN procedure manual for critical care*, ed 6, St Louis, 2011, Saunders.

*23. Castelluci D: Intraaortic balloon pump management. In Wiegand DL-M, editor: *AACN procedure manual for critical care*, ed 6, St Louis, 2011, Saunders.

*24. Puhlman M, Hargraves J: Ventricular assist devices. In Wiegand DL-M, editor: *AACN procedure manual for critical care*, ed 6, St Louis, 2011, Saunders.

25. Abiomed: The AbioCor system. Retrieved from *www.abiomed.com/products/heart-replacement*.

26. Mallick A, Bodenham AR: Tracheostomy in critically ill patients, *Eur J Anaesthesiol* 27:676, 2010.

27. Greene LR, Sposato K: APIC elimination guide: guide to the elimination of ventilator-associated pneumonia. Retrieved from *www.apic.org/Resource_/EliminationGuideForm/18e326ad-b484-471c-9c35-6822a53ee4a2/File/VAP_09.pdf*.

28. Light S: Rapid sequence intubation: stay up to date on this important procedure, *J Am Acad Physician Assistants* 23:37, 2010.

29. Walsh BK, Crotwell DN, Restrepo RD: Capnography/capnometry during mechanical ventilation, *Respir Care* 56:503, 2011.

*30. American Association of Respiratory Care: AARC clinical practice guidelines: endotracheal suctioning of mechanically ventilated patients with artificial airways, *Respir Care* 55:758, 2010.

*31. Sole ML, Su Z, Talbert S, et al: Evaluation of an intervention to maintain endotracheal tube cuff pressure within therapeutic range, *Am J Crit Care* 20:109, 2011.

*32. Chulay M, Seckel MA: Suctioning: endotracheal or tracheostomy tube. In DL-M Wiegand, editor: *AACN procedure manual for critical care*, ed 6, St Louis, 2011, Saunders.

*33. Lusk B, Lash AA: The stress response: psychoneuroimmunology and stress among ICU patients, *Dimens Crit Care Nurs* 24:25, 2005. (Classic)

*34. Thomas LA: Clinical management of stressors perceived by patients on mechanical ventilation, *AACN Clin Issues* 14:73, 2003. (Classic)

35. Jarachovic M, Mason M, Kerber K, et al: The role of standardized protocols in unplanned extubations in a medical intensive care unit, *Am J Crit Care* 20:304, 2011.

*36. Chang L, Wang KK, Yann-Fen C: Influence of physical restraint of unplanned extubation of adult intensive care patient: a case control study, *Am J Crit Care* 17:408, 2008.

*37. Happ MB: Communicating with mechanically ventilated patients: state of the science, *AACN Clin Issues* 12:247, 2001. (Classic)

*38. American Association of Critical-Care Nurses: AACN practice alert: prevention of aspiration. Retrieved from *www.aacn.org/WD/practice/docs/practicealerts/aacn-aspiration-practice-alert.pdf*.

*39. Burns SM: Invasive mechanical ventilation (through an artificial airway): volume and pressure modes. In Wiegand DL-M, editor: *AACN procedure manual for critical care*, ed 6, St Louis, 2011, Saunders.

*40. Burns SM: Noninvasive positive pressure ventilation: continuous positive airway pressure (CPAP) and bilevel positive airway pressure (BiPAP). In DL-M Wiegand, editor: *AACN procedure manual for critical care*, ed 6, St Louis, 2011, Saunders.

*41. Unoki T, Serita A, Grap MJ: Automatic tube compensation during weaning from mechanical ventilation: evidence and clinical implications, *Crit Care Nurs* 28:34, 2008.

42. Ali S, Ferguson ND: High-frequency oscillatory ventilation in ALI/ARDS, *Crit Care Clin* 27:487, 2011.

43. Dickinson S, Park PK, Napolitano LM: Prone-positioning therapy in ARDS, *Crit Care Clin* 27:511, 2011.

44. Park PK, Napolitano LM, Bartlett RH: Extracorporeal membrane oxygenation in adult acute respiratory distress syndrome, *Crit Care Clin* 27:627, 2011.

*45. American Association of Critical-Care Nurses: AACN practice alert: ventilator-associated pneumonia. Retrieved from *ww.aacn.org/WD/Practice/Docs/Ventilator_Associated_Pneumonia_1-2008.pdf*.

46. Institute for Healthcare Improvement: How-to guide: prevent ventilator-associated pneumonia. Retrieved from *www.ihi.org*.

47. FDA Drug Safety Communication: *Clostridium difficile*–associated diarrhea can be associated with stomach acid drugs known as proton pump inhibitors. Retrieved from *www.fda.gov/drugs/drugsafety/ucm290510.htm*.

*48. American Association of Critical-Care Nurses: AACN practice alert: verification of feeding tube placement. Retrieved from *www.aacn.org/wd/practice/content/feeding-tube-practice-alert.pcms?menu=practice*.

49. Vollman KM: Introduction to progressive mobility, *Crit Care Nurse* 30:S3, 2010.

50. Desai SV, Law TJ, Needham DM: Long-term complications of critical care, *Crit Care Med* 39:371, 2011.

*51. Burns SM: Weaning process. In DL-M Wiegand, editor: *AACN procedure manual for critical care*, ed 6, St Louis, 2011, Saunders.

52. American College of Chest Physicians: Home mechanical ventilation resource center. Retrieved from *www.chestnet.org/accp/article/home-mechanical-ventilation-resource-center*.

RESOURCES

American Association of Critical-Care Nurses
www.aacn.org
American Association for Respiratory Care
http://connect.aarc.org/Home
Society of Critical Care Medicine
www.sccm.org

Once you choose hope, anything's possible.
Christopher Reeve

Nursing Management

Shock, Systemic Inflammatory Response Syndrome, and Multiple Organ Dysfunction Syndrome

Maureen A. Seckel

evolve WEBSITE

http://evolve.elsevier.com/Lewis/medsurg

- NCLEX Review Questions
- Key Points
- Pre-Test
- Answer Guidelines for Case Study on p. 1652
- Rationales for Bridge to NCLEX Examination Questions

- Case Studies
  - Patient With Acute Pancreatitis and Septic Shock
  - Patient With Cardiogenic Shock
  - Patient With Sepsis
- Nursing Care Plan (Customizable)
  - eNCP 67-1: Patient in Shock
- Concept Map Creator
- Glossary
- Content Updates

eFigures
- eFig. 67-1: Compensatory stage of shock
- eFig. 67-2: Progressive stage of shock
- eFig. 67-3: Irreversible stage of shock
- eFig. 67-4: Sepsis alert treatment protocol
- eFig. 67-5: Anaphylaxis algorithm

LEARNING OUTCOMES

1. Relate the pathophysiology to the clinical manifestations of the different types of shock: cardiogenic, hypovolemic, distributive, and obstructive.
2. Compare the effects of shock, systemic inflammatory response syndrome, and multiple organ dysfunction syndrome on the major body systems.
3. Compare the collaborative care, drug therapy, and nursing management of patients experiencing different types of shock.
4. Describe the nursing management of a patient experiencing multiple organ dysfunction syndrome.

KEY TERMS

anaphylactic shock, p. 1636
cardiogenic shock, p. 1633
hypovolemic shock, p. 1633
multiple organ dysfunction syndrome (MODS), p. 1649

neurogenic shock, p. 1634
obstructive shock, p. 1637
sepsis, p. 1636
septic shock, p. 1636

shock, p. 1631
systemic inflammatory response syndrome (SIRS), p. 1649

Shock, systemic inflammatory response syndrome (SIRS), and multiple organ dysfunction syndrome (MODS) are serious and interrelated problems (Fig. 67-1). This chapter provides an overview of the different types of shock, SIRS, and MODS, and the related management of each.

SHOCK

Shock is a syndrome characterized by decreased tissue perfusion and impaired cellular metabolism. This results in an imbalance between the supply of and demand for oxygen and nutrients. The exchange of oxygen and nutrients at the cellular level is essential to life. When cells experience hypoperfusion, the demand for oxygen and nutrients exceeds the supply at the microcirculatory level.

Classification of Shock

The four main categories of shock are cardiogenic, hypovolemic, distributive, and obstructive[1,2] (Table 67-1). Although the cause, initial presentation, and management strategies vary

Reviewed by Lori Godaire, RN-BC, MS, CCRN, CNL, Clinical Nurse Leader, Critical Care Services, William W. Backus Hospital, Norwich, Connecticut; Janet E. Jackson, RN, MS, Assistant Professor, Department of Nursing, Bradley University, Peoria, Illinois; and Anna Moore, RN, MS, Associate Professor, J. Sargeant Reynolds Community College, Richmond, Virginia.

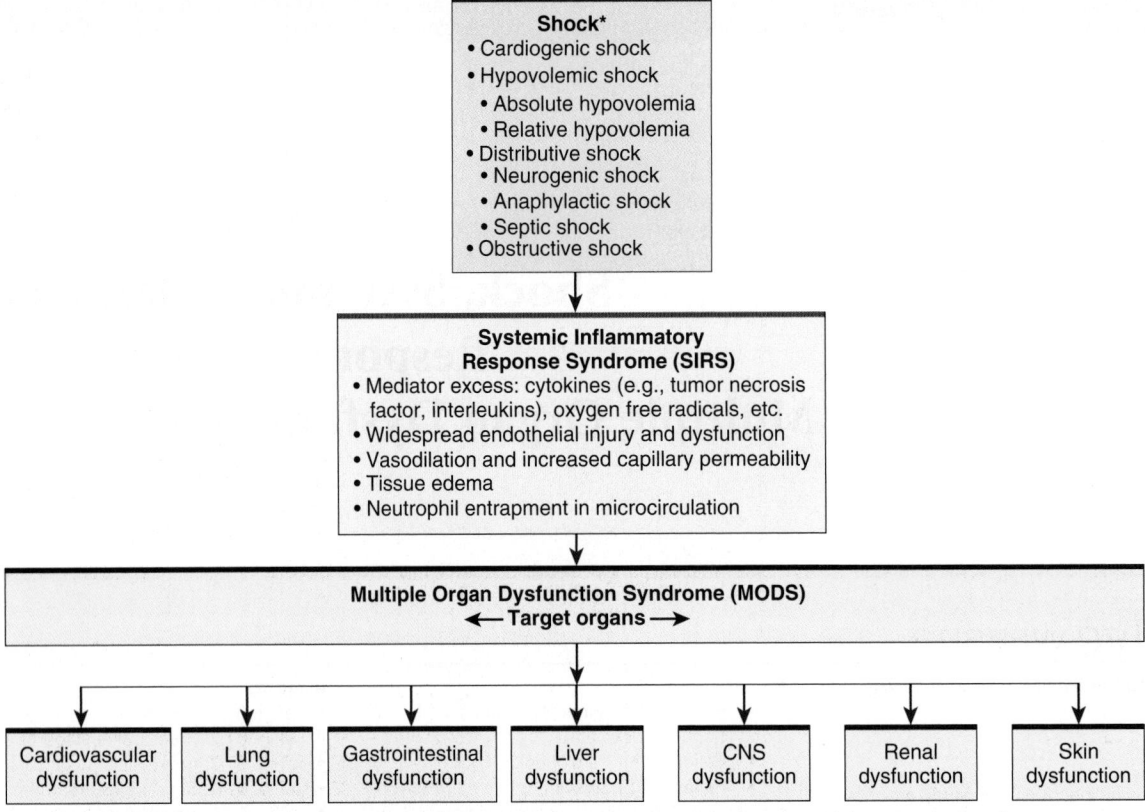

FIG. 67-1 Relationship of shock, systemic inflammatory response syndrome, and multiple organ dysfunction syndrome. *CNS,* Central nervous system. (See Table 67-1 for causes of shock states.)

TABLE 67-1   CLASSIFICATION OF SHOCK STATES

Types and Causes	Examples
Cardiogenic Shock	
• Systolic dysfunction: inability of the heart to pump blood forward	Myocardial infarction, cardiomyopathy, blunt cardiac injury, severe systemic or pulmonary hypertension, myocardial depression from metabolic problems
• Diastolic dysfunction: inability of the heart to fill	Cardiac tamponade, ventricular hypertrophy, cardiomyopathy
• Dysrhythmias	Bradydysrhythmias, tachydysrhythmias
• Structural factors	Valvular stenosis or regurgitation, ventricular septal rupture, tension pneumothorax
Hypovolemic Shock	
Absolute Hypovolemia	
• External loss of whole blood	Hemorrhage from trauma, surgery, GI bleeding
• Loss of other body fluids	Vomiting, diarrhea, excessive diuresis, diabetes insipidus, diabetes mellitus
Relative Hypovolemia	
• Pooling of blood or fluids	Bowel obstruction
• Fluid shifts	Burn injuries, ascites
• Internal bleeding	Fracture of long bones, ruptured spleen, hemothorax, severe pancreatitis
• Massive vasodilation	Sepsis

Types and Causes	Examples
Distributive Shock	
Neurogenic Shock	
• Hemodynamic consequence of spinal cord injury and/or disease at or above T5	Severe pain, drugs, hypoglycemia, injury
• Spinal anesthesia	
• Vasomotor center depression	
Anaphylactic Shock	
• Hypersensitivity (allergic) reaction to a sensitizing substance	Contrast media, blood or blood products, drugs, insect bites, anesthetic agents, food or food additives, vaccines, environmental agents, latex
Septic Shock	
• Infection	Pneumonia, peritonitis, urinary tract, invasive procedures, indwelling lines and catheters
• At-risk patients	Older adults, patients with chronic diseases (e.g., diabetes mellitus, chronic kidney disease, heart failure), patients receiving immunosuppressive therapy or who are malnourished or debilitated
Obstructive Shock	
• Physical obstruction impeding the filling or outflow of blood resulting in reduced cardiac output	Cardiac tamponade, tension pneumothorax, superior vena cava syndrome, abdominal compartment syndrome, pulmonary embolism

for each type of shock, the physiologic responses of the cells to hypoperfusion are similar.

Cardiogenic Shock. Cardiogenic shock occurs when either systolic or diastolic dysfunction of the heart's pumping action results in reduced cardiac output (CO). Causes of cardiogenic shock are listed in Table 67-1. Mortality rates for patients with cardiogenic shock approach 60%.[3] Decreased filling of the heart results in decreased stroke volume.

The heart's inability to pump the blood forward is called *systolic dysfunction.* Systolic dysfunction primarily affects the left ventricle, since systolic pressure is greater on the left side of the heart. When systolic dysfunction affects the right side of the heart, blood flow through the pulmonary circulation is reduced. The most common cause of systolic dysfunction is acute myocardial infarction (MI). Cardiogenic shock is the leading cause of death from acute MI.[4] Causes of diastolic dysfunction are listed in Table 67-1.

Fig. 67-2 describes the pathophysiology of cardiogenic shock. Whether the initiating event is myocardial ischemia, a structural problem (e.g., valvular disorder, ventricular septal rupture), or dysrhythmias, the physiologic responses are similar: the patient experiences impaired tissue perfusion and cellular metabolism.

The early clinical presentation of a patient with cardiogenic shock is similar to that of a patient with acute decompensated heart failure (see Chapter 35). The patient may have tachycardia and hypotension. Pulse pressure may be narrowed due to the heart's inability to pump blood forward during systole and increased volume during diastole. An increase in systemic vascular resistance (SVR) increases the workload of the heart, thus increasing the myocardial oxygen consumption. The heart's inability to pump blood forward also results in a low CO (less than 4 L/minute) and *cardiac index* (less than 2.5 L/min/m²).

On assessment, the patient is tachypneic and has crackles on auscultation of breath sounds because of pulmonary congestion. The hemodynamic profile demonstrates an increase in the pulmonary artery wedge pressure (PAWP), stroke volume variation (SVV), and pulmonary vascular resistance.

Signs of peripheral hypoperfusion (e.g., cyanosis, pallor, diaphoresis, weak peripheral pulses, cool and clammy skin, delayed capillary refill) are seen. Decreased renal blood flow results in sodium and water retention and decreased urine output. Anxiety, confusion, and agitation may develop as cerebral perfusion is impaired. Tables 67-2 and 67-3 describe the laboratory findings and clinical presentation of a patient with cardiogenic shock.

Hypovolemic Shock. Hypovolemic shock occurs after a loss of intravascular fluid volume (see Table 67-1). The volume is inadequate to fill the vascular space. The volume loss may be either an absolute or a relative volume loss. *Absolute hypovolemia* results when fluid is lost through hemorrhage, gastrointestinal (GI) loss (e.g., vomiting, diarrhea), fistula drainage, diabetes insipidus, or diuresis. In *relative hypovolemia,* fluid volume moves out of the vascular space into the extravascular space (e.g., intracavitary space). This type of fluid shift is called *third spacing.* One example of relative volume loss is leakage of fluid from the vascular space to the interstitial space from increased capillary permeability, as seen in burns (see Chapter 25).

In hypovolemic shock the size of the vascular compartment remains unchanged while the volume of blood or plasma decreases. Whether the loss of intravascular volume is absolute or relative, the physiologic consequences are similar. A reduction in intravascular volume results in a decreased venous return to the heart, decreased preload, decreased stroke volume, and decreased CO. A cascade of events results in decreased tissue perfusion and impaired cellular metabolism, the hallmarks of shock (Fig. 67-3).

The patient's response to acute volume loss depends on a number of factors, including extent of injury, age, and general state of health. However, the clinical presentation of hypovolemic shock is consistent (see Table 67-3). An overall assessment of physiologic reserves may indicate the patient's ability to compensate. A patient may compensate for a loss of up to 15% of the total blood volume (approximately 750 mL). Further loss of volume (15% to 30%) results in a sympathetic nervous system (SNS)–mediated response. This response results in an increase in heart rate, CO, and respiratory rate and depth. The stroke volume, central venous pressure (CVP), and PAWP are decreased because of the decreased circulating blood volume.

The patient may appear anxious, and urine output begins to decrease. If hypovolemia is corrected by crystalloid fluid replacement at this time, tissue dysfunction is generally reversible. If volume loss is greater than 30%, compensatory mechanisms may begin to fail and immediate replacement with blood products should be started. Loss of autoregulation in the microcirculation and irreversible tissue destruction occur with loss of more than 40% of the total blood volume.[5,6] Common laboratory studies and assessments that are done include serial measurements of hemoglobin and hematocrit levels, electrolytes, lactate, blood gases, mixed central venous oxygen saturation (SvO₂), and hourly urine outputs (see Table 67-2).

PATHOPHYSIOLOGY MAP

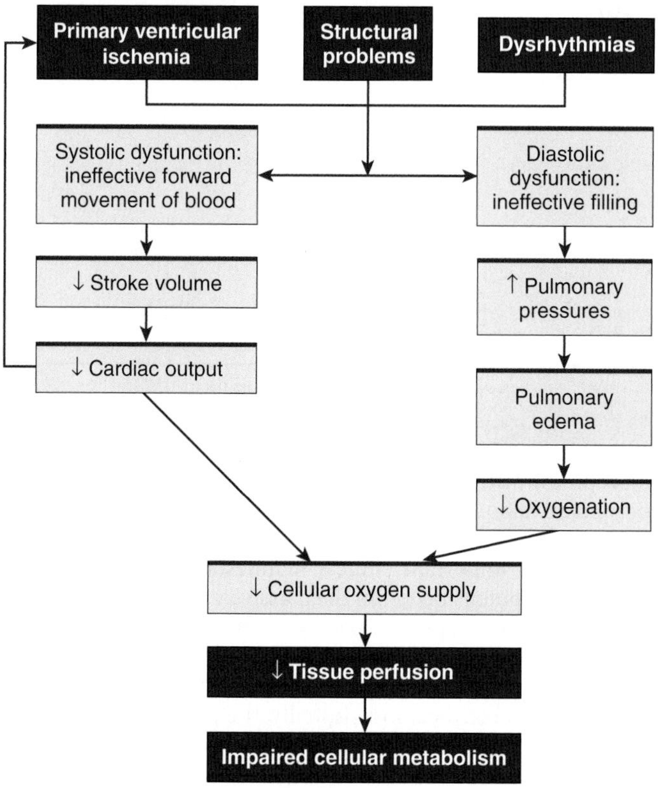

FIG. 67-2 The pathophysiology of cardiogenic shock.

TABLE 67-2   DIAGNOSTIC STUDIES

Laboratory Changes in Shock

Laboratory Study	Finding	Significance of Finding
Red blood cells		
RBC count, hematocrit, hemoglobin	Normal	Remains within normal limits in shock because of relative hypovolemia and pump failure and in hemorrhagic shock before fluid resuscitation.
	↓	Hemorrhagic shock after fluid resuscitation when fluids other than blood are used.
	↑	Nonhemorrhagic shock caused by actual hypovolemia and hemoconcentration.
White blood cells		
WBC count, bands	↑	Infection, septic shock.
DIC screen		Acute DIC can develop within hours to days after an initial assault on the body (e.g., shock).
• Fibrin split products (FSP)	↑	
• Fibrinogen level	↓	
• Platelet count	↓	
• PTT and PT	↑	
• INR	↑	
• Thrombin time	↑	
• D-dimer	↑	
Creatine kinase	↑	Trauma, myocardial infarction in response to cellular damage and/or hypoxia.
Troponin	↑	Increases in myocardial infarction.
BUN	↑	Indicates impaired kidney function caused by hypoperfusion as a result of severe vasoconstriction, or occurs secondary to catabolism of cells (e.g., trauma, infection).
Creatinine	↑	Indicates impaired kidney function caused by hypoperfusion as a result of severe vasoconstriction. Is more sensitive indicator of renal function than BUN.
Glucose	↑	Found in early shock because of release of liver glycogen stores in response to sympathetic nervous system stimulation and cortisol. Insulin insensitivity develops.
	↓	Occurs because of depleted glycogen stores with hepatocellular dysfunction possible as shock progresses.

Laboratory Study	Finding	Significance of Finding
Serum electrolytes		
• Sodium	↑	Found in early shock because of increased secretion of aldosterone, causing renal retention of sodium.
	↓	May occur iatrogenically when excess hypotonic fluid is administered after fluid loss.
• Potassium	↑	Results when cellular death liberates intracellular potassium. Also occurs in acute kidney injury and acidosis.
	↓	Found in early shock because of increased secretion of aldosterone, causing renal excretion of potassium.
Arterial blood gases	Respiratory alkalosis	Found in early shock secondary to hyperventilation.
	Metabolic acidosis	Occurs later in shock when lactate accumulates in blood from anaerobic metabolism.
Base deficit	>−6	Indicates acid production secondary to hypoxia.
Blood cultures	Growth of organisms	May grow organisms in patients who are in septic shock.
Lactate level	↑	Usually increases once significant hypoperfusion and impaired oxygen utilization at the cellular level have occurred. By-product of anaerobic metabolism.
Liver enzymes (ALT, AST, GGT)	↑	Elevations indicate liver cell destruction in progressive stage of shock.

ALT, Alanine aminotransferase; *AST,* aspartate aminotransferase; *BUN,* blood urea nitrogen; *DIC,* disseminated intravascular coagulation; *GGT,* γ-glutamyl transferase; *INR,* international normalized ratio; *PT,* prothrombin time; *PTT,* partial thromboplastin time.

Distributive Shock

Neurogenic Shock. Neurogenic shock is a hemodynamic phenomenon that can occur within 30 minutes of a spinal cord injury at the fifth thoracic (T5) vertebra or above; it can last up to 6 weeks. The injury results in a massive vasodilation without compensation because of the loss of SNS vasoconstrictor tone. This massive vasodilation leads to a pooling of blood in the blood vessels, tissue hypoperfusion, and ultimately impaired cellular metabolism (Fig. 67-4).

In addition to spinal cord injury, spinal anesthesia can block transmission of impulses from the SNS. Depression of the vasomotor center of the medulla from drugs (e.g., opioids, benzo-diazepines) also can decrease the vasoconstrictor tone of the peripheral blood vessels, resulting in neurogenic shock (see Table 67-1).

The most important clinical manifestations in neurogenic shock are hypotension (from the massive vasodilation) and bradycardia (from unopposed parasympathetic stimulation).[7] The patient may not be able to regulate body temperature. Combined with massive vasodilation, the inability to regulate temperature promotes heat loss. Initially, the patient's skin is warm due to the massive dilation. As the heat disperses, the patient is at risk for hypothermia. Later, the patient's skin may be cool or warm depending on the ambient temperature (*poikilothermia*—

TABLE 67-3   CLINICAL PRESENTATION OF TYPES OF SHOCK

	Hypovolemic Shock	Distributive Shock			Obstructive Shock
Cardiogenic Shock		**Neurogenic Shock**	**Anaphylactic Shock**	**Septic Shock**	
Cardiovascular System					
Tachycardia ↓ BP ↓ Capillary refill Chest pain may or may not be present	↓ Preload ↓ Stroke volume ↓ Capillary refill	↓ BP ↓/↑ Temperature Bradycardia	Chest pain Third spacing of fluid	↓/↑ Temperature Myocardial dysfunction Biventricular dilation ↓ Ejection fraction	↓ BP ↓ Preload
Pulmonary System					
Tachypnea Crackles Cyanosis Rhonchi	Tachypnea → bradypnea (late)	Dysfunction related to level of injury	Shortness of breath Edema of larynx and epiglottis Wheezing Stridor Rhinitis	Hyperventilation Crackles Respiratory alkalosis → respiratory acidosis Hypoxemia Respiratory failure ARDS Pulmonary hypertension	Tachypnea → bradypnea (late) Shortness of breath
Renal System					
↑ Na^+ and H_2O retention ↓ Renal blood flow ↓ Urine output	↓ Urine output	Bladder dysfunction	Incontinence	↓ Urine output	↓ Urine output
Skin					
Pallor Cool, clammy	Pallor Cool, clammy	↓ Skin perfusion Cool or warm Dry	Flushing Pruritus Urticaria Angioedema	Warm and flushed → cool and mottled (late)	Pallor Cool, clammy
Neurologic System					
↓ Cerebral perfusion: • Anxiety • Confusion • Agitation	↓ Cerebral perfusion: • Anxiety • Confusion • Agitation	Flaccid paralysis below the level of the lesion Loss of reflex activity	Anxiety Feeling of impending doom Confusion ↓ LOC Metallic taste	Alteration in mental status (e.g., confusion) Agitation Coma (late)	↓ Cerebral perfusion: • Anxiety • Confusion • Agitation
Gastrointestinal System					
↓ Bowel sounds Nausea, vomiting	Absent bowel sounds	Bowel dysfunction	Cramping Abdominal pain Nausea Vomiting Diarrhea	GI bleeding Paralytic ileus	↓ to absent bowel sounds
Diagnostic Findings*					
↑ Cardiac markers ↑ b-Type natriuretic peptide (BNP) ↑ Blood glucose ↑ BUN ECG (e.g., dysrhythmias) Echocardiogram (e.g., left ventricular dysfunction) Chest x-ray (e.g., pulmonary infiltrates)	↓ Hematocrit ↓ Hemoglobin ↑ Lactate ↑ Urine specific gravity Changes in electrolytes		Sudden onset History of allergies Exposure to contrast media	↑/↓ WBC ↓ Platelets ↑ Lactate ↑ Blood glucose ↓ Urine specific gravity ↓ Urine Na^+ Positive blood cultures	Specific to cause of obstruction

*Also see Table 67-2.
ARDS, Acute respiratory distress syndrome; *BUN*, blood urea nitrogen; *LOC*, level of consciousness;

PATHOPHYSIOLOGY MAP

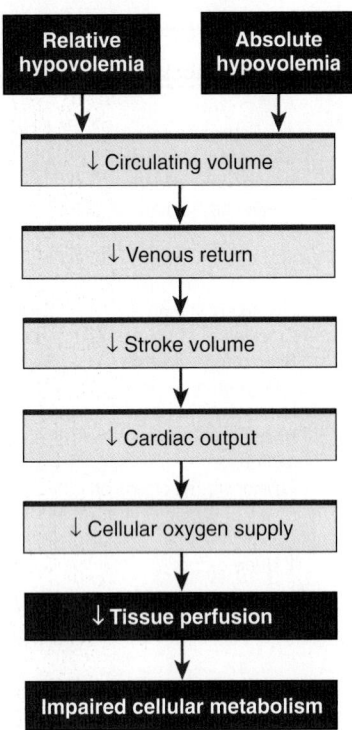

FIG. 67-3 The pathophysiology of hypovolemic shock.

PATHOPHYSIOLOGY MAP

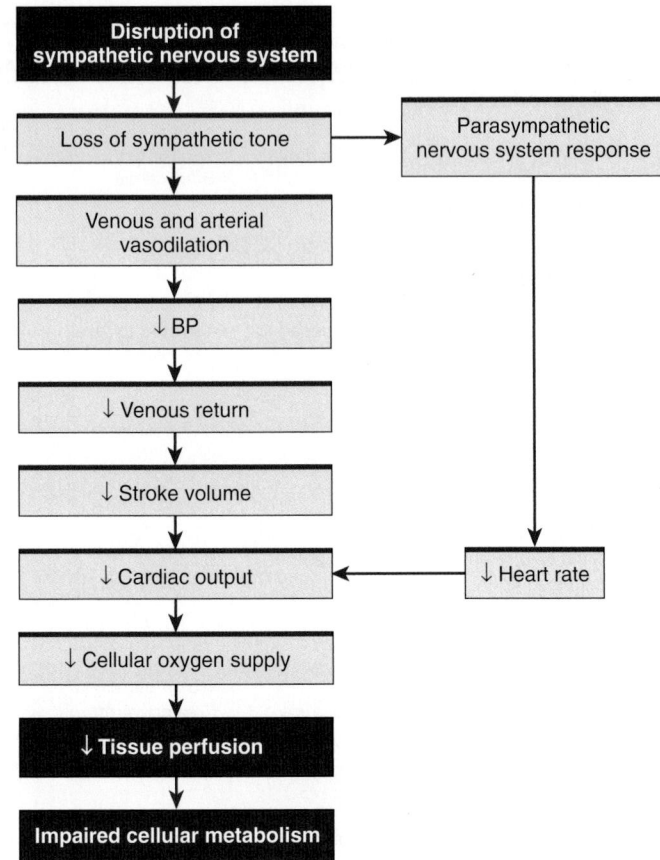

FIG. 67-4 The pathophysiology of neurogenic shock.

taking on the temperature of the environment). In either case, the skin is usually dry. Tables 67-2 and 67-3 further describe the laboratory findings and clinical presentation of a patient with neurogenic shock.

Although spinal shock and neurogenic shock often occur in the same patient, they are not the same disorder. *Spinal shock* is a transient condition that is present after an acute spinal cord injury (see Chapter 61). The patient with spinal shock experiences the absence of all voluntary and reflex neurologic activity below the level of the injury.

Anaphylactic Shock. Anaphylactic shock is an acute, life-threatening hypersensitivity (allergic) reaction to a sensitizing substance (e.g., drug, chemical, vaccine, food, insect venom). The reaction quickly causes massive vasodilation, release of vasoactive mediators, and an increase in capillary permeability. As capillary permeability increases, fluid leaks from the vascular space into the interstitial space. Anaphylactic shock can lead to respiratory distress due to laryngeal edema or severe bronchospasm, and circulatory failure from the massive vasodilation.[8] The patient has a sudden onset of symptoms, including dizziness, chest pain, incontinence, swelling of the lips and tongue, wheezing, and stridor. Skin changes include flushing, pruritus, urticaria, and angioedema. In addition, the patient may be anxious and confused and have a sense of impending doom.

A patient can have a severe allergic reaction, possibly leading to anaphylactic shock, after contact, inhalation, ingestion, or injection with an antigen (allergen) to which the individual has previously been sensitized (see Table 67-1). Parenteral administration of the antigen (allergen) is the route most likely to cause anaphylaxis. However, oral, topical, and inhalation routes can also cause anaphylactic reactions. Tables 67-2 and 67-3

describe the laboratory findings and clinical presentation of a patient in anaphylactic shock. Quick and decisive action is critical to prevent the progression of an allergic reaction to anaphylactic shock. (Anaphylaxis is discussed in Chapter 14.)

Septic Shock. Sepsis is a systemic inflammatory response to a documented or suspected infection (Table 67-4). In as many as 10% to 30% of patients with sepsis, the causative organism is not identified. *Severe sepsis,* defined as sepsis complicated by organ dysfunction, is diagnosed in more than 750,000 patients per year and has mortality rates as high as 28% to 50%.[9-11]

Septic shock is the presence of sepsis with hypotension despite adequate fluid resuscitation, along with inadequate tissue perfusion resulting in tissue hypoxia. The main organisms that cause sepsis are gram-negative and gram-positive bacteria. Parasites, fungi, and viruses can also cause sepsis and septic shock.[12] Fig. 67-5 presents the pathogenesis of septic shock.

When a microorganism enters the body, the normal immune or inflammatory responses are started. However, in severe sepsis and septic shock the body's response to the microorganism is exaggerated. Inflammation and coagulation increase, and fibrinolysis decreases. Endotoxins from the microorganism cell wall stimulate the release of cytokines, including tumor necrosis factor (TNF), interleukin-1 (IL-1), and other proinflammatory mediators that act through secondary mediators such as platelet-activating factor, IL-6, and IL-8.[12] (See Chapter 12 for discussion of the inflammatory response.) The release of platelet-activating factor results in the formation of microthrombi and obstruction of the microvasculature. The combined effects of the mediators

TABLE 67-4	DIAGNOSTIC CRITERIA FOR SEPSIS

Infection, documented or suspected, and some of the following.

General Variables
- Fever (temperature >100.9° F [38.3° C])
- Hypothermia (core temperature <97.0° F [36° C])
- Heart rate >90 beats/min
- Tachypnea
- Altered mental status
- Significant edema or positive fluid balance (>20 mL/kg over 24 hr)
- Hyperglycemia (blood glucose >140 mg/dL) in the absence of diabetes

Inflammatory Variables
- Leukocytosis (WBC count >12,000/µL)
- Leukopenia (WBC count <4000/µL)
- Normal WBC count with >10% immature forms
- Elevated C-reactive protein
- Elevated procalcitonin

Hemodynamic Variables
- Arterial hypotension (SBP <90 mm Hg, MAP <70 mm Hg, or a decrease in SBP >40 mm Hg)

Organ Dysfunction Variables
- Arterial hypoxemia (PaO_2/FIO_2 <300)
- Acute oliguria (urine output <0.5 mL/kg/hr for at least 2 hr despite adequate fluid resuscitation)
- Serum creatinine increase >0.5 mg/dL
- Coagulation abnormalities (INR >1.5 or PTT >60 sec)
- Ileus (absent bowel sounds)
- Thrombocytopenia (platelet count <100,000/µL)
- Hyperbilirubinemia (total bilirubin >4 mg/dL)

Tissue Perfusion Variables
- Hyperlactatemia (>1 mmol/L)
- Decreased capillary refill or mottling

Source: Dellinger RP, Levy MM, Rhodes A, et al: Surviving sepsis campaign: international guidelines for management of severe sepsis and septic shock: 2012, *Crit Care Med* 41:580, 2013.
FIO_2, Fraction of inspired oxygen; *INR*, international normalized ratio; *MAP*, mean arterial pressure; *PaO_2*, partial pressure of arterial oxygen; *PTT*, partial thromboplastin time; *SBP*, systolic blood pressure.

result in damage to the endothelium, vasodilation, increased capillary permeability, and neutrophil and platelet aggregation and adhesion to the endothelium.

Septic shock has three major pathophysiologic effects: vasodilation, maldistribution of blood flow, and myocardial depression. Patients may be euvolemic, but because of acute vasodilation, relative hypovolemia and hypotension occur. In addition, blood flow in the microcirculation is decreased, causing poor oxygen delivery and tissue hypoxia. The combination of TNF and IL-1 is thought to have a role in sepsis-induced myocardial dysfunction. The ejection fraction is decreased for the first few days after the initial insult. Because of a decreased ejection fraction, the ventricles dilate to maintain the stroke volume. The ejection fraction typically improves, and ventricular dilation resolves over 7 to 10 days. Persistence of a high CO and a low SVR beyond 24 hours is an ominous finding and is often associated with an increased development of hypotension and MODS. Coronary artery perfusion and myocardial oxygen metabolism are not primarily altered in septic shock.

In addition to the cardiovascular dysfunction that accompanies sepsis, respiratory failure is common. The patient initially hyperventilates as a compensatory mechanism, resulting in respiratory alkalosis. Once the patient can no longer compensate, respiratory acidosis develops. Respiratory failure develops in 85% of patients with sepsis, and 40% develop acute respiratory distress syndrome (ARDS) (see Chapter 68). These patients need to be intubated and mechanically ventilated. Other clinical signs of septic shock include alteration in neurologic status; decreased urine output; and GI dysfunction, such as GI bleeding and paralytic ileus. Table 67-3 gives the clinical presentation of a patient with septic shock.

Obstructive Shock. Obstructive shock develops when a physical obstruction to blood flow occurs with a decreased CO (Fig. 67-6). This can be caused by restricted diastolic filling of the right ventricle from compression (e.g., cardiac tamponade, tension pneumothorax, superior vena cava syndrome). Other causes include *abdominal compartment syndrome* in which increased abdominal pressures compress the inferior vena cava, thus decreasing venous return to the heart (see Chapter 43). Pulmonary embolism and right ventricular thrombi cause an outflow obstruction as blood leaves the right ventricle through the pulmonary artery. This leads to decreased blood flow to the lungs and decreased blood return to the left atrium.

Patients experience a decreased CO, increased afterload, and variable left ventricular filling pressures depending on the obstruction. Other clinical signs include jugular venous distention and pulsus paradoxus (see Table 37-5). Rapid assessment and treatment are important to prevent further hemodynamic compromise and possibly cardiac arrest (see Fig. 67-6).

Stages of Shock

In addition to an understanding of the underlying pathogenesis of the type of shock that the patient is experiencing, monitoring and management are guided by knowing where the patient is on the shock "continuum." This continuum begins with the initial stage of shock that occurs at a cellular level and is usually not clinically apparent. Metabolism changes at the cellular level from aerobic to anaerobic, causing lactic acid buildup. Lactic acid is a waste product that is removed by the liver. However, this process requires oxygen, which is unavailable because of the decrease in tissue perfusion. Shock is categorized into three clinically apparent but overlapping stages: compensatory stage, progressive stage, and irreversible stage.[5]

Compensatory Stage. In the *compensatory stage* the body activates neural, hormonal, and biochemical compensatory mechanisms in an attempt to overcome the increasing consequences of anaerobic metabolism and to maintain homeostasis. (See eFig. 67-1 on the website for this chapter.) The patient's clinical presentation begins to reflect the body's responses to the imbalance in oxygen supply and demand (Table 67-5).

One of the classic signs of shock is a drop in blood pressure (BP), which occurs because of a decrease in CO and a narrowing of the pulse pressure. The baroreceptors in the carotid and aortic bodies immediately respond by activating the SNS. The SNS stimulates vasoconstriction and the release of the potent vasoconstrictors epinephrine and norepinephrine. Blood flow to the most essential (vital) organs, the heart and brain, is maintained, while blood flow to the nonvital organs, such as kidneys, GI tract, skin, and lungs, is diverted or shunted.

The myocardium responds to the SNS stimulation and the increase in oxygen demand by increasing the heart rate and contractility. However, increased contractility increases myocardial oxygen consumption. The coronary arteries dilate in

PATHOPHYSIOLOGY MAP

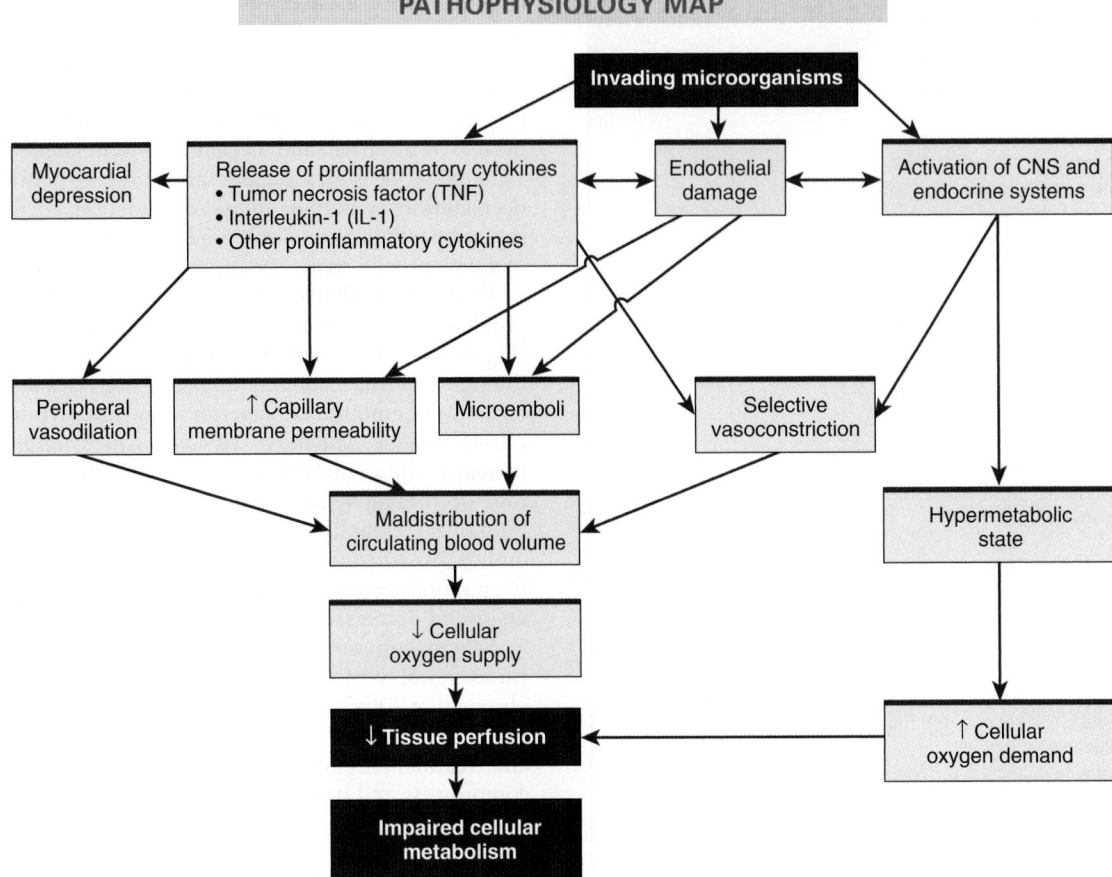

FIG. 67-5 The pathophysiology of septic shock. *CNS,* Central nervous system.

PATHOPHYSIOLOGY MAP

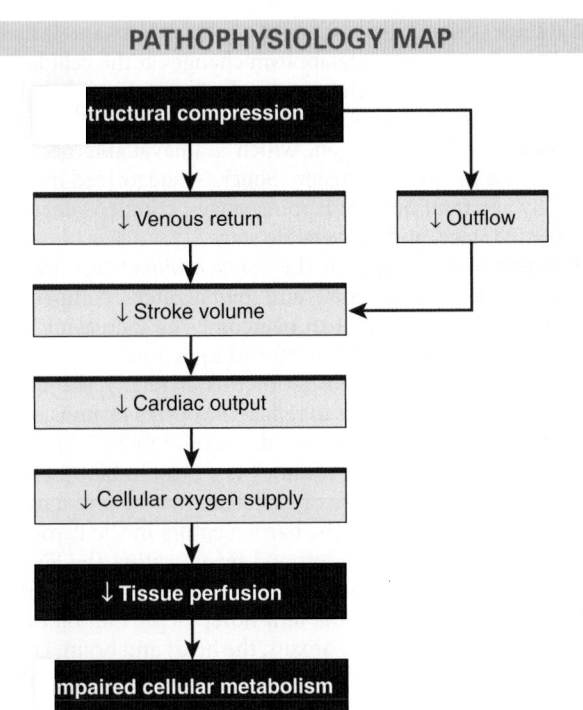

FIG. 67-6 The pathophysiology of obstructive shock.

an attempt to meet the increased oxygen demands of the myocardium.

Shunting blood away from the lungs has an important clinical effect in the patient in shock. Decreased blood flow to the lungs increases the patient's physiologic dead space. *Physiologic dead space* is the anatomic dead space (the amount of air that will not reach gas-exchanging units) and any inspired air that cannot participate in gas exchange. The clinical result of an increase in dead space ventilation is a *ventilation-perfusion mismatch*. Some areas of the lungs that are participating in ventilation will not be perfused because of the decreased blood flow to the lungs. Arterial oxygen levels will decrease, and the patient will have a compensatory increase in the rate and depth of respirations (see Chapter 68).

The shunting of blood from other organ systems also results in clinically important changes. The decrease in blood flow to the GI tract results in impaired motility and a slowing of peristalsis. This increases the risk for the development of a paralytic ileus.

Decreased blood flow to the skin results in the patient feeling cool and clammy. The exception is the patient in early septic shock who may feel warm and flushed because of a hyperdynamic state. Decreased blood flow to the kidneys activates the renin-angiotensin system. Renin stimulates angiotensinogen to produce angiotensin I, which is then converted to angiotensin II (see Fig. 45-4). Angiotensin II is a potent vasoconstrictor that causes both arterial and venous vasoconstriction. The net result is an increase in venous return to the heart and an increase in

TABLE 67-5   MANIFESTATIONS OF STAGES OF SHOCK*

Compensatory Stage	Progressive Stage	Irreversible Stage
Neurologic System		
Oriented to person, place, time	↓ Cerebral perfusion pressure	Unresponsive
Restless, apprehensive, confused	↓ Cerebral blood flow	Areflexia (loss of reflexes)
Change in level of consciousness	↓ Responsiveness to stimuli	Pupils nonreactive and dilated
	Delirium	
Cardiovascular System		
Sympathetic nervous system response:	↑ Capillary permeability → systemic interstitial edema	Profound hypotension
• Release of epinephrine/ norepinephrine (vasoconstriction)	↓ Cardiac output → ↓ BP and ↑ HR	↓ Cardiac output
• ↑ MVO$_2$	MAP <60 mm Hg (or 40 mm Hg drop in BP from baseline)	Bradycardia, irregular rhythm
• ↑ Contractility	↓ Coronary perfusion → dysrhythmias, myocardial ischemia, myocardial infarction	↓ BP inadequate to perfuse vital organs
• ↑ HR	↓ Peripheral perfusion → ischemia of distal extremities, diminished pulses, ↓ capillary refill	
Coronary artery dilation		
Narrowed pulse pressure		
↓ BP		
Respiratory System		
↓ Blood flow to the lungs:	Acute respiratory distress syndrome (ARDS):	Severe refractory hypoxemia
• ↑ Physiologic dead space	• ↑ Capillary permeability	Respiratory failure
• ↑ Ventilation-perfusion mismatch	• Pulmonary vasoconstriction	
• Hyperventilation	• Pulmonary interstitial edema	
• ↑ Minute ventilation (V$_E$)	• Alveolar edema	
• Tachypnea	• Diffuse infiltrates	
	• Tachypnea	
	• ↓ Compliance	
	• Moist crackles	
Gastrointestinal System		
↓ Blood supply	Vasoconstriction and ↓ perfusion → ischemic gut (e.g., stomach, small and large intestines, gallbladder, pancreas)	Ischemic gut
↓ GI motility	• Erosive ulcers	
Hypoactive bowel sounds	• GI bleeding	
↑ Risk for paralytic ileus	• Translocation of GI bacteria	
	• Impaired absorption of nutrients	
Renal System		
↓ Renal blood flow	Renal tubules become ischemic → acute tubular necrosis	Anuria
↑ Renin resulting in release of angiotensin (vasoconstrictor)	↓ Urine output	
↑ Aldosterone resulting in Na$^+$ and H$_2$O reabsorption	↑ BUN/creatinine ratio	
↑ Antidiuretic hormone resulting in H$_2$O reabsorption	↑ Urine sodium	
	↓ Urine osmolality and specific gravity	
	↓ Urine potassium	
	Metabolic acidosis	
Hepatic System		
	Failure to metabolize drugs and waste products	Metabolic changes from accumulation of waste products (e.g., NH$_3$, lactate, CO$_2$)
	Cell death (↑ liver enzymes)	
	Jaundice (decreased clearance of bilirubin)	
	↑ NH$_3$ and lactate	
Hematologic System		
	DIC	DIC progresses
	• Thrombin clots in microcirculation	
	• Consumption of platelets and clotting factors	
Temperature		
Normal or abnormal	Hypothermia or hyperthermia	Hypothermia
Skin		
Pale and cool	Cold and clammy	Mottled, cyanotic
Warm and flushed		

*Also see Table 67-2 and Table 67-3.
DIC, Disseminated intravascular coagulation; *MAP,* mean arterial pressure; *MVO$_2$,* myocardial oxygen consumption; *NH$_3$,* ammonia.

BP. Angiotensin II also stimulates the adrenal cortex to release aldosterone. This results in sodium and water reabsorption and potassium excretion by the kidneys. The increase in sodium reabsorption raises the serum osmolality and stimulates the release of antidiuretic hormone (ADH) from the posterior pituitary gland. ADH increases water reabsorption by the kidneys, thus further increasing blood volume. The increase in total circulating volume results in an increase in CO and BP.

A multisystem response to decreasing tissue perfusion is initiated in the compensatory stage of shock. At this stage the body is able to compensate for the changes in tissue perfusion. If the cause of the shock is corrected, the patient will recover with little or no residual effects. If the cause of the shock is not corrected and the body is unable to compensate, the patient enters the progressive stage of shock.

Progressive Stage. The *progressive stage* of shock begins as compensatory mechanisms fail. (See eFig. 67-2 on the website for this chapter.) Changes in the patient's mental status are important findings in this stage.

The cardiovascular system is profoundly affected in the progressive stage of shock. CO begins to fall, resulting in a decrease in BP and coronary artery, cerebral, and peripheral perfusion. Continued decreased cellular perfusion and resulting altered capillary permeability are the distinguishing features of this stage. Altered capillary permeability allows leakage of fluid and protein out of the vascular space into the surrounding interstitial space. In addition to the decrease in circulating volume, there is an increase in systemic interstitial edema. The patient may have *anasarca* (diffuse profound edema). Fluid leakage from the vascular space also affects the solid organs (e.g., liver, spleen, GI tract, lungs) and peripheral tissues by further decreasing perfusion.

Sustained hypoperfusion results in weak peripheral pulses, and ischemia of the distal extremities eventually occurs. Myocardial dysfunction from decreased perfusion results in dysrhythmias, myocardial ischemia, and possibly MI. The end result is a complete deterioration of the cardiovascular system.

The pulmonary system is often the first system to display signs of critical dysfunction. During the compensatory stage, blood flow to the lungs is already reduced. In response to the decreased blood flow and the SNS stimulation, the pulmonary arterioles constrict, resulting in increased pulmonary artery (PA) pressure. As the pressure within the pulmonary vasculature increases, blood flow to the pulmonary capillaries decreases and ventilation-perfusion mismatch worsens.

Another key response in the lungs is the movement of fluid from the pulmonary vasculature into the interstitial space. As capillary permeability increases, the movement of fluid to the interstitial spaces results in interstitial edema, bronchoconstriction, and a decrease in functional residual capacity. With further increases in capillary permeability, the fluid moves to the alveoli, with resultant alveolar edema and a decrease in surfactant production. The combined effects of pulmonary vasoconstriction and bronchoconstriction are impaired gas exchange, decreased compliance, and worsening ventilation-perfusion mismatch. Clinically, the patient has tachypnea, crackles, and an overall increased work of breathing.

The GI system is also affected by prolonged decreased tissue perfusion. As the blood supply to the GI tract is decreased, the normally protective mucosal barrier becomes ischemic. This ischemia predisposes the patient to ulcers and GI bleeding (see Chapter 42). It also increases the risk of bacterial migration from the GI tract to the blood. The decreased perfusion to the GI tract also leads to a decreased ability to absorb nutrients.

The effect of prolonged hypoperfusion on the kidneys is renal tubular ischemia. The resulting acute tubular necrosis may lead to acute kidney injury. This can be worsened by nephrotoxic drugs (e.g., certain antibiotics, anesthetics, diuretics) (see Chapter 47). The patient has decreased urine output and elevated blood urea nitrogen (BUN) and serum creatinine. Metabolic acidosis occurs from the kidneys' inability to excrete acids (especially lactic acid) and reabsorb bicarbonate.

Other organ systems are also affected by the sustained hypoperfusion in the progressive stage of shock. The loss of the functional ability of the liver leads to a failure of the liver to metabolize drugs and waste products (e.g., lactate, ammonia). Jaundice results from an accumulation of bilirubin. As the liver cells die, enzymes become elevated (e.g., alanine aminotransferase, aspartate aminotransferase, γ-glutamyl transferase). The liver also loses its ability to function as an immune organ. Bacteria that may move from the GI tract are no longer destroyed by the Kupffer cells. Instead, they are released into the bloodstream, thus increasing the possibility of bacteremia.[12]

Dysfunction of the hematologic system adds to the complexity of the clinical picture. The patient is at risk for disseminated intravascular coagulation (DIC), in which consumption of the platelets and clotting factors with secondary fibrinolysis results in clinically significant bleeding from many orifices. These include, but are not limited to, the GI tract, lungs, and puncture sites (see Chapter 31). Altered laboratory values in DIC are presented in Table 67-3.

In this stage, aggressive interventions are necessary to prevent the development of MODS.

Irreversible Stage. In the final stage of shock, the *irreversible stage*, decreased perfusion from peripheral vasoconstriction and decreased CO exacerbate anaerobic metabolism. (See eFig. 67-3 on the website for this chapter.) The accumulation of lactic acid contributes to increased capillary permeability and dilation. Increased capillary permeability allows fluid and plasma proteins to leave the vascular space and move to the interstitial space. Blood pools in the capillary beds secondary to the constricted venules and dilated arterioles. The loss of intravascular volume worsens hypotension and tachycardia and decreases coronary blood flow. Decreased coronary blood flow leads to worsening myocardial depression and a further decline in CO. Cerebral blood flow cannot be maintained, and cerebral ischemia results.

The patient in this stage of shock demonstrates profound hypotension and hypoxemia. The failure of the liver, lungs, and kidneys results in an accumulation of waste products, such as lactate, urea, ammonia, and carbon dioxide. The failure of one organ system affects several other organ systems. In this final stage, recovery is unlikely. The organs are in failure and the body's compensatory mechanisms are overwhelmed (see Table 67-5).

Diagnostic Studies

There is no single diagnostic study to determine whether a patient is in shock. Establishing a diagnosis begins with a history and physical examination. Obtaining a thorough medical and surgical history, and a history of recent events (e.g., surgery, chest pain, trauma), provides valuable data.

Decreased tissue perfusion in shock leads to an elevation of lactate and a base deficit (the amount needed to bring the pH back to normal). These laboratory changes may reflect an increase in anaerobic metabolism. Table 67-2 summarizes other laboratory findings seen in shock.

Additional diagnostic studies include a 12-lead electrocardiogram (ECG), continuous ECG monitoring, chest x-ray, continuous pulse oximetry, and hemodynamic monitoring (e.g., arterial pressure, central venous or PA pressure, $ScvO_2/SvO_2$). (Chapter 66 discusses hemodynamic monitoring.)

Collaborative Care: General Measures

Critical factors in the successful management of a patient experiencing shock relate to the early recognition and treatment of the shock state. Prompt intervention in the early stages of shock may prevent the decline to the progressive or irreversible stage. Successful management of the patient in shock includes the following:

1. Identification of patients at risk for developing shock
2. Integration of the patient's history, physical examination, and clinical findings to establish a diagnosis
3. Interventions to control or eliminate the cause of the decreased perfusion
4. Protection of target and distal organs from dysfunction
5. Provision of multisystem supportive care

Table 67-6 provides an overview of the initial assessment findings and interventions for the emergency care of patients in shock.[13,14] General management strategies begin with ensuring that the patient has a patent airway. Once the airway is established, either naturally or with an endotracheal tube, oxygen delivery must be optimized. Supplemental oxygen and mechanical ventilation may be necessary to maintain an arterial oxygen saturation of 90% or more (PaO_2 greater than 60 mm Hg) to avoid hypoxemia (see Chapter 66). The mean arterial pressure

(MAP) and circulating blood volume are optimized with fluid replacement and drug therapy.

Oxygen and Ventilation. Oxygen delivery depends on CO, available hemoglobin, and arterial oxygen saturation (SaO_2). Methods to optimize oxygen delivery are directed at increasing supply and decreasing demand. Supply is increased by (1) optimizing the CO with fluid replacement or drug therapy, (2) increasing the hemoglobin through transfusion of whole blood or packed red blood cells (RBCs), and/or (3) increasing the arterial oxygen saturation with supplemental oxygen and mechanical ventilation.

Plan care to avoid disrupting the balance of oxygen supply and demand. Space activities that increase oxygen consumption (e.g., endotracheal suctioning, position changes) appropriately for oxygen conservation. Continuous monitoring of $ScvO_2$ by a central venous catheter or mixed venous oxygen saturation (SvO_2) by a PA catheter is helpful. Both reflect the dynamic balance between oxygen supply and demand. Assess these values along with related hemodynamic measures (e.g., arterial pressure–based cardiac output [APCO], oxygen consumption, hemoglobin) to evaluate the patient's response to treatments or activities (see Chapter 66).

Fluid Resuscitation. The cornerstone of therapy for septic, hypovolemic, and anaphylactic shock is volume expansion with administration of the appropriate fluid. Fluid resuscitation should start using one or two large-bore (e.g., 14- to 16-gauge) IV catheters, preferably in the antecubital veins, or a central venous catheter. Both crystalloids (e.g., normal saline or hypertonic solutions) and colloids (e.g., albumin) have a role in fluid resuscitation (Table 67-7; also see Table 17-17). The choice of fluid for resuscitation remains controversial. Currently, isotonic crystalloids, such as normal saline, are used in the initial resus-

---

➕ **TABLE 67-6 EMERGENCY MANAGEMENT**

Shock

Etiology*	Assessment Findings	Interventions
Surgical • Postoperative bleeding • Ruptured organ or vessel • Gastrointestinal bleeding • Aortic dissection • Vaginal bleeding • Ruptured ectopic pregnancy or ovarian cyst **Medical** • Myocardial infarction • Dehydration • Addisonian crisis • Diabetes insipidus • Sepsis • Diabetes mellitus • Pulmonary embolus **Trauma** • Ruptured or lacerated vessel or organ (e.g., spleen) • Fractures, spinal injury • Multiorgan injury	• Restlessness • Confusion • Anxiety • Feeling of impending doom • Decreased level of consciousness • Weakness • Rapid, weak, thready pulses • Dysrhythmias • Hypotension • Narrowed pulse pressure • Cool, clammy skin (warm skin in early onset of septic and neurogenic shock) • Tachypnea, dyspnea, or shallow, irregular respirations • Decreased O_2 saturation • Extreme thirst • Nausea and vomiting • Chills • Pallor • Cyanosis • Obvious hemorrhage or injury • Temperature dysregulation	**Initial** • Assess ABCs. • Stabilize cervical spine as appropriate. • Administer high-flow O_2 (100%) by non-rebreather mask or bag-valve-mask. • Anticipate need for intubation and mechanical ventilation. • Establish IV access with two large-bore catheters (14-16 gauge) or assist with insertion of central line and begin fluid resuscitation with crystalloids (e.g., 30 mL/kg repeated until hemodynamic improvement is noted). • Draw blood for laboratory studies (e.g., blood cultures, lactate, WBC). • Control any external bleeding with direct pressure or pressure dressing. • Assess for life-threatening injuries (e.g., cardiac tamponade, liver laceration, tension pneumothorax). • Consider vasopressor therapy if hypotension persists after fluid resuscitation. • Insert an indwelling bladder catheter and nasogastric tube. • Administer antibiotic therapy after blood cultures if sepsis is suspected. • Obtain 12-lead ECG and treat dysrhythmias. **Ongoing Monitoring** • Level of consciousness • Vital signs, including pulse oximetry; peripheral pulses, capillary refill, skin color and temperature • Respiratory status • Heart rate and rhythm • Urine output

*See Table 67-1 for additional etiologies of shock.
ABCs, Airway, breathing, circulation.

TABLE 67-7 FLUID THERAPY IN SHOCK

Fluid Type	Mechanism of Action	Type of Shock	Nursing Implications
Crystalloids *Isotonic* • 0.9% NaCl (NSS) • Lactated Ringer's (LR)	Fluid primarily remains in the intravascular space, increasing intravascular volume.	Used for initial volume replacement in most types of shock.	Monitor patient closely for circulatory overload. Do not use LR in patients with liver failure. LR may be used if hyperchloremic acidosis develops from use of NSS in fluid resuscitation.
Hypertonic • 1.8%, 3%, 5% NaCl	Fluid remains in the intravascular space, increases serum osmolarity, shifts fluid volume from intracellular space to extracellular space to intravascular space.	May be used for initial volume expansion in hypovolemic shock.	Monitor patient closely for signs of hypernatremia (e.g., disorientation, convulsions). Central line preferred for infusing saline solutions ≥3%, since these may damage veins.
Blood or Blood Products Packed red blood cells Fresh frozen plasma Platelets	Replaces blood loss, increases O$_2$-carrying capability. Replaces coagulation factors. Helps control bleeding caused by thrombocytopenia.	All types of shock.	Same precautions as any blood administration (see Chapter 31).
Colloids Human serum albumin (5% or 25%)	Can increase plasma colloid osmotic pressure. Rapid volume expansion.	All types of shock except cardiogenic and neurogenic shock.	Use 5% solution in hypovolemic patients. Use 25% solution in patients with fluid and sodium restrictions. Monitor for circulatory overload. Mild side effects of chills, fever, and urticaria may develop. More expensive than crystalloids.
dextran (dextran 40)	Hyperosmotic glucose polymer.	Limited use because of side effects, including reducing platelet adhesion, diluting clotting factors.	Increases risk of bleeding. Important to monitor patient for allergic reactions and acute renal failure. Has maximum volume recommendations per manufacturer.

NSS, Normal saline solution.

citation of shock. Lactated Ringer's solution is used cautiously in all shock situations because the failing liver cannot convert lactate to bicarbonate, so serum lactate levels increase. In some cases, hypertonic saline may be considered to expand plasma volume. Colloids are effective volume expanders because the size of their molecules keeps them in the vascular space for a longer time. However, they are costly and no definitive studies have shown that using colloids for resuscitation improves patient outcomes.[15]

The choice of fluid for resuscitation is also based on the type and volume of fluid lost and the patient's clinical status. If the patient does not respond to 2 to 3 L of crystalloids, blood administration and CVP, APCO, or PA pressure monitoring may be started.[16,17] Monitor trends in BP with an automatic BP cuff or an arterial catheter to assess the patient's response. An indwelling bladder catheter monitors urine output and aids in assessing the patient's fluid status during resuscitation.

When large amounts of fluids are required, you must protect the patient against two major complications: hypothermia and coagulopathy. If the patient has persistent hypotension after fluid resuscitation and normalized CVP (8 to 12 mm Hg), a vasopressor (e.g., norepinephrine [Levophed], dopamine [Intropin]) and/or an inotrope (e.g., dobutamine [Dobutrex]) may be added. The goal for fluid resuscitation is restoration of tissue perfusion. Thus decisions on which agent to use should be based on the physiologic goal. Although BP helps determine whether the patient's CO is adequate, an assessment of end-organ perfusion (e.g., urine output, neurologic function, peripheral pulses) provides more relevant information.

SAFETY ALERT
• Warm crystalloid and colloid solutions during massive fluid resuscitation.
• When administering large volumes of packed RBCs, remember that they do not contain clotting factors. Replace these factors based on the clinical situation and laboratory studies.

Drug Therapy. The primary goal of drug therapy for shock is the correction of decreased tissue perfusion. Medications used to improve perfusion in shock are given IV via an infusion pump and central venous line, since many of them have vasoconstrictor properties that would be harmful if the drug extravasated while being infused peripherally (Table 67-8).

Sympathomimetic Drugs. Many of the drugs used in the treatment of shock have an effect on the SNS. Drugs that mimic the action of the SNS are termed *sympathomimetic.* The effects of these drugs are mediated through their binding to α- or β-adrenergic receptors. The various drugs differ in their relative α- and β-adrenergic effects. (See Chapter 33 and Table 33-1.)

Many of the sympathomimetic drugs cause peripheral vasoconstriction and are called vasopressor drugs (e.g., norepinephrine, dopamine, phenylephrine [Neo-Synephrine]). These drugs can cause severe peripheral vasoconstriction and an increase in SVR, further risking tissue perfusion. The increased SVR increases the workload of the heart and can harm a patient in cardiogenic shock by causing further myocardial damage. Use of vasopressor drugs is limited to patients who do not respond to fluid resuscitation. Adequate fluid resuscitation must be achieved before starting vasopressors because the vasoconstric-

TABLE 67-8   DRUG THERAPY

Shock

Drug*	Mechanism of Action	Type of Shock	Nursing Implications
dobutamine (Dobutrex)	↑ Myocardial contractility ↓ Ventricular filling pressures ↓ SVR, PAWP ↑ CO, stroke volume, CVP ↑/↓ HR	Used in cardiogenic shock with severe systolic dysfunction Used in septic shock to increase O₂ delivery and raise ScvO₂/SvO₂ to 70% if Hgb >7 g/dL or Hct ≥30%	Administration via central line is recommended (infiltration leads to tissue sloughing). Do not administer in same line with NaHCO₃. Monitor HR, BP (hypotension may worsen, requiring addition of a vasopressor). Stop infusion if tachydysrhythmias develop.

dopamine (Intropin)	Positive inotropic effects:
	  ↑ Myocardial contractility
	  ↑ Automaticity
	  ↑ Atrioventricular conduction
	↑ HR, CO
	↑ BP, ↑ MAP
	↑ MVO₂
	Can cause progressive vasoconstriction at high doses
		Cardiogenic shock	Administration via central line is recommended (infiltration leads to tissue sloughing).
			Do not administer in same line with NaHCO₃.
			Monitor for tachydysrhythmias.
			Monitor for peripheral vasoconstriction (e.g., paresthesias, coldness in extremities) at moderate to high doses.

epinephrine (Adrenalin)	*Low doses:* β-Adrenergic agonist (cardiac stimulation, bronchodilation, peripheral vasodilation) ↑ HR, contractility, CO ↓ SVR *High doses:* α-Adrenergic agonist (peripheral vasoconstriction) ↑ Stroke volume, SVR ↑ Systolic/↓ diastolic BP, widened pulse pressure ↑ CVP, PAWP	Cardiogenic shock Anaphylactic shock Septic shock requiring additional agent after norepinephrine Cardiac arrest, pulseless ventricular tachycardia, ventricular fibrillation, asystole	Monitor for HR >110 beats/min. Monitor for dyspnea, pulmonary edema. Monitor for chest pain, dysrhythmias secondary to ↑ MVO₂. Monitor for renal failure secondary to ischemia.
hydrocortisone (Solu-Cortef)	Decreases inflammation, reverses increased capillary permeability ↑ BP, HR	Septic shock requiring vasopressor therapy (despite fluid resuscitation) to maintain adequate BP Anaphylactic shock if hypotension persists after initial therapy	Monitor for hypokalemia, hyperglycemia. Consider use as continuous infusion.
norepinephrine (Levophed)	β₁-Adrenergic agonist (cardiac stimulation) α-Adrenergic agonist (peripheral vasoconstriction) Renal and splanchnic vasoconstriction ↑ BP, MAP, CVP, PAWP, SVR ↑/↓ CO	Cardiogenic shock after myocardial infarction Septic shock—first drug of choice for BP unresponsive to adequate fluid resuscitation	Administration via central line is recommended (infiltration leads to tissue sloughing). Monitor for dysrhythmias secondary to ↑ MVO₂ requirements.
phenylephrine (Neo-Synephrine)	α-Adrenergic agonist (peripheral vasoconstriction) Renal, mesenteric, splanchnic, cutaneous, and pulmonary blood vessel constriction ↑ HR, BP, SVR ↑/↓ CO	Neurogenic shock	Monitor for reflex bradycardia, headache, restlessness. Monitor for renal failure secondary to ↓ renal blood flow. Administration via central line is recommended (infiltration leads to tissue sloughing).
nitroglycerin (Tridil)	Venodilation Dilates coronary arteries ↓ Preload, MVO₂, SVR, BP	Cardiogenic shock	Continuously monitor BP and HR, since reflex tachycardia may occur. Glass bottle recommended for infusion.
sodium nitroprusside (Nipride)	Arterial and venous vasodilation ↓ Preload, afterload ↓ CVP, PAWP ↑/↓ CO ↓ BP	Cardiogenic shock with ↑ SVR	Continuously monitor BP. Protect solution from light. Wrap infusion bottle with opaque covering. Administer with D₅W only. Monitor serum cyanide levels and for signs of cyanide toxicity (e.g., metabolic acidosis, tachycardia, altered level of consciousness, seizures, coma, almond smell on breath).
vasopressin (Pitressin, Pressyn)	Antidiuretic hormone Nonadrenergic vasoconstrictor ↑ MAP ↑ Urine output	Shock states (most commonly septic shock) refractory to other vasopressors	Usually administer low dose. Infusions are not titrated. Monitor hemodynamic pressures and urine output.

*Consult individual facility's guidelines, pharmacist, pharmacology references, and drug manufacturer's administration materials for additional information and dosing recommendations.
CO, Cardiac output; *CVP,* central venous pressure; *MAP,* mean arterial pressure; *MVO₂,* myocardial oxygen consumption; *PAWP,* pulmonary artery wedge pressure; *PT,* prothrombin time; *PTT,* partial thromboplastin time; *SVR,* systemic vascular resistance.

tor effects in patients with low blood volume will cause further reduction in tissue perfusion.

The goal of vasopressor therapy is to achieve and maintain a MAP of greater than 65 mm Hg.[9,13] Continuously monitor end-organ perfusion (e.g., urine output, level of consciousness) and serum lactate levels (e.g., every 2 hours for the first 6 hours) to ensure that tissue perfusion is adequate.

Vasodilator Drugs. Patients in cardiogenic shock have decreased myocardial contractility, and vasodilators may be needed to decrease afterload. This reduces myocardial workload and oxygen requirements. Although generalized sympathetic vasoconstriction is a useful compensatory mechanism for maintaining BP, excessive constriction can reduce tissue blood flow and increase the workload of the heart. The rationale for using vasodilator therapy for a patient in shock is to break the harmful cycle of widespread vasoconstriction causing a decrease in CO and BP, resulting in further sympathetic-induced vasoconstriction.

The goal of vasodilator therapy, as in vasopressor therapy, is to maintain the MAP greater than 65 mm Hg. Also monitor hemodynamic parameters (e.g., CVP, APCO, CO, ScvO$_2$/SvO$_2$, PA pressures) so that fluids can be increased or vasodilator therapy decreased if a serious fall in CO or BP occurs. The vasodilator agent most often used for the patient in cardiogenic shock is nitroglycerin (Tridil). Vasodilation may be enhanced with nitroprusside (Nipride) or nitroglycerin in noncardiogenic shock.

Nutritional Therapy. Protein-calorie malnutrition is one of the main manifestations of hypermetabolism in shock. Nutrition is vital to reducing mortality. Enteral nutrition should be started within the first 24 hours.[18] Generally, parenteral nutrition is used if enteral feedings are contraindicated or fail to meet at least 80% of the patient's caloric requirements.[19] (Chapter 40 discusses parenteral and enteral nutrition.) Start the patient on a slow continuous drip of small amounts of enteral feedings (e.g., 10 mL/hr). Early enteral feedings enhance the perfusion of the GI tract and help maintain the integrity of the gut mucosa.

Weigh the patient daily on the same scale at the same time of day. If the patient experiences a significant weight loss, rule out dehydration before adding more calories. Large weight gains are common because of third spacing of fluids. Therefore daily weights serve as a better indicator of fluid status than caloric needs. Serum protein, total albumin, prealbumin, BUN, serum glucose, and serum electrolytes are all used to assess nutritional status.

Collaborative Care: Specific Measures

Cardiogenic Shock. For a patient in cardiogenic shock, the overall goal is to restore blood flow to the myocardium by restoring the balance between oxygen supply and demand. Cardiac catheterization is performed as soon as possible after the initial insult. Specific measures to restore blood flow include angioplasty with stenting, emergency revascularization, and valve replacement (see Chapter 34). Until these interventions are done, the heart must be supported to optimize stroke volume and CO to achieve optimal perfusion (see Tables 67-8 and 67-9).

Hemodynamic management of a patient in cardiogenic shock aims to reduce the workload of the heart through drug therapy and/or mechanical interventions. Drug selection is based on the clinical goal and a thorough understanding of each drug's mechanism of action. Drugs can be used to decrease the workload of the heart by dilating coronary arteries (e.g.,

nitrates), reducing preload (e.g., diuretics), reducing afterload (e.g., vasodilators), and reducing heart rate and contractility (e.g., β-adrenergic blockers).

The patient may also benefit from a circulatory assist device (e.g., intraaortic balloon pump, ventricular assist device [VAD])[20] (see Chapter 66). The goals of this intervention are to decrease the SVR and the left ventricular workload so the heart can heal. A VAD may be used as a temporary measure for the patient in cardiogenic shock who is awaiting heart transplantation. Heart transplantation is an option for a small, select group of patients with cardiogenic shock.

Hypovolemic Shock. The underlying principles of managing patients with hypovolemic shock focus on stopping the loss of fluid and restoring the circulating volume. Fluid resuscitation in hypovolemic shock initially is calculated using a 3:1 rule (3 mL of isotonic crystalloid for every 1 mL of estimated blood loss). Table 67-7 delineates the different types of fluid used for volume resuscitation, the mechanisms of action, and specific nursing implications for each fluid type.

Septic Shock. Patients in septic shock require large amounts of fluid replacement. Volume resuscitation of 30 to 50 mL/kg is usually done with isotonic crytalloids to achieve a target CVP of 8 to 12 mm Hg. Albumin 0.5 to 1 g/kg/dose may be added when patients require substantial volumes. Use of a fluid challenge technique (e.g., to achieve a minimum of 30 mL/kg of crystalloids) is repeated until hemodynamic improvement (e.g., increase in MAP and/or CVP, change in SVV) is noted.[9] (An example of a sepsis alert treatment protocol [eFig. 67-4] is available on the website for this chapter.) Table 67-9 presents predetermined end points of fluid resuscitation. To optimize and evaluate large-volume fluid resuscitation, hemodynamic monitoring with a minimum of a central venous catheter is necessary. The overall goals of fluid resuscitation are to restore the intravascular volume and organ perfusion.

Once the CVP is 8 mm Hg or more, vasopressors may be added. The first drug of choice is norepinephrine. Vasodilation and low CO, or vasodilation alone, can cause low BP in spite of adequate fluid resuscitation. Vasopressin (Pitressin) may be added for patients refractory to vasopressor therapy.[9,10,13] Exogenous vasopressin is used to replace the stores of physiologic vasopressin that are often depleted in septic shock.

DRUG ALERT: Vasopressin (Pitressin)
- Infuse at low doses (e.g., 0.03 U/min).
- Do not titrate infusion.
- Use cautiously in patients with coronary artery disease.

Vasopressor drugs may increase BP but may also decrease stroke volume. An inotropic agent (e.g., dobutamine) is often added to offset the decrease in stroke volume and increase tissue perfusion (see Table 67-8). IV corticosteroids may be considered for patients in septic shock who cannot maintain an adequate BP with vasopressor therapy despite fluid resuscitation.[9] In an attempt to meet the increasing tissue demands coupled with a low SVR, the patient initially demonstrates a normal or high CO. If the patient is unable to achieve and maintain an adequate CO and has unmet tissue oxygen demands, the CO may need to be increased using drug therapy (e.g., dopamine).[9] ScvO$_2$/SvO$_2$ monitoring is used to assess the balance between oxygen delivery and consumption, and the adequacy of the CO[17] (see Chapter 66). If balance is maintained, the tissue demands will be met.

Antibiotics are an important and early component of therapy. They should be started within the first hour of septic shock.

TABLE 67-9   COLLABORATIVE CARE

Shock

Oxygenation	Circulation	Drug Therapies	Supportive Therapies
Cardiogenic Shock • Provide supplemental O_2 (e.g., nasal cannula, non-rebreather mask) • Intubation and mechanical ventilation, if necessary • Monitor $ScvO_2/SvO_2$	• Restore blood flow with thrombolytics, angioplasty with stenting, emergent coronary revascularization • Reduce workload of the heart with circulatory assist devices: IABP, VAD	• Nitrates (e.g., nitroglycerin) • Inotropes (e.g., dobutamine) • Diuretics (e.g., furosemide) • β-Adrenergic blockers (contraindicated with ↓ ejection fraction)	• Treat dysrhythmias

Hypovolemic Shock
• Provide supplemental O_2
• Monitor $ScvO_2/ScvO_2$
	• Restore fluid volume (e.g., blood or blood products, crystalloids)
	• Rapid fluid replacement using two large-bore (14-16 gauge) peripheral IV lines or central venous catheter
	• End points of fluid resuscitation:
	  • CVP 15 mm Hg
	  • PAWP 10-12 mm Hg
		• No specific drug therapy	• Correct the cause (e.g., stop bleeding, GI losses)
			• Use warmed IV fluids, including blood products (if appropriate)

Septic Shock
• Provide supplemental O_2
• Intubation and mechanical ventilation, if necessary
• Monitor $ScvO_2/SvO_2$
	• Aggressive fluid resuscitation (e.g., 30 mL/kg of crystalloids repeated as long as hemodynamic improvement is noted)
	• End points of fluid resuscitation:
	  • CVP 8-12 mm Hg
	  • MAP ≥65 mm Hg
	  • Urine output ≥0.5 mL/kg/hr
	  • Normalized lactate levels
		• Antibiotics as ordered
		• Vasopressors (e.g., norepinephrine)
		• Inotropes (e.g., dobutamine)
		• Anticoagulants (e.g., low-molecular-weight heparin)
			• Obtain cultures (e.g., blood, wound) before beginning antibiotics
			• Monitor temperature
			• Control blood glucose
			• Stress ulcer prophylaxis

Neurogenic Shock • Maintain patent airway • Provide supplemental O_2 • Intubation and mechanical ventilation (if necessary)	• Cautious administration of fluids	• Vasopressors (e.g., phenylephrine) • Atropine (for bradycardia)	• Minimize spinal cord trauma with stabilization • Monitor temperature
Anaphylactic Shock • Maintain patent airway • Optimize oxygenation with supplemental O_2 • Intubation and mechanical ventilation, if necessary	• Aggressive fluid resuscitation with colloids	• Epinephrine (IM or IV) • Antihistamines (e.g., diphenhydramine) • Histamine (H_2)-receptor blockers (e.g., famotidine [Pepcid]) • Bronchodilators: nebulized (e.g., albuterol) • Corticosteroids (if hypotension persists)	• Identify and remove offending cause • Prevent via avoidance of known allergens • Premedicate with history of prior sensitivity (e.g., contrast media)
Obstructive Shock • Maintain patent airway • Provide supplemental O_2 • Intubation and mechanical ventilation, if necessary	• Restore circulation by treating cause of obstruction • Fluid resuscitation may provide temporary improvement in CO and BP	• No specific drug therapy	• Treat cause of obstruction (e.g., pericardiocentesis for cardiac tamponade, needle decompression or chest tube insertion for tension pneumothorax, embolectomy for pulmonary embolism)

CO, Cardiac output; *CVP,* central venous pressure; *IABP,* intraaortic balloon pump; *MAP,* mean arterial pressure; *PAWP,* pulmonary artery wedge pressure; *VAD,* ventricular assist device.

Obtain cultures (e.g., blood, wound exudate, urine, stool, sputum) before antibiotics are started. However, this should not delay the start of antibiotics within the first hour. Broad-spectrum antibiotics are given first, followed by antibiotics that are more specific once the organism has been identified.[9]

Glucose levels should be maintained below 180 mg/dL (10.0 mmol/L) for patients in shock. Intensive glucose control (81 to 108 mg/dL) actually increases mortality.[21] Frequently monitor glucose levels in all patients in septic shock.

Stress ulcer prophylaxis with proton pump inhibitors (e.g., pantoprazole [Protonix]) for patients with bleeding risk factors and venous thromboembolism prophylaxis (e.g., heparin, enoxaparin [Lovenox]) are also recommended for these patients.[9]

Neurogenic Shock. The specific treatment of neurogenic shock is based on the cause. If the cause is spinal cord injury, general measures to promote spinal stability (e.g., spinal precautions, cervical stabilization with a collar) are initially used. Once the spine is stabilized, definitive treatment of the hypotension and bradycardia is essential to prevent further spinal cord damage. Hypotension, which occurs as a result of a loss of sympathetic tone, is associated with peripheral vasodilation and decreased venous return. Treatment involves the use of vasopressors (e.g., phenylephrine) to maintain BP and organ perfusion (see Table 67-8). Bradycardia may be treated with atropine (AtroPen). Infuse fluids cautiously as the cause of the hypotension is not related to fluid loss.[7]

The patient with a spinal cord injury also needs to be monitored for hypothermia caused by hypothalamic dysfunction (see Table 67-9). Although corticosteroids do not have an effect in neurogenic shock, methylprednisolone (Solu-Medrol) is used for patients with a spinal cord injury to prevent secondary spinal cord damage caused by the release of chemical mediators (see Chapter 61).

Anaphylactic Shock. The first strategy in managing patients at risk for anaphylactic shock is prevention. A thorough history is key to avoid the risk factors for anaphylaxis (see Table 67-1). The clinical presentation of anaphylactic shock is dramatic, and immediate intervention is required. (An example of an anaphylaxis algorithm [eFig. 67-5] is available on the website for this chapter.) Epinephrine is the drug of choice to treat anaphylactic shock.[8] It causes peripheral vasoconstriction and bronchodilation and opposes the effect of histamine. IV diphenhydramine (Benadryl) is given to block the massive release of histamine from the allergic reaction.

Maintaining a patent airway is important because the patient can quickly develop airway compromise from laryngeal edema or bronchoconstriction. Nebulized bronchodilators are highly effective. Aerosolized epinephrine can also be used to treat laryngeal edema. Endotracheal intubation or cricothyroidotomy may be necessary to secure and maintain a patent airway.

Hypotension results from leakage of fluid out of the intravascular space into the interstitial space as a result of increased vascular permeability and vasodilation. Aggressive fluid resuscitation, predominantly with colloids, is necessary. IV corticosteroids may be helpful in anaphylactic shock if significant hypotension persists after 1 to 2 hours of aggressive therapy (see Tables 67-8 and 67-9).

Obstructive Shock. The primary strategy in treating obstructive shock is early recognition and treatment to relieve or manage the obstruction (see Table 67-1). Mechanical decompression for pericardial tamponade, tension pneumothorax,

and hemopneumothorax may be done by needle or tube insertion. Obstructive shock from a pulmonary embolism may require thrombolytic therapy. Superior vena cava syndrome, a compression or obstruction of the outflow tract of the mediastinum, may be treated by radiation, debulking, or removal of the mass or cause. A decompressive laparotomy may be indicated for abdominal compartment syndrome for patients with high intraabdominal pressures and hemodynamic instability.

NURSING MANAGEMENT
SHOCK

NURSING ASSESSMENT

Your role is vital in caring for patients who are at risk for developing shock or are in a state of shock. Focus your initial assessment on the ABCs: airway, breathing, and circulation. Next, assess for tissue perfusion. This includes evaluating vital signs, level of consciousness, peripheral pulses, capillary refill, skin (e.g., temperature, color, moisture), and urine output. As shock progresses, the patient's skin becomes cooler and mottled, urine output decreases, peripheral pulses diminish, and neurologic status declines.

To understand the complexity of the patient's clinical status, integrate all of the assessment data. It is essential to obtain a brief history from the patient or caregiver, including a description of the events leading to the shock condition, time of onset and duration of symptoms, and a health history (e.g., medications, allergies, date of last tetanus vaccination, recent travel). In addition, obtain details regarding any care that the patient received before hospitalization.

NURSING DIAGNOSES

Nursing diagnoses for the patient in shock may include, but are not limited to, the following:

- Ineffective peripheral tissue perfusion with risk for decreased cardiac tissue perfusion, ineffective cerebral tissue perfusion, ineffective renal perfusion, impaired liver function, and ineffective GI perfusion *related to* low blood flow or maldistribution of blood
- Anxiety *related to* severity of condition and hypoxemia

Additional information on nursing diagnoses for the patient with shock is presented in eNursing Care Plan 67-1 (available on the website for this chapter).

PLANNING

The overall goals for a patient in shock include (1) evidence of adequate tissue perfusion, (2) restoration of normal or baseline BP, (3) recovery of organ function, (4) avoidance of complications from prolonged states of hypoperfusion, and (5) prevention of health care–acquired complications of disease management and care.

NURSING IMPLEMENTATION

HEALTH PROMOTION. You have an important role in the prevention of shock, beginning with the identification of patients at risk. In general, patients who are older, are immunocompromised, or have chronic illnesses are at an increased risk. Any person who has surgery or trauma is at risk for shock resulting from hemorrhage, spinal cord injury, sepsis, and other conditions (see Table 67-1).

Planning is essential to help prevent shock after you identify an at-risk person. For example, a person with an acute anterior wall MI is at high risk for cardiogenic shock.[22] The primary goal for this patient is to limit the infarct size. This is done by restoring coronary blood flow through percutaneous coronary intervention, thrombolytic therapy, or surgical revascularization. Rest, analgesics, and sedation can reduce the myocardial demand for oxygen. Modify the patient's environment to provide care at intervals that will not increase the patient's oxygen demand. For example, if the patient becomes tired with bathing, perform this care at a time that does not interfere with tests or other activities that may also increase oxygen demand.

A person with a severe allergy to such substances as drugs, shellfish, insect bites, and latex is at increased risk for anaphylactic shock. This risk can be decreased if the patient is carefully questioned about allergies.

SAFETY ALERT
- Always confirm the patient's allergies before administering medications or beginning diagnostic procedures (e.g., computed tomography [CT] scan with contrast media).
- Premedicate (e.g., diphenhydramine, methylprednisolone) patients who need a drug to which they are at high risk for an allergic reaction (e.g., contrast media).
- Encourage patients with allergies to obtain and wear a medical alert tag and report their allergies to their health care providers.
- Instruct patients about the availability of kits that contain equipment and medication (e.g., epinephrine [EpiPen]) for the treatment of acute allergic reactions.

Careful monitoring of fluid balance can help prevent hypovolemic shock. Ongoing monitoring of intake and output and daily weights is important. In addition, monitoring the patient's clinical status is essential because trends in clinical findings are more meaningful than any one piece of clinical information.

Carefully monitor all patients for the development of infection. Progression from an infection to sepsis and septic shock depends on the patient's defense mechanisms. Patients who are immunocompromised are at high risk for opportunistic infections. Strategies to decrease the risk of health care–associated infections (HAIs) include decreasing the number of invasive catheters (e.g., central lines, bladder catheters), using aseptic technique during invasive procedures, and paying strict attention to hand washing. In addition, all equipment must be changed per agency policy and thoroughly cleaned or discarded (if disposable) between patient use.

Evidence-based guidelines are available to reduce the risk of HAIs (e.g., ventilator-associated pneumonia, central line infections, catheter-associated urinary tract infections). These guidelines, called *care bundles,* outline key interventions aimed at reducing infections (see *www.ihi.org/explore/Bundles/Pages/default.aspx*).

ACUTE INTERVENTION. Your role in shock involves (1) monitoring the patient's ongoing physical and emotional status, (2) identifying trends to detect changes in the patient's condition, (3) planning and implementing nursing interventions and therapy, (4) evaluating the patient's response to therapy, (5) providing emotional support to the patient and caregiver, and (6) collaborating with other members of the health team to coordinate care (see Chapter 66).

Neurologic Status. Assess the patient's neurologic status, including orientation and level of consciousness, at least every 1 to 2 hours. The patient's neurologic status is the best indicator of cerebral blood flow. Be aware of the clinical manifestations of neurologic involvement (e.g., changes in behavior, restlessness, hyperalertness, blurred vision, confusion, paresthesias).

Note and report any subtle changes in the patient's mental status (e.g., mild agitation).

Orient the patient to person, place, time, and events on a regular basis. Orientation to the intensive care unit (ICU) environment is particularly important. Minimize noise and light levels to control sensory input. Maintain a day-night cycle of activity and rest as much as possible. Sensory overload and disruption of the patient's diurnal cycle may contribute to delirium (see Chapter 66).

Cardiovascular Status. Most of the therapy for shock is based on information about the patient's cardiovascular status. If the patient is unstable, continuously assess heart rate and rhythm, BP, CVP, and PA pressures, including CO, SVR, and SVV (if available). (Chapter 66 discusses hemodynamic monitoring.) Monitoring trends in hemodynamic parameters provides more important information than single values. Integration of hemodynamic data with physical assessment data is essential in planning strategies to manage the patient with shock.

Patients in shock often have hypotension. There is no definitive research that supports placing patients in the Trendelenburg (head-down) position during hypotensive crisis. Patients in this position may experience compromised pulmonary function and increased intracranial pressure. The Trendelenburg position should not be used to treat hypotension.[23]

Continuously monitor the patient's ECG to detect dysrhythmias that may result from the cardiovascular and metabolic abnormalities associated with shock. Assess heart sounds for an S_3 or S_4 sound or new murmurs. An S_3 sound usually indicates heart failure.

In addition to monitoring the patient's cardiovascular status, give the prescribed therapy to correct the dysfunctions of the cardiovascular system. Assess the patient's response to fluid and medication administration as often as every 10 to 15 minutes. Make appropriate adjustments (e.g., medication titration) as needed. Once tissue perfusion is restored and the patient is stabilized, you can decrease the frequency of monitoring and slowly wean the patient off medications to support BP and tissue perfusion.

Respiratory Status. Frequently assess the respiratory status of the patient in shock to ensure adequate oxygenation, detect complications early, and provide data regarding the patient's acid-base status. Initially monitor the rate, depth, and rhythm of respirations as frequently as every 15 to 30 minutes. Increased rate and depth provide information regarding the patient's attempts to correct metabolic acidosis. Assess breath sounds every 1 to 2 hours and as needed for any changes that may indicate fluid overload or accumulation of secretions.

Use pulse oximetry to continuously monitor oxygen saturation. Pulse oximetry using a patient's finger may not be accurate in a shock state because of poor peripheral circulation. Instead, attach the probe to the ear, nose, or forehead (according to the manufacturer's guidelines). Arterial blood gases (ABGs) provide definitive information on ventilation and oxygenation status and acid-base balance. Initial interpretation of ABGs is often your responsibility. A PaO_2 below 60 mm Hg (in the absence of chronic lung disease) indicates hypoxemia and the need for higher oxygen concentrations or for a different mode of oxygen administration. Low $PaCO_2$ with a low pH and low bicarbonate level may indicate that the patient is attempting to compensate for metabolic acidosis from increasing lactate levels.

A rising $PaCO_2$ with a persistently low pH and PaO_2 indicates the need for advanced pulmonary management. Most patients in shock are intubated and on mechanical ventilation. Maintaining a patent airway and monitoring for ventilator-related complications are critical. (Chapter 66 discusses artificial airways and mechanical ventilation.)

Renal Status. Initially, measure urine output every 1 to 2 hours to assess the adequacy of renal perfusion. Inserting an indwelling bladder catheter facilitates measurements. Urine output below 0.5 mL/kg/hr may indicate inadequate perfusion of the kidneys. Also use trends in serum creatinine values to assess renal function. Serum creatinine is a better indicator of renal function than BUN levels, since BUN is affected by the patient's catabolic state.

Body Temperature and Skin Changes. Monitor temperature every 4 hours if normal. In the presence of an elevated or subnormal temperature, obtain hourly core temperatures (e.g., urinary or PA catheter). Use light covers and control the room temperature to keep the patient comfortably warm. If the patient's temperature rises above 101.5° F (38.6° C) and the patient becomes uncomfortable or experiences cardiovascular compromise, manage the fever with antipyretic drugs (e.g., ibuprofen [Motrin], acetaminophen [Tylenol]) or remove some of the patient's covers.

Monitor the patient's skin (e.g., upper and lower extremities) for signs of adequate perfusion. Changes in temperature, pallor, flushing, cyanosis, diaphoresis, and piloerection may indicate hypoperfusion.

Gastrointestinal Status. Auscultate bowel sounds at least every 4 hours, and monitor for abdominal distention. If a nasogastric tube is present, measure drainage and check for occult blood. Similarly, check all stools for occult blood.

Personal Hygiene. Hygiene is especially important to the patient in shock because impaired tissue perfusion predisposes the patient to skin breakdown and infection. Perform bathing and other nursing measures carefully because a patient in shock is experiencing problems with oxygen delivery to tissues. The increased oxygen demand that occurs during bathing and repositioning of patients with limited oxygen reserves makes the prevention of health care–associated pressure ulcers challenging. Turn the patient at least every 1 to 2 hours and maintain good body alignment to help prevent pressure ulcers. Use a pressure-relieving or pressure-reducing mattress or a specialty bed as needed. Use good clinical judgment in determining priorities of care to limit the demands for increased oxygen. Perform passive range of motion three or four times a day to maintain joint mobility. Monitor trends in oxygen consumption (e.g., SpO_2, $ScvO_2/SvO_2$) during all nursing interventions to assess the patient's tolerance of activity.

Oral care for the patient in shock is essential because mucous membranes may become dry and fragile in the volume-depleted patient. In addition, the intubated patient usually has difficulty swallowing, resulting in pooled secretions in the mouth. Apply a water-soluble lubricant to the lips to prevent drying and cracking. Brush the patient's teeth or gums with a soft toothbrush every 12 hours, and swab the lips and oral mucosa with a moisturizing solution every 2 to 4 hours.[24]

Emotional Support and Comfort. Do not underestimate the effects of fear and anxiety when the patient and caregiver are faced with a critical, life-threatening situation (see Chapter 66). Fear, anxiety, and pain may aggravate respiratory distress and increase the release of catecholamines. When implementing care, monitor the patient's mental state and level of pain. Provide medications to decrease anxiety and pain as appropriate. Continuous infusions of a benzodiazepine (e.g., lorazepam [Ativan])

and an opioid or anesthetic (e.g., morphine, propofol [Diprivan]) are extremely helpful in decreasing anxiety and pain.

Talk to the patient and encourage the caregiver to talk to the patient, even if the patient is intubated, is sedated, or appears comatose. Hearing is often the last sense to decrease, and even if the patient cannot respond, he or she may still be able to hear. If the intubated patient is capable of writing, provide a "magic slate" or a pencil and paper. Alphabet boards or signboards with common requests (e.g., turn, fan, lights) are also useful.

Provide the patient with simple explanations of all procedures before you carry them out, as well as information regarding the current plan of care. If the patient or caregiver asks questions about progress and prognosis, provide simple and honest answers.

Do not overlook the patient's spiritual needs. Patients may desire a visit from a chaplain, priest, rabbi, or minister. One way to provide support is to offer to call a member of the clergy rather than wait for the patient or caregiver to express a wish for spiritual counseling.

Caregivers can have a therapeutic effect on the patient by providing support and comfort. Caregivers (1) link the patient to the outside world; (2) facilitate decision making and advise the patient; (3) assist with activities of daily living; (4) act as liaisons to advise the health care team of the patient's wishes for care; and (5) provide safe, caring, familiar relationships for the patient.[25-27] Most important, caregivers wish to be kept informed of the patient's condition. If possible, the same nurses should continually care for the patient to decrease anxiety, limit conflicting information, and increase trust. If the prognosis becomes grave, support the patient's caregiver when making difficult decisions such as withdrawing life support. The health care team must promote realistic expectations and outcomes. Remember, compassion is as essential as scientific and technical expertise in the total care of the patient and caregiver.

You should ensure that the caregiver is able to spend time with the patient, provided the patient perceives this time as comforting. Explain in simple terms the purpose of any tubes and equipment attached to or surrounding the patient. Inform the caregivers of what they may and may not touch. If possible, place the patient's hands and arms outside the sheets to encourage therapeutic touch. Encourage caregivers to perform simple comfort measures if desired. Provide privacy as much as possible, but assure the patient and caregiver that assistance is readily available should it be needed. Position the call bell in reach of the patient or caregiver at all times.

AMBULATORY AND HOME CARE. Rehabilitation of the patient who has experienced critical illness requires correction of the precipitating cause, prevention or early treatment of complications, and education focused on disease management or prevention of recurrence based on the initial cause of shock. Continue to monitor the patient for indications of complications throughout the recovery period. These may include decreased range of motion, muscle weakness, decreased physical endurance, renal failure following acute tubular necrosis (see Chapter 47), and fibrotic lung disease caused by ARDS (see Chapter 68). Thus patients recovering from shock often require diverse services after discharge. These can include admission to transitional care units (e.g., for mechanical ventilation weaning), rehabilitation centers (inpatient or outpatient), or home health care agencies. Start planning for a safe transition from hospital to home as soon as the patient is admitted to the hospital.

EVALUATION

The expected outcomes for the patient in shock include

- Adequate tissue perfusion with restoration of normal or baseline BP
- Normal organ function with no complications from hypoperfusion
- Decreased fear and anxiety and increased psychologic comfort

Additional information on expected outcomes for the patient with shock is presented in eNursing Care Plan 67-1 (available on the website for this chapter).

SYSTEMIC INFLAMMATORY RESPONSE SYNDROME AND MULTIPLE ORGAN DYSFUNCTION SYNDROME

Etiology and Pathophysiology

Systemic inflammatory response syndrome (SIRS) is a systemic inflammatory response to a variety of insults, including infection (referred to as sepsis), ischemia, infarction, and injury (see Table 67-4). Generalized inflammation in organs remote from the initial insult characterizes SIRS.[12] A systemic inflammatory response can be triggered by many different mechanisms, including the following:

- *Mechanical tissue trauma:* Burns, crush injuries, surgical procedures
- *Abscess formation:* Intraabdominal, extremities
- *Ischemic or necrotic tissue:* Pancreatitis, vascular disease, MI
- *Microbial invasion:* Bacteria, viruses, fungi, parasites
- *Endotoxin release:* Gram-negative and gram-positive bacteria
- *Global perfusion deficits:* Postcardiac resuscitation, shock states
- *Regional perfusion deficits:* Distal perfusion deficits

Multiple organ dysfunction syndrome (MODS) is the failure of two or more organ systems in an acutely ill patient such that homeostasis cannot be maintained without intervention. MODS results from SIRS. These two syndromes represent the ends of a continuum. Transition from SIRS to MODS does not occur in a clear-cut manner[12] (see Fig. 67-1).

Organ and Metabolic Dysfunction. When the inflammatory response is activated, consequences include the release of mediators, direct damage to the endothelium, and hypermetabolism. In addition, vascular permeability increases. This allows mediators and protein to leak out of the endothelium and into the interstitial space. White blood cells begin to digest the foreign debris, and the coagulation cascade is activated (see Chapter 30). Hypotension, decreased perfusion, microemboli, and redistributed or shunted blood flow eventually compromise organ perfusion.

The respiratory system is often the first system to show signs of dysfunction in SIRS and MODS.[9,10,12] Inflammatory mediators have a direct effect on the pulmonary vasculature. The endothelial damage from the release of inflammatory mediators causes increased capillary permeability. This causes movement of fluid from the pulmonary vasculature into the pulmonary interstitial spaces. The fluid then moves to the alveoli, causing alveolar edema. Type I pneumocytes (alveolar cells) are destroyed. Type II pneumocytes are damaged, and surfactant production is decreased. The alveoli collapse. This creates an increase in *shunt* (blood flow to the lungs that does not partici-pate in gas exchange) and worsening ventilation-perfusion mismatch. The end result is ARDS. Patients with ARDS need aggressive pulmonary management with mechanical ventilation. (See Chapter 68 for a complete discussion of ARDS.)

Cardiovascular changes include myocardial depression and massive vasodilation in response to increasing tissue demands. Vasodilation results in decreased SVR and BP. The baroreceptor reflex causes release of *inotropic* (increasing force of contraction) and *chronotropic* (increasing heart rate) factors that enhance CO. To compensate for hypotension, CO increases by an increase in heart rate and stroke volume. Increases in capillary permeability cause a shift of albumin and fluid out of the vascular space, further reducing venous return and thus preload. The patient becomes warm and tachycardic with a high CO and a low SVR. Other signs include decreased capillary refill, skin mottling, increased CVP and PAWP, and dysrhythmias. $ScvO_2$/SvO_2 may be abnormally high because the patient is perfusing areas not consuming much oxygen (e.g., skin, nonworking muscle) while other areas may have blood shunted away from them. Eventually, either perfusion of vital organs becomes insufficient or the cells are unable to use oxygen and their function is further compromised.

Neurologic dysfunction commonly presents as mental status changes with SIRS and MODS. These acute changes can be an early sign of SIRS or MODS. The patient may become confused and agitated, combative, disoriented, lethargic, or comatose. These mental status changes may be due to hypoxemia, the effects of inflammatory mediators, or impaired perfusion.

Acute kidney injury (AKI) is frequently seen in SIRS and MODS. Hypoperfusion and the effects of the mediators can cause AKI. Decreased perfusion to the kidneys activates the SNS and the renin-angiotensin system. The stimulation of the renin-angiotensin system results in systemic vasoconstriction and aldosterone-mediated sodium and water reabsorption. Another risk factor for the development of AKI is the use of nephrotoxic drugs. Antibiotics commonly used to treat gram-negative bacteria (e.g., aminoglycosides) can be nephrotoxic. Careful monitoring of drug levels is essential to avoid the nephrotoxic effects.

The GI tract also plays a key role in the development of MODS. GI motility is often decreased in critical illness, causing abdominal distention and paralytic ileus. In the early stages of SIRS and MODS, blood is also shunted away from the GI mucosa, making it highly vulnerable to ischemic injury. Decreased perfusion leads to a breakdown of this normally protective mucosal barrier, thus increasing the risk for ulceration, GI bleeding, and bacterial movement from the GI tract into circulation.[12]

Metabolic changes are pronounced in SIRS and MODS. Both syndromes trigger a hypermetabolic response. Glycogen stores are rapidly converted to glucose (glycogenolysis). Once glycogen is depleted, amino acids are converted to glucose (gluconeogenesis), reducing protein stores. Fatty acids are mobilized for fuel. Catecholamines and glucocorticoids are released and result in hyperglycemia and insulin resistance. The net result is a catabolic state, and lean body mass (muscle) is lost.

The hypermetabolism associated with SIRS and MODS may last for several days and results in liver dysfunction. Liver dysfunction in MODS may begin long before clinical evidence of it is present. Protein synthesis is impaired. The liver cannot make albumin, one of the key proteins in maintaining plasma oncotic pressure. Consequently, plasma oncotic pressure is altered, and fluid and protein leak from the vascular spaces to the interstitial space. Administration of albumin does not normalize oncotic pressure in these patients at this point.

As the state of hypermetabolism persists, the patient cannot convert lactate to glucose, and lactate accumulates (lactic acidosis). Despite increases in glycogenolysis and gluconeogenesis, eventually the liver is unable to maintain an adequate glucose level and the patient becomes hypoglycemic. Hypoglycemia can also develop due to acute adrenal insufficiency.

DIC may result from dysfunction of the coagulation system. DIC causes simultaneous microvascular clotting and bleeding because of the depletion of clotting factors and platelets in addition to excessive fibrinolysis. (Chapter 31 discusses DIC.)

Electrolyte imbalances are common and result from the hormonal and metabolic changes and fluid shifts. These changes worsen mental status changes, neuromuscular dysfunction, and dysrhythmias. The release of ADH and aldosterone results in sodium and water retention. Aldosterone increases urinary potassium loss, and catecholamines cause potassium to move into the cell, resulting in hypokalemia. Hypokalemia is associated with dysrhythmias and muscle weakness. Metabolic acidosis results from impaired tissue perfusion, hypoxia, and a shift to anaerobic metabolism with a resultant increase in lactate levels. Progressive renal dysfunction also contributes to metabolic acidosis. Hypocalcemia, hypomagnesemia, and hypophosphatemia are common.

Clinical Manifestations of SIRS and MODS

The clinical manifestations of SIRS and MODS are presented in Table 67-10.

NURSING AND COLLABORATIVE MANAGEMENT SIRS AND MODS

The prognosis for the patient with MODS is poor, with mortality rates of 70% to 80% when three or more organ systems fail.[12] The most common cause of death continues to be sepsis. Survival improves with *early, goal-directed therapy.*[9] (An example of a sepsis alert treatment protocol [eFig. 67-4] is available on the website for this chapter.) Therefore the most important goal is to prevent the progression of SIRS to MODS.

A critical part of your role is vigilant assessment and ongoing monitoring to detect early signs of deterioration or organ dysfunction. Collaborative care for patients with SIRS and MODS focuses on (1) prevention and treatment of infection, (2) maintenance of tissue oxygenation, (3) nutritional and metabolic support, and (4) appropriate support of individual failing organs. Table 67-10 summarizes the management for patients with SIRS and MODS.

PREVENTION AND TREATMENT OF INFECTION

Aggressive infection control strategies are essential to decrease the risk for HAIs. Early, aggressive surgery is recommended to remove necrotic tissue (e.g., early debridement of burn tissue) that can provide a culture medium for microorganisms. Aggressive pulmonary management, including early ambulation, can reduce the risk of infection. Strict asepsis can decrease infections related to intraarterial lines, endotracheal tubes, indwelling bladder catheters, IV lines, and other invasive devices or procedures. Daily assessment of the ongoing need for invasive lines and other devices is an important strategy to prevent or limit HAIs.

Despite aggressive strategies, infection may develop. Once an infection is suspected, begin interventions to treat the cause. Send appropriate cultures and initiate broad-spectrum antibiotic therapy, as ordered. Therapy is adjusted based on the causative organism, if necessary.

MAINTENANCE OF TISSUE OXYGENATION

Hypoxemia frequently occurs in patients with SIRS and MODS. These patients have greater oxygen needs and decreased oxygen supply to the tissues. Interventions that decrease oxygen demand and increase oxygen delivery are essential. Sedation, mechanical ventilation, analgesia, and rest may decrease oxygen demand and should be considered. Oxygen delivery may be optimized by maintaining normal levels of hemoglobin (e.g., transfusion of packed RBCs) and PaO_2 (80 to 100 mm Hg), using individualized tidal volumes with positive end-expiratory pressure, increasing preload (e.g., fluids) or myocardial contractility to enhance CO, or reducing afterload to increase CO.

NUTRITIONAL AND METABOLIC NEEDS

Hypermetabolism in SIRS or MODS can result in profound weight loss, cachexia, and further organ failure. Protein-calorie malnutrition is one of the primary signs of hypermetabolism in SIRS and MODS. Total energy expenditure is often increased 1.5 to 2.0 times the normal metabolic rate. Because of their relatively short half-life, monitor plasma transferrin and prealbumin levels to assess hepatic protein synthesis.

The goal of nutritional support is to preserve organ function. Providing early and optimal nutrition decreases morbidity and mortality rates in patients with SIRS and MODS. The enteral route is preferred, but if it cannot be used or cannot meet caloric needs, parenteral nutrition should be initiated or added.[18,19] (Chapter 40 discusses enteral and parenteral nutrition.) Attention to glycemic control with a goal of 140 to 180 mg/dL using insulin infusions is important in these patients.[21]

SUPPORT OF FAILING ORGANS

Support of any failing organ is a primary goal of therapy. For example, the patient with ARDS requires aggressive oxygen therapy and mechanical ventilation (see Chapter 68). DIC should be treated appropriately (e.g., blood products) (see Chapter 31). Renal failure may require dialysis. Continuous renal replacement therapy is better tolerated than hemodialysis, especially in a patient with hemodynamic instability (see Chapter 47).

A final consideration may be that further interventions are futile. It is important to maintain communication between the health care team and, in most cases, the patient's caregiver regarding realistic goals and likely outcomes for the patient with MODS. Withdrawal of life support may be the best option for the patient.

TABLE 67-10 MANIFESTATIONS AND MANAGEMENT OF SIRS AND MODS

Manifestations	Management
Respiratory System	
Development of ARDS (see Chapter 68):	Prevention
• Severe dyspnea	Optimize O₂ delivery and minimize O₂ consumption
• Tachypnea	Mechanical ventilation (see Chapter 66)
• PaO₂/FIO₂ ratio <200	• Positive end-expiratory pressure
• Bilateral fluffy infiltrates on chest x-ray	• Lung protective modes (e.g., pressure-control inverse ratio ventilation, low tidal volumes)
• PAWP <18 mm Hg	• Permissive hypercapnia
• Ventilation-perfusion (V/Q) mismatch	• Positioning (e.g., continuous lateral rotation therapy, prone positioning)
• Pulmonary hypertension	
• Increased minute ventilation	
• Decreased compliance	
• Refractory hypoxemia	
Cardiovascular System	
Myocardial depression	Volume management
Massive vasodilation	• Central venous or PA catheter for hemodynamic monitoring
↓ SVR, BP	
↓ MAP	• APCO for minimally invasive hemodynamic monitoring
↑ HR, stroke volume	
↑ CO	• ↑ Preload via volume replacement
Systolic, diastolic dysfunction	• Arterial pressure monitoring
Biventricular failure	• Maintain MAP >65 mm Hg
	Vasopressors
	Intermittent or continuous ScvO₂/SvO₂ monitoring
	Balance O₂ supply and demand
	Continuous ECG monitoring
	Circulatory assist devices
	Venous thromboembolism prophylaxis
Central Nervous System	
Acute change in neurologic status	Evaluate for hepatic or metabolic encephalopathy
Fever	
Hepatic encephalopathy	Optimize cerebral blood flow
Seizures	↓ Cerebral O₂ requirements
Confusion, disorientation, delirium	Prevent secondary tissue ischemia
Failure to wean, prolonged rehabilitation	Calcium channel blockers (reduce cerebral vasospasm)
Endocrine System	
Hyperglycemia → hypoglycemia	Provide continuous infusion of insulin and glucose to maintain blood glucose 140-180 mg/dL (7.77-10.0 mmol/L)

Manifestations	Management
Renal System	
Prerenal: Renal hypoperfusion	Diuretics
• BUN/creatinine ratio >20:1	• Loop diuretics (e.g., furosemide [Lasix])
• ↓ Urine Na⁺ <20 mEq/L	• May need to increase dosage due to ↓ glomerular filtration rate
• ↑ Urine specific gravity >1.020	
• ↑ Urine osmolality	Continuous renal replacement therapy (see Chapter 47)
Intrarenal: Acute tubular necrosis	
• BUN/creatinine ratio <10:1-15:1	
• ↑ Urine Na⁺ >20 mEq/L	
• ↓ Urine osmolality	
• Urine specific gravity ~1.010	
Gastrointestinal System	
Mucosal ischemia	Stress ulcer prophylaxis
• ↓ Intramucosal pH	• Antacids (e.g., Maalox)
• Potential translocation of gut bacteria	• Proton pump inhibitors (e.g., omeprazole [Prilosec])
• Potential abdominal compartment syndrome	• sucralfate (Carafate)
Hypoperfusion → ↓ peristalsis, paralytic ileus	Monitor abdominal distention, intraabdominal pressures
Mucosal ulceration on endoscopy	Dietary consultation
GI bleeding	Enteral feedings
	• Stimulate mucosal activity
	• Provide essential nutrients and optimal calories
Hepatic System	
Bilirubin >2 mg/dL (34 µmol/L)	Maintain adequate tissue perfusion
↑ Liver enzymes (ALT, AST, GGT)	
↑ Serum NH₃	Provide nutritional support (e.g., enteral feedings)
↓ Serum albumin, prealbumin, transferrin	Careful use of drugs metabolized by liver
Jaundice	
Hepatic encephalopathy	
Hematologic System	
↑ Bleeding times, ↑ PT, ↑ PTT	Observe for bleeding from obvious and/or occult sites
↓ Platelet count (thrombocytopenia)	Replace factors being lost (e.g., platelets)
↑ Fibrin split products	Minimize traumatic interventions (e.g., IM injections, multiple venipunctures)
↑ D-dimer	

ALT, Alanine aminotransferase; *APCO,* arterial pressure–based cardiac output; *ARDS,* acute respiratory distress syndrome; *AST,* aspartate aminotransferase; *BUN,* blood urea nitrogen; *CO,* cardiac output; *GGT,* γ-glutamyl transferase; *MAP,* mean arterial pressure; *NH₃,* ammonia; *PA,* pulmonary artery; *PAWP,* pulmonary artery wedge pressure; *PT,* prothrombin time; *PTT,* partial thromboplastin time; *ScvO₂,* oxygen saturation in venous blood; *SvO₂,* oxygen saturation in mixed venous blood; *SVR,* systemic vascular resistance.

CASE STUDY

Shock

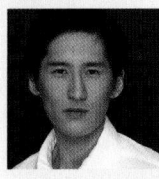

iStockphoto/Thinkstock

Patient Profile

K.L., a 25-yr-old Korean American, was not wearing his seat belt when he was the driver involved in a motor vehicle crash. The windshield was broken, and K.L. was found 15 ft from his car. He was face down, conscious, and moaning. His wife and daughter were found in the car with their seat belts on. They sustained no serious injuries, but were upset. All passengers were taken to the emergency department (ED). The following information pertains to K.L.

Subjective Data

- States, "I can't breathe"
- Cries out when abdomen is palpated

Objective Data

Physical Examination

- Cardiovascular: BP 80/56 mm Hg; apical pulse 138 but no palpable radial or pedal pulses; carotid pulse present but weak
- ECG as follows:

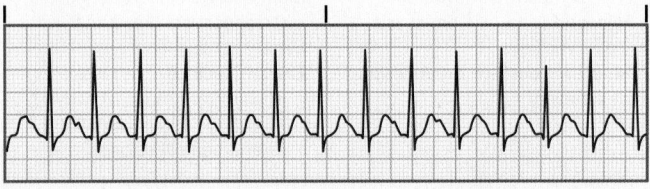

- Lungs: respiratory rate 38 breaths/min; labored breathing with shallow respirations; asymmetric chest wall movement; absence of breath sounds on left side
- Trachea deviated slightly to the right
- Abdomen: slightly distended and left upper quadrant painful on palpation
- Musculoskeletal: open compound fracture of the lower left leg

Diagnostic Studies

- Chest x-ray: Hemothorax and six rib fractures on left side
- Hematocrit: 28%

Collaborative Care *(in the ED)*

- Left chest tube placed, draining bright red blood
- IV access obtained via one peripheral line and right subclavian central line
- Fluid resuscitation started with crystalloids
- High-flow O₂ via non-rebreather mask

Surgical Procedure

- Splenectomy
- Repair of torn intercostal artery
- Repair of compound fracture

Discussion Questions

1. What types of shock is K.L. experiencing? What clinical manifestations did he display that support your answer?
2. What were the causes of K.L.'s shock states? What are other causes of these types of shock?
3. *Priority Decision:* What are the priority nursing responsibilities for K.L.?
4. *Priority Decision:* What ongoing nursing assessment parameters are essential for this patient?
5. What are his potential complications?
6. *Priority Decision:* Based on the assessment data presented, what are the priority nursing diagnoses?
7. *Delegation Decision:* Identify the tasks that could be delegated to unlicensed assistive personnel (UAP).
8. *Evidence-Based Practice:* You are orienting a new graduate RN. He asks you why crystalloids are used instead of colloids for fluid resuscitation. What is your response?

ⓔvolve Answers available at *http://evolve.elsevier.com/Lewis/medsurg.*

▌ BRIDGE TO NCLEX EXAMINATION

The number of the question corresponds to the same-numbered outcome at the beginning of the chapter.

1. A patient has a spinal cord injury at T4. Vital signs include falling blood pressure with bradycardia. The nurse recognizes that the patient is experiencing
   a. a relative hypervolemia.
   b. an absolute hypovolemia.
   c. neurogenic shock from low blood flow.
   d. neurogenic shock from massive vasodilation.

2. A 78-year-old man has confusion and temperature of 104° F (40° C). He is a diabetic with purulent drainage from his right heel. After an infusion of 3 L of normal saline solution, his assessment findings are BP 84/40 mm Hg; heart rate 110; respiratory rate 42 and shallow; CO 8 L/minute; and PAWP 4 mm Hg. This patient's symptoms are most likely indicative of
   a. sepsis.
   b. septic shock.
   c. multiple organ dysfunction syndrome.
   d. systemic inflammatory response syndrome.

3. Appropriate treatment modalities for the management of cardiogenic shock include *(select all that apply)*
   a. dobutamine to increase myocardial contractility.
   b. vasopressors to increase systemic vascular resistance.
   c. circulatory assist devices such as an intraaortic balloon pump.
   d. corticosteroids to stabilize the cell wall in the infarcted myocardium.
   e. Trendelenburg positioning to facilitate venous return and increase preload.

4. The most accurate assessment parameters for the nurse to use to determine adequate tissue perfusion in the patient with MODS are
   a. blood pressure, pulse, and respirations.
   b. breath sounds, blood pressure, and body temperature.
   c. pulse pressure, level of consciousness, and pupillary response.
   d. level of consciousness, urine output, and skin color and temperature.

1. d, 2. b, 3. a, c, 4. d

ⓔvolve

For rationales to these answers and even more NCLEX review questions, visit *http://evolve.elsevier.com/Lewis/medsurg.*

REFERENCES

1. McLean B, Zimmerman JL. Diagnosis and management of shock. In B McLean, JL Zimmerman, editors: *Guide for fundamental critical care support*, ed 4, Mount Pleasant, Ill, 2007, Society of Critical Care Medicine. (Classic)

2. Gallagher JJ: Shock and end points of resuscitation. In KK Carlson, editor: *AACN advanced critical care nursing*, St Louis, 2009, Saunders. (Classic)

3. Patel AK, Hollenberg SM: Cardiovascular failure and cardiogenic shock, *Semin Respir Crit Care Med* 22:598, 2011.

4. McAtee ME: Cardiogenic shock, *Crit Care Nurs Clin North Am* 23:607, 2011.

5. Tuggle D: Optimizing hemodynamics: strategies for fluid and medication titration in shock. In KK Carlson, editor: *AACN advanced critical care nursing*, St Louis, 2009, Saunders. (Classic)

6. Mandel J, Palevsky PM: Treatment of severe hypovolemia or hypovolemic shock in adults, 2012. Retrieved from *www.uptodate.com/contents/treatment-of-severe-hypovolemia-or-hypovolemic-shock-in-adults*.

*7. Casha S, Christie S: A systematic review of intensive cardiopulmonary management after spinal cord injury, *J Neurotrauma* 28:1479, 2011.

*8. Lieberman P, Nicklas RA, Oppenheimer J, et al: The diagnosis and management of anaphylaxis practice parameter: 2010 update, *J Allergy Clin Immunol* 126:477, 2010.

*9. Dellinger RP, Levy MM, Rhodes A, et al: Surviving sepsis campaign: international guidelines for management of severe sepsis and septic shock: 2012, *Crit Care Med* 41:580, 2013.

10. Aitken LM, Williams G, Harvey M, et al: Nursing considerations to complement the surviving sepsis campaign guidelines, *Crit Care Med* 39:1800, 2011.

11. Chalupka AN, Talmor D: The economics of sepsis, *Crit Care Clin* 28:57, 2012.

12. Cheek DJ, Rodgers SC, Schulman CS: Systemic inflammatory response syndrome and multiple organ dysfunction syndrome. In KK Carlson, editor: *AACN advanced critical care nursing*, St Louis, 2009, Saunders. (Classic)

*13. American Association of Critical-Care Nurses: AACN practice alert: severe sepsis. Retrieved from *www.aacn.org/WD/Practice/Docs/Severe_Sepsis_04-2010.pdf*.

14. Strickler J: Halt the downward spiral of traumatic hypovolemic shock, *Nurs 2012 Crit Care* 7:42, 2012.

*15. Perel P, Roberts I, Ker K: Colloids versus crystalloids for fluid resuscitation in critically ill patients, *Cochrane Database Syst Rev* 2:CD000567, 2013.

16. Hata J, Stotts C, Shelsky C: Reduced mortality with noninvasive hemodynamic monitoring of shock, *J Crit Care* 26:e1, 2011.

17. Walley KR: Use of central venous oxygen saturation to guide therapy, *Am J Respir Crit Care Med* 184:514, 2011.

*18. McClave SA, Martindale RG, Vanek VW, et al: Guidelines for the provision and assessment of nutrition support therapy in the adult critically ill patient: Society of Critical Care Medicine and American Society for Parenteral and Enteral Nutrition, *J Parenter Enteral Nutr* 33:277, 2009.

19. Luehrs Hayes G, McKinzie BP, Moore Bullington W, et al: Nutritional supplements in critical illness, *AACN Adv Crit Care* 22:301, 2011.

20. Myers TJ: Temporary ventricular assist devices in the intensive care unit as a bridge to decision, *AACN Adv Crit Care* 23:55, 2012.

21. NICE-SUGAR Study Investigators. Intensive versus conventional glucose control in critically ill patients, *N Engl J Med* 360:1283, 2009.

*22. Wright RS, Anderson JL, Adams CD, et al: 2011 ACCF/AHA focused update of the guidelines for the management of patients with unstable angina/non-ST-elevation myocardial infarction (updating the 2007 guideline), *J Am Coll Cardiol* 57:1920, 2011.

23. Flynn Makic MB, VonRueden KT, Rauen CA, et al: Evidence-based practice habits: putting more sacred cows out to pasture, *Crit Care Nurse* 31:31, 2011.

*24. American Association of Critical-Care Nurses: AACN practice alert: oral care for patients at risk for ventilator-associated pneumonia, 2010. Retrieved from *www.aacn.org/WD/Practice/Docs/Oral_Care_in_the_Critically_Ill.pdf*.

*25. American Association of Critical-Care Nurses: AACN practice alert: family presence during resuscitation and invasive procedures, 2010. Retrieved from *www.aacn.org/WD/Practice/Docs/PracticeAlerts/Family%20Presence%2004-2010%20final.pdf*.

*26. American Association of Critical-Care Nurses: AACN practice alert: family presence: visitation in the adult ICU, 2011. Retrieved from *www.aacn.org/WD/practice/docs/practicealerts/family-visitation-adult-icu-practicealert.pdf*.

*27. Redekopp MA, Leske JS: Family visitation and partnership. In NC Molter, editor: *Protocols for practice: creating healing environments*, ed 2, Sudbury, Mass, 2007, Jones & Bartlett. (Classic)

RESOURCES

Additional resources for this chapter are listed after Chapter 66 on p. 1630 and Chapter 69 on p. 1694.

*Evidence-based information for clinical practice.

What oxygen is to the lungs, such is hope to
the meaning of life.
Emil Brunner

Nursing Management
Respiratory Failure and
Acute Respiratory Distress Syndrome

Richard Arbour

evolve WEBSITE

http://evolve.elsevier.com/Lewis/medsurg

- NCLEX Review Questions
- Key Points
- Pre-Test
- Answer Guidelines for Case Study on
  p. 1671
- Rationales for Bridge to NCLEX
  Examination Questions

- Case Studies
  - Patient With Acute Respiratory Failure
    and Ventilatory Management
  - Patient With Pulmonary Embolism and
    Respiratory Failure
- Nursing Care Plans (Customizable)
  - eNCP 68-1: Patient With Acute
    Respiratory Failure

- Concept Map Creator
- Glossary
- Content Updates

eTable
- eTable 68-1: Predisposing Factors for
  Acute Respiratory Failure

LEARNING OUTCOMES

1. Compare the pathophysiologic mechanisms and clinical manifestations that result in hypoxemic and hypercapnic respiratory failure.
2. Differentiate between the nursing and collaborative management of the patient with hypoxemic or hypercapnic respiratory failure.
3. Relate the pathophysiologic mechanisms and the clinical manifestations associated with acute lung injury and acute respiratory distress syndrome (ARDS).

4. Select appropriate nursing and collaborative management strategies for the patient with ARDS.
5. Prioritize measures to prevent or reverse complications that may result from acute respiratory failure or ARDS.

KEY TERMS

acute lung injury (ALI), p. 1665
acute respiratory distress syndrome
   (ARDS), p. 1665
alveolar hypoventilation, p. 1657

hypercapnia, p. 1654
hypercapnic respiratory failure, p. 1655
hypoxemia, p. 1654
hypoxemic respiratory failure, p. 1655

hypoxia, p. 1658
refractory hypoxemia, p. 1666
shunt, p. 1656
work of breathing (WOB), p. 1659

This chapter discusses the etiology, pathophysiology, and clinical manifestations of acute respiratory failure and acute respiratory distress syndrome (ARDS). Nursing and collaborative management of patients with respiratory failure and ARDS focuses on interventions to promote adequate oxygenation and ventilation while addressing the underlying causes.

ACUTE RESPIRATORY FAILURE

The major function of the respiratory system is gas exchange. This involves the transfer of oxygen (O_2) and carbon dioxide (CO_2) between atmospheric air and circulating blood within the pulmonary capillary bed (Fig. 68-1). *Respiratory failure* results when one or both of these gas-exchanging functions are inadequate (e.g., insufficient O_2 is transferred to the blood or inadequate CO_2 is removed from the lungs). Diseases that interfere with adequate O_2 transfer result in hypoxemia. This causes a decrease in arterial O_2 (PaO_2) and saturation (SaO_2). Insufficient CO_2 removal results in hypercapnia. This causes an increase in arterial CO_2 (PaCO_2).[1-4]

Arterial blood gases (ABGs) are used to assess changes in pH, PaO_2, PaCO_2, bicarbonate, and SaO_2. Pulse oximetry is used intermittently or continuously to assess arterial O_2 saturation (SpO_2).

Reviewed by Susan J. Eisel, RN, MSEd, Associate Professor of Nursing, Mercy College of Ohio, Toledo, Ohio; Eleanor Fitzpatrick, RN, MSN, CCRN, Clinical Nurse Specialist, Thomas Jefferson University Hospital, Philadelphia, Pennsylvania; and Amanda Jones Moose, RN, BSN, Nursing Faculty, Caldwell Community College and Technical Institute, Taylorsville, North Carolina.

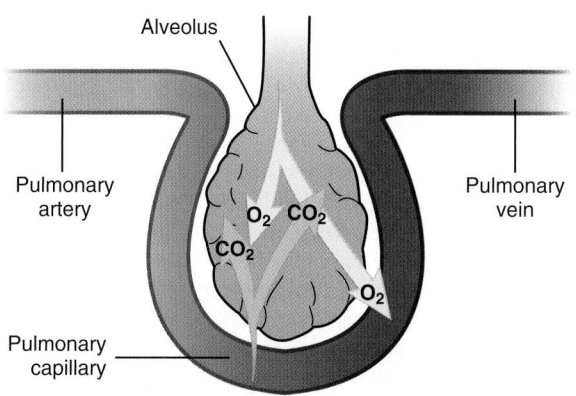

FIG. 68-1 Normal gas exchange unit in the lung.

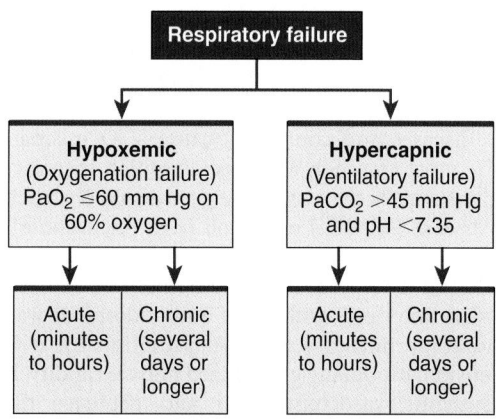

FIG. 68-2 Classification of respiratory failure.

Respiratory failure is not a disease but a symptom of an underlying pathologic condition affecting lung function, O_2 delivery, cardiac output (CO), or the baseline metabolic state. It is a condition that occurs because of one or more diseases involving the lungs or other body systems (Table 68-1 and eTable 68-1 [available on the website for this text]). Respiratory failure is classified as hypoxemic or hypercapnic (Fig. 68-2). Hypoxemic respiratory failure is also referred to as *oxygenation failure* because the primary problem is inadequate O_2 transfer between the alveoli and the pulmonary capillaries. Although no universal definition exists, hypoxemic respiratory failure is commonly defined as a PaO_2 less than 60 mm Hg when the patient is receiving an inspired O_2 concentration of 60% or more. This definition incorporates two important concepts: (1) the PaO_2 level indicates inadequate O_2 saturation of hemoglobin, and (2) this PaO_2 level exists despite administration of supplemental O_2 at a percentage (60%) that is about three times that in room air (21%).[5-7]

Hypercapnic respiratory failure is also referred to as *ventilatory failure* because the primary problem is insufficient CO_2 removal. Hypercapnic respiratory failure is commonly defined as a $PaCO_2$ greater than 45 mm Hg in combination with acidemia (arterial pH less than 7.35). This definition incorporates three important concepts: (1) the $PaCO_2$ is higher than normal, (2) there is evidence of the body's inability to compensate for this increase (acidemia), and (3) the pH is at a level where a further decrease may lead to severe acid-base imbalance. (See Chapter 17 for a discussion of acid-base balance.) Numerous disorders can compromise lung ventilation and subsequent carbon dioxide removal (see Table 68-1 and eTable 68-1).

Many patients experience both hypoxemic and hypercapnic respiratory failure.[6-9] Always interpret data within the context of your assessment findings and the patient's baseline. For example, a person with chronic lung disease may have a baseline $PaCO_2$ higher than "normal."

Etiology and Pathophysiology

Hypoxemic Respiratory Failure. Four physiologic mechanisms may cause hypoxemia and subsequent hypoxemic respiratory failure: (1) mismatch between ventilation (V) and perfusion (Q), commonly referred to as V/Q mismatch; (2) shunt; (3) diffusion limitation; and (4) alveolar hypoventilation. The most common causes are V/Q mismatch and shunt.

Ventilation-Perfusion Mismatch. In normal lungs the volume of blood perfusing the lungs each minute (4 to 5 L) is approximately equal to the amount of gas that reaches the alveoli each

minute (4 to 5 L). In a perfectly matched system, each portion of the lung would receive 1 mL of air (ventilation) for each 1 mL of blood flow (perfusion). This match of ventilation and perfusion would result in a V/Q ratio of 1:1, which is expressed as V/Q = 1. When the match is not 1:1, a *V/Q mismatch* occurs.

Although this example implies that ventilation and perfusion are ideally matched in all areas of the lung, this situation does not normally exist. In reality, some regional mismatch occurs. At the lung apex, V/Q ratios are greater than 1 (more ventilation

TABLE 68-1	**CAUSES OF HYPOXEMIC AND HYPERCAPNIC RESPIRATORY FAILURE***
Hypoxemic Respiratory Failure	**Hypercapnic Respiratory Failure**
Respiratory System	**Respiratory System**
• Acute respiratory distress syndrome	• Asthma
• Pneumonia	• COPD
• Toxic inhalation (e.g., smoke inhalation)	• Cystic fibrosis
• Hepatopulmonary syndrome (e.g., low-resistance flow state, V/Q mismatch)	**Central Nervous System**
	• Brainstem injury or infarction
• Massive pulmonary embolism (e.g., thrombus emboli, fat emboli)	• Sedative and opioid overdose
	• Spinal cord injury
• Pulmonary artery laceration and hemorrhage	• Severe head injury
• Inflammatory state and related alveolar injury	**Chest Wall**
	• Thoracic trauma (e.g., flail chest)
	• Kyphoscoliosis
	• Pain
Cardiac System	• Severe obesity
• Anatomic shunt (e.g., ventricular septal defect)	**Neuromuscular System**
• Cardiogenic pulmonary edema	• Myasthenia gravis
	• Critical illness polyneuropathy
• Shock (decreasing blood flow through pulmonary vasculature)	• Acute myopathy
	• Toxin exposure or ingestion (e.g., tree tobacco, acetylcholinesterase inhibitors, carbamate or organophosphate poisoning)
• High cardiac output states: diffusion limitation	• Amyotrophic lateral sclerosis
	• Phrenic nerve injury
	• Guillain-Barré syndrome
	• Poliomyelitis
	• Muscular dystrophy
	• Multiple sclerosis

*List is not all-inclusive.

than perfusion). At the lung base, V/Q ratios are less than 1 (less ventilation than perfusion). Because changes at the lung apex balance changes at the base, the net effect is a close overall match (Fig. 68-3).

Many diseases and conditions cause V/Q mismatch (Fig. 68-4). The most common are those in which increased secretions are present in the airways (e.g., chronic obstructive pulmonary disease [COPD]) or alveoli (e.g., pneumonia), and in which bronchospasm is present (e.g., asthma).[5-8] V/Q mismatch may also result from alveolar collapse *(atelectasis)* or as a result of pain. Pain interferes with chest and abdominal wall movement and compromises ventilation. Additionally, it increases muscle tension, producing generalized muscle rigidity. Pain also causes systemic vasoconstriction and activates the stress response. Finally, it increases O_2 consumption and CO_2 produc-

tion.[10] In this case, increased O_2 demand and CO_2 production may increase ventilation demands. All these conditions result in limited airflow *(ventilation)* to alveoli but have no effect on blood flow *(perfusion)* to the gas exchange units (see Fig. 68-1). The consequence of the imbalance is V/Q mismatch.

A pulmonary embolus affects the perfusion portion of the V/Q relationship. The embolus limits blood flow but has no effect on airflow to the alveoli, again causing V/Q mismatch[11] (see Fig. 68-4). If large enough, the embolus can cause hemodynamic compromise due to the blockage of a large pulmonary artery.

O_2 therapy is an appropriate first step to reverse hypoxemia caused by V/Q mismatch because not all gas exchange units are affected. O_2 therapy increases the PaO_2 in blood leaving normal gas exchange units, thus causing a higher than normal PaO_2. The well-oxygenated blood mixes with poorly oxygenated blood, raising the overall PaO_2 of blood leaving the lungs. The optimal approach to treating hypoxemia caused by a V/Q mismatch is directed at the cause.

Shunt. A **shunt** occurs when blood exits the heart without having participated in gas exchange. A shunt can be viewed as an extreme V/Q mismatch (see Fig. 68-4). There are two types of shunt: anatomic and intrapulmonary. An *anatomic shunt* occurs when blood passes through an anatomic channel in the heart (e.g., a ventricular septal defect) and bypasses the lungs. An *intrapulmonary shunt* occurs when blood flows through the pulmonary capillaries without participating in gas exchange. Intrapulmonary shunt is seen in conditions in which the alveoli fill with fluid (e.g., acute respiratory distress syndrome [ARDS], pneumonia).

O_2 therapy alone is often ineffective in increasing the PaO_2 if hypoxemia is due to shunt. Patients with shunt are usually more hypoxemic than patients with V/Q mismatch. They often require mechanical ventilation and a high fraction of inspired O_2 (FIO_2) to improve gas exchange.

Diffusion Limitation. *Diffusion limitation* occurs when gas exchange across the alveolar-capillary interface is compromised by a process that thickens, damages, or destroys the alveolar membrane or affects blood flow through the pulmonary capillaries (Fig. 68-5). Diffusion limitation is worsened by disease states affecting the pulmonary vascular bed such as severe COPD or recurrent pulmonary emboli. Some disease states cause the alveolar-capillary interface to become thicker (fibrotic), which slows gas transport. These include pulmonary fibrosis, interstitial lung disease, and ARDS.[12,13]

V/Q	PaO₂	PaCO₂
3.3	132	28
1.0	108	39
0.63	89	42

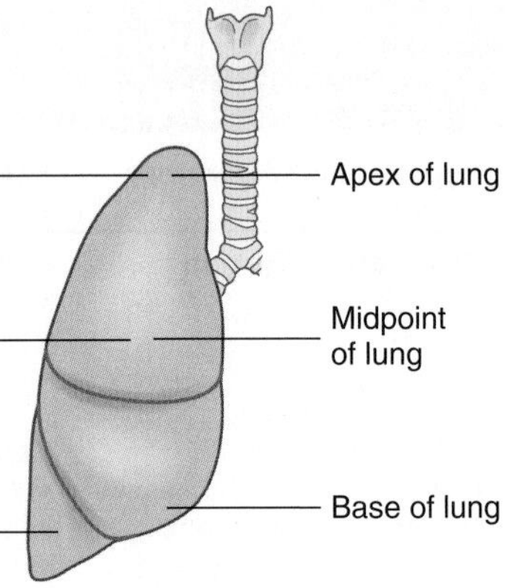

- Apex of lung
- Midpoint of lung
- Base of lung

FIG. 68-3 Regional V/Q differences in the normal lung. At the lung apex, the V/Q ratio is 3.3, at the midpoint 1.0, and at the base 0.63. This difference causes the PaO_2 to be higher at the apex of the lung and lower at the base. Values for $PaCO_2$ are the opposite (i.e., lower at the apex and higher at the base). Blood that exits the lung is a mixture of these values.

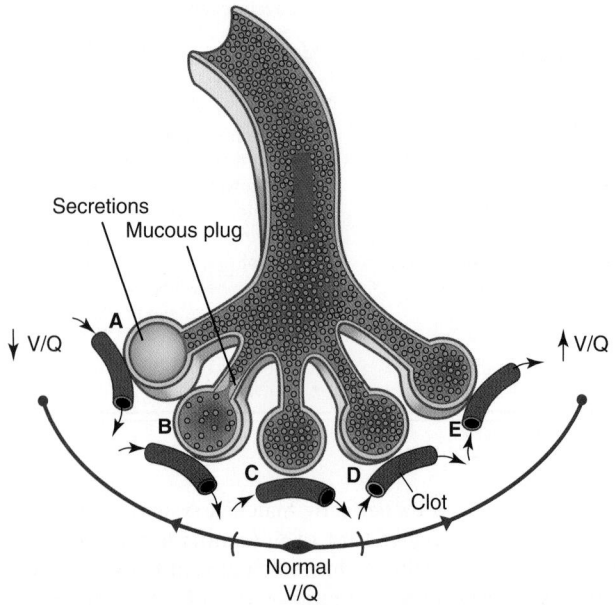

FIG. 68-4 Range of ventilation-to-perfusion (V/Q) relationships. **A,** Absolute shunt, no ventilation because of fluid filling the alveoli. **B,** V/Q mismatch, ventilation partially compromised by secretions in the airway. **C,** Normal lung unit. **D,** V/Q mismatch, perfusion partially compromised by emboli obstructing blood flow. **E,** Dead space, no perfusion because of obstruction of the pulmonary capillary.

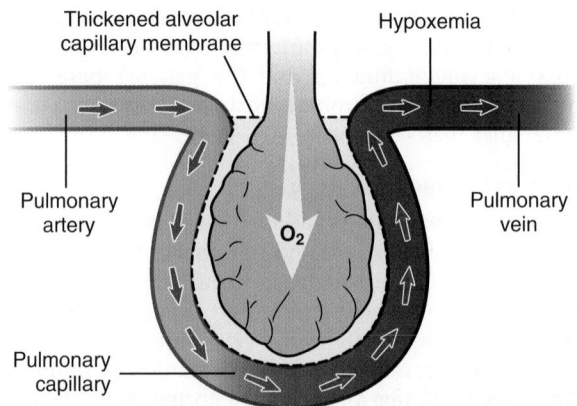

FIG. 68-5 Diffusion limitation. Exchange of CO_2 and O_2 cannot occur because of the thickened alveolar-capillary membrane.

The classic sign of diffusion limitation is hypoxemia that is present during exercise but not at rest. During exercise, blood moves more rapidly through the lungs, decreasing the time for diffusion of O_2 across the alveolar-capillary interface. Diffusion limitation may also occur in a high CO state (e.g., hepatopulmonary syndrome) or other disease states (e.g., inflammatory response seen with pancreatitis or severe brain trauma) unrelated to lung tissue damage. In this situation, CO is markedly elevated and vascular resistance is low. Blood circulates through the pulmonary capillary bed rapidly, allowing less time for gas exchange to occur.[14]

Alveolar Hypoventilation. Alveolar hypoventilation is a generalized decrease in ventilation that results in an increase in the $PaCO_2$ and a consequent decrease in PaO_2. Alveolar hypoventilation may be the result of restrictive lung diseases, central nervous system (CNS) diseases, chest wall dysfunction, acute asthma, or neuromuscular diseases. Although alveolar hypoventilation is primarily a mechanism of hypercapnic respiratory failure, it is mentioned here because it can also cause hypoxemia.[15]

Interrelationship of Mechanisms. Frequently, hypoxemic respiratory failure is caused by a combination of two or more of the following: V/Q mismatch, shunt, diffusion limitation, and alveolar hypoventilation. For example, the patient with acute respiratory failure secondary to pneumonia may have a combination of V/Q mismatch and shunt. In this case, inflammation, edema, and hypersecretion of exudate within the bronchioles and gas exchange units obstruct the airways (V/Q mismatch) and fill the alveoli with exudate (shunt). Additional contributing factors to hypoxemic respiratory failure include increases in O_2 demand such as with severe anxiety or agitation and unrelieved pain.

Hypercapnic Respiratory Failure. Hypercapnic respiratory failure results from an imbalance between ventilatory supply and ventilatory demand. *Ventilatory supply* is the maximum ventilation (gas flow in and out of the lungs) that the patient can sustain without developing respiratory muscle fatigue. *Ventilatory demand* is the amount of ventilation needed to keep the $PaCO_2$ within normal limits. Normally, ventilatory supply far exceeds ventilatory demand. Therefore people with normal lung function can engage in strenuous exercise, which greatly increases CO_2 production without an increase in $PaCO_2$. Patients with lung disease such as severe COPD do not have this advantage and cannot effectively increase lung ventilation in response to exercise or metabolic demands.

Hypercapnia occurs when ventilatory demand exceeds ventilatory supply and $PaCO_2$ cannot be sustained within normal limits. Hypercapnia reflects substantial lung dysfunction. Hypercapnic respiratory failure is sometimes called *ventilatory failure* because the primary problem is the respiratory system's inability to remove sufficient CO_2 to maintain a normal $PaCO_2$. Hypercapnic respiratory failure is also described as acute or chronic respiratory failure. For example, an episode of respiratory failure may represent an acute decompensation in a patient whose underlying lung function has deteriorated to the point that some degree of decompensation is always present (chronic respiratory insufficiency).

Many different diseases can cause a limitation in ventilatory supply (see Table 68-1 and eTable 68-1). These diseases can be grouped into four categories: (1) abnormalities of the airways and alveoli, (2) abnormalities of the CNS, (3) abnormalities of the chest wall, and (4) neuromuscular conditions.[16,17]

Airway and Alveoli Abnormalities. Patients with asthma, COPD, and cystic fibrosis are at high risk for hypercapnic respiratory failure because the underlying pathophysiology of these conditions results in airflow obstruction and air trapping. Ultimately respiratory muscle fatigue and ventilatory failure occur due to the additional work needed to inspire adequate tidal volumes against increased airway resistance and air trapped within the alveoli.[18-21]

Central Nervous System Abnormalities. A variety of CNS problems may suppress the drive to breathe. A common example is an overdose of a respiratory depressant drug (e.g., opioids, benzodiazepines). In a dose-related manner, CNS depressants decrease CO_2 reactivity in the brainstem. This allows arterial CO_2 levels to rise. A brainstem infarction or severe head injury may also interfere with normal function of the respiratory center in the medulla. Patients with these conditions are at risk for respiratory failure because the medulla does not alter the respiratory rate in response to a change in $PaCO_2$. CNS dysfunction may also include high-level spinal cord injuries that limit nerve supply to the respiratory muscles of the chest wall and diaphragm. Apart from direct brainstem dysfunction, metabolic or structural brain injury resulting in decreased or loss of consciousness may interfere with the patient's ability to manage secretions or adequately protect his or her airway.

Chest Wall Abnormalities. Several conditions prevent normal movement of the chest wall and limit lung expansion. In patients with flail chest, fractures prevent the rib cage from expanding normally because of pain, mechanical restriction, and muscle spasm. In patients with kyphoscoliosis, the change in spinal configuration compresses the lungs and prevents normal expansion of the chest wall. In patients with severe obesity, the weight of the chest and abdominal contents may limit lung expansion. These conditions place patients at risk for respiratory failure because they limit lung expansion or diaphragmatic movement and consequently gas exchange.

Neuromuscular Conditions. Various types of neuromuscular diseases may result in respiratory muscle weakness or paralysis (see Table 68-1). For example, patients with Guillain-Barré syndrome, muscular dystrophy, myasthenia gravis (acute exacerbation), or multiple sclerosis are at risk for respiratory failure because the respiratory muscles are weakened or paralyzed as a result of the underlying neuromuscular condition. Therefore they are unable to maintain normal $PaCO_2$ levels.[15-17]

Neuromuscular disorders may be acquired as a consequence of exposure to toxins (e.g., carbamate/organophosphate pesticides, chemical nerve agents) that interfere with the nerve supply to muscles and lung ventilation. Respiratory muscle weakness may also result from muscle wasting during a critical illness, peripheral nerve damage, and/or prolonged effects of neuromuscular blocking agents.

In summary, respiratory failure may occur in three of these categories (CNS, chest wall, neuromuscular conditions) despite the presence of normal lungs. Respiratory failure occurs because the medulla, chest wall, peripheral nerves, or respiratory muscles are not functioning normally. The patient may have no damage to lung tissue but may be unable to inspire a tidal volume sufficient to remove CO_2 from the lungs.

Tissue Oxygen Needs. Remember that even though PaO_2 and $PaCO_2$ determine the definition of respiratory failure, the major cause of respiratory failure is the lung's inability to meet the O_2 needs of the tissues. This failure may occur because of inadequate O_2 delivery to the tissues or because the tissues cannot use the O_2 delivered to them. It may also occur as a result of the stress response and dramatic increases in tissue O_2 consumption.

Tissue O_2 delivery is determined by cardiac output and the amount of O_2 carried in the hemoglobin. Therefore respiratory failure places the patient at greater risk if there are coexisting heart problems or anemia. Failure of O_2 use most commonly occurs in septic shock. Adequate O_2 may be delivered to the tissues, but impaired O_2 extraction or diffusion limitation exists at the cellular level. This results in an abnormally high amount of O_2 returning in the venous blood because it is not used at the tissue level. (Chapter 67 discusses shock.) Acid-base alterations (e.g., alkalosis, acidosis) may also interfere with O_2 delivery to peripheral tissues (see Chapter 17).

Clinical Manifestations

Respiratory failure may develop suddenly (minutes or hours) or gradually (several days or longer). A sudden decrease in PaO_2 or a rapid rise in $PaCO_2$ implies a serious condition, which can rapidly become a life-threatening emergency. An example is the patient with asthma who develops severe bronchospasm and a marked decrease in airflow, resulting in rapid respiratory muscle fatigue, acidemia, and respiratory failure.

A more gradual change in PaO_2 and $PaCO_2$ is better tolerated because compensation can occur. An example is the patient with COPD who develops a progressive increase in $PaCO_2$ over several days after a respiratory tract infection. Because the change occurred over several days, there is time for renal compensation (e.g., retention of bicarbonate), which minimizes the change in arterial pH. The patient will have compensated respiratory acidosis.[3,4] (See Chapter 17 for a discussion of renal compensation for acid-base disorders.)

Manifestations of respiratory failure are related to the extent of change in PaO_2 or $PaCO_2$, the rapidity of change (acute versus chronic), and the patient's ability to compensate for this change. When the patient's compensatory mechanisms fail, respiratory failure occurs. Because clinical manifestations vary, it is important to watch trends in ABGs, pulse oximetry, and assessment findings to fully evaluate the extent of change. Frequently, the first indication of respiratory failure is a change in the patient's mental status. Mental status changes often occur early, before ABG results are obtained. This is because the brain is very sensitive to variations in O_2 and CO_2 levels and acid-base balance. Restlessness, confusion, agitation, and combative behavior suggest inadequate O_2 delivery to the brain and should be fully investigated.

You may detect manifestations of respiratory failure that are specific (primary) (arising from the respiratory system) or nonspecific (secondary) (arising from other body systems) (Table 68-2). Understanding the significance of these manifestations is critical to your ability to detect the onset of respiratory failure and evaluate the effectiveness of treatment.

Tachycardia, tachypnea, and mild hypertension can be early signs of respiratory failure consequent to physiologic stress and elevated catecholamine levels. Such changes can indicate an attempt by the heart and lungs to compensate for decreased O_2 delivery. A severe morning headache may suggest that hypercapnia occurred during the night. Hypercapnia causes cerebral vasodilation, increased cerebral blood flow, and a mild increase in intracranial pressure (ICP) that produces a headache. At night the respiratory rate is slower and the lungs of patients at risk for respiratory failure may remove less $PaCO_2$.[22] Rapid,

TABLE 68-2	**MANIFESTATIONS OF HYPOXEMIA AND HYPERCAPNIA***

Specific	Nonspecific
Hypoxemia	
Respiratory	*Cerebral*
Dyspnea	Agitation
Tachypnea	Disorientation
Prolonged expiration (I:E = 1:3, 1:4)	Restless, combative behavior
Nasal flaring	Delirium
Intercostal muscle retraction	Confusion
Use of accessory muscles in respiration	↓ Level of consciousness
↓ SpO_2 (<80%)	Coma (late)
Paradoxic chest or abdominal wall movement with respiratory cycle (late)	*Cardiac*
	Tachycardia
	Hypertension
	Skin cool, clammy, and diaphoretic
	Dysrhythmias (late)
	Hypotension (late)
Cyanosis (late)	*Other*
	Fatigue
	Inability to speak in complete sentences without pausing to breathe
Hypercapnia	
Respiratory	*Cerebral*
Dyspnea	Morning headache
Use of tripod position	Disorientation
Pursed-lip breathing	Progressive somnolence
↓ Respiratory rate or rapid rate with shallow respirations	Elevated intracranial pressure (if monitored)
↓ Tidal volume	Coma (late)
↓ Minute ventilation	*Cardiac*
	Dysrhythmias
	Hypertension
	Tachycardia
	Bounding pulse
	Neuromuscular
	Muscle weakness
	↓ Deep tendon reflexes
	Tremors, seizures (late)

*List is not all-inclusive.
I:E, Inspiratory:expiratory ratio.

shallow breaths suggest that tidal volume may be inadequate to remove CO_2 from the lungs. Cyanosis is an unreliable indicator of hypoxemia and is a late sign of respiratory failure because it does not occur until hypoxemia is severe (PaO_2 of 45 mm Hg or less).

Consequences of Hypoxemia and Hypoxia. *Hypoxemia* occurs when the amount of O_2 in arterial blood is less than the normal value (normal PaO_2 is 80 to 100 mm Hg). Hypoxia occurs when the PaO_2 falls sufficiently to cause signs and symptoms of inadequate oxygenation (see Table 68-2). Hypoxemia can lead to hypoxia if not corrected. If hypoxia or hypoxemia is severe, the cells shift from aerobic to anaerobic metabolism. Anaerobic metabolism uses more fuel, produces less energy, and is less efficient than aerobic metabolism. The waste product of anaerobic metabolism is lactic acid. This is more difficult to remove from the body than CO_2 because it has to be buffered with sodium bicarbonate. When the body does not have enough sodium bicarbonate to buffer the lactic acid produced by anaerobic metabolism, metabolic acidosis, tissue and cellular dysfunction, and cell death may occur. Blood pressure (BP) and cardiac output can fall, and vasoactive or inotropic agents are often less effective in an acidotic environment.

Hypoxia and metabolic acidosis have adverse effects on the vital organs, especially the heart and CNS. The heart tries to compensate for the decreased O_2 level in the blood by increasing the heart rate and cardiac output. A cardiovascular hyperdynamic state may also occur due to catecholamine release that is associated with the physiologic stress response. As the PaO_2 decreases and acidosis increases, the myocardium becomes dysfunctional and cardiac output may decrease. In addition, angina and dysrhythmias may occur. All of these result in a further decrease in O_2 delivery.

Permanent brain damage may occur if the hypoxia is severe and prolonged. Renal function may also be impaired. Sodium retention, edema, acute tubular necrosis, and uremia may occur. Gastrointestinal (GI) system alterations include tissue ischemia, increased permeability of the intestinal wall, and possible migration of bacteria from the GI tract into circulation.

Specific Clinical Manifestations. The patient in respiratory failure may have a rapid, shallow breathing pattern or a respiratory rate that is slower than normal. Both changes predispose the patient to insufficient CO_2 removal. The patient may increase the respiratory rate in an effort to blow off accumulated CO_2. This breathing pattern requires a substantial amount of work and can lead to respiratory muscle fatigue. A change from a rapid rate to a slower rate in a patient in acute respiratory distress such as that seen with acute asthma suggests extreme progression of respiratory muscle fatigue and increased probability of respiratory arrest.[5-7,9]

The patient's position is an indication of the effort associated with work of breathing (WOB), or the effort used for muscle contraction during inhalation to accomplish lung ventilation. The patient may be able to lie down (mild distress), be able to lie down but prefer to sit (moderate distress), or be unable to breathe unless sitting upright (severe distress). A common position used by patients with moderate to severe COPD is to sit with the arms propped on the overbed table or on the knees. This so-called *tripod position* helps decrease the WOB, since propping the arms increases the anteroposterior diameter of the chest and changes pressure in the thorax (Fig. 68-6).

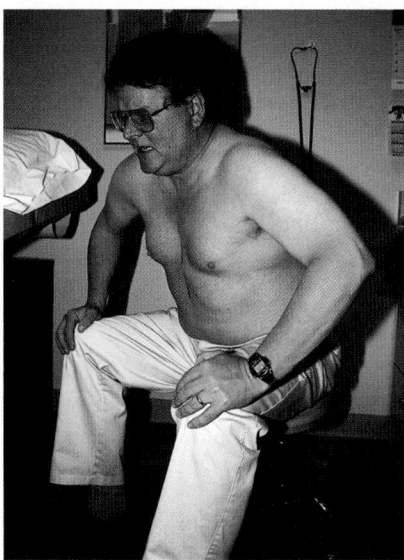

FIG. 68-6 Tripod positioning is used to increase chest and lung expansion and decrease work of breathing for patients with COPD or asthma.

Patients may use pursed-lip breathing (see Table 29-13). This increases SaO_2 because it slows respirations, allows more time for expiration, and prevents the small bronchioles from collapsing, thus helping air exchange. Another assessment parameter is the number of pillows the patient needs to breathe comfortably when lying flat. This is termed *orthopnea* and is documented as one-, two-, three-, or four-pillow orthopnea.

The person who is experiencing dyspnea is working hard to breathe and may be able to speak only a few words at a time between breaths. The patient's ability to speak indicates the severity of dyspnea. The patient may speak in sentences (mild or no distress), short phrases (moderate distress), or only words (severe distress). The number of words is also a clue. The patient may have "two-word" or "three-word" dyspnea, signifying that only two or three words can be spoken before pausing to breathe. There may also be a change in the onset of fatigue with walking. An additional assessment parameter is how far the patient is able to walk without stopping to rest.

The *inspiratory (I) to expiratory (E) (I:E) ratio* may change in patients in respiratory distress. Normally, the I:E ratio is 1:2, which means that expiration is twice as long as inspiration. The ratio may increase to 1:3 or 1:4, which signifies airflow obstruction and that more time is required to empty the lungs.

You may observe *retraction* (inward movement) of the intercostal spaces or the supraclavicular area and use of the accessory muscles (e.g., sternocleidomastoid) during inspiration or expiration. Use of the accessory muscles signifies moderate distress. Paradoxic breathing indicates severe distress. Normally, the thorax and abdomen move outward on inspiration and inward on exhalation. During *paradoxic breathing,* the abdomen and chest move in the opposite manner—outward during exhalation and inward during inspiration. Paradoxic breathing results from maximal use of the accessory muscles of respiration. The patient may also be diaphoretic from the WOB.

Perform auscultation to assess the patient's baseline breath sounds and any changes from baseline. Note and document the presence and location of any abnormal breath sounds. Crackles (generally heard on inspiration) may indicate pulmonary edema. Rhonchi (generally heard on expiration) indicate additional lung secretions and may be symptomatic of pneumonia or COPD. Absent or diminished breath sounds may indicate atelectasis, pleural effusion, or impaired inspiratory effort and hypoventilation. Bronchial breath sounds over the lung periphery often indicate lung consolidation from pneumonia. A pleural friction rub may also be heard in the presence of pneumonia that involves the pleura.

A thorough nursing assessment may result in early detection of respiratory insufficiency, allowing interventions to be started sooner and preventing respiratory failure. Patients with end-stage (severe) chronic lung disease may have low PaO_2 values or elevated $PaCO_2$ levels and crackles as their "normal" baseline. It is especially important to monitor specific and nonspecific signs of respiratory failure in patients with COPD because a small change can cause significant decompensation (see Table 68-2). Immediately report any change in mental status (e.g., agitation, confusion, decreased level of consciousness). This may indicate the onset of rapid deterioration in clinical status and the need for mechanical ventilation.

Diagnostic Studies

After physical assessment, the most common diagnostic studies used to evaluate respiratory failure are chest x-ray and ABG analysis. A chest x-ray helps to identify possible causes of respiratory failure (e.g., atelectasis, pneumonia). ABGs determine the levels of $PaCO_2$, PaO_2, bicarbonate, and pH. In respiratory failure, ABGs are used to evaluate oxygenation (PaO_2) and ventilation ($PaCO_2$) status and acid-base balance. Pulse oximetry monitors oxygenation status, but reveals little about lung ventilation. A catheter may be inserted into an artery to obtain blood for ABGs and monitor BP.

Other diagnostic studies that may be done include a complete blood cell count, serum electrolytes, urinalysis, and electrocardiogram (ECG). Blood and sputum cultures are obtained as necessary to determine sources of possible infection. If pulmonary embolus is suspected, a CT scan or V/Q lung scan may be done. For the patient in severe respiratory failure requiring endotracheal intubation, end-tidal CO_2 ($ETCO_2$) may be used to assess tube placement within the trachea immediately after intubation. (Chapter 66 discusses intubation.) $ETCO_2$ monitoring *(capnography)* and transcutaneous CO_2 monitoring may also be used during ventilator management to assess trends in lung ventilation.[23] Although not commonly done in acute situations, pulmonary function tests may be performed.

In severe respiratory failure, central venous or PA pressure monitoring or arterial pressure–based CO monitoring is used to measure hemodynamic parameters (e.g., central venous pressure, PA pressures, CO, stroke volume variation, central/mixed venous O_2 saturation [$ScvO_2$/SvO_2]). These data help to determine the adequacy of tissue perfusion and the patient's response to treatment measures. Hemodynamic monitoring can also determine whether the accumulation of fluid in the lungs is the result of heart or lung problems. It can also provide feedback on the physiologic effects of mechanical ventilation on hemodynamic status.[24] (Chapter 66 discusses hemodynamic monitoring in detail.)

NURSING AND COLLABORATIVE MANAGEMENT ACUTE RESPIRATORY FAILURE

Because many different problems cause respiratory failure, specific care of these patients varies. This section discusses general assessment and collaborative care measures that apply to patients with acute respiratory failure. In acute care settings, collaboration between nursing and other health care team members (e.g., respiratory therapists) is essential.

NURSING ASSESSMENT
Table 68-3 presents subjective and objective data that should be obtained from the patient with acute respiratory failure.

NURSING DIAGNOSES
Nursing diagnoses for the patient with acute respiratory failure may include, but are not limited to, the following:
- Impaired gas exchange *related to* alveolar hypoventilation, intrapulmonary shunting, V/Q mismatch, and diffusion impairment
- Ineffective airway clearance *related to* excessive secretions, decreased level of consciousness, presence of an artificial airway, neuromuscular dysfunction, and pain
- Ineffective breathing pattern *related to* neuromuscular impairment of respirations, pain, anxiety, decreased level of consciousness, respiratory muscle fatigue, and bronchospasm

---

TABLE 68-3 NURSING ASSESSMENT

Acute Respiratory Failure

Subjective Data
Important Health Information
Past health history: Chronic lung disease; potential occupational exposures to lung toxins; tobacco use (pack-years); alcohol or drug use; previous hospitalizations related to lung disease; thoracic or spinal cord trauma; severe obesity; altered consciousness; age (physiologic and chronologic)
Medications: Use of home O_2, inhalers (bronchodilators), home nebulization, over-the-counter medications; immunosuppressant (e.g., corticosteroid) therapy, CNS depressants
Surgery or other treatments: Previous intubation and mechanical ventilation; recent thoracic or abdominal surgery

Functional Health Patterns
Health perception–health management: Exercise, self-care activities; immunizations (flu, pneumonia, hepatitis)
Nutritional-metabolic: Eating habits; bloating, indigestion; weight gain or loss; change in appetite; use of vitamins or herbal supplements
Activity-exercise: Fatigue, dizziness; dyspnea at rest or with activity, wheezing, cough (productive or nonproductive); sputum (volume, color, viscosity); palpitations, swollen feet; change in exercise tolerance
Sleep-rest: Changes in sleep pattern; use of CPAP
Cognitive-perceptual: Headache, chest pain or tightness; chronic pain
Coping–stress tolerance: Anxiety, depression, hopelessness; risk of drug, alcohol, or nicotine withdrawal

Objective Data
General
Restlessness, agitation

Integumentary
Pale, cool, clammy skin or warm, flushed skin; peripheral and central cyanosis; peripheral dependent edema

Respiratory
Shallow, increased respiratory rate progressing to decreased rate; use of accessory muscles with evidence of retractions, altered I:E ratio; increased diaphragmatic excursion or asymmetric chest expansion; paradoxic chest and abdominal wall movement; tactile fremitus, crepitus, or deviated trachea on palpation; absent, diminished, or adventitious breath sounds; pleural friction rub; bronchial or bronchovesicular sounds heard in other than normal location; inspiratory stridor

Cardiovascular
Vital signs: Tachycardia progressing to bradycardia, dysrhythmias, extra heart sounds (S_3, S_4); bounding pulse; hypertension progressing to hypotension; pulsus paradoxus; jugular venous distention; pedal edema

Gastrointestinal
Abdominal distention, ascites, epigastric tenderness, hepatojugular reflex

Neurologic
Somnolence, confusion, slurred speech, restlessness, delirium, agitation, tremors, seizures, coma; asterixis, decreased deep tendon reflexes; papilledema

Possible Diagnostic Findings
↓/↑ pH, ↑/↓ $PaCO_2$, ↑/↓ bicarbonate, ↓ PaO_2, ↓ SaO_2, ↓ PEFR, ↓ tidal volume, ↓ forced vital capacity, ↓ minute ventilation, ↓ negative inspiratory force; abnormal serum electrolytes, hemoglobin, hematocrit, and white blood cell count; abnormal findings on chest x-ray; abnormal central venous or pulmonary artery pressures, cardiac output

CPAP, Continuous positive airway pressure; *I:E,* inspiratory:expiratory; *PEFR,* peak expiratory flow rate.

Additional information on nursing diagnoses for the patient with acute respiratory failure is presented in eNursing Care Plan 68-1 (available on the website for this chapter).

PLANNING

The overall goals for the patient with acute respiratory failure include (1) normal ABG values or values within the patient's baseline, (2) normal breath sounds or breath sounds within the patient's baseline, (3) no dyspnea or breathing patterns within the patient's baseline, (4) independent maintenance of the airway, and (5) effective cough and ability to clear secretions.

PREVENTION

As part of the plan of care for any patient who may be at risk for respiratory failure, prevention and early recognition of respiratory distress are important. Prevention involves a thorough history and physical assessment to identify the patient at risk for respiratory failure and then the initiation of appropriate nursing interventions. These include teaching the patient about deep breathing and coughing, use of incentive spirometry, and ambulation. Prevention of atelectasis, pneumonia, and complications of immobility, as well as optimization of hydration and nutrition, can potentially decrease the risk of respiratory failure in the acutely or critically ill patient.

RESPIRATORY THERAPY

The major goals of care for acute respiratory failure include maintaining adequate oxygenation and ventilation. Interventions include O_2 therapy, mobilization of secretions, and positive pressure ventilation (PPV) (Table 68-4).

OXYGEN THERAPY. The primary goal of O_2 therapy is to correct hypoxemia. If hypoxemia is secondary to V/Q mismatch, supplemental O_2 administered at 1 to 3 L/minute by nasal cannula, or 24% to 32% by face mask or Venturi mask, should improve the PaO_2 and SaO_2. Hypoxemia secondary to an intrapulmonary shunt is usually not responsive to high O_2 concentrations. In this case, the patient usually requires PPV. PPV provides O_2 therapy and humidification, decreases WOB, and reduces respiratory muscle fatigue. In addition, PPV assists in opening collapsed airways and decreasing shunt. PPV is provided via an endotracheal tube (most frequently) or noninvasively by means of a tight-fitting mask.[25,26] (Chapter 66 discusses mechanical ventilation in detail.)

The patient with acute respiratory failure must be able to tolerate the type of O_2 delivery system chosen. For example, a face mask may cause anxiety from feelings of claustrophobia. The anxiety can cause dyspnea, increase O_2 consumption and CO_2 production, and cause the patient to remove the O_2 device. The selected O_2 delivery system must also maintain PaO_2 at 55 to 60 mm Hg or higher and SaO_2 at 90% or higher at the lowest O_2 concentration possible.

High O_2 concentrations replace the nitrogen gas normally present in the alveoli, thus causing instability and atelectasis. In intubated patients, exposure to 60% or higher FIO_2 for longer than 48 hours poses a significant risk for O_2 *toxicity*. In nonintubated patients the risk is less clear. The effects of prolonged exposure to high levels of O_2 include increased pulmonary capillary permeability, decreased surfactant production and surfactant inactivation, and fibrotic changes in the alveoli. (Chapter 29 and Table 29-20 discuss O_2 delivery devices.)

Another possible risk of O_2 therapy is specific to patients with chronic hypercapnia (e.g., patients with COPD). Chronic

TABLE 68-4 COLLABORATIVE CARE

Acute Respiratory Failure

Diagnostic
- Vital signs
- History and physical examination
- Arterial blood gases
- Pulse oximetry
- Chest x-ray
- CBC
- Serum electrolytes and urinalysis
- ECG
- Blood and sputum cultures (if indicated)
- Hemodynamic parameters: CVP, SVV, PAWP

Collaborative Therapy
Respiratory Therapy
- O_2 therapy
- Mobilization of secretions
  - Effective coughing
  - Incentive spirometry
  - Hydration and humidification
  - Chest physiotherapy
  - Airway suctioning
  - Ambulation
  - Positioning: head of bed elevated to assist lung ventilation; tripod positioning for optimal comfort and efficiency during breathing
- Positive pressure ventilation
  - Noninvasive positive pressure ventilation
  - Intubation with positive pressure ventilation

Drug Therapy
- Relief of bronchospasm (e.g., albuterol [Proventil])
- Reduction of airway inflammation (corticosteroids)
- Reduction of pulmonary congestion (e.g., furosemide [Lasix], morphine)
- Treatment of pulmonary infections (e.g., antibiotics)
- Reduction of severe anxiety, pain, and agitation (e.g., lorazepam [Ativan], fentanyl [Sublimaze], morphine)

Medical Supportive Therapy
- Management of the underlying cause of respiratory failure
- Maintenance of adequate cardiac output
- Maintenance of adequate hemoglobin concentration

Nutritional Therapy
- Enteral nutrition support
- Parenteral nutrition support

CVP, Central venous pressure; *PAWP,* pulmonary artery wedge pressure; *SVV,* stroke volume variation.

hypercapnia blunts the response of chemoreceptors in the medulla to elevated CO_2 levels as a respiratory stimulant. In this situation, hypoxia stimulates respirations. Provide O_2 to patients with chronic hypercapnia through a low-flow device such as a nasal cannula at 1 to 2 L/minute or a Venturi mask at 24% to 28%. Closely monitor patients for changes in mental status, respiratory rate, and ABG results until their PaO_2 level has reached their baseline normal value.

MOBILIZATION OF SECRETIONS. Retained pulmonary secretions may cause or exacerbate acute respiratory failure. This occurs because the movement of O_2 into the alveoli and removal of CO_2 are blocked. Secretions can be mobilized through effective coughing, adequate hydration and humidification, chest physiotherapy (physical therapy), airway suctioning, and ambulation when possible.

Effective Coughing and Positioning. If secretions are obstructing the airway, encourage the patient to cough. The patient with a

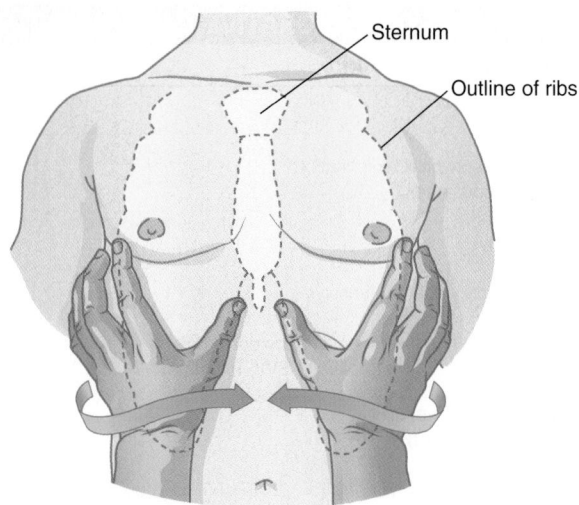

— Sternum

— Outline of ribs

FIG. 68-7 Augmented coughing is performed by placing one or both hands on the anterolateral base of the lungs. After the patient takes a deep inspiration and at the beginning of expiration, move the hand(s) forcefully upward. This increases abdominal pressure and aids in producing a forceful cough.

neuromuscular weakness from a disease or exhaustion may not be able to generate sufficient airway pressures to produce an effective cough. *Augmented coughing (quad coughing)* may be of benefit to these patients. Perform augmented coughing by placing one or both hands on the anterolateral base of the lungs (Fig. 68-7). As the patient ends a deep inspiration and begins the expiration, move your hands forcefully upward, increasing abdominal pressure and facilitating the cough. This measure helps increase expiratory flow and thereby facilitates secretion clearance.

Some patients may benefit from therapeutic cough techniques. *Huff coughing* is a series of coughs performed while saying the word "huff" (see Table 29-23). This technique prevents the glottis from closing during the cough. Patients with COPD generate higher flow rates with a huff cough than is possible with a normal cough. The huff cough is effective in clearing only the central airways, but it may assist in moving secretions upward.

The staged cough also assists in mobilizing secretions. To perform the *staged cough,* the patient assumes a sitting position, breathes three or four times in and out through the mouth, and coughs while bending forward and pressing a pillow inward against the diaphragm.

Positioning the patient upright, either by elevating the head of the bed at least 45 degrees or by using a reclining chair or chair bed, helps maximize thoracic expansion, thereby decreasing dyspnea and improving secretion mobilization. A sitting position improves pulmonary function and assists in venous pooling in dependent body areas such as the lower extremities. When lungs are upright, ventilation and perfusion are best in the lung bases.

Lateral or side-lying positioning may be used in patients with disease involving only one lung. This position, termed *good lung down,* allows for improved V/Q matching in the affected lung. Pulmonary blood flow and ventilation are optimal in dependent lung areas. This position also allows secretions to drain out of the affected lung to the point where they may be removed by suctioning. For example, in patients with significant right-sided pneumonia, optimal positioning would be to place them on their left side to maximize ventilation and perfusion in the "good" lung and facilitate secretion removal from the affected lung (postural drainage). All patients should be side-lying if there is any possibility that the tongue will obstruct the airway or that aspiration may occur. Keep an oral or nasal airway at the bedside for use if necessary. Airway control with endotracheal intubation and PPV is indicated when patients cannot maintain their airway and lung ventilation.

Hydration and Humidification. Thick and viscous secretions are difficult to expel. Adequate fluid intake (2 to 3 L/day) keeps secretions thin and easier to remove. If the patient is unable to take sufficient fluids orally, IV hydration is used. Thoroughly assess the patient's cardiac and renal status to determine whether he or she can tolerate the IV fluid volume and avoid heart failure and pulmonary edema. Regularly assess for signs of fluid overload by clinical evaluation (e.g., crackles, dyspnea) and invasive monitoring (e.g., increased central venous pressure). These considerations would also apply to the patient with renal dysfunction.

An appropriate humidification device is an adjunct in secretion management. Aerosols of sterile normal saline, administered by a nebulizer, may be used to liquefy secretions. O_2 may also be given by aerosol mask to thin secretions and facilitate their removal. Aerosol therapy may induce bronchospasm and severe coughing, causing a decreased PaO_2. Frequent assessment of patient tolerance to therapy is critical. Mucolytic agents such as nebulized acetylcysteine (Mucomyst) mixed with a bronchodilator may be used to thin secretions. A side effect of these drugs is bronchospasm so they are used only in special situations (e.g., during bronchoscopy to remove thick, copious secretions).

Chest Physiotherapy. Chest physiotherapy is indicated in patients who produce more than 30 mL of sputum per day or have evidence of severe atelectasis or pulmonary infiltrates. Postural drainage, percussion, and vibration to the affected lung segments assist in moving secretions to the larger airways where they are removed by coughing or suctioning. Positioning affects oxygenation. Patients may not tolerate head-down or lateral positioning because of extreme dyspnea or hypoxemia caused by V/Q mismatch. (Chest physiotherapy is discussed in Chapter 29 on p. 594.)

Airway Suctioning. Nasopharyngeal, oropharyngeal, or nasotracheal suctioning (blind suctioning without a tracheal tube in place) is done if the patient is unable to expectorate secretions. Suctioning through an artificial airway (e.g., endotracheal tube) is also performed as needed (see Chapters 27 and 66). A minitracheostomy (or mini-trach) is used to suction patients who have difficulty mobilizing secretions and when blind suctioning is difficult or ineffective. The *mini-trach* is a 4-mm indwelling plastic cuffless cannula inserted through the cricothyroid membrane. It is used to instill sterile normal saline solution to elicit a cough and to perform suctioning. Contraindications for a mini-trach include an absent gag reflex, history of aspiration, and the need for long-term mechanical ventilation. At all times, suction cautiously and closely monitor the patient for complications (e.g., hypoxia, increased ICP, dysrhythmias).

POSITIVE PRESSURE VENTILATION. If intensive measures fail to improve ventilation and oxygenation and the patient continues to show signs of acute respiratory failure, ventilatory assistance is needed. PPV may be provided invasively through orotracheal or nasotracheal intubation or noninvasively through a nasal or face mask.[22,26]

Noninvasive positive pressure ventilation (NIPPV) is used for patients with acute or chronic respiratory failure. During NIPPV, a mask is placed tightly over the patient's nose or nose and mouth and the patient breathes spontaneously while PPV

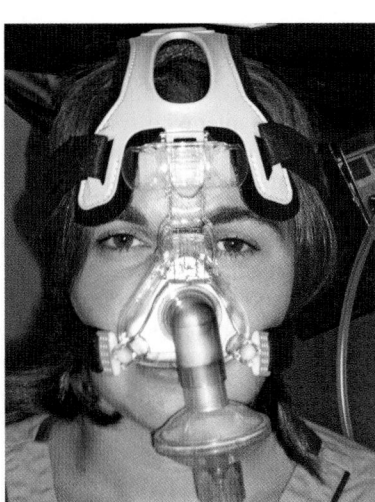

FIG. 68-8 Noninvasive bilevel positive pressure ventilation. A mask is placed over the nose or nose and mouth. Positive pressure from a mechanical ventilator assists the patient's breathing efforts, decreasing the work of breathing.

is delivered. With NIPPV, it is possible to decrease the WOB without the need for endotracheal intubation. Bilevel positive airway pressure (BiPAP) is a form of NIPPV in which different positive pressure levels are set for inspiration and expiration (Fig. 68-8). Continuous positive airway pressure (CPAP) is another form of NIPPV in which a constant positive pressure is delivered to the airway during inspiration and expiration.[27-30]

NIPPV is most useful in managing chronic respiratory failure in patients with chest wall and neuromuscular disease (see Table 68-1). NIPPV has been used in patients with hypoxemic respiratory failure (e.g., ARDS, cardiogenic pulmonary edema), but with less success. NIPPV may also be used for patients who refuse endotracheal intubation but still want some palliative ventilatory support (e.g., patients with end-stage COPD).[31,32] NIPPV is not appropriate for patients who have excessive secretions, decreased level of consciousness, high O_2 requirements, facial trauma, or hemodynamic instability. NIPPV is also used postextubation to avoid reintubation. (Chapter 66 discusses artificial airways, PPV, CPAP, and BiPAP in detail.)

DRUG THERAPY

Goals of drug therapy for patients in acute respiratory failure include (1) relief of bronchospasm; (2) reduction of airway inflammation and pulmonary congestion; (3) treatment of pulmonary infection; and (4) reduction of severe pain, anxiety, and restlessness.

RELIEF OF BRONCHOSPASM. Relief of bronchospasm increases alveolar ventilation. Short-acting bronchodilators, such as metaproterenol (Alupent) and albuterol (Ventolin), reverse bronchospasm. Side effects of these β-adrenergic agonist drugs include tachycardia and hypertension. Prolonged use can increase the risk of dysrhythmias and cardiac ischemia. Monitor ECG and vital signs for any changes with administration of these drugs. Give these drugs using a hand-held nebulizer or a metered-dose inhaler with a spacer. In acute bronchospasm these drugs may be given at 15- to 30-minute intervals until a response occurs. The bronchodilator effects of these medications can sometimes worsen hypoxemia by redistributing the inspired gas to areas of decreased perfusion. Administering the bronchodilator with an oxygen-enriched gas mixture usually reduces this effect.[6,7] (Chapter 29 discusses nursing management related to bronchodilators.)

REDUCTION OF AIRWAY INFLAMMATION. Corticosteroids (e.g., methylprednisolone [Solu-Medrol]) may be used in conjunction with bronchodilating agents for bronchospasm and inflammation. When given IV in acute asthma, corticosteroids speed resolution of airway inflammation and edema. Inhaled corticosteroids require 4 to 5 days for optimum therapeutic effects and are not used for acute respiratory failure.

DRUG ALERT: IV Corticosteroids
- Monitor potassium levels, since corticosteroids exacerbate hypokalemia caused by diuretics.
- Prolonged use causes adrenal insufficiency.

REDUCTION OF PULMONARY CONGESTION. Pulmonary interstitial fluid can accumulate because of direct or indirect injury to the alveolar capillary membrane (e.g., ARDS) or from heart failure. The result is decreased alveolar ventilation and hypoxemia. IV diuretics (e.g., furosemide [Lasix]), morphine, and nitroglycerin (Tridil) are used to decrease the pulmonary congestion caused by heart failure. If atrial fibrillation is also present, calcium channel blockers (e.g., diltiazem [Cardizem]) and β-adrenergic blockers (e.g., metoprolol [Lopressor]) are used to decrease heart rate and improve CO. (Chapter 35 discusses heart failure.)

TREATMENT OF PULMONARY INFECTIONS. Pulmonary infections (e.g., pneumonia, acute bronchitis) result in excessive mucus production; fever; increased O_2 consumption; and inflamed, fluid-filled, or collapsed alveoli. Alveoli that are fluid filled or collapsed cannot participate in gas exchange. Pulmonary infections can either cause or exacerbate acute respiratory failure. IV antibiotics, such as azithromycin (Zithromax) or ceftriaxone (Rocephin), are often given to treat infections. Chest x-rays help identify the location and extent of a suspected infectious process. Sputum cultures help determine the type of organisms causing the infection and their sensitivity to antimicrobial medications.[33]

REDUCTION OF SEVERE ANXIETY, PAIN, AND AGITATION. Anxiety, restlessness, and agitation result from hypoxia. In addition, fear caused by the inability to breathe and a sense of loss of control may increase anxiety. Anxiety, pain, and agitation increase O_2 consumption, which may worsen the hypoxemia. Anxiety, pain, and agitation also increase CO_2 production, affect ventilator management, and increase morbidity. Several strategies can assist the patient in reducing anxiety and pain.

Sedation and analgesia with drug therapy such as propofol (Diprivan) (used for mechanically ventilated patients), benzodiazepines (e.g., lorazepam [Ativan], midazolam [Versed]), and opioids (e.g., morphine, fentanyl [Sublimaze]) are used to decrease anxiety, agitation, and pain. Continued agitation increases the patient's WOB, O_2 consumption, CO_2 production, and risk of injury (e.g., unplanned extubation). Patients receiving these agents are best managed by following an evidence-based protocol that includes a regular "sedation holiday" for ongoing assessment.[34,35] (Sedation holiday is discussed in Chapter 66 on p. 1601.)

SAFETY ALERT
- Monitor patients closely for cardiopulmonary depression when giving any sedative or analgesic agents.
- Agitation is often caused by pain, hypoxemia, electrolyte imbalance, evolution of brain injury, and adverse drug reactions.
- Assess and aggressively treat all potentially reversible causes of agitation.
- Sedative and analgesic agents may have a prolonged effect in critically ill patients, delay weaning from mechanical ventilation, and contribute to increased length of stay.

Address treatable causes of agitation (e.g., hypoxemia, pain, hypercapnia). Patients who breathe asynchronously with mechanical ventilation may also benefit from adjustment of ventilator flow rates and other settings. Patients who remain asynchronous with mechanical ventilation despite aggressive sedative and analgesic dosing may require neuromuscular blockade (paralysis) with agents such as vecuronium (Norcuron) or cisatracurium (Nimbex). These drugs relax skeletal muscles by interfering with neuromuscular transmission and, ultimately, provide synchrony with mechanical ventilation. Neuromuscular blockade may also decrease the patient's risk of lung injury related to excessive inspiratory/intrathoracic pressures. In this way, the ventilator can provide optimal respiratory support. Remember that a patient receiving neuromuscular blockade can appear to be asleep but still possibly be awake and in pain. For this reason, both aggressive sedation and analgesia are essential.

SAFETY ALERT
- Provide concurrent sedation and analgesia to the point of unconsciousness for patients receiving neuromuscular blockade. This eliminates patient awareness, assures patient comfort, and avoids the terrifying experience of being awake and in pain while paralyzed.
- Use neuromuscular blockade for the shortest duration and in the lowest dose possible to avoid complications (e.g., myopathy).

Monitoring levels of sedation in patients receiving neuromuscular blockade is challenging. Noninvasive electroencephalogram-based technology may help guide sedative and analgesic therapy in these patients.[36] Levels of drug paralysis are monitored primarily by clinical assessment of ventilation and whether goals of care are being met. A frequent adjunct to monitoring paralysis is use of a peripheral nerve stimulator (see Fig. 66-19). Clinical assessment is essential to determine the adequacy of sedation, analgesia, and neuromuscular blockade in critically ill patients.

MEDICAL SUPPORTIVE THERAPY

Goals and related interventions to maximize O_2 delivery are essential to improving the patient's oxygenation and ventilation status. The primary goal is to treat the underlying cause of the respiratory failure. Other supportive goals include maintaining an adequate CO and hemoglobin concentration.

TREATING THE UNDERLYING CAUSE. Interventions are directed toward reversing the disease process that caused the acute respiratory failure. Patients with hypoventilation need to be diagnosed and treated rapidly. Patients with V/Q mismatch, shunting, or diffusion limitation are managed differently depending on the underlying cause. In all patient situations, monitoring treatment effects, including trends in ABGs and changes in respiratory status, is an ongoing process.

MAINTAINING ADEQUATE CARDIAC OUTPUT. CO reflects the blood flow reaching the tissues. BP and mean arterial pressure (MAP) are important indicators of the adequacy of CO. Always interpret BP and MAP readings within the context of the physical assessment to determine adequacy of CO and tissue perfusion. Usually a systolic BP of 90 mm Hg or more or a MAP greater than 60 mm Hg is adequate to maintain perfusion to the vital organs. At these levels, changes in mental status may be attributed to the level of O_2 and CO_2 rather than decreased cerebral perfusion. In a patient with chronic, uncontrolled hypertension, a systolic BP of 90 to 100 mm Hg is often inadequate to maintain systemic and cerebral perfusion. Cerebral perfusion may not only tolerate but may require a higher BP and MAP to prevent episodes of brain ischemia or hypoperfusion to other organs.

Decreased CO is treated by administration of IV fluids, medications, or both. (Chapter 67 discusses drugs used to treat decreased CO and shock.) CO can also be decreased by changes in intrathoracic or intrapulmonary pressures from PPV. Patients experiencing exacerbation of COPD or asthma and those receiving PPV are at risk of alveolar hyperinflation, increased right ventricular afterload, and excessive intrathoracic pressures. These changes can result in limited blood flow from the right side of the heart through the pulmonary vasculature to the left side of the heart and can cause hemodynamic compromise. In addition, blood return from the systemic circulation to the right side of the heart may be impaired, further decreasing preload. Each of these physiologic effects can lead to severe hemodynamic compromise. Consequently, closely monitor BP and clinical indicators of adequate CO and tissue perfusion with initiation of or changes in mechanical ventilation.

MAINTAINING ADEQUATE HEMOGLOBIN CONCENTRATION. Hemoglobin is the primary carrier of O_2 to the tissues. Delivery of O_2 to the tissues is compromised in anemic patients. A hemoglobin of 9 g/dL (90 g/L) or higher typically ensures adequate O_2 saturation of the hemoglobin for tissue oxygenation. Monitor the patient for signs of blood loss (e.g., hypotension, melena). Transfusion with packed red blood cells may be used if an adequate hemoglobin level is not maintained and the patient is symptomatic.

NUTRITIONAL THERAPY

Maintenance of protein and energy stores is especially important in patients with acute respiratory failure. The hypermetabolic state in critical illness increases the caloric requirements needed to maintain body weight and muscle mass. Thus nutritional depletion causes a loss of muscle mass, including the respiratory muscles, and may prolong recovery. The dietitian, in collaboration with the health care team, determines the optimal method of feeding and optimal caloric and fluid requirements. During the acute manifestations of respiratory failure, the risk of aspiration typically prevents oral intake. Ideally, enteral or parenteral nutrition is started within 24 hours in malnourished patients and within 3 days in well-nourished patients. When acute manifestations subside, the patient may resume oral intake as able.

EVALUATION

The expected outcomes are that the patient with respiratory failure will

- Maintain a patent airway with effective removal of secretions
- Achieve normal or baseline respiratory rate and rhythm, and breath sounds
- Maintain adequate oxygenation as indicated by normal or baseline ABGs
- Experience normal hemodynamic status

Additional outcomes are presented in eNursing Care Plan 68-1 (available on the website for this chapter).

GERONTOLOGIC CONSIDERATIONS

RESPIRATORY FAILURE

Older adults are the fastest-growing age-group in the United States, a trend that is increasingly reflected within the patient populations in acute and critical care settings. Multiple factors contribute to an increased risk of respiratory failure in older adults. The reduction in ventilatory capacity that accompanies aging places the older adult at risk for respiratory failure. Physiologic aging of the lung includes alveolar dilation, larger air spaces, and loss of surface area for gas exchange. Diminished elastic recoil within the airways, decreased chest wall compliance, and decreased respiratory muscle strength also occur. In older adults the PaO_2 falls further and the $PaCO_2$ rises to a higher level before the respiratory system is stimulated to alter the rate and depth of breathing. This delayed response can contribute to the development of respiratory failure. In addition, a history of tobacco use is a risk factor that can accelerate age-related respiratory changes. Poor nutritional status and less available physiologic reserve in the cardiopulmonary and autonomic nervous systems increase the risk of additional disease states such as pneumonia and heart disease. These may further compromise respiratory function and lead to respiratory failure. Poor nutrition can also result in a decrease in muscle mass and related respiratory drive.[31,37]*

Older adults are more vulnerable to delirium, health care–associated infections, and the adverse effects of polypharmacy. Delirium is an independent risk factor for increased mortality and morbidity rates in critically ill patients. It can complicate ventilator management and weaning by interfering with patient cooperation. Delirium associated with agitation increases CO_2 elimination and O_2 consumption, increases the risk for unplanned extubation and device removal, and extends length of hospital stay and ventilator days.[38,39] (Delirium is discussed in Chapters 60 and 66.)

Adjust assessment parameters for age-related changes. For example, heart rate and BP generally increase with age and the related changes in the cardiovascular system. Therefore you need to know the patient's baseline vital signs. Compare these with the ongoing physical assessment findings to appropriately evaluate changes in cardiopulmonary function in the older adult.

ACUTE RESPIRATORY DISTRESS SYNDROME

Acute respiratory distress syndrome (ARDS) is a sudden and progressive form of acute respiratory failure in which the alveolar-capillary interface becomes damaged and more permeable to intravascular fluid (Fig. 68-9). ARDS exists on a continuum. One way to assess the degree of impairment in gas exchange is to measure the PaO_2/FIO_2 (P/F) ratio. Under normal circumstances (e.g., PaO_2 85 to 100 mm Hg; FIO_2 0.21 [room air]), the P/F ratio would be greater than 400 (e.g., 95/0.21 = 452). With the onset and progression of lung injury and impairment in O_2 delivery through the alveolar-capillary interface, the PaO_2 may remain lower than expected despite increased FIO_2.

The term **acute lung injury (ALI)** is used when the P/F ratio is 200 to 300 (e.g., 86/0.4 = 215). The term *ARDS* is used when the P/F ratio is less than 200 (e.g., 80/0.8 = 100). In both cases, the alveoli fill with fluid, resulting in severe dyspnea, hypoxemia refractory to supplemental O_2, reduced lung compliance, and diffuse pulmonary infiltrates.[40]

The incidence of ARDS in the United States is estimated at more than 150,000 cases annually. Despite supportive therapy, the mortality rate from ARDS is approximately 50%. Patients who have both gram-negative septic shock and ARDS have a mortality rate of 70% to 90%.

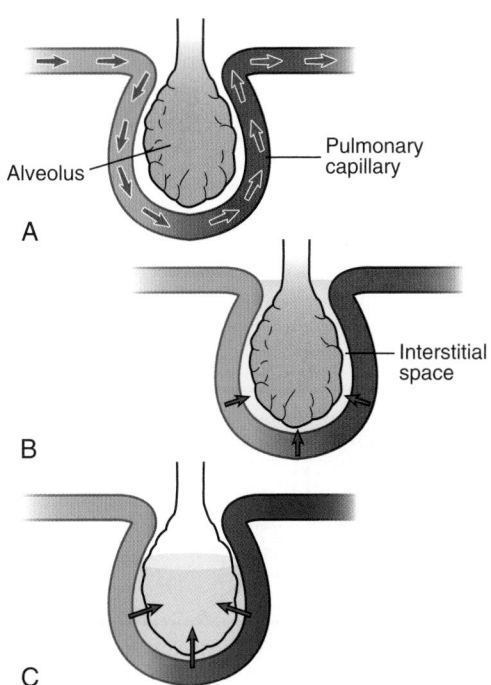

FIG. 68-9 Stages of edema formation in acute respiratory distress syndrome. **A,** Normal alveolus and pulmonary capillary. **B,** Interstitial edema occurs with increased flow of fluid into the interstitial space. **C,** Alveolar edema occurs when the fluid crosses the blood-gas barrier.

TABLE 68-5	**PREDISPOSING CONDITIONS TO ARDS**
Direct Lung Injury	**Indirect Lung Injury**
Common Causes	
Aspiration of gastric contents or other substances	Sepsis (especially gram-negative infection)
Viral or bacterial pneumonia	Severe massive trauma
Sepsis	
Less Common Causes	
Chest trauma	Acute pancreatitis
Embolism: fat, air, amniotic fluid, thrombus	Anaphylaxis
Inhalation of toxic substances	Cardiopulmonary bypass
Near-drowning	Disseminated intravascular coagulation
O_2 toxicity	Nonpulmonary systemic diseases
Radiation pneumonitis	Opioid drug overdose (e.g., heroin)
	Severe head injury
	Shock states
	Transfusion-related acute lung injury (e.g., multiple blood transfusions)

Etiology and Pathophysiology

Table 68-5 lists conditions that predispose patients to the development of ARDS. Patients with multiple risk factors are three or four times more likely to develop ARDS.

The most common cause of ARDS is sepsis. Direct lung injury may cause ARDS (Fig. 68-10), or ARDS may develop because of the systemic inflammatory response syndrome (SIRS) (see Fig. 67-1). SIRS may have an infectious or a noninfectious etiology. It is characterized by widespread inflammation or clinical responses to inflammation after a variety of physiologic insults, including severe trauma, gut ischemia, and lung injury.[41,42] ARDS may also develop as a consequence of

PATHOPHYSIOLOGY MAP

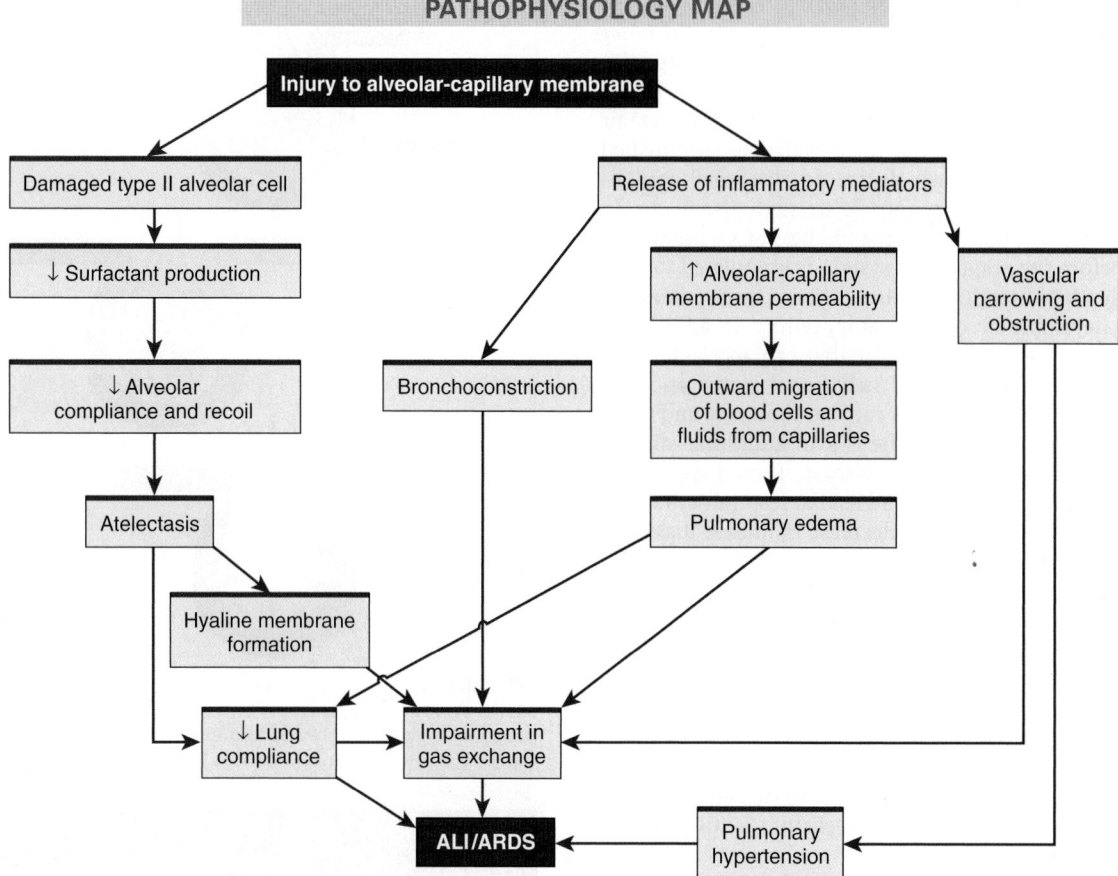

FIG. 68-10 Pathophysiology of acute lung injury *(ALI)* and acute respiratory distress syndrome *(ARDS)*.

multiple organ dysfunction syndrome (MODS). MODS results from organ system dysfunction that progressively increases in severity and ultimately results in multisystem organ failure. (Chapter 67 discusses SIRS and MODS.)

An exact cause for the damage to the alveolar-capillary interface is not known, but it is thought to be caused by stimulation of the inflammatory and immune systems, which causes an attraction of neutrophils to the pulmonary interstitium. The neutrophils release biochemical, humoral, and cellular mediators that produce changes in the lung. These include increased pulmonary capillary membrane permeability, destruction of elastin and collagen, formation of pulmonary microemboli, and pulmonary artery vasoconstriction[41,42] (see Fig. 68-10). (Chapters 12 and 14 discuss these mediators.)

The pathophysiologic changes in ARDS are divided into three phases: (1) injury or exudative phase, (2) reparative or proliferative phase, and (3) fibrotic phase.

Injury or Exudative Phase. The *injury or exudative phase* occurs approximately 1 to 7 days (usually 24 to 48 hours) after the initial direct lung injury or host insult. Initially, engorgement of the peribronchial and perivascular interstitial space produces interstitial edema. Next, fluid from the interstitial space crosses the alveolar membrane and enters the alveolar space. Intrapulmonary shunt develops because the alveoli fill with fluid, and blood passing through them cannot be oxygenated (see Figs. 68-4 and 68-9).

Alveolar type I and II cells (which produce surfactant) are damaged by the changes caused by ARDS. This damage, in addition to further fluid and protein accumulation, results in sur-

factant dysfunction. The function of *surfactant* is to maintain alveolar stability by decreasing alveolar surface tension and preventing alveolar collapse. Decreased synthesis of surfactant and inactivation of existing surfactant cause the alveoli to become unstable and collapse *(atelectasis)*. Widespread atelectasis further decreases lung compliance, compromises gas exchange, and contributes to hypoxemia.

Also during this stage, necrotic cells, protein, and fibrin form hyaline membranes that line the alveoli. Hyaline membranes contribute to the development of fibrosis and atelectasis, leading to a decrease in gas exchange capability and lung compliance.

The primary pathophysiologic changes that describe the *injury or exudative phase* of ARDS are interstitial and alveolar edema (noncardiogenic pulmonary edema) and atelectasis. Severe V/Q mismatch and shunting of pulmonary capillary blood result in hypoxemia unresponsive to increasing concentrations of O_2 (termed refractory hypoxemia). Diffusion limitation, caused by hyaline membrane formation, worsens the hypoxemia. As the lungs become less compliant because of decreased surfactant, pulmonary edema, and atelectasis, the patient must generate higher airway pressures to inflate "stiff" lungs. Reduced lung compliance greatly increases the patient's WOB. During ventilator management at this stage, increasing inspiratory and plateau pressures may be needed to deliver a controlled ventilation because of worsening lung compliance.[41-43]

Hypoxemia and the stimulation of juxtacapillary receptors in the stiff lung parenchyma *(J reflex)* initially cause an increase in respiratory rate and a decrease in tidal volume. This breathing pattern increases CO_2 removal, producing respiratory alkalosis. CO increases in response to hypoxemia, a compensatory effort to increase pulmonary blood flow. However, as atelectasis, pulmonary edema, and pulmonary shunt increase, compensation fails, and hypoventilation, decreased CO, and decreased tissue O_2 perfusion eventually occur.

Reparative or Proliferative Phase. The *reparative or proliferative phase* of ARDS begins 1 to 2 weeks after the initial lung injury. During this phase, there is an influx of neutrophils, monocytes, and lymphocytes and fibroblast proliferation as part of the inflammatory response. The proliferative phase is complete when the diseased lung is characterized by dense, fibrous tissue. Increased pulmonary vascular resistance and pulmonary hypertension may occur in this stage because fibroblasts and inflammatory cells destroy the pulmonary vasculature. Lung compliance continues to decrease as a result of interstitial fibrosis. Hypoxemia worsens because of the thickened alveolar membrane, causing diffusion limitation and shunting. If the reparative phase persists, widespread fibrosis results. If the reparative phase is stopped, the lesions will resolve.

Fibrotic Phase. The *fibrotic phase* of ARDS occurs approximately 2 to 3 weeks after the initial lung injury. This phase is also called the *chronic* or *late phase* of ARDS. By this time, the lung is completely remodeled by collagenous and fibrous tissues. The diffuse scarring and fibrosis result in decreased lung compliance. In addition, the surface area for gas exchange is significantly reduced because the interstitium is fibrotic, and therefore hypoxemia continues. Pulmonary hypertension results from pulmonary vascular destruction and fibrosis.

Clinical Progression

Progression of ARDS varies among patients. Some survive the acute phase of lung injury. Pulmonary edema resolves, and complete recovery occurs in a few days. The chance for survival is poor in those who enter the fibrotic (chronic or late) stage, which requires long-term mechanical ventilation. It is not known why injured lungs repair and recover in some patients, and in others ARDS progresses. Several factors seem to be important in determining the course of ARDS, including the nature of the initial injury, extent and severity of coexisting diseases, and pulmonary complications (e.g., pneumothorax, O_2 toxicity).

Clinical Manifestations and Diagnostic Studies

The initial presentation of ARDS is often subtle. At the time of the initial injury, and for several hours to 1 or 2 days afterward, the patient may not experience respiratory symptoms or may exhibit only dyspnea, tachypnea, cough, and restlessness. Chest auscultation may be normal or reveal fine, scattered crackles. ABGs usually indicate mild hypoxemia and respiratory alkalosis caused by hyperventilation. (Table 68-6 presents the findings that support a diagnosis of ALI and ARDS.) Respiratory alkalosis results from hypoxemia and the stimulation of juxtacapillary receptors. The chest x-ray may be normal or reveal minimal scattered interstitial infiltrates. Edema may not show on the x-ray until there is a 30% increase in fluid content in the lung.

As ARDS progresses, symptoms worsen because of increased fluid accumulation and decreased lung compliance. Respiratory distress becomes evident as WOB increases. Tachypnea and intercostal and suprasternal retractions may be present. Pulmonary function tests in ARDS reveal decreases in compliance,

TABLE 68-6	DIAGNOSTIC FINDINGS IN ALI AND ARDS

Refractory Hypoxemia
Acute lung injury: PaO_2/FIO_2 ratio between 200-300
Acute respiratory distress syndrome: PaO_2/FIO_2 ratio <200

Chest X-Ray
New bilateral interstitial and alveolar infiltrates

Pulmonary Artery Wedge Pressure
≤18 mm Hg or no clinical evidence of heart failure

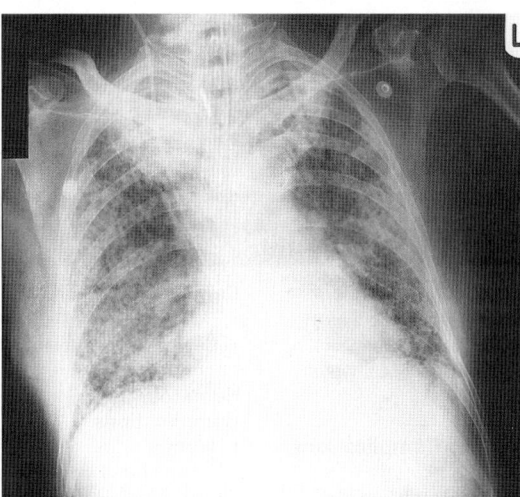

FIG. 68-11 Chest x-ray of a patient with acute respiratory distress syndrome (ARDS). The x-ray shows new, bilateral, diffuse, homogeneous pulmonary infiltrates without cardiac failure, fluid overload, chest infection, or chronic lung disease.

lung volumes, and *functional residual capacity* (FRC, the amount of air remaining in the lungs at the end of normal expiration). Tachycardia, diaphoresis, changes in mental status, cyanosis, and pallor may be present. Chest auscultation usually reveals scattered to diffuse crackles and rhonchi. The chest x-ray shows diffuse and extensive bilateral interstitial and alveolar infiltrates. A central venous or PA catheter may be inserted. PA wedge pressure does not increase in ARDS because the cause is noncardiogenic (not related to the heart).

Hypoxemia despite increased FIO_2 by mask, cannula, or endotracheal tube is a hallmark of ARDS. ABGs may initially demonstrate a normal or decreased $PaCO_2$ despite severe dyspnea and hypoxemia. Hypercapnia signifies that respiratory muscle fatigue and hypoventilation are occurring, interfering with optimum gas exchange.

As ARDS progresses, it is associated with profound respiratory distress requiring endotracheal intubation and PPV. The chest x-ray is often termed *whiteout* or *white lung* because consolidation and infiltrates are widespread throughout the lungs, leaving few recognizable air spaces (Fig. 68-11). Pleural effusions may also be present. Severe hypoxemia, hypercapnia, metabolic acidosis, and manifestations of target organ dysfunction may develop if therapy is not promptly started.

Complications

Complications may develop as a result of ARDS itself or its treatment. (Table 68-7 lists the common complications of

ARDS.) The major cause of death in ARDS is MODS, often accompanied by sepsis. The vital organs most commonly involved are the kidneys, liver, and heart. The organ systems most often involved are the CNS, hematologic system, and GI system.

Ventilator-Associated Pneumonia. A frequent complication of ARDS is ventilator-associated pneumonia (VAP), occurring in as many as 68% of patients with ARDS. Risk factors include impaired host defenses, contaminated equipment, invasive monitoring devices, aspiration of GI contents (especially in patients receiving enteral feedings), and prolonged mechanical ventilation. Strategies to prevent VAP include strict infection control measures (e.g., strict hand washing, sterile technique during endotracheal suctioning, frequent mouth care and oral hygiene) and a ventilator bundle protocol[44-48] (Table 68-8). (Chapter 28 discusses pneumonia, and Chapter 66 discusses VAP.)

Barotrauma. *Barotrauma* may result from rupture of overdistended alveoli during mechanical ventilation. The high peak airway pressures required may predispose patients with ARDS to this complication. Barotrauma results in alveolar air reaching locations where it is not usually found. This can lead to pulmonary interstitial emphysema, pneumothorax, subcutaneous emphysema, pneumoperitoneum, pneumomediastinum, pneumopericardium, and tension pneumothorax.[49] (Chapter 28 discusses pneumothorax.)

To avoid barotrauma and minimize the risk associated with elevated plateau and peak inspiratory pressures, the patient with ARDS is often ventilated with smaller tidal volumes (e.g., 6 mL/kg) and varying amounts of positive end-expiratory pressure (PEEP) to minimize O_2 requirements and intrathoracic pressures. This approach, called the Acute Respiratory Distress Syndrome Clinical Network (ARDSNet) protocol, reduces mortality rate and the number of ventilator days for these patients. One result of this protocol is an elevation in $PaCO_2$. This is termed *permissive hypercapnia* because the $PaCO_2$ is allowed to rise above normal limits. It is generally well tolerated as long as the rise in $PaCO_2$ is gradual to allow systemic and brain circulation to compensate, the pH is 7.2 or higher, and the patient does not have preexisting ICP elevation.[49-51]

TABLE 68-7 COMPLICATIONS ASSOCIATED WITH ARDS

Infection
- Catheter-related infection (e.g., central and peripheral IV catheters, urinary catheters)
- Sepsis

Respiratory Complications
- O_2 toxicity
- Pulmonary barotrauma (e.g., pneumothorax, pneumomediastinum, subcutaneous emphysema)
- Pulmonary emboli
- Pulmonary fibrosis
- Ventilator-associated pneumonia

Gastrointestinal Complications
- Paralytic ileus
- Pneumoperitoneum
- Stress ulceration and hemorrhage
- Hypermetabolic state, dramatically increased nutrition requirements

Renal Complications
- Acute kidney injury

Cardiac Complications
- Dysrhythmias
- Decreased cardiac output

Hematologic Complications
- Anemia
- Disseminated intravascular coagulation
- Thrombocytopenia
- Venous thromboembolism

Endotracheal Tube Complications
- Laryngeal ulceration
- Tracheal malacia
- Tracheal stenosis
- Tracheal ulceration

Central Nervous System and Psychologic Complications
- Delirium
- Sleep deprivation
- Posttraumatic stress disorder

TABLE 68-8 COMPONENTS OF A VENTILATOR BUNDLE

- Elevation of head of the bed 30 to 45 degrees
- Daily "sedation holidays" and assessment of readiness for extubation (see Chapter 66)
- Peptic ulcer disease prophylaxis (see Chapter 42)
- Venous thromboembolism prophylaxis (see Chapter 38)
- Daily oral care with chlorhexidine (0.12%) solution (see Table 66-9)

Source: Institute for Healthcare Improvement: Implement the IHI ventilator bundle. Retrieved from *www.ihi.org/knowledge/Pages/Changes/ImplementtheVentilator Bundle.aspx.*

EVIDENCE-BASED PRACTICE

Translating Research Into Practice

How Effective Is Subglottic Secretion Drainage on Ventilator-Associated Pneumonia?

Clinical Question
In critically ill patients on mechanical ventilation (P), how effective is subglottic secretion drainage (I) on the incidence of ventilator-associated pneumonia (VAP) and length of stay (O)?

Best Available Evidence
- Systematic review and meta-analysis of randomized controlled trials (RCTs)

Critical Appraisal and Synthesis of Evidence
- Sixteen RCTs (*n* = 1709) of critically ill intubated patients receiving intermittent or continuous subglottic secretion drainage. Outcomes were VAP rate, intubation duration, length of ICU and hospital stay, and mortality.
- Subglottic secretions pool immediately above the endotracheal tube cuff.
- Subglottic drainage decreased VAP incidence by 52% and shortened duration on mechanical ventilation by 2 days. Earlier extubation may be related to the 3-day decrease in patient length of ICU stay.
- Subglottic drainage did not affect length of hospital stay or mortality rate.

Conclusion
- Draining subglottic secretions has many positive patient outcomes, including decreased VAP incidence.

Implications for Nursing Practice
- Consult with health care team members regarding the importance of subglottic drainage for patients on mechanical ventilation.

Reference for Evidence
Leasure R, Stirlen J, Lu S: Prevention of ventilator-associated pneumonia through aspiration of subglottic secretions: a systematic review and meta-analysis, *Dimens Crit Care Nurs* 31:102, 2012.

P, Patient population of interest; *I,* intervention or area of interest; *O,* outcomes of interest (see p. 12).

Volutrauma. *Volutrauma* occurs in patients with ARDS or other clinical states requiring mechanical ventilation and large tidal volumes (e.g., 10 to 15 mL/kg) to ventilate noncompliant lungs. Volutrauma results in *alveolar fractures* (damage or tears in the alveoli) and movement of fluids and proteins into the alveolar spaces. To limit this complication, smaller tidal volumes or pressure-control ventilation is recommended in patients with ARDS (see Chapter 66).

Stress Ulcers. Critically ill patients with acute respiratory failure are at high risk for stress ulcers. Bleeding from stress ulcers occurs in 30% of patients with ARDS who require PPV, a higher incidence than other causes of acute respiratory failure. Management strategies include correction of predisposing conditions such as hypotension, shock, and acidosis. Prophylactic management includes antiulcer agents such as proton pump inhibitors (e.g., pantoprazole [Protonix]), and mucosal-protecting agents (e.g., sucralfate [Carafate]). Early initiation of enteral nutrition also helps prevent mucosal damage (see Chapters 40 and 66).

Renal Failure. Renal failure can occur from decreased renal tissue oxygenation because of hypotension, hypoxemia, or hypercapnia. Renal failure may also result from the administration of nephrotoxic drugs (e.g., vancomycin [Vancocin]) used to treat ARDS-related infections.

NURSING AND COLLABORATIVE MANAGEMENT ACUTE RESPIRATORY DISTRESS SYNDROME

The collaborative care for acute respiratory failure (see Table 68-4) and the nursing care plan for acute respiratory failure (eNursing Care Plan 68-1, available on the website for this chapter) apply to patients with ARDS. The following section discusses additional collaborative care measures for the patient with ARDS (Table 68-9).

TABLE 68-9 COLLABORATIVE CARE

Acute Respiratory Distress Syndrome

Diagnostic
See Table 68-6

Collaborative Therapy
Respiratory Therapy
- O_2 administration
- Lateral rotation therapy
- Positive pressure ventilation with PEEP
- Prone positioning
- Permissive hypercapnia
- Alternative modes of mechanical ventilation: pressure-control inverse ratio ventilation, airway pressure release ventilation, high-frequency ventilation (see Chapter 66)

Supportive Therapy
- Identification and treatment of underlying cause
- Hemodynamic monitoring
- Inotropic and vasopressor medications
  - dopamine (Intropin)
  - dobutamine (Dobutrex)
  - norepinephrine (Levophed)
- Diuretics
- IV fluid administration
- Sedation/analgesia
- Neuromuscular blockade

PEEP, Positive end-expiratory pressure.

NURSING ASSESSMENT

Because ARDS causes acute respiratory failure, the subjective and objective data that you should obtain from someone with ARDS are the same as those for acute respiratory failure (see Table 68-3).

NURSING DIAGNOSES

Nursing diagnoses for the patient with ARDS may include, but are not limited to, those described for acute respiratory failure (see p. 1660).

PLANNING

Patients with ARDS are cared for in critical care units. With appropriate therapy, the overall goals include a PaO_2 of 60 mm Hg or higher and adequate lung ventilation to maintain normal pH. The goals for a patient recovering from ARDS include (1) PaO_2 within normal limits for age or baseline values on room air, (2) SaO_2 greater than 90%, (3) patent airway, and (4) clear lungs on auscultation.

OXYGEN ADMINISTRATION. The primary goal of O_2 therapy is to correct hypoxemia. O_2 administered via a face mask or nasal cannula is inadequate to treat refractory hypoxemia that is associated with ARDS. Initially use masks with high-flow systems that deliver higher O_2 concentrations to maximize O_2 delivery. Continuously monitor SpO_2 to assess the effectiveness of O_2 therapy. The general standard for O_2 administration is to give the patient the lowest concentration that results in a PaO_2 greater than 60 mm Hg. The patient's risk for O_2 toxicity increases when the FIO_2 exceeds 60% for more than 48 hours. Patients with ARDS need intubation with mechanical ventilation to maintain the PaO_2 at acceptable levels.

POSITIVE PRESSURE VENTILATION. Endotracheal intubation and PPV provide additional respiratory support. However, even with these interventions it may be necessary to maintain the FIO_2 at 60% or higher to maintain a PaO_2 of at least 60 mm Hg. During PPV, it is common to apply PEEP at 5 cm H_2O to compensate for loss of glottic function caused by the endotracheal tube. In patients with ARDS, higher levels of PEEP (e.g., 10 to 20 cm H_2O) may be used. PEEP increases FRC and opens up collapsed alveoli. PEEP is typically applied in 3 to 5 cm H_2O increments until oxygenation is adequate with FIO_2 less than or equal to 60%. PEEP may improve V/Q in respiratory units that collapse at low airway pressures, thus allowing the FIO_2 to be lowered.

However, PEEP is not a benign therapy. The additional intrathoracic and intrapulmonic pressures can compromise venous return to the right side of the heart, thereby decreasing preload, CO, and BP. High levels of PEEP cause hyperinflation of the alveoli, compression of the pulmonary capillary bed, reduction in blood return to the left side of the heart, and a dramatic reduction in BP. In addition, high levels of PEEP or excessive inspiratory pressures can result in barotrauma and volutrauma.

If hypoxemic respiratory failure persists in spite of high levels of PEEP, alternative modes and therapies may be used. These include airway pressure release ventilation, pressure-control inverse ratio ventilation, high-frequency ventilation, and permissive hypercapnia (low tidal volumes that allow $PaCO_2$ to increase slowly).[49-51] (Chapter 66 provides additional information on mechanical ventilation and PEEP.)

Extracorporeal membrane oxygenation (ECMO) and extracorporeal CO_2 removal (ECCO$_2$R) pass blood across a gas-exchanging membrane outside the body and then return oxygenated blood back to the body. ECCO₂R with PPV allows the lungs to heal while the lungs are not functional.[52,53]

Positioning Strategies. Some patients with ARDS have a marked improvement in PaO₂ when turned from the supine to the prone position (e.g., PaO₂ 70 mm Hg supine, PaO₂ 90 mm Hg prone) with no change in FIO₂[54] (Fig. 68-12). The response may be sufficient to allow a reduction in FIO₂ or PEEP.

In the early phases of ARDS, fluid moves freely throughout the lung. Because of gravity, this fluid pools in dependent regions of the lung. As a result, some alveoli are fluid filled (dependent areas), whereas others are air filled (nondependent areas). In addition, when the patient is supine, the heart and mediastinal contents place more pressure on the lungs than in the prone position. Thus the supine position changes pleural pressure and predisposes the patient to atelectasis. If you turn the patient from supine to prone, air-filled, nonatelectatic alveoli in the ventral (anterior) portion of the lung become dependent. Perfusion may be better matched to ventilation. Not all patients respond to prone positioning with an increase in PaO₂, and there is no reliable way of predicting who will respond. Prone positioning may be considered for patients with refractory hypoxemia who do not respond to other strategies to increase PaO₂.[54]

Other positioning strategies to consider for patients with ARDS include continuous lateral rotation therapy (CLRT) and kinetic therapy. CLRT provides continuous, slow, side-to-side turning of the patient by rotating the actual bed frame less than 40 degrees. The bed's lateral movement is maintained for 18 of

every 24 hours to simulate postural drainage and to help mobilize pulmonary secretions. In addition, the bed may also contain a vibrator pack that provides chest physiotherapy. This feature assists with secretion mobilization and removal (Fig. 68-13). Kinetic therapy is similar to CLRT in that patients are rotated side-to-side 40 degrees or more. It is important to obtain baseline assessments of the patient's pulmonary status (e.g., respiratory rate and rhythm, breath sounds, ABGs, SpO₂) and continue to monitor the patient throughout the therapy.

MEDICAL SUPPORTIVE THERAPY

MAINTENANCE OF CARDIAC OUTPUT AND TISSUE PERFUSION. Patients on PPV and PEEP frequently experience decreased CO. One cause is decreased venous return from the PEEP-induced increase in intrathoracic pressure. Impaired contractility and decreased preload can also decrease CO. Hemodynamic monitoring (e.g., CVP, CO, ScvO₂, SvO₂) via central venous or pulmonary artery pressure, or arterial pressure-based CO monitoring, is essential. This allows you to see trends, detect changes, and adjust therapy as needed. An arterial catheter also provides continuous monitoring of BP and sampling of blood for ABGs. If the CO falls, it may be necessary to administer crystalloid fluids or colloid solutions or to lower PEEP. Use of inotropic drugs such as dobutamine (Dobutrex) or dopamine (Intropin) may also be necessary. (Chapter 66 discusses hemodynamic monitoring in detail.)

Packed red blood cells are used to increase hemoglobin and thus the O₂-carrying capacity of the blood. The hemoglobin level is usually kept around 9 to 10 g/dL (90 to 100 g/L) with an SpO₂ of 90% or more (when PaO₂ is greater than 60 mm Hg).

MAINTENANCE OF NUTRITION AND FLUID BALANCE. Maintenance of nutrition and fluid balance is challenging in the patient with ARDS. Consult with a dietitian to determine optimal caloric needs. Enteral or parenteral feedings are started to meet the high energy requirements of these patients. Enteral formulas enriched with omega-3 fatty acids may improve the clinical outcomes of patients with ARDS.[5]

Increasing pulmonary capillary permeability results in fluid in the lungs and causes pulmonary edema. At the same time, the patient may be volume depleted and thus at risk for hypo-

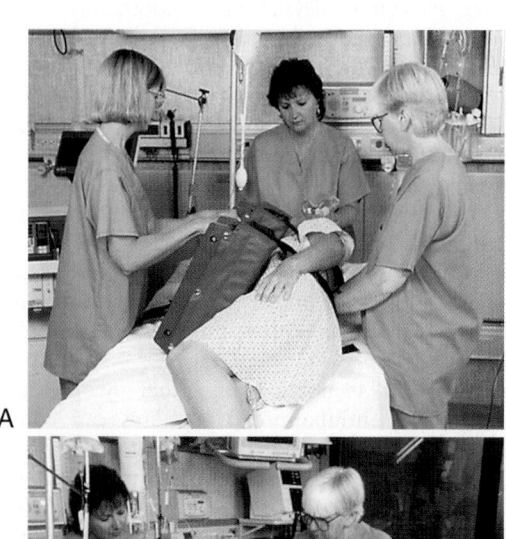

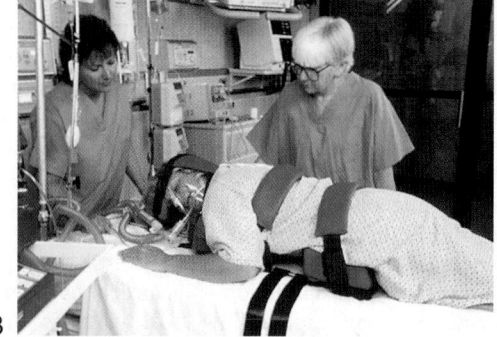

FIG. 68-12 A, Turning patient prone on Vollman Prone Positioner. **B,** Patient lying prone on Vollman Prone Positioner. (©2006 Hill-Rom Services, Inc. Reprinted with permission. All rights reserved.)

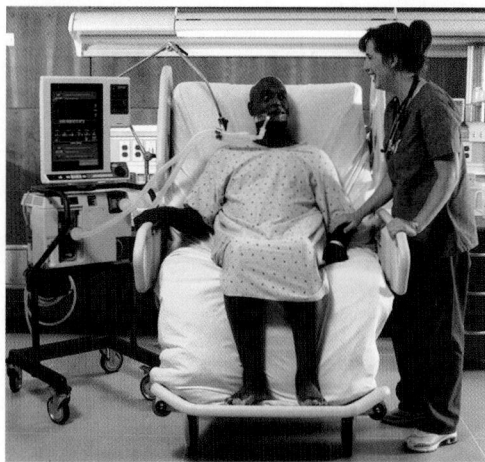

FIG. 68-13 TotalCare SpO2RT Bed System offers continuous lateral rotation therapy and percussion and vibration therapies. Patients can easily and quickly be repositioned. (©2006 Hill-Rom Services, Inc. Reprinted with permission. All rights reserved.)

tension and decreased CO from mechanical ventilation and PEEP. Monitor hemodynamic parameters (e.g., CVP, stroke volume variation), daily weights, and intake and output to assess the patient's fluid status. Controversy exists as to the benefits of fluid replacement with crystalloids versus colloids. Critics of colloid replacement believe that proteins in colloids may leak into the pulmonary interstitium, increasing the movement of fluid into the alveoli. Advocates of colloid replacement believe that colloids help keep fluid from leaking into the alveoli. The patient is often placed on fluid restriction, and diuretics are used as necessary.

EVALUATION

The expected outcomes for the patient with ARDS are similar to those for a patient with acute respiratory failure (see p. 1664).

CASE STUDY

Acute Respiratory Distress Syndrome

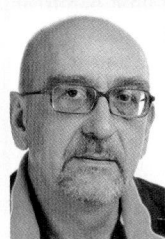

Patient Profile

J.N. is a 55-yr-old white man who was admitted 12 hr ago to a surgical ICU after emergent surgery for an acutely ischemic bowel.

Past Medical History

- Lumbar spine surgery 5 yr ago
- Chronic back pain controlled with oxycodone (Oxy-Contin) 15 mg PO tid

The surgical procedure involved extensive abdominal surgery to repair a perforated colon, irrigate the abdominal cavity, and provide hemostasis. During surgery his systolic BP dropped to 70 mm Hg. Seven units of packed red blood cells and 4 L of 0.9% saline were infused. He is receiving 60% O_2 via an aerosol face mask.

iStockphoto/Thinkstock

Postoperative Orders

- Continuous ECG and pulse oximetry monitoring
- Infuse 0.9% saline at 125 mL/hr via a central venous IV catheter
- Monitor hourly urine output via indwelling bladder catheter
- Pain management via a continuous IV infusion of morphine

J.N.'s pulmonary status worsens. He needs progressively higher FIO_2. Emergent endotracheal intubation and mechanical ventilation are needed. Sedation, analgesia, and neuromuscular blockade are started to achieve anxiolysis, pain control, and ventilator synchrony. Postintubation chest x-ray reveals a pneumothorax, requiring the emergent placement of a chest tube. Immediately after chest tube placement, his O_2 saturation decreased significantly below baseline to 80%-82%. No significant changes were evident in ventilation or lung compliance, and he remained synchronous with mechanical ventilation. ABGs showed $PaCO_2$ increased to 52 mm Hg and PaO_2 decreased to 44 mm Hg. J.N. was tachycardic during and immediately after chest tube insertion. A 10-mg bolus of morphine is given followed by an increase in the continuous infusion. After 30 min, his O_2 saturation improved to 90%-91% and ABGs showed improved oxygenation (PaO_2 63 mm Hg) and ventilation ($PaCO_2$ 45 mm Hg).

Postoperative Day 1

J.N.'s lung function continues to worsen and his hypoxemia is refractory to 100% FIO_2 and high levels of PEEP. He experiences kidney and liver failure. There is little hope of weaning him from mechanical ventilation. He has an advance directive that indicates he does not want to be kept alive by artificial means.

Subjective Data

- Patient is sedated and paralyzed. Unable to communicate.
- His wife and two adult children are at the bedside and voicing concerns and questions regarding his progress.

Objective Data
Physical Assessment

- *General:* Sedated, paralyzed, well-nourished man; head of bed elevated 45 degrees; skin cool with moderate diaphoresis

- *Respiratory:* No accessory muscle use, retractions, or paradoxic breathing; respiratory rate 18 breaths/min and in phase with ventilator; SpO_2 85%; fine crackles at lung bases
- *Cardiovascular:* BP 100/60 mm Hg
- ECG as follows:

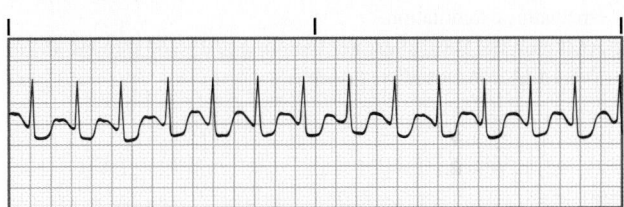

- Equal apical-radial pulse; weak peripheral pulses; temperature 101° F (38.3° C) rectally
- *Gastrointestinal:* Surgical dressing dry and intact; colostomy draining serosanguineous drainage
- *Urologic:* Indwelling bladder catheter draining concentrated urine less than 30 mL/hr

Diagnostic Findings

- ABGs: pH 7.15, PaO_2 59 mm Hg, $PaCO_2$ 57 mm Hg, HCO_3 16 mEq/L, O_2 saturation 86%
- PaO_2/FIO_2 ratio <200
- Chest x-ray: new bilateral, scattered interstitial infiltrates compatible with an ARDS pattern as interpreted by the radiologist

Discussion Questions

1. How does the pathophysiology of ARDS predispose the patient to refractory hypoxemia?
2. What clinical manifestations does J.N. exhibit that support a diagnosis of ARDS?
3. What are the possible causes of ARDS in J.N.?
4. What are the possible complications that J.N. is at risk for developing secondary to ARDS?
5. What are possible reasons for J.N.'s sudden decline in pulmonary status during and immediately after chest tube insertion?
6. ***Evidence-Based Practice:*** You are orienting a new nurse who asks you why you offered J.N.'s family the opportunity to stay at the bedside while the chest tube was placed. How would you respond?
7. What are possible reasons for improved oxygenation and CO_2 levels after administration of additional opioid analgesia?
8. ***Priority Decision:*** What priority interventions should be implemented to improve J.N.'s respiratory status and hypoxemia?
9. ***Priority Decision:*** Based on the assessment data presented, what are the priority nursing diagnoses?
10. ***Delegation Decision:*** When developing the plan of care for J.N., what tasks can you delegate to unlicensed assistive personnel (UAP)?
11. What information should you provide to J.N.'s caregiver(s) given his decline in cardiopulmonary function?
12. Given the guidelines in the patient's advance directive, what ethical/legal issues might you encounter in this patient scenario?

BRIDGE TO NCLEX EXAMINATION

The number of the question corresponds to the same-numbered outcome at the beginning of the chapter.

1. Which signs and symptoms differentiate hypoxemic respiratory failure from hypercapnic respiratory failure *(select all that apply)*?
   a. Cyanosis
   b. Tachypnea
   c. Morning headache
   d. Paradoxic breathing
   e. Use of pursed-lip breathing

2. The O_2 delivery system chosen for the patient in acute respiratory failure should
   a. always be a low-flow device, such as a nasal cannula or face mask.
   b. administer continuous positive airway pressure ventilation to prevent CO_2 narcosis.
   c. correct the PaO_2 to a normal level as quickly as possible using mechanical ventilation.
   d. maintain the PaO_2 at greater than or equal to 60 mm Hg at the lowest O_2 concentration possible.

3. The most common early clinical manifestations of ARDS that the nurse may observe are
   a. dyspnea and tachypnea.
   b. cyanosis and apprehension.
   c. hypotension and tachycardia.
   d. respiratory distress and frothy sputum.

4. Maintenance of fluid balance in the patient with ARDS involves
   a. hydration using colloids.
   b. administration of surfactant.
   c. fluid restriction and diuretics as necessary.
   d. keeping the hemoglobin at levels above 9 g/dL (90 g/L).

5. Which intervention is most likely to prevent or limit barotrauma in the patient with ARDS who is mechanically ventilated?
   a. Decreasing PEEP
   b. Increasing the tidal volume
   c. Use of permissive hypercapnia
   d. Use of positive pressure ventilation

1. a, b, d, 2. d, 3. a, 4. c, 5. c

ℰvolve

For rationales to these answers and even more NCLEX review questions, visit *http://evolve.elsevier.com/Lewis/medsurg*.

REFERENCES

1. Kaynar AM: Respiratory failure. Retrieved from *http://emedicine.medscape.com/article/167981-overview*.
2. Myers TR, Tomasio L: Asthma: 2015 and beyond, *Respir Care* 56:1389, 2011.
3. Nee PA, Al-Jubouri MA, Gray AJ, et al: Critical care in the emergency department: acute respiratory failure, *Emerg Med J* 28:94, 2011.
4. Byrd RP: Respiratory acidosis. Retrieved from *http://emedicine.medscape.com/article/301574-overview*.
5. Harman EH: Acute respiratory distress syndrome. Retrieved from *http://emedicine.medscape.com/article/165139-overview*.
6. Morris MJ: Asthma. Retrieved from *http://emedicine.medscape.com/article/296301-overview*.
7. Jackson DJ, Sykes A, Mallia P, et al: Asthma exacerbations: origin, effect and prevention, *J Allergy Clin Immunol* 128:1165, 2011.
8. Evensen AE: Management of COPD exacerbations, *Am Fam Physician* 81:607, 2010.
9. Abbatecola AM, Fumagalli A, Bonardi D, et al: Practical management problems of chronic obstructive pulmonary disease in the elderly: acute exacerbations, *Curr Opin Pulm Med* 17(Suppl 1):S49, 2011.
10. Patel SB, Kress JP: Sedation and analgesia in the mechanically ventilated patient, *Am J Respir Crit Care Med* 185:486, 2012.
11. Ouellette DR: Pulmonary embolism. Retrieved from *http://emedicine.medscape.com/article/300901-overview*.
12. Cortes I, Penuelas O, Esteban A: Acute respiratory distress syndrome: evaluation and management, *Minerva Anesthesiol* 78:343, 2012.
13. Demirijian BJ: Emphysema. Retrieved from *http://emedicine.medscape.com/article/298283-overview*.
14. Hemprich U, Papadakos PJ, Lachmann B: Respiratory failure and hypoxemia in the cirrhotic patient including hepatopulmonary syndrome, *Curr Opin Anaesthesiol* 23:133, 2010.
15. Racca F, Del Sorbo L, Mongini T, et al: Respiratory management of acute respiratory failure in neuromuscular diseases, *Minerva Anesthesiol* 76:51, 2010.
16. Mokhlesi B: Obesity hypoventilation syndrome: a state-of-the-art review, *Respir Care* 55:1347, 2010.
17. Fayyaz J: Hypoventilation syndromes. Retrieved from *http://emedicine.medscape.com/article/304381-overview*.
18. Tzani P, Aiello M, Elia D, et al: Dynamic hyperinflation is associated with a poor cardiovascular response to exercise in COPD patients, *Respir Res* 12:150, 2011.
19. Ortiz JR, Neuzil KM, Victor JC, et al: Influenza-associated cystic fibrosis pulmonary exacerbations, *Chest* 137:852, 2010.
20. Zemanick ET, Harris JK, Conway S, et al: Measuring and improving respiratory outcomes in cystic fibrosis lung disease: opportunities and challenges to therapy, *J Cystic Fibrosis* 9:1, 2010.
21. Brulotte CA, Lang ES: Acute exacerbations of chronic obstructive pulmonary disease in the emergency department, *Emerg Med Clin North Am* 30:223, 2012.
22. Boldrini R, Fasano L, Nava S: Noninvasive mechanical ventilation, *Curr Opin Crit Care* 18:48, 2012.
23. Restrepo RD, Hirst KR, Wittnebel L, et al: AARC clinical practice guideline: transcutaneous monitoring of carbon dioxide, *Respir Care* 57:1955, 2012.
24. Boerrigter B, Trip P, Bogaard HJ, et al: Right atrial pressure affects the interaction between lung mechanics and right ventricular function in spontaneously breathing COPD patients. Retrieved from *http://www.ncbi.nlm.nih.gov/pmc/articles/PMC3260236/pdf/pone.0030208.pdf*.
25. Russell R, Anzueto A, Weisman I: Optimizing management of chronic obstructive pulmonary disease in the upcoming decade, *Int J COPD* 6:47, 2011.
26. Donahoe M: Acute respiratory distress syndrome: a clinical review, *Pulm Circ* 1:192, 2011.

*27. Keenan SP, Sinuff T, Burns KEA, et al: Clinical practice guidelines for the use of noninvasive positive-pressure ventilation and noninvasive positive airway pressure in the acute care setting, *Can Med Assoc J* 183:E195, 2011.

28. Gursel G, Aydogdu M, Tasyurek G, et al: Factors associated with noninvasive ventilation response in the first day of therapy in patients with hypercapnic respiratory failure, *Ann Thorac Med* 7:92, 2012.

29. Brown LK: Hypoventilation syndromes, *Clin Chest Med* 31:249, 2010.

30. Antonelli M, Azoulay E, Bonten M, et al: Year in review in intensive care medicine 2010, Part III: ARDS and ALI, mechanical ventilation, noninvasive ventilation, weaning, endotracheal intubation, lung ultrasound and paediatrics, *Intens Care Med* 37:394, 2011.

31. Schortgen F, Follin A, Piccari L, et al: Results of noninvasive ventilation in very old patients, *Ann Intens Med* 2:5, 2012.

32. Muir JF, Lamia B, Molano C, et al: Respiratory failure in the elderly patient, *Semin Respir Crit Care Med* 31:634, 2010.

33. Pomares X, Monton C, Espasa M, et al: Long-term azithromycin therapy in patients with severe COPD and repeated exacerbations, *Int J COPD* 6:449, 2011.

*34. DeGrado JR, Anger KE, Szumita PM, et al: Evaluation of a local ICU sedation guideline on goal-directed administration of sedatives and analgesics, *J Pain Res* 4:127, 2011.

*35. Devabhakthuni S: Analgosedation: a paradigm shift in intensive care unit sedation practice, *Ann Pharmacol* 46:530, 2012.

*36. Arbour R, Waterhouse J, Seckel MA, et al: Correlation between the sedation-agitation scale and the bispectral index in ventilated patients in the intensive care unit, *Heart Lung* 38:336, 2009.

37. Permpogkosol S: Iatrogenic disease in the elderly: risk factors, consequences and prevention, *Clin Interven Aging* 6:77, 2011.

*38. Cerejeira J, Mukaetova-Ladinski EB: A clinical update on delirium: from early recognition to effective management. Retrieved from *www.ncbi.nlm.nih.gov/pmc/articles/PMC3169311/pdf/NRP2011-875196.pdf*.

*39. Schreier AM: Nursing care, delirium and pain management for the hospitalized older adult, *Pain Manag Nurs* 11:177, 2010.

40. Villar J: What is the acute respiratory distress syndrome? *Respir Care* 56:1539, 2011.

41. Horlander KT: Imaging in acute respiratory distress syndrome. Retrieved from *http://emedicine.medscape.com/article/362571-overview*.

42. Raghavendran K, Napolitano LM: Definition of ALI/ARDS, *Crit Care Clin* 27:429, 2011.

43. Collins SR, Blank RS: Approaches to refractory hypoxemia in acute respiratory distress syndrome: current understanding, evidence and debate, *Respir Care* 56:1573, 2011.

*44. Crimlisk JT, Gustavson KA, Silva J: Translating guidelines into practice: ventilator-associated pneumonia prevention strategies in an acute rehabilitation unit, *Dimens Crit Care Nurs* 31:118, 2012.

*45. Morris AC, Hay AW, Swann DG, et al: Reducing ventilator-associated pneumonia in intensive care: impact of implementing a care bundle, *Crit Care Med* 39:2218, 2011.

*46. Sole ML, Penoyer DA, Bennett M, et al: Oropharyngeal secretion volume in intubated patients: the importance of oral suctioning, *Am J Crit Care* 20:e141, 2011.

47. Maselli DJ, Restrepo MI: Strategies in the prevention of ventilator-associated pneumonia, *Ther Adv Respir Dis* 5:131, 2011.

*48. Ames NJ: Evidence to support tooth brushing in critically ill patients, *Am J Crit Care* 20:242, 2011.

49. Soo Hoo GW: Barotrauma and mechanical ventilation. Retrieved from *http://emedicine.medscape.com/article/296625-overview*.

50. Hess DR: Approaches to conventional mechanical ventilation of the patient with acute respiratory distress syndrome, *Respir Care* 56:1555, 2011.

51. Pierrakos C, Karanikolas M, Scoletta S, et al: Acute respiratory distress syndrome: pathophysiology and therapeutic options, *J Clin Med Res* 4:7, 2012.

52. Raoof S, Goulet K, Esan A, et al: Severe hypoxemic respiratory failure, part 2: Nonventilatory strategies, *Chest* 137:1437, 2010.

53. Combes A, Bacchetta M, Brodie D, et al: Extracorporeal membrane oxygenation for respiratory failure in adults, *Curr Opin Crit Care* 18:99, 2012.

54. Dickinson S, Park PK, Napolitano LM: Prone-positioning therapy in ARDS, *Crit Care Clin* 27:511, 2011.

*Evidence-based information for clinical practice.

RESOURCES

Resources for this chapter are listed after Chapter 66 on p. 1630.

69

*One of the tests of leadership is the ability to
recognize a problem before it becomes an emergency.*
Arnold H. Glasow

Nursing Management

Emergency, Terrorism, and Disaster Nursing

Linda Bucher

℮volve WEBSITE

http://evolve.elsevier.com/Lewis/medsurg

- NCLEX Review Questions
- Key Points
- Pre-Test
- Answer Guidelines for Case Study on
  p. 1692

- Rationales for Bridge to NCLEX
  Examination Questions
- Case Study
  - Patient With Musculoskeletal Trauma
- Concept Map Creator
- Glossary
- Content Updates

eTables
- eTable 69-1: Trauma Verification Levels
- eTable 69-2: Biologic Agents of Terrorism
- eTable 69-3: Chemical Agents of
  Terrorism by Target Organ or Effect

LEARNING OUTCOMES

1. Apply the steps in triage, the primary survey, and the secondary survey to a patient experiencing a medical, surgical, or traumatic emergency.
2. Relate the pathophysiology to the assessment and collaborative care of select environmental emergencies (e.g., hyperthermia, hypothermia, submersion injury, bites).
3. Relate the pathophysiology to the assessment and collaborative care of select toxicologic emergencies.
4. Select appropriate nursing interventions for victims of violence.
5. Differentiate among the responsibilities of health care providers, the community, and select federal agencies in emergency and mass casualty incident preparedness.

KEY TERMS

emergency, p. 1691
family presence (FP), p. 1678
frostbite, p. 1684
heat cramps, p. 1682
heat exhaustion, p. 1682

heatstroke, p. 1683
hypothermia, p. 1684
jaw-thrust maneuver, p. 1677
mass casualty incident (MCI), p. 1691
primary survey, p. 1676

secondary survey, p. 1678
submersion injury, p. 1686
terrorism, p. 1690
triage, p. 1675

This chapter presents an overview of triage and care of emergency patients not addressed elsewhere in this book. Common emergency situations discussed include heat- and cold-related emergencies, submersion injuries, bites and stings, and various types of poisonings. The chapter concludes with a discussion of terrorism, followed by a description of a mass casualty incident, and the methods of responding to the incident.

The emergency management of various medical, surgical, and traumatic emergencies is discussed throughout the textbook. Tables summarize emergency management of specific problems. Table 69-1 lists each emergency management table by title, chapter number, and page.

Most patients with life-threatening or potentially life-threatening problems arrive at the hospital through the emergency department (ED). More patients report to the ED for less urgent conditions. Every year more than 136 million people visit EDs. This number is increasing for a variety of reasons, including (1) the inability to see a primary care provider, (2) an aging population, (3) shorter hospital stays resulting in frequent readmissions, (4) acute mental health crises, and (5) lack of health insurance (or a primary care provider). These factors, plus the increase in ED closures, result in chronic overcrowding and long wait times.[1,2]

Emergency nurses care for patients of all ages and with a variety of problems. However, some EDs specialize in certain

Reviewed by Janet E. Jackson, RN, MS, Assistant Professor, Department of Nursing, Bradley University, Peoria, Illinois; Lisa A. Webb, RN, MSN, CEN, Instructor of Nursing, Charleston Southern University, Charleston, South Carolina; and Amber Young, RN, MSN, Instructor of Nursing, Bellin College, School of Nursing, Green Bay, Wisconsin.

patient populations or conditions, such as pediatric ED or trauma ED. (See eTable 69-1 for the resources at various levels of trauma designated facilities.) The Emergency Nurses Association (ENA) is the specialty organization aimed at advancing emergency nursing practice. The ENA provides standards of care for nurses working in the ED, and a certification process that allows nurses to become certified emergency nurses (CENs).[3]

CARE OF EMERGENCY PATIENT

Recognition of life-threatening illness or injury is one of the most important goals of emergency nursing. Initiation of interventions to reverse or prevent a crisis is often a priority before a medical diagnosis is made. This process begins with your first contact with a patient. Prompt identification of patients requiring immediate treatment and determination of appropriate interventions are essential nurse competencies.

Triage

Triage, a French word meaning "to sort," refers to the process of rapidly determining patient acuity. It is one of the most important assessment skills needed by emergency nurses.[4,5] Most often, you will confront multiple patients who have a variety of problems. The triage process works on the premise that patients who have a threat to life must be treated before other patients.

A *triage system* identifies and categorizes patients so that the most critical are treated first. The ENA and American College of Emergency Physicians support the use of a five-level triage system.[6] The *Emergency Severity Index* (ESI) is a five-level triage system that incorporates concepts of illness severity and resource utilization (e.g., electrocardiogram [ECG], laboratory work, radiology studies, IV fluids) to determine who should be treated first[5] (Table 69-2). The ESI includes a triage algorithm that directs you to assign an ESI level to patients coming into the ED. (The triage algorithm can be found in the ESI Implementation Handbook available at *www.ahrq.gov/research/esi.*) Initially, assess the patient for any threats to life (ESI-1) (e.g., Is the patient dying?) or presence of a high-risk situation (ESI-2)

✚ TABLE 69-1 EMERGENCY MANAGEMENT

Emergency Management Tables

Title	Chapter	Page
Abdominal Trauma	43	973
Acute Abdominal Pain	43	971
Acute Soft Tissue Injury	63	1507
Anaphylactic Shock	14	214
Chemical Burns	25	457
Chest Pain	34	750
Chest Trauma	28	541
Cocaine and Amphetamine Toxicity	11	164
Depressant Drug Overdose	11	164
Diabetic Ketoacidosis	49	1177
Dysrhythmias	36	793
Electrical Burns	25	456
Eye Injury	22	390
Fractured Extremity	63	1518
Head Injury	57	1372
Hyperthermia	69	1683
Hypothermia	69	1685
Inhalation Injury	25	456
Sexual Assault	54	1302
Shock	67	1641
Spinal Cord Injury	61	1474
Stroke	58	1398
Submersion Injuries	69	1687
Thermal Burns	25	455
Thoracic Injuries	28	542
Tonic-Clonic Seizures	59	1423

TABLE 69-2 FIVE-LEVEL EMERGENCY SEVERITY INDEX (ESI)

Definition	Level				
	ESI-1	ESI-2	ESI-3	ESI-4	ESI-5
Stability of vital functions (ABCs)	Unstable	Threatened	Stable	Stable	Stable
Life threat or organ threat	Obvious	Likely but not always obvious	Unlikely but possible	No	No
How soon patient should be seen by physician	Immediately	Within 10 min	Up to 1 hr	Could be delayed	Could be delayed
Expected resource intensity	High resource intensity Staff at bedside continuously Often mobilization of team response	High resource intensity Multiple, often complex diagnostic studies Frequent consultation Continuous monitoring	Medium to high resource intensity Multiple diagnostic studies (e.g., multiple laboratory studies, x-rays) or brief observation Complex procedure (e.g., IV fluids, medications)	Low resource intensity One simple diagnostic study (e.g., x-ray) or simple procedure (e.g., sutures)	Low resource intensity Examination only
Examples	Cardiac arrest, intubated trauma patient, overdose with bradypnea, severe respiratory distress	Chest pain probably resulting from ischemia, multiple trauma unless responsive	Abdominal pain or gynecologic disorders unless in severe distress, hip fracture in older patient	Closed extremity trauma, simple laceration, cystitis	Cold symptoms, minor burn, recheck (e.g., wound), prescription refill

Modified and reprinted with permission. Copyright 1999, Richard C. Wuerz, MD, and David R. Eitel, MD.
ABCs, Airway, breathing, circulation.

TABLE 69-3 EMERGENCY ASSESSMENT: PRIMARY SURVEY

Assessment	Interventions
Airway With Simultaneous Cervical Spine Stabilization and/or Immobilization	
• Assess for respiratory distress. • Assess airway for patency. • Check for loose teeth or foreign bodies. • Assess for bleeding, vomitus, or edema.	• Open airway. • Use jaw-thrust maneuver. • Remove or suction any foreign bodies. • Insert oropharyngeal or nasopharyngeal airway, endotracheal tube, cricothyroidotomy. • Immobilize cervical spine using rigid cervical collar and cervical immobilization device. Secure forehead to backboard.
Breathing	
• Assess ventilation. • Scan chest for signs of breathing. • Look for paradoxic movement of the chest wall during inspiration and expiration. • Note use of accessory muscles or abdominal muscles. • Observe and count respiratory rate. • Note color of nail beds, mucous membranes, skin. • Auscultate lungs. • Assess for jugular venous distention and position of trachea.	• Give supplemental O_2 via appropriate delivery system (e.g., non-rebreather mask). • Ventilate with bag-valve-mask with 100% O_2 if respirations are inadequate or absent. • Prepare to intubate if severe respiratory distress (e.g., agonal breaths) or arrest. • Have suction available. • If absent breath sounds, prepare for needle thoracostomy and chest tube insertion.
Circulation	
• Check carotid or femoral pulse. • Palpate pulse for quality and rate. • Assess skin color, temperature, and moisture. • Check capillary refill. • Assess for external bleeding. • Measure blood pressure.	• If absent pulse, initiate cardiopulmonary resuscitation and advanced life-support measures. • If shock symptoms or hypotensive, start two large-bore (14- to 16-gauge) IVs and initiate infusions of normal saline or lactated Ringer's solution. • Control bleeding with direct pressure and pressure dressings, if appropriate. • Administer blood products if ordered. • Consider autotransfusion if isolated chest trauma. • Consider use of a pneumatic antishock garment or pelvic splint in the presence of pelvic fracture with hypotension. • Obtain blood samples for type and crossmatch.
Disability *Brief Neurologic Assessment*	
• Assess level of consciousness by determining response to verbal and/or painful stimuli (e.g., AVPU, Glasgow Coma Scale). • Assess pupils for size, shape, equality, and reactivity.	• Periodically reassess level of consciousness, mental status, pupil size and reactivity.
Identify Deformities	
• Inspect extremities for any obvious deformities. • Determine range of movement and strength in extremities.	• Immobilize (e.g., splint) any obvious deformities.
Brief Pain Assessment	
• Assess pain (e.g., PQRST [see Table 34-7]).	• Periodically reassess pain using standardized pain scale.
Exposure and Environmental Control	
• Assess full body for additional or related injuries	• Remove clothing for adequate examination. • Keep patient warm with blankets, warmed IV fluids, overhead lights to prevent heat loss, if appropriate. • Maintain privacy.

AVPU, A = alert, *V* = responsive to voice, *P* = responsive to pain, and *U* = unresponsive.

(e.g., Is this a high-risk patient who should not wait to be seen?). Next, evaluate patients who do not meet the criteria for ESI-1 or ESI-2 for the number of anticipated resources they may need. Assign patients to ESI level 3, 4, or 5 based on this determination. Normal vital signs are required for patients assigned to ESI level 3. Patients with abnormal vital signs may be reassigned to ESI level 2.[5] (For practice using the ESI triage system, see the ESI Implementation Handbook available at *www.ahrq.gov/research/esi.*)

After you complete the initial focused assessment to determine the presence of actual or potential threats to life, proceed with a more detailed assessment. A systematic approach to this assessment decreases the time needed to identify potential threats to life and limits the risk of overlooking a life-threatening condition. A primary and secondary survey is the approach used for all trauma patients. For nontrauma patients, the primary survey is followed by a focused assessment. (Focused assessments are discussed in Chapter 3.)

Primary Survey

The **primary survey** (Table 69-3) focuses on airway, breathing, circulation (ABC), disability, and exposure or environmental control. It aims to identify life-threatening conditions so that appropriate interventions can be started. You may identify life-

TABLE 69-4	POTENTIAL LIFE-THREATENING CONDITIONS FOUND DURING PRIMARY SURVEY*

Airway
- Inhalation injury (e.g., fire victim)
- Obstruction (partial or complete) from foreign bodies, debris (e.g., vomitus), or tongue
- Penetrating wounds and/or blunt trauma to upper airway structures

Breathing
- Anaphylaxis
- Flail chest with pulmonary contusion
- Hemothorax
- Pneumothorax (e.g., open, tension)

Circulation
- Direct cardiac injury (e.g., myocardial infarction, trauma)
- Pericardial tamponade
- Shock (e.g., massive burns, hypovolemia)
- Uncontrolled external hemorrhage
- Hypothermia

Disability
- Head injury
- Stroke

*List is not all-inclusive.

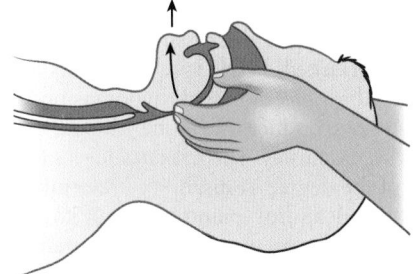

FIG. 69-1 Jaw-thrust maneuver is the recommended procedure for opening the airway of an unconscious patient with a possible neck or spinal injury. With the patient lying supine, kneel at the top of the head. Place one hand on each side of the patient's head, resting your elbows on the surface. Grasp the angles of the patient's lower jaw and lift the jaw forward with both hands without tilting the head.

threatening conditions related to ABCs (Table 69-4) at any point during the primary survey. When this occurs, start interventions immediately, before moving to the next step of the survey.

A = Airway With Cervical Spine Stabilization and/or Immobilization. Nearly all immediate trauma deaths occur because of airway obstruction. Saliva, bloody secretions, vomitus, laryngeal trauma, dentures, facial trauma, fractures, and the tongue can obstruct the airway. Patients at risk for airway compromise include those who have seizures, near-drowning, anaphylaxis, foreign body obstruction, or cardiopulmonary arrest. If an airway is not maintained, obstruction of airflow, hypoxia, and death will result.

Primary signs and symptoms in a patient with a compromised airway include dyspnea, inability to speak, gasping (agonal) breaths, foreign body in the airway, and trauma to the face or neck. Airway maintenance should progress rapidly from the least to the most invasive method. Treatment includes opening the airway using the 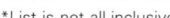 jaw-thrust maneuver (avoiding hyperextension of the neck) (Fig. 69-1), suctioning and/or removal of foreign body, insertion of a nasopharyngeal or an oropharyngeal airway (in unconscious patients only), and endotracheal intubation. If intubation is impossible because of airway obstruction, an emergency cricothyroidotomy or tracheotomy is performed (see Chapter 27). Ventilate patients with 100% O$_2$ using a bag-valve-mask (BVM) device before intubation or cricothyroidotomy.[7]

Rapid-sequence intubation is the preferred procedure for securing an unprotected airway in the ED. It involves the use of sedation (e.g., midazolam [Versed]) or anesthesia (e.g., etomidate [Amidate]) and paralysis (e.g., succinylcholine [Anectine]). These drugs aid intubation and reduce the risk of aspiration and airway trauma.[7] (See Chapter 66 for more information on intubation.)

Suspect cervical spine trauma in any patient with face, head, or neck trauma and/or significant upper chest injuries. Stabilize the cervical spine (head maintained in a neutral position) and/or immobilize during assessment of the airway. At the scene of

the injury, the cervical spine is immobilized with a rigid *cervical collar* (C-collar) and a *cervical immobilization device* (CID) (also known as "head blocks"). Finally, secure the patient's forehead to the backboard. Do not use sandbags because the weight of the bags could move the head if the patient is logrolled.

B = Breathing. Adequate airflow through the upper airway does not ensure adequate ventilation. Many conditions cause breathing changes, including fractured ribs, pneumothorax, penetrating injury, allergic reactions, pulmonary emboli, and asthma attacks. Patients with these conditions may have a variety of signs and symptoms, including dyspnea (e.g., pulmonary emboli), paradoxic or asymmetric chest wall movement (e.g., flail chest), decreased or absent breath sounds on the affected side (e.g., pneumothorax), visible wound to chest wall (e.g., penetrating injury), cyanosis (e.g., asthma), tachycardia, and hypotension.

Every critically injured or ill patient has an increased metabolic and oxygen demand and should have supplemental O$_2$. Administer high-flow O$_2$ (100%) via a non-rebreather mask and monitor the patient's response. Life-threatening conditions (e.g., flail chest, tension pneumothorax) can severely and quickly compromise ventilation. Interventions may include BVM ventilation with 100% O$_2$, needle decompression, intubation, and treatment of the underlying cause.

C = Circulation. An effective circulatory system includes the heart, intact blood vessels, and adequate blood volume. Uncontrolled internal or external bleeding places an individual at risk for hemorrhagic shock (see Chapter 67). Check a central pulse (e.g., carotid) because peripheral pulses may be absent due to direct injury or vasoconstriction. If you feel a pulse, assess the quality and rate. Assess the skin for color, temperature, and moisture. Altered mental status and delayed capillary refill (longer than 3 seconds) are common signs of shock. Take care when evaluating capillary refill in cold environments because cold delays refill.

Insert IV lines into veins in the upper extremities unless contraindicated, such as in a massive fracture or an injury that affects limb circulation. Insert two large-bore (14- to 16-gauge) IV catheters and start aggressive fluid resuscitation using normal saline or lactated Ringer's solution (see Chapter 67 for more information on hypovolemic shock and fluid resuscitation).

Apply direct pressure with a sterile dressing followed by a pressure dressing to any obvious bleeding sites. Obtain blood samples for typing to determine ABO and Rh group. Give type-specific packed red blood cells if needed. In an emergency (life-threatening) situation, give uncrossmatched blood if immediate transfusion is warranted. Pelvic splints or belts for pelvic fracture may be used for bleeding with hypotension.[8]

D = Disability. Conduct a brief neurologic examination as part of the primary survey. The patient's level of consciousness is a measure of the degree of disability. Determine the patient's response to verbal and/or painful stimuli to assess level of consciousness. A simple mnemonic to remember is *AVPU:* *A* = alert, *V* = responsive to voice, *P* = responsive to pain, and *U* = unresponsive. In addition, use the Glasgow Coma Scale (GCS) to determine the level of consciousness (see Table 57-5). Finally, assess the pupils for size, shape, equality, and reactivity.

E = Exposure or Environmental Control. Remove all trauma patients' clothing to perform a thorough physical assessment. This often requires cutting off the patient's clothing. Be careful not to cut through any area that may provide forensic evidence (e.g., bullet hole). Once the patient is exposed, use warming blankets, overhead warmers, and warmed IV fluids to limit heat loss, prevent hypothermia, and maintain privacy.

Secondary Survey

The secondary survey begins after addressing each step of the primary survey and starting any lifesaving interventions. The secondary survey is a brief, systematic process that aims to identify *all* injuries[9] (Table 69-5).

F = Full Set of Vital Signs, Focused Adjuncts, Facilitate Family Presence. Obtain a full set of vital signs, including blood pressure (BP), heart rate, respiratory rate, O_2 saturation, and temperature after the patient is exposed. If the patient has sustained or is suspected of having sustained chest trauma, or if the BP is abnormally high or low, obtain the BP in both arms.

At this point, determine whether to proceed with the secondary survey or to perform additional interventions. The input of other health care team members often influences this decision. The following focused adjuncts are considered for patients who sustain significant trauma or require lifesaving interventions during the primary survey:

- Continuously monitor ECG for heart rate and rhythm.
- Continuously monitor O_2 saturation and end-tidal carbon dioxide (if appropriate) (see Chapter 66).
- Obtain portable chest x-ray to confirm exact placement of tubes (e.g., endotracheal, gastric).
- Insert an indwelling catheter to decompress the bladder, monitor urine output, and check for hematuria. Do not insert an indwelling catheter if blood is present at the urinary meatus (e.g., urethral tear) or if scrotal hematoma or perineal ecchymosis is present. Men with a high-riding prostate gland on rectal examination are at risk for a urethral injury. The physician may order a retrograde urethrogram before inserting a catheter.
- Insert orogastric or nasogastric tube to decompress and empty the stomach, reduce the risk of aspiration, and test the contents for blood. Place an orogastric tube in a patient with significant head or facial trauma, since a nasogastric tube could enter the brain.
- Facilitate laboratory and diagnostic studies (e.g., type and crossmatch, complete blood count and metabolic panel, blood alcohol, toxicology screening, arterial blood gases [ABGs], coagulation profile, cardiac markers, pregnancy [urine], x-rays, computed tomography [CT] scans, ultrasound).
- Determine the need for tetanus prophylaxis.

Facilitating family presence (FP) completes this step of the secondary survey. Research supports the benefits for patients, caregivers, and staff of allowing FP during resuscitation and invasive procedures.[10,11] Patients report that caregivers provide comfort, serve as advocates for them, and help remind the health care team of their "personhood." Caregivers who wish to be present during invasive procedures and resuscitation view themselves as active participants in the care process. They also believe that they comfort the patient and that it is their right to be with the patient. Nurses report that family members serve as "patient helpers" (e.g., provide support) and "staff helpers" (e.g., act as a translator).[10] It is essential to assign a member of the health care team to explain care delivered and answer questions should a caregiver request FP during resuscitation or invasive procedures.

G = Give Comfort Measures. Provision of comfort measures is of paramount importance when caring for patients in the ED. Pain is the primary complaint of most patients who come to the ED.[12] Many EDs have developed pain management guidelines to treat pain early, beginning at triage. Pain management strategies should include a combination of pharmacologic (e.g., nonsteroidal antiinflammatory drugs, IV opioids) and nonpharmacologic (e.g., imagery, distraction, positioning) measures. You play a pivotal role in ongoing pain management because of your frequent contact with patients. General comfort measures such as providing verbal reassurance, listening, reducing stimuli (e.g., dimming lights), and developing a trusting relationship with the patient and caregiver should be provided to all patients in the ED. Additional measures include splinting, elevating, and icing injured extremities as appropriate.

H = History and Head-to-Toe Assessment. The history of the incident, injury, or illness provides clues to the cause of the crisis (e.g., Were the injuries self-inflicted?) and suggests specific assessment and interventions. The patient may not be able to give a history. However, caregivers, friends, witnesses, and prehospital personnel can often provide necessary information. Prehospital information focuses on the mechanism and pattern of injury, injuries suspected, vital signs, treatments initiated, and patient responses.

Details of the incident are extremely important because the mechanism of injury and injury patterns can predict specific injuries. For example, a restrained front-seat passenger may have a head injury or knee, femur, or hip fractures from hitting the dashboard and an abdominal injury from the seat belt. If there were deaths at the scene, the patient is at high risk for significant injury.

Patients who jump from buildings or bridges may have bilateral calcaneal (heel) fractures, bilateral wrist fractures, and lumbar spine compression fractures. They are also at risk for aortic tears. Older patients who have climbed ladders and fallen may have had a stroke or myocardial infarction that led to the fall.

Prehospital personnel provide a detailed description of the patient's general condition, level of consciousness, and apparent injuries. An experienced ED team can complete a history within 5 minutes of the patient's arrival. If the patient is emergently ill, obtain a thorough history from caregivers or friends after the

TABLE 69-5 EMERGENCY ASSESSMENT: SECONDARY SURVEY

Assessment	Interventions
Full Set of Vital Signs Establish baseline vital signs	• Obtain vital signs: temperature, heart rate, respiratory rate, oxygen saturation, BP bilaterally.
Focused Adjuncts Determine need for additional procedures	• Initiate continuous ECG, O_2 saturation, and end-tidal carbon dioxide monitoring. • Insert urinary catheter (if not contraindicated). • Insert gastric tube. • Obtain blood for laboratory studies. • Arrange for diagnostic studies (e.g., chest x-ray). • Provide tetanus prophylaxis, if appropriate.
Facilitate Family Presence Determine caregiver's desire to be present during invasive procedures and/or cardiopulmonary resuscitation	• Assign team member to support caregivers.
Give Comfort Measures Assess, treat, and reassess for pain, anxiety	• Provide emotional support to patient and caregiver. • Provide additional comfort measures as appropriate (e.g., distraction, ice, position of comfort, warm blanket, analgesia).
History and Head-to-Toe Assessment *History*	• Obtain details of the incident/illness, mechanism and pattern of injury, length of time since incident occurred, injuries suspected, treatment provided and patient's response, level of consciousness. • Use the mnemonic **AMPLE** to determine **A**llergies, **M**edication history, **P**ast health history (e.g., preexisting medical/psychiatric conditions, last menstrual period), **L**ast meal, and **E**vents/Environment preceding illness or injury.
Head, Neck, and Face	• Note general appearance, including skin color. • Examine face and scalp for lacerations, bone or soft tissue deformity, tenderness, bleeding, and foreign bodies. • Inspect eyes, ears, nose, and mouth for bleeding, foreign bodies, drainage, pain, deformity, ecchymosis, lacerations. • Palpate head for depressions of cranial or facial bones, contusions, hematomas, areas of softness, bony crepitus. • Examine neck for stiffness, pain in cervical vertebrae, tracheal deviation, distended neck veins, bleeding, edema, difficulty swallowing, bruising, subcutaneous emphysema, bony crepitus.
Chest	• Observe rate, depth, and effort of breathing, including chest wall movement and use of accessory muscles. • Palpate for bony crepitus, subcutaneous emphysema. • Auscultate breath sounds. • Obtain 12-lead ECG and chest x-ray. • Inspect for external signs of injury: petechiae, bleeding, cyanosis, bruises, abrasions, lacerations, old scars.
Abdomen and Flanks	• Look for symmetry of abdominal wall and bony structures. • Inspect for external signs of injury: bruises, abrasions, lacerations, punctures, old scars. • Auscultate for bowel sounds. • Palpate for masses, guarding, femoral pulses. • Note type and location of pain, rigidity, or distention of abdomen.
Pelvis and Perineum	• Gently palpate pelvis. • Assess genitalia for blood at the meatus, priapism, ecchymosis, rectal bleeding, anal sphincter tone. • Determine ability to void.
Extremities	• Inspect for signs of external injury: deformity, ecchymosis, abrasions, lacerations, swelling. • Observe skin color and palpate skin for pain, tenderness, temperature, and crepitus. • Evaluate movement, strength, and sensation in arms and legs. • Assess quality and symmetry of peripheral pulses.
Inspect Posterior Surfaces	• Logroll and inspect and palpate back for deformity, bleeding, lacerations, bruises.

patient is taken to the treatment area. The history should include the following questions:

- What is the chief complaint? What caused the patient to seek attention?
- What are the patient's subjective complaints?
- What is the patient's description of pain (e.g., location, duration, quality, character)?
- What are the witnesses' (if any) descriptions of the patient's behavior since the onset?
- What is the patient's health history? The mnemonic *AMPLE* is a memory aid that prompts you to ask about the following:

  A: Allergies to drugs, food, latex, environment
  M: Medication history
  P: Past health history (e.g., preexisting medical or psychiatric conditions, previous hospitalizations or surgeries, smoking history, recent use of drugs or alcohol, tetanus immunization, last menstrual period, baseline mental status)
  L: Last meal
  E: Events or environmental factors leading to the illness or injury

Head, Neck, and Face. Assess the patient for general appearance, skin color, and temperature. Check the eyes for extraocular movements. A disconjugate gaze is an indication of neurologic damage. Battle's sign, or bruising directly behind the ear(s), may indicate a fracture of the base of the posterior portion of the skull. "Raccoon eyes," or periorbital ecchymosis, is usually an indication of a fracture of the base of the frontal portion of the skull. Check the ears for blood and cerebrospinal fluid (see Chapter 57 and Fig. 57-13). Do not block clear drainage from the ear or nose.

Assess the airway for foreign bodies, bleeding, edema, and loose or missing teeth. Check for the ability to open the mouth and swallow. Inspect the neck for bruising, edema, bleeding, or distended neck veins. Palpate the trachea to determine whether it is midline. A deviated trachea may signal a life-threatening tension pneumothorax. Subcutaneous emphysema may indicate laryngotracheal disruption. A stiff or painful neck may signify a fracture of one or more cervical vertebrae. Protect the cervical spine using a C-collar and supine positioning if indicated.

Chest. Inspect the chest for paradoxic chest movements and large sucking chest wounds. Palpate the sternum, clavicles, and ribs for deformity, point tenderness, and crepitus. Auscultate breath sounds and heart sounds. In addition to tension pneumothorax and open pneumothorax, evaluate the patient for rib fractures, pulmonary contusion, blunt cardiac injury, and hemothorax. Obtain a chest x-ray and 12-lead ECG, particularly on a patient with known or suspected heart disease. The ECG is done to detect dysrhythmias and signs of myocardial ischemia or infarction.

Abdomen and Flanks. The abdomen and flanks are more difficult to assess. Frequent evaluation for subtle changes in the abdomen is essential. Motor vehicle collisions and assaults can cause blunt trauma. Penetrating trauma tends to injure specific, solid organs (e.g., spleen) based on their trajectory. Stabilize impaled objects (e.g., knife), since they need to be removed in a controlled environment such as an operating room. Decreased bowel sounds may indicate a temporary paralytic ileus. Bowel sounds in the chest may indicate a diaphragmatic rupture. Percuss the abdomen for distention (e.g., tympany [excessive air], dullness [excessive fluid]) and palpate for tenderness.

If you suspect intraabdominal hemorrhage, a *focused abdominal sonography for trauma* (FAST) to identify blood in the peritoneal space (hemoperitoneum) is preferred. This procedure is noninvasive and performed quickly at the bedside.[13] However, a FAST cannot rule out a retroperitoneal bleed. If one is suspected, a CT scan is usually ordered.

Pelvis and Perineum. Gently palpate the pelvis to determine stability. Do not rock the pelvis. Pain may indicate a pelvic fracture and the need for an x-ray. Inspect the genitalia for bleeding, priapism, and obvious injuries. Assess for bladder distention, hematuria, dysuria, or inability to void. The physician may perform a rectal examination to check for blood, a high-riding prostate gland (e.g., urethral injury), and loss of sphincter tone (e.g., spinal cord injury).

Extremities. Assess the upper and lower extremities for point tenderness, crepitus, and deformities. Splint injured extremities above and below the injury to decrease further soft tissue injury and pain. Grossly deformed, pulseless extremities should be realigned by the physician and then splinted. Check pulses before and after movement or splinting of an extremity. A pulseless extremity is a time-critical vascular or orthopedic emergency. Immobilize and elevate injured extremities, and apply ice packs. Prophylactic antibiotics are ordered for open fractures.

Also, assess extremities for *compartment syndrome*. This occurs as pressure and swelling increase inside a section of an extremity (e.g., anterior compartment of lower leg) over several hours. This compromises the viability of the extremity muscles, nerves, and arteries. Potential causes of compartment syndrome include crush injuries, fractures, edema (e.g., burns), and hemorrhage.

I = Inspect Posterior Surfaces. The trauma patient should always be logrolled (while maintaining cervical spine immobilization) to inspect the patient's posterior surfaces and whenever movement is needed. This often requires three to four or more people with one person supporting the head. Inspect the back for ecchymosis, abrasions, puncture wounds, cuts, and obvious deformities. Palpate the entire spine for misalignment, deformity, and pain.

Intervention and Evaluation

Once the secondary survey is complete, record all findings. Provide tetanus prophylaxis based on vaccination history and the condition of any wounds[14] (Table 69-6).

Regardless of the patient's chief complaint, ongoing monitoring and evaluation of interventions are critical. You are responsible for providing appropriate interventions and assessing the patient's response. The evaluation of airway patency and the effectiveness of breathing will always be the highest priority. Monitor respiratory rate and rhythm, O_2 saturation, and ABGs (if ordered) to evaluate the patient's respiratory status. Also, closely monitor the level of consciousness; vital signs; quality of peripheral pulses; urine output; and skin temperature, color, and moisture for key information about circulation and perfusion.

Depending on the patient's injuries or illness, the patient may be (1) transported for diagnostic tests (e.g., CT scan) or to the operating room for immediate surgery; (2) admitted to an intensive care, telemetry, or general unit; or (3) transferred to another facility. You may go with critically ill patients on transports. You are responsible for monitoring the patient during

TABLE 69-6 TETANUS VACCINES AND TIG FOR WOUND MANAGEMENT

Vaccination History	Type of Wound	
	Clean, Minor Wounds	All Other Wounds
Age 11–64 Yr*		
Unknown or <3 doses of tetanus toxoid–containing vaccine	Tdap and recommend catch-up vaccination	Tdap and recommend catch-up vaccination TIG
≥3 doses of tetanus toxoid–containing vaccine and <5 yr since last dose	No indication	No indication
≥3 doses of tetanus toxoid–containing vaccine and 5–10 yr since last dose	No indication	Tdap preferred (if not yet received) or Td
≥3 doses of tetanus toxoid–containing vaccine and >10 yr since last dose	Tdap preferred (if not yet received) or Td	Tdap preferred (if not yet received) or Td
Age ≥65 Yr		
Unknown or <3 doses of tetanus toxoid–containing vaccine	Td or Tdap and recommend catch-up vaccination. Tdap preferred if patient has close contact with children <12 mo of age	Td or Tdap and recommend catch-up vaccination. Tdap preferred if patient has close contact with children <12 mo of age TIG
≥3 doses of tetanus toxoid–containing vaccine and <5 yr since last dose	No indication	No indication
≥3 doses of tetanus toxoid–containing vaccine and 5–10 yr since last dose	No indication	Td or Tdap. Tdap preferred if patient has close contact with children <12 mo of age
≥3 doses of tetanus toxoid–containing vaccine and >10 yr since last dose	Tdap preferred (if not yet received) or Td	Td or Tdap. Tdap preferred if patient has close contact with children <12 mo of age

Source: Centers for Disease Control and Prevention: Disaster information: tetanus prevention after a disaster. Retrieved from *www.bt.cdc.gov/disasters/disease/tetanus.asp.*
*Pregnant women: As part of standard wound management care to prevent tetanus, a tetanus toxoid–containing vaccine might be recommended for wound management in a pregnant woman if ≥5 yr have elapsed since last receiving Td. If a tetanus booster is indicated for a pregnant woman who previously has not received Tdap, Tdap should be administered (at any gestational age).
Td, Tetanus-diphtheria toxoid absorbed; *Tdap,* tetanus toxoid, reduced diphtheria toxoid, and acellular pertussis vaccine; *TIG,* tetanus immune globulin (human).

EVIDENCE-BASED PRACTICE

Applying the Evidence

F.P. is a 76-yr-old woman admitted to the emergency department with new-onset atrial fibrillation with a rapid ventricular response (heart rate of 148 beats/min). She has mild shortness of breath and palpitations. As you administer a bolus dose of diltiazem (Cardizem) and prepare the continuous drip, she shares with you that she is concerned about her pets. F.P. lives alone and states that she "must go home" but will "return in the morning" to continue her treatment. She asks you to stop her medication and help her prepare to leave.

Best Available Evidence	Clinician Expertise	Patient Preferences and Values
Atrial fibrillation results in a decrease in cardiac output because of ineffective atrial contractions and/or a rapid ventricular response. Thrombi (clots) can form in the atria and may pass to the brain, causing cerebral embolic events. Ventricular rate control (heart rate <100 beats/min) is a priority for patients with atrial fibrillation. If drugs or cardioversion do not convert atrial fibrillation to normal sinus rhythm, long-term anticoagulation therapy is needed.	You know that the goals of treatment for this patient include rate control, prevention of stroke, and conversion to sinus rhythm, if possible. F.P. is at risk for complications the longer her heart rate remains elevated and she delays treatment of her dysrhythmia.	Patient's concerns for her pets are greater than her concerns for her current health situation.

Your Decision and Action

You and F.P. fully explore options for the care of her pets. None are acceptable to F.P. You then explain the risk she is taking should she leave the emergency department. F.P. states she understands and will sign the papers needed to be able to leave. You inform the physician and prepare the leaving "Against Medical Advice" papers.

Reference for Evidence

Wann LS, Curtis AB, January CT, et al: 2011 ACCF/AHA/HRS focused update on the management of patients with atrial fibrillation (updating the 2006 guideline): a report of the American College of Cardiology Foundation/American Heart Association task force on practice guidelines, *J Am Coll Cardiol* 57:223, 2011.

transport, notifying the health care team should the patient's condition become unstable, and initiating basic and advanced life-support measures as needed.

Post–Cardiac Arrest Hypothermia

Many patients arrive at the ED in cardiac arrest. Patients with nontraumatic, out-of-hospital cardiac arrest benefit from a combination of good chest compressions and rapid defibrillation (see Appendix A), therapeutic hypothermia, and supportive care. Therapeutic hypothermia for 24 hours after the return of spontaneous circulation (ROSC) decreases mortality rates and improves neurologic outcomes in many patients.[15] It is recommended for all patients who are comatose or who do not follow commands after ROSC.[16]

Therapeutic hypothermia involves three phases: induction, maintenance, and rewarming. The induction phase begins in the ED. The goal core temperature is 89.6° to 93.2°F (32° to 34°C). A variety of methods are used to cool patients. These include cold saline infusions and cooling devices (e.g., Arctic Sun). Patients require intubation and mechanical ventilation, invasive monitoring (e.g., arterial and central pressures), and continuous assessment during this therapy.[15] Protocols are used to direct the care of these patients. (Sample protocols and procedures are available at *www.med.upenn.edu/resuscitation/hypothermia/protocols.shtml.*)

Death in the Emergency Department

Unfortunately, a number of patients will not benefit from the skill, expertise, and technology available in the ED. It is important for you to deal with your feelings about sudden death so that you can help caregivers begin the grieving process (see Chapter 10).

Recognize the importance of certain hospital rituals to help caregivers grieve. These can include collecting the belongings, arranging for an autopsy (e.g., coroner's case), viewing the body, and making mortuary arrangements. The death must seem real so that the caregivers can begin to accept the death. You play a significant role in providing comfort to the surviving loved ones after a death in the ED. Whenever possible, provide an area for privacy and, if appropriate, arrange for a visit from a chaplain.[17]

Many patients who die in the ED could potentially be candidates for *non-heart-beating donation*. Certain tissues and organs (e.g., corneas, heart valves, skin, bone, kidneys) can be harvested from patients after death. Approaching caregivers about donation after an unexpected death is distressing to both the staff and caregivers. For many, however, the act of donation may be the first positive step in the grieving process. *Organ procurement organizations* (OPOs) assist in the process of screening potential donors, counseling donor families, obtaining informed consent, and harvesting organs from patients who are on life support or who die in the ED.[18]

GERONTOLOGIC CONSIDERATIONS

EMERGENCY CARE

The proportion of the population over age 65 is growing, with most leading active lives. Overall, people older than 65 account for 24% of all ED visits.[19] Regardless of a patient's age, aggressive interventions are warranted for all injuries or illnesses unless the patient has a preexisting terminal illness, an extremely low chance of survival, or an advance directive indicating a different course of action.

The older population is at high risk for injury because of many of the anatomic and physiologic changes that occur with aging (e.g., reduced visual acuity, limited neck rotation, slower gait, reduced reaction time). Of the injury-related admissions for people over 65 years old, most are for fractures, with many of these resulting from falls.[19] The most common causes of falls in older adults are generalized weakness, environmental hazards (e.g., loose mats, furniture), cardiovascular syncope (e.g., dysrhythmias), and orthostatic hypotension (e.g., side effect of medications, dehydration). When assessing a patient who has fallen, determine whether the physical findings may have caused the fall or may be due to the fall itself. For example, a patient may come to the ED with acute confusion. The confusion may be due to a myocardial infarction or stroke that caused the patient to fall, or the patient may have suffered a head injury as a result of a fall from tripping on a rug.

Understanding the physiologic and psychosocial aspects of aging will improve the care delivered to older adults in the ED (see Chapter 5). Unfortunately, many older adults dismiss symptoms as simply "normal for their age." It is important to fully investigate any complaint by an older adult.

ENVIRONMENTAL EMERGENCIES

Increased interest in outdoor activities such as running, hiking, cycling, skiing, and swimming has increased the number of environmental emergencies seen in the ED. Illness or injury may be caused by the activity, exposure to weather, or attack from various animals or humans. Specific environmental emer-

TABLE 69-7	**RISK FACTORS FOR HEAT-RELATED EMERGENCIES**

Age
- Infants
- Older adults

Environmental Conditions
- High environmental temperatures
- High relative humidity

Preexisting Illness
- Cardiovascular disease
- Cystic fibrosis
- Dehydration
- Diabetes mellitus
- Obesity
- Previous stroke or other central nervous system lesion
- Skin disorders (e.g., large burn scars)

Prescription Drugs
- Anticholinergics
- Antihistamines
- Antiparkinsonian drugs
- Antispasmodics
- β-Adrenergic blockers
- Butyrophenones
- Diuretics
- Phenothiazines
- Tricyclic antidepressants

Alcohol

Street Drugs
- Amphetamines
- Jimson weed
- Lysergic acid diethylamide (LSD)
- Phencyclidine (PCP)
- 3,4-Methylenedioxymethamphetamine (MDMA, Ecstasy)

Adapted from Howard PK, Steinmann RA, editors: *Sheehy's emergency nursing*, ed 6, St Louis, 2010, Mosby.

gencies discussed in this section include heat-related emergencies, cold-related emergencies, submersion injuries, bites, and stings.

HEAT-RELATED EMERGENCIES

Brief exposure to intense heat or prolonged exposure to less intense heat leads to heat stress. This occurs when thermoregulatory mechanisms such as sweating, vasodilation, and increased respirations cannot compensate for exposure to increased ambient temperatures. Ambient temperature is a product of environmental temperature and humidity. Strenuous activities in hot or humid environments, clothing that interferes with perspiration, high fevers, and preexisting illnesses predispose individuals to heat stress (Table 69-7). Table 69-8 presents the management of heat-related emergencies.

Heat Cramps

Heat cramps are severe cramps in large muscle groups fatigued by heavy work. Cramps are brief and intense and tend to occur during rest after exercise or heavy labor. Nausea, tachycardia, pallor, weakness, and profuse diaphoresis are often present. The condition is seen most often in healthy, acclimated athletes with inadequate fluid intake. Cramps resolve rapidly with rest and oral or parenteral replacement of sodium and water. Elevation, gentle massage, and analgesia minimize pain associated with heat cramps. Instruct the patient to avoid strenuous activity for at least 12 hours. Discharge teaching should emphasize salt replacement during strenuous exercise in hot, humid environments. You can also recommend the use of commercially prepared electrolyte solutions (e.g., sports drinks).

Heat Exhaustion

Prolonged exposure to heat over hours or days leads to heat exhaustion. This is a clinical syndrome characterized by fatigue, nausea, vomiting, extreme thirst, and feelings of anxiety (see

✚ TABLE 69-8 EMERGENCY MANAGEMENT

Hyperthermia

Etiology	Assessment Findings	Interventions
Environmental • Lack of acclimatization • Physical exertion, especially during hot weather • Prolonged exposure to extreme temperatures	**Heat Cramps** • Severe muscle contractions in exerted muscles • Thirst	**Initial** • Manage and maintain ABCs. • Provide high-flow O_2 via non-rebreather mask or BVM. • Establish IV access and begin fluid replacement for significant heat injury. • Place patient in a cool environment.
Trauma • Head injury • Spinal cord injury	**Heat Exhaustion** • Pale, ashen skin • Fatigue, weakness • Profuse sweating	• For patient with heatstroke, initiate rapid cooling measures: remove patient's clothing, place wet sheets over patient, and place in front of fan; immerse in a cool water bath; administer cool IV fluids or lavage with cool fluids.
Metabolic • Dehydration • Diabetes • Thyrotoxicosis	• Extreme thirst • Altered mental status (e.g., anxiety) • Hypotension • Tachycardia • Weak, thready pulse • Temperature 99.6°-104°F (37.5°-40°C)	• Obtain 12-lead ECG. • Obtain blood for electrolytes and CBC. • Insert urinary catheter.
Drugs • Amphetamines • Antihistamines • β-Adrenergic blockers • Diuretics • Phenothiazines • Tricyclic antidepressants	**Heatstroke** • Hot, dry skin • Altered mental status (e.g., ranging from confusion to coma) • Hypotension • Tachycardia	**Ongoing Monitoring** • Monitor ABCs, temperature and vital signs, level of consciousness. • Monitor heart rhythm, O_2 saturation, and urine output. • Replace electrolytes as needed.
Other • Alcohol • Cardiovascular disease • CNS disorders	• Weakness • Temperature >104°F (40°C)	• Monitor urine for development of myoglobinuria. • Monitor clotting studies for development of disseminated intravascular coagulation.

ABCs, Airway, breathing, circulation; *BVM,* bag-valve-mask.

Table 69-8). Hypotension, tachycardia, elevated body temperature, dilated pupils, mild confusion, ashen color, and profuse diaphoresis are also present. Hypotension and mild to severe temperature elevation (99.6° to 104°F [37.5° to 40°C]) are caused by dehydration.[20] Heat exhaustion usually occurs in individuals engaged in strenuous activity in hot, humid weather, but it also occurs in sedentary individuals.

Begin treatment by placing the patient in a cool area and removing constrictive clothing. Monitor the patient for ABCs, including cardiac dysrhythmias (caused by electrolyte imbalances). Initiate oral fluid and electrolyte replacement unless the patient is nauseated. Do not use salt tablets because of potential gastric irritation and hypernatremia. Initiate a 0.9% normal saline IV solution if oral solutions are not tolerated. An initial fluid bolus may be needed to correct hypotension. However, correlate fluid replacement to clinical and laboratory findings. Place a moist sheet over the patient to decrease core temperature through evaporative heat loss. Consider hospital admission for the older adult, the chronically ill, or those who do not improve within 3 to 4 hours.

Heatstroke

Heatstroke, the most serious form of heat stress, results from failure of the hypothalamic thermoregulatory processes. It is a medical emergency. Increased sweating, vasodilation, and increased respiratory rate (the body's attempt to lower temperature) deplete fluids and electrolytes, specifically sodium. Eventually, sweat glands stop functioning, and core temperature increases rapidly, within 10 to 15 minutes. The patient has a core temperature greater than 104°F (40°C), altered mentation, absence of perspiration, and circulatory collapse. The skin is hot, dry, and ashen. A range of neurologic symptoms occur

(e.g., hallucinations, loss of muscle coordination, combativeness) because the brain is extremely sensitive to thermal injuries. Cerebral edema and hemorrhage may occur as a result of direct thermal injury to the brain and decreased cerebral blood flow.

Death from heatstroke is directly related to the amount of time that the patient's body temperature remains elevated.[20] Prognosis is related to age, baseline health status, and length of exposure. Older adults and individuals with diabetes mellitus, chronic kidney disease, cardiovascular disease, pulmonary disease, or other physiologic compromise are particularly vulnerable.

Collaborative Care. Treatment of heatstroke focuses on stabilizing the patient's ABCs and rapidly reducing the core temperature. Administration of 100% O_2 compensates for the patient's hypermetabolic state. Ventilation with a BVM or intubation and mechanical ventilation may be required. Correct fluid and electrolyte imbalances and initiate continuous ECG monitoring for dysrhythmias.

Various cooling methods are available, such as removing clothing, covering with wet sheets, and placing the patient in front of a large fan (evaporative cooling), immersing the patient in a cool water bath (conductive cooling), and administering cool fluids or lavaging with cool fluids.[20] Whatever method is selected, closely monitor the patient's temperature and control shivering. Shivering increases core temperature (because of the associated heat generated by muscle activity) and complicates cooling efforts. Chlorpromazine (Thorazine) IV is the drug of choice to control shivering. Aggressive temperature reduction should continue until core temperature reaches 102°F (38.9°C).[20] Antipyretics are not effective in this situation because the elevated temperature is not related to infection.

Monitor the patient for signs of *rhabdomyolysis* (a serious syndrome caused by the breakdown of skeletal muscle). The muscle breakdown leads to myoglobinuria, which places the kidneys at risk for acute kidney injury. Carefully monitor the urine for color (e.g., tea colored), amount, pH, and myoglobin. Finally, obtain clotting studies to monitor the patient for signs of disseminated intravascular coagulation (see Chapter 31).

Patient and caregiver teaching focuses on how to avoid future problems. Provide essential information regarding proper hydration during hot weather and physical exercise. Instruct patients on the early signs of and interventions for heat-related stress.

COLD-RELATED EMERGENCIES

Cold injuries may be localized (frostbite) or systemic (hypothermia). Contributing factors include age, duration of exposure, environmental temperature, homelessness, preexisting conditions (e.g., diabetes mellitus, peripheral vascular disease), medications that suppress shivering (e.g., opioids, psychotropic agents, antiemetics), and alcohol intoxication. Alcohol causes peripheral vasodilation, increases sensation of warmth, and depresses shivering. Smokers have an increased risk of cold-related injury because of the vasoconstrictive effects of nicotine.

Frostbite

Frostbite is true tissue freezing that results in the formation of ice crystals in the tissues and cells. Peripheral vasoconstriction is the initial response to cold stress and results in a decrease in blood flow and vascular stasis. As cellular temperature decreases and ice crystals form in intracellular spaces, the organelles are damaged and the cell membrane destroyed. This results in edema. Depth of frostbite depends on ambient temperature, length of exposure, type and condition (wet or dry) of clothing, and contact with metal surfaces. Other factors that affect severity include skin color (dark-skinned people are more prone to frostbite), lack of acclimatization, previous episodes, exhaustion, and poor peripheral vascular status.

Superficial frostbite involves skin and subcutaneous tissue, usually the ears, nose, fingers, and toes. The skin appearance ranges from waxy pale yellow to blue to mottled, and the skin feels crunchy and frozen. The patient may complain of tingling, numbness, or a burning sensation. Handle the area carefully and never squeeze, massage, or scrub the injured tissue because it is easily damaged. Remove clothing and jewelry because they may constrict the extremity and decrease circulation. Immerse the affected area in a water bath (98.6° to 104° F) [37° to 40° C].[20] Use warm soaks for the face. The patient often experiences a warm, stinging sensation as tissue thaws. Blisters form within a few hours (Fig. 69-2). The blisters should be debrided and a sterile dressing applied. Avoid heavy blankets and clothing because friction and weight can lead to sloughing of damaged tissue. Rewarming is extremely painful. Residual pain may last weeks or even years. Administer analgesia and tetanus prophylaxis as appropriate (see Table 69-6). Evaluate the patient with superficial frostbite for systemic hypothermia.

Deep frostbite involves muscle, bone, and tendon. The skin is white, hard, and insensitive to touch. The area has the appearance of deep thermal injury with mottling gradually progressing to gangrene (Fig. 69-3). The affected extremity is immersed in

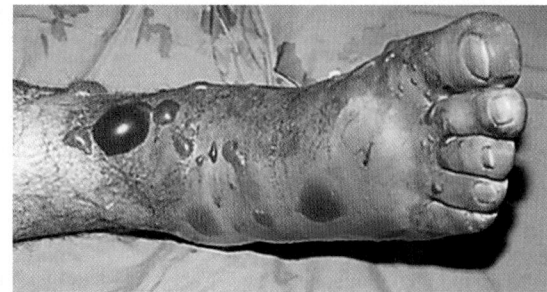

FIG. 69-2 Edema and blister formation 24 hours after frostbite injury occurring in an area covered by a tightly fitted boot.

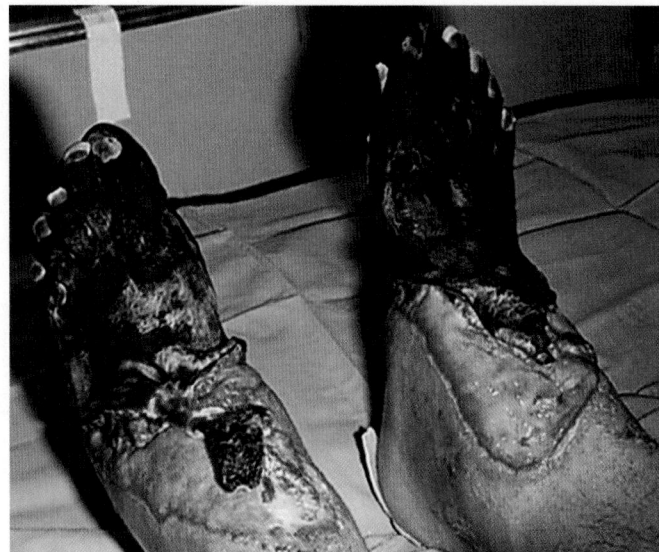

FIG. 69-3 Gangrenous necrosis 6 weeks after the frostbite injury shown in Fig. 69-2.

a circulating water bath (98.6° to 104° F) [37° to 40° C]) until flushing occurs distal to the injured area.[20] After rewarming, the extremity should be elevated to reduce edema. Significant edema may begin within 3 hours, with blistering in 6 hours to days. IV analgesia is required in severe frostbite because of the pain associated with tissue thawing. Provide tetanus prophylaxis and evaluate the patient for systemic hypothermia. Amputation may be required if the injured area is untreated or treatment is unsuccessful. The patient may be admitted to the hospital for observation with bed rest, elevation of the injured part, and prophylactic antibiotics if the wound is at risk for infection.

Hypothermia

Hypothermia, defined as a core temperature below 95° F (35° C), occurs when heat produced by the body cannot compensate for heat lost to the environment.[20] Most body heat is lost as radiant energy, with the greatest loss from the head, thorax, and lungs (with each breath). Wet clothing increases evaporative heat loss to five times greater than normal; immersion in cold water (e.g., near drowning) increases evaporative heat loss to 25 times greater than normal. Environmental exposure to freezing temperatures, cold winds, and wet terrain plus physical exhaustion, inadequate clothing, and inexperience predisposes individuals to hypothermia. Older adults are more prone to hypothermia because of decreased body fat, dimin-

✚ TABLE 69-9 EMERGENCY MANAGEMENT

Hypothermia

Etiology	Assessment Findings	Interventions

Environmental
 • Inadequate clothing for environmental temperature
 • Prolonged exposure to cold
 • Prolonged immersion or near-drowning
 	
 Metabolic
 • Hypoglycemia
 • Hypothyroidism
 	
 Health Care Associated
 • Administration of neuromuscular blocking agents
 • Blood administration
 • Cold IV fluids
 • Inadequate warming or rewarming in the ED or operating room
 	
 Other
 • Alcohol
 • Barbiturates
 • Phenothiazines
 • Shock
 • Trauma
	• Core body temperature:
	   • *Mild hypothermia:* 93.2°–96.8°F (34°–36°C)
	   • *Moderate hypothermia:* 86°–93.2°F (30°–34°C)
	   • *Severe hypothermia:* ≤86°F (≤30°C)
	 • Shivering, diminished or absent at core body temperatures ≤86°F (30°C)
	 • Hypoventilation
	 • Hypotension
	 • Altered mental status (ranging from confusion to coma)
	 • Areflexia (absence of reflexes)
	 • Pale, cyanotic skin
	 • Blue, white, or frozen extremities
	 • Dysrhythmias: bradycardia, atrial fibrillation, ventricular fibrillation, asystole
	 • Fixed, dilated pupils
		Initial
		 • Remove patient from cold environment.
		 • Manage and maintain ABCs.
		 • Provide high-flow O₂ via non-rebreather mask or BVM.
		 • Anticipate intubation for diminished or absent gag reflex.*
		 • Establish IV access with two large-bore catheters for fluid resuscitation
		 • Rewarm patient:
		   • *Passive:* Remove wet clothing, apply dry clothing and warm blankets, use radiant lights.
		   • *Active external:* Apply heating devices (e.g., air or fluid-filled warming blankets), use warm water immersion.
		   • *Active internal:* Provide warmed IV fluids; heated, humidified O₂. Peritoneal lavage with warmed fluids. Extracorporeal circulation (e.g., cardiopulmonary bypass, rapid fluid infuser, hemodialysis).
		 • Obtain 12-lead ECG.
		 • Anticipate need for defibrillation.*
		 • Warm central trunk first in patients with severe hypothermia to limit rewarming shock.
		 • Assess for other injuries.
		 • Keep patient's head covered with warm, dry towels or stocking cap to limit loss of heat.
		 • Treat patient gently to avoid increased cardiac irritability.
		
		 Ongoing Monitoring
		 • Monitor ABCs, temperature, level of consciousness, vital signs.
		 • Monitor O₂ saturation, heart rate and rhythm.
		 • Monitor electrolytes, glucose.

*NOTE: Medications and defibrillation may not be effective with core temperatures <86°F (30°C).
ABCs, Airway, breathing, circulation; *BVM,* bag-valve-mask.

ished energy reserves, decreased basal metabolic rate, decreased shivering response, decreased sensory perception, chronic medical conditions, and medications that alter body defenses.

Hypothermia mimics cerebral or metabolic disturbances causing ataxia, confusion, and withdrawal, so the patient may be misdiagnosed. Peripheral vasoconstriction is the body's first attempt to conserve heat. As cold temperatures persist, shivering and movement are the body's only mechanisms for producing heat.

Assessment findings in hypothermia are variable and depend on core temperature (Table 69-9). Patients with *mild hypothermia* (93.2° to 96.8°F [34° to 36°C]) have shivering, lethargy, confusion, rational to irrational behavior, and minor heart rate changes. *Moderate hypothermia* (86° to 93.2°F [30° to 34°C]) causes rigidity, bradycardia, slowed respiratory rate, BP obtainable only by Doppler, metabolic and respiratory acidosis, and hypovolemia. Shivering diminishes or disappears at core temperatures of 86°F (30°C).[19]

As core temperature drops, basal metabolic rate decreases two or three times. The cold myocardium is extremely irritable, making it vulnerable to dysrhythmias (e.g., atrial and ventricular fibrillation). Decreased renal blood flow decreases glomerular filtration rate, which impairs water reabsorption and leads to dehydration. The hematocrit increases as intravascular volume decreases. Cold blood becomes thick and acts as a thrombus, placing the patient at risk for stroke, myocardial infarction, pulmonary emboli, and renal failure. Decreased blood flow leads to hypoxia, anaerobic metabolism, lactic acid accumulation, and metabolic acidosis.

Severe hypothermia (at or below 86°F [30°C]) makes the person appear dead and is a potentially life-threatening situation. Metabolic rate, heart rate, and respirations are so slow that they may be difficult to detect. Reflexes are absent, and the pupils fixed and dilated. Profound bradycardia, ventricular fibrillation, or asystole may be present. Every effort is made to warm the patient to at least 86°F (30°C) before the person is pronounced dead.[20] The cause of death is usually refractory ventricular fibrillation.

Collaborative Care. Treatment of hypothermia focuses on managing and maintaining ABCs, rewarming the patient, correcting dehydration and acidosis, and treating cardiac dysrhythmias (see Table 69-9). Use passive or active external rewarming for mild hypothermia. *Passive* or *spontaneous rewarming* involves moving the patient to a warm, dry place; removing damp clothing; using radiant lights; and placing warm blankets on the patient. *Active external* or *surface rewarming* involves fluid- or air-filled warming blankets, or warm (98.6° to 104°F [37° to 40°C]) water immersion.[20] Closely monitor the patient for marked vasodilation and hypotension during rewarming.

Use *active internal* or *core rewarming* for moderate to severe hypothermia. This refers to the application of heat directly to the core. Techniques include (1) heated (up to 111.2°F [44°C]), humidified O₂; (2) warmed IV fluids (up to 98.6°F [37°C]); (3) peritoneal lavage with warmed fluids (up to 113°F [45°C]); and (4) extracorporeal circulation with cardiopulmonary bypass, rapid fluid infuser, or hemodialysis.[20]

Gentle handling is essential to prevent stimulation of the cold myocardium. Carefully monitor core temperature during rewarming procedures. Rewarming places the patient at risk for *afterdrop*, a further drop in core temperature. This occurs when cold peripheral blood returns to the central circulation. Rewarming shock can produce hypotension and dysrhythmias. Thus patients with moderate to severe hypothermia should have the core warmed before the extremities. Discontinue active rewarming once the core temperature reaches 89.6° to 93.2°F (32° to 34°C).[19]

Patient teaching focuses on how to avoid future cold-related problems. Essential information includes dressing in layers for cold weather, covering the head, carrying high-carbohydrate foods for extra calories, and developing a plan for survival should an injury occur.

SUBMERSION INJURIES

Submersion injury results when an individual becomes hypoxic as the result of submersion in a substance, usually water. More than 50,000 submersion events and approximately 4000 deaths from drowning occur each year in the United States. Most of the victims are children younger than 5 years of age or boys and men between ages 15 and 25. The primary risk factors for submersion injury include inability to swim, use of alcohol or drugs, trauma, seizures, hypothermia, stroke, and child neglect.

Drowning is death from suffocation after submersion in water or other fluid. *Near-drowning* is survival from a potential drowning. *Immersion syndrome* occurs with immersion in cold water. This leads to stimulation of the vagus nerve and potentially fatal dysrhythmias (e.g., bradycardia, cardiac arrest).

Some near-drowning victims do not aspirate water (i.e., *dry drowning*) but do develop potentially life-threatening bronchospasm and airway obstruction. Near-drowning victims who do aspirate water develop pulmonary edema. Regardless of what type of fluid is aspirated, the end result is acute respiratory distress syndrome[20] (see Chapter 68). The osmotic gradient caused by aspirated fluid leads to fluid imbalances in the body. Hypotonic freshwater is rapidly absorbed into the circulatory system through the alveoli. Freshwater is often contaminated with chlorine, mud, or algae. This causes the breakdown of lung surfactant, fluid seepage, and pulmonary edema. Hypertonic saltwater draws fluid from the vascular space into the alveoli, impairing alveolar ventilation and resulting in hypoxia. Fig. 69-4 shows the pulmonary effects of saltwater and freshwater aspiration. The body attempts to compensate for hypoxia by shunting blood to the lungs. This results in increased pulmonary pressures and deteriorating respiratory status. More and more blood is shunted through the alveoli. However, the blood is not adequately oxygenated, and hypoxemia worsens. This can result in cerebral injury, edema, and brain death.

Table 69-10 lists the assessment findings of a patient with a submersion injury. Aggressive resuscitation efforts (e.g., airway and ventilation management), especially in the prehospital phase, improve survival of near-drowning victims.[20]

Collaborative Care

Treatment of submersion injuries focuses on correcting hypoxia and fluid imbalances, supporting basic physiologic functions, and rewarming when hypothermia is present. Initial evaluation involves assessment of airway, cervical spine, breathing, and circulation. Table 69-10 lists other interventions.

PATHOPHYSIOLOGY MAP

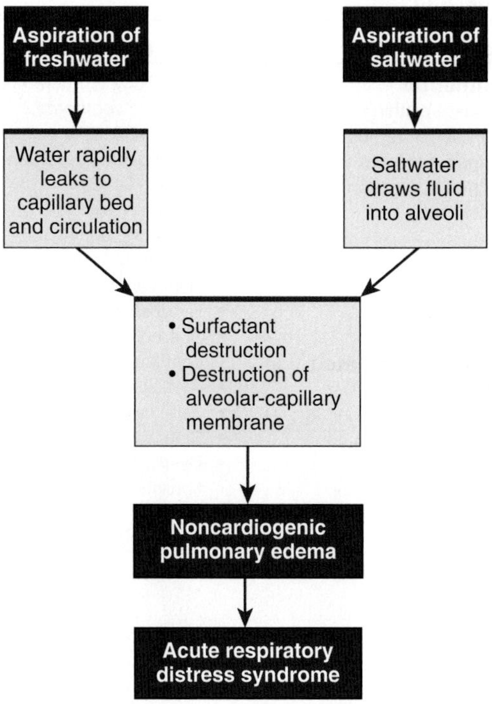

FIG. 69-4 Pathophysiology of submersion injury.

Mechanical ventilation with positive end-expiratory pressure or continuous positive airway pressure is used to improve gas exchange across the alveolar-capillary membrane when significant pulmonary edema is present. Ventilation and oxygenation are the primary techniques for treating respiratory failure (see Chapters 66 and 68). Mannitol (Osmitrol) or furosemide (Lasix) is used to treat cerebral edema or decrease free water.

Deterioration in neurologic status suggests cerebral edema, worsening hypoxia, or profound acidosis. Near-drowning victims may also have head and neck injuries that cause prolonged alterations in the level of consciousness. Complications can develop in patients who are essentially free of symptoms immediately after the near-drowning episode. This *secondary drowning* refers to delayed death from drowning due to pulmonary complications. Consequently, observe all victims of near-drowning in a hospital for a minimum of 23 hours.[20] Additional observation is needed for patients who have co-morbidities (e.g., heart disease).

Patient teaching focuses on water safety and how to minimize the risks for drowning. Remind patients and caregivers to lock all swimming pool gates; use life jackets on all watercrafts, including inner tubes and rafts; and learn water survival skills (e.g., swimming lessons). Emphasize the dangers of combining alcohol and drugs with swimming and other water sports.

STINGS AND BITES

Animals, spiders, snakes, and insects cause injury and even death by biting or stinging. Morbidity is a result of either direct tissue damage or lethal toxins. Direct tissue damage is a product of animal size, characteristics of the animal's teeth, and strength of the jaw. Tissue is lacerated, crushed, or chewed, while teeth, fangs, stingers, spines, or tentacles release toxins that have local

✚ TABLE 69-10 EMERGENCY MANAGEMENT

Submersion Injuries

Etiology	Assessment Findings	Interventions
• Inability to swim or exhaustion while swimming • Entrapment or entanglement with objects in water • Loss of ability to move secondary to trauma, stroke, hypothermia, myocardial infarction (MI) • Poor judgment due to alcohol or drugs • Seizure while in water	**Pulmonary** • Ineffective breathing • Dyspnea • Respiratory distress • Respiratory arrest • Crackles, rhonchi • Cough with pink-frothy sputum • Cyanosis **Cardiac** • Tachycardia • Bradycardia • Dysrhythmia • Hypotension • Cardiac arrest **Other** • Panic • Exhaustion • Coma • Coexisting illness (e.g., MI) or injury (e.g., cervical spine injury) • Core temperature slightly elevated or below normal depending on water temperature and length of submersion	**Initial** • Manage and maintain ABCs. • Assume cervical spine injury in all near-drowning victims and stabilize or immobilize cervical spine. • Provide 100% O₂ via non-rebreather mask or BVM. • Anticipate need for intubation and mechanical ventilation if airway is compromised (e.g., absent gag reflex). • Establish IV access with two large-bore catheters for fluid resuscitation and infuse warmed fluids if appropriate. • Obtain 12-lead ECG. • Assess for other injuries. • Remove wet clothing and cover with warm blankets. • Obtain temperature and begin rewarming if needed. • Obtain cervical spine and chest x-rays. • Insert gastric tube and urinary catheter. **Ongoing Monitoring** • Monitor ABCs, vital signs, level of consciousness. • Monitor O₂ saturation, heart rate and rhythm. • Monitor temperature and maintain normothermia. • Monitor for signs of acute respiratory failure. • Monitor for signs of secondary drowning.

ABCs, Airway, breathing, circulation; *BVM,* bag-valve-mask.

or systemic effects. Death associated with animal bites is due to blood loss, allergic reactions, or lethal toxins. Injuries caused by select insects, ticks, animals (e.g., dogs, cats), and humans are described here.

Hymenopteran Stings

The *Hymenoptera* family includes bees, yellow jackets, hornets, wasps, and fire ants. Stings can cause mild discomfort or life-threatening anaphylaxis (see Chapter 67). Venom may be cytotoxic, hemolytic, allergenic, or vasoactive. Symptoms may begin immediately or be delayed up to 48 hours. Reactions are more severe with multiple stings.[20] Most hymenopterans sting repeatedly. However, the domestic honey bee stings only once, usually leaving a barbed stinger with an attached venom sac in the skin so that release of venom continues. African honey bees (killer bees), which look like domestic bees, have migrated into North America. If threatened, these bees aggressively swarm and can repeatedly sting their victims (e.g., humans, animals). These attacks can be fatal.

SAFETY ALERT: Hymenopteran Stings
• Remove the stinger using a scraping motion with a fingernail, knife, or needle.
• Avoid using tweezers because they may squeeze the stinger and release more venom.
• Remove rings, watches, or any restrictive clothing around the sting site.

Symptoms vary from stinging, burning, swelling, and itching to edema, headache, fever, syncope, malaise, nausea, vomiting, wheezing, bronchospasm, laryngeal edema, and hypotension. Treatment depends on the severity of the reaction. Treat mild reactions with elevation, cool compresses, antipruritic lotions, and oral antihistamines. More severe reactions require intramuscular or IV antihistamines (e.g., diphenhydramine [Bena-

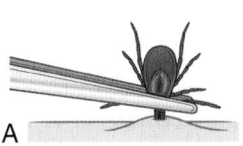 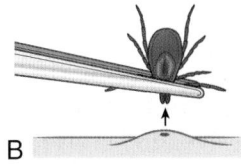

FIG. 69-5 Tick removal. **A,** Use tweezers to grasp the tick close to the skin. **B,** With a steady motion, pull the tick's body up and away from the skin. Do not be alarmed if the tick's mouthparts remain in the skin. Once the mouthparts are removed from the rest of the tick, it can no longer transmit disease.

dryl]), subcutaneous epinephrine, and corticosteroids (e.g., dexamethasone [Decadron]). Chapter 14 discusses allergic reactions and related patient teaching.

Tick Bites

Ticks live throughout the United States, but are most common in the northwestern, Rocky Mountain, and northeastern regions. Emergencies associated with tick bites include Lyme disease, Rocky Mountain spotted fever, and tick paralysis. The infected tick or the release of neurotoxin causes the disease. Ticks release neurotoxic venom as long as the tick head attaches to the body. Therefore safe removal of the tick is essential for effective treatment. Use forceps or tweezers to grasp the tick close to the point of attachment and pull upward in a steady motion (Fig. 69-5). After you remove the tick, clean the skin with soap and water. Do not use a hot match, petroleum jelly, nail polish, or other products to remove the tick, since these measures may cause a tick to salivate, thus increasing the risk for infection.[21]

Lyme disease is the most common tick-borne disease in the United States. Symptoms appear within days of a bite from the *Ixodid* (hard) tick and result from exposure to the spirochete *Borrelia burgdorferi* that lives on the tick. The initial stage of this disease is characterized by flu-like symptoms (e.g., headache, stiff neck, fatigue) and, in some patients, a characteristic bull's eye rash (i.e., an expanding circular area of redness 5 cm or more in diameter). Treatment at this stage includes doxycycline (Vibramycin). The rash will disappear even if the patient is not treated.

Monoarticular arthritis, meningitis, and neuropathies occur days or weeks after the initial symptoms. Recommended treatment includes ceftriaxone (Rocephin).[20] Chronic arthritis, peripheral radiculoneuropathy, and heart disease characterize the later stage of the disease. These illnesses can last several months to years after the initial skin lesion. (Chapter 65 discusses Lyme disease.)

Rocky Mountain spotted fever is caused by *Rickettsia rickettsii,* a bacterium that is spread to humans by the *Ixodid* tick. It has an incubation period of 2 to 14 days. A pink, macular rash appears on the palms, wrists, soles, feet, and ankles within 10 days of exposure. Other symptoms include fever, chills, malaise, myalgias, and headache. Diagnosis is often difficult in the early stages, and without treatment the disease can be fatal.[20] Antibiotic therapy with doxycycline is the treatment of choice.

Tick paralysis occurs 5 to 7 days after exposure to a neurotoxin introduced by a wood tick or dog tick. Classic symptoms are flaccid ascending paralysis, which develops over 1 to 2 days. Without tick removal, the patient dies as respiratory muscles become paralyzed. Tick removal leads to return of muscle movement, usually within 48 to 72 hours.[20]

Animal and Human Bites

Every year more than 5 million animal bites are reported in the United States. Children are at greatest risk. The most significant problems associated with animal bites are infection and mechanical destruction of skin, muscle, tendons, blood vessels, and bone. The bite may cause a simple laceration or be associated with crush injury, puncture wound, or tearing of multiple layers of tissue. The severity of injury depends on animal size, victim size, and anatomic location of the bite. Animal bites from dogs and cats are most common, with wild or domestic rodents (e.g., squirrels, hamsters) following as the third most frequently reported offenders.

Dog bites usually occur on the extremities. However, facial bites are common in small children. Most victims own the dogs that bite them. Dog bites may involve significant tissue damage with deaths reported, usually in children. A plastic surgeon should evaluate all disfiguring wounds of the face.

Cat bites cause deep puncture wounds that can involve tendons and joint capsules and result in a greater incidence of infection than with dog bites. Septic arthritis, osteomyelitis, and tenosynovitis can occur as a result of cat bites. The most common causative organisms of infections from dog and cat bites are from the *Pasteurella* species (e.g., *P. multocida*). Most healthy cats and dogs carry this organism in their mouths.

Human bites also cause puncture wounds or lacerations (Fig. 69-6). These carry a high risk of infection from oral bacterial flora, most commonly *Staphylococcus aureus, Streptococcus* organisms, and hepatitis virus. Hands, fingers, ears, nose, vagina, and penis are the most common sites of human bites and are frequently a result of violence or sexual activity. Patients with Boxer's fracture (fracture of the fourth or fifth metacarpal) often have concurrent open wounds on the knuckles from striking teeth. The human jaw has great crushing ability, causing laceration, puncture, crush injury, soft tissue tearing, and even

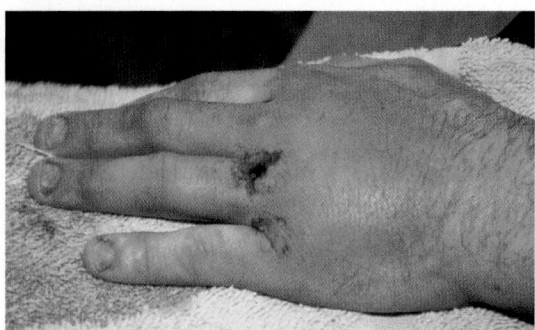

FIG. 69-6 Probable human bite injury, though denied by patient. Human bites cause extensor tendon injuries, fractures, and joint capsule injuries and can harbor foreign bodies.

amputation. Infection rates are as high as 50% when victims do not seek medical care within 24 hours of injury.

Collaborative Care. Initial treatment for animal and human bites includes cleaning with copious irrigation, debridement, tetanus prophylaxis, and analgesics as needed. Prophylactic antibiotics are used for animal and human bites at risk for infection, such as wounds over joints, those greater than 6 to 12 hours old, puncture wounds, and bites of the hand or foot. Individuals at greatest risk of infection are infants, older adults, immunosuppressed patients, alcoholics, diabetics, and people taking corticosteroids.

Leave puncture wounds open. Splint wounds over joints. Lacerations are loosely sutured. However, initial closure is used for facial wounds. The patient is admitted for IV antibiotic therapy when an infection is present. These patients have an increased incidence of cellulitis, osteomyelitis, and septic arthritis. Report animal and human bites to the police as required.

Consideration of rabies postexposure prophylaxis is an essential component in management of animal bites. A neurotoxic virus found in the saliva of some mammals causes rabies. If untreated, the condition is fatal in humans. Consider rabies exposure if an animal attack was not provoked, involves a wild animal, or involves a domestic animal not immunized against rabies. Always provide rabies postexposure prophylaxis when the animal is not found or a carnivorous wild animal causes the bite. Start the regimen with an initial, weight-based dosage of rabies immune globulin (RIG [HyperRab S/D]) to provide passive immunity. Follow this with a series of five injections of human diploid cell vaccine (HDCV [Imovax Rabies]) on days 0, 3, 7, 14, and 28 to provide active immunity.[22] (Rabies is discussed in Chapter 57.)

DRUG ALERT: Rabies Postexposure Prophylaxis
- Administer the calculated dose of RIG via infiltration around the wound edges.
- Administer any remaining volume of RIG intramuscularly at a site distant from the vaccine site (e.g., gluteal site for bite wounds on the arm).
- Administer the HDCV intramuscularly in the deltoid.

POISONINGS

A poison is any chemical that harms the body. More than 5 million cases of human poisonings occur each year in the United States.[23] Poisonings can be accidental, occupational, recreational, or intentional. Natural or manufactured toxins can be ingested, inhaled, injected, splashed in the eye, or absorbed through the skin. Table 69-11 presents common poisons.

TABLE 69-11 COMMON POISONS

Poison	Manifestations	Treatment
Acetaminophen (Tylenol)	*Phase 1* (within 24 hr of ingestion): Malaise, diaphoresis, nausea and vomiting *Phase 2* (24-28 hr after ingestion): Right upper quadrant pain, decreased urine output, diminished nausea, increase in LFTs *Phase 3* (72-96 hr after ingestion): Nausea and vomiting, malaise, jaundice, hypoglycemia, enlarged liver, possible coagulopathies, including DIC *Phase 4* (7-8 days after ingestion): Recovery, resolution of symptoms, LFTs return to normal	Activated charcoal, *N*-acetylcysteine (oral form may cause vomiting, IV form can be used)
Acids and alkalis • *Acids:* Toilet bowl cleaners, antirust compounds • *Alkalis:* Drain cleaners, dishwashing detergents, ammonia	Excess salivation, dysphagia, epigastric pain, pneumonitis; burns of mouth, esophagus, and stomach	Immediate dilution (water, milk), corticosteroids (for alkali burns), induced vomiting is contraindicated
• Aspirin and aspirin-containing medications	Tachypnea, tachycardia, hyperthermia, seizures, pulmonary edema, occult bleeding or hemorrhage, metabolic acidosis	Activated charcoal, gastric lavage, urine alkalinization, hemodialysis for severe acute ingestion, intubation and mechanical ventilation, supportive care
Bleaches	Irritation of lips, mouth, and eyes, superficial injury to esophagus; chemical pneumonia and pulmonary edema	Washing of exposed skin and eyes, dilution with water and milk, gastric lavage, prevention of vomiting and aspiration
Carbon monoxide	Dyspnea, headache, tachypnea, confusion, impaired judgment, cyanosis, respiratory depression	Removal from source, administration of 100% O_2 via non-rebreather mask, BVM, or intubation and mechanical ventilation; consider hyperbaric O_2 therapy
Cyanide	Almond odor to breath, headache, dizziness, nausea, confusion, hypertension, bradycardia followed by hypotension and tachycardia, tachypnea followed by bradypnea and respiratory arrest	Amyl nitrate (nasally), IV sodium nitrate, IV sodium thiosulfate, supportive care
Ethylene glycol	Sweet aromatic odor to breath, nausea and vomiting, slurred speech, ataxia, lethargy, respiratory depression	Activated charcoal, gastric lavage, supportive care
Iron	Vomiting (often bloody), diarrhea (often bloody), fever, hyperglycemia, lethargy, hypotension, seizures, coma	Gastric lavage, chelation therapy (deferoxamine [Desferal])
Nonsteroidal antiinflammatory drugs	Gastroenteritis, abdominal pain, drowsiness, nystagmus, hepatic and renal damage	Activated charcoal, gastric lavage, supportive care
Tricyclic antidepressants (e.g., amitriptyline [Elavil])	*In low doses:* Anticholinergic effects, agitation, hypertension, tachycardia *In high doses:* Central nervous system depression, dysrhythmias, hypotension, respiratory depression	Multidose activated charcoal, gastric lavage, serum alkalinization with sodium bicarbonate, intubation and mechanical ventilation, supportive care; never induce vomiting
Alcohol, barbiturates, benzodiazepines, cocaine, hallucinogens, stimulants	See Chapter 11	See Chapter 11

BVM, Bag-valve-mask; *DIC,* disseminated intravascular coagulation; *LFTs,* liver function tests.

Chapter 11 discusses other poisonings related to the use of illegal drugs such as amphetamines, opioids, and hallucinogens. Poisoning may also be due to toxic plants or contaminated foods. (Chapter 42 discusses food poisoning.)

Severity of the poisoning depends on type, concentration, and route of exposure. Toxins can affect every tissue of the body, so symptoms can be seen in any body system. Specific management of toxins involves decreasing absorption, enhancing elimination, and implementing toxin-specific interventions. Consult the local poison control center 24 hours a day for the most current treatment protocols for specific poisons.[24]

Options for decreasing absorption of poisons include activated charcoal, dermal cleansing, eye irrigation, and, less frequently, gastric lavage. Gastric lavage involves oral insertion of a large-diameter (36F to 42F) gastric tube for irrigation of copious amounts of saline. Elevate the head of the bed or place the patient on the side to prevent aspiration. Patients with an altered level of consciousness or diminished gag reflex are intubated before lavage. Patients who ingest caustic agents, co-ingest sharp objects, or ingest nontoxic substances should not receive lavage. Perform gastric lavage within 1 hour of ingestion of most poisons to be effective.[23] Problems associated with lavage include esophageal perforation and aspiration.

The most common and effective intervention for management of poisonings is administration of activated charcoal orally or via a gastric tube within 1 hour of poison ingestion.[23] Many toxins adhere to charcoal and pass through the gastrointestinal (GI) tract rather than being absorbed into the circulation. Activated charcoal does not absorb ethanol, hydrocarbons, alkali, iron, boric acid, lithium, methanol, or cyanide. Adults receive 50 to 100 g of charcoal. For some toxins (e.g., phenobarbital, digoxin) multiple-dose charcoal may be required.[25] Contraindications to charcoal administration include diminished bowel sounds, ileus, and ingestion of a substance poorly absorbed by charcoal. Charcoal can absorb and neutralize antidotes (e.g., *N*-acetylcysteine [Mucomyst] for acetaminophen toxicity). Do not give these immediately before, with, or shortly after charcoal.[25]

Skin and ocular decontamination involves removal of toxins from skin and eyes using copious amounts of water or saline.[26] Most toxins, with the exception of mustard gas, can be safely removed with water or saline. Water mixes with mustard gas and releases chlorine gas. As a rule, brush dry substances from the skin and clothing before using water. Do not remove powdered lime with water. It should just be brushed off. Wear personal protective equipment (e.g., gloves, gowns, goggles, respirators) for decontamination to prevent secondary exposure. Decontamination procedures are usually done by those specially trained in hazardous material decontamination before the patient arrives at the hospital and again at the hospital, if necessary. Decontamination takes priority over all interventions except those needed for basic life support.

The administration of cathartics, whole-bowel irrigation, hemodialysis, urine alkalinization, chelating agents, and antidotes increases the elimination of poisons. Cathartics, such as sorbitol, are given together with the first dose of activated charcoal to stimulate intestinal motility and increase elimination.[23] Avoid multiple doses of cathartics because of potentially fatal electrolyte abnormalities. Whole-bowel irrigation is controversial and involves administration of a nonabsorbable bowel evacuant solution (e.g., GoLYTELY). Administer the solution every 4 to 6 hours until stools are clear. This process can be effective for swallowed objects, such as cocaine-filled balloons or condoms, and heavy metals such as lead and mercury.[25] There is a high risk of electrolyte imbalance caused by fluid and electrolyte losses with this approach.

Hemodialysis is reserved for patients who develop severe acidosis from ingestion of toxic substances (e.g., aspirin). Other interventions include alkalinization and chelation therapy. Sodium bicarbonate administration raises the pH (greater than 7.5), which is particularly effective for phenobarbital and salicylate poisoning. Vitamin C is added to IV fluids to enhance excretion of amphetamines and quinidine. Chelation therapy is considered for heavy metal poisoning (e.g., edetate calcium disodium [calcium EDTA] for lead poisoning). A limited number of true antidotes are available, and many of these agents are themselves toxic.[25]

Focus patient teaching for toxic emergencies on how the poisoning occurred. Arrange for an evaluation and follow-up by a mental health professional for all patients who experience poisoning because of a suicide attempt or substance abuse. The Occupational Safety and Health Administration should evaluate all poisoning related to an occupational hazard.[27]

VIOLENCE

Violence is the acting out of the emotions of fear and/or anger to cause harm to someone or something. It may be the result of organic disease (e.g., temporal lobe epilepsy), psychosis (e.g., schizophrenia), or antisocial behavior (e.g., assault, murder). The patient cared for in the ED may be the victim or the perpetrator of violence. Violence can take place in a variety of settings, including the home, community, and workplace. EDs have been identified as high-risk areas for *workplace violence*.[28] Measures to protect staff include the use of on-site security personnel and police officers, metal detectors, surveillance cameras, and locked access doors. The ENA supports comprehensive workplace violence prevention plans and recommends that they be implemented and evaluated in every ED.[28]

Family and intimate partner violence (IPV) is a pattern of coercive behavior in a relationship that involves fear; humiliation; intimidation; neglect; or intentional physical, emotional, financial, or sexual injury (see Chapter 54 for information on sexual assault). The ENA encourages ED nurses to become certified *sexual assault nurse examiners* (SANEs). The SANE nurse provides expert emergency care, collects and documents evidence, participates in staff and community education, and advocates for sexual assault and rape victims.[29]

IPV is found in all professions, cultures, socioeconomic groups, age-groups, and genders. Although men can be victims of family violence and IPV, most victims are women, children, and older adults. Each year, more than 5 million women and 3 million men are treated in EDs for *battery* (assault) by spouses, caregivers, or individuals known to them. As many as 20% of battered women are pregnant at the time of the assault.[29]

In the ED, you need to screen for family violence and IPV (e.g., Do you feel safe at home? Is anyone hurting you?). Routine screening for this risk factor is required.[29] Barriers to conducting effective screening include limited privacy in the ED, lack of time, and lack of knowledge about how to ask about family violence and IPV. The development and implementation of policies, procedures, and staff education programs do improve screening practices.[28]

Initiate appropriate interventions for patients who you suspect or find are victims of abuse. These include making referrals, providing emotional support, and informing victims about their options (e.g., safe house, legal rights).[30] See Resources at the end of this chapter for additional information on family violence and IPV.

AGENTS OF TERRORISM

The threat of terrorism is an ongoing concern. Terrorism involves overt actions such as the dispensing of nuclear, biologic, or chemical (NBC) agents as weapons for the express purpose of causing harm. Prompt recognition and identification of potential health hazards are essential in the preparedness of health care professionals.

Biologic agents most commonly used in terrorist attacks include anthrax, smallpox, botulism, plague, tularemia, and hemorrhagic fever. eTable 69-2 (available on the website for this chapter) summarizes general information regarding select biologic agents of terrorism. Anthrax, plague, and tularemia are treated effectively with antibiotics if sufficient supplies are available and the organisms are not resistant. Smallpox can be prevented or the incidence reduced by vaccination, even when first given after exposure. Botulism is treated with antitoxin though several vaccines are being studied. There is no established treatment for most viruses that cause hemorrhagic fever.[31]

Chemicals are also used as agents of terrorism and are categorized according to their target organ or effect.[32] (See eTable 69-3 on the website for this chapter.) For example, sarin is a highly toxic nerve gas that can cause death within minutes of exposure. It enters the body through the eyes and skin and acts by paralyzing the respiratory muscles. Antidotes for nerve agent poisoning include atropine (AtroPen) and pralidoxime chloride (2-PAM chloride). Multiple doses may be needed to reverse the effects of the nerve agents.

Phosgene is a colorless gas normally used in chemical manufacturing. If inhaled at high concentrations for a long enough period, it causes severe respiratory distress, pulmonary edema, and death. Mustard gas is yellow to brown and has a garlic-like odor. The gas irritates the eyes and causes skin burns and blisters. Protocols to treat victims of chemical exposure vary and relate to the specific agent.[32]

Radiologic or nuclear agents represent another category of agents of terrorism. *Radiologic dispersal devices* (RDDs), also known as "dirty bombs," consist of a mix of explosives and radioactive material (e.g., pellets). When the device is detonated, the blast scatters radioactive dust, smoke, and other material into the surrounding environment, resulting in radioactive contamination.[33]

The main danger from an RDD results from the explosion, which can cause serious injuries to the victims. The radioactive materials used in an RDD (e.g., uranium, iodine-131) do not usually generate enough radiation to cause immediate serious illness, except to those victims who are in close proximity to the explosion. However, the radioactive dust and smoke can spread and cause illness if inhaled. Since radiation cannot be seen, smelled, felt, or tasted, you should initiate measures to limit contamination (e.g., covering the patient's nose and mouth) and provide for decontamination (e.g., shower).[33,34]

Ionizing radiation, such as that from a nuclear bomb or damage to a nuclear reactor, represents a serious threat to the safety of victims and the environment. Exposure to ionizing radiation may or may not include skin contamination with radioactive material. Initiate decontamination procedures immediately if external radioactive contaminants are present. *Acute radiation syndrome* (ARS) develops after a substantial exposure to ionizing radiation and follows a predictable pattern.[32,35] (For additional information on ARS, see *www.bt.cdc.gov/radiation/arsphysicianfactsheet.asp.*)

Explosive devices (e.g., TNT, dynamite) that are used as agents of terrorism result in one or more of the following types of injuries: blast, crush, or penetrating. Blast injuries result from the supersonic overpressurization shock wave caused by the explosion. This shock wave primarily damages the lungs, GI tract, and middle ear. Crush injuries (i.e., blunt trauma) often result from explosions in confined spaces causing structural collapse (e.g., falling debris). Some explosive devices contain materials that are projected during the explosion (e.g., shrapnel), leading to penetrating injuries.

EMERGENCY AND MASS CASUALTY INCIDENT PREPAREDNESS

The term emergency usually refers to any extraordinary event (e.g., multi-vehicle crash) that requires a rapid and skilled response and that the community's existing resources can manage. An emergency is differentiated from a mass casualty incident (MCI) in that an MCI is a man-made (e.g., involving NBC agents) or natural (e.g., hurricane) event or disaster that overwhelms a community's ability to respond with existing resources. MCIs usually involve large numbers of victims, physical and emotional suffering, and permanent changes within a community. In addition, MCIs always require assistance from resources outside the affected community (e.g., American Red Cross, Federal Emergency Management Agency [FEMA]) (Fig. 69-7).

When an emergency or an MCI occurs, first responders (e.g., police, emergency medical personnel) are sent to the scene. Triage of victims of an emergency or an MCI differs from the usual triage described earlier. Several systems exist, and many

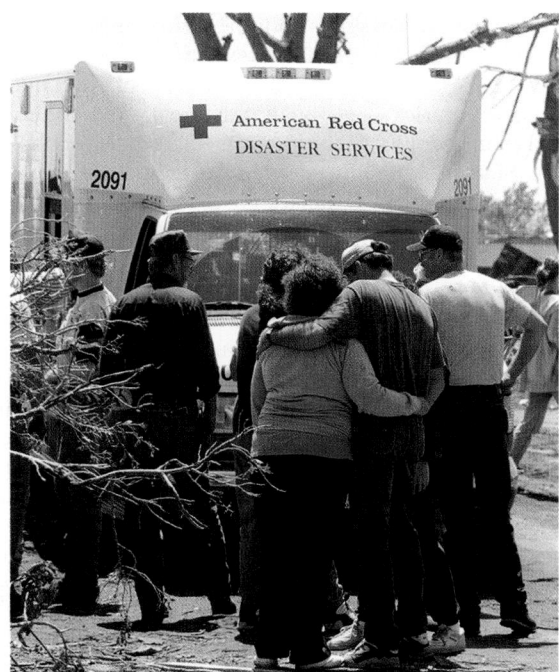

FIG. 69-7 American Red Cross.

ETHICAL/LEGAL DILEMMAS

Good Samaritan

Situation
You are a registered nurse, employed as a charge nurse at a subacute rehabilitation facility. It is midnight and you are driving home from work when you see a motor vehicle collision with a person at the side of the road waving and yelling for help. You stop and call 911 to report the incident. What do you do next?

Ethical/Legal Points for Consideration
- As a licensed health care provider, you are under no legal obligation to stop and render aid.
- If you do stop, you assume an obligation not to leave the scene until sufficiently trained first responders arrive and assume control.
- Between 50 and 75 yr ago, many states moved to encourage trained health care providers to stop and render aid by passing "Good Samaritan" statutes. These statutes, which vary somewhat from state to state, offer immunity from lawsuit for bystanders who offer aid in emergencies except in the case of gross negligence.
- A Good Samaritan must not be in the place of employment or under employment conditions.
- An example of gross negligence might be refusing to assist someone who obviously had a serious hemorrhage in favor of a person with a minor injury because the bleeding person looked old and disheveled.
- Immunity covers only the scene of the accident and not subsequent care under the supervision of health care providers.
- If there is a national disaster, an act of terrorism, or a major emergent need for health care personnel, you may be required to go to an assigned site to offer aid. You would not be covered by the Good Samaritan Act under these circumstances.

Discussion Questions
1. What factors do you think contribute to a health care provider's decision whether to stop to provide aid?
2. What basic aid would you feel comfortable providing if you do not have an emergency or trauma background?
3. Would your professional liability (malpractice) insurance cover you if someone claimed that you acted negligently while providing assistance?

use colored tags to designate both the seriousness of the injury and the likelihood of survival. One system uses green for minor injuries (e.g., sprains) and yellow for urgent, but not life-threatening injuries (e.g., open fractures). Red indicates a life-threatening injury requiring immediate intervention (e.g., shock). Blue indicates those who are expected to die (e.g., massive head trauma), and black identifies the dead.[36]

Triage of victims of an emergency or an MCI must be conducted in less than 15 seconds. In general, two thirds of victims are tagged green or yellow, and the remaining are tagged red, blue, or black. Victims need to be treated and stabilized and, if there is known or suspected contamination, decontaminated at the scene. After this, they are transported to hospitals. Many other victims arrive at hospitals on their own (i.e., walking wounded). The total number of victims a hospital can expect is estimated by doubling the number of victims who arrive in the first hour. Generally, 30% of victims require admission to the hospital, and half of these need surgery within 8 hours.

In addition to the services provided by first responders, many communities have developed *community emergency response teams* (CERTs). CERTs are recognized by FEMA as important partners in emergency preparedness. The CERT training helps citizens understand their personal responsibility in preparing for a natural or man-made disaster. In addition, participants are taught what to expect after a disaster and how to safely help themselves, their family, and their neighbors. Training includes lifesaving skills with emphasis on decision making and rescuer safety. CERTs are an extension of the first responder services. They can offer immediate help to victims and organize untrained volunteers to assist until professional services arrive.[37]

All health care providers have a role in emergency and MCI preparedness. Knowledge of the hospital's *emergency response plan* is essential. This includes individual roles and responsibilities of the members of the response team plus participation in emergency/MCI preparedness drills on a regular basis. Several types of drills can assess a hospital's level of emergency pre-paredness. These include hospital disaster drills, computer simulations, and tabletop exercises. Drills allow health care providers to become familiar with the emergency response procedures.[38]

Response to MCIs often requires the aid of a federal agency. The National Incident Management System (NIMS) is a section within the U.S. Department of Homeland Security. NIMS is responsible for coordinating federal, state, and local government efforts to respond to and manage domestic MCIs.[39] One important aspect of NIMS is the development of the *Incident Command System* (ICS). This standardized organizational structure provides for the management of all incidents. NIMS requires that all emergency services–related disciplines (e.g., hospitals, health care providers, emergency response services) wishing to participate in the emergency management of disasters must be NIMS and ICS trained. You can take courses online and at no cost *(http://training.fema.gov/is/nims.asp)*.

The National Disaster Medical System (NDMS) is a part of the U.S. Department of Health and Human Services, Office of Preparedness and Response. The NDMS expands the nation's medical response capability by organizing and training volunteer disaster medical assistance teams (DMATs). Each DMAT consists of members with a variety of health or medical skills and those with specialized support skills (e.g., communications, logistics, security). DMATs are sent to disaster sites with enough supplies and equipment to remain self-sufficient for 72 hours while providing medical care. DMAT personnel are deployed for a period of 2 weeks.[40]

All disasters result in psychologic stress to the individuals involved immediately after the event. This stress can persist for an extended period and is influenced, in part, by the nature of the event, the individual's age, preexisting coping mechanisms, role in the event, and medical and psychologic history. Many hospitals and DMATs have a *critical incident stress management unit*. This unit arranges group discussions to allow participants to share and validate their feelings and emotions about the experience. This is important for emotional recovery.

CASE STUDY

Trauma

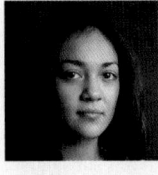
iStockphoto/Thinkstock

Patient Profile
D.F., a 20-yr-old Hispanic female trauma patient, is brought to the ED in an ambulance. She was the driver in a motor vehicle collision and was not wearing a seat belt. Two children in the car were pronounced dead at the scene. The paramedics stated that there was significant damage to the car on the driver's side.

Subjective Data
• Patient asks, "What happened? Where am I?"
• Complains of shortness of breath and leg pain

Objective Data
Physical Examination
• Vital signs: blood pressure 85/40 mm Hg, heart rate 140 beats/min, respiratory rate 36 breaths/min; O₂ saturation 85% with 100% non-rebreather mask
• Decreased breath sounds on left side of chest
• Asymmetric chest wall movement

• Glasgow Coma Score = 14; pupils slightly unequal
• Badly deformed left lower leg with significant swelling and a pedal pulse by Doppler only
• 4-cm head laceration, bleeding controlled

Discussion Questions
1. What are D.F.'s most likely life-threatening injuries?
2. *Priority Decision:* What is the priority of care for D.F.?
3. *Priority Decision:* What interventions does this patient need immediately?
4. What other interventions should you consider?
5. *Delegation Decision:* What activities could you delegate to unlicensed assistive personnel (UAP)?
6. Several family members have arrived in the ED, including the mother of one of the children who died. The second child who died was the patient's child. How should you approach the family?
7. *Priority Decision:* Based on assessment data presented, what are the priority nursing diagnoses? Are there any collaborative problems?
8. *Evidence-Based Practice:* What are the best practice guidelines for fluid resuscitation in patients who are experiencing hypovolemic shock?

BRIDGE TO NCLEX EXAMINATION

The number of the question corresponds to the same-numbered outcome at the beginning of the chapter.

1. An older man arrives in triage disoriented and tachypneic. His skin is hot and dry. His wife states that he was fine earlier today. The nurse's next priority would be to
   a. obtain a detailed medical history from his wife.
   b. assess his vital signs, including a rectal temperature.
   c. determine the kind of insurance he has before treating him.
   d. start supplemental oxygen and have the ED physician see him.

2. A patient has a core temperature of 90° F (32.2° C). The most appropriate rewarming technique would be
   a. passive rewarming with warm blankets.
   b. active internal rewarming using warmed IV fluids.
   c. passive rewarming using air-filled warming blankets.
   d. active external rewarming by submersing in a warm bath.

3. Effective interventions to decrease absorption or increase elimination of an ingested poison include which of the following (select all that apply)?
   a. Hemodialysis
   b. Milk dilution
   c. Eye irrigation
   d. Gastric lavage
   e. Activated charcoal

4. An older woman arrives in the ED complaining of severe pain in her right shoulder. The nurse notes that her clothes are soiled with urine and feces. She tells the nurse that she lives with her son and that she "fell." She is tearful and asks you if she can be admitted. What possibility should the nurse consider?
   a. Paranoia
   b. Possible cancer
   c. Family violence
   d. Orthostatic hypotension

5. A chemical explosion occurs at a nearby industrial site. The first responders report that victims are being decontaminated at the scene and approximately 125 workers will need medical evaluation and care. The nurse receiving this report should know that this will first require activation of
   a. a code blue alert.
   b. a disaster medical assistance team.
   c. the local police and fire departments.
   d. the hospital's emergency response plan.

1. b, 2. b, 3. a, d, e, 4. c, 5. d

ⓔvolve

For rationales to these answers and even more NCLEX review questions, visit *http://evolve.elsevier.com/Lewis/medsurg.*

REFERENCES

1. Gilboy N: Triage. In PK Howard, RA Steinmann, editors: *Sheehy's emergency nursing,* ed 6, St Louis, 2010, Mosby.
2. American College of Emergency Physicians: Emergency department wait times, crowding and access fact sheet, 2012. Retrieved from *www.acep.org/uploadedFiles/ACEP/News_Room/ NewsMediaResources/Media_Fact_Sheets/FINAL%20Wait%20 Times%20Crowding%20and%20Access.pdf.*
3. Emergency Nurses Association: Welcome to BCEN. Retrieved from *www.bcencertifications.org/Pages/default.aspx.aspx.*
4. Rund DA, Rausch TS: *Triage,* St Louis, 1981, Mosby. (Classic)
5. Gilboy N, Tanabe P, Travers DA, et al: *Emergency Severity Index (ESI): a triage tool for emergency department, version 4: Implementation handbook 2012 edition,* AHRQ Pub No. 12-0014, Rockville, Md, 2011, Agency for Healthcare Research and Quality. Retrieved from *www.ahrq.gov/research/esi.*
6. Emergency Nurses Association, American College of Emergency Physicians: Standardized ED triage scale and acuity categorization. Retrieved from *www.ena.org/SiteCollection Documents/Position%20Statements/STANDARDIZEDED TRIAGESCALEANDACUITYCATEGORIZATION.pdf.*
7. O'Neal JV: Airway management. In BB Hammond, PG Zimmermann, editors: *Sheehy's manual of emergency care,* ed 7, St Louis, 2013, Mosby.
8. Cerepani MJ: Orthopedic and neurovascular trauma. In PK Howard, RA Steinmann, editors: *Sheehy's emergency nursing,* ed 6, St Louis, 2010, Mosby.
9. Solheim J: Assessment and stabilization of the trauma patient. In BB Hammond, PG Zimmermann, editors: *Sheehy's manual of emergency care,* ed 7, St Louis, 2013, Mosby.
*10. American Association of Critical-Care Nurses: AACN practice alert: family presence during CPR and invasive procedures.

Retrieved from *www.aacn.org/WD/Practice/Docs/PracticeAlerts/ Family%20Presence%2004-2010%20final.pdf.*
11. Emergency Nurses Association: Family presence at the bedside during invasive procedures and resuscitation. Retrieved from *www.ena.org/SiteCollectionDocuments/Position%20Statements/ FamilyPresence.pdf.*
12. American Society for Pain Management Nursing, Emergency Nurses Association, American College of Emergency Physicians, American Pain Society: Optimizing the treatment of pain in patients with acute presentations. Retrieved from *www.ena.org/SiteCollectionDocuments/Position%20Statements/ Pain_Mgmt_pol.pdf.*
13. Harris C: Abdominal trauma. In BB Hammond, PG Zimmermann, editors: *Sheehy's manual of emergency care,* ed 7, St Louis, 2013, Mosby.
14. Centers for Disease Control and Prevention: Disaster information: tetanus prevention after a disaster. Retrieved from *www.bt.cdc.gov/disasters/disease/tetanus.asp.*
15. Bucher L, Buruschkin R, Kenyon D, et al: Improving outcomes with therapeutic hypothermia, *Nurs Crit Care* 7:22, 2012.
*16. O'Gara P, Kushner FG, Ascheim DD, et al: 2013 ACCF/AHA guideline for the management of ST-elevation myocardial infarction, *J Am Coll Cardiol* 61:e78, 2013.
17. Emergency Nurses Association: End-of-life care in the emergency department. Retrieved from *www.ena.org/ SiteCollectionDocuments/Position%20Statements/EndofLife CareintheEmergencyDepartment.pdf.*
18. United Network for Organ Sharing: Professional education. Retrieved from *www.unos.org/resources/UNOSprofessional Resources.asp.*
19. Samaras N, Chevalley T, Samaras D, et al: Older patients in the emergency department: a review, *Ann Emerg Med* 56:261, 2010.
20. Hammond BB, Zimmermann PG, editors: *Sheehy's manual of emergency care,* ed 7, St Louis, 2013, Mosby.

*Evidence-based information for clinical practice.

21. Centers for Disease Control and Prevention: Tick removal. Retrieved from *www.cdc.gov/lyme/removal/index.html*.

22. Denke NJ: Wound management. In PK Howard, RA Steinmann, editors: *Sheehy's emergency nursing*, ed 6, St Louis, 2010, Mosby.

23. Sturt P: Toxicologic emergencies. In PK Howard, RA Steinmann, editors: *Sheehy's emergency nursing*, ed 6, St Louis, 2010, Mosby.

24. National Capital Poison Control Center: Act fast. Retrieved from *www.poison.org/actFast/1800.asp*.

25. Lehne RA: *Pharmacology for nursing care*, ed 7, St Louis, 2010, Mosby.

26. Egging D: Ocular emergencies. In PK Howard, RA Steinmann, editors: *Sheehy's emergency nursing*, ed 6, St Louis, 2010, Mosby.

27. Occupational Health and Safety Administration: Occupational injury and illness recording and reporting requirements. Retrieved from *www.osha.gov/pls/oshaweb/owadisp.show _document?p_table=FEDERAL_REGISTER&p_id=16312*.

28. Emergency Nurses Association: Violence in the emergency setting. Retrieved from *www.ena.org/SiteCollectionDocuments/ Position%20Statements/Violence_in_the_Emergency_Care _Setting_-_ENA_PS.pdf*.

29. Emergency Nurses Association: Intimate partner and family violence, maltreatment, and neglect. Retrieved from *www .ena.org/SiteCollectionDocuments/Position%20Statements/ Violence_-_Intimate_Partner_and_Family_-_ENA_PS.pdf*.

*30. Nelson HD, Bougatsos C, Blazina I: Screening women for intimate partner violence: a systematic review to update the U.S. Preventive Services Task Force recommendation, *Ann Intern Med* 156:796, 2012.

31. Centers for Disease Control and Prevention: Viral hemorrhagic fevers. Retrieved from *www.cdc.gov/ncidod/dvrd/spb/mnpages/ dispages/vhf.htm*.

32. Andress K: Nuclear, biologic, and chemical agents of mass destruction. In PK Howard, RA Steinmann, editors: *Sheehy's emergency nursing*, ed 6, St Louis, 2010, Mosby.

33. Centers for Disease Control and Prevention: Frequently asked questions about dirty bombs. Retrieved from *www.bt.cdc.gov/ radiation/dirtybombs.asp*.

34. Emergency Nurses Association: Hazardous material exposure. Retrieved from *www.ena.org/SiteCollectionDocuments/Position% 20Statements/Hazardous_Material_Exposure_-_ENA_PS.pdf*.

35. Military Medical Operations Armed Forces Radiobiology Research Institute: Medical management of radiological casualties. Retrieved from *www.usuhs.mil/afrri/outreach/ pdf/3edmmrchandbook.pdf*.

*36. Lerner EB, Schwartz RB, Coule PL, et al: Mass casualty triage: an evaluation of the data and development of a proposed

national guideline, *Disaster Med Public Health Preparedness* 2:S25, 2008. (Classic)

37. Community Emergency Response Team: About CERT. Retrieved from *www.citizencorps.gov/cert/about.shtm*.

*38. Agency for Healthcare Research and Quality: Evidence report/ technology assessment number 95: training of hospital staff to respond to a mass casualty incident. Retrieved from *archive. ahrq.gov/downloads/pub/evidence/pdf/hospmci/hospmci.pdf*.

39. Robinson KS: Emergency preparedness. In PK Howard, RA Steinmann, editors: *Sheehy's emergency nursing*, ed 6, St Louis, 2010, Mosby.

40. US Department of Health and Human Services: Disaster medical assistance teams. Retrieved from *www.phe.gov/ Preparedness/responders/ndms/teams/Pages/dmat.aspx*.

RESOURCES

American College of Emergency Physicians
www.acep.org
American Nurses Association, Disaster Preparedness and Response
www.nursingworld.org/MainMenuCategories/WorkplaceSafety/DPR
American Red Cross
www.redcross.org
American Trauma Society
www.amtrauma.org
Association of Emergency Physicians (AEP)
www.aep.org
Centers for Disease Control and Prevention, Emergency Preparedness and Response
www.bt.cdc.gov
Emergency Nurses Association (ENA)
www.ena.org
Federal Emergency Management Agency (FEMA)
www.fema.gov
National Capital Poison Center
www.poison.org
National Coalition Against Domestic Violence
www.ncadv.org
National Domestic Violence Hotline
www.ndvh.org
National Response Center
www.nrc.uscg.mil/index.htm
US Department of Health and Human Services, Public Health Emergency
www.ndms.dhhs.gov/index.html
US Department of Justice, Office on Violence Against Women
www.ovw.usdoj.gov

CASE STUDY

Managing Multiple Patients

You are working in a 12-bed intensive care unit and have been assigned to care for the following two patients. There is one UAP available to help as needed.

Patients

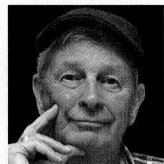

iStockphoto/Thinkstock

R.K. is a 72-year-old white man who was admitted with a massive stroke after collapsing on the street. He is unresponsive, even to painful stimuli. He has an oral endotracheal (ET) tube in place and is receiving mechanical ventilation (assist-control mode, FIO_2 70%, VT 700 mL, respiratory rate 16 breaths/min, PEEP 5 cm H_2O). His chest x-ray revealed right lower lung consolidation. A subclavian central line was placed to monitor CVP and administer fluids. IV antibiotics have been started. His cardiac rhythm on admission was atrial fibrillation with a rapid ventricular response. He is receiving IV diltiazem (Cardizem) and his ventricular response has slowed to 84 bpm. His temperature is elevated despite receiving acetaminophen q 4 hr. He is also receiving enteral feeding at 25 mL/hr via small-bore nasogastric feeding tube and has an external condom catheter for urinary drainage.

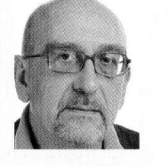

iStockphoto/Thinkstock

J.N. is a 55-year-old white man who was admitted 24 hours ago after emergent surgery for an acutely ischemic bowel. The surgical procedure involved extensive abdominal surgery to repair a perforated colon, irrigate the abdominal cavity, and provide hemostasis. During surgery his systolic BP dropped to 70 mm Hg. Seven units of packed red blood cells and 4 L of 0.9% saline were infused. His pulmonary status worsened within 12 hours of admission to the ICU, requiring an emergent ET intubation. He developed a pneumothorax after intubation and a left-side chest tube was placed at that time. His hypoxemia has rapidly progressed and is currently refractory to 100% FIO_2 and high levels of PEEP. His laboratory test results indicate kidney and liver failure. He has an advance directive that indicates he does not want to be kept alive by artificial means, but he has a full code status. He is currently sedated, paralyzed, and unable to communicate. His urinary catheter is draining concentrated urine <30 mL/hr. He has a central line in place and is receiving 0.9% saline at 125 mL/hr. His most recent ABGs are as follows: pH 7.12, PaO_2 50 mm Hg, $PaCO_2$ 62 mm Hg, HCO_3 17 mEq/L, and O_2 saturation 84%. His PaO_2/FIO_2 ratio is <200 and his chest x-ray shows worsening bilateral interstitial infiltrates compatible with an ARDS pattern.

Management Discussion Questions

1. **Priority Decision:** After receiving report, which patient should you see first? Provide rationale.
2. **Delegation Decision:** Which tasks could you delegate to the UAP *(select all that apply)?*
   a. Record vital signs on R.K. and J.N.
   b. Suction R.K. and J.N.'s ET tubes as needed.
   c. Titrate the diltiazem IV drip downward based on R.K.'s heart rate.
   d. Talk to J.N.'s family regarding his advance directive and current code status.
3. **Priority and Delegation Decision:** As you are assessing J.N., the UAP informs you that R.K. just vomited all over his bed. Which initial action would be most appropriate?
   a. Ask the UAP to give R.K. a bath while you finish assessing J.N.
   b. Turn off the enteral tube feeding on R.K. and auscultate his lungs.
   c. Ask the UAP to inform the health care provider about J.N.'s ABG results while you assess R.K.
   d. Finish assessing R.K. and then suction R.K.'s endotracheal tube to remove any aspirated emesis.

Case Study Progression

R.K.'s lungs are clear to auscultation. Evaluation of his gastrointestinal status reveals minimal bowel sounds and a gastric residual of 200 mL even after his emesis. You elevate the head of his bed to 60 degrees, hold the tube feeding, and notify his health care provider.

4. Which intervention would you expect the health care provider to order for R.K.?
   a. Morphine sulfate 2 mg IV stat
   b. Metoclopramide (Reglan) 10 mg IV q6hr
   c. Restart enteral tube feeding while maintaining HOB elevation at 90 degrees
   d. Hold enteral tube feeding for 1 hour and restart with half-strength fluids at same rate
5. J.N.'s ABG results reflect a worsening of his ARDS. You correctly identify that these results demonstrate
   a. uncompensated respiratory acidosis.
   b. uncompensated respiratory alkalosis.
   c. partially compensated respiratory acidosis.
   d. partially compensated respiratory alkalosis.
6. **Management Decision:** You walk into J.N.'s room and find his wife whispering in his ear with her hand on the ventilator tubing, appearing to be ready to disconnect him from life support. What is your best initial action?
   a. Ask J.N.'s wife to leave the room immediately.
   b. Report the incident to the charge nurse and security immediately.
   c. Ask J.N.'s wife if you could talk to her about her husband's condition.
   d. Report the incident to J.N.'s health care provider to address J.N.'s code status.

A

Basic Life Support for Health Care Providers

Linda Bucher

Basic life support (BLS) consists of a series of actions and skills performed by the rescuer(s) based on assessment findings. The first actions the rescuer performs on finding an adult victim are to assess for responsiveness and to look for signs of breathing. This is done by tapping or shaking the victim's shoulder and asking, "Are you all right?" and scanning the victim's chest for signs of breathing. If the victim does not respond, there is no breathing or abnormal breathing (e.g., agonal gasps), and the rescuer is alone, the rescuer shouts for help. If someone responds, the rescuer sends him or her to activate the *emergency response system* (ERS) and get an *automatic external defibrillator* (AED) (if available). If no one responds, the rescuer activates the ERS, gets an AED (if available), returns to the victim, and begins *cardiopulmonary resuscitation* (CPR) and defibrillation if necessary.[1]

CARDIOPULMONARY RESUSCITATION

Cardiac arrest is characterized by the absence of a pulse and breathing in an unconscious victim. The current approach for CPR is the chest *compressions–airway–breathing* (CAB) sequence.[1]

The first step in CPR is to perform a pulse check by palpating the carotid pulse for at least 5 but no more than 10 seconds.

While maintaining a head-tilt position with one hand on the forehead, locate the victim's trachea using two or three fingers of the other hand. Slide these fingers into the groove between the trachea and the neck muscles where the carotid pulse can be felt. The technique is more easily performed on the side nearest you.

If a pulse is felt, give one rescue breath every 5 to 6 seconds (10 to 12 breaths/minute) and recheck the pulse every 2 minutes (see Fig. A-1 and Airway and Breathing below). If no pulse is felt, initiate CAB.[1]

Chest Compressions

The proper technique for providing chest compressions is shown in Fig. A-2. Chest compression technique consists of fast and deep applications of pressure on the sternum. The victim must be in the supine position when the compressions are performed. The victim must be lying on a flat, hard surface, such as a CPR board (specially designed for use in CPR), a headboard from a unit bed, or, if necessary, the floor. Position yourself close to the side of the victim's chest.

Chest compressions are combined with rescue breathing for an effective resuscitation effort of the adult victim of cardiac arrest. The compression-ventilation ratio for one- or two-rescuer CPR is 30 compressions to 2 breaths (Table A-1).

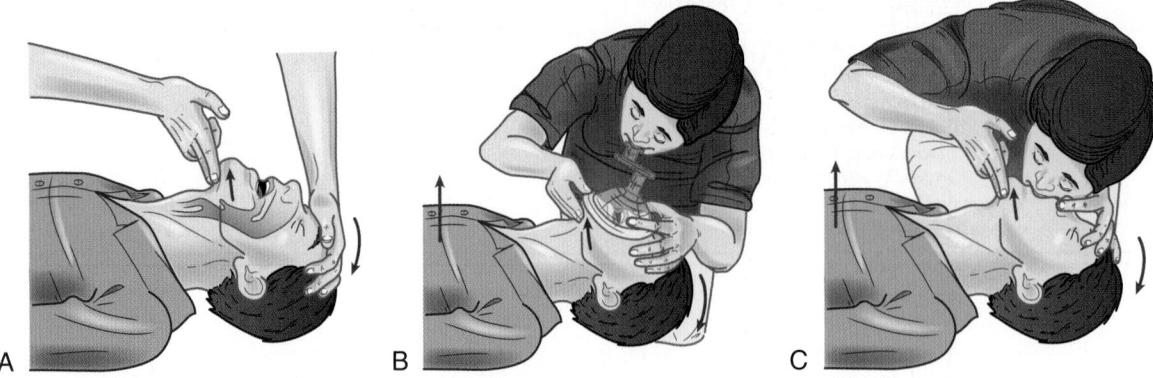

FIG. A-1 The head tilt–chin lift maneuver is used to open the victim's airway to give rescue breaths. **A,** Rescuer places one hand on the victim's forehead and applies firm, backward pressure with the palm to tilt the head back. The chin is lifted and brought forward with the fingers of the other hand. **B,** Mouth-to-barrier device: Rescuer places the device tightly over the victim's mouth and nose and delivers a regular breath. **C,** Mouth-to-mouth technique: Rescuer pinches the victim's nostrils, tightly seals mouth over victim's mouth, and delivers a regular breath. NOTE: Rescuer should observe for a rise in the victim's chest *(blue arrows)*.

Reviewed by Amber Young, RN, MSN, Instructor of Nursing, Bellin College, School of Nursing, Green Bay, Wisconsin.

TABLE A-1	**ADULT ONE- AND TWO-RESCUER BASIC LIFE SUPPORT WITH AUTOMATIC EXTERNAL DEFIBRILLATOR (AED)**

Assess
- Determine unresponsiveness: tap or shake victim's shoulder; shout, "Are you all right?"
- Check for no breathing or abnormal breathing (e.g., gasping).

Activate Emergency Response System (ERS)
- Activate ERS (e.g., call 911) and get the AED (if available) (outside of hospital).
- Call a code and ask for the AED or crash cart (in hospital).

Check for Pulse
- Feel for carotid pulse (5-10 sec).
- If victim has a pulse but is not breathing or not breathing adequately, begin rescue breathing at a rate of 1 breath every 5-6 sec (see Fig. A-1) and recheck circulation every 2 minutes.

Begin High-Quality CPR
- If there is no pulse, expose the victim's chest and immediately begin chest compressions (see Fig. A-2).
- Deliver compressions at a rate of at least 100/minute.
- Compress the chest at least 2 inches.
- Allow for complete chest recoil after each compression.
- Deliver a compression-ventilation ratio of 30 compressions to 2 breaths.
- Minimize interruptions in compressions by delivering the 2 breaths in <10 sec.

Deliver Effective Breaths
- Open airway adequately (see Fig. A-1, *A*).
- Deliver breath to produce a visible chest rise (see Fig. A-1, *B, C*).
- Avoid excessive ventilation.

Integrate Prompt Use of the AED
- Use AED as soon as possible.
- If rhythm is shockable, deliver one shock and then resume chest compressions immediately after delivery of shock.
- If the rhythm is not shockable, resume CPR and recheck rhythm every five cycles.

Continue CPR
- Continue CPR between rhythm checks and shocks, and until ACLS providers arrive or the victim shows signs of movement.

Source: American Heart Association: *BLS for healthcare providers—student manual,* Dallas, 2011, The Association.
ACLS, Advanced cardiovascular life support; *CPR,* cardiopulmonary resuscitation.

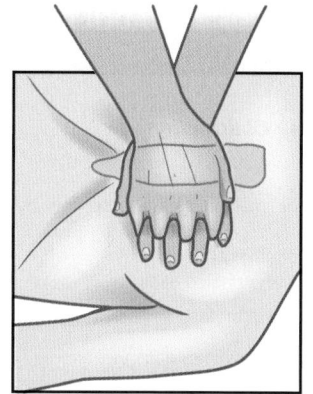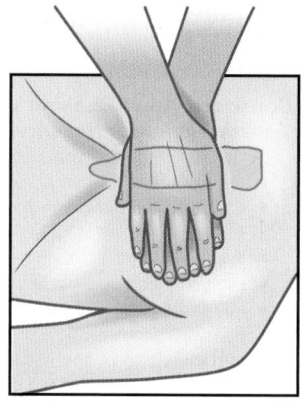
A

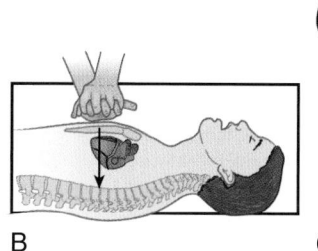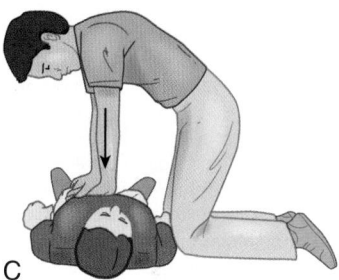
B   C

FIG. A-2 Cardiopulmonary resuscitation. **A,** Position of the hands during chest compressions. **B,** When pressure is applied, the sternum is displaced posteriorly with the heel of the hand. **C,** Arms are kept straight and the rescuer pushes deep (at least 2 in) and fast (a rate of at least 100 compressions per minute).

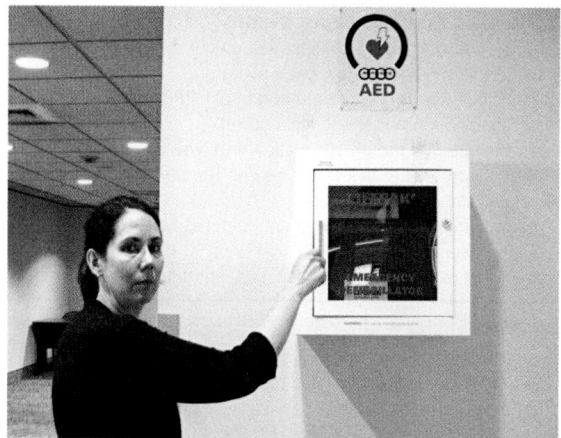

FIG. A-3 Automatic external defibrillator (AED) located in a shopping center.

If the patient has an advanced airway (e.g., endotracheal tube, laryngeal mask airway), do not pause between compressions for breaths.[1]

It is preferable to have two persons performing CPR. One rescuer, positioned at the victim's side, performs chest compressions while the second rescuer, positioned at the victim's head, maintains an open airway and performs ventilations. To maintain the quality and rate of compressions, rescuers should change roles every 2 minutes.[1] Interruptions in CPR should be limited.

Defibrillation

When the AED or advanced cardiovascular life support (ACLS) team arrives, assess the victim's rhythm. If the victim has a shockable rhythm (e.g., ventricular tachycardia, ventricular fibrillation), deliver one shock followed by five cycles of CPR before checking the rhythm again. If the rhythm is not a shockable rhythm, resume CPR and recheck the rhythm every five cycles. CPR should continue between rhythm checks and shocks, and until the ACLS team arrives or the victim shows signs of movement.[1]

The American Heart Association includes training in the use of AEDs with instruction of health care personnel and laypersons in BLS. Survival from cardiac arrest is the highest when immediate CPR is provided and defibrillation occurs within 3 to 5 minutes.[1] AEDs are found in many out-of-hospital, public settings (Fig. A-3).

Airway and Breathing

If a victim has a pulse but is gasping (e.g., agonal breathing) or not breathing, establish an open airway and begin rescue breath-

TABLE A-2   MANAGEMENT OF THE ADULT CHOKING VICTIM

Conscious Adult Choking Victim
Assess Victim for Severe Airway Obstruction
Look for any of the following signs:
- Poor or no air exchange
- Clutching the neck with the hands, making the universal choking sign
- Weak, ineffective cough or no cough at all
- High-pitched noise while inhaling or no noise at all
- Increased respiratory difficulty
- Possible cyanosis

Ask the victim if he or she is choking. If the victim nods yes and cannot talk or has any of the symptoms noted above, severe airway obstruction is present and you must take immediate action.

Abdominal Thrusts (Heimlich Maneuver) With Standing or Sitting Victim (see Fig. A-4)
1. Stand or kneel behind victim and wrap arms around the victim's waist.
2. Make fist with one hand.
3. Place thumb side of fist against victim's abdomen. Position fist midline, slightly above navel and well below breastbone.
4. Grasp fist with other hand and press fist into victim's abdomen with a quick, forceful upward thrust.
5. Give each new thrust with a separate, distinct movement to relieve the obstruction. Caution: If victim is pregnant or obese, give chest thrusts instead of abdominal thrusts. Position hands (as described) over lower portion of the breastbone and apply quick backward thrusts.
6. Repeat thrusts until object is expelled or victim becomes unresponsive.

Unconscious Adult Choking Victim
If you see a choking victim collapse and become unresponsive:
1. Activate the emergency response system.
2. Lower the victim to the ground and begin CPR, starting with compressions (do not check for a pulse).
3. Open the victim's mouth wide each time you prepare to give breaths. Look for the object. If you see the object and can easily remove it, do so with your fingers. If you do not see the object, continue with CPR using the chest compression–airway-breathing sequence (see Table A-1).
4. If efforts to ventilate are unsuccessful, continue with CPR.

Source: American Heart Association: *BLS for healthcare providers—student manual,* Dallas, 2011, The Association.

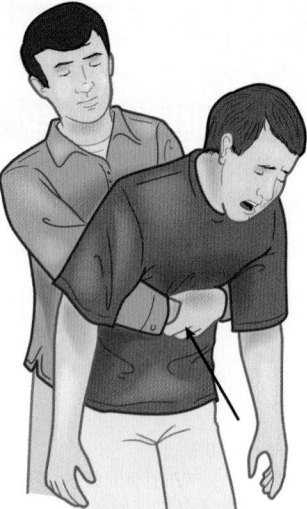

FIG. A-4 Abdominal thrusts (Heimlich maneuver) administered to a conscious (standing) choking victim.

and watch for a rise in the victim's chest. Continue rescue breaths at a rate of 10 to 12 per minute. When the victim has a tracheostomy, give ventilations through the stoma.

If the victim cannot be ventilated, proceed with CPR. When providing the next rescue breaths, look for any objects in the victim's mouth and remove them if visible (Table A-2).

HANDS-ONLY CPR

Hands-only CPR can be used to help adult victims who suddenly collapse from cardiac arrest outside of a health care setting. If you witness this event (as a bystander), you can choose to provide chest compressions only (push fast and deep in the center of the chest) or conventional CPR (described previously). Both methods are effective when done in the first few minutes of an out-of-hospital cardiac arrest.[2]

REFERENCES

1. American Heart Association: *BLS for healthcare providers—student manual,* Dallas, 2011, The Association.
2. American Heart Association: Two steps to staying alive with hands-only CPR. Retrieved from *www.heart.org/HEARTORG/CPRAndECC/HandsOnlyCPR/Hands-Only-CPR_UCM_440559_SubHomePage.jsp.*

RESOURCES

American Heart Association, CPR and Emergency Cardiovascular Care
www.heart.org/cpr
American Heart Association, Hands-Only CPR
http://handsonlycpr.org

ing. Open an adult's airway by hyperextending the head (see Fig. A-1). Use the *head tilt–chin lift maneuver.* This involves tilting the head back with one hand and lifting the chin forward with the fingers of the other hand. Use the *jaw-thrust maneuver* if you suspect a cervical spine injury (see Fig. 69-1). Attempt to ventilate the victim using a mouth-to-barrier (recommended) device (e.g., face mask or bag-valve-mask) or mouth-to-mouth resuscitation[1] (see Fig. A-1, *B, C*).

For mouth-to-mouth resuscitation give ventilations with the victim's nostrils pinched. Take a regular (not deep) breath and tightly seal your lips around the victim's mouth. Give one breath

Nursing Diagnoses

Activity Intolerance
Activity Intolerance, Risk for
Activity Planning, Ineffective
Activity Planning, Risk for Ineffective
Adverse Reaction to Iodinated Contrast Media, Risk for
Airway Clearance, Ineffective
Allergy Response, Risk for
Anxiety
Aspiration, Risk for
Attachment, Risk for Impaired
Autonomic Dysreflexia
Autonomic Dysreflexia, Risk for
Behavior, Disorganized Infant
Behavior, Readiness for Enhanced Organized Infant
Behavior, Risk for Disorganized Infant
Bleeding, Risk for
Blood Glucose Level, Risk for Unstable
Body Image, Disturbed
Body Temperature, Risk for Imbalanced
Breast Milk, Insufficient
Breastfeeding, Ineffective
Breastfeeding, Interrupted
Breastfeeding, Readiness for Enhanced
Breathing Pattern, Ineffective
Cardiac Output, Decreased
Caregiver Role Strain
Caregiver Role Strain, Risk for
Childbearing Process, Ineffective
Childbearing Process, Readiness for Enhanced
Childbearing Process, Risk for Ineffective
Comfort, Impaired
Comfort, Readiness for Enhanced
Communication, Readiness for Enhanced
Confusion, Acute
Confusion, Chronic
Confusion, Risk for Acute
Constipation
Constipation, Perceived
Constipation, Risk for
Contamination
Contamination, Risk for
Coping, Defensive
Coping, Ineffective
Coping, Readiness for Enhanced
Coping, Ineffective Community
Coping, Readiness for Enhanced Community

Coping, Compromised Family
Coping, Disabled Family
Coping, Readiness for Enhanced Family
Death Anxiety
Decision-Making, Readiness for Enhanced
Decisional Conflict
Denial, Ineffective
Dentition, Impaired
Development, Risk for Delayed
Diarrhea
Disuse Syndrome, Risk for
Diversional Activity, Deficient
Dry Eye, Risk for
Electrolyte Imbalance, Risk for
Energy Field, Disturbed
Environmental Interpretation Syndrome, Impaired
Failure to Thrive, Adult
Falls, Risk for
Family Processes, Dysfunctional
Family Processes, Interrupted
Family Processes, Readiness for Enhanced
Fatigue
Fear
Feeding Pattern, Ineffective Infant
Fluid Balance, Readiness for Enhanced
Fluid Volume, Risk for Imbalanced
Fluid Volume, Deficient
Fluid Volume, Excess
Fluid Volume, Risk for Deficient
Gas Exchange, Impaired
Gastrointestinal Motility, Risk For Dysfunctional
Gastrointestinal Motility, Dysfunctional
Gastrointestinal Perfusion, Risk for Ineffective
Grieving
Grieving, Complicated
Grieving, Risk for Complicated
Growth, Risk for Disproportionate
Growth and Development, Delayed
Health, Deficient Community
Health Behavior, Risk-Prone
Health Maintenance, Ineffective
Home Maintenance, Impaired
Hope, Readiness for Enhanced
Hopelessness
Human Dignity, Risk for Compromised
Hyperthermia

Hypothermia
Immunization Status, Readiness for Enhanced
Impulse Control, Ineffective
Incontinence, Functional Urinary
Incontinence, Overflow Urinary
Incontinence, Reflex Urinary
Incontinence, Stress Urinary
Incontinence, Urge Urinary
Incontinence, Risk for Urge Urinary
Incontinence, Bowel
Infection, Risk for
Injury, Risk for
Insomnia
Intracranial Adaptive Capacity, Decreased
Jaundice, Neonatal
Jaundice, Risk for Neonatal
Knowledge, Deficient
Knowledge, Readiness for Enhanced
Latex Allergy Response
Latex Allergy Response, Risk for
Lifestyle, Sedentary
Liver Function, Risk for Impaired
Loneliness, Risk for
Maternal–Fetal Dyad, Risk for Disturbed
Memory, Impaired
Mobility, Impaired Bed
Mobility, Impaired Physical
Mobility, Impaired Wheelchair
Moral Distress
Nausea
Noncompliance
Nutrition, Readiness for Enhanced
Nutrition, Imbalanced: Less Than Body Requirements
Nutrition, Risk for Imbalanced: More Than Body Requirements
Nutrition, Imbalanced: More Than Body Requirements
Oral Mucous Membrane, Impaired
Other-Directed Violence, Risk for
Pain, Acute
Pain, Chronic
Parenting, Impaired
Parenting, Readiness for Enhanced
Parenting, Risk for Impaired
Perioperative Positioning Injury, Risk for
Peripheral Neurovascular Dysfunction, Risk for
Personal Identity, Disturbed
Personal Identity, Risk for Disturbed
Poisoning, Risk for
Post-Trauma Syndrome
Post-Trauma Syndrome, Risk for
Power, Readiness for Enhanced
Powerlessness
Powerlessness, Risk for
Protection, Ineffective
Rape-Trauma Syndrome
Relationship, Ineffective
Relationship, Readiness for Enhanced
Relationship, Risk for Ineffective
Religiosity, Impaired
Religiosity, Readiness for Enhanced
Religiosity, Risk for Impaired
Relocation Stress Syndrome
Relocation Stress Syndrome, Risk for

Renal Perfusion, Risk for Ineffective
Resilience, Impaired Individual
Resilience, Readiness for Enhanced
Resilience, Risk for Compromised
Role Conflict, Parental
Role Performance, Ineffective
Self-Care, Readiness for Enhanced
Self-Care Deficit, Bathing
Self-Care Deficit, Dressing
Self-Care Deficit, Feeding
Self-Care Deficit, Toileting
Self-Concept, Readiness for Enhanced
Self-Directed Violence, Risk for
Self-Esteem, Chronic Low
Self-Esteem, Situational Low
Self-Esteem, Risk for Chronic Low
Self-Esteem, Risk for Situational Low
Self-Health Management, Ineffective
Self-Health Management, Readiness for Enhanced
Self-Mutilation
Self-Mutilation, Risk for
Self-Neglect
Sexual Dysfunction
Sexuality Pattern, Ineffective
Shock, Risk for
Skin Integrity, Impaired
Skin Integrity, Risk for Impaired
Sleep Deprivation
Sleep, Readiness for Enhanced
Sleep Pattern, Disturbed
Social Interaction, Impaired
Social Isolation
Sorrow, Chronic
Spiritual Distress
Spiritual Distress, Risk for
Spiritual Well-Being, Readiness for Enhanced
Spontaneous Ventilation, Impaired
Stress Overload
Sudden Infant Death Syndrome, Risk for
Suffocation, Risk for
Suicide, Risk for
Surgical Recovery, Delayed
Swallowing, Impaired
Therapeutic Regimen Management, Ineffective Family
Thermal Injury, Risk for
Thermoregulation, Ineffective
Tissue Integrity, Impaired
Tissue Perfusion, Ineffective Peripheral
Tissue Perfusion, Risk for Decreased Cardiac
Tissue Perfusion, Risk for Ineffective Cerebral
Tissue Perfusion, Risk for Ineffective Peripheral
Transfer Ability, Impaired
Trauma, Risk for
Unilateral Neglect
Urinary Elimination, Impaired
Urinary Elimination, Readiness for Enhanced
Urinary Retention
Vascular Trauma, Risk for
Ventilatory Weaning Response, Dysfunctional
Verbal Communication, Impaired
Walking, Impaired
Wandering

Laboratory Reference Intervals

The tables in this appendix list some of the most common tests, their reference intervals (formally referred to as normal values), and possible etiologies of abnormal results. Laboratory results may vary depending on different techniques or different laboratories. Possible etiologies are presented in alphabetic order. Abbreviations appearing in the tables are defined as follows:

mEq = milliequivalent
mm Hg = millimeter of mercury
mm = millimeter
mOsm = milliosmole

L = liter
dL = deciliter (10^{-1} liter)
mL = milliliter (10^{-3} liter)
μL = microliter (10^{-6} liter, 10^{-3} milliliter)
fL = femtoliter (10^{-15} liter, 10^{-12} milliliter)

g = gram
mg = milligram (10^{-3} gram)
mcg = microgram (10^{-6} gram)
ng = nanogram (10^{-9} gram)
pg = picogram (10^{-12} gram)

U = unit
μU = microunit
IU = international unit

mmol = millimole (10^{-3} mole)
μmol = micromole (10^{-6} mole)
nmol = nanomole (10^{-9} mole)
pmol = picomole (10^{-12} mole)
kPa = kilopascal
μkat = microkatal

Source: Burtis CA, Ashwood ER, Bruns DE: *Tietz textbook of clinical chemistry and molecular diagnostics*, ed 5, St Louis, 2013, Elsevier.

TABLE C-1 SERUM, PLASMA, AND WHOLE BLOOD CHEMISTRIES

Test	Reference Intervals		Possible Etiology	
	Conventional Units	SI Units	Higher	Lower
Acetone			Diabetic ketoacidosis, high-fat diet, low-carbohydrate diet, starvation	
• Quantitative	<2.0 mg/dL	<344 μmol/L		
• Qualitative	Negative	Negative		
Albumin	3.5-5.0 g/dL	35-50 g/L	Dehydration	Chronic liver disease, malabsorption, malnutrition, nephrotic syndrome
Aldolase	1.5-8.1 U/L	1.5-8.1 U/L	Skeletal muscle disease	Renal disease
α₁-Antitrypsin	78-200 mg/dL	0.78-2.0 g/L	Acute and chronic inflammation, arthritis	Chronic lung disease (early onset), malnutrition, nephrotic syndrome
α₁-Fetoprotein	<10 ng/mL	<10 mcg/L	Cancer of testes, ovaries, and liver	
Ammonia	15-45 mcg N/dL	11-32 μmol N/L	Severe liver disease	
Amylase	30-122 U/L (method dependent)	0.51-2.07 μkat/L	Acute and chronic pancreatitis, mumps (salivary gland disease), perforated ulcers	Acute alcoholism, cirrhosis of liver, extensive destruction of pancreas
Bicarbonate	22-26 mEq/L	22-26 mmol/L	Compensated respiratory acidosis, metabolic alkalosis	Compensated respiratory alkalosis, metabolic acidosis
b-Type natriuretic peptide (BNP)	<100 pg/mL	<100 pmol/L	Heart failure	
Bilirubin			Biliary obstruction, impaired liver function, hemolytic anemia, pernicious anemia	
• Total	0.2-1.2 mg/dL	3-21 μmol/L		
• Indirect	0.1-1.0 mg/dL	1.7-17.0 μmol/L		
• Direct	0.1-0.3 mg/dL	1.7-5.1 μmol/L		

Continued

Reviewed by Julie Dittmer, RN, MSN, Eastern Iowa Community College, Bettendorf, Iowa.

TABLE C-1 SERUM, PLASMA, AND WHOLE BLOOD CHEMISTRIES—cont'd

| Test | Reference Intervals | | Possible Etiology | |
	Conventional Units	SI Units	Higher	Lower
Blood gases*				
• Arterial pH	7.35-7.45	7.35-7.45	Alkalosis	Acidosis
• Venous pH	7.32-7.43	7.32-7.43		
• $PaCO_2$	35-45 mm Hg	4.66-5.98 kPa	Compensated metabolic alkalosis	Compensated metabolic acidosis
• $PvCO_2$	38-55 mm Hg	5.06-7.32 kPa	Respiratory acidosis	Respiratory alkalosis
• PaO_2	80-100 mm Hg	10.6-13.33 kPa	Administration of high concentration of oxygen	Chronic lung disease, decreased cardiac output
• PvO_2	38-42 mm Hg	5.04-5.57 kPa		
Calcium (total)	8.6-10.2 mg/dL	2.15-2.55 mmol/L	Acute osteoporosis, hyperparathyroidism, vitamin D intoxication, multiple myeloma	Acute pancreatitis, hypoparathyroidism, liver disease, malabsorption syndrome, renal failure, vitamin D deficiency
Calcium (ionized)	4.64-5.28 mg/dL	1.16-1.32 mmol/L		
Carbon dioxide (CO_2)	23-29 mEq/L	23-29 mmol/L	Same as bicarbonate	
Carotene	10-85 mcg/dL	0.19-1.58 µmol/L	Cystic fibrosis, hypothyroidism, pancreatic insufficiency	Dietary deficiency, malabsorption disorders
Chloride	96-106 mEq/L	96-106 mmol/L	Metabolic acidosis, respiratory alkalosis, corticosteroid therapy, uremia	Addison's disease, diarrhea, metabolic alkalosis, respiratory acidosis, vomiting
Cholesterol	<200 mg/dL	<5.2 mmol/L	Biliary obstruction, hypothyroidism, idiopathic hypercholesterolemia, renal disease, uncontrolled diabetes	Extensive liver disease, hyperthyroidism, malnutrition, corticosteroid therapy
• High-density lipoproteins (HDLs)	Male: >40 mg/dL Female: >50 mg/dL	>1.04 mmol/L >1.3 mmol/L		
• Low-density lipoproteins (LDLs)	*Recommended:* <100 mg/dL *Near optimal:* 100-129 mg/dL (2.6-3.34 mmol/L) *Moderate risk for CAD:* 130-159 mg/dL (3.37-4.12 mmol/L) *High risk for CAD:* >160 mg/dL (>4.14 mmol/L)	*Recommended:* <2.6 mmol/L *Near optimal:* 2.6-3.34 mmol/L *Moderate risk for CAD:* 3.37-4.12 mmol/L *High risk for CAD:* >4.14 mmol/L		
Copper	80-155 mcg/dL	12.6-24.3 µmol/L	Cirrhosis	Wilson's disease
Cortisol	8 AM: 5-23 mcg/dL 8 PM: <10 mcg/dL	0.14-0.63 µmol/L <0.28 µmol/L	Cushing syndrome, pancreatitis	Adrenal insufficiency, panhypopituitary states
Creatine	0.2-1.0 mg/dL	15.3-76.3 µmol/L	Active rheumatoid arthritis, biliary obstruction, hyperthyroidism, renal disorders, severe muscle disease	Diabetes mellitus
Creatine kinase (CK)	*Male:* 20-200 U/L *Female:* 20-180 U/L	Male: 20-200 U/L Female: 20-180 U/L	Musculoskeletal injury or disease, myocardial infarction, severe myocarditis, exercise, numerous IM injections	
• CK-MB	<4%-6% of total CK	<0.4-0.6	Acute myocardial infarction	
Creatinine	0.6-1.3 mg/dL	53-115 µmol/L	Severe renal disease	
Ferritin	10-250 ng/mL	10-250 mcg/L	Sideroblastic anemia, anemia of chronic disease (infection, inflammation, liver disease)	Iron-deficiency anemia
Folate (folic acid)	5-16 ng/mL	11-36 nmol/L	Hypothyroidism	Alcoholism, hemolytic anemia, inadequate diet, malabsorption syndrome, megaloblastic anemia
Gamma-glutamyl transferase (GGT)	0-30 U/L	0-0.5 µkat/L	Liver disease, infectious mononucleosis, pancreatitis, hyperthyroidism	Hypothyroidism
Glucose (fasting)	70-99 mg/dL	3.9-5.5 mmol/L	Acute stress, Cushing disease, diabetes mellitus, hyperthyroidism, pancreatic insufficiency	Addison's disease, hepatic disease, hypothyroidism, insulin overdosage, pancreatic tumor, pituitary hypofunction
Haptoglobin	26-185 mg/dL	260-1850 mg/L	Infectious and inflammatory processes, malignant neoplasms	Hemolytic anemia, mononucleosis, toxoplasmosis, chronic liver disease

TABLE C-1 SERUM, PLASMA, AND WHOLE BLOOD CHEMISTRIES—cont'd

| Test | Reference Intervals | | Possible Etiology | |
	Conventional Units	**SI Units**	**Higher**	**Lower**
Insulin (fasting)	4-24 µU/mL	29-172 pmol/L	Acromegaly, adenoma of pancreatic islet cells, untreated mild case of type 2 diabetes	Inadequately treated type 1 diabetes mellitus
Iron, total	50-175 mcg/dL	9.0-31.3 µmol/L	Excessive RBC destruction	Iron-deficiency anemia, anemia of chronic disease
Iron-binding capacity	250-425 mcg/dL	44.8-76.1 µmol/L	Iron-deficient state, polycythemia	Cancer, chronic infections, pernicious anemia
Lactic acid (L-Lactate)	6.3-22.5 mcg/dL	0.7-2.5 mmol/L	Acidosis, heart failure, shock	
Lactic dehydrogenase (LDH)	140-280 U/L	0.83-2.5 µkat/L	Heart failure, hemolytic disorders, hepatitis, metastatic cancer of liver, myocardial infarction, pernicious anemia, pulmonary embolus, skeletal muscle damage	
Lactic dehydrogenase isoenzymes				
• LDH_1	18%-33%	0.18-0.33	Myocardial infarction, pernicious anemia	
• LDH_2	28%-40%	0.28-0.40	Pulmonary embolus, sickle cell crisis	
• LDH_3	18%-30%	0.18-0.30	Malignant lymphoma, pulmonary embolus	
• LDH_4	6%-16%	0.06-0.16	Systemic lupus erythematosus, pulmonary infarction	
• LDH_5	2%-13%	0.02-0.13	Heart failure, hepatitis, pulmonary embolus and infarction, skeletal muscle damage	
Lipase	31-186 U/L	0.5-3.2 µkat/L	Acute pancreatitis, hepatic disorders, perforated peptic ulcer	
Magnesium	1.5-2.5 mEq/L	0.75-1.25 mmol/L	Addison's disease, hypothyroidism, renal failure	Chronic alcoholism, severe malabsorption
Osmolality	275-295 mOsm/kg	275-295 mmol/kg	Chronic renal disease, diabetes mellitus	Addison's disease, diuretic therapy
Oxygen saturation (arterial) (SaO_2)	>95%	>0.95	Polycythemia	Anemia, cardiac decompensation, respiratory disorders
pH	See Blood gases			
Phenylalanine	0.8-1.8 mg/dL	48-109 µmol/L	Phenylketonuria	
Phosphatase, acid	0-0.6 U/L	0-90 µkat/L	Advanced Paget's disease, cancer of prostate, hyperparathyroidism	
Phosphatase, alkaline	38-126 U/L	0.65-2.14 µkat/L	Bone diseases, marked hyperparathyroidism, obstruction of biliary system, rickets	Excessive vitamin D ingestion, hypothyroidism
Phosphorus (phosphate)	2.4-4.4 mg/dL	0.78-1.42 mmol/L	Healing fractures, hypoparathyroidism, renal disease, vitamin D intoxication	Diabetes mellitus, hyperparathyroidism, vitamin D deficiency
Potassium	3.5-5.0 mEq/L	3.5-5.0 mmol/L	Addison's disease, diabetic ketosis, massive tissue destruction, renal failure	Cushing syndrome, diarrhea (severe), diuretic therapy, gastrointestinal fistula, pyloric obstruction, starvation, vomiting
Progesterone (Female)				
• Follicular phase	15-70 ng/dL	0.5-2.2 nmol/L	Adrenal hyperplasia, choriocarcinoma of ovary, pregnancy, cysts of ovary	Threatened abortion, hypogonadism, amenorrhea, ovarian tumor
• Luteal phase	200-2500 ng/dL	6.4-79.5 nmol/L		
• Postmenopause	<40 ng/dL	1.28 nmol/L		
Prostate-specific antigen (PSA)	<4 ng/mL	<4 mcg/L	Prostate cancer	

Continued

TABLE C-1   SERUM, PLASMA, AND WHOLE BLOOD CHEMISTRIES—cont'd

Test	Reference Intervals		Possible Etiology	
	Conventional Units	SI Units	Higher	Lower
Proteins			Burns, cirrhosis (globulin fraction), dehydration	Liver disease, malabsorption
• Total	6.4-8.3 g/dL	64-83 g/L		
• Albumin	3.5-5.0 g/dL	35-50 g/L		
• Globulin	2.0-3.5 g/dL	20-35 g/L		
• Albumin/globulin ratio	1.5:1-2.5:1	1.5:1-2.5:1	Multiple myeloma (globulin fraction), shock, vomiting	Malnutrition, nephrotic syndrome, proteinuria, renal disease, severe burns
Sodium	135-145 mEq/L	135-145 mmol/L	Dehydration, impaired renal function, primary aldosteronism, corticosteroid therapy	Addison's disease, diabetic ketoacidosis, diuretic therapy, excessive loss from GI tract, excessive perspiration, water intoxication
Testosterone	*Male:* 280-1100 ng/dL	*Male:* 10.4-38.17 nmol/L		Hypofunction of testes, hypogonadism
	Female: 15-70 ng/dL	*Female:* 0.52-2.43 nmol/L	Polycystic ovary, virilizing tumors	
T_4 (thyroxine), total	4.6-11.0 mcg/dL	59-142 nmol/L	Hyperthyroidism, thyroiditis	Cretinism, hypothyroidism, myxedema
T_4 (thyroxine), free	0.8-2.7 ng/dL	10-35 pmol/L		
T_3 uptake	24%-34%	0.24-0.34	Hyperthyroidism	Hypothyroidism
T_3 (triiodothyronine), total	*Ages 20-50:* 70-204 ng/dL	1.08-3.14 nmol/L	Hyperthyroidism	Hypothyroidism
	Ages >50: 40-181 ng/dL	0.62-2.79 nmol/L		
Thyroid-stimulating hormone (TSH)	0.4-4.2 μU/mL	0.4-4.2 mU/L	Myxedema, primary hypothyroidism, Graves' disease	Secondary hypothyroidism
Transaminases				
• Aspartate aminotransferase (AST)	10-30 U/L	0.17-0.51 μkat/L	Liver disease, myocardial infarction, pulmonary infarction, acute hepatitis	
• Alanine aminotransferase (ALT)	10-40 U/L	0.17-0.68 μkat/L	Liver disease, shock	
Transferrin	190-380 mg/dL	1.9-3.8 g/L		
Transferrin saturation (%)	15%-50%	15%-50%		
Triglycerides	<150 mg/dL	<1.7 mmol/L	Diabetes mellitus, hyperlipidemia, hypothyroidism, liver disease	Malnutrition
Troponins (cardiac)			Myocardial infarction	
• Troponin T (cTnT)	<0.5 ng/mL (<0.5 mcg/L)			
• Troponin I (cTnI)	<0.1 ng/mL (<0.1 mcg/L)			
Urea nitrogen (BUN)	6-20 mg/dL	2.1-7.1 mmol/L	Increase in protein catabolism (fever, stress), renal disease, urinary tract infection	Malnutrition, severe liver damage
Uric acid	*Male:* 4.4-7.6 mg/dL	*Male:* 262-452 μmol/L	Gout, gross tissue destruction, high-protein weight reduction diet, leukemia, renal failure	Administration of uricosuric drugs
	Female: 2.3-6.6 mg/dL	*Female:* 137-393 μmol/L		
Vitamin A (retinol)	30-80 mcg/dL	1.05-2.80 μmol/L	Excess ingestion of vitamin A	Vitamin A deficiency
Vitamin B_{12} (cobalamin)	200-835 pg/mL	148-616 pmol/L	Chronic myeloid leukemia	Strict vegetarianism, malabsorption syndrome, pernicious anemia, total or partial gastrectomy
Vitamin C (ascorbic acid)	0.4-2.0 mg/dL	23-114 μmol/L	Excessive ingestion of vitamin C	Connective tissue disorders, hepatic disease, renal disease, rheumatic fever, vitamin C deficiency
Zinc	70-120 mcg/dL	10.7-120 μmol/L		Alcoholic cirrhosis

*Because arterial blood gases are influenced by altitude, the value for PaO_2 decreases as altitude increases. The lower value is normal for an altitude of 1 mile.
$PaCO_2$, Partial pressure of CO_2 in arterial blood; $PvCO_2$, partial pressure of CO_2 in venous blood; PaO_2, partial pressure of oxygen in arterial blood; PvO_2, partial pressure of oxygen in venous blood; *RBC*, red blood cell; SaO_2, arterial oxygen saturation.

TABLE C-2 HEMATOLOGY

Test	Reference Intervals		Possible Etiology	
	Conventional Units	SI Units	Higher	Lower
Bleeding time	2-7 min	120-420 sec	Defective platelet function, thrombocytopenia, von Willebrand disease, aspirin ingestion, vascular disease	
Activated partial thromboplastin time (aPTT)	25-35 sec*	25-35 sec*	Deficiency factors I, II, V, VIII, IX, X, XI, XII; hemophilia, liver disease; heparin therapy	
Prothrombin time (Protime, PT)	11-16 sec*	11-16 sec*	Warfarin therapy; deficiency of factors I, II, V, VII, and X; vitamin K deficiency; liver disease	
Fibrinogen	200-400 mg/dL	2-4 g/L	Burns (after first 36 hr), inflammatory disease	Burns (during first 36 hr), DIC, severe liver disease
Fibrin split (degradation) products	<10 mcg/mL	<10 mg/L	Acute DIC, massive hemorrhage, primary fibrinolysis	
D-Dimer	<250 ng/mL	<250 mcg/L	DIC, myocardial infarction, deep vein thrombosis, unstable angina	
Erythrocyte count† (altitude dependent)	Male: 4.3-5.7 × 10^6/µL Female: 3.8-5.1 × 10^6/µL	Male: 4.3-5.7 × 10^{12}/L Female: 3.8-5.1 × 10^{12}/L	Dehydration, high altitudes, polycythemia vera	Anemia, leukemia, posthemorrhage
Red blood indices				
• Mean corpuscular volume (MCV)	80-100 fL	80-100 fL	Macrocytic anemia	Microcytic anemia
• Mean corpuscular hemoglobin (MCH)	27-34 pg	27-34 pg	Macrocytic anemia	Microcytic anemia
• Mean corpuscular hemoglobin concentration (MCHC)	32%-37%	0.32-0.37	Spherocytosis	Hypochromic anemia
Erythrocyte sedimentation rate (ESR)	<30 mm/hr (some gender variation)	<30 mm/hr (some gender variation)	*Moderate increase:* acute hepatitis, myocardial infarction; rheumatoid arthritis *Marked increase:* acute and severe bacterial infections, malignancies, pelvic inflammatory disease	Malaria, severe liver disease, sickle cell anemia
Hematocrit† (altitude dependent)	Male: 39%-50% Female: 35%-47%	Male: 0.39-0.50 Female: 0.35-0.47	Dehydration, high altitudes, polycythemia	Anemia, hemorrhage, overhydration
Hemoglobin† (altitude dependent)	Male: 13.2-17.3 g/dL Female: 11.7-15.5 g/dL	Male: 132-173 g/L Female: 117-155 g/L	COPD, high altitudes, polycythemia	Anemia, hemorrhage
Hemoglobin, glycosylated (A1C)	4.0%-6.0%	4.0%-6.0%	Poorly controlled diabetes mellitus	Sickle cell anemia, chronic renal failure, pregnancy
Platelets (thrombocytes)	150-400 × 10^3/µL	150-400 × 10^9/L	Acute infections, chronic granulocytic leukemia, chronic pancreatitis, cirrhosis, collagen disorders, polycythemia, postsplenectomy	Acute leukemia, DIC, thrombocytopenic purpura
Reticulocyte count	0.5%-1.5% of RBC	0.5%-1.5% of RBC	Hemolytic anemia, polycythemia vera	Hypoproliferative anemia, macrocytic anemia, microcytic anemia
White blood cell count†	4.0-11.0 × 10^3/µL	4.0-11.0 × 10^9/L	Inflammatory and infectious processes, leukemia	Aplastic anemia, side effects of chemotherapy and irradiation
WBC differential				
• Segmented neutrophils	50%-70%	0.50-0.70	Bacterial infections, collagen diseases, Hodgkin's lymphoma	Aplastic anemia, viral infections
• Band neutrophils	0%-8%	0-0.08	Acute infections	
• Lymphocytes	20%-40%	0.20-0.40	Chronic infections, lymphocytic leukemia, mononucleosis, viral infections	Corticosteroid therapy, whole body irradiation
• Monocytes	4%-8%	0.04-0.08	Chronic inflammatory disorders, malaria, monocytic leukemia, acute infections, Hodgkin's lymphoma	
• Eosinophils	0%-4%	0-0.04	Allergic reactions, eosinophilic and chronic granulocytic leukemia, parasitic disorders, Hodgkin's lymphoma	Corticosteroid therapy
• Basophils	0%-2%	0-0.02	Hypothyroidism, ulcerative colitis, myeloproliferative diseases	Hyperthyroidism, stress

*Values depend on reagent and instrumentation used.
†Components of complete blood count (CBC).
COPD, Chronic obstructive pulmonary disease; *DIC,* disseminated intravascular coagulation; *RBC,* red blood cell; *WBC,* white blood cell.

TABLE C-3 SEROLOGY-IMMUNOLOGY

Test	Reference Intervals		Possible Etiology	
	Conventional Units	**SI Units**	**Higher**	**Lower**
Antinuclear antibody (ANA)	Negative at 1:40 dilution	Negative at 1:40 dilution	Chronic hepatitis, rheumatoid arthritis, scleroderma, systemic lupus erythematosus	
Anti-DNA antibody	<70 IU/mL	<70 IU/mL	Systemic lupus erythematosus	
Anti-Sm (Smith)	Negative	Negative	Systemic lupus erythematosus	
C-reactive protein (CRP)	6.8-820 mcg/dL	68-8200 mcg/L	Acute infections, any inflammatory condition, widespread malignancy	
Carcinoembryonic antigen (CEA)	*Nonsmoker:* <3 ng/mL *Smoker:* <5 ng/mL	*Nonsmoker:* <3 mcg/L *Smoker:* <5 mcg/L	Carcinoma of colon, liver, pancreas; chronic cigarette smoking; inflammatory bowel disease; other cancers	
Complement, total hemolytic (CH_{50})	75-160 U/mL	75-160 kU/L		Acute glomerulonephritis, systemic lupus erythematosus, rheumatoid arthritis, subacute bacterial endocarditis
Direct Coombs or direct antihuman globulin test (DAT)	Negative	Negative	Acquired hemolytic anemia, drug reactions, transfusion reactions	
Fluorescent treponemal antibody absorption (FTA-Abs)	Negative or nonreactive	Negative or nonreactive	Syphilis	
Hepatitis A antibody	Negative	Negative	Hepatitis A	
Hepatitis B surface antigen (HB_sAg)	Negative	Negative	Hepatitis B	
Hepatitis C antibody	Negative	Negative	Hepatitis C	
Monospot or monotest	Negative	Negative	Infectious mononucleosis	
Rheumatoid factor (RF)	Negative or titer <1:17	Negative or titer <1:17	Rheumatoid arthritis, Sjögren's syndrome, systemic lupus erythematosus	
RPR	Negative or nonreactive	Negative or nonreactive	Syphilis, systemic lupus erythematosus, rheumatoid arthritis, leprosy, malaria, febrile diseases, IV drug abuse	
VDRL	Negative or nonreactive	Negative or nonreactive	Syphilis	

RPR, Rapid plasma regain test; *VDRL,* Veneral Disease Research Laboratory test.

TABLE C-4 URINE CHEMISTRY

Test	Specimen	Reference Intervals Units	Reference Intervals SI Units	Possible Etiology Higher	Possible Etiology Lower
Acetone	Random	Negative	Negative	Diabetes mellitus, high-fat and low-carbohydrate diets, starvation	
Aldosterone	24 hr	3-30 mcg/day (low sodium diet increases threefold to fivefold)	0.08-0.83 nmol/day	*Primary aldosteronism:* adrenocortical tumors *Secondary aldosteronism:* cardiac failure, cirrhosis, large dose of ACTH, salt depletion	ACTH deficiency, Addison's disease, corticosteroid therapy
Amylase	24 hr	1-17 U/hr	1-17 U/hr	Acute pancreatitis	
Bence Jones protein	Random	Negative	Negative	Multiple myeloma	
Bilirubin	Random	Negative	Negative	Liver disorders	
Calcium	24 hr	100-250 mg/day	2.5-6.3 mmol/day	Bone tumor, hyperparathyroidism	Hypoparathyroidism, malabsorption of calcium and vitamin D
Catecholamines	24 hr			Pheochromocytoma, progressive muscular dystrophy, heart failure	
• Epinephrine		<20 mcg/day	<109 nmol/day		
• Norepinephrine		15-80 mcg/day	89-473 nmol/day		
Creatine	24 hr	<100 mg/day	<763 μmol/day	Liver cancer, hyperthyroidism, diabetes, Addison's disease, infections, burns, muscular dystrophy, skeletal muscle atrophy	Hypothyroidism
Creatinine	24 hr	0.6-2.0 g/day	5.3-17.7 mmol/day	Anemia, leukemia, muscular atrophy	Renal disease
Creatinine clearance	24 hr	59-137 mL/min/1.73 m^2	0.59-1.37 mL/sec/m^2		Renal disease
Estrogens	24 hr				
• Female				Gonadal or adrenal tumor	Endocrine disturbance, ovarian dysfunction, menopause
• Premenopause		15-80 mcg/day	15-80 mcg/day		
• Postmenopause		<20 mcg/day	<20 mcg/day		
• Male		15-40 mcg/day	15-40 mcg/day		
Glucose	Random	Negative	Negative	Diabetes mellitus, pituitary disorders	
Hemoglobin	Random	Negative	Negative	Extensive burns, glomerulonephritis, hemolytic anemias, hemolytic transfusion reaction	
5-Hydroxyindole acetic acid (5-HIAA)	24 hr	2-7 mg/day	10.5-36.6 μmol/day	Malignant carcinoid syndrome	
Ketone bodies	24 hr	20-50 mg/day	0.34-0.86 mmol/day	Diabetes mellitus, starvation, dehydration	
Metanephrine	24 hr	92-934 mcg/day	500-5100 nmol/day	Pheochromocytoma	
Myoglobin	Random	Negative	Negative	Crushing injuries, electric injuries, extreme physical exertion	
Osmolality	Random	300-1300 mOsm/kg	300-1300 mmol/kg	Dehydration, tubular dysfunction (kidney lost ability to dilute urine)	Tubular dysfunction (kidney lost ability to concentrate urine)
pH	Random	4.0-8.0	4.0-8.0	Urinary tract infection, urine allowed to stand at room temperature	Respiratory or metabolic acidosis
Protein (dipstick)	Random	0-trace	0-trace	Acute and chronic renal disease, especially involving glomeruli; heart failure	
Protein (quantitative)	24 hr	<150 mg/day	<0.15 g/day	Cardiac failure, inflammatory processes of urinary tract, nephritis, nephrosis, strenuous exercise	
Sodium	24 hr	40-220 mEq/day	40-220 mmol/day	Acute tubular necrosis	Hyponatremia
Specific gravity	Random	1.003-1.030	Same as conventional units	Albuminuria, dehydration, glycosuria	Diabetes insipidus
Uric acid	24 hr	250-750 mg/day	1.5-4.5 mmol/day	Gout, leukemia	Nephritis
Urobilinogen	24 hr	0.5-4.0 mg/day	0.8-6.8 μmol/day	Hemolytic disease, hepatic parenchymal cell damage, liver disease	Complete obstruction of bile duct
Vanillylmandelic acid	24 hr	1.4-6.5 mg/day	7-33 μmol/day	Pheochromocytoma	

ACTH, Adrenocorticotropic hormone.

TABLE C-5 FECAL ANALYSIS

| Test | Reference Intervals | | Possible Etiology |
	Conventional Units	SI Units	Higher
Fecal fat	<6 g/24 hr	Same as conventional units	Chronic pancreatic disease, obstruction of common bile duct, malabsorption syndrome
Mucus	Negative	Negative	Mucous colitis, spastic constipation
Pus	Negative	Negative	Chronic bacillary dysentery, chronic ulcerative colitis, localized abscesses
Blood*	Negative	Negative	Anal fissures, hemorrhoids, malignant tumor, peptic ulcer, inflammatory bowel disease
Color			
• Brown			Various color depending on diet
• Clay			Biliary obstruction or presence of barium sulfate
• Tarry			More than 100 mL of blood in gastrointestinal tract
• Red			Blood in large intestine
• Black			Blood in upper gastrointestinal tract or iron medication

*Ingestion of meat may produce false-positive results. Patient may be placed on a meat-free diet for 3 days before the test.

TABLE C-6 CEREBROSPINAL FLUID ANALYSIS

| Test | Reference Intervals | | Possible Etiology | |
	Conventional Units	SI Units	Higher	Lower
Pressure	60-150 mm H_2O	60-150 mm H_2O	Hemorrhage, intracranial tumor, meningitis	Head injury, spinal tumor, subdural hematoma
Blood	Negative	Negative	Intracranial hemorrhage	
Cell count (age dependent)			Inflammation or infections of CNS	
• WBC	0-5 cells/μL	$0-5 \times 10^6$ cells/L		
• RBC	Negative	Negative		
Chloride	118-132 mEq/L	118-132 mmol/L	Uremia	Bacterial infections of CNS (meningitis, encephalitis)
Glucose	40-70 mg/dL	2.2-3.9 mmol/L	Diabetes mellitus, viral infections of CNS	Bacterial infections and tuberculosis of CNS
Protein				
• Lumbar	15-45 mg/dL	0.15-0.45 g/L	Guillain-Barré syndrome, poliomyelitis, trauma	
• Cisternal	15-25 mg/dL	0.15-0.25 g/L	Syphilis of CNS	
• Ventricular	5-15 mg/dL	0.05-0.15 g/L	Acute meningitis, brain tumor, chronic CNS infections, multiple sclerosis	

CNS, Central nervous system.

A

absence (petit mal) seizure seizure characterized by a brief staring spell and a very brief loss of consciousness that usually occurs only in children and rarely continues beyond adolescence.

acromegaly a condition caused by excessive secretion of growth hormone characterized by an overgrowth of the bones and soft tissues.

actinic keratosis a slowly developing, localized thickening and scaling of the outer layers of the skin consisting of hyperkeratotic papules and plaques as a result of chronic, prolonged exposure to the sun; also known as solar keratosis.

acute bronchitis an inflammation of the lower respiratory tract that is usually due to infection.

acute hepatic failure a clinical syndrome characterized by severe impairment of liver function associated with hepatic encephalopathy; also referred to as acute liver failure.

acute kidney injury (AKI) clinical syndrome characterized by a rise in serum creatinine and/or a reduction in urine output.

acute lung injury (ALI) a condition that occurs when the patient's PaO_2/FIO_2 ratio is 200–300 (e.g., 86/0.4 = 215).

acute pancreatitis an acute inflammatory process of the pancreas caused by autodigestion and marked by symptoms of an acute condition of the abdomen and escape of pancreatic enzymes into the pancreatic tissues.

acute respiratory distress syndrome (ARDS) a sudden and progressive form of acute respiratory failure in which the alveolar-capillary membrane becomes damaged and more permeable to intravascular fluid.

acute tubular necrosis (ATN) a type of intrarenal acute injury of the kidney that affects the renal tubules, caused by renal ischemia and nephrotoxic injury.

adhesion a band of scar tissue between or around organs.

adventitious sounds extra breath sounds that are not normally heard, such as crackles, rhonchi, wheezes, and pleural friction rubs.

afterload the peripheral resistance against which the left ventricle must pump.

allergic rhinitis the reaction of the nasal mucosa to a specific allergen.

alopecia partial or complete lack of hair resulting from normal aging, endocrine disorder, drug reaction, anticancer medication, or skin disease.

Alzheimer's disease (AD) a chronic, progressive, degenerative disease of the brain.

amyotrophic lateral sclerosis (ALS) a rare progressive neurologic disorder characterized by loss of motor neurons and by weakness and atrophy of the muscles of the hands, forearms, and legs, spreading to involve most of the body and face.

anaphylactic shock an acute and life-threatening hypersensitivity (allergic) reaction to a sensitizing substance, such as a drug, chemical, vaccine, food, or insect venom.

aneurysm congenital or acquired weakness of the arterial wall resulting in dilation and ballooning of the vessel.

angina chest pain that is a clinical manifestation of reversible myocardial ischemia.

ankylosing spondylitis a chronic inflammatory disease that primarily affects the axial skeleton, including the sacroiliac joints, intervertebral disc spaces, and costovertebral articulations.

ankylosis stiffness or fixation of a joint usually resulting from destruction of articular cartilage and subchondral bone.

aortic dissection the result of a tear in the intimal (innermost) lining of the arterial wall that allows blood to enter between the intima and media, thus creating a false lumen.

aphasia an abnormal neurologic condition in which language function is disordered or absent because of an injury to certain areas of the cerebral cortex.

aplastic anemia a disease with a deficiency of all of the formed elements of blood (specifically red blood cells, white blood cells, and platelets), representing a failure of the cell-generating capacity of bone marrow.

appendicitis an inflammation of the appendix that, if undiagnosed, leads rapidly to perforation and peritonitis.

arterial blood pressure a measure of the pressure exerted by blood against the walls of the arterial system.

arteriovenous fistula (AVF) type of vascular access created most commonly in the forearm with an anastomosis between an artery (usually radial or ulnar) and a vein (usually cephalic).

arteriovenous grafts (AVGs) fistula made of synthetic materials that forms a "bridge" between the arterial and venous blood supplies.

arthritis inflammation of a joint; most prevalent types are osteoarthritis, rheumatoid arthritis, and gout.

arthrocentesis incision or puncture of joint capsule to obtain samples of synovial fluid from within joint cavity or to remove excess fluid.

arthrodesis the surgical fusion of a joint.

arthroplasty surgical reconstruction or replacement of a joint.

arthroscopy insertion of an arthroscope into a joint for visualization or surgery.

ascites an abnormal intraperitoneal accumulation of a fluid containing large amounts of protein and electrolytes as a result of portal hypertension.

asterixis flapping tremor (liver flap) commonly affecting the arms and hands that is a manifestation of hepatic encephalopathy.

asthma a chronic inflammatory lung disease that results in airflow obstruction; characterized by recurring episodes of paroxysmal dyspnea, wheezing on expiration, and/or inspiration caused by constriction of the bronchi, coughing, and viscous mucoid bronchial secretions.

asystole represents the total absence of ventricular electrical activity.

atelectasis an abnormal condition characterized by the collapse of alveoli, preventing the respiratory exchange of carbon dioxide and oxygen in a part of the lungs.

atherosclerosis formation of focal deposits of cholesterol and lipids known as atheromas or plaque, primarily within the intimal wall of arteries, that obstruct circulation.

atrial fibrillation a cardiac dysrhythmia characterized by a total disorganization of atrial electrical activity without effective atrial contraction.

atrial flutter an atrial tachydysrhythmia identified by recurring, regular, sawtooth-shaped flutter waves.

atrophy wasting of muscle, characterized by decreased circumference and flabby appearance leading to decreased function and tone.

aura a sensation of light or warmth or other perception that may be a warning of an attack of a migraine or an epileptic seizure.

auscultation the act of listening for sounds within the body to evaluate the condition of the heart, blood vessels, lungs, pleura, intestines, or other organs.

autoimmunity an inappropriate immune reaction to self-proteins.

azotemia an accumulation of nitrogenous waste products such as blood urea nitrogen (BUN) and creatinine.

B

bariatric surgery a surgical procedure used to treat severe obesity.

Barrett's esophagus a precancerous esophageal disorder characterized by metaplastic cell changes.

basal cell carcinoma a malignant epithelial cell tumor arising from epidermal basal cells that begins as a papule and enlarges peripherally, developing a central crater that erodes, crusts, and bleeds.

Bell's palsy a disorder characterized by a disruption of the motor branches of the facial nerve (cranial nerve [CN] VII) on one side of the face in the absence of any other disease such as a stroke.

benign prostatic hyperplasia (BPH) a nonmalignant, noninflammatory enlargement of the prostate gland caused by an increase in the number of epithelial cells and stromal tissue.

biologic therapy treatment using biologic agents such as interferons, interleukins, monoclonal antibodies, and growth factors to modify the relationship between the host and tumor.

borborygmi audible abdominal sounds produced by hyperactive intestinal peristalsis.

botulism a serious food poisoning caused by GI absorption of the neurotoxin produced by *Clostridium botulinum* that results in disturbed muscle innervation.

brachytherapy radiation delivery system that means "closed" treatment and consists of the implantation or insertion of radioactive materials directly into the tumor or in close proximity to the tumor.

brain abscess an accumulation of pus within the brain tissue that can result from a local or a systemic infection from another source, such as the skull, sinuses, or other structures in the head.

brain attack term used to describe a stroke.

brain death a clinical diagnosis of an irreversible loss of all brain functions, including those of the brainstem.

bursitis inflammation of the bursa.

C

calculus an abnormal stone formed in body tissues by an accumulation of mineral salts.

carboxyhemoglobinemia the presence of carboxyhemoglobin in the blood; occurs with carbon monoxide poisoning.

carcinogens agents capable of producing cellular alterations leading to the development or increasing the incidence of neoplastic growth.

carcinoma in situ a lesion with all the histologic features of cancer except invasion.

cardiac index (CI) a measure of the cardiac output of a patient per square meter of body surface area.

cardiac output (CO) the amount of blood pumped by each ventricle in 1 minute.

cardiac pacemaker an electronic device used to increase the heart rate in severe bradycardia by electrically stimulating the heart muscle.

cardiac reserve the ability to respond to demands (exercise, stress, hypovolemia) by altering cardiac output threefold or fourfold.

cardiac tamponade compression of the heart produced by fluid accumulation in the pericardial sac.

cardiogenic shock shock occurring when either systolic or diastolic dysfunction of the myocardium results in compromised cardiac output.

cardiomyopathy a group of diseases that directly affect the structural or functional ability of the myocardium.

carpal tunnel syndrome a condition caused by compression of the median nerve beneath the transverse carpal ligament within the narrow confines of the carpal tunnel located in the wrist.

cataract an abnormal progressive condition of the lens of the eye characterized by an opacity within the lens.

celiac disease an inborn error of metabolism characterized by the inability to hydrolyze peptides contained in gluten.

cell-mediated immunity immunity that is initiated through specific antigen recognition by T lymphocytes, monocytes/macrophages, and natural killer cells.

cellulitis a diffuse, acute bacterial infection of the skin and subcutaneous tissue characterized most commonly by local heat, redness, pain, and swelling.

central cord syndrome damage to the central spinal cord characterized by microscopic hemorrhage, edema of the central spinal cord, and compression on anterior horn cells.

cerebral edema increased accumulation of fluid in the extravascular spaces of brain tissue that can lead to increased intracranial pressure.

chancre painless indurated lesions found on the penis, vulva, lips, mouth, vagina, and rectum characteristic of syphilis.

cheilosis a disorder of the lips and mouth characterized by bilateral scales and fissures, resulting from a deficiency of riboflavin in the diet.

chemotherapy the treatment of disease with chemical agents.

Cheyne-Stokes respiration an abnormal breathing pattern characterized by alternating periods of apnea and deep, rapid breathing; usually seen as a person nears death.

cholecystitis inflammation of the gallbladder.

cholelithiasis stones in the gallbladder.

chronic bronchitis obstructive pulmonary disease characterized by excessive production of mucus and chronic inflammatory changes in the bronchi.

chronic fatigue syndrome (CFS) a disorder characterized by debilitating fatigue and a variety of associated complaints.

chronic kidney disease (CKD) the presence of kidney damage or decreased glomerular filtration rate for at least 3 months with functional or structural abnormalities, with or without decreased glomerular filtration rate.

chronic kidney disease (CKD) mineral and bone disorder a systemic disorder of mineral and bone metabolism due to progressive deterioration in kidney function.

chronic pancreatitis progressive destruction of the pancreas with fibrotic replacement of pancreatic tissue.

chronic stable angina chest pain that occurs intermittently over a long period with the same pattern of onset, duration, and intensity of symptoms.

cirrhosis chronic progressive disease of the liver characterized by extensive degeneration and destruction of the liver parenchymal cells.

cluster headaches repeated headaches that can occur for weeks to months at a time, followed by periods of remission.

collateral circulation development of arterial branching that occurs within the coronary circulation when occlusion of the coronary arteries occurs slowly over a long period.

coma a profound state of unconsciousness.

community-acquired pneumonia (CAP) a lower respiratory tract infection of the lung parenchyma with onset in the community or during the first 2 days of hospitalization.

compartment syndrome a condition in which elevated intracompartmental pressure within a confined myofascial compartment compromises the neurovascular function of tissues within that space.

complete heart block third-degree atrioventricular heart block in which no impulses from the atria are conducted to the ventricles.

concussion a sudden transient mechanical head injury, such as a blow or explosion, with disruption of neural activity and a change in the level of consciousness.

continuous renal replacement therapy (CRRT) provides a means by which solutes and fluids can be removed slowly and continuously in the hemodynamically unstable patient.

contracture an abnormal, usually permanent condition of a joint, characterized by flexion and fixation.

contusion the bruising of the brain tissue within a focal area without altering the integrity of the pia mater and arachnoid layers.

coronary artery disease (CAD) an abnormal condition that may affect the heart's arteries and produce various pathologic effects, especially the reduced flow of oxygen and nutrients to the myocardium.

cor pulmonale hypertrophy of the right side of the heart, with or without heart failure, resulting from pulmonary hypertension.

crackle short, low-pitched sound consisting of discontinuous bubbling caused by air passing through the airway intermittently occluded by mucus, an unstable bronchial wall, or a fold of mucosa.

crepitation crackling sound or grating sensation as a result of friction between bones.

cretinism hypothyroidism that develops in infancy.

cryosurgery the use of subfreezing temperatures to perform surgery.

curettage scraping of material from the wall of a cavity or other surface; performed to remove tumors or other abnormal tissue or to obtain tissue.

Cushing syndrome a metabolic disorder resulting from the chronic and excessive production of cortisol by the adrenal cortex or by the administration of glucocorticoids in large doses for several weeks or longer.

cystic fibrosis (CF) an autosomal recessive, multisystem disease characterized by altered function of the exocrine glands involving primarily the lungs, pancreas, and sweat glands.

cystitis an inflammatory condition of the urinary bladder characterized by pain, urgency, frequency of urination, and hematuria.

cystocele herniation or protrusion of the urinary bladder through the wall of the vagina, resulting from weakened connective tissue support between the vagina and bladder.

D

death rattle a sound produced by air moving through mucus that has accumulated in the throat of a dying person who has lost the cough reflex.

debridement removal of dirt, foreign objects, damaged tissue, and cellular debris from a wound or a burn to prevent infection and promote healing.

deep vein thrombosis (DVT) a disorder involving a thrombus in a deep vein; most commonly the iliac and femoral veins.

degenerative disc disease (DDD) progressive degeneration that is a normal process of aging; results in the intervertebral discs losing their elasticity, flexibility, and shock-absorbing capabilities.

dehiscence the separation and disruption of previously joined wound edges, typically an abdominal incision.

delirium a state of temporary but acute mental confusion.

dementia a syndrome caused by brain disease, evidenced by chronic personality disintegration, confusion, memory impairment, and deterioration of intellectual capacity and function.

dermatomyositis a disease of the connective tissues characterized by pruritic or eczematous inflammation of the skin and tenderness of the muscles.

diabetes insipidus (DI) a group of conditions associated with deficient production or secretion of antidiuretic hormone (ADH), or a decreased renal response to ADH caused by injury of the neurohypophyseal system.

diabetes mellitus (DM) a multisystem disease related to abnormal insulin production, impaired insulin utilization, or both.

diabetic ketoacidosis (DKA) an acute metabolic complication of diabetes occurring when fats are metabolized in the absence of insulin resulting in formation of acid by-products, such as ketones.

dialysis technique in which substances move from the blood through a semipermeable membrane and into a dialysis solution.

diabetic nephropathy a microvascular complication of diabetes mellitus associated with damage to the small blood vessels that supply the glomeruli of the kidney.

diabetic neuropathy nerve damage caused by the metabolic derangements associated with diabetes mellitus.

dislocation a severe injury of the ligamentous structures that surround a joint resulting in the complete displacement or separation of the articular surfaces of the joint.

disseminated intravascular coagulation (DIC) a grave coagulopathy resulting from the overstimulation of clotting and anticlotting processes in response to disease or injury.

diverticulum a saccular dilation or outpouching of the mucosa through the circular smooth muscle of the intestinal wall.

dysarthria a disturbance in the muscular control of speech resulting from interference in the control and execution over the muscles of speech.

dysmenorrhea abdominal cramping pain or discomfort associated with menstrual flow.

dyspareunia abnormal pain during sexual intercourse.

dysphagia difficulty swallowing.

dysphasia difficulty related to the comprehension or use of language.

dysplastic nevi nevi that are larger than usual with irregular borders and various shades of color; also known as atypical moles.

dyspnea shortness of breath; difficulty breathing that may be caused by certain heart or lung conditions, strenuous exercise, or anxiety.

E

ecchymoses bruising.

ectopic pregnancy the implantation of a fertilized ovum anywhere outside the uterine cavity.

embolic stroke a stroke that occurs when an embolus lodges in and occludes a cerebral artery, resulting in infarction and edema of the area supplied by the involved vessel.

emergence delirium a neurologic alteration in recovery from anesthesia that can include behaviors such as restlessness, agitation, disorientation, thrashing, and shouting.

emphysema an abnormal condition of the pulmonary system characterized by overinflation and destructive changes in alveolar walls.

empyema an accumulation of purulent exudates in a body cavity, especially the pleural space, that results from bacterial infection, such as pleurisy or tuberculosis.

encephalitis an acute inflammation of the brain usually caused by a virus.

endometriosis the presence of normal endometrial tissue in sites outside the endometrial cavity.

endoscopy the direct visualization of a body structure through a lighted instrument (scope).

endotracheal intubation artificial airway created by inserting a tube into the trachea through the mouth or nose, past the larynx, and bypassing the upper airway and laryngeal structures.

enteral nutrition (EN) the administration of a nutritionally balanced, liquefied food or formula through a tube inserted into the stomach, duodenum, or jejunum.

epididymitis acute or chronic inflammation of the epididymis, usually secondary to an infectious process, trauma, or urinary reflux down the vas deferens.

epidural block injection of a local anesthetic into the epidural (extradural) space by either a thoracic or lumbar approach.

epidural hematoma collection of blood between the dura and inner surface of the skull, producing compression of the dura mater and thus of the brain.

epilepsy a condition in which a person has spontaneously recurring seizures caused by a chronic underlying condition.

epistaxis nosebleed.

erectile dysfunction (ED) the inability to attain or maintain an erect penis that allows satisfactory sexual performance.

erythema redness or inflammation of the skin or mucous membranes that result from dilation and congestion of superficial capillaries.

escharotomy incisions into necrotic tissue from a severe burn performed when eschar formation compromises circulation.

esophageal diverticulum saclike outpouching of one or more layers of the esophagus.

esophageal speech a method of swallowing air, trapping it in the esophagus, and releasing it to create sound.

esophageal varices distended, tortuous, fragile veins at the lower end of the esophagus that result from portal hypertension.

esophagitis inflammation of the mucosal lining of the esophagus caused by infection, irritation from a nasogastric tube, or, most commonly, backflow of gastric juice from the stomach.

evisceration the separation and disruption of previously joined wound edges to the extent that an internal organ, typically intestinal contents, protrudes through the wound.

excision and grafting procedure during which eschar is removed down to the subcutaneous

tissue or fascia, depending on the degree of injury; a graft is then placed on clean, viable tissue to achieve good adherence.

exophthalmos protrusion of the eyeballs from the orbits caused by increased fat deposits and fluid in the retroorbital tissues.

external otitis inflammation or infection of the epithelium of the auricle and ear canal.

F

fat embolism syndrome (FES) embolization of fat globules that occurs in a small percentage of patients with fractures.

fibrinolysis a continual process resulting in the dissolution of fibrin to maintain blood in its fluid form.

fibroadenoma a small, painless, round, well-delineated, mobile benign breast tumor commonly found in young women.

fibrocystic changes a benign condition of the breasts characterized by development of excess fibrous tissue, hyperplasia of the epithelial lining of the mammary ducts, proliferation of mammary ducts, and cyst formation.

fibromyalgia a chronic disorder characterized by widespread, nonarticular musculoskeletal pain and fatigue with multiple tender points.

flail chest instability of the chest wall resulting from multiple rib fractures.

focal seizures seizures that begin in a specific region of the cortex and may be confined to one side of the brain and remain partial or focal in nature, or they may spread to involve the entire brain.

fracture a disruption or break in the continuity of the structure of bone.

fremitus vibration of the chest wall produced by vocalization.

frontotemporal lobar degeneration (FTLD) a rare disorder caused by shrinking frontal and temporal lobes of the brain; characterized by disturbances in behavior, sleep, personality, and eventually memory.

frostbite freezing that results in the formation of ice crystals in the tissues and cells.

full-thickness burn destruction of all skin elements and subcutaneous tissues with possible involvement of muscles, tendons, and bones.

G

galactorrhea a milky secretion from the nipple caused by inappropriate lactation.

gastritis inflammation of the gastric mucosa.

gastroenteritis an inflammation of the mucosa of the stomach and small intestine.

gastroesophageal reflux disease (GERD) any clinically significant symptomatic condition or histopathologic alteration presumed to be secondary to reflux of gastric contents into the lower esophagus.

generalized seizures seizures characterized by bilateral synchronous epileptic discharge in the brain with loss of consciousness for a few seconds to several minutes.

genital herpes a sexually transmitted infection caused by the herpes simplex virus type 2 (HSV-2), resulting in painful genital or anal vesicular lesions.

Glasgow Coma Scale assessment tool for altered states of consciousness that evaluates motor responses, verbal responses, and eye opening.

glaucoma a group of disorders characterized by (1) increased intraocular pressure and the consequences of elevated pressure, (2) optic nerve atrophy, and (3) peripheral visual field loss.

glial cells cells in the central nervous system that provide support, nourishment, and protection to neurons.

glomerular filtration rate (GFR) the amount of blood filtered by the glomeruli in a given time.

glomerulonephritis an immune-related inflammation of the glomeruli characterized by proteinuria, hematuria, decreased urine production, and edema.

glycemic index term used to describe the rise in blood glucose levels after a person has consumed a carbohydrate-containing food.

goiter enlargement of the thyroid gland that may be associated with hyperthyroidism, hypothyroidism, or normal thyroid function.

gonorrhea infection of the genitalia, the rectum, and/or the oropharynx by *Neisseria gonorrhoeae,* which, if left untreated, leads to the formation of fibrous tissue and adhesions.

Goodpasture syndrome an example of cytotoxic autoimmune disease characterized by the presence of circulating antibodies against the glomerular basement membrane and alveolar basement membrane.

gout recurrent attacks of acute arthritis associated with increased levels of serum uric acid.

Guillain-Barré syndrome an acute, rapidly progressing, and potentially fatal form of polyneuritis possibly caused by a cell-mediated immunologic reaction directed at the peripheral nerves.

gynecomastia a transient enlargement of one or both breasts in men.

H

heat cramps severe cramps in large muscle groups caused by depletion of both water and salt; usually follow vigorous exertion in an extremely hot environment.

heat exhaustion a clinical syndrome characterized by fatigue, light-headedness, nausea, vomiting, diarrhea, and feelings of impending doom precipitated by prolonged exposure to heat over hours or days.

heatstroke the most serious form of heat stress; results from failure of the central thermoregulatory mechanisms and is considered a medical emergency.

heaves sustained lifts of the chest wall in the precordial area that can be seen or palpated.

hematemesis vomiting of blood that indicates bleeding in the upper GI tract.

hemochromatosis an autosomal recessive disease characterized by increased intestinal iron absorption and, as a result, increased tissue iron deposition.

hemodialysis (HD) dialysis that uses an artificial membrane as the semipermeable membrane through which the patient's blood circulates.

hemolytic anemia an anemia caused by destruction of RBCs at a rate that exceeds production.

hemophilia hereditary bleeding disorders caused by defective or deficient clotting factors.

hemorrhagic stroke a stroke that results from bleeding into the brain tissue itself or into the subarachnoid space or ventricles.

hemorrhoids varicosities in the lower rectum or anus caused by congestion in the veins of the hemorrhoidal plexus.

hemothorax accumulation of blood in the pleural space.

hepatic encephalopathy changes in neurologic and mental function resulting from high levels of ammonia in the blood that a damaged liver cannot detoxify.

hepatitis inflammation of the liver.

hepatorenal syndrome a serious complication of cirrhosis characterized by functional renal failure with advancing azotemia, oliguria, and intractable ascites.

hernia a protrusion of a viscus through an abnormal opening or a weakened area in the wall of the cavity in which it is normally contained.

herniated disc herniation of nuclear material from the intervertebral disc that may compress or place tension on a cervical, lumbar, or sacral spinal nerve root.

hiatal hernia herniation of a portion of the stomach into the esophagus through an opening, or hiatus, in the diaphragm.

histologic grading a categorization of tumors in which the appearance of cells and the degree of differentiation are evaluated pathologically.

Hodgkin's lymphoma a malignant condition characterized by proliferation of abnormal giant, multinucleated cells, called *Reed-Sternberg cells,* which are located in lymph nodes.

hordeolum an infection of the sebaceous glands in the eyelid margin; commonly known as a sty.

hospice a concept of care that provides compassion, concern, and support for the dying person.

human immunodeficiency virus (HIV) a retrovirus that causes HIV infection and acquired immunodeficiency syndrome.

human leukocyte antigens (HLAs) a system consisting of a series of linked genes that occur together on the sixth chromosome in humans and that is used to assess tissue compatibility.

humoral immunity antibody-mediated immunity.

Huntington's disease a genetically transmitted, autosomal dominant disorder that affects both men and women of all races and is characterized by chronic, devastating loss of all neurologic function, resulting in dementia.

hydronephrosis dilation or enlargement of the renal pelvis and calyces resulting from obstruction in the lower urinary tract with backflow of urine to the kidney.

hydrostatic pressure the force that fluid exerts within a compartment.

hydroureter dilation of the renal pelvis due to backflow of urine.

hyperaldosteronism excessive aldosterone secretion caused by an adenoma of the adrenal zona glomerulosa or bilateral adrenal hyperplasia.

hypercapnia greater than normal amounts of carbon dioxide in the blood; also called hypercarbia.

hypercapnic respiratory failure a condition in which the $PaCO_2$ is above normal in combination with acidemia.

hyperopia farsightedness or the inability of the eye to focus on nearby objects.

hyperosmolar hyperglycemic syndrome (HHS) a life-threatening syndrome that can occur in the patient with diabetes who is able to produce enough insulin to prevent diabetic ketoacidosis but not enough to prevent severe hyperglycemia, osmotic diuresis, and extracellular fluid depletion.

hyperparathyroidism a condition involving increased secretion of parathyroid hormone resulting in increased serum calcium levels.

hypertension a common disorder characterized by sustained elevation of blood pressure.

hypertensive crisis a severe and abrupt elevation in blood pressure.

hyperthyroidism a clinical syndrome in which there is a sustained increase in the synthesis and release of thyroid hormones by the thyroid gland.

hypertonic a solution that increases the degree of osmotic pressure on a semipermeable membrane.

hypertrophic scar an inappropriately large, red, raised, and hard scar that occurs when the body produces excess collagen tissue.

hypoparathyroidism a condition of insufficient secretion of the parathyroid glands.

hypopituitarism a rare disorder that involves a decrease in one or more of the pituitary hormones and marked by excessive deposits of fat and persistence or acquisition of adolescent characteristics.

hypothermia a core temperature <95° F (35° C) that occurs when heat produced by the body cannot compensate for heat lost to the environment.

hypothyroidism insufficient circulation of thyroid hormones resulting in a hypometabolic state.

hypotonic a solution that has a lower concentration of solute than another solution, thus exerting less osmotic pressure on a semipermeable membrane.

hypoxemia low oxygen tension in the blood characterized by a variety of nonspecific clinical signs and symptoms.

hypoxemic respiratory failure a condition in which the PaO_2 is 60 mm Hg or less when the patient is receiving an inspired oxygen concentration of 60% or greater.

hypoxia the state in which the PaO_2 has fallen sufficiently to cause signs and symptoms of inadequate oxygenation.

hysterectomy surgical removal of the uterus.

I

ileal conduit urinary diversion procedure in which ureters are implanted into a part of the ileum or colon that has been resected from the intestinal tract and an abdominal stoma is created.

impaired fasting glucose (IFG) an intermediate stage between normal glucose homeostasis and diabetes.

impaired glucose tolerance (IGT)   an intermediate stage between normal glucose homeostasis and diabetes where the blood glucose level is 140 mg/dL (7.8 mmol/L) to 199 mg/dL (11 mmol/L) 2 hours after a meal.

infective endocarditis   an infection of the endocardial surface of the heart.

infertility   the inability to achieve a pregnancy after at least 1 year of regular intercourse without contraception.

inflammatory bowel disease (IBD)   chronic, recurrent inflammatory diseases of the intestinal tract that include ulcerative colitis and Crohn's disease.

insulin resistance   a condition in which body tissues do not respond to the action of insulin.

intensive insulin therapy   multiple daily insulin injections together with frequent self-monitoring of blood glucose.

intermittent claudication   ischemic muscle ache or pain precipitated by a consistent level of exercise, resolves within 10 minutes or less with rest, and is reproducible.

interstitial cystitis   chronic, painful inflammatory disease of the bladder probably associated with an autoimmune or allergic response.

intraaortic balloon pump (IABP)   a temporary circulatory assist device used to enhance the function of a compromised heart by reducing afterload and augmenting the aortic diastolic pressure.

intracerebral hematoma   collection of blood within the parenchyma of the brain, possibly from the rupture of an intracerebral vessel at the time of a head injury.

intracerebral hemorrhage   a type of hemorrhagic stroke in which bleeding within the brain is caused by a rupture of a blood vessel.

intracranial pressure   the hydrostatic force measured in the brain cerebrospinal fluid compartment.

intravenous pyelogram (IVP)   a diagnostic study using an IV contrast medium excreted through the urinary system; used to examine the structure and function of the urinary system.

iron-deficiency anemia   a microcytic hypochromic anemia caused by inadequate supplies of iron needed to synthesize hemoglobin; characterized by pallor, fatigue, and weakness.

irritable bowel syndrome (IBS)   a symptom complex characterized by intermittent and recurrent abdominal pain associated with an alteration in bowel function (diarrhea or constipation).

ischemic stroke   a stroke that results from inadequate blood flow to the brain due to partial or complete occlusion of an artery.

isometric contractions   muscular contraction that increases tension but does not produce movement.

isotonic contractions   muscular contraction with shortening that produces movement.

J

jaundice   a symptom of yellowish discoloration of body tissues that results from an increased concentration of bilirubin in the blood.

jaw-thrust maneuver   a technique used to maintain an open airway that should be used in emergency situations.

K

keloid   an overgrowth of collagenous scar tissue at the site of a skin injury, particularly a wound or a surgical incision; the new tissue is elevated, rounded, and firm.

keratinocytes   cells synthesized from epidermal cells in the basal layer; the cells produce a specialized protein, keratin, that is vital to the protective barrier function of the skin.

keratitis   an inflammation or infection of the cornea; may be caused by a variety of microorganisms or by other factors.

Korotkoff sounds   sounds heard during the taking of a blood pressure reading using a sphygmomanometer and stethoscope.

Korsakoff's psychosis   a form of amnesia often seen in people with chronic alcoholism; characterized by loss of short-term memory and an inability to learn.

Kupffer cells   a type of macrophage found in the liver that removes bacteria and toxins from the blood.

kyphosis   anterior-posterior or forward bending of spine with convexity of curve in posterior direction.

L

lactase deficiency   an inherited abnormality in which the amount of the digestive enzyme lactase is inadequate for the normal digestion of milk products, resulting in the inability to digest lactose.

lacunar stroke   a stroke resulting from occlusion of a small penetrating artery with development of a cavity in the place of the infarcted brain tissue.

leiomyoma   a benign smooth muscle tumor that occurs most commonly within the uterus, stomach, esophagus, or small intestine; uterine fibroid.

leukemia   a broad term given to a group of malignant diseases characterized by diffuse replacement of bone marrow with proliferating leukocyte precursors.

leukopenia   an abnormal decrease in the number of total white blood cells to <4000/μL.

lichenification   the thickening of the skin as a result of proliferation of keratinocytes with accentuation of the normal markings of the skin often caused by repeated scratching of a pruritic lesion.

lithotripsy   the use of sound waves to break renal stones into small particles that can be eliminated from the urinary tract.

lordosis   lumbar spinal deformity resulting in anterior-posterior curvature with concavity in posterior direction.

lumpectomy   breast conserving surgery that involves the removal of the entire tumor along with a margin of normal tissue.

lung abscess   a pus-containing lesion of the lung parenchyma that results in a cavity formed by necrosis of lung tissue.

Lyme disease   a spirochetal infection caused by *Borrelia burgdorferi* and transmitted by the bite of an infected deer tick; characterized by fever, chills, headache, stiff neck, and migratory joint and muscle pain.

lymphedema   accumulation of lymph in soft tissue with swelling resulting from inflammation, obstruction, or removal of lymph channels and nodes.

lymphomas   malignant neoplasms originating in the bone marrow and lymphatic structures resulting in the proliferation of lymphocytes.

M

malabsorption syndrome   a complex of symptoms resulting from disorders in the intestinal absorption of nutrients, characterized by anorexia, weight loss, abdominal bloating, muscle cramps, bone pain, and steatorrhea.

malignant hyperthermia   a rare genetic metabolic disease characterized by hyperthermia with rigidity of skeletal muscles that can result in death.

malignant melanoma   a tumor arising in cells producing melanin, usually the melanocytes of the skin.

malignant neoplasm   a tumor that tends to grow, invade, and metastasize; usually has an irregular shape and is composed of poorly differentiated cells.

Mallory-Weiss tear   a tear that occurs in the esophageal mucosa at the junction of the esophagus and stomach, caused by severe retching and vomiting and results in severe bleeding.

mammoplasty   a change in the size or shape of the breast due to surgery.

mass casualty incident   a human-caused (e.g., biologic warfare) or natural (e.g., hurricane) event or disaster that overwhelms a community's ability to respond with existing resources.

mastalgia   breast pain; can be caused by congestion or "caking" during lactation, an infection, or fibrocystic disease, especially during or before menstruation, or in advanced cancer.

mastectomy   surgical removal of the breast.

mastitis   an inflammatory condition of the breast that occurs most frequently in lactating women, caused by streptococcal or staphylococcal infection.

mean arterial pressure (MAP)   a calculated average of systolic and diastolic blood pressures; calculated by adding the diastolic pressure to one third of the pulse pressure.

medical care–associated pneumonia (MCAP)   pneumonia occurring 48 hours or longer after hospital admission and not incubating at the time of hospitalization.

megaloblastic anemias   a group of disorders caused by impaired DNA synthesis and characterized by the presence of large red blood cells.

melena   black, tarry stools that indicate slow bleeding from an upper GI source.

menarche   the first episode of menstrual bleeding; indicates female has reached puberty.

Ménière's disease   a disease characterized by symptoms caused by inner ear disease including episodic vertigo, tinnitus, fluctuating sensorineural hearing loss, and aural fullness.

meningitis an acute inflammation of the pia mater and the arachnoid membrane surrounding the brain and the spinal cord.

menopause the physiologic cessation of menses associated with declining ovarian function.

metabolic equivalent (MET) a unit of measurement of heat production by the body; used to determine the energy costs of various exercises.

metabolic syndrome a collection of risk factors that increase an individual's chance of developing cardiovascular disease and diabetes mellitus.

metastasis the spread of the cancer from the initial or primary site to a distant site.

migraine headache a recurring headache characterized by unilateral or bilateral throbbing pain and a triggering event or factor; can occur with and without an aura.

mild cognitive impairment (MCI) a state of cognition and functional ability between normal aging and early Alzheimer's disease.

mixed dementia presentation of two or more types of dementia simultaneously.

mitral valve prolapse (MVP) a structural abnormality of the mitral valve leaflets and the papillary muscles or chordae that allows the leaflets to prolapse, or buckle, back into the left atrium during ventricular systole.

multiple myeloma a condition in which malignant neoplastic plasma cells infiltrate the bone marrow and destroy bone.

multiple organ dysfunction syndrome (MODS) the failure of more than one organ system in an acutely ill patient such that homeostasis cannot be maintained without intervention.

multiple sclerosis (MS) a chronic, progressive, degenerative disorder of the central nervous system characterized by disseminated demyelination of nerve fibers of the brain and spinal cord.

murmur a gentle blowing, fluttering, or humming sound heard on auscultation and produced by turbulent blood flow through the heart or the walls of large arteries.

muscular dystrophy (MD) a group of genetically transmitted diseases characterized by progressive symmetric wasting of skeletal muscle without evidence of neurologic involvement.

myasthenia gravis (MG) an autoimmune disease of the neuromuscular junction characterized by the fluctuating weakness of certain skeletal muscle groups.

myasthenic crisis an acute exacerbation of myasthenia gravis triggered by infection, surgery, emotional distress, or overdose or inadequate medication.

myelodysplastic syndrome (MDS) a group of related hematologic disorders characterized by a change in the quantity and quality of bone marrow elements.

myocardial infarction (MI) an irreversible cardiac cellular death caused by sustained myocardial ischemia.

myocarditis a focal or diffuse inflammation of the myocardium.

myopia nearsightedness or the inability of the eye to focus on objects far away.

myxedema the progression of the mental sluggishness, drowsiness, and lethargy of hypothy-roidism to a notable impairment of consciousness or coma that is a medical emergency.

N

nadir the lowest point, such as the blood cell count after it has been depressed by chemotherapy.

narcolepsy a chronic neurologic disorder caused by the brain's inability to regulate sleep-wake cycles normally; results in fleeting urges to sleep throughout the day.

nasal polyps benign mucous membrane masses that form slowly in response to repeated inflammation of the sinus or nasal mucosa and project into the nasal cavity.

nephrolithiasis the formation of stones in the urinary tract.

nephrosclerosis a vascular disease of the kidney characterized by sclerosis of the small arteries and arterioles of the kidney resulting in renal tissue necrosis.

nephrotic syndrome an abnormal condition of the kidney characterized by peripheral edema, massive proteinuria, hyperlipidemia, and hypo-albuminemia.

neurofibrillary tangles tangled bundles of fibers seen in the cytoplasm of abnormal neurons in those areas of the brain most affected by Alzheimer's disease.

neurogenic bladder any type of bladder dysfunction related to abnormal or absent bladder innervation caused by a lesion of the nervous system.

neurogenic bowel loss of voluntary neurologic control over the bowel.

neurogenic shock neurologic syndrome caused by the loss of vasomotor tone caused by spinal cord injury at the fifth thoracic (T5) vertebra or above and characterized by hypotension, bradycardia, and warm, dry extremities.

neuropathic pain pain caused by damage to nerve cells or changes in spinal cord processing of nervous system input.

neurosyphilis an infection of any part of the nervous system by the organism *Treponema pallidum*.

neutropenia an abnormal reduction of the neutrophil count to <1000/μL.

nociception activation of the primary afferent nerves with peripheral terminals that respond to noxious stimuli.

nociceptive pain pain caused by damage to somatic or visceral tissue; occurs abruptly after an injury or disease, persists until healing occurs, and often is intensified by anxiety or fear.

nonalcoholic fatty liver disease (NAFLD) a group of disorders characterized by hepatic *steatosis* (accumulation of fat in the liver) and is not associated with other causes such as hepatitis, autoimmune disease, or consumption of alcohol.

normal pressure hydrocephalus an uncommon disorder characterized by an obstruction in the flow of cerebrospinal fluid; causes a buildup of this fluid in the brain.

nuchal rigidity resistance to flexion of the neck.

nulliparous never having given birth.

nystagmus an abnormal, involuntary, repetitive movement of the eyes.

O

O₂ toxicity a condition of oxygen overdosage caused by prolonged exposure to a high level of oxygen.

obese the classification used to describe individuals with body mass index values ≥30 kg/m².

obstructive shock develops when a physical obstruction of blood flow occurs with decreased cardiac output.

obstructive sleep apnea (OSA) a condition characterized by partial or complete upper airway obstruction during sleep.

oliguria producing <400 mL of urine in 24 hour.

oncogenes potentially cancer-inducing genes.

oncotic pressure the osmotic pressure of a colloid in solution.

orchitis an acute inflammation of the testis.

orthostatic hypotension abnormally low blood pressure occurring when an individual suddenly assumes a standing position.

osteoarthritis a slowly progressive, noninflammatory disorder of the diarthrodial (synovial) joints.

osteochondroma primary benign bone tumor characterized by an overgrowth of cartilage and bone near the end of the bone at the growth plate.

osteomalacia a rare condition of adult bones associated with vitamin D deficiency, resulting in decalcification and softening of bone.

osteomyelitis a severe infection of the bone, bone marrow, and surrounding soft tissue.

osteon cylindrical-shaped structural units that fit closely together in compact bone, creating a dense bone structure.

osteopenia bone loss that is more than normal (a T-score between −1 and −2.5), but not yet at the level for a diagnosis of osteoporosis.

osteoporosis a metabolic bone disease characterized by low bone mass and structural deterioration of bone tissue, leading to increased bone fragility and pathologic fractures.

osteosarcoma a primary bone tumor that is extremely aggressive and rapidly metastasizes to distant sites; usually occurs in the metaphyseal region of the long bones of the extremities.

osteotomy removing or adding a wedge or slice of bone to change its alignment and shift weight bearing, thereby correcting deformity and relieving pain.

ostomy a surgical procedure in which an opening is made to allow the passage of urine from the bladder or intestinal contents from the bowel through an incision or stoma surgically created in the wall of the abdomen.

otosclerosis a hereditary condition in which irregular ossification occurring on the footplate of the stapes in the oval window results in decreased hearing acuity.

P

Paget's disease of the bone a skeletal bone disorder in which there is excessive bone resorption followed by replacement of normal marrow by vascular, fibrous connective tissue and new bone that is larger, disorganized, and weaker.

Paget's disease of the breast   a breast malignancy characterized by a persistent lesion of the nipple and areola with or without a palpable mass.

palliative care   an approach that improves the quality of life of patients and their families who face problems associated with life-threatening illness.

palpation   a physical examination technique in which the examiner feels the texture, size, consistency, and location of certain body parts with the hands.

pancytopenia   a marked decrease in the number of red blood cells, white blood cells, and platelets.

paracentesis   a procedure in which fluid is withdrawn from a cavity of the body.

paralytic ileus   the lack of intestinal peristalsis.

paraplegia   paralysis characterized by motor and/or sensory loss in the lower limbs and trunk.

parasomnias   unusual and often undesirable behaviors that occur with sleep or during arousal from sleep, such as enuresis (bed-wetting), hallucinations, and eating.

parenteral nutrition (PN)   the administration of nutrients by a route (e.g., bloodstream) other than the GI tract.

Parkinson's disease (PD)   a disease of the basal ganglia characterized by a slowing down in the initiation and execution of movement, increased muscle tone tremor at rest, and impaired postural reflexes.

paroxysmal nocturnal dyspnea (PND)   sudden attacks of respiratory distress that awaken the sleeper, usually after several hours of sleep in a reclining position.

partial-thickness burn   varying degrees of epidermal and dermal skin injury in which some skin elements remain viable for regeneration.

pelvic inflammatory disease (PID)   an infectious condition of the pelvic cavity that may involve infection of the fallopian tubes, ovaries, and pelvic peritoneum.

peptic ulcer disease (PUD)   erosion of the GI mucosa that results from the digestive action of HCl acid and pepsin.

percussion   a physical examination technique in which the examiner taps the body with the fingertips or fist.

percutaneous coronary intervention (PCI)   a common intervention for coronary artery disease in which a catheter equipped with an inflatable balloon tip is inserted into a narrowed coronary artery and the balloon is inflated.

pericardiocentesis   a procedure in which a 16- to 18-gauge needle is inserted into the pericardial space to remove fluid for analysis and to relieve cardiac pressure.

pericarditis   a condition caused by inflammation of the pericardial sac.

perimenopause   a normal life transition that begins with the first signs of change in menstrual cycles and ends after cessation of menses.

peripheral artery disease (PAD)   the progressive narrowing and degeneration of the arteries of the neck, abdomen, and extremities.

peripheral stem cell transplantation   the transplantation of stem cells obtained from the peripheral blood in an outpatient procedure;

often takes more than one procedure to obtain enough stem cells.

peritoneal dialysis (PD)   dialysis using the peritoneal membrane as the semipermeable membrane.

peritonitis   the inflammation of the peritoneum.

pernicious anemia   a progressive megaloblastic macrocytic anemia resulting from inadequate gastric secretion of intrinsic factor necessary for absorption of cobalamin.

pertussis   a highly contagious infection of the lower respiratory tract with a gram-negative bacillus, *Bordetella pertussis.*

petechiae   small purplish lesions.

phantom limb sensation   the perception of sensations or pain in an amputated limb.

pharmacogenetics   the study of variability of responses to drugs due to variations in single genes.

pharmacogenomics   the study of variability of responses to drugs due to variations in and interactions of multiple genes.

pheochromocytoma   a rare condition characterized by a tumor of the adrenal medulla that produces excessive catecholamines causing persistent or intermittent hypertension.

phimosis   a constriction of the uncircumcised foreskin around the head of the penis making retraction difficult.

pleural effusion   an abnormal accumulation of fluid in the intrapleural spaces of the lungs.

pleural friction rub   a creaking or grating sound from roughened, inflamed surfaces of the pleura rubbing together, evident during inspiration, expiration, or both and no change with coughing.

pleurisy (pleuritis)   inflammation of the pleura.

pneumoconiosis   a general term for lung diseases caused by inhalation and retention of dust particles.

pneumonia   an acute inflammation of the lungs, often caused by inhaled pneumococci of the species *Streptococcus pneumoniae.*

pneumothorax   a collection of air or gas in the pleural space causing the lung to collapse.

point of maximal impulse (PMI)   the site on the chest wall where the thrust or pulsation of the left ventricle is most prominent.

polycystic kidney disease (PKD)   a genetic kidney disorder in which the cortex and the medulla are filled with thin-walled cysts that enlarge and destroy surrounding tissue.

polycythemia   an abnormal condition with excessive levels of red blood cells.

polymyositis   diffuse, idiopathic, inflammatory myopathies of striated muscle, producing bilateral weakness usually most severe in the proximal or limb-girdle muscles; some forms of polymyositis are associated with malignancy.

portal hypertension   increased venous pressure in the portal circulation caused by compression and destruction of the portal and hepatic veins and sinusoids.

positive end-expiratory pressure (PEEP)   a ventilatory maneuver in which positive pressure is applied to the airway during exhalation.

postural drainage   the use of various positions to promote gravity drainage of bronchial secretions.

prediabetes   impaired glucose tolerance; occurs when a 2-hour plasma glucose level is higher than normal but lower than that considered diagnostic for diabetes.

prehypertension   a disorder characterized by a systolic blood pressure of 120 to 139 mm Hg and a diastolic blood pressure of 80 to 89 mm Hg.

preload   the volume of blood in the ventricles at the end of diastole before the next contraction.

premature atrial contraction (PAC)   contraction originating from an ectopic focus in the atrium in a location other than the sinus node.

premature ventricular contraction (PVC)   a contraction originating in an ectopic focus in the ventricles.

premenstrual syndrome (PMS)   a common disorder in women in which a group of physical and psychologic symptoms occur during the last few days of the menstrual cycle and before the onset of menstruation.

presbycusis   hearing loss associated with aging.

presbyopia   a hyperopic shift to farsightedness resulting from a loss of elasticity of the lens of the eye.

pressure ulcer   a localized area of tissue necrosis caused by unrelieved pressure that occludes blood flow to the tissues.

primary hypertension   an elevated systemic arterial pressure for which no cause can be found and which is often the only significant clinical finding.

Prinzmetal's angina   a variant angina; occurs at rest, usually in response to reversible, severe spasm of a major coronary artery.

prostatitis   an acute or chronic inflammation of the prostate gland, usually as a result of infection.

pruritus   itching.

psoriasis   a chronic skin disorder characterized by circumscribed red patches covered by thick, dry, silvery, adherent scales.

pulmonary edema   an acute, life-threatening situation in which the lung alveoli become filled with serous or serosanguineous fluid, caused most commonly by heart failure.

pulmonary embolism   a thromboembolic occlusion of the pulmonary vasculature resulting from thrombi in the venous circulation or right side of the heart that travel as emboli until lodging in the pulmonary vessels.

pulmonary hypertension   elevated pulmonary pressure resulting from an increase in pulmonary vascular resistance to blood flow through small arteries and arterioles.

pulse pressure   the difference between the systolic and diastolic pressures.

pursed-lip breathing   a technique of exhaling against pursed lips to prolong exhalation, preventing bronchiolar collapse and air trapping.

pyelonephritis   a diffuse pyogenic infection of the renal parenchyma and collecting system.

pyrosis   a burning sensation in the epigastric or substernal area; heartburn.

R

radical prostatectomy   the surgical removal of the entire prostate gland, seminal vesicles, and part of the bladder neck (ampulla).

Raynaud's phenomenon an episodic vasospastic disorder of small cutaneous arteries, most frequently involving the fingers and toes.

rectocele the herniation or protrusion of the rectum through the wall of the vagina resulting from weakened connective tissue support between the vagina and rectum.

refractive error a defect in the ability of the lens of the eye to focus an image accurately on the retina, as occurs in nearsightedness and farsightedness.

renal artery stenosis a partial occlusion of one or both renal arteries and their major branches; is a major cause of abrupt-onset hypertension.

repetitive strain injury (RSI) a cumulative trauma disorder resulting from prolonged, forceful, or awkward movements resulting in strain of tendons, ligaments, and muscles, causing tiny tears that become inflamed.

restless legs syndrome (RLS) the unpleasant sensory and motor abnormalities of one or both legs; characterized by an irritating sensation of uneasiness, tiredness, and itching deep within the muscles of the leg.

retinal detachment a separation of the retina from the retinal pigment epithelium in the back of the eye, allowing the vitreous humor to leak between the two layers.

retinopathy the process of microvascular damage of the retina; may develop slowly or rapidly.

rheumatic fever an inflammatory disease of the heart that potentially involves all layers.

rheumatic heart disease (RHD) the resulting damage to the heart muscle and heart valves from rheumatic fever, a chronic condition characterized by scarring and deformity of the heart valves.

rheumatoid arthritis (RA) a chronic, systemic autoimmune disease characterized by inflammation of connective tissue in the diarthrodial (synovial) joints, typically with periods of remission and exacerbation.

rhinoplasty the surgical reconstruction of the nose.

rhonchi the continuous rumbling, snoring, or rattling sounds from obstruction of large airways with secretions.

S

sarcoma a malignant tumor that originates from embryonal mesoderm that becomes connective tissue, muscle, bone, and fat.

scleroderma a disorder of connective tissue characterized by fibrotic, degenerative, and occasionally inflammatory changes in the skin, blood vessels, synovium, skeletal muscle, and internal organs.

scoliosis a lateral S-shaped curvature of the thoracic and lumbar spine.

secondary hypertension elevated blood pressure associated with any of several primary diseases, such as renal, pulmonary, endocrine, and vascular disease.

seizure a paroxysmal, uncontrolled electrical discharge of neurons in the brain that interrupts normal function leading to a sudden, violent involuntary series of contractions of a group of muscles.

sepsis a systemic inflammatory response to infection.

septic arthritis infectious or bacterial arthritis caused by invasion of the joint cavity with microorganisms; bacterial inflammation of a joint may be caused by the spread of bacteria through the bloodstream from an infection elsewhere in the body or by contamination of a joint during trauma or surgery.

septic shock the presence of sepsis with hypotension despite adequate fluid resuscitation along with the presence of tissue perfusion abnormalities.

severely obese the classification used to describe individuals with body mass index values >40 kg/m².

sexually transmitted infections (STIs) infectious diseases transmitted most commonly through sexual intercourse or genital contact.

shock a syndrome characterized by decreased tissue perfusion and impaired cellular metabolism resulting in an imbalance between the supply of and demand for oxygen and nutrients.

sickle cell disease (SCD) a group of inherited, autosomal recessive disorders characterized by the presence of an abnormal form of hemoglobin in the erythrocyte.

silent ischemia an asymptomatic ischemia that may damage the heart.

Sjögren's syndrome an autoimmune disease that targets moisture-producing glands, leading to the common symptoms of xerostomia (dry mouth) and keratoconjunctivitis sicca (dry eyes).

Somogyi effect a condition in which an excessive dose of insulin causes blood glucose levels to decline during sleep, triggering the release of counterregulatory hormones that increase the blood glucose levels, resulting in high blood glucose levels at morning testing; indicates a need for reduced dose of insulin.

spermatogenesis the formation of sperm.

spider angiomas small, dilated blood vessels with a bright red center point the size of a pinhead from which small blood vessels radiate.

spinal shock the immediate failure of all spinal cord function at the time of injury below the level of cord damage resulting in flaccid paralysis, loss of reflexes, and loss of sympathetic innervation.

spondyloarthropathies a group of interrelated multisystem inflammatory disorders that affect the spine, peripheral joints, and periarticular structures.

status epilepticus a state of continuous seizure activity or a condition in which seizures recur in rapid succession without return to consciousness between seizures.

steatorrhea a greater than normal amount of fat in the feces.

stenosis a constriction or narrowing.

stent an expandable meshlike structure designed to maintain vessel patency by compressing the arterial walls and resisting vasoconstriction.

strabismus a condition in which the individual cannot consistently focus both eyes simultaneously on the same object.

stricture an abnormal temporary or permanent narrowing of the lumen of a hollow organ.

stroke the death of brain cells that occurs when there is ischemia to a part of the brain or hemorrhage into the brain.

subarachnoid hemorrhage a stroke resulting from intracranial bleeding into the cerebrospinal fluid–filled space between the arachnoid and pia mater membranes on the surface of the brain.

subdural hematoma a collection of blood between the dura mater and the arachnoid layer of the meninges of the brain that is generally of venous origin, usually caused by injury.

submersion injury hypoxia resulting from submersion in a substance, usually water.

sudden cardiac death (SCD) unexpected death from cardiac causes.

sundowning a condition in which the individual becomes more confused and agitated in the late afternoon or evening.

surfactant a lipoprotein that lowers the surface tension in the alveoli, reduces the amount of pressure needed to inflate the alveoli, and decreases the tendency of the alveoli to collapse.

syndrome of inappropriate antidiuretic hormone (SIADH) a condition associated with overproduction or oversecretion of ADH.

synovectomy the surgical removal of synovial membrane.

syphilis the infection of organs and tissues of the body by *Treponema pallidum*.

systemic inflammatory response syndrome (SIRS) a systemic inflammatory response to a variety of insults, including infection, ischemia, infarct, and injury.

systemic lupus erythematosus (SLE) a chronic multisystem inflammatory disorder associated with abnormalities of the immune system.

systolic failure a type of ventricular failure caused by impaired contractile function, increased afterload, or mechanical abnormalities.

T

teletherapy radiation therapy administered by a machine positioned at some distance from the patient; the most common form of radiation therapy treatment.

tenesmus the painful spasmodic contraction of the anal sphincter and a persistent desire to empty the bowel.

tension pneumothorax a rapid accumulation of air in the pleural space causing severely high intrapleural pressures with resultant tension on the heart and great vessels.

tension-type headache a headache characterized by a bilateral feeling of pressure around the head.

tetanus lockjaw; an extremely severe polyradiculitis and polyneuritis affecting spinal and cranial nerves that results from the effects of a potent neurotoxin released by the anaerobic bacillus *Clostridium tetani*.

tetraplegia the paralysis of the arms, legs, and trunk occurring with spinal cord damage at C8 or above.

thalassemia an autosomal recessive genetic disorder of inadequate production of normal hemoglobin.

thoracentesis a surgical procedure done to remove fluid from the pleural space.

thoracotomy a surgical opening into the thoracic cavity.

thrombocytopenia a reduction of the platelet count.

thrombocytosis a condition marked by excessive platelets; a disorder that occurs with inflammation and some malignant disorders.

thrombotic stroke a stroke resulting from thrombosis or narrowing of the blood vessel.

thyroiditis an inflammatory process in the thyroid gland.

thyrotoxicosis (also called thyrotoxic crisis) a hypermetabolic state caused by excessive circulating levels of T_4, T_3, or both.

tinnitus a subjective noise sensation, often described as ringing, heard in one or both ears.

tonic-clonic seizure a seizure characterized by loss of consciousness and falling to the ground, followed by stiffening of the body for 10 to 20 seconds and subsequent jerking of the extremities for another 30 to 40 seconds.

tracheostomy a surgical opening into the trachea through which an indwelling tube may be inserted.

tracheotomy a surgical incision into the trachea for the purpose of establishing an airway; performed below a blockage by a foreign body, tumor, or edema of the glottis.

traction the application of a pulling force to an injured or diseased part of the body or an extremity while countertraction pulls in the opposite direction.

transurethral resection of the prostate (TURP) a surgical procedure involving the removal of prostate tissue with the use of a resectoscope inserted through the urethra.

triage a system that identifies and categorizes patients so the most critical are treated first.

trigeminal neuralgia a neurologic condition of the trigeminal facial nerve characterized by paroxysms of flashing, stablike pain radiating along the course of a branch of the nerve from the angle of the jaw.

trigger point a circumscribed hypersensitive area within a tight band of muscle that is caused by acute or chronic muscle strain.

tuberculosis (TB) an infectious disease caused by *Mycobacterium tuberculosis;* usually involves the lungs, but also occurs in the larynx, kidneys, bones, adrenal glands, lymph nodes, and meninges and can be disseminated throughout the body.

tumor angiogenesis the process of the formation of blood vessels within the tumor itself.

tumor-associated antigens the altered cell surface antigens found on cancer cells.

U

ulcerative colitis a chronic inflammatory bowel disease that causes ulceration of the colon and rectum.

unstable angina (UA) an angina that is new in onset, occurs at rest, or has a worsening pattern.

uremia the presence of excessive amounts of urea and other nitrogenous waste products in the blood; renal function declines to the point that symptoms develop in multiple body systems.

urethritis inflammation of the urethra.

urinary incontinence (UI) an uncontrolled leakage of urine; can be caused by anything that interferes with bladder or urethral sphincter control, including confusion or depression, infection, atrophic vaginitis, urinary retention, restricted mobility, fecal impaction, or drugs.

urinary retention the inability to empty the bladder despite micturition, or the accumulation of urine in the bladder because of an inability to urinate.

urosepsis a urinary tract infection that has spread into the systemic circulation; life-threatening condition requiring emergency treatment.

urticaria a pruritic skin eruption characterized by transient wheals of varying shapes and sizes with well-defined erythematous margins and pale centers; usually an allergic phenomenon.

uterine prolapse the downward displacement of the uterus into the vaginal canal as a result of impaired pelvic support.

V

Valsalva maneuver a maneuver that involves contraction of the chest muscles on a closed glottis with simultaneous contraction of the abdominal muscles.

varicose veins the dilated, tortuous subcutaneous veins most frequently found in the saphenous system.

vascular dementia the loss of cognitive function resulting from ischemic, ischemic-hypoxic, or hemorrhagic brain lesions caused by cardiovascular disease.

vasectomy the bilateral surgical ligation or resection of the vas deferens performed for the purpose of sterilization.

ventricular assist device (VAD) a device that is applied externally or internally into the path of flowing blood to augment or replace the action of the ventricle of the heart.

ventricular fibrillation a severe derangement of the heart rhythm characterized on electrocardiogram (ECG) by irregular undulations of varying contour and amplitude.

ventricular tachycardia (VT) a condition that occurs when an ectopic focus or foci fire repetitively and the ventricle takes control as the pacemaker.

vertigo a sensation that a person or objects around the person are moving or spinning; usually stimulated by movement of the head.

vesicants agents that when accidentally infiltrated into the skin cause severe local tissue breakdown and necrosis.

viral load the quantity of viral particles in a biologic sample.

Virchow's triad three important factors in the etiology of venous thrombosis: (1) venous stasis, (2) damage of the endothelium (inner lining of the vein), and (3) hypercoagulability of the blood.

viremia large amounts of virus in the blood, resulting from initial infection with a virus.

W

Wernicke's encephalopathy an inflammatory, hemorrhagic, degenerative condition of the brain resulting from a deficiency of thiamine; is seen in association with chronic alcoholism.

wheezes a form of rhonchus characterized by a continuous high-pitched squeaking sound caused by rapid vibration of bronchial walls.

window period a time period of 2 months after HIV infection during which an infected individual will not test positive for HIV-antibody.

ILLUSTRATION CREDITS

CHAPTER 1

Fig. 1-4, Courtesy Elizabeth Burkhart, RN, MPH, PhD, Chicago, Ill. **Fig. 1-6,** Courtesy Kathryn Bowles. From Moser DK, Riegel B: *Cardiac nursing: a companion to Braunwald's heart disease,* St Louis, 2008, Saunders. **Fig. 1-7,** Adapted from Courtlandt CD, Noonan L, Leonard GF: Model for improvement—part 1: A framework for health care quality, *Pediatric Clinics of North America* 56:757, 2009.

CHAPTER 2

Fig. 2-1, From McGinnis JM, Williams-Russo P, Knickman JR: The case for more active policy attention to health promotion, *Health Affairs* 21:78, 2002. **Fig. 2-2,** From *www.cdc.gov/vitalsigns.* **Fig. 2-9,** From Giger JN: *Transcultural nursing,* ed 6, St Louis, 2013, Mosby.

CHAPTER 3

Figs. 3-1, 3-4, Courtesy Linda Bucher, RN, PhD, CEN, CNE, Staff Nurse, Virtua Memorial Hospital, Mt. Holly, N.J. **Fig. 3-3,** From Seidel HM, Ball JW, Dains JE, Flynn JA: *Mosby's guide to physical examination,* ed 7, St Louis, 2011, Saunders.

CHAPTER 4

Figs. 4-2, 4-3, 4-4, Courtesy Linda Bucher, RN, PhD, CEN, CNE, Staff Nurse, Virtua Memorial Hospital, Mt. Holly, N.J.

CHAPTER 5

Fig. 5-1, From Woog P: *The chronic illness trajectory framework: the Corbin and Strauss nursing model,* New York, 1992, Springer. **Fig. 5-7,** Adapted from Fulmer T: The geriatric nurse specialist role: a new model, *Nursing Management* 22:91, 1991. © Copyright Lippincott Williams & Wilkins, *http://lww.com.* **Fig. 5-10,** Redrawn from Benzon J: Approaching drug regimens with a therapeutic dose of suspicion, *Geriatric Nursing* 12(4):1813, 1991.

CHAPTER 8

Fig. 8-4, Modified from LaFleur Brooks M: *Exploring medical language: a student-directed approach,* ed 8, St Louis, 2012, Mosby. **Fig. 8-5,** From Goldman L, Schafer AI: *Goldman's Cecil medicine,* ed 24, Philadelphia, 2012, Saunders.

CHAPTER 9

Fig. 9-1, Developed by McCaffery M, Pasero C, Paice JA. Modified from M McCaffery, C Pasero: *Pain: clinical manual,* ed 2, St Louis, 1999, Mosby. **Fig. 9-7,** From DeLee JC, Drez D, Miller MD: *DeLee and Drez's orthopaedic sports medicine: principles and practices,* ed 3, Philadelphia, 2009, Saunders.

CHAPTER 10

Fig. 10-1, Courtesy Kathleen A. Pollard, RN, MSN, CHPN, Phoenix, Ariz. **Fig. 10-4,** From Rick Brady, Riva, Md.

CHAPTER 12

Fig. 12-5, From Bale S, Jones V: *Wound care nursing: a patient-centered approach,* ed 2, St Louis, 2006, Mosby. **Fig. 12-6,** From Hayden RJ, Jebson PJL: Wrist arthrodesis, *Hand Clinics,* 21(4): 631-640, 2005. **Figs. 12-7, 12-8,** Reproduced with kind permission from Dr. C. Lawrence, Wound Healing Research Unit, Cardiff. In S Bale, V Jones, editors: *Wound care nursing: a patient-centered approach,* ed 2, St Louis, 2006, Mosby. **Fig. 12-9,** Courtesy Robert B. Babiak, RN, BSN, CWOCN, San Antonio, Tex. **Fig. 12-10,** From Perry AG, Potter PA, Elkin MK: *Nursing interventions and clinical skills,* ed 5, St Louis, 2012, Mosby.

Fig. 12-11, From Abai B, Zickler RW, Pappas PJ, et al: Lymphorrhea responds to negative pressure wound therapy, *Journal of Vascular Surgery* 45(3):610-613, 2007.

CHAPTER 13

Figs. 13-1, 13-2, Adapted from *The New Genetics.* National Institute of General Medical Science. National Institutes of Health. US Department of Health and Human Services.

CHAPTER 14

Figs. 14-8, 14-9, From Morison MJ: *Nursing management of chronic wounds,* Edinburgh, 2001, Mosby. **Fig. 14-13,** From McKenry L, Tessier E, Hogan M: *Mosby's pharmacology in nursing,* St Louis, 2006, Mosby.

CHAPTER 15

Fig. 15-5, From Emond R, Welsby P, Rowland H: *Colour atlas of infectious diseases,* ed 4, Edinburgh, 2003, Mosby. **Fig. 15-6,** From Friedman-Kien AE: *Color atlas of AIDS,* Philadelphia, 1989, Saunders. **Fig. 15-7,** Set of slides published in 1992 by Jon Fuller, MD and Howard Libman, MD at Boston University School of Medicine, Boston, Mass. **Fig. 15-8,** From the Centers for Disease Control and Prevention. Courtesy Jonathan W.M. Gold, MD, New York. **Fig. 15-9,** From James WD, Berger T, Elston D: *Andrews' diseases of the skin: clinical dermatology,* ed 11, St Louis, 2011, Saunders.

CHAPTER 16

Fig. 16-1, Adapted from Kumar V, Abbas AK, Fausto N, et al: *Robbins and Cotran pathologic basis of disease,* ed 8, Philadelphia, 2010, Saunders. **Fig. 16-3,** Adapted from Stevens A, Lowe J: *Pathology: an illustrated review in colour,* ed 2, London, 2000, Mosby. **Fig. 16-4,** Adapted from Fidler IT: The pathogenesis of cancer metastasis: the "seed and soil" hypothesis revisited, *Nature Reviews. Cancer* 3:453-458, 2003. **Fig. 16-7,** From Shimizu N, Masuda H, Yamanaka H, et al: Fluorodeoxyglucose positron emission tomography scan of prostate cancer bone metastases with flare reaction after endocrine therapy, *Journal of Urology* 161(2): 609, 1999. **Fig. 16-11,** From Weinzweig N, Weinzweig J: *The mutilated hand,* Philadelphia, 2005, Mosby. **Figs. 16-12, 16-13,** Courtesy Jormain Cady, Virginia Mason Medical Center, Seattle, Wash. **Fig. 16-18,** From Forbes CD, Jackson WF: *Colour atlas and text of clinical medicine,* ed 3, London, 2003, Mosby.

CHAPTER 17

Fig. 17-1, Modified from Copstead-Kirkhorn LC, Banasik JL: *Pathophysiology,* ed 4, St Louis, 2010, Mosby. **Figs. 17-4, 17-6, 17-7,** From Patton KT, Thibodeau GA: *Anatomy and physiology,* ed 8, St Louis, 2013, Mosby. **Fig. 17-14,** From McCance KL, Huether SE: *Pathophysiology: the biologic basis for disease in adults and children,* ed 6, St Louis, 2010, Mosby.

CHAPTER 18

Fig. 18-1, Courtesy Susan R. Volk, RN, MSN, CCRN, CPAN, Staff Development Specialist, Christiana Care Health System, Newark, Del.

CHAPTER 19

Fig. 19-1, Courtesy Greg McVicar. **Fig. 19-2,** Courtesy Swedish Edmonds Hospital, Edmonds, Wash. Photograph by Amy Wesley. **Fig. 19-4,** Courtesy The Methodist Hospital, Houston, Tex. Photograph by Donna Dahms, RN, CNOR. **Fig. 19-5,** Courtesy Covidien, Mansfield, Mass.

CHAPTER 20

Fig. 20-5, Courtesy Christine R. Hoch, RN, MSN, Nursing Instructor, Delaware Technical Community College, Newark, Del.

CHAPTER 21

Figs. 21-1, 21-3, 21-6, Modified from Patton KT, Thibodeau GA: *Anatomy and physiology,* ed 8, St Louis, 2013, Mosby. **Fig. 21-4,** From Kanski JJ: *Clinical ophthalmology: a synopsis,* ed 2, New York, 2009, Butterworth-Heinemann. **Fig. 21-5,** From Newell FW: *Ophthalmology: principles and concepts,* ed 7, St Louis, 1992, Mosby. **Fig. 21-7, B, C,** from Swartz MH: *Textbook of physical diagnosis: history and examination,* ed 6, Philadelphia, 2010, Saunders.

CHAPTER 22

Figs. 22-1, 22-2, 22-3, 22-4, 22-5, 22-8, Courtesy Cory J. Bosanko, OD, FAAO, Eye Centers of Tennessee, Crossville, Tenn. **Fig. 22-9,** From Flint P, Haughey B, Lund V, Niparko JK, editors: *Cummings otolaryngology: head and neck surgery,* ed 5, St Louis, 2010, Mosby.

CHAPTER 23

Fig. 23-2, From Patton KT, Thibodeau GA, Douglas M: *Essentials of anatomy and physiology,* St. Louis, 2012, Mosby. **Figs. 23-3, 23-6,** From Habif TP: *Clinical dermatology: a color guide to diagnosis and therapy,* ed 5, St Louis, 2009, Mosby. **Figs. 23-4, 23-8,** From Gawkrodger D, Ardern-Jones MR: *Dermatology,* ed 5, Edinburgh, 2012, Churchill Livingstone. **Figs. 23-5, 23-7, 23-10,** From Graham-Brown R, Bourke J, Cunliffe T: *Dermatology: fundamentals of practice,* Edinburgh, 2008, Mosby Ltd. **Fig. 23-9,** From Hurwitz S: *Clinical pediatric dermatology: a textbook of skin disorders of childhood and adolescence,* ed 2, Philadelphia, 1993, Saunders.

CHAPTER 24

Figs. 24-1, 24-11, From Habif TP: *Clinical dermatology: a color guide to diagnosis and therapy,* ed 5, St Louis, 2010, Mosby. **Fig. 24-2,** From The Skin Cancer Foundation, New York, N.Y. **Figs. 24-3, 24-12,** From Graham-Brown R, Bourke J, Cunliffe T: *Dermatology: fundamentals of practice,* Edinburgh, 2008, Mosby Ltd. **Figs. 24-4, 24-8,** From Swartz MH: *Textbook of physical diagnosis: history and examination,* ed 6, Philadelphia, 2010, Saunders. **Figs. 24-5, 24-9,** From Gawkrodger D, Ardern-Jones MR: *Dermatology,* ed 5, Edinburgh, 2012, Churchill Livingstone. **Fig. 24-6,** From Habif TP: *Clinical dermatology: a color guide to diagnosis and therapy,* ed 4, St Louis, 2004, Mosby. **Figs. 24-7, 24-10,** From James WD, Berger T, Elston DMD: *Andrews' diseases of the skin,* ed 11, Philadelphia, 2011, Saunders. **Fig. 24-13,** Courtesy Peter Bonner, Placitas, N. Mex. **Fig. 24-14,** From Pastorek N, Bustillo A: Deep plane facelift, *Facial Plastic Surgery Clinics of North America* 13:433-449, 2005.

CHAPTER 25

Figs. 25-1, 25-2, 25-8, 25-9, 25-11, 25-12, Courtesy Judy A. Knighton, Toronto, Canada. **Fig. 25-6,** From American Association of Critical-Care Nurses: *AACN advanced critical care nursing,* St Louis, 2009, Mosby. **Fig. 25-14,** Courtesy Linda Bucher, RN, PhD, CEN, CNE, Staff Nurse, Virtua Memorial Hospital, Mt. Holly, N.J.

CHAPTER 26

Fig. 26-1, Redrawn from Price SA, Wilson LM: *Pathophysiology: clinical concepts of disease processes,* ed 6, St Louis, 2003, Mosby. **Figs. 26-2, 26-3, 26-8, 26-9,** Redrawn from Thompson JM, McFarland GK, Hirsch JE, Tucker SM: *Mosby's clinical nursing,* ed 5, St Louis, 2002, Mosby. **Fig. 26-4, A,** From Dantzker DR, Bone RC, George RB, editors: *Pulmonary and critical care medicine,* vol 1, St Louis, 1993, Mosby. **Fig. 26-4, B,** From Albertine KH, Williams MC, Hyde DM: Anatomy of the lungs. In RJ Mason, VC Broaddus, JF Murray, et al, editors: *Murray and Nadel's textbook of respiratory medicine,* ed 4, Philadelphia, 2005, Saunders. **Fig. 26-10,** Redrawn from Beare PG, Myers JL: *Adult health nursing,* ed 3, St Louis, 1998,

Mosby. **Fig. 26-11, A,** Courtesy Olympus America Inc, Melville, N.Y. **Fig. 26-12,** Redrawn from Du Bois RM, Clarke SW: *Fiberoptic bronchoscopy in diagnosis and management,* Orlando, 1987, Grune & Stratton.

CHAPTER 27

Fig. 27-1, A, Courtesy Boston Medical, Westborough, Mass. **Fig. 27-1, B,** From Roberts JR, Hedges JR: *Clinical procedures in emergency medicine,* ed 5, Philadelphia, 2009, Saunders. **Fig. 27-4,** From Potter PA, Perry AG: *Basic nursing: essentials for practice,* ed 7, St Louis, 2011, Mosby. **Fig. 27-5, D,** Courtesy Dale Medical Products, Inc, Plainville, Mass. **Fig. 27-8,** Courtesy Passy-Muir, Inc, Irvine, Calif. **Fig. 27-11,** From Eggers G, Flechtenmacher C, Kurzen J, Hassfeld S: Infiltrating basal cell carcinoma of the neck 34 years after irradiation of an haemangioma in early childhood. A case-report, *Journal of Cranio-maxillofacial Surgery* 33:199, 2005. **Fig. 27-12, A,** Courtesy Wade Hampton.

CHAPTER 28

Fig. 28-2, From Damjanov I, Linder J: *Anderson's pathology,* ed 10, St Louis, 1996, Mosby. **Fig. 28-3,** From Kumar V, Abbas AK, Aster JC, Fausto N: *Robbins and Cotran pathologic basis of disease,* ed 8, Philadelphia, 2010, Saunders. **Fig. 28-8,** From Atrium Medical Corporation, Hudson, N.H. **Fig. 28-9, A,** Courtesy and © Copyright Becton, Dickinson and Company. **Fig. 28-11,** From the teaching collection of the Department of Pathology, University of Texas Southwestern Medical School, Dallas, Tex. In V Kumar, AK Abbas, JC Aster, N Fausto, editors: *Robbins and Cotran pathologic basis of disease,* ed 8, Philadelphia, 2010, Saunders.

CHAPTER 29

Fig. 29-1, Adapted from McCance KL, Huether SE, editors: *Pathophysiology: the biologic basis for disease in adults and children,* ed 6, St Louis, 2010, Mosby. **Fig. 29-3,** Redrawn from Price SA, Wilson LM: *Pathophysiology: clinical concepts of disease processes,* ed 6, St Louis, 2003, Mosby. **Fig. 29-4,** Modified from National Heart, Lung, and Blood Institute: *Expert Panel Report 3: Guidelines for the diagnosis and management of asthma.* National Asthma Education and Prevention Program, The Institute, 2007. **Figs. 29-5, 29-7,** From Potter PA, Perry AG, Stockert P, Hall A: *Basic nursing: essentials for practice,* ed 7, St. Louis, 2011, Mosby. **Figs. 29-12, 29-13,** Courtesy Nellcor Puritan Bennett, Inc, Pleasanton, Calif. **Fig. 29-15,** Courtesy Smiths Medical North America. **Fig. 29-17, C,** From Kumar V, Abbas AK, Aster JC, Fausto N: *Robbins and Cotran pathologic basis of disease,* ed 8, Philadelphia, 2010, Saunders.

CHAPTER 30

Figs. 30-1, 30-2, Modified from Patton KT, Thibodeau GA: *Anatomy and physiology,* ed 8, St Louis, 2013, Mosby. **Fig. 30-7,** Modified from Herlihy B, Maebius N: *The human body in health and illness,* ed 4, Philadelphia, 2011, Saunders.

CHAPTER 31

Fig. 31-4, Modified from McCance KL, Huether SE: *Pathophysiology: the biologic basis for disease in adults and children,* ed 6, St Louis, 2010, Mosby. **Figs. 31-6, 31-8, 31-10,** From Forbes CD, Jackson WF: *Colour atlas and text of clinical medicine,* ed 3, London, 2003, Mosby. **Fig. 31-12,** Modified from McKinney ES, James SR, Murray SS, Nelson K: *Maternal-child nursing,* Philadelphia, 2000, Saunders. **Fig. 31-13,** From Hoffman AV, Pettit JE: *Color atlas of clinical hematology,* ed 4, Philadelphia, 2009, Mosby. **Fig. 31-15,** From Cotran RS, Kumar V, Abbas AK: *Robbins pathologic basis of disease,* ed 6, Philadelphia, 1999, Saunders.

CHAPTER 32

Figs. 32-9, 32-12, From Drake RL, Vogl AW, Mitchell AWM: *Gray's anatomy for students,* ed 2, Philadelphia, 2010, Churchill Livingstone. **Fig. 32-10,** From Otto C: *Textbook of clinical echocardiography,* ed 3, St Louis, 2004, Saunders. **Fig. 32-11,** From Libby P et al: *Braunwald's heart disease: a textbook of cardiovascular medicine,* ed 8, St Louis, 2008, Saunders.

CHAPTER 33

Fig. 33-2, From Kumar V, Cotran RS, Robbins SL: *Robbins basic pathology,* ed 8, Philadelphia, 2007, Saunders. **Fig. 33-3,** From US Department of Health and Human Services: *Seventh report of the Joint National Committee on Prevention, Detection, Evaluation, and Treatment of High Blood Pressure (JNC 7),* Washington, DC, 2003, National Institutes of Health. **Fig. 33-4,** From Kliegman RM, Behrman RE, Jenson HB, Stanton B: *Nelson textbook of pediatrics,* ed 18, Philadelphia, 2011, Saunders.

CHAPTER 34

Fig. 34-7, From Zipes DB, Libby P, Bonow RO, Braunwald E: *Braunwald's heart disease: a textbook of cardiovascular medicine,* ed 7, St Louis, 2005, Saunders. **Fig. 34-10,** From Kumar V, Abbas AK, Aster JC, Fausto N: *Robbins and Cotran pathologic basis of disease,* ed 8, Philadelphia, 2010, Saunders.

CHAPTER 35

Fig. 35-2, Modified from Huether SE, McCance KL: *Understanding pathophysiology,* ed 3, St Louis, 2004, Mosby. **Fig. 35-3,** Modified from Urden LD, Stacy KM, Lough ME: *Critical care nursing: diagnosis and management,* ed 6, St Louis, 2010, Mosby. **Fig. 35-6,** Used with permission from Honeywell HomMed.

CHAPTER 36

Fig. 36-5, Modified from Wesley K: *Basic dysrhythmias and acute coronary syndromes,* ed 4, St Louis, 2011, Mosby JEMS. **Fig. 36-10,** Modified from Urden LD, Stacy KM, Lough ME: *Critical care nursing: diagnosis and management,* ed 6, St Louis, 2010, Mosby. **Fig. 36-21,** Courtesy Medtronic Physio-Control, Redmond, Wash. **Figs. 36-22,** *A,* **36-24,** *A,* **36-25,** Courtesy Medtronic, Inc., Minneapolis, Minn. **Fig. 36-29,** From Bucher L, Melander S: *Critical care nursing,* Philadelphia, 1999, Saunders.

CHAPTER 37

Fig. 37-1, Modified from Patton KT, Thibodeau GA: *The human body in health and disease,* ed 5, St Louis, 2010, Mosby. **Figs. 37-2, 37-4,** From Damjanov I, Linder J: *Pathology: a color atlas,* St Louis, 2000, Mosby. **Fig. 37-5,** From Guzzetta CE, Dossey BM: *Cardiovascular nursing: holistic practice,* St Louis, 1992, Mosby. **Fig. 37-7,** From McCance KL, Huether SE: *Pathophysiology: the biologic basis for disease in adults and children,* ed 6, St Louis, 2010, Mosby. **Figs. 37-8, 37-11, 37-12,** From Kumar V, Abbas AK, Aster JC, Fausto N: *Robbins and Cotran pathologic basis of disease,* ed 8, Philadelphia, 2010, Saunders. **Fig. 37-9,** From Crawford MH, DiMarco JP, Paulus WJ: *Cardiology,* ed 3, Edinburgh, 2010, Mosby Ltd. **Fig. 37-10,** From Bonow RO, Mann DL, Zipes DP, Libby P: *Braunwald's heart disease: a textbook of cardiovascular medicine,* ed 9, Philadelphia, 2012, Saunders.

CHAPTER 38

Figs. 38-3, 38-13, From Kamal A, Brockelhurst JC: *Colour atlas of geriatric medicine,* ed 2, 1991, Mosby-Year Book-Europe. **Fig. 38-4,** Courtesy Jo Menzoian, Boston, Mass. **Fig. 38-8,** From Damjanov I, Linder J, editors: *Anderson's pathology,* ed 10, St Louis, 1996, Mosby. **Fig. 38-10,** From Etufugh CN, Phillips TJ: Venous ulcers, *Clinics in Dermatology,* 25(1):125, 2007. **Fig. 38-12,** From Goldman MP, Guex JJ, Weiss RA: *Sclerotherapy: treatment of varicose and telangiectatic leg veins,* ed 5, Philadelphia, 2011, Mosby.

CHAPTER 39

Fig. 39-2, From Patton KT, Thibodeau GA: *Anatomy and physiology,* ed 8, St Louis, 2013, Mosby. **Figs. 39-9, 39-10,** From Drake RL, Vogl W, Mitchell AWM: *Gray's anatomy for students,* ed 2, Edinburgh, 2010, Churchill Livingstone. **Fig. 39-11,** From Given Imaging, Inc, Norcross, Ga.

CHAPTER 40

Fig. 40-1, US Department of Agriculture, Center for Nutrition Policy and Promotion: Guidance on Use of USDA's MyPlate and Statements about Amounts of Food Groups Contributed by Foods on Food Product Labels, Washington, DC. **Fig. 40-2,** US Department of Health and Human Services, Nutrition Facts Label, Silver Spring, Md. **Fig. 40-3,** From Morgan SL, Weinsier RL: *Fundamentals of clinical nutrition,* ed 2, St Louis, 1998, Mosby. **Fig. 40-4,** From Kamal A, Brockelhurst JC: *Color atlas of geriatric medicine,* ed 2, St Louis, 1991, Mosby. **Fig. 40-5,** Adapted from Ukleja A, Freeman KL, Gilbert K, and the ASPEN Board of Directors: Standards for nutrition support: adult hospitalized patients, *Nutrition in Clinical Practice* 25:403, 2010. **Fig. 40-7,** Redrawn from Mahan LK, Arlin M: *Krause's food, nutrition, and diet therapy,* ed 8, Philadelphia, 1992, Saunders.

CHAPTER 41

Fig. 41-6, From Shermak MA: Contouring the epigastrium, *Aesthetic Surgery Journal* 25:506, 2005.

CHAPTER 42

Fig. 42-1, Modified from McKenry L, Tessier E, Hogan M: *Mosby's pharmacology in nursing,* ed 22, St Louis, 2006, Mosby. **Fig. 42-4,** Modified from Doughty DB, Jackson DB: *Mosby's clinical nursing series: gastrointestinal disorders,* St Louis, 1993, Mosby. **Figs. 42-6, 42-8, 42-9,** Modified from Price SA, Wilson LM: *Pathophysiology: clinical concepts of disease processes,* ed 6, St Louis, 2003, Mosby. **Figs. 42-10, 42-15,** From Kumar V, Abbas AK, Aster JC, Fausto N: *Robbins and Cotran pathologic basis of disease,* ed 8, Philadelphia, 2010, Saunders.

CHAPTER 43

Fig. 43-6, Courtesy David Bjorkman, MD, University of Utah School of Medicine, Department of Gastroenterology. In McCance KL, Huether SE: *Pathophysiology: the biologic basis for disease in adults and children,* ed 6, St Louis, 2010, Mosby. **Fig. 43-8,** Modified from McCance KL, Huether SE: *Pathophysiology: the biologic basis for disease in adults and children,* ed 6, St Louis, 2010, Mosby. **Fig. 43-14,** *A and B,* From Zitelli BJ, McIntire SC, Nowalk AJ: *Zitelli and Davis' atlas of pediatric physical diagnosis,* ed 6, Philadelphia, 2012, Saunders. **Fig. 43-14,** *C,* From Swartz MH: *Textbook of physical diagnosis: history and examination,* ed 6, Philadelphia, 2010, Saunders. **Fig. 43-16,** From Townsend CM, Beauchamp RD, Evers BM, et al: *Sabiston textbook of surgery: the biological basis of modern surgical practice,* ed 19, Philadelphia, 2012, Saunders.

CHAPTER 44

Figs. 44-1, 44-8, 44-13, From Butcher GP: *Gastroenterology: an illustrated colour text,* London, 2004, Churchill Livingstone. **Figs. 44-2, 44-3,** From McCance KL, Huether SE: *Pathophysiology: the biologic basis for disease in adults and children,* ed 6, St Louis, 2010, Mosby. **Figs. 44-4, 44-10,** *B,* **44-14,** From Kumar V, Abbas AK, Aster JC, Fausto N: *Robbins and Cotran pathologic basis of disease,* ed 8, Philadelphia, 2010, Saunders. **Figs. 44-5, 44-7,** Adapted from Huether SE, McCance KL: *Understanding pathophysiology,* ed 5, St Louis, 2012, Mosby. **Fig. 44-10,** *A,* From Kumar V, Abbas AK, Fausto N: *Robbins and Cotran pathologic basis of disease,* ed 7, Philadelphia, 2005, Saunders. **Fig. 44-12,** From Stevens A, Lowe J: *Pathology: illustrated review in colour,* ed 2, London, 2000, Mosby.

CHAPTER 45

Fig. 45-3, Modified from Thibodeau GA, Patton KT: *The human body in health and disease,* ed 4, St Louis, 2005, Mosby. **Fig. 45-4,** Modified from Herlihy B, Maebius N: *The human body in health and disease,* ed 4, Philadelphia, 2011, Saunders. **Fig. 45-5,** Modified from Thibodeau GA, Patton KT: *Anatomy and physiology,* ed 6, St Louis, 2007, Mosby. **Figs. 45-6, 45-8,** From Brundage DJ: *Renal disorders,* St Louis, 1992, Mosby. **Fig. 45-10, A,** Courtesy Circon Corporation, Santa Barbara, Calif.

CHAPTER 46

Figs. 46-2, 46-4, From Kumar V, Abbas AK, Aster JC, Fausto N, et al: *Robbins and Cotran pathologic basis of disease,* ed 8, Philadelphia, 2010, Saunders. **Fig. 46-5, A,** From Stevens A, Lowe JS, Scott I: *Core pathology: illustrated review in color,* ed 3, London, 2009, Mosby Ltd. **Figs. 46-5, B,** and **46-6,** From Bullock N, Doble A, Turner W, Cuckow P: *Urology: an illustrated colour text.* London, 2008, Churchill Livingstone. **Fig. 46-7, A,** From Brundage DJ: *Renal disorders,* St Louis, 1992, Mosby. **Figs. 46-7, B, and 46-8, 46-9, B,** From Kumar V, Abbas AK, Fausto N: *Robbins and Cotran pathologic basis of disease,* ed 7, Philadelphia, 2005, Saunders. **Fig. 46-9, A,** From Stevens A, Lowe J: *Pathology: illustrated review in colour,* ed 2, London, 2000, Mosby. **Figs. 46-12, 46-14, 46-15,** Courtesy Lynda Brubacher, Virginia Mason Hospital, Seattle, Wash.

CHAPTER 47

Fig. 47-1, From Stevens A, Lowe J: *Pathology: illustrated review in colour,* ed 2, London, 2000, Mosby. **Fig. 47-6,** Courtesy Mary Jo Holechek, Baltimore, Md. **Fig. 47-7,** Courtesy Baxter Healthcare Corporation, McGaw Park, Ill. **Figs. 47-9, 47-11, B, C,** Courtesy Dr. Stephen Van Voorst, MD. **Fig. 47-10, A,** Courtesy Quinton Instrument Co., Seattle, Wash. **Fig. 47-13,** From NxStage Medical, Inc, Lawrence, Mass.

CHAPTER 48

Figs. 48-1, 48-6, Modified from Patton KT, Thibodeau GA: *Anatomy and physiology,* ed 8, St Louis, 2013, Mosby. **Fig. 48-3,** Modified from McCance KL, Huether SE: *Pathophysiology: the biologic basis for disease in adults and children,* ed 6, St Louis, 2010, Mosby. **Fig. 48-8,** From Thibodeau GA, Patton KT: *The human body in health and disease,* ed 4, St Louis, 2005, Mosby.

CHAPTER 49

Figs. 49-11, 49-13, From Kumar V, Abbas AK, Aster JC, Fausto N: *Robbins and Cotran pathologic basis of disease,* ed 8, Philadelphia, 2010, Saunders. **Fig. 49-12,** Modified from Urden LD, Stacy KM, Lough ME: *Critical care nursing: diagnosis and management,* ed 6, St Louis, 2010, Mosby. **Figs. 49-15, 49-16,** From Chew SL, Leslie D: *Clinical endocrinology and diabetes: an illustrated colour text,* Edinburgh, 2006, Churchill Livingstone.

CHAPTER 50

Fig. 50-1, Courtesy Linda Haas, Seattle, Wash. **Fig. 50-3,** Modified from Urden LD, Stacy KM, Lough ME: *Critical care nursing: diagnosis and management,* ed 6, St Louis, 2010, Mosby. **Fig. 50-6,** From Forbes CD, Jackson WF: *Colour atlas and text of clinical medicine,* ed 3, London, 2003, Mosby. **Figs. 50-7, 50-12, 50-13,** From Chew SL, Leslie D: *Clinical endocrinology and diabetes: an illustrated colour text,* Edinburgh, 2006, Churchill Livingstone. **Fig. 50-9,** Courtesy Paul W. Ladenson, MD, The Johns Hopkins University and Hospital, Baltimore, Md. From HM Seidel, JW Ball, JE Dains, GW Benedict, editors: *Mosby's guide to physical examination,* ed 6, St Louis, 2006, Mosby. **Fig. 50-10,** From Seidel HM, Ball JW, Dains JE, Benedict GW: *Mosby's guide to physical examination,* ed 6, St Louis, 2006, Mosby.

CHAPTER 51

Figs. 51-1, 51-2, 51-4, 51-5, 51-7, Modified from Patton KT, Thibodeau GA: *Anatomy and physiology,* ed 8, St Louis, 2013, Mosby. **Fig. 51-3,** Modified from McKenry L, Tessier E, Hogan M: *Mosby's pharmacology in nursing,* St Louis, 2006, Mosby. **Fig. 51-8, A,** From Abrahams P, Marks S, Hutching R: *McMinn's color atlas of human anatomy,* ed 5, Philadelphia, 2003, Saunders. **Fig. 51-8, B,** From Symonds EM, MacPherson MB: *Color atlas of obstetrics and gynecology,* London, 1994, Mosby Wolfe.

CHAPTER 52

Fig. 52-1, Data from American Cancer Society: How to perform a breast self-exam, revised October 2011. *www.cancer.org/Cancer/BreastCancer/MoreInformation/BreastCancerEarlyDetection/breast-cancer-early-detection-acsrecsbse.* **Fig. 52-2,** From Adam A, Dixon AK, Grainger RG, et al: *Grainger and Allison's diagnostic radiology,* ed 5, St Louis, 2008, Churchill Livingstone. **Fig. 52-5,** From Donegan WL, Spratt JS: *Cancer of the breast,* ed 3, Philadelphia, 1988, Saunders. **Fig. 52-7,** From Swartz MH: *Textbook of physical diagnosis: history and examination,* ed 6, Philadelphia, 2010, Saunders. **Fig. 52-10,** Courtesy Brian Davies, MD. From Fortunato N, McCullough S: *Plastic and reconstructive surgery,* St Louis, 1998, Mosby. **Fig. 52-11, A,** Modified from Cameron J: *Current surgical therapy,* ed 5, St Louis, 1995, Mosby. **Fig. 52-11, B,** Courtesy Brian Davies, MD. From Fortunato N, McCullough S: *Plastic and reconstructive surgery,* St Louis, 1998, Mosby.

CHAPTER 53

Fig. 53-1, From Marx J, Walls R, Hockberger R: *Rosen's emergency medicine: concepts and clinical practice,* ed 7, St Louis, 2010, Mosby. **Figs. 53-2, 53-7, 53-8, B,** From Morse S, Moreland A, Holmes K, editors: *Atlas of sexually transmitted diseases and AIDS,* London, 1996, Mosby-Wolfe. **Figs. 53-3, A,** and **53-6,** From Cohen J, Powderly WG: *Infectious diseases,* ed 2, St Louis, 2004, Mosby. **Figs. 53-3, B,** and **53-5,** From Mandell GL, Bennett JE, Dolin R: *Mandell, Douglas, and Bennett's principles and practice of infectious diseases,* ed 7, Philadelphia, 2010, Churchill Livingstone. **Fig. 53-4,** From Forbes CD, Jackson WF. *Color atlas and text of clinical medicine,* ed 3, London, 2003, Mosby. **Figs. 53-8, A, C,** and **53-10, C,** From Centers for Disease Control and Prevention. Courtesy Susan Lindsley. **Fig. 53-9,** From Centers for Disease Control and Prevention. Courtesy Dr. Hermann. **Fig. 53-10, A,** From Centers for Disease Control and Prevention. Courtesy Joe Millar. **Fig. 53-10, B,** From Centers for Disease Control and Prevention. Courtesy Dr. Wiesner.

CHAPTER 54

Fig. 54-3, From Katz V: *Comprehensive gynecology,* ed 5, St Louis, 2007, Mosby. **Fig. 54-4,** From Kumar V, Abbas AK, Aster JC, Fausto N: *Robbins and Cotran pathologic basis of disease,* ed 8, Philadelphia, 2010, Saunders. **Fig. 54-5,** Modified from Stenchever MA, Droegemueller W, Herbst AL, Mishell D Jr: *Comprehensive gynecology,* ed 4, St Louis, 2001, Mosby. **Fig. 54-6,** From McCance KL, Huether SE: *Pathophysiology: the biologic basis for disease in adults and children,* ed 6, St Louis, 2010, Mosby. **Fig. 54-7,** From Symonds EM, McPherson MBA: *Colour atlas of obstetrics and gynecology,* London, 1994, Mosby. **Fig. 54-8,** From Kumar V, Abbas A, Fausto N: *Robbins and Cotran pathologic basis of disease,* ed 7, Philadelphia, 2005, Saunders. **Fig. 54-9,** From Drake RL, Vogl W, Mitchell AWM: *Gray's anatomy for students,* ed 2, Edinburgh, 2010, Churchill Livingstone. **Fig. 54-10,** Modified from Phipps WJ, Sands JK, Marek JF: *Medical-surgical nursing: concepts and clinical practice,* ed 6, St Louis, 1999, Mosby. **Fig. 54-12,** Modified from Seidel HM, Ball JW, Dains JE, Flynn JA: *Mosby's guide to physical examination,* ed 7, St Louis, 2011, Mosby. **Fig. 54-13, B,** From Huffman JW: *Gynecology and obstetrics,* Philadelphia, 1962, Saunders. **Fig. 54-14, B,** From Townsend CM: *Sabiston textbook of surgery,* ed 18, St Louis, 2009, Mosby.

CHAPTER 55

Fig. 55-3, From Townsend CM, Beauchamp RD, Evers BM, Mattox KL: *Sabiston textbook of surgery,* ed 19, Philadelphia, 2012, Saunders. **Fig. 55-5,** From Mettler F: *Essentials of radiology,* ed 2, Philadelphia, 2004, Saunders. **Fig. 55-7,** *B,* From Abeloff MD, Armitage JO, Niederhuber JE, Kastan MB, editors: *Abeloff's clinical oncology,* ed 4, 2008, Churchill Livingstone. **Fig. 55-10,** From Swartz MH: *Textbook of physical diagnosis,* ed 6, Philadelphia, 2010, Saunders. **Fig. 55-11,** From Seidel HM, Ball JW, Dains JE, Flynn JA: *Mosby's guide to physical examination,* ed 7, St Louis, 2011, Mosby.

CHAPTER 56

Figs. 56-1, 56-8, 56-9, 56-10, Modified from Thibodeau GA, Patton KT: *Anatomy and physiology,* ed 8, St Louis, 2013, Mosby. **Fig. 56-2,** Modified from Thibodeau GA, Patton KT: *Anatomy and physiology,* ed 6, St Louis, 2007, Mosby. **Fig. 56-6,** From Herlihy B: *The human body in health and illness,* ed 4, St Louis, 2011, Saunders. **Fig. 56-7,** Redrawn from McCance KL, Huether SE: *Pathophysiology: the biologic basis for disease in adults and children,* ed 6, St Louis, 2010, Mosby. **Figs. 56-11, 56-12,** Courtesy DaiWai Olson, RN PhD, CCRN, Dallas, Tex. **Fig. 56-14,** From Chipps E, Clanin N, Campbell V: *Neurologic disorders,* St Louis, 1992, Mosby. **Fig. 56-15,** From Fuller G, Manford M: *Neurology: an illustrated colour text,* ed 3, New York, 2010, Churchill Livingstone.

CHAPTER 57

Fig. 57-4, Modified from McCance KL, Huether SE: *Pathophysiology: the biologic basis for disease in adults and children,* ed 6, St Louis, 2010, Mosby. **Fig. 57-7,** Modified from Copstead-Kirkhorn LC, Banasik JL: *Pathophysiology,* ed 5, St Louis, 2013, Mosby. **Fig. 57-9,** Courtesy Meg Zomorodi, RN, PhD, CNL, Raleigh, N.C. **Fig. 57-13,** *C,* From Bingham BJG, Hawke M, Kwok P: *Clinical atlas of otolaryngology,* St Louis, 1992, Mosby. **Fig. 57-15,** From Copstead-Kirkhorn LC, Banasik JL: *Pathophysiology,* ed 4, St Louis, 2010, Mosby. **Fig. 57-16,** From Kumar V, Abbas AK, Aster JC, Fausto N: *Robbins and Cotran pathologic basis of disease,* ed 8, Philadelphia, 2010, Saunders. **Fig. 57-17,** From Stevens A, Lowe J: *Pathology: illustrated review in colour,* ed 2, London, 2000, Mosby.

CHAPTER 58

Fig. 58-3, From Kumar V, Abbas AK, Aster JC, Fausto N: *Robbins and Cotran pathologic basis of disease,* ed 8, Philadelphia, 2010, Saunders. **Fig. 58-11,** Modified from Hoeman SP: *Rehabilitation nursing,* ed 2, St Louis, 1995, Mosby. **Fig. 58-12,** From Forbes CD, Jackson WF: *Colour atlas and text of clinical medicine,* ed 3, London, 2003, Mosby.

CHAPTER 59

Fig. 59-4, From Stevens A, Lowe J: *Pathology: illustrated review in colour,* ed 2, London, 2000, Mosby. **Fig. 59-7,** From Lehne RA: *Pharmacology for nursing care,* ed 8, St Louis, 2013, Saunders. **Fig. 59-8,** From Aminoff MJ, Daroff RB: *Encyclopedia of the neurological sciences,* Waltham, Mass., 2003, Academic Press. **Fig. 59-11,** From Sanders DB, Massey JM: Clinical features of myasthenia gravis. In AG Engel, editor: *Neuromuscular junction disorders: handbook of clinical neurology,* New York, 2008, Elsevier.

CHAPTER 60

Fig. 60-5, From Roberts GS: *Neuropsychiatric disorders,* London, 1993, Mosby-Wolfe. **Fig. 60-6,** Modified from Stern TA: *Massachusetts General Hospital comprehensive clinical psychiatry,* Philadelphia, 2008, Mosby.

CHAPTER 61

Fig. 61-1, Modified from Patton KT, Thibodeau GA: *Anatomy and physiology,* ed 8, St Louis, 2013, Mosby. **Fig. 61-2,** Courtesy Joe Rothrock, Media, Pa. **Fig. 61-3,** From Forbes CD, Jackson WF: *Color atlas and text of clinical medicine,* ed 3, London, 2003, Mosby. **Fig. 61-4,** Modified from Marciano FF, Greene KA, Apostolides PJ, et al: Pharmacologic management of spinal cord injury: review of the literature, *BNI Quarterly* 11(2):11, 1995. In KL McCance, SE Huether, editors: *Pathophysiology: the biologic basis for disease in adults and children,* ed 5, St Louis, 2006, Mosby. **Fig. 61-5,** *A, B, C,* From Copstead-Kirkhorn LC, Banasik JL: *Pathophysiology,* ed 5, St Louis, 2014, Mosby. **Fig. 61-7,** From American Spinal Injury Association/International Medical Society of Paraplegic (ASIA/IMOSP): *International standards for neurological functional classification of spinal cord injury patients* (revised), Chicago, 2002, The Association. **Figs. 61-8, 61-12,** Courtesy Michael S. Clement, MD, Mesa, Ariz. **Fig. 61-11,** Modified from Urden LD, Stacy KM, Lough ME: *Priorities in critical care nursing,* ed 6, St Louis, 2012, Mosby.

CHAPTER 62

Fig. 62-1, *A,* From Herlihy B, Maebius N: *The human body in health and illness,* ed 4, Philadelphia, 2011, Saunders. **Figs. 62-1,** *B,* **62-6,** From Patton KT, Thibodeau GA: *Anatomy and physiology,* ed 8, St Louis, 2013, Mosby. **Fig. 62-5,** From Patton KT, Thibodeau GA, Douglas M: *Essentials of anatomy and physiology,* St Louis, 2012, Mosby. **Fig. 62-7,** *A,* From Wilson SF, Giddens JF: *Health assessment for nursing practice,* ed 5, St Louis, 2013, Mosby. **Fig. 62-7,** *B,* From Barkauskas V, Baumann L, Stoltenberg-Allen K, et al: *Health and physical assessment,* ed 2, St Louis, 1998, Mosby. **Fig. 62-8,** From Zitelli BJ, McIntire SC, Nowalk AJ: *Zitelli and Davis' atlas of pediatric physical diagnosis,* ed 6, St Louis, 2012, Mosby. **Fig. 62-9,** From Miller MD, Howard RF, Plancher KD: *Surgical atlas of sports medicine,* Philadelphia, 2003, Saunders.

CHAPTER 63

Fig. 63-2, From Buttaravoli P: *Minor emergencies,* ed 3, Philadelphia, Saunders, 2012. **Fig. 63-4,** *A,* From David Lintner, MD, Houston, Tex., *www.drlintner.com.* **Fig. 63-4,** *B, C,* Courtesy Peter Bonner, Placitas, N. Mex. **Figs. 63-9, 63-20,** Courtesy Mary Wollan, RN, BAN, ONC, Spring Park, Minn. **Fig. 63-12,** From Maher AB, Salmond SW, Pellino T, editors: *Orthopaedic nursing,* ed 3, Philadelphia, 2002, Saunders. **Fig. 63-13,** *A,* Courtesy Howmedica, Inc, Allendale, Pa. **Fig. 63-13,** *B,* From Canale ST, Beaty JH: *Campbell's operative orthopaedics,* ed 12, Philadelphia, 2013, Mosby. **Fig. 63-14,** From Jeremy Lewis, MD. Dallas, Tex. **Fig. 63-15,** From Browner BD, Jupiter JB, Levine AM, Trafton P: *Skeletal trauma: fractures, dislocations, ligamentous injuries,* ed 4, Philadelphia, 2009, Saunders. **Fig. 63-16,** Mettler FA: *Essentials of radiology,* ed 2, Philadelphia, 2005, Saunders. **Fig. 63-21,** Courtesy R.A. Weinstein, Denver, Colo.

CHAPTER 64

Fig. 64-2, From Thibodeau GA, Patton KT: *The human body in health and disease,* ed 5, St Louis, 2010, Mosby. **Fig. 64-3,** From Damjanov I, Linder J: *Anderson's pathology,* ed 10, St Louis, 1996, Mosby. **Figs. 64-6, 64-7,** From Canale ST, Beaty JH: *Campbell's operative orthopaedics,* ed 12, Philadelphia, 2013, Mosby. **Fig. 64-9,** *A,* From Phillips N: *Berry & Kohn's operating room technique,* ed 12, St Louis, 2013, Mosby. **Fig. 64-9,** *B,* Courtesy MA Mir. In Kanski JJ: *Clinical diagnosis in ophthalmology,* St Louis, 2006, Mosby.

CHAPTER 65

Fig. 65-1, *D,* From Forbes CD, Jackson WF: *Color atlas and text of clinical medicine,* ed 3, London, 2003, Mosby. **Figs. 65-3,** *D,* From Canale ST, Beaty JH: *Campbell's operative orthopaedics,* ed 12, Philadelphia, 2013, Mosby. **Fig. 65-6,** Courtesy John Cook, MD. From Goldstein, BG, Goldstein AE: *Practical dermatology,* ed 2, St Louis, 1997, Mosby. **Fig. 65-7,** From Marx J, Hockberger R, Walls R: *Rosen's emergency medicine,* ed 7, Philadelphia, 2009, Mosby. **Fig. 65-8,** From Kim DH, Henn J, Vaccaro AR, Dickman C: *Surgical anatomy and techniques to the spine,* Philadelphia, 2006, Saunders. **Figs. 65-10, 65-13,** From Firestein GS, Budd RC, Gabriel SE, McInnes IB: *Kelley's textbook of rheumatology,* ed 9, Philadelphia, 2012, Saunders. **Fig. 65-12,** From Zitelli BJ, Davis HW: *Atlas of pediatric physical diagnosis,* ed 4, St Louis, 2002, Mosby.

CHAPTER 66

Fig. 66-1, From Avera Health, Sioux Falls, S. Dak. **Fig. 66-2,** Courtesy Spacelabs Medical, Redmond, Wash. **Fig. 66-5,** From Darovic GO, Vanriper S, Vanriper J: Fluid-filled monitoring systems. In GO Darovic: *Hemodynamic monitoring,* ed 2, Philadelphia, 1995, Saunders. **Figs. 66-6, 66-9, 66-10,** Modified from Urden LD, Stacy KM, Lough ME: *Critical care nursing: diagnosis and management,* ed 6, St Louis, 2010, Mosby. **Fig. 66-14,** *A,* From Beare PG, Myers JL: *Adult health nursing,* ed 3, St Louis, 1998, Mosby.

CHAPTER 67

Figs. 67-2, 67-3, 67-4, 67-5, Modified from Urden LD, Stacy KM, Lough ME: *Critical care nursing: diagnosis and management,* ed 6, St Louis, 2010, Mosby.

CHAPTER 68

Fig. 68-6, From Wilson SF, Giddens JF: *Health assessment for nursing practice,* ed 4, St Louis, 2009, Mosby. **Fig. 68-7,** From American Association of Critical Care Nurses: *AACN advanced critical care nursing,* St Louis, 2009, Mosby. **Fig. 68-8,** Courtesy Richard Arbour, RN, MSN, CCRN, CNRN, CCNS, FAAN and Anna Kirk, RN, MSN. **Fig. 68-11,** From Cohen J, Powderly WG: *Infectious diseases,* ed 2, St Louis, 2004, Mosby.

CHAPTER 69

Figs. 69-2, 69-3, Courtesy Cameron Bangs, MD. From Auerbach PS, Donner HJ, Weiss EA: *Field guide to wilderness medicine,* ed 2, St Louis, 2003, Mosby. **Fig. 69-6,** From Roberts JR, Hedges JR: *Clinical procedures in emergency medicine,* ed 5, Philadelphia, 2009, Saunders. **Fig. 69-7,** Photo used with the permission of the American Red Cross.

NOTE: Disorder names and key terms are in **boldface**. Page numbers in **boldface** indicate main discussions. Page numbers followed by f, t, or b indicate figures, tables, and boxes, respectively.

ABG	arterial blood gas	DKA	diabetic ketoacidosis
ACE	angiotensin-converting enzyme	DM	diabetes mellitus; diastolic murmur
ACLS	advanced cardiac life support	DRE	digital rectal examination
ACS	acute coronary syndrome	DVT	deep vein thrombosis
ACTH	adrenocorticotropic hormone	ECF	extracellular fluid
ADH	antidiuretic hormone	ECG	electrocardiogram
AED	automatic external defibrillator	ED	emergency department; erectile dysfunction
AIDS	acquired immunodeficiency syndrome	EEG	electroencephalogram
AKA	above-knee amputation	EMG	electromyogram
AKI	acute kidney injury	EMS	emergency medical services
ALI	acute lung injury	ENT	ear, nose, and throat
ALL	acute lymphocytic leukemia	ERCP	endoscopic retrograde cholangiopancreatography
ALS	amyotrophic lateral sclerosis	ERT	estrogen replacement therapy
AMI	acute myocardial infarction	ESKD	end-stage kidney disease
ANA	antinuclear antibody	ESR	erythrocyte sedimentation rate
ANS	autonomic nervous system	ET	endotracheal
AORN	Association of periOperative Room Nurses	FEV	forced expiratory volume
APD	automated peritoneal dialysis	FRC	functional residual capacity
aPTT	activated partial thromboplastin time	FUO	fever of unknown origin
ARDS	acute respiratory distress syndrome	GCS	Glasgow Coma Scale
ATN	acute tubular necrosis	GERD	gastroesophageal reflux disease
BCLS	basic cardiac life support	GFR	glomerular filtration rate
BKA	below-knee amputation	GH	growth hormone
BMI	body mass index	GI	glycemic index
BMR	basal metabolic rate	GTT	glucose tolerance test
BMT	bone marrow transplantation	GU	genitourinary
BPH	benign prostatic hyperplasia	GYN, Gyn	gynecologic
BSE	breast self-examination	HAI	health care–associated infection
BUN	blood urea nitrogen	HAV	hepatitis A virus
CABG	coronary artery bypass graft	Hb, Hgb	hemoglobin
CAD	coronary artery disease; circulatory assist device	HBV	hepatitis B virus
CAPD	continuous ambulatory peritoneal dialysis	Hct	hematocrit
CAVH	continuous arteriovenous hemofiltration	HCV	hepatitis C virus
CBC	complete blood count	HD	hemodialysis, Huntington's disease
CCU	coronary care unit; critical care unit	HDL	high-density lipoprotein
CDC	Centers for Disease Control and Prevention	HF	heart failure
CIS	carcinoma in situ	HIV	human immunodeficiency virus
CKD	chronic kidney disease	H&P	history and physical examination
CLL	chronic lymphocytic leukemia	HPV	human papillomavirus
CML	chronic myelocytic leukemia	HSCT	hematopoietic stem cell transplantation
CMP	cardiomyopathy	IABP	intraaortic balloon pump
CN	cranial nerve	IBS	irritable bowel syndrome
CNS	central nervous system	ICP	intracranial pressure
CO	cardiac output	I&D	incision and drainage
COPD	chronic obstructive pulmonary disease	IE	infective endocarditis
CPAP	continuous positive airway pressure	IFG	impaired fasting glucose
CPR	cardiopulmonary resuscitation	IGT	impaired glucose tolerance
CRRT	continuous renal replacement therapy	INR	international normalized ratio
CRNA	certified registered nurse anesthetist	IOP	intraocular pressure
CSF	cerebrospinal fluid	IPPB	intermittent positive-pressure breathing
CT	computed tomography	ITP	idiopathic thrombocytopenic purpura
CVA	cerebrovascular accident; costovertebral angle	IUD	intrauterine device
CVAD	central venous access device	IV	intravenous
CVI	chronic venous insufficiency	IVP	intravenous push; intravenous pyelogram
CVP	central venous pressure	JVD	jugular venous distention
D&C	dilation and curettage	KS	Kaposi sarcoma
DDD	degenerative disk disease	KUB	kidney, ureters, and bladder (x-ray)
DI	diabetes insipidus	KVO	keep vein open
DIC	disseminated intravascular coagulation	LAD	left anterior descending
DJD	degenerative joint disease	LDL	low-density lipoprotein